A TEXTBOOK OF RADIOLOGY AND IMAGING

A TEXTBOOK OF RADIOLOGY AND IMAGING

EDITED BY
DAVID SUTTON
MD, FRCP, FRCR, DMRD, MCAR (Hon)
Consulting Radiologist, St Mary's Hospital, London and
The National Hospitals for Nervous Diseases, London, UK

FOURTH EDITION

VOLUME 1

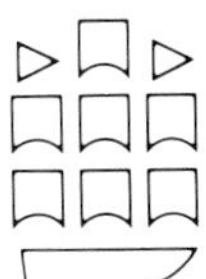

CHURCHILL LIVINGSTONE
EDINBURGH LONDON MELBOURNE AND NEW YORK 1987

CHURCHILL LIVINGSTONE
Medical Division of Longman Group UK Limited

Distributed in the United States of America by Churchill Livingstone Inc., 1560 Broadway, New York, N.Y. 10036, and by associated companies, branches and representatives throughout the world.

First edition 1969
Second edition 1975
Third edition 1980
Fourth edition 1987

ISBN 0 443 03329 3

British Library Cataloguing in Publication Data
Textbook of radiology and imaging. — 4th ed.
1. Imaging systems in medicine 2. Diagnosis
I. Sutton, David, 1917
616.07'54 R857.06

Library of Congress Cataloging in Publication Data
Main entry under title:

A Textbook of radiology and imaging.

Includes bibliographies and index.
1. Diagnosis, radioscopic. 2. Diagnostic imaging.
I. Sutton, David, 1917 . [DNLM: 1. Radiology.
2. Radionuclide Imaging. WN 100 T355]
RC78.S89 1986 616.07'57 85-23951

Printed and bound in Great Britain by
William Clowes Limited, Beccles and London.

PREFACE

Apart from a complete update of all areas of the book, the major feature of this new edition is the integration of different imaging techniques into the general text wherever desirable. Techniques are also, as in previous editions, dealt with separately in dedicated chapters in the latter part of the text. It is hoped that this approach will enable the student to judge the relative value of individual imaging techniques in a specific clinical context, as well as to study these techniques as a whole.

Imaging has featured prominently in the major medical advances of the last decade. MRI is undoubtedly the most exciting new technique, and although few radiologists are fortunate enough as yet to be involved in this new field of imaging, it behoves us all to learn what it now has to offer. It is clearly destined to play an increasing role in the future.

Ultrasound has also made major advances in recent years and its increasingly important role in imaging diagnosis is emphasized in this new edition. In CT the fourth generation scanners have improved resolution and accuracy both in neuroradiology and body scanning. DSA has now an accepted place in angiography and is being used as much for arterial as for venous injections. Interventional radiological techniques have also gained wider acceptance and entered new areas in the last five years. These major advances are dealt with either in the regional chapters or in those devoted to techniques. Other new features of this edition are chapters on the paediatric chest and abdomen.

In any book of this size there is an inevitable time lag between writing and publication. Though the publishers have done their best to reduce this to a minimum, the student must bear this in mind when studying for his examinations and boards and should supplement his reading by reference to the current literature.

London, 1987 D.S.

CONTRIBUTORS

M. A. Al-Kutoubi
MD, DMRD, FRCR
Consultant Radiologist, St Mary's Hospital; Teacher in Radiology, University of London, London, UK

Ian Beggs
MB, FRCR, DMRD
Consultant Radiologist, Royal Infirmary, Edinburgh, UK

J. O. M. C. Craig
FRCSIre, FRCSEng, FRCR
Consultant Radiologist, St Mary's Hospital; Teacher of Diagnostic Radiology, University of London, London, UK

K. C. Dewbury
BSc, MB, FRCR, DMRD
Consultant Radiologist, Southampton General Hospital, Southampton, UK

Robert Dick
FRCR, FRACR
Consultant Radiologist and Chairman, Division of Radiology, Royal Free Hospital and School of Medicine, London, UK

Claire M. Dicks-Mireaux
BA, MB, MRCP, DMRD, FRCR
Consultant Radiologist, The Hospital for Sick Children, Great Ormond Street; Senior Lecturer and Honorary Consultant, St Bartholomew's Hospital Medical College, London, UK

Robert M. Donaldson
MD, MRCP, FACC
Consultant Cardiologist, National Heart Hospital, London, UK

David Edwards
MB, FRCP, FRCR
Director, Department of Radiology, University College Hospital; Teacher in Radiology, University of London, London, UK

Stuart Field
MA, DMRD, FRCR
Consultant Radiologist, Canterbury Hospital, Canterbury, Kent, UK

W. StC. Forbes
MA, MB BCh, DRCOG, DMRD, FRCR
Consultant Radiologist, Hope Hospital, Salford; Lecturer, Department of Diagnostic Radiology, University of Manchester, Manchester, UK

I. H. Gravelle
BSc, FRCPEdin, FRCR, DMRD
Consultant Radiologist, University Hospital of Wales; Clinical Teacher, University of Wales College of Medicine, Cardiff, UK

R. H. S. Gregson
BSc, DMRD, FRCR
Consultant Radiologist and Clinical Teacher in Radiology, University of Nottingham, Nottingham, UK

James F. Griffin
MB, BCh, FFRRCSIre
Consultant Radiologist, St Vincent's Hospital, Elm Park and Royal Victoria Eye and Ear Hospital, Dublin, Eire

J. H. Highman
FRCR, FRCP
Consultant Radiologist, St Mary's Hospital, Samaritan Hospital for Women and the Western Ophthalmic Hospital; Recognized Teacher in Radiology, University of London, London, UK

Ivan Hyde
FRCPEdin, FRCR, DMRD, DCH
Consultant Radiologist, Southampton General Hospital, Southampton, UK

Ian Isherwood
MRCP, FRCR, FFRCSIre(Hon)
Professor of Diagnostic Radiology, University of Manchester, Manchester, UK

Philip Jacobs
TD, DMRD, FRCP, FRCR
Consulting Radiologist, Royal Orthopaedic Hospital, Birmingham, Birmingham General Hospital, Birmingham Accident Hospital and Warwickshire Orthopaedic Hospital for Children, UK

Jeremy P. R. Jenkins
Mb ChB, MRCP, DMRD, FRCR
Senior Research Fellow, Magnetic Resonance Imaging

Unit, Department of Diagnostic Radiology, University of Manchester; Honorary Consultant Radiologist, Manchester Royal Infirmary, Manchester, UK

Brian E. Kendall
MB, FRCP, FRCR, DMRD
Consultant Radiologist The National Hospitals for Nervous Diseases, The Hospital for Sick Children and The Middlesex Hospital, London, UK

John W. Laws
CBE, FRCP, FRCR
Director of Radiology, King's College Hospital, London, UK

William R. Lees
FRCR
Consultant Radiologist, The Middlesex Hospital and King Edward VII Hospital for Officers; Honorary Senior Clinical Lecturer, University of London, London, UK

N. A. Lewtas
MB, FRCP, FRCR
Consulting Radiologist, Sheffield Area Health Authority(T), Sheffield, UK

Glyn A. S. Lloyd
MA, DM, FRCR
Director, Radiology Department, Royal National Throat Nose and Ear Hospital; Consultant Radiologist, Moorfields Eye Hospital, London, UK

Richard Mason
FRCS, MRCP, FRCR
Consultant Radiologist, The Middlesex Hospital, London, UK

Ivan F. Moseley
BSc, MD, FRCR, FRCP
Consultant Radiologist, National Hospital, Queen Square and Moorfields Eye Hospital, London, UK

Janet Murfitt
MRCP, DMRD, FRCR
Consultant Radiologist, The London Hospital, Whitechapel, London, UK

R. O. Murray
MBE, MD, FRCP, FRCR, DMR, FACR(Hon), FRACR(Hon)
Consulting Radiologist, Royal National Orthopaedic Hospital, London, UK

Jonathan S. Olney
MB, BS, FRCR
Senior Registrar, Lysholm Department of Radiology, The National Hospitals for Nervous Diseases, London, UK

Michael C. Pearson
MA, MRCP, FRCR
Consultant Radiologist, Brompton Hospital and London Chest Hospital, London, UK

Peter D. Phelps
MD, FRCS, FRCR, DMRD
Consultant Radiologist, Walsgrave Hospital, Coventry; Honorary Consultant Radiologist, Royal National Throat Nose and Ear Hospital, London, UK

Maurice J. Raphael
MA, MD, FRCP, FRCR, DMRD
Consultant Radiologist, National Heart Hospital and The Middlesex Hospital, London, UK

Peter Renton
FRCR, DMRD
Consultant Radiologist, Royal National Orthopaedic Hospital, University College Hospital, Hospital for Tropical Diseases and University College Dental Hospital; Honorary Senior Lecturer, University College and the Institute of Orthopaedics, London, UK

E. Rhys Davies
MA, FRCP, FRCR, FFRRCSIre(Hon)
Professor of Radiodiagnosis, University of Bristol; Honorary Consultant Radiologist, University of Bristol; Honorary Consultant Radiologist, Bristol and Weston Health District, Bristol, UK

Michael L. Rigby
MD, MRCP
Consultant Paediatric Cardiologist, Cardiothoracic Institute, Brompton Hospital, London, UK

Michael B. Rubens
FRCR, DMRD
Consultant Radiologist, National Heart Hospital and London Chest Hospital; Honorary Senior Lecturer, Cardiothoracic Institute, University of London, London, UK

Donald Shaw
MA, MSc, DMRD, FRCP, FRCR
Consultant Radiologist, Hospitals for Sick Children, London, UK

Keith C. Simpkins
MB BS, FRCP(Lond), FRCPEdin, FRCR, FRACR(Hon)
Consultant Radiologist, The General Infirmary at Leeds; Senior Clinical Lecturer in Diagnostic Radiology, University of Leeds, Leeds, UK

F. Starer
FRCPEd, FRCR
Consultant Radiologist, Westminster Hospital and Westminster Children's Hospital, London, UK

Dennis J. Stoker
FRCP, FRCR
Consultant Radiologist, Royal National Orthopaedic Hospital and St George's Hospital; Director of Radiological Studies, Institute of Orthopaedics, University of London, London, UK

G. R. Sutherland
FRCR, FRCPEdin, MRCPGlasg
Consultant Radiologist in Administrative Charge, Stobhill General Hospital and associated hospitals; Honorary Clinical Lecturer, University of Glasgow, Glasgow, UK

David Sutton
MD, FRCP, FRCR, DMRD, MCAR(Hon)
Consulting Radiologist, St Mary's Hospital and the National Hospitals for Nervous Diseases, London, UK

Brian M. Thomas
MB, FRCP, FRCR
Consultant Radiologist, University College Hospital and St Mark's Hospital for Diseases of the Rectum and Colon; Teacher in Radiology, University College, London, UK

Iain Watt
MRCP, FRCR
Consultant Radiologist, Bristol Royal Infirmary; Clinical Lecturer in Radiodiagnosis, University of Bristol, Bristol, UK

CONTENTS

VOLUME 1

PART 1: Bones and Joints

PART 2: The Chest

PART 3: The Cardiovascular System

PART 8: Modern Imaging

PART 1

BONES AND JOINTS

CHAPTER 1

CONGENITAL SKELETAL ANOMALIES: SKELETAL DYSPLASIAS; CHROMOSOMAL DISORDERS

CONGENITAL SKELETAL ANOMALIES

Very many congenital skeletal anomalies have been described. In a study of 57 000 Birmingham infants (live and stillborn) 2.3% were malformed (i.e. had macroscopic abnormalities of structure attributable to faulty development and present at birth). Some minor abnormalities are only discovered coincidentally or are never noticed. In many of these the skeleton is affected and often is the only system implicated. Many orthopaedic conditions acquired in childhood have been wholly or partially eradicated. Therefore, congenital abnormalities are assuming increasing importance and present tremendous challenges to orthopaedic surgeons. However, only those of importance to the radiologist will be dealt with in this section.

UPPER LIMB

A short glossary of descriptive terms in common use is presented here.

Adactyly, absence of fingers
Amelia, absence of limbs
Brachydactyly, short phalanges
Brachymesophalangy, short middle phalanges
Clinodactyly, incurving of a finger, usually the fifth, in the coronal plane
Hemimelia, absence of part of a hand
Hyper- or hypophalangism, the presence of a greater or lesser number of phalanges
Longitudinal defect, absence of part of the limb along its longitudinal axis. This may be pre-axial (radial), post axial (ulnar) or central
Macrodactyly, enlargement of a digit
Oligodactyly, absence of fingers
Phocomelia, absence of the proximal parts of a limb
Polydactyly, increased number of digits. May be pre- or postaxial
Symphalangism, fusion of phalanges in one digit
Syndactyly, fusion of adjacent digits. May involve soft tissues and/or bone.
(after Poznanski)

The lesions may be grouped into:

1. Failure of differentiation, e.g. syndactyly
2. Failure of development, which may be transverse, e.g. aphalangy, or longitudinal
3. Duplications
4. Overgrowth, as in neurofibromatosis
5. Generalized dysplasias
6. Congenital (Streeter's) bands.

Some lesions are solitary and of no significance, i.e. isolated clinodactyly, while others occur in combination, so that clinodactyly is also seen as part of major syndromes, e.g. trisomy 21. Radial defects especially are associated with other anomalies, e.g. with atrial septal defects in the Holt–Oram syndrome. Some defects are attributable to drugs, such as thalidomide (Distaval) administered to the mother in the first three months of pregnancy. This may cause damage to the growing nerve, and it may be that the sensory nerve is the tissue organiser (McCredie, 1975). Epanutin, used in the treatment of maternal epilepsy, may cause hypoplasia of distal phalanges *in utero*. Many lesions are genetically inherited so that the harmless *congenital broad thumb* may be seen in different generations of the same family. Other defects may represent sporadic mutations to the gene.

Sprengel's shoulder. This deformity consists of an abnormally high scapula. The deformity is due to failure of the shoulder girdle to descend from its embryonic position in the neck, a process which is normally completed by the end of the third fetal month. The lesion is usually unilateral though it may be bilateral. Other congenital anomalies are frequently associated.

Radiographs show the characteristic elevated scapula. The scapula may be normal in shape, but usually there is some shortening of its vertebral border with the result that it approaches the shape of an equilateral triangle. Rotation of the scapula may often be observed; generally the inferior angle rotates towards the spine though rotation in the opposite direction may occur.

From the upper part of the vertebral border or from the superior angle, an accessory bone — the omovertebral or suprascapular bone — may be found uniting this part of scapula to the spine (Fig. 1.1). This structure may be represented only by fibrous tissue or cartilage and, if bony, may vary greatly in size and radio-opacity.

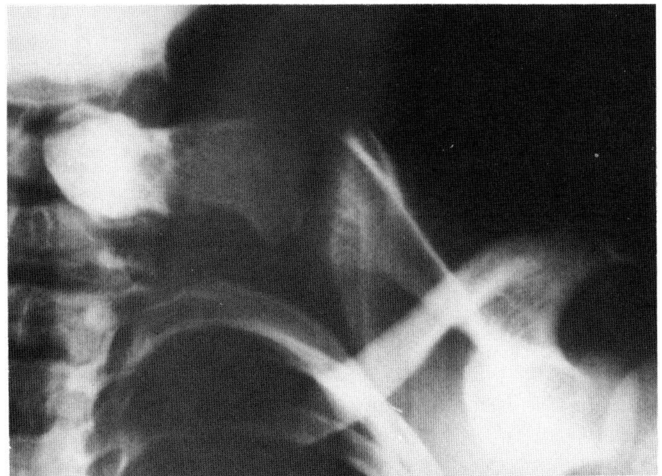

Fig. 1.1 The scapula is elevated and a large omovertebral bone is shown.

Other anomalies which frequently co-exist include cervical spina bifida, the Klippel–Feil anomaly, cervical ribs and other rib lesions, scoliosis and hemivertebrae.

No difficulties in diagnosis should arise. In old *paralytic* lesions the scapula may be raised. If not evident from the history, the correct diagnosis should be suspected by noting the hypoplasia of bones typical of a paralytic lesion.

Congenital dislocation of the shoulder. True congenital dislocation of the shoulder is rare though the term is often wrongly used for acquired dislocations at birth. A true congenital dislocation is posterior and subspinous.

Supracondylar process of the humerus. The supracondylar process is a bony, beak-shaped downward projection from the antero-medial surface of the humerus some 5–7 cm above the medial epicondyle (Fig. 1.2). It varies in size from a few millimetres to a centimetre or more. The process is a developmental anomaly found in up to 1% of subjects. The lesion may be accompanied by severe median nerve symptoms — probably caused by an abnormal ligament pressing the nerve against the spur.

Radius and ulna. Radial defects are much more common than ulnar and may occur in isolation or as part of major syndromes, in which case they are usually bilateral. Radial defects may occur with:

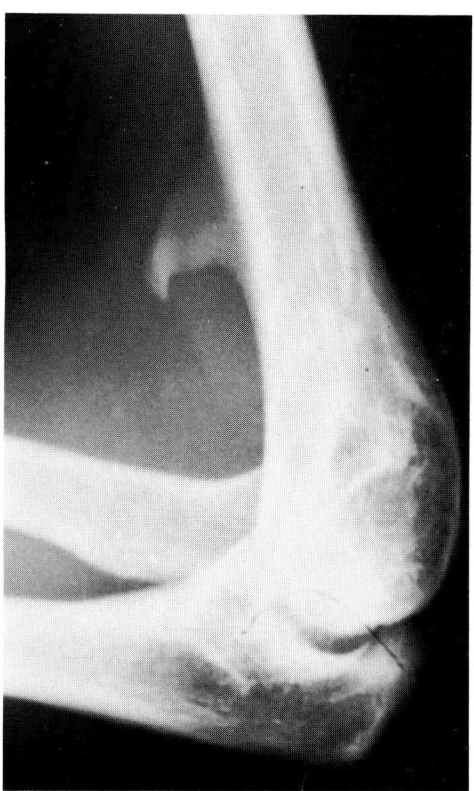

Fig. 1.2 Supracondylar process of the humerus.

Ectodermal dysplasia
Holt–Oram syndrome
Fanconi syndrome
Thrombocytopenia — absent radius syndrome
Trisomy 18
Thalidomide embryopathy
Renal, ear and oesophageal anomalies

The defect may range from hypoplasia of the thumb to complete absence of the radius, scaphoid, trapezium and thumb. The limb is shortened and a radial club hand results, with the hand deviated to the side of the absent bone.

Synostosis of the radius and ulna may be seen at the upper end and is usually associated with dislocation of the radial head (Fig. 1.3). This lesion has marked hereditary tendencies.

Patella cubiti. This term signifies the presence of a large sesamoid bone — a homologue of the patella — in the triceps tendon. The existence of the lesion is very doubtful. The reported radiographic appearances are much more likely to be due to post-traumatic ossification.

Madelung's deformity. This lesion is much commoner in girls and it is generally bilateral. It usually presents during adolescence. The cardinal abnormality is defective development of the inner third of the epiphysis of the lower end of the radius. As a consequence the radial shaft is bowed so increasing the interosseous space. The lower end

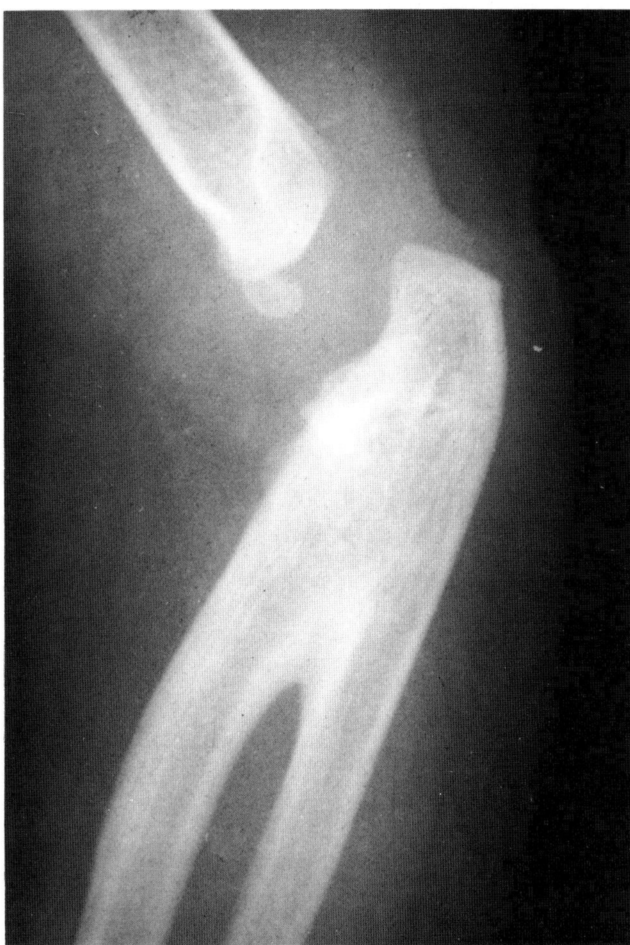

Fig. 1.3 Proximal radio-ulnar synostosis.

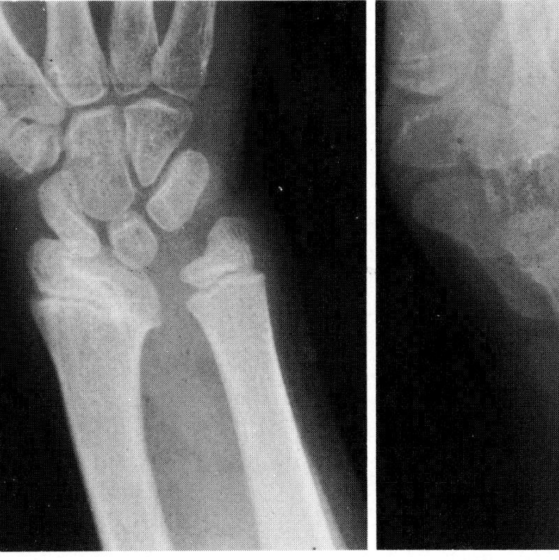

Fig. 1.4 **Fig. 1.5**

Fig. 1.4, 1.5 Madelung's deformity — defective development of the inner third of the radial epiphysis, increase in interosseous space, backward projection of the ulna and anterior displacement of the hand.

of the ulna is subluxed backwards. The hand and carpus project forward at the wrist joint to produce a bayonet-like appearance in a lateral view (Figs. 1.4 and 1.5).

The lesion may be part of the *Leri–Weil syndrome* (dyschondrosteosis, see below) and *Turner's syndrome*. Similar appearances may follow trauma or infection to the growing epiphyseal plate.

Hand and wrist lesions. Very many congenital abnormalities (and normal variants) may be found in the hands and feet. Specialist monographs should be consulted (see end of chapter).

Carpal fusions may occur in isolation or as part of a syndrome. In isolation they are usually transverse, e.g. lunate-triquetrum and capitate-hamate, and are much commoner in Blacks. In syndromes, they are usually proximo-distal and occur in *Apert's syndrome, dyschondrosteosis, chondro-ectodermal dysplasia, Holt–Oram syndrome* and *Turner's syndrome*. Similar appearances may follow trauma, infection and rheumatoid disease.

Polydactyly. Polydactyly is more common in Negroes. It may be postaxial (ulnar) and may range from a minor ossicle to complete duplication of the little finger. Pre-axial lesions (radial) range from minor partial duplication of the thumb distal phalanx to complete thumb duplication. On occasion the hand may be duplicated. Syndactyly may be associated with polydactyly.

Polydactyly may be associated with *Ellis–van Creveld disease* (*chondro-ectodermal dysplasia*), *Laurence-Moon-Biedl disease* (polysyndactyly, mental defect, obesity and retinitis pigmentosa), *trisomy 13*, and *asphyxiating thoracic dysplasia* (all post-axial) and with *Holt–Oram syndrome* and *Fanconi's anaemia* (pre-axial).

Syndactyly occurs in *Apert's syndrome, Fanconi's anaemia, Laurence–Moon–Biedl syndrome, trisomy 13* and *trisomy 18*. (For fuller list consult specialist texts; see references at end of chapter.)

Os styloideum. This ossicle may be found between the capitate and trapezium and the bases of the second and third metacarpals. It may fuse with the bases of the second or third metacarpal forming a styloid process. Patients complain of its presence — a hard, localized protruberance at the back of the wrist easily seen radiographically in a lateral or tangential projection.

THE LOWER LIMB

Congenital dislocation of the hip. This is a very important condition because success in its treatment depends upon early recognition. The incidence of hip instability at birth is 5–10/1000, and of frank dislocation 1–1.5/1000. One third of cases of congenital dislocation of the hip are detected late but these often have a family history of the disease.

Instability and dislocation is usually unilateral (L:R = 11:1) but both hips may be involved (unilateral to bilateral = 11:4). Females are more commonly affected (M:F = 1:5). 60% of affected children are first-born. These children are far more likely to have been breech presentations (breech:vertex = 6:1), possibly because the abnormal lie does not permit reduction *in utero*. Children born by caesarian section are thus also more likely to have associated instability and dislocation. A family or twin history is also common; a subsequent child has a 6% risk of involvement.

Congenital dislocation of the hip is more commonly found in the winter (winter:summer = 1.5:1), possibly because of tight swaddling of children in a position of dislocation in winter.

It is emphasized that radiology in the early stage — helpful as it often is — is only ancillary to clinical methods based on hearing a click as the femoral head slips over the acetabular roof into its socket. The child is laid on its back with the hips flexed to a right angle and the knees *flexed*. Starting with the knees together, the hips are slowly *abducted* and, if one is dislocated, somewhere in the 90° arc of abduction the head of the femur slips back into the acetabulum with a visible and palpable movement described by Ortolani as a 'click'. This test is reliable for babies approaching the age of 1 year. Barlow has devised a more reliable modification which he uses for the newborn.

Radiographic signs. At the Royal National Orthopaedic Hospital, London, it is considered that there are both absolute and relative indications for X-ray.

Absolute indications (If any one of these is present, the hips should be examined radiologically).

1. Family history of congenital dislocation of hip
2. Neonatal hip instability
3. Limb shortening
4. Limitation of hip abduction in flexion.

Relative indications (If any two of these are present, the hips should be examined radiologically).

1. Breech presentation
2. First-born child
3. Caesarian section
4. Other congenital anomalies
5. Excessive fetal moulding.

An early diagnosis may be difficult to make from a standard anteroposterior radiograph of the hips because in the first few weeks of life the difference between a normal and dislocated hip may be slight. At birth, neither femoral head is ossified.

Sometimes poor development of the acetabulum is obvious in cases of congenital dislocation of the hip. In our experience the acetabular angle is increased in congenital dislocations even in the neonatal period. The acetabular angle is the angle subtended by a line drawn through the centres of both Y-cartilages (Hilgenreiner's line) and a line parallel to the acetabular roof.

Occasionally, at birth, a notch above the acetabulum may be present (Fig. 1.6) and even in the absence of the femoral head, congenital dislocation of the hip can then be diagnosed.

The eventual position of the femoral head and its relationship to the acetabulum can often be inferred from a film of the hips in the neutral position. The site of the nonossified epiphysis may be inferred as lying superior to the epiphyseal plate. This in turn lies at right angles and proximal to the femoral neck (Fig. 1.6).

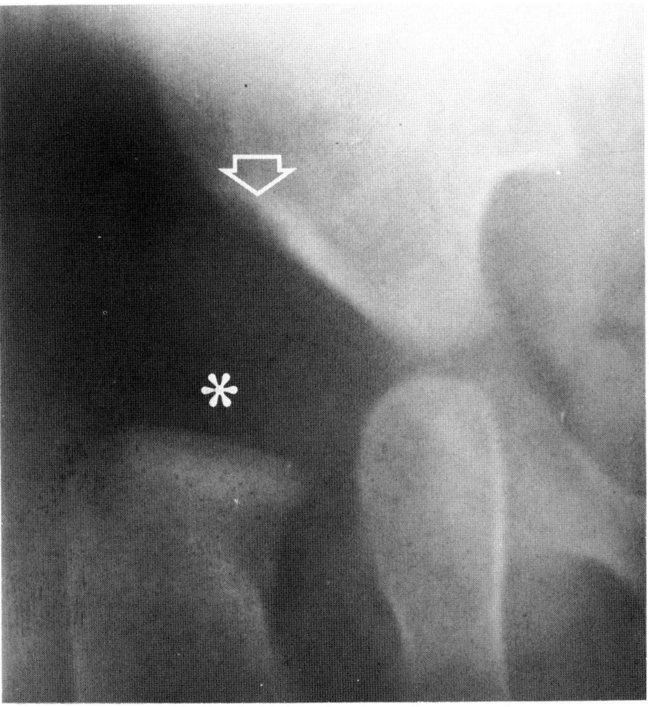

Fig. 1.6 A small defect with marginal sclerosis is seen above the acetabulum (arrow) in a neonate who later was shown to have a congenitally dislocated femoral head. The * marks the site of the projected femoral head.

Andren and von Rosen described an anteroposterior projection with the hips and knees fully extended, both legs abducted to 45° and the femora fully internally rotated. The baby must lie symmetrically on the table top and immobilization may be aided by a lightly applied compression band. The test may fail if the baby is grasped too firmly above the hips because reduction of the dislocation may occur.

Von Rosen and Andren state that a line drawn through the shaft of an undislocated femur will point to the outer lip of the acetabulum and will, if extended, cross the spine at the level of the lumbo-sacral junction. On the other hand, if the hip is in dislocation, a similar line will point

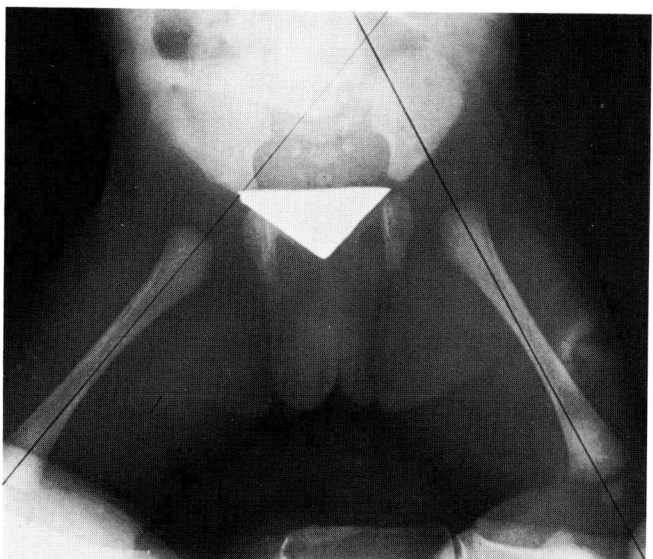

Fig. 1.7 Congenital dislocation of the left hip. On the normal right side a line through the long axis of the femur crosses the spine at the level of the lumbo-sacral articulation. On the dislocated side the spine is crossed at a higher level and the line through the long axis of the femur passes outside the acetabular rim. In practice it is unusual to find such a pronounced degree of dislocation in newborn infants.

outside the acetabulum and will cross the spine at a higher level (Fig. 1.7).

The degree of ossification of the acetabular roof must influence these measurements to some extent. It is our experience that in an undislocated hip, the line through the long axis of an abducted femur will pass well within the acetabular contour.

Radiographically one will see restricted abduction of the femoral shaft in congenital dislocation. The authors believe that abduction of 45° with the femur in internal rotation is difficult to attain or to maintain in the presence of a dislocation. It seems that the success of the Andren and von Rosen technique depends at least partially on this fact.

In few babies are the femoral capital epiphyses ossified at birth. If they are, then the diagnosis of dislocation is simplified. Retarded ossification of the femoral ossific nuclei is a traditional sign of congenital dislocation of the hip. In some early cases, however, the femoral ossific nucleus may appear to be larger on the dislocated than on the normal side. Some incongruous findings are probably explicable by the lesion being essentially bilateral.

Seen later, from the age of 6 months onwards, the radiological diagnosis is usually easy (Fig. 1.8). The femoral head will be displaced upwards and outwards and delayed ossification of its epiphyses will be observed. The acetabulum will be shallower than that of the normal hip and its roof will not be set horizontally but will slope upwards and outwards. Use of the many lines and coordinates described in this condition is not necessary, provided heed is paid to the possibility of a bilateral dislocation.

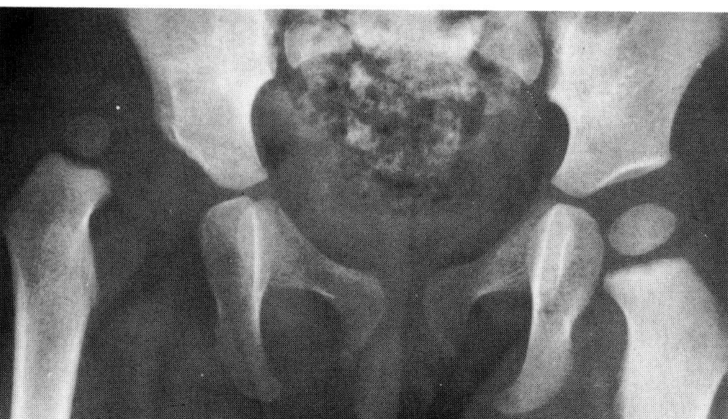

Fig. 1.8 Congenital dislocation of the right hip. *Note* sloping acetabular roof, delayed ossification of the femoral capital epiphysis and false acetabulum formation.

During management the radiologist will be asked to decide whether reduction has been attained or maintained. This decision may be very difficult to make on radiographs taken through plaster. In such cases tomography may give the required information — three sections using a multisection box will suffice.

Reduction may be impossible to obtain or the hip may be unstable. In such cases arthrography may be used to study the disposition of soft tissue structures of the joint.

The technique is described in Chapter 4. Possible abnormal findings are:

1. The fibrocartilaginous rim of the acetabulum, called the limbus, may become inverted into the joint, and form a barrier to stable reduction. In an arthrogram of a normal hip a thorn-like projection marks a small gap between the outer part of the limbus and the capsular attachment (see Fig. 4.68). When the limbus is inverted, the 'thorn' is lost and the filling defect caused by the limbus is seen (Fig. 1.9).

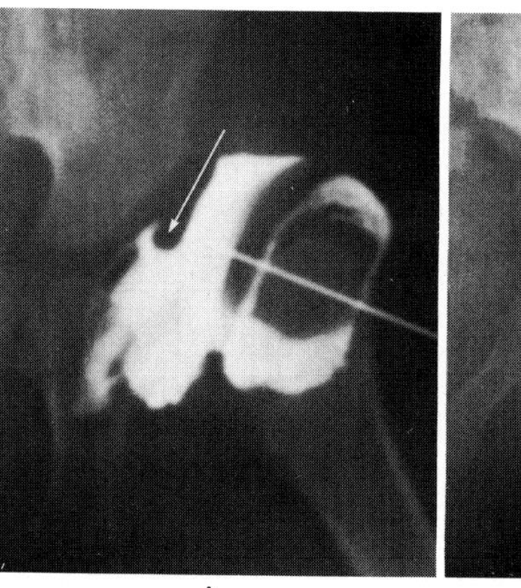

A

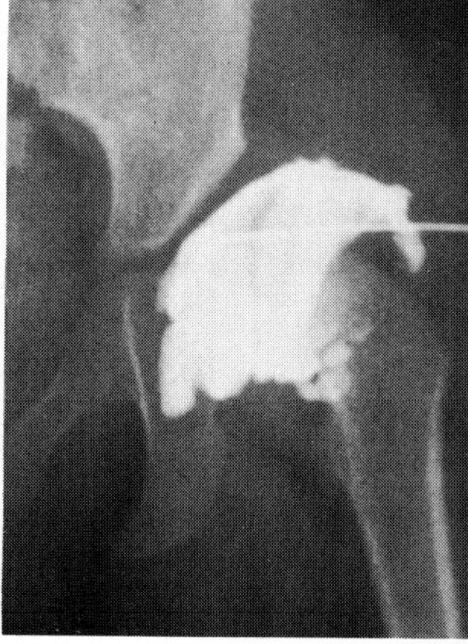

B

Fig. 1.9 A. Arthrogram of left hip shows filling defect caused by inverted limbus (arrow); **B**. Appearances following limbectomy. (Courtesy of Mr A. C. Clark.)

2. The capsule of the joint may be constricted and an hour-glass appearance may result. This finding is visible on arthrography. It is found only in cases treated in prolonged abduction plasters.

3. The ligamentum teres may become so large that it may offer a barrier to reduction. A hypertrophic ligamentum teres may be visible on the arthrogram but estimation of its size by this means is unreliable.

4. The psoas tendon may become contracted and a notch for the tendon is seen inferiorly.

5. The fibro-fatty material occupying the floor of the acetabulum may be increased and may thus prevent stable reduction.

6. Arthrography is of particular service in deciding whether complete reduction of a dislocation has been achieved. There are times when this information is not possible from examination of plain films, especially so when the femoral ossific nucleus appears to be set eccentrically on the femoral neck.

The primary cause of unstable reduction of a dislocated femoral head has long been debated. Excessive anteversion of the femoral neck is often seen and the condition often necessitates a de-rotation osteotomy for reduction to be maintained. The femoral neck of a normal baby is usually anteverted to 35°; this diminishes to 15° in the adult. In congenital dislocation, the femoral neck may be anteverted to 70–80°. The presence of anteversion is revealed by comparing radiographs taken in the neutral position with those in full internal rotation of the hips. In the neutral view, the anteverted femoral neck will be foreshortened; in internal rotation the femoral neck will be shown well separated from the upper femoral shaft (Fig. 1.10). Various specialized techniques are available for measuring the degree of anteversion.

In neglected dislocations, the misplaced femoral head may produce a depression on the side of the ilium above the acetabulum, constituting a false acetabulum. This may vary in size from a shallow depression to a deep socket. The original acetabular socket becomes progressively more shallow.

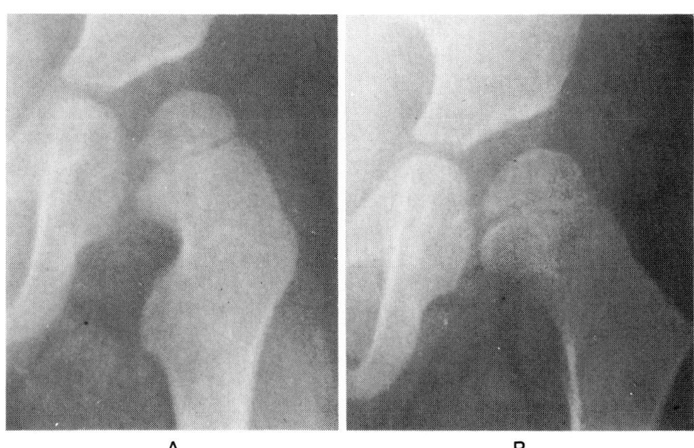

Fig. 1.10 **A**. Shows foreshortening of the anteverted femoral head in the neutral A.P. position; **B**. In internal rotation, the femoral neck is well visualized.

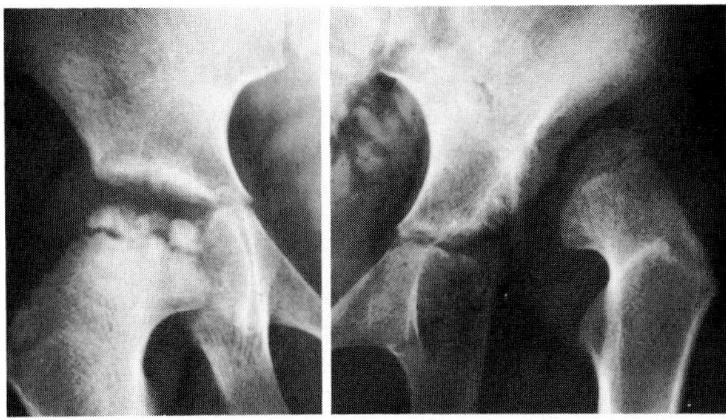
Fig. 1.11 This child presented with a congenital dislocation of the left hip and Perthes' disease of the right hip.

Osteochondritis may complicate a congenital dislocation of the hip, particularly after vigorous methods of reduction. Not all cases of osteochondritis are attributable to the complications of treatment for there does appear to be a true association between congenital dislocation and Perthes' disease of the hip (Fig. 1.11)

PROXIMAL FEMORAL ABNORMALITIES

Idiopathic coxa vara of childhood: proximal femoral focal deficiency (PFFD)

Two types of idiopathic coxa vara are recognized:

1. A congenital form, generally present at birth (Fig. 1.12), sometimes associated with other congenital lesions.

2. An infantile form, not present at birth, recognized around the age of 4 years and often bilateral (33%).

PFFD (congenitally short femur) consists of failure of normal development of a lesser or greater part of the proximal femur. Some distal femur, by definition, is always present, thus distinguishing it from femoral agenesis.

Coxa vara is included as part of the PFFD spectrum if the varus is associated with congenital femoral shortening present from birth, i.e. Type 1 above. If PFFD is severe, coxa vara cannot arise at all, even in congenital cases.

The mean angle of the neck on the shaft at 1 year of age is 148°, decreasing to 135° at 5 years and 120° in the elderly. Coxa vara is present when the angle is less than normal, but certainly if below 110°.

Radiographic findings: *Coxa vara*. The lesion is usually bilateral (Fig. 1.12) though it may be unilateral. Coxa vara will be evident. The femoral head will be situated low in the acetabulum and its outline may appear woolly. Secondary deformity of the acetabulum may result from the

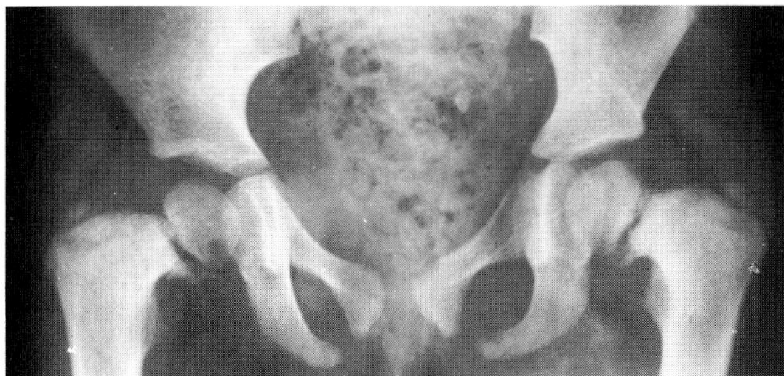

Fig. 1.12 Bilateral congenital coxa vara. *Note* triangular fragments of bone near the inferior surfaces of the femoral necks.

malposed femoral head. A triangular fragment of bone may be seen at the lower part of the femoral neck. This wedge of bone, commoner in the infantile cases, is bounded by two clear bands forming an inverted V (Fig. 1.13). The inner band is the epiphyseal line. The outer one is, of course, abnormal. Some writers have regarded it as an area of osteochondritis, others as a stress fracture. In later cases the greater trochanter will be found to curve in a beak-like fashion and it may articulate with the ilium. Not all these features are necessarily present in every case.

Acquired coxa vara may be found in rickets, fibrous dysplasia, osteogenesis imperfecta, cleidocranial dysplasia, Perthes' disease and following slipped epiphysis.

In some cases which appear to have PFFD with no proximal femur in which to have coxa vara, arthrography of the hip may reveal a cartilaginous neck and head with varus deformity.

Radiographic findings: *PFFD.* (Fig. 1.14A and B) A short femur is demonstrated at birth which is laterally situated and proximally displaced. The distal femur is by definition present. Ossification of the proximal portion is delayed. When varus appears it is subtrochanteric, i.e. bowing is present. A spectrum of proximal deficiencies exists.

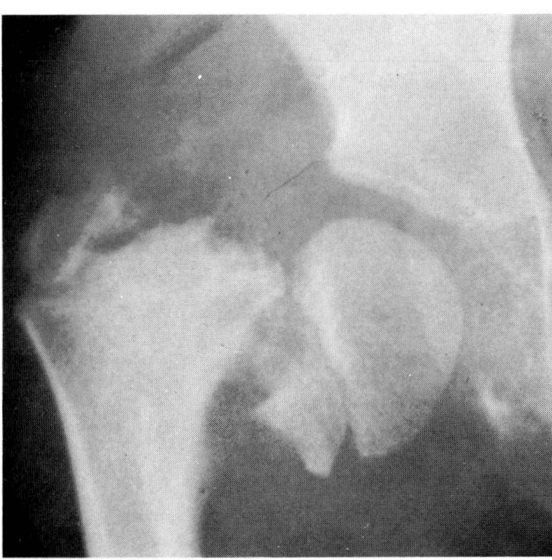

Fig. 1.13 Congenital coxa vara: extreme coxa vara with some slip of the epiphysis. A triangular fragment of bone is well shown.

Anomalies of the patella. The patella is frequently bipartite and sometimes multipartite. The upper, outer part is always involved. The anomaly is often bilateral and well corticated all round, thus helping to distinguish it from a fissure fracture. Not all cases, however, are bilateral.

In the *nail patella syndrome* the patella may be rudimentary or hypoplastic and set laterally (see Fig. 1.21).

The patella may be dislocated due to a variety of congenital causes, e.g. hypoplasia of the lateral femoral condyle, external rotation of the tibia and malattachment of the ilio-tibial tract. The displacement is invariably outwards.

Congenital dislocation of the knee. This is a rare lesion known also as *congenital genu recurvatum* and due to intra-uterine degeneration of the quadriceps muscles. At first only hyperextension of the knee may be found, later the tibia may be pulled up in front of the femoral condyles. The patella is often small or absent in this condition.

Congenital pseudarthrosis of the tibia and fibula. This condition was formerly regarded as a birth fracture but it is now realized that an underlying bony abnormality is always present. The pseudarthrosis of the tibia is seen at the junction of the middle and lower thirds. Often a similar lesion is found in the fibula.

Radiological examination of early cases may show a radiolucent zone in the affected area. Later a pathological fracture will occur and the severed ends of the bone become sclerotic. Still later, the proximal part becomes cupped and the distal part pointed, so forming a pseudarthrosis (Fig. 1.15).

This uncommon lesion is notoriously resistant to treatment. Amputation is often needed after a succession of unsuccessful attempts to obtain union.

Neurofibromatosis is usually given as the most frequent cause of this condition. Associated stigmata of neurofibromatosis have not been found in many of our cases. Another association is with fibrous dysplasia.

Very rarely a similar lesion has been found affecting the forearm bones.

The foot and ankle. Congenital anomalies of the foot are found which correspond to those in the hand.

Accessory bones of the foot. Supernumerary centres of ossification are more common in the foot than in the hand. They should be identified to distinguish them from fractures. They may themselves fracture and be a cause of pain, or may be involved in arthritis or infections. More than 50 have been described but most of them are rarities. The incidence rises to 30% in adults as they become radiologically visible. The os tibiale externum is found in some 7% of feet, the os trigonum in 5% and the os pero-

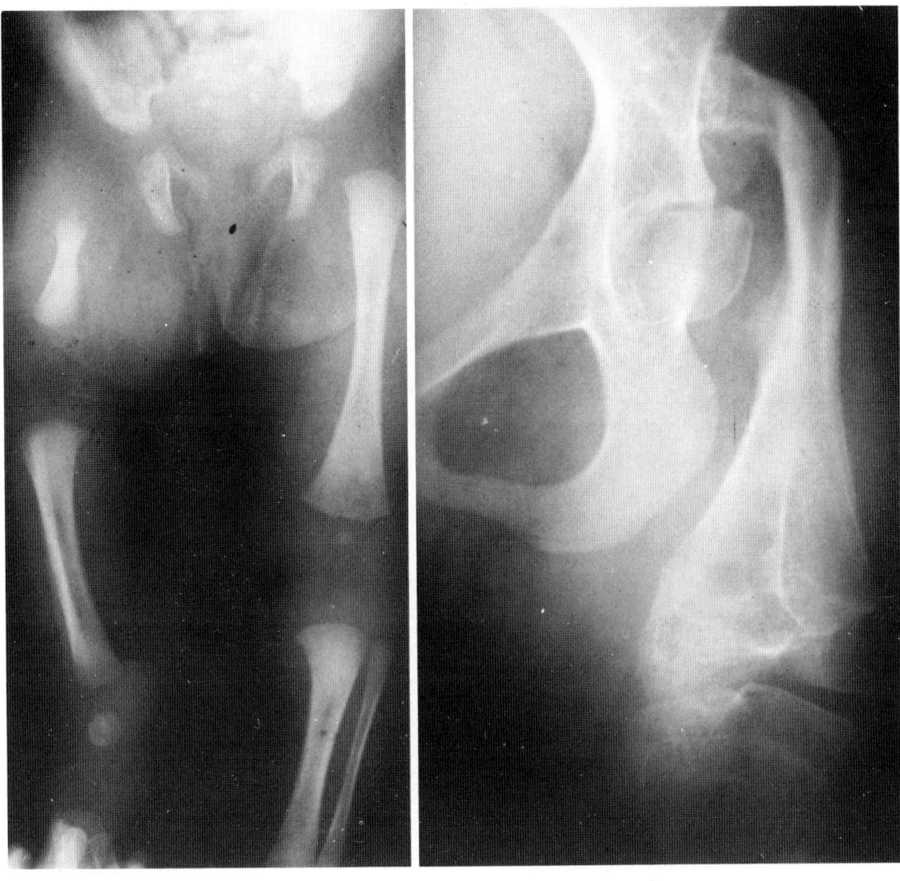

Fig. 1.14 A. Proximal focal femoral deficiency. Only a hypoplastic portion of the distal femur is apparent; **B.** Hypoplasia of the proximal femur with gross varus deformity and a normally located femoral head.

neum in 8% but surveys differ as to their incidence. Two sesamoids are regularly seen at the head of the great toe metatarsal. The medial is bipartite in one third of cases, the lateral in only 5%. A bipartite sesamoid is larger than its normal counterpart and corticated all round, while a fractured sesamoid shows non-corticated fracture parts.

Congenital talipes equino-varus (*congenital club foot*). This condition is nearly always idiopathic but club foot is sometimes associated with other bony abnormalities. The osseous type is associated with defects or absence of the tibia. Absence of some toes or of bones of the foot may be seen.

The idiopathic type is of limited interest to the radiologist. The three cardinal abnormalities are 1) adduction of the forefoot, 2) inversion of the foot and 3) plantar flexion of the foot. Radiologically medial displacement of the navicular and cuboid in relation to the heads of the talus and calcaneum will be seen. The calcaneum will rotate medially under the talus. Plantar flexion will be seen by posterior displacement of the calcaneum.

Ossification of the talus and navicular may be retarded. Usually secondary hypoplasia of the bones of the tarsus and of the soft tissues is seen.

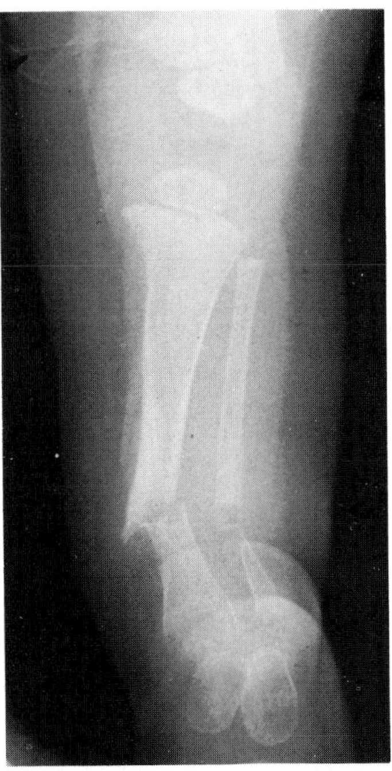

Fig. 1.15 Typical congenital pseudarthrosis of the tibia and fibula. This child had neurofibromatosis though other stigmata of neurofibromatosis are not always found in this condition.

Congenital dislocation of the ankle. This is a rare abnormality always associated with obvious bony abnormalities.

Ball and socket ankle joint. In this condition the ankle joint is abnormally shaped and its range of movement increased. It is usually compensatory for rigid mid-tarsal and subtaloid joints generally caused by tarsal fusions. In such cases inversion and eversion of the ankle compensate for the loss of these movements at the mid-tarsal and subtaloid joints.

Some cases are seen in patients with a short leg — in a few no underlying cause is seen.

Radiographic features are characteristic. The trochlear surface of the talus, normally convex anteroposteriorly and concave from side to side, loses this concavity and approaches the shape of a sphere. The mortice of the talus becomes correspondingly moulded into a cup-like cavity to form a ball and socket articulation (Fig. 1.16).

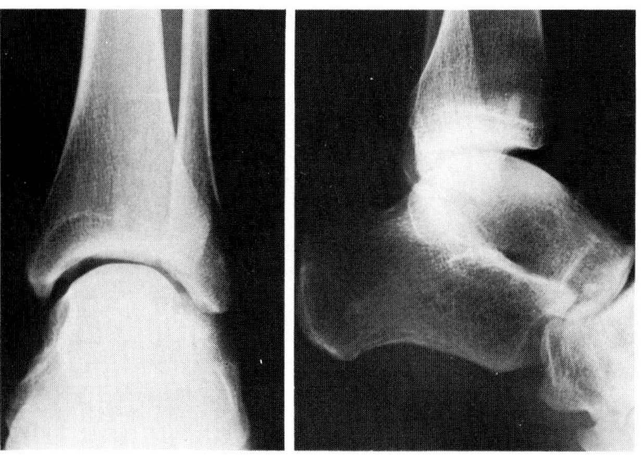

Fig. 1.16 Ball and socket ankle associated with talonavicular fusion.

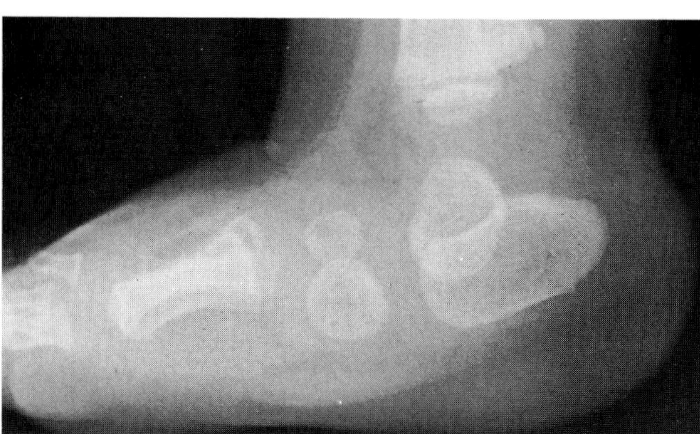

Fig. 1.17 Congenital vertical talus. *Note* vertical position of the talus and elevation both of the calcaneum and of the forefoot.

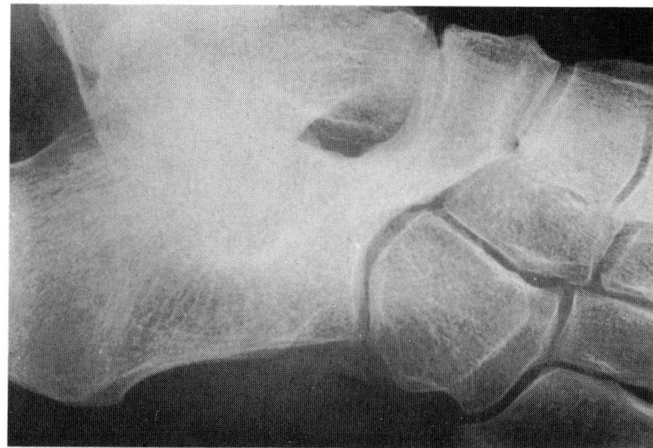

Fig. 1.18 Calcaneo-navicular bar.

Congenital vertical talus. This is a rare cause of congenital flat foot in children. The lesion is, in effect, a congenital dislocation of the talo-navicular joint, a feature that would be obvious were the navicular ossified at birth.

The radiographic appearances are diagnostic. The talus is vertical, its long axis following that of the tibial shaft. The vertical displacement of the talus remains constant whether the patient is standing or recumbent. The bones of the forefoot and the calcaneum are raised and the typical rocker bottom foot is caused (Fig. 1.17). When the navicular becomes ossified its shape will be seen to appear normal except for a little constriction of its waist. It will be seen obviously dislocated and lying in contact with the body of the talus.

In some other forms of flat foot the talus is displaced downwards but the talo-navicular joint is not dislocated.

Congenital fusions. Painful flat foot (the peroneal spastic flat foot) may be due to fusion of certain tarsal bones (Figs. 1.18 and 1.19). If the union is cartilaginous or fi-

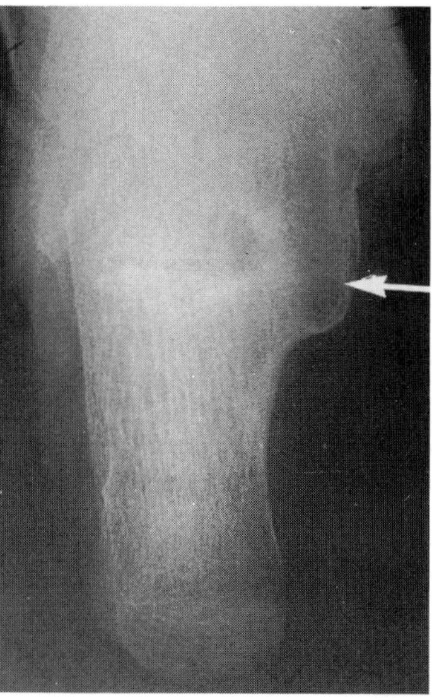

Fig. 1.19 Talo-calcaneal synostosis.

brous, it is not seen radiologically but flattening of the longitudinal arch of the foot may be seen. Bony union is not directly demonstrable before adolescence but appears with ossification of the cartilaginous link between the bones. Fusion of the medial facet of the subtalar joint is the most common. It is well seen on an axial view of the foot. Calcaneo-navicular fusion is shown on oblique views of the foot (Fig. 1.18). Coalition has been described between all the bones of the hind foot. Restriction of movement at the subtalar joint causes abnormal movement and lipping at the calcaneo-navicular joint, seen together with longitudinal arch flattening and obliteration of subtalar joints on the lateral view of the foot. These changes result in a local increase in uptake with isotope bone scanning. CT scanning, when available, will also show foot fusions.

THE PELVIS

Naegele and Robert pelvis. Both are very rare but of obstetric importance. The *Naegele* pelvis is characterized by absence of one wing of the sacrum with ankylosis of the sacro-iliac joint on the affected side. The *Robert* pelvis is a bilateral Naegele pelvis. Both types are further discussed in the section on obstetric radiology.

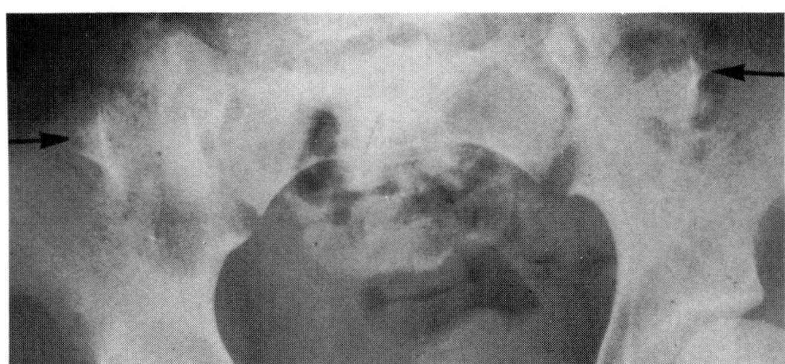

Fig. 1.20 Nail-patella syndrome. Iliac horns are seen (arrows).

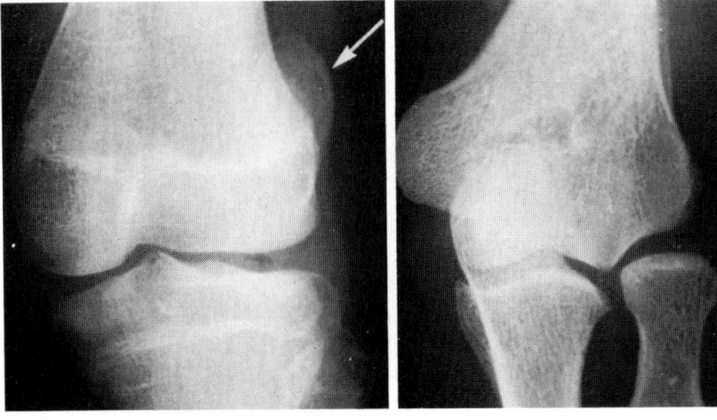

Fig. 1.21 **Fig. 1.22**

Fig. 1.21 A small laterally placed patella is shown.
Fig. 1.22 Hypoplasia of the capitellum is shown.

Iliac horns . These are bony processes projecting dorsally from the outer surface of the wings of each ilium. They may occur alone or be associated with the syndrome of rudimentary or absent patellae, deformity of the elbows (hypoplasia of capitellum and radial head) and dystrophy of the nails (*Nail-patella syndrome — Fong's lesion*) (Figs 1.20–1.22).

THE SPINE

Spinal anomalies range from gross defects, incompatible with life, to minor anomalies which are no more than anatomical variants. Some of these may be mistaken for fractures, e.g. the unfused accessory ossification centres at the tips of inferior articular facets or those related to the anterosuperior part of the margins of vertebral bodies. Fractures rarely are seen at such sites and have ragged rather than smooth edges.

Coronal cleft vertebra. This anomaly is seen in vertebral bodies of newborn infants due to failure of fusion of two ossification centres. In about half the cases more than one vertebral body is affected. The abnormality has been seen on prenatal radiographs — it occurs more frequently in male infants.

The cleft is seen on a lateral radiograph as a linear or oval defect between a small posterior and larger anterior ossification centre (Fig. 1.23). The anteroposterior diameter of the affected vertebral body is often increased. The cleft consolidates in a few months. They are of no importance except that they are seen in some dysplasias.

Butterfly vertebra. This anomaly, sometimes called 'anterior spina bifida', is due to persistence of fetal notochordal remnants. In the affected vertebra, the upper and lower surfaces are deeply concave or V-shaped so that the vertical dimension of the vertebral body in the midline is much reduced. In the frontal projection, it is seen that vertebrae above and below are moulded into the deficient centres of the affected vertebra (Fig. 1.24).

Malfusions of appendages. Epiphyses of the spinous processes, transverse processes and articular facets may remain unfused. The abnormality is without importance except that fractures may be mimicked.

Hemivertebra. They may cause scoliosis unless an equal number appear on each side. In the thoracic region, a hemivertebra will bear a rib. Multiple hemivertebrae may cause dwarfism.

Congenital vertebral fusions. Many forms of congenital vertebral fusion may be found. Complete fusion of the bodies and neural arches may occur or the fusion may be limited to parts of the bodies or neural arches. At times it may not be possible to decide whether a fusion is developmental or postinflammatory. Fusion of neural arches, however, is almost always a developmental anomaly. The anteroposterior diameter of congenital block vertebrae may be reduced and an anterior concavity may be found. These

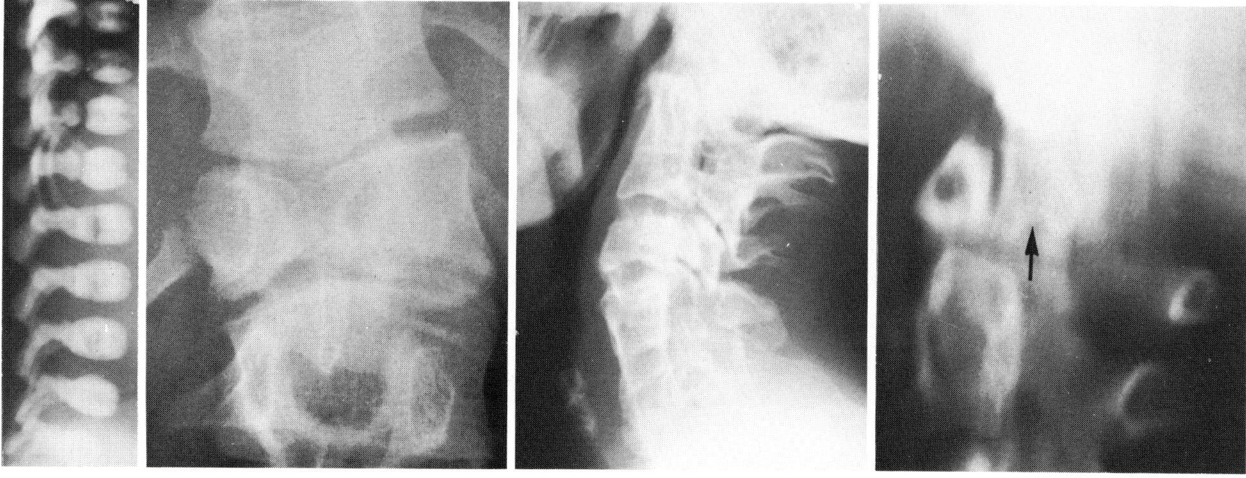

Fig. 1.23 Fig. 1.24 Fig. 1.25 Fig. 1.26

Fig. 1.23 Coronal cleft vertebra. (Courtesy of Dr K. A. Rowley.)

Fig. 1.24 Butterfly vertebra. Upper and lower surfaces of affected vertebra are V-shaped, and contiguous vertebrae are moulded into the deficient centre.

Fig. 1.25 Klippel-Feil syndrome. Cervical fusions are seen with a short neck.

Fig. 1.26 Os odontoideum. This separate ossicle is possibly the result of previous odontoid peg fracture.

features may also be found in old post-infective fusions. However, a posterior concavity in addition is diagnostic of a congenital fusion. Complete vertebral fusions are often called 'block vertebrae'. They may be of no clinical significance, but frequently disc degeneration above or below the fused vertebrae develops due to altered mechanics in the spine. Such lesions are relatively common in the cervical spine where a more severe anomaly, the *Klippel–Feil syndrome*, may be seen (Fig. 1.25). In this condition, many cervical vertebrae are fused, the neck is short, its movements limited and hair grows low on to the neck. Often there is torticollis and atrophy of facial musculature. Other congenital anomalies, such as spina bifida, rib lesions and Sprengel's shoulder, usually co-exist.

Separate odontoid (*os odontoideum*). The odontoid peg may sometimes be completely detached from the body of the second cervical vertebra, and be situated in the region of the foramen magnum (Fig. 1.26). Neurological symptoms may be associated.

It has been shown that in some cases at least the separate ossicle results from a fracture in childhood of the base of the odontoid peg, with subsequent non-union. The lesion is thus not always 'congenital'.

Cervical rib. This is a common anomaly. The supplementary rib usually arises from the seventh cervical vertebra, rarely from the sixth and very rarely from the fifth.

The diagnosis is straightforward, though it may be necessary to count all the ribs in order to distinguish a rudimentary first thoracic rib from a cervical rib. Cervical ribs arise from cervical transverse processes. These slope downwards from the neural arch in the cervical spine but upwards in the thoracic spine. Cervical ribs vary greatly in size and shape and clinical symptoms bear little relation to the radiographic abnormality. A very small cervical rib element may have a fibrous attachment to the first thoracic rib which causes much disability, whereas a large cervical rib may be asymptomatic.

Sacralization and lumbarization. It is often difficult to give a definite level to a particular vertebral body in the lumbar region, especially if the lumbo-sacral region is transitional. Again, it may be necessary to count all the vertebral bodies from C1 down. It has been said that the transverse processes of L3 are the lowest (most caudal) which lie truly transversely, while those for L4 are inclined upwards. Various permutations occur. Small, or absent ribs on T12 may occur with large transverse processes on L5 which fuse with the sacrum (sacralization of L5). This is known as cranial shift. Caudal shift implies the presence

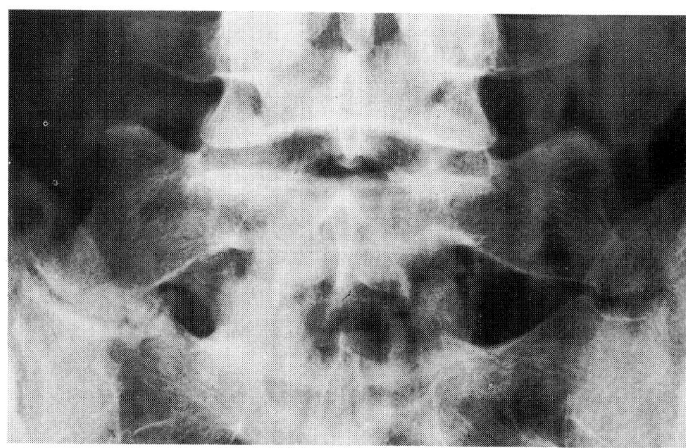

Fig. 1.27 Bilateral sacralization. Osteoarthritic changes are seen round the pseudarthrosis on the right side.

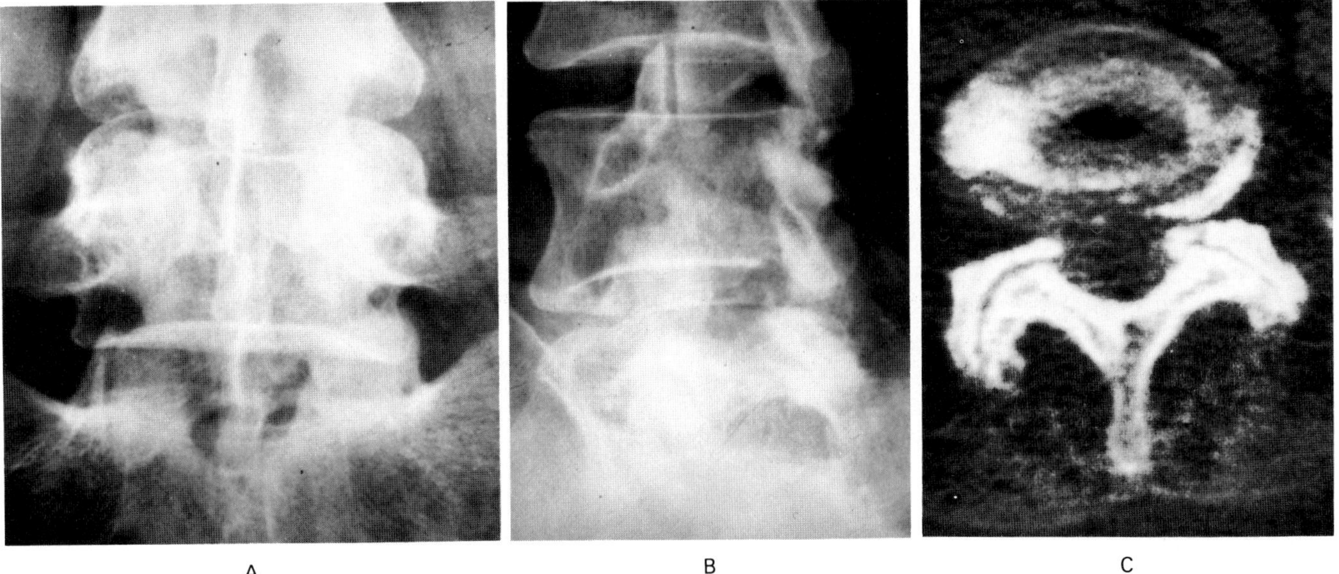

A B C

Fig. 1.28 (**A** and **B**) The facet joints are no longer symmetrical and show features of degeneration. (**C**) The CT scan shows gross new bone formation around narrowed facet joints. There is marked bony encroachment upon the exit foramina, especially the left. Gas is seen in the disc (vacuum phenomenon).

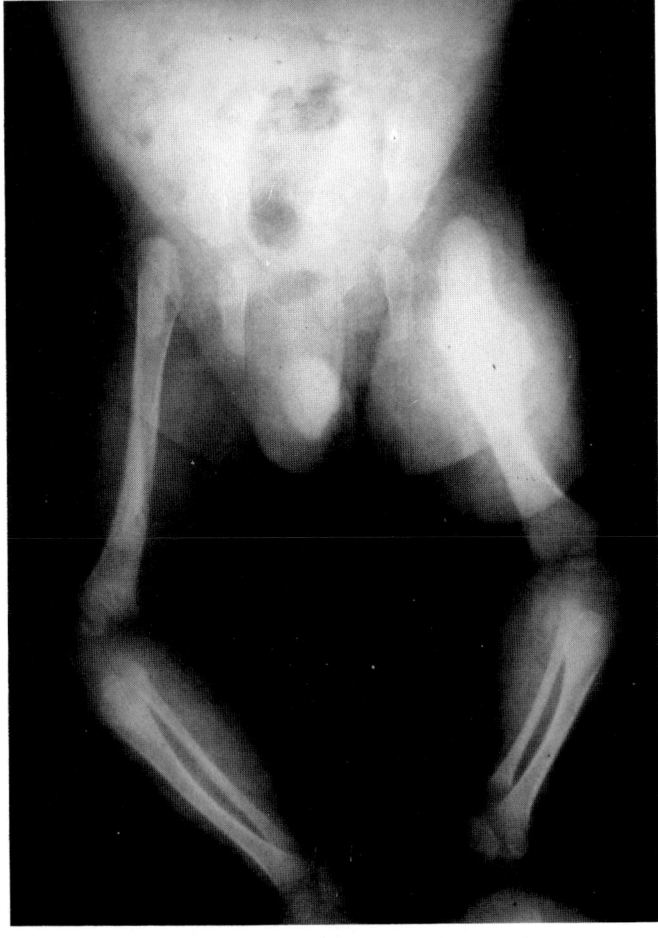

A

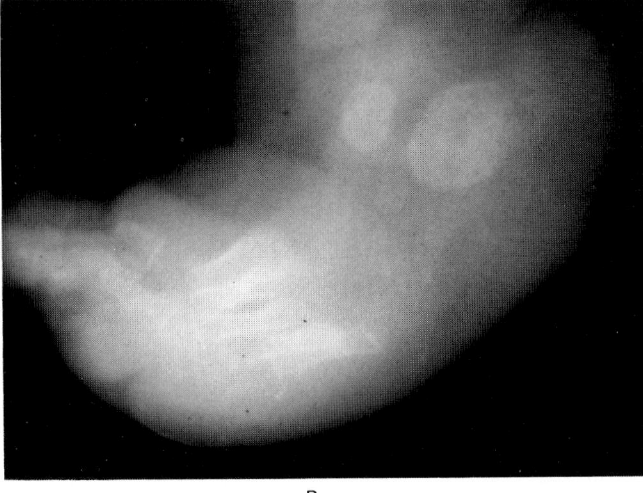

B

Fig. 1.29 Arthrogryposis multiplex congenita. (**A** and **B**) Dislocations of the hip joints are accompanied by hypoplasia of the muscles. Club foot is present. There is also evidence of birth trauma.

of ribs on L1 and lumbarization of S1, that is, it comes to bear free-floating transverse processes. A rudimentary disc is then seen between S1 and S2.

The sacralized transverse process may form a pseudarthrosis with the ilium and degenerative sclerosis may appear around the false joint (Fig. 1.27). This may be a site of low back pain.

Anomalies of lumbo-sacral facets (trophism). The facet joints in the lumbar spine may be clearly seen in the anteroposterior projection. They should be symmetrical. With degeneration, the lower lumbar facet joints cease to be symmetrical, so that often one joint is seen and the other at that level is no longer seen (Fig. 1.28A). This rotational change is associated with much new bone around narrowed facet joints and adjacent laminae, often with symptoms of nerve root impingement. The changes are well demonstrated with CT scanning (Fig. 1.28B), when the acquired asymmetry of the entire neural arch is seen as well as the local new bone formation.

Spina bifida. Incomplete fusion of neural arches is a common finding. In most cases only a minor midsagittal defect in the neural arch is seen. The rather misleading term 'spina bifida occulta' is applied to this condition. There is no true breach in such cases; the radiolucent area represents merely non-ossified cartilage. In children many of these areas become ossified as growth progresses.

True breaches in the neural arch do, of course, occur, and they may be accompanied by a meningocele protruding posteriorly and usually in the lumbar region. Occasionally, in the thorax and in the sacral region, the sac may protrude laterally and anteriorly through the intervertebral foramina and sacral foramina respectively. Other vertebral and rib anomalies are very frequent in the severe forms of spina bifida. The presence of hydrocephalus is a common feature in marked spina bifida.

Foot deformities, such as pes cavus, may be associated with spina bifida. Likewise, perforating ulcers causing absorption of metatarsal heads, neuropathic joints and spontaneous fractures accompanied by excessive callus may all occur. Metaphyseal fractures are sometimes seen in this condition.

In cases of alimentary reduplications, the possibility of associated malformations of the spine should be borne in mind. The reduplications or *neurenteric cysts* may be associated with severe anterior and posterior spina bifida, hemivertebra, absent vertebra or diastematomyelia. In some cases no vertebral deformity is demonstrable.

ARTHROGRYPOSIS MULTIPLEX CONGENITA

This lesion is characterized by congenital failure of muscle development and by joint lesions such as club foot, club hand, congenital dislocation of the hip and congenital genu recurvatum. This disease is probably overdiagnosed since it provides a useful diagnostic repository for lesions of children with multiple skeletal abnormalities.

It is important to be sure that muscle bundles are deficient before this diagnosis is made. Radiographically, muscle shadows are represented by mere strands of water density running through the soft tissues of an extremity that appear to consist solely of fat (Fig. 1.29A and B). Sometimes other skeletal abnormalities are associated, e.g. fusion of carpal bones.

DYSPLASIAS OF BONE

An immediate hindrance to the understanding of this group of lesions is the difficulty in defining the conditions. The authors will follow Rubin's divisions and propose this simplified version:

Dysplasia, a disturbance in bone form or modelling intrinsic to bone.
Dysostosis, a disturbance in bone form or modelling associated with a disturbance of ectodermal or other mesenchymal tissue.
Dystrophy, a disturbance in bone form or modelling of nutritional or metabolic origin.

Not all conditions about to be considered will fit tidily into the above categories. Some conditions are frankly incorrectly designated according to this grouping.

The diagnosis of these lesions is mainly radiological and often entirely so. The radiologist will observe such features as alteration in bone density and in the size and shape of the bones. He will also observe the distribution of the lesion and the parts of the bones affected. The following tables (Tables 1.1 and 1.2) are presented with the intention of helping the radiologist who sees few of these lesions to reach a differential diagnosis. He will then be able to proceed to more detail in the text and, if necessary, to refer to larger volumes. The classification is based entirely on radiographic appearances. Accurate diagnosis is now of prime importance and not merely an academic exercise. Genetic counselling is, of course, a well-established speciality depending on accurate diagnosis. In other fields such as the mucopolysaccharidoses new lines of therapy are being evaluated.

CLEIDOCRANIAL DYSPLASIA (CCD)

(Synonym: *cleidocranial dysostosis*)

This is a benign hereditary condition which is inherited as an autosomal dominant and which is recognised during childhood. The disease has considerable variation of expression.

Radiological features. Changes are widespread.

Clavicles. There may be total (in 10% of cases) or partial absence of the clavicle (Fig. 1.30). The outer end is absent more frequently than the inner, both to an extremely variable extent. Central defects also occur. The clavicles may also be normal. The scapulae tend to be small and high, and the glenoid fossae are small.

Table 1.1 Bone dysplasias and allied lesions.

Main radiographic features	Dysplasia	Some differentiating and characteristic features
Disseminated developmental defects	(1) Cleidocranial dysplasia	Defects in clavicles, skull, teeth, sometimes congenital coxa vara.
	(2) Acro-osteolysis	Destruction of distal phalanges. Osteoporosis. Basilar invagination.
Disseminated developmental defects and increase in bone density	(1) Pycnodysostosis	Combined features resembling cleidocranial dysplasia and osteopetrosis.
Reduction in bone density	(1) Osteogenesis imperfecta	Multiple fractures, blue sclerae, otosclerosis, dental changes.
	(2) Fibrogenesis imperfecta ossium	Seen in older subjects. May be fractures. Secondary trabeculae resorbed, coarsened 'fish-net' pattern of primary trabeculae.
Areas of increased and reduced bone density	(1) Fibrous dysplasia	May be monostotic and show one feature only. Pigmentation of skin in some and precocious puberty in some females. Femur affected in all polyostotic cases. Epiphyses spared. Skull and facial bones affected in many.
Increase in bone density		
(a) Generalized	(1) Osteopetrosis (Albers-Schönberg disease)	Splaying of bone ends, anaemia. Liver and spleen may be enlarged.
(b) Large local areas	(1) Melorheostosis (Leri's disease)	Appearance of molten wax flowing down the side of a candle.
	(2) Craniometaphyseal dysplasia	Extra density in bone shafts and skull base in infants.
(c) Disseminated areas	(1) Osteopoikilosis	Lesions have characteristic appearances. Of no clinical significance.
	(2) Osteopathia striata	
Bone density normal: main change in bone structure		
(a) Epiphyseal lesions	(1) Dysplasia epiphysealis punctata	Some shortening of tubular bones. Mental changes. Cataract.
	(2) Dysplasia epiphysealis hemimelica	Limited to part of an epiphysis especially to lower fibula and talus.
	(3) Dysplasia epiphysealis multiplex	Some secondary metaphyseal irregularity: spine, pelvis normal.
(b) Metaphyseal lesions (see also Table 1.4)	(1) Metaphyseal dysplasia (Pyle)	Symmetrical expansion of metaphyses of long bones and clavicles — in adults.
	(2) Metaphyseal dysostosis	Splaying and irregularity of metaphyses. Severe Jansen type, milder Schmid type. Intermediate forms also.
(c) Diaphyseal lesions (see also Table 1.4)	(1) Diaphyseal dysplasia (Engelmann's disease)	Symmetrical fusiform thickening of long bones. Mild sclerosis of skull in some.
(d) Metaphyseal and diaphyseal lesions		
(i) extra-osseous	(1) Diaphyseal aclasia	Splaying of bone ends. Often associated with a short bowed ulna.
(ii) endosteal	(2) Dyschondroplasia (Ollier)	Columns of unossified cartilage which may be partially calcified extend from the metaphysis into the shaft of the bone. Epiphyseal changes absent or slight, spine not affected (cf. chondro-osteo-dystrophy).
Dwarfism and various changes in epiphyses and metaphyses		
(a) Short-limbed dwarfs (see Table 1.2)		
(b) Short trunk dwarf	(1) Spondyloepiphyseal dysplasia including Morquio-Brailsford	Gross platyspondyly, protrusion of central tongue of bone from vertebral body
(c) Short limb and short trunk (may not be marked)	(1) Dysostosis multiplex (gargoylism) (not a dysplasia)	Biconvex vertebrae with beak-like protrusion of lower part. Swollen tapering bones especially in arms. Visceral manifestations.
Elongation of tubular bones	(1) Arachnodactyly	Distal bones affected more than proximal. Visceral changes, e.g. eye and heart. Similar changes may be found in homocystinuria but osteoporosis, mental retardation, vascular thrombosis and cutaneous flushes may be seen in homocystinuria but not arachnodactyly.
Soft tissue dysplasia	(1) Myositis ossificans progressiva (fibrodysplasia ossificans progressiva)	Hypoplasia of thumbs and great toes.

Table 1.2 Short limb dwarfs.

Main radiographic feature	Dwarf	Some differentiating and characteristic features
Short limb dwarf: proximal bones affected more than distal bones (i.e. rhizomelic)	Achondroplasia	Depressed bridge of nose, square-shaped ilia, proximity of epiphyses to metaphyses. Reduction in interpedicular distance from L1 to L5.
Very short limbs. Failure of ossification of vertebral column and pubis.	Achondrogenesis	Distal ends of femora may bow outwards. Lethal.
More severe than achondroplasia. Some similarity to thanatophoric dwarf.	Homozygous achondroplasia	Both parents have achondroplasia. Lethal.
Very short curved bones. Proximal bones especially.	Thanatophoric dwarfism	Extreme platyspondyly, posterior arches normal. Large 'disc spaces'. Lethal.
Gross metaphyseal enlargement — dumb-bell bones especially in femora.	Metatrophic dwarfism	Platyspondyly but posterior arches normal. Kyphoscoliosis occurs from 6 months onwards.
Short limbs, clubbed feet. Hitch-hiker's thumb.	Diastrophic dwarfism	Cystic inflammation of the pinna in first few days in 80%. Progressive scoliosis.
Short limbs — distal limbs affected more than proximal (i.e. acromelic). Polydactyly.	Chondroectodermal dysplasia (Ellis-van Creveld syndrome)	Narrow elongated thorax, short ribs, enlarged anterior ends. Trident acetabular roof. Proximal femoral epiphyses ossified at birth.
A high thorax in A.P. and lateral planes. High clavicle.	Asphyxiating thoracic dystrophy	Short iliac wings, horizontal acetabular roof, trident pelvis.
(a) Symmetrical shortening of long bones and metaphyseal flaring. (b) Asymmetrical shortening of long bones. In both (a) and (b), punctate calcification in and around epiphyses.	Chondrodysplasia punctata (a) rhizomelic type (b) Conradi-Hunermann type	(a) Microcephaly and mental defect. Lethal. (b) Normal intelligence.
Short bones with fractures and deformities of many types.	Osteogenesis imperfecta (severe type)	Some cases have slender bones. Osteoporosis. Lethal.
Lack of ossification of skull. Short bones with gross flaring of metaphyses.	Hypophosphatasia (severe form)	Severe forms are lethal.
Angulation of femora above middle of diaphyses. Angulation of tibiae near lower third.	Campomelic dwarfism	Dislocated femora. Hypoplastic scapulae. Lethal.
Limbs only slightly shortened. Prominent epiphyses.	Hypochondroplasia	Skull normal. Interpedicular distances reduce from L1 to L5.
Flared metaphyses. Short metacarpals and phalanges. Signs not evident until 1 year of age.	Pseudoachondroplasia	Ossification defects at the ventral upper and lower borders of vertebral bodies, subsequently becoming almost normal.
Rhizomelic shortening of long bones. Short iliac wings. Delayed ossification of pubic bones, epiphyses of knees, talus, calcaneum. Vertebral bodies flattened posteriorly.	Spondyloepiphyseal dysplasia congenita	Myopia, retinal detachment, cataract, cleft palate, hearing loss.
Shortening of forearm bones and tibiae and fibulae.	Dyschondrosteosis	Madelung's deformities.

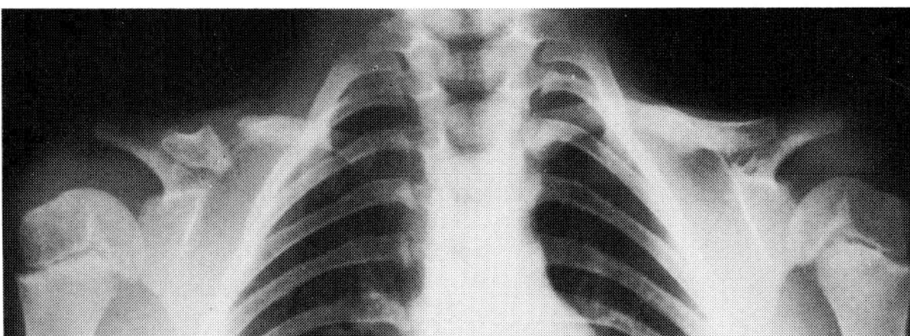

Fig. 1.30 Cleidocranial dysplasia: clavicular defects especially on the right side.

Thorax. The thorax is usually narrow, the ribs are short and directed obliquely downwards. Respiratory distress may occur in the newborn. The sternum is incompletely ossified. Failure of fusion of neural arches occurs with delay in maturation of vertebral bodies, which retain an infantile biconvex shape. Supernumerary or bifid ribs also occur.

Skull. In the newborn, mineralization is delayed. The facial bones are small but the mandible normal in size. The fontanelles remain open late and the sutures are widened. The bodies of the sphenoids are hypoplastic. Many Wormian bones are seen. Frontal and parietal bossing may be present and basilar invagination may occur (Fig. 1.31).

Pelvis. Pelvic bones are commonly affected. Delayed and imperfect ossification of the pubic bones is a recognized finding (Fig. 1.32) and congenital coxa vara is frequently seen.

Teeth. See Chapter 52.

Hands. Anomalies of the hand are very common. The second and fifth metacarpals are long and have supernumerary ossification centres at their bases. The middle phalanges of the second and fifth fingers are short. Cone epiphyses and distal phalangeal tapering are found.

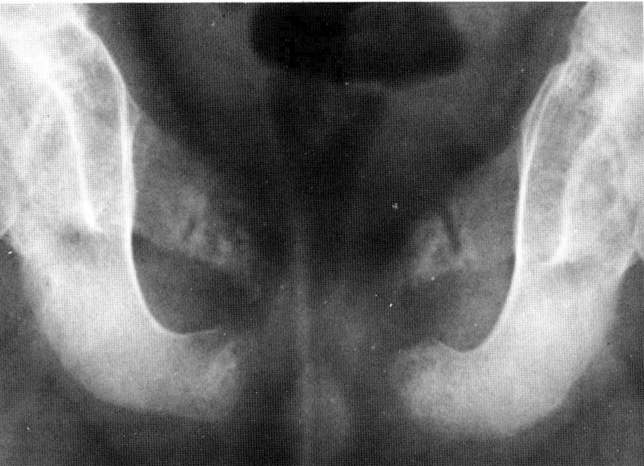

Fig. 1.32 Cleidocranial dysplasia. Failure of ossification of the symphysis pubis is demonstrated.

Short fibulae, congenital pseudarthrosis of the femur, genu valgum and obliquity of the articular space of the ankle joint are among many reported associations.

PYCNODYSOSTOSIS

This condition has been confused with cleidocranial dysplasia (because of some similar clavicular and skull changes) and osteopetrosis (because of the generalized in-

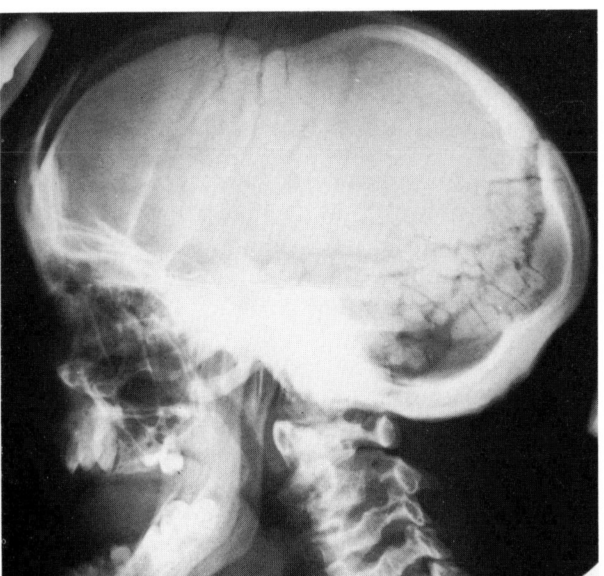

Fig. 1.31 Cleidocranial dysplasia — skull. *Note* delayed mineralisation in fronto-parietal region and Wormian bones posteriorly. Facial bones are small but the mandible is normal. Delayed dentition is also seen.

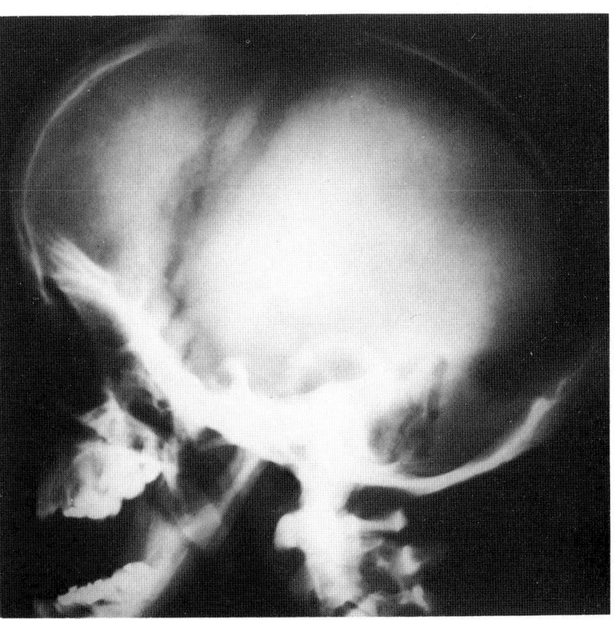

Fig. 1.33 Pycnodysostosis. The skull shows failure of sutural fusion and sclerosis of the base. The angle of the mandible is obtuse and the maxilla hypoplastic (Courtesy of Dr A. Thomas.)

crease in diffuse bone density). It is inherited as an autosomal recessive disease, and parental consanguinity is often present. The patients are short (below 150 cm; not a prominent feature of CCD). The skeleton is susceptible to fractures. The disease is rare and the patients are found in all races. The French painter Toulouse-Lautrec is believed to have suffered from this disease.

Radiographic features. *Skull.* There is brachycephaly with wide sutures and persistence of open fontanelles into adult life (Fig. 1.33). Wormian bones are seen. The calvarium, base of skull and especially the orbital rims are very dense. The facial bones are small and the maxilla hypoplastic (Fig. 1.33). The mandible has no angle — it is obtuse (see Chapter 52).

Limbs. Normal modelling of long bones is usually seen. The cortices are dense but the medullary canals not completely obliterated. The distal phalanges show acro-osteolysis.

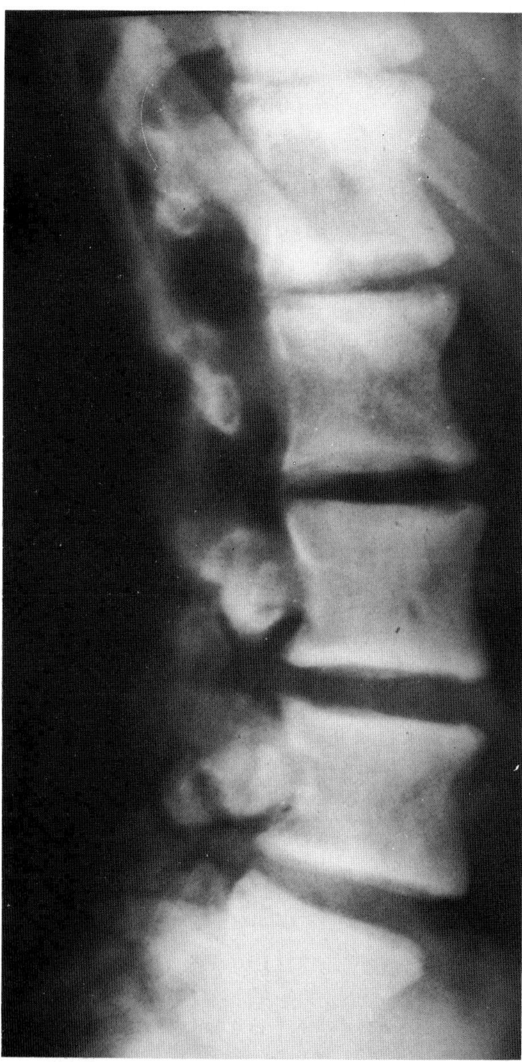

Fig. 1.34 Pycnodysostosis. Increased density of spool-shaped vertebral bodies with multiple pars fractures. (Courtesy of Dr A. Thomas.)

Thorax. Hypoplasia of the lateral ends of the clavicles is present to a varying degree. The ribs are dense overall.

Spine. Failure of fusion of the neural arches and spondylolisthesis are found. In adults the vertebral bodies resemble spools, with large anterior and posterior defects. The bones are uniformly dense (Fig. 1.34).

Hands. Acro-osteolysis occurs, often with irregular distal fragments of the distal phalanges.

ACRO-OSTEOLYSIS

(Eponym: *Hajdu–Cheney syndrome*)

Acro-osteolysis means disintegration of bone of the tips of the fingers and toes. This specific syndrome is inherited as an autosomal dominant. Other features include spinal osteoporosis, Wormian bones in children and basilar invagination causing posterior fossa symptoms. Other types of inherited phalangeal resorption exist.

There are many other causes of resorption of distal phalanges (Table 1.3). In some, resorption has a characteristic pattern and is accompanied by other features of the disease. Thus, in hyperparathyroidism, tuft resorption is accompanied by subperiosteal bone resorption around the cortices of middle phalanges.

Table 1.3 Atrophic changes in distal phalanges

Atrophy of distal phalanges may be seen in disorders due to many causes:

Congenital	Many forms of phalangeal agenesis may be found as congenital familial disorders.
Dysplastic	Cleidocranial dysplasia. Pycnodysostosis. Acro-osteolysis.
Infective	In acute infections usually only one digit affected — diagnosis obvious. Leprosy — neurotrophic factors contributory. Sarcoid.
Trauma	Frostbite. Electrical injuries.
Poisons	Ergot — peripheral arterial spasm and gangrene. Polyvinyl tank cleaners.
Metabolic	Hyperparathyroidism.
Vascular	Scleroderma with secondary Raynaud's phenomenon. Occlusive vascular disease. Pseudoxanthoma elasticum.
Neurotrophic	Tabes, syringomyelia. Diabetes — vascular and infective changes may be contributory.
Neoplastic	Kaposi's sarcoma where diffuse cutaneous and visual lesions are seen (disease of Eastern and Central Europe and Africa).
Miscellaneous	Psoriasis, pityriasis rubra, epidermolysis bullosa, reticulohistiocytosis. Ainhum. Neurofibromatosis. Progeria.

Some patients have neurological lesions, e.g. in syphilis, syringomyelia and diabetes. In some conditions, such as rheumatoid arthritis and psoriasis, peripheral vascular deficiency has been shown to occur in the region of tuft resorption.

OSTEOGENESIS IMPERFECTA

(Synonym: *fragilitas ossium*. Eponyms: *Vrolik — congenital recessive form; Lobstein — dominant form*)

This is a relatively rare disorder manifested by increased fragility of bones and osteoporosis, as well as dental abnormalities (see Ch. 52), lax joints and thin skin. Osteoblasts are abnormal and diminished in number. An immature form of osteoid matrix is formed and the thinned trabeculae formed are easily broken. Collagen is also defective, so that the sclera, cornea, joints and skin are also abnormal.

Recessive form. Diagnosis of the more severe form of the disease, the congenital recessive form, has been made *in utero*. The children may be stillborn, or die shortly after birth with only rarely less severely affected patients surviving into adult life. These patients often have blue sclerae.

Overall the bones are grossly demineralized with thin cortices. Numerous healed or healing fractures are seen at

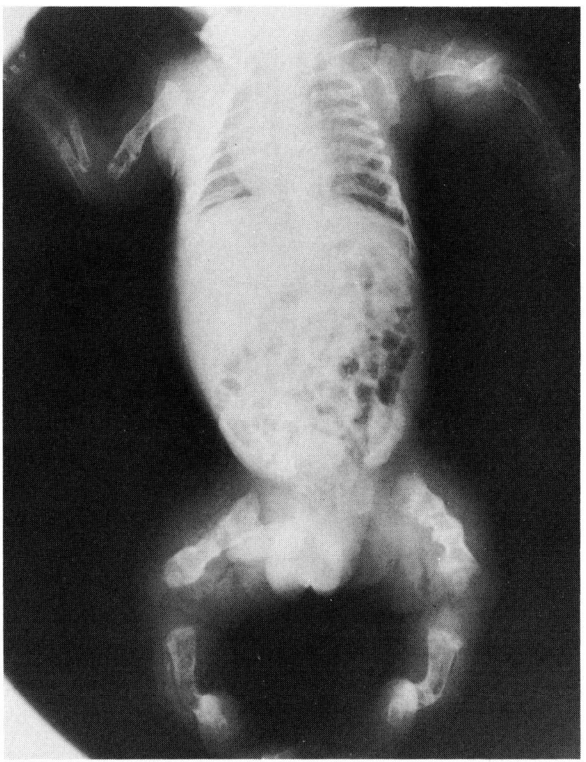

Fig. 1.35 Osteogenesis imperfecta in a neonate — showing multiple fractures and deformities.

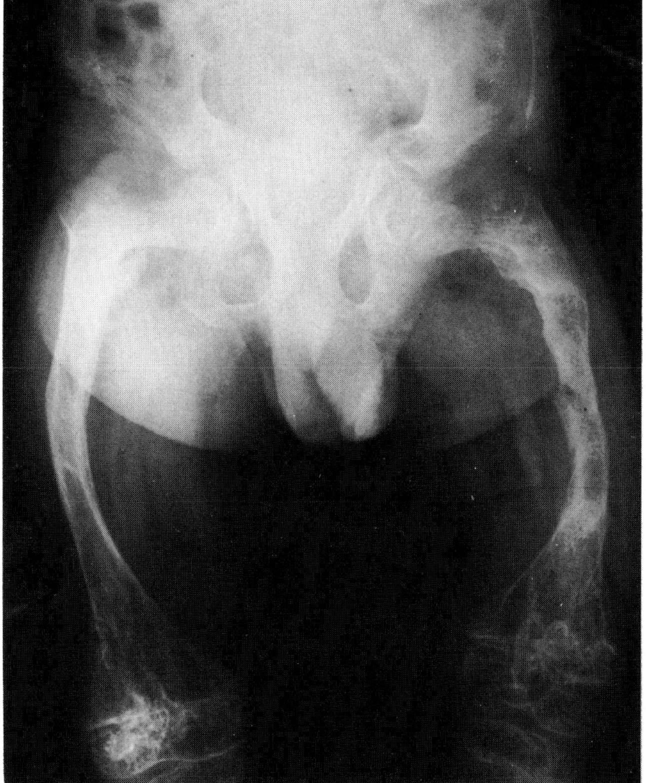

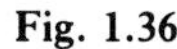

Fig. 1.36

Fig. 1.36 Osteogenesis imperfecta: marked deformities, diminished bone density and recent and old fractures.

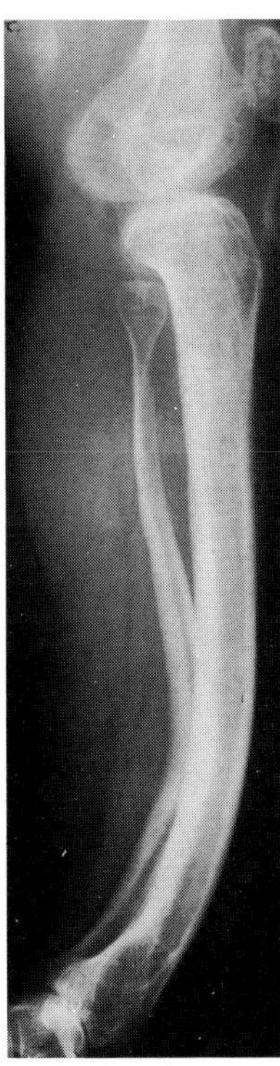

Fig. 1.37

Fig. 1.37 Osteogenesis imperfecta: marked bowing of hypoplastic bones.

birth despite the protection of amniotic fluid. Fractures also occur during delivery. Ribs and long bones are especially affected (Fig. 1.35), and hyperplastic callus may form.

Skull. Mineralization may be so severely retarded that only the petrous bones are calcified, and the vault is barely distinguishable from soft tissues. This may also be seen in hypophosphatasia. Numerous Wormian bones are present.

Spine. Compression of all the vertebral bodies with irregularity and demineralization is seen.

Limbs. Multiple fractures of soft bones *in utero* result in short, thick and bowed long bones with gross callus formation but non-union is also sometimes present. Fairbank (1951) commented on this 'thick bone type', distinguishing it from the 'thin bone type' which is probably not the recessive form even if present at birth. He also described a 'cystic type'. A cystic, grossly honeycomb appearance of bone is found in those recessive patients who survive birth.

Dominant form. This type is more frequent and varies greatly in its expression. Not all of the described changes need to be present.

Fractures may present at any age, but usually in the first 5 years of life. Some patients, however, develop multiple fractures in adult life. These clearly have a benign form of the disease. The fractures occur especially in the long bones of lower limbs and may be incomplete or transverse (Fig. 1.36). Healing again is by the formation of excessive callus, possibly because the periosteum is very loosely attached, and the appearance may simulate osteogenic sarcoma. A sarcomatous degeneration is indeed described but is extremely rare. If the callus does not organize properly the bone ends up broad. Pseudarthroses are also found. Depending on the severity of the disease, however, the long bones are usually gracile, slender, deformed and bowed (Fig. 1.37). These changes, with demineralisation and thin cortices, are characteristic of osteogenesis imperfecta tarda. Bowing results from softening and fractures. Metaphyseal softening results in invagination of the epiphysis into the metaphysis, often with premature fusion.

Skull. Wormian bones persist and the vault is thinned. The base of the skull is indented by the cervical spine so that the temporal and occipital bones bulge (Fig. 1.38A–C). Basilar invagination gives rise to hydrocephalus. Deafness

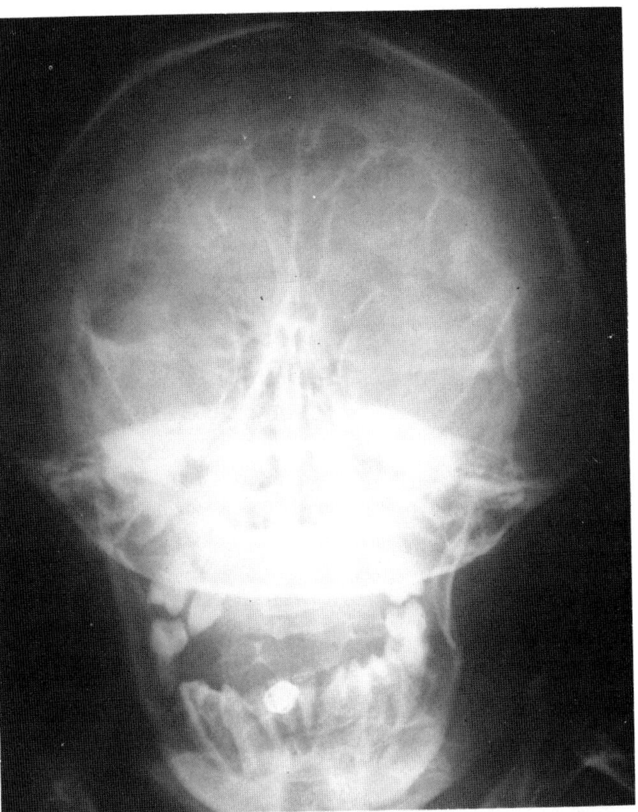

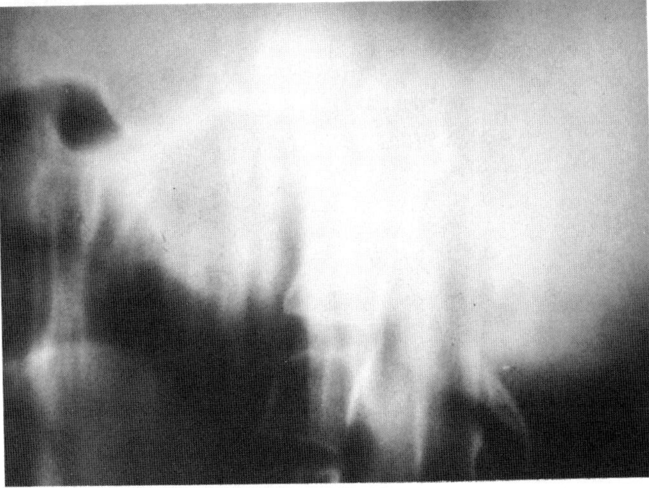

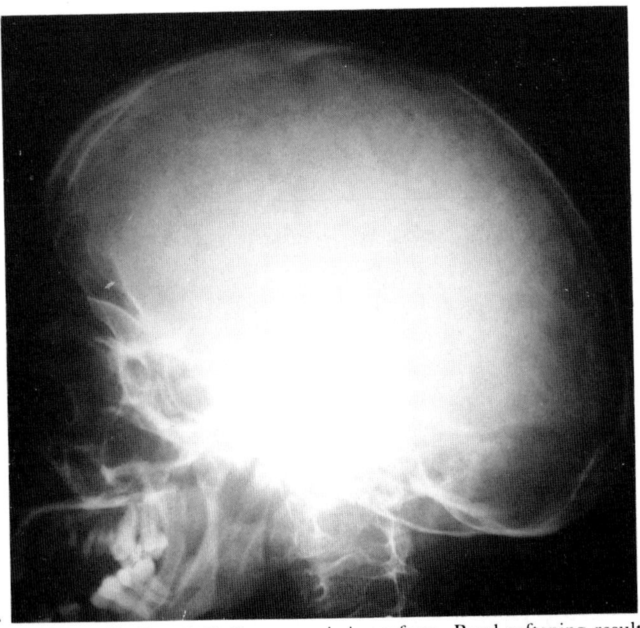

Fig. 1.38 (**A**, **B** and **C**) Osteogenesis imperfecta. Basal softening results in a Tam o'Shanter skull. Tomography shows the gross upward herniation of the odontoid peg. Similar changes are seen in Paget's disease.

is found in adults and may be due to ankylosis of ossicles as well as a form of osteosclerosis.

Axial skeleton. Vertebral bodies are either flattened or have the appearance of 'cod fish' vertebrae. The pelvis shows protrusio acetabuli, and further compression hinders childbirth. The ribs are so soft and thin that the downward pull of the intercostal muscles makes their posterior portion convex *downwards*.

Teeth. Dentinogenesis imperfecta is an associated change (see Ch. 52).

Differential diagnosis

Battered baby syndrome (q.v.). In osteogenesis imperfecta the fractures are often diaphyseal rather than metaphyseal, and the urinary hydroxyproline is often elevated. The differentiation is often of medico-legal significance.

Idiopathic juvenile osteoporosis starts just before puberty and is usually self-limiting. Vertebral compression (Fig. 1.39) and characteristically *metaphyseal* fractures, especially of the lower limb long bones, occur (Fig. 1.40). The calcium balance is negative only in severe cases, otherwise the biochemical findings are normal.

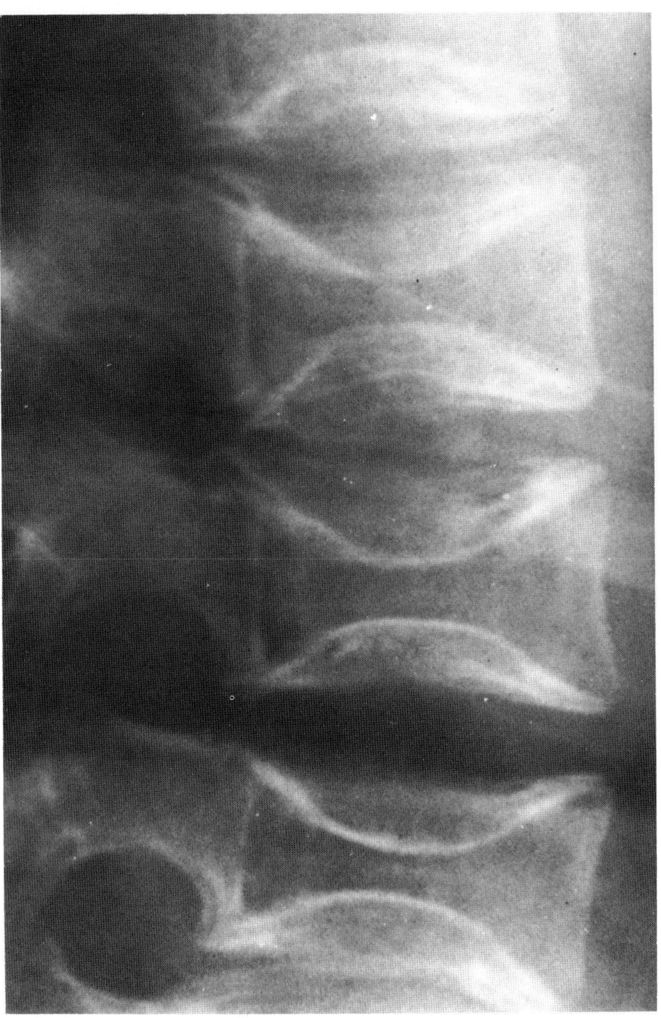

Fig. 1.39 Idiopathic juvenile osteoporosis. Gross vertebral compression affects mainly the central portions of the vertebral bodies.

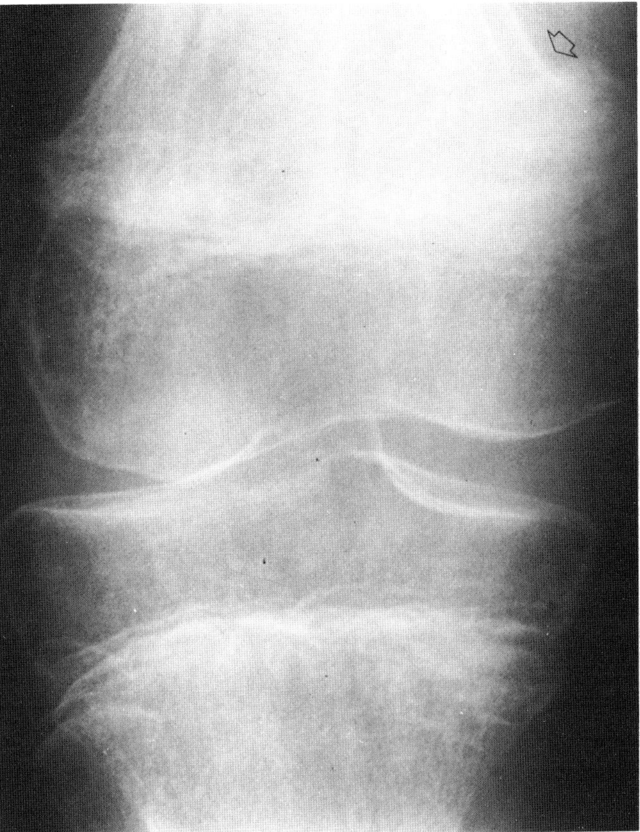

Fig. 1.40 Metaphyseal fractures around the knee (arrow) in idiopathic juvenile osteoporosis distinguish this condition from osteogenesis imperfecta.

FIBROGENESIS OSSIUM IMPERFECTA

This is a rare condition which affects elderly patients and usually presents with pathological fractures. Radiologically, a gross coarsening of trabeculae is present so that the disease looks like Paget's disease (Fig. 1.41A and B). All the bones are affected except the skull. Unlike Paget's disease, the bones retain their usual contour.

OSTEOPETROSIS

(Synonym: *marble bones*. Eponym: *Albers–Schonberg's disease*)

As with osteogenesis imperfecta and many other dysplasias, it is helpful to classify this disease into two forms.

1. A severe, often fatal, early form, manifest in infancy or childhood and inherited in an autosomal recessive form. This has been diagnosed *in utero*.
2. A more benign, tarda form, later in onset, inherited as a dominant, as was Albers-Schonberg's initial case.

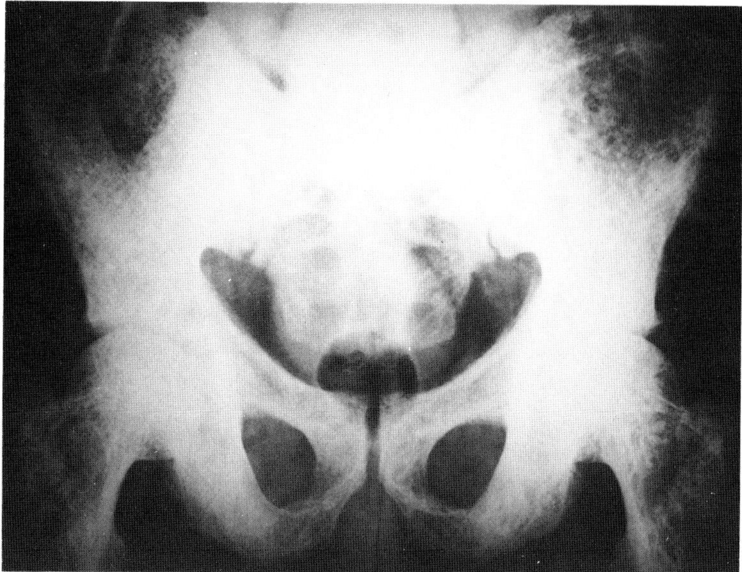

A

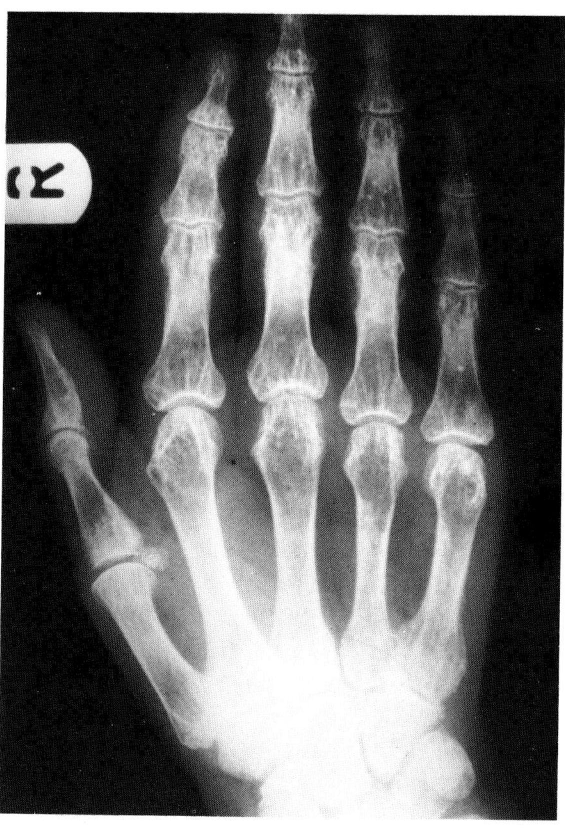

B

Fig. 1.41 Fibrogenesis imperfecta. **A.** and **B.** Marked coarsening of trabeculation occurs throughout the skeleton but the bones retain their contour.

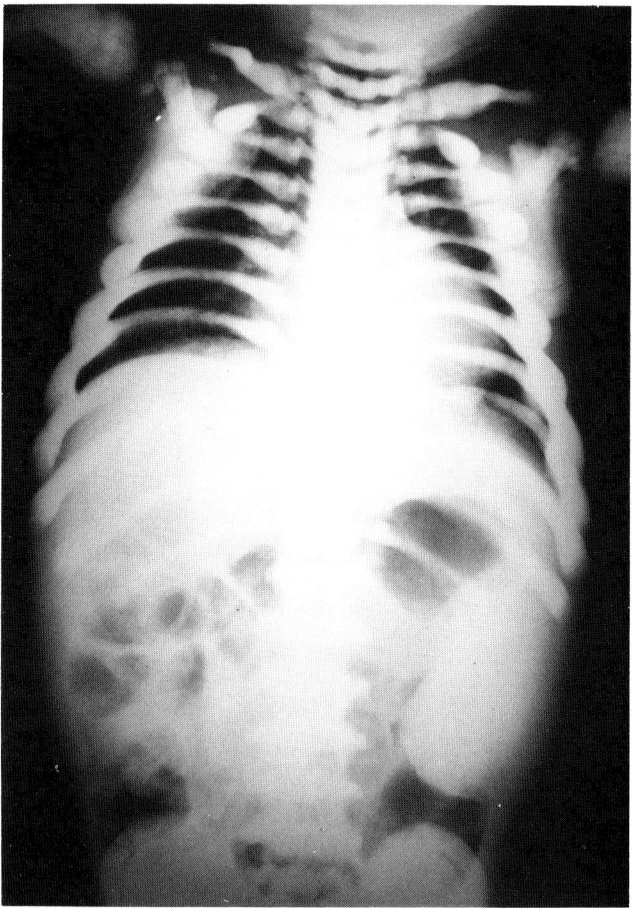

Fig. 1.42 Osteopetrosis. Bone density is uniformly increased apart from a small curved zone of normal bone at the iliac crest metaphysis. The spleen is the site of extramedullary haemopoiesis.

Histologically there is failure of resorption of the primary primitive fetal spongiosa by the vascular mesenchyme. This primitive bone has a higher calcium content on ashing, and appears denser on radiology. The bone is brittle and fractures easily, but heals normally.

Normal bone may be laid down in episodes so that zones of normal and denser bone may be seen, but the marrow is encroached upon and extramedullary haemopoiesis occurs (Fig. 1.42).

In the severe forms of the disease, anaemia and hepatosplenomegaly are found within months of birth and life expectancy is poor.

In the tarda form of the disease, the diagnosis is often made fortuitously when 2–3 fractures occur, perhaps in the space of a year, in an adult patient. The bones may be slightly dense. Modelling abnormalities are seen in both forms with metaphyseal undertubulation.

Dental disease is common (see Ch. 52) with osteomyelitis occurring in the rather compact bone.

Radiological features. Increased density and thickening of long bones, especially metaphyses, can be seen *in utero*. The presence of a 'bone within a bone' differentiates osteopetrosis from the other sclerosing dysplasias. This is due to the cyclical nature of the disease so that the dense shadow of, say, the tibia at the time of formation of abnormal bone is seen within the outline of the current normal or abnormal shadow. The timing of intra-uterine onset

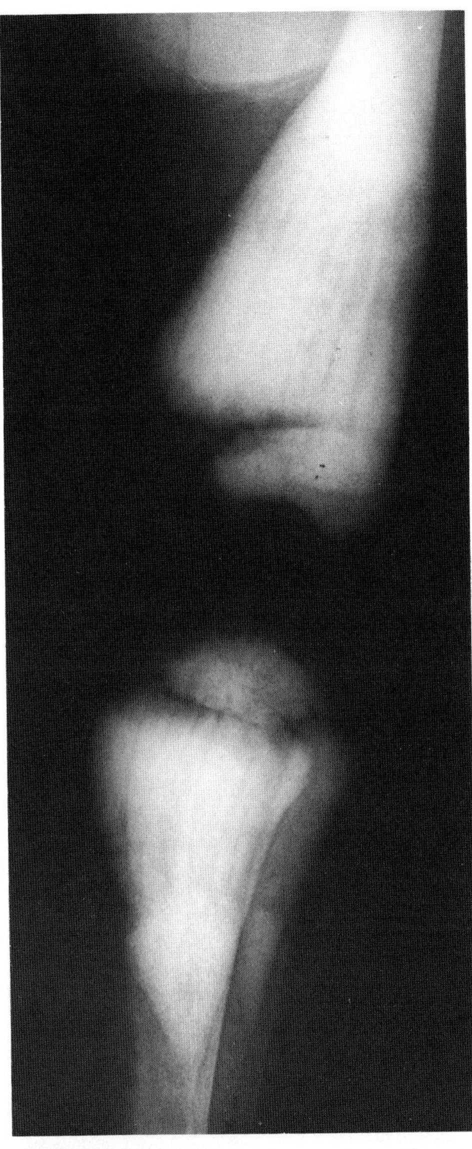

Fig. 1.43 Osteopetrosis. Fine vertical lucencies are seen extending to the metaphyses together with a 'bone within a bone' appearance at the tibial and fibular diaphyses.

of disease can thus be assessed. This 'bone within a bone' may be vertical in the long bone shafts and digits, transverse at the metaphyses or arcuate beneath the iliac crests.

Long bones. Besides the 'Erlenmayer flask' deformity due to failure of metaphyseal remodelling, giving gross distal undertubulation, and the presence of dense bone, vertical fine lucencies extending to the metaphyses are also present (Fig. 1.43), probably due to vascular channels being better seen against dense bone.

Fractures are usually transverse (Fig. 1.44) and heal with normal callus. Residual varus results from proximal femoral fractures. Some diaphyseal remodelling is to be expected and sclerotic bone there can be resorbed so that shafts are not parallel but are almost normal in contour. Skeletal maturation is normal.

Skull. (For dental abnormalities, see Ch. 52). The bones of the skull base are initially affected with sclerosis and thickening prominent in the floor of the anterior cranial fossa. The cranium is affected to a lesser degree. The sphenoid and frontal sinuses and mastoids are under- or non-pneumatised. Neural foramina are encroached upon and blindness results in serious cases. Bone softening with hydrocephalus does not appear to be a problem.

Spine. Platyspondyly does not seem to occur, but spondylolisthesis does. In vertebral bodies, an appearance like a rugger jersey spine may be seen due to the inserted shadow of an earlier, more dense body (Fig. 1.45).

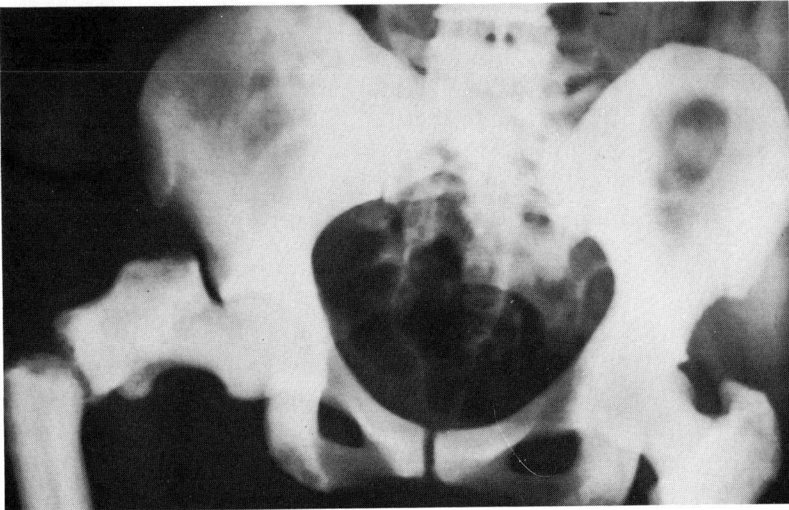

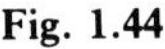

Fig. 1.44

Fig. 1.44 Osteopetrosis: spontaneous fracture in upper end of right femur.

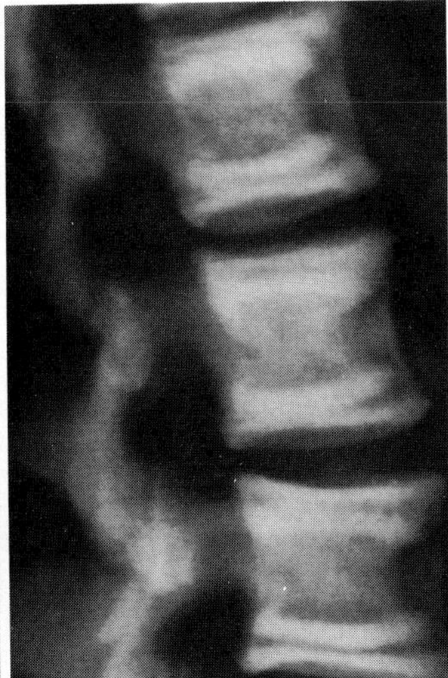

Fig. 1.45

Fig. 1.45 Osteopetrosis. Note inset of an earlier vertebra within each vertebral body.

In the adult form of the disease, the bones are roughly normal in shape. The medulla in the proximal skeleton is primarily involved and the periphery spared.

HYPEROSTOSIS CORTICALIS GENERALISATA FAMILIARIS

(Synonym: *Endosteal hyperostosis*. Eponyms: *van Buchem — recessive form*; *Worth — autosomal dominant form*)

Both recessive and dominant forms of this condition have been described, and the recessive type tends to be more severe in its manifestations.

Clinically, the mandible and forehead are prominent. Cranial nerve palsies occasionally result. There is no increased incidence of fracture and patients are of normal intelligence.

Radiological findings. *Skull*. There is thickening and increased sclerosis of the skull vault with loss of cortico-medullary differentiation. The base is also sclerotic. The sinuses may remain pneumatised or may be obliterated. The mandible is especially large and sclerotic, and this may be the only abnormality in the dominant form. A hard bony lump of the palate — the 'torus palatinus' — may occasionally be present.

Long bones. Endosteal new bone encroaches on the medulla in affected cases. The diaphysis is always affected but the new bone may reach bone ends. Externally there is no thickening, as opposed to craniometaphyseal dysplasia, but occasionally exostoses may be seen.

Axial skeleton. A 'reverse rugger-jersey' appearance with a central dense band in the vertebral body may be diagnostic.

MELORHEOSTOSIS

(Eponym: *Leri's disease*)

This is a very rare lesion affecting both sexes; no familial trend has been reported. Though the condition has not been observed in a child under the age of 3 years, there is strong presumptive evidence that it is present at birth. The condition is, therefore, probably a dysplasia rather than an acquired disorder.

Patients may complain of pain and of restricted movements of joints but the condition is often asymptomatic.

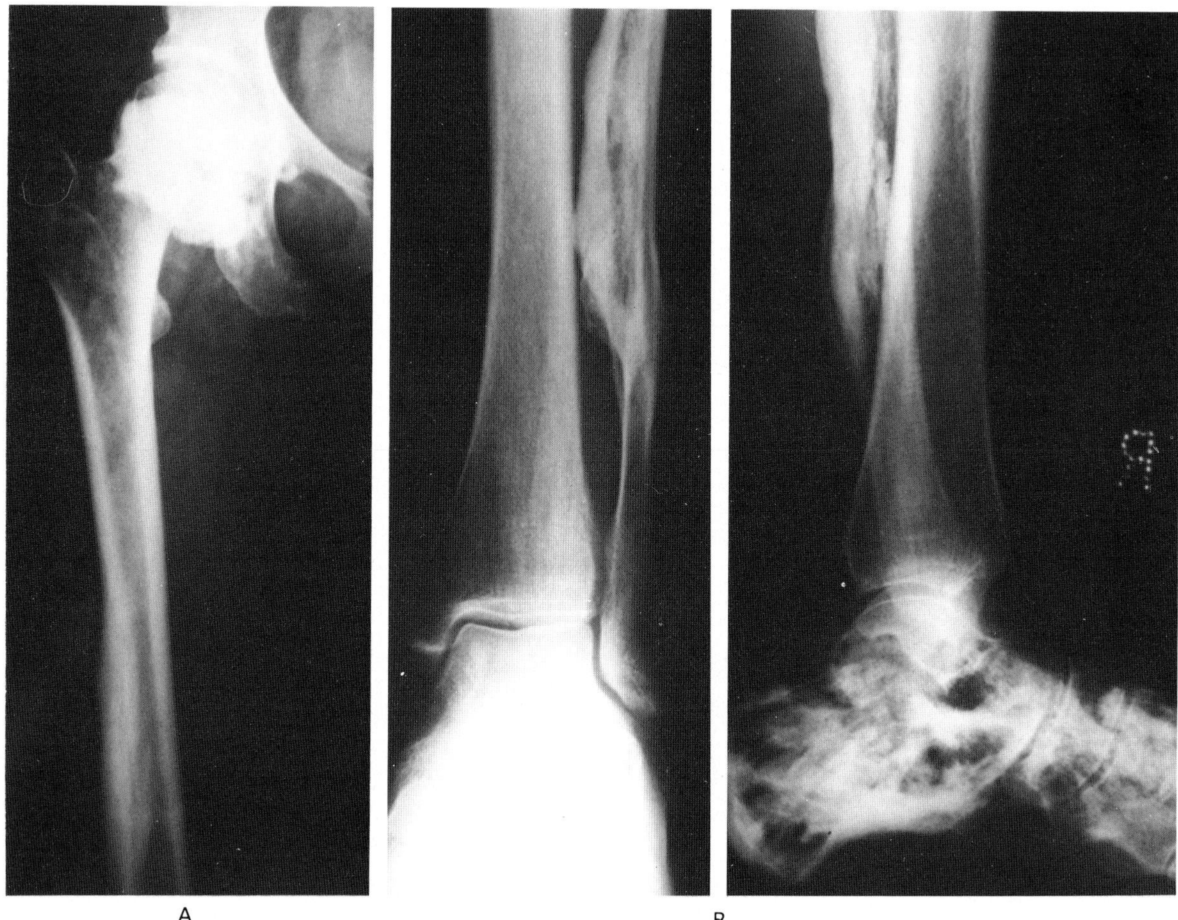

Fig. 1.46 (**A** and **B**) Melorheostosis. Exuberant dense new bone is seen both on the outside of the bone and within the cortex. At the hip joint new bone is seen bridging the joint space.

Some cases are associated with skin lesions, such as scleroderma, and with vascular anomalies; joint contractures may be found in some patients.

The condition is characterized by the presence of dense irregular bone running down the cortex of a long bone. Both the internal and external aspects of the cortex may be affected. Dense areas tend to be overgrown and bowing may result. Murray and McCredie (1979) have pointed out that the distribution of the new bone corresponds to a sclerotome, the segmental root nerve innervation of a bone.

The new bone has been likened to molten wax running down the side of a burning candle (Fig. 1.46). The lesions tend to be segmental and unilateral, though both limbs on one side of the body may be affected. Occasionally the condition is bilateral but never symmetrical. Some lesions are progressive. The lower limbs are most commonly affected. Premature epiphyseal fusion may result so that an affected limb may be larger or smaller than normal.

The skull, spine and ribs are rarely affected. Ectopic bone may be found in soft tissues around joints between affected bones.

OSTEOPOIKILOSIS

(Synonym: *osteopathia condensans disseminata*)

This is usually an incidental radiological finding but some patients have associated skin nodules. The lesions are familial. It affects both sexes equally and is characterized by the presence of multiple dense radio-opaque spots which are round, oval or lanceolate, and tend to be situated parallel to the axis of the affected bone. They are usually uniform in density but may have relatively clear central zones. Any bone may be affected. They occur especially frequently in the ends of long bones and around joints, in the carpus and tarsus, and in the pelvis (Fig. 1.47). This lesion must be differentiated from serious conditions such as tuberous sclerosis and metastases, but their distribution, around joints, and the infrequency of the nodules increasing in size or number under observation, distinguishes this benign condition from metastases.

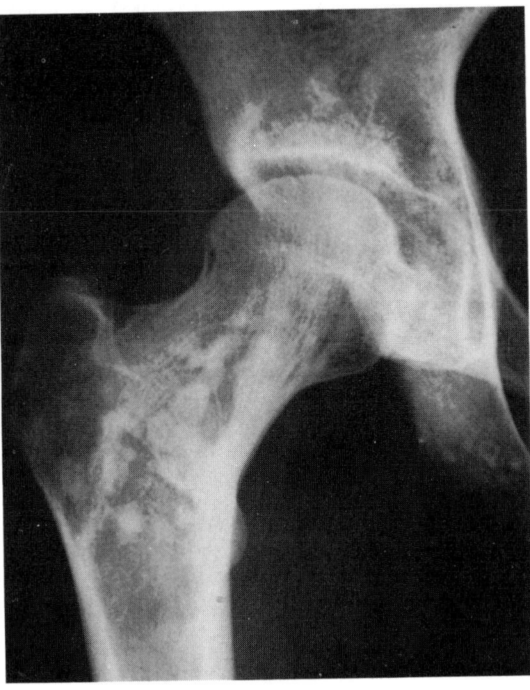

Fig. 1.47 Osteopoikilosis.

OSTEOPATHIA STRIATA

(Eponym: *Voorhoeve's disease*)

In this asymptomatic disorder sclerotic striations are found in the long bones, especially of the lower limbs, affecting both bone ends and diaphyses (Fig. 1.48).

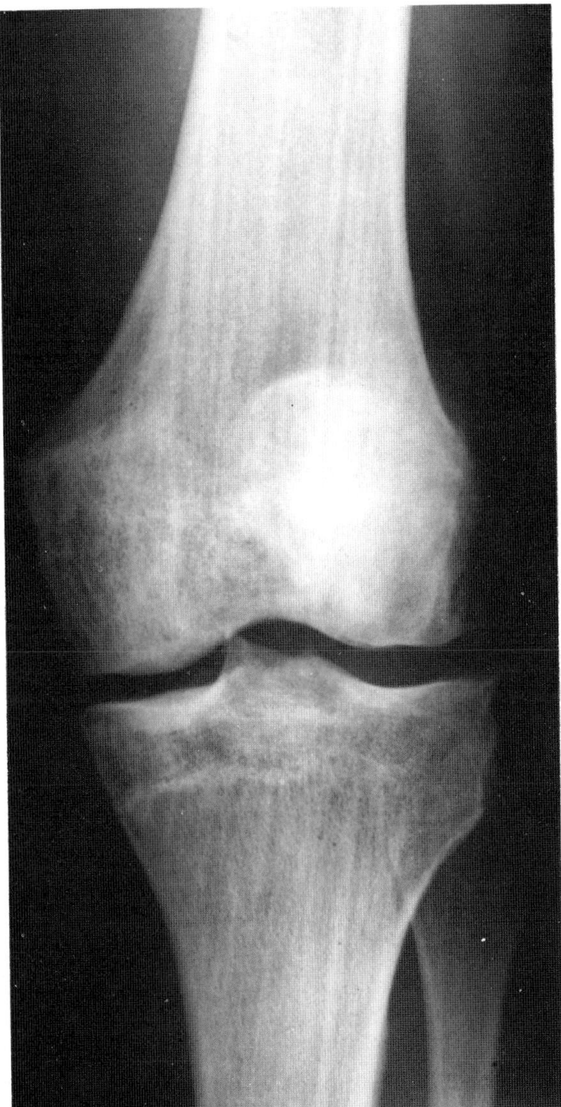

Fig. 1.48 Vertical striation extends to the articular surfaces in osteopathia striata.

Similar striations may be found in association with cranial stenosis. This syndrome is inherited as an autosomal dominant. The head is enlarged with increased density of the skull vault, base and mandible, with hypoplasia of the facial sinuses. Deafness results, often from nerve compression. Elsewhere, scoliosis and defects in the neural arches are found.

FIBROUS DYSPLASIA

This is a disease of unknown aetiology. It is probably more common in women. The disease is found in two forms, monostotic and polyostotic. With polyostotic disease, over 50% of the skeleton may be involved, but symmetry is unusual and the lesions tend to be unilaterally distributed. The lesions are usually found incidentally or following pathological fracture. Deformity may occasionally be marked. The alkaline phosphatase is elevated but does not correlate with the extent of the disease. The age of onset is in the second and third decades, but polyostotic disease may present in the first decade. The lesions often cease growing with skeletal maturity but may be seen in old age. Monostotic lesions are more likely to enlarge in adult life. Prognosis is worse when the lesions occur early in life.

Pathologically, medullary bone is replaced by well-defined areas of fibrous tissue, and cysts containing blood to serous fluid. These appear similar on radiographs. The fibrous tissue then undergoes varying degrees of abnormal ossification so that some of the lesions show an increase in density, dependent on the extent of ossification. This increase in density may thus be patchy, giving a cottonwool appearance, or homogenous, giving a ground glass appearance.

Radiologically, the lesions have a smooth dense margin of varying degrees of width, often so wide as to resemble a 'rind' of orange. The bone is expanded and the cortex scalloped and thinned but intact. Lesions tend to be multilocular and expand down the medulla rather than cause great cortical expansion (Figs 1.49 and 1.50). Unlike Paget's disease, the bone ends are not necessarily affected

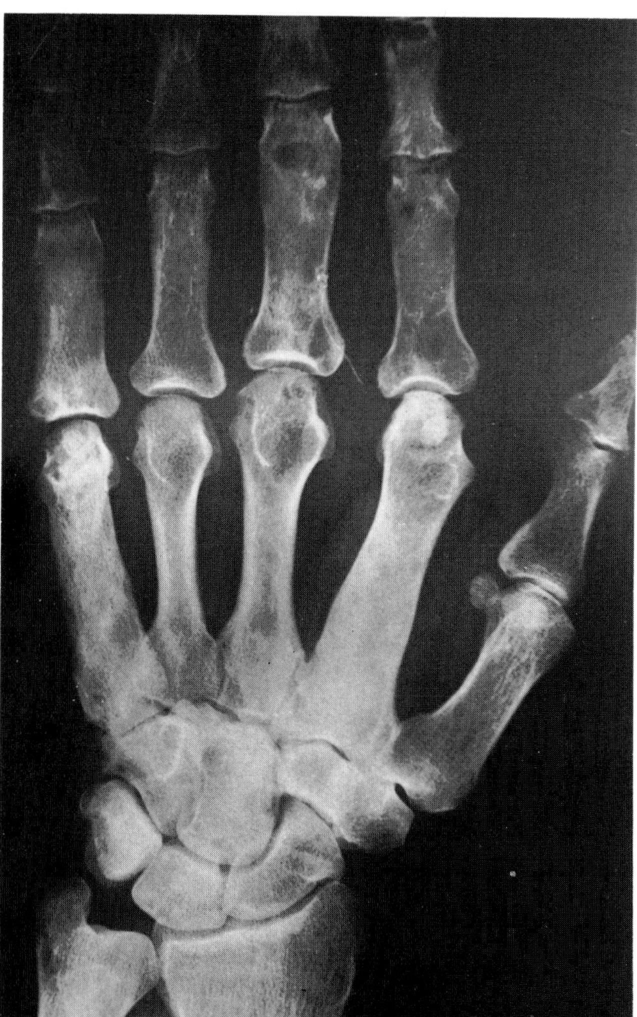

Fig. 1.49 Fibrous dysplasia, showing variable appearances in metacarpals and proximal phalanges.

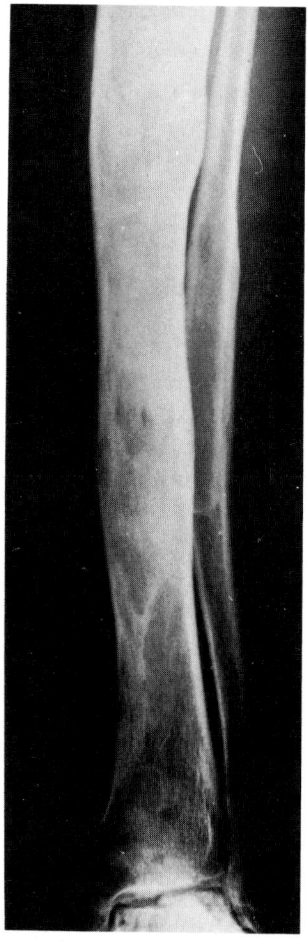

Fig. 1.50 Fibrous dysplasia. Tibia and fibula showing irregular expansion, ground-glass appearance in upper part of the tibia and cystic changes in the lower end.

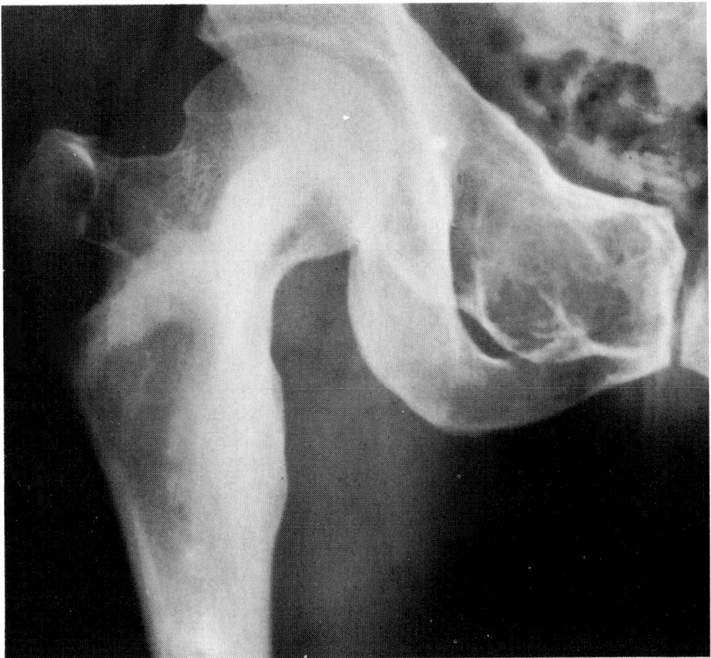

Fig. 1.51 Fibrous dysplasia: large expanding lesion in superior pubic ramus and sclerosis in upper end of the femur.

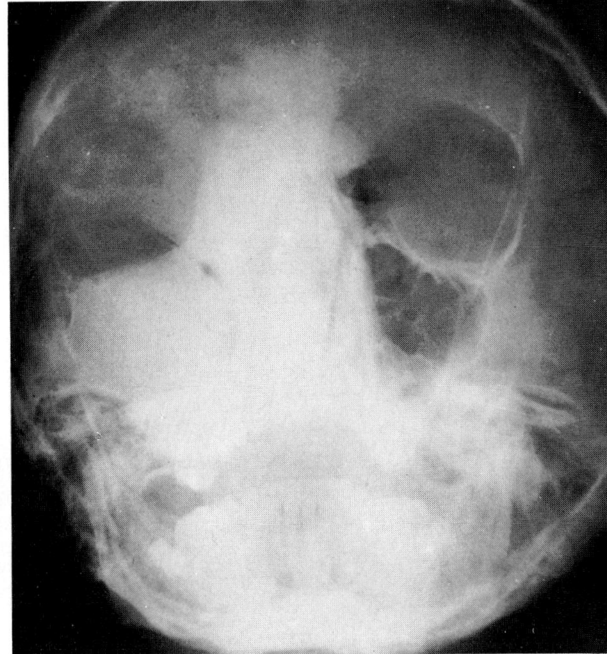

Fig. 1.52 Fibrous dysplasia: involvement of maxilla and facial bones on right side.

and lesions tend to be diametaphyseal. Bone ends may be involved after fusion and epiphyses may be involved in the child.

Any bone may be affected though involvement of the spine is uncommon. Vertebral collapse is unusual unless cystic degeneration occurs. Lesions there do not really need to be diagnosed by biopsy as appearances here, as elsewhere, are usually characteristic.

The pelvis (Fig. 1.51), femur and ribs are commonly involved. In the skull, the frontal, sphenoid, parietal and maxillary bones and mandible are often affected (Fig. 1.52). In the *femur*, deformity due to softening, expansion and fracture give an appearance likened to a 'shepherd's crook' (Fig. 1.53). Limb length discrepancies result. Lesions there are well-defined and expanded with well-defined margins and may be lucent, dense or a mixture of the two, with small flecks of density due to ossification.

In the *skull*, a grossly expanded sclerotic hyperostosis of the sphenoid may resemble a meningioma. Orbital fissures may be encroached upon and proptosis may result. Obliteration and bony expansion of the facial sinuses give a grotesque mask-like facial appearance. In the vault, lesions tend to be grossly expansile, sclerotic, but localised (blister lesion).

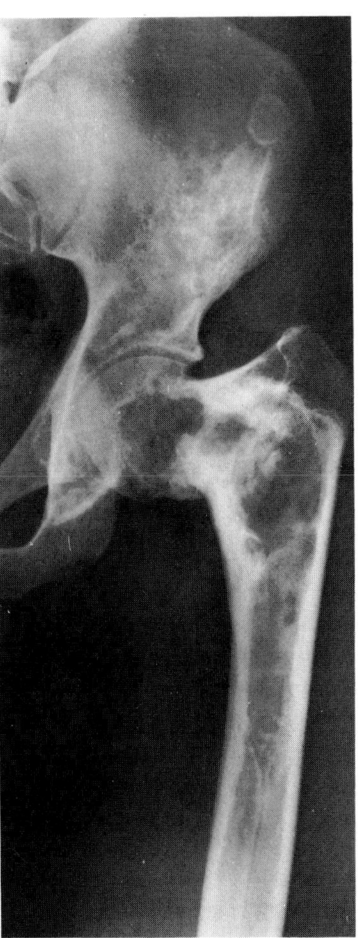

Fig. 1.53 Fibrous dysplasia: marked coxa vara secondary to cystic changes in the femoral neck. Sclerotic changes also in left ilium.

The lesions show increased uptake on radio-isotope scans. Fractures should thus be assessed on plain radiographs.

Complications. (a) Fractures, deformity and irregularity of limb length have been mentioned. Nerve palsies may occur in the skull. (b) Endocrine complications. *Albright's syndrome* consists of skin pigmentation, usually on the side of the bone lesions, fibrous dysplasia (usually polyostotic) and precocious puberty. This occurs usually in females, and only rarely in males. Most patients with skin pigmentation and polyostotic disease do not have associated endocrine disease and, in females, only 50% have precocious puberty.

Hyperthyroidism, *acromegaly*, *Cushing's syndrome*, *gynecomastia* and *parathyroid enlargement* have all been reported in association with polyostotic fibrous dysplasia. (c) Sarcomatous degeneration occurs in less than 1% of patients, usually to fibrosarcoma (Fig. 1.54). Some, but not all of these patients give a history of previous irradiation.

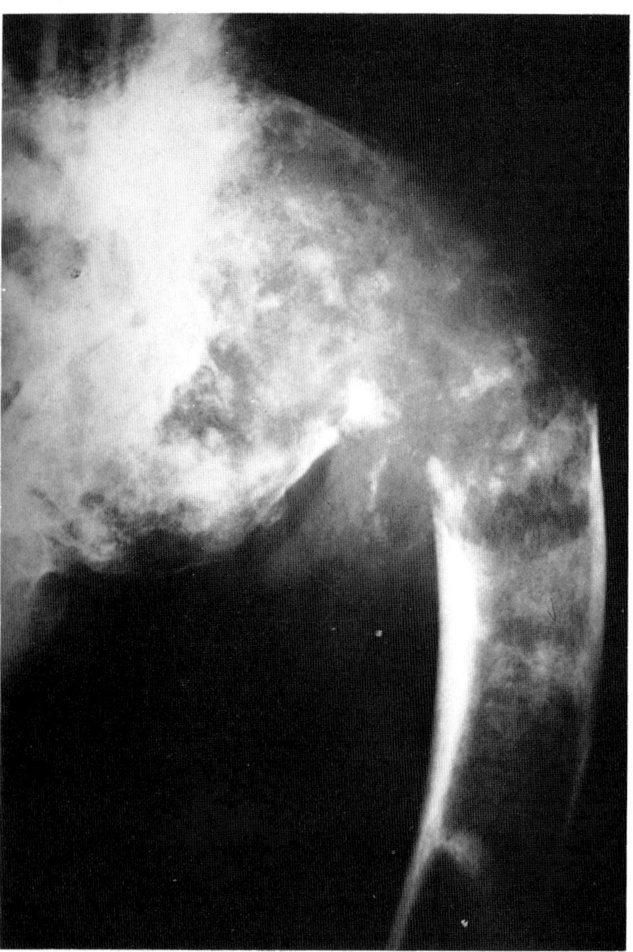

Fig. 1.54 A pathological fracture with irregular bone destruction due to malignant degeneration is superimposed upon fibrous dysplasia.

CHONDRODYSTROPHIA CALCIFICANS CONGENITA

(Synonyms: *dysplasia epiphysealis punctata: stippled epiphyses*)

This disease exists in two forms.

1. The less severe *dominant* form. Even in this form, early fatal disease may occur. The condition is characterized in infancy by stippling or punctate calcification of the tarsus and carpus, long bone epiphyses, vertebral transverse processes and the pubic bones. The resulting epiphyses in later life are often mis-shapen, and deformities with asymmetric limb shortening result. The spine often ends up scoliotic. If the infants survive, life expectancy is normal.

2. The more severe *recessive* form, which usually results in death in the first year and mental defect in survivors. Stippling is present as above but is if anything more gross, also occurring in the trachea. Long bones show gross symmetrical shortening and metaphyseal irregularity. In this form the vertebral bodies show a vertical radiolucency on the lateral view which does not occur in the dominant type (Fig. 1.55). In survivors, there is marked retardation of epiphyses.

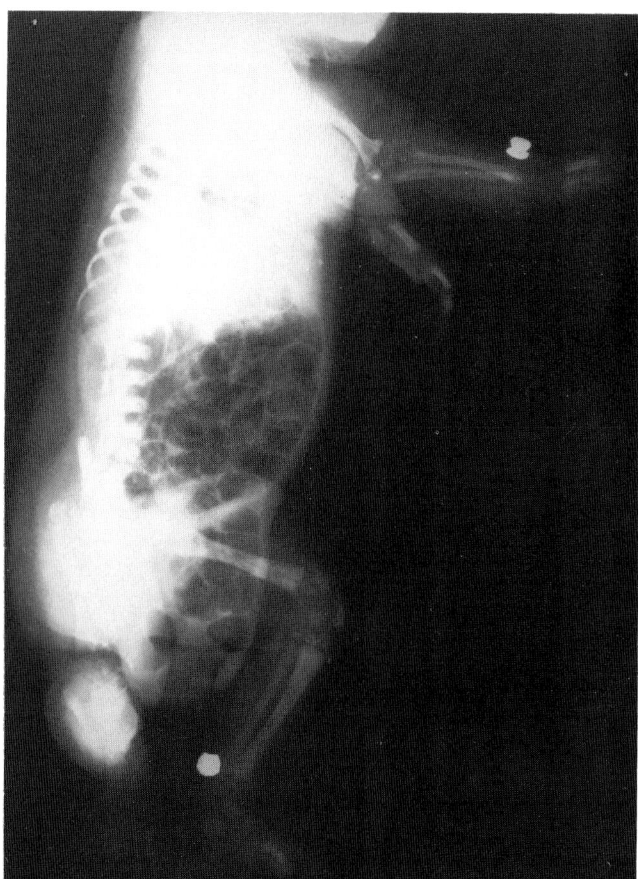

Fig. 1.55 Chondrodysplasia calcificans congenita. Clefts of the vertebral bodies are prominent in this case together with stippled epiphyses and punctate calcifications around the joints and in the tracheal cartilages.

MULTIPLE EPIPHYSEAL DYSPLASIA

(Synonym: *dysplasia epiphysealis multiplex*)

'his condition, which is transmitted as an autosomal domi-ant, primarily affects epiphyses. Dwarfism of the short-mb type may be seen, but this feature is not usually pro-ounced and may even be overlooked unless the patient is ompared with unaffected members of the family. The con-ition may express itself in various ways, so much so that ome writers subdivide the disease into a severe form (*Fair-ank*) characterized by small epiphyses, and a mild type *Ribbing*) characterized by flat epiphyses. It is improbable hat such subdivisions are of use because much overlap nay occur within families and even within the same patient.

In order of frequency, the epiphyses affected are those of the hips, shoulders, ankles, knees, wrists and elbows.

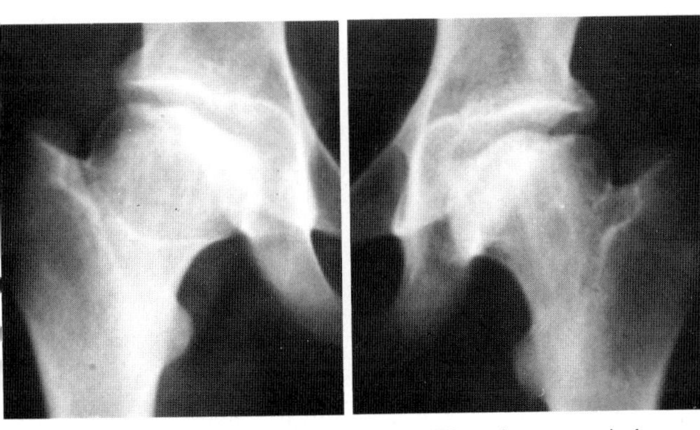

Fig. 1.56 Dysplasia epiphysealis multiplex. There is symmetrical flattening and irregularity of both femoral heads. Joint spaces are preserved but degeneration may supervene.

Epiphyses tend to appear late and are fragmented and flattened (Figs 1.56–1.59); the deformities persist throughout life and cause premature osteoarthritis. No characteristic changes are found in the metaphyses but they may be widened to conform to the deformed contiguous epiphyses. Secondary changes in contour are often seen in the glenoid and acetabular fossae. The carpal and tarsal bones may be affected and digits and toes may be 'stubby'. The skull is not affected. Some features may be characteristic but none is constant.

a. *Lower tibial epiphysis*. The lateral part of the lower tibial epiphysis is thinned compared with the medial part; the trochlear part of the talus is shaped to conform to the abnormal mortice. Thus the articular surface of the ankle joint becomes oblique from the lateral to the medial side (Fig. 1.57). The fibula may appear elongated. This deformity is found in roughly half of all cases.

b. The double layered patella (Fig. 1.58) is characteristic but is found in few cases.

c. *The femoral and tibial condyles* may be square and angular and the intercondylar notch shallow (Fig. 1.59). Flattening of the femoral and tibial condyles causes an appearance of widening of the joint.

Spinal changes are seldom pronounced and may be absent. The appearances in the spine, if present, resemble osteochondritis. Only the anterior parts of the vertebral bodies are wedged in contradistinction to the true platyspondyly of spondyloepiphyseal dysplasia. The latter condition may in other ways be difficult to differentiate from multiple epiphyseal dysplasia. Some cases of chondrodystrophia calcificans congenita may survive and their pattern may later resemble that of multiple epiphyseal dysplasia.

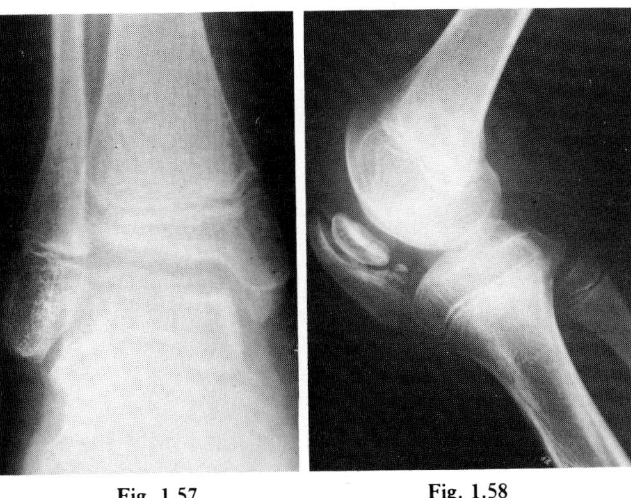

Fig. 1.57 **Fig. 1.58**

Fig. 1.57 Dysplasia epiphysealis multiplex, showing thinning of the outer part of the lower tibial epiphysis. This is seen in about half of all cases.
Fig. 1.58 Knee of same patient as Figure 1.57. Marked fragmentation of the patella.

DYSPLASIA EPIPHYSEALIS HEMIMELICA

(Synonym: *tarso-epiphyseal aclasis*. Eponym: *Trevor's disease*)

In this rare condition irregular overgrowth of part of an epiphysis or epiphyses lying on one side of a single limb is seen (Fig. 1.60). The leg is commonly affected but the arm may be. Sometimes both an arm and a leg may be involved and bilateral lesions have been recorded. If more than one epiphysis is affected then the same part, i.e. the medial or lateral, of the other epiphysis is abnormal.

Hyperplasia of the affected epiphysis may lead to a lesion that is indistinguishable radiologically and histologically from an osteochondroma. The lesions may be easily palpable. Such a feature is relatively common in the lower end of the fibula and adjacent talus (Fig. 1.60). The terms 'tarso-epiphyseal aclasis' and 'Trevor's disease' have been applied to this individual lesion.

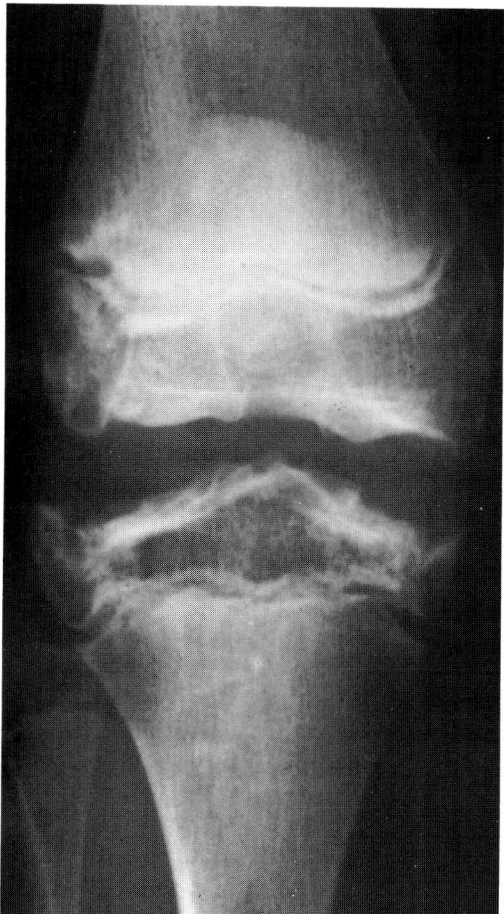

Fig. 1.59 Dysplasia epiphysealis multiplex: angular condyles and flat intercondylar notch. This is a characteristic appearance though not always present.

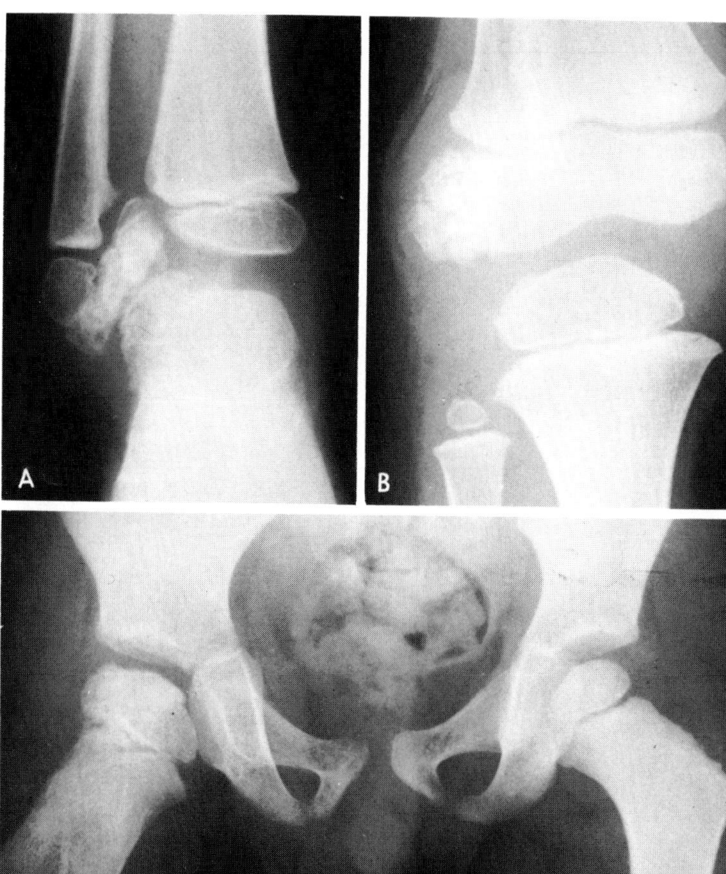

Fig. 1.60 Dysplasia epiphysealis hemimelica. **A.** shows lesion between the lower end of the fibula and the talus; **B.** and **C.** show involvement of outer part of the lower femoral and femoral capital epiphyses respectively.

(FAMILIAL) METAPHYSEAL DYSPLASIA
(Eponym: *Pyle's disease*)

This is an extremely rare condition. The original description was of a child with splaying of the metaphyses of the long bones and knock knees. Inheritance is autosomal recessive. This disease is not to be confused with craniometaphyseal dysplasia, which has been split off from it. The condition is benign.

Radiological findings. *Long bones*. There is marked metaphyseal widening (Erlenmeyer flask) and the widening extends to adjacent diaphyses. Cortices are thinned and the bones look demineralized. Changes are maximal at the knee with valgus deformity (Fig. 1.61). The wrists and the medial ends of the clavicles are similarly severely affected. The long bone midshafts appear spindle-shaped in comparison with the widened metaphyses. The phalanges and metacarpals also show undertubulation.

Axial skeleton. Ischial and pubic bones are expanded and appear demineralized. The anterior ends of the ribs are expanded. Platyspondyly is mild if present. The skull is not always involved but there may be minor, patchy sclerosis.

CRANIOMETAPHYSEAL DYSPLASIA

This condition, now separated from Pyle's disease (see Table 1.4), is inherited both in a more severe autosomal recessive form and in a more benign dominant form.

In this disease, the skull is severely affected, and more so in the recessive type. The skull is enlarged with bone sclerosis. Sclerosis is especially prominent in the base and around sutures (Fig. 1.62). Sinuses are obliterated and the bridge of the nose expanded, giving hypertelorism. Compression of optic, facial and auditory cranial nerves results.

Changes in the long bones are of metaphyseal widening (Fig. 1.63), but not to the extent seen in Pyle's disease in which, it will be remembered, the skull is minimally involved.

Table 1.4 Distinguishing features of craniotubular dysplasias

	Metaphyseal dysplasia	Craniometaphyseal dysplasia	Craniodiaphyseal dysplasia	Diaphyseal dysplasia
SKULL: thickening	±	+++	+++	±
density	±	+++	+++	±
LONG BONE EXPANSION:				
diaphysis	±	–	+++	++
metaphysis	+++	++	+	–
density	–	–	+++	++

(After Beighton & Cremin, 1980)

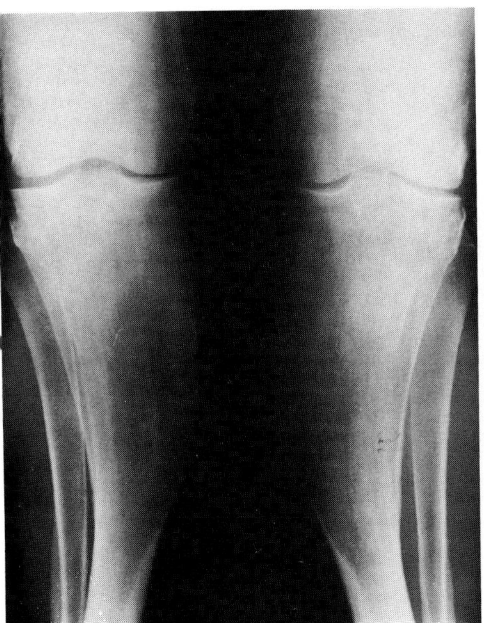

Fig. 1.61

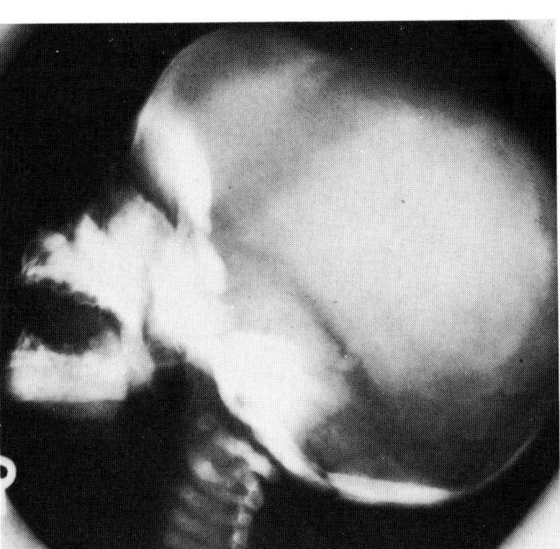

Fig. 1.62

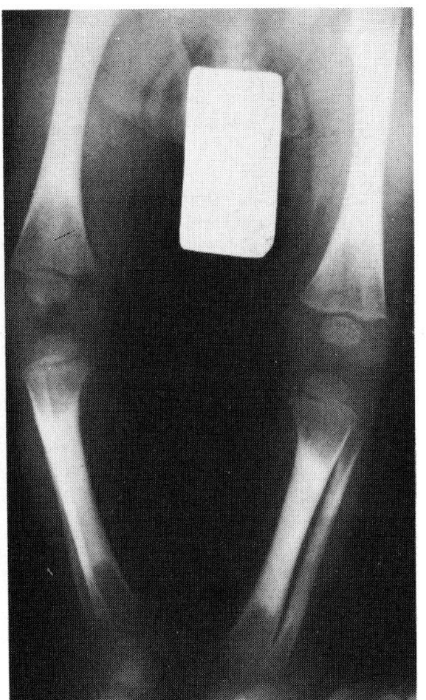

Fig. 1.63

Fig. 1.61 Metaphyseal dysplasia: Pyle's disease in an adult, showing fusiform expansion of the bone ends but no sclerosis. (Courtesy of Dr W. J. A. Gibson.)

Fig. 1.62 Craniometaphyseal dysplasia in an infant showing extra density in the base of the skull and in the jaw. (Courtesy of Dr W. J. A. Gibson.)

Fig. 1.63 Craniometaphyseal dysplasia in an infant showing extra density in the diaphyses of the femora and tibiae. No expansion is seen in the ends of the bones. (Courtesy of Dr W. J. A. Gibson.)

DIAPHYSEAL DYSPLASIA

(Synonym: *progressive diaphyseal dysplasia*. Eponyms: *Camurati 1922; Engelmann 1929*)

In this rare disease, which is inherited as an autosomal dominant, there is diminution of muscle mass associated with leg pains, muscle weakness and abnormal gait. Skull changes are not marked but the usual cranial stenoses may result.

Radiological changes. *Long bones*. Gross symmetrical fusiform expansion of the diaphyses is found and new bone is laid down internally and externally so that an expanded sclerotic lesion is seen (Fig. 1.64). Epiphyses are not involved. The hands and feet are usually normal.

Axial skeleton. There may be a mild sclerosis of the skull base and mandible. This is not a prominent feature. The ribs and pelvis are less often affected.

CRANIODIAPHYSEAL DYSPLASIA

This condition has been split off from diaphyseal dysplasia. Changes predominate in the skull with cranial enlargement and gross depression of the bridge of the nose. This causes obstruction of the nasal passages. Blindness and deafness are also present.

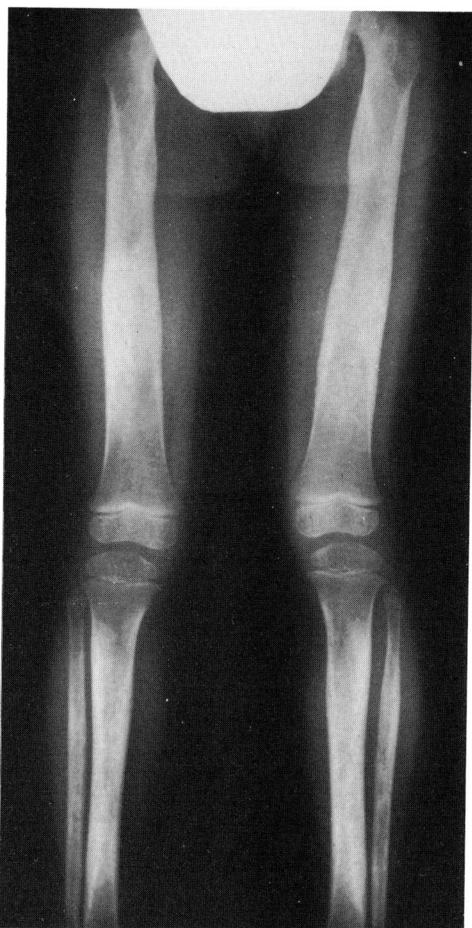

Fig. 1.64 Progressive diaphyseal dysplasia (Engelmann's disease).

Radiological features. *Skull.* There is thickening and increased density of the whole of the skull, including the mandible which becomes grosser than in the other skull–long bone dysplasia. The sinuses are non-pneumatised.

Long bones. Marked diaphyseal thickening with new bone laid down both periosteally and endosteally results in a tubular long bone. Metaphyses and epiphyses are relatively spared. Hand bones are similarly affected.

Axial skeleton. Involvement is mild and not inevitable.

METAPHYSEAL DYSPLASIA

(Synonyms: *metaphyseal dysostosis; metaphyseal chondrodysplasia*)

Many lesions are now recognized under the above heading and the subject is very confused because some writers include conditions in which the lesion is not confined to the metaphyses. The spine, diaphyses and epiphyses should be unaffected in this group of lesions. Unfortunately, the subject is additionally complicated by the patient who regarded as having a classical metaphyseal dysplasia later develops changes elsewhere. Some well-defined groups are:

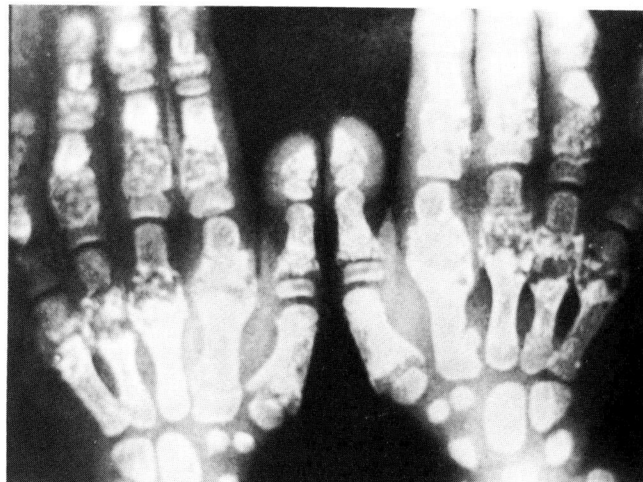

Fig. 1.65 Metaphyseal dysostosis (Jansen). (Courtesy of Dr W. H. D. De Hass.)

1. *Jansen's metaphyseal dysplasia*. Grossly irregular mineralization is seen in the metaphyses of tubular bones (Fig. 1.65). A large gap is seen between the epiphyses and disordered metaphyses. This is a spot radiographic diagnosis. However, a late follow-up of Jansen's original patient showed very few residual changes.
2. *Schmid* described a much milder type that is relatively common (Fig. 1.66). Metaphyses of long bones are cupped and resemble rickets. No biochemical changes are found. The patient may be wrongly diagnosed as suffering from vitamin D resistant rickets and consequently injudiciously given large doses of vitamin D.
3. Other types named after *Pena* and *Vaandrager* show intermediate involvement of metaphyses, less than in the Jansen type but more than in the Schmid type (Fig. 1.67). Such lesions may resemble Ollier's disease.
4. Some cases of metaphyseal dysplasia are associated with *pancreatic insufficiency* and *neutropenia* (Burke type).
5. *McKusick* described a syndrome of sparse hair, metaphyseal lesions and dwarfism in Amish families — '*cartilage–hair hypoplasia*'.
6. Sometimes metaphyseal changes are associated with lesions of the spine — such conditions should be designated '*spondylometaphyseal dysplasia*'.

DIAPHYSEAL ACLASIS

(Synonym: *hereditary multiple exostoses*)

This disease is inherited and familial. Some 60% of those affected have an involved parent. The remainder are presumably mutants to the gene. The sex incidence is equal. Lesions within the family are not necessarily of the same severity.

Fig. 1.66

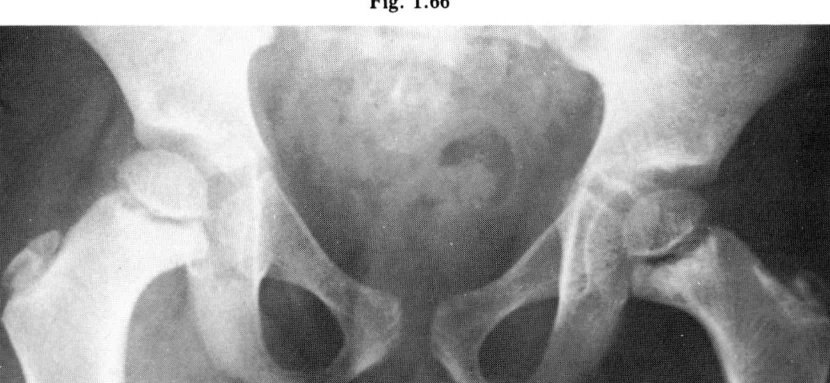

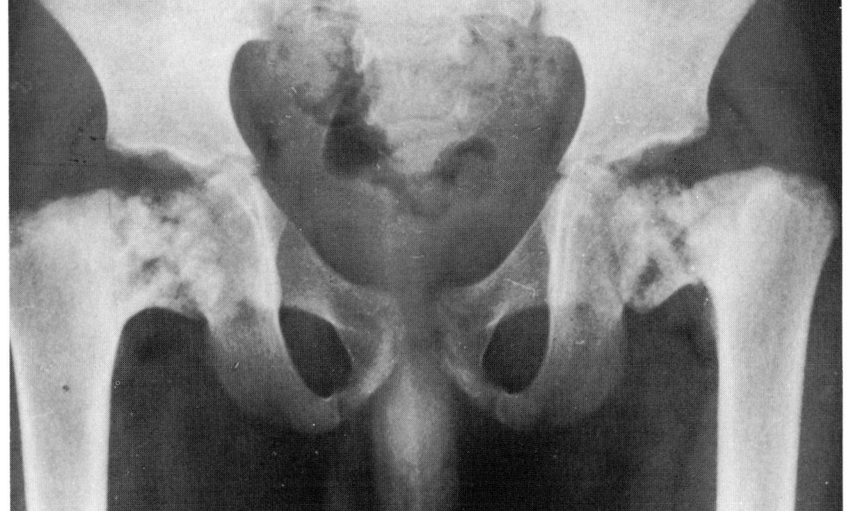

Fig. 1.67

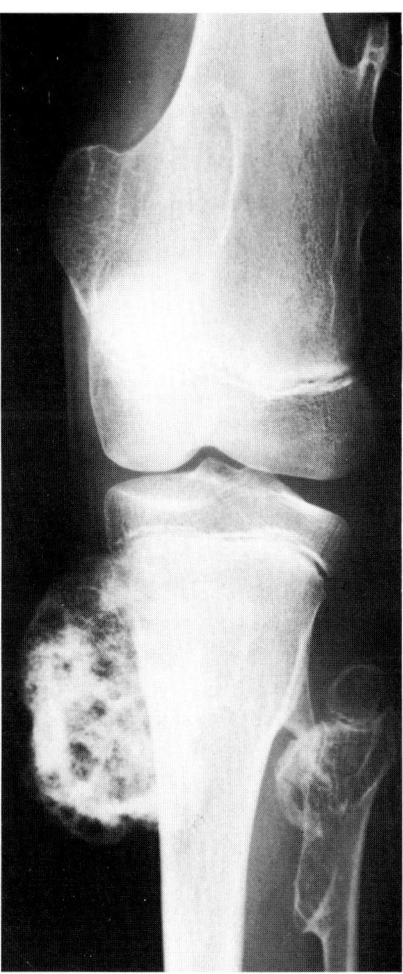

Fig. 1.68

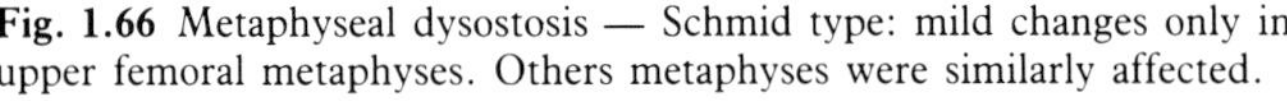

Fig. 1.66 Metaphyseal dysostosis — Schmid type: mild changes only in upper femoral metaphyses. Others metaphyses were similarly affected.

Fig. 1.67 Metaphyseal dysostosis: coxa vara and much metaphyseal irregularity. The epiphyseal involvement is illusory and caused by overlap of the abnormal metaphyses. (Courtesy of Dr M. W. Guirguis.)

Fig. 1.68 Diaphyseal aclasia: exostoses and expansion of metaphyses. Note cauliflower-like exostosis arising from the upper medial part of the tibia.

The bones chiefly affected are the long bones, especially in the metaphyseal regions of the shoulders, hips, knees and ankles, which become irregularly expanded and club-shaped. Upon these local enlargements of the shaft are projected osseous excrescences — exostoses — which are round or pointed. Their cortex merges with that of the shaft and their cancellous bone merges with the cancellous bone of the shaft, that is, they do not lie upon cortex. Exostoses are also found on the vertebral bodies and on the medial border of the scapula. The epiphyses are not involved.

Exostoses may be seen as small metaphyseal projections in infants and their growth may be observed. With growth, they come to point away from the adjacent joint (Fig. 1.68). During skeletal growth, the bony exostoses are covered by a cartilage cap which undergoes spotty calcification, and with increasing maturity the cartilaginous mass becomes increasingly dense and a smooth margin can be discerned. By the time growth ceases, the cartilage has usually completely ossified. The exostoses and the metaphyseal clubbing are separate lesions though the former may be superimposed on the latter.

Increase in transverse width is often accompanied by shortening so that deformities result. These changes are especially common at the radius and ulna so that Madelung deformity results (Fig. 1.69). Metacarpal bowing, radio-ulnar synostosis and radial head dislocation may also be found. Ollier's disease gives a similar appearance.

Lesions may be apparent early on in life, especially if it is known that one parent is affected. Lesions of subcutaneous bones, such as the tibia, often present early. Nerve compression occurs and paraplegia may result if the vertebral column is affected (Fig. 1.70A, B and C). Some lesions may present with a dull ache, but pain and rapid

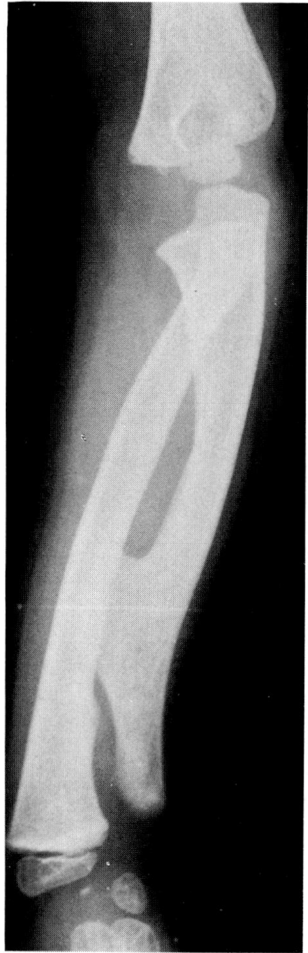

Fig. 1.69 Diaphyseal aclasia: typical deformity of bones of the forearm.

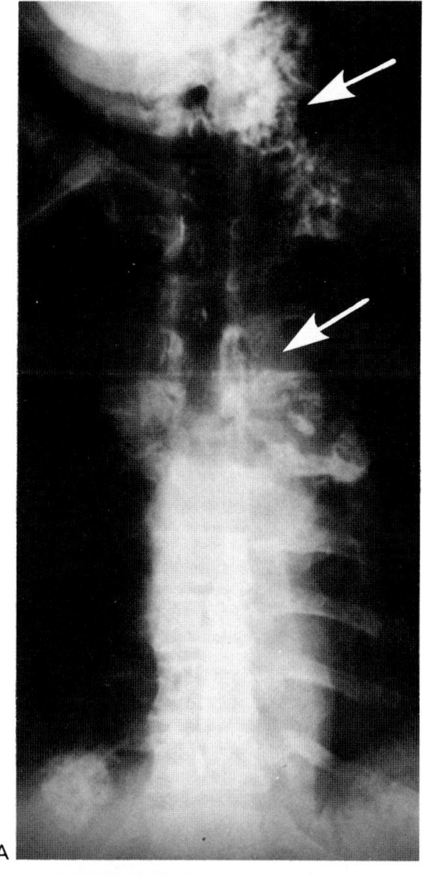

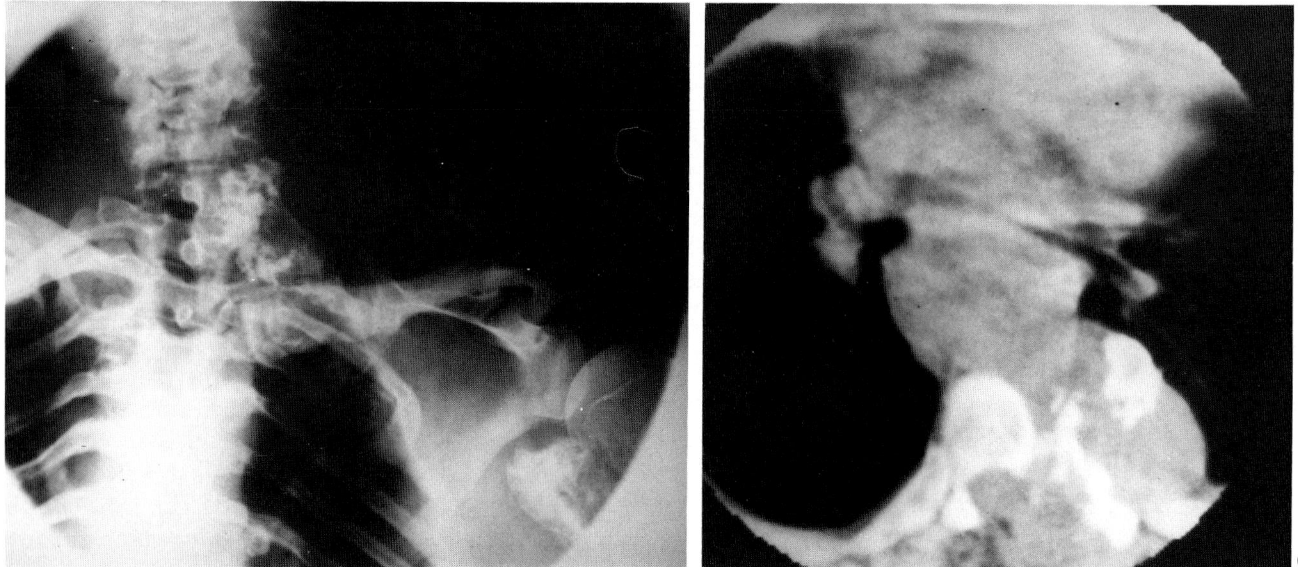

Fig. 1.70 A. and **B.** Diaphyseal aclasis. Exostoses (arrows) are seen associated with the spine in this patient who developed paraplegia. **C.** CT scan showing intrathoracic and spinal masses.

growth raise the possibility of malignant degeneration. The incidence of chondrosarcoma in diaphyseal aclasis is said to be around 10%, and these are often around the hip.

ACHONDROPLASIA

This is the most common type of disproportionate dwarfism. In these, one part of a limb shows relatively greater shortening. If proximal, rhizomelia is present; if medial, mesomelia; if distal, acromelia. In recent years many conditions, such as thanatophoric dwarfism, have been split off from achondroplasia so that a truly homogenous picture now emerges. Inheritance is autosomal dominant but most cases (85%) seem to be due to mutation of the gene, probably in older fathers. The patients have normal intelligence though a lack of muscle tone at birth suggests retardation.

The children have classical features at birth. Trident hands with short stubby fingers, a depressed nasal bridge with a prominent forehead and a disproportionally large skull, and prominent buttocks due to lumbar lordosis are all seen. The large head can obstruct labour. Limb bones are short with rhizomelic pattern.

Radiological findings. *Long bones*. The tubular bones are short, appear relatively widened and have prominent muscle insertions. The humeri and femora are affected more than distal bones (rhizomelia). The fibulae are long and bowed. The epiphyses are deformed by their insertion into V-shaped defects at the metaphyses. The epiphyses themselves have V-shaped distal ends with deep intercondylar notches. The appearances are similar to those seen with local premature fusion after infection, trauma or irradiation. The joint spaces appear widened owing to the proximity of epiphyses and metaphyses.

Retardation of ossification and a reduced anteroposterior diameter cause the upper ends of the femora of babies to appear relatively radiolucent. A defect is present in older

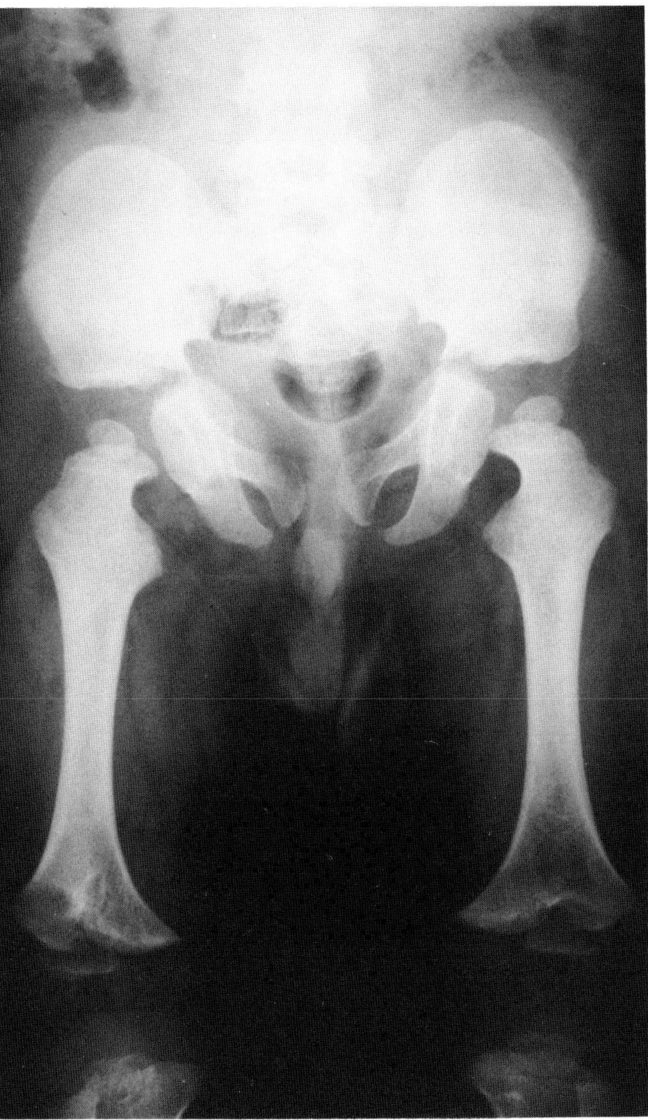

Fig. 1.71 Achondroplasia: square iliac blades with horizontal acetabular roofs. Note also the narrow interpedicular distances in the lumbo-sacral region and the defects at the distal femoral metaphyses into which the epiphyses insert.

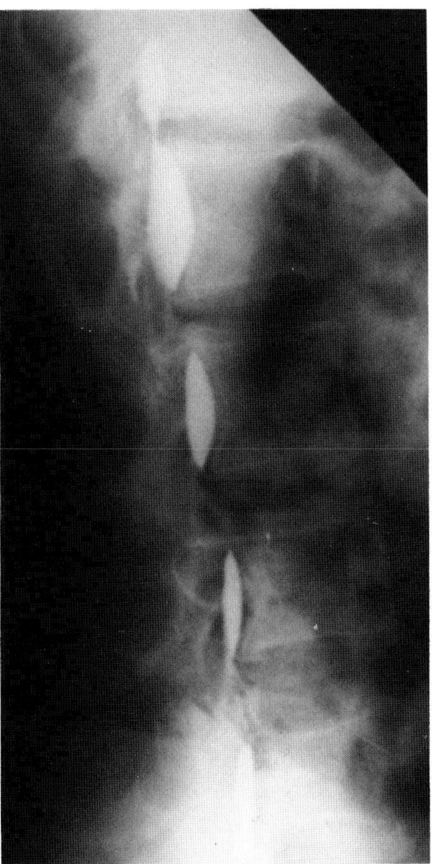

Fig. 1.72 Achondroplasia. There is posterior scalloping of the vertebral bodies and the defects fill with contrast. Similar changes occur in neurofibromatosis.

children at the site of the epiphysis of the tibial tubercle due to an excess of uncalcified cartilage at this age.

Pelvis. The pelvis is small and its diameters reduced. The iliac blades especially are reduced and rather square — the 'tombstone' appearance. The acetabula are set posteriorly and the acetabular roofs are horizontal (Fig. 1.71). L5 is deeply set and excessive pelvic tilt causes prominence of buttocks and an illusion of lordosis. The sacro-sciatic notch is narrow with a prominent medially directed spur. The pelvic inlet resembles a champagne glass.

Spine. The anteroposterior diameters of vertebral bodies are often short but the height of vertebral bodies is insignificantly reduced. In the thoraco-lumbar region a vertebral body or two may appear wedged or bullet-nosed. In some a thoraco-lumbar vertebral body may resemble that found in Hurler's syndrome. Scalloping at the back of vertebrae may be seen (Fig. 1.72)

The spinal canal in the lumbar region tapers caudally so that the interpedicular distances decrease from L1 to L5 (Figs 1.71 and 1.72). The lateral view will also show the small spinal canal. Severe symptoms from disc protrusions are liable to develop in later life — the spinal stenosis in the lumbo-sacral region is an important predisposing facto and can be confirmed by radiculography or CT.

Skull changes are mandatory to the diagnosis c achondroplasia. The calvarium is large but the base i shortened. The sella may be small. The foramen magnun is characteristically small and funnel-shaped — hydrocepha lus may occur and it is attributed to this mechanical cause

Chest. The ribs are short, the anterior ends widened an the sternum short and broad. The scapulae have peculia shapes losing their sharp angles; the glenoid fossae ar small in relation to the humeral heads.

Hands and feet. Tubular bones of the hands and feet ap pear short and wide, but carpal and tarsal bones are littl affected (Fig. 1.73). The trident hand, in which all th fingers are almost of equal length and diverge from on another in two pairs plus the thumb is often found.

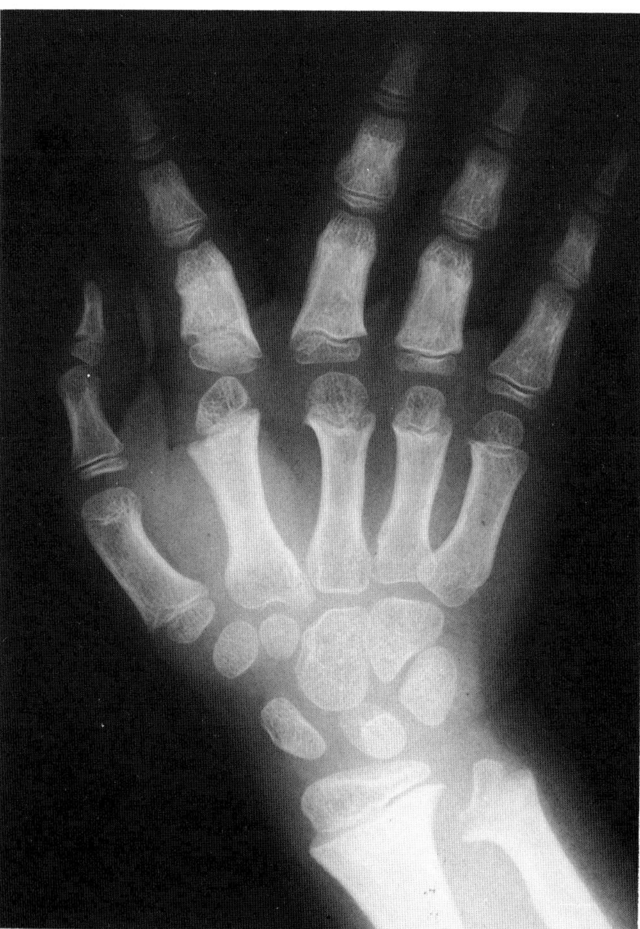

Fig. 1.73 Trident hand in achondroplasia.

HYPOCHONDROPLASIA

This is a condition which has been separated from classica achondroplasia, though there are some features in com mon. The skull is never affected, and the patients ar either normal or mildly reduced in height. The disease i inherited as a dominant. The abdomen and buttocks ar prominent, as in achondroplasia, and the legs are bowe in childhood.

Radiologically, there is rhizomelia with a short, broa femoral neck. The distal fibula is overgrown compare

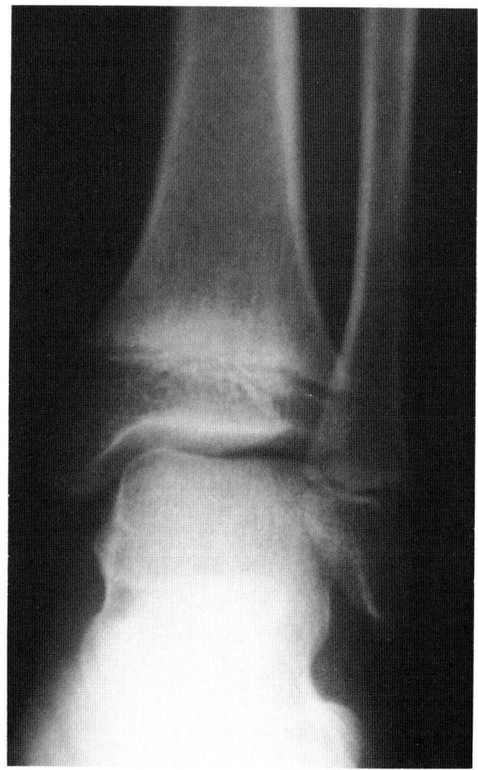

Fig. 1.74 Overgrowth of the distal fibula in hypochondroplasia.

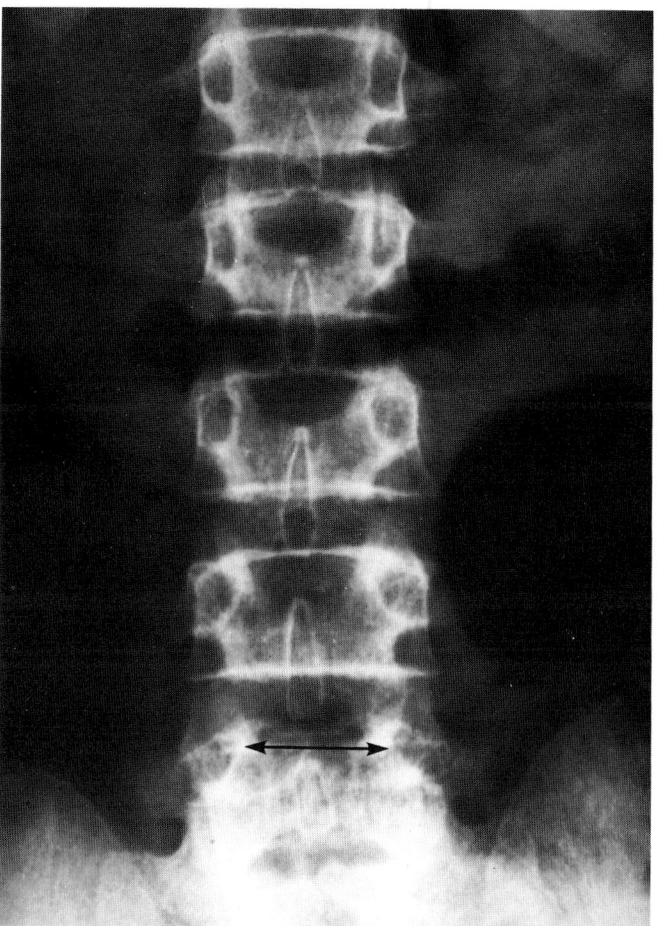

Fig. 1.75 Hypochondroplasia: a narrowed interpedicular distance (→) at L5 in the same patient as Figure 1.74.

with the distal tibia (Fig. 1.74). The iliac bones are smaller than normal but not as markedly reduced as in achondroplasia. The interpedicular distances narrow from L1 to L5 and the pedicles are short, so that spinal stenosis results (Fig. 1.75). The lumbar lordosis is increased.

PSEUDOACHONDROPLASIA

This condition is a short-limbed dwarfism occurring in both recessive and dominant forms of mild or marked severity, so that some patients are barely affected and some are grossly deformed. In all patients, however, the skull is normal, distinguishing this condition from achondroplasia. Changes are also not seen in the first year of life.

Spine. Vertebral bodies may be flat and irregular with central anterior 'tongues' (Fig. 1.76A). In adult life appearances vary from near normal to platyspondyly and scoliosis. The spine in multiple epiphyseal dysplasia is barely affected.

Long bones. The epiphyses are delayed in appearance and markedly irregular (Fig. 17.6B), again differing from achondroplasia. Metaphyses are broad and spurred. After fusion, epiphyseal dysplasia of varying degrees of severity is found.

Pelvis. The acetabulum is irregular and premature osteoarthritis of the hips occurs. The ilia are large and the pubes and ischia short

Hands. In severe cases, the tubular bones are short and stubby with delay in ossification of irregular epiphyses and carpal bones (Fig. 1.76C). In the adult the metacarpals end up shortened. Shortening of radius and ulna may be marked and both bones at the wrist may be hypoplastic centrally, giving a 'V' appearance.

DIASTROPHIC DWARFISM

This is an autosomal recessive short limb form of dwarfism characterised by multiple dislocations and increasing scoliosis (Fig. 1.77). The term 'diastrophic', meaning twisted, indicates the serious deformities to be expected in these patients whose mentalities are unimpaired. Cystic changes in the antihelix of the ear are common.

Club foot, congenital dislocation of the hip and other joints, and joint contractures are found.

The long bones are broad and short. Ulnar deviation of the hand is found. The first metacarpal is characteristically shortened, proximally placed and the thumb abducted, giving the classical 'hitch-hiker's thumb'. A similar deformity of the great toe may be found.

Lesions in the cervical spine are common, the odontoid may be rudimentary. The rest of the spine is generally not affected except for gross scoliosis.

THANATOPHORIC DWARFISM

This has only relatively recently been separated from achondroplasia and is the commonest fatal neonatal dysplasia.

Radiological findings. *Limbs*. There is rhizomelic dwarfism but the long bones are bowed. The metaphyses are irregular and the epiphyses of the knee are absent at birth. Short, wide metacarpals and phalanges are shown.

Axial skeleton. There is marked platyspondyly but the posterior vertebral elements are normal so that on an anterior view the vertebral bodies resemble the letter H (Fig. 1.78). The pelvis shows poor mineralisation of ischium and pubis, and small square iliac blades. The skull often shows lateral temporal bulging (cloverleaf skull) due to craniostenosis.

The ribs are short and flared anteriorly.

The infants are stillborn or die shortly after birth.

METATROPHIC DWARFISM

The striking feature of this remarkable condition is the reversal of the distribution of the dwarfism as growth pro-

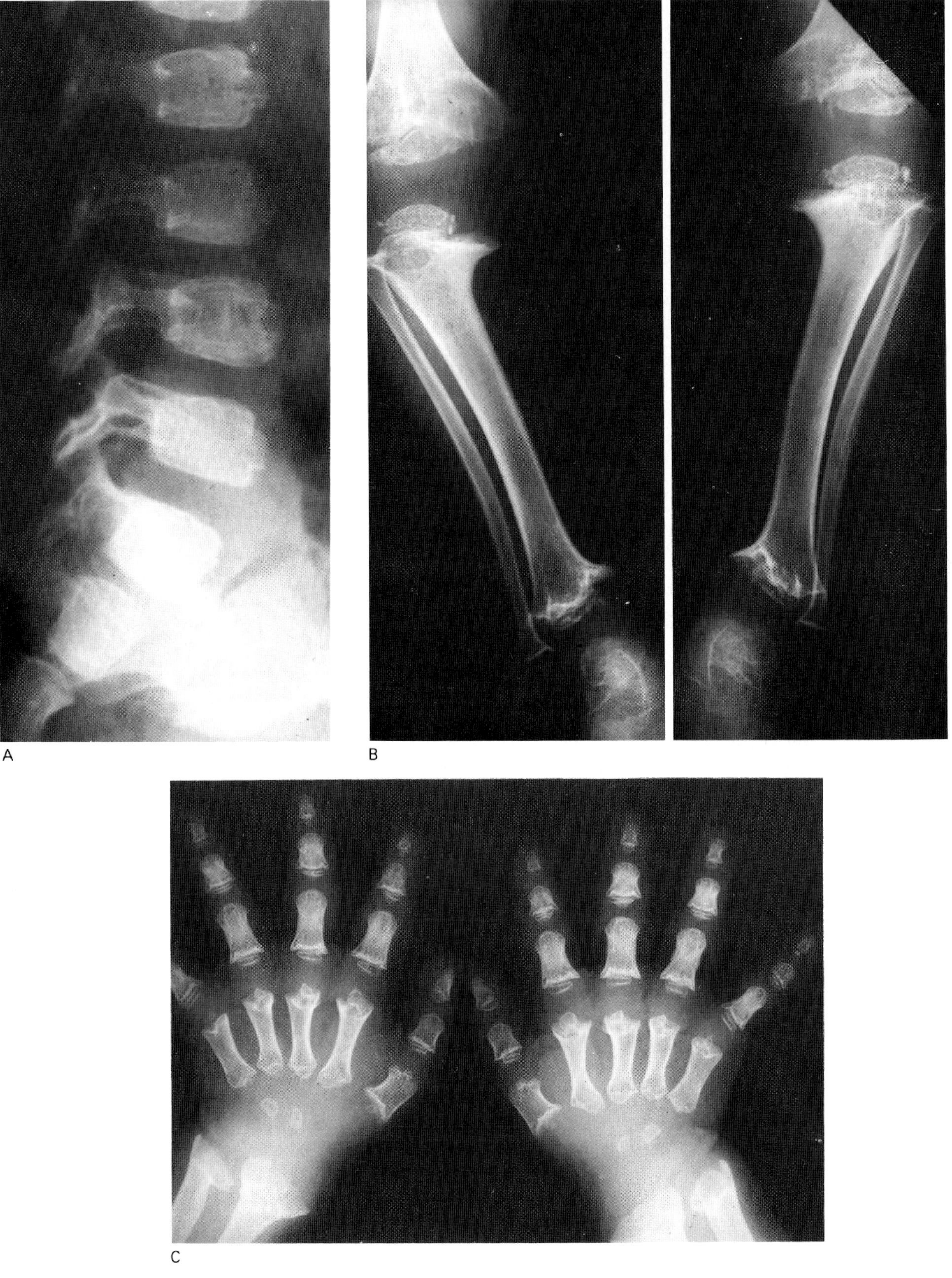

Fig. 1.76 Pseudoachondroplasia. **A.** Tongue-like projections of the vertebral bodies with superior and inferior defects. **B.** Long bones — irregular epiphyses and metaphyses with tilt deformities. **C.** Hands — the radius and ulna are flared at the metaphyses, the carpal bones delayed and irregular, and the metacarpals short. The phalanges are stubby and the epiphyses angular and irregular.

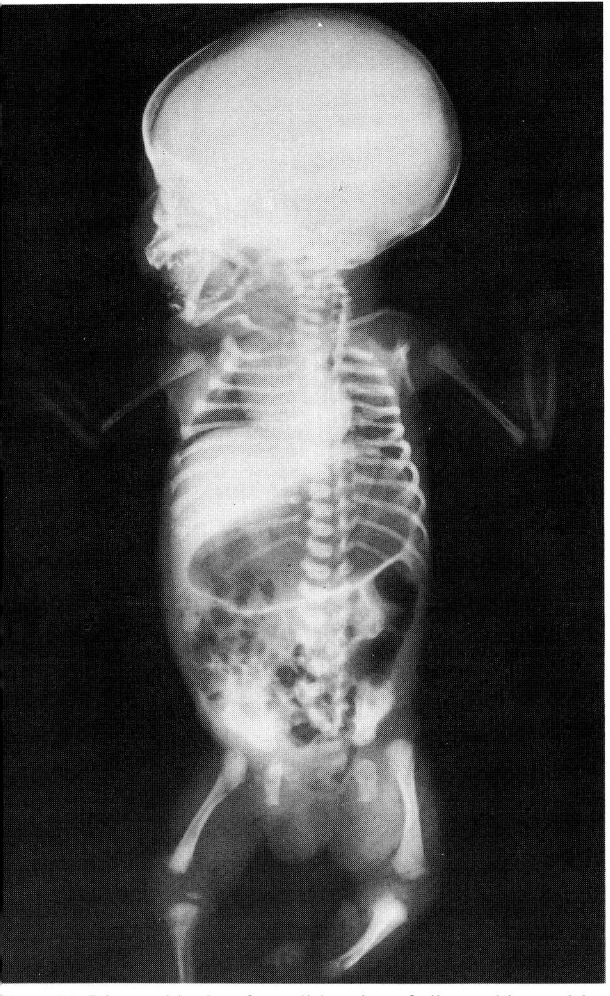

Fig. 1.77 Diastrophic dwarfism: dislocation of elbows, hips and knees. This baby had changes in the cervical spine and cystic changes in the antihelix of the ear. (Courtesy of Dr R. West.)

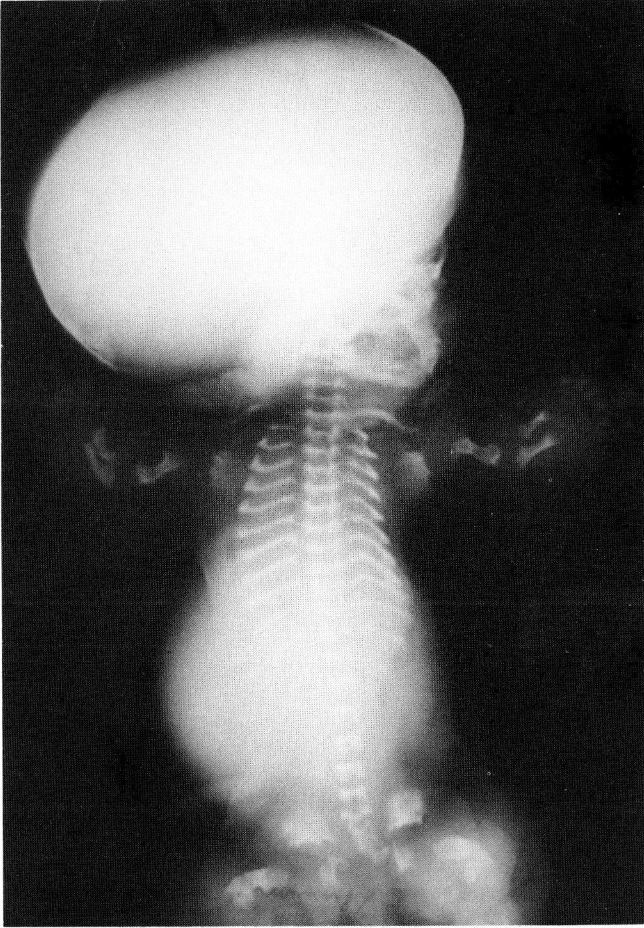

Fig. 1.78 Thanatophoric dwarfism: a grossly constricted chest with non-aeration of the lungs in a stillborn child. Note the shortened and curved long bones and the shelf-like and spurred acetabula. H-shaped vertebral bodies are seen caudally.

proceeds. Initially the limbs are very short and the trunk of normal dimensions. If the child survives, the trunk becomes relatively more shortened than the limbs because of severe kyphoscoliosis. One meaning of the prefix 'meta' is transformation, hence the term 'metatrophic dwarfism', i.e. transformation from a short limb to a short trunk dwarf. Many of these patients have a caudal tail-like appendage near the coccyx.

In early life remarkable flaring of the ends of long bones will be seen — the bone thus resembles a dumb-bell (Fig. 1.79). The ribs are short and the volume of the thorax is diminished as in asphyxiating thoracic dystrophy. Extreme platyspondyly of vertebral bodies is seen; the posterior arches are unaffected. The pelvis resembles that of achondroplasia.

Should the baby survive, a severe kyphoscoliosis will develop and the limb changes become less striking. At this stage the condition will resemble the Morquio–Brailsford chondro-osteodystrophy (mucopolysaccharidosis IV). A diagnosis of late metatrophic dwarfism might be considered in supposed cases of Morquio-Brailsford lesions in whom mucopolysaccharides are absent from the urine.

ASPHYXIATING THORACIC DYSPLASIA
(Eponym: *Jeune disease*)

Most, but not all, patients with this disease die in infancy from respiratory distress. In contradistinction to thanatophoric dwarfism, the spine is normal and the long bones are not curved and only a little shortened.

The thorax is stenotic. The ribs are short and horizontal and the clavicles highly placed (Fig. 1.80).

Polydactyly is present in many cases and epiphyses are present at the knee.

Inheritance is autosomal recessive. In those patients who survive, renal failure may result, even if bone changes revert to normal.

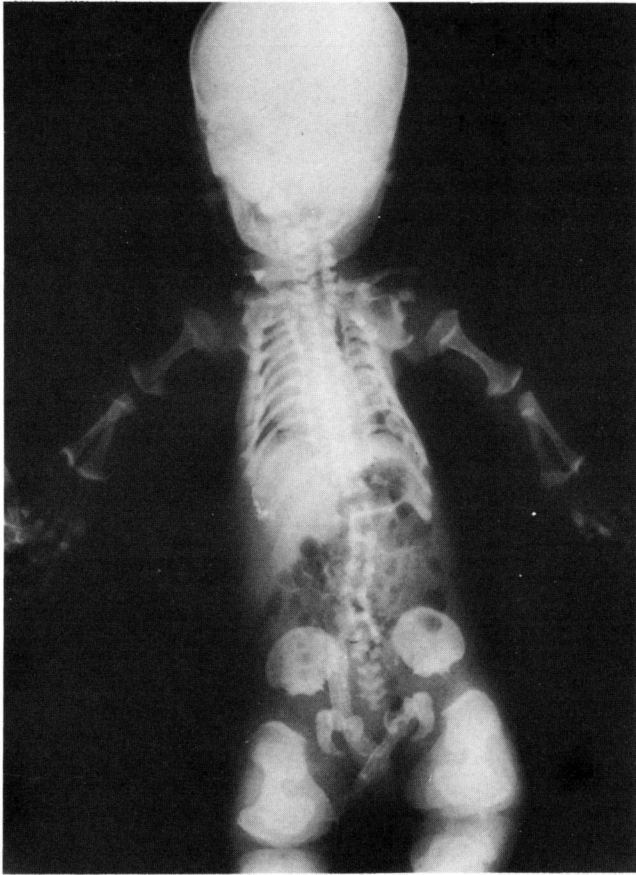

Fig. 1.79 Metatrophic dwarfism — newborn baby. In this stage the limbs are relatively more shortened than the spine. Note dumb-bell femora and humeri. The pelvis is that of achondroplasia. Note the small thoracic cage.

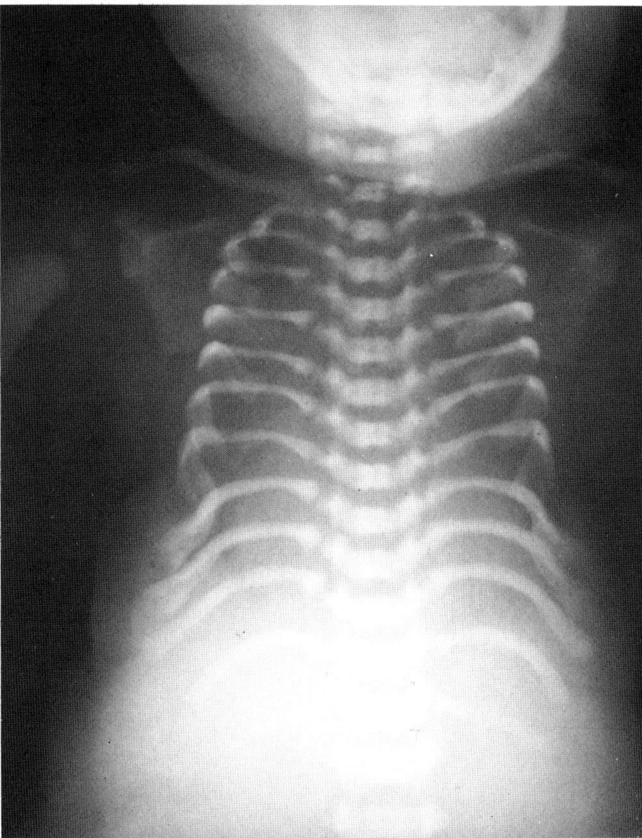

Fig. 1.80 Asphyxiating thoracic dystrophy: short horizontal ribs with high clavicles but a normal spine. The scapulae are hypoplastic.

CHONDROECTODERMAL DYSPLASIA
(Eponym: *Ellis–van Creveld disease*)

Neonates are seen with limb shortening which especially affects mid and distal segments. A narrow rib cage and polydactyly occur. Some 50% of patients have congenital cardiac defects which may be fatal.

Radiographic features. *Limbs.* In the limbs, the paired long bones are short and the metaphyses dome-shaped (Fig. 1.81). At the proximal tibia the developing epiphysis is situated over the abnormal medial tibial plateau and is defective laterally. Valgus deformity results. Post-axial polysyndactyly is present (Fig. 1.82).

Axial skeleton. The skull and spine are normal. The rib cage resembles that seen in asphyxiating thoracic dystrophy. The acetabulum has a medial spur in the region of the triradiate cartilage.

The ectodermal dysplasia, with partial or total absence of teeth, and abnormal hair and nails is not seen in asphyxiating thoracic dystrophy.

DYSCHONDROSTEOSIS
(Eponym: *Leri–Weil disease*)

Inherited as a autosomal dominant, the patients are short in stature with a mesomelic type of dwarfism. There is hypoplasia of the inner aspect of the distal radius and the ulna is therefore prominent. It is subluxed dorsally (*Madelung deformity*). The carpal bones herniate proximally into the deficiency caused by the hypoplastic radius (Fig. 1.83).

The medial aspect of the tibia is similarly defective.

Fig. 1.81 Ellis-van Creveld disease — long bones. Mesomelic dwarfism is associated with dome-shaped metaphyses and hypoplasia of the lateral tibial plateau.

Fig. 1.82 Ellis-van Creveld disease. Polysyndactyly is present, together with anomalies of carpal segmentation.

Fig. 1.83 Dyschondrosteosis. **A.** There is separation of the hypoplastic distal radius and ulna with proximal herniation of the carpus. **B.** The lateral view shows the posterior situation of the ulna and hypoplasia of the proximal radius.

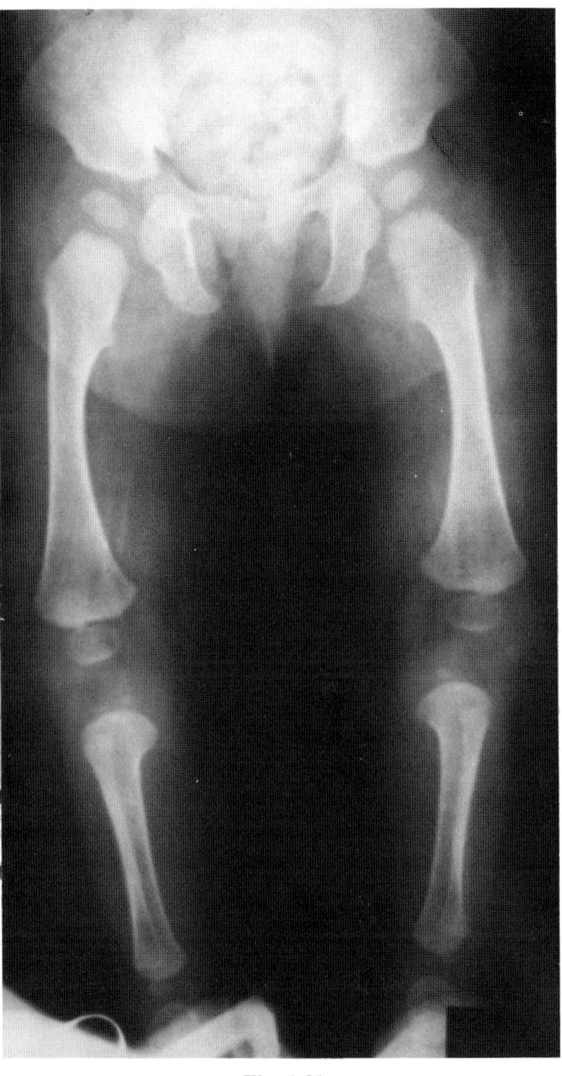

Fig. 1.81

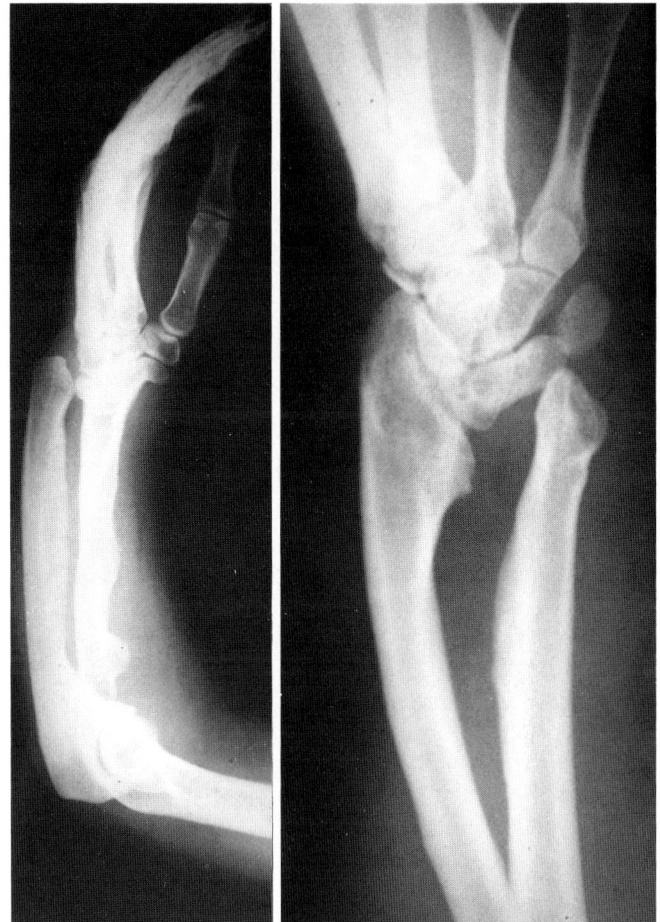

Fig. 1.83 A Fig. 1.83 B

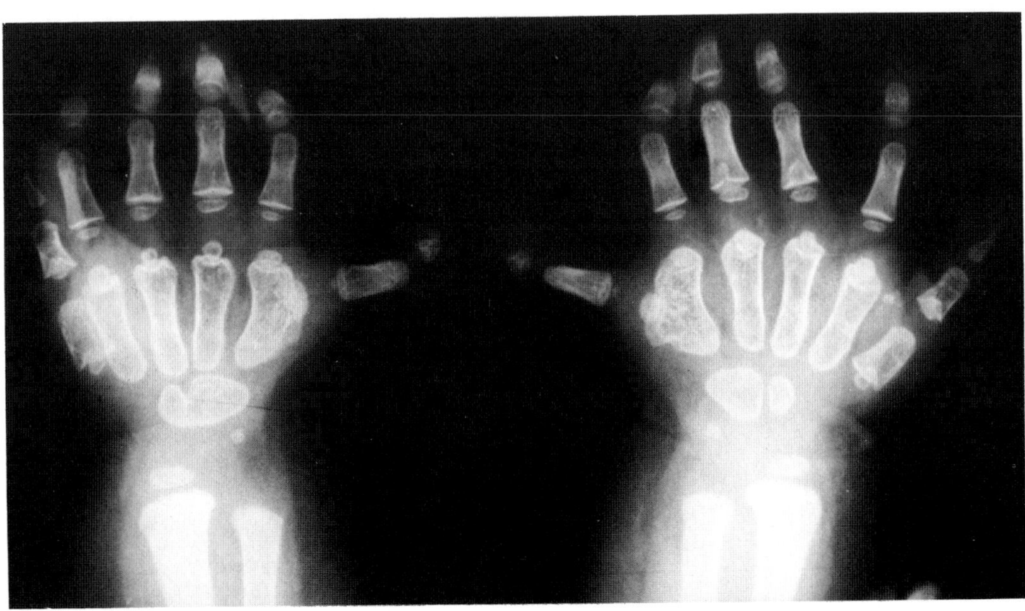

Fig. 1.82

MUCOPOLYSACCHARIDOSES AND MUCOLIPOIDOSES

The above terms embrace an extremely complex group of disorders. All members of the group are associated with an abnormality in mucopolysaccharide or glycoprotein metabolism.

Types of mucopolysaccharidoses are:

1. Hurler (gargoylism)
2. Hunter
3. Sanfilippo
4. Morquio–Brailsford
5. Scheie
6. Maroteaux–Lamy

The *Hunter* type is inherited as an X-linked recessive, the rest as autosomal recessives. Some are severe, others relatively mild. They have various degrees of mental retardation, corneal clouding and skeletal changes.

Skeletal changes include macrocephaly, J-shaped sella, thickened calvaria, oar-shaped ribs, hook-shaped vertebral bodies (Fig. 1.84). The ilia are widely flared, femoral ossific nuclei fragmented and coxa valga is usual. The proximal ends of the metacarpals taper and in older children the distal ends of the radius and especially the ulna slope towards each other (Fig. 1.85). Different degrees of these changes may be found in all these lesions.

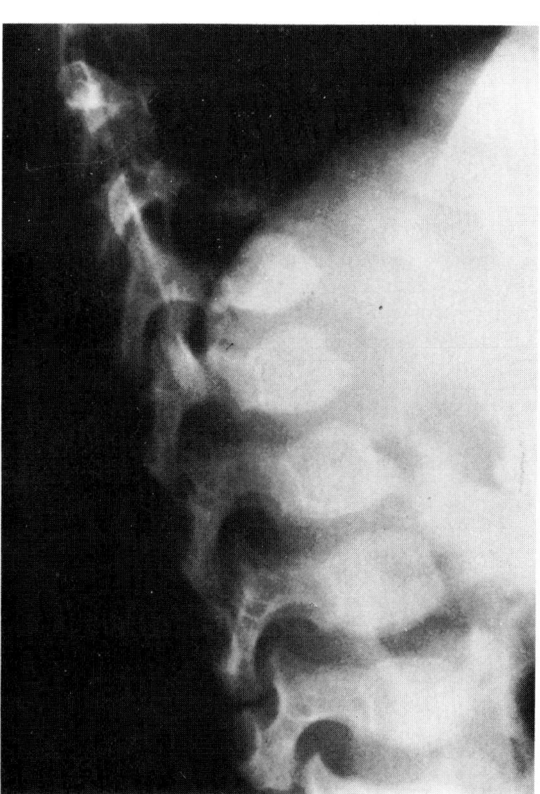

Fig. 1.84 Vertebrae of mucopolysaccharidosis I (gargoylism). Note hook-shaped vertebra and convex upper and lower surfaces. (Courtesy of Dr Roy Astley.)

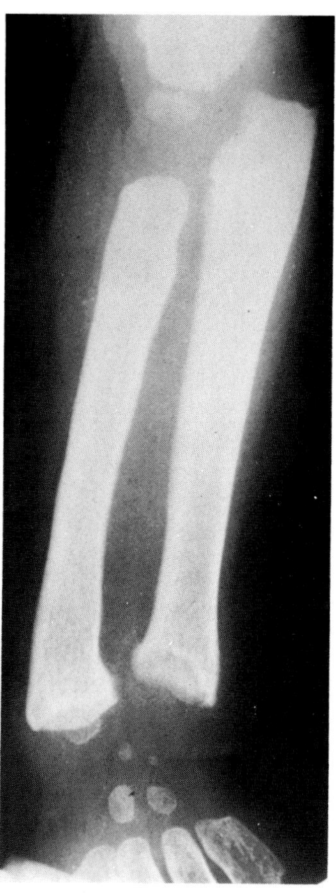

Fig. 1.85 Mucopolysaccharidosis I: expanded shafts of radius and ulna and tapering bone ends. Expansion of metacarpals is also seen. (Courtesy of Dr Roy Astley.)

Type 4 is somewhat different and it will be considered separately. The most that can be expected of the radiologist is to suggest a diagnosis of mucopolysaccharidosis and niceties of nosology are the province of the clinician, geneticist and biochemist. The same considerations apply to the mucolipoidoses.

MUCOPOLYSACCHARIDOSES IV

(Synonyms: *Morquio–Brailsford dystrophy*; *dyschondroplasia*; *spondyloepiphyseal dysplasia*)

This condition presents with dwarfism due mainly to shortness of the spine and to a marked kyphosis. The tubular bones are also widely affected. The lesion may be familial and the clinical picture is fairly characteristic. The patient will be dwarfed, kyphotic, knock-kneed and flat-footed. He stands with hips and knees flexed in a crouching position, and waddles like a duck when walking. The changes are usually first observed at about the age of 4 years. Mentality is unimpaired.

Radiographic features. Spinal changes are the dominant feature. The vertebrae are flat, and in childhood tend to have a characteristic form. The upper and lower surfaces of the vertebral body are defective and a central tongue of bone protrudes forwards (Fig. 1.86). This appearance is seen best in the lower dorsal and upper lumbar region. Later, as growth proceeds, the defect becomes repaired. One dorso-lumbar vertebra may be smaller than its fellows and displaced posteriorly, causing a marked kyphosis.

As a rule, tubular bones are not markedly affected but may be short and rather wide with somewhat irregular metaphyses. The epiphyses are markedly irregular and fragmented, notably those of the femoral heads. The joint spaces are increased and the joint surfaces, e.g. of the acetabulum and glenoid, are shallow and irregular.

The pelvis tends to be narrow, or shaped like that of an ape (Fig. 1.87). In the hands and feet the tubular bones are short and stubby, and some irregularity of the carpal and tarsal bones is also found.

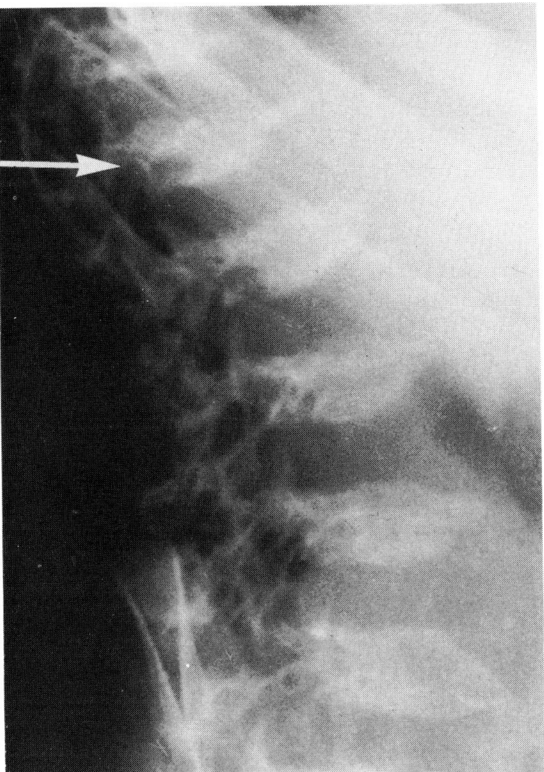

Fig. 1.86 Mucopolysaccharidosis IV: spine, showing flattening of vertebral bodies and forward protrusion of central tongue of bone. Note posterior displacement of dorso-lumbar vertebra (arrow).

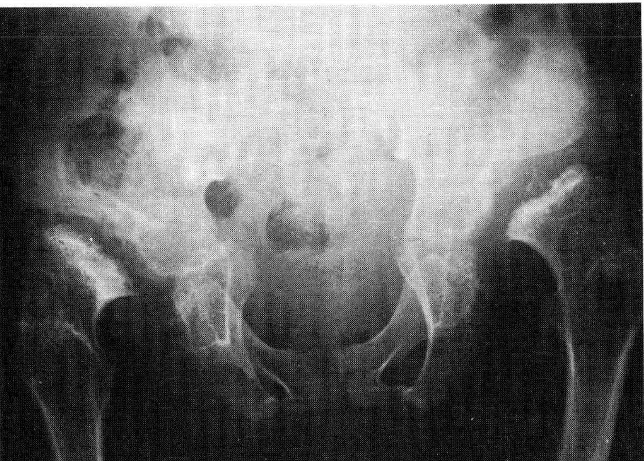

Fig. 1.87 Mucopolysaccharidosis IV: simian pelvis, fragmented maldeveloped femoral capital epiphyses with associated metaphyseal irregularity. Shallow acetabula with dislocation of both femoral heads shown also, a feature sometimes seen in this condition.

SPONDYLOEPIPHYSEAL DYSPLASIA

The term 'spondyloepiphyseal dysplasia' is used to embrace a group of conditions characterized by platyspondyly and dysplasia of other bones. The degrees of spinal and tubular bone involvement and the amount of dwarfism vary between the different groups.

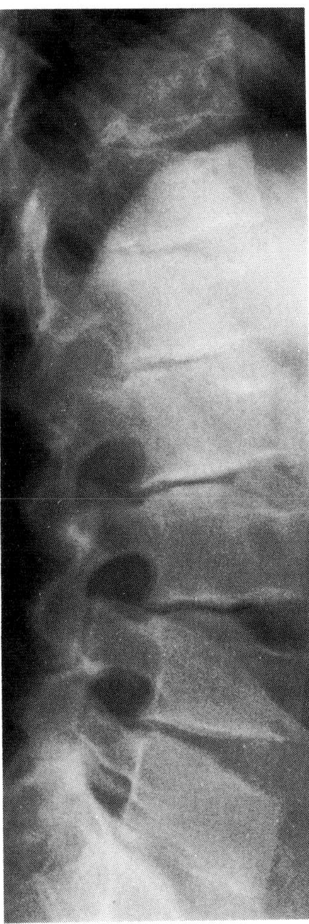

Fig. 1.88 Spondyloepiphyseal dysplasia X-linked recessive form, showing characteristic platyspondyly. Mounds of bone are seen on the superior and inferior parts of the posterior parts of the vertebral bodies. Gas is seen in the prematurely degenerate discs.

A. An X-linked variety — *SED tarda*. This type has a distinctive spinal lesion. Mounds of dense bone are found on the superior and inferior surfaces of the posterior parts of the vertebral end-plates (Fig. 1.88). The tubular bones are not much affected and may resemble those of mild cases of dysplasia epiphysealis multiplex (Fig. 1.89). The iliac wings are characteristically small. Hip degeneration frequently occurs prematurely.

B. Dominant variety — *SED congenita*. In these the platyspondyly is maximal in the thoracic spine. Lesions of tubular bones are severe and early osteoarthritis may be expected. The hands are unaffected. Retinal detachment is common.

C. Recessive variety. The platyspondyly is generalized and the severe wedging of the dominant form is not found.

HYPOPHOSPHATASIA

This is a genetically determined metabolic disease included in this section on account of its manifestations. Several subgroups have been described dependent on the age of onset and severity of symptoms. They are characterized by (a) low or absent serum alkaline phosphatase; (b) phosphoethanolamine in the urine and plasma; (c) hypercalcaemia in severe forms.

In the severe type, gross general failure of ossification of the skeleton is seen (Fig. 1.90). These babies do not survive. Some less severe forms present as severe rickets. If they survive the radiographic picture may resemble that of Ollier's disease. An adult form of this condition is characterized by osteoporosis and a tendency to fractures.

ARACHNODACTYLY

(Eponym: *Marfan's syndrome*)

This condition is inherited as an autosomal dominant. Clinically, the long bones are lengthened. Muscle weakness, hypermobility and lens dislocations are found. A high arched palate, depressed sternum and scoliosis occur. Cardiovascular lesions include aortic dissections, atrial septal defects and mitral valve lesions.

Radiographic features. The tubular bones are elongated and slender, the distal bones being much more affected than the proximal ones. The hands and feet are especially elongated (Fig. 1.91) and occasionally their bones have extra epiphyses. Kyphosis and scoliosis are frequent findings. Some scalloping of the back of vertebral bodies may be seen.

The diagnosis is usually straightforward. Estimation of the metacarpal index will aid the diagnosis in doubtful cases. This index is estimated by measuring the lengths of the second, third, fourth and fifth metacarpals and dividing their breadths taken at the exact mid-points. The resulting figures, from each of the four metacarpals, are added together and divided by four. In normal adult subjects the metacarpal index varies from 5.4 to 7.9; in arachnodactyly the range varies from 8.4 to 10.4.

HOMOCYSTINURIA

This lesion has some similarity to Marfan's syndrome but is inherited as an autosomal recessive. A definite biochemical abnormality has been demonstrated. Absence of the enzyme cystathionine synthesase results in an excess of

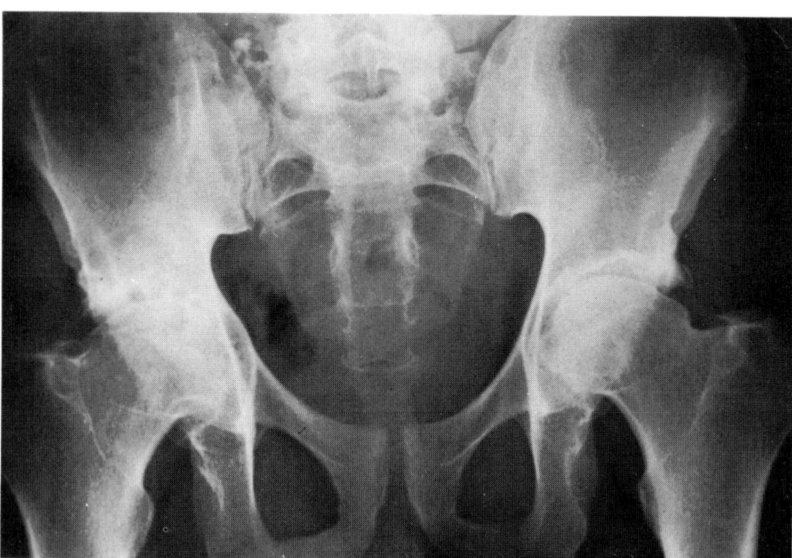

Fig. 1.89 Pelvis of Figure 1.88. Some, but not gross, osteoarthritis is seen with some bilateral acetabular protrusion. The iliac wings are characteristically small in this condition.

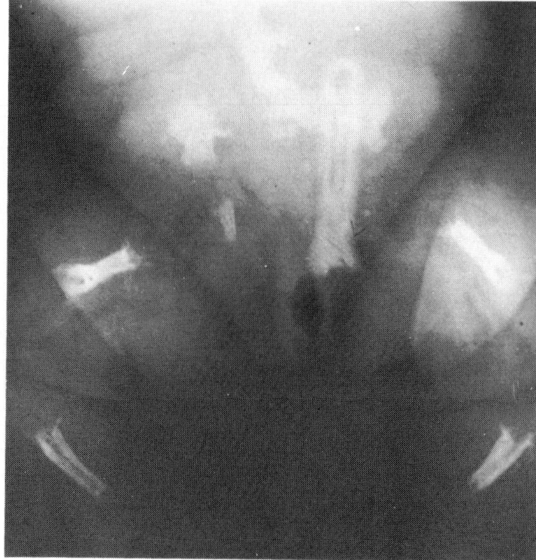

Fig. 1.90 Hypophosphatasia in newborn; gross failure of ossification of bones of the legs and of the pelvis.

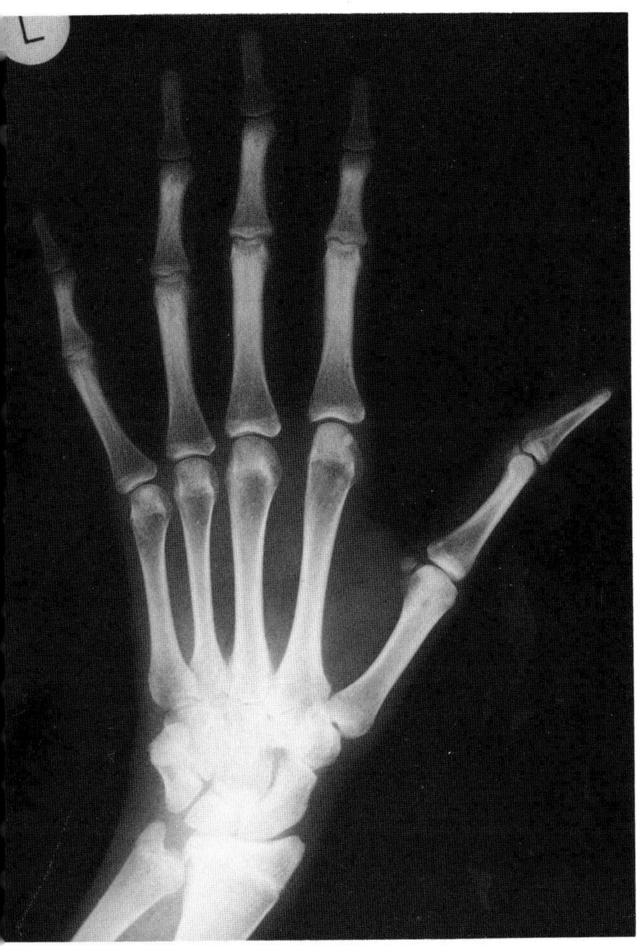

Fig. 1.91 Marfan's syndrome. Elongation of metacarpals and phalanges is demonstrated.

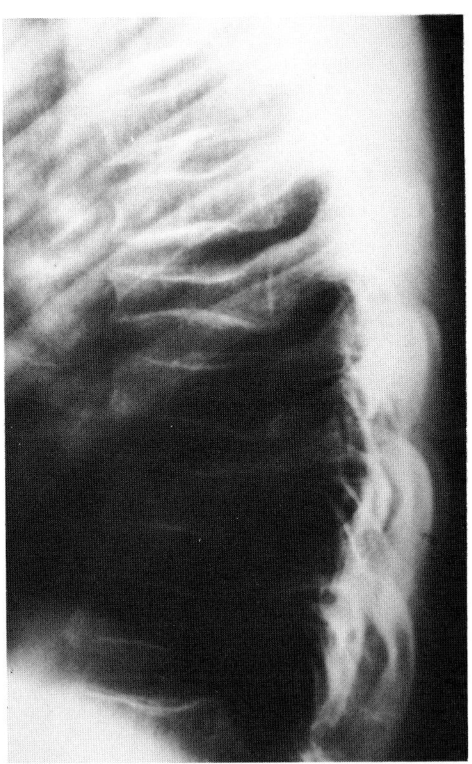

Fig. 1.92 Homocystinuria. Osteoporosis is associated with platyspondyly of the thoracic spine.

urinary homocystine. The most important feature is that thrombosis of arteries and veins is liable, especially after catheterization. Fatalities have been reported.

Osteoporosis in the spine, with posterior scalloping of the vertebral bodies (Fig. 1.92), differentiate this condition radiologically from Marfan's syndrome. Epiphyses and carpal bones tend to be enlarged and metaphyses broadened (Fig. 1.93), but arachnodactyly is less marked. Also these patients tend to have pes cavus and grosser sternal lesions than in Marfan's syndrome. Cardiac and aortic lesions are less common.

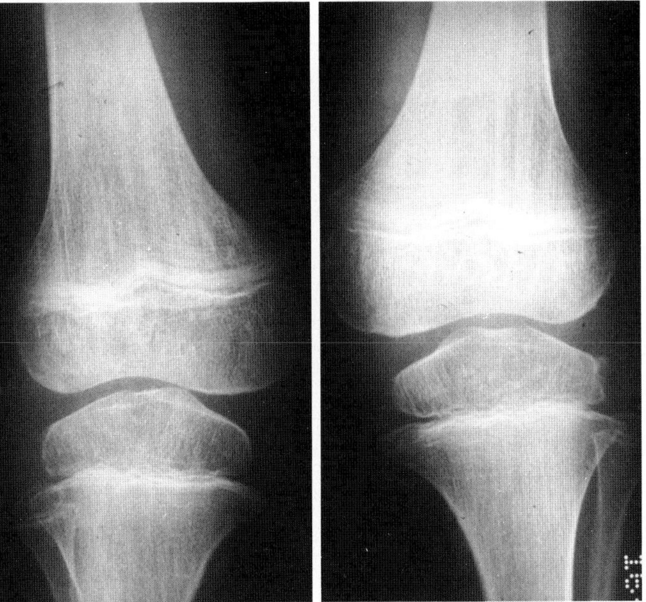

Fig. 1.93 Homocystinuria. Metaphyseal flaring is associated with bulbous enlargement of the epiphyses at the knee.

ACHONDROGENESIS

This is an uncommon lethal form of infantile dysplasia characterized by a large deformed head with gross underdevelopment of the limbs and a large squat abdomen.

Radiologically, the long bones are extremely short, irregular and grossly undermineralised (Fig. 1.94). The pelvis is barely visualized at birth or *in utero* (Type I). In type II, the limb bones are still short and metaphyses irregular, but slightly better mineralized. The vertebral bodies, however, may be non-mineralized, especially caudally.

The diseases are both inherited as autosomal recessives.

Fig. 1.94 Achondrogenesis. Gross shortening of the long bones is seen. The metaphyses are irregular and the epiphyses around the knee delayed in appearance. Poor mineralization of the caudal vertebral bodies, sacrum and pubic bones characterize Type II achondrogenesis.

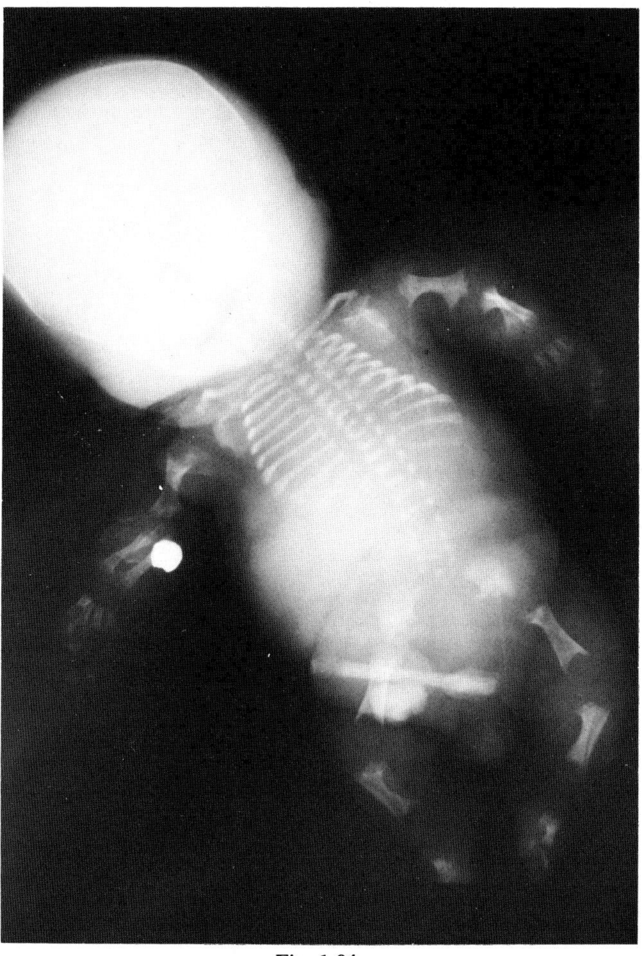

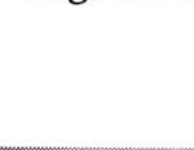

Fig. 1.94

Fig. 1.95 Fibrodysplasia ossificans progressiva; soft tissue ossification (arrows).

Fig. 1.96 Fibrodysplasia ossificans progressiva. Extensive new bone had been deposited in many soft tissues. Disuse osteoporosis of the bones is seen. (Courtesy of Mr T. McSweeney.)

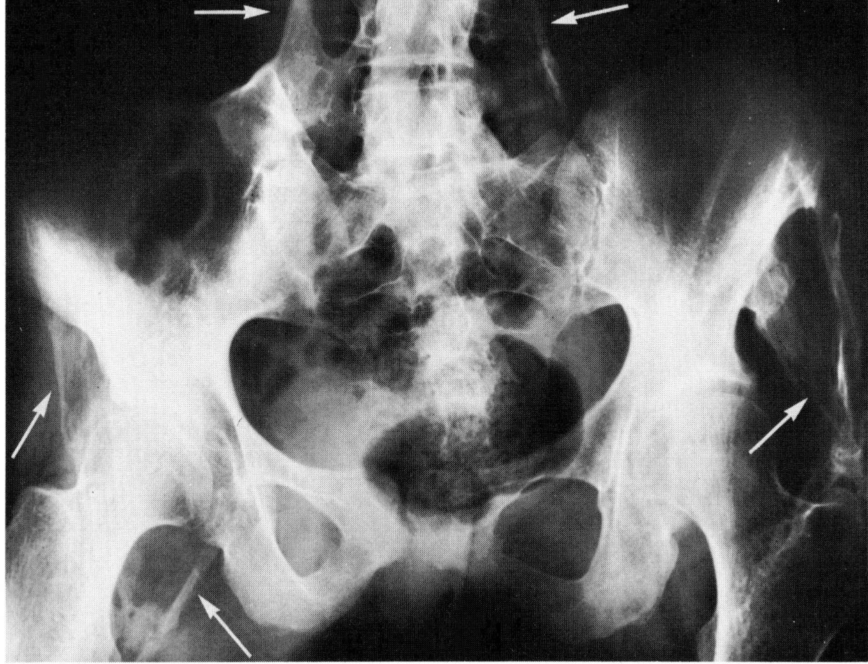

Fig. 1.95

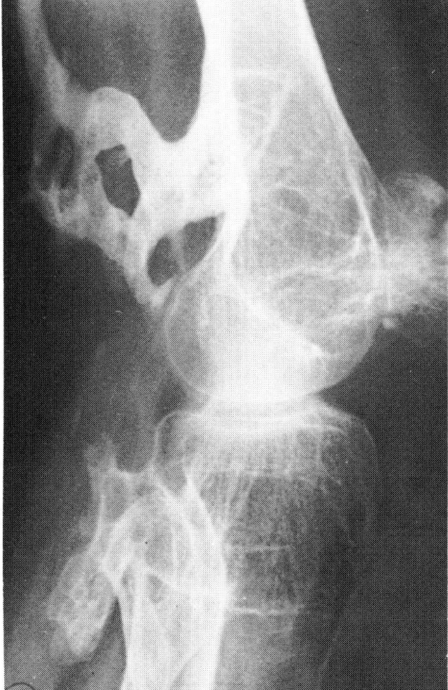

Fig. 1.96

FIBRODYSPLASIA OSSIFICANS PROGRESSIVA

(Synonym: *myositis ossificans progressiva*. Eponym: *Munchmeyer's disease*)

The disease process primarily involves the connective tissues rather than muscle fibres. Soft tissue swellings begin *in utero* or early on in life. These painful swellings affect the neck and upper trunk. Ossification commences in the lumps within months and is aggravated by surgical biopsy. Large masses of bone form in voluntary muscles which may extend to the normal skeletal structures and resemble exostoses (Figs. 1.95 and 1.96). Movements become restricted.

Skeletal involvement is present at birth. 75% have involvement of the great toe, with fusion and microdactyly or hallux valgus (Fig. 1.97). 50% have thumb hypoplasia and little finger clinodactyly. Femoral necks and mandibular condyles are broad. Cervical vertebral bodies are hypoplastic and fused.

Inheritance is probably autosomal dominant but most cases are sporadic as few patients survive to reproduce.

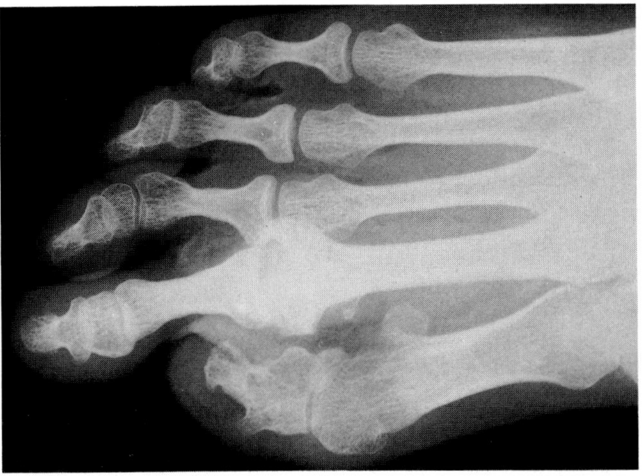

Fig. 1.97 Fibrodysplasia ossificans progressiva: developmental anomaly of the great toe. (Osteochondritis of the second metatarsal is also present.)

CHROMOSOMAL DISORDERS

Normally a human cell has 22 pairs of autosomes and two sex chromosomes. Some well-defined clinical syndromes are caused by abnormalities of the sex chromosomes. Nine clinical syndromes that result from anomalies of the autosomes have been described. Four of these have fairly well-defined radiological patterns: mongolism, trisomy 17–18, trisomy 13–15 and the *cri-du-chat* syndrome.

MONGOLISM

(Eponym: *Down's syndrome*. Synonym: *trisomy 21*)

This condition is associated with an extra chromosome in the 21–22 group. The clinical diagnosis of older children suffering from mongolism is usually easy. In a baby the diagnosis may not be evident clinically, but it is, of course, of great human importance. The newborn mongol has a large ilium with a flat acetabular roof; an elongated tapering ischium develops after a few months. Caffey and Ross expressed these features quantitatively. They described the 'iliac index' obtained by adding the 'iliac angle' to the 'acetabular angle' (Fig. 1.98). These angles are obtained by first drawing a horizontal line through corresponding points of the articulation at the centre of each acetabulum. A line is

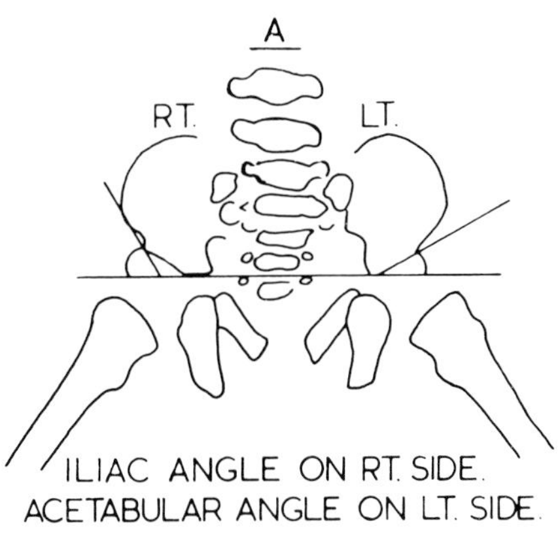

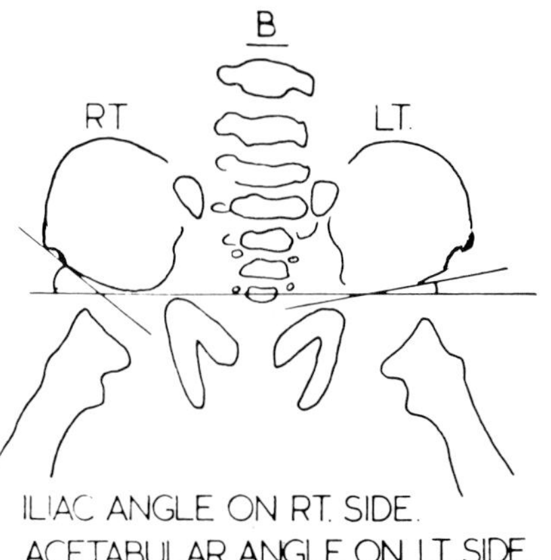

Fig. 1.98 Normal neonatal pelvis (**A**) and neonatal pelvis of a mongol (**B**). *Note* the protuberant ilium and flat acetabulum of the mongol and consequent reduction in the iliac and acetabular angles compared with the normal.

then drawn between the most lateral part of the ilium and the outer part of the acetabular roof. The angle between this line and the horizontal is called the iliac angle. The acetabular angle is given by the intersection of a line between the outer and the inner lips of the acetabulum with the same horizontal line.

Caffey and Ross and, later, Astley concluded that the iliac index affords a useful though not infallible means of diagnosis of mongolism in the first few weeks of life. Astley suggests the following criteria:

1. If the iliac index is under 60, mongolism is very probable.
2. If the index is over 78, mongolism is probably absent.
3. If the iliac index lies between 60 and 78, only a qualified report can be given. Between 68 and 60, mongolism is probable, but 10% of normals occur in this range. Between 68 and 78 mongolism is unlikely, but 6% of mongols do occur in this range.

Many other skeletal and visceral anomalies have been described in this disease, though none of them is invariably present. Some of the following anomalies have been only recently recognized:

a. Brachycephaly, hypoplasia of the nasal bones, maxillae and sphenoids, and absent frontal sinuses. Instability of the atlanto-axial joint and abnormalities in the upper cervical spine may be found.

b. The interorbital distance is decreased in most mongols, indicating orbital hypotelorism.

c. Extra ossification centres for the manubrium sterni are found in 90% of mongols between the ages of 1 and 4 years; this sign is seen in 20% of normal children of the same age group.

d. Many mongols have only 11 pairs of ribs.

e. The middle and distal phalanges of the fifth digits are often hypoplastic and curve inwards.

f. The lumbar vertebrae are often greater in height than in width, a reversal of normal ratio, and they show concave anterior surfaces. Thus a lateral view of the lumbar spine may be of diagnostic help. This is not diagnostic of mongolism but may be found in many children with delayed motor development.

g. Congenital heart disease is frequently found in mongols, as is an aberrant right subclavian artery.

h. An increased incidence of duodenal stenosis and atresia and of Hirschsprung's disease may be found in mongols.

TRISOMY 17–18

An extra chromosome is found in the 17–18 (E) group in this condition. These babies are mentally defective and have an average life span of 90 days, though some have survived for 10 years. Radiographic appearances include:

a. *Hand*. The most characteristic clinical and radiographic changes are found in the hand. The first metacarpal and thumb are short. Ulnar deviation of the fingers is seen and a gap is found between the bases of the second and third digits.

b. *Skull*. The vault is thin, the occiput prominent and the maxilla and mandible hypoplastic.

c. *Chest*. The thorax is asymmetrical. Hypoplasia or absence of the medial thirds of the clavicles may be found. The ribs are gracile and anomalies of segmentation may be found in the sternum. Congenital heart lesions are frequent.

d. *Abdomen*. A variety of renal abnormalities have been reported. Malrotation of the bowel may be found.

e. *Pelvis*. Anterior rotation of the iliac bones may be seen, giving an appearance of narrowing in the anteroposterior view. This is the reverse of the deformity in the mongol and is thus called the 'anti-mongoloid pelvis'.

TRISOMY 13–15

The extra chromosome is in the 13–15 group in this condition. The babies are mentally defective and usually have hideous craniofacial abnormalities of the arrhinocephalic type. Radiographic manifestations are not individually characteristic. Main findings include:

a. *Skull*. Hypotelorism, diminished ossification of the vault, clefts and absence of midline structures.

b. *Chest*. Malformed ribs and congenital heart lesions.

c. *Abdomen*. Abdominal and genito-urinary lesions are frequent.

d. *Hand*. Syndactyly, polydactyly and narrow distal phalanges.

CRI-DU-CHAT SYNDROME

No extra chromosome occurs in this condition but partial deletion of the short arm of chromosome 5 is found. The condition is so called on account of the high pitched cry that is similar to that of a distressed kitten. Patients are severely retarded mentally, but tend to live longer than those with trisomy 17–18 and 13–15. Radiographic findings are not characteristic but include:

a. Hypertelorism and microcephaly.
b. Faulty development of long bones.
c. A pelvic lesion in which the acetabular angle is normal but the iliac angle increased.

In addition to the four conditions noted, five other autosomal lesions have been reported but they have rather indefinite features. Autosomal abnormalities also occur in Fanconi's pancytopenia, ataxia telangiectasia, Bloom's syndrome and in the haemopoietic cells of many patients with chronic myeloid leukaemia.

ABNORMALITIES OF THE SEX CHROMOSOMES

The basic defect in this group is failure of sex chromosomes to separate from each other in cell division. For practical purposes Turner's syndrome is the only one of importance to the radiologist. Not all patients with Turner's syndrome have an abnormal sex chromosome pattern, nor do all individuals with the characteristic chromosomal pattern have Turner's syndrome.

TURNER'S SYNDROME

The essential components of this condition are agenesis of the gonads, webbing of the neck and cubitus valgus. The syndrome is confined to females. Mental deficiency, congenital cardiac and aortic lesions and anomalies of the kidneys such as malrotation are often associated. Sometimes males are found with a similar body configuration, *viz.*, short stature and a webbed neck. However, these boys have a normal chromosomal pattern and they tend to get auricular septal defects and pulmonary stenosis rather than coarctation of the aorta that may be associated with Turner's syndrome.

Radiological findings. The skeletal features are inconstant and non-specific. Density of the skeleton is reduced, especially of the hands and feet. General osteoporosis is frequent in older patients. The metacarpals may be short, especially the fourth (Fig. 1.99) and accelerated fusion of the epiphysis may be found. The so-called 'metacarpal sign' is an expression of the shortening of the fourth metacarpal. Normally a line extending tangentially from the distal ends of the fourth and fifth metacarpals should pass distally to the head of the third metacarpal. If the fourth metacarpal is short, as in Turner's syndrome, such a line will either just touch or pass through the head of the third metacarpal. This sign may be seen in some normal subjects.

The increase in the carrying angle of the elbow is better assessed clinically than radiologically. However, a radial tilt of the articular surface of the trochlea may be evident. The medial tibial condyle is depressed and beak-like and the medial femoral condyle may project downwards (as in Blount's disease) (Fig. 1.100).

Maldevelopment of the clavicles and slender ribs are often seen. Kyphosis and scoliosis are frequently found. Hypoplasia of the atlas and odontoid peg may be seen. In many females the pelvic inlet is android, the pubic arch narrowed and the sacro-sciatic notches small.

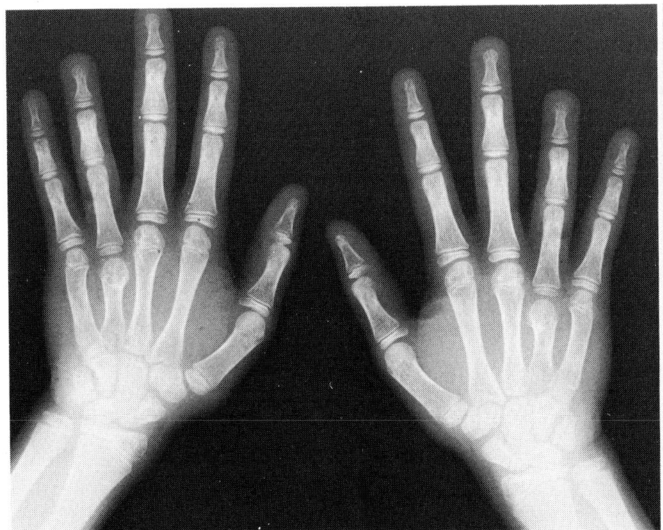

Fig. 1.99 Turner's syndrome: typical shortening of fourth metacarpals.

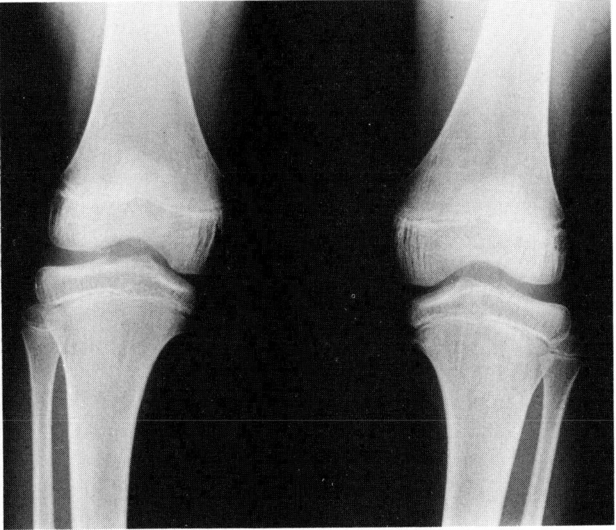

Fig. 1.100 Turner's syndrome — knees: depression of medial tibial condyles and small beaks on medial corners of metaphyses.

REFERENCES AND SUGGESTIONS FOR FURTHER READING

Andren, L., Von Rosen, S. (1958) The diagnosis of dislocation of the hip in newborns and the primary results of immediate treatment. *Acta Radiologica, Stockholm*, **49**, 89–95.

Astley, R. (1963) Chromosomal abnormalities in childhood with particular reference to Turner's syndrome and mongolism. *British Journal of Radiology*, **36**, 2–10.

Baker, S. L., Dent, C. E., Friedman, M., Watson, L. (1966) Fibrogenesis imperfecta ossium. *Journal of Bone & Joint Surgery*, **48B**, 804–825.

Beighton, P., Cremin, B. J. (1980) *Sclerosing Bone Dysplasias*. Berlin: Springer Verlag.

Caffey, J., Ross, S. (1956) Mongolism (mongoloid deficiency) during

early infancy — some newly recognized diagnostic changes in the pelvic bones. *Paediatrics*, **17**, 643–651.
Fielden, P., Russel, J. G. B. (1970) Coronally cleft vertebra. *Clinical Radiology*, **21**, 327–328.
Houang, M. T. W., Brenton, D. P., Renton, P., Shaw, D. G. (1978) Idiopathic juvenile osteoporosis, *Skeletal Radiology*, **3**, 17–23.
Jacobs, P. (1962) Some uncommon deformities of the ankle and foot. *British Journal of Radiology*, **35**, 776–782.
Jacobs, P. (1966) Detection of early congenital dislocation of the hip. *Proceedings of the Royal Society of Medicine*, **59** (No. 12), 1225–1229.
James, A. E., Jr., Merz, T., Janower, M. L., Dorst, J. P. (1971) Radiology of the most common autosomal disorders. *Clinical Radiology*, **22**, 417–431.
Kaufmann, H. J. (1973) Progress in pediatric radiology. In: *Intrinsic Diseases of Bones*. Basel: Karger.
Levinson, E. D., Ozonoff, M. B., Royen, P. M. (1977) Proximal femoral focal deficiency. *Radiology*, **125**, 197–203.
McCredie, J., McBride, W. G. (1973) Some congenital abnormalities possibly due to embryonic peripheral neuropathy. *Clinical Radiology*, **24**, 204–211.
McCredie, J. (1975) Congenital fusion of bones — radiology, embryology and pathogenesis. *Clinical Radiology*, **26**, 47–57.
Murray, R. O., McCredie, J. (1979) Melorheostosis and the sclerotomes. *Skeletal Radiology*, **4**, 57–71.
Murray, R. O., Jacobson, H. G. (1977) *The Radiology of Skeletal Disorders*. 2nd edn. Edinburgh: Churchill Livingstone.
Poznanski, A. K. (1984) *The Hand in Radiologic Diagnosis*. 2nd edn. Philadelphia: Saunders.
Rubin, P. (1964) *Dynamic Classification of Bone Dysplasias*. Chicago: Year Book Medical Publishers.
Spranger, J. W., Langer, L. O., Wiedemann, H. R. (1974) *Bone Dysplasias*. Philadelphia: Saunders.
Warrick, C. K. (1973) Some aspects of polyostotic fibrous dysplasia. *Clinical Radiology*, **27**, 125–138.
Wynne-Davies, R., Fairbank, T. J. (1976) *Fairbank's Atlas of General Affections of the Skeleton*. 2nd edn. Edinburgh: Churchill Livingstone.

CHAPTER 2

PERIOSTEAL REACTION; BONE AND JOINT INFECTIONS; SARCOID

PERIOSTEAL NEW BONE FORMATION
(Periosteal reaction)

The use of these terms does not imply a post-inflammatory aetiology as does the term 'periostitis'. New bone is laid down in many conditions with different aetiologies (Table 2.1). In some the periosteum is physically elevated by tumour, haemorrhage or infection. Vascular abnormalities, viruses and auto-immune diseases may all cause new bone deposition. In some cases the cause of new bone formation is unclear. New bone may be deposited locally, around a solitary focus of disease, or may be generalized. In some systemic conditions, new bone is laid down in characteristic sites.

In its simplest form the new bone is seen as a linear density separated from the bony shaft by a clear zone, often later obliterated as the new bone merges with the cortex. This new bone is frequently missed or wrongly diagnosed. Difficulty is caused by bones such as the fibula which have naturally irregular outlines. Insertions of interosseous membranes, ligaments and tendons in other bones also cause confusion.

There are many types of periosteal reaction and, while certain patterns can be discerned, it is safer to assume that the type of periosteal reaction cannot accurately be correlated with the underlying disease.

Tumours and periosteal new bone

A tumour, having broken through the cortex, elevates the periosteum and new bone forms beneath it. If the tumour is slowly growing, the elevated periosteal new bone may remain intact and even take over the function of the destroyed cortex. If tumour growth is cyclical, as in Ewing's sarcoma, successive layers of periosteal new bone are laid down, giving a lamellated or onion skin appearance. If tumour growth is rapid, the periosteal new bone becomes disorganized and remains intact at the tumour margins only. Buttressing and elevation of periosteal new bone at tumour margins leads to a so-called *Codman's triangle* which is usually indicative of a malignant tumour; however in an aneurysmal bone cyst Codman's triangle merely indicates rapidity of progression.

In Ewing's sarcoma and in hypertrophic osteoarthropathy (see Ch. 4) the layers of new bone are characteristically fine and thinner than the spaces between them. New bone in osteogenic sarcoma, parosteal sarcoma and secondary deposits tends to be coarser and less well defined, so that the spicules are thicker than the intervening spaces. In osteogenic sarcoma, also, new bone may be perpendicular to the shaft and, originating from a finite focus of disease, resembles a sunray — so-called '*sunray spiculation*'. This may also be found with angioma and thalassaemia, but is then generally more orderly and better organized. Meningioma may resemble osteogenic sarcoma more closely, but the site is characteristic. Vertical spicules ('*hair-on-end*') are also found in Ewing's sarcoma but in keeping with the more diffuse nature of the underlying tumour are not usually 'sunray', but extend for a considerable distance along the bone, and are more delicate. Vertical spiculation may result from bony deposition along the elevated and stretched fibres connecting periosteum to bone, the Sharpey fibres.

Vascular insufficiency and periosteal new bone

Venous stasis causes changes in the lower limb especially at the diaphysis and distal metaphysis of the tibia and fibula. The periosteal new bone which is formed may be lamellar or irregular. Changes may be seen in the presence of chronic ulceration (Fig. 2.1), but also in its absence, so that an ulcer is not essential. Indeed, the periosteal new bone often extends far proximally from an ulcer. Phleboliths may be present and varicosities may also be seen in subcutaneous tissues which appear thickened and oedematous.

A florid and exuberant periosteal reaction occurs infrequently in polyarteritis nodosa. Arterial occlusion and skin ulceration are found and the periosteal reactions often occur around affected parts and in relation to skin lesions.

Thyroid acropachy (lit. 'Thickening of the extremities')
This occurs in patients who have been treated for thyro-

Table 2.1 Causes of periosteal new bone formation

Physiological	In neonates, especially in prematurity
Congenital	Tuberous sclerosis
Dysplastic	Melorheostosis, Engelmann's disease
Traumatic	Local subperiosteal trauma, fractures including March fracture. Unrecognized skeletal trauma (Caffey's 'battered baby syndrome')
Infective	Acute — osteomyelitis — staphylococcal, streptococcal, pneumococcal, etc. Chronic — Brodie's abscess, tuberculosis, syphilis (congenital and acquired), yaws; also from nearby infection, e.g. varicose ulcer; ribs in pulmonary and pleural infections
Hypo- and *hypervitaminosis*	Rickets, scurvy, hypervitaminosis A
Endocrine	Thyroid acropachy, hyperparathyroidism in healing phase; secondary hyperpara-thyroidism in renal osteodystrophy
Vascular	Haemophilia and other bleeding diseases. Myeloid metaplasia probably due to associated thrombocytopenia. Erythroblastic anaemias. Leukaemias. Varicose veins (before ulceration occurs). Hypertrophic pulmonary osteoarthropathy (probably of vascular aetiology) and pachydermoperiostosis
Collagen diseases	Polyarteritis nodosa
Reticuloses	Hodgkin's disease, etc.
Neoplastic	Primary benign — meningioma, angioma, osteoid osteoma malignant — osteogenic sarcoma, fibrosarcoma, Ewing's tumour, etc. Secondary — any metastatic bony deposit may be associated with periosteal reaction
Primary joint lesions	Ankylosing spondylitis, juvenile chronic arthritis (Still's disease), Reiter's syndrome, rheumatoid arthritis, osteoarthritis (femoral neck only)
Miscellaneous	Infantile cortical hyperostosis (Caffey), histiocytosis

Trauma and *inflammation* are the commonest causes of periosteal reaction both in adults and in children. *Primary malignant neoplasms* are rare but nearly always cause periosteal reaction. Periosteal reaction is occasionally seen in *metastases*. In adults, less common causes such as *reticuloses*, *hypertrophic pulmonary osteoarthropathy* and *varicose ulceration* may cause diagnostic difficulty. In neonates, *congenital syphilis* and *infantile cortical hyperostosis* must be remembered. Later, *scurvy*, *leukaemia* and *erythroblastic anaemias* (in immigrants) are possible causes. *Ewing's tumour* and *metastases from neuroblastoma* are other childhood causes which may prove diagnostically elusive.

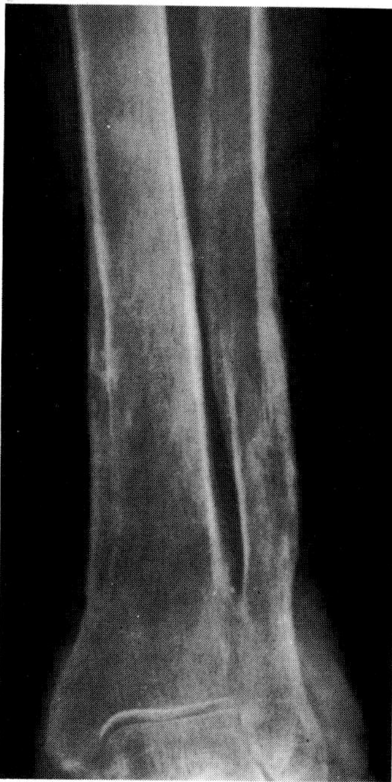

Fig. 2.1 Marked periosteal reaction due to varicose ulceration.

toxicosis and end up myxoedematous. The hands are more commonly affected than the feet. The distal ends of paired long bones are less often affected. The distribution is similar to hypertrophic osteoarthropathy but the new bone is more likely to be shaggy, spiculated and perpendicular to the shaft rather than lamellar. The overlying soft tissues are often grossly thickened (Fig. 2.2).

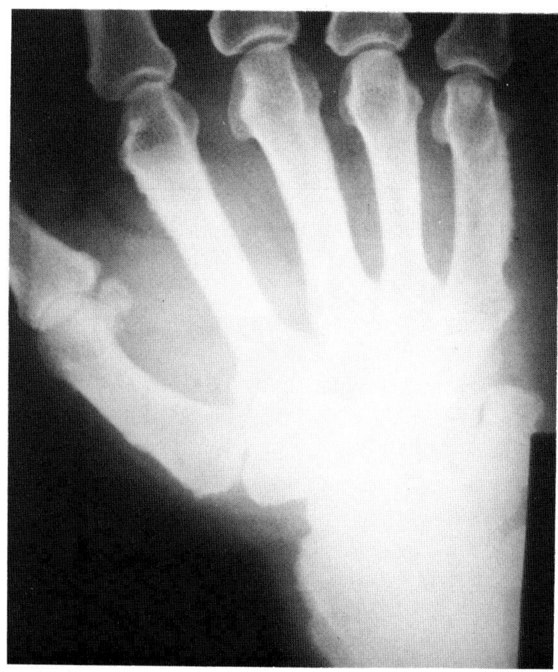

Fig. 2.2 Coarse periosteal reaction is applied to the metacarpal shafts in thyroid acropachy.

INFECTION

OSTEOMYELITIS

n invading organism may attack bone by direct invasion om an infected wound, or from an infected joint, or it ay gain access by haematogenous spread from distant ci, usually in the skin. Haematogenous osteomyelitis sually occurs during the period of growth, though less ften in neonates and infants; but all ages may be affected nd cases are even found in old age. In infants, *Streptococ- us* usually causes osteomyelitis. In adults, *Staphylococcus* more common.

It is important to understand the blood supply to bone efore describing blood-borne infection. The blood supply a long bone is via (1) the nutrient artery. This is the ajor source of blood supply throughout life. It supplies e marrow and most of the inner cortex; (2) Periosteal essels. These supply the outer cortex; (3) Metaphyseal and piphyseal vessels.

In the infant, vessels penetrate the epiphyseal plate in oth directions. Metaphyseal infections can thus pass to the piphysis and then the joint. Acute pyogenic arthritis is herefore a relatively common sequel of osteomyelitis in nfants. The periosteum in infants is very loosely attached o underlying bone. Pus easily elevates periosteum and so an extend to the epiphyseal plate along the shaft. In situ- tions where the metaphysis is intracapsular, such as the ip, metaphyseal infection also results in septic arthritis.

In childhood, between 2 and 16 years, few vessels cross the epiphyseal plate though the periosteum is still relatively loosely attached. The epiphysis and joint are thus less frequently infected. The metaphyseal vessels terminate instead in slow-flowing sinusoids which promote blood-borne infective change (Fig. 2.3).

In the adult, after the epiphyseal plate has fused, metaphyseal and epiphyseal vessels are again connected so that septic arthritis can occur again. Periosteum, however, is well bound down and articular infections via a metaphyseal route are less likely.

The formation of pus in the bone deprives local cortex and medulla of its blood supply. Dead bone is resorbed by *granulation tissue*. Pieces of dead bone, especially if cortical or surrounded by *pus*, are not resorbed and remain as *sequestra* (Figs. 2.4 and 2.5). As sequestra are devitalized they remain denser than surrounding vital bone which becomes demineralized due to hyperaemia and immobilization. Absorption of sequestra is also facilitated by the presence of an *involucrum*. The involucrum forms beneath vital periosteum which has been elevated by pus. As periosteum is poorly attached in infants, involucrum formation is greater and so is the resorption of dead bone, and healing.

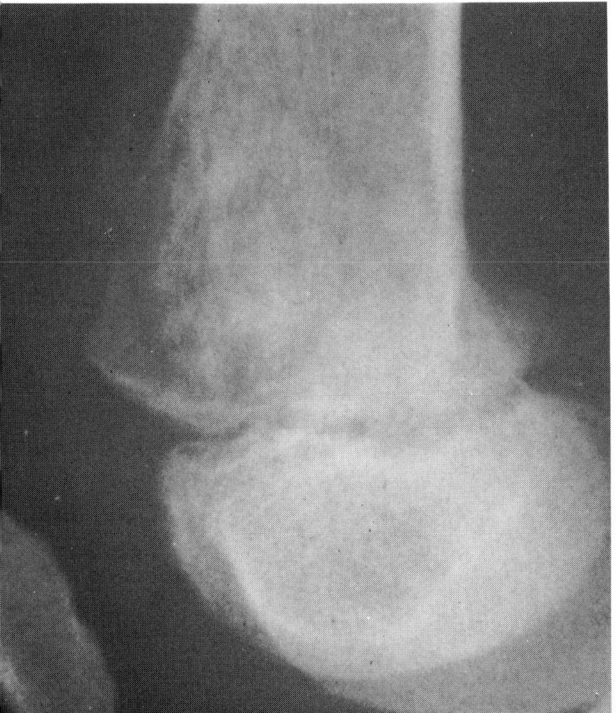

ig. 2.3 Infective focus in metaphysis in early osteomyelitis. This area f destruction is more pronounced than usual.

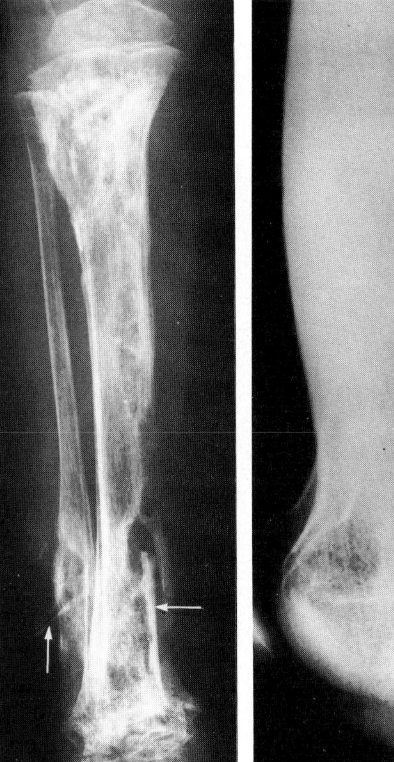

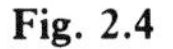

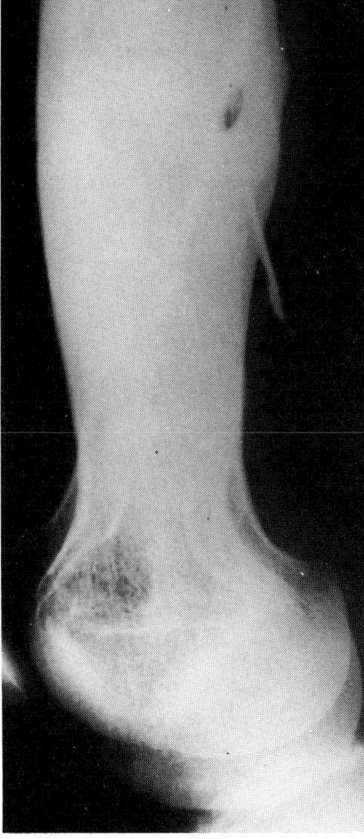

Fig. 2.4 **Fig. 2.5**

Fig. 2.4 Advanced osteomyelitis involving the whole of the right tibia and lower end of the fibula. Note sequestrum in tibia (arrow) and further sequestrum being extruded from the fibula (arrow).

Fig. 2.5 Chronic osteomyelitis with sequestrum extruding from a posterior cavity.

In areas of dead periosteum, defects in the involucrum occur. These *cloacae* allow pus and sequestra to escape, sometimes to the skin via a sinus. The track and its deep connection to bone can then be demonstrated by sinography using a water-soluble contrast medium.

Radiological findings. These depend to some extent on the age of the patient.

Soft tissue changes may be immediately apparent, especially in infants, and on CT scanning. Swelling, with oedema and blurring of fat planes is seen — in distinction to the soft tissue masses around tumours, where the displaced fat planes are preserved. Osteoporosis may be visualized within 10–14 days of onset of symptoms. In children this is usually metaphyseal.

An involucrum is usually visualized after 3 weeks and is more prolific in infants and children than in adults (Fig. 2.6). The rapid escape and decompression of pus which results prevents vascular compression and infarction, and promotes healing. It may be necessary to use tomography or tangential views to obtain an adequate projection of the stripped periosteum. Tomography is invaluable in detecting sequestra. These are seen as fragments of dense bone within areas of local bone destruction. Treatment by antibiotics and/or surgical decompression affects the course of the disease so that often little apart from new bone may be found during the course of the disease.

With adequate treatment in infants and children, a return to more or less normal appearances with growth is to

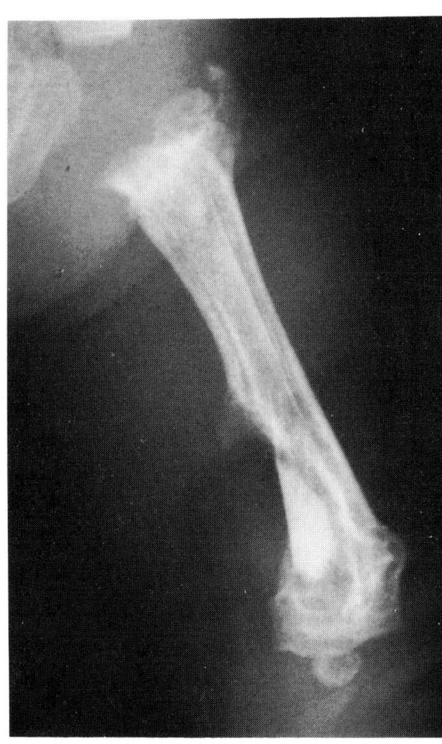

Fig. 2.6 Osteomyelitis of femur and septic arthritis of the hip in neonate. Note dislocation of hip, involucrum, cloaca and sequestrum.

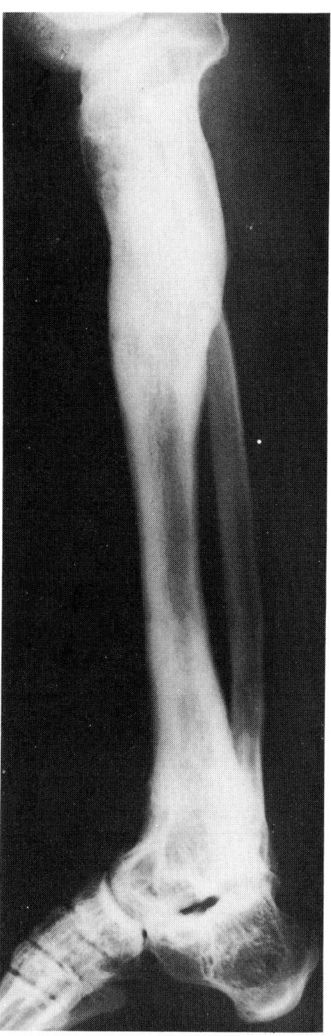

Fig. 2.7 Chronic osteomyelitis of both ends of tibia and a complicating ankylosis of the ankle joint.

Table 2.2 Haematogenous osteomyelitis of tubular bones

	Infant	Child	Adult
Localization	Metaphyseal with epiphyseal extension	Metaphyseal	Epiphyseal
Involucrum	Common	Common	Not common
Sequestration	Common	Common	Not common
Joint involvement	Common	Not common	Common
Soft tissue abscess	Common	Common	Not common
Pathological fracture	Not common	Not common	Common*
Fistulae	Not common	Variable	Common

* In neglected cases

(Reproduced from *Diagnosis of Bone and Joint Disorders* by kind permission of Drs D. Resnick and G. Niwayama, and W. B. Saunders, publishers)

be expected, unless the epiphyseal plate and epiphysis have been damaged, in which case growth abnormalities may result. In adults the affected bone often remains sclerotic and irregular in outline (Fig. 2.7). Should chronic sepsis persist, tomography may reveal persistent cloacae and sequestra. The radiographic picture never returns completely to normal in cases discovered late (Table 2.2).

SPECIAL FORMS OF OSTEOMYELITIS

Sclerosing osteomyelitis of Garré. This condition is manifested by gross sclerosis in the absence of apparent bone destruction (Fig. 2.8). True examples of this condition are found occasionally, but some of the cases described in the past were probably examples of *osteoid osteoma*.

Brodie's abscess. This localized form of osteomyelitis is usually found in the cancellous tissue near the end of a long bone, usually the tibia (Fig. 2.9). A well-circumscribed area of bone destruction has a surrounding zone of reactive sclerosis, sometimes accompanied by a periosteal reaction. It may have a finger-like extension into neighbouring bone towards the epiphyseal plate, which, when present, is pathognomonic of infection ('tunnelling') (Fig. 2.10). If a sequestrum is present an osteoid osteoma may be simulated (Fig. 2.11).

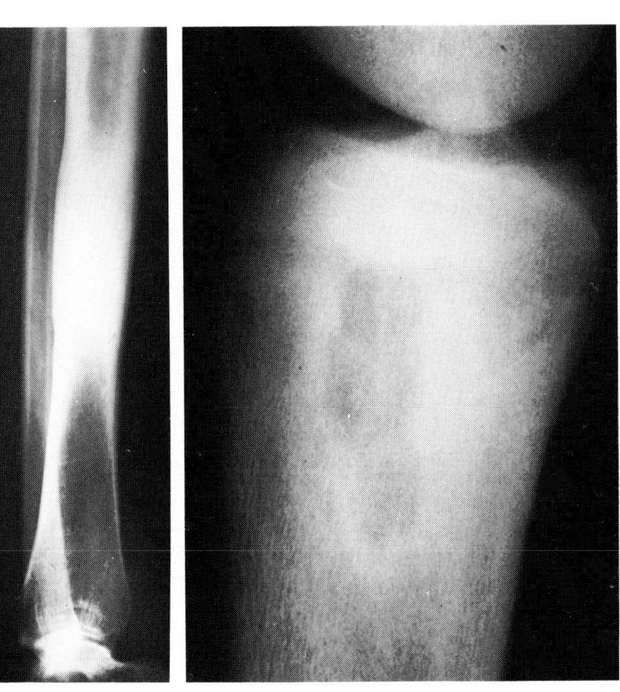

Fig. 2.8 **Fig. 2.9**

Fig. 2.8 Garré's type of osteomyelitis.

Fig. 2.9 Brodie's abscess in upper end of tibia.

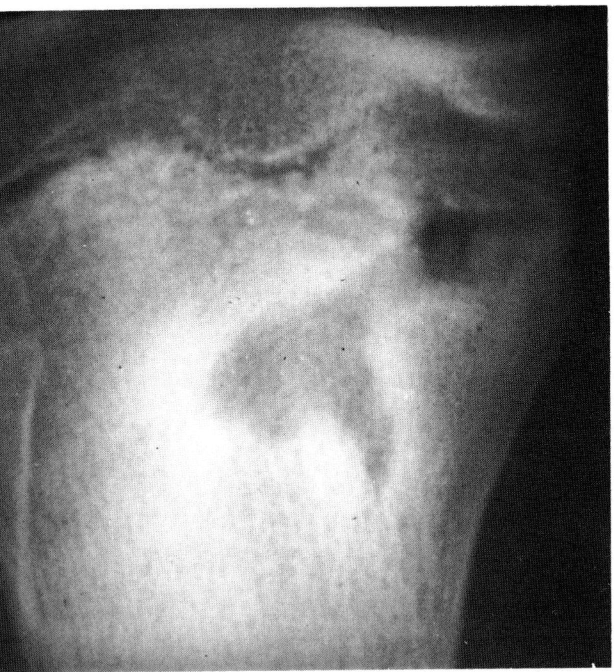

Fig. 2.10 A finger-like process of osteomyelitic bone destruction extends from the main focus. This is tunnelling which usually indicates the presence of chronic infection.

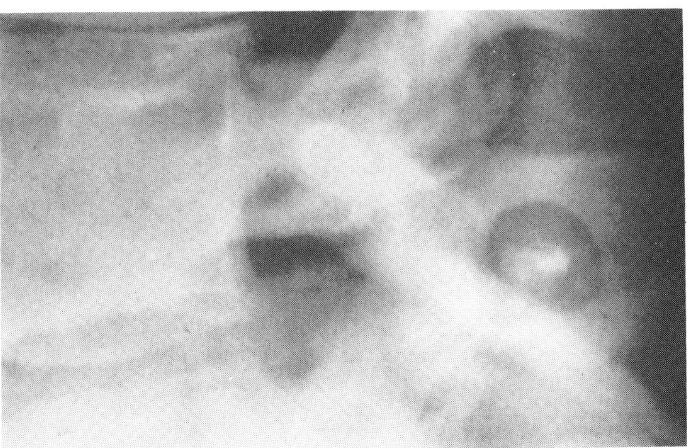

Fig. 2.11 Bone abscess with sequestrum in the spinous process of a lumbar vertebra.

OSTEOMYELITIS IN SPECIAL SITES

Skull. Lesions occur secondary to scalp infection or frontal sinus suppuration (Fig. 2.12). Local and diffuse types are described; both respond rapidly to antibiotics and drainage.

Mandible. Infection may complicate a fracture into the mouth, or it may follow dental extraction. Infection via the pulp canal is probably most common and follows poor oral hygiene and dental decay. Osteomyelitis of the mandible is amenable to treatment because of the relatively rich vascular supply.

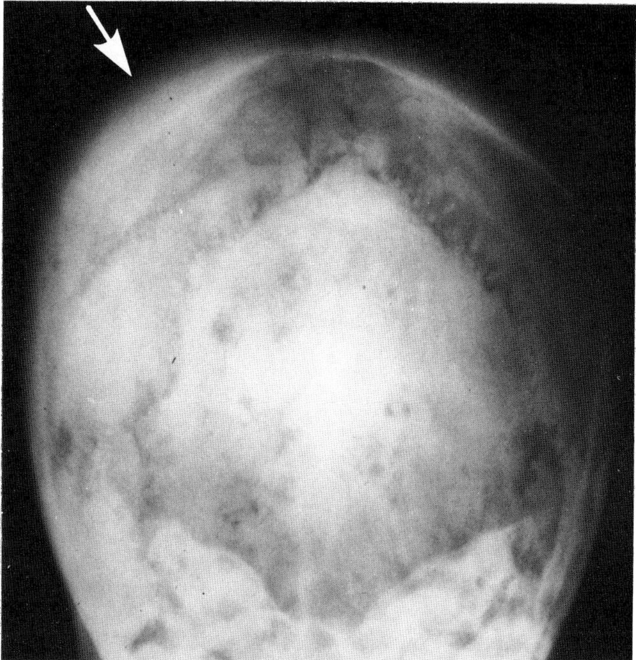

Fig. 2.12 Multiple areas of bone destruction and reactive sclerosis (arrow) are seen in a patient with chronic osteomyelitis.

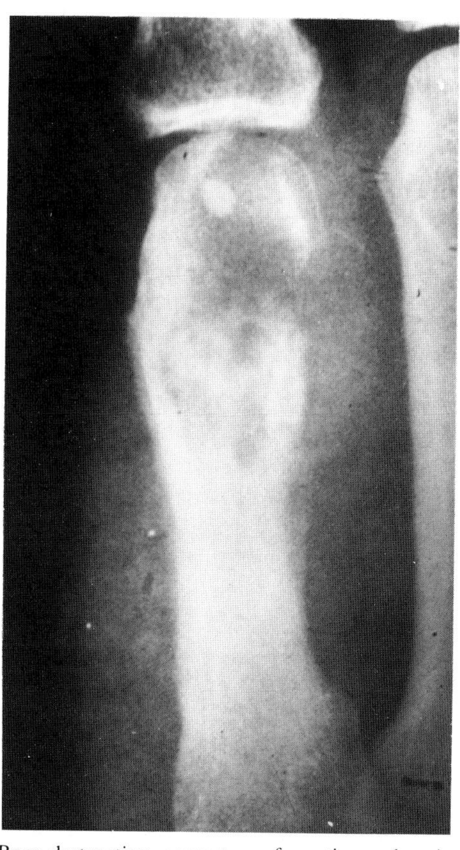

Fig. 2.13 Bone destruction, sequestrum formation and periostitis follow implantation of oral organisms after a bite.

Pelvis. The sacro-iliac joint is occasionally affected. It may be difficult radiologically to differentiate pyogenic from tuberculous lesions. Clinically, pelvic lesions are often accompanied by abscesses from which the causal organism may be isolated. Diagnostic points are that pyogenic infections tend to run a more rapid course, and that the abscess associated with tuberculosis may later calcify. Ankylosis of the sacro-iliac joint may result from either cause.

Osteitis pubis is a low-grade infection round the symphysis pubis which may complicate operations on the prostate and bladder or, occasionally, other pelvic operations. Loss of bone substance and irregularity and sclerosis on both sides of the symphysis is seen. Resolution readily occurs, often with bony fusion across the symphysis pubis.

Hands. Bone infections may follow perforating injuries to the pulp space. The distal phalanx may be involved by osteomyelitis or local pressure may cause ischaemia and avascular necrosis. Infection of tendon sheaths also occurs following perforating injuries, and the infection can spread proximally along the synovial sheaths. Soft tissue swelling, osteoporosis and osteomyelitis result.

A bizarre form of osteomyelitis, often due to oral organisms, follows bite wounds on hands or after punching the face and teeth, with resulting perforation and implantation (Fig. 2.13).

Feet. Puncture wounds of the feet are common in children and in those societies where walking barefoot is common. Soft tissue infections may lead to osteomyelitis, often with destruction of joints. In the tropics, direct implantation by mycetoma results in 'Madura foot' (p. 75). Implantation by thorns leads to a particular lesion.

Complications of osteomyelitis

1. *Amyloid disease* infrequently complicates chronic osteomyelitis.
2. *Malignant changes* can follow long-standing suppurative osteomyelitis with draining sinuses. Increasing severity of symptoms with rapid osteolysis raise the possibility of a tumour, either an *epithelioma* of the sinus tract or, less frequently, an *osteosarcoma*.

The spine

Spinal osteomyelitis is not common, comprising less than 10% of bone infections (Epstein). It is more common in the middle-aged, and in males. Patients often have a history of skin or pelvic infections. Spread of infection is usually to the vertebral body rather than to appendages and is mainly blood-borne, though osteomyelitis may follow spinal surgery. Arterial supply to a vertebral body is both by the nutrient artery which enters through the foramen on the back of the vertebral body and by smaller perforating vessels which penetrate the cortex from surrounding soft tissues. Spread of disease from the pelvis is facilitated through Batson's vertebral venous plexus, which is a valveless system of veins joining the pelvis with the rest of the axial skeleton via the spinal canal. Flow in this valveless system ebbs back and forth with changes in intra-abdominal pressure. Vertebral bodies are very vascular, especially below end-plates where large sinusoids with a sluggish blood flow potentiate infection. Spinal osteomyelitis is most common in the lumbar region and least common in the cervical and sacral spines. The most common causative organism is *Staphylococcus*, but *Esch. coli* and *Salmonella* are also encountered.

Radiological findings. Infection usually starts anteriorly beneath the end-plate. Plain film changes lag behind symptoms by 2–3 weeks, when a focus of osteolysis becomes visible and the cortex becomes blurred or vanishes. Perforation may be anterior, beneath the anterior longitudinal ligament, facilitating vertical spread, or into the disc which is then rapidly destroyed and loses height (Fig. 2.14). The adjacent end-plate then also loses density and vertebral destruction begins in the body above or below. Collapse of the body also potentiates loss of disc height with herniation of remaining disc material into the softened body. In most patients only two bodies are involved, and only rarely is the infection confined to one vertebral body.

Collapse of a vertebral body is accompanied by soft tissue masses which are easily seen against air in the larynx, trachea or lung (Fig. 2.15). Blurring or displacement of the psoas shadows also occurs. Kyphosis and cord compression may also follow.

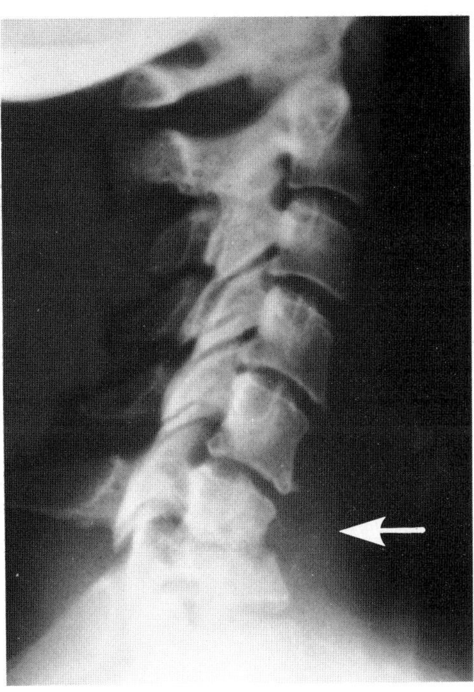

Fig. 2.15 End-plate destruction with discal loss and a kyphosis is associated with facet subluxation and a large anterior soft tissue mass (←).

Reparative processes can begin as early as 4–6 weeks after onset of radiological change if treatment is effective. Sclerotic new bone is formed around the disc, in the bodies and at vertebral margins (Fig. 2.16). Dense spurs bridge discs peripherally. Ankylosis across discs may result in fu-

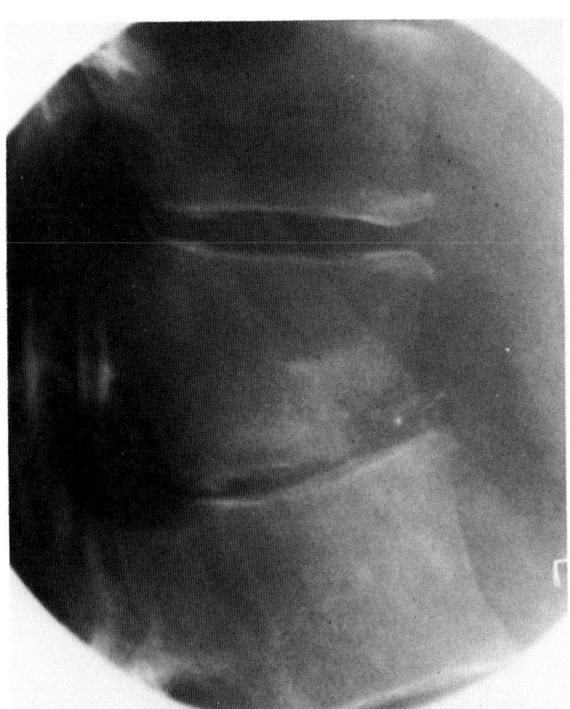

Fig. 2.14 Anterior destruction of a vertebral body is accompanied by rapid loss of the disc and adjacent end-plates.

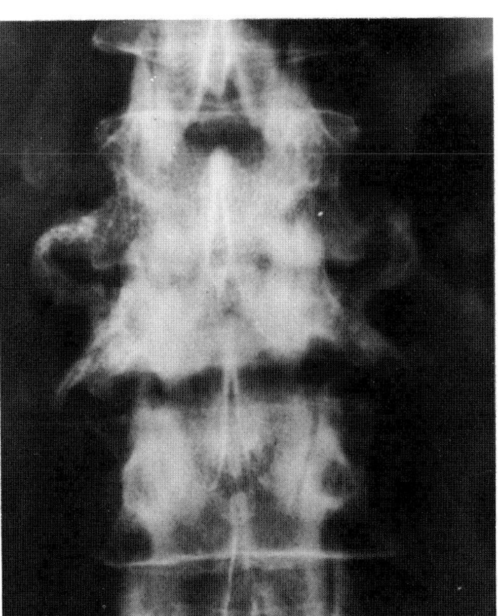

Fig. 2.16 Reparative change in chronic osteomyelitis with marked sclerosis and bony bridging around discs.

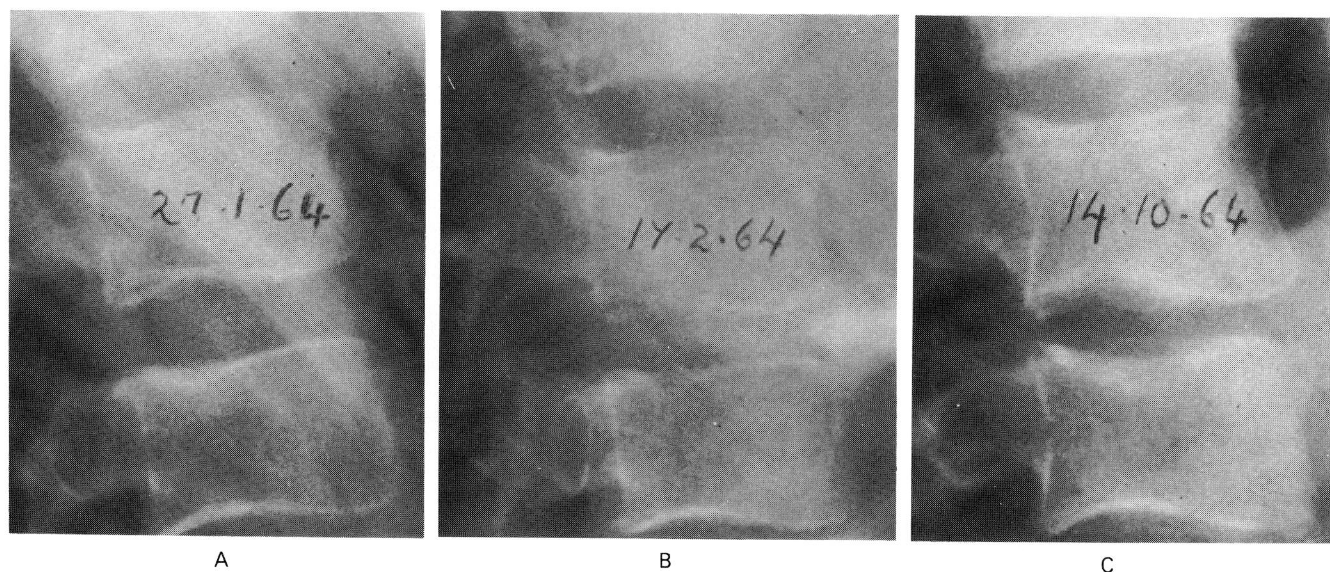

A B C

Fig. 2.17 A., B. and **C.** Discitis, showing progressive loss of disc without any bone involvement. Tomography did not show evidence of bone destruction. The patient was a 14-year-old boy who presented with a febrile illness and pains in the back. He was asymptomatic before the loss of L2–L3 disc became apparent.

sion of bodies. If this occurs after skeletal maturity, the sagittal diameters of vertebral bodies are not likely to be reduced. 'Ivory' vertebrae and soft tissue calcification are occasionally found.

Infective discitis

Perforating blood vessels still supply the disc in children and young adults so that in these age groups a primary infection of the discs can occur. Changes are most common in the lumbar spine (Fig. 2.17). Disc narrowing is followed by blurring and erosion of end-plates and later by marked reactive sclerosis.

OSTEOMYELITIS IN DIABETES

Infection occurs in both soft tissue and bone. Soft tissue infection may follow a puncture through anaesthetic skin and presents with swelling and loss of fat planes due to oedema. In the presence of gas-producing organisms, spherical lucencies are seen extending proximally. Anaesthetic ulcers show as soft tissue defects, usually over pressure points such as the metatarsal heads, and over the tips and proximal interphalangeal joints of the commonly associated claw toes. Initially painless, the ulcers involve underlying bones with the development of osteomyelitis. Sepsis may be superimposed on a neuropathic lesion, so

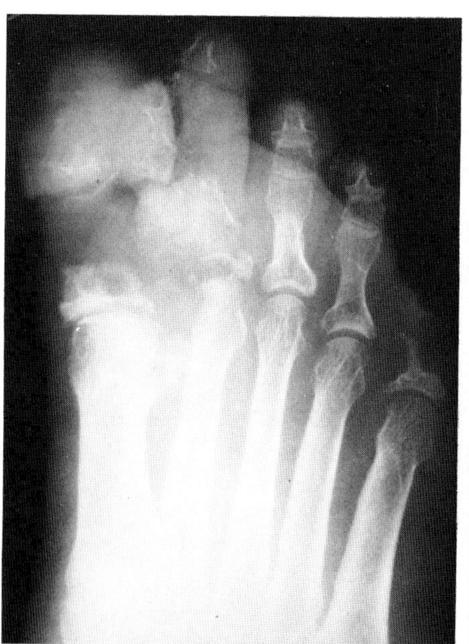

A

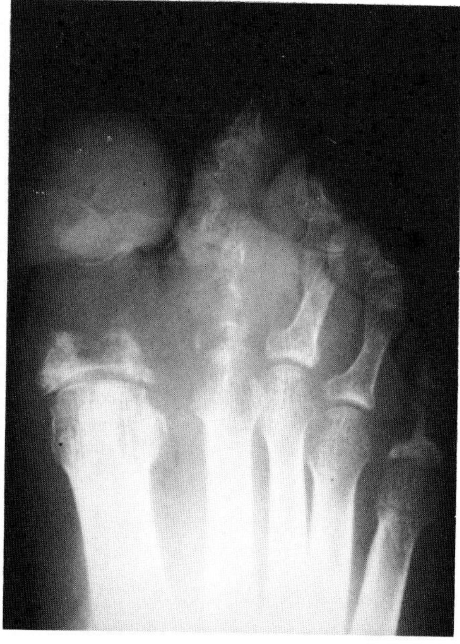

B

Fig. 2.18 A. and **B.** The changes at the little toe are those of neuropathic bone resorption. The cloudy resorption of bone with osteoporosis and soft tissue swelling at the first and second toes indicate superimposed osteomyelitis.

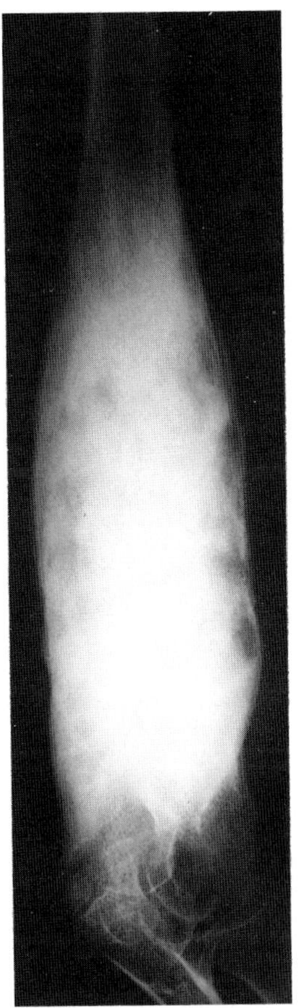

Fig. 2.19

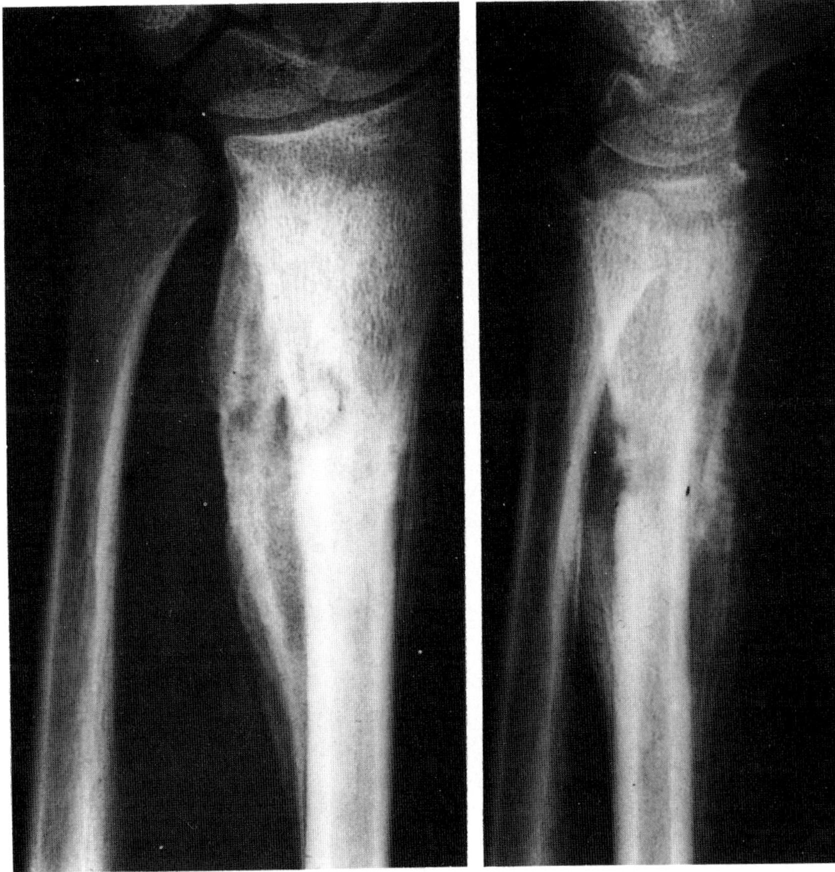

Fig. 2.20

Figs. 2.19 and 2.20 Gross reactive sclerosis with new bone formation at multiple sites is found in chronic granulomatous disease.

that osteoporosis and destruction are accelerated (Fig. 2.18). If skin ulceration is absent, osteomyelitis is unlikely to be seen.

CHRONIC GRANULOMATOUS DISEASE OF CHILDHOOD

This is a group of disorders in which the leucocytes are unable to respond normally to infections, especially to those organisms which cause chronic low-grade infections. Leucocytes are able to engulf bacilli but cannot destroy them so that toxins are still produced. A chronic inflammatory process results. A spectrum of disease is seen, ranging from a severe form in males to a more mild form in females. Chronic inflammation occurs in lung, liver, spleen, retroperitoneum and bladder base as well as in the gut. Bones are commonly affected. Widespread small foci of osteolysis may be found often abutting on to epiphyseal plates. The lesions heal with florid formation of new bone, both endosteally and superficially, so that sclerosis and expansion result, often resembling malignant tumours (Figs. 2.19 and 2.20). The lesions are usually multifocal.

SEPTIC ARTHRITIS

Joint infections occur at any age, but especially in children. Staphylococci, streptococci and pneumococci are common causative organisms. Usually only one joint is affected. If more than one joint is infected, an immune defect should be suspected or the possibility of steroid administration queried.

A joint may be contaminated by:

1. Direct intervention — following surgery, aspiration or perforating injury.
2. Spread from adjacent bone. As has already been stated, metaphyseal infections lead to joint infections if the metaphysis is intra-articular. Such a situation is seen in the hip, as well as in the distal femur, tibia and radius. Moreover, as will be remembered, blood vessels cross the epiphyseal plate in infancy so that for both reasons septic arthritis of the hip in infancy (described by Tom Smith) is relatively common. Changes of osteomyelitis precede those of arthritis.
3. Haematogenous spread. Direct infection of synovium by septic emboli.

Radiological features. Initially synovial thickening and effusion distend the joint. Fat lines are displaced but may

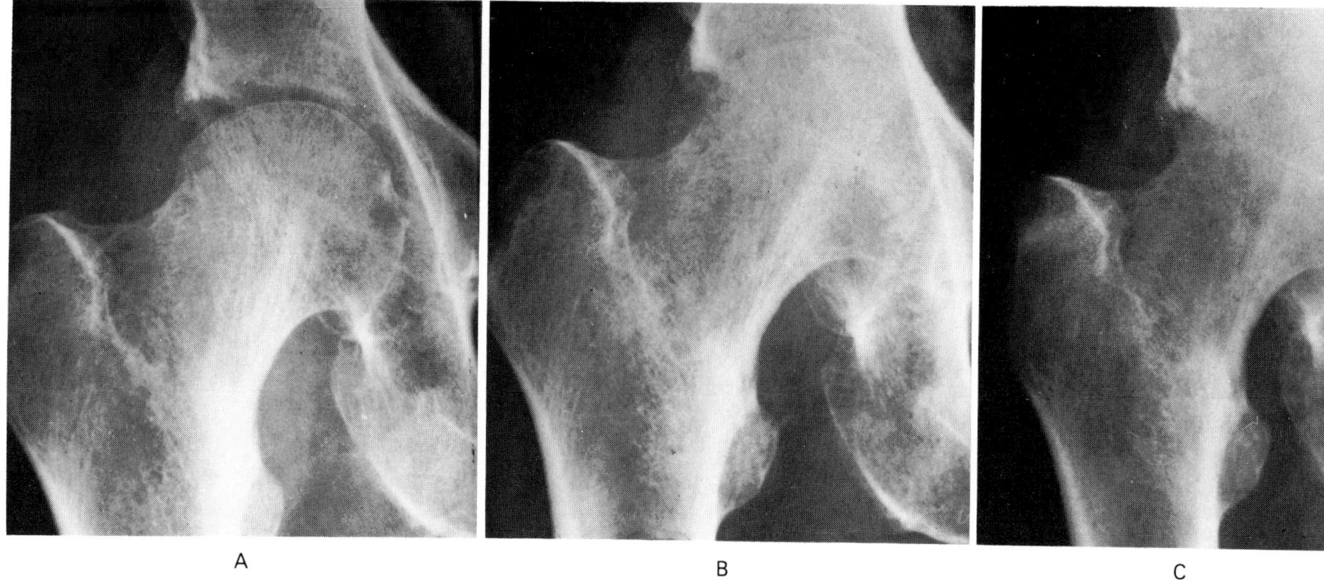

Fig. 2.21 A., B. and **C.** Pyogenic arthritis of the hip: rapid progression of the lesion during a period of 1 month.

be blurred by oedema. Demineralization follows hyperaemia and immobilization. When infection begins to destroy cartilage, joint narrowing becomes apparent. In pyogenic arthritis, cartilage is rapidly destroyed early in the course of the disease (Fig. 2.21), which is not the case in tuberculous arthritis. The articular cortex becomes blurred and then eroded, both peripherally and centrally, and subarticular bone is later destroyed. Severe cases are characterized by massive destruction, separation of bone ends, subluxation and dislocation.

During recovery, bones recalcify and in severe cases fibrous and bony ankylosis may result. Dystrophic calcification may be seen on occasion following pyogenic arthritis. Marginal erosions persist but their outlines become well-demarcated and sclerotic.

Arthritis of the hip in infants (Tom Smith arthritis). The hip joint in infants is especially susceptible to infection as explained above. In neonates sepsis may be transmitted via the umbilical vessels, often due to *Streptococcus*, but infection may be directly introduced following blood sampling at the groin. In infants, because of lax muscles around the hip and the cartilaginous nature of the acetabulum, an effusion may dislocate the hip (Fig. 2.22). This can be assessed even if the ossific nucleus has not appeared. In any case, gross metaphyseal destruction is soon apparent with cortical and medullary erosions. Gross sequestration rapidly occurs and an involucrum may involve the entire femur. The femoral shaft generally heals, but the femoral head and neck may be totally destroyed, never to appear. Deformity and shortening inevitably result. In older children, such change is less likely as the epiphyseal plate is not crossed by vessels. The femoral head, even if severely affected, then reconstitutes with a flattened mushroom-like appearance similar to old Perthes' disease or slipped epiphysis. Because of vascular compression, osteonecrosis may actually complicate infection.

The definitive diagnosis is usually bacteriological; immediate aspiration of synovial contents is indicated in order

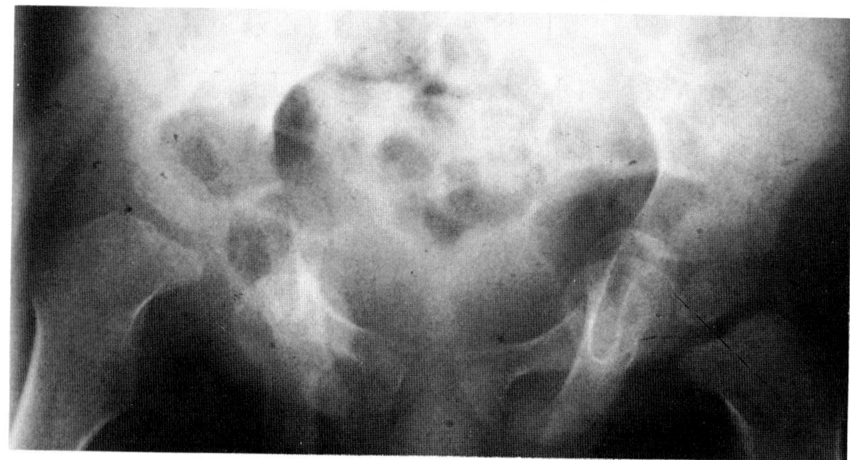

Fig. 2.22 Septic dislocation of the right hip.

o isolate the causal organism. The condition usually responds rapidly to antibiotics so that severe destructive lesions, which were once commonplace, are now seldom een. Occasionally, however, rapid and progressive cartiage destruction may be found despite antibiotic therapy.

Gonococcal arthritis. The incidence of this condition has been overestimated in the past. In most cases of arthritis associated with urethritis, the gonococcus is not found in he synovial fluid or in the urethral discharge. Moreover, he condition does not respond to penicillin. Thus most cases previously regarded as gonococcal joints were undoubtedly examples of *Reiter's syndrome*. The occurrence of an occasional true gonococcal arthritis is not disputed; n such cases the radiographic appearances will be indistinguishable from those of other pyogenic arthritis lesions.

TUBERCULOSIS OF BONES AND JOINTS

Though the incidence of skeletal tuberculosis has fallen markedly in recent years, the disease has not yet been eradicated. Thus the condition still occurs much more frequently than do primary bone tumours, even though the florid lesions and crippling deformities, so common in the past, are now seldom seen. This is true of our local population, but roughly one third of our present-day patients are immigrants to Britain. The latter tend to produce unusual disease patterns which will later be described.

Haematogenous spread of infection to the skeleton is assumed to be from the lung and may occur at the time of primary infection or later from post-primary foci. Chest radiography, however, shows active disease in less than 50% of cases, the organism presumably having lain dormant and become active later. The bacillus lodges in the spongiosa of the metaphysis of a long bone, but the vertebral column is affected in 50% of cases. Lesions are usually single, though multifocal cystic osseous tuberculosis is described. Children are most commonly affected, but no age is exempt.

Certain features are relatively common. The tuberculous reaction is destructive and accompanied by pus which may later become calcified. Calcification of abscesses is rarely seen currently if antibiotic treatment is adequate. In contradistinction to pyogenic osteomyelitis, neither sequestration nor periostitis is a prominent feature. Abscesses often point to the skin and a sinus track may be demonstrated after injection of contrast medium.

Radiographic appearances. The diagnosis is usually made after considerable delay and radiographic changes are seen at presentation, in contrast to pyogenic infections where radiographic changes occur 2–3 weeks after clinical presentation. Changes in synovial tuberculosis may be even longer delayed.

The metaphysis is the site of election; an oval or rounded focus will be found which soon crosses the epiphyseal line (Figs. 2.23 and 2.24). Its outline may be sharply defined or it may fade imperceptibly into surrounding bone. No surrounding sclerosis is to be expected. Sequestra are small and are absorbed by granulation tissue. Though slight periosteal reaction may be found if the local lesion is subcortical, this is not a prominent feature. The initial focus may sometimes be sited in the epiphysis.

Lesions of the diaphysis are rare, and even rarer is the

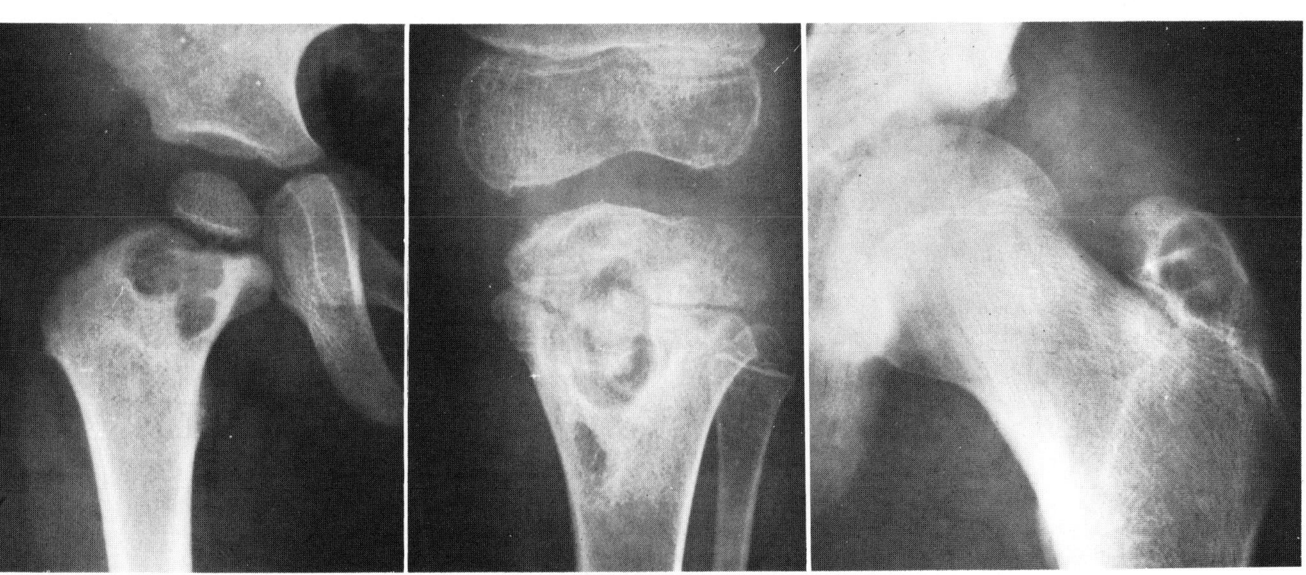

Fig. 2.23 Fig. 2.24 Fig. 2.25

Fig. 2.23 TB of femur: large metaphyseal focus.

Fig. 2.24 TB of knee the metaphyseal lesion has extended across the epiphyseal line. The sequestrum is more prominent than usual but it was absorbed completely during healing.

Fig. 2.25 TB focus in greater trochanter. This type is less common than a surface erosion.

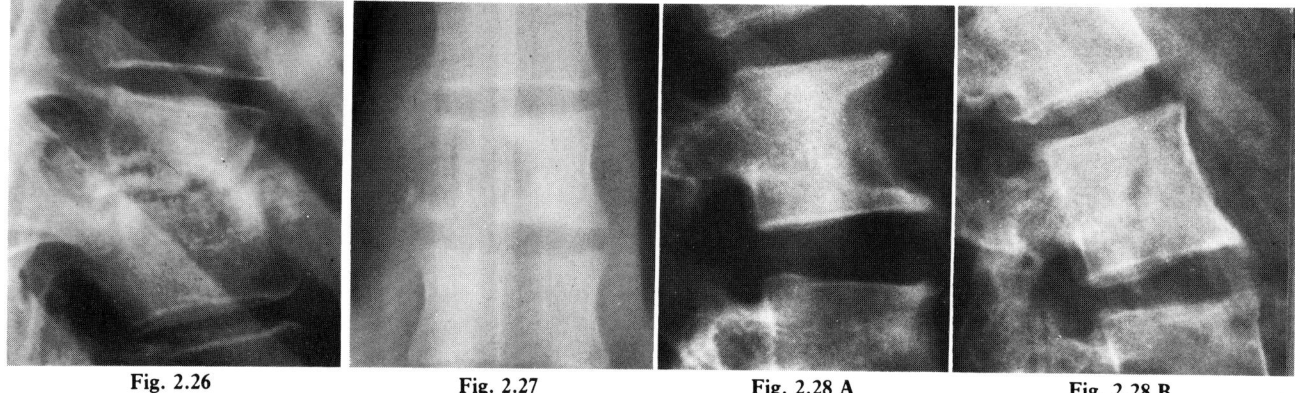

Fig. 2.26 Fig. 2.27 Fig. 2.28 A Fig. 2.28 B

Fig. 2.26 Pott's disease: erosion of adjacent vertebral bodies, destruction of disc and mottled calcification anterior to the spine.

Fig. 2.27 Tomographic section of central tuberculous lesion extending to the right side of the vertebral body.

Fig. 2.28 **A.** and **B.** Anterior subperiosteal type of Pott's disease, before and after conservative treatment.

multiple cystic type of lesion. This latter is best described as 'disseminated bone tuberculosis' in order to avoid confusion with the condition known as 'osteitis tuberculosa multiplex cystoides' — a manifestation of sarcoidosis.

LESIONS OF INDIVIDUAL BONES

Greater trochanter. This is a common site, particularly in adolescents and young adults. The lesion may start in the bone or in the overlying bursa. The erosion may be deep, but often it is superficial and difficult to detect; sometimes it may be cystic (Fig. 2.25). Lesions tend to recur and reactivation may be hard to detect radiographically. The lesion may spread to the hip joint, but more often it remains localized.

The spine. Roughly half the cases of osteoarticular tuberculosis seen in this country occur in the spine. Most lesions occur in or below the mid-dorsal spine and involvement of the cervical and upper dorsal spine is uncommon. All ages may be affected.

Radiographic appearances. (Figs. 2.26, 2.27 and 2.28). Vertebral bodies may be first affected in three places — at the upper or lower disc margin, in the centre, and anteriorly under the periosteum. The marginal type corresponds to the metaphyseal lesions of long bones. Destructive foci are found in the anterior corners of adjacent vertebral bodies. The disc substance is eroded. Two or more vertebrae may be attacked. Tomography may show the lesion to be more extensive than it appears from examination of routine films. Since the anterior parts of the vertebrae are most affected, a local kyphos or gibbus will appear, and some scoliosis may also occur. Abscesses form early and are easily seen in the dorsal region in contrast to the radiolucent lungs. In the lumbar region, lateral bulging of the psoas outlines may be demonstrable. Radiographs must be exposed during suspended respiration if abscesses are to be clearly defined. Abscesses may track widely and may become calcified. Abscesses may sometimes be intraosseous and subsequently calcify (Fig. 2.29). Rib crowding may be seen, even on a chest radiograph, if vertebral bodies collapse.

It is often difficult to differentiate between tuberculous and pyogenic spondylitis, especially if the patient is white. Clearly, tuberculosis must always be suspected if the patient is of African or Asian origin. Reactive new bone formation is much less pronounced in tuberculous disease, so that sclerotic osteophytes are unusual. Discs are destroyed early with simple infections and later, or infrequently not at all, in tuberculosis. Calcification, where present, indicates tuberculosis.

The lesions generally respond rapidly to antibiotics, and the gross destructive lesions formerly seen are no longer to be expected. Quiescence is evidenced by return of bone detail and density, and by the eroded bony margins becoming sharply defined. Later, consolidation will occur to a greater or lesser degree. Before antibiotics were introduced, gross destructive lesions were common and the affected vertebral bodies frequently became fused.

In the less common central type of vertebral tuberculosis, an abscess forms in the centre of the vertebral body. It usually extends peripherally later, and thereafter resembles the marginal type of infection. Tomography may be necessary to demonstrate these lesions in the early stages. The subperiosteal type of infection begins anteriorly under the periosteum and spreads under the anterior common ligament. Disc destruction may be late, and the anterior erosions may be difficult to detect. The patient suffers severe symptoms in relation to the minor radiographic abnormalities. Lateral tomography may be of great service in identifying this type of lesion.

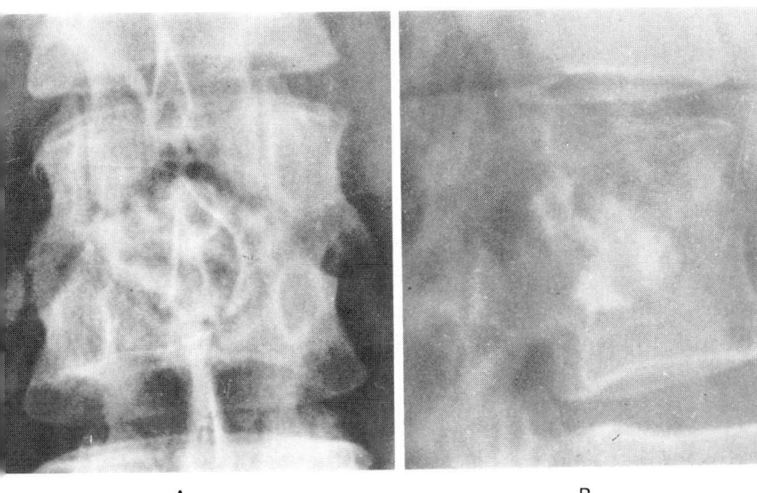

Fig. 2.29 A. and **B.** Old Pott's disease: healing with calcified intra-osseous abscess — AP and lateral views.

The *aneurysmal effect* may be found in Pott's disease associated with an anterior paravertebral abscess between D4 and D10. Aortic pulsation, transmitted through an anterior paraspinal abscess between D4 and D10 may cause the vertebral bodies to become deeply concave anteriorly (Fig. 2.28). This process does not affect the intervertebral discs. An aneurysm causes similar changes by direct pulsation.

In the coloured races, tuberculous spondylitis has a somewhat different presentation. Often, only one vertebra is involved with conspicuous preservation of adjacent discs, even if the body is totally destroyed or flattened. Occasionally, vertebra plana results (Fig. 2.30). Sclerosis and new bone formation is a feature of the disease in coloured patients, as in pyogenic spondylitis. More importantly, the posterior elements are frequently involved, especially in the lumbosacral and thoraco-lumbar junctions, often with huge abscesses (Fig. 2.31). The cervical spine is also more frequently involved than in the white races, with dysphagia or paraplegia as complications. Multiple lesions are also more common. Involvement of the spinal column also follows gibbus formation or extrusion of granulation tissue into the canal.

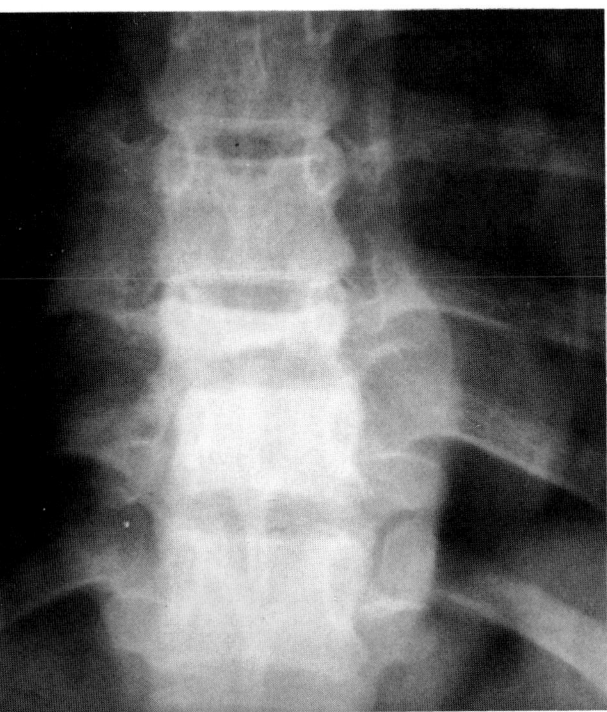

Fig. 2.30 Flattening of the vertebral body is accompanied by a paraspinal swelling but there is relative discal sparing. Adjacent end-plates are also relatively intact.

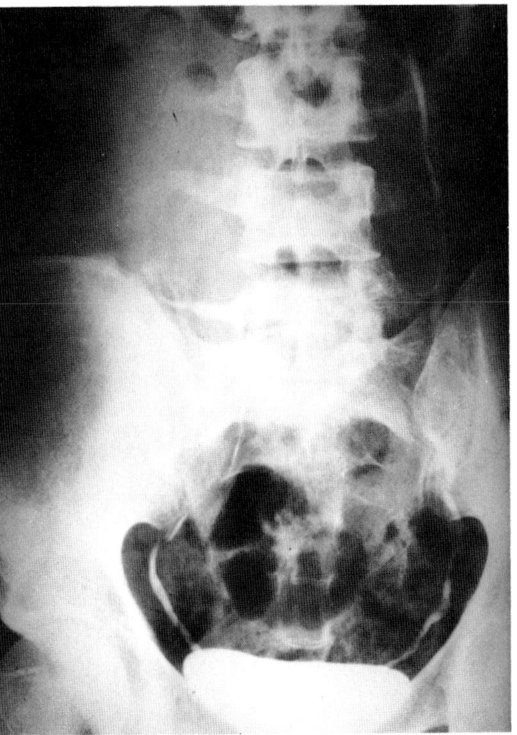

Fig. 2.31 A large abscess displaces the right ureter medially and destroys the right transverse process and adjacent part of the body of L5. 1.42 litres of tuberculous pus were removed at operation.

Tuberculous dactylitis. This lesion is sometimes seen in our immigrant population. The affected phalanx is characteristically widened by medullary expansion, whereas in syphilitic dactylitis the bone is widened by the production of cortical new bone. This differentiation is not always apparent. However, one rare type of tuberculous dactylitis, *spina ventosa* (the first lesion to be described radiographically in a child), does produce a characteristic appearance. Spina ventosa means literally 'a short bone inflated with air' (Fig. 2.32).

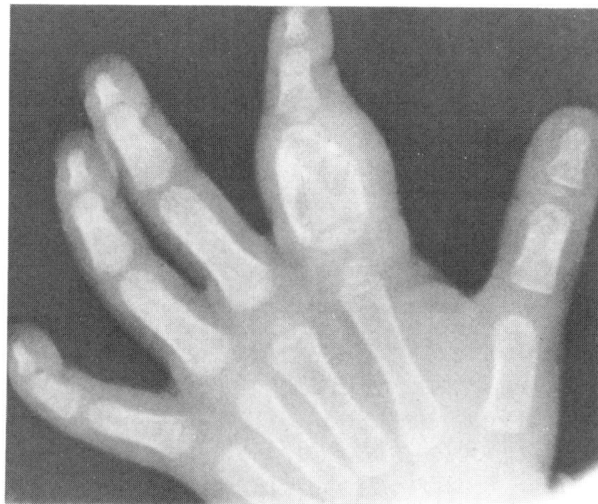

Fig. 2.32 Typical spina ventosa of the proximal phalanx of the forefinger. (Courtesy of Dr D. J. Mitchell.)

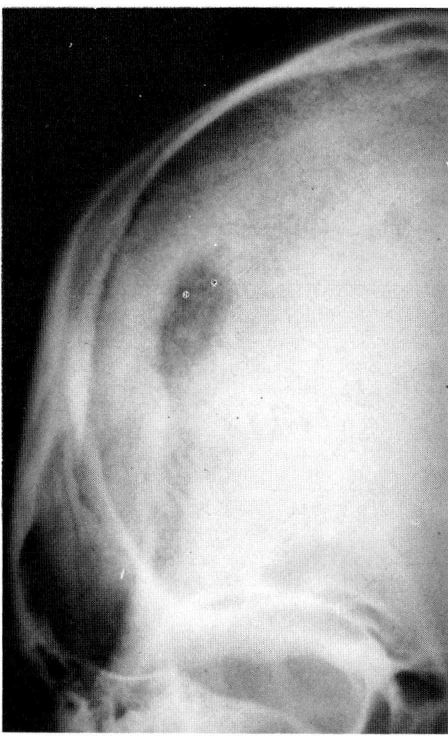

Fig. 2.33 Tuberculosis of the skull vault. The fairly well-defined lytic lesion was a solitary finding but these changes are often multiple. Note the gross tunnelling.

The skull. Tuberculous lesions are rare in the skull other than in immigrants. They may be localized and well-defined, resembling eosinophilic granuloma, or they may be more diffuse (Fig. 2.33) Overlying cold abscesses are generally associated.

Calcaneum. This bone is sometimes affected. The lesion may be confined to the body or tuberosity of the bone and it may then mimic a simple cyst. Some cases become more diffuse and collapse of diseased bone results.

JOINT LESIONS

Tuberculous arthritis is second in frequency to spondylitis and usually affects major joints — the *hip* and *knee* especially. Multifocal infection is rare. Infection may be synovial or secondary to bony disease. The latter is facilitated as the epiphyseal plate apparently offers little resistance to tuberculosis.

Early radiographic signs in synovial lesions are non-specific and will be manifested by capsular thickening, synovial effusion and surrounding osteoporosis. A radiograph of the opposite joint may be needed to enable one to detect these early changes (Fig. 2.34). Later, continued hyperaemia will cause accelerated maturation of bone ends and epiphyses if the infection occurs in children. Bony trabeculae become blurred and the cortex thinned.

The bone ends eventually become affected. Either the entire articular cortex becomes blurred or local marginal or surface erosions may appear (Fig. 2.35). Loss of joint space will ultimately occur, but this is not as prominent a feature as it is in pyogenic arthritis. Sometimes one-half of a joint will be affected and bony erosions seen on contiguous bony surfaces.

Should the primary focus be bony, a combination of the signs of a synovial infection and metaphyseal and epiphyseal destructive foci will result.

The advent of antibiotics has changed the picture considerably. Patients usually respond well to treatment so that only the earlier phases are now seen. Formerly such sequelae as subluxation and ankylosis of joints, severe bone atrophy and tracking abscesses were common.

LESIONS OF INDIVIDUAL JOINTS

Hip. This is a common site; lesions may arise in the acetabulum, synovium, femoral epiphysis or metaphysis. Sometimes infection spreads to the hip from foci in the greater trochanter or ischium. Hip lesions were characterized by much destruction but such gross changes are now seldom seen. All degrees of bone loss of the femoral head and neck could be found. A frequent finding was the pointed 'bird's beak' appearance (Fig. 2.36). Expansion and destruction within the acetabulum sometimes led to intrapelvic protrusion of the hip joint.

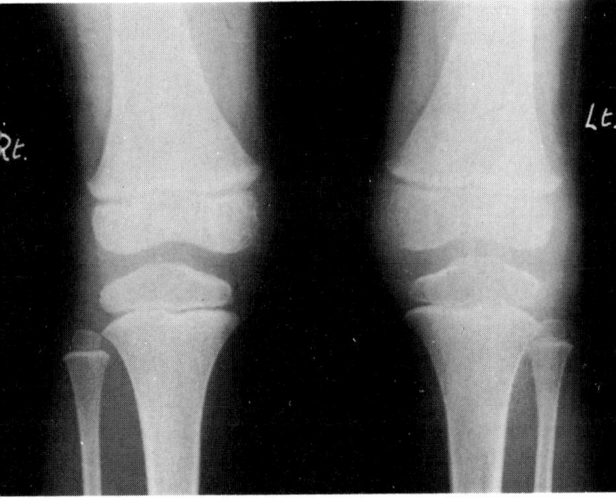

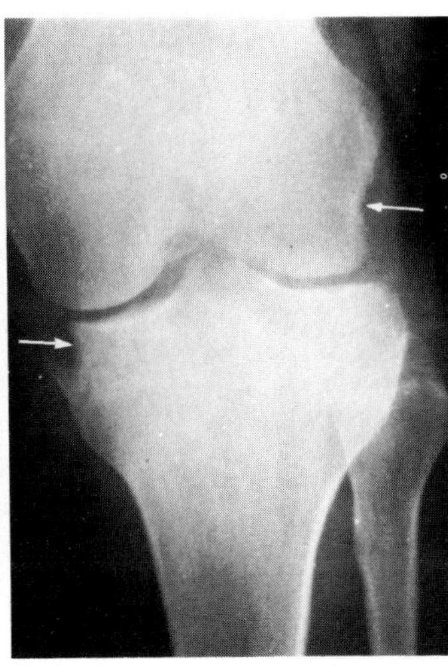

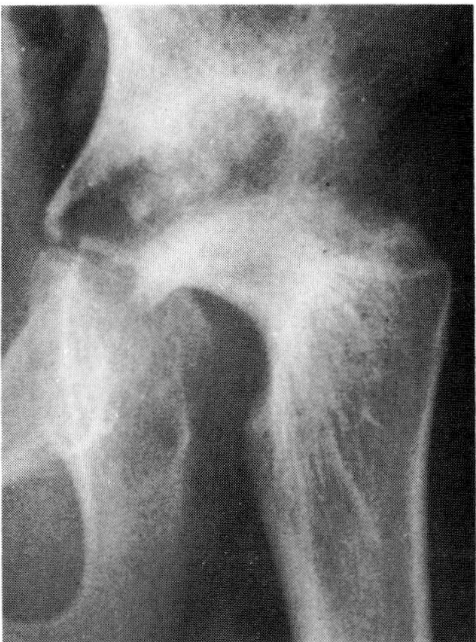

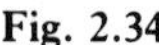

Fig. 2.34 **Fig. 2.35** **Fig. 2.36**

ig. 2.34 Synovial TB of left knee. Note synovial effusion, steoporosis, blurring of trabeculae and accelerated maturation of bone nds (normal right knee for comparison).

ig. 2.35 TB erosions of margins of medial tibial condyle and lateral emoral condyle (arrows).

ig. 2.36 Late TB of hip showing 'bird's beak' appearance.

Knee. With synovial infection in childhood, effusion, steoporosis and accelerated skeletal maturation are seen Fig. 2.34). Overgrowth leads to modelling abnormalities, vith big bulbous squared epiphyses, so that the appearance esembles that seen in juvenile chronic arthritis and aemophilia.

Ankle. Lesions are usually first manifested by a 'woolliness' of articular surfaces, but sometimes a bone focus nay be seen early. In considering differential diagnosis, it hould be noted that rheumatoid arthritis seldom attacks he ankle except in late cases.

Shoulder. The humeral head, the glenoid or both may e affected (Fig. 2.37). Sometimes a lesion in the humeral ead is large and cystic in appearance and may resemble an osteoclastoma. Should the glenoid be involved also, the two conditions will be differentiated since an osteoclastoma does not cross the joint.

Some tuberculous shoulder lesions run a relatively benign course without pus formation — *caries sicca*. In such cases a relatively small pitted erosion is seen on the humeral head (Fig. 2.38). These may resemble degenerative changes.

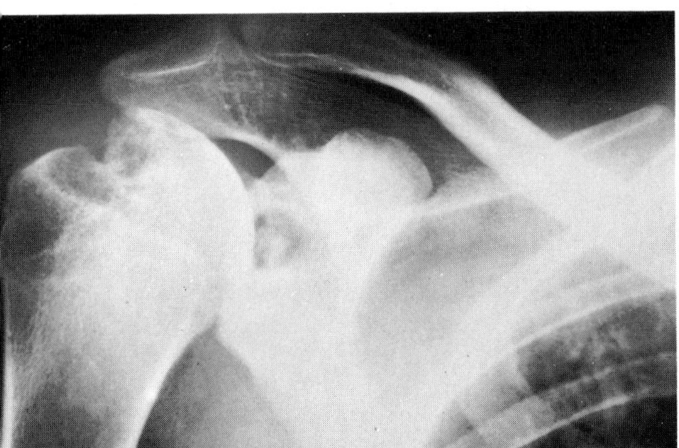

Fig. 2.37 TB of shoulder. Note lesions of humerus and glenoid and in the lung.

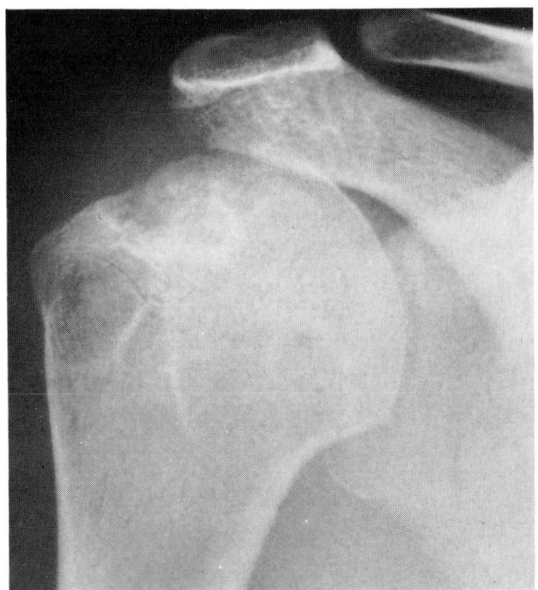

Fig. 2.38 Caries sicca of the humeral head. The term 'caries sicca' means 'dry rot'.

Elbow (Fig. 2.39). Lesions present as a general blurring of articular cortex and osteoporosis. Later the sigmoid fossa becomes deepened. In tuberculous lesions of the elbow there may be a little periostitis affecting adjacent bones. Lesions of the elbow particularly resemble rheumatoid arthritis but rheumatoid lesions are seldom confined to the elbow.

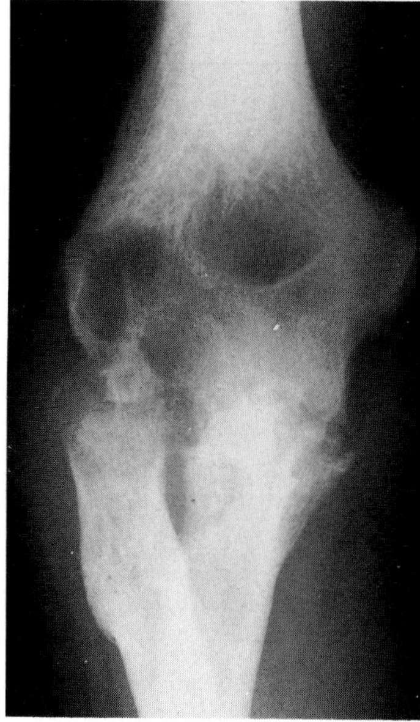

Fig. 2.39 TB elbow: marked general destruction and a large focus in the capitellum.

Wrist and carpus (Figs. 2.40 and 2.41). All carpal bones tend to be attacked in the adult whereas more localized lesions are the tendency in children. This is possibly due to the relatively thicker articular cartilage in the latter. With cartilage destruction the carpal bones become crowded and even if initially one bone is the focus of irregularity, the destructive process soon involves adjacent bones. Intense demineralisation is found throughout the carpus and dist radius and ulna, within the confines of synovium. Demi eralization is often also pronounced at distal small join of the hand with relative preservation of metacarpal an phalangeal shaft density. These joints are however n eroded as in rheumatoid arthritis.

Sacro-iliac joints (Fig. 2.42). This joint is affected mo often in young adults that in children. Sometimes the co dition is bilateral. Subarticular erosions cause widening joint space. The infection is usually associated with absce formation over the back of the joint and, later, pus ma calcify. Tuberculous infection of the spine is a freque accompaniment.

SYPHILIS OF BONES AND JOINTS

Very few cases of syphilis of bone are now seen in Britai Yet up to the time of the last war it was a condition th merited serious consideration in the differential diagnos of most conditions of bone. In this section merely a sum mary of the findings is presented and illustrations are se lected with a view to emphasizing the protean pattern the lesions.

CONGENITAL SYPHILIS

Lesions may be found in infants whose serological reaction are negative, especially when the mother is receiving trea

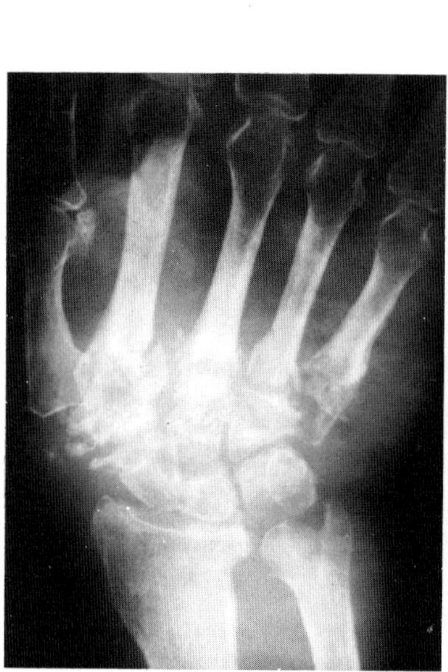

Fig. 2.40

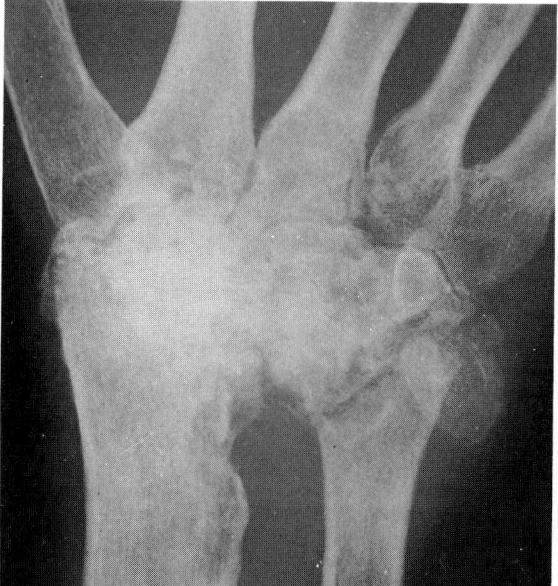

Fig. 2.41

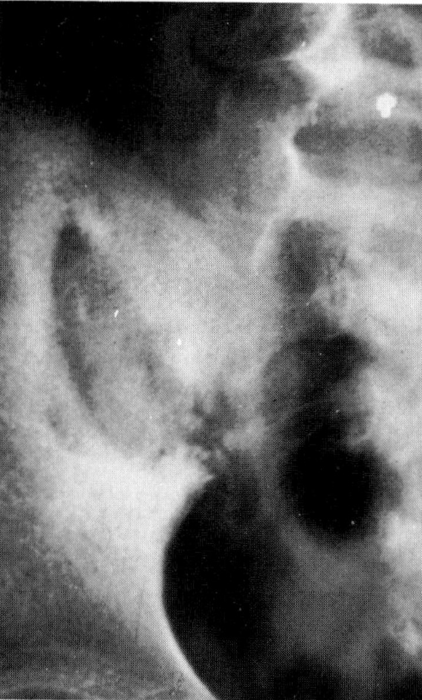

Fig. 2.42

Fig. 2.40 There is soft tissue swelling around the wrist with evidence of a widespread synovial abnormality. Bone and cartilage are destroyed. Osteoporosis is seen at the metacarpophalangeal joints. The metacarpal shafts however remain normal in density. The fifth metacarpal shaft has a periosteal reaction.

Fig. 2.41 Tuberculosis wrist and carpus — late case: gross destruction of the wrist and carpus and calcified abscess shown.

Fig. 2.42 Tuberculous sacro-iliac joint: extensive destructive lesion.

ment. They may appear early, i.e. from birth to 4 years, or later, i.e. between the ages of 5 and 15 years.

Radiographic appearances. The lesions may be widespread and are usually symmetrical. Generally they are best shown in the lower ends of the radius and ulna and around the knee.

Periostitis. This is the commonest feature and is seen either as a thin layer or as more marked laminated layers. Marked thickening on the convexity of a diaphysis may be seen in later cases as, for example, in the so-called 'sabre tibia'.

Metaphysitis. This lesion has also been called 'osteochondritis' — a term best avoided, since in common usage it connotes epiphyseal lesions. Syphilis does not attack epiphyses. The normal radiographic white lines at bone ends are widened due to delay in ossification. This sign is not specific, since it may be seen in other disease causing delay in growth such as osteopetrosis and also in heavy metal poisoning. Beneath the white line a translucent zone may be found (Fig. 2.43). There may be irregularity of metaphyses and metaphyseal fractures may occur.

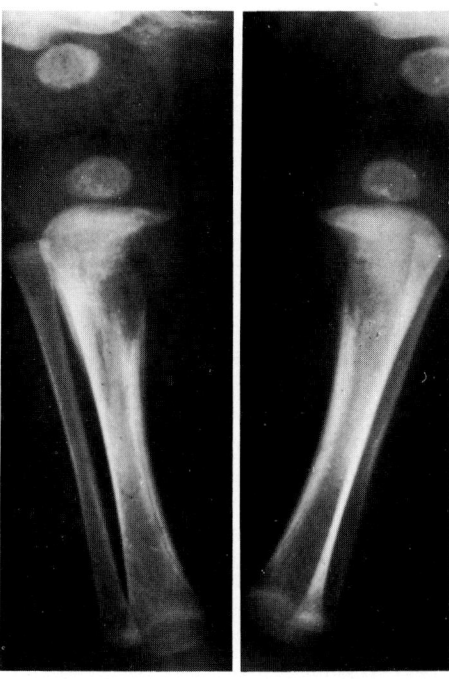

Fig. 2.44 Congenital syphilis, showing osteomyelitis of upper medial ends of both tibiae. Note periostitis on the upper, outer part of the right tibia.

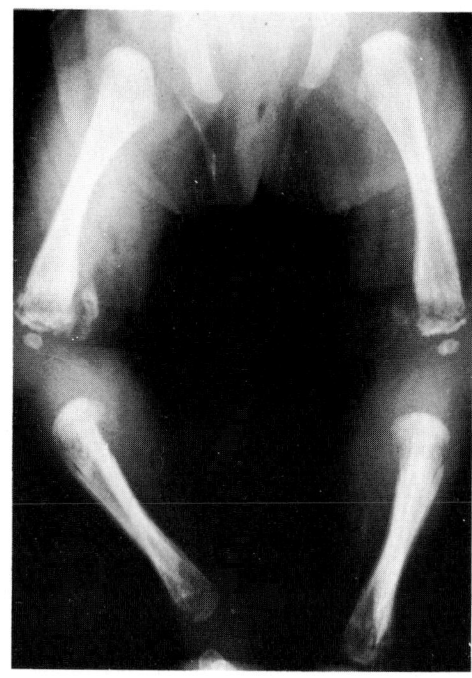

Fig. 2.43 Congenital syphilis: some increased density with subjacent translucent zones of lower ends of femora. Metaphyseal fractures are shown.

Osteitis or osteomyelitis. Erosions on the upper medial surfaces of the tibiae are very characteristic of congenital syphilis (Fig. 2.44). Sometimes more diffuse osteomyelitis of single bones is seen. Syphilis is a productive lesion so sclerosis will be found frequently in such lesions.

Syphilitic dactylitis is rare and may be differentiated with certainty from tuberculous dactylitis (also rare) only by serological tests. The bony widening in syphilis is due to periosteal proliferation, whereas in tuberculous dactylitis it is due to expansion of the medulla.

Skull lesions may be purely sclerotic or may present as a combination of sclerosis and osteolysis. In purely sclerotic lesions, new bone may be laid down in the frontal and parietal regions, so producing the 'hot cross bun' skull.

ACQUIRED SYPHILIS

Any bone may be affected by this condition. Radiological manifestations comprise periostitis and osteomyelitis.

Periostitis. This sign may be seen as a simple laminated periosteal reaction or by a more exuberant lace-like appearance. Bony spiculation at right-angles to the shaft is rare but, when it occurs, it may mimic a neoplastic lesion.

Osteomyelitis. This may occur as a localized or as a diffuse lesion. The localized lesion is termed a gumma (Fig. 2.45) but a more diffuse lesion is often referred to as 'gummatous osteitis' (Figs. 2.46 and 2.47). Sclerosis is generally found; irregularity of bone trabeculation is often apparent. Syphilis causes a combination of destruction and proliferation of bone.

It is important to remember the possibility of syphilis when presented with an atypical bony lesion (Fig. 2.48). This applies especially should symptoms seem relatively slight compared with a rather florid radiographic picture. Syphilitic lesions respond readily to specific therapy.

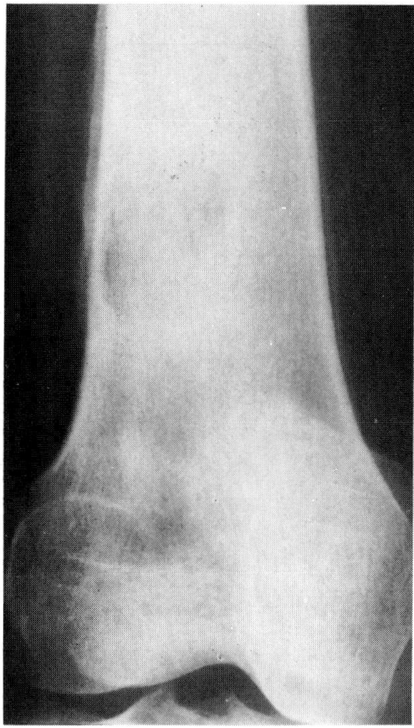

Fig. 2.45 Gumma of the lower femoral shaft. Note bone destruction and periosteal reaction.

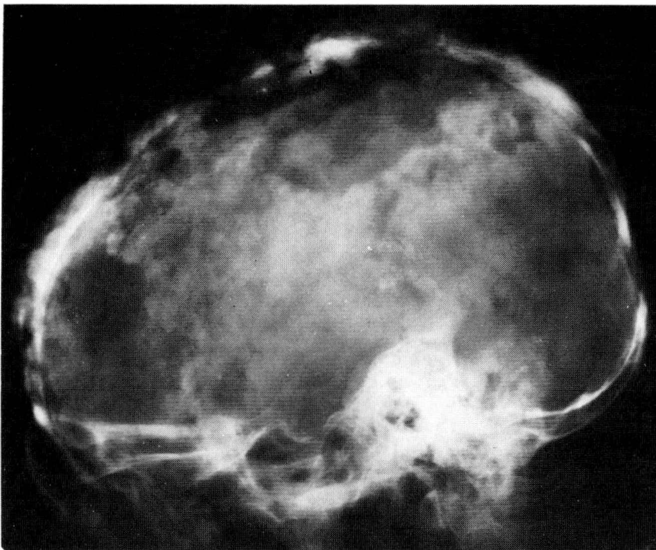

Fig. 2.47 Gummatous osteomyelitis of the skull.

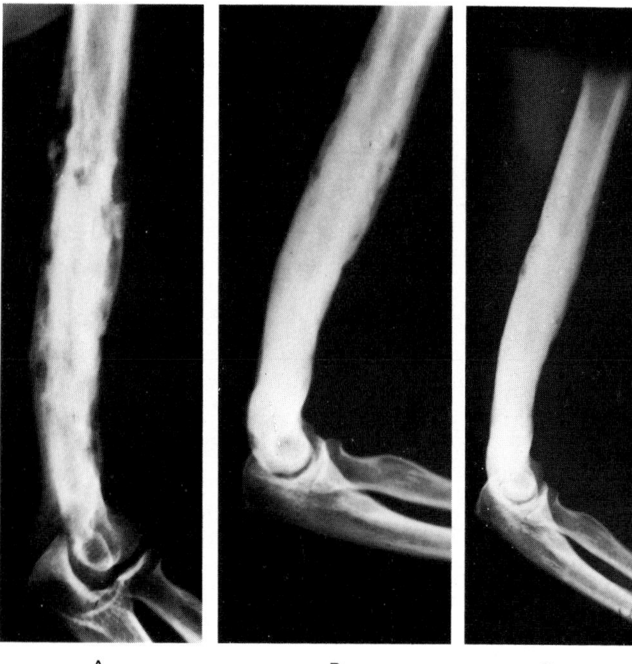

A B C

Fig. 2.46 A., B. and **C.** Syphilitic osteomyelitis of the humerus. Films taken at intervals of 3 months showing a favourable response to therapy. (Courtesy of Dr W. Fowler.)

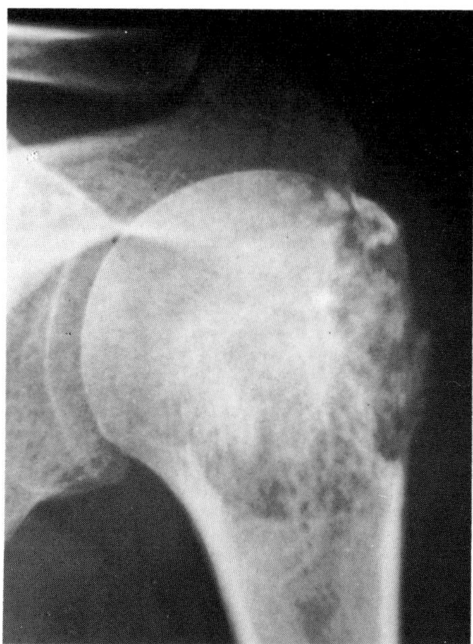

Fig. 2.48 Proven syphilitic osteitis of upper end of the humerus.

RADIO-ISOTOPE SCANNING IN BONE INFECTION

Skeletal scintigraphy in infection should precede plain film examination. Plain radiographic changes are not seen for up to 10–14 days with simple infections, though in tuberculous disease changes are usually present at first presentation. Using scintigraphy, however, the diagnosis of osteomyelitis can be confirmed as early as 48 hours after the onset of the disease, even if clinical signs are equivocal. Early aggressive treatment may prevent gross bone destrucion and, indeed, if treatment is given early enough, on the basis of a positive scan, bone destruction need never develop.

Standard techniques involve the use of ^{99m}technetium-labelled phosphonate and phosphate compounds. The accretion of isotope in bone is related to blood flow as well as to local bone turnover. This allows two separate sets of images to be obtained in osteomyelitis.

1. A 'blood pool' image of the painful area immediately after injection. This shows increased local radioactivity, if positive, in areas of increased blood flow.

2. Delayed skeletal scintigraphic images at 3–4 hours. By this time absorption of isotope on to bone crystal has taken place. This gives a skeletal image with local accentuation in areas of increased blood flow and bone turnover (Fig. 2.49A). This also differentiates osteomyelitis from cellulitis.

Using these techniques it can safely be said that not only is scanning more sensitive in detecting infective foci earlier, but it is nearly always accurate — positive or negative. It is however non-specific in that tumours and infection may give similar appearances. Technetium uptake is, however, limited if blood vessels are occluded in the infective process by tamponade or thrombus.

^{67}Gallium-labelled citrate scans may be used when the technetium scan is negative in patients with clinical osteomyelitis, or even in conjunction with a technetium scan. Gallium concentrates avidly at a site of infection following local accumulation of leucocytes and proteins which are labelled *in vivo*. The radiation dose is higher however and the image poorer. Gallium scans are also probably more helpful in follow-up of active osteomyelitis as such scans are negative earlier than technetium scans when disease becomes quiescent. Technetium scans remain positive for some time even in inactive disease, as the mode of uptake depends on a different physiological process. Gallium scans cannot distinguish with accuracy between cellulitis and osteomyelitis.

Similar results may be obtained with *in vitro* indium-labelled leucocytes which are reinjected into the patient (Fig. 2.49B).

BONE BIOPSY IN INFECTION

This heading can be extended to malignant disease since bone biopsy by needle is performed in the diagnosis of both infections and tumours. Generally in our radiological practice the spine is most frequently biopsied; open biopsy for tissue and bacteriological diagnosis is clearly a much more serious procedure and is generally not the first technique to be used.

As far as infection is concerned, successful biopsy (1) confirms the presence of infection and excludes tumour or other causes of a radiological lesion; (2) distinguishes the organism, both by direct microscopic examination of the aspirate and after culture; and (3) allows correct antibiotic treatment after appropriate sensitivities have been established.

Fig. 2.49 A. Technetium scan. Increase in uptake of the proximal femur and acetabulum following infection around a prosthesis. **B.** Indium scan of the same patient shows the soft tissue infection in the sinus track as well as the bony change.

Fig. 2.49 A

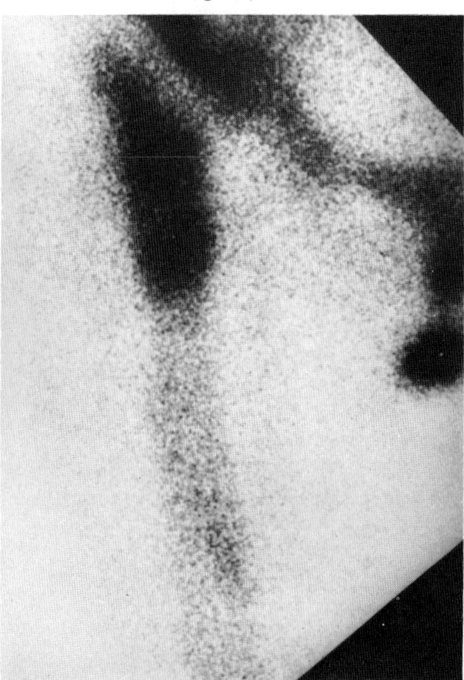

Fig. 2.49 B

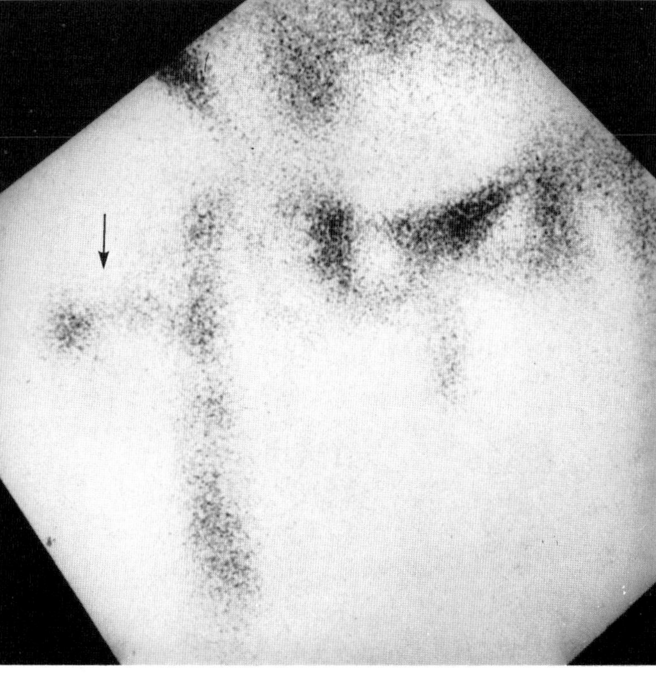

General anaesthesia is unnecessary unless in infancy, or if non-cooperation is expected. Sedation and analgesia are adequate. Analgesia should be both intravenous and local including infiltration of local anaesthesia down to the periosteum.

Biopsy is best performed using biplane fluoroscopy. The use of plain films for one plane delays the procedure considerably. Many types of biopsy needles are available. Some are of very large bore and consist of pointed trochars in a cannula which are used to enter bone, when the pointed trochar is replaced by a trephine with a cutting edge. Certainly hard bone needs a rigid biopsy needle. Infections of bone or disc, however, tend to be soft and in practice a fine aspiration needle is often all that is needed. Complications using a fine needle are usually minor. Pneumothorax and bleeding in the chest, or bleeding from abdominal organs, are not usually a serious problem. Usually the preference of the histologist governs the size of the sample the radiologist needs to obtain.

SARCOIDOSIS

This disease is a non-caseating granulomatous disorder commoner in young adult males and especially in Black patients. Changes in the skeleton are moderately common, occurring in up to 15% of cases. The hands and feet are far more commonly affected but any bone may be involved. Lesions in the skull, vertebrae and long bones have all been described. Though the granulomas usually cause lysis of bone, often resembling tuberculosis, sclerosis occasionally results. Radionuclide scanning detects early bone lesions with greater sensitivity than plain radiographs.

Radiological findings. The changes in the bones include:

1. Punched-out, well-defined areas of lucency in the phalanges (Fig. 2.51). These are probably due to deposition of sarcoid tissue but, as in granulomatous leprosy (see below), the nutrient foramina are also said to be enlarged.
2. A more diffuse reticular lace-like pattern of resorption permeating the bone, described as a lattice-like appearance (Fig. 2.50).
3. Resorption of distal phalanges (Fig. 2.51) and of cortical bone along phalangeal shafts. Cortical resorption vaguely resembles that seen in hyperparathyroidism.
4. Sclerosis, which may be widely disseminated (Fig. 2.52).
5. Periosteal reaction.
6. Soft tissue nodules — far commoner than bone changes.
7. Periarticular calcification due to the hypercalcaemia which occurs in 20–45% of cases of sarcoid.

Sarcoid arthritis. An arthritis is a common joint manifestation of sarcoid, occurring in up to 37% of patients, most commonly in females. In the acute form joint destruction does not occur but, in chronic disease a destructive arthropathy of large joints does rarely occur due to local granulomas.

Fig. 2.50 Sarcoid: coarsened trabeculation of middle phalanx with marked bone resorption and spontaneous fracture. Absorption of the tuft of the distal phalanx is also seen.

Fig. 2.51 Sarcoid: foot of same patient as in Figure 2.54, showing typical pseudocysts and absorption of tufts of distal phalanges.

Fig. 2.52 Multiple foci of sclerosis are a recognised, if uncommon, feature of sarcoid.

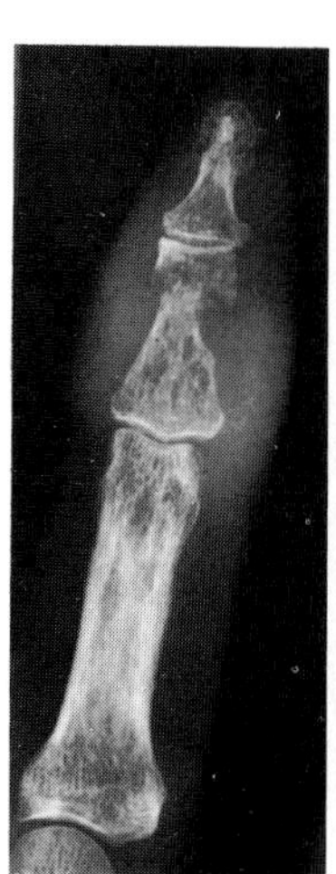

Fig. 2.50

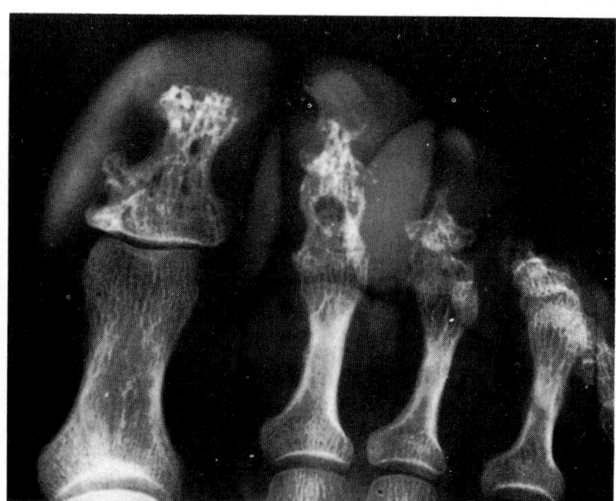

Fig. 2.51

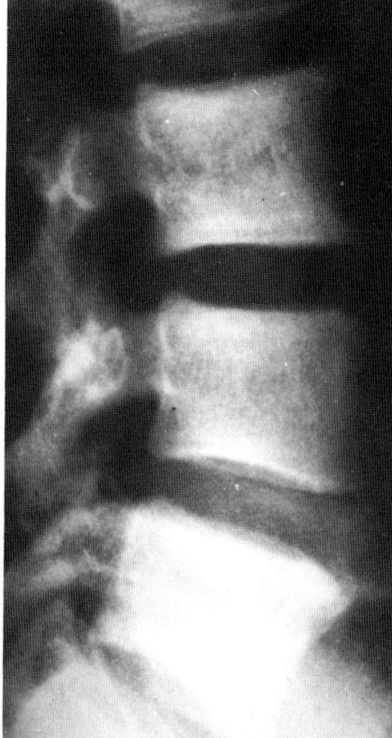

Fig. 2.52

RARE BONE INFECTIONS

BRUCELLOSIS

(Synonyms: *undulant fever*; *Malta fever*)

This disease is more prevalent in Britain than had been thought. Transmission is from unpasteurized milk or by direct contact with affected animals. *Brucella melitensis* infects sheep, *Br. abortus* infects cattle and *Br. suis* pigs.

The bones are affected in 10% of cases, most often the spine and especially in the lumbar region. Widespread granulomatous lesions may be present.

a. *Spinal lesions*. These bear a marked resemblance to other forms of osteomyelitis. Focal sclerosis develops to a marked degree around areas of bone destruction beneath the end-plate (Fig. 2.53A and B). The disc is rapidly destroyed and adjacent vertebrae rapidly affected. Healing is by gross sclerosis, fusion and the production of extremely large, coarse and shaggy bridging osteophytes. Small paravertebral abscesses are seen which do not calcify.

b. *Changes in other bones*. The radiographic appearances resemble those of subacute osteomyelitis and Brodie's abscesses such as are found in low grade pyogenic infections.

c. *Changes in joints*. These resemble the changes of synovial tuberculosis. In advanced cases erosive lesions may be seen.

In obscure and atypical bone infections, it is always advisable to test samples of the blood and of the synovial fluid of affected joints for the agglutination reaction for brucellosis, and also for the typhoid and paratyphoid group of bacilli.

ACTINOMYCOSIS

Bony lesions due to this disease are rarely seen. They usually result from direct extension of soft tissue lesions. The lesion may be suspected clinically and radiographically but final diagnosis is reached only by isolation of the causal fungus. Manifestations may be seen in the following sites:

a. *Mandible*. Chronic osteomyelitis arises by direct spread from oral infections and infected cervical glands. The lesion appears to be irregularly destructive, and in some cases a honeycomb appearance is found.

b. *Ribs and thoracic spine*. Destructive foci and periosteal reaction in these bones arise from pleuro-pulmonary lesions.

c. *Right side of the pelvis and lumbar spine*. Infection spreads to these bones from ileocaecal foci. Spinal lesions are usually accompanied by paravertebral abscesses. The disc is usually spared.

Very rarely destructive metastatic foci are found in other bones.

HYDATID (ECHINOCOCCUS) DISEASE

Hydatid disease is rare in Britain and in less than 2% of affected patients is bone involved. The pelvis, spine and proximal long bones are usually involved. The disease in man follows ingestion of ova. The few that bypass the lungs and liver enter bone via the systemic circulation. The disease is found in the Middle East and Asia, but also in sheep-farming areas in the United Kingdom, other European countries and the USA.

The enlarging cysts in bone absorb trabeculae and spread along the medulla, thinning the cortex and expanding the bone. Later the cystic lesions become well-defined so that fibrous dysplasia may be simulated in long bones.

Around the hip joint both the acetabulum and femoral head and neck are destroyed by large cystic lesions (Fig. 2.54). Fusion may result.

In the spine the cysts break out of the cortex, forming large paraspinal masses which do not calcify but do cause

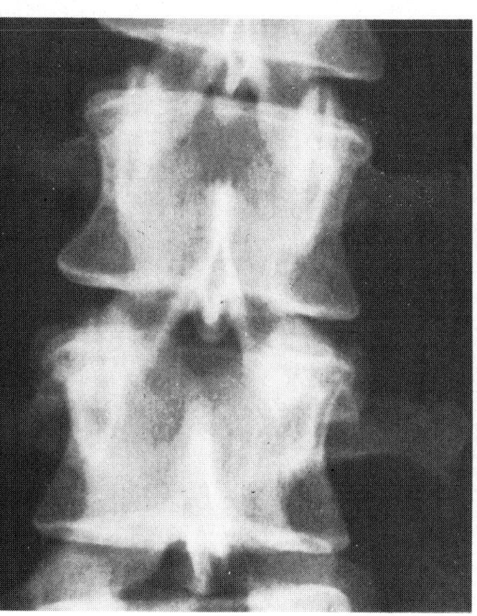

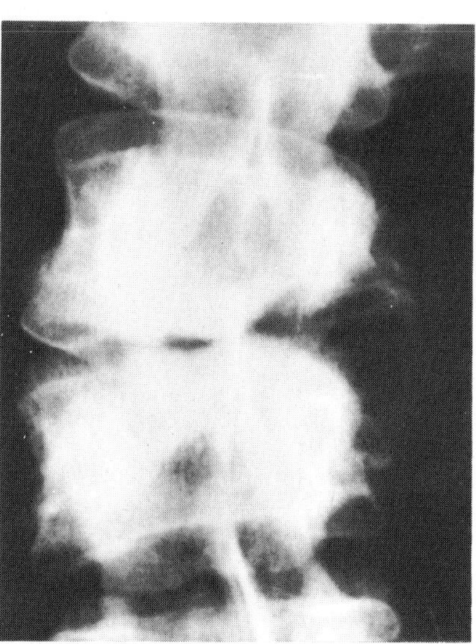

B

Fig. 2.53 A. Brucellosis: reduction of disc space at L2–L3 — no bony involvement. (Courtesy of Dr O. Bauerova.) **B.** Brucellosis — 3 months later; destructive changes L2 and L3, sclerosis and lipping between L2 and L3 seen on original radiograph. (Courtesy of Dr. O. Bauerova.)

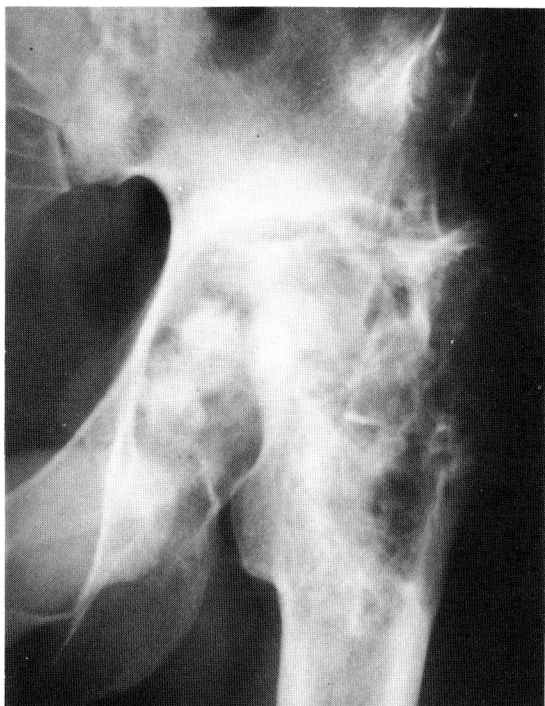

Fig.2.54 Bone destruction with the formation of large cysts around both sides of the hip joint are a classical feature of osseous hydatid. Sequestra can be seen.

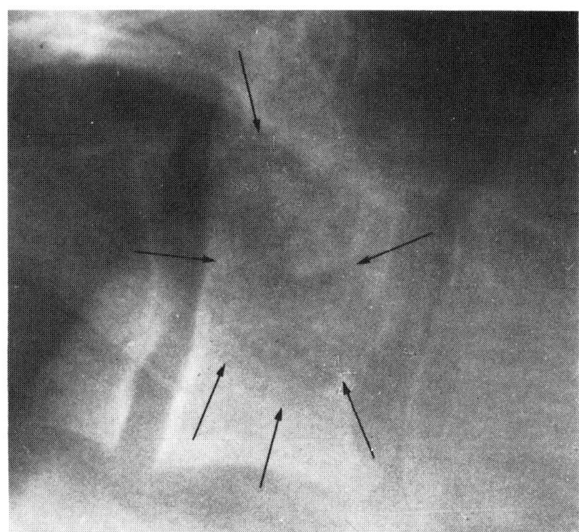

Fig. 2.55 Hydatid disease. The patient was a young man who attended hospital on account of spinal compression. A large hydatid cyst was found in the vertebral body (arrows). Note the preservation of discs above and below the affected vertebra.

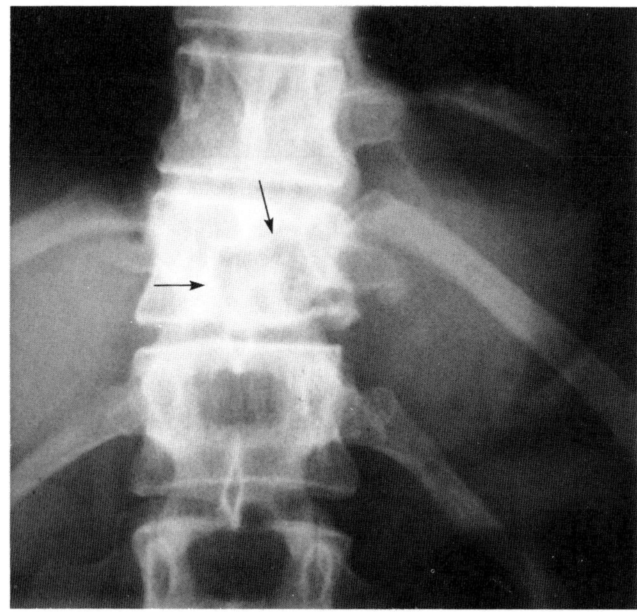

A

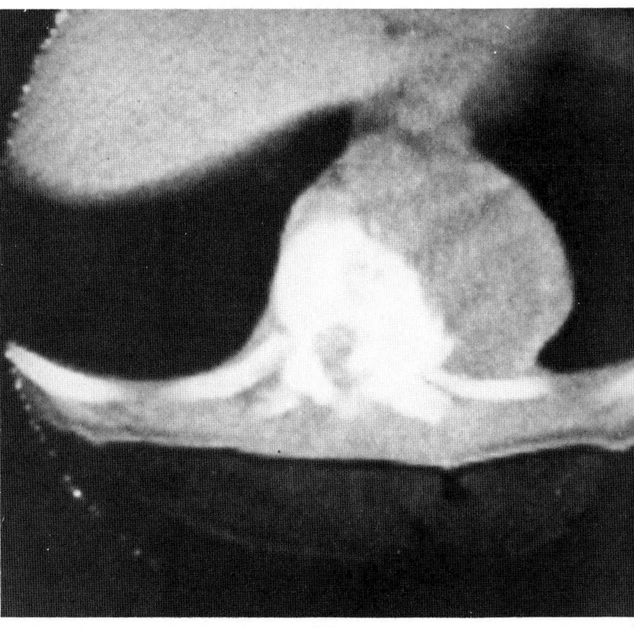

B

Fig. 2.56 A. This patient had never been outside England but has hydatid disease of the spine. Note the large paraspinal soft tissue mass. **B.** CT scan of same patient.

paraplegia (Figs. 2.55 and 2.56). The appearance may resemble dumb-bell tumours in neurofibromatosis.

TROPICAL CONDITIONS

YAWS (treponematosis)

This disease, which has more or less been eradicated, may still be seen in chronic cases. It was prevalent in the West Indies, East Indies and parts of tropical Africa and South America, and is due to a non-venereal infection by *Treponema pertenue*. As the disease is not transmitted to the fetus, congenital yaws does not occur but children become infected. Infection usually occurs through a cut or abrasion. Bony changes are seen in the secondary and tertiary stages; these are usually indistinguishable radiologically.

Any bone may be involved. The distribution may be random, but there is a tendency to symmetry. In the early stages, multiple small rarified areas of bone destruction are shown with overlying periosteal new bone (Fig. 2.57). The hand may be especially affected. Larger areas of destruction occur in the skull and long bones, often with marked surrounding reactive sclerosis and new bone formation. Periostitis along the shaft and softening of bone due to osteitis lead to the sabre tibia deformity.

In the skull gummatous lesions cause foci of osteolysis while slowly growing masses arising from the premaxilla produce a dense hyperostosis known as *goundou*. *Gangosa*, another manifestation of yaws, is an ulceration of the face causing severe necrosis of subjacent bone.

LEPROSY

This disease has a widespread geographical distribution, occurring in Egypt, Africa, Asia, the West Indies and Pacific Islands. It is also seen in Britain's immigrant population. The lesions seen radiologically mostly affect the hands, feet and face, and are caused by infection by *Mycobacterium leprae*. This bacillus is of low infectivity and prolonged exposure is needed. The nature of the disease depends on host resistance. The incidence of bony change in leprosy may be around 15%. Three types of bony lesions are found:

1. Specific changes of osteitis leprosa (15%). *M. leprae* is usually found in the marrow of lepers with lepromatous

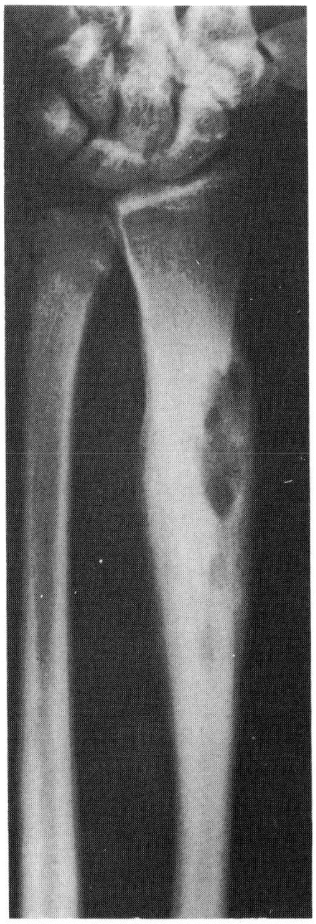

Fig. 2.57 Yaws: moderately early stage showing destructive areas and much periosteal new bone formation. The appearances of the small destructive foci in yaws have been likened to the effects of a borer beetle. (Courtesy of Dr A.G. Davies.)

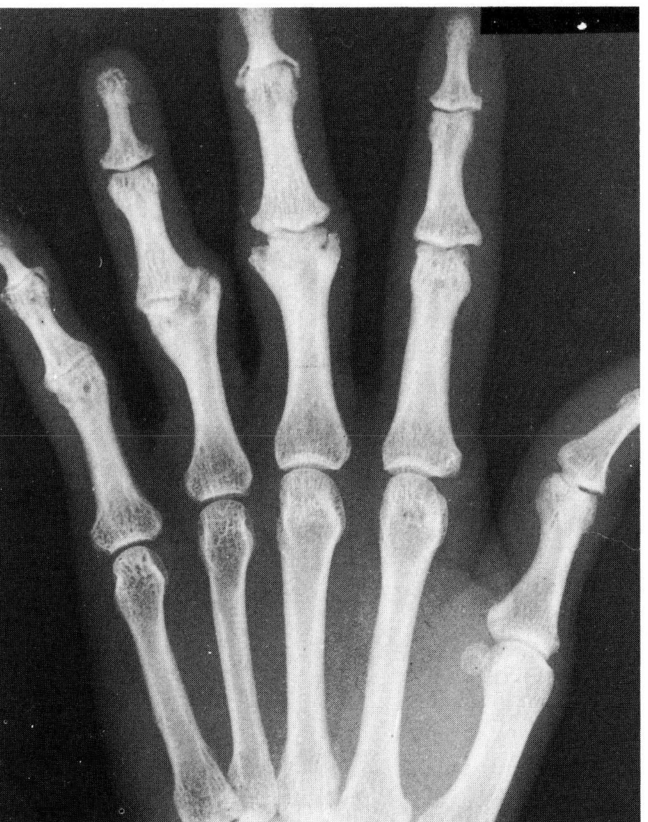

Fig. 2.58 Leprosy. Some small 'cysts' are seen, e.g. in the head of the proximal phalanx of the fifth finger — this condition is sometimes called 'osteitis multiplex cystica leprosa'. The end result of leprous granulomata are seen in the heads of the proximal phalanges of the third and fourth fingers. (Courtesy of Dr D.E. Paterson.)

leprosy but only a minority have visible bony change. Granulomas cause areas of focal cortical or medullary bone destruction and, if subarticular, the joint surfaces collapse and deformity results. The lesions may be rounded or may infiltrate, giving a lace-like pattern just as in sarcoid. In addition, medullary nutrient foramina enlarge (Fig. 2.58).

2. Non-specific leprous osteitis (50%). In these patients Hansen bacilli are rarely found in the marrow. Clear-cut resorption of the bone occurs at distal phalanges and metatarsophalangeal joints, giving a 'licked candy stick' appearance with bone loss both longitudinally and circumferentially (Fig. 2.59). In addition, Charcot-like changes take place in the tarsus. These patients have abnormal, thickened nerves and arterial occlusions. Abnormal stance potentiates this bone resorption in the denervated weight-bearing foot.

With anaesthesia, plantar ulceration and bone and soft tissue infections are superimposed, so that pyogenic osteomyelitis is common in these patients. This does not usually show sequestrum and involucrum formation. These changes are superimposed upon those of the neuropathic osteopathy.

3. A diffuse osteoporosis is seen which is non-specific.

Thickening of the nerves has been demonstrated by perineural injection of lipiodol. Nerve calcification is occasionally seen.

TROPICAL ULCER

This common lesion found throughout the tropics may also be seen in immigrants to Britain. Chronic indolent skin ulcers cause secondary bone changes usually in the tibia or fibula. Periostitis is seen early in various forms, e.g. linear, onion layer, lacework and spicular. The latter type may

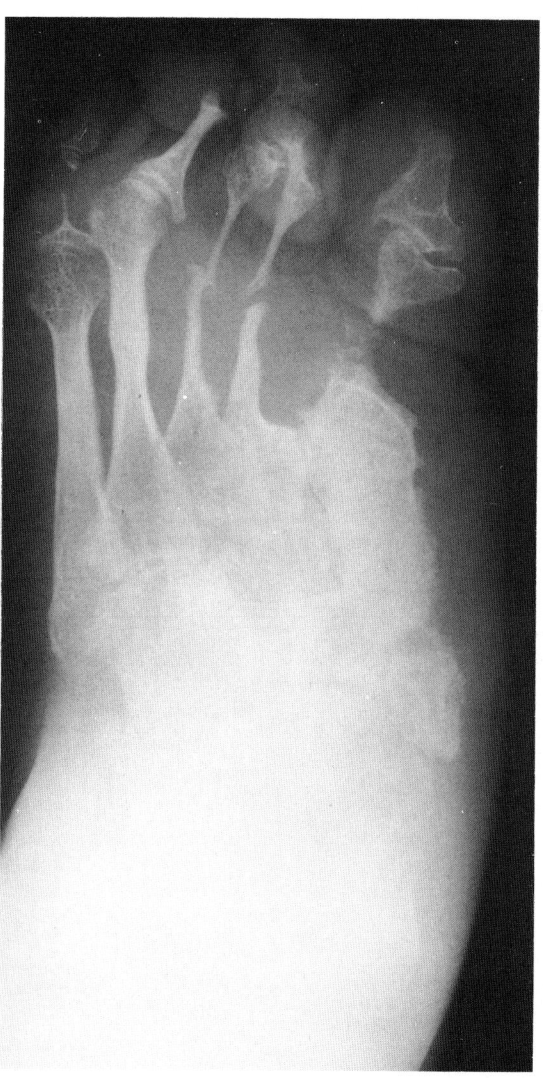

Fig. 2.59 Well-defined longitudinal and circumferential bone resorption with no evidence of superadded osteomyelitis in leprosy. Charcot-like changes are evident in the tarsus.

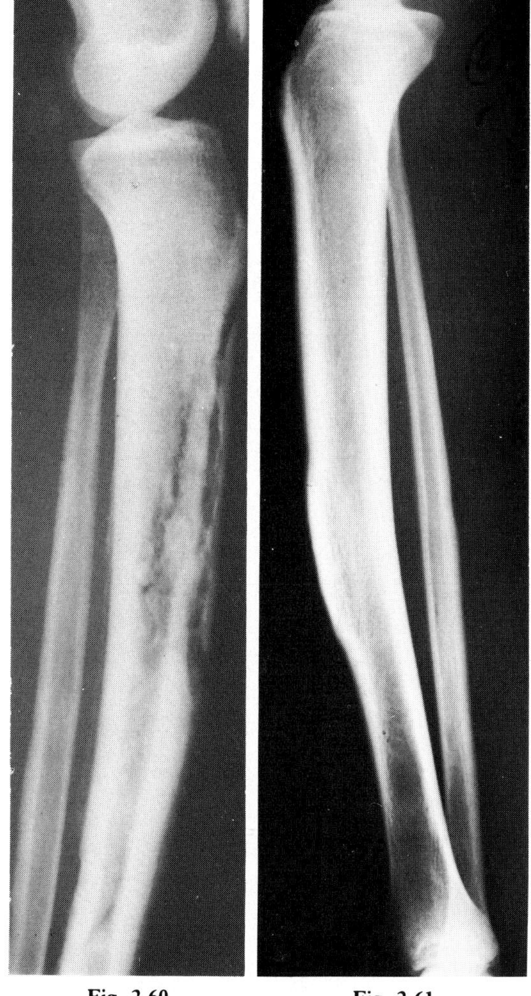

Fig. 2.60 **Fig. 2.61**

Fig. 2.60 Tropical ulcer. Extensive osteomyelitis is seen in the underlying tibia.

Fig. 2.61 Tropical ulcer: osteoma-like lesion on the front of the tibial shaft — a late sequel of tropical ulcer.

CHAPTER 3

AVASCULAR NECROSIS OF BONE: OSTEOCHONDRITIS: MISCELLANEOUS BONE LESIONS

OSTEONECROSIS

(Synonyms: *aseptic necrosis, avascular necrosis, bone infarction*)

The term 'osteonecrosis' implies that a segment of bone has lost its blood supply so that the cellular elements within it die. The phrase 'aseptic necrosis' indicates that infection generally plays no part in the process, though a sequestrum is also necrotic and avascular.

Pathology. Ischaemia of bone follows occlusion of arteries or veins and is therefore dependent on the anatomy of the blood supply to a given bone (a rise in venous pressure eventually arrests arterial supply). Ischaemia results in death of haemopoietic tissue within 6–12 hours; of the osteoclasts, osteoblasts and osteocytes within 12–48 hours; and of marrow fat in 2–5 days. Empty osteocyte lacunae indicate death of bone. Dead bone at this stage is radiologically normal since the trabecular framework remains intact.

Revascularization is seen at the live marrow-dead marrow interface. The necrotic zone is invaded by capillaries, fibroblasts and macrophages. Fibrous tissue replaces dead marrow and in turn may calcify. New osteoblasts lay down fresh woven bone on the devitalised trabeculae. This advancing front of neo-vascularization and ossification has been termed 'creeping substitution' (Phemister).

At bone ends, cartilage receives nutrition from synovial fluid. Cartilage and subcartilaginous bone are not therefore necessarily affected.

Radiological changes are thus:

1. *Acute stage*. No changes are visible.

2. *Intermediate stage*. Disuse, for instance following immobility, leads to a generalised osteoporosis, except in devitalised avascular bone which is now devoid of osteoclasts and osteocytes. Avascular areas therefore remain normal in density while immobile but vascular bone loses density. The avascular proximal pole of the scaphoid thus remains dense after waist of scaphoid fractures.

3. *Late stage*. At large joints — hip, shoulder, knee — structural failure in subarticular bone at areas of maximal stress results in cortical microfractures followed by collapse and trabecular compression. This results in a flattened articular surface with increased subarticular density as trabeculae are compressed into a smaller space.

In the diametaphysis and subarticular regions, the infarcted area is surrounded by a serpiginous line of sclerosis representing the advancing front of new bone laid down on the old trabecular framework. The central area within the infarct may look relatively lucent, or may actually be the site of osteoclastic resorption, but may also contain foci of added density representing dystrophic calcification in debris.

In some diseases following infarction, a 'bone within a bone' or 'split cortex' is seen as a linear density lying within and parallel to the healthy cortex. This probably represents the old infarcted cortex left behind by processes of growth and remodelling beneath the vital periosteum. This change is seen in Gaucher's and in sickle-cell disease, and following osteomyelitis.

Epiphyseal abnormalities. Infarcts at growth plates, for instance in the hands and at the vertebral end-plates in sickle-cell disease, cause local arrest of growth or may result in 'cone' epiphyses or premature fusion. The latter also occurs after irradiation, infection or trauma.

Infarcted bone, e.g. following irradiation is susceptible to fractures. This is seen in the ribs following irradiation for breast cancer and in the femoral necks after pelvic irradiation, though less commonly nowadays.

Causes of osteonecrosis (Table 3.1)

Vascular insufficiency to bone is of three types.

1. *Interruption to the flow of blood* to bone most commonly follows trauma with tearing of blood vessels.

2. *Emboli or sludging*. This occurs in sickle-cell disease where abnormal red cells aggregate; in pancreatitis where fat emboli obstruct vessels; and in decompression disease where possibly gas bubbles occlude small vessels. A vasculitis, in collagen disorders and following irradiation, also occludes small vessels.

3. *Intra-osseous compression of vessels* occurs in Gaucher's disease where masses of Gaucher cells pack marrow spaces.

Table 3.1 Conditions associated with spontaneous aseptic bone necrosis

**Alcoholism	*Haemopoietic disorders	Obesity
Arthropathy	Haemophilia	**Pancreatitis
**Rheumatoid arthritis	Gaucher's disease	Peripheral neuropathy
Psoriasis	Histiocytosis	Peripheral vascular disease
Neuropathic	Polycythaemia	Periarteritis nodosa
Osteoarthrosis	*Hypercorticism	Pregnancy
Clotting defects	Hypercholesterolaemia	**Systemic lupus erythematosus
Convulsive disorders	**Hyperlipaemia	*Thermal injuries
*Cushing's syndrome	Hypertension	Burns
*Decompression syndrome	**Hypertriglyceridaemia	Electrical
**Diabetes	**Hyperuricaemia	Frostbite
Endocarditis	Immobilisation	*Trauma
**Fat embolism	*Immunosuppresive therapy	
Giant cell arteritis	*Irradiation	
Gonorrhoea	Microfractures	
**Gout	Mitral insufficiency	
*Haemoglobinopathy	Myxoedema	

* Generally accepted contributory factor
** Commonly reported associated factor

(Reproduced from *Aseptic Necrosis of Bone* by kind permission of Excerpta Medica, Amsterdam)

The role of drugs in avascular necrosis. Steroids and non-steroidal anti-inflammatory drugs are associated with bone necrosis.

Pain relief and euphoria associated with prolonged dosage leads to overuse of often already damaged joints and a Charcot-type lesion results with bone loss and eburnation. Similar changes may follow alcohol abuse. In addition, steroids cause vasculitis and marked subcortical osteoporosis which further potentiates bone collapse.

OSTEOCHONDRITIS (OSTEOCHONDROSIS)

Osteochondritis is a disease of epiphyses, beginning as necrosis and followed by healing. The term 'osteochondritis' is used to describe the lesions but is a misnomer, as there is (i) no inflammation and (ii) cartilage is not primarily involved. Over 40 sites have been described and all have eponyms which are too closely associated with the lesions to be currently abandoned (Table 3.2).

The mechanism of pathological change is not identical at all sites. Some, such as Perthes' disease, are generally regarded as being due to vascular occlusion. The mechanism for this is not clearly understood, especially as in some patients an osteochondritis affects more than one epiphysis. At other sites — the tibial tubercle and the lower pole of patella — tendons avulse bone which subsequently necroses. Vertebra plana follows eosinophil granuloma. Adolescent kyphosis may follow discal herniation into end-plate defects.

Table 3.2 Eponymous osteochondritides

Disease	Cause	Site
Legg-Calvé-Perthes	Primary aseptic necrosis	Femoral head
Kohler	? primary aseptic necrosis ? necrosis following fracture	Tarsal navicular
Freiberg	? primary aseptic necrosis ? necrosis following fracture	Metatarsal head
Kienböck	? necrosis following fracture ? primary aseptic necrosis	Lunate
Osgood-Schlatter	Necrosis following partial avulsion of patellar tendon	Tibial tubercle
Sinding-Larsen	Necrosis following partial avulsion of patellar tendon	Lower pole of patella
Siever	Necrosis following partial avulsion of tendo achilles	Calcaneal apophysis
Calvé	Eosinophil granuloma	Vertebral body
Scheuermann	Disc herniation through defective end-plate	Ring-like epiphysis of vertebra

(Reproduced from Aseptic Necrosis of Bone by kind permission of Dr Mary Catto and Excerpta Medica, Amsterdam)

Epiphyseal areas of necrosis eventually heal and are converted into normal bone. In some sites, especially at the femoral head, prominent metaphyseal changes are also present.

OSTEOCHONDRITIS OF THE FEMORAL CAPITAL EPIPHYSIS

(Synonym: *coxa plana*; Eponyms: *Waldenstrom (1909), Legg (1910), Calvé (1910), Perthes (1910)*)

This condition is commoner in boys than girls (M:f = 4:1) and most cases are between four and nine years of age at presentation. Girls have an earlier age of onset and a worse prognosis.

Bilateral disease is even more common in boys (M:F = 7:1) but the disease is rarely symmetrical, being less severe in the second hip to be affected. If symmetry is present, hypothyroidism or multiple epiphyseal dysplasia should be excluded. There is no increased familial incidence, but parents of affected children are often elderly. Many of the affected children have a below average birth weight and, at presentation, show skeletal growth retardation in the hands. This is especially seen in boys. There is an increased incidence of associated congenital anomalies, including congenital heart disease, pyloric stenosis, hernia, renal anomalies and undescended testicle.

Clinical features. Symptoms are usually longstanding in classical disease, with a limp and pain in the hip being most apparent. The limp is of the antalgic type, sparing the stiff, affected hip. Fixed flexion and adduction may result with shortening and muscle wasting. The feet rarely may be abnormal with subtalar stiffness and associated osteochondritis of the tarsal navicular.

Pathological features. Between three and eight years of age, the main blood supply to the femoral capital epiphysis is from the superior and inferior branches of the medial femoral circumflex artery which, at this age, lie beneath the periosteum and only later become incorporated into bone. This late change would prevent vessel compression if an effusion were present in the joint, but ischaemia occurs if the vessel is unprotected.

Following ischaemia, the ossific nucleus of the epiphysis necroses, causing growth arrest. The overlying cartilage, which is supplied by synovial fluid, survives and thickens, especially in the non-weight-bearing regions, medially and laterally. Creeping substitution eventually occurs in the ossific nucleus which thus becomes denser, the process usually reaching the dome from the peripheral and deep parts of the epiphysis.

Radiological features

1. *Lateral displacement of the femoral head.* Early on, and in the irritable hip syndrome, displacement of the femoral head (Waldenstrom's sign) is seen (Fig. 3.1A). The femoral head may be displaced laterally by 2–5 mm, possibly due to effusion or to thickening of the ligamentum teres. Later, the superior part of the joint may also be widened.

2. *A subcortical fissure in the femoral ossific nucleus.* This sign is seen early on in the disease but is transient. It is best seen in the 'frog' lateral view, and on traction, when lowered pressure in the abducted joint 'pulls' off the cortical fragment from the underlying bone. The resulting defect may fill with gas ('vacuum sign'). This change initially occurs anteriorly — another reason for the 'frog' lateral view (Fig. 3.1B).

3. *Reduction in size of the ossific nucleus of the epiphysis.* This is found in some 50% of cases and is due to growth retardation. The medial joint space then seems wider.

4. *Increase in density of the femoral ossific nucleus.* This is due to trabecular compression, dystrophic calcification in debris and creeping substitution (see above) (Figs. 3.2 and 3.3).

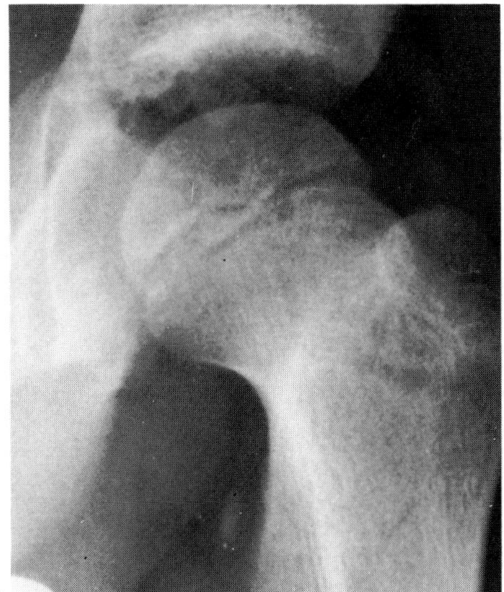

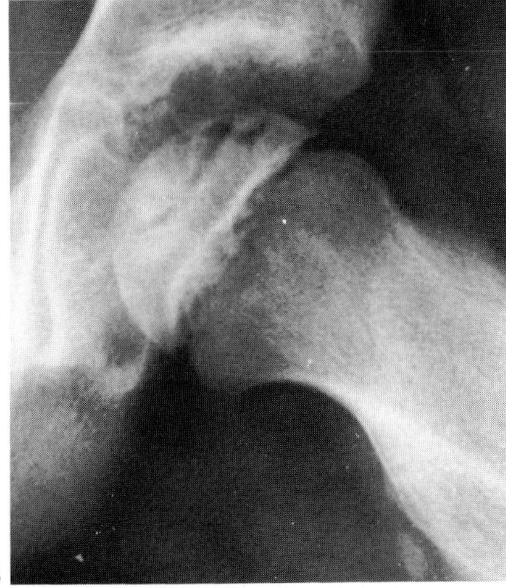

Fig. 3.1 A. Perthes' disease, showing increased joint space in AP view. **B.** Fissures in the femoral head are shown well in the frog view.

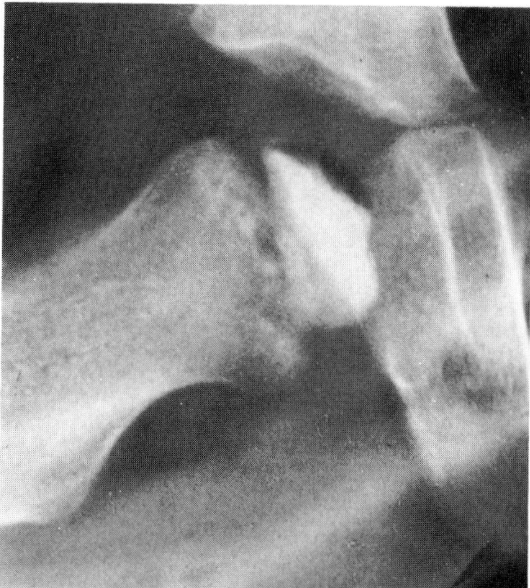

Fig. 3.2 Perthes' disease: intra-epiphyseal gas with flattening and sclerosis of the femoral head.

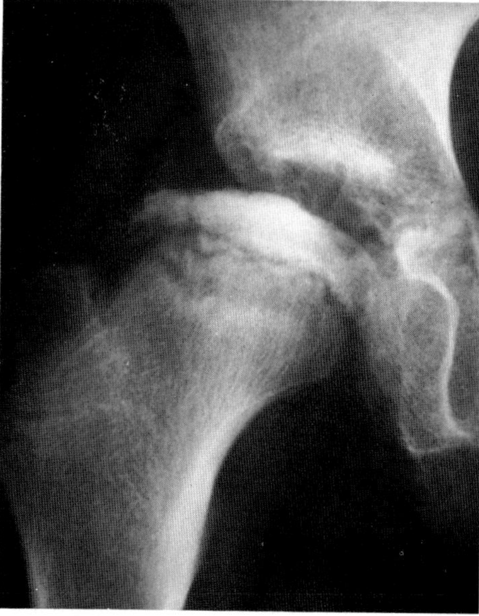

Fig. 3.3 Perthes' disease. The femoral head is flat, broad, irregular in outline, sclerotic and fissured. Metaphyseal broadening and irregularity is also present.

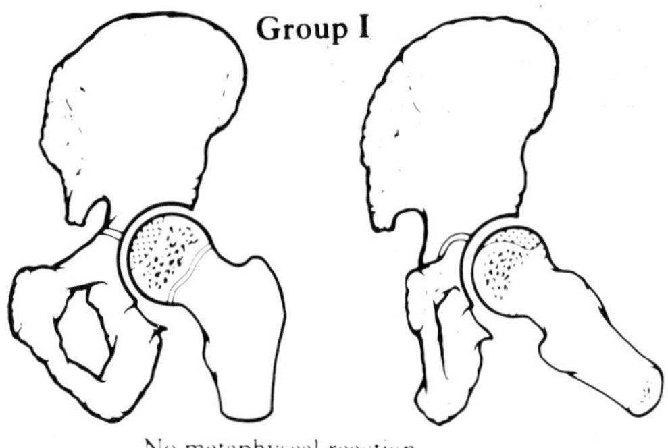

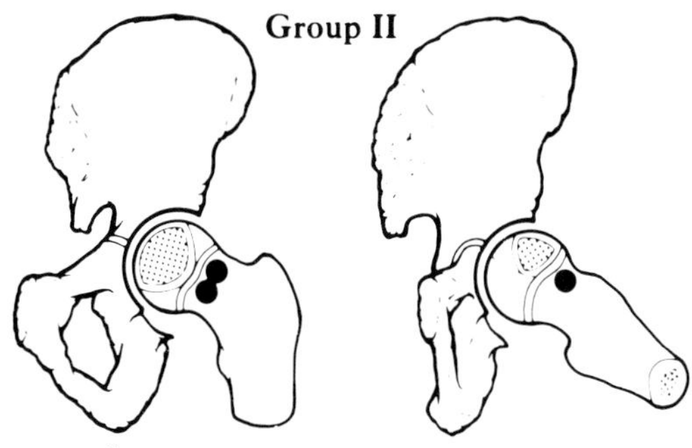

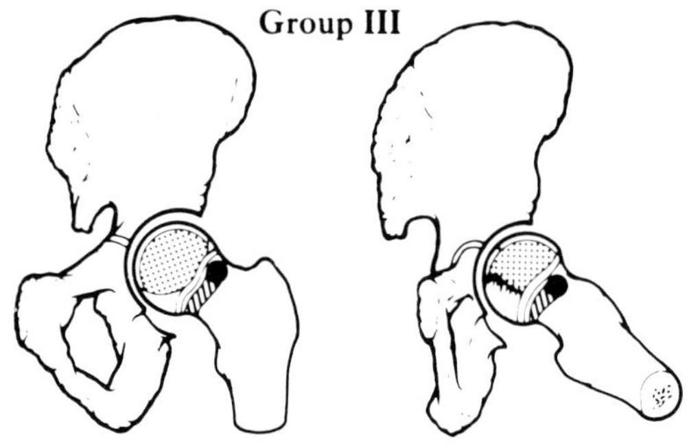

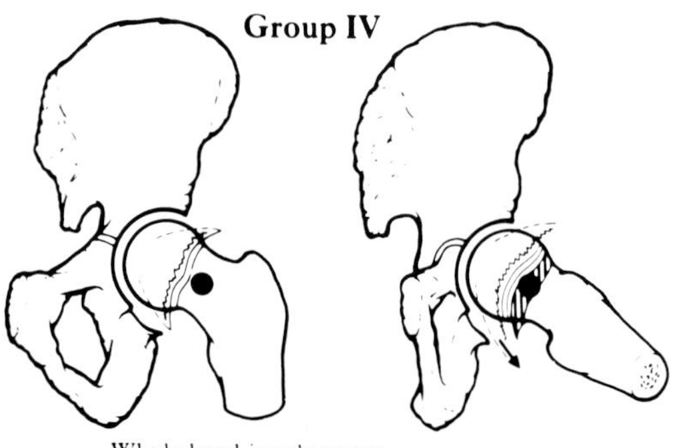

Fig. 3.4 Catterall classification of Perthes' disease. (Reproduced by kind permission of Mr A. Catterall FRCS.)

Catterall has grouped Perthes' disease depending on the degree of epiphyseal involvement as assessed radiologically (Fig. 3.4). Prognosis depends on the degree of radiological involvement.

Group I The anterior part of the epiphysis only is involved. Collapse does not occur. Normal bone lies above the epiphyseal plate. Healing occurs from the periphery of the defect.

Group II More of the anterior part of the epiphysis is affected. The involved segment collapses and a dense sequestrum forms. Only the unaffected segment retains its height and reaches the epiphyseal plate normally. Metaphyseal changes are minor. The involved segment heals by ossification from the periphery.

Group III Only a small normal portion, usually posterior, remains. Subchondral fissuring is prominent, sparing only the posterior aspect of the nucleus. Speckled ossification occurs in the cartilage around the nucleus. Metaphyseal changes are more general and imply a worse prognosis.

Collapse of the head is greater in Group III and the head more deformed.

Group IV The whole epiphysis is involved and flattened to a thin dense line. All quadrants are flattened and a 'mushroom' deformity results. If the head remains in the acetabulum it may regenerate. If lateral subluxation occurs the head ends up flatter. As all the dense bone must be removed before healing occurs, the duration of the disease is longer.

Stages of the disease occur within each group.

There is an *initial* phase of onset, with widening of the joint space and increased density of all or part of the ossific nucleus, which is followed by collapse of part or all of the nucleus, according to group. *Repair* removes the fragmented, crushed, necrotic bone. *Healing* shows as an increase in size and re-ossification (Fig. 3.5). *Remodelling* then occurs and is aided when the femoral head is completely contained within the acetabulum. Uncovering of the lateral margin of the femoral head has a bad prognosis.

The metaphyseal lesion leads to an abnormal femoral neck. The most severely involved cases have a broad, short neck, that is, the neck length/width ratio is lower than normal (Fig. 3.6).

Prognosis. The prognosis in untreated disease is proportional to the degree of epiphyseal involvement. Thus, Group I and Group II patients have a good prognosis.

The irritable hip syndrome

A few patients with this syndrome (up to 7%) develop changes of Perthes' disease. The affected children present with acute hip pain and often fever and a raised ESR. Most cases resolve with simple bed rest, but prolonged immobilisation and traction may be necessary. Other causes of acute hip pain — infection or juvenile arthritis — must also be excluded.

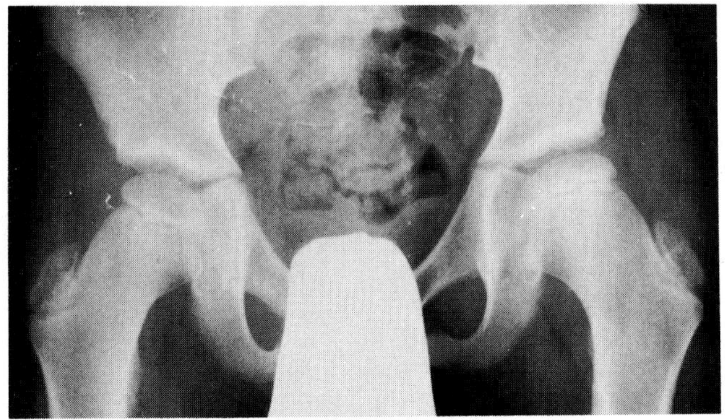

Fig. 3.5 Perthes' disease — healing phase: residual flattening of femoral capital epiphysis and widening of the femoral neck on left side.

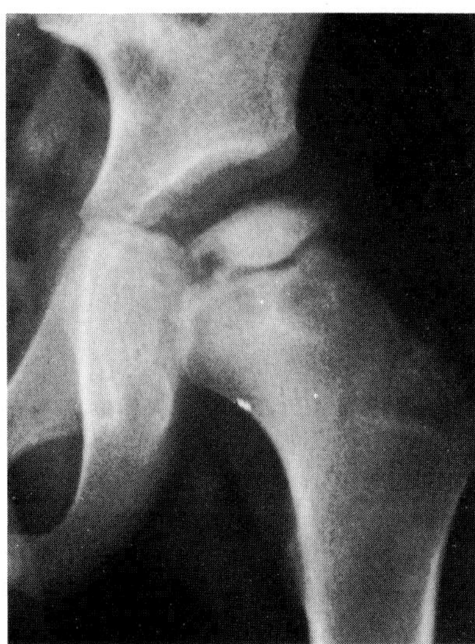

Fig. 3.6 Perthes' disease: condensation of femoral capital epiphysis and cystic appearance in metaphysis.

RADIO-ISOTOPE BONE SCANNING IN ASEPTIC NECROSIS OF THE FEMORAL HEAD

Technetium scan images of bone depend in part on blood flow to bone. Avascular areas, therefore, are seen as scan defects. Nuclide scanning of a painful hip distinguishes a 'cold' area in infarction from an area of increased uptake in infective or inflammatory disease. It seems logical to scan all children with acutely painful hips.

In the early stage, when no radiological abnormality is yet visible in the child with an avascular lesion, a defect is seen in the femoral head image on isotope scanning. In the early case, the size of the defect on the scan correlates well with the eventual size of the defect on the radiograph, which only becomes assessable some 6–9 months after the initial nuclide scan (Fig. 3.7).

In cases of established disease, correlation of the scan defect with radiological change is less helpful, as revascularization gives a local increase in activity, so that the defect size is underestimated.

Prognosis in an early case can be assessed from the defect size on the early scan, so that a small defect has a good prognosis.

OSTEOCHONDRITIS OF THE TIBIAL TUBERCLE

(Synonyms: *Osgood's disease, Schlatter's disease*)

The presentation is of a child of 12–15 years with pain and

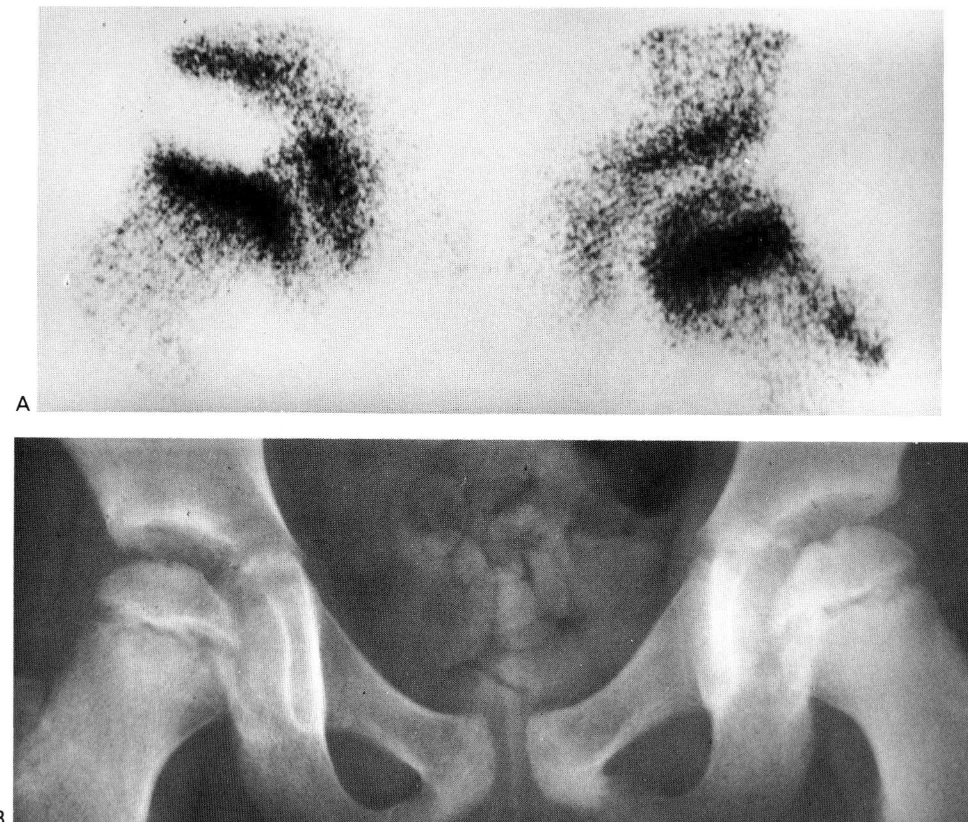

Fig. 3.7 Perthes' disease. **A.** The lateral aspect of the femoral head does not show up on radio-isotope scanning. **B.** The involved area on X-ray looks smaller than on the scan.

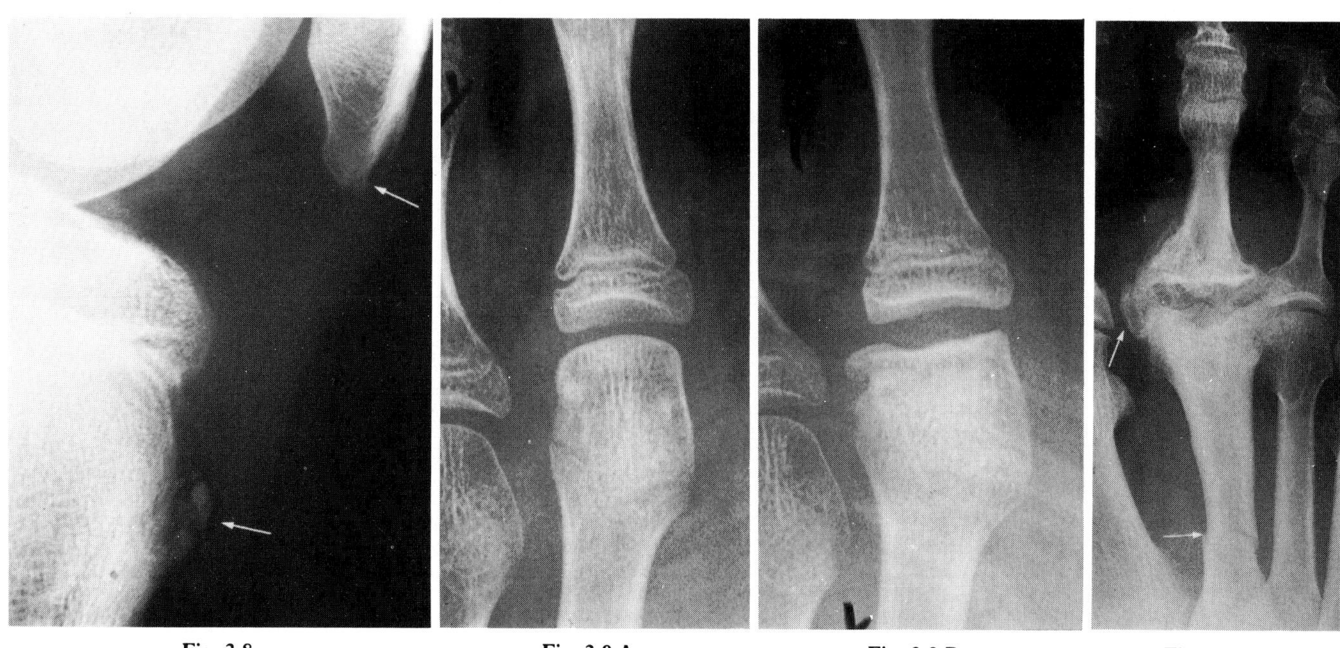

Fig. 3.8 **Fig. 3.9 A** **Fig. 3.9 B** **Fig. 3.10**

Fig. 3.8 Osgood–Schlatter's disease. Note also some osteochondritis of the epiphysis of the lower pole of the patella.

Fig. 3.9 Osteochondritis of second metatarsal head. **A.** minimal change of increased density of the epiphysis. **B.** later stage of flattening of the epiphysis, increased joint space and loose body separation.

Fig. 3.10 Osteochondritis of second metatarsal head — advanced case. Note loose body (upper arrow). The patient sustained a spontaneous fracture (lower arrow). (Courtesy of Mr H. I. C. Bowie.)

oft tissue swelling in the region of a prominent and tender ibial tuberosity. It is more commonly seen in boys but girls are affected at an earlier age. There is often a history of sports, especially involving the quadriceps. The disease s an example of a traction injury.

The tibial tuberosity develops at about seven years of age, either as a downward prolongation of the epiphysis, or independently. It therefore has no 'classical' appearance but a spectrum exists. The apophysis is the insertion of the patellar tendon.

The diagnosis is essentially clinical and is confirmed radiologically by a soft tissue lateral film of the area. This demonstrates local soft tissue swelling over an often fragmented and dense tuberosity (Fig. 3.8). The other knee should also be examined radiologically, especially to compare the soft tissues. The condition is usually self-limiting and rest brings relief of symptoms.

The tubercle fuses to the shaft at 15 years, but occasionally remains unfused and fragmented. Examination of soft tissues will rule out on-going disease.

OSTEOCHONDRITIS OF THE METATARSAL HEAD

(Synonyms: *Freiberg's infraction, Köhler's disease*)

The second metatarsal head is one of the most frequently involved though the lesion may affect other metatarsals. The condition is commoner in girls. Its usual age incidence is between 10 and 15 years but cases sometimes begin in adult life. In some there is a history of frank trauma, in others chronic trauma may be associated, e.g. girls wearing high heels for the first time.

Radiographic appearances. Condensation, increased density (Fig. 3.9) and fragmentation of the epiphysis are seen. The joint space may be increased in size and the opposing bone surfaces greatly splayed. Gradual thickening of the metatarsal neck and shaft occurs. Quite often a bony fragment becomes completely detached from the epiphysis and forms a loose body in the joint (Fig. 3.9 and 3.10). For this reason, the lesion is sometimes classified as a form of osteochondritis dissecans.

OSTEOCHONDRITIS OF THE TARSAL NAVICULAR

(Synonym: *Köhler's disease*)

The ossific nucleus for the navicular appears at around $1\frac{1}{2}$ to 2 years in girls and $2\frac{1}{2}$ to 3 years in boys. Minor variations occur with multiple centres of ossification and some irregularity being a normal finding in the painless foot. As in Osgood-Schlatter's disease, the combination of pain and radiological change is needed for the diagnosis to be made. The disease is much more common in boys. Age incidence is 3–10 years, with the peak between 5–6 years, and the disease appears earlier in the female — as does the ossific nucleus itself. The process is thought to be ischaemic in origin. 15–20% are bilateral.

Radiographic appearances. Irregularity of the outline of the navicular and fissure formation are early signs. Later, fragmentation and condensation with resultant increased bony density will be noted. The bone may appear as a mere dense disc and sometimes an even denser core may appear (Fig. 3.11). No loss of cartilage on either side of the bone occurs. The onset of regeneration is shown by the production of new bone round the compressed disc. Gradually, complete recovery of shape and texture of the navicular occurs, the whole process taking up to two years.

OSTEOCHONDRITIS OF THE VERTEBRAL BODY

(Synonyms: *Calvé's disease, vertebra plana*)

This condition is very rare. It is manifested by collapse and increased density of a vertebral body; the adjacent disc spaces are normal or increased in width (Fig. 3.12). Recovery to normal shape follows, but it may be incomplete.

Most cases may be shown to be a manifestation of histiocytosis. Regeneration is expected but histiocytosis may be complicated by paraplegia. Leukaemia, Ewing's sarcoma, metastases, Tb, etc. may cause similar appearances and should always be excluded before a diagnosis of Calvé's disease is accepted. Most authorities do not accept the condition of Calvé's disease as being a disease entity caused by ischaemic necrosis.

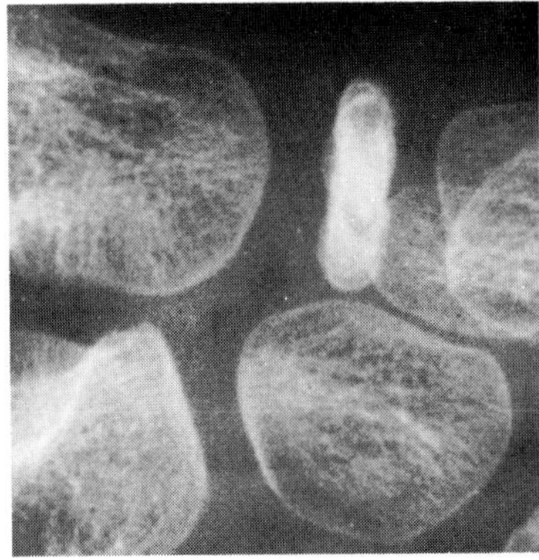

Fig. 3.11

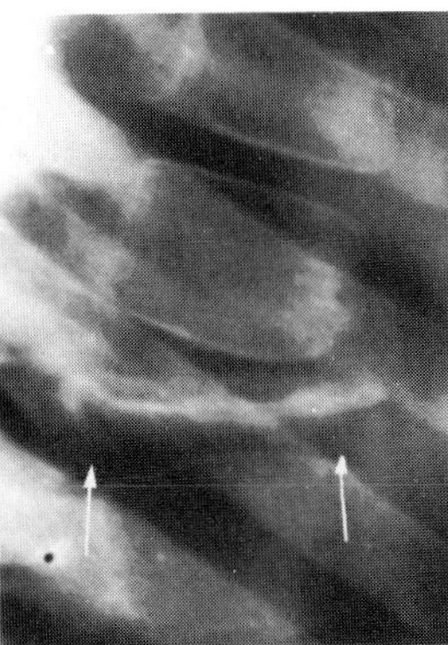

Fig. 3.12

Fig. 3.11 Osteochondritis of the tarsal navicular.

Fig. 3.12 Calvé's disease (vertebra plana) of a mid-thoracic vertebral body. Complete regeneration occurred. No evidence of histiocytosis was found on biopsy.

ADOLESCENT KYPHOSIS

(Synonyms: *vertebral epiphysitis, osteochondritis of vertebral epiphyseal plates*. Eponym: *Scheuermann's disease*)

The term adolescent kyphosis is best used since the pathogenesis is controversial. Scheuermann considered that the lesion was due to avascular necrosis of the ring apophysis. It has since been shown that the ring apophysis does not contribute to longitudinal growth of the vertebral body but acts as a site of annular and ligamentous attachment. Longitudinal growth occurs at the end-plates which differ from subarticular bone at joints elsewhere in that spongy bone lies beneath the cartilage, rather than a firm cortex. Schmorl suggested that discal herniation occurred into bony defects in the end-plates, resulting in irregularity. In addition, pre-existing osteoporosis may predispose to discal herniation.

Pathologically, no evidence of avascular necrosis is found. Discal material and cartilage are found herniated into the vertebral body (Schmorl's nodes) and the cartilage–bone interface may be completely disrupted. The anterior longitudinal ligament is markedly shortened and taut. Anterior vertebral compression follows growth plate disruption and disc narrowing, leading to progressive kyphosis.

The condition affects both sexes; it usually begins at puberty, having a peak incidence from 15 to 16 years. The mid and lower thoracic spine is the region most commonly affected and usually several adjacent vertebrae are involved (Fig. 3.13). Less frequently the lesion may be found in the lumbar spine (Fig. 3.14) and in the upper thoracic spine. Sometimes changes are confined to a single vertebra.

Radiographic appearances. Irregularity is seen affecting first the anterosuperior and anteroinferior parts of the vertebral bodies; this irregularity may spread backwards to involve the whole surface. Subjacent cancellous bone becomes crumbled and later wedging of vertebral bodies and kyphosis appear. Some scoliosis may also be seen. Schmorl's nodes are seen and disc spaces become narrowed. Sometimes a small paraspinal bulge is observed at the level of the lesion.

The radiographic picture tends to remain static for a while. Improvement is slow and consolidation may take several years. Radiographic recovery is often incomplete: various degrees of irregularity and wedging of thoracolumbar vertebrae may be permanent. Indeed, evidence of old adolescent kyphosis is one of the most frequent abnormalities seen in spinal radiographs.

Diagnosis of established cases is straightforward, but detection of early cases may not be possible and serial follow-up X-rays will be necessary. Lesions implicating single vertebrae may be mistaken for Pott's disease, and, in the past, many cases of adolescent kyphosis were treated in sanatoria, having been misdiagnosed as Pott's disease. No constitutional effects are found in adolescent kyphosis and the vertebral defects are bounded by sclerotic rims, which are not seen in tuberculous lesions. Pott's disease is often accompanied by large fusiform paravertebral swellings. Such appearances are not found in adolescent kyphosis although, in the latter, a little localized soft tissue swelling may be seen on either side of the vertebral bodies.

Residual wedging in late cases may be indistinguishable from that caused by a previous compression fracture. Such cases often perplex those engaged in medico-legal work. The ring apophysis may be displaced by discal herniation, never to unite. It is then seen as a triangular fragment of bone adjacent to the end-plate. At discography, the contrast-filled disc is shown to extend between the vertebral body and the detached fragment of bone, which is well corticated all round.

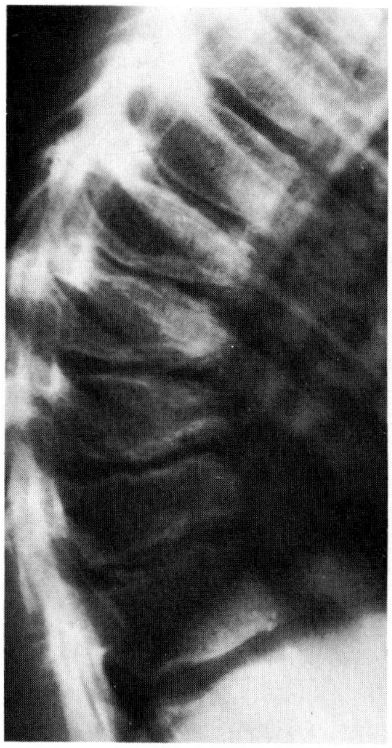

Fig. 3.13

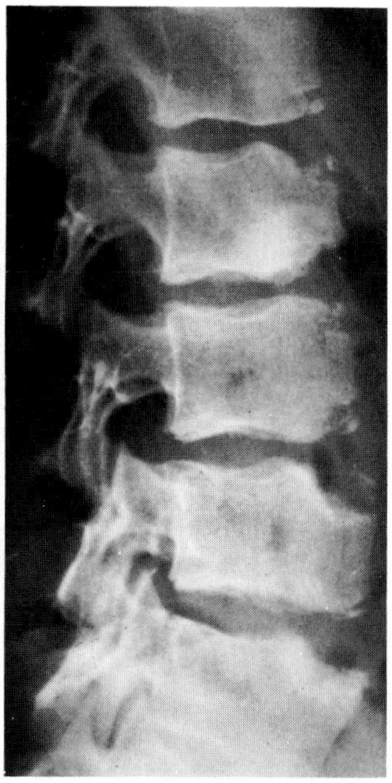

Fig. 3.14

Fig. 3.13 Adolescent kyphosis (advanced case).

Fig. 3.14 'Osteochondritis' of lumbar vertebral bodies.

OSTEOCHONDRITIS AT OTHER SITES

'Osteochondritis' of varying degrees of histological accuracy has been described in around 40 sites. The great majority are found at the hip and spine, especially if more dubious entities, such as Siever's disease and Blount's disease, are excluded.

The next most common sites are the tarsal navicular, inferior pole of the patella, metatarsal heads and in the humerus — capitellum and medial condyle, as well as olecranon.

The humeral osteochondritides are of interest in that they are post-traumatic and occur classically in juvenile baseball pitchers ('Little Leaguers'). Similar changes are not seen in cricketers, where the missile is delivered from the top of an arc, rather than being thrown.

Capitellum — Osteochondritis of the capitellum is uncommon. The radiographic pattern (Fig. 3.15 A, B and C) is similar to that of osteochondritis in other situations. It

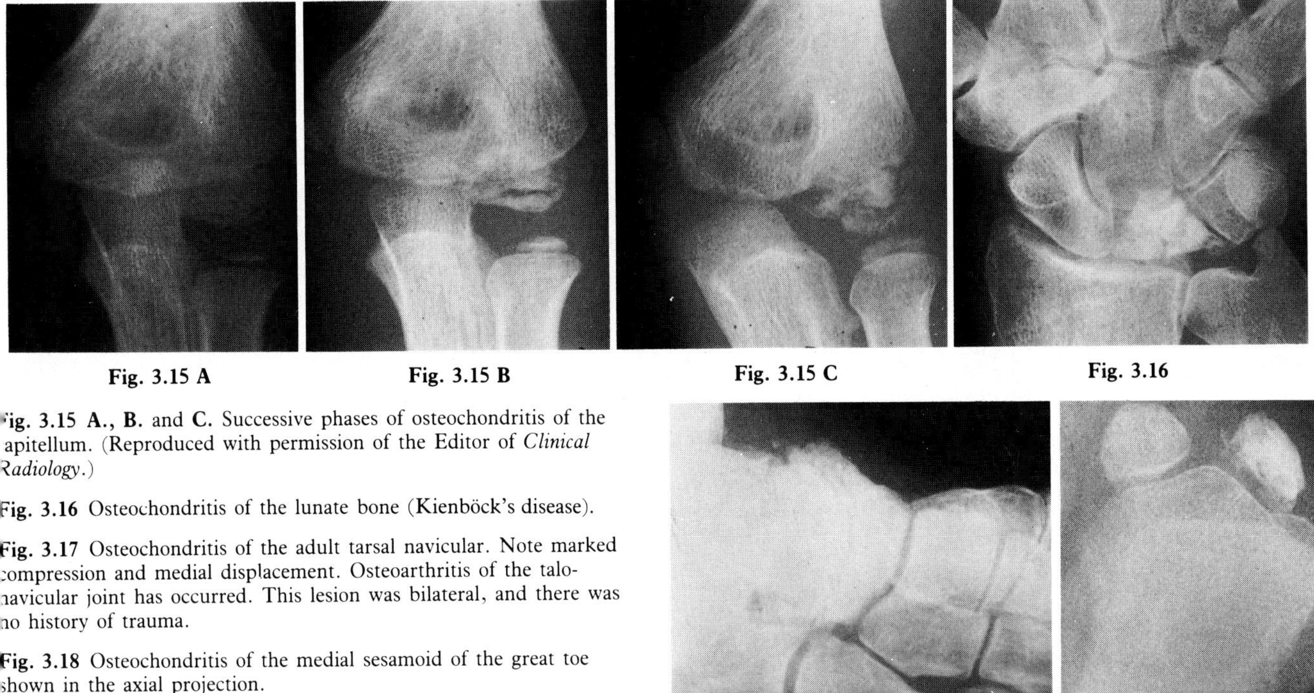

Fig. 3.15 A Fig. 3.15 B Fig. 3.15 C Fig. 3.16

Fig. 3.15 A., B. and C. Successive phases of osteochondritis of the capitellum. (Reproduced with permission of the Editor of *Clinical Radiology*.)

Fig. 3.16 Osteochondritis of the lunate bone (Kienböck's disease).

Fig. 3.17 Osteochondritis of the adult tarsal navicular. Note marked compression and medial displacement. Osteoarthritis of the talonavicular joint has occurred. This lesion was bilateral, and there was no history of trauma.

Fig. 3.18 Osteochondritis of the medial sesamoid of the great toe shown in the axial projection.

Fig. 3.17 Fig. 3.18

is not always possible to differentiate the condition from osteochondritis dissecans of the capitellum.

Patella — primary centre (Köhler's disease). This is a difficult diagnosis to make because the patella normally ossifies in an irregular manner. There may be differences in mineralization of the two patellae in asymptomatic children. Consequently, a diagnosis of osteochondritis of the primary ossification centre of the patella must be primarily clinical.

Secondary centre (Sinding-Larsen's disease). This is a fairly common lesion affecting an accessory ossification centre for the lower pole of the patella. Some are associated with Osgood-Schlatter's disease. This condition is also almost always due to an avulsion strain by the patellar ligament.

Tibia vara (osteochondritis of the medial tibial condyle — Blount's disease). This change may be seen from the first to the twelfth year of age, but is most common in the earlier age group. As the name implies, the abnormality is usually to be seen on the medial aspect of the knee joint. An irregular defect is often present on the medial aspect of the proximal tibial metaphysis beneath which a large and prominent spur sticks out, almost at right-angles. The adjacent aspect of the tibial epiphysis may be defective, and a local femoral spur may also be seen. The overall effect is a varus deformity. The lateral aspect of the proximal tibial metaphysis is straight, and not bowed as in physiological bow legs. Occasionally the defect is found laterally resulting in tibia valga, with a lateral spur.

The changes are possibly related to early onset of walking, with excessive pressure on the medial and posterior aspects of the proximal tibia because of the obliquity of the femur on the tibia.

OSTEOCHONDRITIS IN ADULT BONES

Often a closer link with trauma is seen in adult osteochondritis than in juvenile cases, but this is not always so. Such sites subject to trauma include the *scaphoid*, the *carpal lunate* (Kienbock's disease) (Fig. 3.16), the *tarsal navicular* (Fig. 3.17), and the *medial sesamoid bone of the great toe* (Fig. 3.18).

OSTEOCHONDRITIS DISSECANS

In this condition fragments of articular cartilage, with or without subchondral bone, become partially or completely detached at characteristic sites. The separated fragment is avascular in contradistinction to that at an osteochondral fracture, and the 'bed' of the defect remains vital, in contradistinction to avascular necrosis.

Sites of election are the medial femoral condyle, the capitellum of the humerus and the trochlear surface of the talus. Other sites include the lateral femoral condyle, the patella, the femoral head, the shoulder and the head of a metatarsal, especially the first. The lesion is twice as common in males as females and about one third of all cases are bilateral. In some patients several epiphyses are affec-

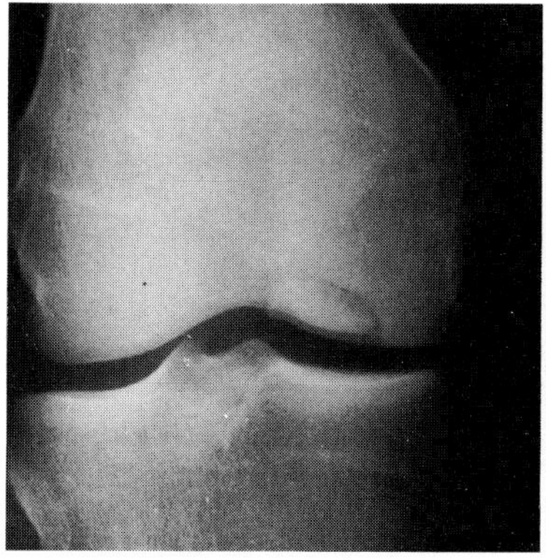

Fig. 3.19 A

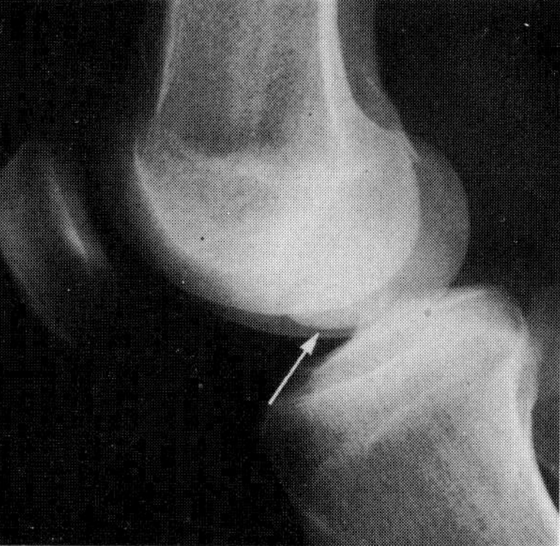

Fig. 3.19 B

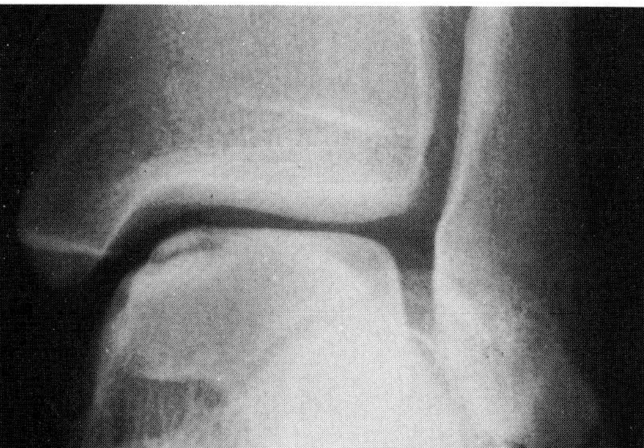

Fig. 3.20

Fig. 3.19 (**A** and **B**) Osteochondritis dissecans of the medial femoral condyle (AP and lateral views).

Fig. 3.20 Osteochondritis dissecans of the medial part of the articular surface of the talus.

ted. The condition is not always symptomatic. The lesion characteristically occurs in adolescence and early adult life though it may be found in middle and in old age. It is the commonest cause of a loose body in the joint of a young adult.

The present tendency is to emphasize the role of trauma in the aetiology of this lesion. Aichroth noted a history of frank trauma in many, a history of high athletic achievement in others and mechanical abnormalities of the knee in some. The other school of thought believes the condition to be due to cartilaginous softening secondary to vascular occlusion. It is probable that trauma is responsible for most cases, but not all.

Radiographic features. In early cases it may be necessary to take several views of the joint in different degrees of obliquity in order to demonstrate the lesion adequately. Tomography is often helpful, particularly in lesions involving the elbow where often the patient cannot fully extend the joint. Arthrography also is often useful.

When separation of the fragment is being established, one will see a radiolucent ring surrounding the bony fragment when viewed 'en face'; the loosening fragment may be seen opposite a pit in the bone when viewed 'en profile' (Figs. 3.19A and B, 3.20). The loose fragments are usually small and ovoid in shape though they may be larger and irregular (Fig. 3.21).

The fragment may become completely separated and form an intra-articular loose body. If entirely cartilaginous in content, the image of the loose body will not be seen on routine radiographs but it may be demonstrable by arthrography. If not removed surgically, the loose body may grow and calcify later; it is able to obtain adequate nourishment from synovial fluid even when it is completely detached from its parent bone. On the other hand, the fragment may not become free, but it may become incorporated in the parent bone or it may become absorbed leaving a residual gap in the underlying bone.

CAISSON DISEASE

(Synonym: *dysbaric osteonecrosis*)

Exposure to a hyperbaric atmosphere, whether working in a caisson in tunnel construction or in deep sea diving, may result in decompression sickness — 'the bends' — and in the late complication of osteonecrosis. The lesions are liable to appear if the worker is too rapidly decompressed. It is thought that nitrogen becomes liberated from bone marrow in which it is held in high concentration due to its solubility in fat. Bubbles of liberated nitrogen cause bone infarcts by occluding small blood vessels. The subject has naturally become very important of late in Britain and in other countries because of extensive oil exploration.

It was believed up to relatively recently that bone changes occurred only in those workers who had experi-

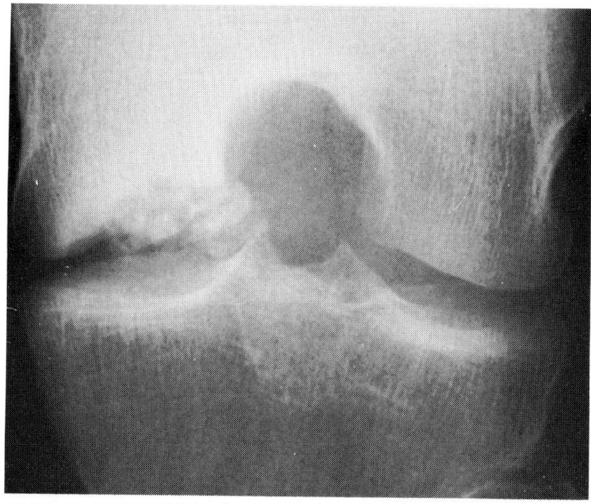

Fig. 3.21 Osteochondritis dissecans of medial femoral condyle. The lesion is larger than usual.

nced decompression sickness. However, it is now known hat a history of previous decompression sickness is not necessary for the occurrence of osteonecrosis.

Radiographic findings. Lesions may be juxta-articular or in the head, neck or shaft of a bone. The juxta-articular lesions may be asymptomatic when first seen or they may later cause symptoms. The lesions in the head and neck or shaft of a bone are asymptomatic.

1. Juxta-articular lesions — these are seen most commonly in the humerus, sometimes in the upper end of the femur but never around the knee or other joints. They are recognized as:

(a) Dense areas on the articular cortex (Fig. 3.22).

(b) Spherical, blotchy opacities near the articular cortex.

(c) A linear opacity on the periphery of the humeral head that may affect two thirds of the joint surface, though it is generally smaller (Fig. 3.23).

(d) A transradiant subcortical band that may underlie as much as two thirds of the articular cortex (Fig. 3.24).

(e) Collapse of part of the articular cortex.

(f) Sequestration of part of the cortex.

(g) Secondary osteoarthritis (Fig. 3.25).

2. Head, neck and shaft lesions are most frequently seen in the lower ends of the femoral and tibial shafts. They cause the following appearances:

(a) Dense areas — small, multiple, bilateral, ill-defined opacities resembling bone islands in the upper ends of the femoral and humeral shafts and in the femoral neck.

(b) Irregular calcified areas — typical in the distal part of the femoral shafts (Fig. 3.26) and in the proximal parts of the shafts of the humeri and tibiae.

Malignant changes have rarely been reported in such infarcts, usually in the form of malignant fibrous histiocytoma (Fig. 3.27).

(c) Transradiant areas that may be corticated — in the head and neck of the humerus and in the femoral neck.

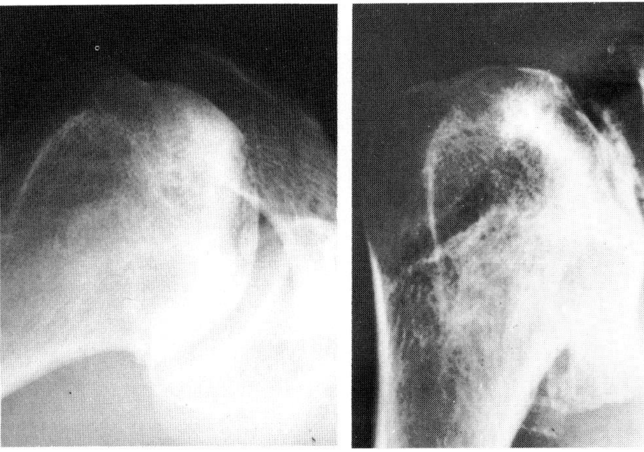

Fig. 3.24 **Fig. 3.25**

Fig. 3.24 Caisson disease. The humeral head shows a subcortical band of radiolucency with underlying sclerosis. The articular surface is collapsing.

Fig. 3.25 Caisson disease: gross secondary osteoarthritis.

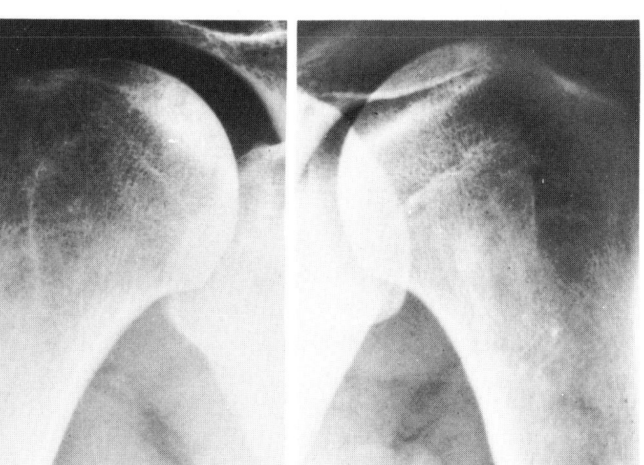

Fig. 3.22 **Fig. 3.23**

Fig. 3.22 Caisson disease: subarticular sclerotic areas.

Fig. 3.23 Caisson disease: subarticular dense band.

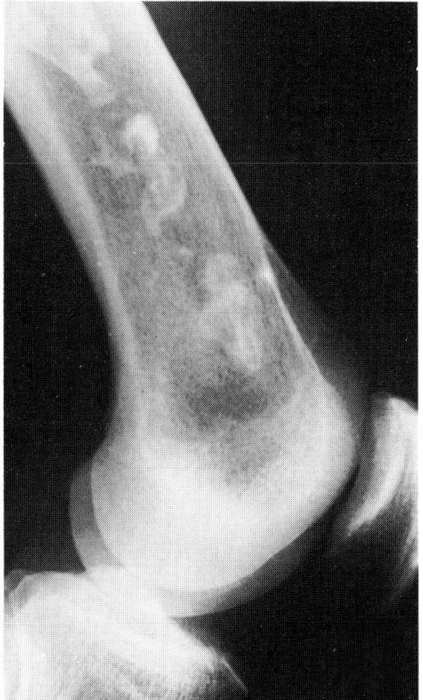

Fig. 3.26 Caisson disease.

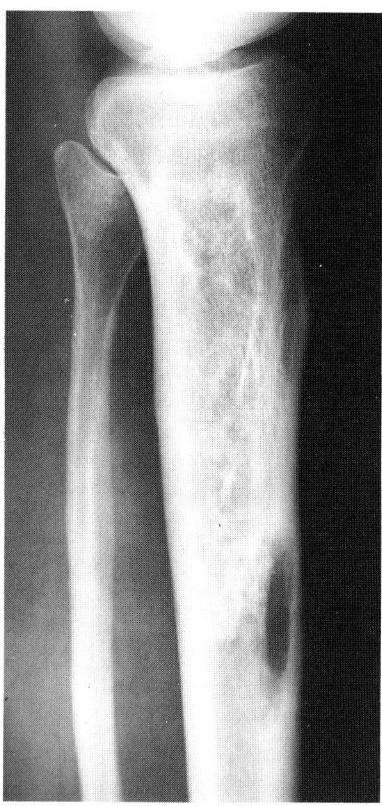

Fig. 3.27 Changes of medullary infarction are associated with an area of osteolysis due to fibrosarcoma.

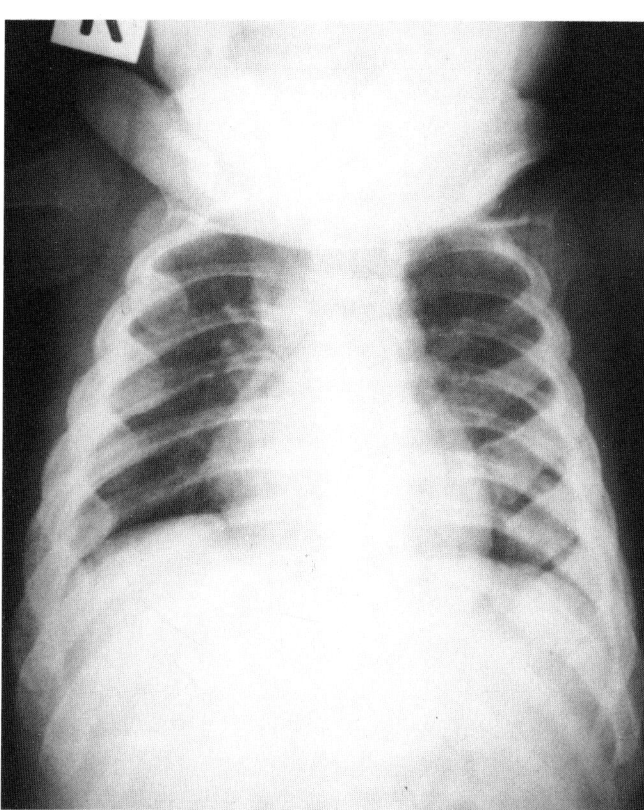

Fig. 3.28 Caffey's disease. Gross periostitis affects the ribs and the mandible is also thickened. (Courtesy of Dr Ann Barrington, Sheffield.)

INFANTILE CORTICAL HYPEROSTOSIS (CAFFEY'S DISEASE)

The cause of this disease is unknown. Many affected children have high fever, most have raised sedimentation rates and occasionally pleural exudates are found. However, an infective agent has never been identified. Occasionally the disease has been reported in siblings, cousins and twins.

The condition has been diagnosed *in utero*. Usually, however, the babies are well for several weeks before the onset. The average age at onset is 9 weeks and cases do not apparently start after the age of 5 months.

Three features common to all these patients are hyperirritability, soft tissue swelling and bony cortical thickening. The soft tissue swellings may be very painful, but are deeply situated and not accompanied by surface warmth or discolouration. Such swellings appear before bony changes are demonstrable and they disappear long before the bone lesions resolve. Sometimes the swellings may recur at their original site or new swellings may appear at other sites. The disease is characterized by the patchy distribution of the lesions and by remissions and relapses.

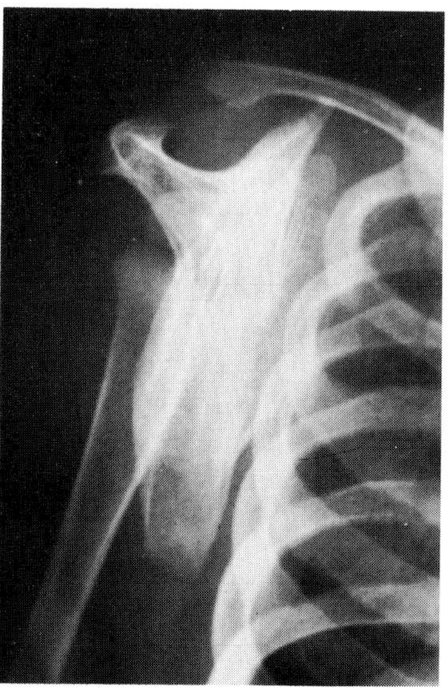

Fig. 3.29 Infantile cortical hyperostosis: massive cortical thickening of the scapula. (Courtesy of Mr T. McSweeney.)

Bones commonly affected are the *mandible*, *ribs* (Fig. 3.28), *clavicle*, *scapula* (Fig. 3.29) and the *ulna*, but any tubular bones except the phalanges may be affected. The condition may also be found in the *skull* and *pelvis* but not in the spine. Lesions are confined to the shafts of the bones, and the epiphyses and metaphyses are not affected. This distribution affords a ready differentiation from rickets, scurvy and congenital syphilis.

Radiologically, marked periosteal proliferation and cortical thickening are seen in bones beneath the soft tissue swellings. The cortical hyperostosis may be massive. Patients usually recover after several weeks or months; in about 12 months bones will usually have returned to normal.

Caffey also describes a chronic form in which symptoms and signs may persist for some years. Even in these, complete recovery is the rule, though in some there may be residual deformities. Cross-union may be found in paired bones.

The diagnosis is made from the symptoms, radiological features and distribution of the lesions. Should an individual bone be affected, however, the diagnosis from inflammatory and neoplastic lesions would be difficult. Differential diagnoses include unrecognized skeletal trauma, syphilis and hypervitaminosis A.

PROGERIA

This is an extremely rare condition of unknown aetiology. Affected infants and children have retarded development and premature old age, and they rapidly resemble old wizened dwarfs. All are similar; there are no gradations of this condition.

Radiological findings. The long bones are thin and slender and constricted in places (Fig. 3.30). The clavicles are small and may shrink and completely disappear. The fontanelles of the skull remain open. Wormian bones and hypoplasia of the maxillae and mandibles are usual findings.

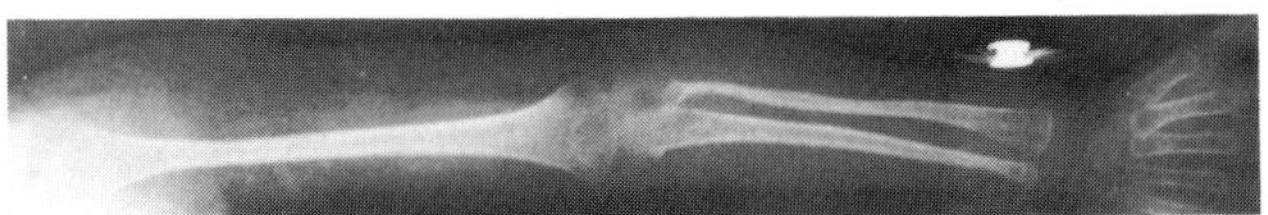

Fig. 3.30 Progeria: very thin slender bones showing some constrictions. (Courtesy of Dr P. P. Franklyn.)

Atrophy of the distal phalanges of the fingers and toes is seen. Cross-union may be found in paired bones. Much vascular calcification is frequently seen.

PAGET'S DISEASE
(Synonym: *osteitis deformans*)

Sir James Paget first described this disease in 1876. Its origin is not definitely known. Nonetheless current thinking is that a 'slow' virus may be the initiating factor. Though no virus has been isolated, histological changes are seen that are present in viral infections.

There is variation in the distribution of the disease. It is common in the United Kingdom, parts of the United States, Australia and New Zealand, but uncommon in the Far and Middle East and Scandinavia. Within Britain there appear to be some regional differences in the incidence, while in Australia the incidence seems to be related to recent immigration, the disease being more common in first generation Australians. There is an increased familial incidence but this could be compatible either with a viral aetiology or a familial predisposition.

The incidence of the disease as judged by pathological and radiological surveys in 3–4% of the population. Men are slightly more affected than women. Paget's disease is predominantly found in the elderly. Monostotic disease is not common, its incidence being 10–20%. Overall, the condition is found most commonly in the sacrum and lumbar spine, followed by the skull, pelvis and right femur. Apart from the skull, the weight-bearing and persisting red marrow areas are most commonly involved, though multiple rib and upper limb lesions are uncommon. No bone is exempt. Lesions of the fibula are very rare.

The radiographic appearances are explained by the underlying pathological processes.

1. An initial phase of increased osteoclastic activity results in bone resorption. This early phase is osteolytic and is not commonly seen radiologically; still less in established disease. It may persist in the skull, as osteoporosis circumscripta (Fig. 3.31), possibly because the vault is non-weight-bearing. Radio-isotope scanning is at this stage more sensitive that conventional radiology. The bone at this stage is soft and brittle.

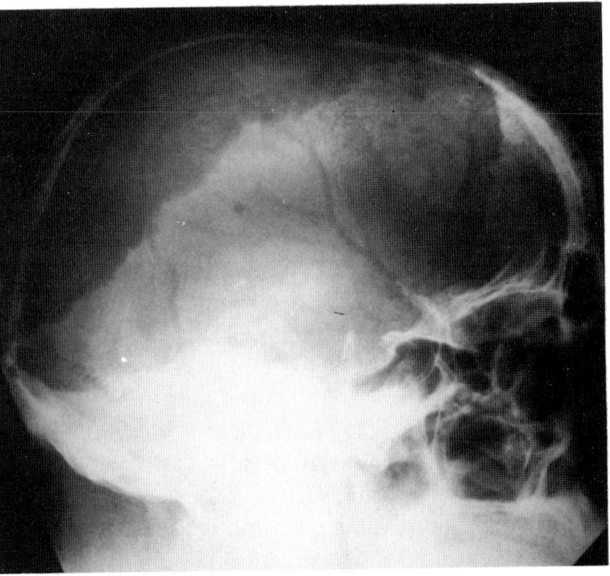

Fig. 3.31 Osteoporosis circumscripta. A well-defined osteolytic lesion affects most of the skull vault.

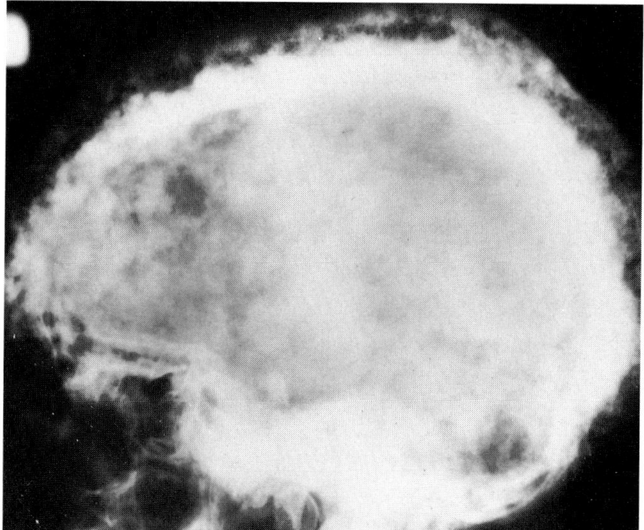

Fig. 3.32 Paget's disease of skull: marked thickening of calvarium. Note the well-demarcated intracranial border of the inner table. Marked sclerosis of the base of the skull is also present.

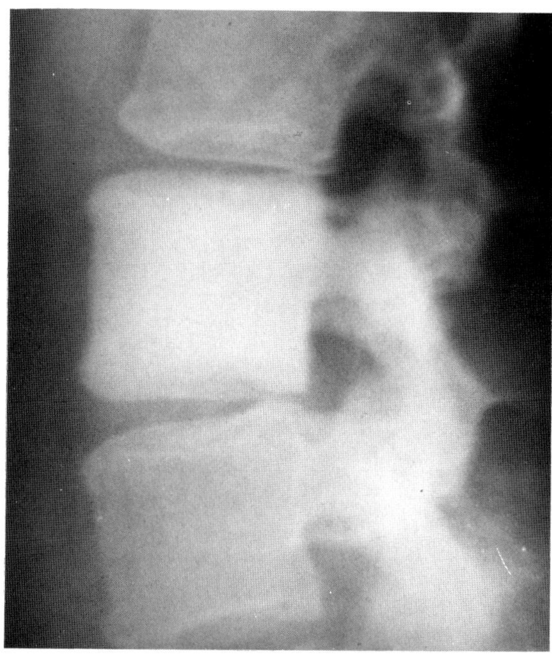

Fig. 3.33 Paget's disease: increase in size and density of a lumbar vertebral body which shows pure sclerosis.

2. Mixed phase (spongy type with coarse irregular trabeculation). Increased resorption of bone is followed by increased formation of abnormally coarsened trabeculae of increased volume (Fig. 3.32). Haversian systems are destroyed and replaced by new bone with a characteristic mosaic pattern. The margin between cortex and medulla is lost. Even newly laid down bone is rapidly resorbed, but Paget's bone is usually sharply demarcated from normal bone.

3. Sclerotic phase (amorphous appearance) (Fig. 3.33). Osteoclastic activity declines and osteoblastic activity proceeds so that disorganised new bone of increased density replaces lytic areas. Eventually osteoblastic activity and blood flow also decline and the disease becomes quiescent. At this stage radio-isotope studies may not be positive.

Isotopic bone scanning is thus of value during early activity when it will pick up lesions which may not be radiologically detectable, while in the quiescent phase the presence of disease is best shown by conventional means. The total body scan detects disease in sites not routinely examined, such as the foot, but such sites are not commonly affected. The scan does however provide a quick overview of the skeleton and is useful in assessing change or malignant degeneration, so that follow-up is probably best performed by scanning. Changes in distribution and qualitative changes in uptake in individual bones may indicate healing or presage onset of malignant disease, fractures or arthritis. Such areas can then be examined conventionally.

Radiological features. *Long bones.* The lesion is almost always seen extending to one end of a long bone however much the diaphysis is affected (Fig. 3.34). The diagnosis of Paget's disease should not be made in the absence of subarticular involvement. One exception to this rule is in the tibia, where the anterior cortex is the site of disease extending to the tibial tubercle (Fig. 3.35). The fibula is rarely involved.

Paget's disease thus seems to start at the site of previous epiphyses or apophyses and as it extends to the other bone end it is demarcated from normal bone by a V-shaped zone of transition (Fig. 3.34). Sometimes the advancing front of the lesion may cause an oval, cystic appearance, e.g. in the anterior cortex of the tibia.

Long bones increase in cortical width and the femur and tibia may be bowed. Bones also increase in length and this may result in bowing if only one of paired long bones is affected. Paget's disease may cause more bony enlargement than is seen in any other disease.

Pelvis. In early stages slight loss of normal trabeculation with coarsening of those remaining may be seen, but often the change is subtle. Thickening and loss of clarity of the ileo-pectineal line and the teardrop also indicate the disease. The pelvis is often enlarged, especially in the ischiopubic regions. Narrowing of the hip joint space, especially in a medial direction, leads to protrusio with deformity of the pelvic brim. Secondary osteoarthritis then develops (Fig. 3.36).

Vertebrae. All three forms of the disease may be found in the vertebrae. The neural arch and pedicles may be involved as well as the vertebral body, and all parts are enlarged. The width of the body is increased and so is thus the interpedicular distance, even if the pedicles are en-

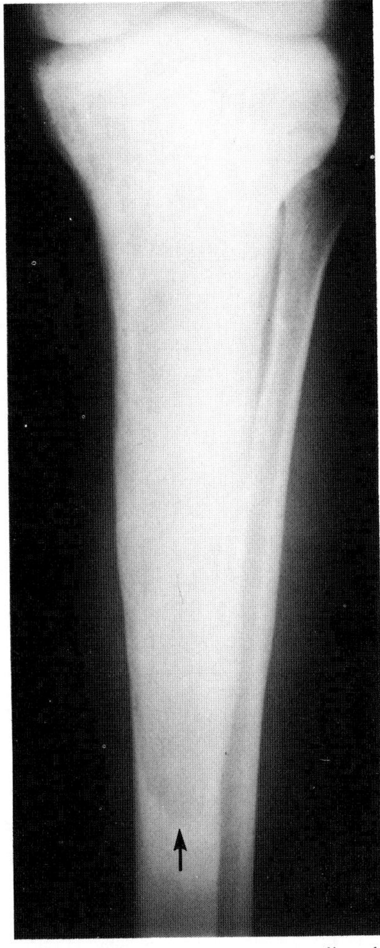

Fig. 3.34 Paget's disease. Changes are seen extending downwards from the proximal tibia, ending with a flame-shaped border (↑).

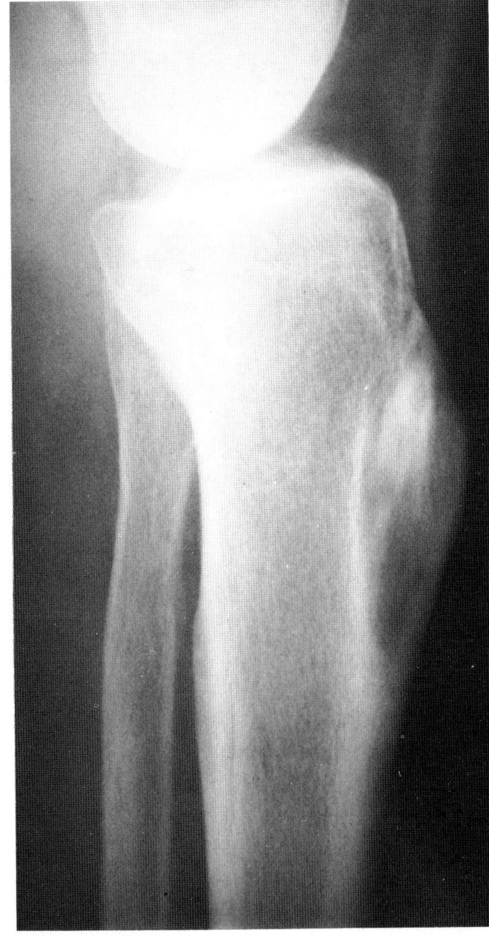

Fig. 3.35 Paget's disease is confined to the region of the tibial tubercle.

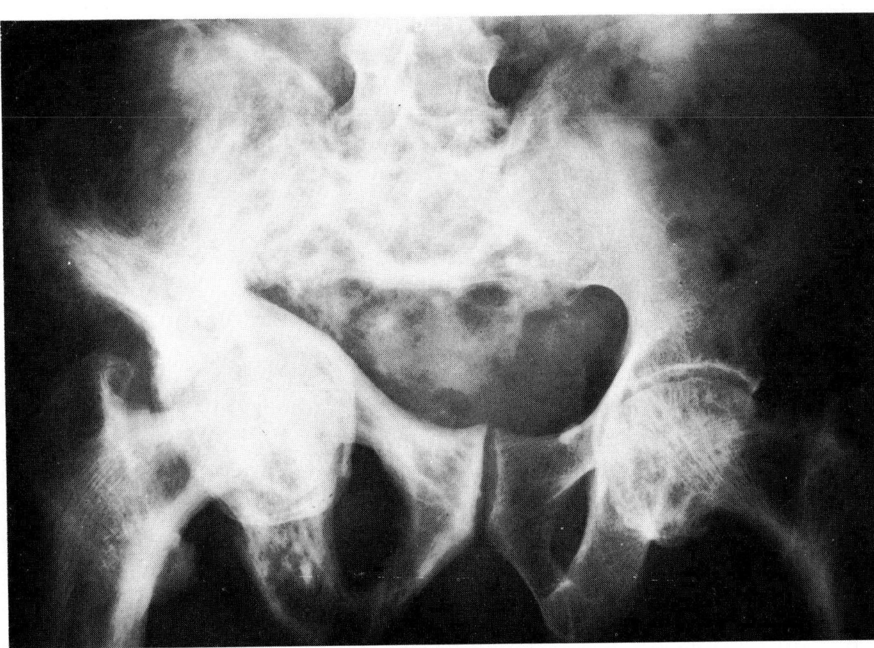

Fig. 3.36 Pelvis in Paget's disease. There is a combination of spongy and amorphous bone. Note the striated appearance of the left femoral head and neck. Marked deformity of the pelvic inlet and acetabular protrusion on the right side are shown. There is enlargement of the right pubis and ischium.

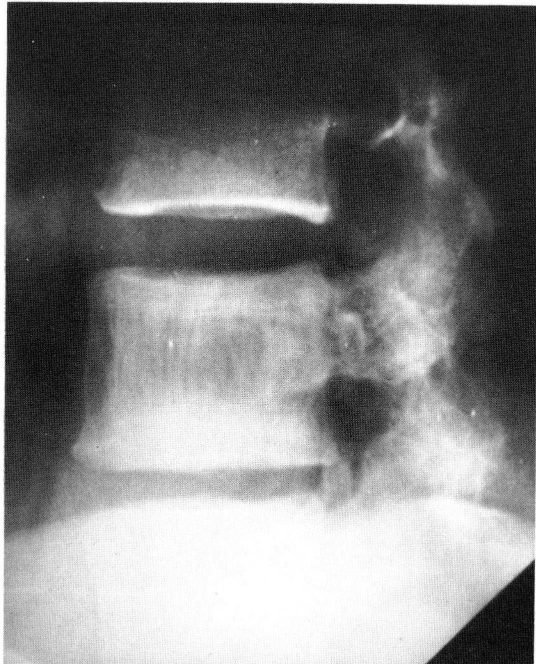

Fig. 3.37 Picture-frame appearance in a vertebral body witth Paget's disease. The appendages are also enlarged.

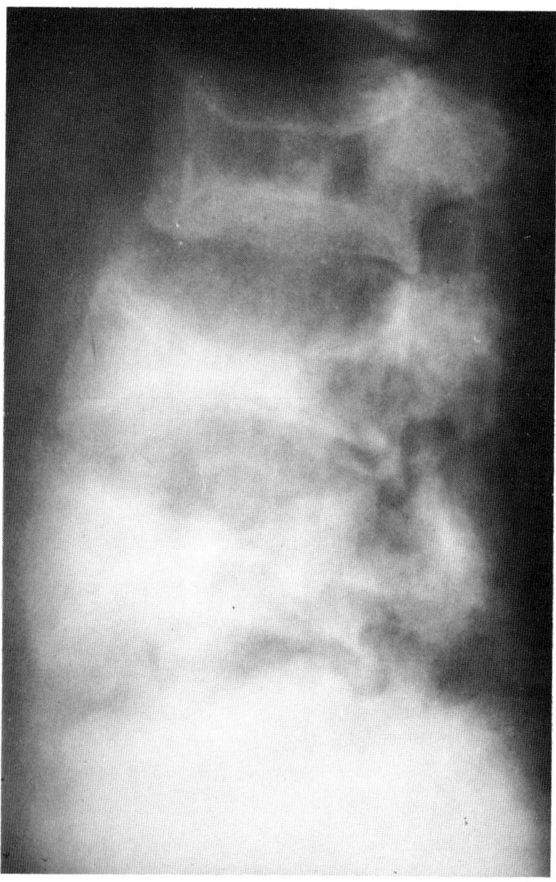

Fig. 3.38 Paget's disease: vertebral collapse and expansion together with abnormal bone texture.

larged. A characteristic, if infrequent, finding is a picture frame appearance with condensed thickened end-plates and vertebral margins enclosing a cystic spongiosa (Fig. 3.37). The condensed end plates are not seen with haemangioma and involvement of posterior elements is also less common. Enlargement is unusual in both haemangiomas and metastatic disease.

Collapse is common and may cause spinal nerve compression. This is due to bone softening. Vertebral enlargement distinguishes this from osteoporotic or malignant disease (Fig. 3.38).

Skull. In the skull the disease begins as a destructive process affecting the outer table and sparing the inner table (Fig. 3.31). The full picture of osteoporosis circumscripta is rarely seen. In the reparative stage, sclerosis of the inner table is pronounced and later the diploic spaces and the outer table become thickened. A classic, widespread cotton wool effect results (Fig. 3.32). The cranial cavity is not encroached upon.

Dental abnormalities include loss of lamina dura and hypercementosis (see Ch. 52).

Complications of Paget's disease

A. *Marginal (incremental) or incomplete transverse fractures.* These fractures resemble pseudofractures in osteomalacia, but are found in different sites. They are usually found on the thickened convex surface of the bowed bone where they may be multiple (Fig. 3.39). The edges are jagged and sclerosed. They may heal at the surface. Occasionally such a fracture may become complete (see below). These lesions may actually be the site of a dilated perforating periosteal artery supplying the hypervascular bone.

B. *Pathological fractures* are the commonest complication of Paget's disease and are most often seen in the early stages of the disease. Usually transverse, they are more common in women (Fig. 3.40). Often multiple, they are most common in the upper femur and upper tibia. Callus forms around the pathological fracture and shows features of Paget's disease. The distal bone becomes intensely demineralised until union occurs, but healing is poorer in Paget's disease than in normal bone. Sarcoma may follow a pathological fracture or be revealed by it.

Bone may also be avulsed at sites of muscle insertions.

C. *Osteoarthritis* occurs at major joints (see above). Paget's disease does not generally cause much pain but the onset of degenerative joint disease may be painful. Neoplastic disease must then also be excluded.

D. *Skull complications.* Cranial nerve palsies result when foramina are encroached upon. The second, fifth, seventh and eighth nerves are especially involved. Vascular compromise also causes blindness. Deafness may result from involvement of the ossicles or cochlea or compression of the eighth nerve.

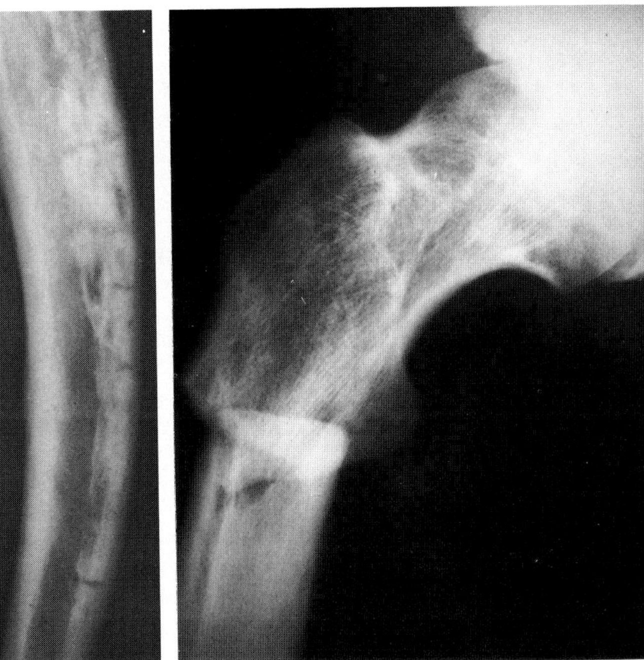

Fig. 3.39 Fig. 3.40

Fig. 3.39 Paget's disease, showing multiple cortical marginal fractures.

Fig. 3.40 Paget's disease. A transverse fracture affects the pathological bone.

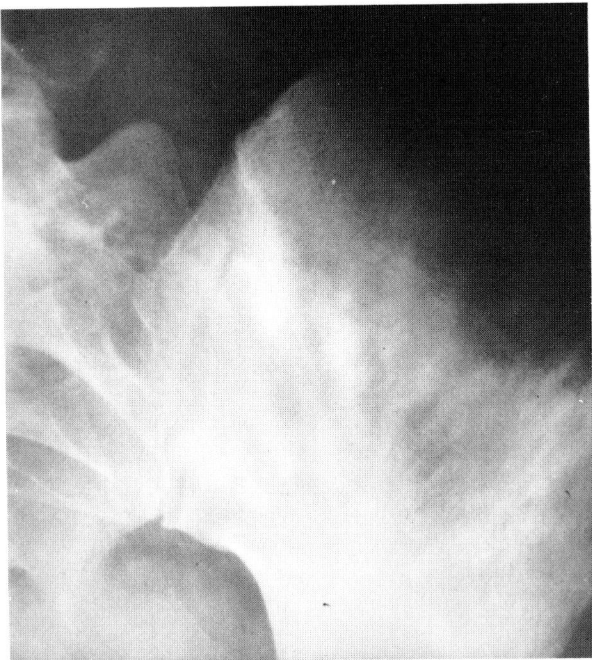

Fig. 3.41 Tuberous sclerosis: flame-shaped areas of sclerosis in the iliac blades.

Basilar invagination may cause brain stem compression. CSF obstruction can lead to hydrocephalus. Stretching of vertebral arteries may give rise to vertebro-basilar insufficiency.

E. *Cardiovascular complications*. In early phases of the disease bone is hypervascular. Cardiac output is increased and, if much of the skeleton is actively involved, cardiomegaly, cardiac ischaemia and high output failure result. Systemic hypertension and calcification of the media of the arteries also result. These phenomena are not purely due to the age at which Paget's disease occurs but are related to the extent of the disease and its activity.

F. *Malignant degeneration*. Osteogenic sarcoma and, to a lesser extent, fibrosarcoma, chondrosarcoma and malignant fibrous histiocytoma may arise as complications of Paget's disease (see Ch. 5, p. 157).

Differential diagnosis. Most difficulties arise in monostatic cases. Sometimes a full bone survey will reveal evidence of Paget's disease elsewhere, but often it will prove negative. A solitary dense vertebra or vertebra nigra may cause diagnostic difficulties because osteosclerotic metastases and reticuloses can cause identical appearances. The amorphous type of Paget's disease in the pelvis, especially if little bone enlargement is evident, may be difficult to differentiate from prostatic secondaries. Elevation of the serum acid phosphatase will be found in the latter lesion. The diagnostic difficulties may be compounded by second-

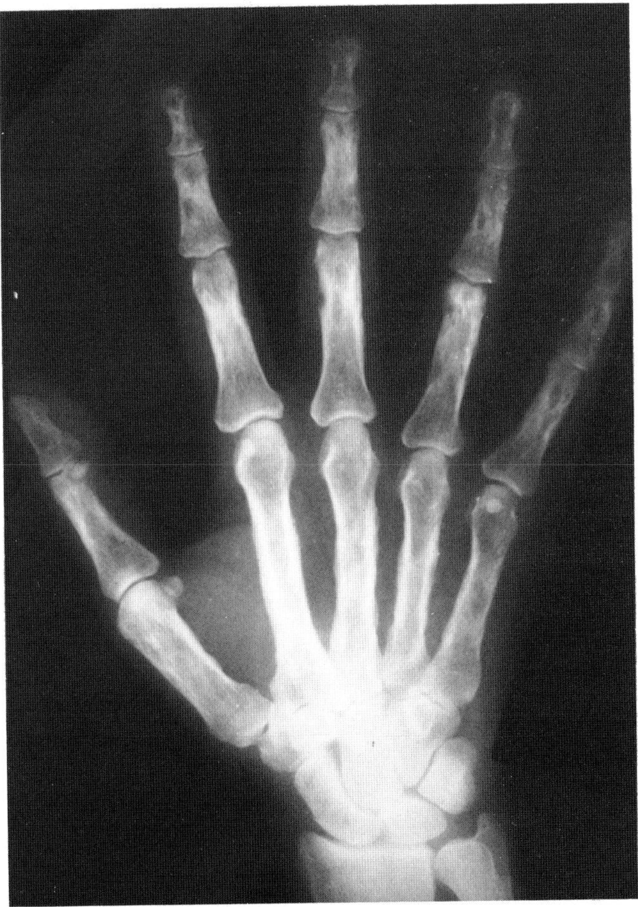

Fig. 3.42 Tuberous sclerosis — hands: cyst-like defects are seen in the bones, both beneath the fingernails and more proximally. Cortical defects and periostitis are also present.

ary deposits that occasionally cause much enlargement of bone.

The spongy type of Paget's disease seldom causes diagnostic difficulties. Rarely it may resemble hyperparathyroidism and renal osteodystrophy. An angioma of a vertebral body may resemble Paget's disease, but an angioma will not produce the typical widening of the bone seen in Paget's disease. In difficult cases, a bone survey may show evidence of Paget's disease in other sites.

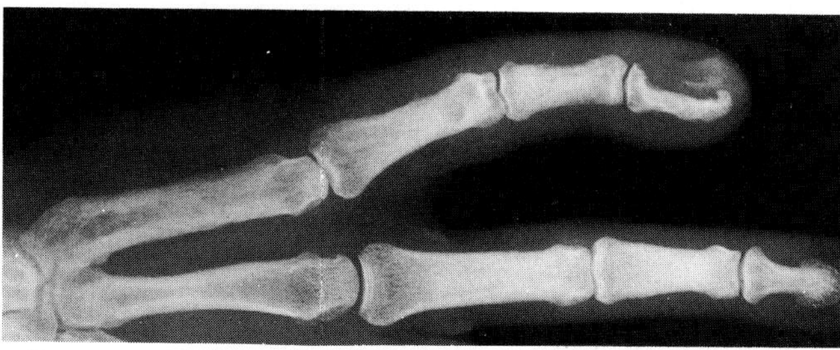

Fig. 3.43 Tuberous sclerosis. Note periosteal thickening of fifth metacarpal, cysts in head of proximal phalanx and pressure erosion of distal phalanx by subungual tumour. (Courtesy of Dr L. Langton.)

LEONTIASIS OSSEA

This term is used in two senses; specifically for an isolated progressive sclerosing hyperostosis of the skull, and descriptively when diseases such as Paget's disease and fibrous dysplasia affect the skull and facial bones. Whether or not the condition is ever a specific entity is debatable. It could well be that the isolated lesion is really a form of fibrous dysplasia.

TUBEROUS SCLEROSIS

(Synonym: *epiloia*. Eponyms: *von Recklinghausen 1862*, *Bourneville 1880*)

The classical clinical manifestations are a triad of epilepsy, mental retardation and adenoma sebaceum. The disease is inherited as an autosomal dominant condition but most cases are sporadic. Pathologically, hamartomas are formed in many of the body tissues, brain, eyes, lungs, kidneys and gastrointestinal tract.

In the skeleton, the commonest finding is that of poorly defined areas of sclerosis, affecting the skull, spine and pelvis. In the skull, woolly areas of density may be due to osteosclerosis, or to tuberous calcifications within the brain. CT scanning rapidly differentiates between the two. Sclerosis also affects vertebral bodies. In the pelvis, the iliac blades are the sites of flame-shaped densities which do not resemble metastases (Fig. 3.41), or more nodular densities which do simulate malignancy.

Periostitis may be found on long bones, metatarsals and, to a lesser extent, metacarpals. In the hands, rather than the feet, cysts occur in phalanges (Fig. 3.42). These may be related to subungual fibromas and are well demarcated (Fig. 3.43).

REFERENCES AND SUGGESTIONS FOR FURTHER READING

Aichroth, P. (1971) Osteochondritis dissecans of the knee — a clinical survey. *Journal of Bone and Joint Surgery*, **55B**, 440–447.

Catterall, A. (1971) The natural history of Perthes' disease. *Journal of Bone and Joint Surgery*, **53B**, 37–53.

Catterall, A. (1982) *Legg-Calvé-Perthes' Disease*. London: Churchill Livingstone.

Davidson, J. K. (Ed) (1975) *Aseptic Necrosis of Bone*. Amsterdam: Excerpta Medica.

Edeiken, J., Hodes, P. J., Libshitz, H. L. & Weller, M. H. (1967) Bone ischaemia. *Radiologic Clinics of North America*, Vol. V (No. 3), 515–529.

Fisher, R. L., Roderique, J. W., Brown, D. C., Danigelis, J. A., Ozonoff, M. B. & Sziklas, J. J. (1980) The relationship of isotopic bone imaging guiding the prognosis in Legg-Perthes' disease. *Clinical Orthopaedics*, **150**, 23–29.

Hamdy, R. C. (1981) *Paget's Disease of Bone*. New York: Praeger.

Harrison, M. H. M. H., Turner, M. H. & Jacobs, P. (1976) Skeletal immaturity in Perthes' disease. *Journal of Bone and Joint Surgery*, **58B**, 37–40.

McCallum, R. I. & Walder, D. N. (1966) Bone lesions in compressed air workers. *Journal of Bone and Joint Surgery*, **48B**, 207–235.

Murray, R. O. & Jacobson, H. G. (1977) *The Radiology of Skeletal Disorders*. 2nd edn. Edinburgh: Churchill Livingstone.

Resnick, D. & Niwayama, G. (1981) *Diagnosis of Bone and Joint Disorders*. Philadelphia: W. B. Saunders.

Serafini, A. N. (1976) Paget's disease of bone. *Seminars in Nuclear Medicine*, **VI**, 47–58.

CHAPTER 4

DISEASES OF JOINTS: ARTHROGRAPHY

LESIONS OF JOINTS

RHEUMATOID ARTHRITIS

The diagnosis of rheumatoid arthritis is essentially clinical. Diagnostic criteria have been laid down by the American Rheumatism Association. Classic radiological change of bone loss around involved joints is not necessarily present at the onset of symptoms and a few patients (5–10%) do not develop this change in the first three years of the disease. In most cases, however, radiological change is evident within six months of the onset, possibly modified by treatment and activity. The disease is seen at all ages, but especially from 20–55 years, with smaller peaks in childhood and in the elderly. One type may have an acute onset with lesions affecting many peripheral joints and with systemic upset. A more insidious type may involve fewer joints, often the larger central joints. Prognosis may be related to the levels of rheumatoid factor, those with lower titres having a better outcome. Women are more commonly affected (M:F = 1:3).

The joints most typically involved are the small joints, especially the metatarso-phalangeal and metacarpo-phalangeal and carpal joints, but any joint, including the temporo-mandibular and cricoarytenoid may be affected. The axial skeleton is later and less often affected, with the exception of the cervical spine. Sites of ligamentous and tendinous insertions (entheses) are also infrequently involved. The tendency at the peripheral joints is to symmetry and often identical digits on either side of the body are affected. Asymmetry of distribution may follow unilateral paralysis or weakness, when under-utilization of a limb may prevent the onset of rheumatoid disease in that limb. Conversely, asymmetry may follow over-use of a limb which often is more severely involved. This is seen especially in males and in those performing heavy manual occupations. In general, excess physical activity leads to more severe forms of joint disease.

Radiological findings

Joint changes may be summarized as follows:

1. Soft tissue changes
2. Osteoporosis
3. Joint space changes and alignment deformities
4. Periostitis
5. Erosions
6. Secondary osteoarthritis

Changes 1,2,4 and 5 may be seen at entheses, that is, metabolically active sites of ligamentous and tendinous insertions into bone. Rheumatoid arthritis is a systemic disease, and other body systems may be involved, e.g. lung parenchyma and pleura.

1. SOFT TISSUE CHANGES. These changes are best assessed clinically but may also be shown radiologically in the hand (Fig. 4.1), knee or foot and other joints. Soft tissue swelling is due to oedema of periarticular tissues and synovial inflammation in bursae, joint spaces and along tendon sheaths. Joint distention also follows an increase in synovial fluid.

In the hand, fusiform swelling due to capsular distention and local oedema may be seen over the interphalangeal joints and over the second and fifth metacarpophalangeal joints. Soft tissue swelling over the third and fourth metacarpophalangeal joints is seen as a local increase in density and occasionally as a soft tissue projection into adjacent web spaces. Soft tissue swelling over the ulnar styloid can be due to local involvement of the extensor carpi ulnaris tendon sheath. Changes at the radial styloid are related to local radio-carpal joint synovial hypertrophy.

Soft tissue changes are less well demonstrated in the foot. Changes over the first and fifth metatarsophalangeal joints reflect synovitis in the bursae over the first and fifth metatarsal heads, but swelling over the remaining metatarsophalangeal joints may be seen as fusiform increases in density.

The Achilles tendon inserts into the back of the calcaneum below its upper margin. It is sharply demarcated anteriorly by the pre-Achilles fat pad and more inferiorly,

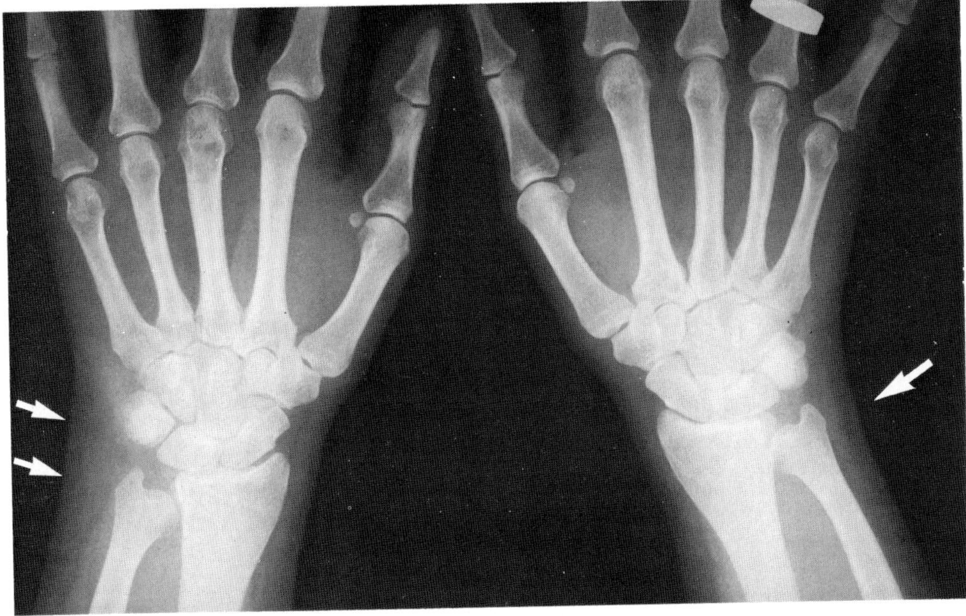

Fig. 4.1 Marked soft tissue swelling is present over the right ulnar styloid and adjacent carpus in an early case of rheumatoid arthritis with no local erosion.

by the retrocalcaneal bursa. Local synovitis thickens the bursa and oedema obliterates the fat and blurs out the tendon, which also thickens. Similar changes occur inferiorly, at the plantar fascial origin at the base of the calcaneum.

Distension of the capsule of the knee joint is shown on the anteroposterior radiograph as a lateral bulging of the normally poorly seen fat lines over the distal femur. On a lateral view of the knee the suprapatellar pouch is distended and its surrounding fat lines blurred. Posteriorly, a distended joint capsule may give a local increase in density and in this way a Baker's cyst is often identified. This can be confirmed by ultrasound or arthrography.

On the lateral view of the elbow, the anterior and posterior fat planes are displaced in a direction vertical to the long axis of the joint, but may be obliterated by local oedema.

Swelling around an affected joint is symmetrical while in gout the swelling is eccentric. In rheumatoid arthritis, however, a rheumatoid nodule may cause a localized eccentric swelling, but these often occur at pressure points.

2. OSTEOPOROSIS. Assessment of osteoporosis depends in part on film quality and comparison between normal and abnormal joints in the same patient may be helpful. Interpretation is subjective and changes are seen only after loss of 25–50% of mineral. Differences in assessment of osteoporosis may exist, both between different observers and between the same observer at different times.

Osteoporosis in rheumatoid arthritis is of two types:

Generalized. This may be due to steroids or limitation of movement due to pain, or muscle wasting. This type is uncommon and occurs late in the course of the disease. It may also reflect coincidental bone loss in post-menopausal females, commonly affected by this disorder.

Local osteoporosis around joints occurs earlier and is due to synovial inflammation and hyperaemia.

Osteoporosis increases in incidence with the duration of the disease and the age of the patient. Some 30% of patients show it at presentation but by 2 years, 80% are affected.

Osteoporosis is a precursor of erosive disease and may mask early erosions. Generalized or solitary *sclerosis* of one or more distal phalanges (terminal phalangeal sclerosis) is often rendered more prominent because of osteoporosis elsewhere. This occurs in some 35% of patients with rheumatoid arthritis and other arthropathies and may be present before any other abnormality. In a female, especially, it may prognosticate future disease, but is seen in some normal patients.

3. JOINT SPACE CHANGES AND ALIGNMENT DEFORMITIES. In the early stage a joint space may be widened by synovial hypertrophy and an effusion. Later on in the disease joint spaces narrow due to cartilage destruction by pannus (Fig. 4.2). Narrowing of joint spaces may, however, be apparent rather than real in the presence of flexion deformities, so that an oblique view is needed to assess the space. Alignment abnormalities at joints may result from local synovitis weakening the capsule and tendinitis preventing normal musculo-tendinous action. Tendons may also rupture in the region of roughened bone. Thus, rotator cuff tears allow upward subluxation of the eroded humeral head.

The classic changes of alignment in the rheumatoid hand are irreversible. Subluxations at metacarpophalangeal joints

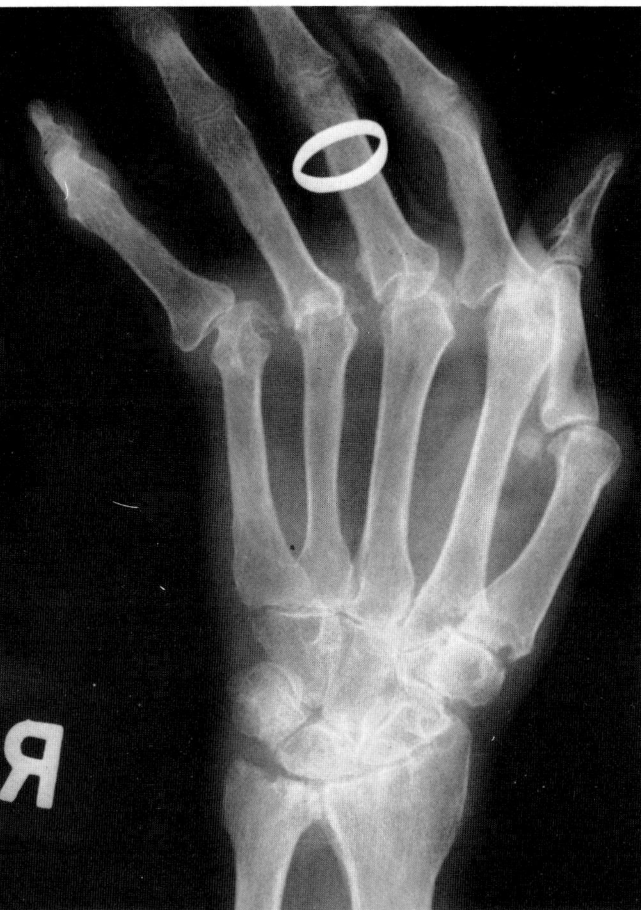

Fig. 4.2 Gross rheumatoid arthritis at the carpus with ulnar deviation, subluxation and joint narrowing at the metacarpo-phalangeal joints. Boutonnière deformities are present at the index and little fingers.

lead to ulnar deviation (Fig. 4.2) which occurs in up to 50% of those with chronic disease. This is also associated with increasing palmar flexion. This change may result from ulnar deviation of extensor tendons.

The boutonnière deformity (Fig. 4.2) results from proximal interphalangeal joint flexion and distal interphalangeal joint extension and the swan-neck deformity from the reverse (proximal interphalangeal joint extension and distal interphalangeal joint flexion). The boutonnière deformity is the more common.

Lateral deviation of the toes similarly may be found. Hallux valgus is especially common. The hallux sesamoids sublux between the first and second metatarsal heads and the transverse arch flattens as local inflammation causes ligamentous laxity.

4. PERIOSTITIS. Local periosteal reactions occur either along the midshaft of a phalanx or metacarpal as a reaction to local tendinitis, or at the metaphysis near a joint affected by synovitis. Such changes are less common in rheumatoid arthritis than in the seronegative arthropathies. They are difficult to identify, may be mistaken for lumbrical impressions and are commoner in the feet (Fig. 4.3). Periostitis in the form of fluffy calcaneal spurs, plantar and posterior, is also less common in rheumatoid arthritis than in the seronegative arthropathies (Fig. 4.4). When present, they are larger and more irregular than the normal small well-corticated spurs of the elderly. Spurs may arise ab initio or may follow healing of erosions.

5. EROSIONS. These are the most important diagnostic change but are not necessarily present when the patient first attends. Their incidence rises from less than 40% of patients at 3 months to up to 90 or 95% at 10 years.

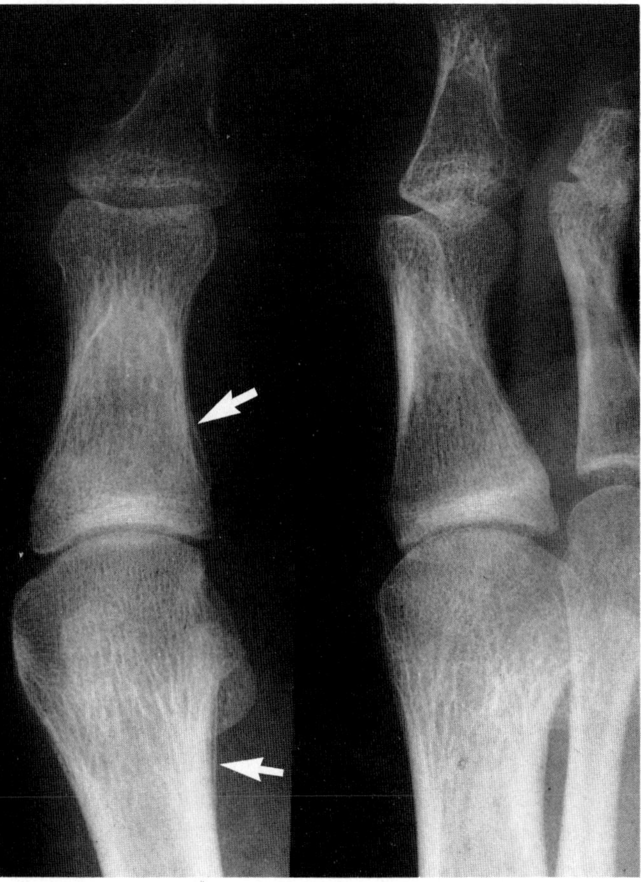

Fig. 4.3 Rheumatoid arthritis with narrowing of the metatarso-phalangeal joint of the great toe and a fine periostitis on the adjacent shafts.

Classical periarticular erosions occur at the so-called 'bare areas' of bone between the edge of the articular cartilage and the attachment of the joint capsule (Fig. 4.5). In the hand, these bare areas are larger on the proximal surface of the joint, i.e. at the metacarpal head, than at the local phalangeal base. Cartilage, moreover, is thicker over the centre of a metacarpal head than at the periphery and is thicker reciprocally at the periphery of the base of the proximal phalanx. This anatomy predisposes to the distri-

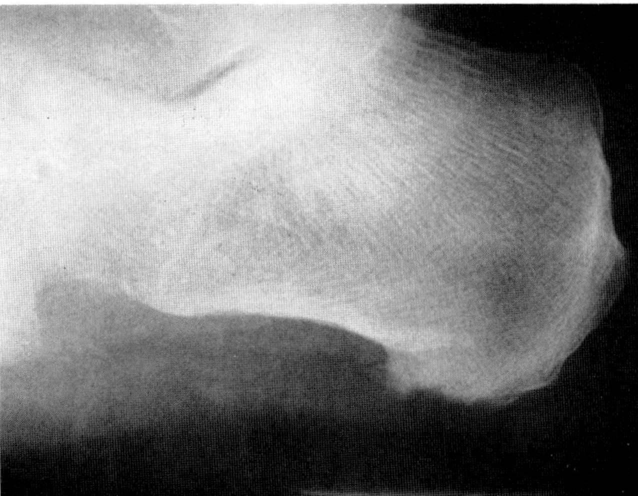

Fig. 4.4 Irregularity and erosion in the region of the plantar spur distinguishes this painful lesion from the normal benign spur, which is seen in around 20% of the population.

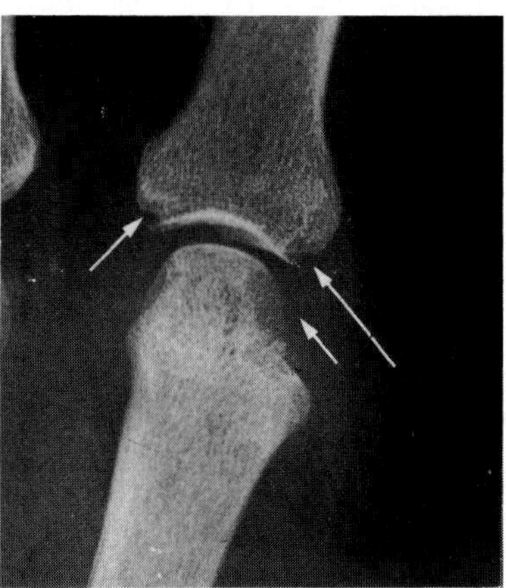

Fig. 4.5 Early rheumatoid arthritis showing marginal erosions (arrows).

bution of joint erosions. At the distal interphalangeal joints, the bare areas are larger on the proximal than on the distal joint surfaces (Fig. 4.6).

Erosions in rheumatoid arthritis should be sought for at the common sites. Supplementary views, such as the Norgaard 'ball-catcher' view (supine 25 degrees oblique view), may be needed. Erosions appear earlier and are more often seen in the feet, 90% of which will eventually be eroded, than in the hands (75%), and most often at the fifth metatarsophalangeal joint. The hallux metatarsophalangeal joint is the least often involved. Erosions affect typically the lateral side of the fifth metatarsal but the medial side of the others.

The metatarsal head erodes before the base of the distal phalanx, presumably as cartilage is thinner peripherally at that site. In the hand, the second and third metacarpophalangeal joints are the earliest affected, initially on the

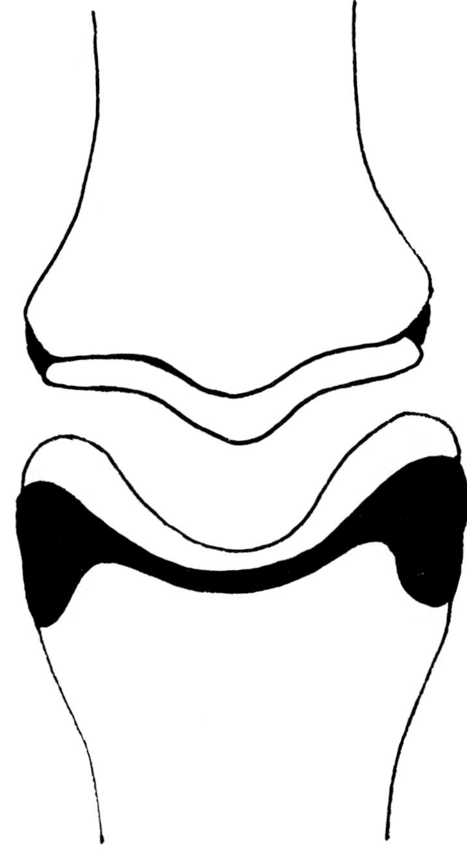

Fig. 4.6 Bare areas at a distal interphalangeal joint (after Martel). The black areas represent bone which is not covered by either synovium or cartilage. The bare areas are larger proximally. Cartilage is uneven, being thicker proximally at the periphery of the joint and thicker centrally at the base of the distal phalanx.

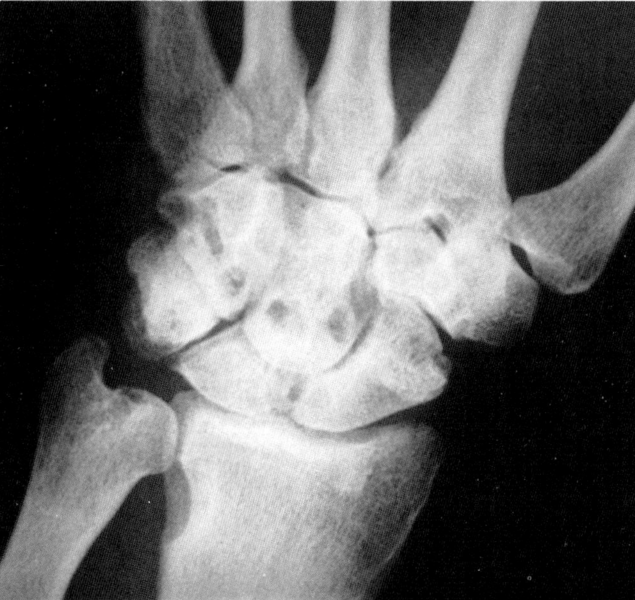

Fig. 4.7 Rheumatoid arthritis. Apart from the carpal changes, there are also erosions at the distal radioulnar joint, proximal to the triangular cartilage at the distal ulna, and at the ulnar styloid tip.

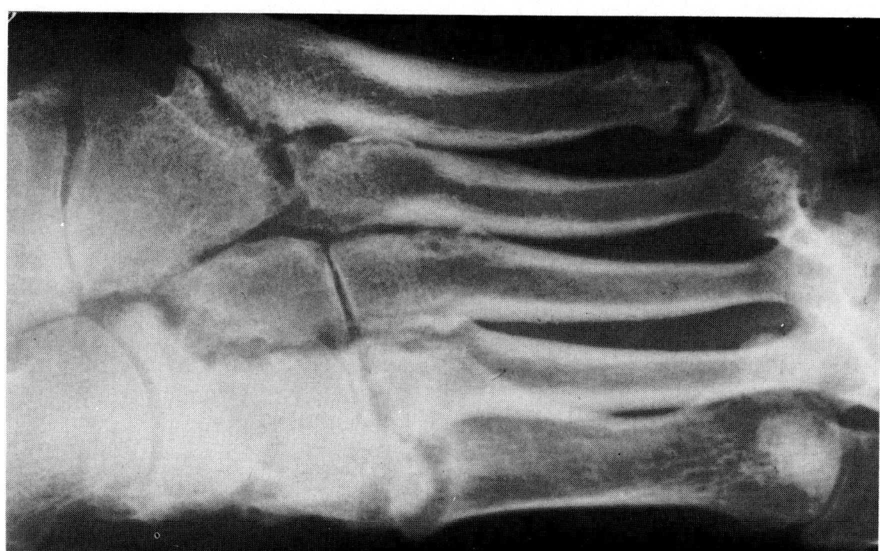

Fig. 4.8 Rheumatoid arthritis: very pronounced destructive changes in the tarsus and in metatarsal heads.

radial aspects. More distal erosions are inconstant, and the terminal interphalangeal joints are usually spared. At the distal ulna, erosions occur (1) at the tip of the ulnar styloid, (2) proximal to the insertion of the triangular cartilage and (3) laterally, adjacent to the extensor carpi ulnaris tendon sheath (Fig. 4.7). Wrist erosions also occur at the radial styloid and at the proximal compartment of the distal radio-ulnar joint (Fig. 4.7). Carpal erosions occur throughout the wrist. An erosion is, for example, commonly seen on the lateral scaphoid at its waist. Carpal disease may be followed by fusion, but this is uncommon elsewhere in adult rheumatoid arthritis. On occasion, massive carpal destruction may be found in the presence of virtually normal peripheral joints.

Tarsal erosions, other than at the posterior and inferior surfaces of the calcaneum, are uncommon and are also less common in rheumatoid arthritis than in the seronegative spondyloarthropathies (Fig. 4.8). In rheumatoid arthritis, erosions are usually seen at or above the insertion of the tendo-achillis into the back of the calcaneum.

Erosions are first seen as an area of local demineralization beneath the cortex which in turn becomes fuzzy and eventually vanishes, leaving irregular underlying trabeculae. The destroyed area increases in size and, as pannus spreads over articular surfaces, the entire articular cortex may be destroyed, leaving a pointed bone end. Chronic trauma, in weight-bearing or due to abnormal tendon alignment, may further collapse articular surfaces. Steroids and analgesics also modify the disease so that neuropathic type destructive changes may result. Healing rarely reverses erosions so that a normal appearance infrequently returns. Usually the margins of healed erosions become corticated and they do not enlarge on follow-up.

Erosive change is less common at the larger joints but often bone destruction is greater owing to the greater stresses placed on knees, elbows and shoulders. On occasion, intra-osseous defects, up to 2–3 cm in diameter, may be seen beneath joint surfaces. These large cysts or *geodes* (Fig. 4.9) may be the result of patients maintaining normal activity or even excess activity under the influence of analgesics. They may be filled with pannus, or synovial fluid pumped into bone through microfractures on the bone surface. Such connections can be demonstrated at arthrography, when the geode can be shown to communicate with the joint. An alternative form of change at large articular surfaces is a superficial surface irregularity with a little reactive sclerosis in the presence of much joint narrowing. This change is seen at the elbow, knee and hip. In the hip joint it is characteristically the medial joint space which is narrowed and eroded (as opposed to the superior in osteoarthritis). Muscle pull on adjacent irregular articular surfaces leads to medial migration of the femoral head and

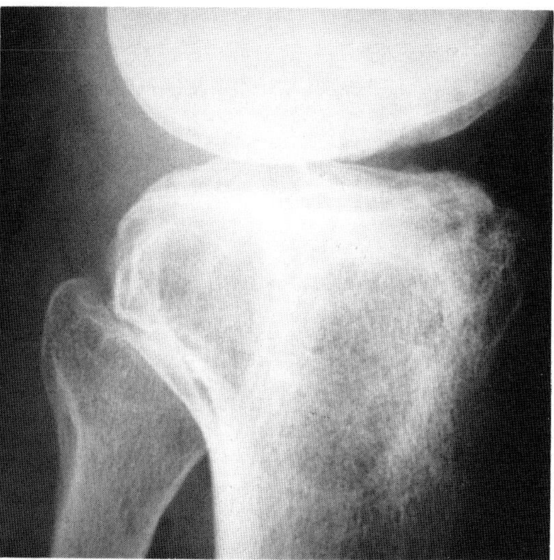

Fig. 4.9 A large cyst is seen beneath the articular surface of the tibia in rheumatoid arthritis.

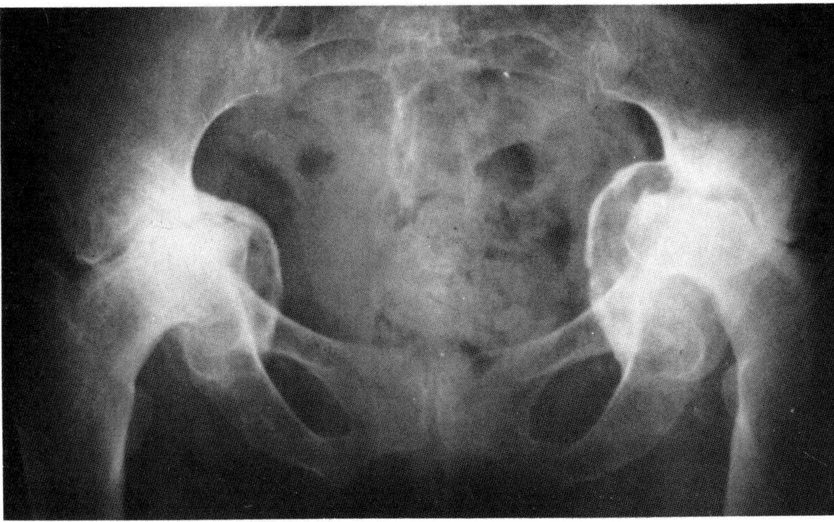

Fig. 4.10 Rheumatoid pelvis: extreme protrusio with medial migration and erosion of the femoral heads. Compare this film with Fig. 4.38B (protrusio in osteoarthritis).

acetabular resorption, causing protrusio acetabuli. This is classical, but not pathognomonic of rheumatoid arthritis, as it also occurs in osteoarthritis, in conditions with bone softening, and in an idiopathic inherited form. Gross loss of bone, especially at the femoral head, may result in a 'bird's beak' appearance (Fig. 4.10). Marked loss of bone around articular surfaces is also common at the elbow (Fig. 4.11) and shoulder, and deformities of alignment follow. Bone loss at the acromio-clavicular joint may often be seen on a chest radiograph with pointing of adjacent bone ends and scalloping of the undersurface of the acromion (Fig. 4.12). Erosions of the superior aspects of the upper ribs are seen in patients with longstanding disease and muscle wasting, and are probably due to the adjacent scapula rubbing on the rib.

RHEUMATOID CHANGES IN THE AXIAL SKELETON. *Sacro-iliac joints*: Changes are less common and less severe than in seronegative disease but may be seen in up to 30% of those with longstanding disease. The changes are more common in women (cf. ankylosing spondylitis) and rarely end in fusion. The erosions are mainly in the lateral side of the joint, associated with mild joint space narrowing and little reactive sclerosis. Mild changes are also found infrequently at the symphysis pubis.

Spinal changes. Rheumatoid changes are common in the cervical spine but uncommon in the thoracic and lumbar regions. This has been said to be due to the presence in the neck of the synovium-lined uncovertebral joints of Luschka, so that pannus from these joints extends to erode the disc annulus and lateral and posterior disc-bone borders.

Osteoporosis, disc narrowing and end-plate irregularity are seen (Fig. 4.13) with only a little reactive new bone formation at the *upper* cervical vertebrae. Osteoarthritis in distinction is seen more inferiorly. Facet joint erosions may result in subluxation (Fig. 4.14), so that nerve entrapment

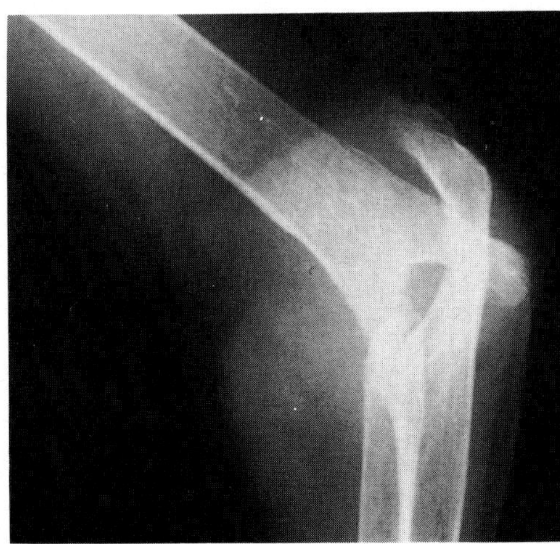

Fig. 4.11 Rheumatoid arthritis: marked bone absorption shown. At this stage the patient was free from pain.

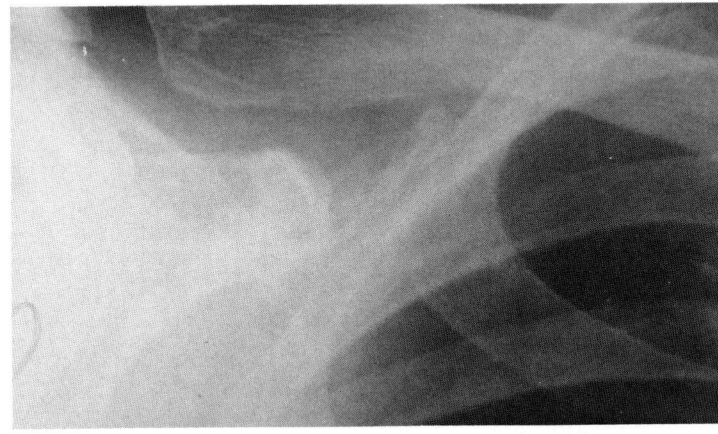

Fig. 4.12 Widening of the right acromio-cavicular joint with well-demarcated margins distinguishes rheumatoid arthritis from hyperparathyroidism. The erosion of the third and fourth ribs superiorly may be seen in both conditions.

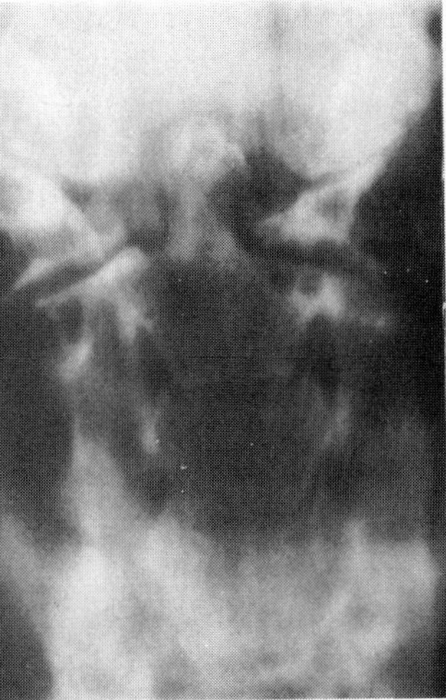

Fig. 4.13

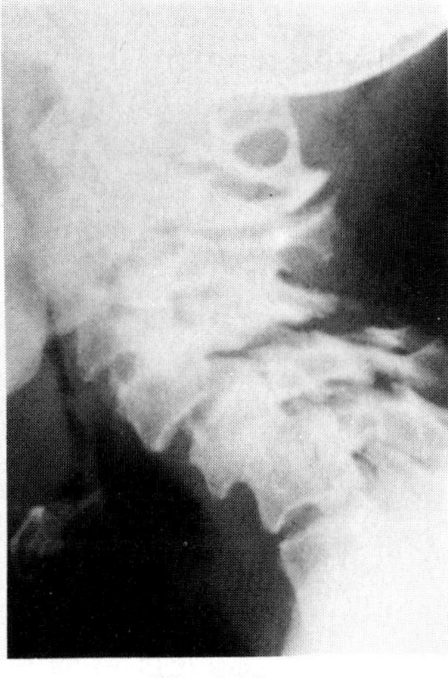

Fig. 4.14

ig. 4.13 Rheumatoid arthritis of cervical spine — tomographic section owing erosions of the left atlanto-axial articulation, similar changes fect the right side and also the occipito-atlanto joints and the dontoid peg.

ig. 4.14 Rheumatoid arthritis cervical spine — gross bizarre estruction. Subluxation of C4 on C5 and of C5 on C6 is seen. Note ross destruction in the spinous processes and posterior arches.

ollows. Subluxation and erosion also occur at the synovial oint between the odontoid peg and arch of atlas, and are otentiated by laxity of ligaments around the peg. Separation in flexion of more than 2.5 mm in adults or 5 mm n children is held to be abnormal. This instability can be een in up to 30% of patients with chronic rheumatoid arthritis. The eroded odontoid may also fracture.

Erosions at the joints between occipital condyles and lateral masses of the atlas may result in upward displacement of C1 and C2, and this may be fatal (Fig. 4.13). Resorption of bone at non-articular surfaces occurs in the cervical pine at the spinous processes which become short, sharp nd tapered in patients with chronic disease (Fig. 4.14).

Changes in the thoracic and lumbar regions are less common. Occasionally disc narrowing at one or two levels is ssociated with local end-plate 'erosions' and reactive sclerosis. Similar changes may be seen in seronegative arthropathies. These local changes may be post-traumatic, esulting from acquired apophyseal joint instability, or they may be 'enthesopathies', resulting from locally inflamed oft tissues.

Erosions at other sites of musculo-tendinous insertions re much less common than in seronegative disease and, f marked, the diagnosis should be questioned.

6. SECONDARY OSTEOARTHRITIS. Weight-bearing joints affected by rheumatoid arthritis often develop secondary osteoarthritis. Indeed, at the hips, osteoarthritic change may be superimposed on a previously unrecognized rheumatoid rthritis. Reactive sclerosis and new bone formation in osteoarthritis is not marked in those whose underlying disease has characteristic features of osteoporosis and bone destruction.

ARTHRITIS IN CHILDREN

There are many causes of polyarthritis in children, the most common being viral infections. It is now recognized that chronic childhood polyarthritis is a heterogenous group of disorders, the generic term for which is 'juvenile chronic polyarthritis' (Table 4.1).

Table 4.1 Classification of juvenile chronic polyarthritis

1. Adult-type rheumatoid arthritis (with IgM rheumatoid factor)
2. Polyarthritis with ankylosing spondylitis-type sacro-iliitis
3. Still's disease
   a) systemic
   b) polyarticular
   c) pauci-articular, with or without chronic iridocyclitis
4. Psoriatic arthropathy
5. Arthritis associated with ulcerative colitis or regional enteritis (as in adults)
6. Polyarthropathies associated with other disorders, such as systemic lupus erythematosus or familial Mediterranean fever, etc.

(Reproduced by kind permission of Dr B. M. Ansell)

Arthritides due to juvenile ankylosing spondylitis, psoriasis, inflammatory bowel disease and systemic lupus erythematosus all form definite subgroups. These may account for up to 40% of the total. Some 10% of the total eventually have a seropositive form of disease similar to, or identical with, adult rheumatoid arthritis, that is, an essentially peripheral erosive polyarthritis. The remaining patients have seronegative juvenile chronic arthritis for which definite clinical and histological diagnostic criteria exist.

Children with seronegative juvenile chronic arthritis may be further subdivided:

1. Acute systemic onset type (true Still's disease) with constitutional symptoms and hepatosplenomegaly, but little or no joint involvement.
2. Pauci-articular (four or less joints involved) affecting especially the knees, wrists and ankles. This usually ends up as:
3. Polyarticular disease, which may also present at the onset. Radiological changes are late and the disease is non-erosive.

In the carpus and tarsus the bones show accelerated maturation due to hyperaemia, crowding of bones with joint space narrowing and an abnormal angular shape (Fig. 4.15). In general, early overgrowth of epiphyseal

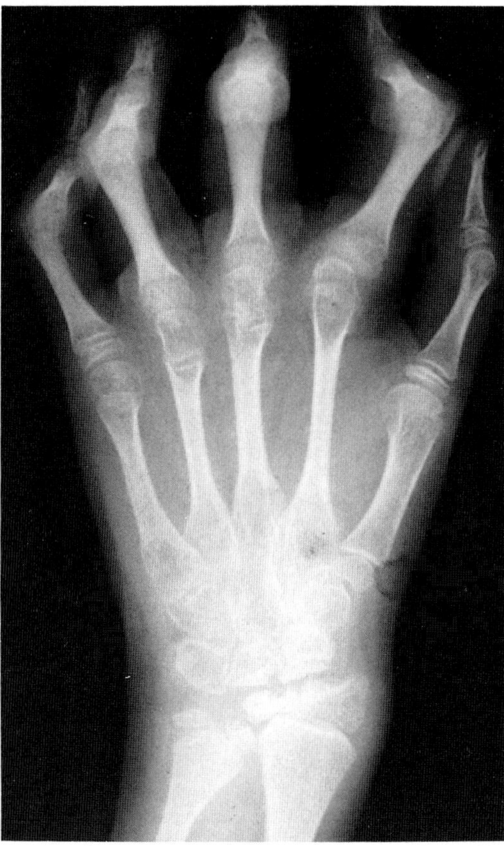

Fig. 4.15 Juvenile chronic arthritis. Accelerated skeletal maturity with modelling abnormalities of the carpal bones and metacarpal heads together with osteoporosis and soft tissue wasting. At the distal radius and ulna the epiphyses are fragmented and overgrown.

centres (Fig. 4.16) with squaring or angulation (Fig. 4.17) leads to premature fusion and eventual hypoplasia. This occurs at metacarpal and metatarsal epiphyses and around the knees, hips, elbows and shoulders. The abnormally modelled bone ends cannot easily be distinguished from the similar changes of synovial tuberculosis or haemophilia. Osteoporosis may result from hyperaemia or steroid administration which, in large doses, also causes undergrowth. Pathological fractures may result. Residual trabeculae along lines of stress are rendered very prominent. At the elbow, marked radial head enlargement may be seen and the paired long bones may bow. The cervical spine is often affected and indeed is the cause of presentation in 2% of cases. Diminution of neck movement is followed by apophyseal joint changes, maximal at C2–C3 where erosions lead to ankylosis. The associated vertebral bodies fail to develop. Atlanto-axial subluxation is said to occur only rarely in those patients with seronegative disease, and neurocentral joint lesions do not occur in seronegative disease.

Juvenile ankylosing spondylitis has a characteristic onset at about 10 years of age. It is five times more common in boys and presents initially with an asymmetric peripheral arthropathy. Sacro-iliac changes develop some 5–15 years later.

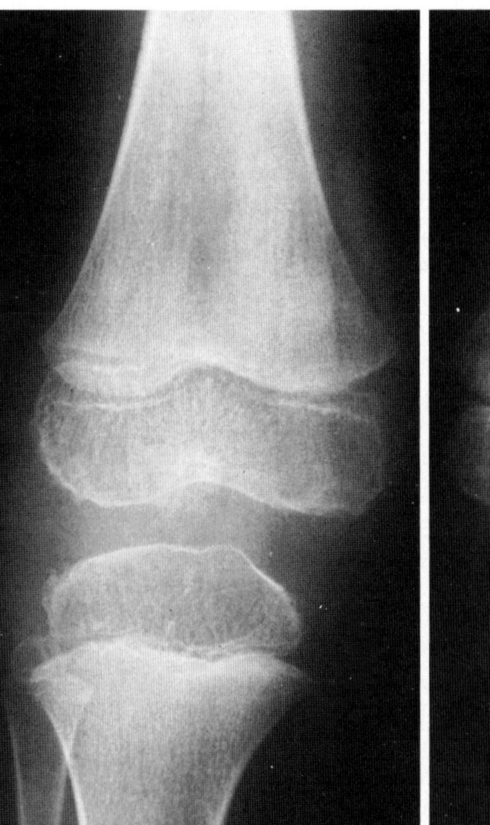

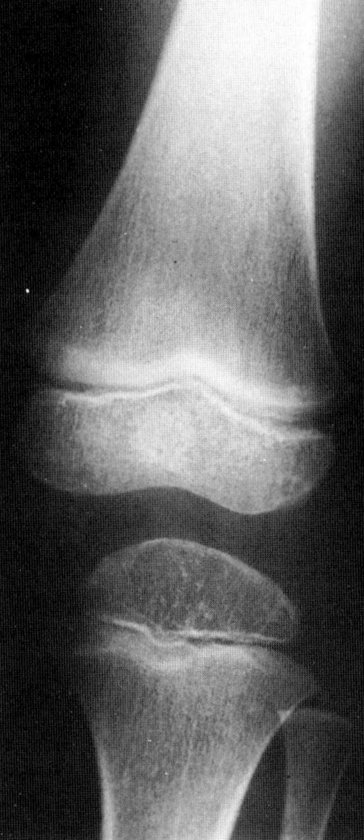

Fig. 4.16 Juvenile chronic arthritis. Monarticular arthritis with soft tissue swelling and overgrowth of the epiphyses at the right knee.

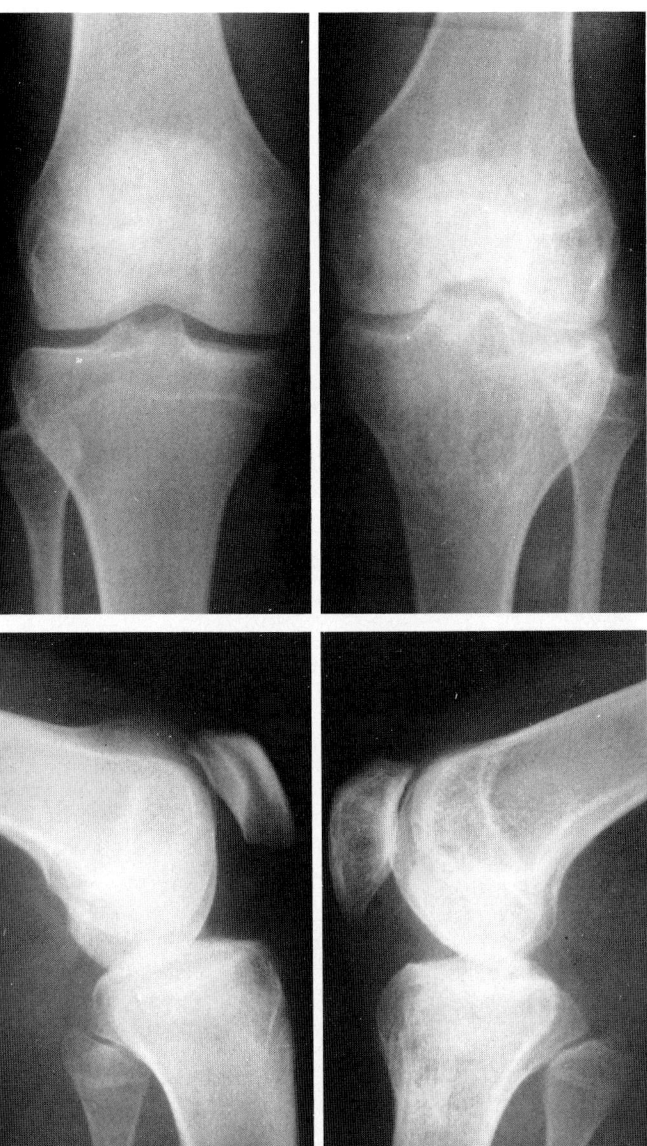

Fig. 4.17 (**A** and **B**) Juvenile chronic arthritis. After five years modelling abnormalities and osteoporosis are seen, but erosive change is not present.

SERONEGATIVE SPONDYLOARTHROPATHIES

This is a group of non-rheumatoid seronegative disorders which have clinical, radiological and familial inter-relationships. There are definite criteria for their diagnosis.

These features include:

1. Absence of rheumatoid factors
2. Peripheral arthropathy
3. Sacro-iliitis with or without ankylosing spondylitis
4. Clinical overlap, including two or more of the following features — psoriatic skin or nail lesions, conjunctivitis, ulceration of mouth, intestines or genitals, genito-urinary infections, erythema nodosum.
5. Increased incidence of the same or any other of these diseases in families.

The diseases which fit into these categories are:

1. Ankylosing spondylitis
2. Psoriatic arthritis
3. Reiter's syndrome
4. Ulcerative colitis
5. Crohn's disease
6. Whipple's disease
7. Behçet's syndrome

The inter-relationships between the diseases are seen in Figure 4.18. Chronic inflammatory bowel disease can for instance be seen to be linked to spondylitis and uveitis, while spondylitis is further linked to aortitis, seronegative arthritis and psoriasis.

This genetic and clinical overlap accounts for the marked radiological overlap of these syndromes, so that spondylitis is seen in many of these conditions. Nonetheless, differences in the type of spondylitis seen in these diseases also exist.

PSORIATIC ARTHRITIS

An association between psoriasis and arthritis was described as long ago as 1822. Some 10% of patients develop arthritis before the skin lesions appear, in 25% the two develop simultaneously and in 65% psoriasis preceeds arthritis often by up to 35 years. It seems that about 5% of patients with psoriasis develop an arthritis but 15–30% of these are seropositive and have a radiological appearance identical with that of rheumatoid disease. The remainder have a 'pure' pattern of psoriatic arthropathy, or a mixture of the two types. Normal bone mineralization is regarded as a solid diagnostic criterion for psoriatic arthritis, but is in fact not particularly common, especially in chronic or severe disease.

The hands are as frequently affected by erosive change as are the feet in psoriatic arthropathy in contradistinction to the patterns of Reiter's disease. Nail changes are related to resorption of the distal phalanges but no definite correlation exists between nail lesions and interphalangeal joint erosions. Erosions have a predilection for the distal interphalangeal joints (Fig. 4.19), and especially the interphalangeal joint of the great toe. Erosive changes are asymmetrical, even late in the disease, unlike rheumatoid arthritis, and especially if the metacarpophalangeal joints are involved. Joint narrowing may never occur. One ray only may be affected.

Erosions are modified by proliferation of adjacent new bone at the interphalangeal joints and especially around erosions on the calcaneum, where large, irregular fluffy painful spurs form both posteriorly and inferiorly. Such erosions are not found as often as in Reiter's syndrome (these changes are uncommon in rheumatoid arthritis).

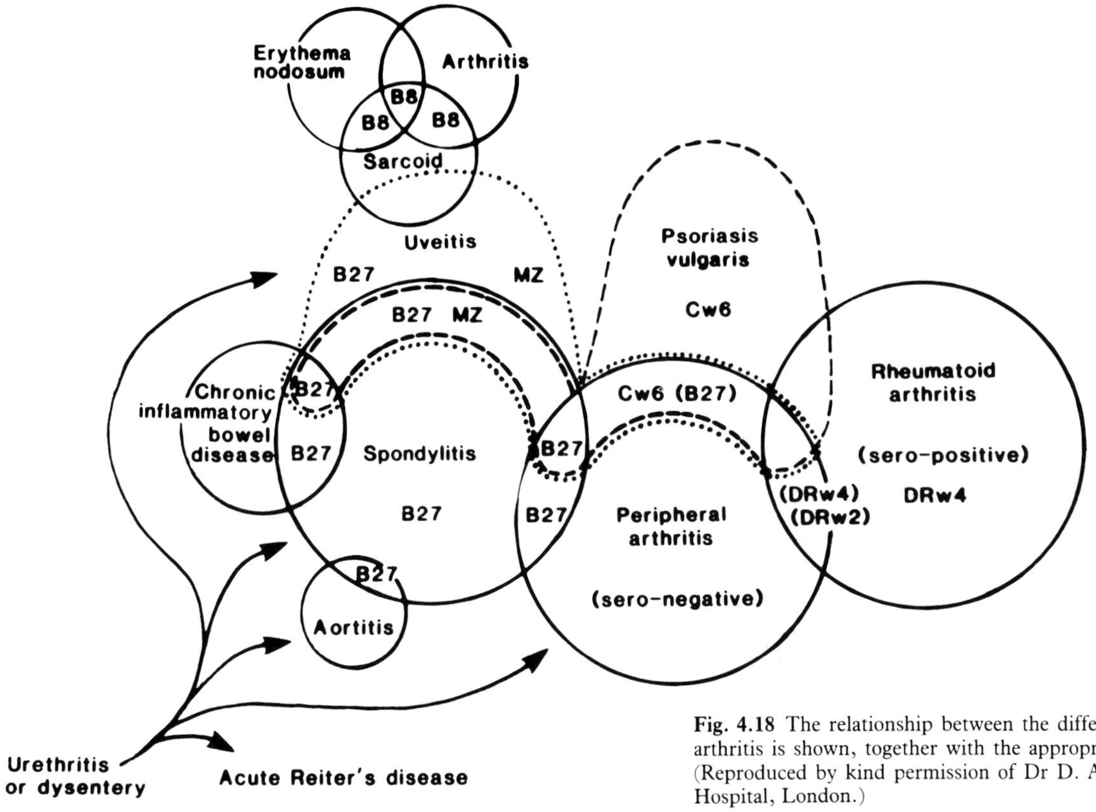

Fig. 4.18 The relationship between the different manifestations of arthritis is shown, together with the appropriate tissue markers. (Reproduced by kind permission of Dr D. A. Brewerton, Westminster Hospital, London.)

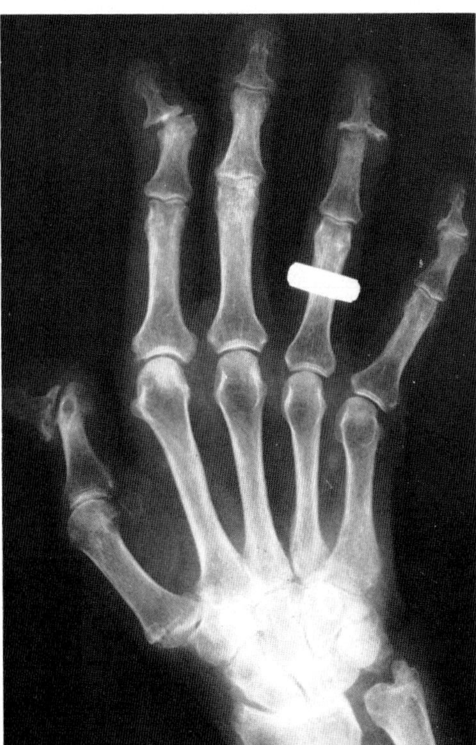

Fig. 4.19 Psoriasis. Erosive changes with overlying soft tissue swelling are predominantly at the distal interphalangeal joints. The erosions are initially peripheral and splaying of the distal phalangeal bases results.

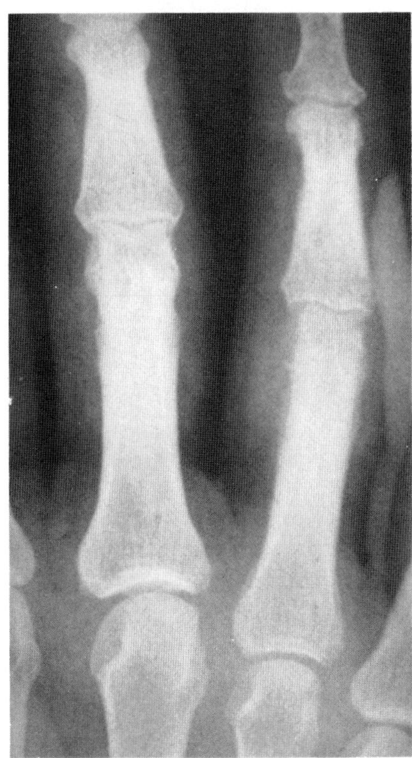

Fig. 4.20 Psoriatic arthritis. Sausage-like swelling is associated with a fuzzy periostitis. Note the normal adjacent finger with normal muscle insertions. (Courtesy of Dr R. Allen, King's College Hospital.)

Late changes in the hands include osseous fusion of the interphalangeal joints, and a 'cup-and-pencil' appearance at affected joints, leading to arthritis mutilans, but not ulnar deviation.

Periostitis in psoriatic arthritis occurs along the shafts of the tubular bones on hands and feet (Fig. 4.20).

Involvement of the larger joints is not common, but sacro-iliitis may be seen in up to 50% of those with psoriatic arthritis. Usually symmetrical, erosions, joint widening and sclerosis are seen but fusion is less common than in ankylosing spondylitis.

Paravertebral ossification may be the only feature of an osteopathy, even occurring in the absence of sacro-iliac or digital disease. This is unusual in ankylosing spondylitis but is seen in as many as 20% of psoriatics. New bone is attached to the vertebral body along its mid portion and not at the margins, as in ankylosing spondylitis, and may appear to even 'float free', separate from the bodies, with a vertical orientation (Fig. 4.27). These *syndesmophytes* should be distinguished from the more horizontally directed degenerative osteophytes. Vertebral squaring is uncommon in psoriatic spondylitis (Fig. 4.21).

REITER'S SYNDROME

This occurs most commonly in young adult males and is usually sexually transmitted. The classic triad in Great Britain consists of a male patient with arthritis, urethritis and conjunctivitis. Gonococcal arthritis may thus cause confusion, especially if the classic three features of Reiter's syndrome are not all present. In Continental Europe, the similar syndrome, originally described by Reiter in 1916, occurs in association with bacillary dysentery in both sexes.

Skeletal abnormalities will eventually be found in up to 80% of patients. Initial attacks of pain subside, but later recur, leaving progressive change at joints and entheses (the sites of musculotendinous insertion into bone). Reiter's syndrome affects the feet rather than the hands, and also in a more severe form. In the foot, erosions occur at the metatarso-phalangeal joints and the interphalangeal joint of the great toe. Osteoporosis is not a prominent feature of the disorder. Asymmetry occurs, unlike the distribution of rheumatoid arthritis.

Irregular erosions occur at entheses and local fluffy periostitis (Fig. 4.22) presumably represents attempted healing. Periostitis also occurs on the malleoli (Fig. 4.23) and metatarsal shafts, where it may be fine and lamellar in acute cases, or fluffy and irregular in chronic disease. Painful erosions (Fig. 4.23) and reactive spurs are very common around the calcaneum, probably more so than in any other arthropathy, occurring in 20% of patients. In contrast to ankylosing spondylitis, the feet are severely affected.

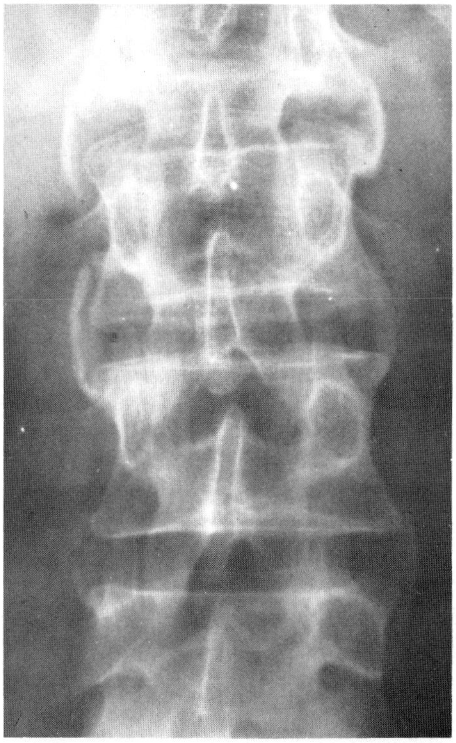

Fig. 4.21 Psoriatic spondylitis. Non-marginal vertical floating syndesmophytes are more typical of psoriasis and are less often seen in ankylosing spondylitis. (Courtesy of Dr J. T. Patton, Manchester.)

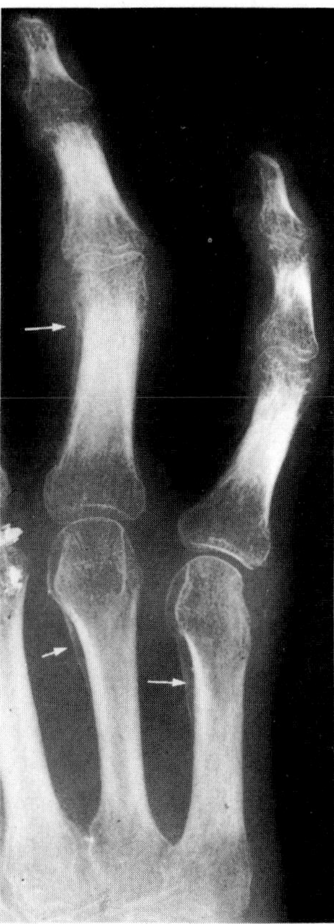

Fig. 4.22 Reiter's syndrome — acute form, showing marked osteoporosis and periosteal reaction (arrows).

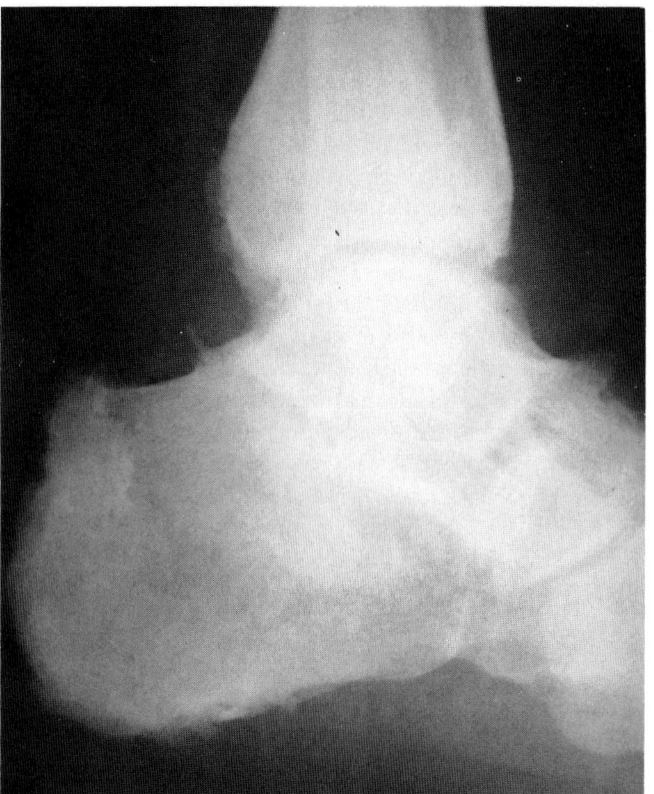

Fig. 4.23 Gross periostitis and erosive change at the distal tibia and on the posterior and plantar aspects of the calcaneum. Note also the hindfoot fusion.

Sacro-iliitis develops late in Reiter's syndrome but may be seen in about half of all cases (Fig. 4.24). The changes are usually bilateral but often asymmetrical, as opposed to almost inevitable symmetry in ankylosing spondylitis. Fusion is also less frequent than in ankylosing spondylitis. Spinal non-marginal or floating syndesmophytes, identical to those seen in psoriatic arthritis, occur, especially around the thoraco-lumbar junction, but less frequently than in psoriatic arthritis.

ANKYLOSING SPONDYLITIS

Ankylosing spondylitis (*Marie Strumpell arthritis, Bechterew disease*) is a seronegative spondylo-arthropathy. Some 90% of patients with this disease have the HLA-B27 antigen or, to put it another way, an individual with this antigen is 300 times as likely to have ankylosing spondylitis as is a person without the antigen. 65% of patients with psoriasis and spondylitis, or inflammatory bowel disease and spondylitis, have HLA B27 but in psoriasis with a peripheral arthropathy there is only a weak association if spondylitis or sacro-iliitis are not present. Thus the antigen is essentially related to the presence of spinal changes.

Histologically, the synovitis of ankylosing spondylitis is identical with that of rheumatoid arthritis; the enthesopathy consists of destruction of ligaments and local bone with subjacent inflammatory infiltrates. The destructive lesion heals by deposition of new bone which joins the eroded ligament, causing healing with bone proliferation at non-articular sites, syndesmophytes at vertebral margins and ossification of joint capsules.

Though the disease may affect children, it is said to occur more often in men in their late teens and twenties but recently it has been realized that women may be affected in equal numbers. The onset is often insidious so that sacro-iliitis is usually seen at presentation. Spondylitis need not be present but develops subsequently, often at the thoraco-lumbar region initially, but sometimes affecting the cervical spine in females. Spinal changes without sacro-iliac changes are very rare in this disease.

Sacro-iliac joints. Though ankylosing spondylitis occasionally causes asymmetrical involvement of the sacro-iliac joints at the onset of the disease, symmetrical change is almost inevitable later on (Fig. 4.25). Erosions, often worse on the iliac side, widen the joint and its hazy margins may resemble the normal adolescent joint. The erosions later show considerable sclerosis, and the joint narrows as irregular new bone bridges the joint space, so that fusion eventually occurs. Joint changes are probably best assessed

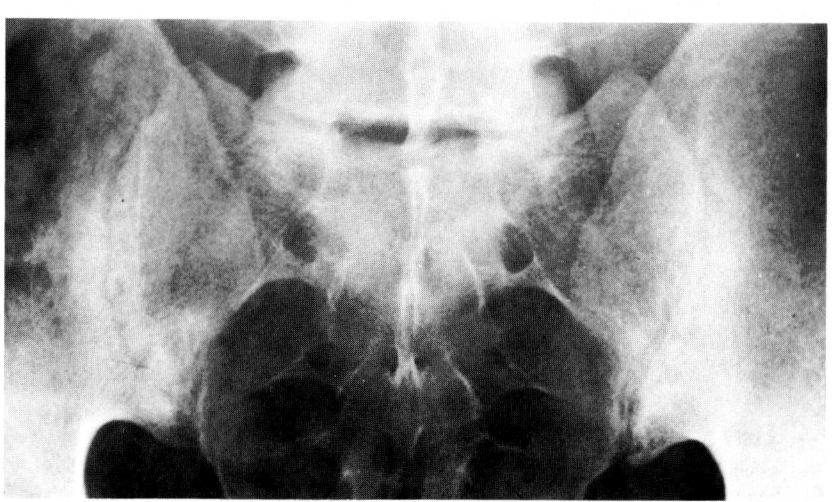

Fig. 4.24 Sacro-iliitis in psoriatic arthritis.

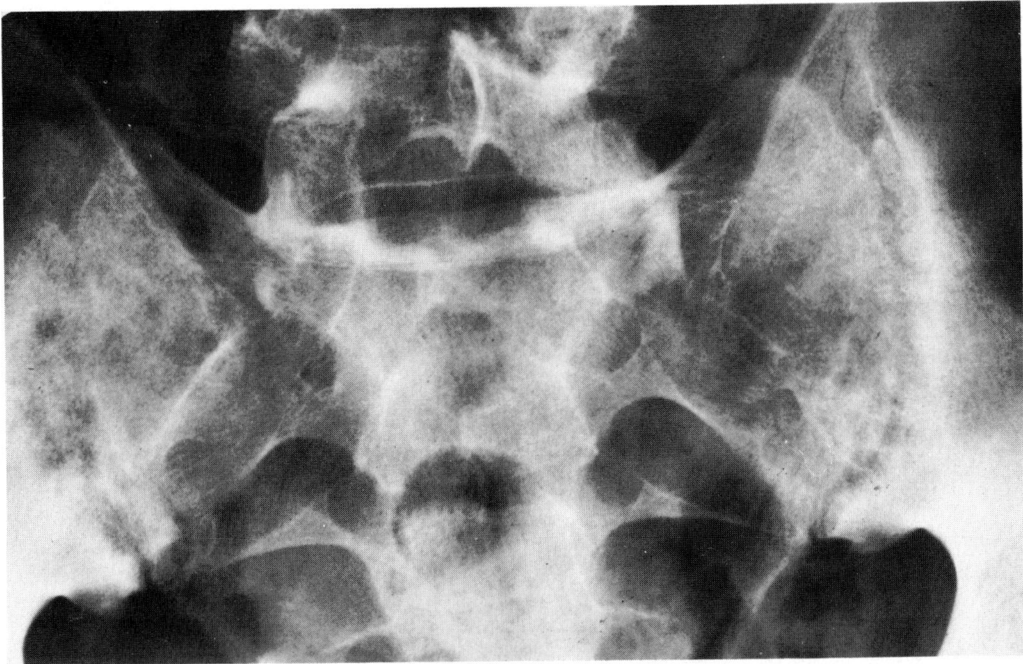

Fig. 4.25 Ankylosing spondylitis — early: serrated margins of sacro-iliac joints and periarticular sclerosis.

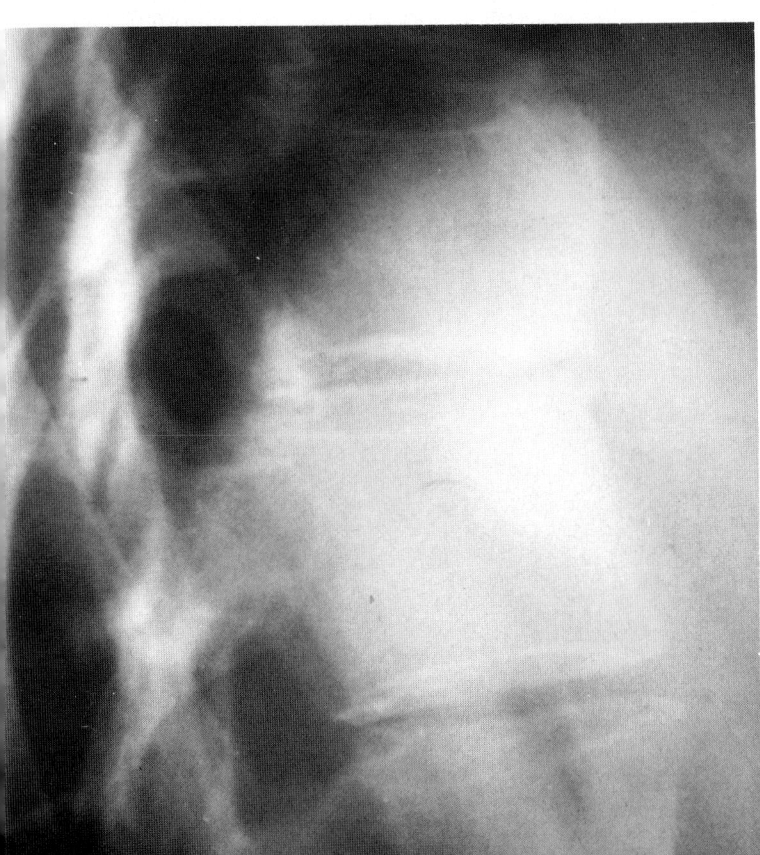

Fig. 4.26 Ankylosing spondylitis. Discal narrowing and adjacent erosions heal with prolific new bone formation. Sclerosis and vertebral squaring result.

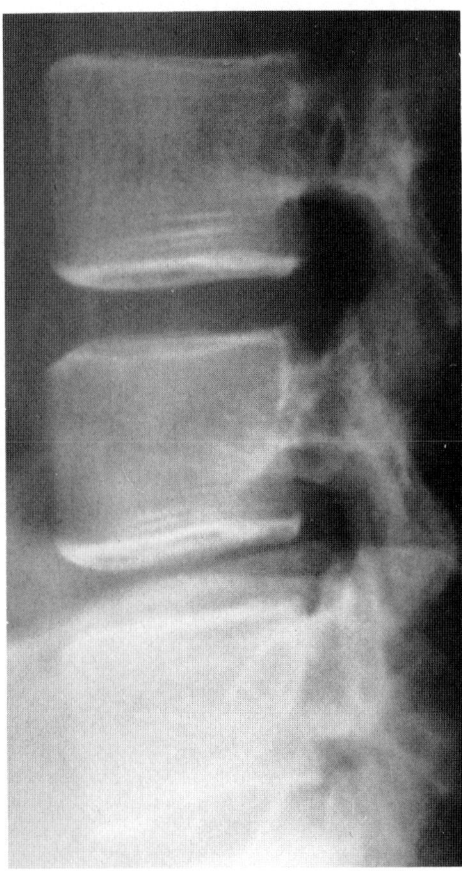

Fig. 4.27 Ankylosing spondylitis: loss of normal anterior concavity of vertebral bodies. Note the growth arrest lines, presumably related to periods of immobilisation in acute disease.

using the prone view of the sacro-iliac joint, though oblique views and tomography are occasionally helpful.

Spinal changes. Erosions of vertebral margins heal by proliferation of sclerotic bone, which stands out in marked contrast to the rest of the vertebral body (Fig. 4.26). These healed erosions of vertebral margins may account for vertebral 'squaring'; an alternative cause is the laying down of new bone anteriorly beneath the longitudinal ligament Both mechanisms may be operative (Fig. 4.27).

Further bony outgrowths in a later stage of healing lea to neat, vertically disposed marginal syndesmophyte which may extend all the way up the spine (Figs. 4.28 an 4.29). The ossification lies in the annulus. Similar well defined bands of ossification may be seen in the interspinou

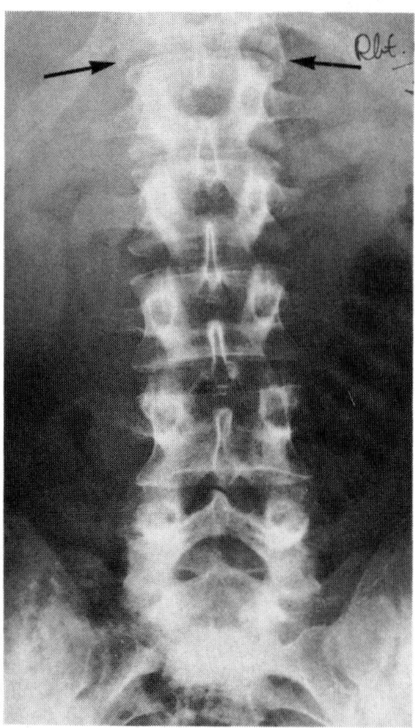

Fig. 4.28

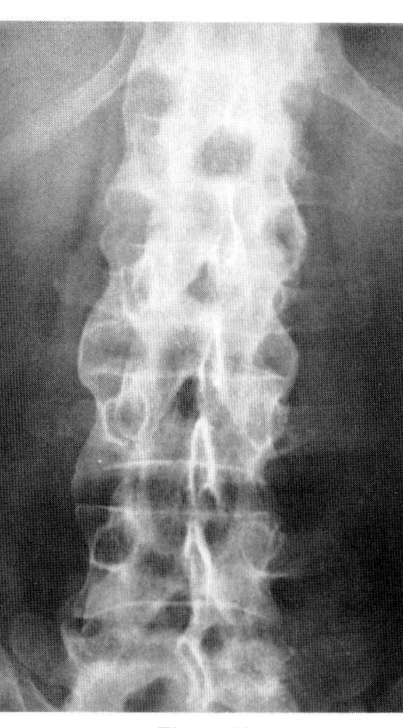

Fig. 4.29

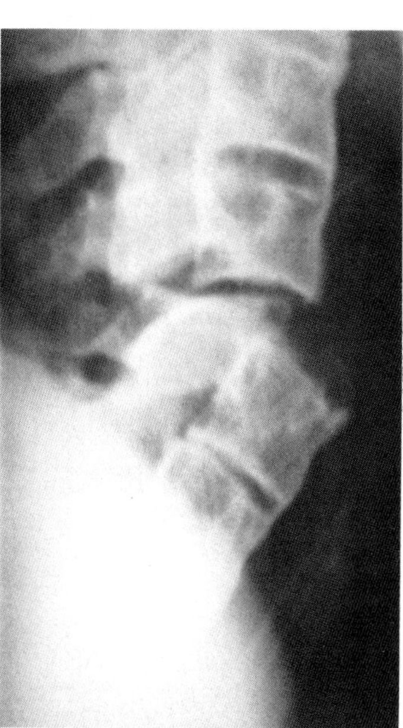

Fig. 4.30

Fig. 4.28 Ankylosing spondylitis: early ligamentous calcification at D12-L1 (arrows). Note changes in sacro-iliac joints.

Fig. 4.29 Ankylosing spondylitis: bamboo spine with marginal syndesmophytes.

Fig. 4.30 Cervical spine in ankylosing spondylitis with fractures through the C4–C5 and C5–C6 discs.

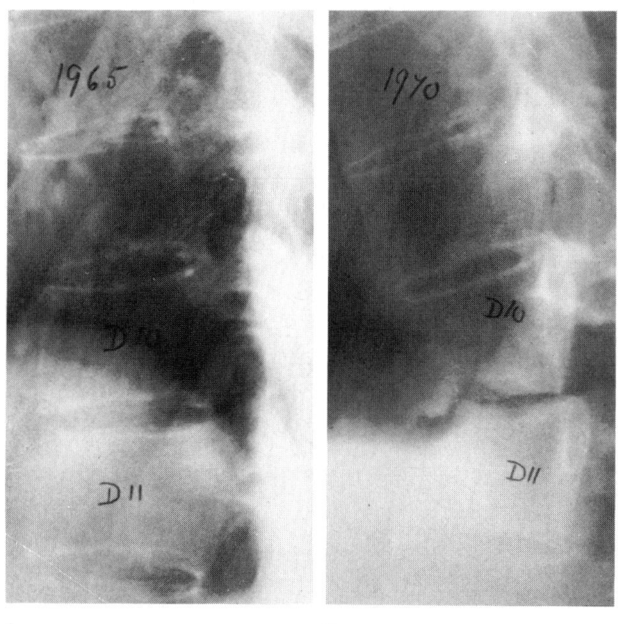

Fig. 4.31 A. and **B.** Ankylosing spondylitis, showing the development of much vertebral destruction — the 'pseudarthrosis' effect.

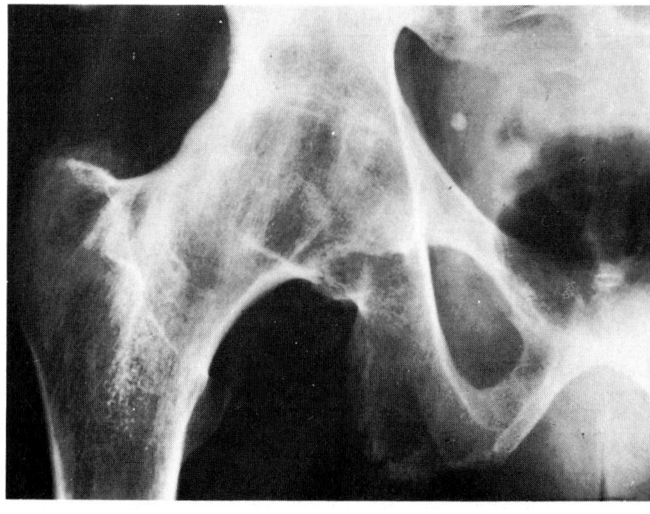

Fig. 4.32 Ankylosing spondylitis. Note bony ankylosis across joint cartilage. Irregularity of the surface of the ischium is also shown.

ligaments and around minor and major joints. If the intervertebral disc is intact at the time of syndesmophyte formation, it often never narrows, but may undergo central calcification. This phenomenon often follows vertebral fusion of any cause. Should the disc bulge, the syndesmophytes may be displaced. Syndesmophytes give the spine a knobbly appearance (Fig. 4.29), likened to a bamboo stick. Erosions at costo-transverse and apophyseal joints also end in fusion. A cauda equina syndrome may result from arachnoiditis when large posterior dural diverticula are occasionally seen at radiculography, with osseous defects in the laminae.

If the patient falls forward on to the head or chest, the rigid spine may snap, often through the porotic bone just beneath the end-plate. Hypermobility may be demonstrated on fluoroscopy. Fractures may also occur through discs (Fig. 4.30).

Occasionally localized destructive lesions of adjacent end-plates are seen with disc narrowing and marked reactive sclerosis (Fig. 4.26). This lesion resembles infective discitis and neuropathy but is probably post-traumatic. An associated pseudarthrosis is usually present at the neural arch at the same level (Fig. 4.31 A and B).

Peripheral joints. Osteoporosis, erosions and joint space narrowing are less prominent than in rheumatoid arthritis, but shaggy periostitis and ankylosis are more common. At the hip, a prominent fringe of new bone may form at the capsule–bone junction. Bony ankylosis may precede or follow prosthetic joint replacement (Fig. 4.32).

Enthesopathies at iliac, ischial and calcaneal sites of ligamentous and tendinous insertions cause erosions followed by marked sclerotic periostitis.

ENTEROPATHIC SPONDYLOARTHROPATHIES

Ulcerative colitis, regional enteritis and Whipple's disease may be associated with joint disease of two distinct types.

1. *Peripheral arthropathy.* Episodes of fleeting asymmetric peripheral arthritis follow the cyclic course of the gut disease and its severity is also proportional to the extent of the lesion. Radiographic change is usually confined to soft tissue swelling and local periostitis. Erosive change and joint narrowing is not common and the findings are not typical of rheumatoid arthritis but are said to occur in up to 10% of those with ulcerative colitis or with regional enteritis, especially if the latter affects the colon. These patients are seronegative and HLA-B27 negative. Sex incidence matches that of the gut disease.

2. *Sacro-iliitis and spondylitis.* Pelvic and spinal changes identical to those of ankylosing spondylitis are seen. These do not correlate with gut disease activity but may precede its onset and continue to worsen even if, for instance, the colon is totally removed. These patients (usually male) have a high level of HLA-B27 antigen.

Attempts have been made to use both isotope scanning and CT in the investigation of sacro-iliitis, but the results have proved equivocal or inconsistent. Simple X-ray remains the most practical method of assessment.

DIFFUSE IDIOPATHIC SKELETAL HYPEROSTOSIS (DISH)

(Forestier's disease, senile ankylosing spondylitis)

This condition was originally thought to affect the spine only. The current title clearly indicates that the condition is a generalized one, in which extensive ossification is found at many sites. It is usually seen in elderly males (M:F = 3:1). Some studies show an increased incidence of HLA-B27 in patients with DISH.

In the spine, dense ossification is found in the cervical (Fig. 4.33) and especially the lower thoracic regions. Bone is laid down often in continuity anteriorly and, in the thoracic region, on the right side, as the left-sided aortic pulsation presumably prevents its deposition. The thick, flowing, corticated plaques may indent the oesophagus. This florid exuberance is grosser than that seen in degenerative change. While continuity might also be seen following spinal infections, in DISH it is superimposed on a background of normal vertebrae and discs. On the other hand, osteoarthritis shows underlying bone and disc disease. In contradistinction to ankylosing spondylitis, the sacro-iliac joints show neither erosions or ankylosis. The

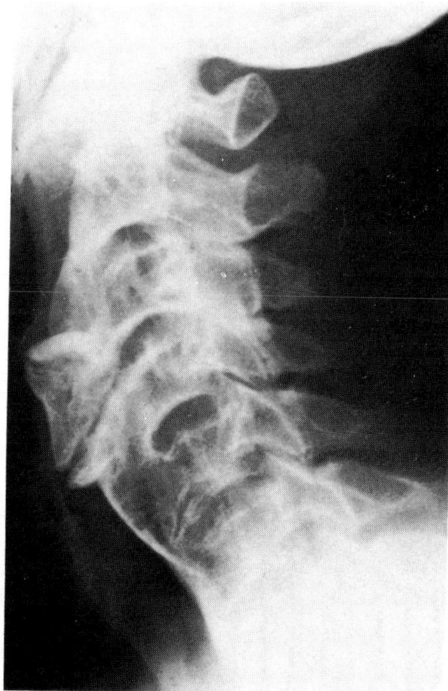

Fig. 4.33 Senile ankylosing hyperostosis — this is an extreme example of this common lesion. Tremendous new bone formation has arisen. The outlines of the original vertebral bodies and disc spaces are preserved.

patients may, however, complain of spinal stiffness and low back pain. Florid neo-ossification is also seen at extraspinal sites, around the iliac crests, ischia and above the acetabulum, at the sites of ligamentous or tendinous insertions into bone.

Similar changes are found in the foot, especially on the calcaneum, where florid spur formation is sometimes seen. The new bone is generally well-defined and not related to local erosive or degenerative change. Fusion between the paired long bones may occasionally occur.

OSTEOARTHRITIS (OSTEOARTHROSIS, DEGENERATIVE ARTHRITIS, HYPERTROPHIC ARTHRITIS)

Osteoarthritis is a degenerative condition affecting articulations, especially those which bear weight or those subjected to much 'wear and tear'. The disease may be considered primary when no underlying cause can be discerned, or secondary if the joint is abnormal in form ab initio or is subjected to unusual stresses. In terms of end stage appearances and treatment the difference is probably academic.

Though there may be differences in the radiological appearances of osteoarthritis at different joints, degenerative disease has a number of specific features wherever it occurs.

Joint space narrowing

The width of a joint space seen radiologically is due to the radiolucent cartilage; joint space narrowing is therefore the result of cartilage destruction. Often in a given joint a predictable pattern of joint narrowing may be expected. This depends on the anatomy of the joint and the usual direction of stresses placed upon it. Cartilage softening and fibrillation (Fig. 4.34A) leads to denudation of the bony surfaces. These changes characteristically occur in areas of excessive weight-bearing. Though presumably excessive in a particular patient, however, the forces are not necessarily pathologically high, that is, not necessarily higher than the forces acting on joint surfaces in patients who do not develop osteoarthritis. Nutrition of cartilage is actually dependent on the pumping action of synovial fluid which occurs when joint pressure rises; cartilage wasting and joint narrowing may also follow immobilization, as in poliomyelitis, though these non-weight bearing joints do not develop osteoarthritis.

Joint space remodelling

Joint narrowing due to cartilage destruction is followed by loss of underlying bone in stressed areas, and formation of new bone and cartilage in non-stressed areas and at joint margins. Often the two processes occur simultaneously. Change in the contour of articular surfaces, and in their anatomic relationships result, so that joint alignment alters (Fig. 4.35).

Beneath areas of cartilage destruction, eburnation results (Figs. 4.34B and 4.35). Localized increase in density is presumably due to (1) stress-induced new bone formation and (2) trabecular collapse. Flattening and sclerosis result. New bone formation arises in areas of low stress, at joint margins — peripheral osteophytosis — or within the joint — central osteophytosis. Peripheral osteophytes develop because of bony transformation of capsular and ligamentous attachments to joint margins. It may be that a narrowed joint results in peripheral capsular laxity and local periosteal elevation, or the local alteration of stresses consequent upon joint narrowing results in what is essentially remodelling, with osteophytic new bone formed in response to new lines of force and even preventing further malalignment. Buttressing osteophytes may thus be seen on the narrower side of a degenerate disc.

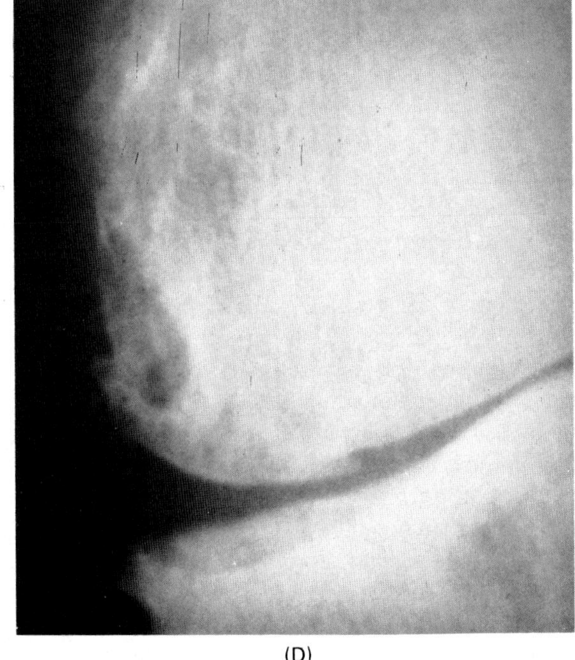

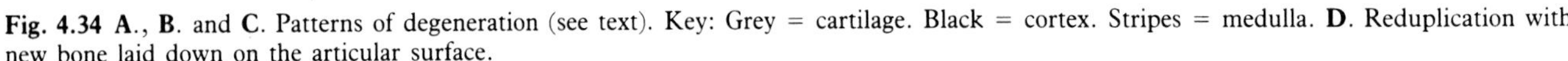

(A) Fibrillation (B) Eburnation (C) Reduplication (D)

Fig. 4.34 A., **B.** and **C.** Patterns of degeneration (see text). Key: Grey = cartilage. Black = cortex. Stripes = medulla. **D.** Reduplication with new bone laid down on the articular surface.

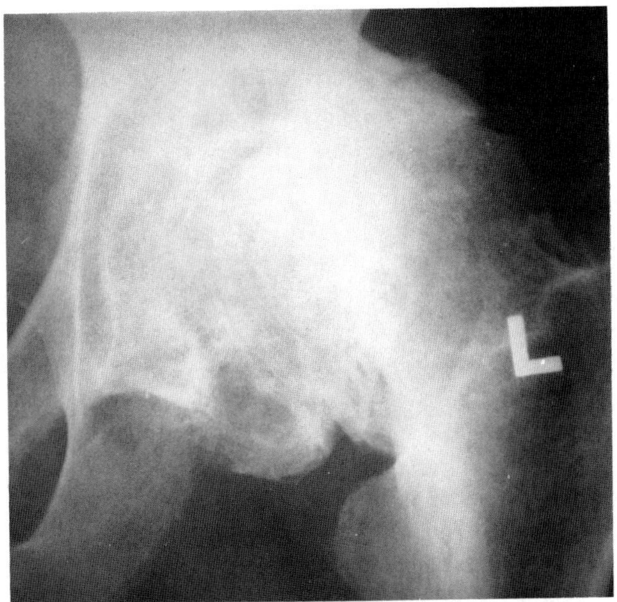

Fig. 4.35 Osteoarthritis of the hip: lateral migration of the femoral head with loss of bone superiorly and marked new bone formation, both on the medial aspect of the head and at the adjacent part of the acetabulum. A superior acetabular cyst is present.

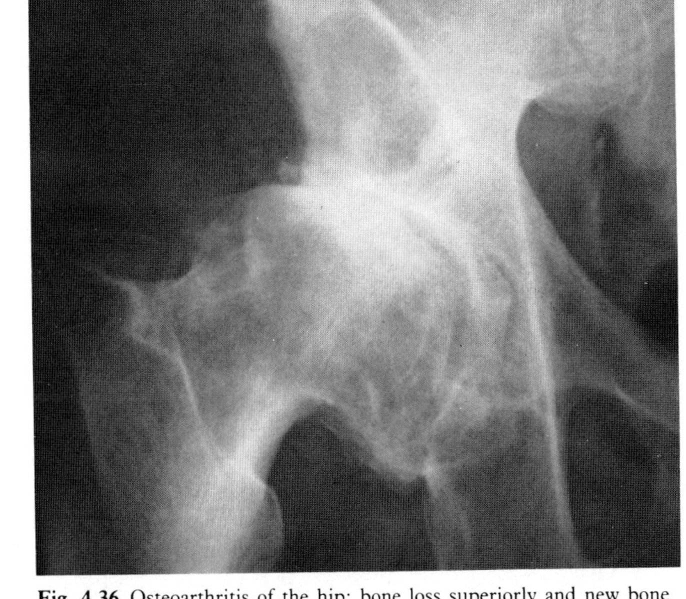

Fig. 4.36 Osteoarthritis of the hip: bone loss superiorly and new bone formation medially is accompanied by a large acetabular geode.

New bone may also be seen within a joint as a phenomenon of 'reduplication' (Fig. 4.34C and D). Cartilage remnants ossify, giving rise to an irregular bony surface.

Cyst or geode formation in subarticular regions occurs in osteoarthritis as well as in rheumatoid arthritis and is found in the weight-bearing areas, often associated with joint narrowing, eburnation and collapse of bone (Fig. 4.36). They are not true 'cysts', i.e. epithelium-lined defects in bone, but possibly result from intrusion of synovial fluid through cracks in the cartilage-denuded articular surfaces. On occasion, communication between the cyst and joint space can be demonstrated at arthrography. Usually, however, a communication is not shown as the crack has been obliterated. An alternative aetiology postulates subchondral bone collapse, possibly avascular in nature, as local blood supply can be compromised by high pressures in the joint.

Loose bodies

These are formed by detachment of osteophytes, crumbling of articular surfaces or ossification of cartilage debris. Osteoporosis and bony ankylosis are not manifestations of degenerative disease. Indeed, hypertrophic new bone is seldom seen in patients who are osteoporotic. Osteoporotic patients often fracture their femoral necks, but do not form masses of new bone about their hips. Conversely, patients with florid osteophytosis tend to have good bone density and fewer femoral neck fractures. When osteoarthritis results in pain and immobility, osteoporosis and soft tissue wasting may secondarily result.

OSTEOARTHRITIS IN PARTICULAR JOINTS

The hip joint

Murray has shown that only 35% of cases have no underlying radiologically determinable abnormality. Many patients who develop premature osteoarthritis — in their 40s — are found to have a pre-existing abnormality. Some result from childhood: congenital dysplasias, congenital dislocation of the hip, acetabular dysplasia, Perthes' disease or slipped epiphysis. The underlying cause is often recognizable. Others occur later: Paget's disease, scoliosis, rheumatoid arthritis and variants and aseptic necrosis of any cause.

There is no 'typical' appearance for osteoarthritis of the hip; rather, groups of different patterns may be defined. The appearances are complicated by analgesic therapy which may result in a neuropathic-type appearance with eburnation and rapid loss of bone (Fig. 4.37).

Patterns of osteoarthritis of the hip

These depend on the direction of migration of the femoral head which may be displaced superiorly (78%) (Fig. 4.38A), or medially (22%) (Fig. 4.38B). Superior migration may occur laterally (Figs. 4.35 and 4.36), medially (Fig. 4.38C) or in an intermediate direction with narrowing of the appropriate segments of the joint.

Medial migration may lead to protrusio acetabuli (Fig. 4.38B), lateral migration to lateral acetabular restraining osteophytes and new bone within the medial aspect of the acetabulum (Figs. 4.35 and 4.36). Capsular traction leads to buttressing new bone formation, usually

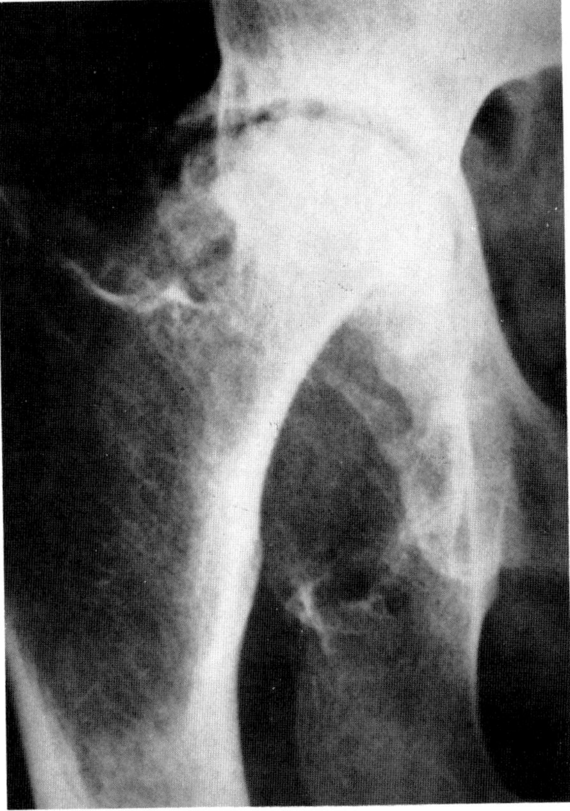

Fig. 4.37 Loss of the femoral head and deepening of the acetabulum may be the end-stage of osteoarthritis.

on the medial, rather than the lateral, aspect of the femoral neck (Fig. 4.35).

The end result is often a femoral head which shows bone loss in weight-bearing areas and bone proliferation in non-weight-bearing areas (Fig. 4.36). The acetabulum may be deepened following medial migration or shows new bone medially and supero-laterally following lateral migration of the femoral head.

The shoulder joint

Osteoarthritis does not usually occur at the glenohumeral articulation in the absence of a predisposing factor, e.g. the use of crutches, or secondary to acromegaly, or with the malalignment that follows a chronic rotator cuff tear. Golding has shown that degenerative changes in the shoulder joint are closely linked with soft tissue degeneration. Radiological manifestations include cupping and sclerosis of the greater tuberosity, cysts or irregular sclerosis along the anatomical neck (at the site of the capsular insertion) (Fig. 4.39); later atrophy of the tuberosities and upward subluxation of the humeral head occur. Occasionally, however, examples of the more classical type of osteoarthritis are seen in the shoulder, manifested by osteophytosis, sclerosis and marked loss of cartilage space (Fig. 4.40). Changes are commonly seen at the acromio-clavicular joint, with irregularity, sclerosis and cyst formation at the articular surfaces.

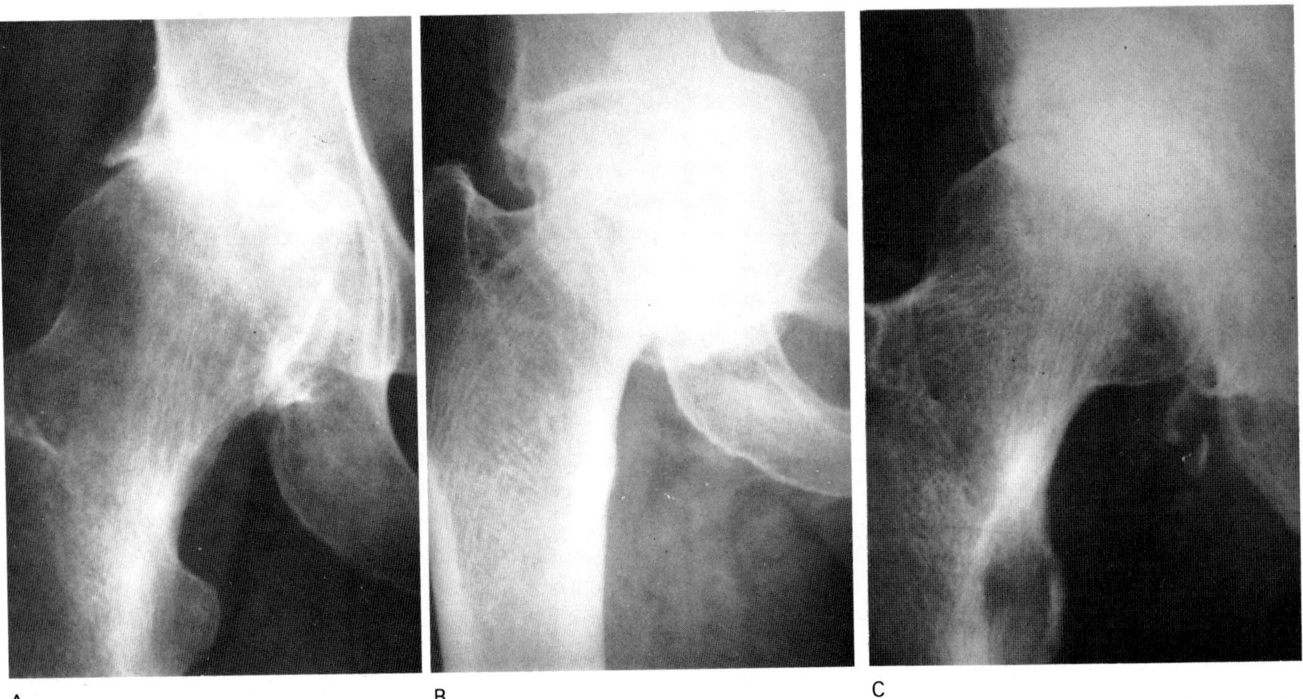

Fig. 4.38 Patterns of osteoarthritis. **A**. Superior migration of the femoral head. There is new bone on the medial aspect of the acetabulum. **B**. Osteoarthritis associated with protrusio acetabuli. **C**. Migration of the femoral head is in a superomedial direction.

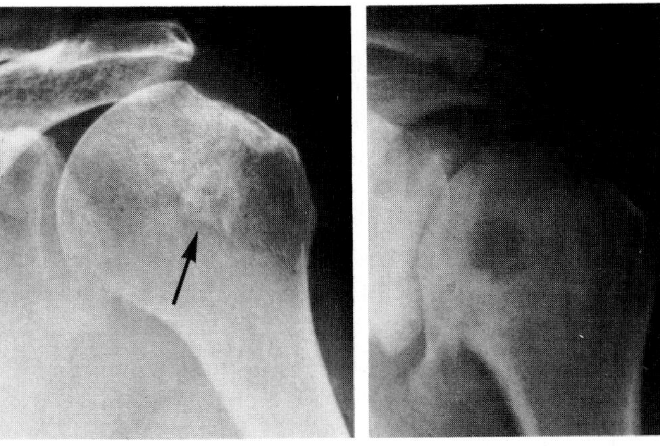

Fig. 4.39 Fig. 4.40

Fig. 4.39 Osteoarthritis of the shoulder. Note excavation of upper part of the anatomical neck with local sclerosis, and cysts seen *en face* (arrow).

Fig. 4.40 Osteoarthritis of the shoulder — 'classical type': loss of joint space, eburnation, cyst formation and osteophytosis shown.

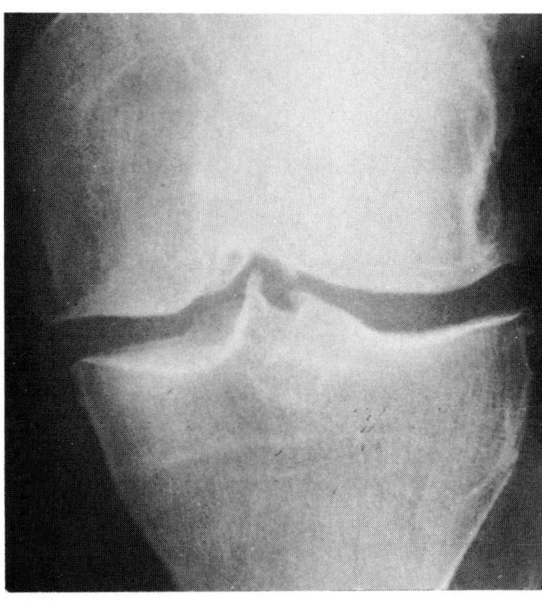

Fig. 4.42 Early osteoarthritis of the knee. Note spiking of the tibial spines and marginal osteophytic formation.

The knee joint

This is the most commonly affected joint in clinical practice. It consists of three compartments: a medial and lateral tibio-femoral and the patello-femoral. The bone most commonly involved in osteoarthritic change is the patella, which is especially subjected to large loads when the knee is flexed in a squatting position. Joint narrowing, osteophytosis and articular irregularity can be seen at the patello-femoral compartment on the lateral and skyline views, especially at the lateral facet of the patella, and the patella often migrates outwards. The lateral view also shows a scalloped defect of the anterior distal femur, especially in severely affected females (Fig. 4.41).

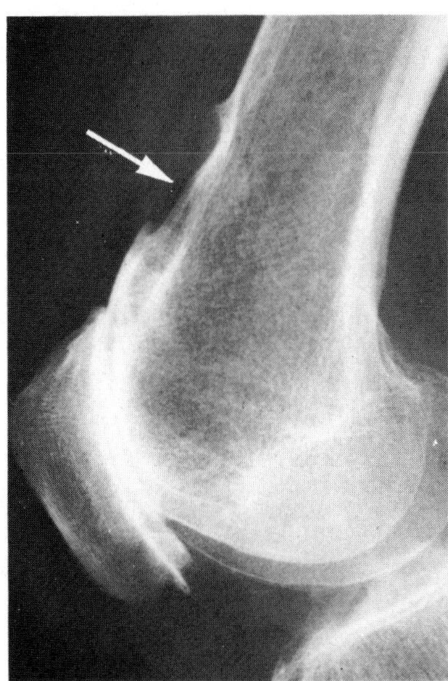

Fig. 4.41 Osteoarthritis of the patello-femoral joint. There is a groove on the lower anterior part of the femoral shaft (arrow).

Spiking of the tibial spines and osteophytes on the articular margins are seen in early disease (Fig. 4.42). Joint narrowing affecting one or other compartment results in valgus or varus deformity, best seen in erect anteroposterior views, with gross buttressing osteophytosis on the side of the narrowing. The opposite compartment may then be widened. Varus deformity is more common and is possibly related to the more common medial meniscus abnormalities. Osteoarthritis of the knees is also more common in the obese. The fabella may also be enlarged and irregular in osteoarthritis.

The hands

The carpo-metacarpal joint of the thumb and the trapezio-scaphoid joint are commonly affected, especially in women (Fig. 4.43). These joints are seldom involved in rheumatoid arthritis. In contrast to the changes in rheumatoid arthritis, the distal interphalangeal joints are most commonly affected in osteoarthritis, but any joint may be involved. Narrowing may affect all, or a few, distal interphalangeal joints with large osteophytes on the distal phalangeal bases and overlying soft tissue swelling. There may be small peri-articular ossicles in the adjacent soft tissues (Fig. 4.44).

EROSIVE OSTEOARTHRITIS

Patients are typically seronegative and complain of episodic pain due to a symmetric arthritis of the interphalangeal joints and, less commonly, metacarpophalangeal and carpometacarpal joints. Bone density remains good but the joints show a mixture of marked joint narrowing and erosion with

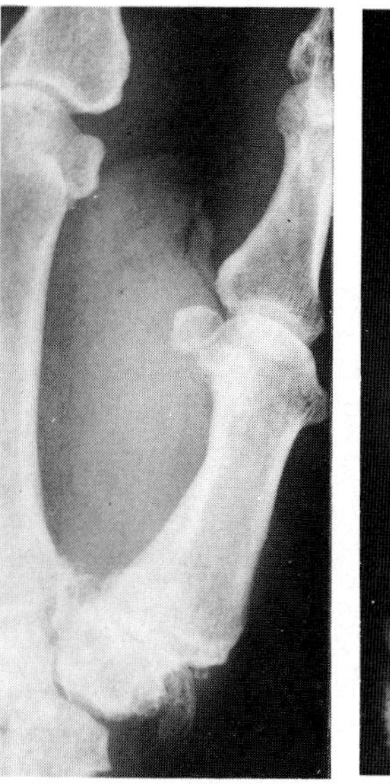

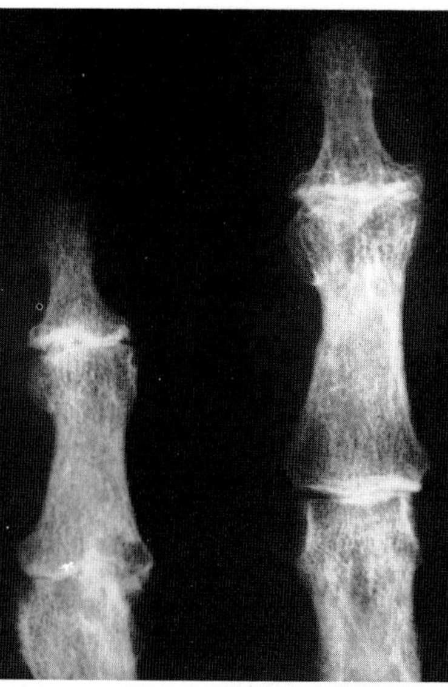

Fig. 4.43 Fig. 4.44

Fig. 4.43 Severe osteoarthritis of the carpo-metacarpal joint of the thumb.

Fig. 4.44 Osteoarthritis: joint narrowing and osteophyte formation with broadening of the bone underlying the Heberden's nodes.

florid base of phalanx new bone formation. The erosions spread across the entire joint surface, which then collapses (Fig. 4.45). Fusion at interphalangeal joints or marked deformity may result. Pathologically, the synovium is inflamed and some patients seem to develop rheumatoid arthritis later.

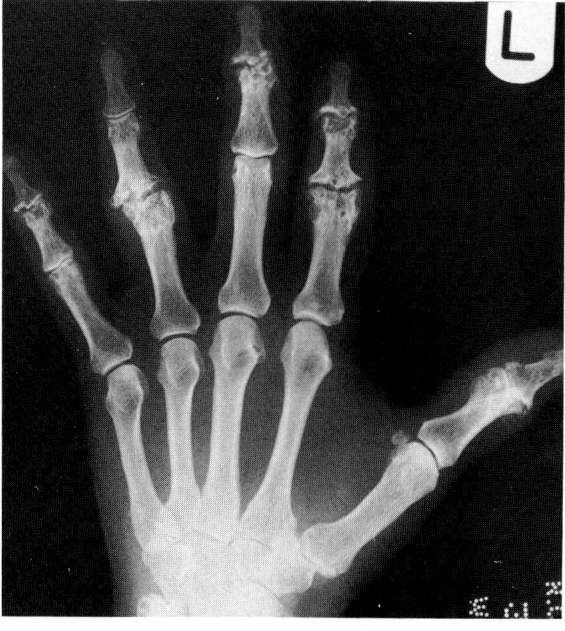

Fig. 4.45 Erosive osteoarthritis of the interphalangeal joints. Appearance of destruction around some proximal and distal IP joints.

SPINAL DEGENERATIVE DISEASE

Changes in the spine are of two basic types.

a. True osteoarthritic changes at intervertebral facet joints and unco-vertebral joints in the cervical spine.
b. New bone formation at vertebral margins usually associated with disc degeneration. These two types are often associated, since disc disease may result from abnormal mobility posteriorly, and vice versa.

Though the structure of a disc and its surrounding vertebral end plates differs anatomically from that at a synovial articulation, the radiological appearance of degeneration at both sites is similar. The space between two opposing bones becomes narrowed and marginal new bone formation, 'articular' irregularity and sclerosis appear. Later, malalignment may result. In the spine the marginal new bone results from elevation of the paraspinal ligaments following disc narrowing. New bone forms beneath the displaced and elevated ligaments. The outgrowths, osteophytes, are generally laterally rather than vertically directed as is seen in syndesmophytes. Osteophytes also develop on the concavity of a scoliosis, no doubt also secondary to ligamentous redundancy, but act as a buttress, similar to the restraining osteophytes in hip degeneration.

Disc degeneration alters mobility at the apophyseal joints, where degenerative changes become manifest by joint space narrowing and sclerosis. Facet slip at these joints results in encroachment on exit foramina, and new bone around them may narrow the spinal canal. Compressive symptoms result. Degenerative instability, scoliosis and spondylosis may also result.

Cervical spine. Additional synovial joints, the uncovertebral or neurocentral joints of Luschka are found from C3 down and are easily recognized on the anteroposterior view. As elsewhere, disc degeneration results in narrowing of these joints with osteophytic lipping. In the adult, maximal movement between flexion and extension occurs around the level of the disc between the fifth and sixth cervical vertebral bodies and it is here that the earliest and also most severe degenerative changes are to be found. Changes are next most common around the C6–C7 disc, but degeneration is less common superiorly.

Oblique views confirm the level of degeneration, and show encroachment on exit foramina at levels affected by disc narrowing (Figs. 4.46 and 4.47).

Posterior vertebral body osteophytosis, disc narrowing and longitudinal ligament laxity may all cause cord compression.

Thoracic spine. Degeneration in the thoracic spine is not usually severe or significant, though girdle-type pain may result, or even long tract signs if disc material herniates posteriorly.

Minor disc narrowing and osteophytosis is usually present anteriorly, especially in the elderly, often in association with a smooth kyphos.

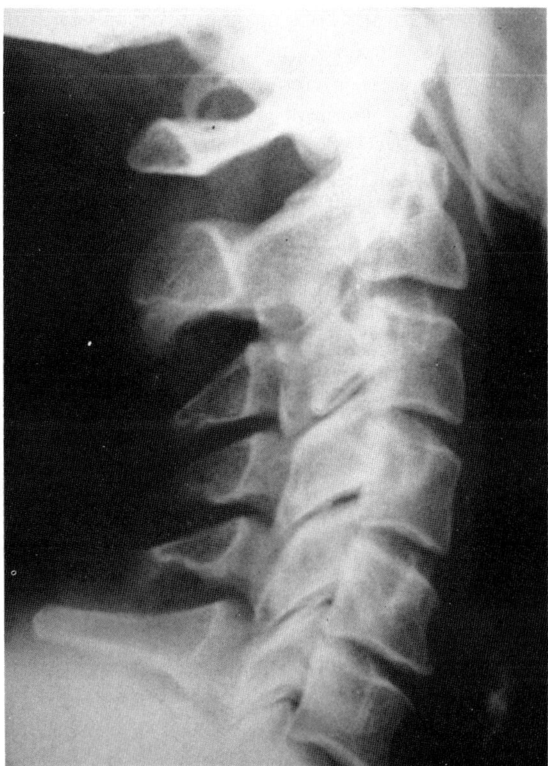

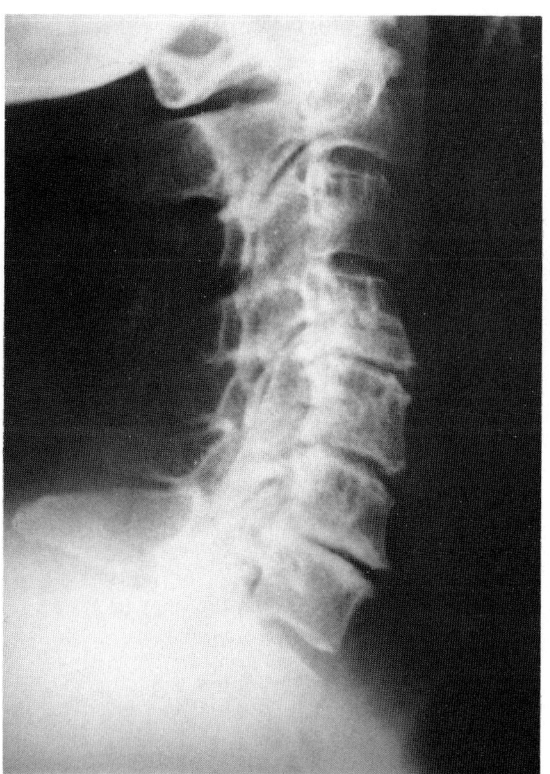

Fig. 4.46 Cervical spondylosis. **A**. There is early narrowing of the C5–C6 disc and the beginnings of anterior osteophytosis. **B**. Disc degeneration is now pronounced with both anterior and posterior osteophytes.

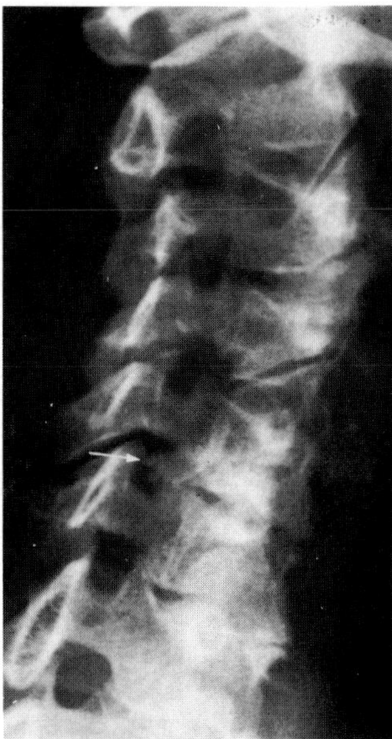

Fig. 4.47 Oblique projection of cervical spine showing large osteophytic protrusions into the C5–C6 intervertebral foramen (arrow).

Lumbar spine. Disc narrowing most commonly affects the L4–L5 and L5–S1 discs. When the radiograph is initially inspected the number of lumbar type vertebral bodies should be noted. The first sacral body may be totally or partially lumbarized, with a narrow disc between S1 and S2. A unilateral pseudarthrosis between the S1 transverse process and the iliac crest may be the seat of degeneration. Facet joint degeneration may cause osteophytic encroachment into the spinal canal and exit foramina (trophism). Slip at the facets narrows the exit foramina further. Disc degeneration may result in fissuring and gas is seen in the disc space — a 'vacuum' phenomenon, as well as calcification on occasion.

Facet and disc degeneration may result in vertebral slip without pars defects. With an excessive lordosis, contact between 'kissing' spinous processes may result in soft tissue entrapment and local pain (Fig. 4.48A and B).

RADIO-ISOTOPE SCANNING IN ARTHRITIS

Isotope scans using ^{99m}technetium-phosphate compounds will usually be positive in diseased joints. Exceptions are seen in joints in which the disease is inactive, as in fused sacro-iliac joints, and, surprisingly, in some cases of osteoarthritis. Because of their sensitivity, positive scans antedate even clinical activity as well as radiological change

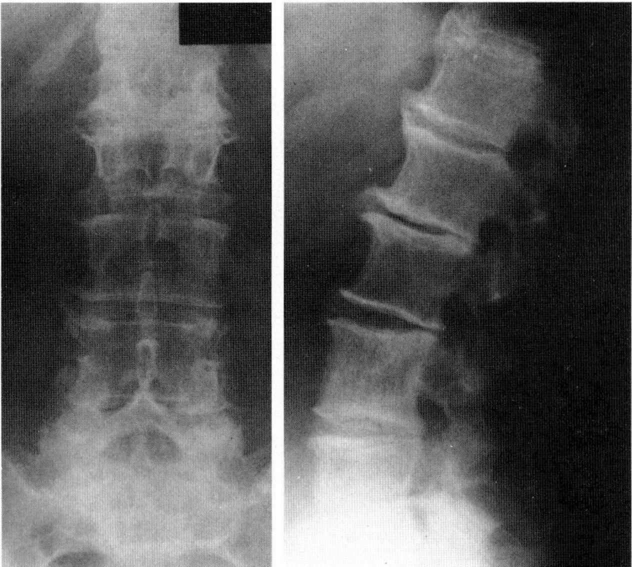

Fig. 4.48 Lumbar spondylosis. There is discal narrowing and a vacuum phenomenon is present in the degenerate discs. Marginal osteophytes are present. Inferiorly the facet joints show features of degeneration and, with the increase in lordosis, the spinous processes are in contact.

and indicate further sites of involvement in patients with established joint disease elsewhere. Using high resolution gamma cameras even the smallest joints can be successfully imaged. The areas of increased uptake indicate a joint abnormality but not the type of lesion. The distribution of the disease may indicate the underlying process and, in rheumatoid arthritis, scanning is probably more helpful than conventional radiography, especially in the early case where bone changes are minimal. Changes are maximal in the appendicular skeleton, especially at the wrist.

Rheumatoid variants may usually be distinguished from true rheumatoid arthritis by their different distribution pattern. Again, scanning is probably more sensitive than radiography. It is less specific than radiography in distinguishing subgroups within the seronegative arthritides, possibly because of overlap of syndromes, and also because inactive burnt-out disease is not registered. Scanning is probably also of value in long term follow-up of patients in recording response to therapy. Nonetheless, it is likely that scanning will remain an adjunct to conventional radiology. It cannot stage disease processes as other than active or inactive, whereas the conventional radiographs show the degree of anatomical change. Taken in correlation with clinical assessment, scanning is theoretically more effective than conventional radiology. Old habits however die hard.

GOUT

Gout is a metabolic disease in which joint changes predominate. It begins by causing acute attacks of arthritis which last for a few days and then clear completely. Traditionally, the great toe is the favourite site, but involvement of other joints is just as frequent. A remission will occur lasting perhaps two years to be followed by a further attack of greater severity and lasting a little longer. Attacks become increasingly frequent and more severe and the original monarticular lesion becomes polyarticular. Earlier attacks recover completely but later ones do not. Thus, it

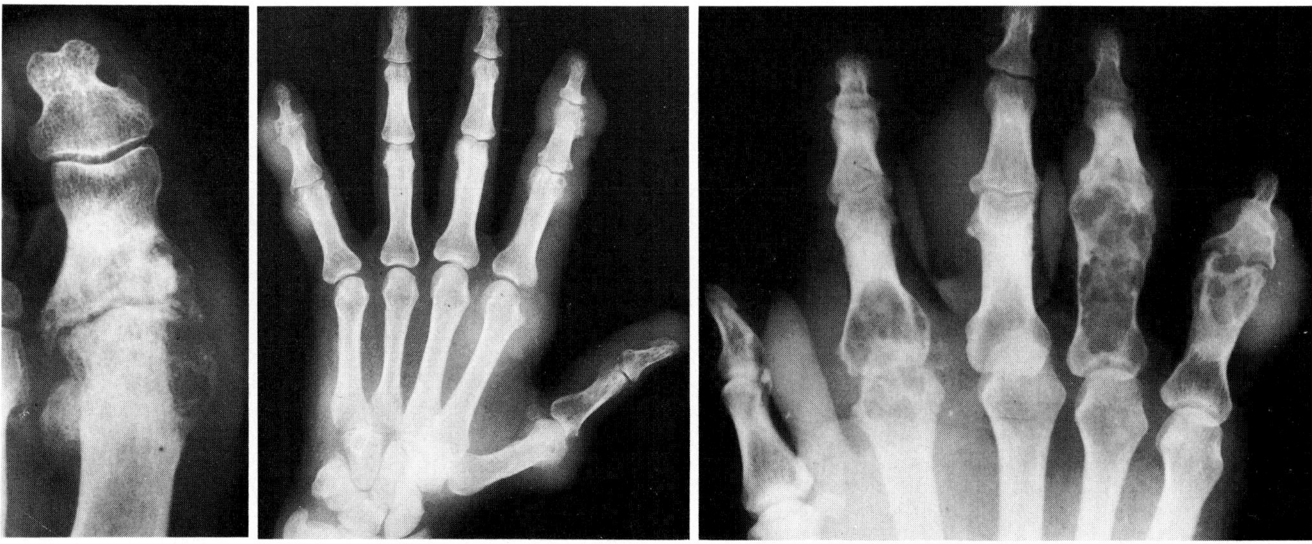

Fig. 4.49 **Fig. 4.50** **Fig. 4.51**

Fig. 4.49 Gout. Erosion on medial part of first metacarpal extends away from the joint surface.

Fig. 4.50 Gout. Note eccentric soft tissue swellings, some erosions away from the joint surface. Involvement of the distal IP joints (second and fifth in this patient) is quite common in gout.

Fig. 4.51 Very advanced gout. Note eccentric soft tissue swellings, intra-osseous tophi extending to bone ends and lack of osteoporosis.

s usually several years before radiographic signs of gout become manifest. Rarely, radiological changes of gout have been reported in young people. It is much commoner in he male.

Radiographic findings. a. *Erosions*. These are caused by deposition of *sodium biurate* and are typically punched-out n appearance. They tend to appear near joint margins. As they enlarge, they tend to involve more of the cortex of the shaft rather than the articular surface (Figs. 4.49 and 4.50). Large erosions extend to the articular cortex and diffusely n the shafts (Fig. 4.51). Erosions seen *en face* in carpal bones produce a spotty effect. Erosions rarely are found in bones remote from joints. In the hand, gout tends to attack the distal and proximal interphalangeal joints whereas rheumatoid arthritis affects the metacarpo-phalangeal and proximal interphalangeal joints.

b. *Cartilage destruction*. This is a relatively late manifestation. Usually much bony destruction is seen before cartilage loss supervenes.

c. *Osteoporosis* is not seen except in advanced cases which have been immobilized.

d. *Osteophytosis*. There is no tendency to form osteophytes though some splaying and spurring of opposing bony surfaces may be seen round a damaged joint.

e. *Tophi*. These are shown as soft tissue swellings eccentric in distribution in contradistinction to the fusiform soft-tissue swellings of rheumatoid arthritis (Fig. 4.51).

Eventually, both soft tissue and intra-osseous tophi may become calcified (Fig. 4.52) but this is uncommon.

Differential diagnosis. Differentiation between gout and *multiple enchondromata* may be difficult radiographically.

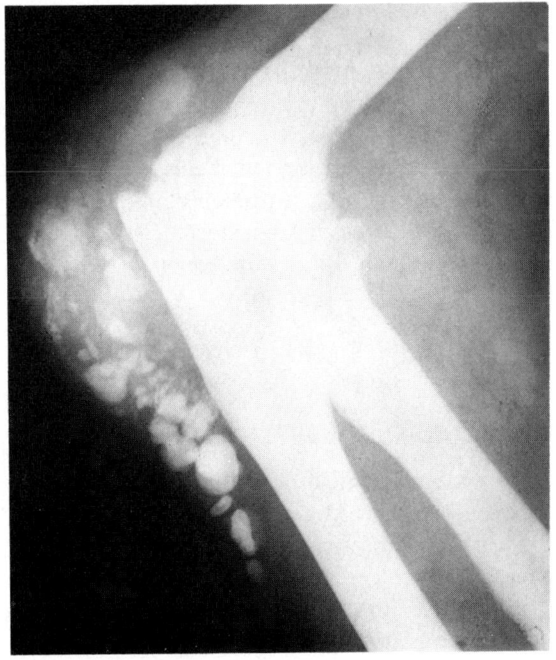

Fig. 4.52 Gout: large calcified tophi in olecranon bursa.

The tendency of multiple enchondromata to spare bone ends is an important diagnostic point. The clinical findings and history readily differentiate the two conditions.

In practice, the most frequent difficulty is in differentiating gout from *rheumatoid arthritis*. Important points are the longer latent period of gout, its eccentric, often gross soft tissue swellings and tendency to attack distal interphalangeal joints. Osteoporosis is found much more frequently in rheumatoid arthritis. Rheumatoid erosions are not so sharply defined as those of gout. Calcified tophi are, of course, diagnostic of gout. In difficult cases, differentiation will be made by laboratory tests revealing a raised blood uric acid.

HYPERTROPHIC (PULMONARY) OSTEOARTHROPATHY

This condition was originally thought to be associated solely with intrathoracic disease, but it is now known to be associated with intra-abdominal and other diseases. The word 'pulmonary' is best avoided in the title. The vast majority of cases are associated with intrathoracic neoplasms, mainly bronchogenic carcinoma, up to 12% of which have hypertrophic osteoarthropathy, with the exception of oat-cell carcinomas. Hypertrophic osteoarthropathy is also associated with secondary lung tumours. Its highest incidence is found with fibrous mesothelioma of the pleura. Hypertrophic osteoarthropathy is more common with peripherally seated tumours.

Hypertrophic osteoarthropathy is also observed with bronchiectasis, rarely with tuberculosis and congenital cyanotic heart disease, and it may also be found with chronic liver and gut inflammatory disorders. Even though hypertrophic osteoarthropathy is usually accompanied by clubbing, the latter should be separated on clinical, radiological and pathological grounds.

Periostitis is seen earliest at the distal third of the radius and ulna (Fig. 4.53), then the distal tibia and fibula, and then the humerus and femur, metacarpals, metatarsals and proximal and middle phalanges (Fig. 4.54). Distal phalanges and the axial skeleton are rarely affected.

Radiologically, soft tissue swelling may be seen over distal phalanges if clubbing is present, but the underlying bone is normal. In the long bones, periostitis affects the distal diaphyses but the bone ends are uninvolved. A single, fine layer, or multiple layers of periosteal new bone, giving an onion skin appearance, may be seen. On occasion the periostitis may be shaggy. The new bone merges with the cortex in longstanding cases. Endosteal new bone is not seen.

Occasionally joint pain and swelling are related to an underlying arthritis, usually of larger joints. Radiologically osteoporosis and effusions may be recognised but erosions do not apparently occur.

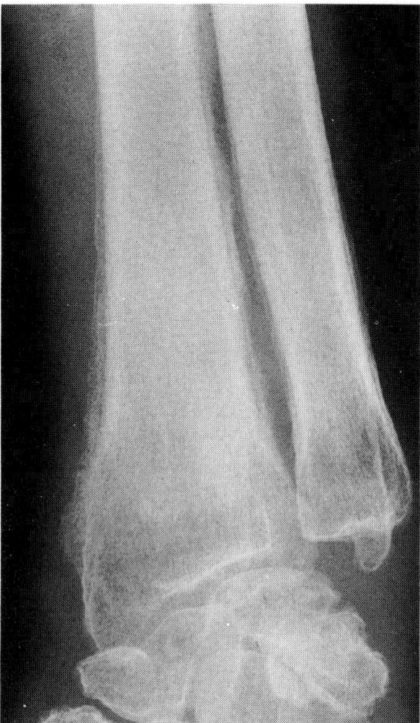

Fig. 4.53 Hypertrophic pulmonary osteoarthropathy: exuberant periosteal reaction of the radius and ulna. In this patient, changes in the bones of the hands were minimal.

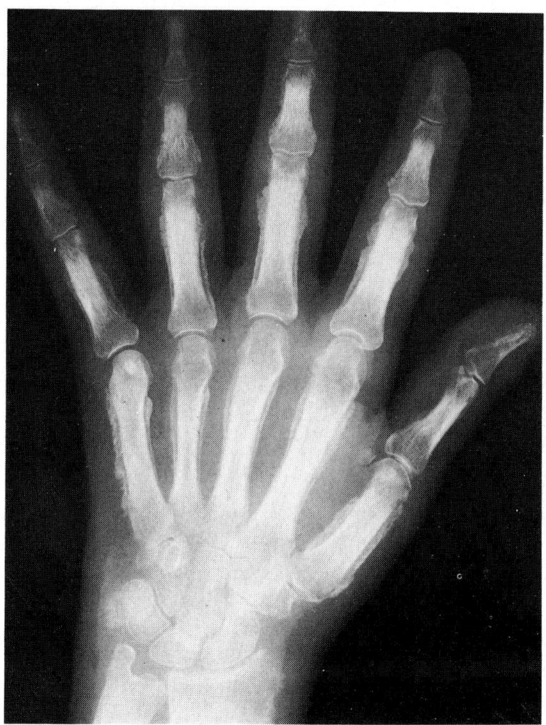

Fig. 4.54 Hypertrophic pulmonary osteoarthropathy secondary to pulmonary neoplasm.

Radio-isotope scanning in hypertrophic osteoarthropathy

Hypertrophic osteoarthropathy is a disease in which blood flow to the limb is increased and new bone is formed. As expected, scanning is an accurate and sensitive means of detecting disease, and the changes are seen before those on the plain films. Increased uptake is seen symmetrically along the shafts of affected long bones paralleling the cortices and thus differing from focal or widespread metastatic foci. With treatment of the underlying condition, both film and scan changes regress. Increased uptake on scan is also seen around affected joints.

PACHYDERMOPERIOSTOSIS

In this condition radiological changes identical with those seen in hypertrophic osteoarthropathy present early in life, often after puberty. Though the periosteal new bone is similar to that seen in hypertrophic osteoarthropathy, it is often coarser and may extend further along the shafts to the epiphyses. A familial history is present in over 50% of cases and males are said to be more commonly affected. No related chest disease is found. The skin of the face, especially the forehead, becomes thickened and greasy with acne and hyperhydrosis.

SYSTEMIC LUPUS ERYTHEMATOSUS

This disorder is more common in young females and in black patients. It is associated with a 'butterfly' skin rash over the cheeks, with pleurisy, pericarditis, glomerulonephritis and psychiatric disorders. It may be precipitated by drugs.

Systemic lupus erythematosus may present with a symmetrical peripheral arthropathy in which erosive change is infrequent. Soft tissue swelling and osteoporosis are seen, but erosive change is minimal and uncommon. Soft tissue calcification also occurs around joints and in blood vessels. Alignment deformities of the hands are more typical, so that ulnar deviation and swan-neck deformities are seen, which are reversible, voluntarily and involuntarily.

Avascular necrosis is common, being found in the hips, knees and shoulder joints. It probably follows steroid therapy but, in view of the high incidence (10%), may be due to the disease alone. C1–C2 subluxation may be found.

PROGRESSIVE SYSTEMIC SCLEROSIS

This is a widespread disorder of connective tissue which often presents with Raynaud's phenomenon due to small vessel occlusion. Fibrosis of the skin, especially over distal phalanges, leads to resorption of the distal phalanges and then progressively of the middle and proximal phalanges. Soft tissue calcification is seen, especially over distal phalanges and around joints. Fibrosis may lead to contractures

Fig. 4.55). These changes may be preceded by or accompanied with a polyarthritis similar to rheumatoid arthritis in at least 10% of patients. Osteoporosis, joint space narrowing, erosions and subluxations may be seen. Changes of an erosive arthropathy in association with calcification should suggest the presence of progressive systemic sclerosis.

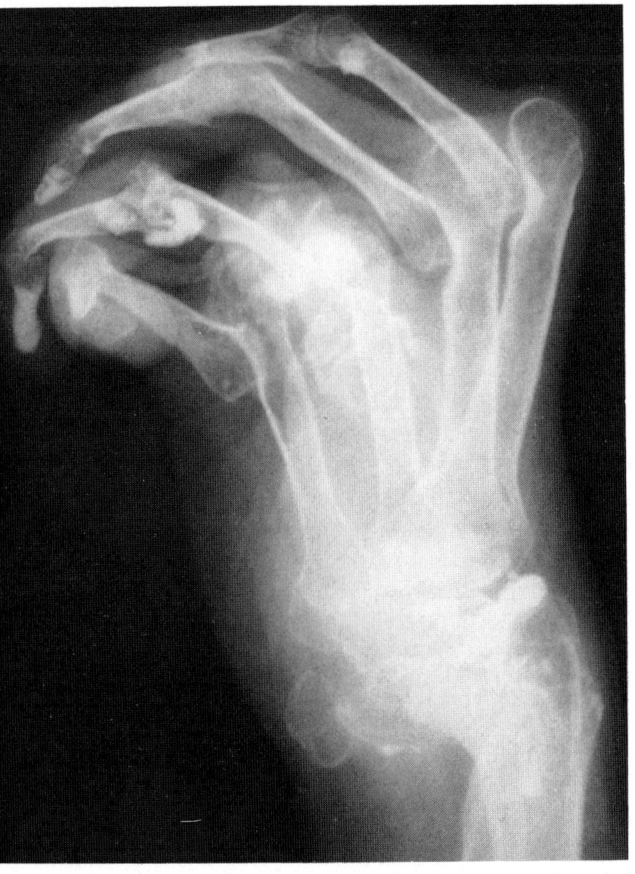

Fig. 4.55 Scleroderma. Contractures result in pressure resorption of bone at metacarpal necks. Para-articular calcification is prominent, as is distal phalangeal sclerosis.

JACCOUD'S ARTHROPATHY

Jaccoud, in 1867, described a syndrome in a 29-year-old man of episodic polyarthritis and rheumatic fever. The patient eventually developed endocarditis, mixed aortic valve disease and heart failure. The arthropathy does not involve synovium but causes capsular fibrosis. Deformities of the hands and feet, that are initially reversible, occur. Lateral deviation of the hands and feet may be seen when these parts are examined without weight-bearing. When pressed down on to the cassette surface the deformities vanish. The joint spaces are mainly preserved. True erosions are not found, but so-called 'hook' erosions of the metacarpal heads are produced, possibly because of local capsular pressure (see Fig. 4.55). The combination of ulnar deviation and metacarpal 'erosions' then simulates rheumatoid arthritis. The deviation, initially reversible, becomes irreversible. The patients are seronegative for rheumatoid arthritis.

MIXED CONNECTIVE TISSUE DISEASE

This is a so-called 'overlap syndrome' comprising a mixture of features of rheumatoid arthritis, dermatomyositis, systemic lupus erythematosus and progressive systemic sclerosis. Antibodies are present to the soluble ribonuclearprotein portion (RNP) of extractable nuclear antigen (ENA) in the high titres. Unlike systemic lupus erythematosus, involvement of the brain and kidney is mild.

Osteoporosis, soft tissue swelling and joint space narrowing are found at affected joints. The distribution also may mimic rheumatoid arthritis, but distal interphalangeal joints may be affected and the peripheral arthropathy may be asymmetrical. Erosive change is not inevitably present at these sites, which are a mixture of the sites of rheumatoid arthritis and psoriasis. The distal phalanges may show soft tissue loss, distal tuft bone resorption and calcification suggesting progressive systemic sclerosis. Ulnar drift as in systemic lupus erythematosus or rheumatoid is also seen. Pericardial and pleural effusions may be shown by chest radiography.

ARTHROGRAPHY

Radiological visualization of intra-articular structures is achieved by the injection of iodine-based water-soluble contrast media, or a suitable gas, or both, into the joint.

KNEE JOINT

Arthrography of the knee is of most value in the diagnosis of meniscal lesions. It is as accurate as arthroscopy in experienced hands and requires neither hospitalization nor anaesthesia. The examination takes 15 minutes and the patient walks away.

Technique. Single contrast techniques using a water-soluble medium, such as Conray 280, or air, or carbon dioxide alone may be used. Gas alone is used if there is a history of major allergic reaction. A double contrast technique is more aesthetically satisfying, though recent work indicates that it is not necessarily more accurate than a single contrast technique using a water-soluble medium.

The skin over the lateral pole of the patella is anaesthetized. The patella is pulled laterally and a No. 19 gauge needle introduced into the joint, between the patella and the lateral femoral condyle. An effusion, if present must be aspirated. 20 ml of air rapidly injected distends the suprapatellar pouch, confirming the intra-articular location of the needle. 4 ml of contrast medium are then instilled, or 6 ml if an effusion has been present. The joint is then distended with air or carbon dioxide, the latter being absorbed more rapidly. Up to 100 ml of gas may need to be injected to give adequate distention of the joint compartments. The knee is then examined fluoroscopically under stress, widening first the medial, then the lateral compartment. Serial films are taken during meniscal rotation so that both menisci are completely examined. Most modern screening machines have an arthrography programme enabling 8–10 spot films to be taken of each meniscus on one film. Where available, a 0.3 mm focal spot should be used. The knee should be as near the film as possible.

Fluoroscopy enables the meniscus always to be examined in its optimal position. This generally occurs when the beam is parallel to the medial tibial plateau. Often the lateral meniscus is best examined with a degree of flexion. The posterior aspects of the menisci *must* be examined. They are seen when, during rotation, the condyles are almost overlapping.

Lateral views of the knee in flexion against resistance *may* demonstrate the synovium *around* the anterior cruciate ligament. Normal synovium does not, however, imply that the contained ligament is intact. Only a gross disruption is therefore diagnostic.

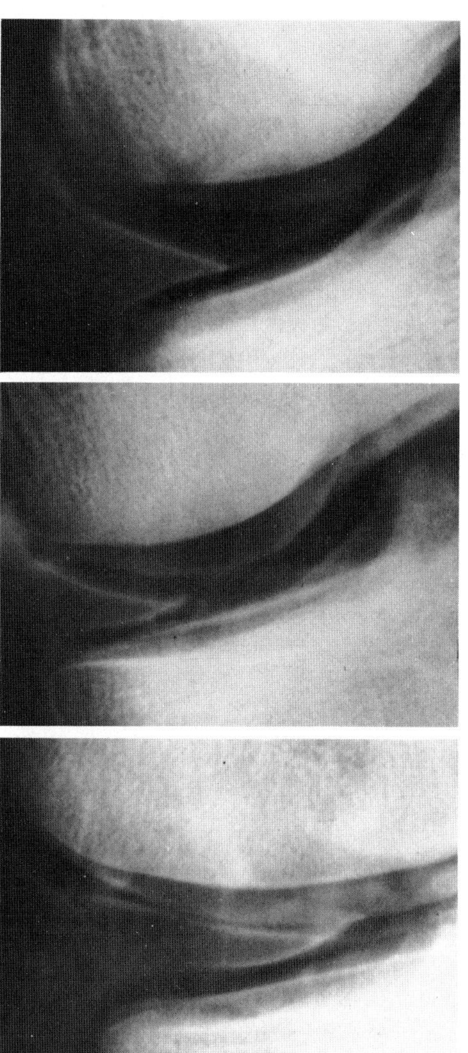

Fig. 4.56 Medial meniscus from front to back. The posterior horn is larger than the anterior horn. The normal meniscus is triangular in shape. (Reproduced by kind permission of Dr D. J. Stoker, and Chapman & Hall, publishers.)

The normal arthrogram

The meniscus is seen to be triangular in cross-section and its surface smooth (Fig. 4.56). The local articular cartilage and underlying bone are clearly shown. The joint space can also be assessed for loose bodies and lateral stress may demonstrate collateral ligament laxity.

The lateral meniscus has, from the midline of the knee posteriorly, a smooth peripheral crescentic defect representing a tunnel, the superior and inferior margins of which are fairly mobile. In this synovium-lined tunnel runs the popliteus tendon sheath (Fig. 4.57). Failure of meniscal involution *in utero* leaves an abnormally large discoid meniscus (Fig. 4.58).

Tears are seen as interruptions in the normal meniscus that fill with air, contrast medium, or both. They are potentiated by contralateral stressing of the joint. Tears are

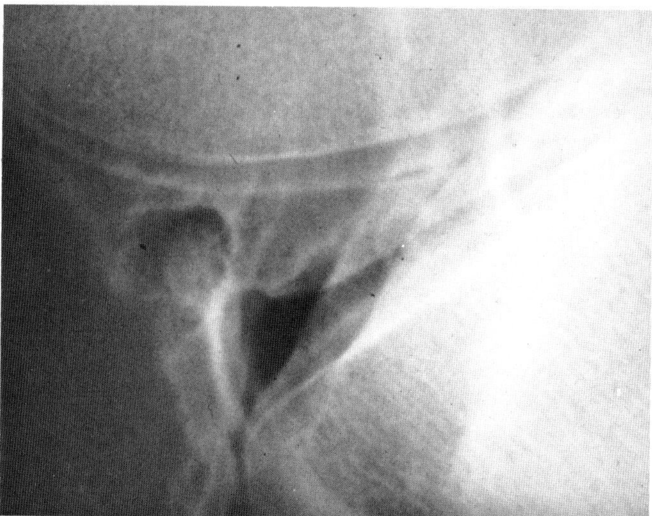

Fig. 4.57 Posterior horn of the lateral meniscus shows peripheral defect through which runs the popliteus tendon sheath. The superior and inferior struts around the defect are intact.

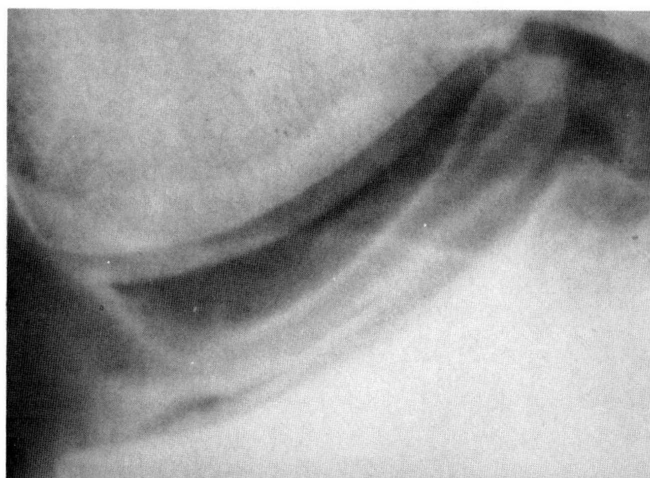

Fig. 4.58 Discoid meniscus. The meniscus extends medially to the midline of the joint and has a bulbous internal aspect.

more common in the medial meniscus than in the lateral by 3:1 and especially in the posterior horn of the medial meniscus. Thus, this region must be very carefully examined.

Tears may be classified as follows (Fig. 4.59):

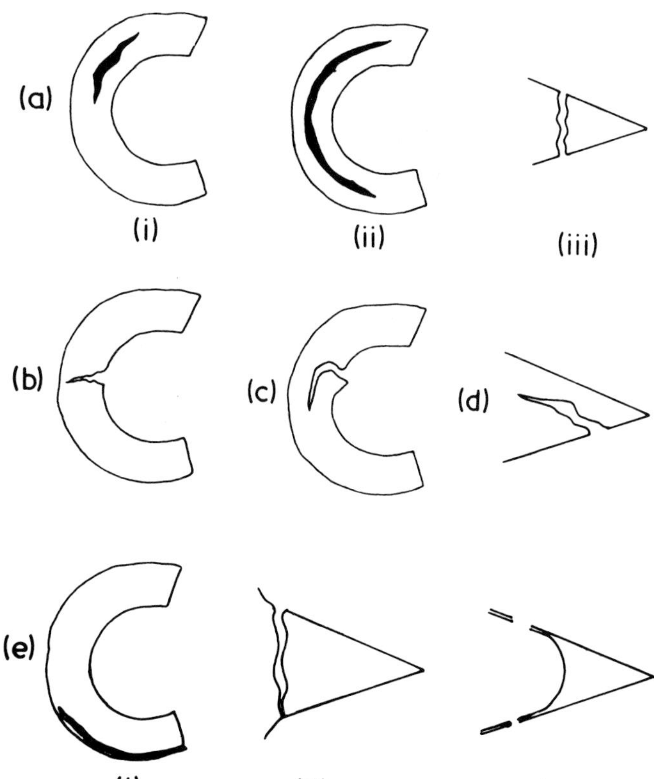

Fig. 4.59 Types of meniscal tear (see text). (Reproduced by kind permission of Dr D. J. Stoker and Chapman & Hall, publishers.)

1. *Vertical tears* — Limited or bucket handle (Figs. 4.59A and 4.60).

These are the commonest type in the young adult and especially affect the posterior horn of the medial meniscus.

2. *Radial tears* (Fig. 4.59B). This type of tear is difficult to identify and is especially common in the lateral meniscus.

3. *Complex tears* (Figs. 4.59C and 4.61). A mixture of (1) and (2).

4. *Horizontal cleavage tears* (Figs. 4.59D and 4.62). These may follow meniscal degeneration and are more often seen in the elderly.

5. *Peripheral detachment* (Figs. 4.59E and 4.63). This resembles a vertical tear in the medial meniscus. At the lateral meniscus it is seen as a tear of one or other of the struts across the fossa for the popliteus tendon sheath, so

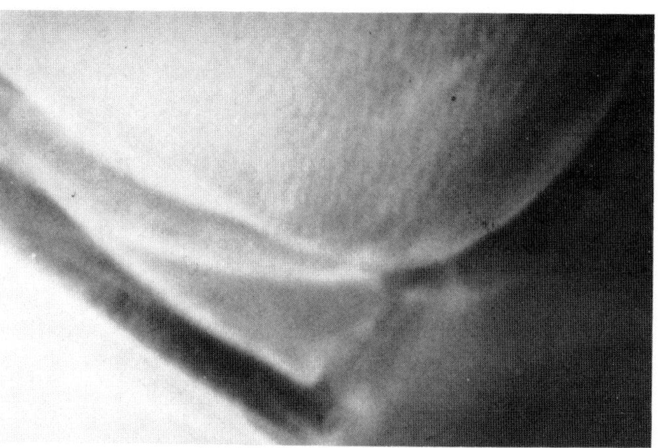

Fig. 4.60 There is a vertical peripheral tear of the medial meniscus. (Reproduced by kind permission of Dr D. J. Stoker and Chapman & Hall, publishers.)

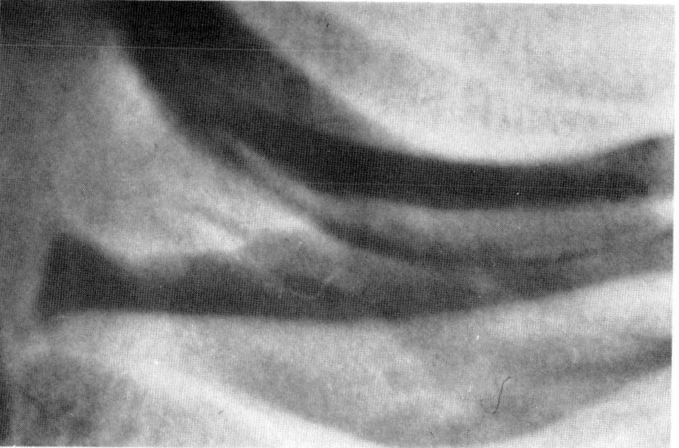

Fig. 4.61 A complex tear which has horizontal and oblique components is seen. The internal portion of the meniscus is no longer present but may be intact 'on the horizon', indicating a local defect. (Reproduced by kind permission of Dr D. J. Stoker and Chapman & Hall, publishers.)

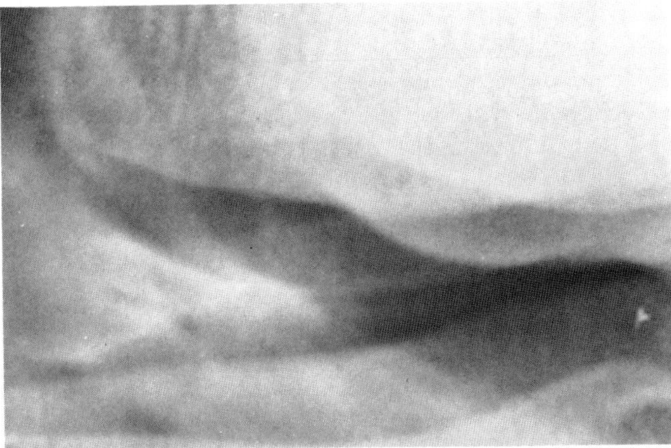

Fig. 4.62 There is a horizontal tear of the inferior surface of the meniscus similar to that seen in Figure 4.61. (Reproduced by kind permission of Dr D. J. Stoker and Chapman & Hall, publishers.)

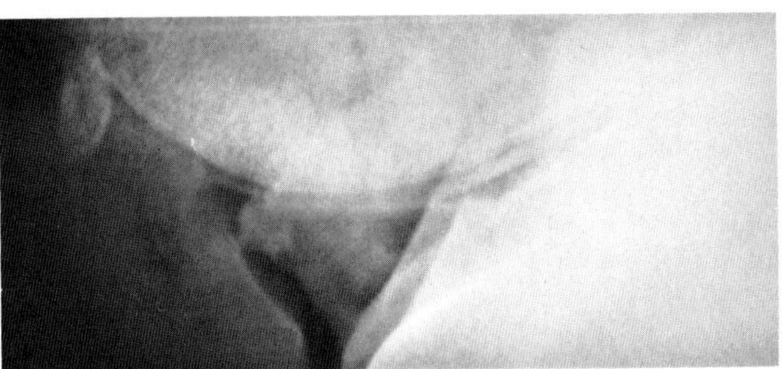

Fig. 4.63 Peripheral detachment of the lateral meniscus. The struts seen in Figure 4.57 are no longer visible and the meniscus is hypermobile.

that the meniscus is hypermobile and not attached peripherally.

Sometimes a torn medial fragment is displaced centrally and cannot be identified. In that case the remaining fragment is hypoplastic and its internal portion may absorb contrast medium, causing opacification. This phenomenon may be seen if the examination is prolonged or if the cartilage is irregular and degenerate.

Defects in articular cartilage and chondromalacia patellae may occasionally be confirmed, the latter by using skyline views.

Baker's cysts may be associated with congenital plicae (septa) in the suprapatellar pouch, but they are also seen with joint disease. Should they rupture, synovial fluid is released into the calf muscles which become painful and swollen, giving a clinical picture resembling deep vein thrombosis. Rupture of a Baker's cyst may be diagnosed by injecting 20 ml of contrast into the joint, which is then exercised. Leak of contrast confirms rupture (Fig. 4.64).

Following attempted meniscectomy, symptoms referable to a torn meniscus may recur. Arthrography is of value in showing how much meniscus remains; the posterior horn of the medial meniscus is the part most frequently left behind, and it may suffer further tears (Fig. 4.65).

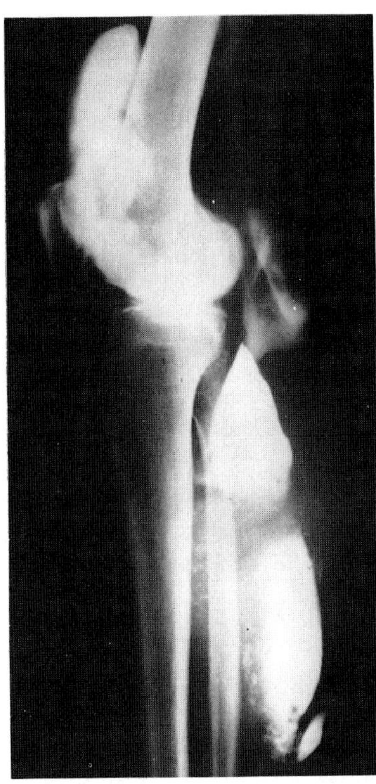

Fig. 4.64 Rupture of a Baker's cyst is demonstrated. This is probably chronic as the cavity in the calf has a smooth margin. (Courtesy of Dr A. R. Taylor.)

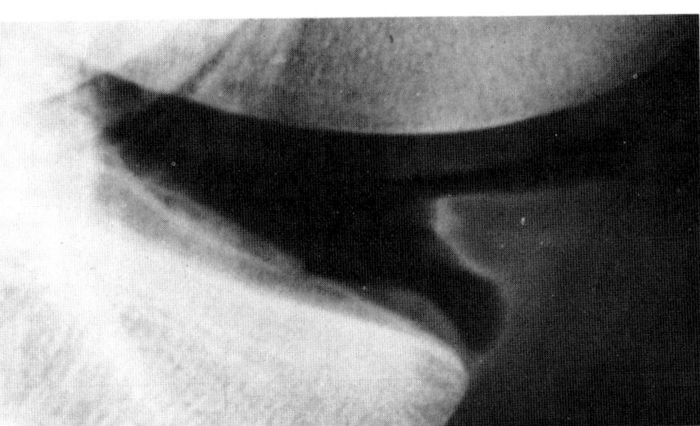

Fig. 4.65 A posterior horn remnant is seen after meniscectomy. Its internal aspect is irregular. (Reproduced by kind permission of Dr D. J. Stoker and Chapman & Hall, publishers.)

SHOULDER JOINT

Arthrography is used especially to demonstrate rotator cuff and long head of biceps tears, but also to demonstrate loose bodies and to assess joint volumes in restrictive capsulitis.

Technique. With the patient supine on the screening table, and the opposite shoulder elevated 45 degrees, the beam passes straight through the gleno-humeral joint space. The humeral head is shown in profile. The needle-tip of the syringe containing local anaesthesia is placed and left in the soft tissues over the cortex of the articular surface of the humeral head. A fine spinal needle (23 gauge) is then advanced adjacent to the anaesthetic needle till its tip lies in the bone of the humeral head just medial to its articular cortex. The needle is not withdrawn, as the bevel will be in the joint space if the tip is in the bone. 6 ml of contrast medium are injected into the joint. It should flow very freely and not remain at the needle tip after a test injection. 20 ml of air are then injected. The joint should take this easily. If air does not enter freely, either the needle is misplaced or a restrictive capsulitis is present. In this case, further injection of air ruptures the joint, often with relief of symptoms.

Interpretation. The normal shoulder has an intact Mahoney's line (cf. Shenton's line) and a space of 1–1.5 cm between the humeral head and the acromion. This space consists, from above down, of the subacromial bursa, the rotator cuff, the long head of biceps and the shoulder joint space proper. The two synovial spaces are thus separate (Fig. 4.66). With chronic rotator cuff tears, the defect in the tendon allows the humeral head to sublux upward and contrast fills the subacromial bursa from the gleno-humeral joint, that is, it comes to lie beneath the acromion, which may be scalloped by the elevated humeral head (Fig. 4.67).

On an axial view, contrast is shown to extend inferiorly, below the line of the anatomical neck.

The normal joint also shows a normal subcoracoid recess and an axillary recess.

Foreign bodies are especially easily shown in the shoulder.

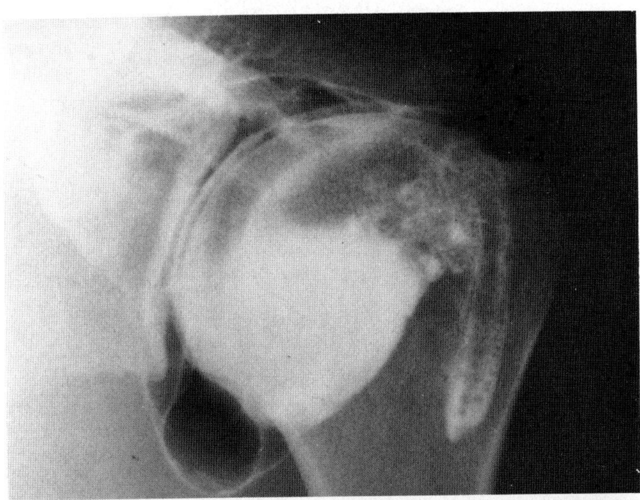

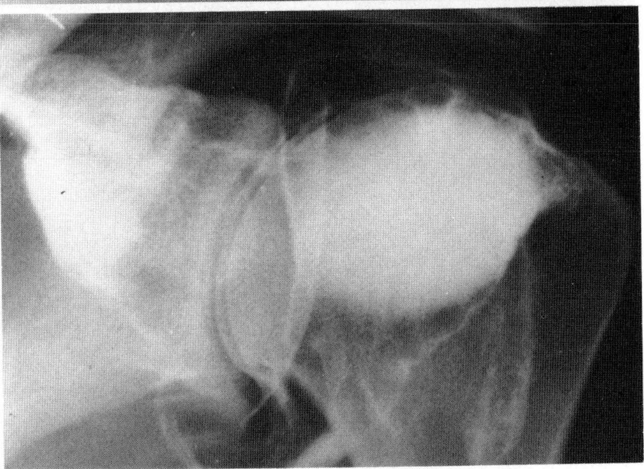

Fig. 4.66 The normal shoulder arthrogram shows a clear space between the acromion and the joint capsule. The long head of biceps is demonstrated as well as the infraglenoid and subcoracoid recesses.

ANKLE JOINT

Indications. Investigation of ligamentous injuries is the main indication but arthrography is seldom used in British practice in studying this joint.

Technique. The injection is performed under image intensification with the ankle joint in a true lateral position so that the malleoli are in line and perpendicular to the table top. This is easily achieved using pads. The foot is plantar-flexed, and a fine needle inserted anteriorly into the joint space midway between the malleoli. Only 2–3 ml of contrast need be injected, followed by 5 ml of air if desired. Anteroposterior, lateral and oblique radiographs are taken. Rapid tomography may help if loose bodies are being looked for.

Interpretation. In the normal arthrogram, contrast medium may extend upwards for 1 cm into the inferior tibio-fibular joint. In ligamentous and capsular ruptures, contrast medium will seep into adjacent tissues and into tendon sheaths.

ELBOW JOINT

Indications. This is usually performed in the search for loose bodies.

Technique. The elbow is placed on the screening table in the lateral position, radial side uppermost, flexed to 90°. The radial head can be felt to rotate between pronation and supination. A fine needle (22 gauge) is used, first to anaesthetize the skin, and then to inject the joint. It is inserted above the radial head and enters the joint easily while screening. Injection of 2 ml of contrast and 4–5 ml of air is made under fluoroscopic control. Unfortunately, when air is used, bubbles can be a problem. Again, after anteroposterior, lateral and oblique views, tomography may help but, if not rapidly carried out, contrast becomes diluted and smeary.

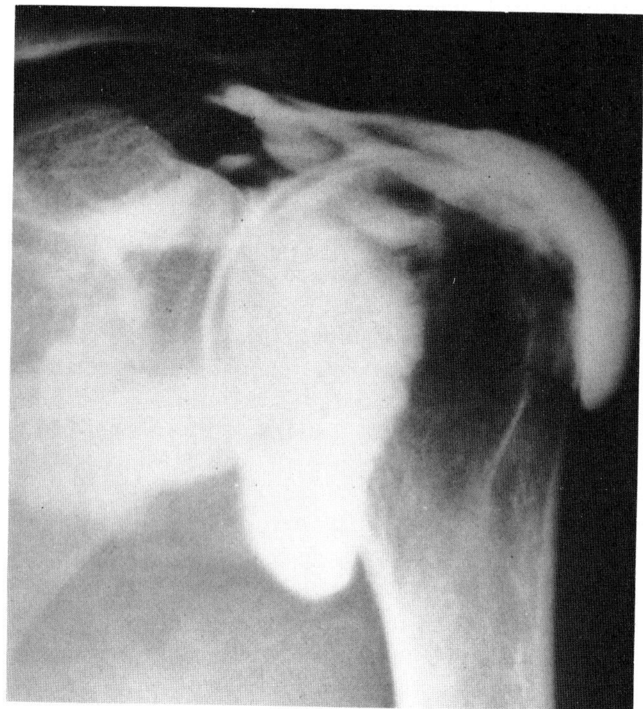

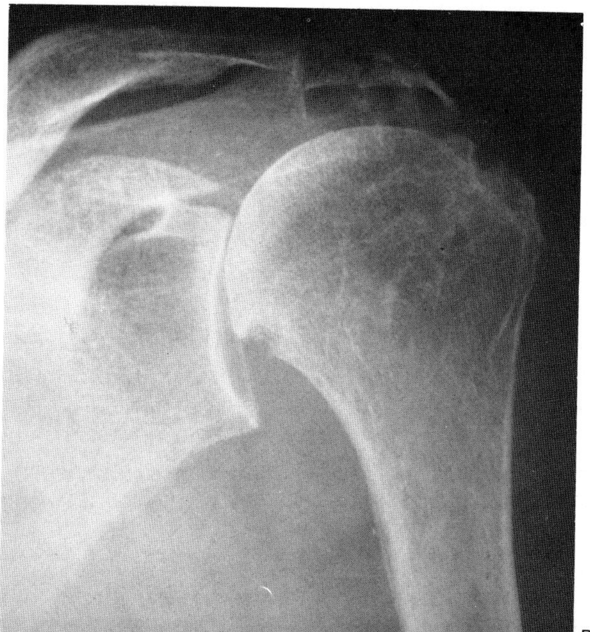

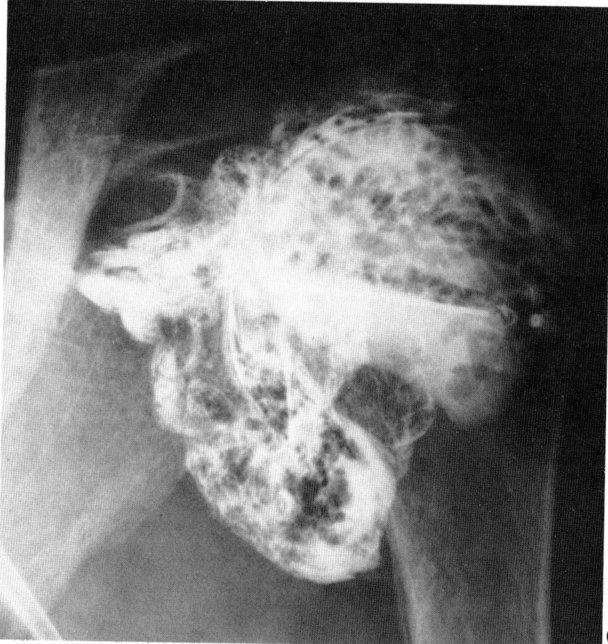

Fig. 4.67 Abnormalities at shoulder arthrography. **A**. A rupture of the rotator cuff is seen at shoulder arthrography with contrast filling the subacromial space. **B**. Rheumatoid arthritis. Erosions and upward subluxation of the humeral head. **C**. Arthrogram of **B**. Numerous 'millet seeds' float freely within the joint. There is also a rotator cuff tear.

Interpretation. Capsular ruptures are shown by spreading of contrast medium into adjacent soft tissues. Intra-articular loose bodies are outlined by contrast medium.

OTHER JOINTS

Arthrography has been used occasionally in the investition of lesions of the wrist and the temporomandibular joints, but the indications are few.

HIP JOINT

Indications

1. Evaluation of hip dysplasias — congenital dislocation of the hip, proximal focal femoral deficiency, epiphyseal dysplasias.
2. Evaluation of Perthes' disease.
3. Evaluation of dislocations associated with paralysis or joint laxity.
4. Assessment of synovial infection, inflammation or tumours.
5. Localization of loose bodies.
6. The assessment of pain following total hip replacement.

Technique. The technique varies with the age of the patient. In **infants** the joint is punctured under suitable anaesthesia — a general anaesthetic is used in those under 10 years. Various approaches — superolateral, inferomedial (where there is redundant capsule) and anterior are available, using fluoroscopic control. The anterior seems to be preferred, with the needle aiming for the lateral aspect of the femoral head, avoiding the femoral artery.

Synovial fluid should always be aspirated before contrast medium is injected, as contrast medium is bacteriocidal. If the needle is intra-articular, a test injection of contrast flows freely away from the needle, otherwise it remains

·und the needle tip. Excessive contrast medium need not : injected; in infants 1–2 ml is adequate.

Anatomy of the infant hip. The plain radiograph may ıow a shallow acetabulum and a small, or no, ossific nu- eus for the proximal femoral epiphysis. The rest of the ucent' joint space is, of course, taken up by articular car- lage and this is demonstrated after contrast medium has een injected. The ossific nucleus lies centrally within the herical cartilage (Fig. 4.68A and B).

The acetabular cartilaginous labrum deepens the acet- bulum and has a triangular, sharply pointed prominence n its superolateral aspect, the limbus. This is covered by ynovium and is lax. If medially displaced into the joint, prevents normal location of the femoral head. Contrast nedium on the lateral aspect of the normal limbus lies in recess resembling a rose thorn. Superomedially, the acet- bular cartilage is continued as the transverse ligament vhich causes a further constriction of the capsule. The rose horn and the transverse ligament mark the lateral and nedial extents of the acetabular cartilage. The capsule is constricted around the mid portion of the neck by a lucent band representing a bundle of muscle fibres, the zona orbicularis. The normal ligamentum teres is not identified, but its fossa in the head is.

The cartilage of the head should fit congruously within that of the acetabulum and contrast should be parallel with and evenly distributed between them, indicating that the joint space is even throughout (Fig. 4.68A).

Hip arthrography in children should be performed under fluoroscopic control and, if possible, videotape recordings made during manipulation of the hip, as well as taking static films. The head should be contained at all times within the congruous acetabulum and its movement not restricted.

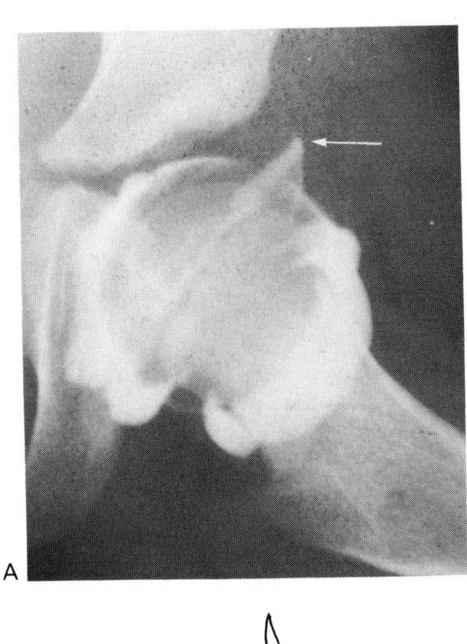

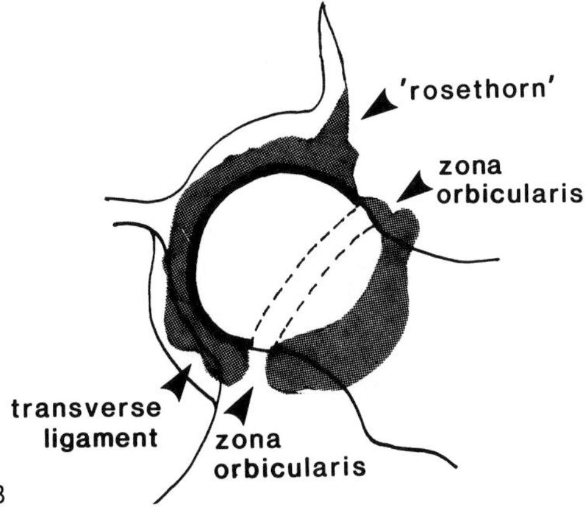

Fig. 4.68 A. Arthrogram of the hip showing 'rose-thorn' appearance of normal limbus (arrow). The rose-thorn is larger than usual.
B. Diagrammatic representation of the normal hip arthrogram (see text).

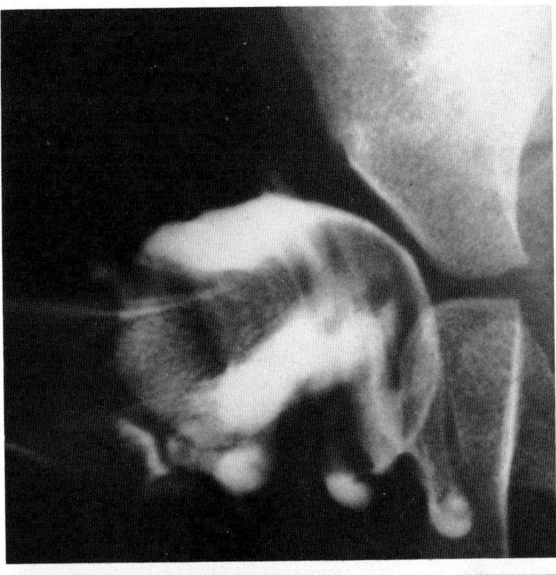

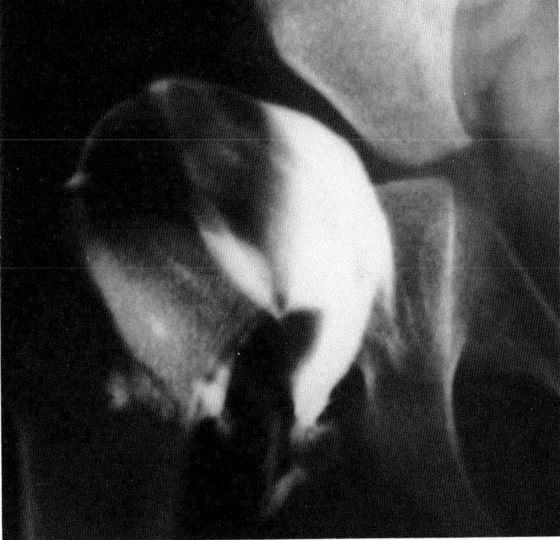

Fig. 4.69 Hip arthrogram in a child. The acetabulum is dysplastic. The ossific nucleus is seen within the largely cartilaginous head. **A**. In abduction the femoral head is congruous with the acetabular cartilage. **B**. In the neutral position the femoral head is incongruous with pooling of contrast medially.

Congenital dislocation of the hip. With partial dislocation, or subluxation, movement is excesive and the lateral aspect of the head is uncovered. The limbus and rose thorn are elevated and laterally displaced. Contrast pools medially with distention of the medial joint space. Manipulation of the hip under screen control in congenital dislocation of the hip shows the positions in which the femoral head and acetabular fossa are congruous (Fig. 4.69A) and incongruous (Fig. 4.69B). This information aids the surgeon in planning the operation required to facilitate joint development.

With total dislocation, the cartilaginous femoral head is totally uncovered, the limbus is medially and posteriorly displaced and may prevent reduction (Fig. 1.9). Contrast medium again pools medially. Lateral subluxation of the head and medial displacement of the limbus narrows the capsule, giving a so-called 'hour-glass' constriction.

Perthes' disease. It must be understood that the ossific nucleus is not the entire femoral head and, in Perthes' disease, the cartilaginous outline of the femoral head is essentially normal and not flat, irregular and fragmented, as the ossific nucleus may be. Arthrography does not diagnose Perthes' disease but determines (1) size and shape of articular cartilage, (2) presence or absence of congruity.

In early Perthes' disease, even though the ossific centre is abnormal, the arthrogram is usually normal. Later, the cartilaginous femoral head may alter in shape, flattening superiorly and becoming irregular, but enlarging laterally. The acetabular cartilage may become elevated superolaterally, the head being no longer 'covered' and the joint surfaces no longer congruous. Contrast pools medially. These findings are especially seen in abduction and indicate a poor prognosis, with incongruity leading to eventual osteoarthritis (Fig. 4.70A, B and C). Such patients may benefit from osteotomy. A more normal cartilaginous outline in the later stages of disease carries a good prognosis.

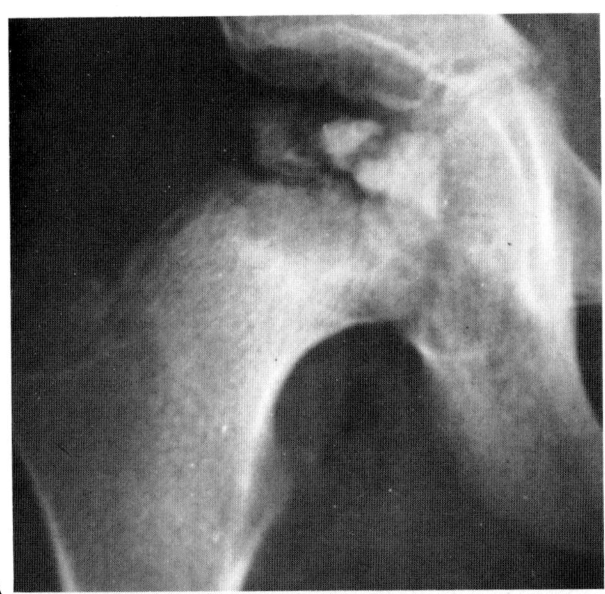
A

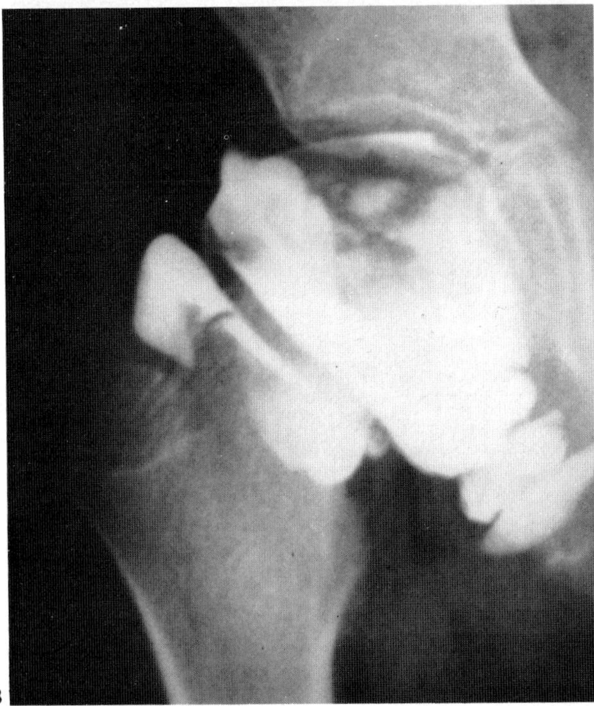
B

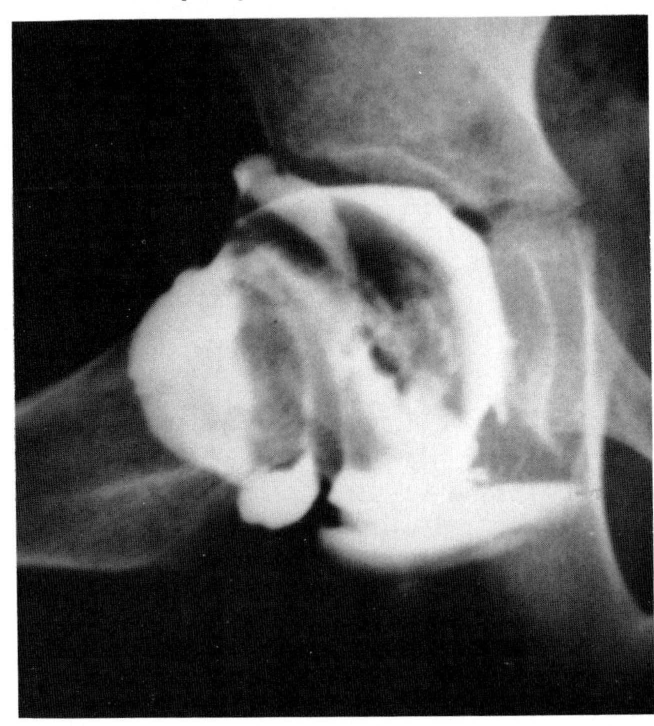
C

Fig. 4.70 **A**. Gross Perthes' disease of the femoral head. **B**. The outline of the cartilaginous epiphysis is somewhat dome-shaped with slight flattening and broadening laterally. The lateral aspect of the femoral head is uncovered but in the neutral position is in congruity. **C**. In abduction there is pooling of contrast medially within the joint.

Hip arthrography in adults. *Indications*. Most adult hip arthrograms are performed to assess either loosening or infection of a prosthesis. These patients complain of pain of increasing severity, often years after hip replacement. Such complications arise in up to 20% of patients, and 5% are infected.

Methyl methacrylate cement causes thermal necrosis of bone. A 1 mm zone of lucency is thus to be expected at the cement-bone interface, especially around the cup of the acetabular prosthesis. Lucency between cement and metal or bone and metal is less prominent and may result from movement during insertion of the prosthesis, pressure on weight-bearing or osteoclastic stimulation. Excessive or progressive widening of the interface lucency, or settling of the prosthesis into bone or cement may indicate loosening or infection with resorption of bone.

Technique. Following local anaesthetic infiltration and avoiding the line of the femoral artery, a fine spinal needle is inserted vertically under fluoroscopic control onto the neck of the prosthetic femoral component. Placement is achieved when metal touches metal. Fluid must be aspirated before contrast is instilled as the contrast medium is bacteriocidal. Infection is best diagnosed by isolation of an organism from aspirate or joint washings. Up to 20 ml of contrast are injected. Large bursae and the new joint capsule may fill. If these are small, however, only 7–10 ml may be needed. The hip is then exercised passively. Anteroposterior and frog lateral views are taken before and after contrast. Loosening is shown by tracking of contrast between interfaces (Fig. 4.71). This is especially seen at the femoral component, but a thin (less than 1 mm) smear of contrast around the cup does not necessarily indicate loosening, especially if the contrast does not cover the entire cup. Subtraction techniques aid visualization of contrast medium around the prosthesis.

Infection also causes bone resorption at interfaces, but occasionally sinuses develop. Sinograms then show a connection with the prosthesis (Fig. 4.72). Bone resorption is usually more severe and focal.

Synovial lesions or loose bodies may also be demonstrated by arthrography (Fig. 4.73). The needle is again inserted vertically over the central part of the femoral neck.

ISOTOPE BONE SCANNING AND PROSTHETIC LOOSENING

Following insertion of a prosthesis, increased uptake of tracer is to be expected in the surrounding bone. This is

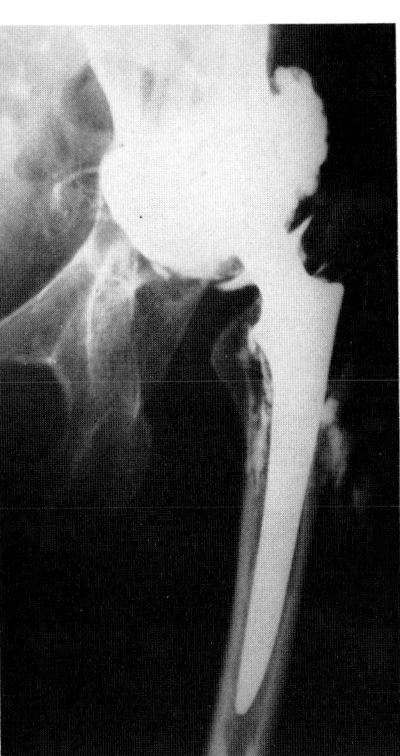

Fig. 4.71

Fig. 4.71 Loosening of the hip prosthesis is demonstrated at arthrography. Contrast surrounds the acetabular component and tracks down the femoral stem. There is also a defect in the bone through which contrast escapes into the soft tissues.

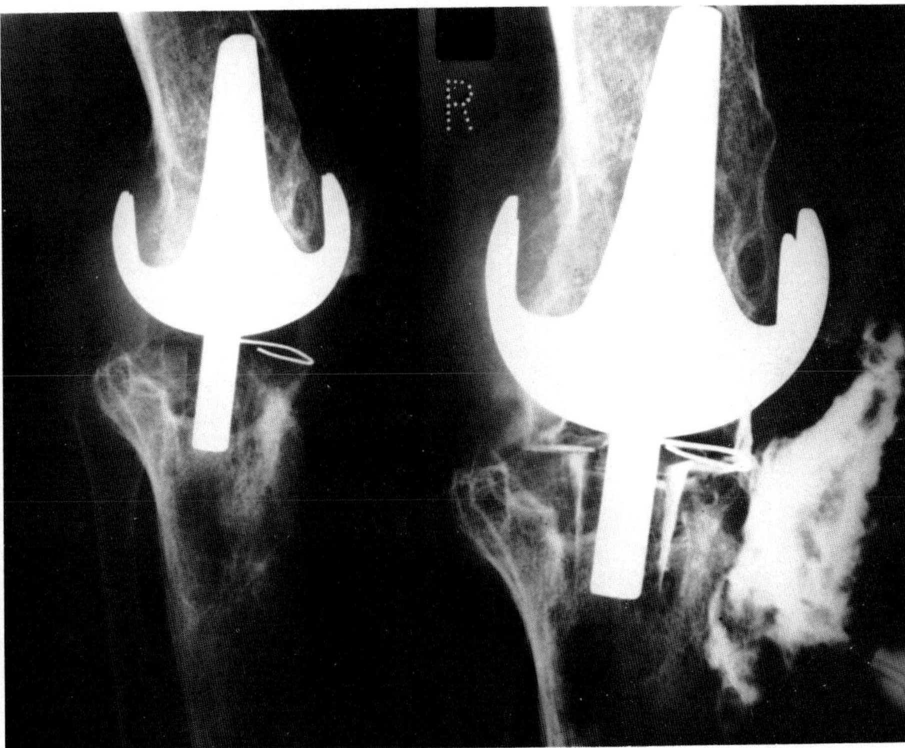

Fig. 4.72

Fig. 4.72 Sinogram following total knee replacement demonstrates the track extending from the skin through to the joint and contrast outlines the tibial portion of the prosthesis, indicating loosening probably associated with infection.

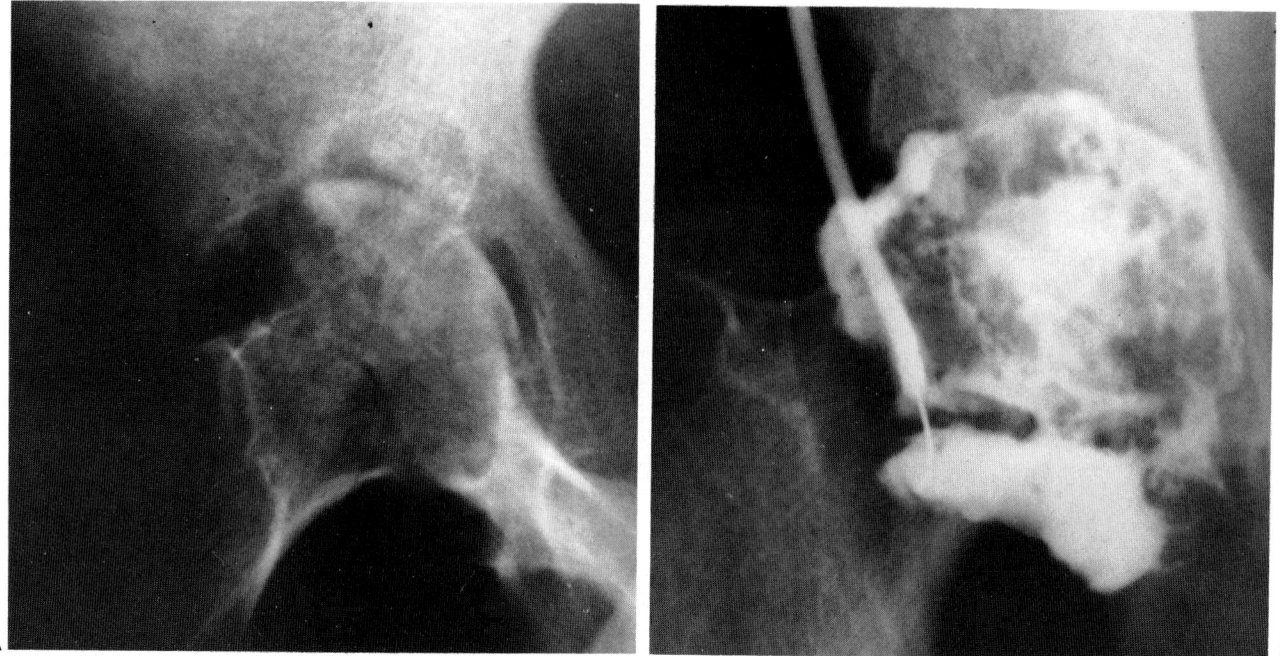

Fig. 4.73 Synovial tuberculosis. **A**. The plain film shows bone and cartilage destruction on both sides of the joint. **B**. The arthrogram shows gross irregular synovial hypertrophy. The geode does not fill.

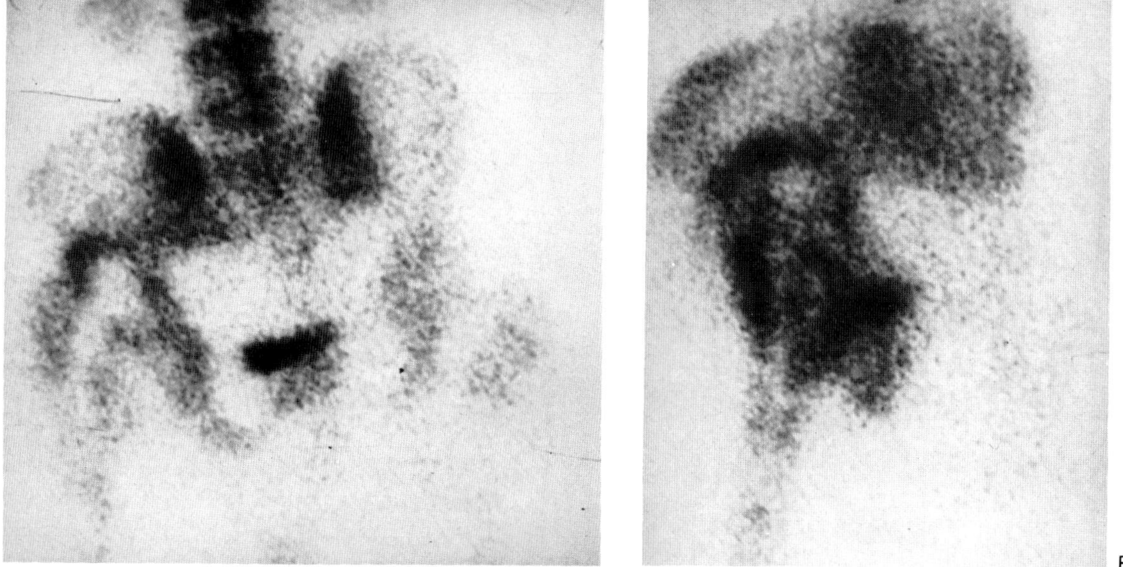

Fig. 4.74 Technetium bone scan. **A**. Anterior scan of pelvis. **B**. Oblique scan of right hip. The prosthesis can be seen as a defect on the scan, and there is increased uptake around it, especially at the femoral component.

uniformly distributed and lasts for up to one year, after which no increase is to be seen. No conclusion as to abnormality can be drawn in this early stage. After this time, *focal* increase in uptake using ^{99m}technetium-labelled phosphate tracers can be assumed to represent infection or loosening, or both. Such uptake is most commonly found at the tip of the femoral prosthetic stem and along its lateral margin (Fig. 4.74).

Differentiation between loosening and infection cannot be made using ^{99m}technetium scans, though a negative technetium scan probably rules out these factors as a cause of hip pain. Differential scanning using ^{67}gallium citrate in addition to technetium is said to differentiate between loosening and infection. Gallium localizes well in leukocytes at the site of infection. This change is best seen 24 hours after injection, when the vascular phase of increased local uptake is over. A positive technetium but negative gallium scan indicates loosening alone, while if both are positive, infection is probably present.

JOINT REPLACEMENTS

Joint replacement is now very widely practiced, and many different types of prosthesis are currently in use, particularly for hip joints. The radiologist should be familiar with the appearances of these prostheses, and many are illustrated in Figures 4.75–4.80. Also included are some examples of knee, shoulder, and elbow replacements (Figs 4.81–4.83).

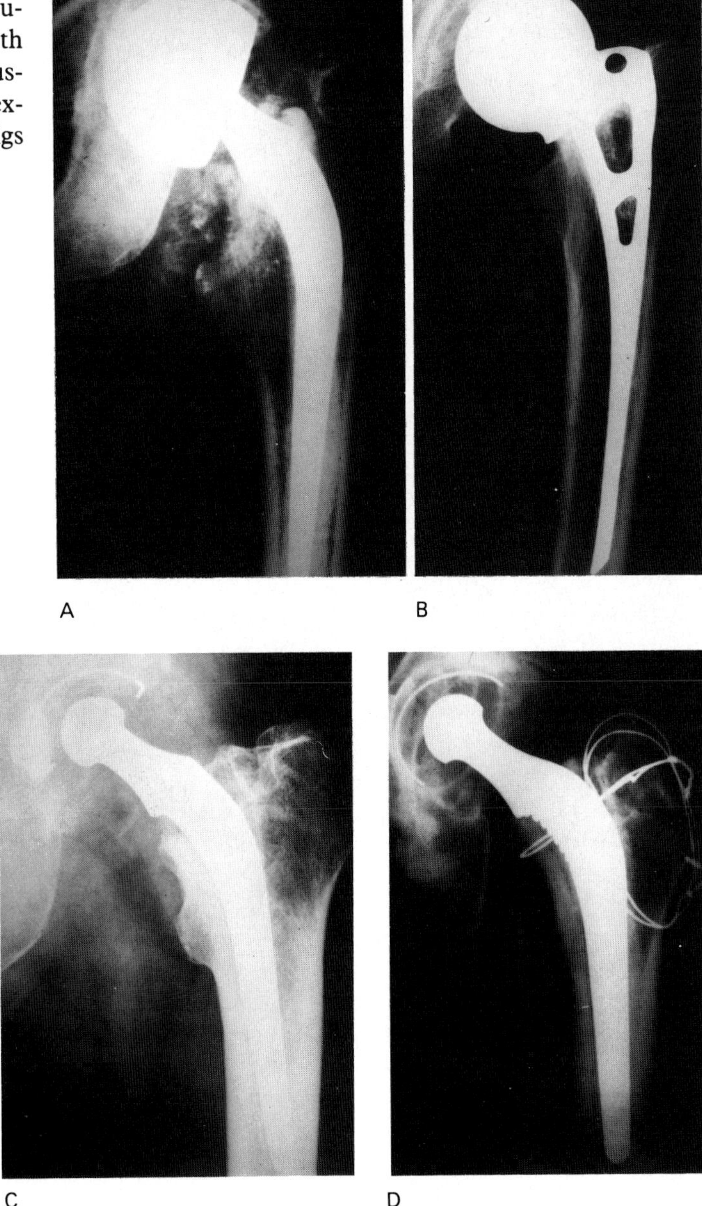

Fig. 4.75 Hip replacements. **A**. Austin-Moore; **B**. Bateman; **C**. Charnely; **D**. Charnley (heavy duty).

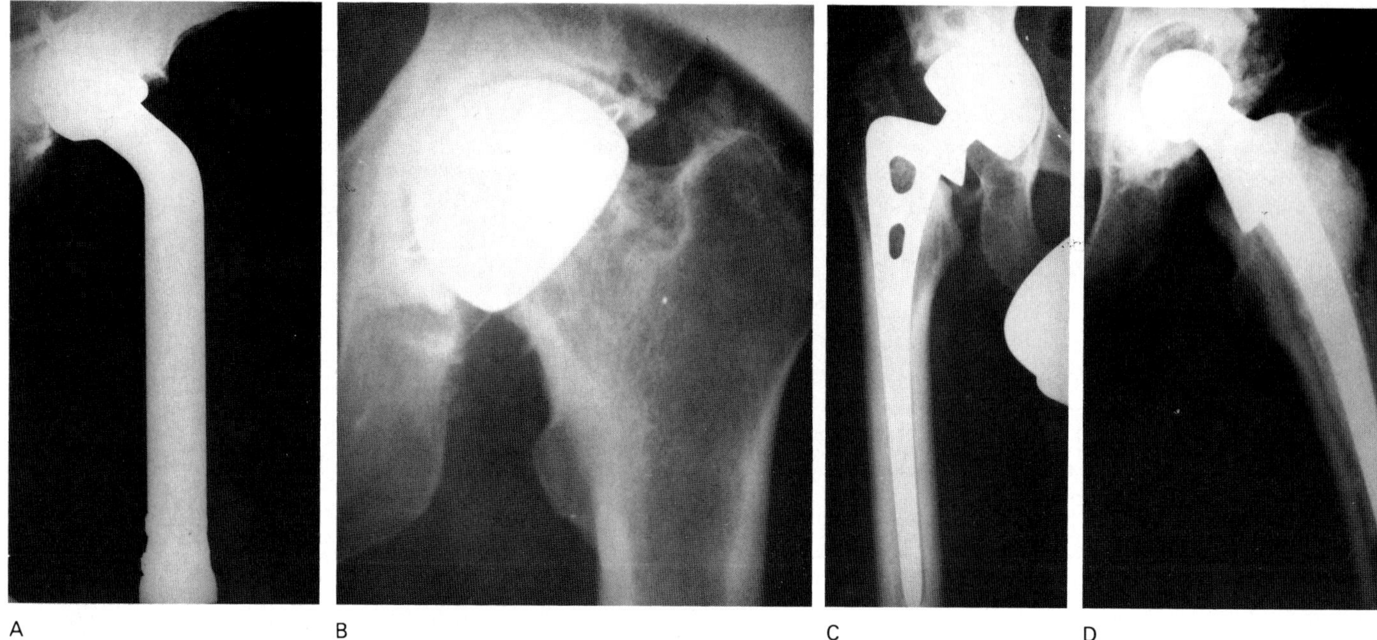

Fig. 4.76 Hip replacements. **A**. Custom-built (tumour replacement); **B**. Double-cup arthroplasty; **C**. Double-cup Monk; **D**. Howse.

Fig. 4.78 Hip replacements. **A**. McKee–Arden; **B**. McKee–Arden with mesh acetabulum; **C**. McKee–Farrar.

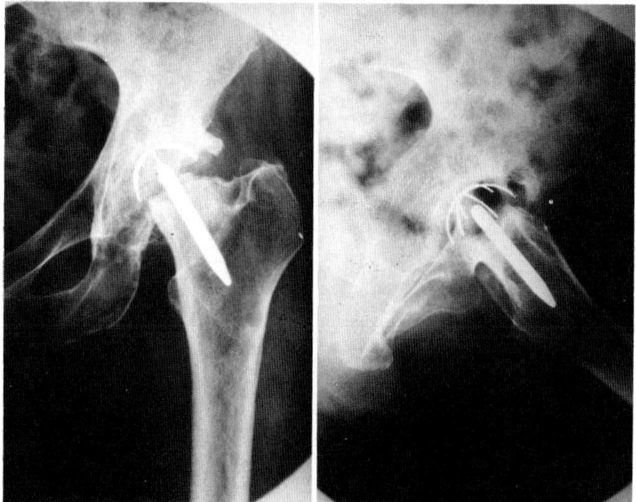

Fig. 4.77 Judet arthroplasty.

Fig. 4.79 Hip replacements. **A**. Minneapolis with McKee cup; **B**. Minneapolis; **C**. Monk hard top.

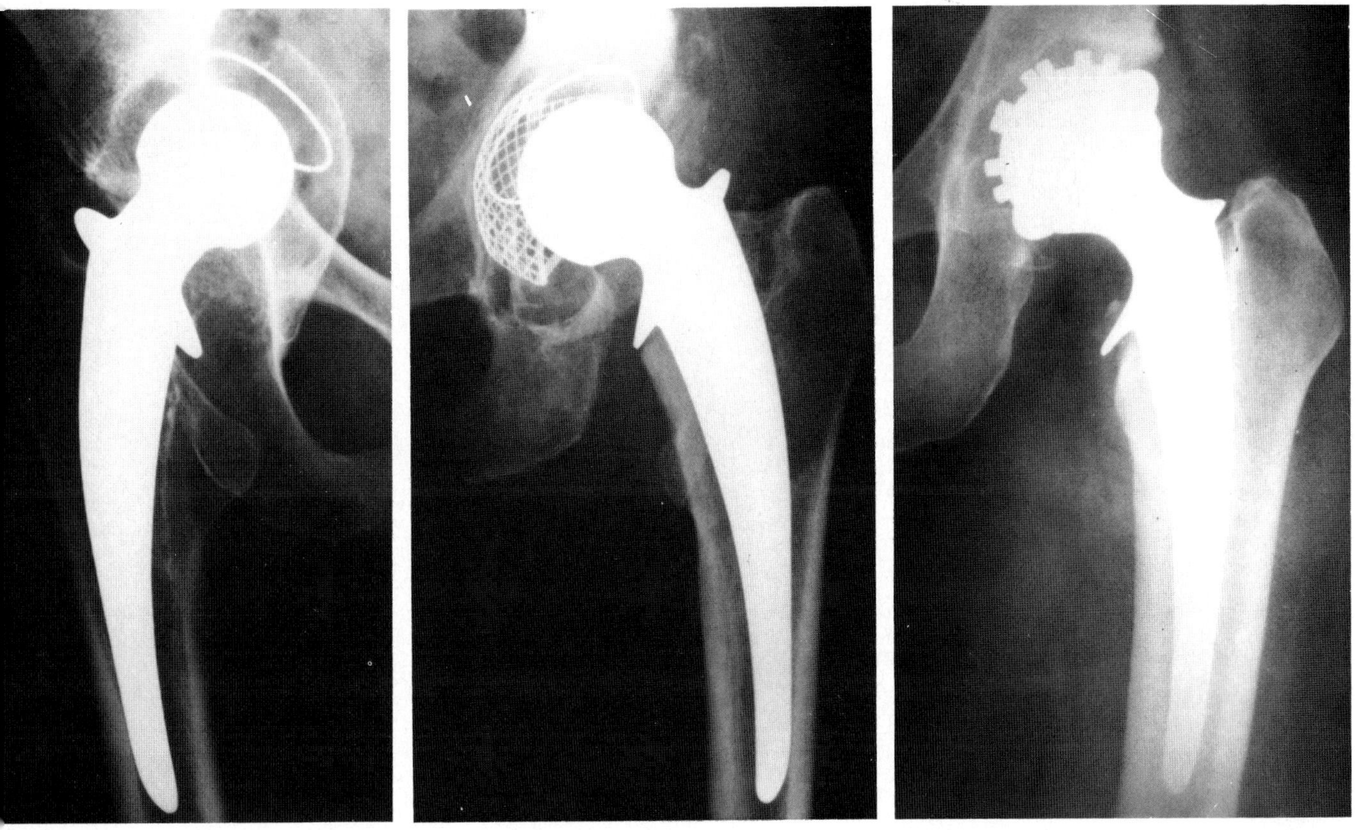

B

C

g. 4.78

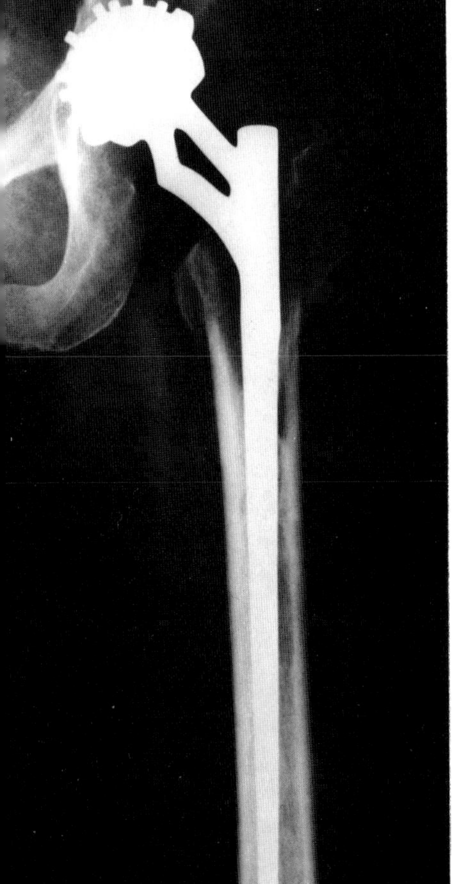

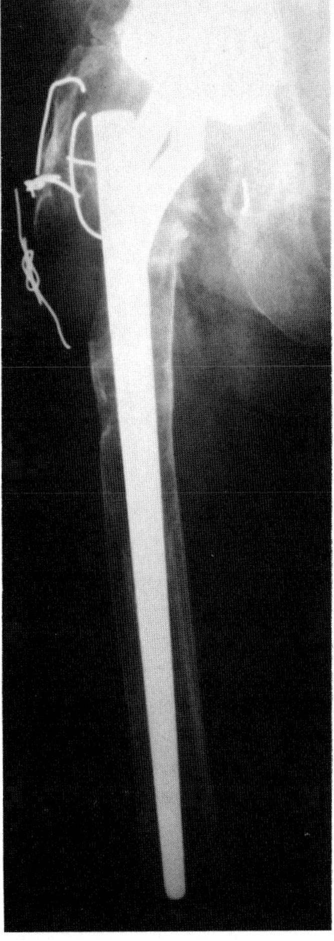

B

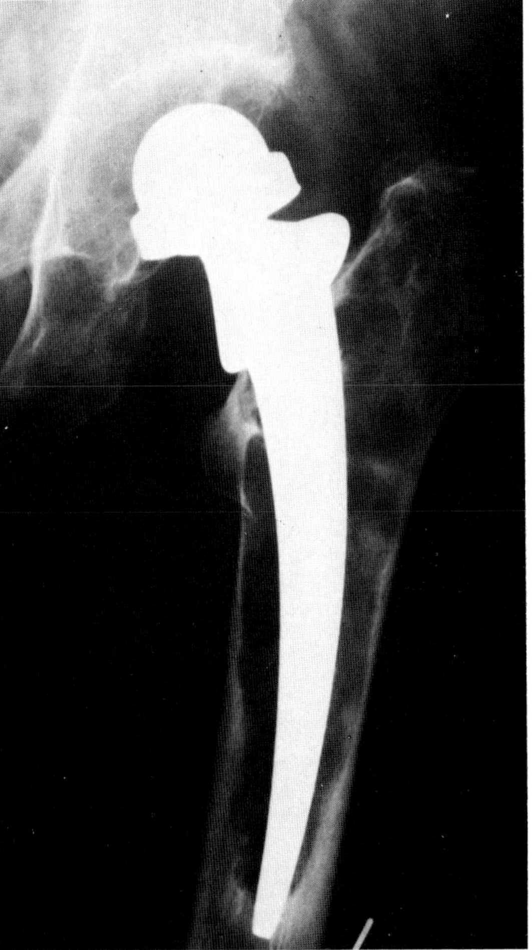

C

ig. 4.79

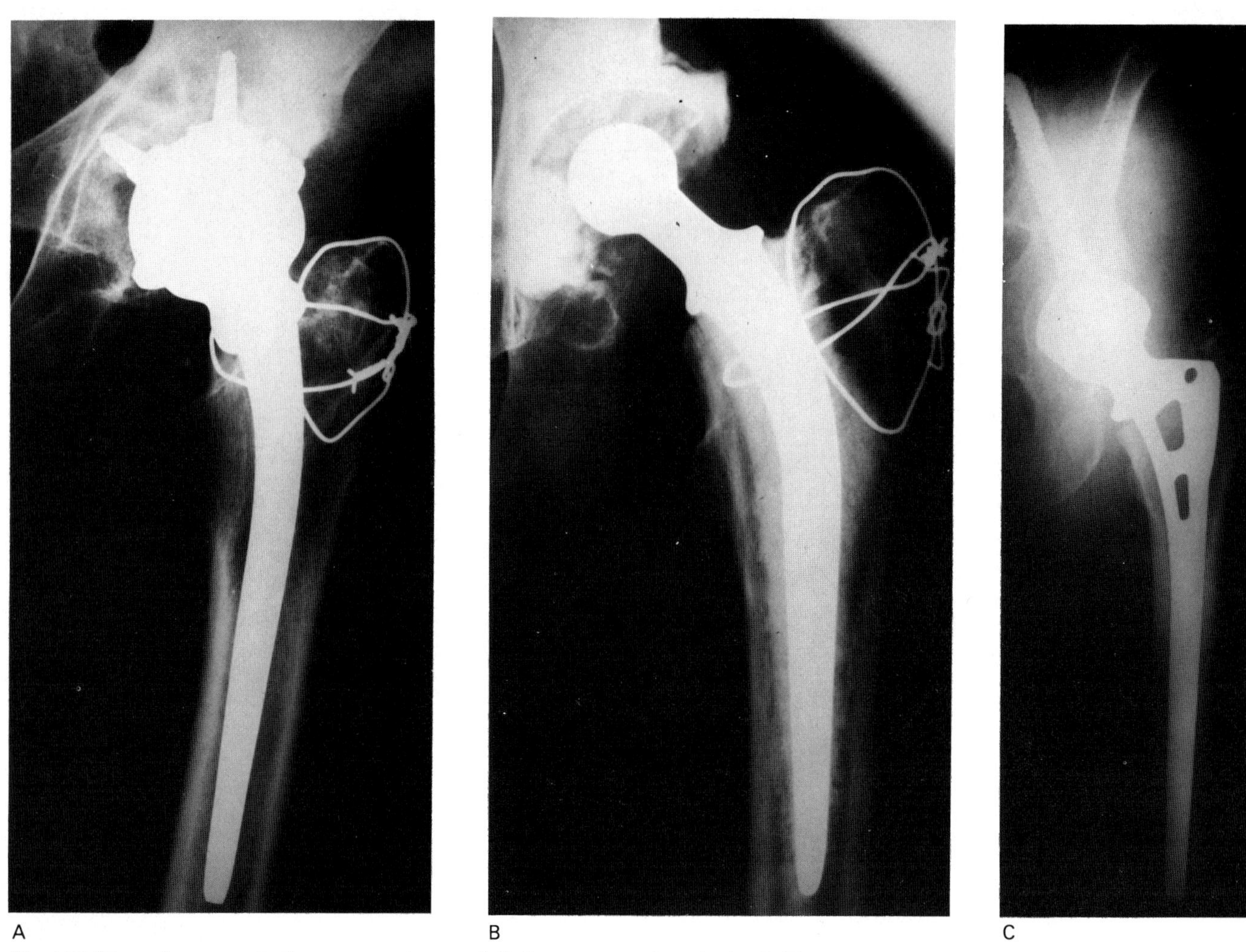

Fig. 4.80 Hip replacements. **A**. Stanmore metal-to-metal; **B**. Stanmore metal-to-plastic; **C**. Ring.

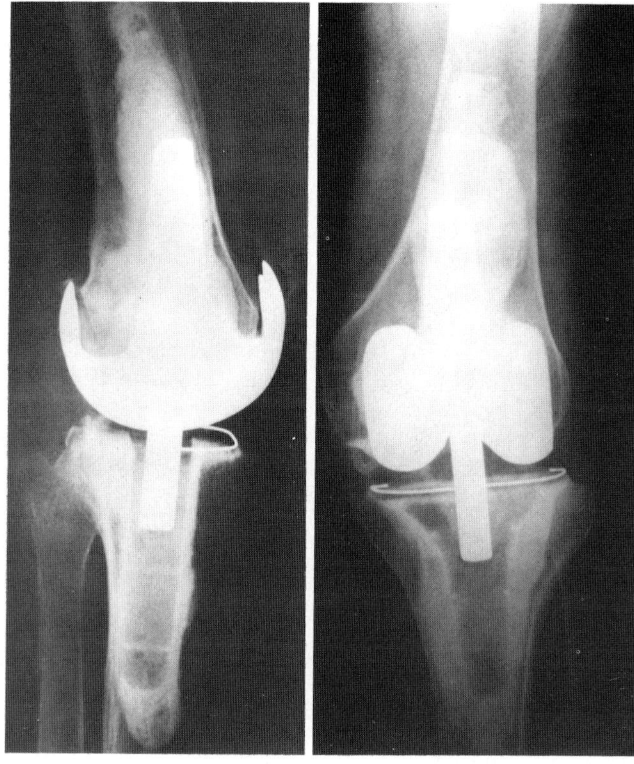

A

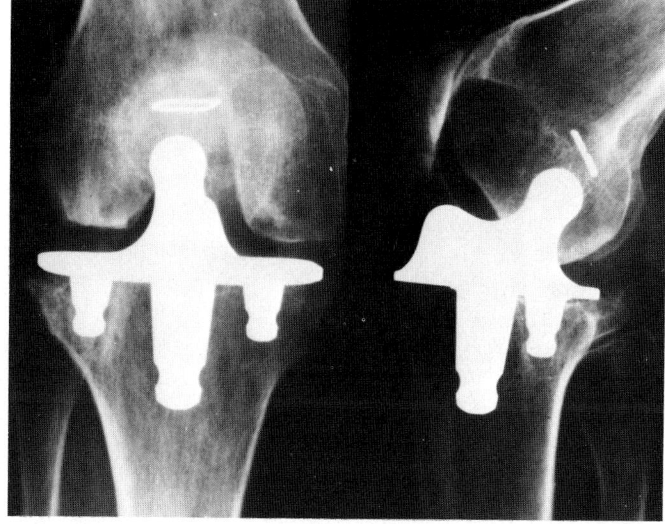

B

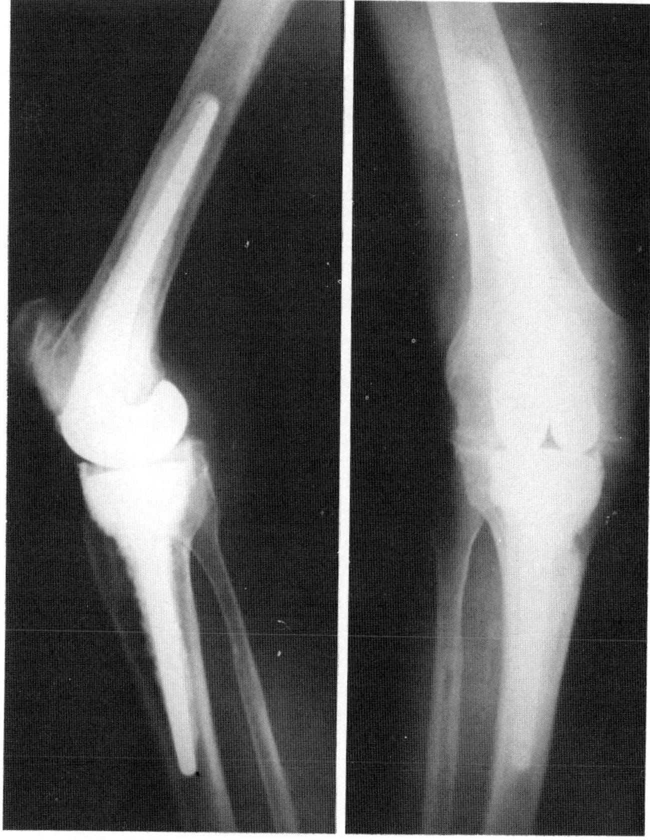

C

Fig. 4.81 Knee replacements. **A.** Attenborough; **B**. Deane; **C**. Shiers.

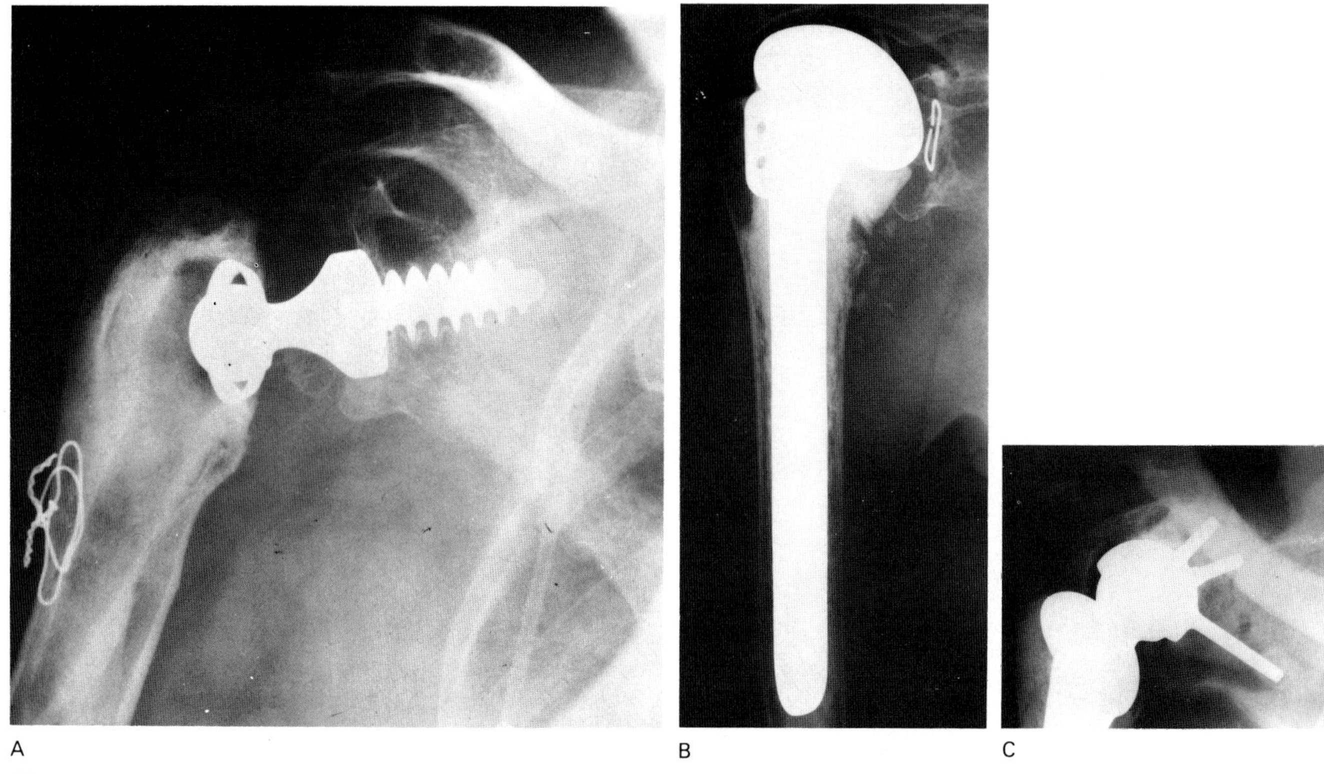

Fig. 4.82 Shoulder replacements. **A**. Kessel; **B**. Neer; **C**. Stanmore.

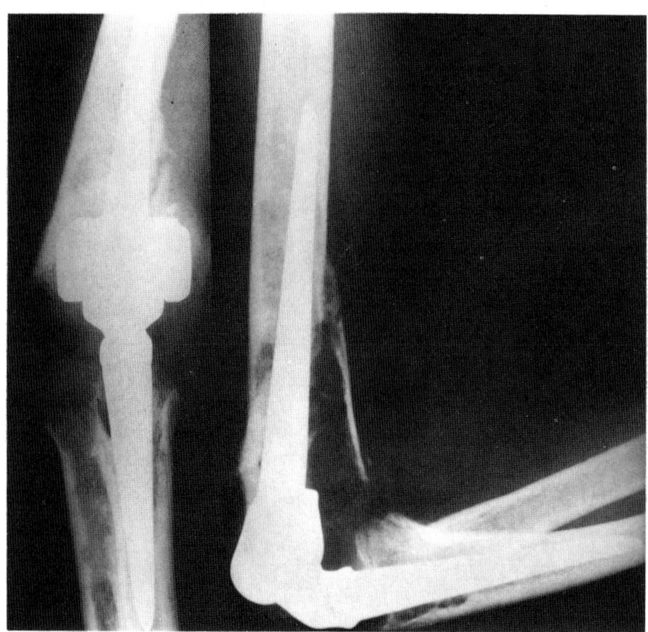

Fig. 4.83 McKee elbow prosthesis.

REFERENCES AND SUGGESTIONS FOR FURTHER READING

Ansell, B. M. (1980) *Rheumatic Disorders in Childhood*. London: Butterworths.

Ansell, B. M. & Kent, P. A. (1977) Radiological changes in juvenile chronic polyarthritis. *Skeletal Radiology*, **1**, 129–144.

Ball, J. (1979) Spondyloarthritides: aspects of pathology. *Rheumatology and Rehabilitation*, **18**, 10–213.

Bergs, H., Remans, J., Drieskens, L., Kiebooms, L. & Polderman, J. (1978) Diagnostic value of SI joint scintigraphy with ^{99m}technetium pyrophosphate in sacro-iliitis. *Annals of Rheumatic Disorders*, **37**, 190–194.

Boriazon, G.S., Seigel, R., Kuhns, L.R., Good, A.E., Rapp, R. & Martel, W. (1981) CT in the evaluation of SI arthritis. *Radiology*. **139**, 437–440.

Boyle, J. A. & Buchanan, W. W. (1971) *Clinical Rheumatology*. Oxford: Blackwell.

Brewerton, D. A, (1967) A tangential radiographic projection for demonstrating involvement of metacarpal heads in rheumatoid arthritis. *British Journal of Radiology*, **40**, 233–234.

Brewerton, D. A. (1979) Symposium on the spondyloarthritides — genetic aspects. *Rheumatology & Rehabilitation*, **18**, 204–209.

Copeman, W. S. C. (1978) *Copeman's Textbook of the Rheumatic Diseases*. Ed. J. T. Scott, 5th edn. Edinburgh: Churchill Livingstone.

Curry, H. L. F., Key, J. J., Mason, R. M. & Swettenham, K. V. (1966) Significance of radiological calcification of joint cartilage. *Annals of Rheumatic Diseases*, **25**, 295–305.

Golding, F. C. (1962) The shoulder — the forgotten joint. *British Journal of Radiology*, **35**, 149–158.

Goldman, A. B. (1981) Hip arthrography. *Radiologic Clinics of North America*, **19**, 329–348.

Goodman, N. (1967) The significance of terminal phalangeal sclerosis. *Radiology*, **69**, 709–712.

Grech, P. (1977) *Hip Arthrography*. London: Chapman & Hall.

Greenfield, G. B., Schorsch, H. & Shkolinick, A. (1967) The various roentgen appearances of pulmonary hypertrophic osteoarthropathy. *American Journal of Roentgenology*, **101**, 927–931.

Lazarus, J. H. & Galloway, J. K. (1973) Pachydermoperiostosis. *American Journal of Roentgenology*, **18**, 308–313.

Lawson, J. P. (1982) Connective tissue diseases. *Seminars in Roentgenology*, Vol. XVII, pp. 25–28.

Martel, W., Stuck, K. J., Dworin, A. M. & Hylland, R. G. (1980) Erosive osteoarthritis and psoriatic arthritis: a radiological comparison in the hand, wrist and foot. *American Journal of Roentgenology*, **134**, 125–135.

Moll, J. M. H., Haslock, I. & Wright, V. (1978) Seronegative spondyloarthritides. In Scott, J. T. (ed.) *Textbook of the Rheumatoid Diseases*, 5th edn. Edinburgh: Churchill Livingstone.

Murphy, W. A. & Staple, T. W. (1973) Jaccound's arthropathy reviewed. *American Journal of Roentgenology*, **118**, 300–307

Murray, R. O. (1965) The aetiology of primary osteoarthritis of the hip. *British Journal of Radiology*, **38**, 810–824.

Norgaard, F. (1970) The earliest radiological changes in polyarthritis of the rheumatoid type. *Symposium Ossium*, pp. 72–74. Edinburgh: Livingstone.

Patton, J. T. (1976) Differential diagnosis of inflammatory spondylitis. *Skeletal Radiology*, **1**, 77–85.

Peter, J. P., Pearson, C. M. & Marmor, L. (1966) Erosive osteoarthritis of the hands. *Arthritis and Rheumatism*, **9**, 365–387.

Reing, C. M., Richin, P. F. & Kenmore, P. I. (1979) Differential bone scanning in the evaluation of a painful total joint replacement. *Journal of Bone and Joint Surgery*, **61A**, 933–936.

Resnick, D., Shaul, R. & Robins, J. M. (1975) Diffuse idiopathic skeletal hyperostosis: Forestier's disease with extraspinal manifestations. *Radiology*, **115**, 513–524.

Resnick, D. & Niwayama, G. (1981) *Diagnosis of Bone and Joint Disorders*. Philadelphia: W. B. Saunders.

Ropes, M. W., Bennett, G. A., Cobb, S., Jacox, R. & Jesser, R. A. (1959) 1958 revision of diagnostic criteria for rheumatoid arthritis. *Bulletin of the Rheumatic Diseases*, **9**, 175–176.

Sholkoff, S. D., Glickman, M. G. & Steinbach, H. L. (1970) Roentgenology of Reiter's syndrome. *Radiology*, **97**, 497–503.

Simon, M. A. (1981) Radioisotope evaluation of skeletal disease. *Journal of Bone and Joint Surgery*, **63-A**, 673–681.

Solokoff, L. (1969) *The Biology of Degenerative Joint Disease*. Chicago; London: University of Chicago Press.

Stoker, D. J. (1980) *Knee Arthrography*. London: Chapman & Hall.

Weissberg, D. R., Resnick, D., Taylor, A., Becker, M. & Alazraki, N. (1978) Rheumatoid arthritis and its variants. Analysis of scintigraphic, radiographic and clinical examinations. *American Journal of Roentgenology*, **131**, 665–673.

CHAPTER 5

TUMOURS AND TUMOUR-LIKE CONDITIONS OF BONE(1)

INTRODUCTION

Bone tumours present problems to the radiologist which vary from simple to impossible. Whilst benign and innocuous lesions, such as fibrous cortical defects are common, being said to occur in about 30% of normal children, primary malignant tumours of bone are relatively rare and are responsible only for about 1% of all deaths from neoplasia. Consequently most radiologists will see comparatively few cases in their working life times and, even in referral centres, considerable difficulty often arises in making a differential diagnosis.

Three important questions require to be answered: *First*, is the lesion neoplastic or infective? *Second*, is it benign or malignant? *Third*, is it a primary or secondary neoplasm? In many circumstances these three problems can be resolved without hesitation. In others, notably those in which cartilaginous tissue is involved, great difficulty may be experienced. It must never be forgotten that it is much more common for malignancy in bones to be metastatic rather than primary. It is important to appreciate the principle that a radiological diagnosis should be made prior to biopsy. An apparently simple radiological diagnosis may not be confirmed histologically and vice versa. Biopsy itself may significantly alter radiological features, particularly in the cases of scintigraphy and angiography. It is also important to remember that although the pathologist should be regarded as the final arbiter in the diagnosis of a lesion, fully representative material must be available for opinion and this may require sectioning the whole lesion. In some benign conditions, such as non-ossifying fibroma or an osteochondroma, it may be considered unnecessary to resort to pathological confirmation, and a conservative attitude, or treatment by a minor surgical procedure may be adopted. On the other hand if a more radical course is being considered such as radiotherapy or surgical resection, radiology serves not only to provide a diagnosis but also to delineate soft tissue and bony involvement, thereby permitting procedural planning. Inadequate investigations have occasionally been responsible for erroneous diagnoses of benign lesions as malignant, resulting in unnecessary surgical procedures, including especially such iatrogenic disasters as amputation.

Many different types of bone tumour are now recognized varying greatly in their mode of clinical presentation, pathology and behaviour. Their aetiology remains obscure. But some seem superimposed upon pre-existing disease such as Paget's disease and bone infarctions. An accepted incidence of both benign and malignant neoplams is known to follow radiation therapy.

Classification of bone tumours

It would be convenient to classify bone tumours according to their cell of origin or histogenesis and in the past many attempts have been made to do this. However, it is generally accepted that this is not possible in the light of present knowledge. Histologically the exact cell of origin of a tumour is not always certain and typing may depend only on the cell or cells which predominate in the developed lesion. In some cases a single tumour may produce several major different types of cell line (for example, osteosarcoma), in others undifferentiated small round cells may be a predominant histological feature permitting only a broad collective diagnosis of malignant round cell tumour of bone. A number of inter-related connective tissue cells are present in bone and from this skeletal connective tissue the majority of bone tumours appear to arise. Other bone tumours are related to non-osseous components of the skeleton, including blood vessels and nerves. Those associated with haematopoietic and lymphoreticular elements are discussed elsewhere (Ch. 7).

A classification of bone tumours is suggested in Table 5.1. Whilst most bone tumours find a place in this classification it must be appreciated that occasionally definitive histological typing cannot be made, particularly with anaplastic or pleomorphic lesions. Non-neoplastic tumours, (the word tumour is literally synonymous with a swelling), abscess, haematoma and so forth, have been included since they must feature in the differential diagnosis. Never forget that a radiologically unusual metastasis is commoner, particularly with older patients, than a primary tumour.

Table 5.1 Classification of primary tumours of bone

	Benign	Malignant
A. Presumed to arise from skeletal tissue		
Bony origin?	Bone island Ivory osteoma Osteoid osteoma Osteoblastoma	Osteosarcoma Parosteal osteosarcoma
Cartilaginous?	Chondroma Chondroblastoma Chondromyxoid fibroma	Chondrosarcoma Dedifferentiated chondrosarcoma Mesenchymal chondrosarcoma
Fibrous?	Fibrous cortical defect Non-ossifying fibroma	Fibrosarcoma
	Desmoplastic fibroma Fibromatosis [Differentiate from — Fibrous dysplasia	Fibrous histiocytoma
	Atypical Paget's disease Hyperparathyroid brown tumour]	Paget's sarcoma
Giant cell containing?	Giant cell tumour Aneurysmal bone cyst	Malignant giant cell tumour
B. Presumed to arise from other tissues in bones		
Blood vessels?	Haemangioma Cystic angiomatosis Haemangiomatosis [Massive osteolysis/vanishing bone disease] Glomus tumour [Haemangiopericytoma]	Angiosarcoma
Nerves?	Neurofibroma Neurilemmoma	Neurofibrosarcoma Neuroblastoma
Fat?	Lipoma [Intra-osseous and parosteal]	Liposarcoma
Notocord?	—	Chordoma
Epithelium?	Implantation dermoid	Adamantinoma
Lymphoid/haemato-poietic? (See Ch. 7)	—	Leukaemias Lymphomas Plasmacytoma Myelomatosis
C. Presumed to arise from joints		
	Intraosseous ganglion Pigmented villonodular synovitis Synovial chondromatosis [Differentiate from — Osteoarthritic cyst Rheumatoid geode]	Synovioma
D. No known origin		
	Solitary bone cyst	Malignant round cell tumours (including Ewing's, neuroblastomas, reticulosarcoma)
E. Non-neoplastic tumours		
(a tumour is a swelling!)	Brodie's abscess Haematoma Infarction Histiocytosis	

GENERAL PRINCIPLES OF RADIOLOGICAL DIAGNOSIS OF BONE TUMOURS

Before attempting to interpret the radiological features of a bone tumour the radiologist should consider both the *age* of the patient and the *clinical history*. Many of the tumours to be described are found in fairly constant age groups. The history may be less useful since many of these lesions present with common non-specific features of pain, swelling or pathological fracture. However even these factors may not be present since lesions not infrequently are discovered as a chance finding. The sex incidence in primary bone tumours is of little diagnostic value, although clearly the sex of the patient is of relevance in interpretation of skeletal metastases.

The basis of diagnosis will be plain X-ray films and these will be supplemented as necessary by tomography, computerized tomography, scintigraphy and angiography.

1. Is the lesion solitary or multiple? With the exception of multiple osteochondromata of diaphyseal aclasia and multiple cartilage tumours in dyschondroplasia most primary bone tumours are solitary.

In the first instance ^{99}technetium MDP bone scan is the investigation of choice to establish whether or not the lesion is unifocal (Fig. 5.1). Other abnormal foci then may be subjected to radiographic examination and, in the vast number of cases, are detected satisfactorily. Difficulties will be experienced in myelomatosis or with metastasis from some of the less common tumours, such as cholangiocarcinoma and the cervix uteri, when most lesions are photon deficient. A more time consuming and expensive radiographic skeletal survey then may be justified. Never forget to take an X-ray of the chest whether or not a plain film skeletal survey has been undertaken. The diagnosis becomes easier if a bronchial carcinoma or an obvious metastasis can be detected.

2. What type of bone is involved? It is of some value to differentiate between flat bones and tubular bones since, for example, lesions in the axial skeleton or proximal ends of long bones are in the sites of persistent haematopoietic tissue and should always raise the possibility of a metastasis or a reticulosis. Osteoid osteoma is very rare in membrane bone and should not enter, for practical purposes, the differential diagnosis of a lesion in the vault. Similarly a radiolucency in the mandible is more likely to be myeloma than metastasis. Although no part of the skeleton is exempt from involvement by a primary bone tumour a large proportion are found in the pelvis and in the long bones particularly around the hips and knees.

3. Where is the lesion within the bone? Many benign tumours tend to appear in characteristic sites, for example, non-ossifying fibroma and fibrous cortical defects are by definition in the cortex, eccentrically towards the metadiaphysis of a long bone. Chondroblastoma occurs in an epiphysis or apophysis. Giant cell tumour is almost invariably

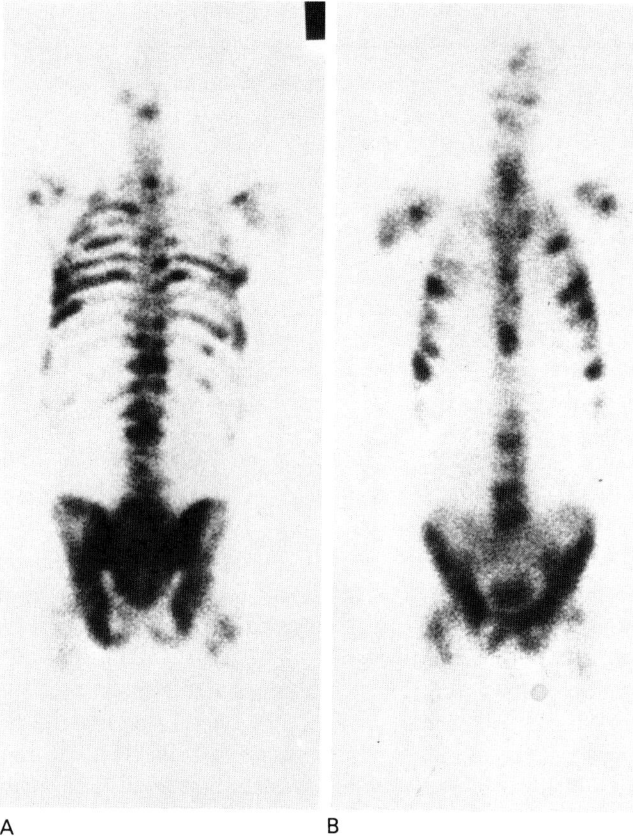

Fig. 5.1 Multiple skeletal metastases are demonstrated on a whole body isotope bone scan. The primary tumour was carcinoma of the breast in a middle-aged woman. Note the predominantly axial distribution of the lesions, many of which were not apparent on plain X-rays. **A**. PA view **B**. AP view.

immediately sub-articular and eccentric in location. Most tumours of cartilaginous origin, except those which are associated with an osteochondroma, have a medullary location.

4. Plain film features. Never settle for anything less than perfect plain films. It is most important that soft tissue detail is not lost on an over-exposed film, because a soft tissue tumour extension typically presents a well-defined margin, whereas soft tissue swelling associated with inflammation is ill-defined. Similarly soft tissue calcification or ossification may be overlooked. Do not settle for underpenetrated films since the inner texture of a tumour, for example the ground glass quality of fibrous dysplasia, may be overlooked, or the radiolucent focus of an osteoid osteoma may be not visualized. Take films 'around the clock'. Simply because periosteal new bone cannot be visualized on a standard AP and lateral film does not mean that it will not be present on an oblique. A skull unit is a satisfactory means of obtaining these additional films with peripheral lesions. Is the pattern of bone change destructive, proliferative or both? Correlating the size of the lesion with the length of history may be a guide as to its rapidity of growth and similarly follow-up films permit an assessment of its aggressive potential or malignancy. Tumours of osteoblastic origin are commonly, but not always, bone producing. Consequently areas of increased density and/or surrounding new bone formation extending into soft tissue are likely to be evident. Cartilaginous tumours are mainly radiolucent but small foci of calcification represent an important hallmark. Fibrosarcoma, on the other hand, tends to be purely destructive and to stimulate virtually no reactive bone formation.

5. What do the margins of the lesion look like? Is there a narrow or wide zone of transition between apparent tumour and normal bone? A wide zone of transition suggests an aggressive tumour or infection. Is the zone of transition marked with bone reaction or not? A thin rim of sclerosis is present characteristically around a non-ossifying fibroma, whereas extensive sclerosis is typical of a cortical osteoid osteoma. These findings are, of course, not constant and ill-defined sclerosis with a widened zone of transition may occur in such benign conditions as histiocytosis. Examine the cortex: is it resorbed from within indicating medullary lesions as cartilaginous tumours or myelomatosis? Peripheral cortical lesions on the other hand, with the exception of 'saucerisation' of Ewing's sarcoma, are caused more commonly by pressure or direct invasion from abnormalities in adjacent soft tissues. If the margins of such a defect are smooth the lesion is usually benign, such as a neurofibroma, or non-neoplastic as in the case of anterior erosions of the vertebral bodies by an aortic aneurysm. Conversely an irregular margin may suggest invasion by a malignant soft tissue lesion, for example, metastasis or direct invasion by carcinoma of the antrum or lymphoma. Finally is there an associated soft tissue mass? The presence of a soft tissue mass can frequently be shown in relation to malignant bone tumours, although oblique views may be necessary to delineate them. An ill-defined soft tissue mass is almost invariably associated with an inflammatory lesion. Examine the margin of the soft tissue lesion to see whether or not there is a thin shell of bone as occurs in some aggressive types of aneurysmal bone cysts, particularly those arising in the spine.

Further imaging investigations

Tomography. All further investigations are performed in order to delineate or elicit differential characteristics of a lesion already demonstrated by plain films. Tomography has been superseded largely by computerized tomography (CT). The object of a tomogram is to delineate either the characteristic radiological features summarized above or to assist demarcation of the intra- and extra-osseous extent of the abnormality.

Scintigraphy should be performed as the first additional investigation in most instances. High resolution gamma camera images using ^{99m}technetium-labelled diphosphonate compounds probably provide the optimal images. Two phases of the bone scan should be recorded. Firstly by counting the first three hundred thousand events after the injection a blood pool scan is obtained whilst the radiopharmaceutical is still largely in the intravascular or perivascular extracellular fluid space. Two to three hours later the skeleton is imaged when the radiopharmaceutical has localized in bone and is in the delayed or bone scan phase. The blood pool phase is vital and should never be overlooked. Scintigraphy may be used to assess the primary presenting lesion and also to detect whether it is monostotic or accompanied by other skeletal lesions, such as metastases.

Examine the blood pool phase; is the lesion vascular as in an aneurysmal bone cyst or avascular as in most cartilage tumours? Does the lesion itself accumulate radiopharmaceutical, suggesting that it is being bound into a fibrous, cartilaginous or bone-forming matrix, or is the lesion essentially photon deficient with increased activity surrounding it suggesting either a heterogenous tumour or a host reaction? Does the lesion extend beyond the confines demonstrated by plain film, remembering that the apparent extent of intra-osseous involvement can be artefactually slightly greater because the scan may not distinguish between bone-forming tumour and a rim of reactive host response? If the lesion is photon rich, **check the lungs** since metastases from an osteosarcoma are frequently detectable by bone scanning. Finally are there any lesions elsewhere? If so, radiograph them.

Computerized tomography has a most important part to play both in the assessment of the primary presenting lesion and in the detection of potential metastatic dissemination. CT will give an impression of the predominant variety of tissue present particularly if there is fat or calcification. It will not, however, necessarily indicate whether or not those tissues are benign. Examine the intra-osseous extent of the tumour looking for subtle changes in medullary fat. Examine also extra-osseous extent and soft tissue relationships. Contrast medium enhancement is of little value, since most tumours do not helpfully enhance. However, the vascular nature of a tumour may be detected and the relationship of the soft tissue component of the tumour to blood vessels be assessed. Without doubt more metastases are detected by CT, or whole lung tomography, than is possible with routine plain film examinations.

Angiography has been the subject of fashion but, in recent years, has fallen into disrepute. The initial hope that it would, in isolation, distinguish reliably between benign and malignant lesions has foundered. No characteristic angiographic feature of malignancy exists. However, two signs, encasement and tumour vessels, occur with much greater frequency in malignant tumours. Encasement results from the vessel being surrounded by tumour and hence is shown by a localized segment of narrowing. Tumour vessels are defined as structures pursuing a random course with an irregular branching pattern. Angiography should be used in the differential, rather than in the absolute, diagnosis of a lesion, as for example, to distinguish between tumour and infection. A malignant round cell tumour has an intrinsically abnormal vascular pattern, whereas osteomyelitis is characterized by an increased number of normal arterial branches and enlarged periosteal veins. Similarly angiography may be used to distinguish between tumours since osteosarcomas are highly vascular, whereas most chondrosarcomas are hypovascular. It is arguable, however, whether angiography now contributes significantly to the assessment of primary tumours and their extent, since much of the information obtainable on angiogram may be obtained by scintigraphy and CT. Angiography, however, may still be necessary in order to delineate involvement of major vessels by extension of a tumour into soft tissue when prosthetic or other limb conservation surgery is being considered.

Other investigations. On occasions virtually the whole spectrum of radiological investigations will be necessary to differentiate between tumours or to gauge their extent. For example, lymphography may be necessary in order to detect local nodal involvement or arthrography to demonstrate the degree of synovial involvement in synovial chondromatosis or pigmented villonodular synovitis.

SECONDARY NEOPLASTIC INVOLVEMENT OF BONE

The later stages of many malignant neoplasms are associated almost inevitably with metastases and the skeleton is very commonly affected. The radiographic presence of such lesions very often lags behind their detectability by scintigraphy. Post-mortem studies also have shown that their incidence is much higher than may be detected by either examination. Bony metastases are present in approximately 25% of all deaths from malignant disease. Any primary tumour may metastasize to bone, but in women the most important carcinoma is breast from which secondary deposits develop in about two thirds of cases. In men approximately 80% of cases of carcinoma of the prostate and a quarter of tumours of the lung and kidney may be expected to produce bone metastases. A metastasis, indeed, may be the presenting feature of the disease.

It should be clear therefore that bony metastases are common, whereas primary bone tumours are relatively rare. Secondary deposits are here described first to emphasize their relative frequency.

Clinical features. Whilst a bone metastasis may present as a pathological fracture, usually they produce only vague pain or are entirely occult. Biopsy of a metastasis may indicate the site of origin of a previously unsuspected primary tumour. Usually the more malignant the primary tumour, the more rapidly does secondary spread occur. Some tumours, however, may present with a metastasis years before the primary lesion is clinically apparent and indeed the metastasis itself may remain virtually unchanged radiologically for a long time. This sequence may be observed particularly with carcinoma of the thyroid or kidney. A latent period often separates the removal of a primary tumour, particularly from the breast, and the subsequent development of skeletal metastases.

The *spine, pelvis* and *ribs* are the most common sites of involvement together with the proximal ends of the *humeri* and *femora* and, less often, the *skull* (Fig. 5.1). These areas correspond to sites of persistent haematopoiesis in the adult, malignant spread usually occurring by a haematogenous route. Local spread to the lumbar spine and pelvis may be expected from tumours arising in the pelvis, notably carcinoma of the cervix. Some metastases have a predictable distribution, the majority of renal cell carcinoma metastases occurring in the lumbar spine and pelvis. They have a rather characteristic radiological appearance (see below). Metastases distal to the knee and elbow are rather rare and usually arise from a primary tumour of the bronchus or pelvic organs, particularly colon and bladder. Partial or complete collapse of a vertebral body with the secondary features of spinal cord compression is by no means rare.

Blood chemistry studies may be of some value. The *serum alkaline phosphatase* is always raised in the presence of multiple bony metastases, but remains normal in myelomatosis. With widespread osteolytic destruction the *serum calcium* usually is elevated and in the case of carcinoma of the prostate a marked rise in the *serum acid phosphatase* level is characteristic.

Some metastases respond to treatment with, for example, hormone therapy. Under these circumstances both radiography and scintigraphy are needed in order to monitor the progress of such lesions. Remember that it is inadequate simply to document the number and extent of metastases; it is a radiologist's duty to draw the clinician's attention to those metastases which may be considered hazardous, for example those associated with significant vertebral body collapse (and the possible development of cord compression) or in long bones of the lower limb (with the potential for disabling fracture). In the latter circumstance prophylactic nailing of the femur is preferable to protracted recumbency in a Thomas splint in terms of acceptability for a patient with a limited life expectancy.

Radiological features. The majority of metastases are predominantly osteolytic. Typically they arise in the medulla and progressively extend in all directions destroying the cortex,

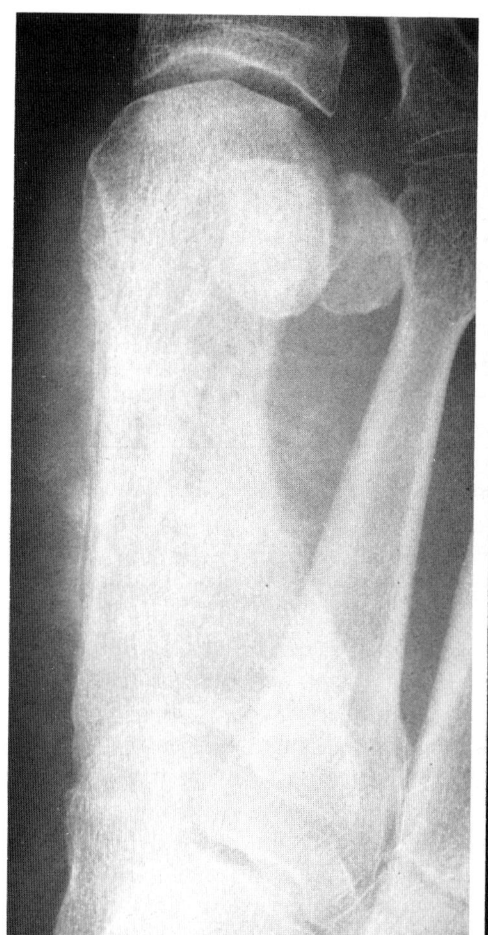

Fig. 5.2 Two examples of solitary metastases producing bone in the adjacent soft tissues. **A**. carcinoma of the colon in a great toe metatarsal and **B**. transitional cell carcinoma of the bladder in the mid tibia.

usually without the development of much periosteal reaction. Soft tissue extension is relatively uncommon. Some metastases, particularly those from bronchial carcinoma may appear eccentric and primarily destroy cortex, especially in the femur. Others are predominantly osteoblastic, including those derived from the prostate, stomach and carcinoid. They produce dense and often well-circumscribed areas of increased radio-opacity. Such lesions are usually associated with only mild discomfort and are less subject to pathological fracture. A small group of metastases are accompanied by tumour bone formation; these include osteosarcoma, liposarcoma, transitional cell carcinoma (of either bladder or kidney) and some adenocarcinomas of the colon (Fig. 5.2).

The diagnosis of metastases is usually simplified by the multiplicity of these lesions. The greatest difficulty may arise when a lesion is apparently solitary after full examination scintigraphically or radiographically of the remainder of the skeleton and chest. Remember that unusual primary tumours are often responsible for unusual metastases and, further, that a metastasis can simulate closely almost any known primary bone tumour!

Breast. Not only is this the most common primary tumour in women but its metastases show an unusual affinity for bone. Bone scanning demonstrates a significant incidence of bone metastases at the time of diagnosis, roughly in proportion to the degree of malignancy. The lesions are usually osteolytic, commonly being multiple and several centimetres in diameter. Diffuse infiltration, however, may cause an apparently coarse trabecular pattern without an obvious localized area of bone destruction. The condition should be suspected in the presence of vertebral compression fractures in older females. Differentiation of these from osteoporotic collapse may be difficult although in the latter evidence of focal areas of bone destruction is usually lacking. Multiple lytic lesions also may resemble myelomatosis, but in that condition the margins of the lucencies are sharply defined with endosteal scalloping and the serum alkaline phosphatase is usually normal. About 10% of metastases from carcinoma of the breast produce osteoblastic lesions and in another 10% the lesions are mixed (Fig. 5.3). Sclerosis may occur in lytic lesions following successful hormone or radiation therapy. Difficulty may be experienced in differentiating between intense disuse osteoporosis following radiotherapy and metastatic disease. This problem arises particularly around the shoulder where the bones inevitably have been included in the radiation field. The lesions of intense disuse osteoporosis, however, tend to be sharply defined and elipsoid in the long axis of bone. Similarly multiple rib fractures secondary to radiation therapy

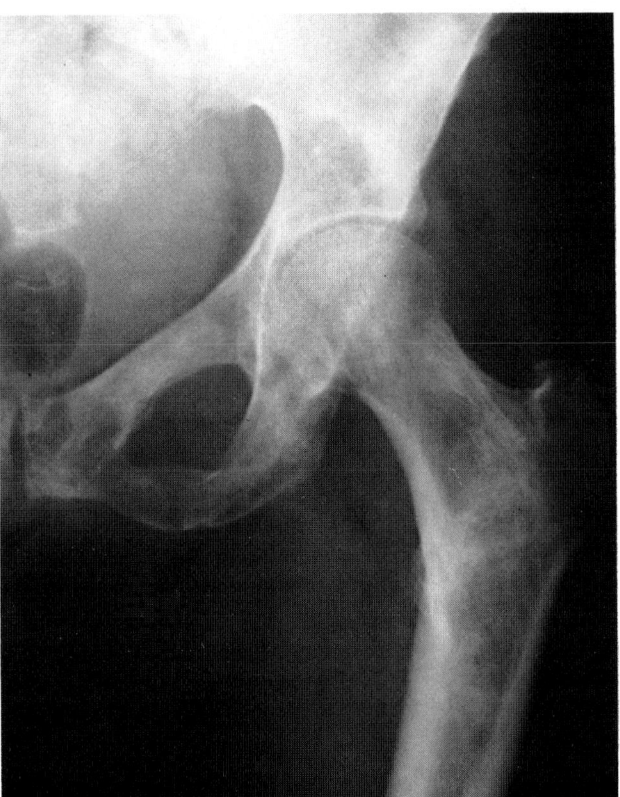

Fig. 5.3 Mixed skeletal metastases from carcinoma of the breast in a middle-aged woman.

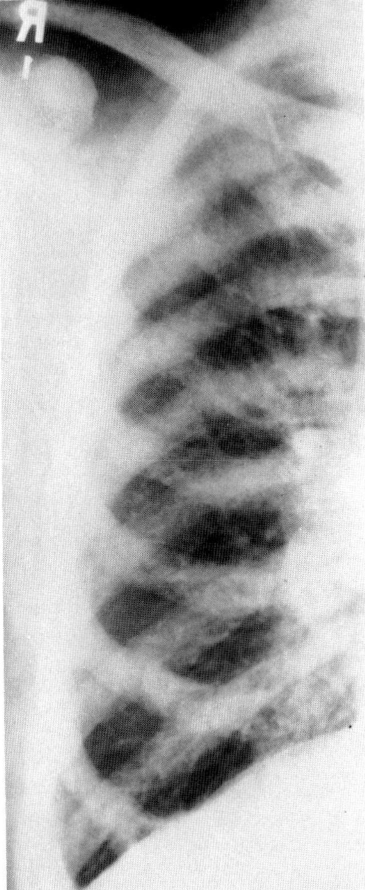

Fig. 5.4 Carcinoma of prostate — extensive sclerosis is present in the ribs and clavicle due to widespread metastasis in an elderly male patient.

should not be mistaken for metastases. The fractures often occur at the edge of the radiation field and consequently tend to be in a line, a distribution observed also in osteomalacia.

Prostate. This is the commonest secondary bone tumour in men and in contrast to breast deposits almost all these metastases are osteoblastic (Fig. 5.4). They appear as round or oval areas of increased density, particularly in the pelvis and spine, growing slowly and merging so that widespread and diffuse increase in bone density may ensue. Periosteal new bone formation and/or apparent expansion of bone may occur so that the differentiation from Paget's disease may be difficult. The deposits may be demonstrated to regress with hormone therapy. In some patients metastases from the prostate may be osteolytic and expansile (Fig. 5.5). They may even be solitary. If the carcinoma involves the base of the bladder some metastases may be associated with new bone formation in the adjacent soft tissue resembling an osteosarcoma.

Kidney. Renal cell carcinoma is characteristically responsible for solitary bone metastases with a marked predelection for the pelvis and lumbar spine. Even when multiple their number seldom exceeds six. These lesions are typically expansile with a crenellated margin and usually have a typical radiological appearance (Fig. 5.6). They are richly vascular, as demonstrated scintigraphically or angiographically. Since these tumours grow slowly, renal cell carcinoma is often associated with a relatively good prognosis, particularly following excision of the affected kidney and a solitary deposit. Transcatheter embolization may prove to be a useful addition to management.

Lung. In men this tumour is second only to the prostate in causing a high proportion of cases which develop skeletal metastases, such bone lesions occurring eventually in about

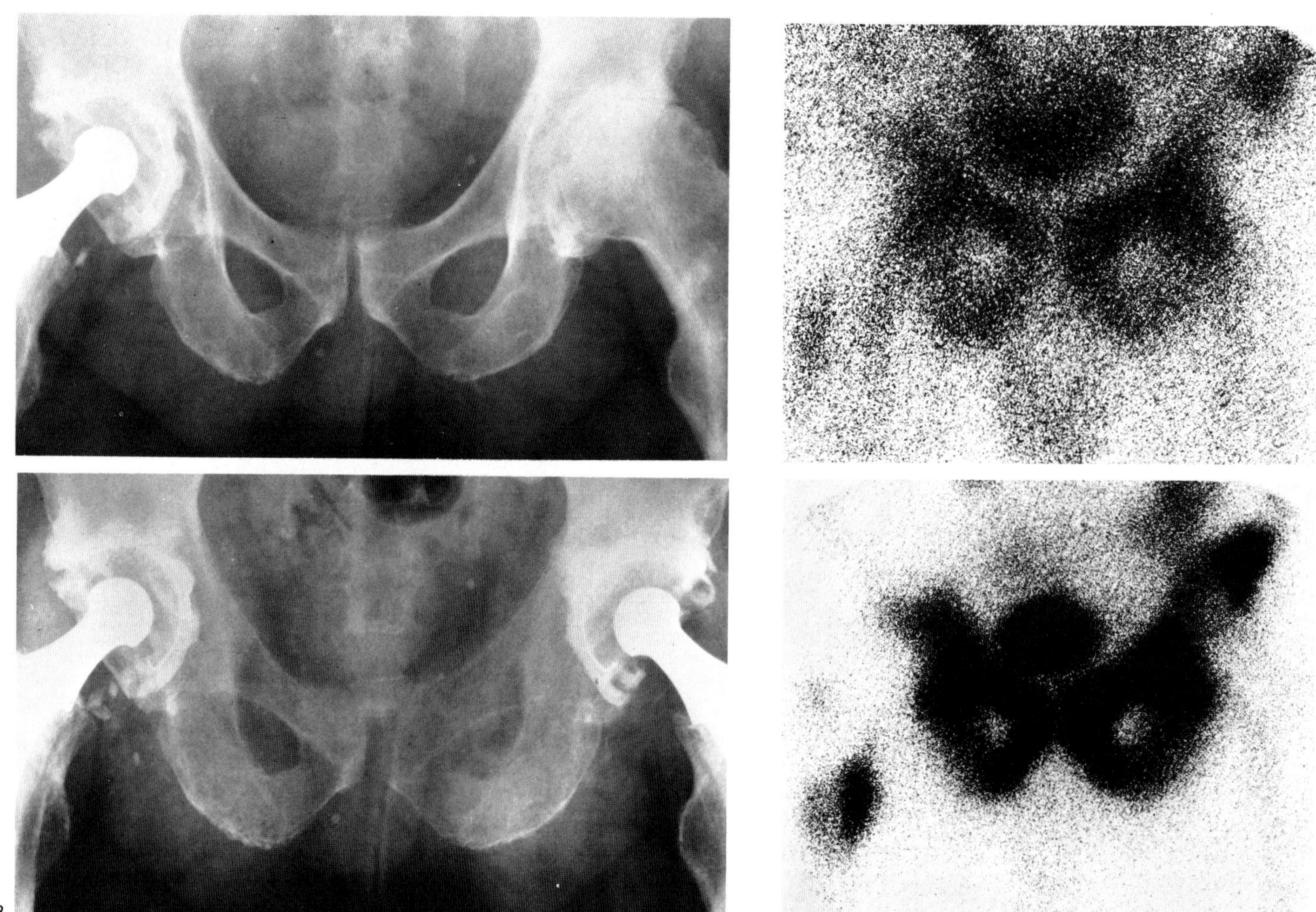

Fig. 5.5 Carcinoma of the prostate with expansile lytic metastases. **A**. a view of the pelvis before the onset of symptoms reveals no abnormality in the pubic rings. **B**. 5 years later the patient was complaining of severe pain in the groin. Note the ill-defined trabecular pattern, expansion of bone and ill-definition of cortex which has developed since the previous picture. **C**. Blood pool phase of a bone scan and **D**. delayed image reveals a marked increase in activity.

Note the abnormality in the lesser trochanter of the right femur. These features could not be distinguished from active aggressive Paget's disease on purely scintigraphic grounds except that the lesion in the right femur has not started at a joint. The diagnosis was established by biopsy and the presence of a very high acid phosphatase level in the blood.

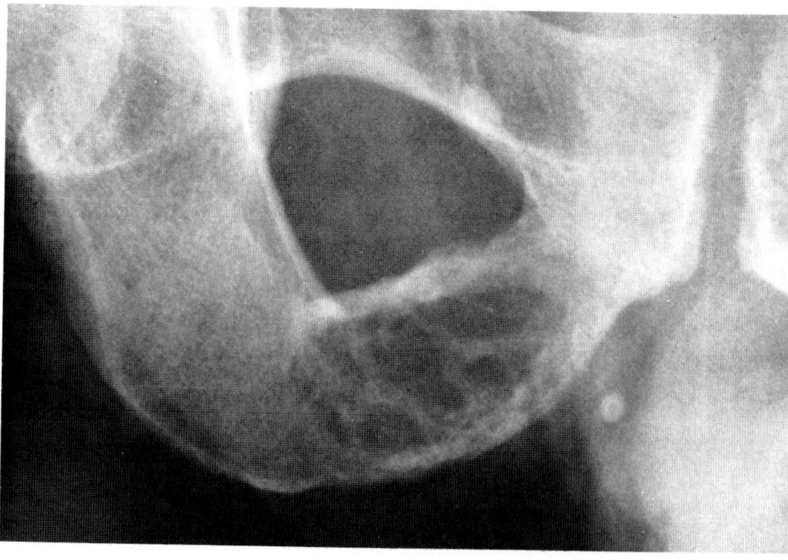

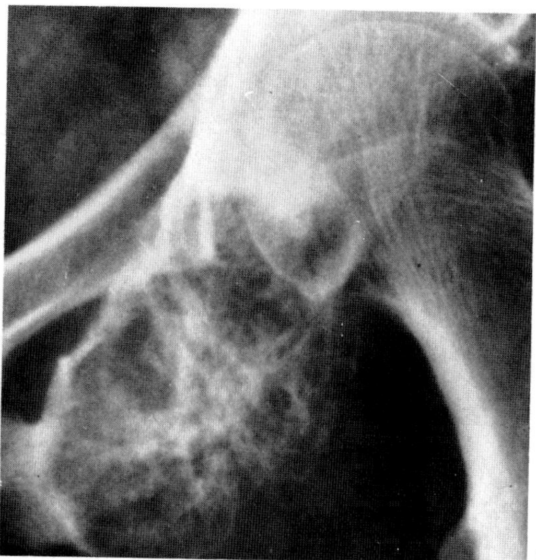

Fig. 5.6 A. and **B.** Two examples of solitary metastases from renal cell carcinoma. In both cases these metastases were the presenting abnormality. Both are expansile and have crenellated margins, with trabeculation in the lesion.

a third. These metastases are almost always osteolytic and can be unusual, occurring in the small bones of the hand or eccentrically in the cortex of a long bone.

Alimentary tract. Carcinoma of the stomach and colon, and carcinoid, may metastasize to bone in both sexes. Metastases from the stomach and carcinoid are often osteoblastic and may be multiple. The bone forming characteristic of colonic metastases has been already emphasised.

Sympathetic nervous sytem is a presumed site of origin of neuroblastoma which in childhood rapidly metastasizes to bone, usually causing extensive destructive lesions, although on occasions such deposits may be osteoblastic. Even at post-mortem the primary tumour may be difficult to identify, but commonly it is situated in the medulla of an adrenal gland. A solitary metastasis may present the radiological characteristics of a malignant round cell tumour with an ill-defined destructive focus in medullary bone and layered periosteal new bone formation. More usually, however, the destruction is extensive involving the metaphyses of long bones and causing widening of the sutures of the skull. Thus it may not be possible to differentiate the condition radiologically from leukaemia.

Other primary tumours often produce bizarre and atypical radiological patterns. In particular the metastases from thyroid carcinoma are classically expansile, osteolytic and often solitary (Fig. 5.7).

INVASION AND DESTRUCTION OF BONE BY EXTRA-OSSEOUS PRIMARY MALIGNANT TUMOURS

Lesions of this type are rare compared with skeletal metastases, but may be observed in association with direct spread of such lesions as carcinoma of the cervix or bladder, and also from carcinoma of the paranasal sinuses. Malignant tumours adjacent to bone may cause resorption of the cortex with a permeative pattern but lower grade malignancies, including tendon sheath abnormalities, may produce well-defined cortical defects suggesting pressure erosion. Destruction of adjacent bones should suggest a lesion originating in soft tissues. An important example is involvement of the upper ribs by bronchial carcinoma (Pancoast tumour) in patients being assessed for neck, brachial plexus or shoulder pain (Fig. 5.8).

BONE TUMOURS PRESUMED TO ARISE FROM SKELETAL TISSUE — BONE FORMING

BONE ISLAND (also known as enostosis)

Although no evidence exists to suggest that this is a true bony neoplasm, confusion may arise on occasions. The lesions may be single or multiple, are always medullary in location and consist of normal, compact lamellar bone. The lesion is uniformly dense but the margins may be ill-defined showing radiating spiculation into the surrounding medullary cavity with a narrow zone of transition (Fig. 5.9). Bone islands may grow up to the age of skeletal maturity and occasionally thereafter. Exceptionally they may regress. Periosteal new bone and cortical expansion do not occur. On an isotope bone scan they may show a slight increase in activity, the degree being related to their size. No blood pool abnormality becomes evident. In elderly patients it may be necessary to differentiate these sclerotic lesions from osteoblastic metastases.

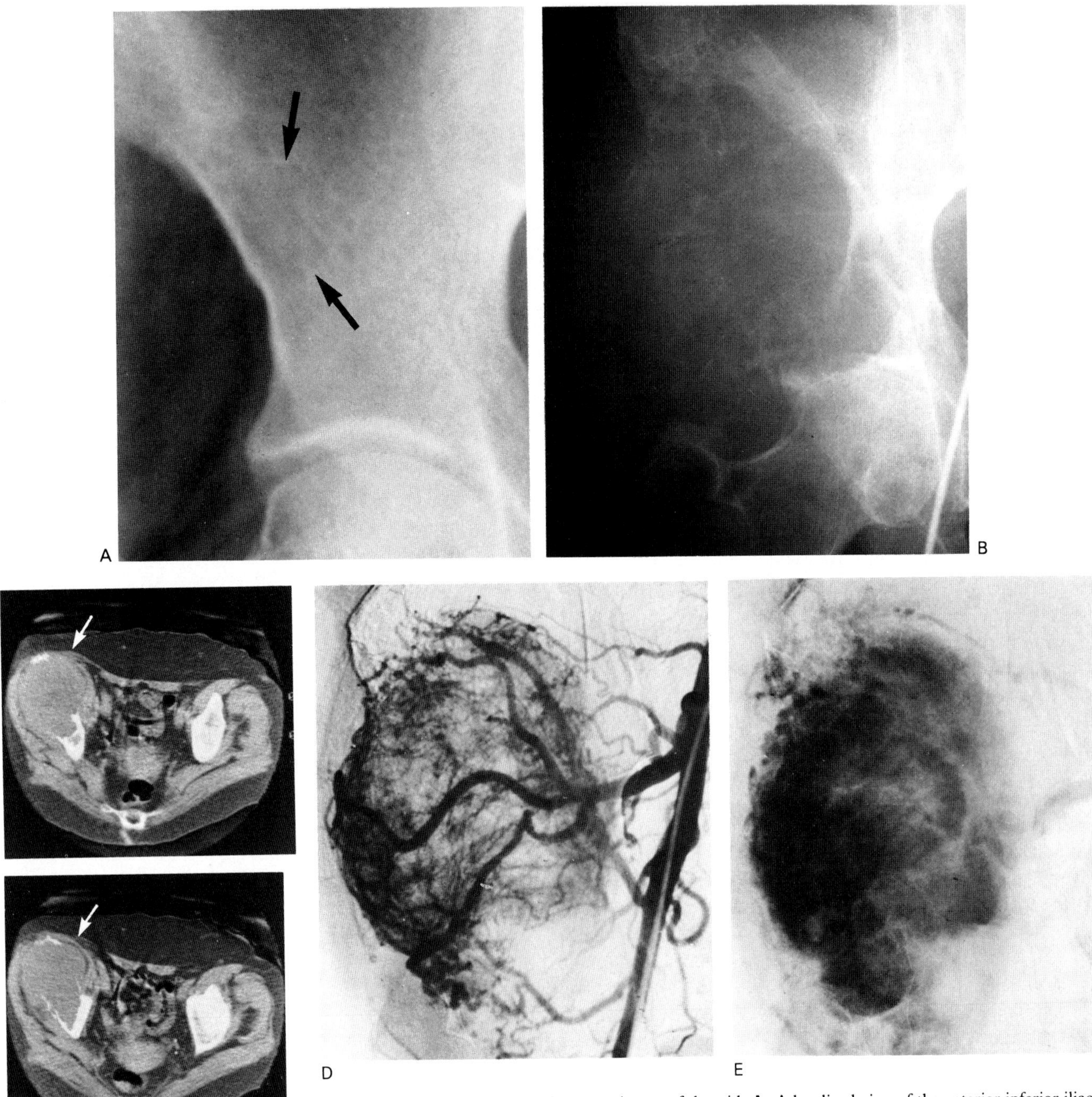

Fig. 5.7 Metastasis from carcinoma of thyroid. **A**. A localized view of the anterior inferior iliac crest shows a small radiolucent defect with a faint sclerotic margin (arrows). **B**. 5 years later a very large destructive bone lesion is present with relatively well-defined margins and apparent strands of calcification within the lesion. **C**. CT scan confirms the very extensive nature of the tumour and shows soft tissue planes to be preserved (arrow). The strands of calcification are shown to be residual bone anteriorly and posteriorly and not new bone in the metastasis. **D**. and **E**. Common iliac arteriography (substraction images) demonstrates the very vascular nature of this metastasis. Note the increase in number of abnormal vessels with changing calibre, the dense tumour blush and early venous filling.

OSTEOMA

True osteomas are rather rare, arising principally from skull, paranasal sinuses and mandible (Fig. 5.10). They are benign, slow growing tumours consisting entirely of well-differentiated bone. They have a broad base with a smooth well defined margin. Two types are recognized. The dense variety, the so-called ivory osteoma, and the trabeculated or spongy variety more commonly occurring in the cranial vault. Whilst varying in size few are larger than 2.5 cm in diameter. The tumour itself is asymptomatic, but growth from the inner table of the skull may produce raised intracranial pressure or other symptoms similar to those of

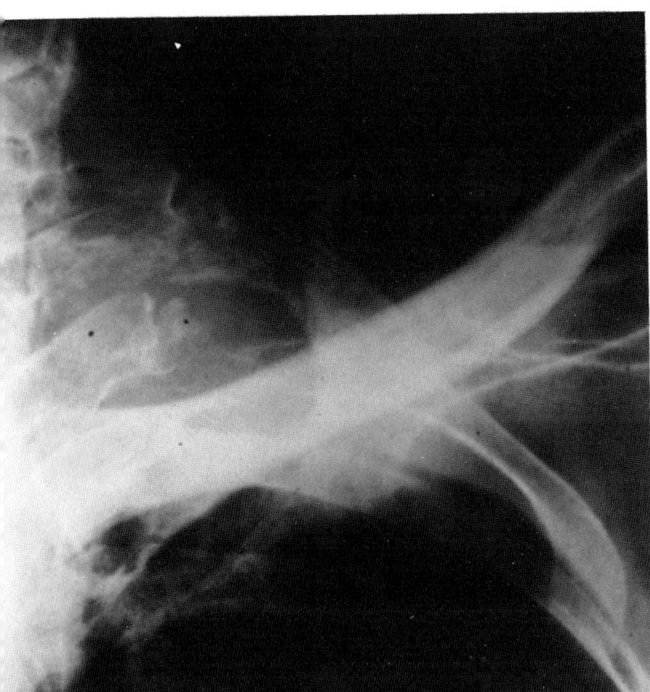

Fig. 5.8 Pancoast tumour — carcinoma of the apex of the lung — invading and destroying the first and second ribs.

a meningioma. Growth within the paranasal sinuses may interfere with nasal drainage, causing a mucocoele or even perforation of the cribriform plate to cause pneumocephalus. The rarer, spongy variety is shown histologically to contain moderate quantities of fibrous tissue and may be a variant of fibrous dysplasia.

Further investigation is rarely necessary apart from documenting the secondary effects of the lesion, such as a mucocoele from obstruction to drainage of a paranasal sinus. Scintigraphically the increased activity reflects the size of the lesion as in the case of a bone island.

When craniofacial osteomas are detected the possibility of Gardner's syndrome should be considered, particularly if lesions are present in the mandible. The presence of osteomas elsewhere in the skeleton, soft tissue tumours of connective tissue origin and polyposis coli establish the diagnosis.

OSTEOID OSTEOMA

Unlike other bone tumours this lesion has a definite male preponderance of the order of three to one. The majority of cases present in the second and third decades. The typical history is of localized, intermittent bone pain of several weeks or months duration, occurring especially at night with dramatic relief by aspirin. Many patients, however, suffer non-specific symptoms and aspirin relief is not necessarily constant. There may be sufficient pain to provoke muscle wasting from limitation of movement. Growth disparities may develop in the immature skeleton, including failure of tubulation and leg length discrepancy. Difficulty in diagnosis sometimes causes these patients to be referred to psychiatrists in the belief that their symptoms are functional. The natural history of this tumour is uncertain since most cases are treated by immediate surgical excision but it appears probable that untreated lesions eventually undergo spontaneous involution.

The diaphyses of long bones are the sites of predeliction with at least half of all cases occurring in the femur, especially its proximal end and the tibia, although virtually any bone may be affected, even the skull on rare occasions. When the spine is involved the tumour is almost always situated in the neural arch and not the vertebral body. The symptoms of spinal involvement may mimic those of an adolescent disc protrusion and indeed painful scoliosis in a child or adolescent with muscle spasm demands careful scrutiny of the neural arches at the apex of the concavity to exclude the presence of this particular tumour.

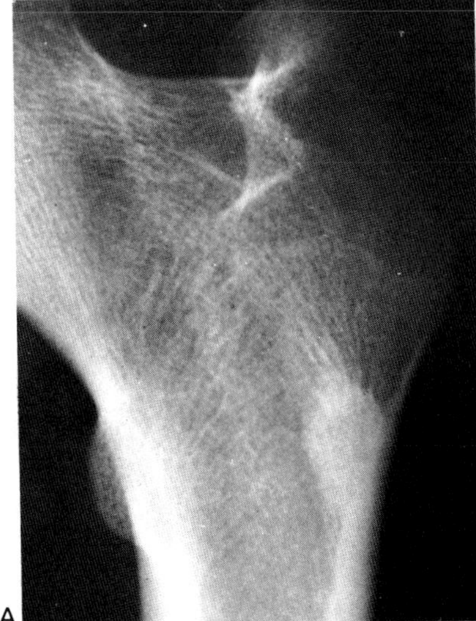

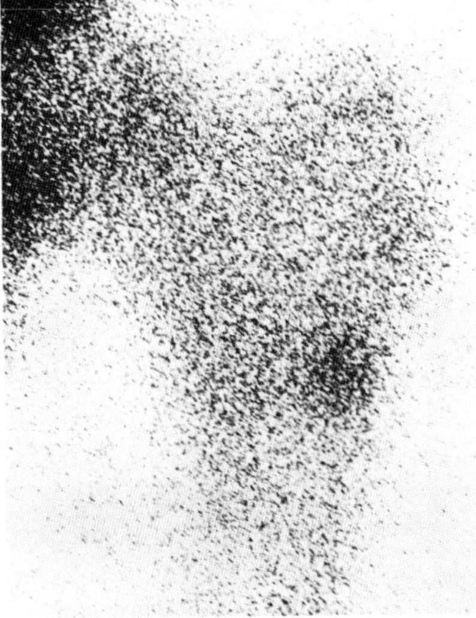

Fig. 5.9 Bone island — enostosis. **A**. A dense area of endosteal sclerosis present in the upper femoral shaft, discovered by chance following injury. **B**. A bone scan reveals slight increase in activity localized to the area of sclerosis. Biopsy confirmation.

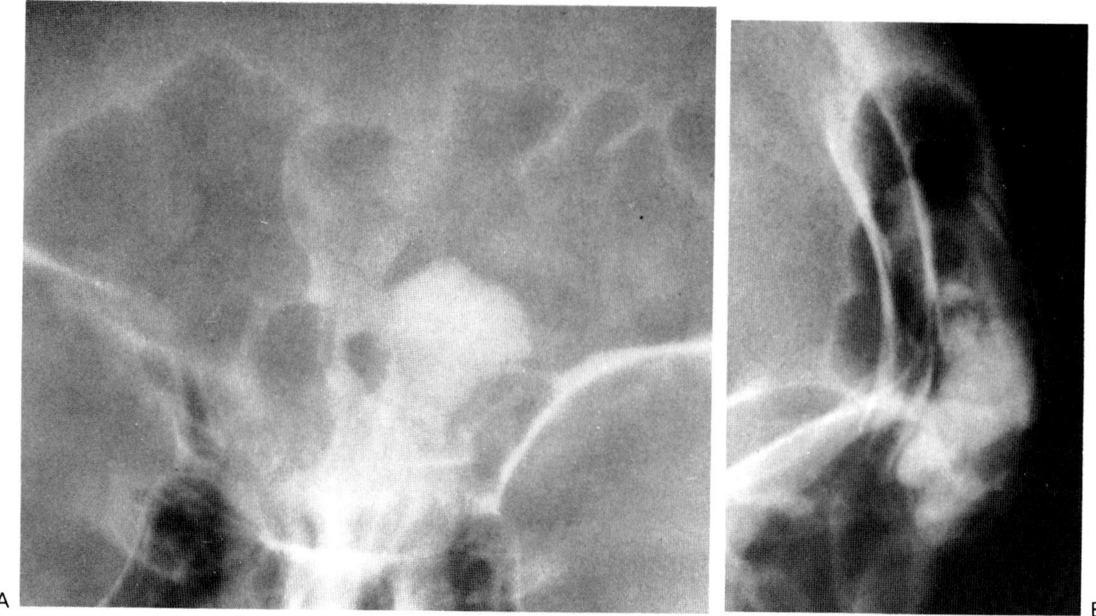

Fig. 5.10 Ivory osteomas of the frontal sinus. A typical, compact, rounded, dense opacity is demonstrated on (**A**) the frontal view. **B**. In another patient a larger lesion has moulded to the shape of the sinus.

Radiological features. The lesion comprises a round or oval area of radiolucency with a sclerotic margin. This radiolucency usually contains a small dense opacity known, on this side of the Atlantic, as the nidus (Fig. 5.11). In North America the word nidus, meaning nest, is employed more correctly for the radiolucency itself. While the overall size of the lesion varies up to about 2.5 cm in diameter the width of the central density rarely exceeds 1 cm. The lesion is surrounded by a variable degree of dense sclerosis. The extent of this density depends on the actual site of the tumour within the affected bone. It is minimal when the tumour lies in the spongy bone of the medulla, particularly close to joints (Fig. 5.12). Occasionally no peripheral density may be evident and the small central opacity appears to lie within an area of radiolucency. More commonly the lesion is sited in relation to cortical bone and is surrounded by dense sclerosis which may be extensive and extend into the medulla. When the lesion is adjacent to the periosteum in children new bone formation is particularly florid. In the last two instances the reactive new bone may be so dense that the lesion itself is obscured on plain radiographs.

Provided that the essential features of the radiolucency and its central density are demonstrated, the diagnosis usually is established radiologically with little difficulty. When the lesion is surrounded by dense sclerosis further investigation is necessary, requiring over-penetrated films, tomography (either conventional or CT) and bone scintigraphy. Because of the extensive sclerosis it is important not to overcount the bone scan since the focal area of increased activity due to the osteoid osteoma may be obscured. In the case of a medullary osteoid osteoma with little or no radiological abnormality on conventional films, bone scinti-

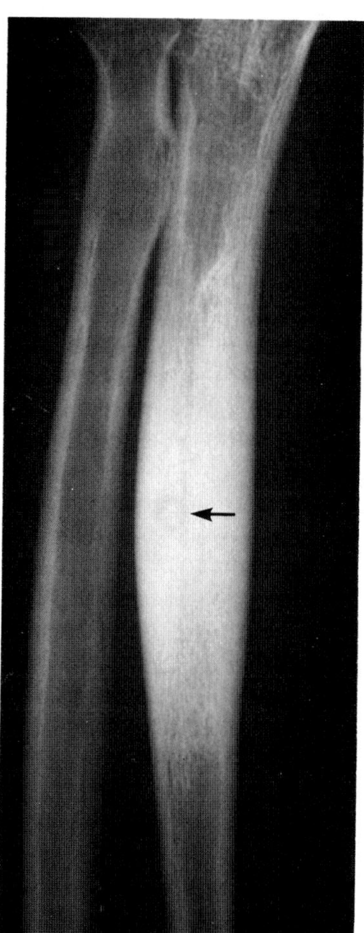

Fig. 5.11 Osteoid osteoma of the ulna in a 13-year-old male. The appearances are typical with a well-defined area of radiolucency (arrow) containing a dense nidus. Extensive cortical sclerosis is present around the lesion.

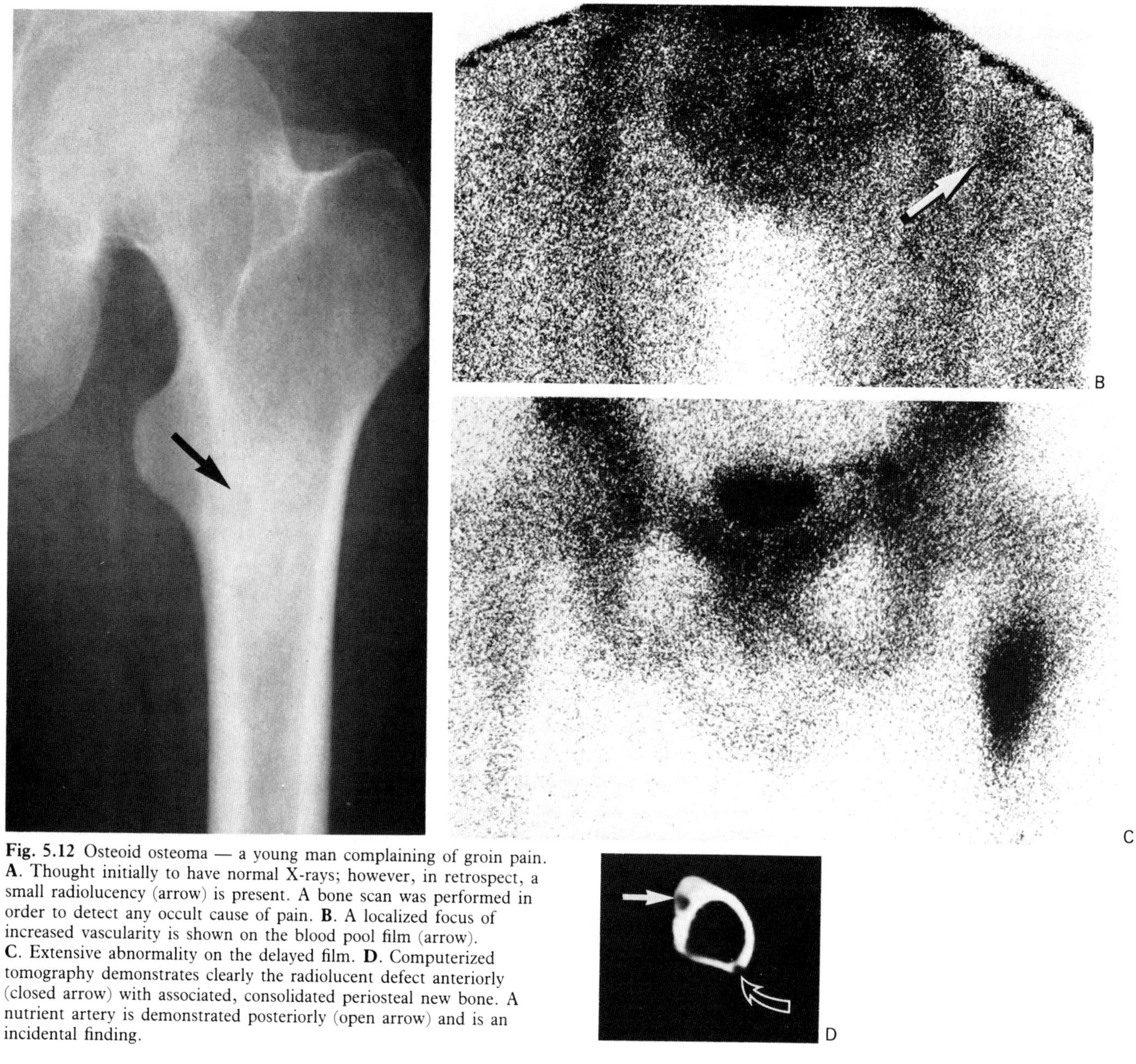

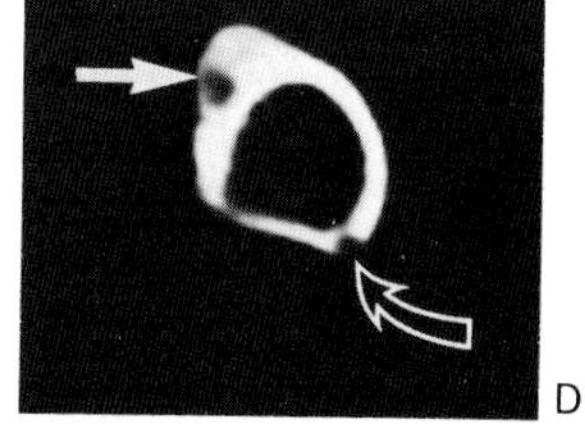

Fig. 5.12 Osteoid osteoma — a young man complaining of groin pain. **A**. Thought initially to have normal X-rays; however, in retrospect, a small radiolucency (arrow) is present. A bone scan was performed in order to detect any occult cause of pain. **B**. A localized focus of increased vascularity is shown on the blood pool film (arrow). **C**. Extensive abnormality on the delayed film. **D**. Computerized tomography demonstrates clearly the radiolucent defect anteriorly (closed arrow) with associated, consolidated periosteal new bone. A nutrient artery is demonstrated posteriorly (open arrow) and is an incidental finding.

graphy remains the most important means of detecting the presence of a lesion. An intense focal abnormality is evident in the blood pool image and intense activity persists in the delayed image. So constant are these findings that scintigraphy should be undertaken in any young person with bone pain and apparently normal radiographs. These scintigraphic abnormalities correspond to the highly vascular nature of the neoplasm which may be demonstrated by angiography, particularly by the tumour blush evident in the late venous phase. Angiography, however, has been supplanted by scintigraphy to a large extent in the investigation of these lesions. The presence of the lesion and its exact site may require localisation with computerized tomography.

The pain produced by these tumours is relieved immediately by surgical excision and the reactive new bone slowly undergoes remodelling. If, however, removal of the tumour is incomplete, not only will the pain persist but the lesion will recur. It should be appreciated that, on rare occasions, osteoid osteoma may be multifocal, in that more than one opacity is contained within a single area of radiolucency. Some lesions near joints in childhood may be associated with synovitis, with resulting diffuse hyaline cartilage thinning and disuse osteoporosis.

Osteoid osteoma must be differentiated from osteoblastoma (described below) and other causes of chronic cortical thickening. These include, chronic sclerosing osteomyelitis, foreign body granulomas ('blackthorn'), polyarteritis nodosa and subperiosteal haematoma, particularly along the shin. In general the distinction between osteoid osteoma and chronic osteomyelitis is straightforward. In osteomyelitis the area of radiolucency tends to be more irregular, although a sequestrum may be confused with a nidus. Whereas the central opacity of an osteoid osteoma is almost always round or slightly oval, the majority of osteomyelitic sequestra are irregular and often linear in shape. Scintigraphy shows a diffuse increase in activity both in the blood pool and the delayed phases. Angiography fails to opacify a sequestrum, although it does demonstrate enlarged periosteal veins typical of infection.

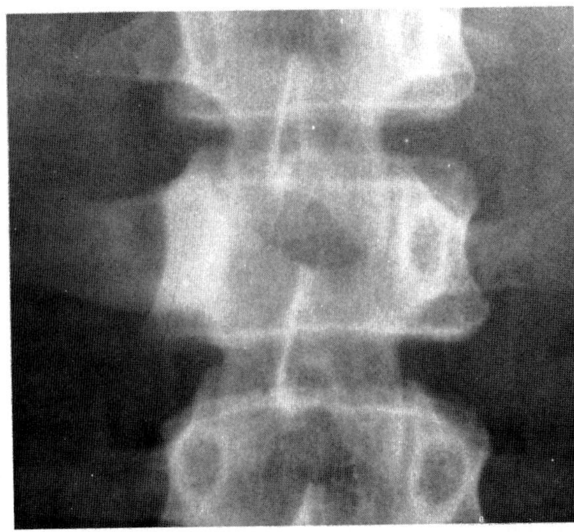

Fig. 5.13 Osteoblastoma of the right transverse process and pedicle of L3. An ill defined radiolucency is shown within a sclerotic and expanded transverse process and pedicle.

OSTEOBLASTOMA

This tumour is now accepted as a distinct entity, although a considerable overlap undoubtedly exists with osteoid osteoma. Indeed the situation is confused by the occasional osteoid osteoma which is larger than usual and may be referred to as giant osteoid osteoma. Both osteoblastoma and osteoid osteoma superficially have similar histological characteristics. The tumour is, in almost all circumstances, benign, but may be aggressive (see below). It is accompanied often by a long, insidious, history of pain, one in ten patients suffering worsening of the pain at night. Aspirin relief is not a feature. No definite sex incidence has been recognized but at least 80% of the patients are under the age of 30. Whilst any bone may be involved, the majority of lesions occur in the spine and flat bones, particularly the vertebral appendages. Again, as in the case of osteoid osteoma, the last location may stimulate a scoliosis; indeed in one series as many as 50% of the patients had a scoliosis, some with positive neurological signs. On the other hand many of these tumours develop in the small bones of the hands and feet and even, rarely, the skull.

Pathologically the lesion is larger than an osteoid osteoma, irregular in shape, friable and haemorrhagic. Abundant osteoid tissue is present with broad, widely spread trabeculae, in relation to which are numerous osteoblasts and osteoclasts. Many thin-walled capillaries account for the marked vascularity of the tumour.

Radiological features. An area of radiolucency is typical, being considerably larger than that of an osteoid osteoma and of the order of 2–10 cm in diameter (Fig. 5.13). As previously suggested difficulty may arise on occasions in distinguishing this appearance from an exceptionally large osteoid osteoma. The margins of the radiolucency show considerable irregularity, even though they are usually sharply demarcated. This margin, however, may sometimes be ill-defined and not easily distinguishable from a malignant lesion, particularly an osteosarcoma. A giant cell tumour may be considered when the lesion is subarticular in location. Cortical expansion and exquisite thinning is common so that only a fine opaque shell may remain. This appearance simulates the cortical expansion caused by an aneurysmal bone cyst, but may be distinguished easily by the total absence of bone reaction and the poorly defined margin of the latter tumour. The majority of osteoblastomas enlarge slowly with consequent remodelling of bone around the lesion. The degree of associated bone sclerosis varies considerably but may be profound though not usually sufficient to obscure the primary lesion as in osteoid osteoma. Calcification or ossification of osteoid tissue within the tumour may cause a punctate increase in density (Fig. 5.14) best appreciated on tomography or CT. Further calcification and ossification may occur following radiotherapy. Calcification is never annular as in a cartilage tumour. Scintigraphically these lesions are extremely active both in the blood pool and delayed phases of a bone scan. On the delayed phase the lesion may seem very extensive reflecting the secondary bone sclerosis. If angiography is undertaken the radiolucency may be shown to contain an increased number of vessels with a blush and small lakes of contrast medium, but encasement and other features suggestive of malignancy are not present.

In the vast majority of patients the prognosis is excellent once total excision of the tumour has been achieved. On some occasions, however, an osteoblastoma behaves in an aggressive fashion, particularly after incomplete removal or radiotherapy. Not only is the lesion radiographically aggressive with soft tissue masses containing ill-defined calcification and ossification but a similar pattern of aggression is visible also under the microscope. On rare occasions the lesion behaves frankly as an osteosarcoma with pulmonary metastasis.

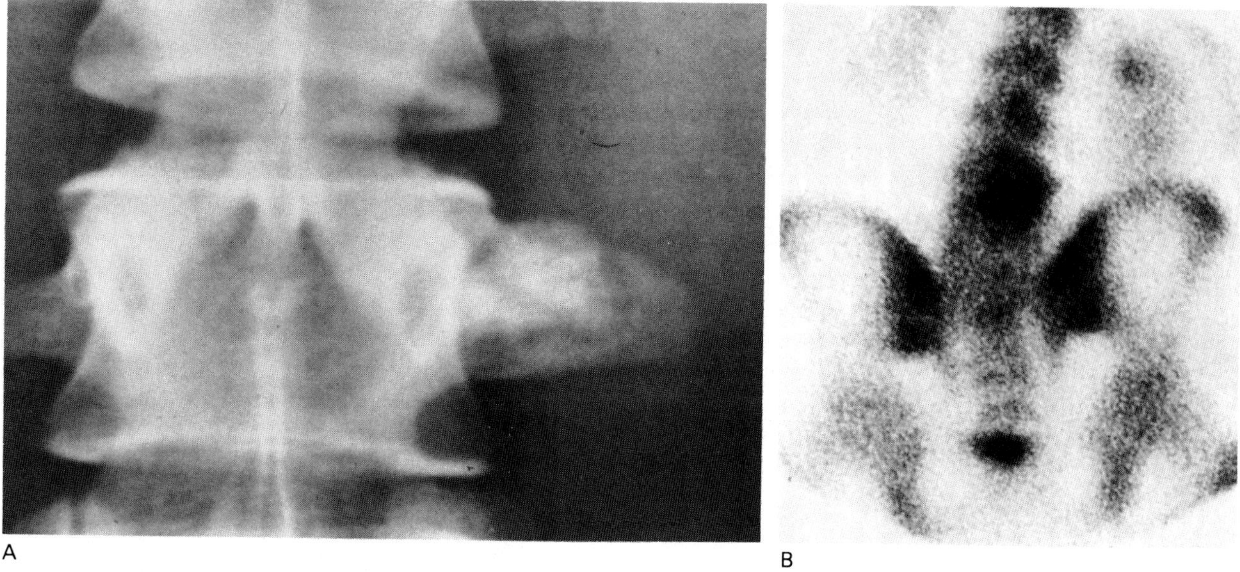

Fig. 5.14 Osteoblastoma of the left transverse process of L3. **A.** In this example the central area exhibits calcification. Expansion is present with diffuse sclerosis. **B.** Note on the bone scan (which has been reversed for ease of comparison) the extensive area of increased activity corresponding to the whole of the osteoblastoma on the plain film. Note also the scoliosis with which these patients may present.

OSTEOSARCOMA

Osteosarcoma is the commonest primary malignant bone tumour. Characteristically it is histologically pleomorphic, but two diagnostic features are, firstly, its ability to produce osteoid tissue, without necessarily the development of a cartilaginous precursor, and, secondly, the presence of abundant alkaline phosphatase histochemically within the tumour cells. The osteoid tissue may undergo a variable degree of ossification. However, because of the pleomorphic nature of the sarcoma a dominant cell line may modify the appearance. If osteoblasts predominate tumour bone formation will result, whereas, if cells of cartilage origin are present, extensive calcification may be a presenting feature. Terms such as osteoblastic (Fig. 5.15), chondroblastic (Fig. 5.16), fibroblastic and anaplastic or telangectatic (Fig. 5.17), are often applied. No convincing evidence has been established that these pathological subgroups have much influence on prognosis. Nonetheless, each has slightly different radiological characteristics. Osteosarcoma arising in relation to the periosteum and secondary to other conditions is considered below.

Osteosarcoma presents usually with localized pain or swelling, particularly around the knee in an adolescent or young adult. Not infrequently the lesion is recognized first on account of a pathological fracture (Fig. 5.18). Advanced tumours may be found in an emaciated, pyrexial patient, when the unwary may consider a diagnosis of chronic osteomyelitis. A slight male preponderance exists, the peak incidence occurring between 10 and 25 years of age. Many of the tumours occurring in older age groups are associated with Paget's disease (see below). Although any bone may

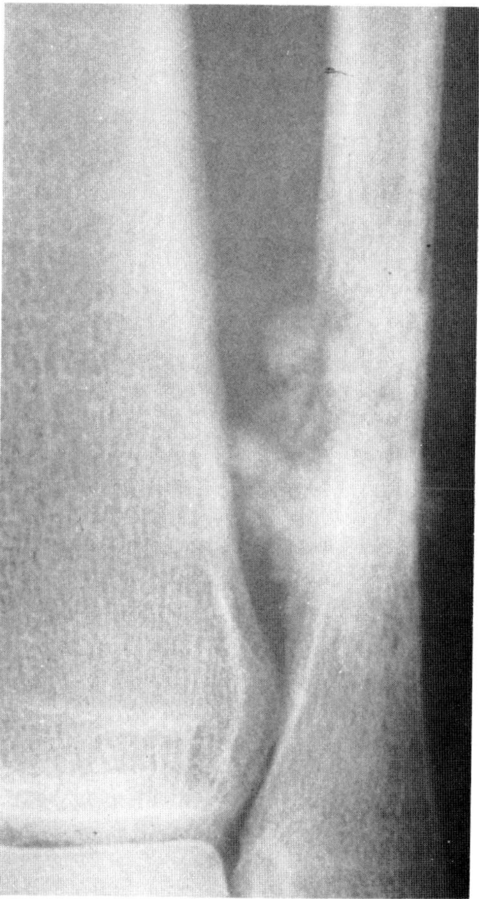

Fig. 5.15 Osteosarcoma of the distal fibula — predominantly osteoblastic. Amorphous calcification/ossification is present in the soft tissues with cortical destruction and a little periosteal new bone formation.

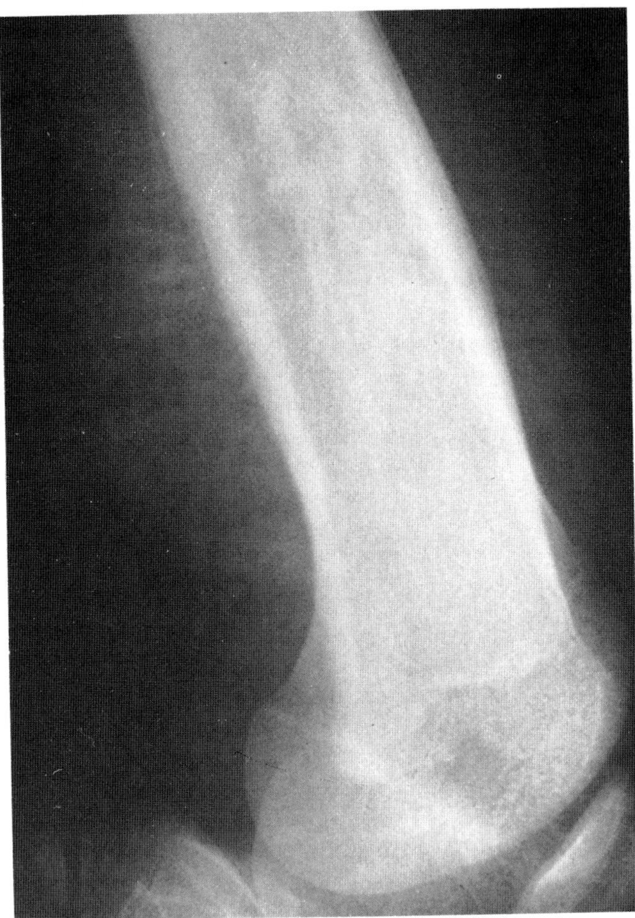

Fig. 5.16 Osteosarcoma of the distal femur — predominantly chondroblastic. Note the well-defined soft tissue mass and radiating spiculation of calcification within it. Sclerosis and lysis are present within the medullary cavity which is slightly expanded.

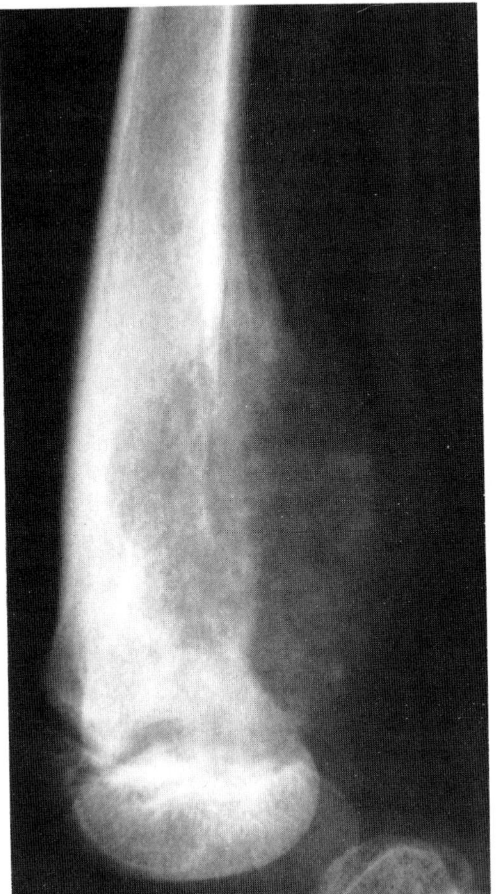

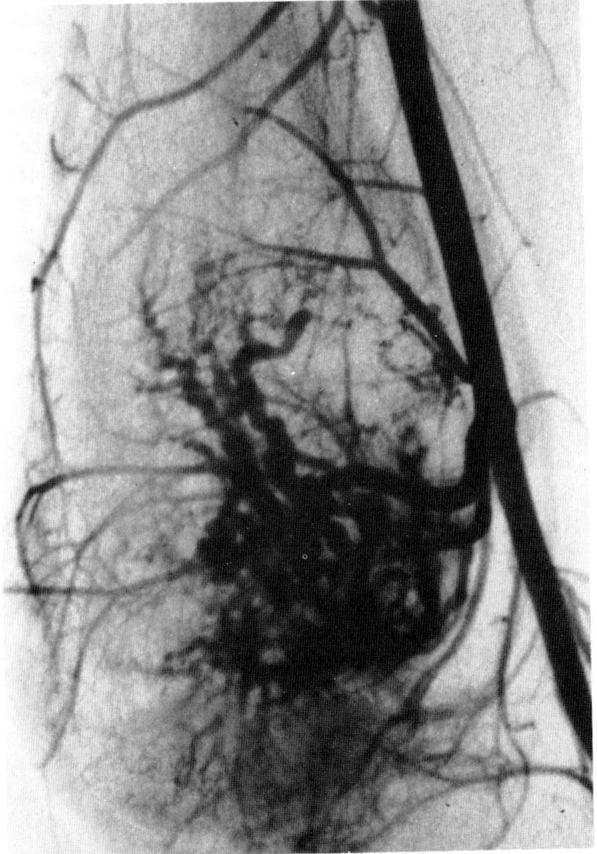

be involved rather more than half of all osteosarcomas are located around the knee involving the metadiaphyses of the distal end of the femur and the proximal end of the tibia. Indeed the vast majority of osteosarcomas arise in those sites in long bones which are exhibiting the greatest longitudinal growth. About 10% of tumours arise in the diaphysis. These have a similar age and sex incidence to ordinary osteosarcoma (see below). Orthodox teaching suggested that epiphyseal involvement occurs late, metaphyseal cartilage acting as a temporary barrier to spread of the tumour. Although the truth of this statement appears to be supported by the evidence of plain films, investigation by scintigraphy, angiography and histology has indicated

Fig. 5.17 Telangectatic osteosarcoma of the distal femur. **A**. A predominantly radiolucent defect is shown on plain film which (**B**) angiographically is shown to contain large, tortuous, pathological vessels. Well marked Codman's triangles are present together with sclerosis in the shaft of the bone, surrounding the lesion.

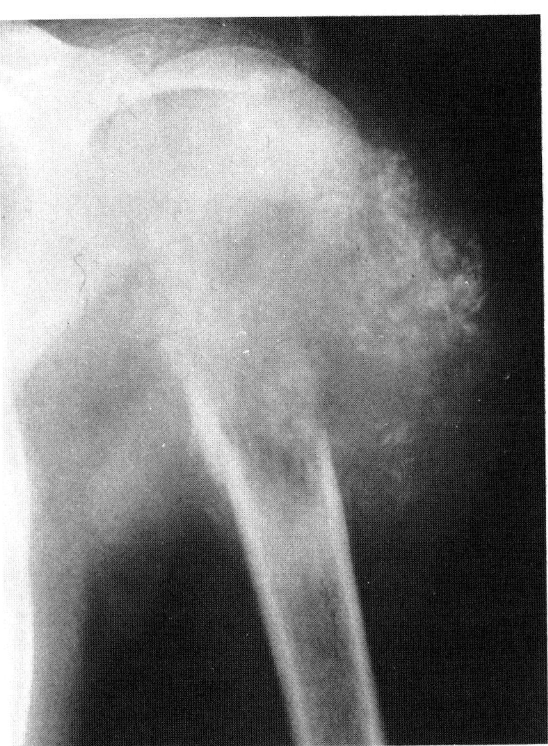

Fig. 5.18 An advanced osteosarcoma of the proximal humerus presents with a pathological fracture. A large well defined soft tissue mass contains calcification and ossification. Codman's triangles are present. Extensive tumour in the medulla has caused both bone destruction and bone formation.

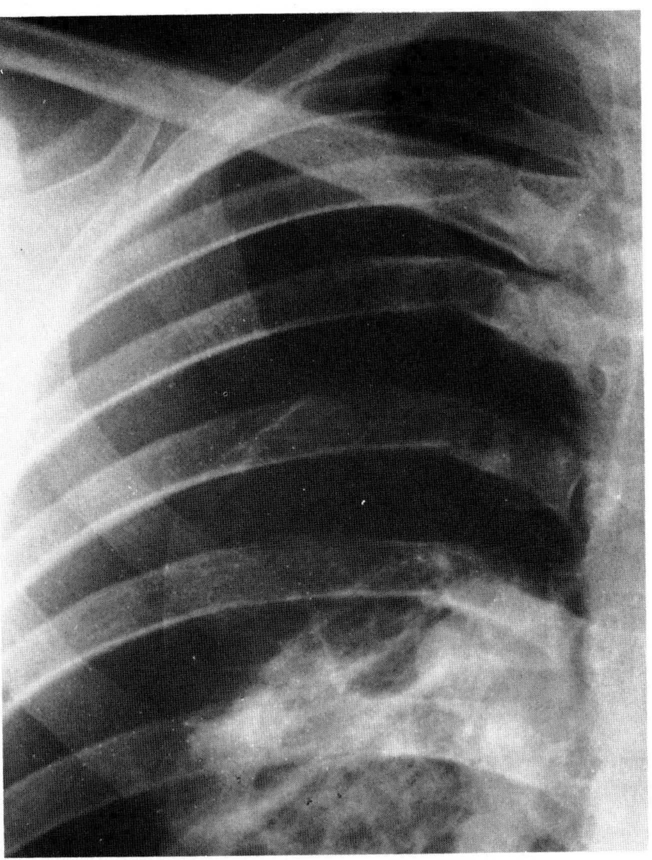

Fig. 5.19 Osteosarcoma — metastasis in the lungs presents with a pneumothorax.

that in many cases epiphyseal involvement occurs earlier. It is exceptional, however, for a joint cavity to be involved.

The lesion commonly arises eccentrically in the medullary cavity with ill-defined cortical destruction and soft tissue involvement. The pleomorphic nature of the histology may on occasion cause misleading biopsy results, since if the sample is taken from areas rich in cartilaginous elements, a misdiagnosis of chondrosarcoma may occur. Metastatic spread occurs by the haematogenous route so that a diligent search for pulmonary metastases should be undertaken. Pulmonary metastasis is associated with an unusually high incidence of pneumothorax (Fig. 5.19). Indeed any lung lesion arising in a patient with osteosarcoma should be regarded with suspicion (Fig. 5.20). Lymphatic spread is relatively rare. In the later stages metastases may develop in bone; population surveys have suggested that these deposits are themselves metastatic from the pulmonary lesions.

Imaging features. On *plain films* an eccentric area of bone destruction usually is present in the metadiaphysis adjacent to the knee joint, being associated typically with cortical destruction and a well-defined extension of the lesion into soft tissues. Elevation of the periosteum is associated with new bone formation, the so-called Codman's triangles. The epiphysis usually appears normal radiologically. The soft tissue mass may contain calcification which may show either an amorphous or a spiculated appearance. A mixture of sclerosis and bone destruction is present usually within the bony lesion. It is unusual for a lesion to be purely lytic. *Scintigraphically* increased vascularity is constant in the blood pool phase of a bone scan with an extensive abnormality on the delayed images (Fig. 5.21). The extent of the tumour, as delineated by a bone scan, may be greater than that shown on plain film, being due in part to a surrounding rim of reactive bone. Scintigraphy may confirm epiphyseal spread of the tumour, but an apparent increase in activity in an adjacent joint should not be mistaken for synovial involvement. Scintigraphy also may detect the presence of lung metastases, although this procedure is not reliable if purely fibroblastic lesions are present or if the metastases have been treated. A cerebral metastasis may not be observed with a bone scan. *Computerized tomography* demonstrates to advantage those features on the plain films and is particularly useful for delineating the intra- and extra-osseous extent of tumour (Figs 5.21c, 5.22d). It is the most sensitive means of detecting pulmonary metastases (Fig. 5.20b). The *angiographic features* suggest an aggressive tumour and again

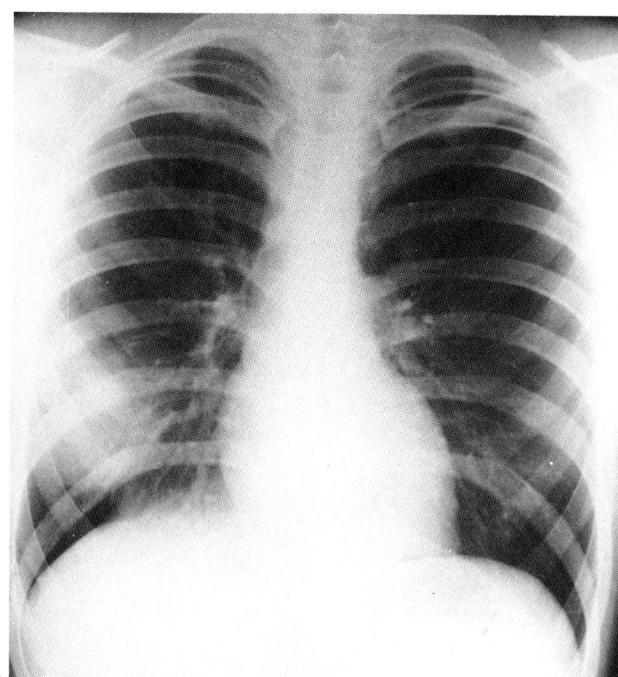

Fig. 5.20 Metastasis from osteosarcoma presents with (**A**) an encysted pleural effusion on the right after several months apparently disease-free after amputation. **B**. A CT scan demonstrates the encysted effusion in the horizontal fissure with calcification dorsally due to metastasis. This feature had not been appreciated on conventional tomography. A second metastasis is shown in the right lower lobe, again not obvious on plain films. (W 200, L + 16).

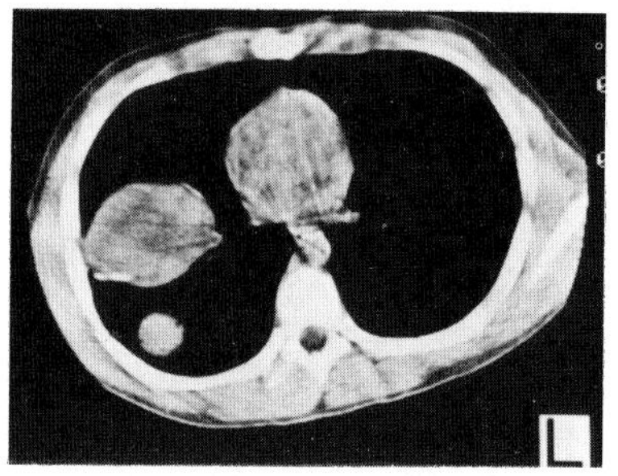

Fig. 5.21 Osteoblastic osteosarcoma of the proximal tibia. **A**. Plain film reveals patchy increased density in much of the upper tibia. Note a little new bone laterally. **B**. A scan in the early blood pool (left) and delayed phases (right) demonstrates an extensive abnormality. Note the activity is more uniform and extensive than the apparent involvement shown on the plain film. The distal extent of the tumour is confirmed however by (**C**) a CT scan which shows a subtle change in marrow attenuation below the level of the apparent tumour on plain film. An example of how CT may be used to gauge the extent of marrow involvement.

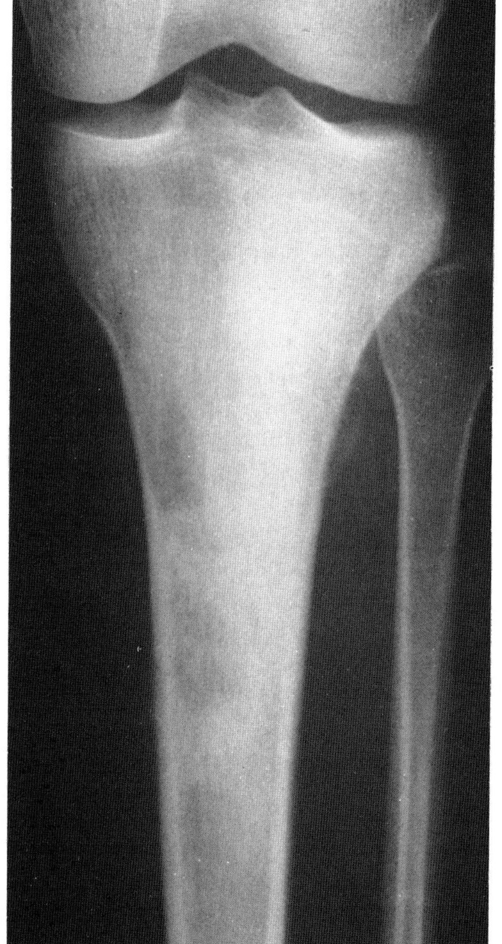

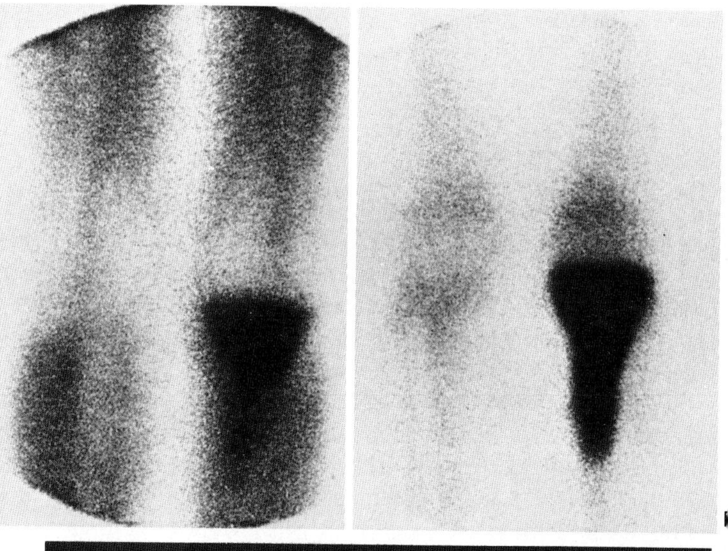

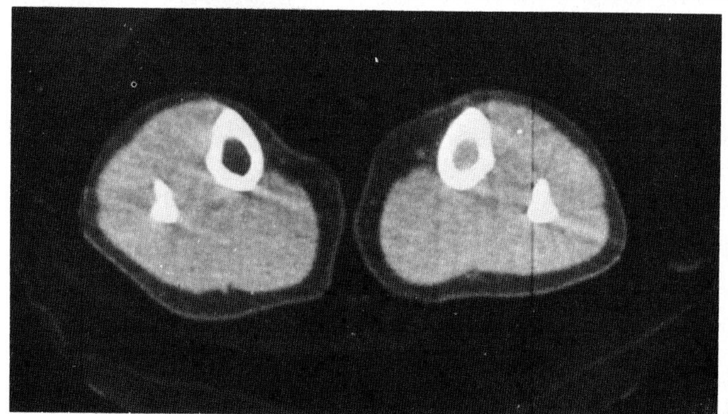

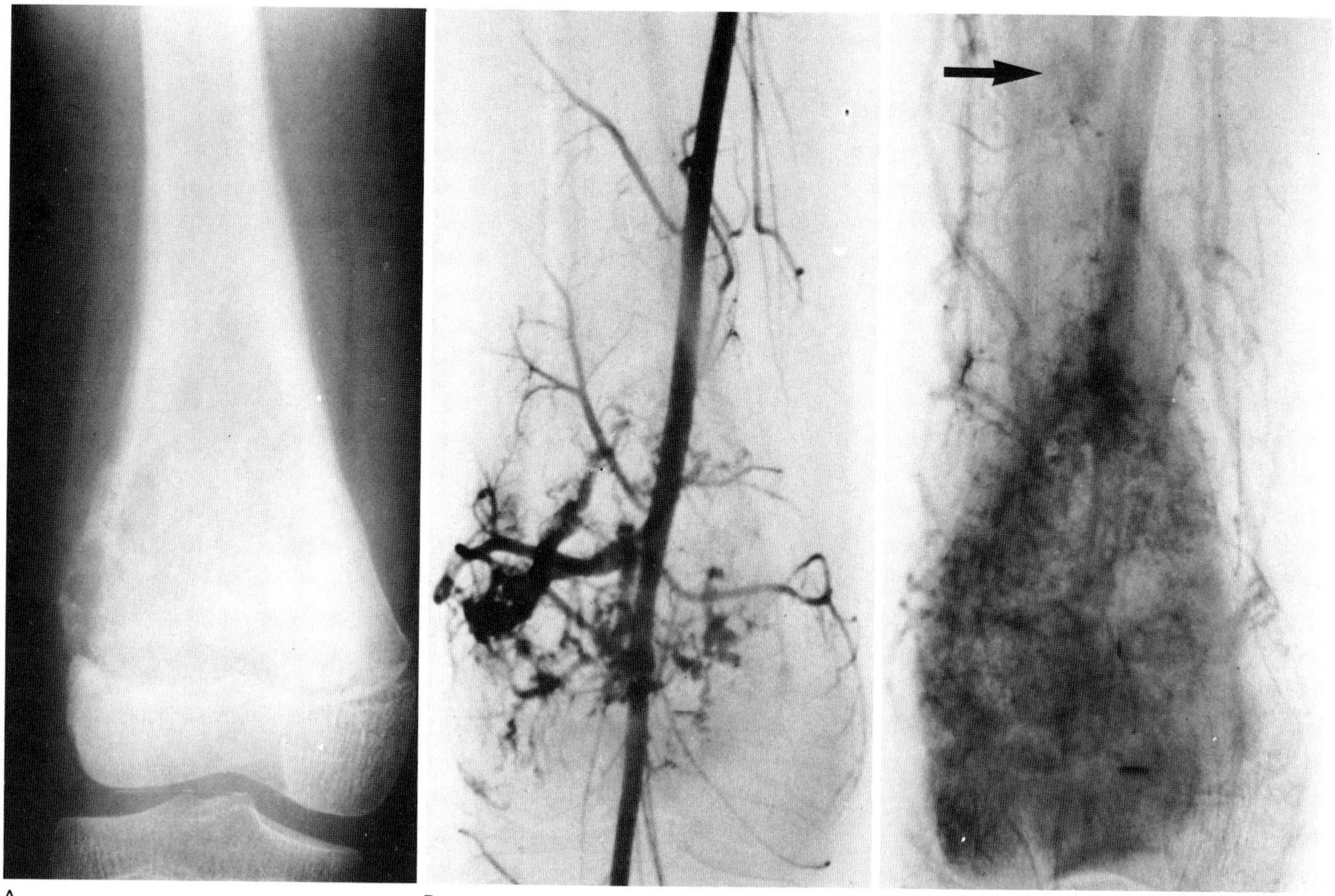

Fig. 5.22 Osteosarcoma of the distal femur of a young woman. **A**. The full intraosseous extent is difficult to assess on the plain film. **B**. An arteriogram demonstrates a very extensive pathological circulation and (**C**) on the late capillary phase note that the tumour extends into the epiphysis, almost to the articular surface, and that there is a satellite or 'skip' lesion in the proximal femoral shaft (arrow). This latter lesion is confirmed by (**D**) CT and is shown to be bone-forming (the upper image shows an attenuation of 94 EMI units in the lesion, the lower image is at L12, W200).

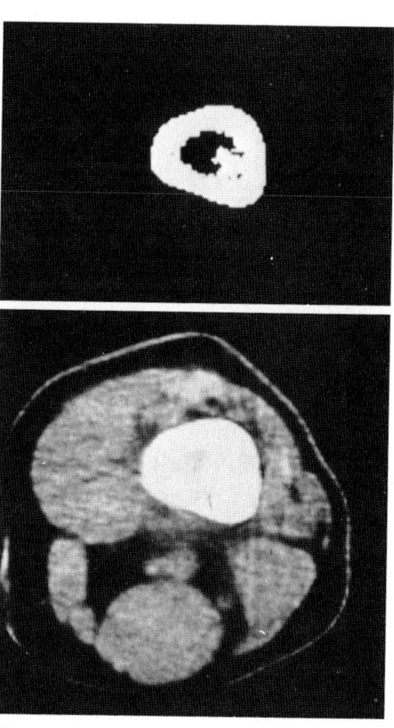

may be used to establish the extent of tumour, if treatment by prosthetic replacement is being considered (Figs 5.22, 5.23).

Differential diagnosis is either from other neoplasms, including malignant round cell tumours and metastases, or from chronic bone infections, including tuberculosis and mycetoma. In the case of infections the aetiology may be suggested by diffuse swelling of soft tissues, disproportionately extensive new bone formation and widespread photon activity on a bone scan.

SPECIAL TYPES OF OSTEOSARCOMA

Diaphyseal. A few of these tumours (approximately 10%) arise in the diaphyses of long bones and their appearances may cause diagnostic confusion. Whilst most resemble

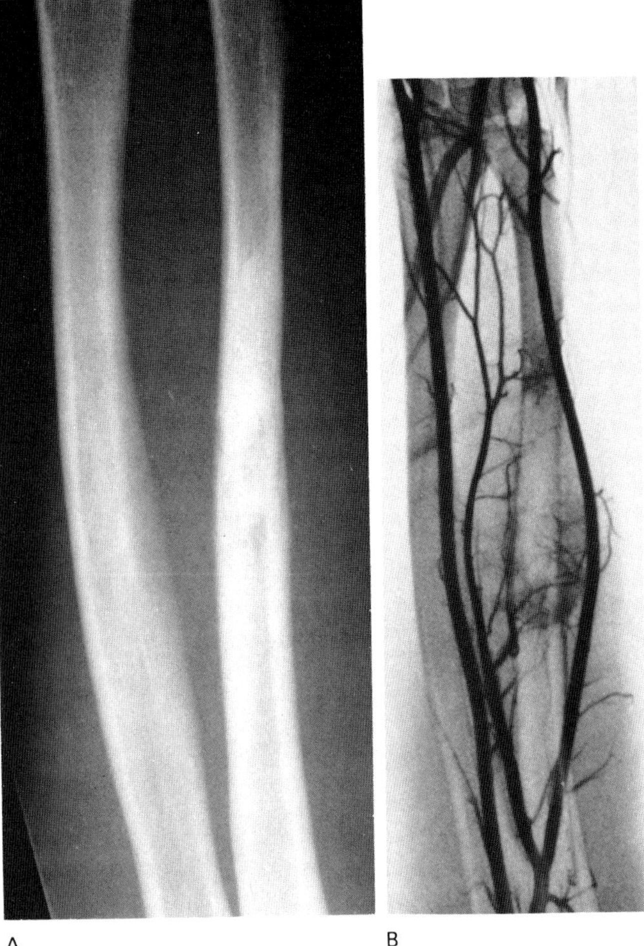

Fig. 5.23 Osteoblastic osteosarcoma. A middle-aged woman presented with pain and swelling in the mid ulna. **A**. A radiograph shows ill-defined sclerosis and cortical destruction. **B**. An angiogram demonstrates an egg-shaped soft tissue mass with displacement of both the ulnar and interosseous arteries. The extra-osseous extent of the tumour was thereby delineated.

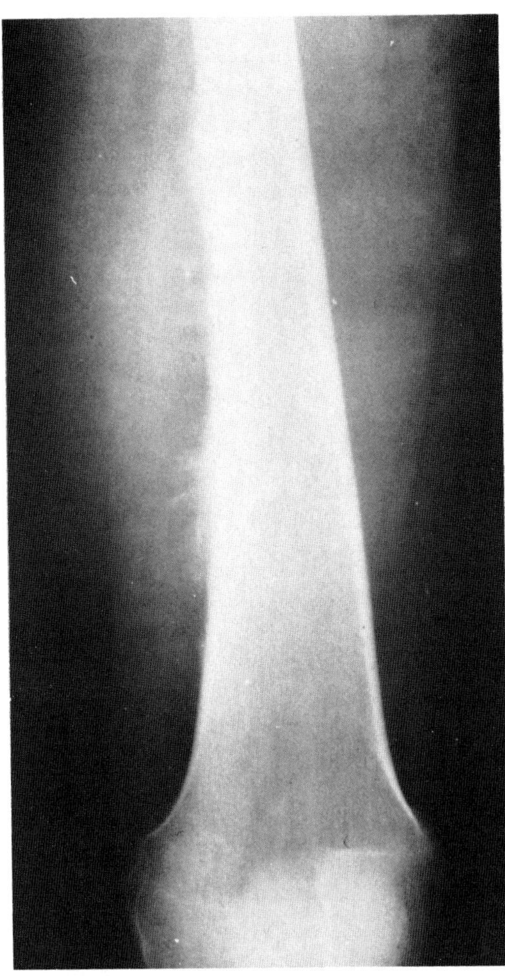

Fig. 5.24 Diaphyseal osteosarcoma of the mid shaft of the femur. Note the radiating spiculation of bone, Codman's triangles and well defined soft tissue mass.

those of osteosarcoma elsewhere (Fig. 5.24) others are purely lytic or indeed purely sclerotic (Fig. 5.25) and an accurate pre-biopsy diagnosis may not be possible. Exceptionally some early cases have been detected as lytic areas confined entirely within a cortex.

Central osteosarcoma. Similar diagnostic difficulty may arise when a lesion presents in the metadiaphysis as an area of dense sclerosis which may be thought initially to represent a large bone island. Specific characteristics on plain films to suggest malignant disease are absent. Scintigraphy and angiography however, will demonstrate much more aggressive features.

Multifocal osteosarcoma is extremely rare and occurs only in childhood. The condition is rapidly fatal with pulmonary metastases and is characterized by a marked elevation of serum alkaline phosphatase. Radiologically symmetrical and densely sclerotic lesions have a predilection for metaphyses and flat bones. Unlike ordinary osteosarcoma epiphyseal and soft tissue involvement occurs early.

Soft tissue osteosarcoma. On rare occasions the tumour arises purely in soft tissue (Fig. 5.26). Various sites of origin have been described, including breast and kidney. Usually, however, the lesion is para-articular. The ill-defined amorphous nature of the soft tissue opacification may suggest tumour bone rather than calcification. Scintigraphy and angiography are usually inconclusive. The differential diagnosis is from post-traumatic myositis ossificans. This entity also can produce markedly abnormal features with scintigraphy and angiography particularly early in its evolution. Histological examination of both entities also is fraught with diagnostic pitfalls in inexperienced hands. However, myositis ossificans may be demonstrated to regress with time and so, if possible, a watching brief is advocated.

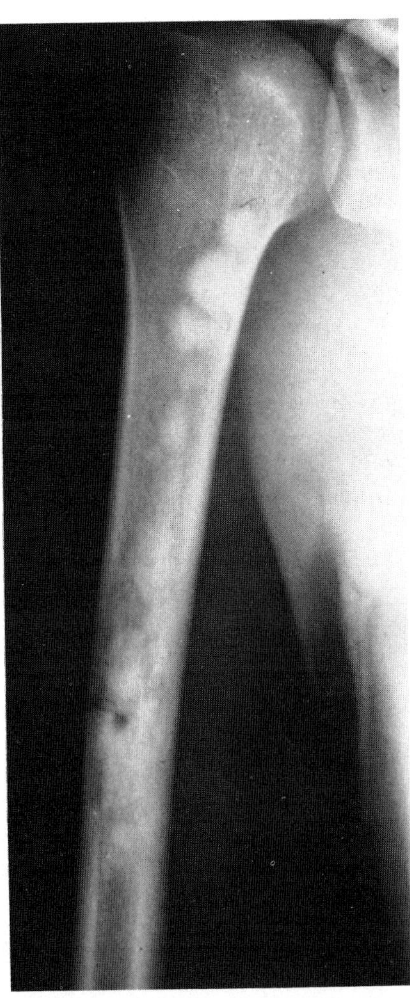

Fig. 5.25 Diaphyseal osteosarcoma. A pathological fracture is present in the mid humerus with extensive endosteal sclerosis and cortical destruction from the medullary aspect. Tumour is present to the neck of the humerus with areas of dense sclerosis and surrounding faint radiolucency. These 'skip' lesions do not represent isolated tumour, the shaft was involved continuously. This variety carries a poor prognosis.

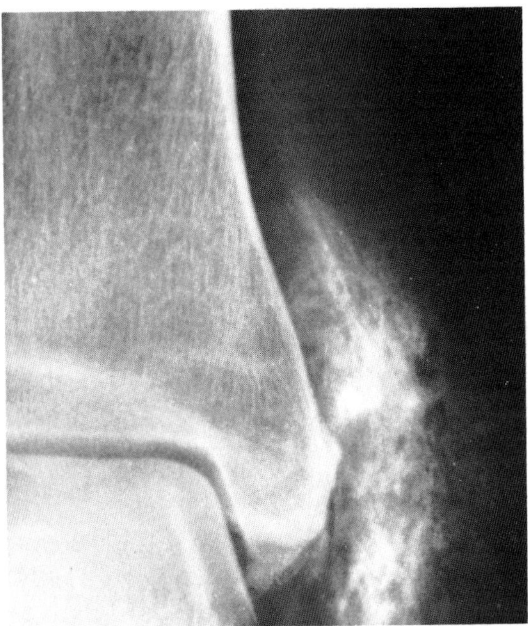

Fig. 5.26 Soft tissue osteosarcoma. An elderly vicar complained of an enlarging soft tissue mass adjacent to the medial malleolus of his right ankle. Note the amorphous soft tissue ossification and calcification and normal bone underlying the lesion.

RADIATION INDUCED SARCOMA

Radiation therapy. Sarcomas arise in bone following radiation typically when the total dose has exceeded 3000 rads, often after a latent interval of 7–10 years. Whilst most are fibrosarcomas a few osteosarcomas do occur. The diagnosis is not difficult radiologically but they often have a predominantly lytic nature and are markedly aggressive. They arise in predictable sites, based on radiation fields, for example in the pelvis following treatment of gynaecological cancer (Fig. 5.27), or around the shoulder as a result of radiation therapy for the common carcinoma of the breast.

The ingestion of radioactive material. Radium and radiomesothorium were introduced in America in 1914 in the preparation of luminous paint. In applying this to watch dials ingestion of the radioactive material occurred through pointing the paint brush with the lips. The subsequent development of osteosarcoma was first reported in 1931 although more usually areas of bone destruction and sclerosis are due to infarction. A long latent interval between ingestion and tumour development is typical. Thorium is, of course, associated with abdominal neoplasia (see Ch. 26).

PAROSTEAL OSTEOSARCOMA

Some confusion in nomenclature relates to osteosarcomas arising in or near the periosteum. For practical purposes these may be divided into two groups: *parosteal osteosarcoma* which will be described; and periosteal osteosarcoma which is similar in most ways to an ordinary osteosarcoma except that it arises close to the periosteum.

Parosteal osteosarcoma comprises some 1% of all malignant primary bone tumours and about 4% of osteosarcomas. Clinically it occurs in patients who are older, at least 50% being over the age of 30. The tumour is slow growing by comparison and has a much better prognosis. In low grade lesions the histology may not immediately suggest a neoplasm at all.

Radiological features. Typically a dense tumour surrounds a long bone, particularly a femur or a tibia. The tumour bone may be extensive, ranging between 2 and 10 cm in length and as much as 5 cm in transverse breadth. The margins are sharply defined but tend to undulate. Whilst the peripheral margin may be clear cut it may be difficult to demonstrate separation of the lesion from un-

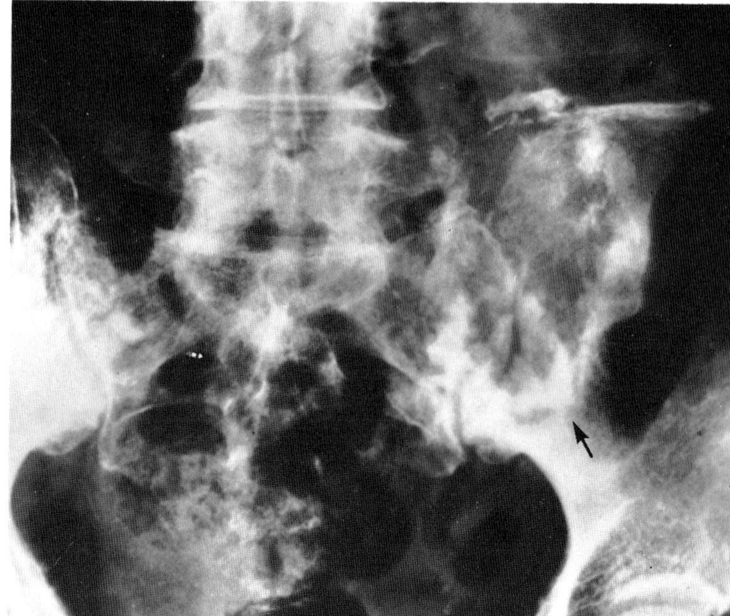

Fig. 5.27 Radiation sarcoma arising in the posterior iliac crest on the left, in an elderly lady treated 6 years previously for carcinoma of the cervix. The lesion is purely osteolytic with ill-defined surrounding sclerosis (arrows).

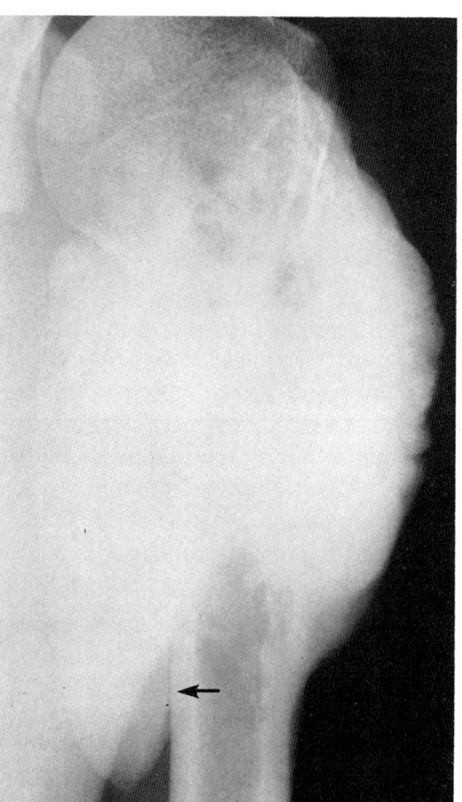

Fig. 5.28 Parosteal osteosarcoma of the proximal humerus. A well-defined mass of dense tumour bone surrounds the humeral shaft. A typical radiolucent line is present between the tumour bone and the proximal shaft infero-medially (arrow). The underlying bone seems normal.

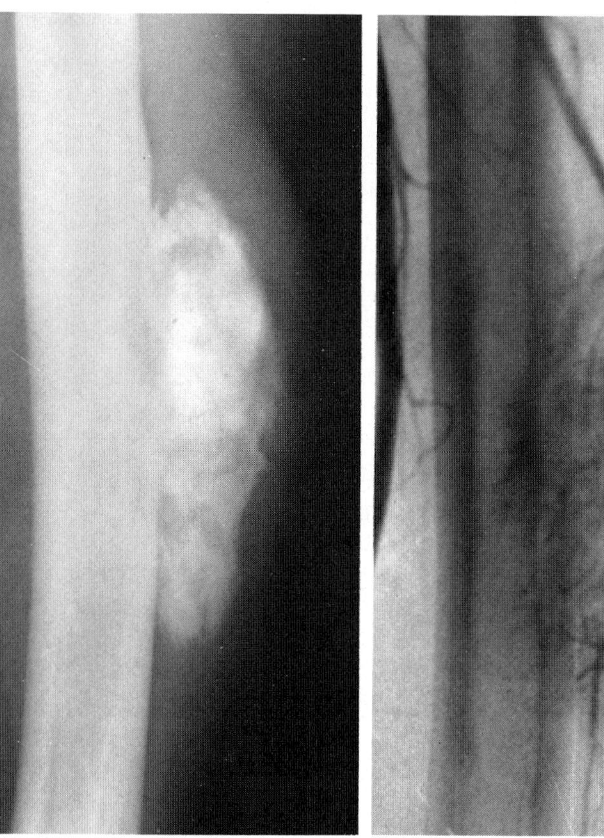

Fig. 5.29 Parosteal osteosarcoma arising from anterior aspect of the femur (**A**) is shown (**B**) angiographically to be unremarkable apart from a slight increase in number of branches going into the tumour. The lesion was of very low grade malignancy at biopsy.

derlying bone. This feature is important since the characteristic radiological sign is a zone of radiolucency between the tumour and the host bone (Fig. 5.28). Penetrated films, tomography or CT may be required in order to demonstrate this sign. The tumour appears usually to be attached to bone by a broad pedicle. Endosteal sclerosis may occur. Scintigraphically the blood pool image usually is unremarkable although considerable increase in activity is evident in the delayed phase. Some evidence suggests that the malignancy of this tumour is reflected by the degree of abnormal vascularity on an angiogram (Fig. 5.29).

The condition must be differentiated from subperiosteal haematoma and other benign causes of periosteal new bone formation.

A

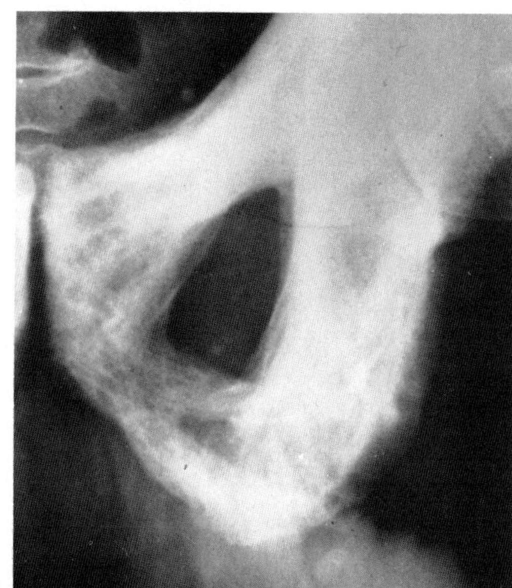

B

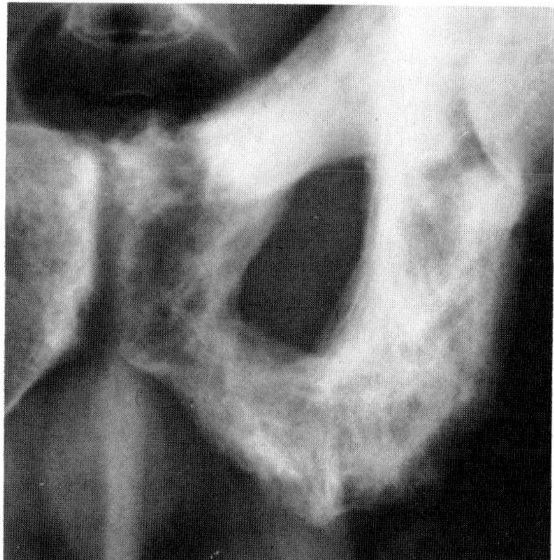

Fig. 5.30 Paget's sarcoma of the body of the pubis. **A**. No malignancy was seen in this man at initial presentation with polyostotic Paget's disease. **B**. 3 years later, however, he complained of local pain with the development of a purely lytic destructive lesion involving the body of the pubis.

SARCOMA IN PAGET'S DISEASE

Malignant tumours are said to arise in bone affected by Paget's disease in about 1% of cases. It is difficult to gauge the exact incidence, since many cases of Paget's disease are asymptomatic or diagnosed by chance. The possibility of a sarcoma arising in Paget's disease should be considered when alteration occurs in the character of bone pain, either an increase in severity or more precise localization; or if a pathological fracture develops. The presence of a soft tissue mass and a further rise in the serum alkaline phosphatase may be observed. Sarcomas may occur in the polyostotic or monostotic disease though there seems to be a particular predilection for the humerus in the latter circumstance. Overall the skull, pelvis and long bones are typical sites with a small but definite incidence of multifocal tumours (Fig. 5.30). Men are more commonly affected, even allowing for the increased male incidence of Paget's disease. Histologically the tumours may be classified as osteosarcoma, fibrosarcoma and chondrosarcoma. However, the tumour is very aggressive and the outlook is very poor. Radiologically, in order of frequency, the lesion is lytic, mixed or sclerotic and the tumour grows rapidly with an extensive soft tissue mass. The margins of the lesion within bone are usually ill-defined, frequently with extensive cortical destruction. Periosteal new bone formation is relatively uncommon. It should be remembered that bone in Paget's disease is susceptible to metastatic involvement, both from Paget's sarcoma elsewhere and from other primary neoplasms.

BONE TUMOURS PRESUMED TO ARISE FROM SKELETAL TISSUE — CARTILAGE FORMING

Benign cartilage lesions divide into two main groups, central and peripheral. The former includes chondroma (with which must be considered the generalized dysplasia of bone — dyschondroplasia), benign chondroblastoma and chondromyxoid fibroma. The malignant counterpart of chondroma is a central chondrosarcoma. As yet there are no reports of the malignant transformation of chondroblastoma and chondromyxoid fibroma. The peripheral lesion to be considered is an osteochondroma, or cartilage capped exostosis, which in its multiple form also constitutes a general bone dysplasia (diaphyseal aclasia). The cartilage cap of these lesions is a potential site for the development of chondrosarcoma. The majority of chondrosarcomas, however, arise with no evidence whatever of a pre-existing benign tumour.

CHONDROMA

Nearly all of these tumours are benign in their clinical presentation and in their radiological and histological appearances, yet all must be regarded as the site of potential malignancy. It is very unusual for the common chondromatous lesions which occur in the hands and feet to become malignant but every flat or long bone cartilage tumour should be regarded as a potential risk if the patient survives long enough. The development of increasing pain, the demonstration, on serial films, of alteration in the radiological appearances or the late development of a pathological fracture are in themselves sufficient to justify anxiety. The transition from benign to malignant in the histological spectrum may be very difficult and contentious. These tumours are notoriously insensitive to radiotherapy. Local recurrence is very high unless there is meticulous surgical removal and cartilage tumours have the habit of becoming more aggressive with each subsequent episode of surgical or therapeutic interference. It must be emphasized the exact time of change from benign to malignant is extremely hard to establish and it is possible that those which are frankly malignant have been so since their inception. Whilst most cartilage tumours arise in conjunction with bone it is important to note that they may occur in soft tissues particularly tendon sheaths and in relation to synovium. They may even occur intracerebrally and when present at the base of the skull should be considered in the differential diagnosis of chordoma.

Single tumours are common. Approximately half are found in the hands, in the medullary cavity of the phalanges, less commonly in metacarpals. About 10% occur in the small bones of the feet. Long bones, particularly the femur, humerus and tibia, are involved in 20% of cases, the remainder occurring in flat bones particularly the pelvis, scapula and vertebral bodies. It is in these areas that the potential danger of malignant transformation is greatest.

Clinical features. The age of onset is usually later than with bone forming tumours. Since these lesions grow slowly they are rarely symptomatic and are often uncovered through examinations for other indications particularly trauma. However, the patient may have noted on direct questioning a localized hard swelling for many years. Pathological fracture is not uncommon. To restate, low grade pain or swelling of recent onset should cause the possibility of chondrosarcoma to be considered.

Radiological features. Cartilaginous tissue is not radio-opaque. The characteristic feature is of a single well-defined demarcated zone of radiolucency in the medulla. In the small bones of the hand and feet tumours are particularly likely to expand and thin the overlying cortex (Fig. 5.31) but without its destruction or the development of a periosteal reaction other than that following a fracture. The zone of transition is narrow and sclerotic. The endosteal margin may be scalloped. As in all neoplasms of cartilaginous origin, flecks of calcification frequently are present within the tumour, especially as they become more mature and may assume a pathognomonic 'pop-corn' or annular configuration. Calcification also may be observed together with ossification, in healing callus following a pathological fracture. Lesions rarely extend to the ends of the affected bones and are often situated in the distal portions. Very few other osteolytic lesions in the bones of the hands are likely to cause diagnostic difficulty, apart from the rare implantation dermoid cyst in a terminal phalanx or perhaps fibrous dysplasia. These cartilaginous tumours are unremarkable scintigraphically or angiographically and their low vascularity is readily demonstrated. Unless they have fractures they are unlikely to be striking on the delayed phase of a bone scan. A marked increase of photon activity should raise the possibility of a chondrosarcoma.

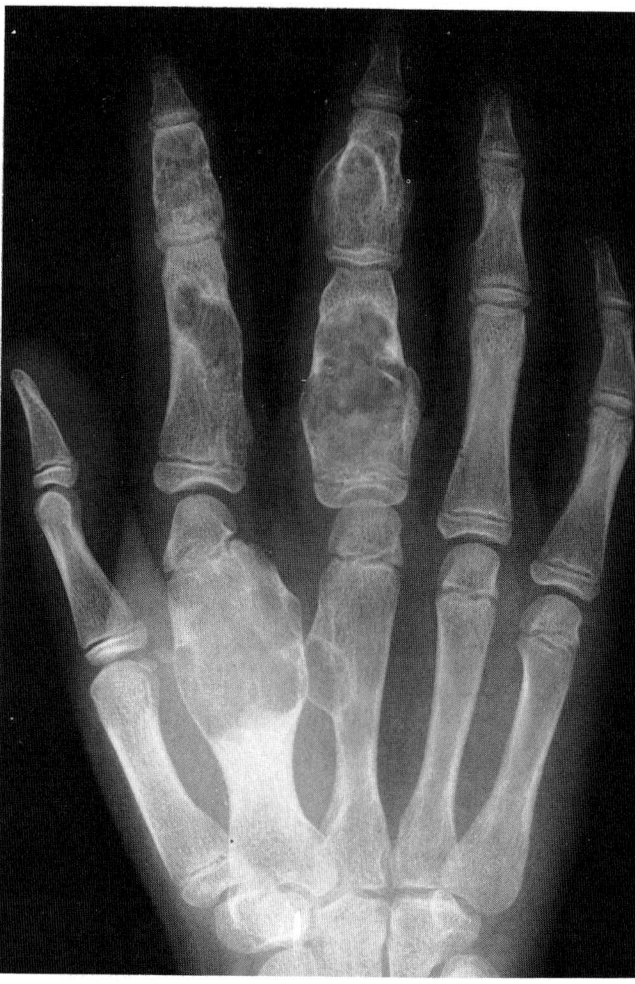

Fig. 5.31 Multiple chondromas in the hand. This child presented with painless swelling. Note the cortical expansion and thinning, well-defined defects, patchy amorphous calcification and moulding abnormalities indicating slow growth.

Less commonly, but infinitely more importantly, chondromas develop in the medullary cavities of long bones and must be distinguished from other medullary osteolytic lesions. Here again the presence of speckled calcification is a great help, but is not entirely specific as it may be observed also in osteosarcoma or even, indeed, in fibrosarcoma on rare occasions. The tumour margin is usually harply defined and accompanied by some evidence of sclerosis. The tumour erodes the cortex from within with a clear cut edge. The cortex, however, remains intact and the development of an enlarging lesion may cause eccentric expansion of bone due to organized periosteal new bone. Most of these tumours are discovered in adult life and therefore differentiation from other osteolytic lesions, such as bone cysts and non-ossifying fibromas, offers less difficulty because of the patient's age. Evidence of extension of the lesion or irregularity of the margin (particularly in the presence of periosteal new bone formation or a soft tissue mass) will immediately suggest a chondrosarcoma. Bone scans and angiograms are unrewarding, although computerized tomography may serve to delineate the extent of the larger intramedullary lesion more clearly.

It is necessary to distinguish the central variety of chondroma from unimportant areas of amorphous calcification arranged in a roughly linear fashion in the medullary canal, often described as 'cartilage rests'. The localized stippled nature of these opacities and the absence of any other radiological abnormality indicates the latter diagnosis. These lesions are scintigraphically and angiographically inert. On the other hand differentiation of a central chondroma from a medullary bone infarct may be more difficult. A helpful feature is the curvilinear peripheral calcification around the infarct rather than the annular calcification with a true cartilage tumour. Both lesions may be associated with subsequent malignant complications, dedifferentiated chondrosarcoma from chondroma (see below) and fibrosarcoma or malignant fibrous histiocytoma from the wall of an infarct.

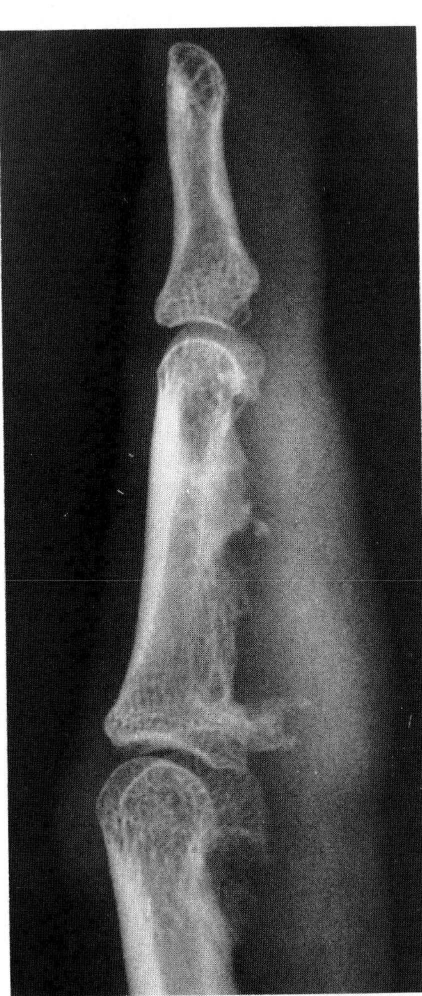

Fig. 5.32 Juxtacortical chondromas arising on the volar aspect of the proximal and middle phalanges of the index finger. Obvious pressure defects are present with new bone formation at the margins. Punctate calcification is present in the middle of the proximal lesion.

SPECIAL TYPES OF CHONDROMA

Juxtacortical chondroma is a rare benign cartilage tumour usually arising in young adults, related to the cortex of a long bone, most commonly the humerus or femur. The presenting complaint is of a slowly enlarging hard mass which may not be tender (Fig. 5.32). Radiologically a well-defined soft tissue mass may contain calcification and be bordered by a thin, but usually incomplete, shell of overlying bone. Pressure erosion of the underlying cortex usually provokes a variable sclerotic reaction. The presence of calcification within the lesion makes the diagnosis of a cartilage containing tumour relatively easy. On the other hand if calcification is absent the mass may have to be distinguished from non-ossifying fibroma, periosteal lipoma or neurofibroma.

Multiple enchondromas. The individual lesions of the bone dysplasia described by Ollier are now known as dyschondroplasia and are essentially neoplastic in type corresponding to the descriptions already given. Cartilage tumours found in dysplasias may be extremely gross and cause complete destruction of the bones of the hand. In addition to the multiple cartilage tumours columns of dysplastic cartilage frequently cause considerable tubulation anomalies and growth deformities of limbs. Although recognized in the literature to be subject to chondrosarcomatous change this complication has been uncommon in the experience of the authors.

Maffucci's syndrome is the rare association of dyschondroplasia with cavernous haemangiomas in the soft tissues, the latter being characterized by soft tissue masses containing phleboliths (Fig. 5.33). Chondrosarcomatous metaplasia is a recognized hazard of this entity and probably develops in about 20% of cases.

CHONDROBLASTOMA

This relatively rare tumour arises in almost all instances within an epiphysis, 50% occurring in the second decade of life. Presentation is of pain around the joint, usually of mild proportions and of months or even years duration. Joint movement often is limited. Most of these tumours

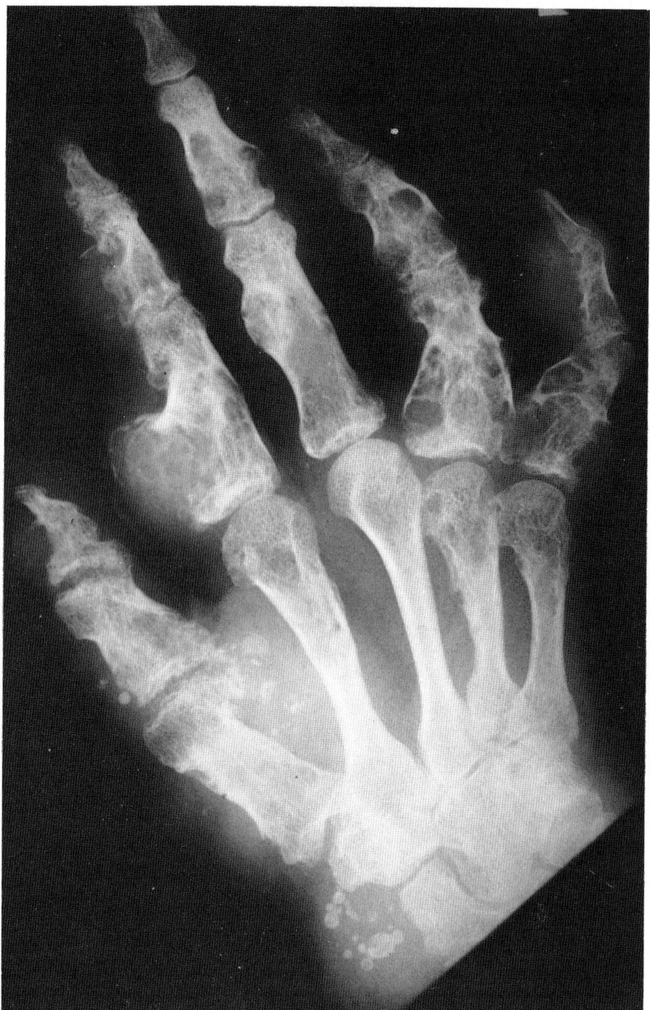

Fig. 5.33 Maffucci's syndrome (female aged 23). Numerous chondromas in this case of dyschondroplasia are accompanied by soft tissue swelling which contains phleboliths indicating haemangiomas. These skeletal lesions are more liable than ordinary chondromas to undergo malignant change transformation.

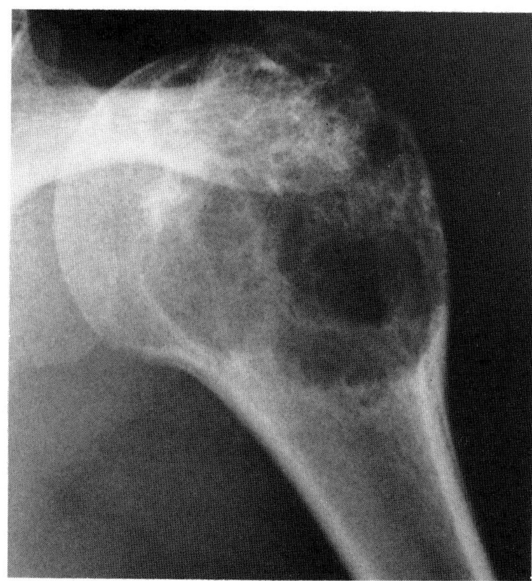

Fig. 5.34 Chondroblastoma. A purely lytic lesion in a characteristic site, involves the apophysis of the tuberosities of the humerus. A faint sclerotic reaction is present between the chondroblastoma and underlying bone. Note the organized periosteal new bone formation in the upper shaft.

occur in epiphyses of long bones, especially around the hips, knees or shoulders, but some have been observed in apophyses. Histologically the appearances are distinctive, cartilage cells being interspersed with foci of calcification and giant cells. This lesion has been considered as a giant cell tumour variant.

Radiologically a well-defined, radiolucent, oval lesion within an epiphysis is characteristic, often with a thin rim of sclerosis and cortical expansion (Figs 5.34, 5.35). The endosteal margin is well defined. Not infrequently the tumour traverses the growth plate to involve the metaphysis. Stippled calcification occurs in about a quarter of mature examples and in a smaller number an adjacent periosteal reaction may be present. The extreme vascularity of these lesions is confirmed by the blood pool phase of the bone scan or by angiography. The delayed phase of a bone scan is not helpful. Computerized tomography may be of value in assessing the extent of those few lesions which expand rapidly into the soft tissues. No incidence of spontaneous malignant transformation, however, has been recorded.

CHONDROMYXOID FIBROMA

This tumour is predominantly chondroid, but contains myxomatous tissue and giant cells in addition. Histologically it may be mistaken for a chondrosarcoma. The presenting complaints are non-specific, usually localized pain and swelling often of many months duration. The peak age incidence is in young adults around 20–30 years of age with no particular sex incidence. Typically the lesion occurs around the knee joint in two thirds of cases, with an especial affinity for the proximal end of the tibia. Flat bones and short bones have been affected.

Radiologically the predominant feature is a radiolucent, eccentric, space occupying lesion which is situated in the metaphysis. The margin within bone is usually well defined with surrounding sclerosis (Fig. 5.36). The sharpness of the margin between the lesion and the sclerosis contrasts with the rather ill-defined margin between the sclerosis and host bone. In many cases the cortex is expanded considerably (Fig. 5.37), the peripheral bony margin often becoming hazy and poorly defined. This aggressive appearance may be so marked that the possibility of malignant change may be considered. Calcification within the lesion is very uncommon, unlike other cartilaginous neoplasms. Whilst scintigraphy in the blood pool phase of a bone scan or an-

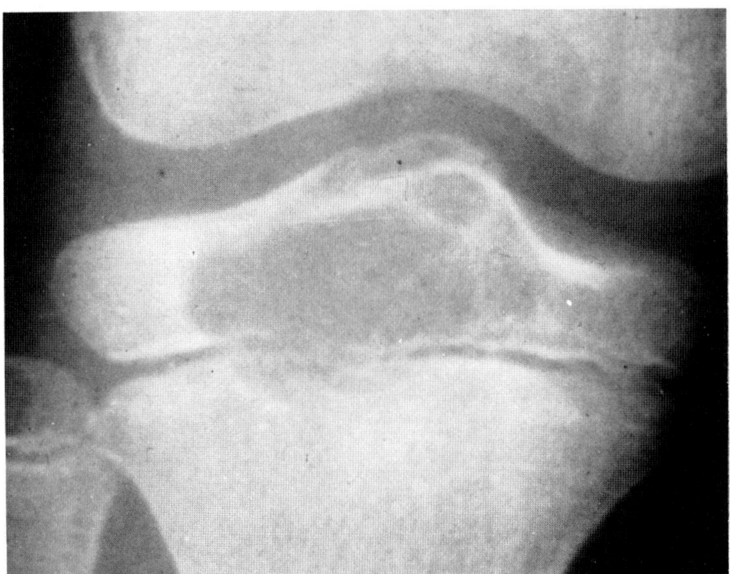

Fig. 5.35 Chondroblastoma in the proximal epiphysis of the tibia. The tumour has thinned the overlying cortex and extends across the growth plate into the upper metaphysis.

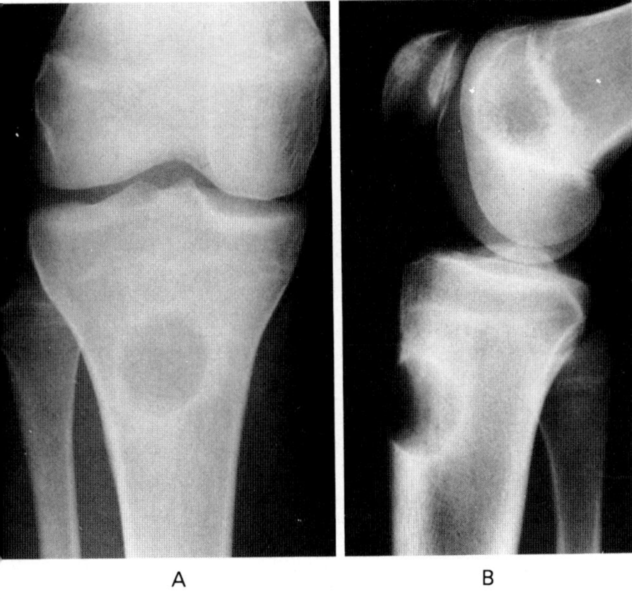

Fig. 5.36 Chondromyxoid fibroma of the proximal tibia. Note the extremely well-defined radiolucent defect with a sclerotic margin on the endosteal aspect. **A**. AP view. **B**. Lateral view.

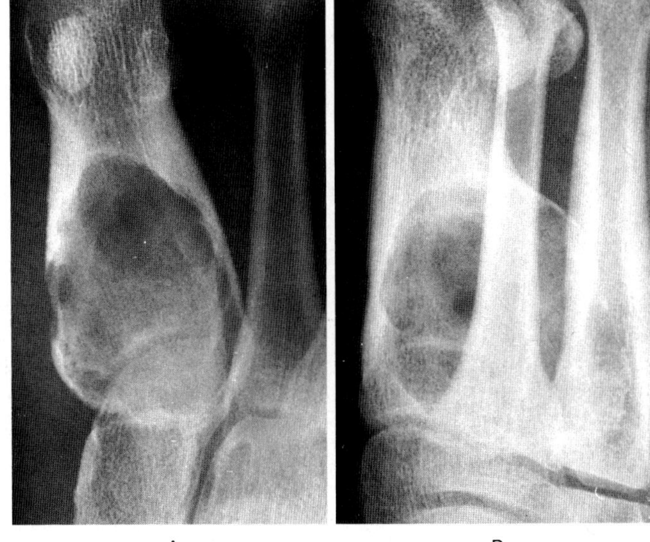

Fig. 5.37 Chondromyxoid fibroma — great toe metatarsal. **A**. and **B**. The tumour is eccentric in position with extreme cortical expansion and thinning. The endosteal margin is well defined and faintly sclerotic. No calcification is present.

giography may reveal a slight increase in perfusion to the lesion the vascular pattern is unremarkable. When the bone scan does show increased activity it is usually localized to the reactive sclerosis rather than to the lesion itself. CT may be necessary to delineate a cortical margin in the expanded soft tissue mass.

This tumour is undoubtedly very closely related to benign chondroblastoma and indeed aneurysmal bone cysts, since all three contain giant cells. Histological differentiation is reasonably well established, but unrepresentative biopsy material may create confusion. Radiologically confusion will only occur when these lesions occur in childhood, although the site of chondroblastoma and the ill-defined endosteal margin of an aneurysmal bone cyst normally will suggest the correct diagnosis.

OSTEOCHONDROMA (CARTILAGE CAPPED EXOSTOSIS)

This lesion is essentially an osseous outgrowth arising from bony cortex. Usually it grows slowly during childhood and adolescence with endochondral ossification, the central spongiosa merging with that of the bone from which it is derived. Very occasionally the lesion involutes with increasing age and finally results only in a minor abnormality of tubulation. It is usual for growth to cease with skeletal maturity. Although commonly solitary the tumours may be multiple, when the condition is recognized as the deforming congenital bone dysplasia known as diaphyseal aclasia (Ch. 1). The importance of this relatively common benign tumour, and its place among bone tumours, relates to the cartilage cap with which it is covered. This structure may be very prominent and in this tissue lies the very small risk of malignancy in the form of chondrosarcoma. This risk is probably less than 1% but may be significantly higher (of the order of 10%) in diaphyseal aclasia.

These tumours arise mainly in tubular bones near the metaphyses related to the sites of tendinous attachments. They are particularly common around the knee and the proximal end of the humerus. They may be either sessile or pedunculated. The latter type always grow away from the metaphysis being directed towards the diaphysis. Flat bones also may be affected, the pelvis and scapula being equally involved. In the pelvis these lesions are almost invariably of the sessile type, attention being drawn to the lesion by palpation of the mass. Tumours on the medial aspect of the scapula may grate against and deform the ribs. Rare lesions related to the laminae of vertebral bodies may produce neurological signs.

Both types occur equally in the sexes and may be entirely asymptomatic, apart from their cosmetic effect. Presentation usually follows minor trauma. They may interfere with footwear comfort and can cause localized neural or vascular compression. Such symptoms are unlikely to develop until the later stages of growth, at or around puberty, but are promptly relieved by surgical excision. If this procedure is complete, recurrence is virtually unknown. Surgical removal should be undertaken if any increase in pain or size of the lesion occurs, particularly after growth has ceased. Features of this type may indicate chondrosarcomatous change in the cartilage cap.

Radiological features. Osteochondromas have a characteristic appearance which is readily recognized. With a pedunculated tumour it is particularly easy to identify the continuation of its cortex with that of the underlying bone from which it arises and the merging of its trabecular pattern into the medullary cavity through the cortical defect (Fig. 5.38). In young adults the cartilage cap may not be visualised on plain films, although seen clearly on CT. As age progresses calcification becomes apparent within the

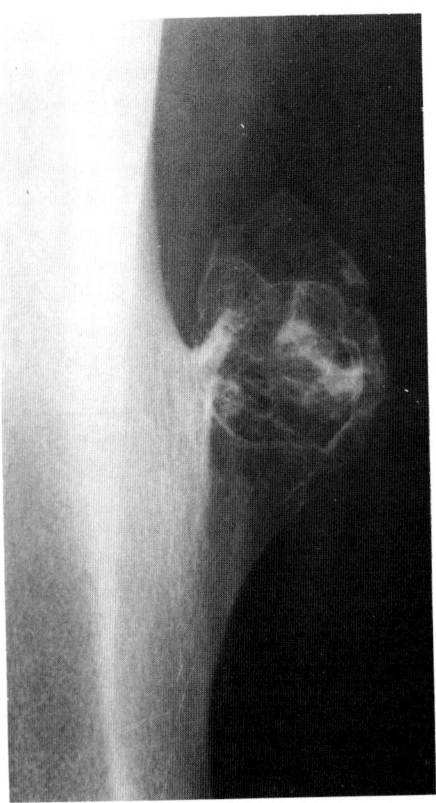

Fig. 5.38

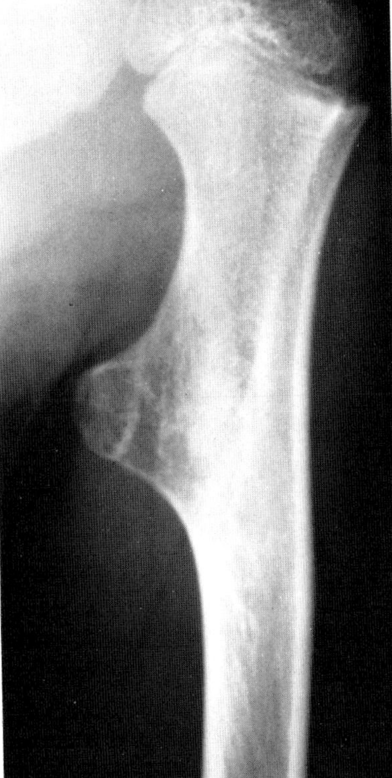

Fig. 5.39A

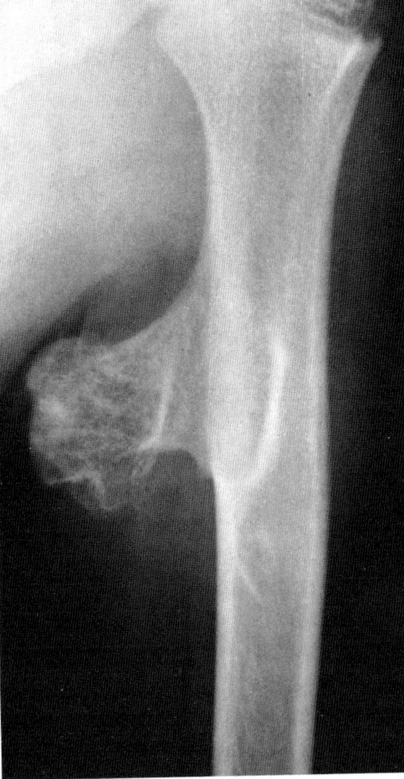

Fig. 5.39B

Fig. 5.38 Osteochondroma of the distal femur. The cortex is continuous with that of the underlying bone and trabecular bone merges with that of the femur. A well-defined cartilage cap contains calcification and is directed away from the joint.

Fig. 5.39 A. and **B**. A pedunculated osteochondroma exhibits growth over a 2-year period in the humerus of a child. Such growth is common and stops usually at, or soon after, puberty.

artilaginous element of the tumour, causing an increase n punctate or curvilinear radiodensity. Thus the developed esion in the adult is likely to show irregular calcification. Growth of osteochondromas usually occurs until skeletal naturation is complete (Fig. 5.39), ceasing thereafter. Rarely osteochondromas may be shown to regress Fig. 5.40). Pedunculated tumours vary in size, but may e up to 8 or 10 cm in length and are typically directed way from the nearest joint. Flat and sessile types are more ommonly related to flat bones, particularly the pelvis, and nay grow to a substantial size, be of considerable irregu-arity and become very dense. In such cases the resem-lance to a cauliflower may be striking! Provided that the harply defined peripheral margin is preserved, and serial xaminations reveal no increase in size, their benign nature nay be assumed. Any change in radiological appearance, articularly with the development of poor definition of the nargin, even in one part of the lesion, is highly suggestive of chondrosarcoma particularly if accompanied by a history of an insiduous increase in local pain. Local resection and istological studies then become essential because of the

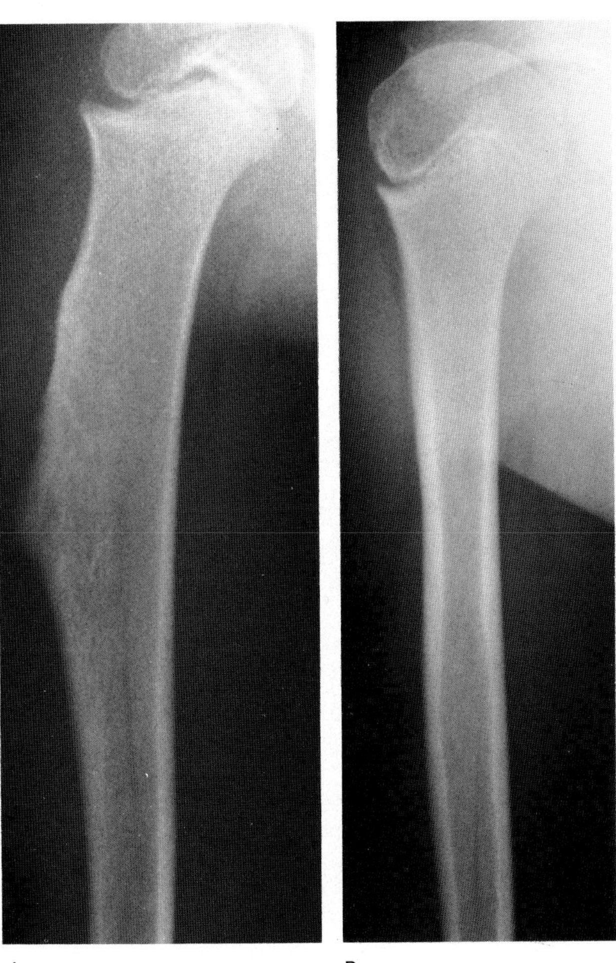

Fig. 5.40 A. and **B**. Osteochondromas may be shown to regress rarely, remodelling resulting in normal appearances. Here an osteochondroma of the proximal humerus cannot be visualized 6 years later.

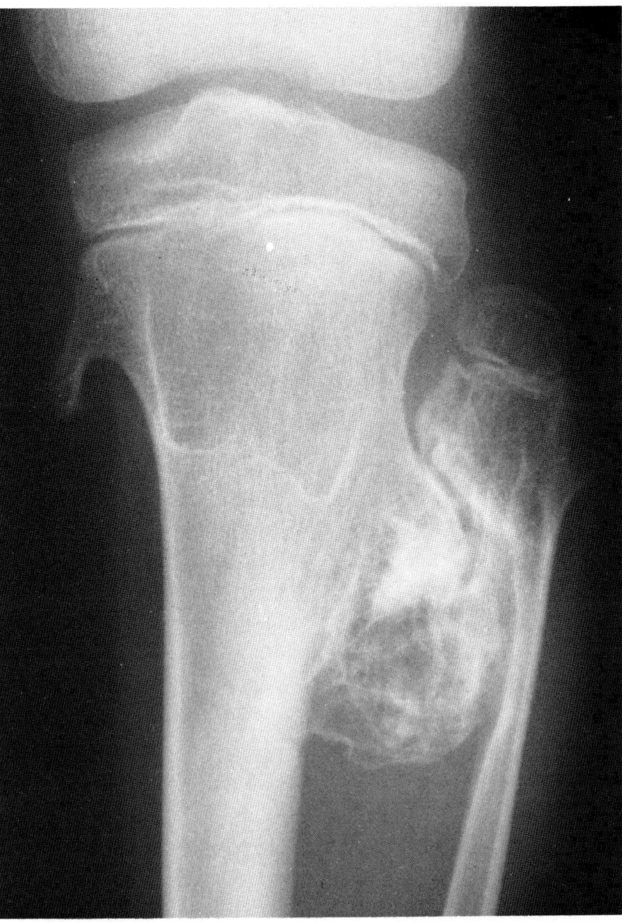

Fig. 5.41 Diaphyseal aclasia — multiple osteochondromas are present in the proximal tibia and fibula. A large sessile lesion of the proximal tibia has caused widening of the intraosseous space and secondary moulding abnormalities both of the tibia and fibula.

short-comings of further radiological investigation in detecting chondrosarcoma (see below). The individual lesions of diaphyseal aclasia are those of any osteochondroma. However, their multiplicity results in considerable moulding abnormality and deformity (Fig. 5.41).

CHONDROSARCOMA

Differentiation of this malignant member of the group of cartilage forming tumours is to be made from osteosarcoma with which it may be confused. Chondrosarcoma forms a spectrum of malignancy, but usually they develop later in life than osteosarcoma and carry a much better prospect of survival because metastases often occur very late. A very high grade (aggressively malignant) chondrosarcoma, however, behaves in a fashion very similar to an osteosarcoma.

The **clinical problem,** therefore, is not so much that of metastatic dissemination but of local recurrence. Failure to provide adequate and early excision is attended by the subsequent necessity of further and more difficult surgical procedures. Some evidence, indeed, exists that each surgical insult causes the tumour to become even more aggressive. Certain pleomorphic osteosarcomas demonstrate cartilage formation, but the established chondrosarcoma is associated with cartilage which is mature in its development. Although some of this cartilaginous tissue may ossify, no direct ossification, unlike an osteosarcoma, takes place in the absence of a chondroid precursor. In addition these cells are histochemically negative for the production of alkaline phosphatase, a substance always indicative of increased osteoblastic activity.

As has been indicated previously chondrosarcomas may develop in a cartilaginous lesion previously thought to be benign. Malignancy may arise in the cartilage cap of an osteochondroma or in a long or flat bone (Fig. 5.42). Chondrosarcoma of the hand or foot is distinctly unusual. The lesions of dyschondroplasia, particularly if associated with the haemangiomas of Maffucci's syndrome, are also subject to malignant change. Nonetheless the incidence of what might be called secondary chondrosarcoma is far less common than those apparently arising de novo. Indeed only 10% of these neoplasms arise from a recognizable precursor, usually the cartilage cap of an osteochondroma, especially in patients suffering from diaphyseal aclasia.

Primary chondrosarcoma occurs mainly between the ages of 30 and 70 years and is relatively rare distal to the elbow and knee joints, the pelvis and ribs being the most common sites, followed closely by the proximal end of the femur. Because of this distribution virtually all chondromas arising in flat and long bones should be regarded as potentially malignant ab initio. Diagnosis may be delayed on account of slow growth or relatively mild symptomatology. The tumour, therefore, may be very large when it is first recognised.

Prognosis for chondrosarcoma is relatively good if complete surgical excision is possible before dissemination, metastases only occurring in the later stages by the haematogenous route. Because of the risks of local recurrence, already stressed, it may be necessary to undertake amputation. The histological spectrum of chondrosarcoma varies widely. Difficulties with differentiation arise, at the benign end of the spectrum, from a benign chondroma, and at the aggressive end, from an osteosarcoma. In consequence, the interpretation of a highly skilled pathologist is essential. Particularly in the case of less aggressive chondrosarcoma,

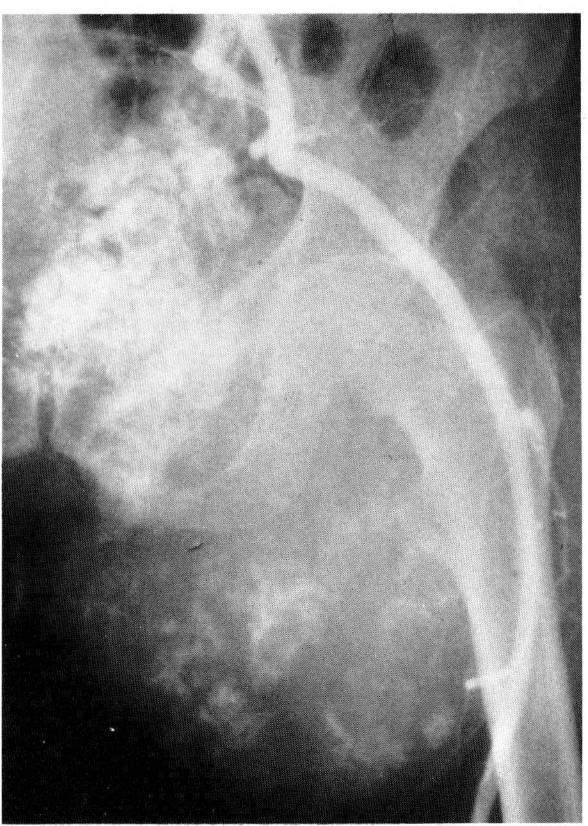

Fig. 5.42 Chondrosarcoma arising from the superior pubic ramus on the left. A huge mass is present containing extensive calcification. The femoral artery is displaced by the mass but note the absence of any pathological circulation. This is typical of a low-grade chondrosarcoma.

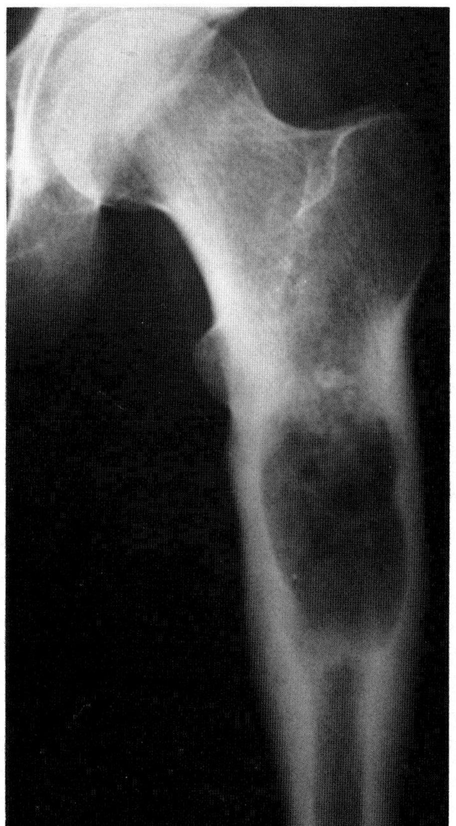

Fig. 5.43 Central chondrosarcoma. The destructive lesion in the femoral shaft has smooth well-defined margins, but in the upper portion, some characteristic punctate calcification is visible. The tumour is of a slow-growing type since organized periosteal new bone has thickened the cortex around the lesion.

ituated in sites of easy access, such as the proximal end f the femur, prosthetic replacement is an effective and osmetic surgical treatment.

Radiological features. When a chondrosarcoma arises rom a previous cartilaginous lesion the diagnosis is sually straightforward. In the case of osteochondroma articular attention should be paid to areas of local cortical lestruction with ill-defined margins. In addition, it may be ossible to demonstrate an associated soft tissue mass repesenting abnormal cartilage growth. These features are lemonstrated more clearly by CT. The radiological demnstration of cartilage within such a mass by punctate or urvilinear calcification may be absent, as this characterstic feature tends to occur in the more mature parts of hese tumours. Similarly the central chondroma which beomes malignant tends clinically to grow silently, spreading vithin the medullary cavity to produce irregular medullary lestruction. Uneven infiltration makes it difficult to deternine the margin between normal and abnormal tissue. Irregular calcification is likely to be present in the older and central parts of the tumour. These more organized zones may be destroyed by newer malignant infiltration indicating the dedifferentiated form of chondrosarcoma.

As growth proceeds slowly, the tumour causes smooth, scalloped erosions on the endosteal aspect of the cortex. An overlying lamellar periosteal reaction is not rare especially if the degree of malignancy is low grade. In consequence the ultimate thickness of the cortex around the tumour may exceed that in the unaffected portion of the bone, the appearance then being that of a localized fusiform expansion (Fig. 5.43). Pathological fractures are quite common and may draw initial attention to these tumours. The malignant nature of the lesion is unequivocal when actual penetration of the cortex occurs, with the development of an associated and clearly defined soft tissue mass, within which calcification, or even ossification, may occur (Fig. 5.44).

Primary chondrosarcoma, particularly in its early stages, presents difficult diagnostic problems as the pre-

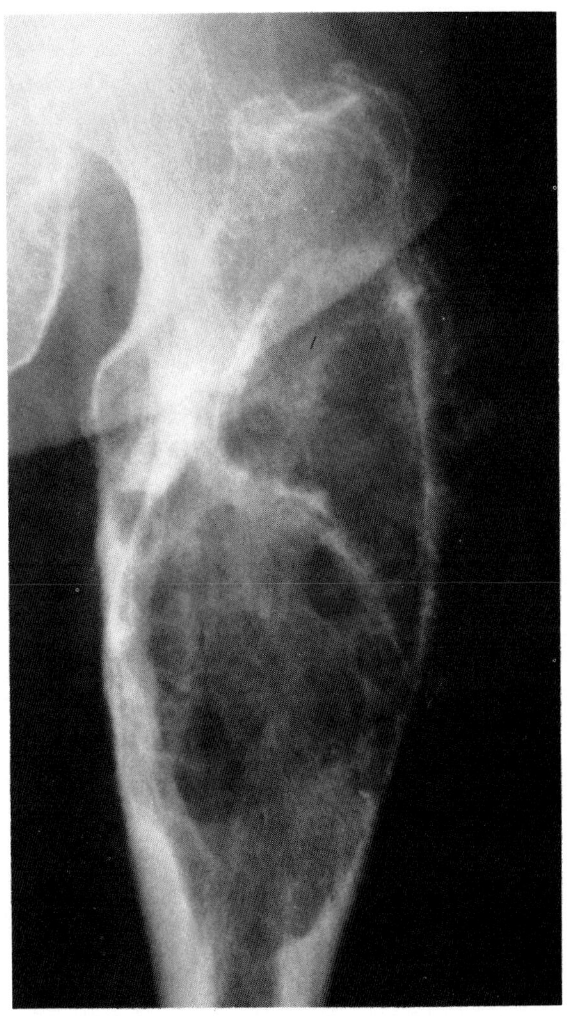

A

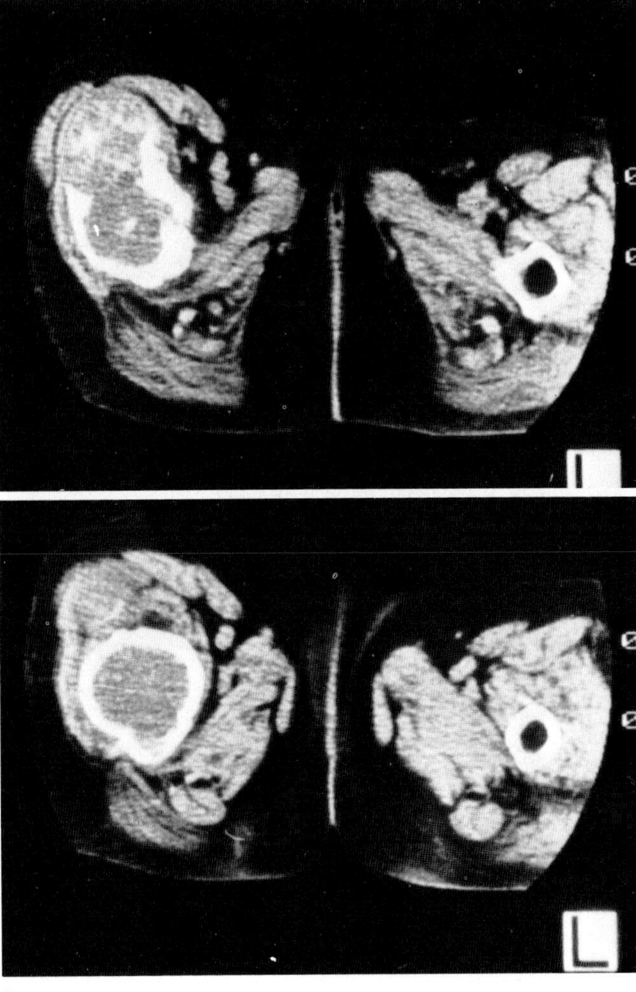

B

Fig. 5.44 A. and **B**. Central chondrosarcoma. The tumour is more aggressive than in Figure 5.43, and has extended into soft tissues. This is confirmed by CT showing extension anterior to the femoral shaft (W200, L25). Calcification is present both in the soft tissue mass and within the shaft lesion.

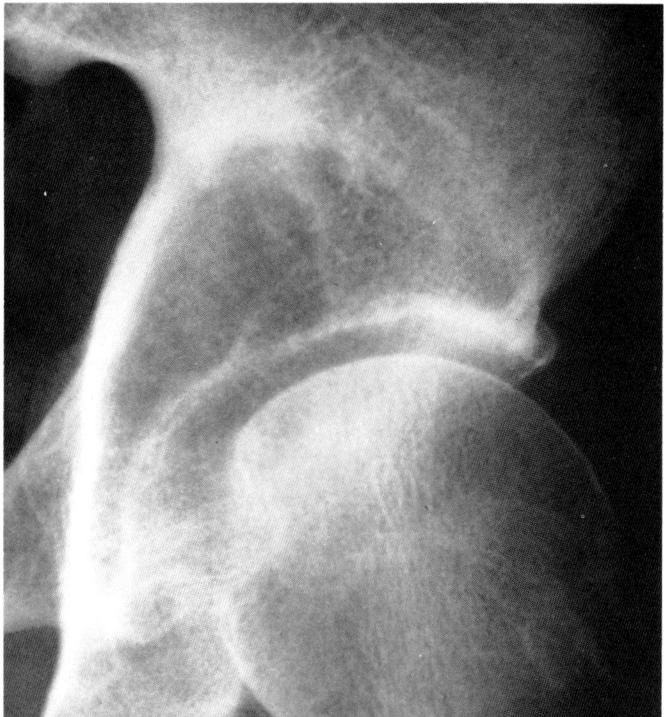

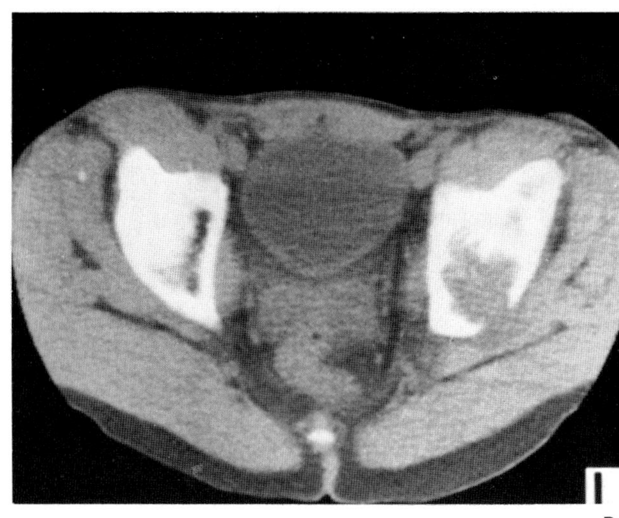

Fig. 5.45 Chondrosarcoma arising in the acetabulum of a 45-year-old male. **A**. The tumour is purely lytic. Cortical thickening is shown medially. **B**. CT demonstrates disruption of the cortex posteriorly, with a localized soft tissue mass beneath the glutei and faint calcification within the lesion (W400, L20).

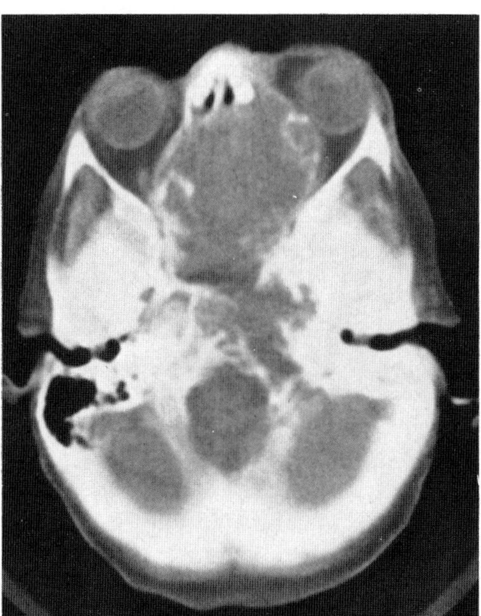

Fig. 5.46 Chondrosarcoma arising in the sphenoid bone of an adult female patient. A large soft tissue tumour extends from the nasal cavity to the middle fossa. A thin sclerotic margin outlines the mass which contains faint punctate calcification. Note the displacement of the eyeballs (W400, L40).

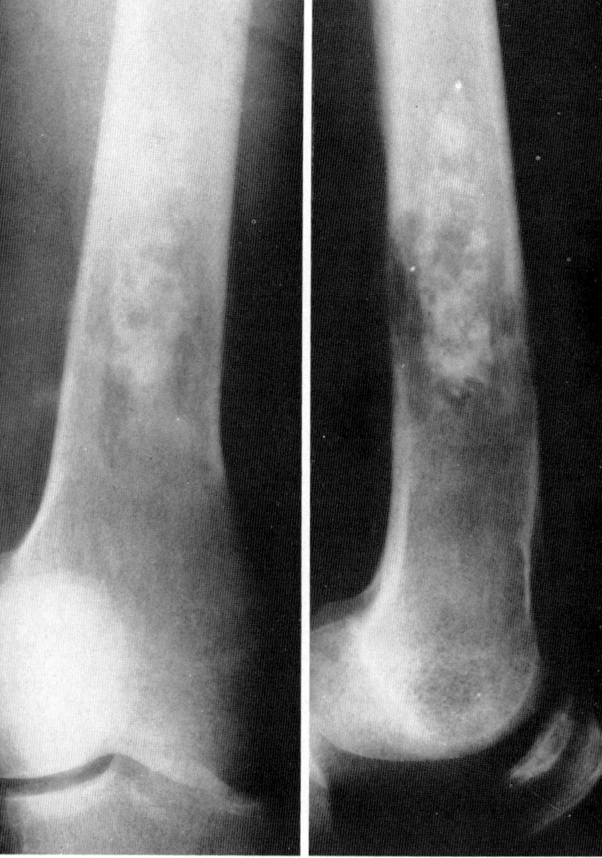

Fig. 5.47 Dedifferentiated chondrosarcoma. A chondrosarcoma is present centrally within the distal femoral shaft characterized by slight expansion and amorphous calcification. In addition an area of osteolysis is present with cortical destruction around the lower half of the tumour. The latter represents a high-grade malignancy arising in conjunction with a pre-existing relatively low-grade tumour.

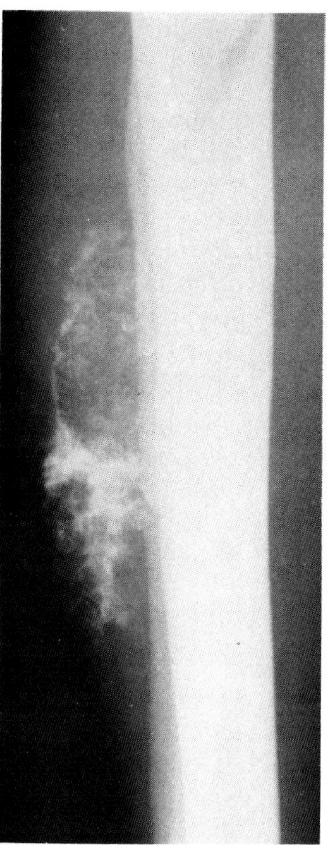

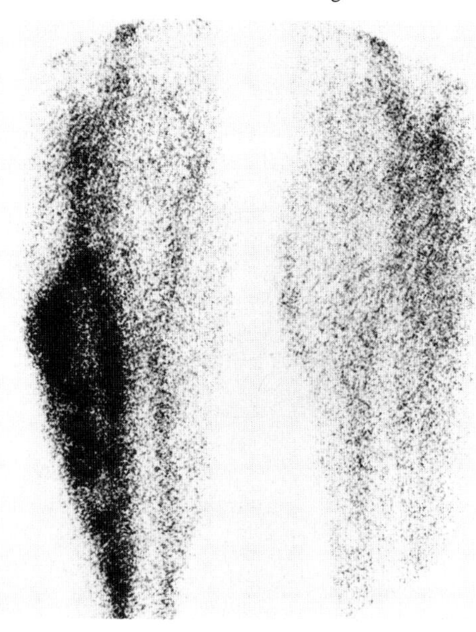

Fig. 5.48 Mesenchymal chondrosarcoma. A hard mass had been present in this middle-aged man's calf for 8 years. Recently it had increased in size. A soft tissue radiograph (**A**) shows extensive calcification in a well-defined tumour mass. **B**. The blood pool phase of a bone scan reveals a marked increase in vascularity throughout the lesion which is intensely active on (**C**) the delayed images (top right). Note also the presence of multiple metastases particularly in vertebrae and the pelvis. **D**. A femoral arteriogram confirms the markedly abnormal vascularity with pathological vessels throughout the tumour mass. The similarity between the extent of the abnormality shown angiographically and on the blood pool phase of the bone scan is striking.

A

B

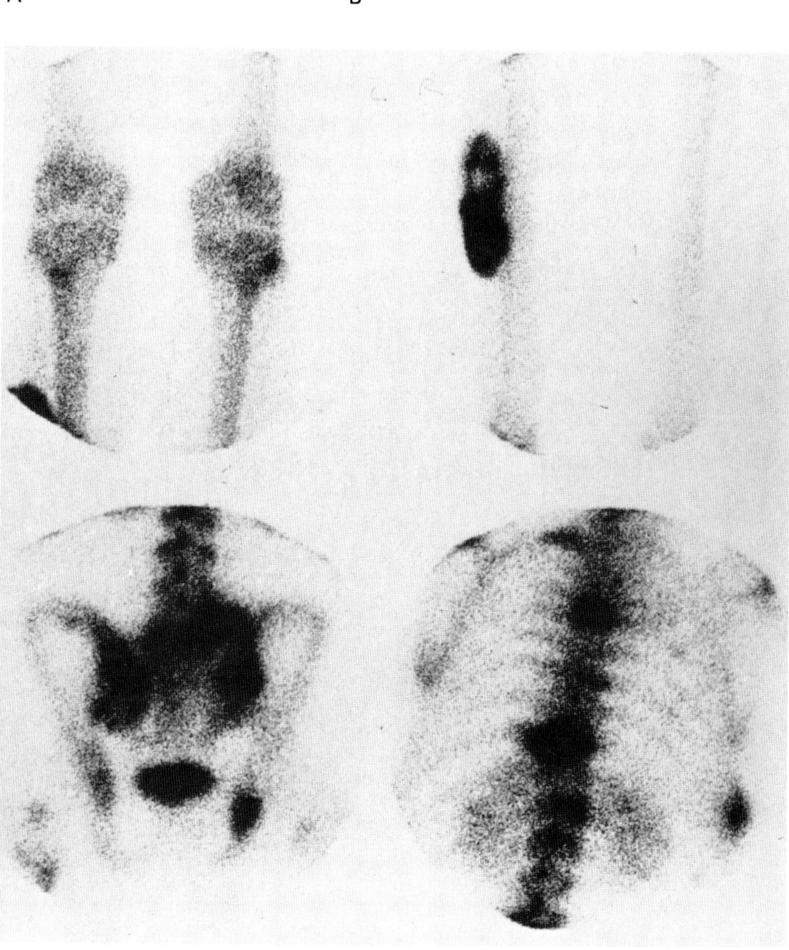

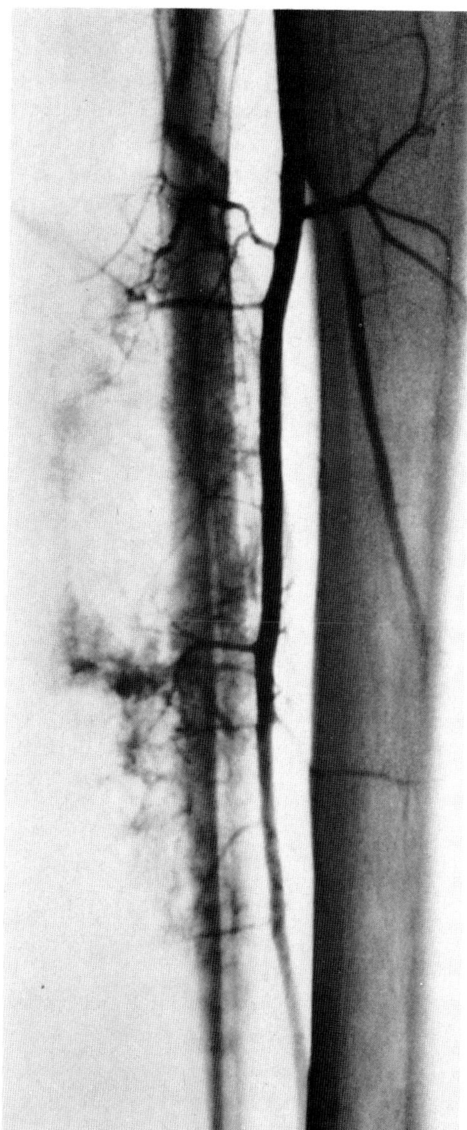

D

senting symptoms of minor pain or discomfort may be accompanied by only minimal radiological change. This may be a poorly defined area of medullary translucency with possibly a little periosteal reaction or the presence of an abnormal soft tissue mass. The acetabulum is sometimes the site of the development of these rather nebulous and difficult lesions (Fig. 5.45). The first radiological evidence of its presence may be a soft tissue mass projecting into the pelvic cavity. The cortex of flat bones tends to be thinner than that of long bones and chondrosarcomas of the ribs or the pelvis penetrate it at an early stage. This feature may be demonstrated more clearly by CT. Hence these tumours are especially liable to grow to a substantial size over a prolonged period, particularly if in a clinically occult area. Rapid growth naturally indicates a more aggressive type of malignancy. As may be expected the more mature cartilage elements frequently progress to calcification and ossification and larger tumours are frequently lobulated or cauliflower-like. Very rarely a chondrosarcoma may arise in soft tissues, including tendon sheath and meninges. Cranial lesions also can arise from the sphenoid (Fig. 5.46) and clivus.

Radiologically no criteria of malignancy are absolute. The demonstration of increase in size and ill-defined margins on plain film is highly suggestive. Destruction of organized existing cartilage calcification is indicative also of local infiltration. The demonstration of cortical disruption is helpful. Scintigraphically most of these neoplasms tend to have a slight increase in activity only on the delayed phase of a bone scan, but high grade chondrosarcomas may demonstrate an increase in the blood pool image. Angiographically minor vascular displacement usually is evident with scanty new vessels in the majority. Only when the tumour is of particularly high grade malignancy is the type of increased perfusion and new vessel formation similar to that associated with an osteosarcoma.

DEDIFFERENTIATED CHONDROSARCOMA

Reference has been made above to malignant cartilaginous tumours of relatively low grade malignancy, as indicated by extensive calcification of the cartilaginous components undergoing relatively rapid and sinister deterioration. In such instances the radiological diagnosis may be suggested when an area of osteolytic destruction develops adjacent to the chondrosarcoma (Fig. 5.47) and which, may, indeed destroy part of the calcified portion of the original tumour. The age, sex and clinical features otherwise are comparable to those of an orthodox chondrosarcoma and the diagnosis of these fulminating lesions depends essentially on histological study. These dedifferentiated forms may exhibit the microscopic appearance of a frank osteosarcoma, fibrosarcoma or, not uncommonly, a malignant fibrous histiocytoma with its characteristic storiform pattern of the tumour cells (see below).

MESENCHYMAL CHONDROSARCOMA

This malignant cartilage tumour is rare. Histologically it is characterized by the presence of more or less differentiated cartilage together with highly vascular spindle cell or round cell mesenchymal tissue. About a third of these tumours arise in the soft tissues especially in the extremities (thigh and calf). The soft tissue mass frequently shows irregular calcification (Fig.5.48).

Radiologically this lesion shows a rapid increase in size with highly aggressive features including increased vascularity scintigraphically and the early detection of metastases. The condition affects adults at an earlier age than most chondrosarcomas although in general the age group is older than that of osteosarcoma.

REFERENCES AND SUGGESTIONS FOR FURTHER READING

See end of Chapter 7.

CHAPTER 6

TUMOURS AND TUMOUR-LIKE CONDITIONS OF BONE(2)

BONE TUMOURS PRESUMED TO ARISE FROM SKELETAL TISSUE — FIBROUS TUMOURS

1. FIBROUS CORTICAL DEFECT

Fibrous cortical defects are extremely common, occurring in up to a third of normal children between the ages of 2 and 15 years. Characteristically they occur around the knee especially in the distal postero-medial femoral cortex. They are almost always discovered by chance and are not known to be symptomatic.

Radiologically they are blister-like expansions of the cortex with a thin shell of overlying bone (Fig. 6.1). They may be slightly lobulated, but are always sharply defined (Fig. 6.2) and have a fine sclerotic margin particularly when seen in profile. Because of their characteristic site they are radiolucent when observed in a frontal view of the knee. An oblique projection will always show its cortical situation and these lesions fill in as the skeleton matures. Bone scans are unremarkable, revealing only a minimal increase in activity on the delayed phase in proportion to the size of the lesion.

The differential diagnosis, when the lesion occurs in its typical site, is from adductor trauma (cortical avulsion syndrome). This abnormality is attributed to chronic low grade traction on the adductor tubercle, corresponding to the insertion of the adductor magnus muscle. It causes irregularity of the femoral cortex, sometimes with a radiolucency, but often with irregular calcification. Because these lesions are almost certainly of traumatic origin an abnormal

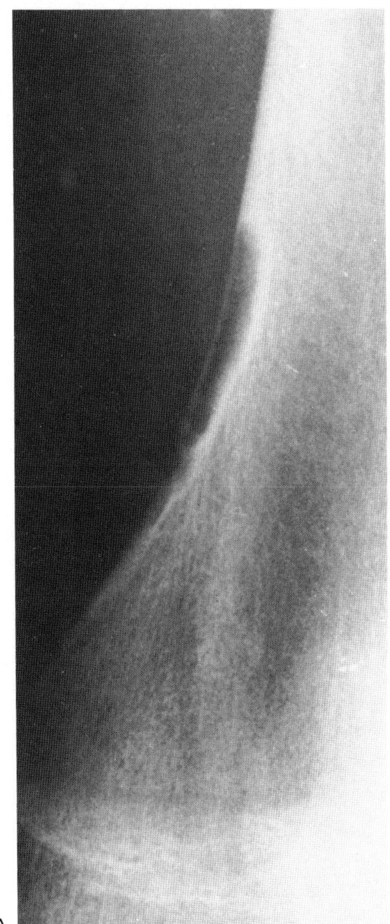

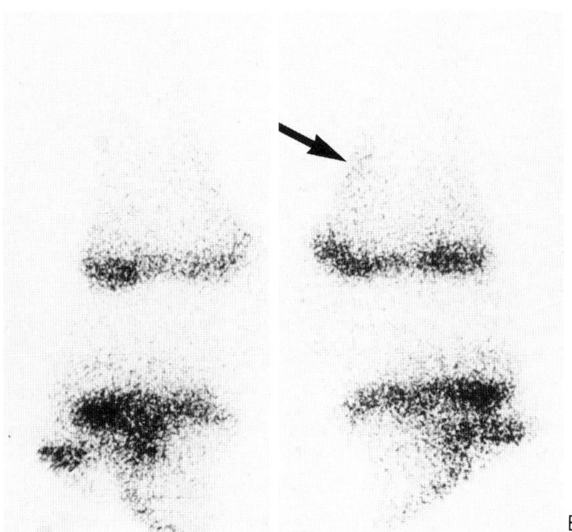

Fig. 6.1 Fibrous cortical defect arising in posteromedial aspect of the distal medial femur. **A**. The abnormality is confined to the cortex with a very fine shell of overlying bone and a sharply defined endosteal margin; **B**. A bone scan demonstrates a slight increase in activity (arrow) at the site of the lesion.

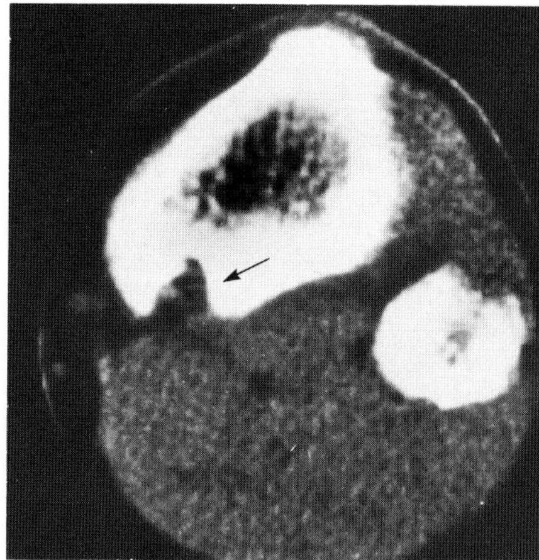

Fig. 6.2 Fibrous cortical defect in the upper medial tibia is shown on CT. Note the purely cortical position of the defect and its sharply defined margin. The thin shell of overlying bone is not seen completely because of the partial volume effect.

increase in activity is evident on a bone scan and a slight increase in vascularity on an angiogram. The typical site and lack of endosteal abnormality should prevent the misdiagnosis of a sarcoma.

2. NON-OSSIFYING FIBROMA

The lesion is similar to a fibrous cortical defect except that it is much larger and characteristically occurs in a slightly older age group between 10 and 20 years. The vast majority occur around the knee joint, the distal end of the femur being the most common site. The lesion occasionally presents with a pathological fracture (Fig. 6.3). Usually it is not symptomatic.

The radiological findings reveal an area of increased radiolucency which is sharply defined in the metadiaphysis,

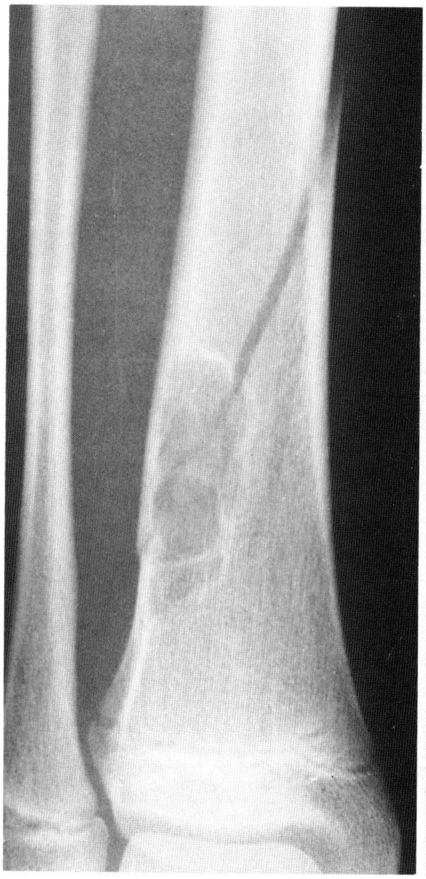

Fig. 6.3

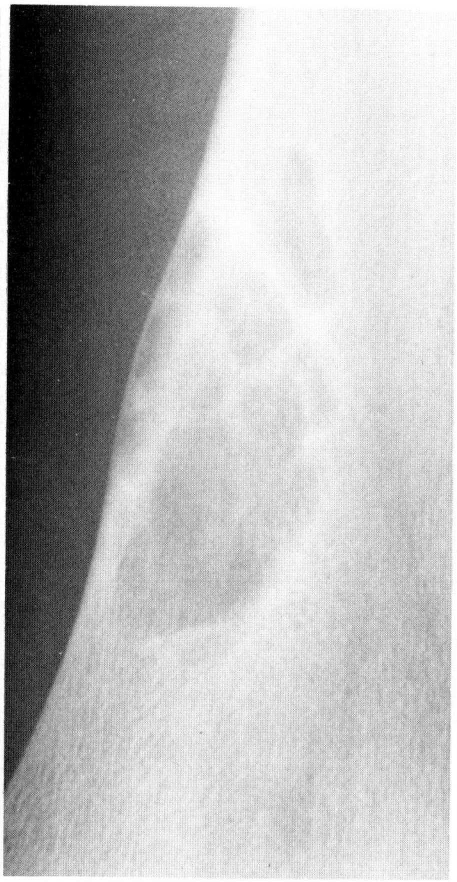

Fig. 6.4

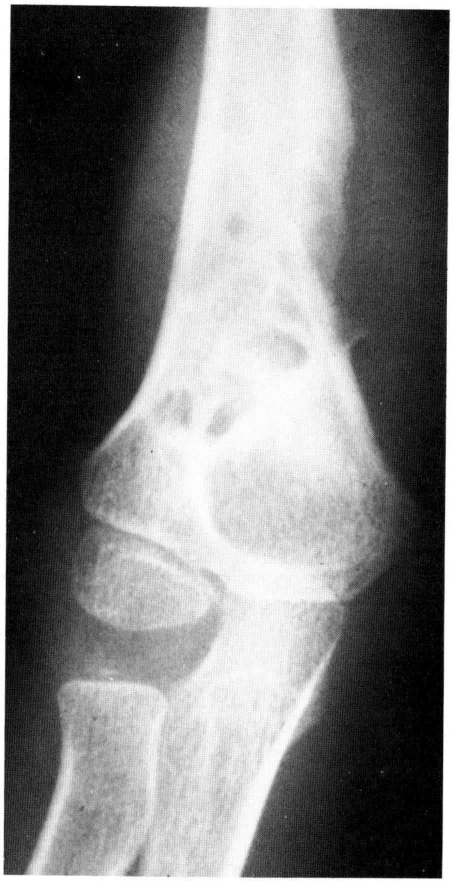

Fig. 6.5

Fig. 6.3 Non-ossifying fibroma of the distal tibia presenting with a fracture. The well-defined outline and eccentric position of the tumour are demonstrated together with sharply defined sclerotic margins.

Fig. 6.4 Non-ossifying fibroma — a localized view of a lesion in the distal medial femur shows a slight cortical expansion, sharply-edfined sclerotic margins and a lobulated outline. This appearance is very similar to a fibrous cortical defect, and no clear distinction can be made sometimes between these two tumours.

Fig. 6.5 Desmoplastic fibroma. A destructive, lobulated space occupying lesion is present in the distal metadiaphysis of the humerus. Bone expansion is present with sclerotic margins around the tumour. A soft tissue component has caused consolidated periosteal new bone formation.

ıe margins are smooth and sharp, with a rather lobulated ppearance, and are defined by a thin zone of reactive sclersis (Fig. 6.4). In larger bones such as the tibia and fibula he lesion may be eccentric and appropriate oblique views vill show its relationship to one of the cortices. However, ı more slender bones, such as the fibula, the whole width f the bone may be involved. On the outer margin the corex is usually slightly expanded but remains intact and hinned. Scintigraphically only a minimal increase in acivity can be detected on the delayed phase scan, the degree f increased activity reflecting solely the size of the lesion nless there has been a pathological fracture. Angiography s unremarkable and usually unnecessary since the plain ilm appearances are sufficiently characteristic to permit a onfident radiological diagnosis. As in fibrous cortical deect the natural history is for the lesion to regress, initially y an increase in the surrounding zone of sclerosis and laterly by replacement with normal bone.

The differential diagnosis, particularly when the whole width of the bone is involved, is from a solitary bone cyst or monostotic fibrous dysplasia. Differentiation from the former may be very difficult on all radiological grounds whereas distinction from monostotic fibrous dysplasia is relatively straightforward due to the avidity of the latter for bone seeking radiopharmaceuticals (see Ch. 66).

3. DESMOPLASTIC FIBROMA

This rare tumour exhibits dense fibrous tissue simulating desmoid tumours of the abdominal wall. Relatively few occur in bone and then usually in young adults. Pain is a constant presenting feature. The lesion is often tender. The majority arise in the metadiaphysis of long bones (Fig. 6.5), although the pelvis and spine are other sites of predilection.

Radiologically they tend to be large, solitary and destructive, with an expanded and irregular sclerotic margin. There may be a slight increase in density within the lesion so that superficially it may resemble monostotic fibrous dysplasia. Slight irregularity of the margin may suggest an aneurysmal bone cyst when the lesion is purely osteolytic.

Multiple fibromatous tumours are present in **congenital generalized fibromatosis** in which half the patients have associated bony abnormalities. This rare childhood condition demonstrates multiple, rounded, corticated, cystic metaphyseal lesions often with sharply defined sclerotic margins. These fibromatous foci tend to regress with increasing age and have an excellent prognosis. However, some patients have associated involvement of skin, muscle, heart and lungs; the outlook in this group is poor.

4. FIBROSARCOMA

Although this is the least common of the malignant primary tumours arising in skeletal connective tissue, representing about 5% of all, individual lesions vary widely in their appearances and to this extent can create diagnostic difficulties. This variation corresponds to a wide range of histological characteristics but the degree of malignancy and the radiological features correlate reasonably well. Many of the characteristics lie between those of osteosarcoma and chondrosarcoma. For example, the age of presentation has a mean of about 35 years of age and survival is also between the poor outlook of osteosarcoma and the better prognosis of chondrosarcoma.

Presentation is usually due to low grade pain, sometimes swelling, usually present for less than a year. In many the precipitating factor may be a pathological fracture (Fig. 6.6). Whilst a few of these tumours arise primarily in soft tissue and cause secondary bony changes, the majority develop primarily in bone and may be either medullary or periosteal in location. A medullary lesion is considerably more common and usually arises in the metaphyseal area. Approximately 80% occur around the knee. It is less usual for a flat bone to be involved. The rarer periosteal type has a more widespread distribution, but still has a predilection for long bones where any portion of the shaft may be affected. This type tends to develop a clinically palpable mass in the earlier stages.

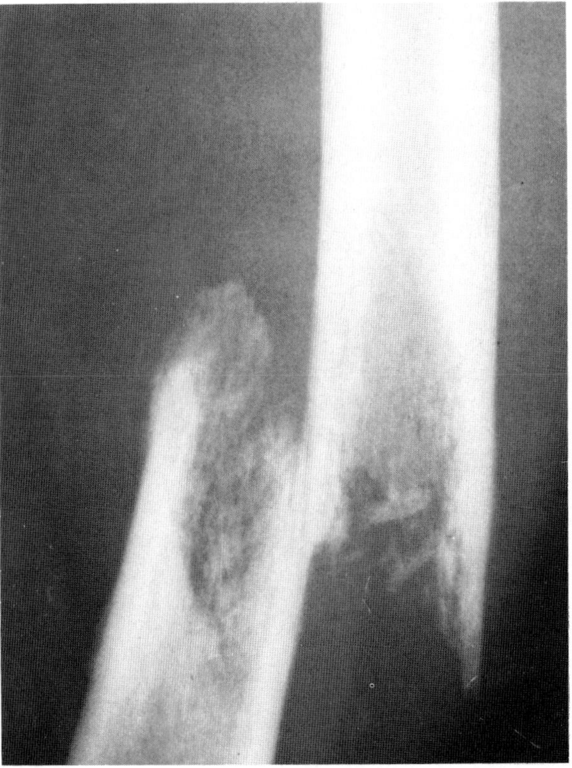

Fig. 6.6 Fibrosarcoma — presenting with pathological fracture of the femur in a woman of 50. Ill-defined bone destruction, particularly of the medulla, is associated with very minor periosteal new bone formation and no sclerosis. The cortex has been thinned on the endosteal surface.

Radiological features. The tumour is essentially osteolytic, provokes little new bone formation and usually lacks calcification or ossification. The medullary variety is characterized usually by an irregular area of radiolucency. The zone of transition may vary from being relatively narrow, indicating a well-differentiated tumour, to being diffuse and permeative, suggesting a highly aggressive tumour (Fig. 6.7). In the latter circumstance densities resembling calcification may be present within the tumour. These, in fact, represent residual dead bone rather than new bone. With very low grade tumours a minimal degree of sclerosis may surround the radiolucency. Slowly growing tumours may thin and expand the cortex, but with a diffuse infiltrative pattern it is more usual for actual destruction to occur. The subsequent soft tissue extensions are without calcification or ossification and periosteal new bone formation is unremarkable. This feature may differentiate the tumour from osteosarcoma or chondrosarcoma. The periosteal, on the other hand, frequently does exhibit shaggy ill-defined periosteal new bone arising from the underlying cortex. Destruction of the outer side of the cortex frequently takes place, but the erosion is usually clearly defined, almost as though a piece of bone has been removed surgically. In this respect, the appearance of a sharp margin, considerable variance is shown from the poor definition of the edge of most malignant tumours. Consequently the impression may be gained of a benign periosteally related tumour, such as a lipoma. Secondary involvement of bone may result also from a fibrosarcoma arising in soft tissue. The resulting abnormality is comparable to any other cortical pressure erosion — a shallow, clearly defined cortical excavation becoming evident.

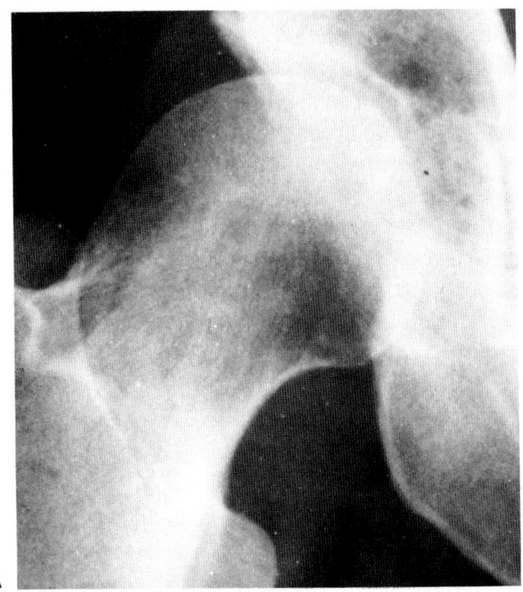

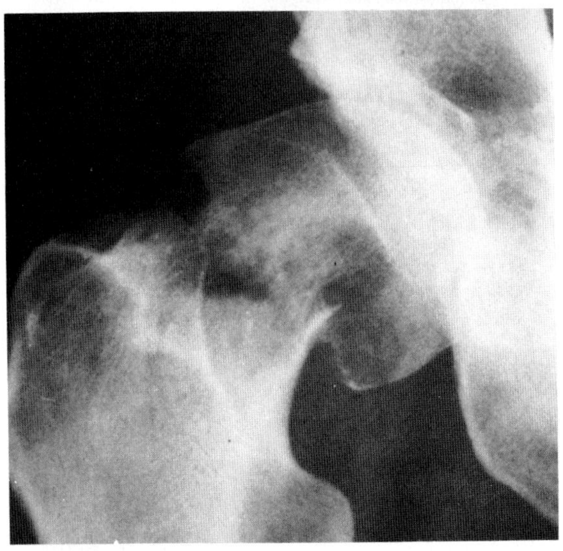

Fig. 6.7 Fibrosarcoma arising in the medulla of the femoral head and neck. This 35-year-old man presented with poorly localized pain in the hip. **A.** At presentation an ill-defined area of bone destruction on the medial aspect of the femoral head and neck. The cortex is preserved with no new bone formation; **B.** 3 months later a pathological fracture has occurred through the destructive lesion.

As with the plain film appearances, angiography roughly mirrors the degree of malignancy of the tumour. Relatively low grade fibrosarcomas are associated only with a slight increase in the number of arteries and evidence of tumour vessel encasement. At the other extreme the appearances may be indistinguishable from an osteosarcoma, although it is rare for a very florid malignant circulation to be present. Arteriography remains necessary in the assessment of soft tissue lesions in order to delineate, with CT, not only the extent of the tumour but also evidence of major vessel involvement. The increase in arterial vascularity shown on angiography can be detected also on the blood pool phase of a bone scan. The delayed phase of a bone scan is variable, depending on the degree of bone response and the amount of periosteal new bone formation. Metastatic dissemination from fibrosarcoma usually is not detectable with a bone seeking agent.

Fibrosarcoma also may arise in the fibrous wall of a medullary infarct and, in addition, is one of the histological patterns associated with Paget's sarcoma. To differentiate fibrosarcoma of bone from other malignancies is by no means straightforward. The major differential is from osteosarcoma and chondrosarcoma. Moreover, the more aggressive, ill-defined varieties may be indistinguishable from malignant round cell tumours, including particularly non-Hodgkin's lymphoma (reticulum cell sarcomas).

5. MALIGNANT FIBROUS HISTIOCYTOMA

Of late a group of tumours have been separated, mainly from fibrosarcomas, on the basis of histological and clinical findings. These aggressive, often metastasising, tumours are probably of histiocytic origin. They occur in an older population, usually around 55 years of age, affected individuals complaining chiefly of pain, swelling or of a slowly enlarging mass. The majority develop in soft tissues. The rela-

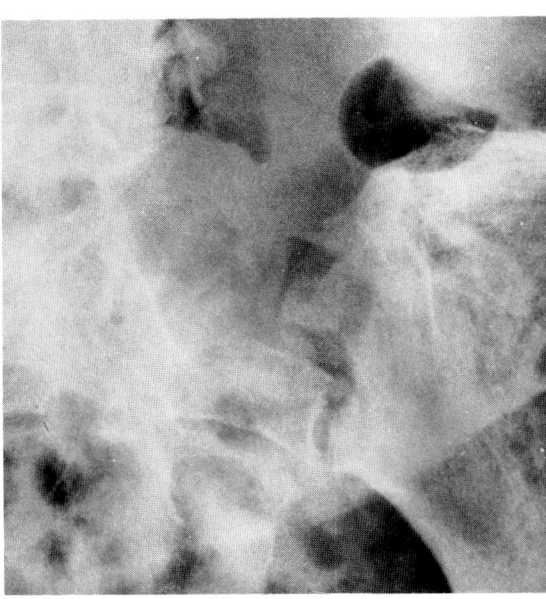

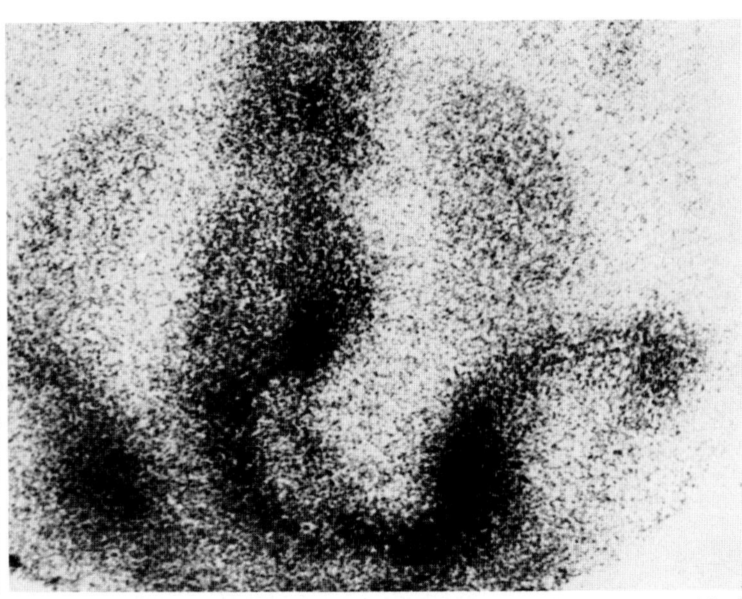

Fig. 6.8 Malignant fibrous histiocytoma arising in the sacral ala of a 60-year-old woman. **A**. A purely destructive, lytic lesion is present with slight sclerosis around its margins. Note that the lower border of L5 has also been destroyed together with part of the iliac wing; **B**. An isotope bone scan shows the tumour to be photon deficient but a rim of increased activity corresponds to reactive bone sclerosis.

tively small number arising in bone have a predeliction for the femur and the ends of the tibia and humerus. Others arise in the pelvis and ribs.

The radiological features are primarily those of an ill-defined, purely osteolytic lesion with early cortical destruction, frequently in a permeative fashion, often with some expansion. To this extent they resemble fibrosarcomas of an aggressive type. Occasionally punctate, soft tissue calcification is present and a small proportion exhibit periosteal reaction and endosteal sclerosis (Fig. 6.8). A soft tissue mass often develops early. Angiographically areas of avascularity and hypervascularity are typical, including the demonstration of new vessels and encasement. Scintigraphy is not typically informative. Many cases present with multiple skeletal lesions and the initial impression is the likelihood of skeletal metastases rather than of a primary or multifocal bone tumour. As with fibrosarcoma, malignant round cell tumours require consideration in differential diagnosis.

6. ADAMANTINOMA OF LONG BONE

This rather unusual neoplasm is almost invariably located in the tibial shaft. Only a few isolated instances of the involvement of other long bones have been recorded. **Clinically** localized pain and swelling usually has been present for several years. On examination a soft tissue, possibly cystic, swelling is palpated. The age range varies from 15 to 55 years. Histologically difficulty may arise in differentiating this lesion from metastatic adenocarcinoma or squamous cell carcinoma, since the glandular and fibrous component of the tumour may suggest an epithelial derivation.

Radiologically an eccentric area of destruction usually involves the anterior portion of the tibial shaft. Slight expansion and cortical thinning, with a cystic or multiloculated appearance, are customary (Fig. 6.9). Periosteal reaction is not marked, but cortical destruction may be extensive. The margin of the tumour varies from being sharply and clearly defined, with a slight sclerotic margin, to a hazy zone of transition several millimetres in width, comparable to that observed in giant cell tumours. Some of these tumours may be 15 or more centimetres in length with satellite lesions.

Adamantinoma probably has a relationship to ossifying fibroma, which may be itself a localized form of fibrous dysplasia, in which it has been observed to develop as a late complication. Whilst the radiological appearances of adamantinoma are not pathognomonic, the location and the clinical history should help to suggest the diagnosis. The tumour continues to grow at a slow rate, but is characterised by local recurrence and eventual metastasis to lung. Extensive local resection is the usual form of treatment.

BONE TUMOURS PRESUMED TO ARISE FROM SKELETAL TISSUE — GIANT CELL CONTAINING

A group of tumours rich in giant cells were confused in the older literature. This group now has been subdivided, on histological and radiological grounds, into giant cell tumour ('osteoclastoma') and the giant cell tumour variants. The latter include chondroblastoma (p. 159), chondromyxoid fibroma (p. 160) and aneurysmal bone cyst (see below). However, all these variants exhibit some areas

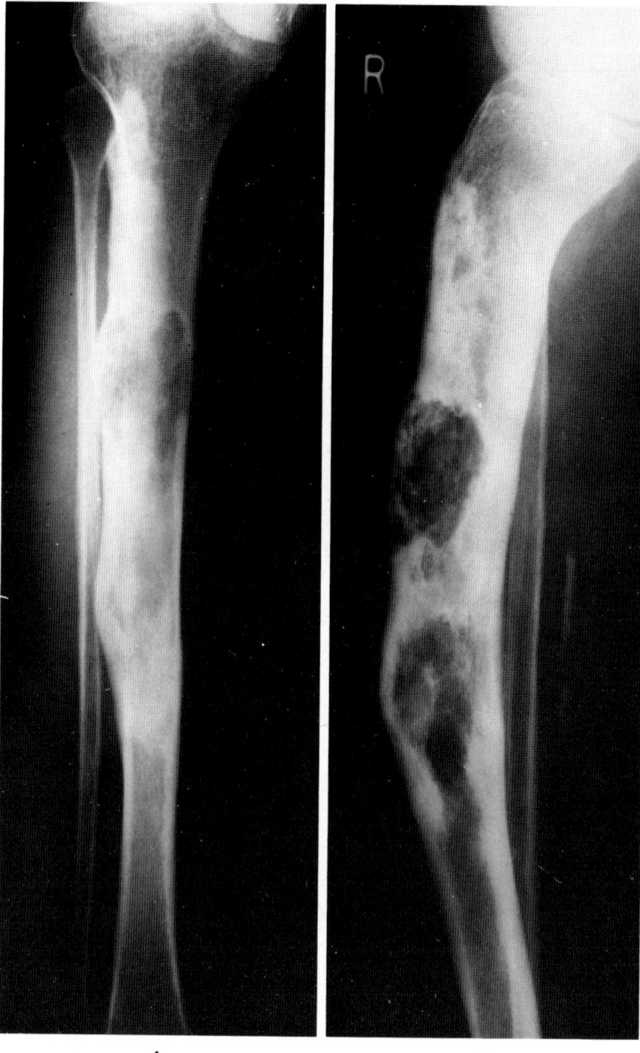

Fig. 6.9 Adamantinoma of the tibia. Eccentric areas of bone destruction are present anteriorly with thinning of the cortex. The cortex is expanded. In addition to this abnormality sclerosis and ill-defined cortical thickening are present throughout the whole of the tibia which is also bowed. These features are due to associated fibrous dysplasia (or a close variety sometimes known as ossifying fibroma which occurs only at this site). **A**. AP view. **B**. Lateral view.

which are histologically identical. In consequence, whilst broadly clear cut radiological and histological categorisation is possible, a definite overlap exists. In some series the 'brown' tumours of hyperparathyroidism also have been included in this category.

1. GIANT CELL TUMOUR (OSTEOCLASTOMA)

These tumours conform to a fairly constant clinical and radiological pattern. As with many other tumours the initial presentation is of localized pain and swelling, some presenting following trauma or as an incidental finding. Histologically richly vascular tissue contains plump spindle cells and numerous giant cells containing 50 to 100 nuclei. The tumour forms neither bone nor cartilage. It is locally aggressive and likely in more than half of instances to recur in spite of extensive curettage or excision with or without radiotherapy.

A variable proportion are deemed malignant. Malignancy seems to be divided between those which are initially extremely aggressive and others that become so following surgical or therapeutic intervention. Sometimes confusion arises because the extreme aggressiveness of the tumour histologically and radiologically, does not correlate with the subsequent development of actual distant metastases to lung. A small group of undoubtedly malignant, metastatic giant cell tumours has been recognized, often with a dominant fibrosarcomatous stroma. Attempts at histological and radiological grading have had only limited prognostic value.

The majority of patients present between the ages of 20 and 40 years. Only about 3% of cases develop in immature skeletons, distinguishing these patients from those with aneurysmal bone cysts, in whom the tumour maximally occurs prior to epiphyseal fusion. Giant cell tumours are multifocal in about 0.5% of cases, often in the hands. The solitary lesion shows a predilection for bones adjacent to the knee joint and the distal end of the radius; the sacrum and pelvis are occasionally involved. Histological review of a number of cases in which spinal lesions have been

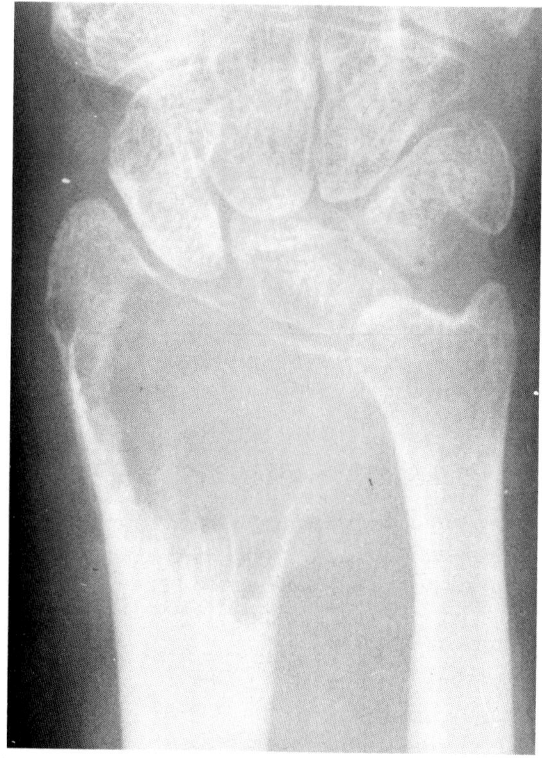

Fig. 6.10 Giant cell tumour arising in the distal radius of an adult male patient. A characteristic, eccentric, immediately subarticular position makes this diagnosis very probable. The margins are ill-defined with no sclerotic reaction.

detected has indicated that the correct diagnosis is much more commonly an aneurysmal bone cyst. Facial bones appear to be exempt.

Radiological features. A zone of radiolucency typically is situated immediately beneath the articular cortex, being sited eccentrically at the end of a long bone (Fig. 6.10). The only exception to this rule is when the lesion arises in a former apophysis, notably the greater trochanter. Unless complicated by a fracture the lesion does not contain calcification or ossification, although in about 40% of cases it is characterized by a 'soap-bubble' pattern of trabeculation. The margins are purely osteolytic and, with the exception of tumours arising in the femoral condyles, a sclerotic margin is evident rarely. Characteristically, therefore, the margin is hazy and ill-defined with no bone reaction (Fig. 6.11). More aggressive lesions are associated with evidence of widening of the zone of transition. The overlying cortex may be expanded and exquisitely thinned with a crenellated outline usually without the development of periosteal new bone formation, except as a response to a pathological fracture. The tumour may produce a well-defined extension into the adjacent soft tissues, without evidence of calcification or new bone formation. As the lesion enlarges the whole width of bone may become involved, causing an increased susceptibility to fracture. The presence of such a soft tissue mass does not, of necessity, indicate a sarcoma. This complication is inferred by a rapid change in size or character of the tumour on sequential radiographs.

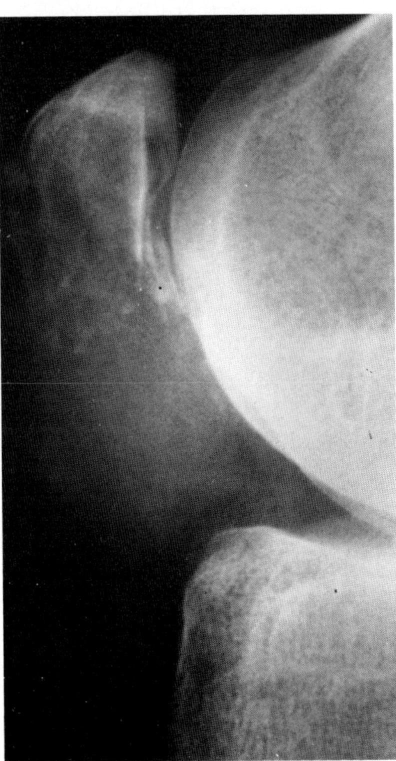

Fig. 6.11 Giant cell tumour of the patella. Giant cell tumours can arise in almost any bone but those around the knee are particularly affected. Note the immediately subarticular, eccentric position of the tumour which is purely osteolytic with no sclerotic reaction. The epiphyses have fused.

Angiographically, and on the blood pool phase of a bone scan, vascularity is markedly increased, typically with an increased number of vessels, arteriovenous shunting and tumour staining. Many exhibit encasement. These features do not correlate with either clinical aggressiveness or sarcomatous change and may be extremely difficult to distinguish from those observed in other giant cell containing tumours, particularly aneurysmal bone cysts. The delayed phase of a bone scan is usually normal. CT may be necessary to delineate fully the soft tissue extent of the tumour.

Many of the rather more aggressive giant cell containing tumours in the younger age group may in fact be giant cell rich osteosarcomas (Fig. 6.12). It is possible that some of the reported metastasising malignant giant cell tumours may be of this type. Usually, however, little difficulty arises in differential diagnosis, the eccentric, purely lytic and subarticular location of the tumour being characteristic. Differential diagnosis includes aneurysmal bone cysts and chondroblastoma. The 'brown' tumours of hyperparathyroidism and monostotic fibrous dysplasia require consideration.

In spite of apparently successful curettage and packing with bone chips these tumours have a tendency to recur even years after initial treatment and plain film follow up is necessary. Secondary sarcomatous change may occur also following radiotherapy after intervals of several years. Treated tumours may be difficult to judge radiologically because of regression in the form of sclerosis on the one hand and continued evolution on the other. Total excision is the preferable means of therapy. On rare occasions the tumour may cross a joint or extend from one bone to another.

2. ANEURYSMAL BONE CYST

The exact aetiology of this tumour is unknown, but the descriptive name is derived from the macroscopic appearances of a blood filled, expansile, sponge-like tumour containing numerous giant cells. Some reports have suggested that aneurysmal bone cyst is not a true neoplasm, since it has been shown to arise in association with other abnormalities of the skeleton, particularly non-ossifying fibroma, fibrous dysplasia and chondromyxoid fibroma. Such lesions have been described as 'secondary' aneurysmal bone cysts. They have been recorded also following a fracture. Whatever the aetiology aneurysmal bone cyst has a close relationship to all the giant cell variants.

In the main these tumours present in childhood or early adolescent life, with a predilection for the long bones and the lumbar spine. Those arising in the spine occur slightly later, between 10 and 20 years of age. The neural arch is more commonly involved than the body, half of these cases

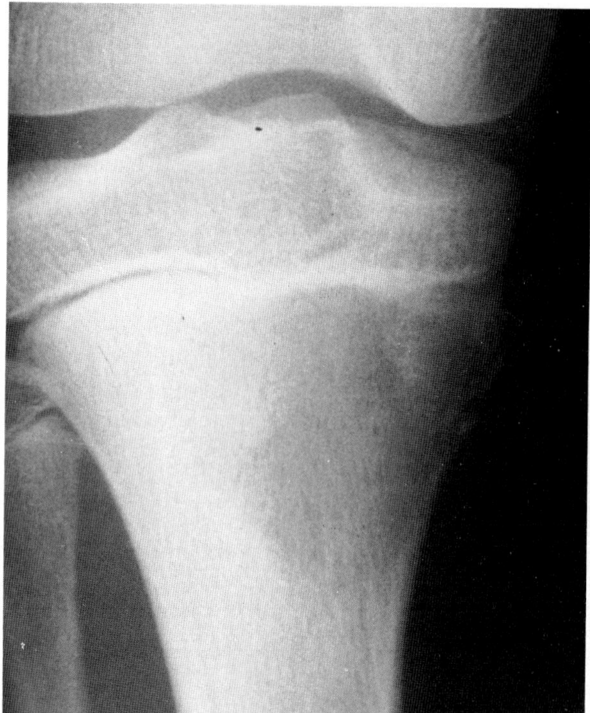

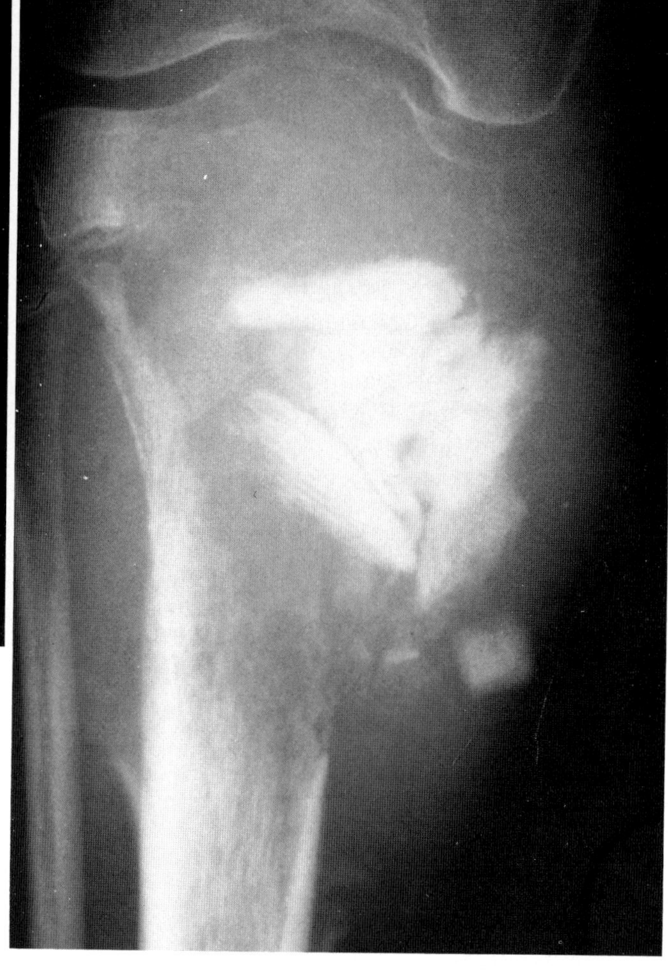

A

Fig. 6.12 Giant cell rich osteosarcoma **A**. A radiograph of this boy at presentation demonstrates an eccentric, purely osteolytic lesion in the upper tibial metaphysis. The cortex has been breeched but there is no periosteal new bone and only very faint surrounding sclerosis. **B**. 6 months later, following curettage and packing with bone chips, the flagrantly aggressive nature of this tumour is obvious. Note now the Codman's triangle on the lateral aspect of the tibial shaft and a substantial soft tissue mass that contains ossification.

involving more than one vertebra. The prognosis is entirely benign apart from secondary neurological lesions due to spinal canal compression.

Radiological features. Typically an area of bone resorption occurs with slight or marked expansion (Fig. 6.13), the size of the lesion varying between 2 and in gross examples as much as 20 cms in diameter. The overlying cortex is thinned and may be expanded (Fig. 6.14) to such a degree that in places it can be identified only by tomography or CT. The endosteal margin is relatively well-defined against cortex, and an ill-defined zone of transition is usual between the lesion and medullary bone, occasionally with slight sclerosis. A margin of this type is similar to that observed in giant cell tumour. Sometimes it is scalloped or irregular. Angiographically many features are common to giant cell tumour, in particular a rich increase in vessels with diffuse opacification and early venous filling. This appearance may be shown in the blood pool phase of a bone scan. The absence of any particular feature on the delayed scan demonstrates the failure of the tumour to calcify or form bone.

Most lesions evolve slowly. However a few show a highly aggressive radiological pattern and may increase alarmingly in size, even doubling in a few weeks. The possibility of a very malignant vascular tumour such as an angiosarcoma may then be entertained.

Differentiation from giant cell tumour is aided by the age of the patient as three-quarters of aneurysmal bone cysts occur before epiphyseal fusion has occurred and their widespread anatomical distribution contrasts with the majority of giant cell tumours occurring around the knee and wrist. Therefore difficulty is likely to arise only when the abnormality occurs after epiphyseal closure or when it is situated at the end of a long bone. Aneurysmal bone cyst rarely extends to the articular surface and is often central compared to the subarticular eccentric nature of giant cell tumour. The spinal lesions need to be differentiated from osteoblastoma and osteoid osteoma. The bone forming nature of these latter two tumours together with their associated sclerotic reactions provide valuable differential diagnostic signs.

Aneurysmal bone cysts are treated by curettage or radiotherapy, the latter method being particularly valuable in spinal lesions where surgery may be considered hazard-

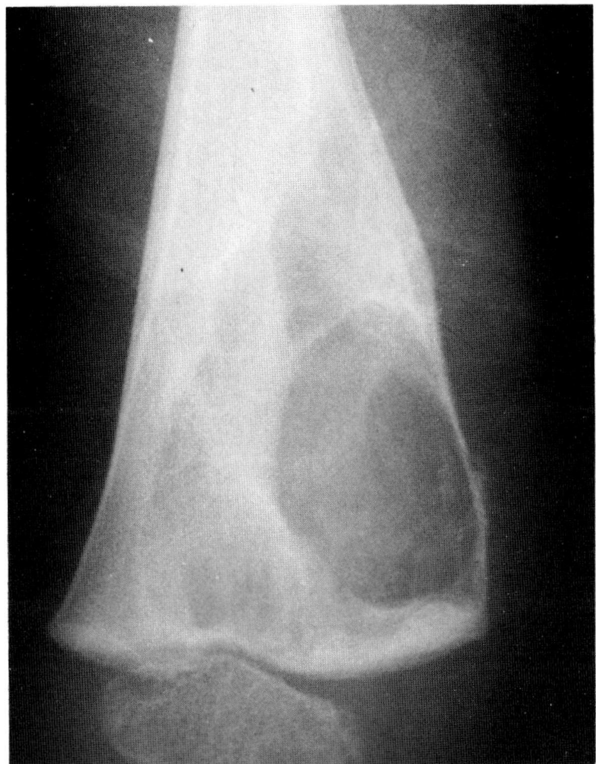

Fig. 6.13 Aneurysmal bone cyst (male aged two). This film was taken because of an asymptomatic swelling and shows the characteristic features of metaphyseal involvement, cortical expansion and thinning, with a relatively well-defined endosteal margin.

ous. An increasing role, however, has developed for transcatheter embolisation in the successful management of these tumours. Aneurysmal bone cyst is a particularly good example of the importance of radiological investigation being complete before biopsy is undertaken, since these lesions, not surprisingly, bleed considerably and the preoperative demonstration of the vascular nature of this tumour may save some embarrassment!

TUMOURS PRESUMED TO ARISE FROM OTHER TISSUES IN BONE — BLOOD VESSELS

1. HAEMANGIOMA

Intraosseous haemangiomas are benign and slow-growing. Malignancy is virtually unknown. Many of these benign vascular neoplasms are asymptomatic, their presence being detected incidentally in the course of an examination for some other purpose. However, the autopsy incidence is about 10%. A few cause swelling and mild pain. Vertebral lesions tend to become symptomatic during pregnancy. Occasionally significant neurological deficits may occur secondary to the collapse of an involved vertebral body with or without an extra-osseous soft tissue tumour component. The age of presentation is between 10 and 45 years.

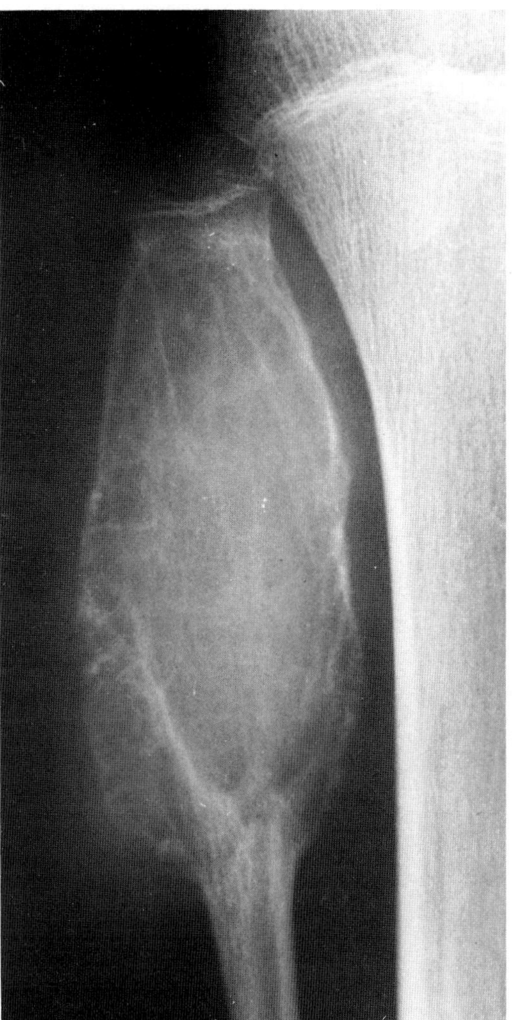

Fig. 6.14 Aneurysmal bone cyst of the proximal fibula. Considerably greater expansion has occurred in this example. The cortex is now very thin though apparently intact. The zone of transition between the lesion and adjacent bone is narrow but ill-defined. Note apparent multiple septa with the lesion.

Haemangiomas are either cavernous, with large thin-walled vessels occurring particularly in vertebrae and the skull, or capillary with fine capillary loops tending to spread in a sun-burst pattern. Typically the tumour is solitary, the commonest site being a thoracic or lumbar vertebral body.

Radiologically plain films show increased translucency with a characteristic fine vertical striation (Fig. 6.15). Half the lesions involve purely the vertebral body, the other half extending into the posterior elements. A small proportion have an associated soft tissue mass. The overall size of the vertebral body often is within normal limits, a helpful differential feature from Paget's disease.

The remainder of the skeleton is affected in approximately half of cases, the skull and long bones being sites of predilection. Although these tumours may present a

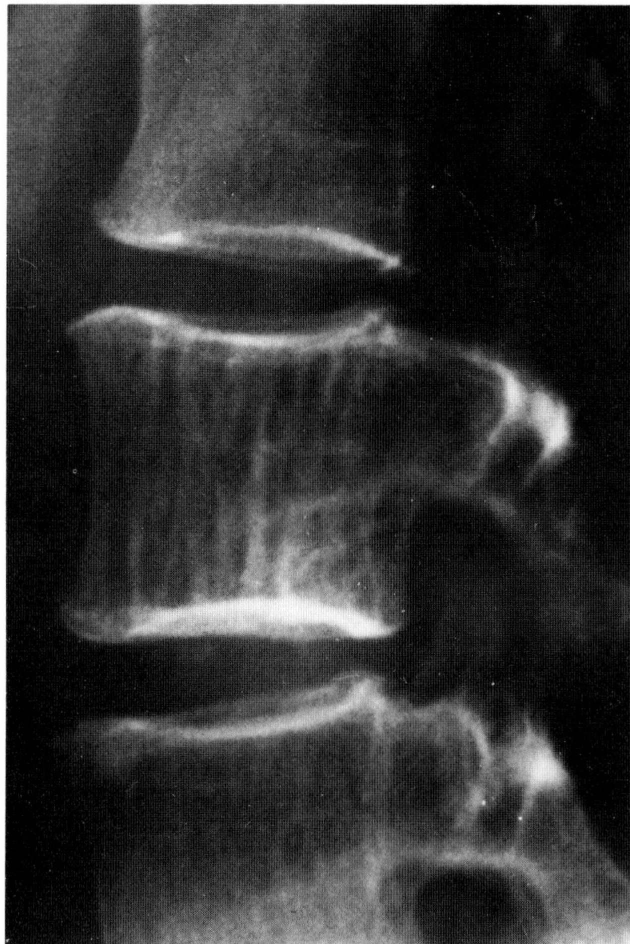

Fig. 6.15 Haemangioma of the vertebral body of L3. The whole body is marked by the characteristic vertical striation, which in this example does not extend into the pedicles.

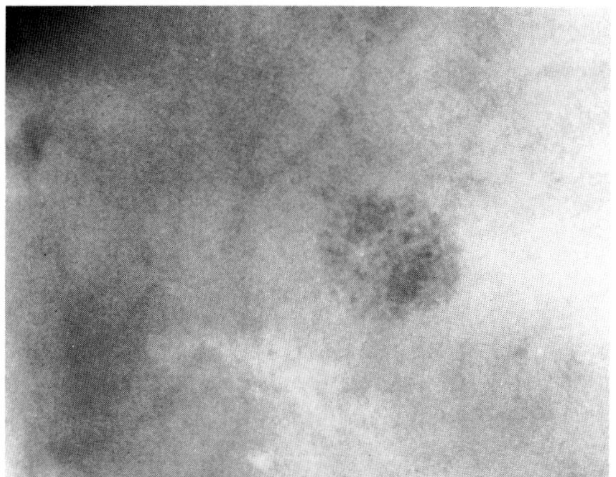

Fig. 6.16 Haemangioma of the skull is shown on a localized view of the temporal fossa. Note the purely osteolytic lesion with stippled radiodensities.

striated appearance in long bones and ribs, as in the vertebral lesions, the radiological changes in these other areas are usually very different, tending to be osteolytic with sclerotic margins and, often causing some cortical expansion. The osteolytic component has a soap-bubble appearance within which a sun-burst or stippled radiodensity may be evident, possibly extending into the soft tissues with radiating spicules of bone. This pattern may be encountered with a capillary haemangioma, particularly in the skull and pelvis (Fig. 6.16). In some cases localized cortical thickening, from which peripheral bone spicules may extend, simulates an osteosarcoma. However closer scrutiny and appropriate further investigation resolves any difficulty.

Soft tissue cavernous haemangiomas may be recognised by well-defined circular calcifications due to phleboliths (Fig. 6.17). This is one component of Maffucci's syndrome, the other being multiple chondromas (see Fig. 5.33).

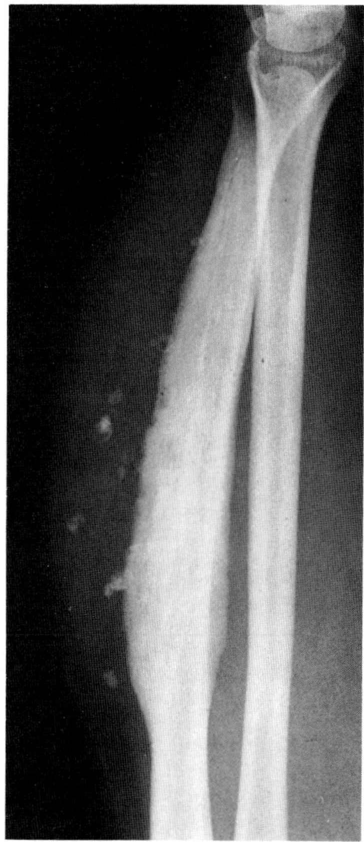

Fig. 6.17 Cavernous haemangioma of the soft tissues of the forearm is diagnosed by the presence of soft tissue swelling within which there are phleboliths. The presence of extensive consolidated periosteal new bone and bowing of the ulna suggest an intimate relationship with the periosteum.

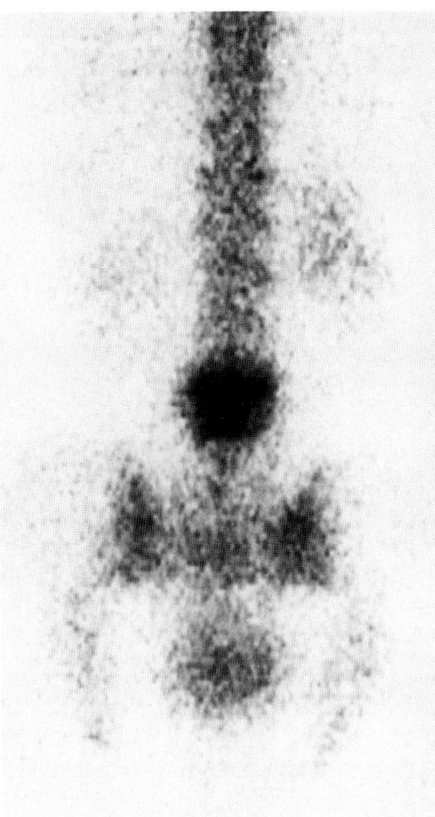

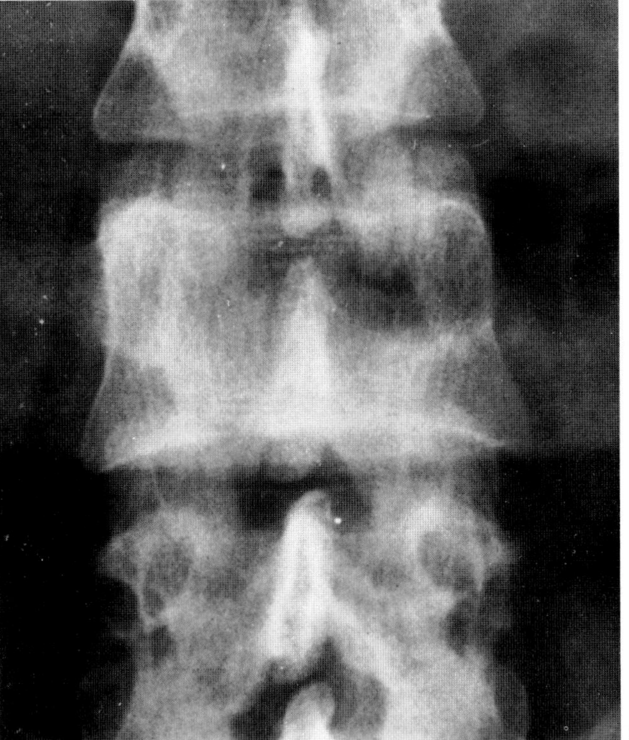

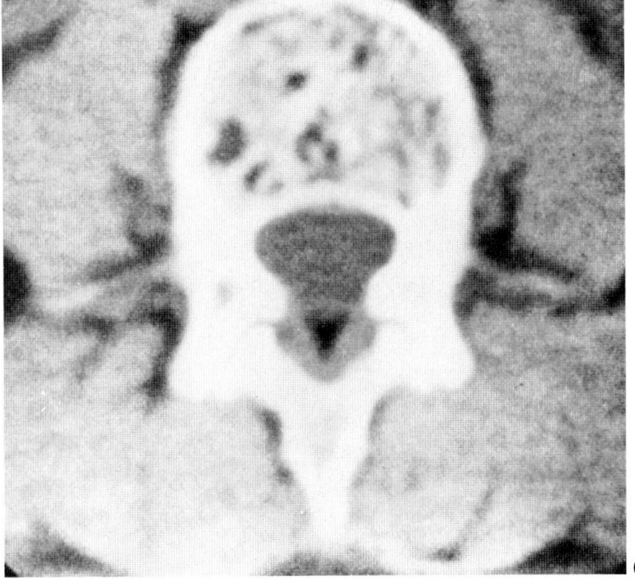

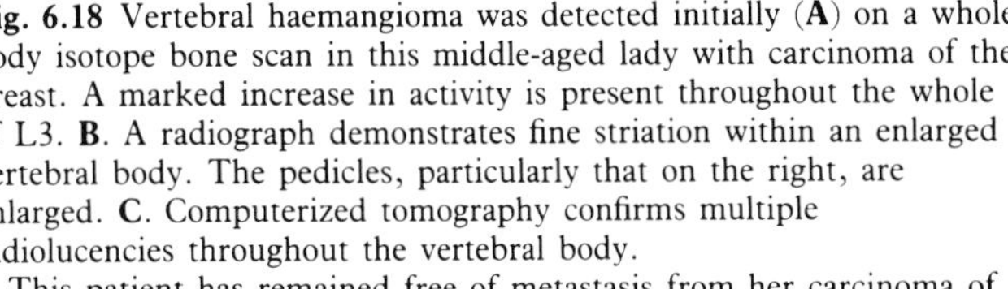

Fig. 6.18 Vertebral haemangioma was detected initially (**A**) on a whole body isotope bone scan in this middle-aged lady with carcinoma of the breast. A marked increase in activity is present throughout the whole of L3. **B**. A radiograph demonstrates fine striation within an enlarged vertebral body. The pedicles, particularly that on the right, are enlarged. **C**. Computerized tomography confirms multiple radiolucencies throughout the vertebral body.

This patient has remained free of metastasis from her carcinoma of the breast to date.

Scintigraphically the bone lesion shows increased activity on the delayed phase of a bone scan (Fig. 6.18). Both bone and soft tissue lesions may be detected by a blood pool scan (Fig. 6.19). The appearance of increased activity in a vertebral tumour cannot therefore be used to distinguish between Paget's disease, a sclerotic metastasis or a haemangioma. On occasions the soft tissue mass arising from a vertebral lesion may require delineation with spinal angiography if surgical resection is considered. It may be important to demonstrate the artery of Adamkiewicz in order that surgical excision or transcatheter embolisation does not result in paraplegia. Some lesions respond well to radiotherapy, particularly those in vertebrae.

2. VANISHING BONE DISEASE (Gorham's disease)

This relatively rare syndrome is a variant of angiomatosis of bone in which vascular proliferation predominates. Its origin is unknown. It is recognized usually in childhood, but more than one third of patients are over the age of 35. Progressive weakness and limitation of movement of the affected area characterize the onset. Pain is not an early feature, although obviously occurring with a pathological fracture. After a period of months or years the limb becomes useless or flail. The course is unpredictable, either stabilising or progressing fatally with the development of chylothorax.

Radiologically an ill-defined area of radiolucency may be observed in a single bone, but this destructive process progresses slowly to involve adjacent bones without respect

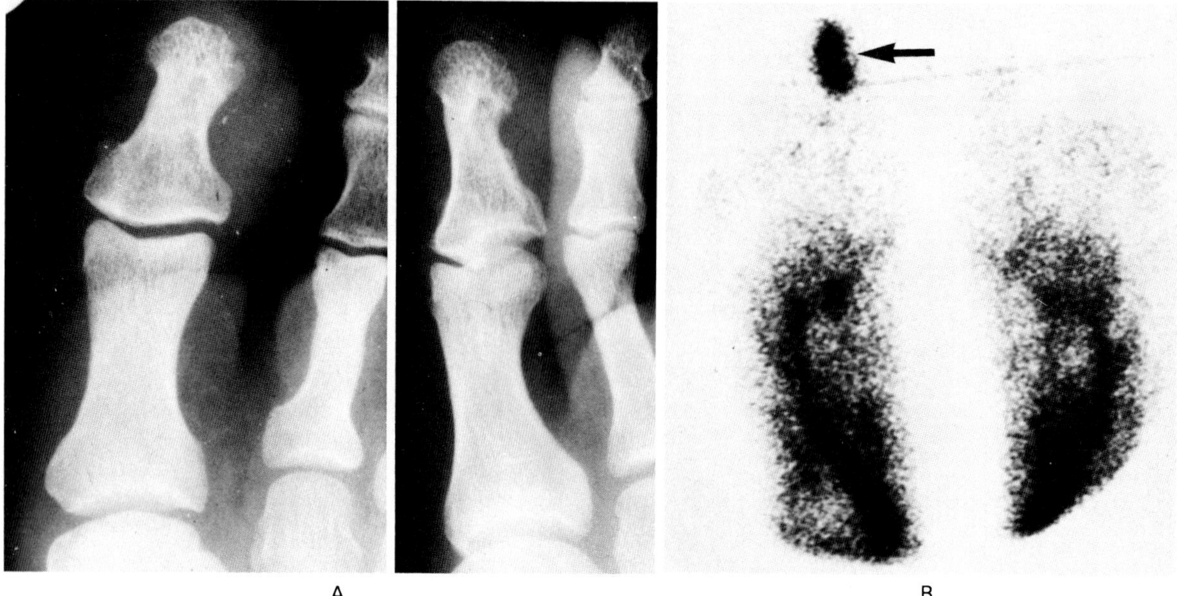

Fig. 6.19 Soft tissue cavernous haemangioma of the great toe. This patient complained of a swollen great toe with a purple area of discolouration. **A**. A plain film reveals soft tissue swelling and pressure erosion of the plantar aspect of the distal phalanx. **B**. A blood pool scan confirms an intense focus of activity (arrow) corresponding to the cavernous haemangioma.

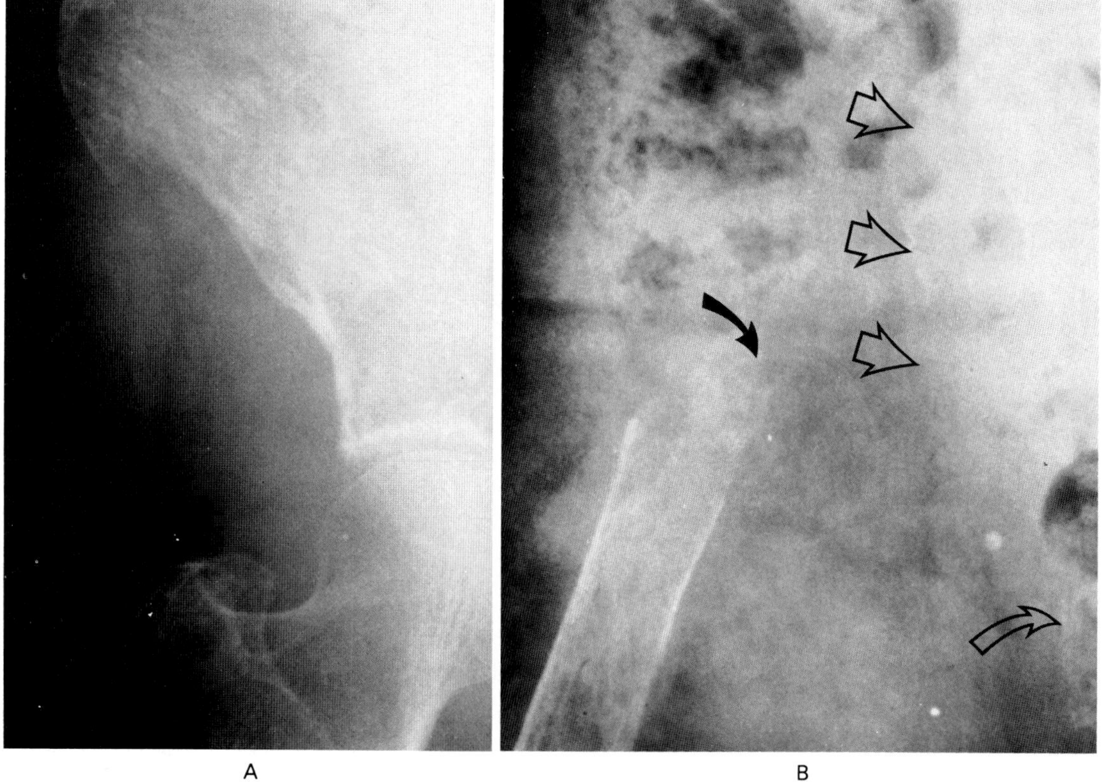

Fig. 6.20 Vanishing bone disease. A 70-year-old lady presented with poorly localised pain in her right hip. **A**. A radiograph at presentation reveals ill-defined destruction at the anterior inferior iliac spine. **B**. 9 months later there is total destruction of the whole of the hemipelvis and hip joint. Note the faint outline of the residual femoral head (arrow), pathological fracture of the femoral neck and the articular surfaces of the sacrum and symphysis pubis which no longer articulate with bone (open arrows).

or intervening joints (Fig. 6.20). Symptoms, however, may be so insidious that extensive absorption of many adjacent bony structures may be revealed at the initial examination. Arteriography and lymphography have shown no connection of these lesions to either the vascular or lymphatic circulations.

The radiological appearance is consequently that of a diffuse increase in translucency with progressive absorption of the affected structures. In the course of the process, deformity is likely to develop and may be crippling. Although local recurrence is a major hazard, slow progression is the rule.

Similar massive osteolysis may occur with tumorous masses of lymphatic origin (**lymphangiomatosis**). Histological differentiation of the cavernous spaces that are found may be difficult and the radiological features are virtually identical.

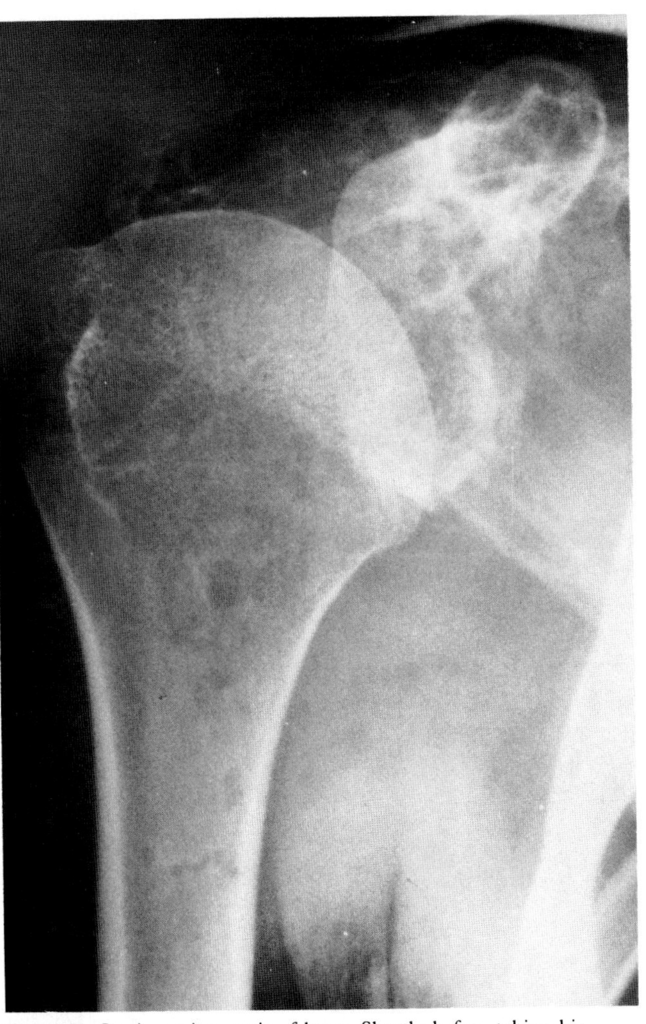

Fig. 6.21 Cystic angiomatosis of bone. Shortly before taking his university entrance examination this young man complained of a vague discomfort in his right shoulder. Note multiple well-defined radiolucencies involving the acromion, coracoid, glenoid and upper humeral shaft. The latter has a rather 'woodworm'-like appearance. Lesions were present elsewhere in the skeleton but he had no soft tissue abnormality.

3. CYSTIC ANGIOMATOSIS OF BONE

This rare entity is probably due to a hamartomatous malformation of primitive vessels. It may be difficult to distinguish the tissue of origin. Some lesions are clearly related to blood vessels, others to lymphatics. Among numerous synonyms, *cystic angiomatosis* is the most descriptive term.

The condition may be recognised in childhood or adolescence in the virtual absence of symptoms, other than mild bony swellings or, occasionally, a pathological fracture. The diagnostic radiological abnormalities may be discovered incidentally. Broadly two groups of patients are affected, those with and those without visceral and/or cutaneous involvement. The former have multiple angiomatous lesions in abdominal viscera, brain, muscle, lungs and lymph nodes, and although these lesions are histologically innocent, death may be caused from anaemia or bleeding. The prognosis in the latter group is excellent.

Radiologically multiple sharply defined radiolucent lesions involve both cortex and medulla (Fig. 6.21). An initial impression of myeloma may be given. The skull, flat bones and proximal ends of long bones are affected particularly. Scintigraphically activity may be increased around the lesions. Angiography is usually normal, but in those cases which have differentiated more closely along lymphatic lines a connection with deep lymphatics by lymphography may be demonstrated.

4. GLOMUS TUMOUR

This rare, highly differentiated, benign vascular tumour affects soft tissues more than bone. It creates, however, pressure erosion usually of a terminal phalanx, particularly the subungual portion (Fig. 6.22). A few lesions may originally arise in bone. Typically an extremely sharp margin is associated with a well-marked sclerotic rim. Clinically they are exquisitely tender and have many episodes of stabbing pain, particularly with the rarer and less differentiated haemangiopericytoma. Angiographically the lesion is richly vascular and so may be detected on a blood pool scan or on the early phase of a bone scan. The correct clinical diagnosis is usually established with little difficulty by the classic triad of pain, tenderness and sensitivity to cold.

5. ANGIOSARCOMA

(*Haemangioendothelial sarcoma*)

Primary malignant vascular tumours in bone are rare. None have been observed to arise from a benign precursor.

Radiologically the lesions are purely lytic, rapidly fatal with metastatic spread to the lungs often being present at the time the diagnosis is made. The destructive areas have irregular endosteal margins with slight expansion or coarse loculation occasionally giving a rather soap-bubble appearance. Distinction of this lesion from a highly vascular (telangectatic) osteosarcoma may require expert histological differentiation particularly as both occur in a similar age group and have strikingly abnormal angiographic appearances. A clue may be derived from the multifocal nature of angiosarcoma occurring in about one third of cases.

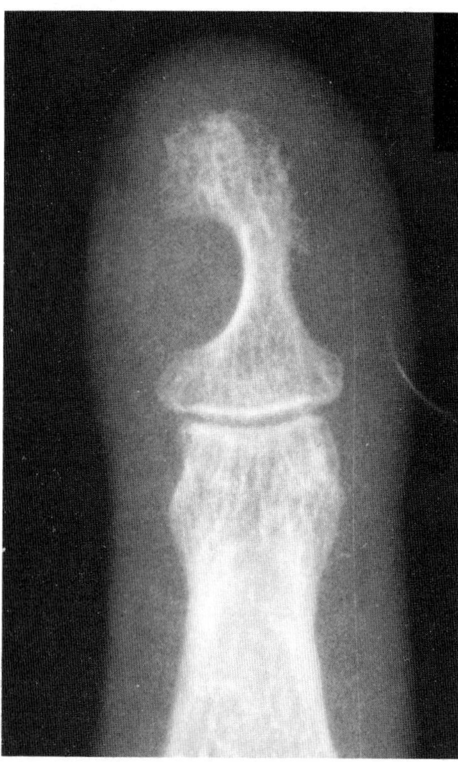

Fig. 6.22 Glomus tumour. Intermittent swelling of the index finger had been present for many years and had, intermittently, been exquisitely painful. A discrete soft tissue mass caused a pressure erosion on the radial side of the terminal phalanx.

TUMOURS PRESUMED TO ARISE FROM OTHER TISSUES IN BONE — NERVE TISSUE

1. NEUROFIBROMA AND NEURILEMMOMA

There is no clear distinction between these two tumours. It is thought that neurilemmoma or Schwannomas arise from a specific cell, the Schwann cell, whereas neurofibromas come from non-specific cells in nerve sheath. When these lesions enlarge in intimate relation to bone the latter undergoes pressure erosion resulting in an osseous defect. Radiological differentiation between such lesions is not possible. However there is some histological importance since neurilemmomas are usually solitary and never undergo malignant change whereas neurofibromas are often multiple and may become sarcomatous. Tumours arise at any age, and in either sex, usually giving rise to symptoms only as the result of nerve pressure or occasionally pathological fracture. Nerve pressure arises typically when the tumour is located within an osseous canal. Neurilemmomas have a predilection for the mandible whereas neurofibromas are more intimately related to the spinal canal.

Radiological features. The presence of a benign lesion within the spinal canal may be evident from erosion of a pedicle or widening of an exit foramen (Fig. 6.23). The

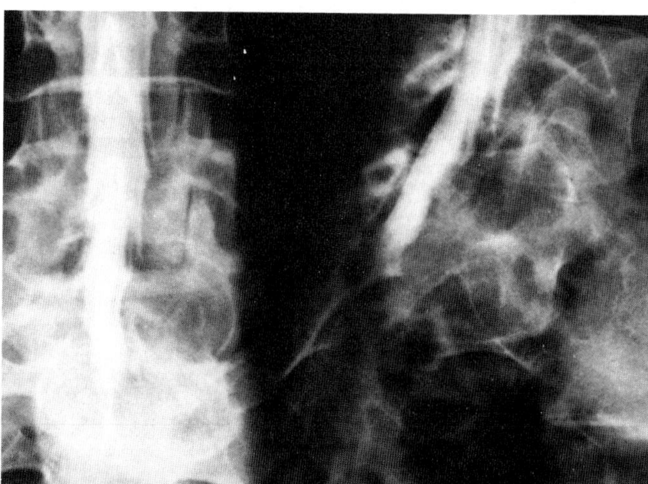

B

Fig. 6.23 Neurofibroma arising in the exit foramen of the first sacral segment. The patient presented with sciatic pain and (**A**) two views from a water soluble radiculogram reveal amputation of the S1 nerve root sheath, displacement of the S1 and S2 roots and a large well-defined rounded radiolucency with sclerotic margins in the exit foramen; **B**. Frontal tomograms confirm a large bony defect (arrow), compared with the normal right foramen.

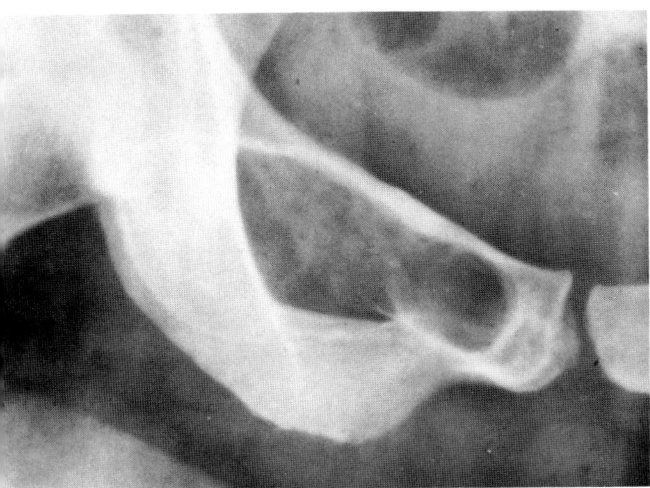

Fig. 6.24 Neurofibroma arising in the obturator ring has caused considerable pressure erosion of both pubic rami, particularly the superior one. The margins of the pressure defect are sharply defined.

width of the interpedicular distance also may be increased. A soft tissue mass projecting through the enlarged foramen is typical of the so-called dumb-bell tumour. Neurofibromas represent the majority of tumours arising within the internal auditory canal. Discrete pressure erosions on the surface of bone may be observed elsewhere in the skeleton (Fig. 6.24) but as these tumours are able to grow away from bone they are usually not symptomatic. Neurofibromas cause notches at the inferior surface of ribs but should not be confused with those in coarctation of the aorta since they vary both in size and in distribution, not principally affecting the fourth to eighth ribs. All erosive lesions are rounded and clearly defined with a discrete sclerotic margin. An axial view or CT, however, may be necessary to demonstrate that they have predominantly a soft tissue origin. Because of the predilection of neurofibromas to arise in nerve roots many appear in the sacrum and are detected during the investigation of low back pain and sciatica (Figs 6.25 and 6.23).

2. NEUROFIBROMATOSIS

Neurofibromatosis is often noticed at birth or soon after. Typical clinical manifestations are café-au-lait spots and multiple cutaneous tumours. Larger soft tissue masses or growth disparities also may become apparent. These include scoliosis, pseudoarthrosis of long bones (particularly the tibia) and hemihypertrophy. Scoliosis, usually of short segment distribution, often occurs in the thoracic spine. In addition numerous abnormalities arise related to the neural canal including generalized dilatation with scalloping of

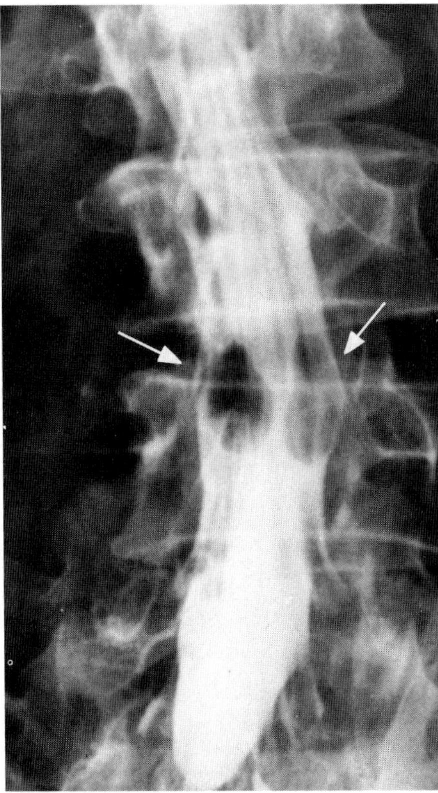

Fig. 6.25 Multiple neurofibromas in the cauda equina. This middle-aged patient was investigated for low back pain by radiculography. Two large ovoid neurofibromas are shown in close relationship to the L4 and L5 roots.

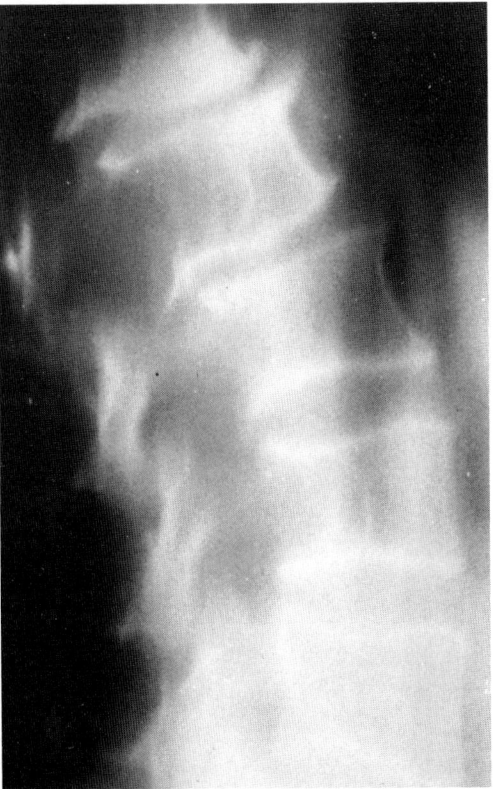

Fig. 6.26 Neurofibromatosis. A lateral tomogram of the lumbar spine demonstrates typical posterior scalloping, part of the general dysplasia of the neural canal and its contents found in this condition.

vertebral bodies (Fig. 6.26), internal meningoceles and dysraphic anomalies (see Ch. 58). Abnormal rib tubulation results in an appearance likened to 'ribbon shaped'. A particularly common abnormality is defective ossification of the posterior superior wall of the orbit. Pseudarthrosis of the tibia is characterized by marked absorption of the fracture margins such that they become pointed (Fig. 6.27). Similar lesions may occur in the radius or clavicle. A number of published reports suggest that malignant sarcomatous change is relatively common, of the order of 5 to 12% of affected patients. The radiological appearances then become that of an infiltrating diffuse destructive process (Fig. 6.28).

Many extraskeletal manifestations of neurofibromatosis occur because of the neuroectodermal and mesodermal derivation of the tissue. Gliomas of the optic nerves, phaeochromocytomas, aneurysms of cerebral and renal arteries, and acoustic neurilemmomas are well recognized. Similarly the incidence of fibrous tumours of bone is increased,

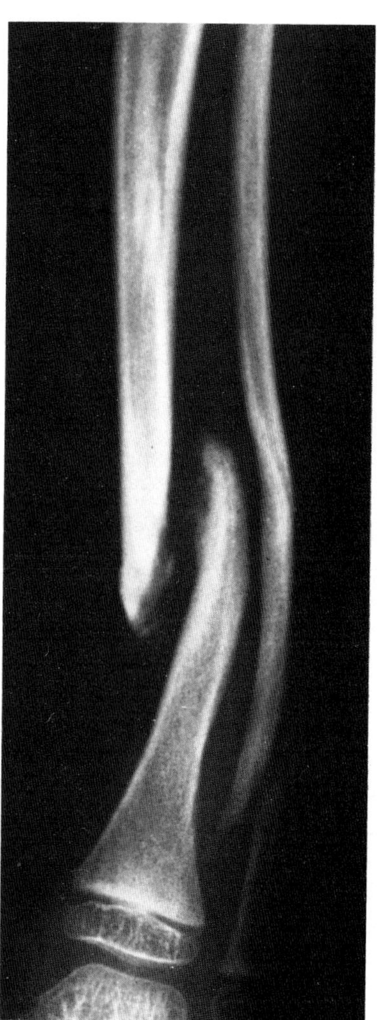

Fig. 6.27 Neurofibromatosis. Pseudoarthroses of the tibia and fibula shown in an infant. Bowing of bone and absence of any evidence of bone repair are typical.

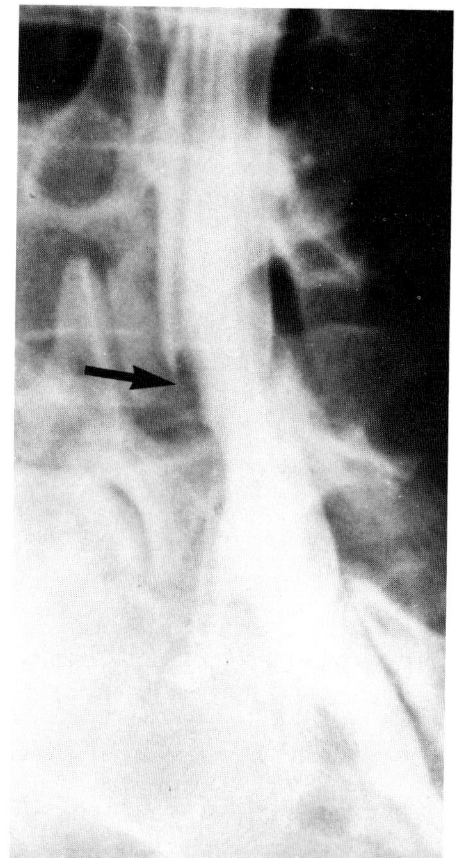

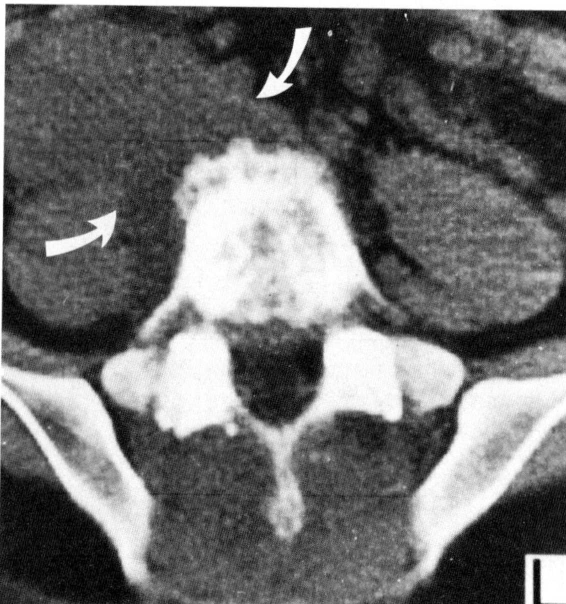

Fig. 6.28 Neurofibrosarcoma. A man in his 40s complained of progressive back and thigh pain. **A**. Water soluble radiculogram demonstrates amputation of L5 root sheath with a rather lobulated indentation of the thecal sac. Preliminary plain films were normal. **B**. CT at the level of L5 demonstrates a soft tissue mass (arrows) displacing and invading the right psoas which, on other sections, was shown to extend into the exit foramen. Osteophyte is present on the vertebral body together with osteoarthritis of the L5–S1 facet joints. L60, W400.

particularly around the knee where radiologically they seem identical to non-ossifying fibromas and fibrous cortical defects.

TUMOURS PRESUMED TO ARISE FROM OTHER TISSUES IN BONE — FATTY TISSUE

1. LIPOMA AND LIPOSARCOMA

Although fat represents one of the normal connective tissue elements within bone, **intra-osseous lipoma** are exceedingly rare. The few that have been observed usually cause an oval lytic lesion within a long bone and bear a distinct resemblance to non-ossifying fibroma (Fig. 6.29). A sharply defined discrete sclerotic margin is associated with bone expansion and trabeculation. Periosteal new bone formation is not a feature. If calcification is present within the lesion then a bone scan may show increased activity. **Parosteal lipomas** on the other hand present a much more characteristic appearance with strands of ossification forming around the radiolucent fatty lobules of this rare tumour (Fig. 6.30). They tend to be very slow in growth and produce minor symptoms. Marked periosteal new bone formation does occur, with an obvious, but well-defined, soft tissue mass.

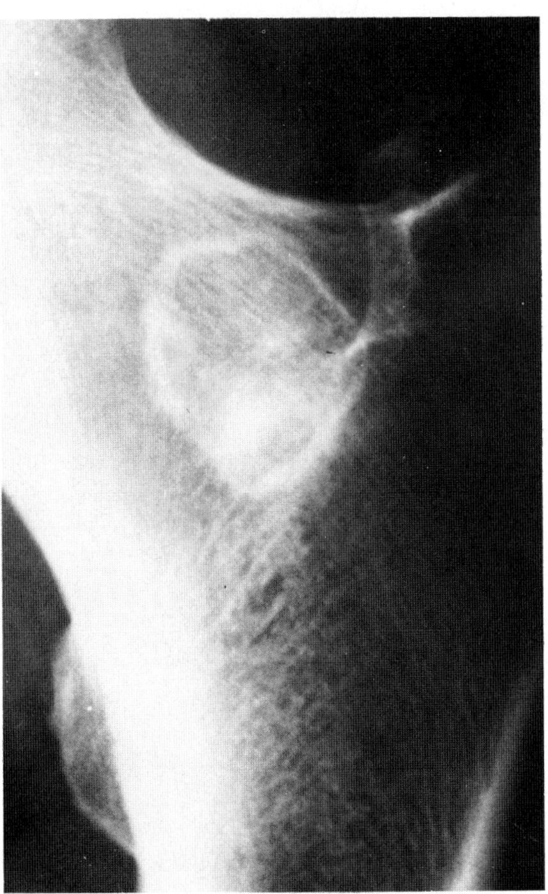

Fig. 6.29 Intra-osseous lipoma. Discovered incidentally in the intertrochanteric region of a young patient. The lesion is oval with sclerotic margins and contains areas of patchy calcification. The appearances cannot be distinguished easily from a benign fibrous tumour or chondroma.

A more aggressive nature, however, must be considered when the soft tissue element fails to contain fatty lucencies possibly indicating the presence of a **parosteal liposarcoma. Intra-osseous liposarcoma** has been described but is exceedingly rare and produces an ill-defined lytic area usually in the femur or tibia, which is extremely vascular either on angiogram or the blood pool phase of a bone scan. Rapid extension into the soft tissues, and early pulmonary metastasis, is usual.

The characteristic radiolucencies of soft tissue **lipomas** are discussed in Chapter 53, and **lipomas** in the lumbar canal are considered in Chapter 58. **Macrodystrophia lipomatosa** is a rare form of localised gigantism of a hand or foot accompanied by an overgrowth of the associated mesenchymal elements, particularly fat.

TUMOURS PRESUMED TO ARISE FROM OTHER TISSUES IN BONE — NOTOCHORD

1. CHORDOMA

The notochord extends, during embryological development, from the coccyx to the buccopharyngeal membrane and is the precursor of the vertebrae and intervertebral discs. Chordoma is a destructive bone tumour believed to arise from notochord cell rests within vertebral bodies. All are locally malignant with a strong tendency to recur after attempted excision even where this has been possible. The lesions are slow growing and become apparent due to pressure symptoms with or without localized pain. The extreme ends of the axial skeleton are involved, approximately half the lesions arising in the sacrum and/or coccyx, the others in the basi-occipital and hypophyseal regions of the skull. A vertebral origin is found only in 15% of patients. Adjacent vertebrae may be involved. A fatal outcome results from a local extension, metastatic spread being unusual.

The usual clinical presentation is of a male patient aged between 40 and 70, the clinical symptoms and signs depending on the site of obstruction. Constipation is often a feature of those arising from the sacrum.

Radiological features. In the sacral area the tumour typically arises in the midline and involves the fourth or fifth sacral vertebrae (Fig. 6.31). The lesion is purely lytic, relatively well-defined, usually being oval or slightly lobulated. It may contain areas of calcification. The sacral margins may occasionally be sclerotic. The soft tissue structures within the pelvis are displaced anteriorly. Tumours arising at the basi-occipital or hypophyseal regions are accompanied by erosion and destruction of the dorsum sellae and clivus. Once again a lobulated or rounded area of bone destruction is associated with a large soft tissue mass displacing nasopharynx anteriorly and sometimes

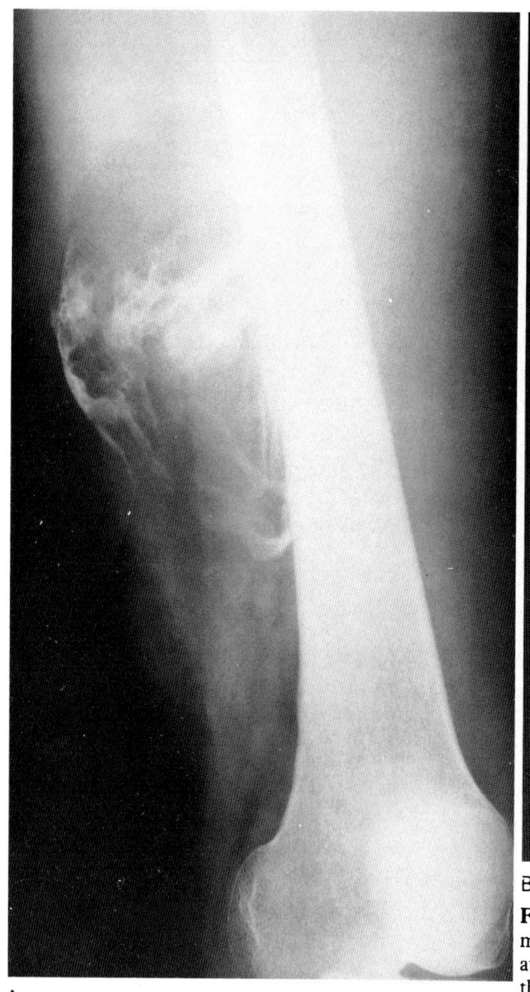
A

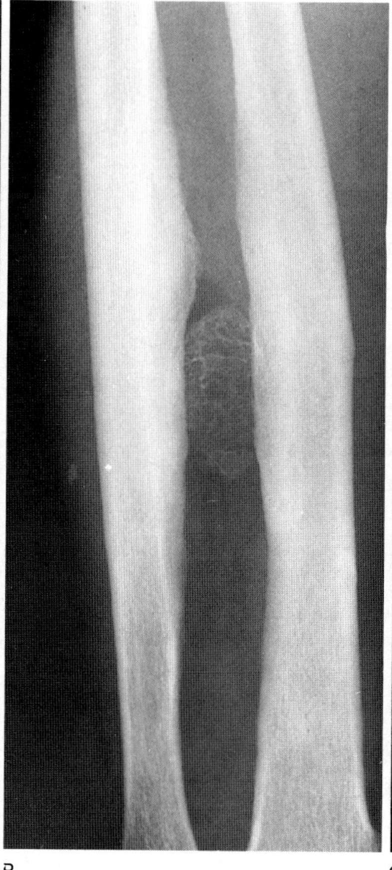
B

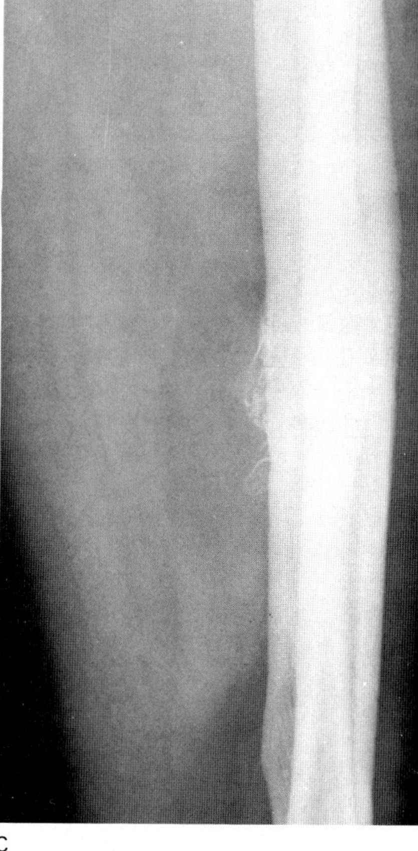
C

Fig. 6.30 Parosteal lipoma. Two examples are shown of parosteal lipomas arising in middle-aged patients. Both presented with a painless, rather firm mass, apparently attached to bone. **A.** A large lesion arising on the lateral aspect of the femur. Note the strands of ossification surrounding the radiolucent areas of fat. **B.** and **C.** A more discrete tumour arises from the interosseous membrane of the forearm. A fatty radiolucency is present together with ossification in the soft tissues and some periosteal new bone formation.

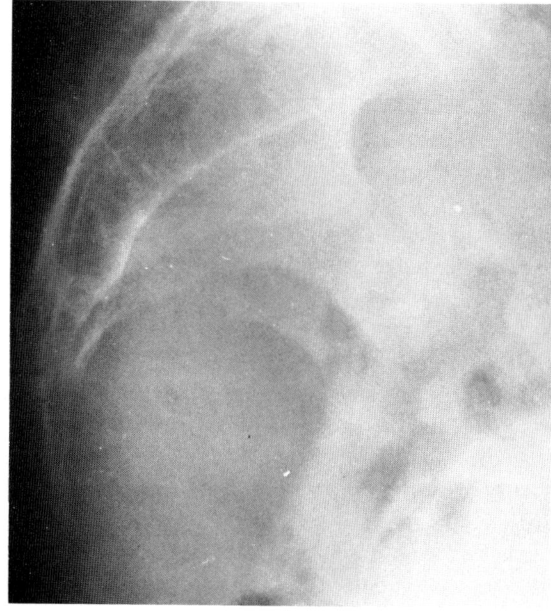
A

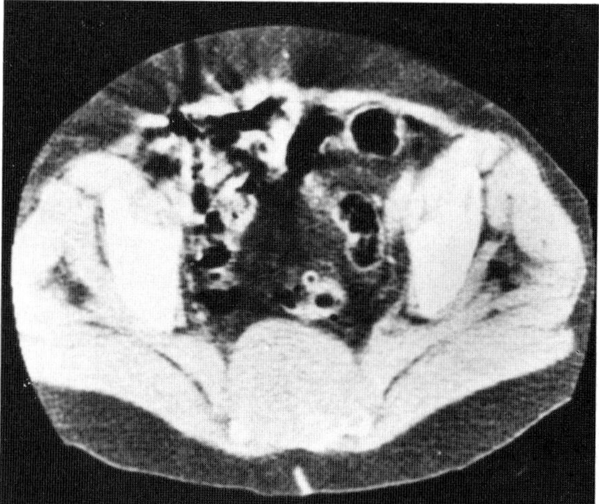
B

Fig. 6.31 Chordoma of the distal sacrum. **A.** A lateral film demonstrates a large soft tissue mass displacing bowel anteriorly. The anterior cortex of the distal sacral vertebrae are ill-defined and the coccyx is not seen;
B. Computerized tomography demonstrates the typical well-defined soft tissue mass extending anteriorly from the sacrum. The anterior cortex of the sacrum has been destroyed. Chordomas usually exhibit an apparent disproportion between the size of the soft tissue mass and the extent of the bony involvement. L20, W200.

containing amorphous calcification. Here the differential diagnosis is from chondrosarcoma whereas in the sacrum the possibility of plasmacytoma should be considered.

TUMOURS PRESUMED TO ARISE FROM OTHER TISSUES IN BONE — EPITHELIAL ORIGIN

IMPLANTATION DERMOID CYSTS

These rare lesions almost always follow a penetrating wound when it is assumed that epithelial cells are carried into the underlying bony structure. Typically they arise in distal phalanges of adolescents or young adults, the left middle finger being the single commonest site. The lesion grows slowly over many years.

Radiologically a well-defined translucency results, with slight expansion and sharply defined margins around which a minimal sclerotic reaction may be visible (Fig. 6.32). Subungual fibromas represent the only serious differential diagnostic possibility. A glomus tumour is almost invariably extra-osseous.

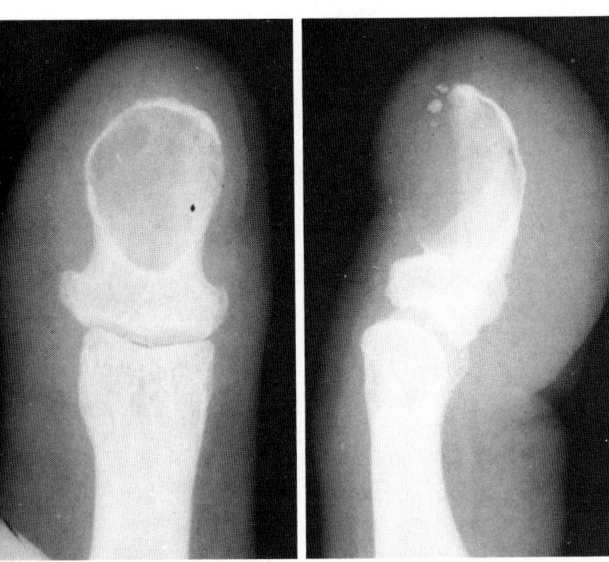

Fig. 6.32 Implantation dermoid cyst. A cystic lesion in the terminal phalanx of the thumb was found in an elderly female many years after a penetrating injury. The sharp definition of its margins and the location of the lesion are characteristic.

TUMOURS RELATED TO JOINTS

1. SYNOVIAL CHONDROMATOSIS
(Osteochondromatosis)

This is a relatively unusual synovial disease, commonly regarded as a benign neoplasm, in which metaplastic cartilage formation occurs throughout the synovium. Typically young and middle-aged adults are affected with a male preponderance and an affinity for large joints, in particular the knee. Minimal pain, swelling and limitation of movement are the usual presenting complaints. Cartilaginous lesions develop throughout the synovium, though mainly in the proliferative layer, later becoming pedunculated and separating into the joint space. When large enough they undergo ossification. This condition undoubtedly progresses in phases, with episodes of intrasynovial disease and the shedding of loose bodies (Fig. 6.33).

In the early stages the only abnormality which may be detected on plain film is an apparent joint effusion. This may be delineated by CT when a slight increase in density may be observed. Arthrography, however, demonstrates not only an irregular, nodular synovium (Fig. 6.34) but also cartilaginous loose bodies. Calcification and ossification of the cartilaginous masses results in numerous oval or rounded opacities often of similar size demonstrated on plain film. Serial examination may show these to be fairly constant in position. Scintigraphy using bone seeking radio-

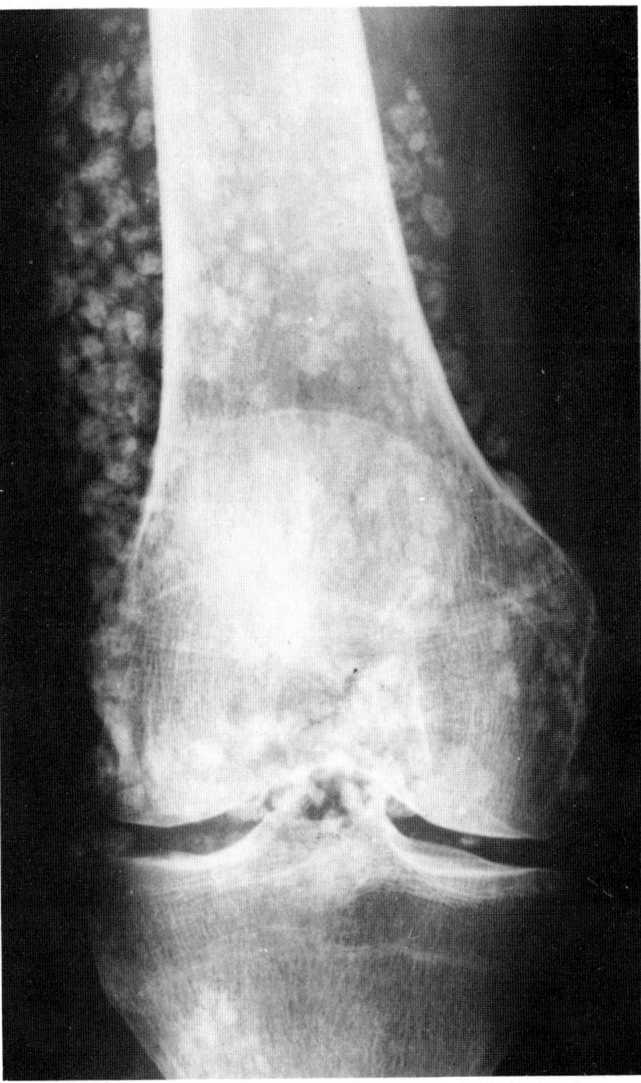

Fig. 6.33 Synovial chondromatosis. Hundreds of calcified lesions are shown in relation to the synovium, all of them approximately the same size. Nearly all were loose bodies.

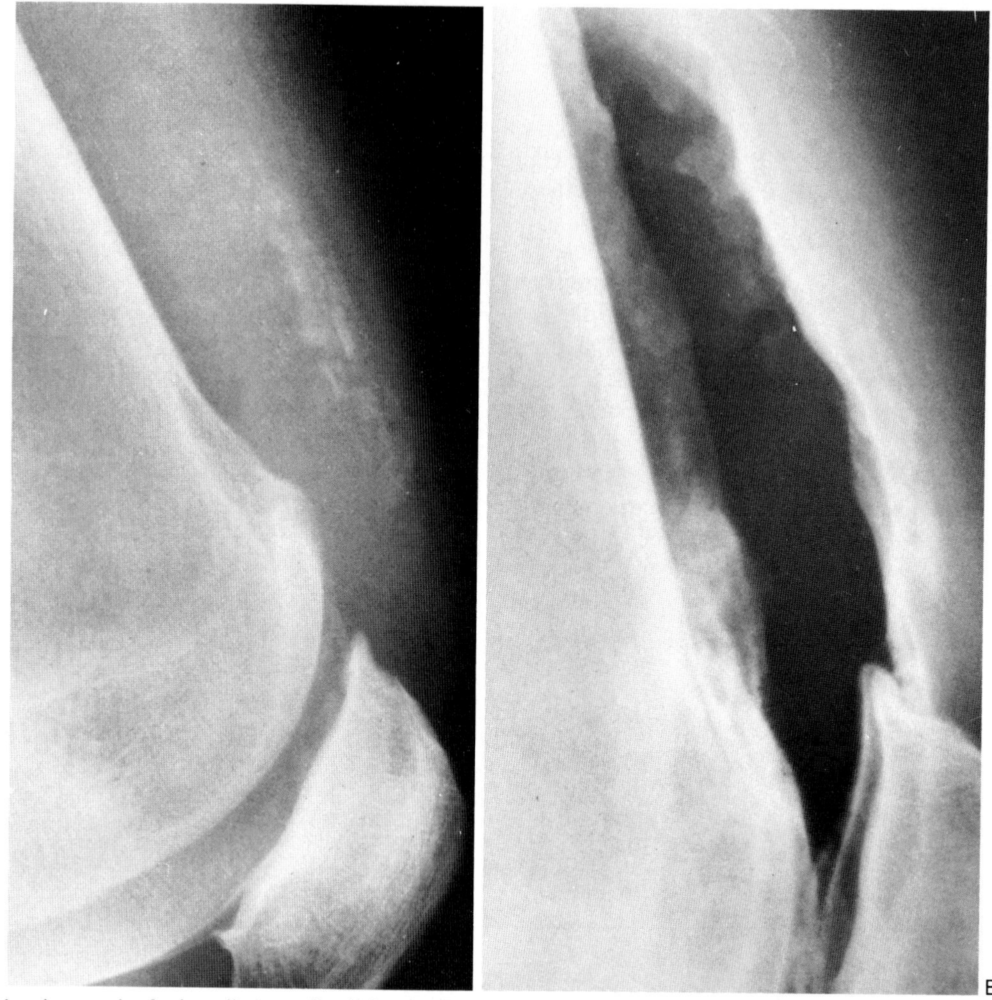

Fig. 6.34 Synovial chondromatosis. **A**. A preliminary film before knee arthrography demonstrates calcification in the thickened suprapatellar pouch. **B**. A localized view of the knee arthrogram demonstrates both nodular synovial thickening and intrasynovial calcification.

pharmaceutical often demonstrates an appreciable increase in activity localized particularly in the larger masses, suggesting that active ossification and calcification are occurring. Eventually extensive capsular distension may result in marginal bony erosions occurring characteristically at the insertion of joint capsule with clearly defined margins. Degenerative arthritis always occurs at a later stage in the evolution of the disease. Synovial chondromatosis also occurs in tendon sheaths and bursae. Chondrosarcoma is an extremely rare occurrence.

2. PIGMENTED VILLONODULAR SYNOVITIS

The aetiology of this uncommon disorder of synovium is still not known. It is generally regarded as a benign neoplasm. The disease may be monoarticular or polyarticular, the latter being very rare. Adolescents and young adults are affected, usually complaining of local pain and swelling, occasionally with cystic masses related to a large joint, usually the knee or hip. Histologically proliferation of villonodular masses of synovial tissue is associated with the deposition of haemosiderin, a feature which may be detected by increased tissue attenuation on CT.

Radiologically synovial thickening usually is evident, particularly with soft tissue exposures. Features which suggest the diagnosis are sharply defined para-articular erosions with sclerotic margins, particularly if these lesions are present on both sides of the affected joint (Fig. 6.35). As in gout integrity of the articular surfaces and preservation of the width of the joint space are maintained until relatively late in the disease. Disuse osteoporosis is not an initial feature. Calcification within the synovial mass is exceedingly rare, unlike malignant synovioma. Arthrographically the thickening of the synovium is confirmed usually being diffuse in larger joints, such as the knee, whereas in small joints, particularly metacarpal phalangeal joints, the thickening is nodular (Fig. 6.36). The synovium of tendon sheaths and bursae also may be affected by this disease (Fig. 6.37).

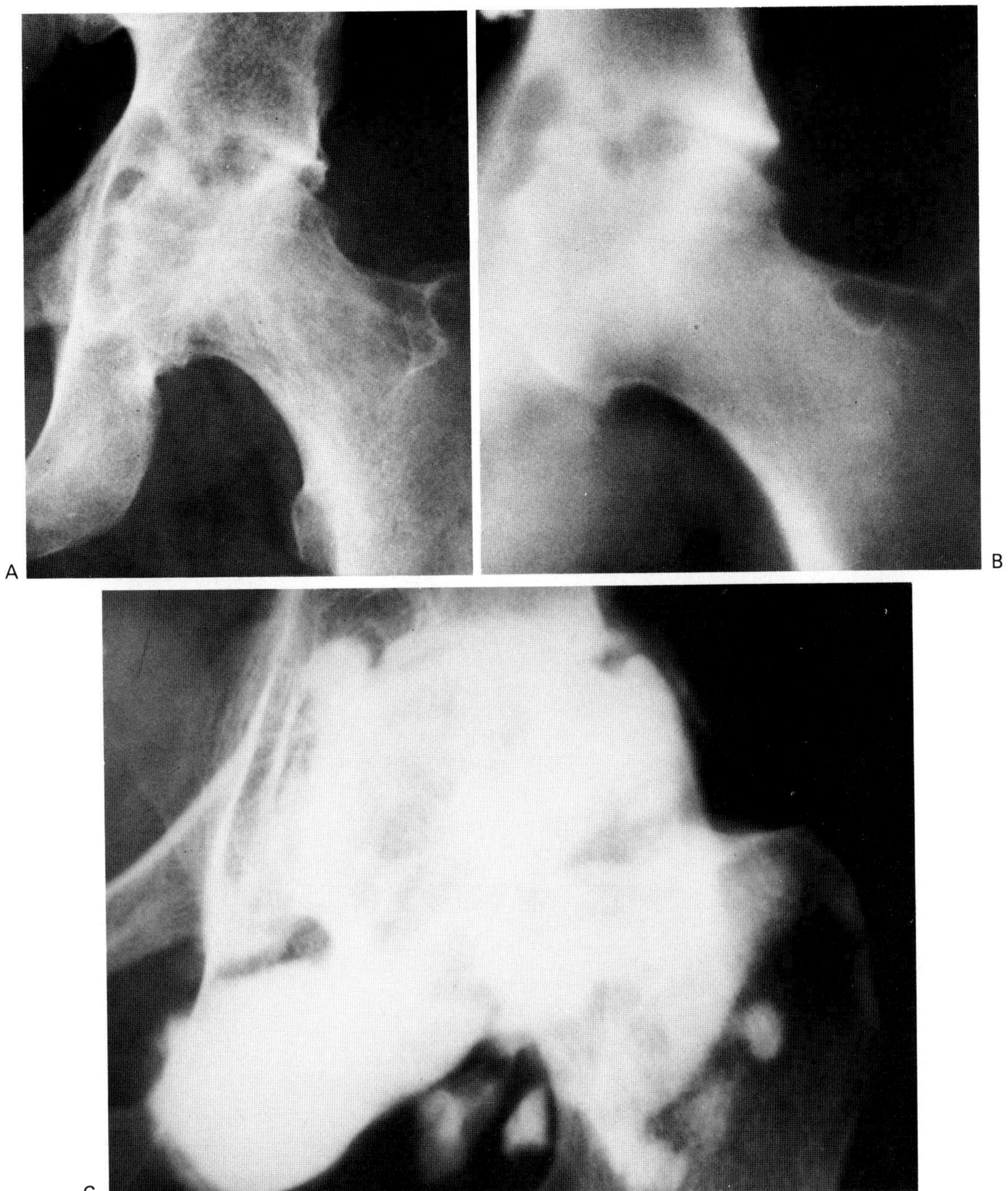

Fig. 6.35 Pigmented villonodular synovitis of the hip. **A**. Plain film illustrates sharply defined radiolucent defects involving the acetabulum and the femoral head and neck. **B**. The sharply defined nature of the lesions is confirmed on tomography. Note the sclerotic margins. This patient has relatively advanced disease and joint space narrowing is present. **C**. A hip arthrogram from another patient demonstrates a capacious hip joint with sacculation extending into the soft tissues and contrast medium outlining defects on the femoral head and acetabulum.

3. SYNOVIOMA

This is a highly malignant tumour growing rapidly with early metastases to lymph nodes, unlike most other musculoskeletal tumours. Young adults are most commonly affected, the mean age being 35. The lesion arises in soft tissue adjacent to synovial structures of joints, tendon sheaths and bursae. 70% of cases involve the lower extremities, particularly around the knee. Clinically a soft tissue mass or ill-defined swelling is present in nearly three quarters of patients, associated with local pain.

Radiologically a soft tissue mass is shown associated with a joint, about one patient in five demonstrating calcification of an amorphous nature. Ossification does not occur unlike the later stages of synovial chondromatosis. About 10% of cases are associated with bone involvement shown radiologically by irregular bone destruction particularly at capsular attachments (Fig. 6.38).

This tumour may occasionally arise in the synovial lining of tendon sheaths producing a similar soft tissue mass. Sec-

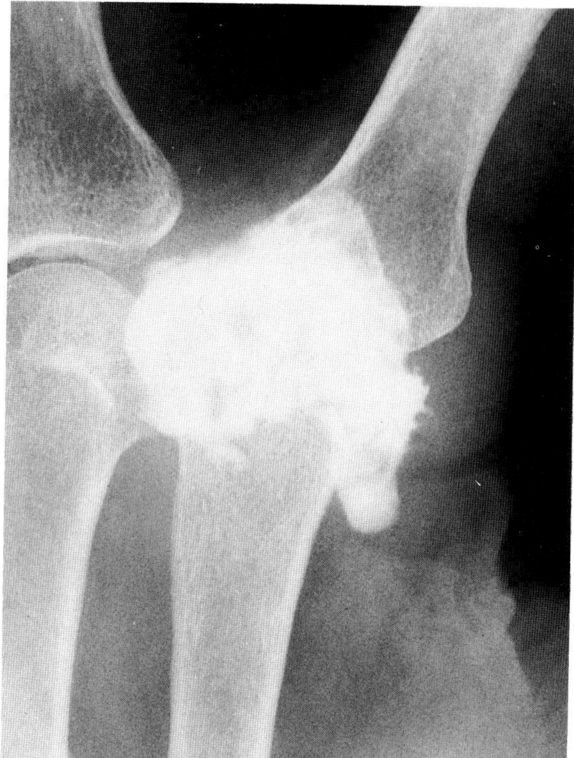

Fig. 6.36 Pigmented villonodular synovitis of the index finger metacarpo-phalangeal joint. An arthrogram confirms an enlarged joint space and thickened nodular synovium.

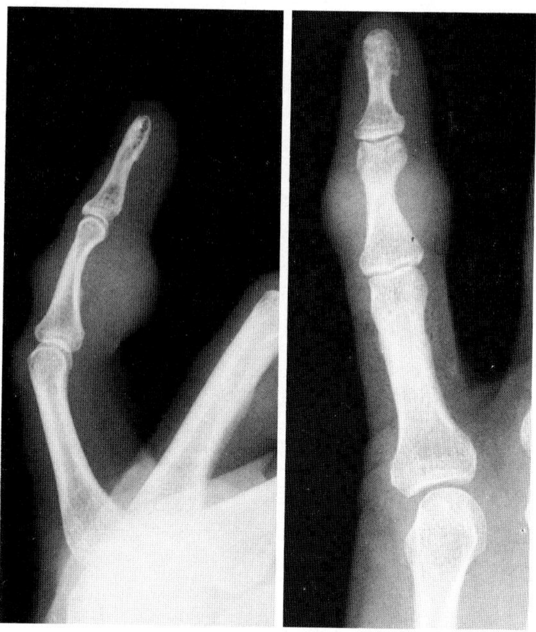

Fig. 6.37 A. and **B.** Pigmented villonodular synovitis of the flexor tendon sheath of the middle finger. A sharply circumscribed soft tissue mass has caused slight pressure erosion of the middle phalanx.

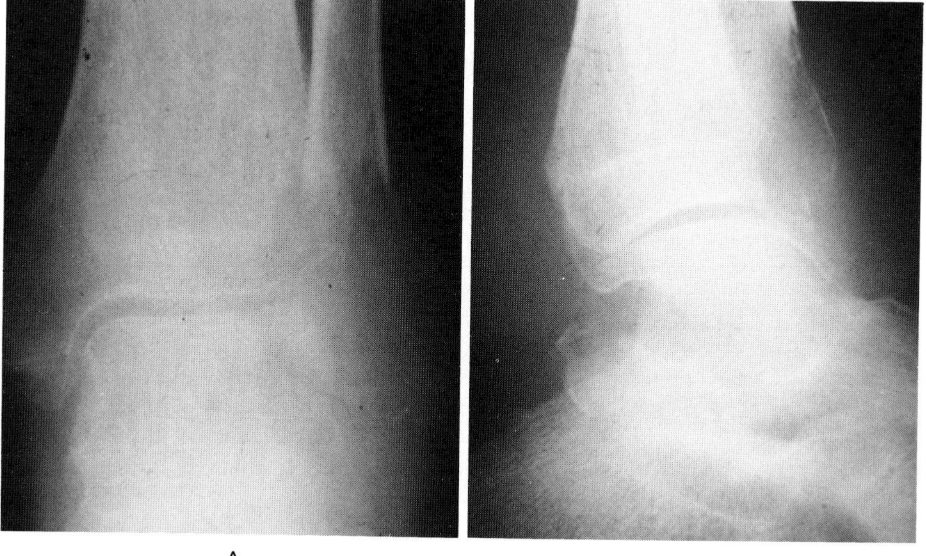

Fig. 6.38 Malignant synovioma of the ankle. Gross synovial thickening was present with hazy erosion of the capsular attachment. **A.** AP view. **B.** Lateral view.

ɩdary involvement of adjacent bone has been observed ɩrticularly in the feet.

4. INTRA-OSSEOUS GANGLION

his is a relatively uncommon lesion representing ganglion aterial within a long tubular bone, the origin of which unclear. Direct communication with a joint is demonrated rarely. It may, on occasions, be shown to extend om an extra-osseous lesion. Clinically patients are between) and 60 years of age and two thirds complain of local int pain often related to exercise. Most commonly the sion occurs in the tibia around the knee or ankle; hips nd carpus are also common sites.

Radiologically an oval or circular eccentric osteolytic leon is shown which is often expansile with a thin sclerotic m. These may appear multilocular varying between –5 cm in size (Fig. 6.39).

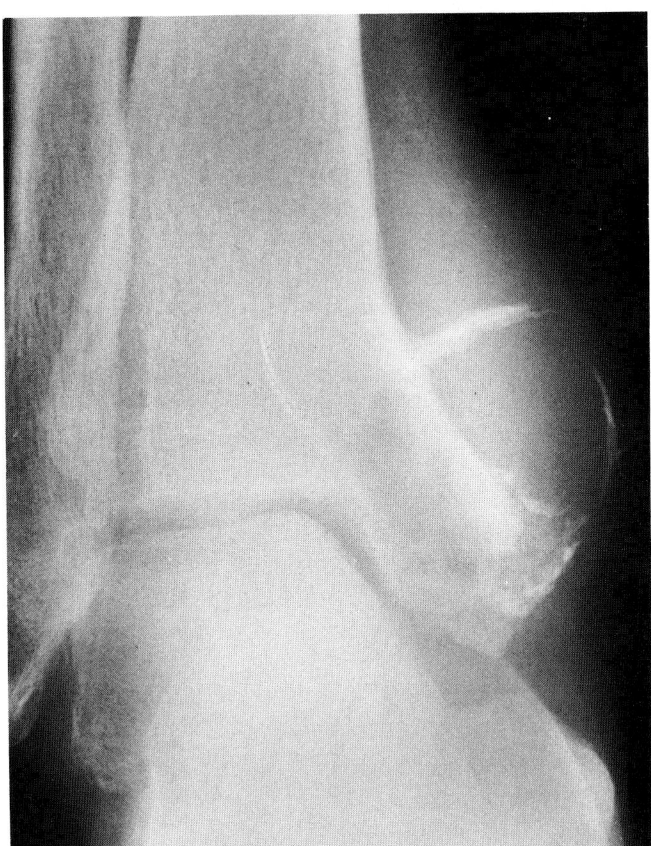

Fig. 6.39 Intra-osseous ganglion. An oval, eccentric, osteolytic lesion arises from the medial malleolus with a thin sclerotic margin.

5. SUBARTICULAR ARTHRITIC CYST AND GEODE

Though not neoplasms these space occupying lesions may ccasionally cause confusion. Described in detail elsewhere Ch. 4) they most usually accompany rheumatoid disase, particularly with secondary degenerative change, oseoarthritis and pyrophosphate arthropathy. The knee and ip are classical sites, the latter may present with a pathoogical fracture. The historical and radiological features f a pre-existing arthropathy should assist the diagnosis toether with their discrete sclerotic margins and close reationship with a joint (Fig. 6.40).

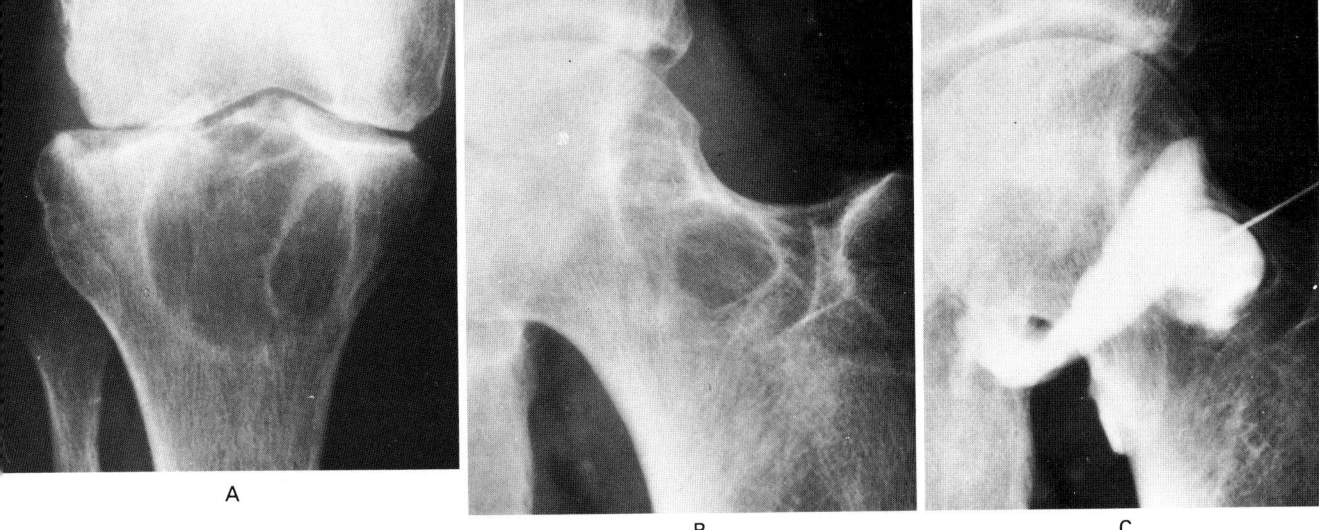

Fig. 6.40 Subarticular geodes. **A.** An elderly lady with rheumatoid arthritis and secondary degenerative arthritis has a typical, large geode immediately beneath the articular surface of the tibia. **B.** A younger man with rheumatoid disease has an oval, well-defined defect in the upper femoral neck. This too has a sclerotic margin. **C.** Aspiration of the defect yielded synovial fluid and injection of contrast medium confirmed communication between the subarticular geode and the joint cavity.

TUMOURS OF NO KNOWN ORIGIN

1. SOLITARY BONE CYST (*Unicameral bone cyst*)

No satisfactory aetiological explanation of this entirely benign lesion is commonly accepted. It seems unlikely that it is a true neoplasm, but is considered here since its diagnosis depends largely on radiological findings which can resemble those of known neoplastic conditions and because of its predilection to recur after treatment.

Solitary bone cysts are always unilocular. The site of origin depends on the patient's age, prior to epiphyseal fusion the majority occur in the proximal humeri and femora (Fig. 6.41). The former being the most usual site. Following skeletal maturation some lesions have been described occurring in such bones as the calcaneus (Fig. 6.42). Solitary bone cysts are commoner in males and develop during skeletal growth. Childhood and early adolescence is therefore the usual time for them to be discovered. More than half present due to a pathological fracture, a few may produce minor discomfort, others are found incidentally.

During the stage of skeletal development the lesion lies close to the metaphysis and often is situated in the midline, extending across the whole shaft. With further skeletal growth normal bone develops between the cyst and metaphysis so that the lesion is seen to be carried further into the diaphysis. Hence those which develop early eventually lie in the middle of the shaft of a bone. The cyst contains clear liquid unless there has been contamination by bleeding following a fracture. It is lined by a thin layer of connective tissue.

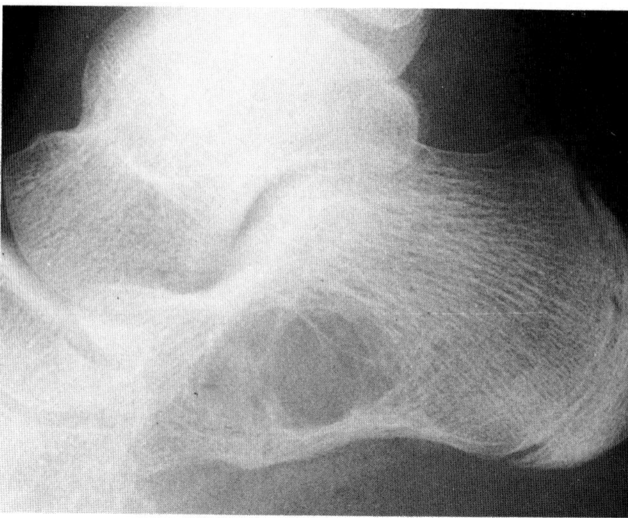

Fig. 6.42 Solitary bone cyst arising in a typical site in the os calcis. The margins in this bone tend to be less well-defined.

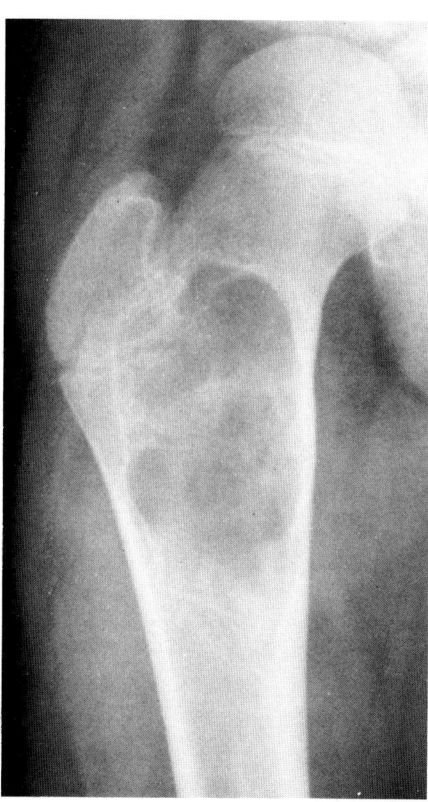

Fig. 6.41 Solitary bone cyst of the proximal femur showing expansion and thinning of the cortex, clearly defined endosteal margins but no calcification or periosteal new bone formation.

Radiologically an area of translucency in the affected metadiaphysis is characteristic. The overlying cortex is often thinned and slightly expanded with no periosteal reaction unless a fracture has occurred. This reaction may be prompted by a minor cortical infarction. The lesion may develop in relation to an apophysis particularly the greater trochanter of the femur. In the earlier stages of growth in the metaphysis cysts tend to have a continuous rounded sharply defined margin on the metaphyseal side but perhaps slightly less demarcation on the diaphyseal side. Sclerotic reaction is usually present around the margin but may be quite discrete. A serpiginous margin may cause the cyst to appear multilocular. As normal bone grows in the metaphysis subsequent examination demonstrates the apparent migration of the lesion along the shaft of the affected bone with an increasing sclerotic reaction around its margins. On bone scanning no abnormality develops in the blood pool phase, in contrast to aneurysmal bone cysts. The delayed image demonstrates increased activity only around the margins of the lesion, unlike fibrous dysplasia (Fig. 6.43). The only serious differential diagnostic possibility is a chondroma, but no calcification occurs in a simple bone cyst unless callus has formed from a fracture.

The prognosis depends partly on the patient's age. Before the age of 10 recurrences are frequent whereas after that age primary healing usually occurs even after fractures. Because of the risk of pathological fracture the majority of patients are treated by curettage and packing with bone chips. Some lesions have been reported to regress satisfactorily after injection with steroids.

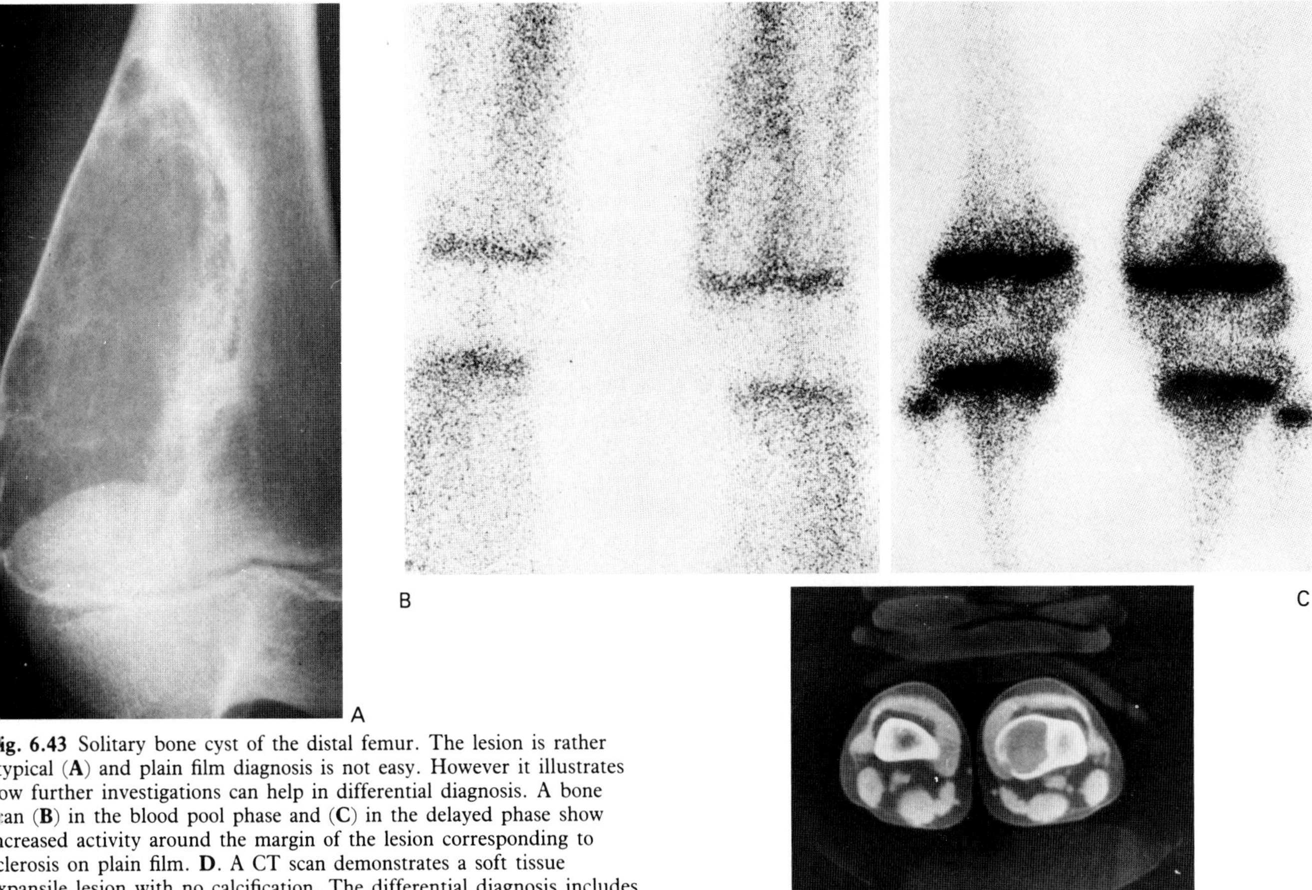

ig. 6.43 Solitary bone cyst of the distal femur. The lesion is rather typical (A) and plain film diagnosis is not easy. However it illustrates ow further investigations can help in differential diagnosis. A bone an (B) in the blood pool phase and (C) in the delayed phase show ıcreased activity around the margin of the lesion corresponding to clerosis on plain film. D. A CT scan demonstrates a soft tissue xpansile lesion with no calcification. The differential diagnosis includes neurysmal bone cyst, fibrous dysplasia (monostotic) and a chondroma. neurysmal bone cyst is vascular in the blood pool phase of a bone can, fibrous dysplasia markedly so on the delayed scan. Calcification ıay be expected on CT in a chondroma. L40, W400.

2. EWING'S SARCOMA — MALIGNANT ROUND CELL TUMOURS

group of highly malignant tumours involving bone is haracterized histologically by numerous small round cells. Vithin this group are included Ewing's sarcoma, metatatic neuroblastoma, non-Hodgkin's lymphoma and undifferentiated tumours. Pathological distinction may be xtremely difficult, even with the benefit of electron microscopy and histochemical techniques. In the final analysis he differentiation may depend on histological classification n spite of its difficulties and shortcomings. It is clear that hese entities show considerable overlap, but Ewing's arcoma is sufficiently distinctive to require definitive lescription.

Clinically pain of several weeks or months duration is ccompanied by localized tender swelling. The majority of patients are between 5 and 30 years of age. This rapidly progressive malignant tumour is characterized by pyrexia, anaemia and a raised ESR. These clinical symptoms and signs may simulate closely osteomyelitis but occur also in non-Hodgkin's lymphoma (reticulum cell sarcoma). It should be emphasised that the child with a Ewing's tumour is ill, in contrast to those with such benign lesions as eosinophilic granuloma which may cause similar radiological appearances. Histologically the malignant round cells typically contain glycogen granules. The lesion is most often found in a long bone, the diaphysis being more commonly affected than a metaphysis. In about 40% of cases, however, the axial skeleton is involved, particularly the pelvis and ribs. No bone is exempt. Metastatic spread occurs early to lungs and to other bones where the radiological and histological findings are virtually identical. The time delay between the discovery of the primary lesion and the development of secondary deposits suggest that this tumour does indeed originate in bone, unlike some other malignant round cell tumours.

Radiologically the appearances are inconclusive. The lesion is essentially destructive, ill-defined and principally involves the medullary cavity. Cortical erosions and overlying periosteal reactions occur early, indeed a periosteal reaction may be the only sign of abnormality (Figs 6.44

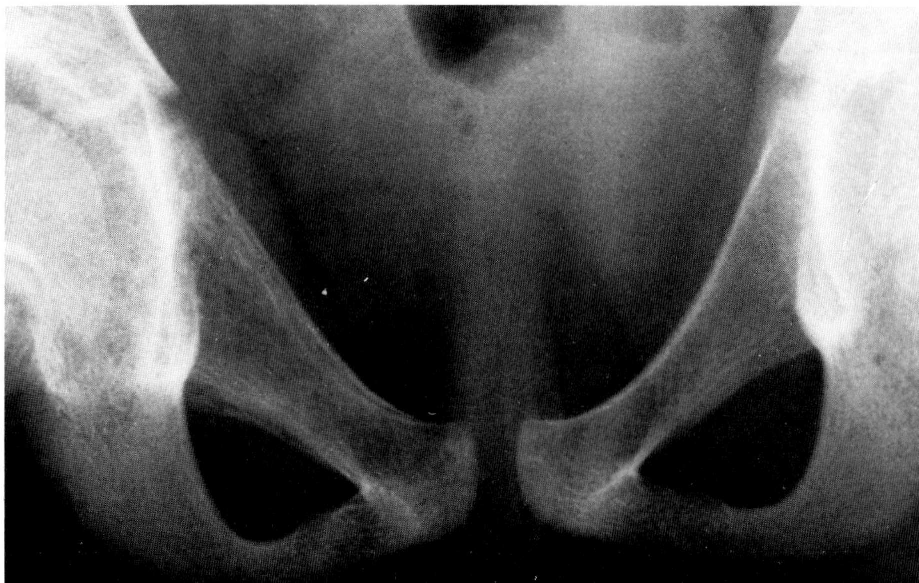

Fig. 6.44 Ewing's sarcoma. The only abnormal sign here is of lamellar periosteal new bone arising from the superior pubic ramus on the right.

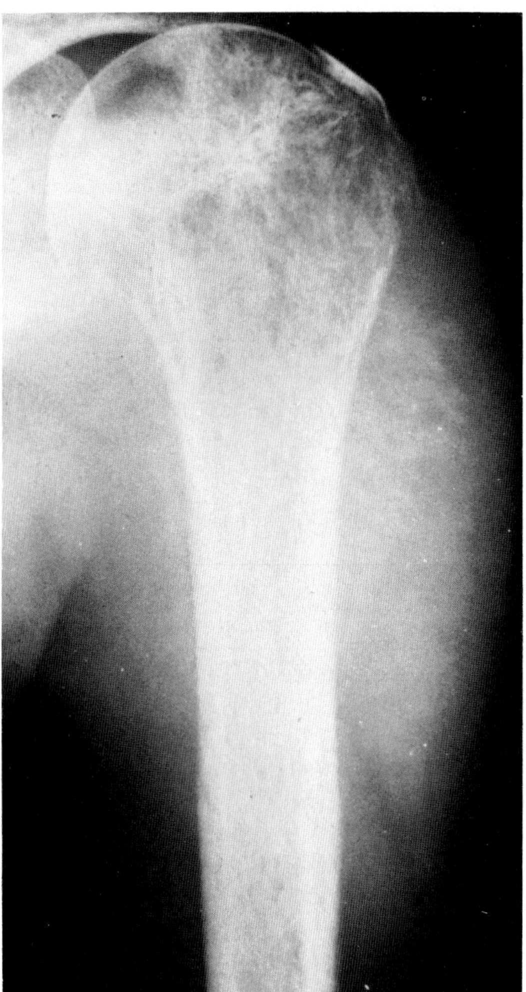

Fig. 6.45 Ewing's sarcoma. This tumour is much more advanced with a well-defined soft tissue mass, Codman's triangles, ossification and calcification in the soft tissues and ill-defined bony destruction. The radiological distinction from osteosarcoma is difficult.

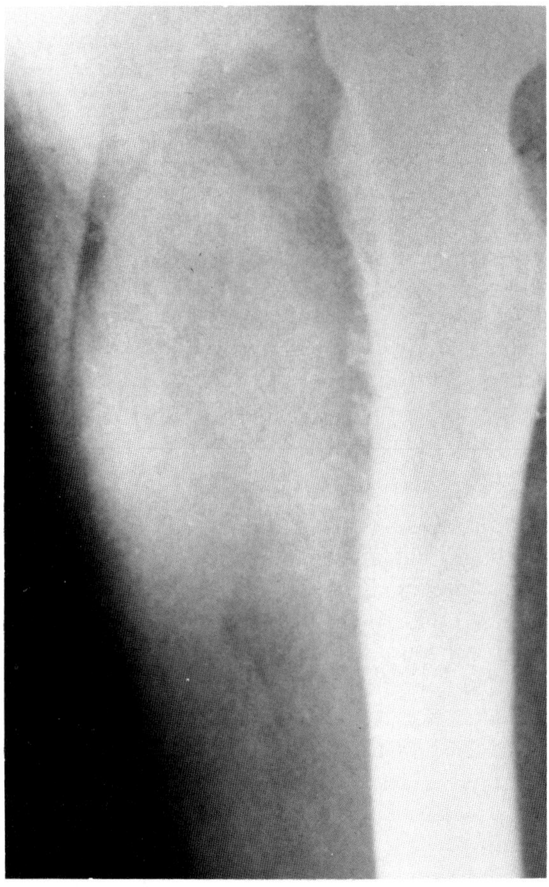

Fig. 6.46 Ewing's sarcoma arising primarily in the soft tissues of the thigh. A well-marked erosion ('saucerization') defect has been caused with periosteal new bone formation.

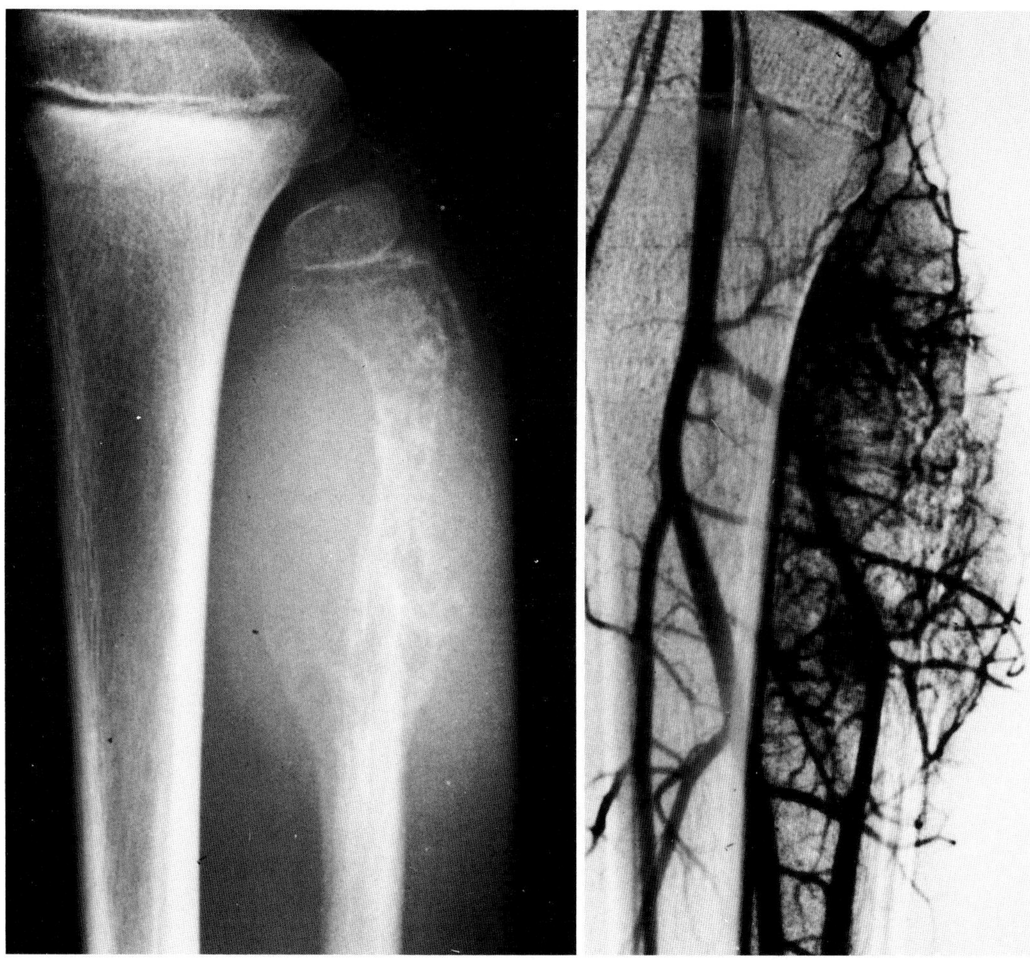

Fig. 6.47 Ewing's sarcoma of bone arising in the proximal fibula of an -year-old. A. An advanced tumour is shown on plain films, with Codman's triangles, a soft tissue mass and ill-defined bone destruction. B. The subtraction print of femoral arteriogram demonstrates a very abnormal circulation with a large soft tissue mass. C. A bone scan, in the delayed phase, demonstrates increased activity where new bone formation is present on plain films. The lesion itself is photon deficient. Osteosarcoma may present similar appearances.

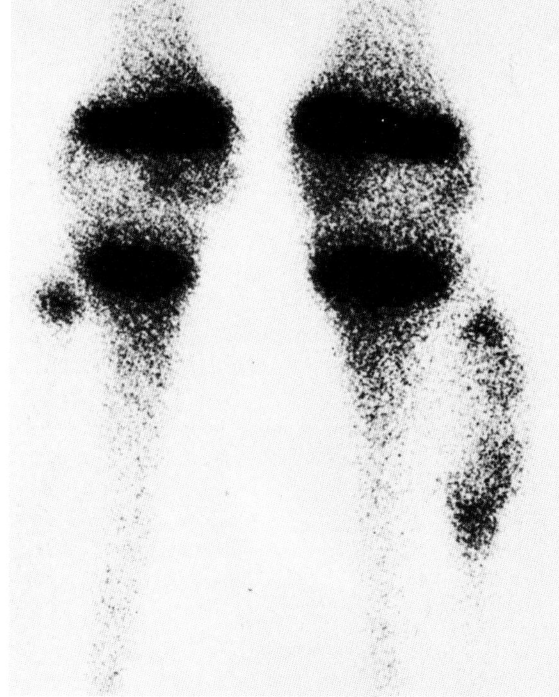

and 6.45). Although the onion-peel lamellar type of periosteal reaction is classically associated with this lesion it is observed only infrequently. Onion-peel periosteal reaction occurs in many other lesions, including osteosarcoma and infection. Elevation of periosteal new bone at the margins of cortical erosions (Codman triangles), may emphasize the shallow cortical erosions; known as 'saucerization' defects they offer a highly suspicious diagnostic feature (Fig. 6.46). The tumour is highly vascular and grows rapidly. Angiographically the extensive soft tissue component and abnormal circulation is obvious (Fig. 6.47). The blood pool phase of a bone scan also demonstrates increased vascularity, but, in the delayed phase, an increase in activity is evident only at the margins of the tumour with bone and in periosteal new bone. These modalities and CT are

necessary to delineate the soft tissue extent of the tumour, which often is much greater than may be appreciated on plain films. A whole body isotope bone scan is also of value in detecting recurrences and metastases. The differential diagnosis may be difficult. Osteosarcoma may present almost identical radiological features and benign conditions; histiocytosis and aggressive osteomyelitis (particularly from *Staphylococcus*) require consideration.

REFERENCES AND SUGGESTIONS FOR FURTHER READING

See end of Chapters 7.

CHAPTER 7

DISORDERS OF THE LYMPHORETICULAR SYSTEM AND OTHER HAEMOPOIETIC DISORDERS

This important group of disorders is responsible for some of the most bizarre radiological abnormalities encountered in the skeleton and may be subdivided conveniently into diseases affecting:

1. the red blood cells
2. the white blood cells
3. the lymphoreticular system, and
4. the coagulation mechanism.

DISEASES PRIMARILY INVOLVING RED BLOOD CELLS

In the infant, the tissue responsible for the formation of red blood cells extends throughout the medullary cavities of the whole skeleton. During the first few months of life these cells are also produced by the spleen and liver, this function being described as *extramedullary erythropoiesis*. The physiological requirement for erythrocyte production diminishes progressively during the years of growth and the corresponding redundancy of erythroblastic tissue is met firstly by a cessation of this function in the liver and spleen and secondly by a regression of the red marrow areas in the peripheral skeleton. By the age of 20 years, this activity is normally confined to the proximal ends of the femora and humeri and to the axial skeleton, consisting of the spine, the thoracic cage, the diploic space of the skull and the shoulder and pelvic girdles. The residual areas of fatty non-haematopoietic marrow in the appendicular skeleton, as well as the liver and spleen, may be reactivated to their original function should the need arise. Such a response occurs normally after a severe haemorrhage, but these episodes are insufficiently prolonged to cause radiological changes.

Chronic haemolytic anaemias, however, in which red blood cells suffer extensive destruction, are followed in many instances by such a degree of marrow hyperplasia that striking skeletal abnormalities result. The great majority of these diseases are congenital and hereditary in origin. The red blood cells are abnormal in shape, in fragility and in the type of haemoglobin which they contain. The clinical picture is that of any chronic anaemia. Dyspnoea, pallor, fatigue and weakness are often accompanied by jaundice due to the circulating end-products of erythrocyte destruction. If extramedullary haematopoiesis occurs, the liver and spleen may be enlarged, particularly the latter, and especially when the anaemia is profound. Cardiac enlargement may occur and result in cardiac failure, many of the more severely affected patients dying before puberty.

Radiological changes in the skeleton, resulting from marrow hyperplasia, vary greatly with the severity of the affection. In children, where much or all of the marrow has a haematopoietic function, the changes are widespread and are usually demonstrated most easily in the extremities and the skull. To some degree, such hyperplasia of the marrow takes place at the expense of destruction of many of the medullary trabeculae. This process is followed by thinning and expansion and even perforation of the overlying cortex. In many of the affected patients this hyperplasia achieves its compensatory object, so that a state of erythrocytic balance is reached. The areas of bone destruction then become the scene of attempted repair, firstly by formation of fibrous tissue and secondly by the development of reactive bone sclerosis. The latter thickens the remaining trabeculae and, in some instances, the endosteal aspect of the cortex, to produce an overall increase in bone density. As age advances, the peripheral bones, now in a state of balance, tend to revert to a normal appearance, but some residual increase of density may remain as a permanent stigma. Evidence of continued erythropoiesis to a greater degree than normal, is confined then to the physiological red marrow areas.

Extramedullary haematopoiesis, in addition to producing evidence of hepatosplenomegaly, may be revealed by the presence of sharply defined paravertebral soft tissue masses of haematopoietic tissue around the thoracic spine (Fig. 7.1).

THALASSAEMIA (*Cooley's anaemia*)

Described by Cooley in 1927, this condition, which means literally 'anaemia of the sea' is known also as *Mediterranean anaemia*, but it is by no means confined to the Mediter-

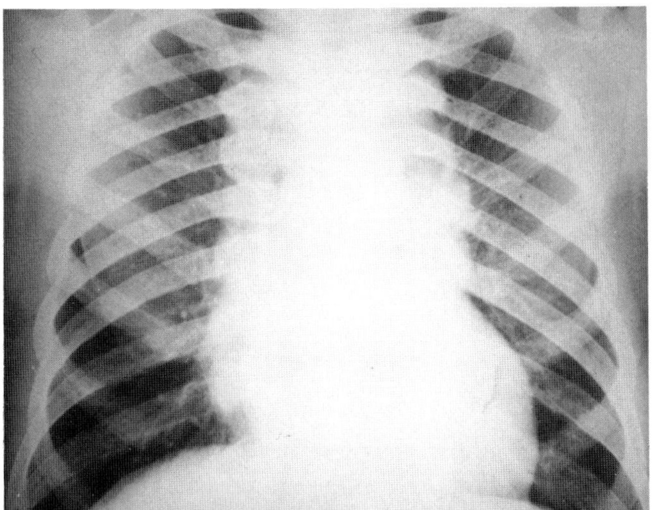

Fig. 7.1 Thalassaemia. Rounded soft-tissue masses due to extramedullary haematapoiesis are present adjacent to the thoracic spine.

ranean countries nor to the races of that region. Its geographical distribution extends eastwards in a broad band through Asia and it is also encountered in West Africa. In such areas the entity is observed sufficiently frequently to be commonplace. It may be encountered anywhere in the world in individuals having a heredity originating from these areas.

The disease is due to abnormalities of the haemoglobin molecule of which many have been established by electrophoresis. Homozygous subjects, who have inherited the trait from both parents, develop the more severe form of the disease, known clinically as *thalassaemia major*, whereas heterozygous subjects, of whom one parent alone carries the trait, develop a minor form. Both forms, however, may vary greatly in severity, so that distinction between them and other haematological variants is of relatively little radiological importance. Severe forms usually become manifest in the first two years of life. Although the majority of these patients die before puberty, some survive to early adult life. Those with less severe disease live correspondingly longer and minimal manifestations may be found only by examination of the blood of individuals who otherwise appear entirely normal. The important clinical features, in addition to those of other anaemias, are dwarfing, delay in development of secondary sexual characteristics, and either 'mongoloid' or 'rodent' facies due to expansion of the underlying facial bones as a consequence of erythroblastic hypertrophy.

Radiological changes. Hyperplasia of the marrow destroys many of the medullary trabeculae and expands and thins the overlying cortex. In children this process is evident especially in the *hands*, when the shafts of the phalanges and metacarpals become biconvex instead of being biconcave (Fig. 7.2). The *feet* are affected in the same way.

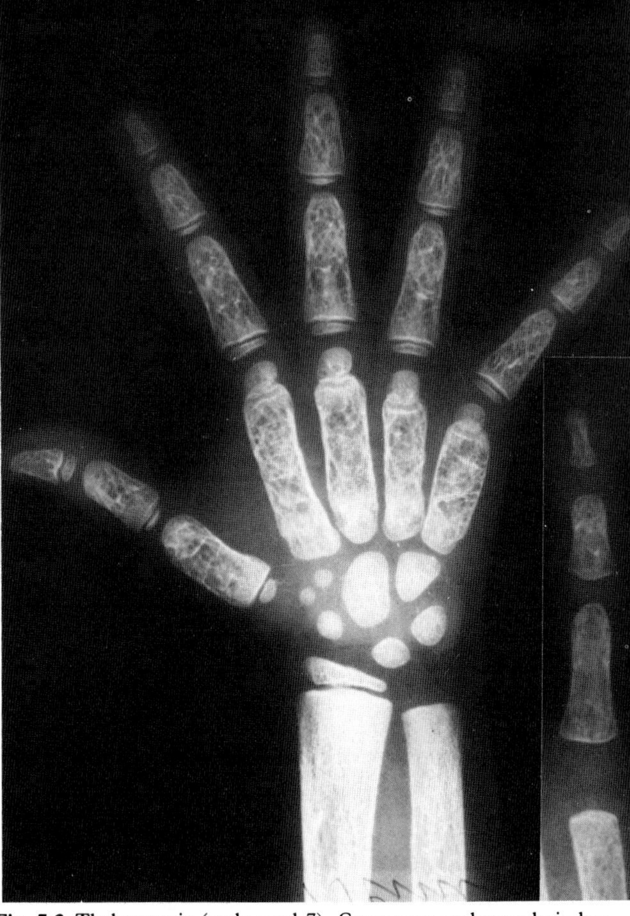

Fig. 7.2 Thalassaemia (male aged 7). Gross marrow hyperplasia has expanded and thinned overlying cortical bone. Medullary trabeculae have been destroyed and the residual ones are coarsened. **Inset** — earl changes of the same type in a finger of a child aged 4.

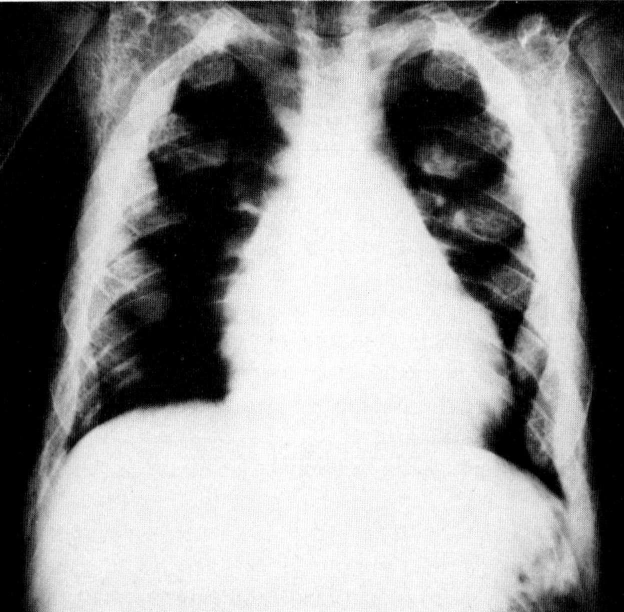

Fig. 7.3 Thalassaemia (male aged 15). A chest film shows gross expansion of bone structures due to marrow hyperplasia. Note particularly involvement of the ribs and scapulae.

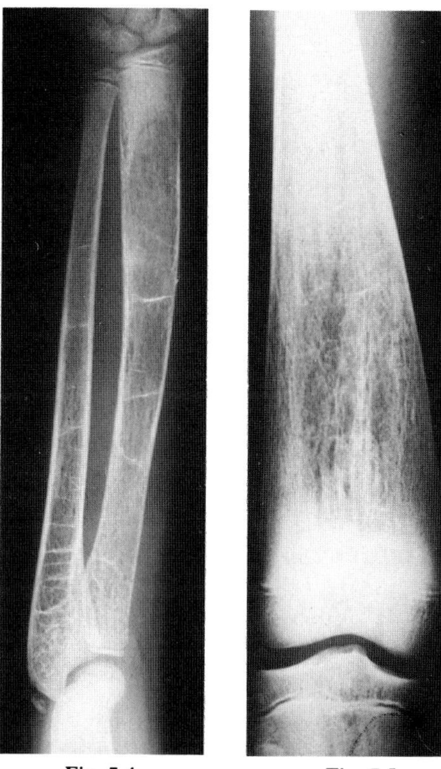

Fig. 7.4 Fig. 7.5

ig. **7.4** Thalassaemia. Considerable bone expansion, cortical thinning nd simplification of trabecular pattern is demonstrated in the forearm f a boy of 15.

ig. **7.5** Thalassaemia. Considerable marrow expansion has produced a ask shape of the distal femur. The coarsened trabecular pattern and ortical thinning are obvious.

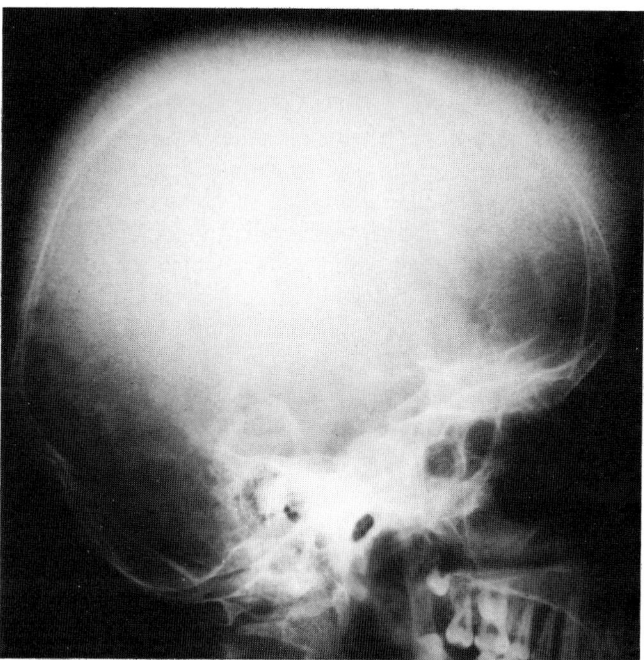

Fig. 7.6 Thalassaemia. Thickening of the outer table of the skull in the frontal area with perpendicular striation — the 'hairbrush sign'.

imilar abnormalities in the *ribs* (Fig. 7.3) and *long bones* Fig. 4.7) may produce apparent failure of modelling with, or example, flask-shaped femora (Fig. 7.5). In the *skull* he diploic space is widened and gross thinning of the outer able may be followed by marked diploic thickening, starting in the frontal region, but usually exempting the occipital bone in which the marrow content is minimal Fig. 7.6). The classical appearance of the 'hairbrush' spicles, is in fact relatively uncommon. These changes appear considerably later than those in the short bones of the xtremities. Development of the air spaces of the skull, specially the maxillary antra and the mastoids, is impaired nd even suppressed as a result of hyperplasia of the marow, accounting for the clinical manifestation of 'rodent' acies, with mal-occlusion of the teeth. The *spine* shows nly diffuse demineralization with the same generalized oarsened trabecular pattern as that observed in the appendicular skeleton. Vertebral collapse is distinctly ncommon.

Osseous abnormalities of this type may be observed also n a number of lesser forms of thalassaemia and its variants, including those associated with other abnormal haemoglobins and the sickle cell trait. In all these conditions, however, the changes tend to be very much less prominent than in thalassaemia major.

SICKLE CELL DISEASE

This chronic haemolytic anaemia is also congenital and hereditary in origin. The erythrocytes, when in a state of hypoxia, become quite abnormal in shape, being unusually long and slender. The abnormal haemoglobin which they contain has a reduced oxygen-carrying capacity. The disease occurs almost exclusively in Black races, especially those in Central Africa or their descendants, who are homozygous for the sickling trait. This trait may be crossed with normal haemoglobin, with abnormal haemoglobins (of which there are several) or with thalassaemia. In these crossed types, the patient is usually less severely affected both clinically and radiologically. Differentiation of the true homozygous state from the variants (of which combination with haemoglobin C is the most common) is of some importance. The former group rarely survive after the age of 30, whereas the latter may have a normal lifespan. The former are characterized clinically by early onset of the severe anaemic picture with frequent skeletal and abdominal crises. These acutely painful episodes, lasting for several days, are due essentially to infarction, attributed to vascular blockage by collections of erythrocytes which have undergone sickling in areas of capillary stasis with resultant hypoxia. The exact mechanism, however, is not finally established but it is suspected that increased viscosity causes stasis with subsequent thrombosis and infarction. Such infarcts may affect many systems. For example, haematuria may occur when a kidney is affected. The fundamental skeletal abnormalities consist of hyperplasia of the marrow with superimposition of areas of necrosis of bone due to infarction and subsequent growth disparities. A further clinical complication, not uncommon in Central Africa, is the development of infection within these infarcts, particularly in lesions developing in the long bones of children.

Radiological changes. The pathological processes occurring in this chronic haemolytic state are reflected by the development of characteristic and diagnostic radiological abnormalities, affecting primarily the erythropoietic skeleton, but also the soft tissues involved by extramedullary haematopoiesis. The frequency with which abnormalities are discovered increases with age. All variants of sickle cell disease produce essentially similar radiological abnormalities.

1. *Marrow hyperplasia* is fundamental, as in any of these haemolytic disorders. In this disease, however, the effects on the skeleton, which are so prominent in thalassaemia major, occur in a very modified form. Sickle cell disease, indeed, even in its worst clinical manifestations, is less severe than thalassaemia major. A generalized osteoporotic appearance is evident throughout the haematopoietic areas of the skeleton, but even in infants and children it is recognized more easily in the axial than the peripheral skeleton. This feature alone is not diagnostic, but, if observed in a Black child, should arouse suspicion of the disorder. Unlike severe thalassaemia, significant modelling abnormalities are uncommon so that the air spaces of the paranasal sinuses are rarely affected. The diploic space of the skull may be widened with consequent bossing. If, as commonly occurs, a state of erythrocytic balance is achieved, diffuse trabecular thickening is likely to develop. Such an appearance may be disclosed incidentally in an adult sickle cell trait carrier in whom the disease has never been symptomatic. In more advanced cases, diagnostic suspicion aroused by this coarse medullary pattern is enhanced by another reactive process. The vascular channels of bone, especially in proximal or middle phalanges, enlarge.

2. *Endosteal apposition of bone.* This inward cortical thickening, representing another response to the disorder of the marrow, is separated occasionally by a thin zone of translucency to result in the appearance in the long bones of 'a bone within a bone'. This sign may be observed in other conditions including Gaucher's disease (q.v.). The medullary cavities, in severe cases, ultimately may be grossly narrowed and almost obliterated, so that a diffuse and generalized increase in bone density results. In the adult, these changes virtually suppress evidence of marrow hyperplasia. To this the bone of the axial skeleton, the spine, pelvis and skull — being persistent red marrow areas — provide notable exceptions, since they remain porotic from childhood into adult life, thus providing an important diagnostic feature, even in the absence of other signs.

3. *Infarction of bones* provides the diagnostic hallmark of this disease. As explained above, infarction of various tissues may be caused by sickling of the erythrocytes during phases of hypoxia and is considered to be the cause of the classical, clinical episodes of sickle cell crises. Unlike thalassaemia, in which infarction is virtually unknown, this type of involvement of the skeleton is common. The consequent radiological abnormalities are comparable to those observed in other systemic disorders such as dysbaric osteonecrosis (caisson disease) and Gaucher's disease. Such infarcts are usually multiple and most commonly affect the femoral and humeral heads (Fig. 7.7), in particular the medullary bone contained within them. Medullary infarcts may be of two varieties, either those with sharply defined margins or those producing diffuse sclerosis. In their mildest form they may be recognized even in an asymptomatic patient. The classical 'snowcap' sign refers to the subarticular area of increased density, particularly in a humeral head, which reflects the revascularization of an area of bone which has been necrotic (Fig. 7.8). At this phase of development bone scans are usually abnormal with increased activity. However, in acute infarction, within 24 hours of the insult, a photon deficiency often is present (Fig. 7.9).

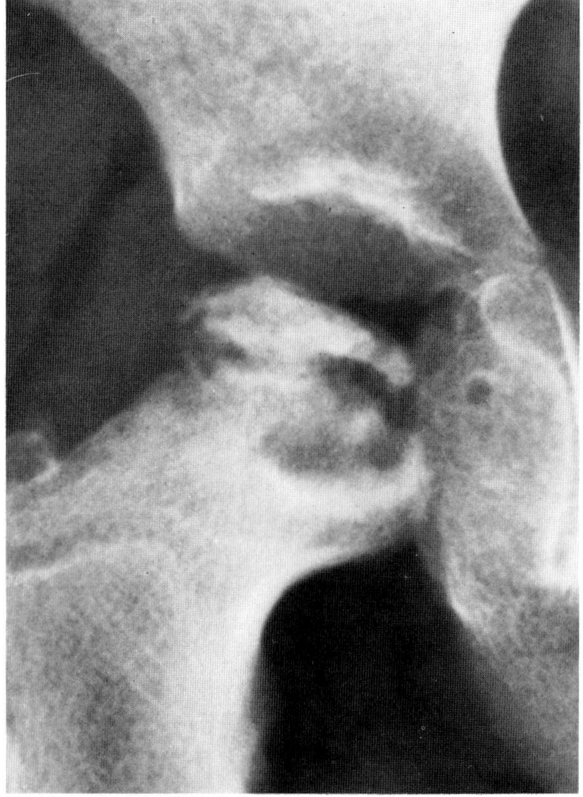

Fig. 7.7 Sickle cell disease. Infarction in the proximal femoral metaphysis has produced a large defect with avascular necrosis of the femoral head. These features are similar to Perthes' disease.

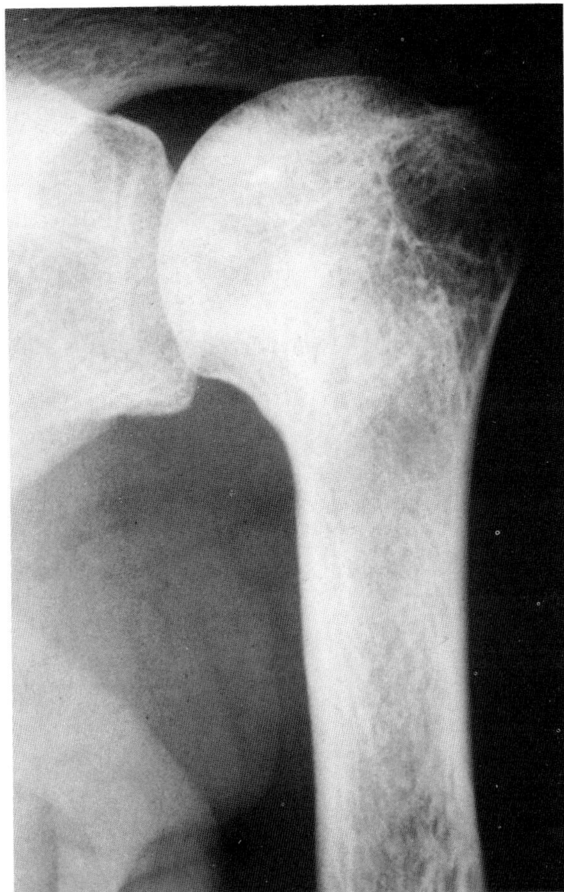

Fig. 7.8 Sickle cell disease. Endosteal bone deposition has resulted in diffuse sclerosis beneath the articular surface (the 'snow-cap' sign) due to medullary infarction. Note the lack of distinction between cortical and medullary bone in the upper humeral shaft, again due to endosteal deposition of bone.

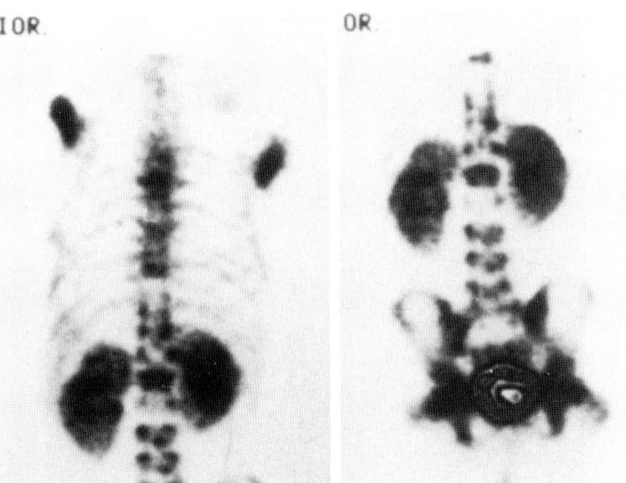

Fig. 7.9 Sickle cell disease. A bone scan performed 16 hours after the onset of severe pain in a boy with known sickle cell disease. Acute infarction of L2 has resulted in a relative photon deficiency in this area. Previous infarctions, in varying phases of evolution, are shown as areas of increased activity (see particularly L1 and mid-thoracic vertebrae).

Repairing bone is brittle, however, and liable to undergo disintegration from minor stresses — varying from 'osteochondritis dissecans' to complete collapse (Fig. 7.10).

Femoral heads so affected in *childhood* present an appearance exactly comparable to Perthes' disease (Fig. 7.7). In young Black children the areas of predilection for infarctions are the small tubular bones of the hands and feet (Fig. 7.11, 7.12), causing destructive changes accompanied by massive and painful soft tissue swellings and periosteal reactions which may be florid and reflect associated infarction of cortical bone. These findings may indicate the correct diagnosis, but other causes of infantile periosteal reactions such as cortical hyperostosis of both the infantile

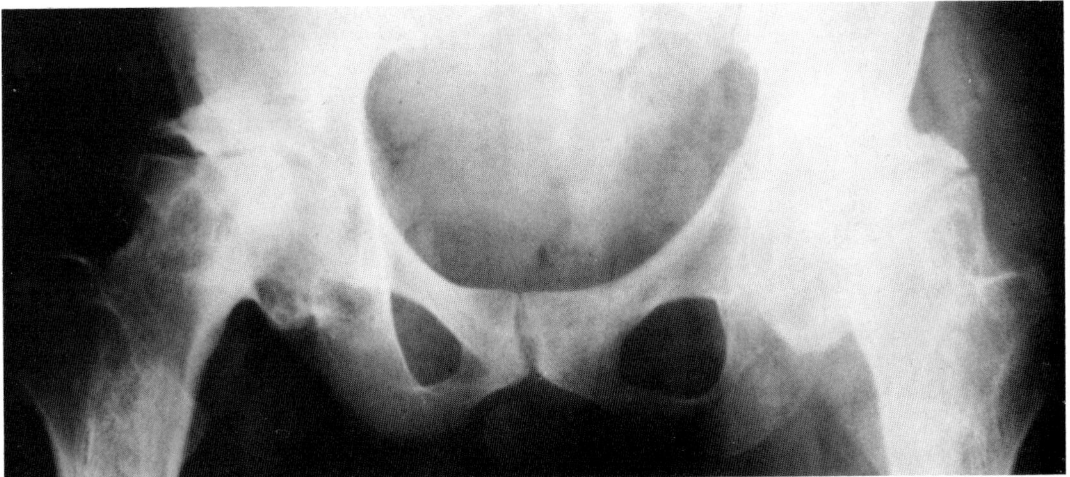

Fig. 7.10 Sickle cell/haemoglobin C disease (male aged 37). Severe degenerative changes in the hips have resulted from previous infarctions. The patient had had numerous skeletal crises in childhood. Endosteal opposition of bone is evident in the femora.

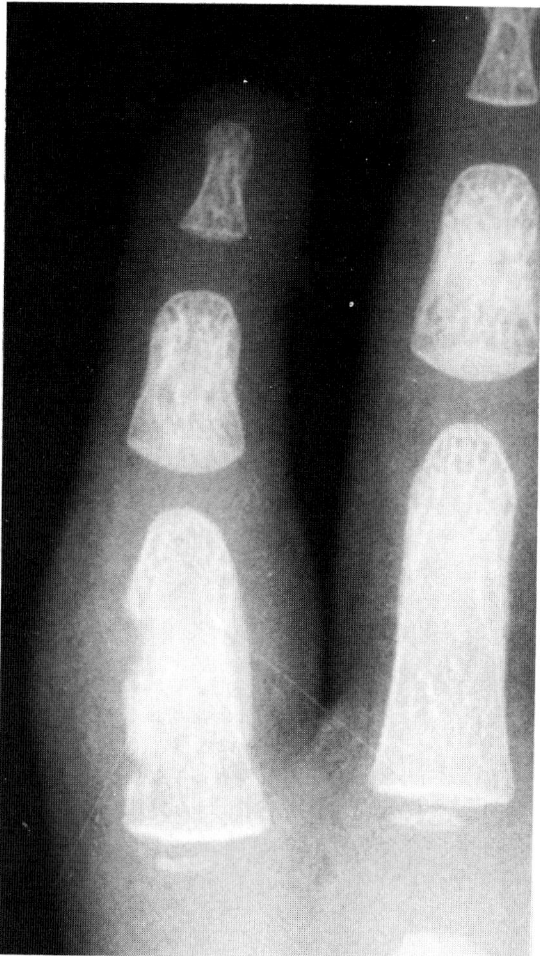

Fig. 7.11 Sickle cell disease. Soft tissue swelling surrounds an expanded proximal phalanx. Medullary expansion is present with simplification of trabecular pattern and penetration of the cortex. The distinction between these changes and osteomyelitis is extremely difficult.

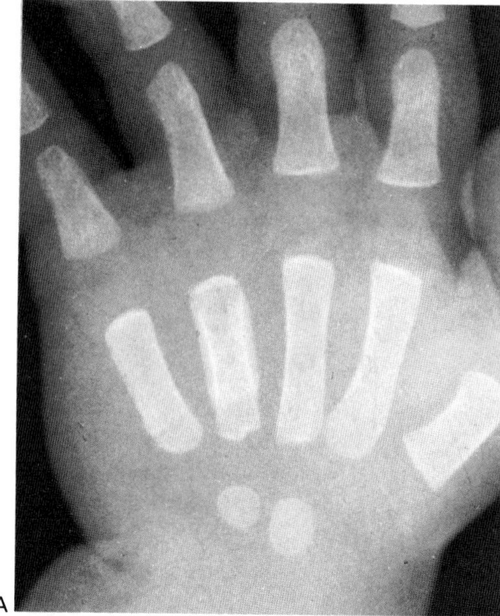

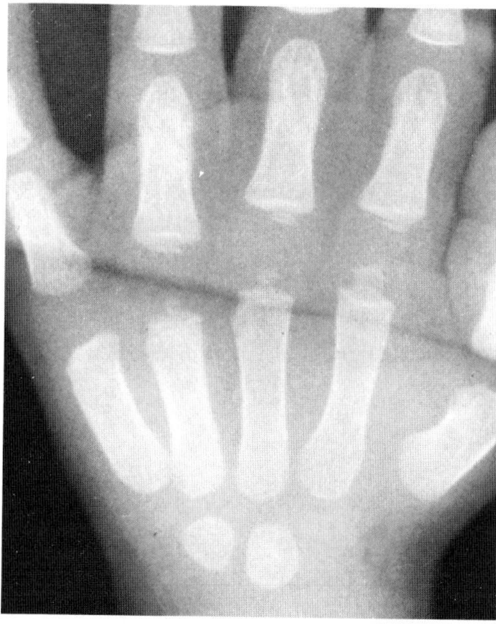

Fig. 7.12 Sickle cell disease, infarction in childhood. **A.** At presentation periosteal new bone formation surrounds the diaphysis of the fourth finger metacarpal. **B.** 10 months later resolution has occurred and growth has proceeded normally. The distinction between infarction and infection may be very difficult. In this case no specific treatment was given.

or traumatic types, or possibly hypervitaminosis A may require consideration. The formation of perpendicular bony spicules on the skull, uncommon even in thalassaemia, is distinctly unusual. More important is a decision concerning the possibility of super added infection, discussed below.

Infarcts of vertebral bodies are responsible for yet another characteristic radiological stigma. Generalized depressions of the central portions of the vertebral plates are common, and again, may be demonstrated in an asymptomatic patient. The depressions are often concave and rounded, simulating an ordinary nucleus pulposis impression on a bone which is already porotic. However, indubitable infarction may be deduced when the centre of the depression is flat and the sides slope obliquely (Fig. 7.13).

The diaphyses of the long bones, especially in the older child and the adolescent, are sites of predilection for infarction. Typically they involve the zones between the mid diaphysis and the metaphyses, the so-called 'intermediate fifths'. When the growth plate is involved significant deformity may occur due to growth arrest. Central metaphyseal defects and lucencies are typical. These in turn may produce fragmentation and deformity of the epiphyses. They may also be the site of pathological fractures. Infarcts may be so massive, causing bone destruction sequestration, reactive sclerosis and even the formation of involucrum, that the pattern becomes highly suggestive of an

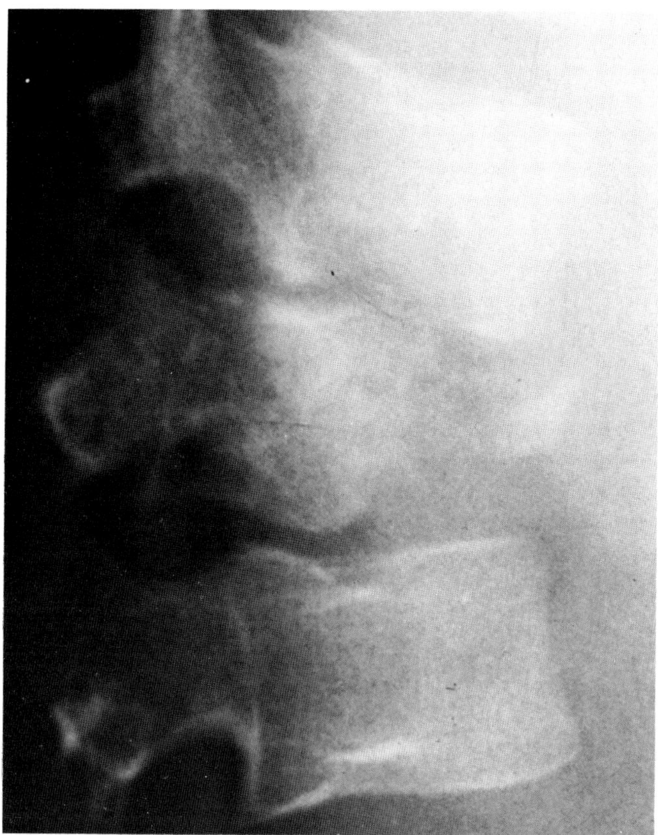

Fig. 7.13 Sickle cell disease. Flat depressions within the vertebral bodies with sloping sides typify metaphyseal infarct ('the vertebral step sign'). Frank destruction of the vertebral body with narrowing of the contiguous disc spaces is due to associated *Salmonella* osteomyelitis.

acute pyogenic osteomyelitis. The added hazard of infection does, in fact, exist.

4. *Superadded infection.* The areas of bone necrosis caused by infarction are especially susceptible to infection, mainly by salmonella organisms of the paratyphoid B group, presumably harboured endemically by the individual and present by coincidence. For these organisms the necrotic bone offers a potential site for their growth. Differentiation between the pure infarct and those which have been infected in this way may be extremely difficult (Fig. 7.14), both radiologically and pathologically, since cultures are often sterile. Such lesions are liable to occur especially in the tubular bones of the hands and feet in infants and in the long bones and the spine of older children (Fig. 7.13). In the adult an occasional septic arthritis, due to the same organism, may be superimposed on an adjacent infarct. With appropriate treatment, either by conservative antibiotic therapy or by active surgical measures, including sequestrectomy, healing usually takes place with remarkable rapidity.

5. *Soft tissue involvement*, as in the case of other chronic haemolytic anaemias, and such disorders of the marrow as Gaucher's disease, is reflected by hepato-splenomegaly caused by extramedullary haematopoiesis. Heterotopic masses of haematopoietic tissue may develop in the dorsal paravertebral areas. Release of iron pigments by accelerated destruction of erythrocytes may precipitate the formation of biliary calculi. Assessment of abnormalities of the soft tissues in relation to any skeletal disorder is a fundamental diagnostic requirement.

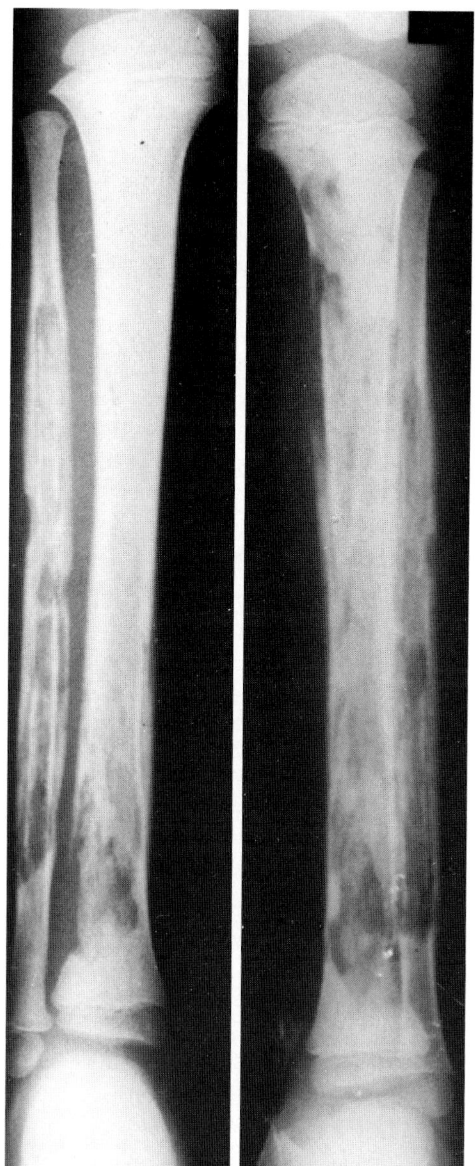

Fig. 7.14 Sickle cell disease with salmonella osteomyelitis. (male Nigerian aged 4). Extreme destructive changes in the long bones have been caused by infection superimposed upon infarction. Numerous sequestra are present. (Courtesy of Mr Geoffrey Walker.)

ERYTHROBLASTOSIS FETALIS
(*Haemolytic disease of the newborn*)

Haemolytic anaemia occurring in the fetus and newborn

results from immunological incompatability between the blood of the mother and the fetus. In Europe and North America this most commonly concerns the Rh factor, although other haematological errors of this type are known. The severity of the affection of the infant may vary widely, from a mild anaemia to icterus neonatorum and fetal hydrops.

The Rh positive erythrocytes of the fetus, crossing the placental barrier in a mother without Rh antigen, stimulates maternal formation of anti-Rh antibodies which traverse the placenta to enter the fetal circulation, there to haemolyse the fetal red blood cells. The danger of infants being affected by this incompatability increases with the number of conceptions but early recognition of the disorder and the adoption of prophylactic measures has greatly reduced its incidence.

Radiological changes. The only characteristic skeletal abnormality is the development of transverse bands of metaphyseal translucencies in the long bones. These translucencies are due to a disturbance of endochondral ossification and are non-specific, since they may occur also with other severe maternal illnesses during pregnancy and also in congenital syphilis. With successful treatment the translucent areas ossify with residual growth lines to mark the episode. In the spine, such growth lines often cause 'ghost shadows' within the vertebral bodies. *Fetal hydrops* may be diagnosed sonographically (Ch. 46) by the detection of growth retardation and subcutaneous oedema. The fetus is displaced by enlargement of the placenta. Spreading of the fetal limbs is due to subcutaneous oedema, with obliteration of the fetal fat line; this may be recognized radiographically.

OTHER CHRONIC ANAEMIAS

The anaemia of infants suffering from **iron deficiency** may produce radiological changes in the skull due to marrow hyperplasia similar to those of the less severe congenital anaemias. An inadequate diet is the usual cause, but malabsorption or abnormal loss of iron may be important factors. The widening of the diploic space and the subsequent bossing of the skull vault are again characteristic, but the disease has never been reported to cause changes sufficiently severe to involve the long bones and facial bones.

Hereditary spherocytosis is an inherited defect in which the red blood cells are of an abnormal round shape. They are trapped in the spleen and prematurely destroyed. The anaemia which results may produce mild changes comparable to the other congenital anaemias. Removal of the spleen eliminates the destructive mechanism and permits the bone structures to revert to a normal appearance.

Fanconi's syndrome of congenital aplastic anaemia with multiple congenital anomalies (not to be confused with the other syndrome described by the same author and concerned with osteomalacia and an abnormal renal tubular mechanism) is of interest in that the haematological changes are unlikely to appear before the age of 2 years. These consist of hypoplastic anaemia, marrow hypoplasia and skin pigmentation. The defect is inherited and congenital abnormalities of the skeleton are associated, e.g. deficient formation of the bones of the thumb, first metacarpal and radius; other abnormalities such as congenital dislocation of the hip and clubfoot also have been observed. These are evident long before the haematological abnormalities become apparent, and the latter are not responsible for any skeletal abnormalities. Some cases have terminated in leukaemia.

POLYCYTHAEMIA

This condition is due to overproduction of red cells. Although occasionally responsible for bone infarction, it produces no characteristic radiological changes in the skeleton. Transition to myeloid metaplasia, especially after radioactive phosphorus therapy, is common and illustrates one of the many common links which may exist between the types of disease now being considered. Pulmonary abnormalities in polycythaemia may occur in the form of increased reticulation or fine mottling.

DISEASES PRIMARILY INVOLVING WHITE BLOOD CELLS

LEUKAEMIA

Children are most commonly affected, and almost invariably by an acute and rapidly fatal form. In adults the disease may also be acute, but it is more commonly chronic. The course of the disease, even with chronic forms, is unlikely to be more than three years. Haematopoietic tissue is widely distributed throughout the skeleton of a child but is confined in the adult to the 'red marrow' areas of the axial skeleton and the proximal ends of the humeri and femora. Thus it is logical that radiological changes in the bones are present more commonly in the younger age-groups. More than half the children affected show skeletal abnormalities, while in adults they are found in fewer than 10% of cases. While the diagnosis usually is confirmed rapidly by examination of the blood and sternal marrow, it is important to appreciate that these bone changes actually may precede the development of a grossly pathological blood picture, especially in the so-called *aleukaemic* type, and may thus provide the earliest indication of the diagnosis.

Differentiation between myeloid and lymphatic types of leukaemia cannot be made with confidence by radiological examination. It has, however, been observed that the myeloid form is most commonly encountered in children, whereas the lymphatic form predominates in adults.

Radiological changes are observed mainly in children and consist of the following:

1. *Metaphyseal translucencies.* In children the most characteristic sign, occurring in 90% of cases, is the presence of bands of increased translucency running transversely across the metaphyses (Figs 7.15 and 7.16). Such bands may be narrow and incomplete in the early stages of the disease, but in the course of a few weeks they may be found to traverse the metaphysis completely and be as much as 5 mm in width. The most rapidly growing areas — knees, wrists and ankles — are commonly affected first, but later the metaphyses of the shoulders, hips and vertebral bodies also may be involved. The abnormality is caused by a disturbance of endochondral bone growth together with the development of leukaemic tissue. Similar growth disturbances may occur in scurvy and in infections, particularly syphilis, but in these conditions they tend to be observed only in the first two years of life. Leukaemia, however, has its peak incidence between the ages of 2 and 5 years, when the presence of this sign should be regarded as diagnostic until proved otherwise. With treatment, temporary remission may occur, and the bands of translucency may resolve.

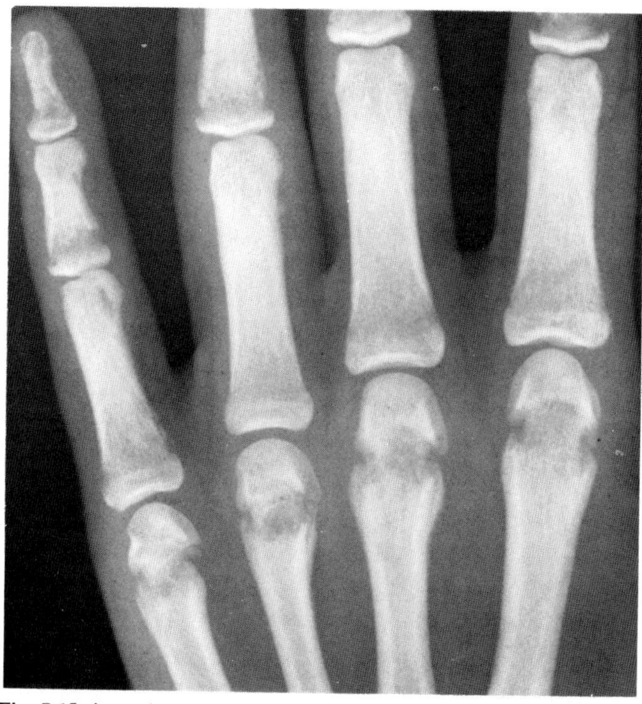

Fig. 7.15 Acute leukaemia. Extensive metaphyseal radiolucencies are present with adjacent periosteal new bone formation.

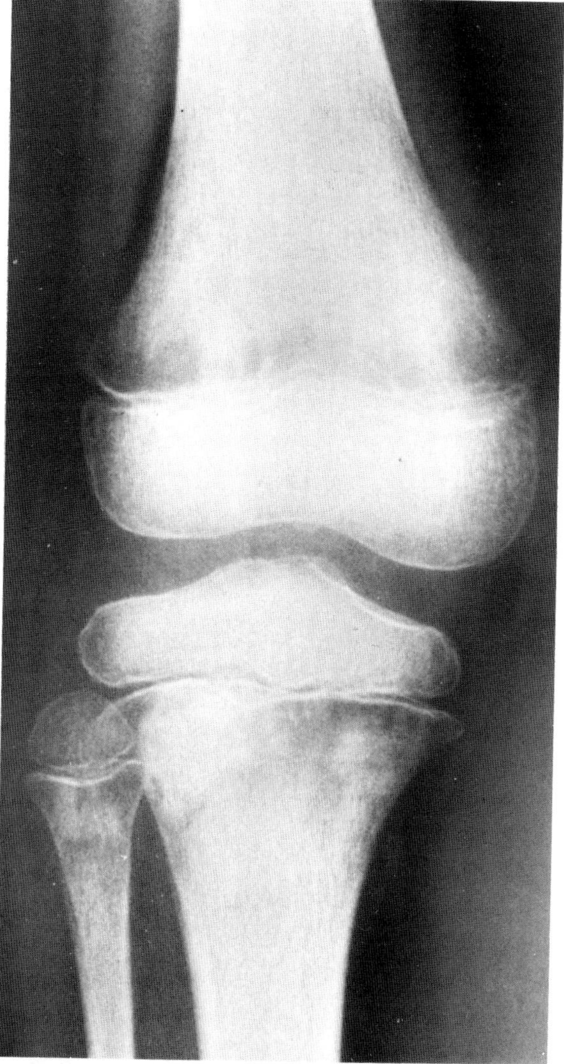

Fig. 7.16 Lymphatic leukaemia. Metaphyseal radiolucencies are present around the knee. Endosteal sclerosis is present adjacent to these lesions, obscuring the cortico-medullary junction. Minor periosteal new bone formation is present in the upper tibia and fibula.

2. *Metaphyseal cortical erosions* on the medial side of the proximal ends of the humeral (Fig. 7.17a) and tibial shafts sometimes occur as an early feature, possibly being evident even before the blood picture has become abnormal. Although such an appearance may be without significance, it should always arouse suspicion of this disease. When it does occur this sign is usually bilateral.

3. *Osteolytic lesions* develop in over half the cases. Usually they are punctate and diffusely scattered, though solitary and larger lesions may occur. While any portion of the skeleton may be involved by such leukaemic deposits, they are commonest in the shafts of the long bones (Fig. 7.18). When the vertebral bodies are involved, collapse often takes place before specific areas of rarefaction can be identified (Fig. 7.17b).

4. *Periosteal reactions* are usually associated clearly with underlying lesions, being due to the leukaemic tissue breaking through cortical bone to separate the cortex and the periosteum.

5. *Osteosclerosis* of the metaphysis is a rare but well-recognized primary manifestation. It may develop during treatment.

In *metastatic neuroblastoma* skeletal changes take place which may be indistinguishable from leukaemia. Separation of the sutures of the skull in the former condition is usually a helpful differentiating sign, but its value has been lessened by occasional demonstration of extensive leukaemic deposits along the cranial sutures, producing an appearance suggestive of suture separation. This is similar to the mechanism in neuroblastoma.

In *adults* skeletal lesions are rare and even the few that are recognized may include cases of *lymphosarcoma* which have reached a terminal leukaemic phase. As has been stressed before, the deposits occur essentially in red marrow areas, so that the changes which do take place include porosis, translucent areas of leukaemic bone destruction, which tend to be oval with the long axis parallel to the shaft, and vertebral destruction and collapse. Periosteal reactions are unusual. Occasionally, generalized osteosclerosis of the marrow area is evident. This is likely to be caused by trabecular thickening during periods of remission and may be patchy in type. In some instances, however, the

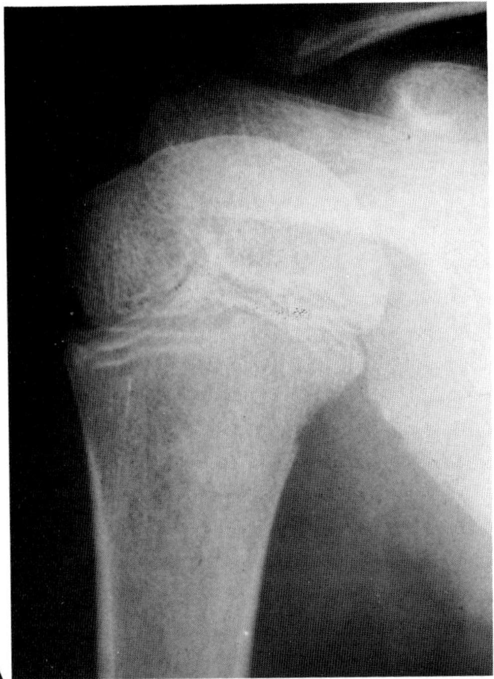

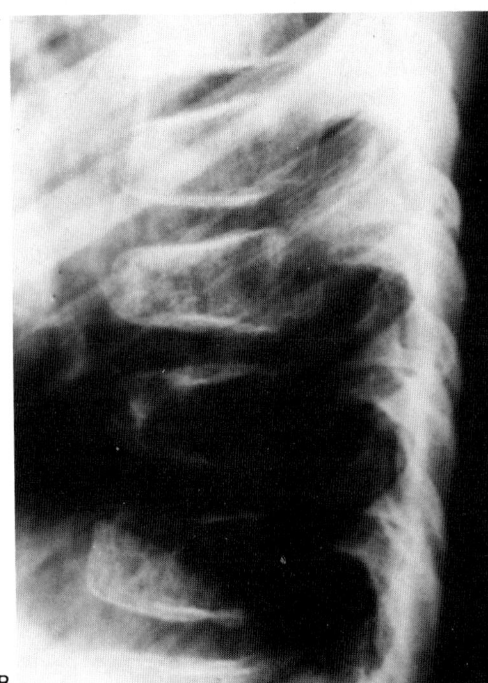

Fig. 7.17 Lymphatic leukaemia. **A**. Erosion of the medial side of the proximal metaphyses of both humeri were present in this 8-year-old. The disease was in an aleukaemic phase, not an uncommon finding even when skeletal changes are present. **B**. The same child complained of back pain. Multiple vertebral collapse is shown with the preservation of disc-space height. Overall bone density is reduced with a simplified trabecular pattern.

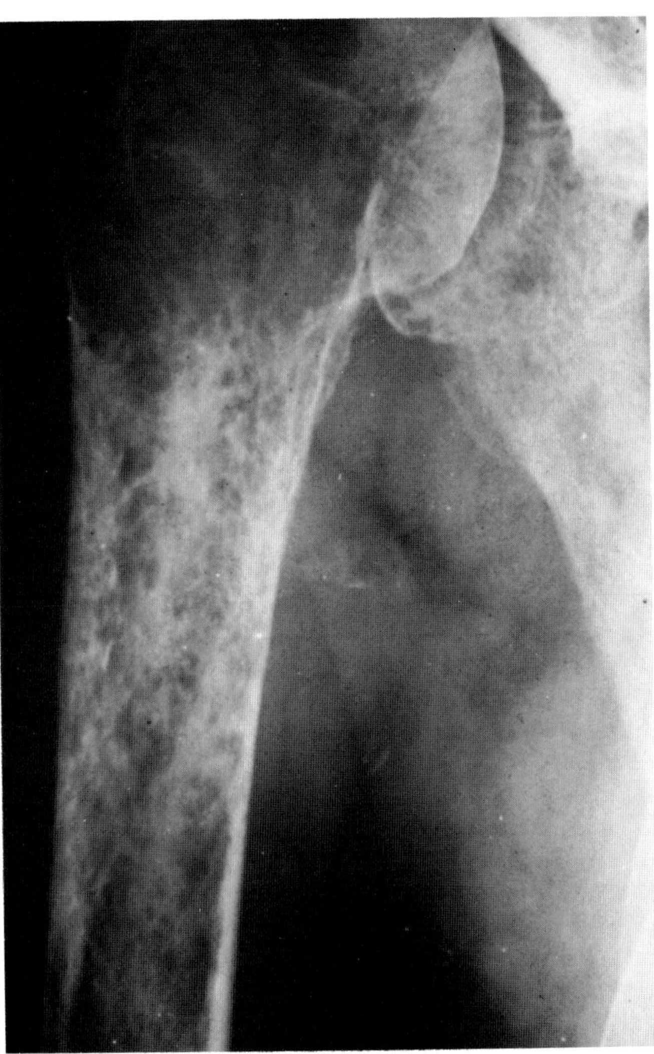

Fig. 7.18 Chronic lymphatic leukaemia — adult type. Diffuse medullary infiltration is shown in the humerus and scapula with cortical erosion.

leukaemic changes may be a secondary and terminal process in myeloid metaplasia.

MYELOID METAPLASIA
(Myelofibrosis and myelosclerosis)

This syndrome is characterized by the triad of myelofibrosis, myeloid metaplasia and features in the peripheral blood film which simulate leukaemia. This relationship between myeloid metaplasia (formerly known as myelofibrosis), myelosclerosis and other diseases including polycythaemia rubra vera and chronic myeloid leukaemia, is intimate. The typical patient is a middle-aged or elderly adult, the primary disorder being metaplasia of the marrow cells to fibrous tissue. The usual presenting complaints are of fatigue and abdominal fullness due to hepatosplenomegaly. Obliteration of the haematopoietic tissue results in progressive anaemia, the appearance of immature red and white cells in the peripheral blood and compensatory splenomegaly. In the later stages of the disease, the fibrous tissue becomes converted to bone and endosteal cortical thickening develops. Polycythaemia may be followed by myeloid metaplasia and it appears probable that nearly half of the developed cases of myeloid metaplasia previously had some form of this blood disorder. Generalized purine hypermetabolism may manifest itself as secondary gout.

Radiological changes. When the sclerotic stage of the disease has been reached, increased density of the bones may be expected. This may be diffuse and widespread in type or patchy in nature. Areas of relative translucency due to fibrosis may persist. The increased density is due to actual new bone deposition on the trabeculae and also to the endosteal cortical thickening. The narrowing of the medullary space becomes clearly visible and is closely resembled by changes in the long bones of the later stages of sickle-cell anaemia. Irregular periosteal reactions, particularly near the ends of long bones, may occur. These may be well organized and continuous with the cortex or separated from it by a zone of translucency. While the red marrow areas (particularly the pelvis) are especially subject to these pathological changes, the whole skeleton may be affected. Density of the skull is associated with obliteration of the diploic space, though some persistent areas of fibrosis may remain translucent. Splenomegaly is almost invariably evident (Fig. 7.19).

Differentiation must be made from other conditions causing a generalized increase of bone density. The congenital sclerosing dysplasias, including osteopetrosis, are likely to be encountered in adult life only as an incidental finding or in association with a pathological fracture. *Fluorosis* is likely to occur in an endemic area. *Mastocytosis* may cause some confusion, but the lesions are usually less diffuse and are accompanied by urticaria pigmentosa. Sclerosing and widespread *metastases*, particularly prostatic, should never be forgotten.

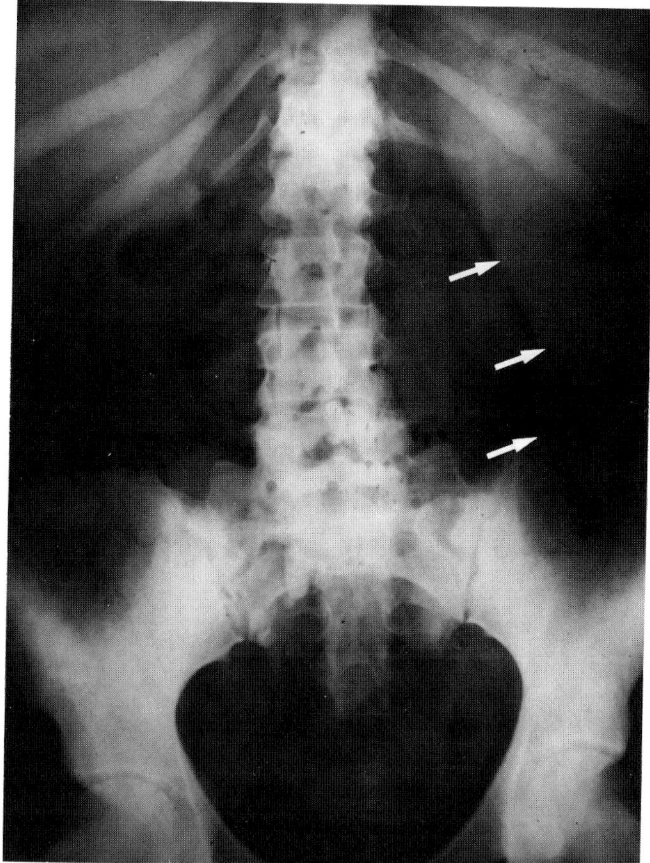

Fig. 7.19 Myeloid metaplasia (female aged 63). All the bones are diffusely dense with lack of distinction between cortical and medullary bone. The spleen is grossly enlarged (arrows).

DISORDERS OF THE LYMPHORETICULAR SYSTEM

Four main groups of disorder will be considered, divided, for convenience as follows:

A. Lymphomas: including Hodgkin's and non-Hodgkin's lymphomas
B. Plasma cell disease: Plasmacytoma and multiple myeloma
C. Histiocytosis
D. Storage disorders: Gaucher's disease and Niemann–Pick disease

THE LYMPHOMAS

The classification of the proliferative disorders of the lymphoreticular system is changing constantly and is based essentially upon histological features detected in lymph nodes. Consequently caution is necessary in extending such classifications to bone or bowel lymphoma. **Malignant lymphoma** is a generic term embracing all previously named tumours including Hodgkin's disease, lymphadenoma, lymphosarcoma, reticulum-cell sarcoma and others.

Malignant lymphomas may be subdivided into two groups: Hodgkin's disease and a group of non-Hodgkin's lymphomas.

HODGKIN'S DISEASE

This defined tumour has an agreed classification on histological grounds, named after Rye. This comprises nodular sclerosing Hodgkin's disease, a complaint of young women involving intrathoracic lymph nodes, and three others, lymphocyte dominant Hodgkin's disease, mixed Hodgkin's disease and lymphocyte depleted Hodgkin's disease. The last three comprise a spectrum with, in order listed, worsening outlook. Bone involvement always implies a less favourable prognosis. It is a feature of widespread disease and has been found at post-mortem in more than half of cases. Skeletal lesions at presentation are far less common. Primary Hodgkin's disease of bone probably does not occur. There is no correlation between the variety of Hodgkin's disease and the nature of the individual bony lesions it produces.

The age of onset varies widely from childhood to old age but the diagnosis is most commonly made in young adults. The red marrow areas, as is common in most of the lymphomas, are the most frequent sites of presentation, the majority of lesions being found in the *spine*, *thoracic cage* and *pelvis*. Bone pain may precede, by several months, the development of these lesions and the importance of serial radiological examination either radiographic or scintigraphic must be stressed.

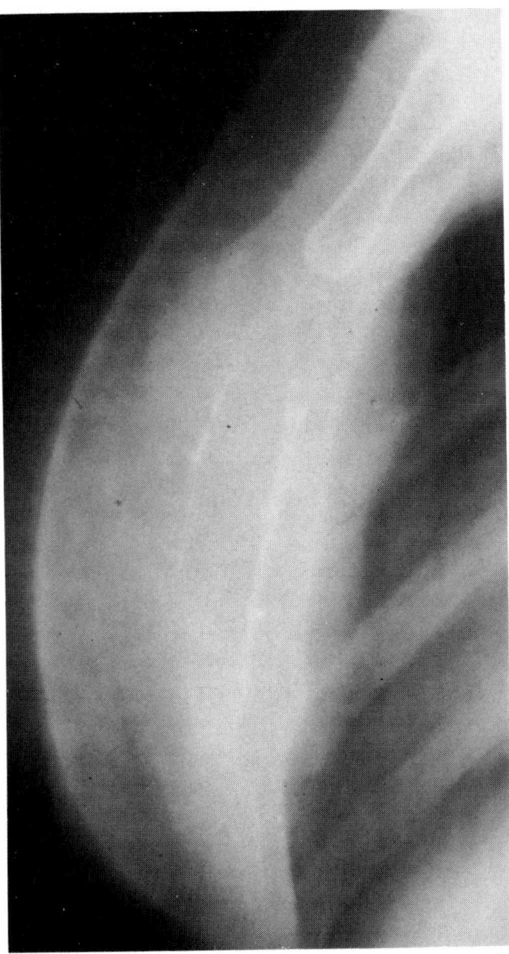

Fig. 7.20 Hodgkin's disease. An expanding, destructive lesion involves the body of the sternum, with anterior and posterior soft tissue masses. Bizarre changes in this bone should always arouse suspicion of a lymphoma.

Radiological changes in the skeleton. The majority of early bone lesions are destructive and often large at the time they are first observed, either from direct involvement from affected soft tissues, particularly lymph nodes, or from infiltration of bone marrow. About a third are essentially osteolytic in type (Fig. 7.20). The majority, about three-fifths, are however of mixed type with patchy sclerosis and destruction (Fig. 7.21). Diffuse trabecular thickening in areas of bone marrow infiltration causes sclerotic lesions in the remainder (Fig. 7.22). Such an appearance may develop in a few months, being preceded by bone pain, and may well show no preliminary bone destruction. It may also follow treatment of a formerly osteolytic lesion. Conversely, some sclerotic lesions may be observed to become osteolytic or normal following treatment (Fig. 7.22). Whereas the osteolytic lesions may thin, displace and erode the overlying cortex and develop associated soft tissue masses, the primary sclerotic lesion does not cause enlargement of the affected bone. Skeletal scintigraphy is a sensitive means of detecting the presence of bony lesions particularly when sclerotic deposits have developed. The method is less reliable when purely lytic lesions are present.

The *spine* is by far the most frequently involved area. A feature which is almost diagnostic is anterior erosion of a vertebral body (Fig. 7.23). This may or may not present reactive sclerosis in its margin and is attributed to involvement of adjacent paravertebral lymph nodes. Several vertebrae may be affected and the osteolytic lesions are likely to collapse. Soft tissue masses will stimulate paravertebral abscesses. The sclerotic type shows a diffuse increase of density, possibly also with some anterior erosion but without increase in size of the affected body. Solitary dense vertebrae, especially in young adults, are suggestive of this disease. When, as commonly occurs, the adjacent ribs are affected, usually by osteolytic lesions, the appearance becomes almost pathognomonic. In all these types the intervertebral discs are usually spared, aiding differentiation from an infection. Even in the rare cases where a disc space does become narrowed, preservation of density of the vertebral end plates usually permits differentiation from an

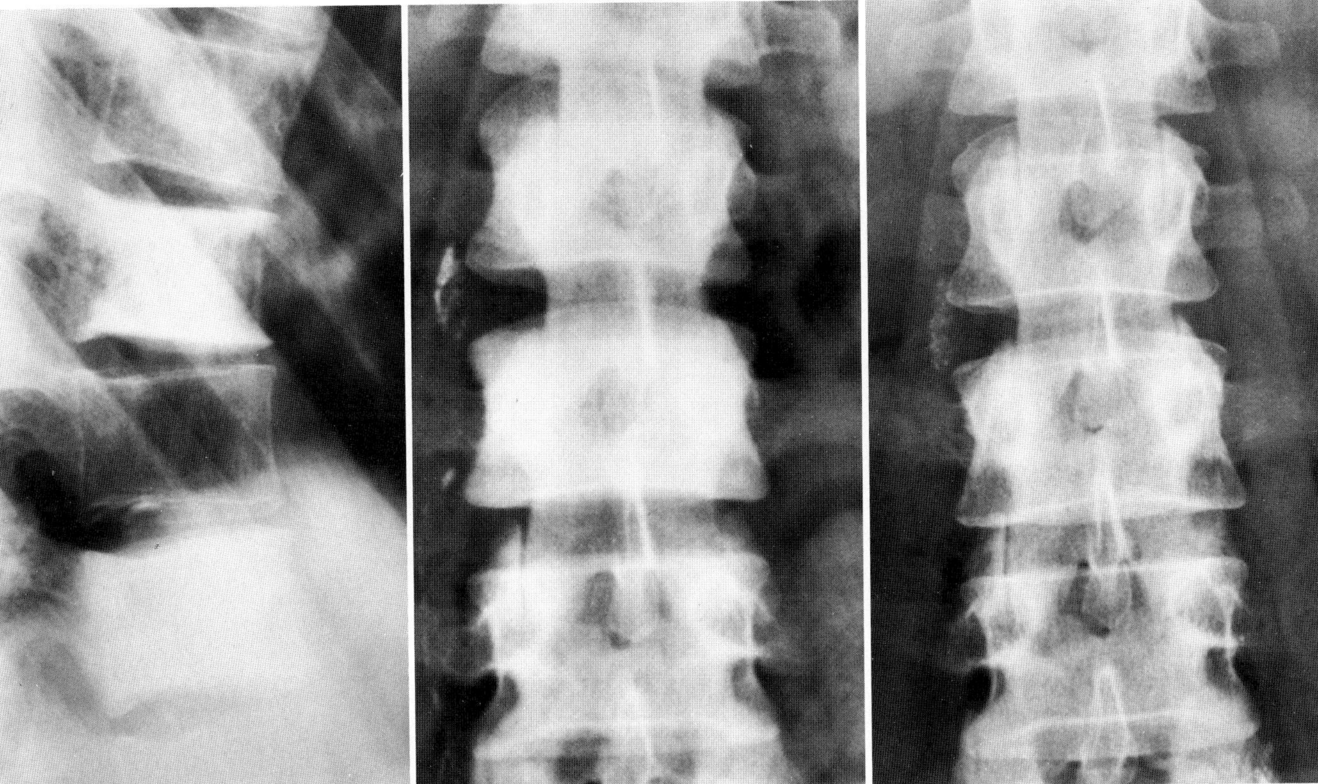

Fig. 7.21 Fig. 7.22A Fig. 7.22B

Fig. 7.21 Hodgkin's disease. The common pattern of endosteal sclerosis and patchy bone destruction is shown in the vertebral body of T9 in an adult male patient. Similar changes are also present at T11. These features are virtually diagnostic.

Fig. 7.22 Hodgkin's disease. **A**. Diffuse sclerosis is present in the bodies of L2 and L3 in a young woman at presentation with the disease. **B**. $2\frac{1}{2}$ years later, following treatment, the appearances have reverted to normal. (Lymphographic contrast medium is present in para-aortic nodes.)

infective discitis where loss of this density is an early diagnostic sign. Lesions in the *ribs* may be found by themselves, sometimes being observed in a chest radiograph. They are usually osteolytic and expanding in type. Similarly the *sternum* is not an infrequent site for a lesion to appear, again usually osteolytic, but sometimes mixed in type with perpendicular spicules of new bone. Presternal oedema is a frequent precursor of such lesions and the presence of retrosternal soft tissue swelling is not uncommon (Fig. 7.20). In the *pelvis* mixed or sclerosing types tend to preponderate. The medial portions of the innominate bones are often dense. Osteolytic lesions, rather nonspecific in appearance, are not uncommon in the ischia and change from either type to the mixed pattern may be observed in serial examinations. In the *long bones* the sites of predilection are the red marrow areas in the proximal portions of the femora and humeri. These are much more often of the osteolytic type and many small translucencies,

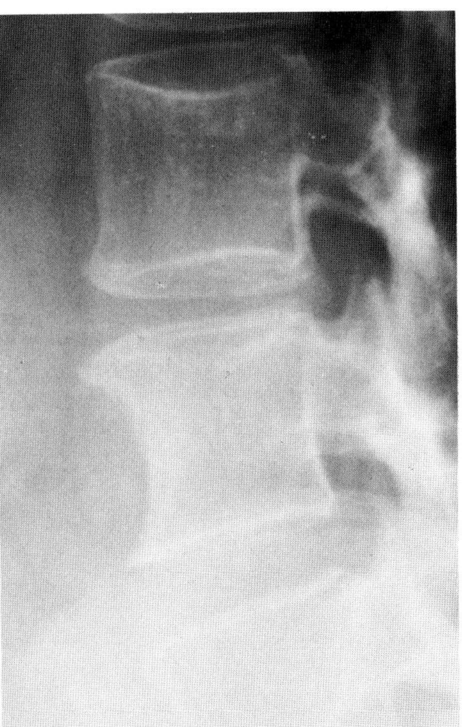

Fig. 7.23 Hodgkin's disease. A typical anterior scalloping of L4 is due to pressure erosion from enlarged lymph nodes. The cortex is preserved, as are the disc spaces.

oval in the long axis of the bone, may extend throughout the marrow cavity and may cause endosteal scalloping of the cortex. While such an appearance is a feature of this disease, it may be observed also in *non-Hodgkin's lymphoma, leukaemia* and *Gaucher's disease*. Fusion of such areas may produce a honeycomb pattern, with coarse residual trabeculation, very like the medullary changes of Gaucher's disease. Organized periosteal reactions are not infrequent. Such a feature is rare in Gaucher's disease. The skull, clavicles and scapulae are sometimes affected. Pathological fractures are uncommon. With sclerosing lesions in elderly individuals, confusion with *Paget's disease* may easily arise, but the characteristic enlargement of the affected bone in that disease will probably be absent. Differentiation, in all these lesions, must be made from *metastases*. Intrathoracic disease may present with hypertrophic osteoarthropathy.

NON-HODGKIN'S LYMPHOMA

This forms a much more difficult spectrum of disease with no simple classification. That commonly used is based on lymph node histology (Rappaport), though the application of such a classification to bone disease may not be reliable. Broadly speaking non-Hodgkin's lymphoma in bone may be divided into three groups. The first, with larger cells histologically, essentially with a poor prognosis, was formerly called *reticulum cell sarcoma*. Another with multiple small round cells, and a much less aggressive nature, was called *lymphosarcoma*. This group merges into a spectrum with other small round cell tumours including *Ewing's sarcoma* and *chronic lymphocytic leukaemia*. The third group is *Burkitt's lymphoma*, which may be distinguished by nature of presentation and the age of patient (q.v.).

It is difficult to assess how many patients actually present with primary skeletal non-Hodgkin's lymphoma; the proportion is probably less than one third, the majority of patients having diffuse disease at diagnosis. Experience suggests that reticulum cell sarcoma may present as a primary bone tumour, although in older patients particularly it can be multifocal and systemic. It is unlikely that lymphosarcoma ever presents primarily in the skeleton.

RETICULUM CELL SARCOMA

This condition represents about 3% of all apparent primary malignant tumours of bone. The customary presentation is of localized pain and swelling, often over a protracted period. The tumour may be asymptomatic to such a degree that many lesions present on account of pathological fracture. Radiological examination is then likely to reveal a large, and hitherto unsuspected, area of bone destruction. Males are affected twice as commonly as females. The majority are observed in the third and fourth decades although presentation during later years is not unusual. The lesions may be multifocal in the older age group. These tumour may be confused with other malignancies including osteo sarcoma, metastasis and malignant round cell tumours. Indeed differentiation between these tumours in a young adult may be extremely difficult, not only on clinical and radiological grounds, but also histologically.

The lesion may arise as an apparently *primary* tumour within bone marrow tending to remain confined to the skeleton, although it may spread to other bones and only at a later stage to lymph nodes and viscera. The latter structures, in contrast, may be involved first in the *extraskeletal* form of reticulum cell sarcoma, which invades the skeleton only in its later stages.

In its primary form the condition is localized to a single bone with a marked predilection for the long bones. Nearly half the cases occur in the vicinity of the knee (Fig. 7.24) often with an associated synovial effusion. The proximal end of the humerus is another common site (Fig. 7.25) and about a third of cases are found in the flat bones of the axia

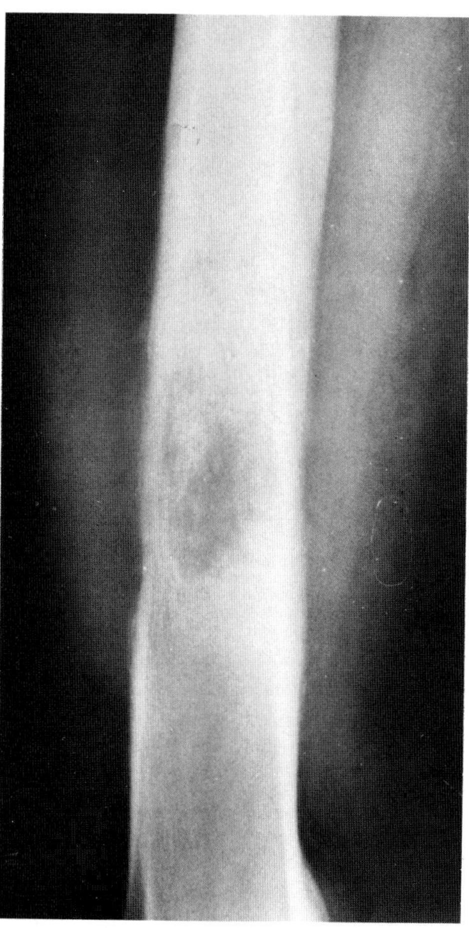

Fig. 7.24 Non-Hodgkin's lymphoma — reticulum cell sarcoma. A purely destructive lesion is present in the distal femur of an adult female patient. The margins are ill-defined with cortical destruction. Periosteal new bone formation is present adjacent to this destruction. These appearances resemble metastasis and osteosarcoma.

skeleton. Spinal, rib and pelvic involvement tends to occur with the extraskeletal form, and in the older age group.

The tumour is extemely radio-sensitive and this treatment alone or combined with amputation has resulted in many long survivals (Fig. 7.26). Even though a primary lesion may have regressed entirely with radiotherapy generalized skeletal dissemination is likely to occur eventually.

Radiological changes. The earliest evidence of the tumour is diffuse medullary destruction of a patchy nature with very poorly defined margins (Fig. 7.25, 7.27). At this stage it may be impossible to differentiate the lesion radiologically from any other aggressive neoplasm. In particular an *osteolytic metastasis* is likely to present the greatest difficulty. The lesion may resemble other primary malig-

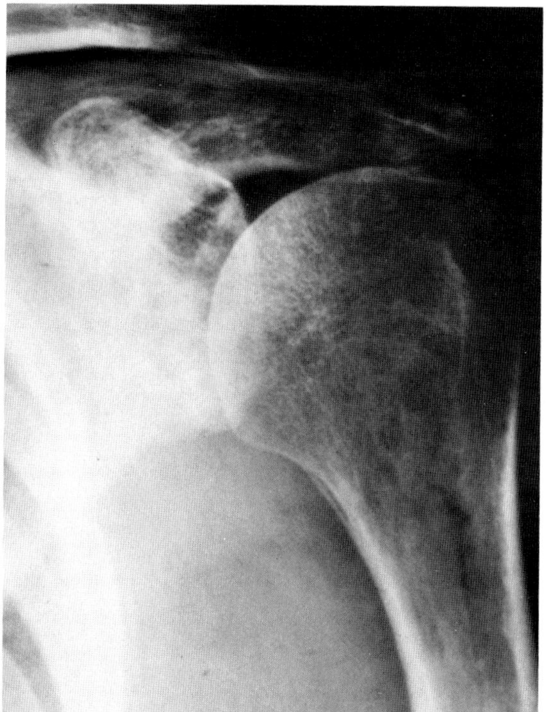

Fig. 7.25 Non-Hodgkin's lymphoma — reticulum cell sarcoma. Diffuse destruction permeates the medulla of the humerus and neck of the scapula.

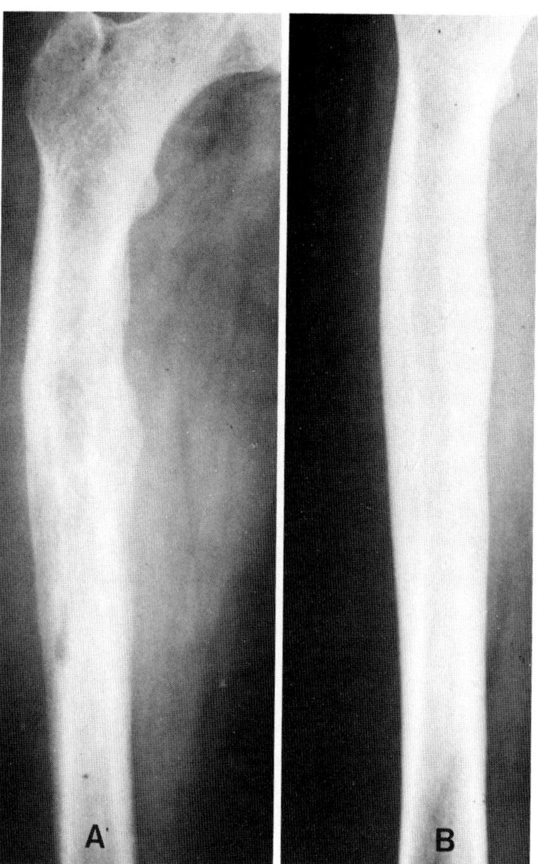

Fig. 7.26 Non-Hodgkin's lymphoma — reticulum cell sarcoma. Advanced changes are shown in the femoral shaft with dramatic resolution 11 months later following local radiotherapy.

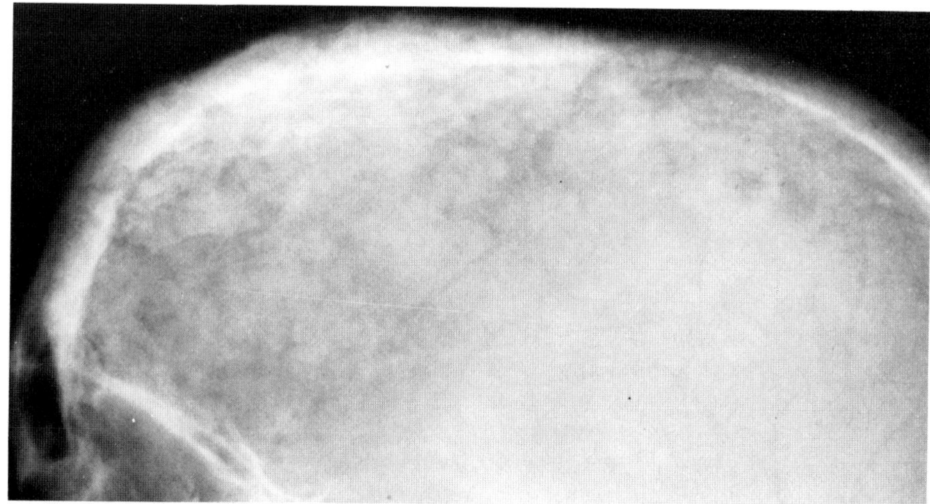

Fig. 7.27 Non-Hodgkin's lymphoma — reticulum cell sarcoma. Extensive patchy destruction of the cranium was present in this adult patient with generalized disease.

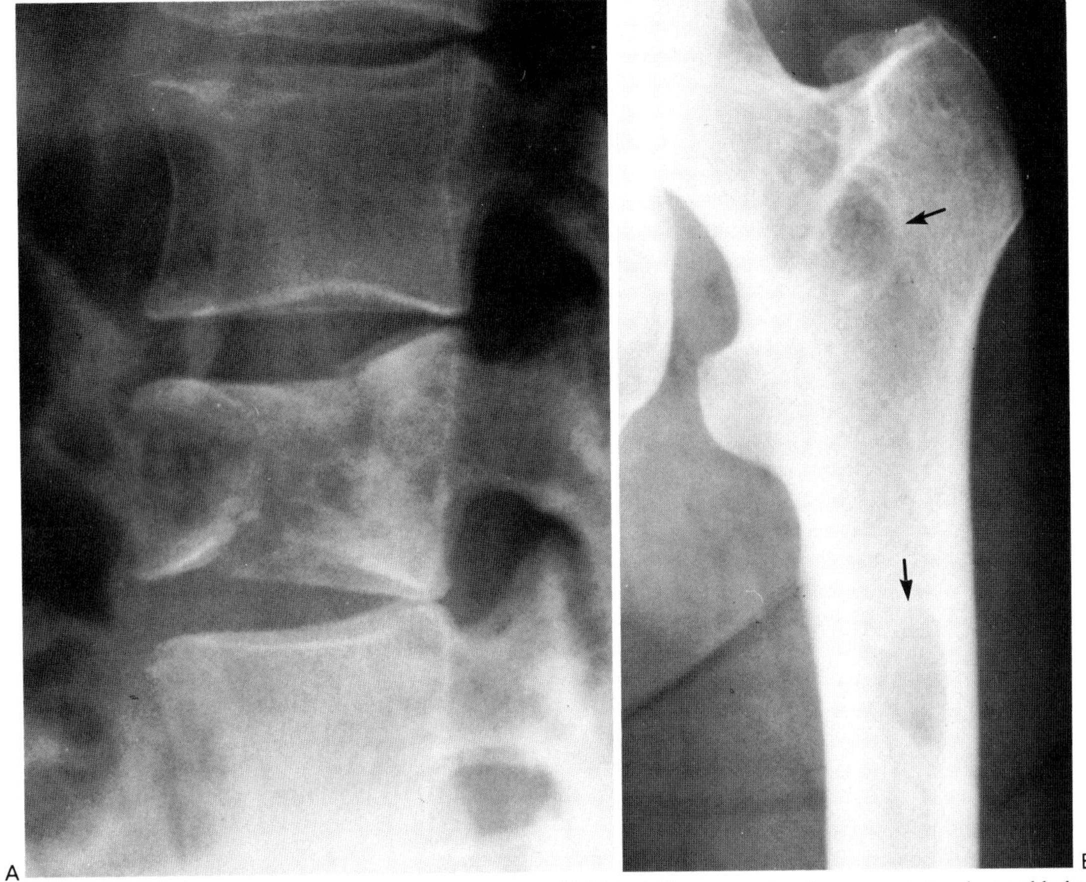

Fig. 7.28 A and **B**. Non-Hodgkin's lymphoma — reticulum cell sarcoma. Multifocal disease was found at presentation in an elderly patient with low back pain. In addition to a pathological fracture of a lumbar vertebral body ill-defined endosteal defects are present in the femoral shaft (arrows).

nant neoplasms stimulating little or no reactive bone formation such as *Ewing's tumour, fibrosarcoma* or *malignant fibrous histiocytoma*. Radiological confusion with osteomyelitis may arise also particularly as overlying periosteal reaction is present in half the cases (Fig. 7.24). Indeed such periosteal reaction may be present before medullary changes become evident. The absence of leukocytosis is of value in excluding such an inflammatory process. *Scintigraphically* the features are unremarkable. Usually increased activity is detected. Multifocal lesions may be found. Radiologically the area of destruction spreads widely through the marrow cavity and remains patchy in nature. Much of the adjacent cortex undergoes resorption with the development of well-defined soft tissue swellings from soft tissue tumour extension. Cortical thickening and reactive sclerosis are not prominent features, although they may occur exceptionally.

In the generalized form of the disease, lesions may be detected throughout the skeleton and each present the same characteristics as a solitary focus (Fig. 7.28). The patient is likely to be over the age of 40. The ultimate degree of osseous destruction attained may be extreme.

LYMPHOSARCOMA

This malignant tumour is rarer than Hodgkin's disease and mainly affects an older age group consisting of patients in the fifth and sixth decades. Nonetheless a number of cases have been observed in children and in these an unexplained male sex preponderance has been found. A proportion of these patients develop frank lymphocytic leukaemia.

The incidence of bone lesions is of the order of 10–20%, although more are detected at post-mortem. Prognostically bone lesions imply a poor outcome. Primary skeletal involvement is probably extremely rare.

Radiological changes in the skeleton resemble very closely those of Hodgkin's disease; other lesions grow more rapidly and are almost always osteolytic in type. Areas of destruction, commonly in red marrow areas, may be large with diffuse and irregular margins, and with scalloping of the inner aspects of the cortex. They may be solitary or multiple and, because of their osteolytic nature, pathological fractures are common. The latter affect especially the femoral and humeral necks and may cause collapse of vertebral bodies. When the lesions are multiple they all tend to be of the same osteolytic type, unlike Hodgkin's disease when all the different types of bone change may be present. Erosion of the cortex is likely to be followed by the formation of large associated soft tissue masses with relatively little periosteal reaction. Such erosions usually take place through an area of cortex which has already been thinned and expanded by underlying pathological process emphasising the radiological similarity of the individual lesions to Ewing's sarcoma.

BURKITT'S TUMOUR

An exceptional and particularly sinister form of lymphoma is common in African children and has been reported in other parts of the world. Large, destructive lesions develop especially in the mandible and maxilla (Fig. 7.29).

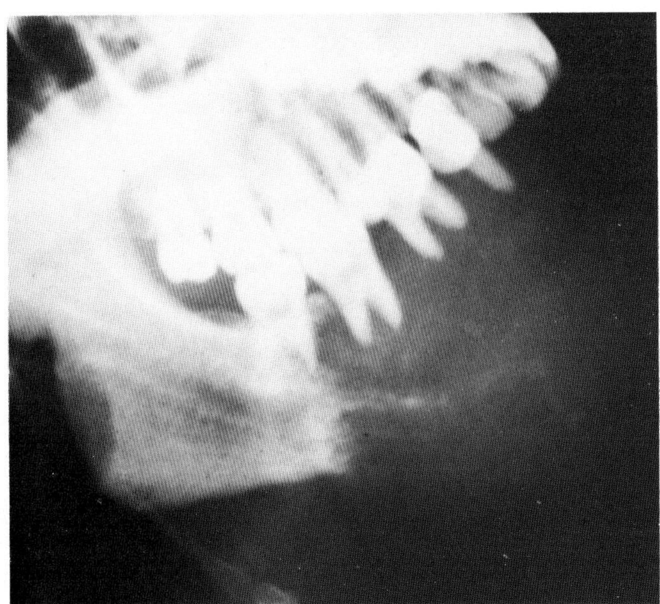

Fig. 7.29 Burkitt's tumour. A large destructive lesion in the mandible of this African child is typical of this form of lymphoma.

Radiologically these lesions are purely osteolytic and grow at an alarming rate. The jaw lesions are characterized by the resorption of the lamina dura with multiple lytic foci which eventually coalesce with radiating spicules of bone. Spinal lesions are characterised by lytic, ill-defined destructive foci with paravertebral masses. In long bones the permeative lytic nature of the tumour, particularly with cortical erosions, may resemble a Ewing's sarcoma. Foci develop in soft tissues particularly the kidneys, ovaries and abdominal lymph nodes.

The disease is associated with a virus (Epstein–Barr) and is especially prevalent in endemic malarial areas. Death usually follows within a few months although remarkable regression can occur following the use of cytotoxic drugs.

MASTOCYTOSIS

The rare condition of urticaria pigmentosa, for long regarded purely as a skin disease, is now known to be associated with enlargement of the liver, spleen and lymph nodes due to the proliferation of mast cells. The disease is relatively benign, but a few instances of leukaemic termination have been recorded. Bone changes are usually identified in early adult life.

Radiological changes. In probably a third of cases, generalized skeletal changes are present. These are diffuse or circumscribed areas of increased density, apparently due to thickening of the medullary trabeculae (Fig. 7.30). It may be difficult to identify the endosteal margin of the cortex. The absorption of some trabeculae and the thickening of others may cause the osseous structures to have a coarse pattern but the generalized increase in density usually predominates. Any bone may be affected. At this stage it is possible to demonstrate only a few mast cells in the bone marrow. The appearance may closely resemble *myelosclerosis*, the *sclerosing types of leukaemia*, *chronic anaemias* and *osteopetrosis*. Occasionally the dense areas are sharply defined, of considerable size and localized to a few areas. Particularly in young adults, differentiation from *Hodgkin's disease* must be made.

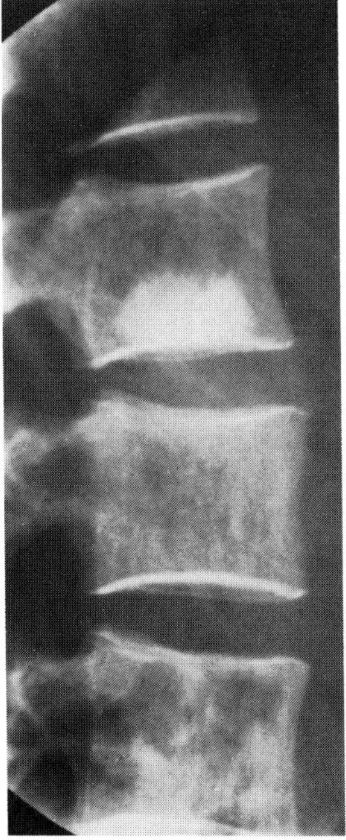

Fig. 7.30 Mastocytosis (male aged 34). A localised area of endosteal sclerosis is present in the body of L1. In addition, ill-defined thinning of trabeculae is demonstrated in L2 and patchier changes in the upper surface of L3.

PLASMA CELL DISEASES

Plasma cells represent the end-product of B-lymphocyte maturation. Pathological proliferation produces either a local tumour (plasmacytoma) or disseminate disease (myelomatosis).

PLASMACYTOMA

This condition is unifocal, causing a localized destructive lesion in the skeleton, in a red marrow area. Many other descriptive terms, such as solitary myeloma, for this localized lesion have been used. Although for many years it may remain localized, and without gross health disturbance, ultimately it undergoes transition to generalized myelomatosis. A latent interval of 5–10 years is usual. Consequently the outlook is better than multiple myelomatosis. In comparison with the latter these lesions are uncommon. The exact incidence is difficult to assess since they are frequently asymptomatic and therefore occult. For example, a plasmacytoma in a rib may be noted incidentally on a routine examination of the chest.

When symptoms occur they are commonly those of bone pain, particularly backache. The vertebral bodies, especially in the thoracolumbar and lumbar regions, are the most common sites for these lesions and are likely to undergo partial collapse. The pelvis, especially the ilium, femur and humerus are the next most commonly involved sites.

The vast majority of affected individuals are between 30 and 60 years of age so that this is almost entirely a disease of late middle age. The differential diagnosis always includes a solitary osteolytic metastasis.

Radiological changes. These lesions arise almost constantly in areas of persistent red marrow function. Bone expansion, which may be considerable with thinning of the overlying cortex, is common but, when a vertebral body is affected, collapse may precede such apparent expansions. The margins are usually well-defined and sharply demarcated and characteristically without a sclerotic reaction (Fig. 7.31). Some tumours, however, do exhibit a sclerotic margin, etching clearly the edge of the lesion, particularly after treatment. It is rarely exuberant and is usually incomplete. Coarse trabecular strands of increased density may give a network appearance in the area of destruction, and,

A

B

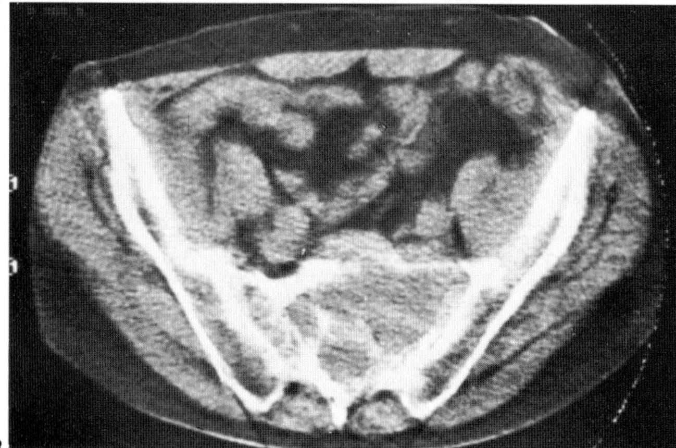

Fig. 7.31 Plasmacytoma of sacrum. **A.** An adult male patient exhibits a well-defined radiolucent defect involving the left sacral ala. **B.** CT scan demonstrated extensive destructive nature of the tumour, seen clearly to cross the mid line. Note the marked cortical thinning with absence of sclerosis or periosteal new bone formation.

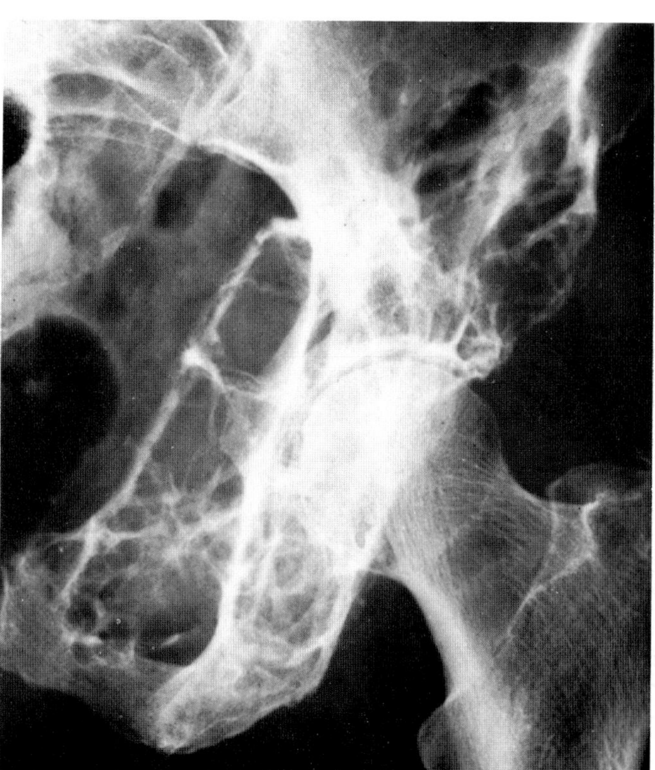

Fig. 7.32 Plasmacytoma of pelvis. This very extensive lesion was unaccompanied by any systemic abnormality. Bone expansion is associated with coarse trabeculation producing a soap bubble appearance.

Exceptionally the lesion may be entirely sclerotic. Large lesions in flat bones may assume a soap bubble appearance (Fig. 7.32).

Differential diagnosis of these tumours, especially if they have been observed incidentally, may be difficult. In view of the age group concerned, the first and most important alternative to be considered is an osteolytic metastasis. In vertebrae, such metastases are likely to involve the pedicles more commonly. If metastatic disease can be excluded, the development of a solitary osteolytic lesion in a vertebral body in a patient of the late middle age should always be considered as a plasmacytoma, until proven otherwise. Chordoma may produce similar features. Plasmacytoma represents one of the many types of vertebral lesions which may cause symptoms of spinal cord or root compression. Other differential diagnoses to be considered, especially with an expanding lytic focus in a rib, are *fibrous dysplasia*, a *'brown' tumour of hyperparathyroidism* and, particularly when the lesion is adjacent to an articular surface, a *giant cell tumour*. Resemblance to a giant cell tumour may be close, however these lesions are found in early adult life and furthermore have a different distribution, commonly affecting the appendicular skeleton, whereas plasmacytoma is more likely to be axial. Scintigraphy and CT afford no specific diagnostic features. Increased activity is observed on the blood pool phase of a bone scan while the delayed phase shows increased activity around the margins. CT confirms the extent of these tumours but does not afford tissue specific information.

MULTIPLE MYELOMATOSIS

The disseminated or generalized form of plasma cell infiltration of bone marrow is known as multiple myelomatosis. This entity may be preceded by an established solitary plasmacytoma or may arise apparently de novo.

It is much more common for the widespread form to present radiologically as a fully developed entity in the over 40 age group. Males are affected twice as often as females. Persistent bone pain or a pathological fracture are usually the first complaints.

Plasma cells have the function of elaborating globulin so that their abnormal proliferation causes elevation of the total serum proteins, due to the production of abnormal immunoglobulins. Such proliferation eventually takes place at the expense of all other marrow functions so that a non-specific leucopenia and secondary anaemia develop. Rouleaux formation of the red blood cells, although not specific, is suggestive of this condition. In about half of cases presence of an abnormal urinary protein constituent, Bence–Jones proteose, may be demonstrated. Abnormal proteinuria causes cast formation in the renal tubules with impairment of renal function. Excretion urography has been alleged to be hazardous in this disease by causing acute tubular obstruction from protein deposition. It is likely that dehydration, as a preliminary to excretion urography, is the more probable culprit. This is accentuated no doubt by the known incidence of hypercalcaemia, hypercalcuria and atypical amyloidosis. The last occurs in about 10% of all cases. The hypercalcaemia and hypercalcuria are unassociated with an elevation of either the serum alkaline phosphatase or phosphate levels.

The pattern of bone destruction may vary from diffuse osteoporosis, through small and almost insignificant areas of translucency, to rounded or oval defects with sharply defined margins. The last, which have long been regarded as characteristic, develop only at a relatively late stage of the disease. Frequently they coalesce to produce even larger areas of osteolysis. In the more advanced stages, many lesions may be present simultaneously which, individually, would present the features of a solitary plasmacytoma. Different portions of the skeleton may show different degrees of involvement, but very often the general pattern, especially when the condition is fully developed, tends to be constant.

Radiological changes. The two cardinal features are generalized reduction in bone density and localized areas of radiolucency in marrow cavities, especially those of the persistent red marrow areas. The axial skeleton, therefore, is affected predominantly. Lesions may be observed also in the shafts of long bones and in the skull. In spite of positive bone marrow aspiration, radiological features may be absent in as many as one third of cases, at least at initial presentation. This group of patients tend to develop generalized osteoporosis.

Since the detection of skeletal lesions is important in management, radiology plays a large part in assessing the extent of disease. Generally speaking a radiographic skeletal survey is superior to scintigraphic investigation, using a bone scanning agent, because the lesions are essentially osteolytic with no bone reaction. A bone scan is superior, however, in detecting lesions in the ribs because the associated fractures are demonstrated more easily.

Diffuse osteoporosis alone can cause suspicion of the disease in an elderly patient. Even though senile osteoporosis may be expected the possibility of myelomatosis always merits consideration, particularly when symptomatic bone pain is present. The smaller areas of radiolucency are poorly demarcated and appear to be irregular accentuations of the generalized osteoporotic process (Fig. 7.33). The rounded and oval defects that develop are characterised by the sharp definition of their edges. Reactive marginal sclerosis tends to be conspicuous by its absence, this feature providing a valuable diagnostic sign from metastases. Typically the cortex is eroded from within sharply defined margins (Fig. 7.34). Exceptionally, however, *sclerosing changes* have been reported. These have varied, some resembling focal lesions of prostatic metastases, some the spiculation of osteosarcoma and some a generalized diffuse increase in density. This very rare form of multiple my-

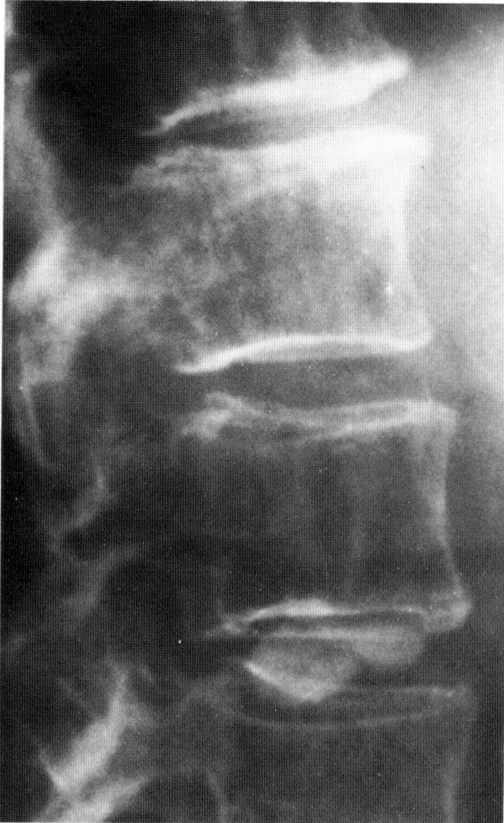

Fig. 7.33 Myelomatosis. Diffuse marrow involvement has resulted in an overall reduction in bone density similar to that seen in osteoporosis. However the rather patchy nature of radiolucencies should raise the possibility of myeloma.

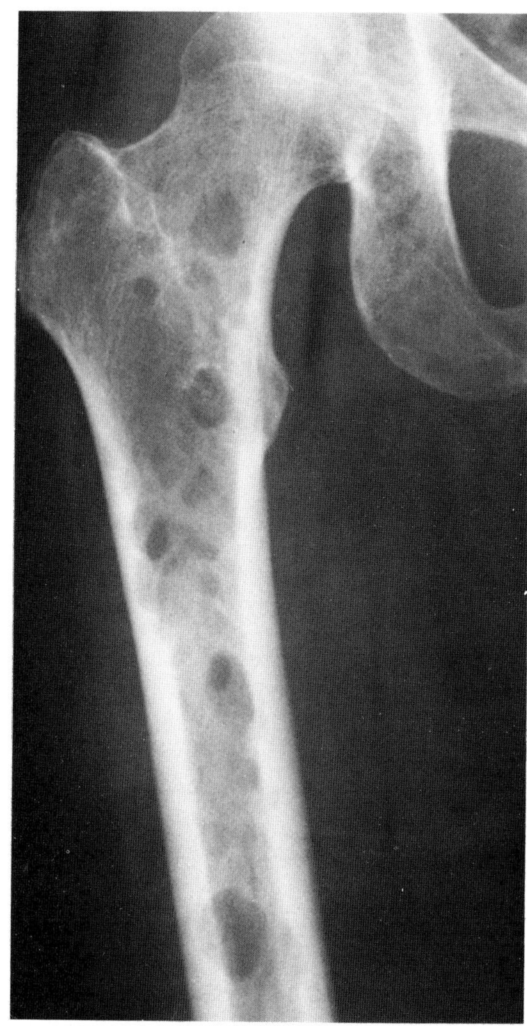

Fig. 7.34 Typical localized lesions of myeloma are demonstrated in the upper femur of an adult female patient. The sharply defined rounded defects with endosteal erosion of the cortex are characteristic.

lomatosis occurs in probably 2% of cases, and frequently is accompanied by a peripheral neuropathy.

Treatment, as in other conditions, may alter these appearances and, during its course, it is common to observe some lesions resolving whilst others evolve.

The *distribution of lesions* is very widespread and destructive foci are commonly located in the long bones in addition to the axial skeleton. Nor are these lesions confined any longer to cancellous structures. Cortical lesions also occur, but they require to be larger than those of cancellous bone before they can be shown in a radiograph. Involvement of the *skull* is quite variable. Diffuse and irregular translucencies with generalized osteoporosis are not uncommon. Such changes eventually become pronounced and extensive. The disease will not always be evident by the presence of the classical 'rain-drop' lesions — circular defects varying in diameter from a few millimetres to 2 or 3 cm — as has been suggested by earlier descriptions. Indeed, the skull sometimes may be totally exempt, even in the presence of many lesions elsewhere in the skeleton. Areas of osteolysis may be observed also in the *mandible*, a site only rarely affected by metastases. These myelomatous lesions, whether in the skull or in any bone, may erode the cortex and extend into the adjacent soft tissues. The resulting soft tissue masses are helpful in differentiating the advanced forms of the disease from the lesions of *metastatic carcinoma* which much less commonly produce extension into the soft tissues. The *spine* is often merely osteoporotic, but as the disease advances, multiple foci of destruction, almost invariably accompanied by some degree of collapse of the affected bodies, are likely to be present. With such collapse, paravertebral soft tissue shadows are common. Differentiation from inflammatory lesions can be made with some confidence as the intervertebral disc spaces and the articular surfaces are not affected. In the sacrum the destructive lesions may attain considerable size without being subjected to sufficient stress to cause collapse. The pedicles and posterior elements are involved less frequently and at a later stage than occurs with metastases. In the thorax a destructive rib lesion with a large associated soft tissue mass is much more suggestive of myelomatosis than of a plasmacytoma. Diffuse involvement, however, is more usual, numerous cystic foci of characteristic appearance being visible. The *clavicles* and *scapulae* may also show these destructive changes. Early diagnosis has been prompted by the recognition in a routine chest radiograph of small diffuse translucencies in the outer ends of the clavicles and in the acromion processes.

The *long bones*, as might be expected, are affected most commonly in the persistent red marrow areas of the proximal ends of the humeri and femora. Lesions, however, are by no means found only in such areas and irregular or punched-out translucencies in the shafts of other bones may be the first radiological manifestation of disease. In some advanced cases lytic defects may be due also to *secondary amyloidosis*, which can complicate many chronic disorders, such as rheumatoid disease and long-standing infections.

Pathological fractures are very often the initiating factor in the diagnosis of the disease. Whilst a compression fracture of a vertebral body may be overlooked despite causing back pain, a fracture of a long bone makes radiographic examination inevitable. These fractures heal remarkably quickly and soundly with massive callus and new bone formation. This response is somewhat surprising in view of the numerous cystic lesions and widespread osteoporosis which are likely to be present without any evidence of reactive sclerosis.

HISTIOCYTOSIS

The basic pathological abnormality in this group of diseases is a proliferation of histiocytic cells occurring particularly in the bone marrow, the spleen, the liver, the lymphatic glands and the lungs. In the more chronic forms these cells may become swollen with lipid deposits, essentially cholesterol (though the blood cholesterol level remains normal) and they present the pathological appearances of 'foam cells'. Some of these become necrotic and are replaced by fibrous tissue.

Various forms of the condition have been regarded in the past as separate entities. These forms are outlined below but it must be emphasized that this sub division is entirely arbitary since histiocytosis essentially presents a spectrum of disease.

EOSINOPHILIC GRANULOMA

This is the most mild expression of histiocytosis. Pathological changes are predominantly bony, although occasionally pulmonary involvement may occur. Children, especially boys, between 3 and 12 years are most commonly affected, although these lesions may be observed in adolescents, young adults and exceptionally the middle aged.

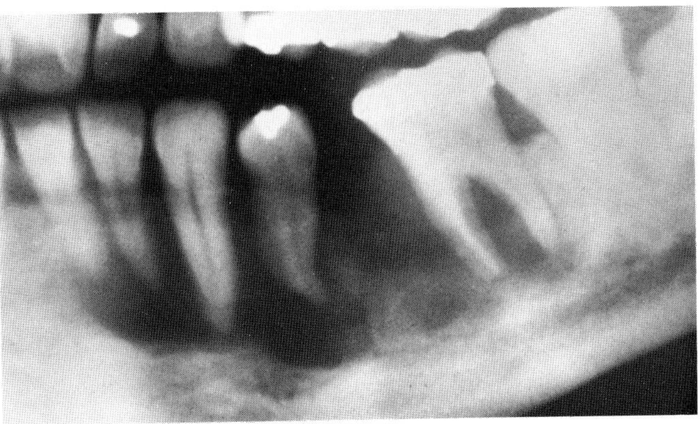

Fig. 7.35 Histiocytosis. A purely osteolytic lesion is present in the mandible, with well-defined, slightly scalloped margins. The lamina dura has been destroyed. The teeth seem to 'float in air'.

Any bone may be affected. A quarter of cases occur in the skull. The skull, pelvis and femora between them account for nearly two thirds of all cases.

Clinically pain and swelling may be accompanied by mild fever. Histologically the eosinophilic infiltration is found around collections of histiocytes. In this relatively mild form necrosis and fibrosis are rare and the appearance of foam cells suggests a more serious variety.

Radiological changes. Translucent areas of bone destruction with sharply defined margins and often of considerable size, are characteristic. The round or oval defects may have scalloped margins (Fig. 7.35). Although in the active phase they provoke no sclerotic margin, the healing phase, which usually develops by spontaneous regression, is marked by peripheral sclerosis round the lesion and slow reconstitution of the bony structure. This healing phase may be accelerated by biopsy, radiotherapy or steroid injection. True expansion is uncommon except in ribs and vertebral bodies. Apparent expansion may result from thickening of the overlying periosteum, especially if the cortex has been partially eroded (Fig. 7.36) or a pathological infarction has occurred. In approximately two thirds of patients the lesions are *solitary*. Differential diagnosis of a solitary lesion of this type may be extremely difficult and is either from a focus of osteomyelitis or, particularly, from Ewing's tumour which has a similar age incidence. In many patients skeletal survey will disclose the presence of other lesions, often entirely asymptomatic, facilitating the diagnosis. Multiple eosinophilic granulomas usually are found to be in different phases of evolution. As one lesion resolves another may appear in a different part of the skeleton. In the skull particularly new lesions of several centimetres in diameter may appear in as many weeks.

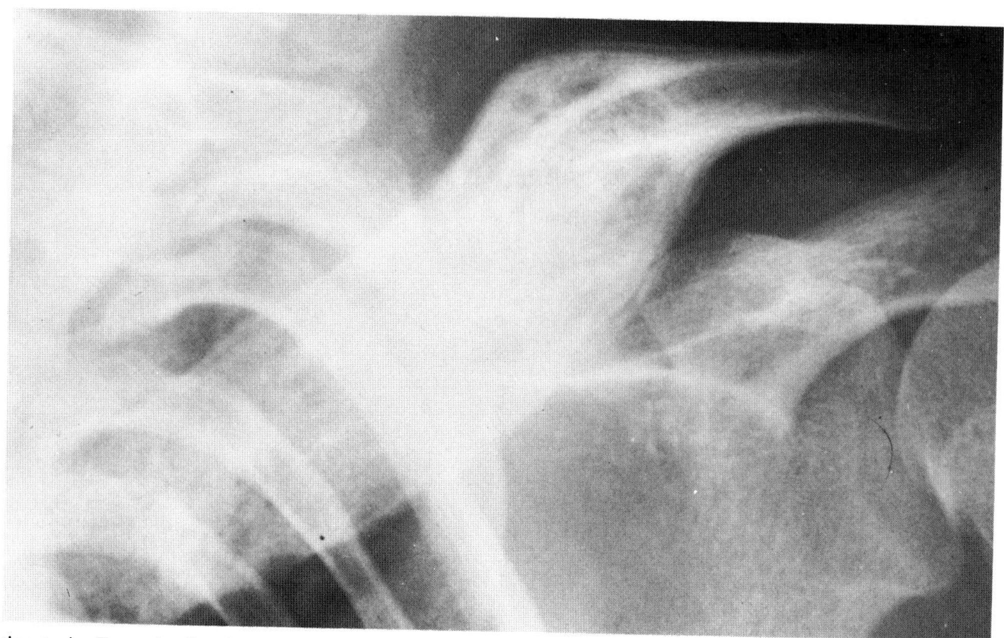

Fig. 7.36 Histiocytosis. Extensive involvement of a bone, here the clavicle, is often associated with layered periosteal new bone causing bony expansion. Ill-defined areas of resorption may be visualised in the lesion. This was the only abnormality found in a young girl over several years' follow-up.

Button sequestra may be observed. Skeletal scintigraphy is a sensitive means of detecting the lesions, particularly in the healing phase, and may be used conveniently in follow-up studies.

Solitary lesions in the spine may collapse, partially or completely, in the latter case presenting the classical appearance of *vertebra plana* (Fig. 7.37). The most commonly affected site is the thoracic spine which is affected more frequently than the lumbar and cervical spine. The lesions at one time were considered to represent an 'osteochondritis' and were named *Calvé's disease*. During the phase of collapse, the walls of the affected vertebral body tend to bulge laterally and paravertebral soft tissue shadows may be evident. The disc spaces on either side remain intact and may even be widened. As healing occurs, remarkably good reconstitution of these vertebral bodies may take place if sufficient years of growth remain. The vast majority of vertebra plana lesions, especially in a relatively healthy child, are caused by an eosinophil granuloma, and confirmatory biopsy is usually unnecessary. Nevertheless exceptions do exist, since the differential diagnosis of collapse of a single vertebral body includes the relative rarities of Ewing's tumour, metastasis from a neuroblastoma, benign osteoblastoma or, most exceptionally, a bizarre and atypical tuberculous focus.

This benign form of histiocytosis occasionally affects long bones and initially has a predilection for the diaphysis (Fig. 7.38). However, metaphyseal involvement may occur again causing confusion with a pyogenic infection. A rare entity, *chronic granulomatous (Landing–Shirkey) disease*, tends to cause skeletal lesions, including those in the metaphyses, which simulate closely the radiological appearance of multiple eosinophil granulomas. This condition is due usually to inherited and inadequate responses of leukocytes to infection.

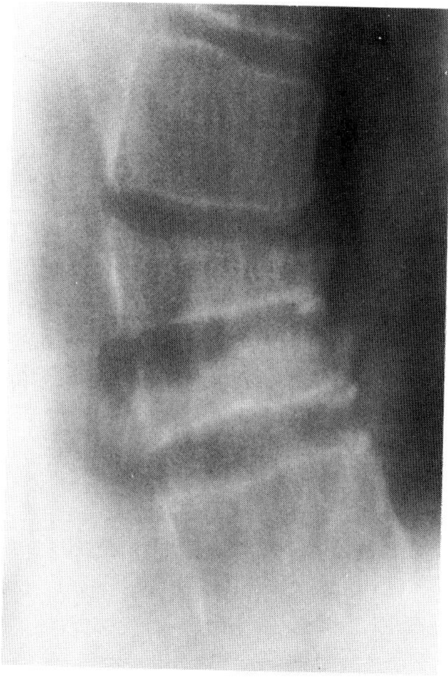

Fig. 7.37 Histiocytosis. Vertebral lesions in the thoracic spine are shown on a lateral tomogram. The bodies of T7 and 8 have collapsed with a slight increase in bone density. Note the relative preservation of the disc spaces.

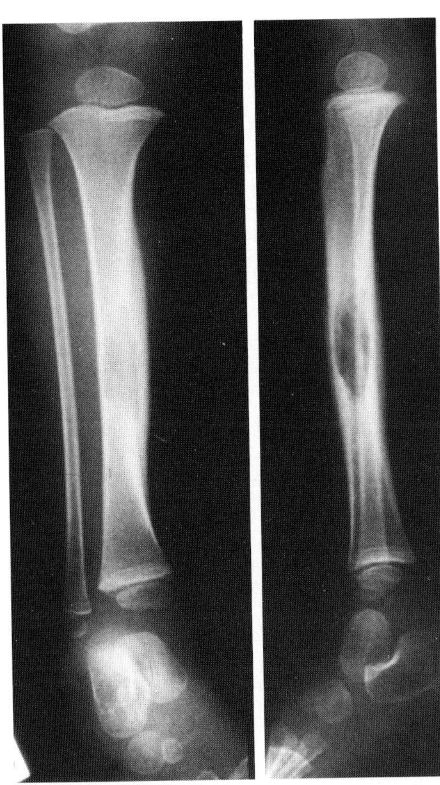

Fig. 7.38 Histiocytosis. A healing diaphyseal lesion exhibits periosteal new bone formation and minimal sclerosis around the margins of the radiolucency.

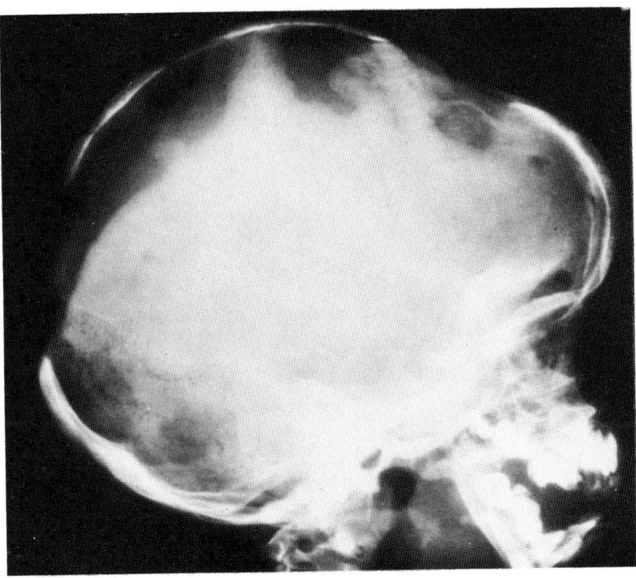

Fig. 7.39 Histiocytosis. Extensive skull involvement in a child with the Hand–Schüller–Christian type of lesion. The areas of destruction in the flat bones of the skull have a map-like configuration.

HAND–SCHÜLLER–CHRISTIAN DISEASE

This is a more chronic form of the disease, with dissemination of lesions in the lungs, lymph nodes, liver and spleen, in addition to virtually constant and early involvement of the skeleton.

The early case reports drew attention to a syndrome consisting of skull defects, exophthalmos and diabetes insipidus, the last two being associated with lesions round the orbit and the hypophysis respectively. This syndrome appears to have arisen by coincidence, since it is most uncommon to encounter the complete triad, and in some patients none of these features are present. Children below the age of 5 years are most frequently affected, though sporadic cases occur at later ages up to middle life. The course of the disease is chronic, often extending over 10 or more years. It is characterized by soreness of the mouth and loose teeth, due to deposits in the gums and jaws, and skin lesions. Abnormalities in the temporal bone are common, with an associated otitis media. The eventual prognosis is good, since spontaneous remission, possibly initiated or accelerated by radiotherapy, takes place in the majority of cases. Over 10%, however, terminate fatally.

Radiological changes. The bone defects are essentially the same as those of eosinophil granulomata, actual differentiation depending on the histological picture. They are, however, very much more numerous and particularly affect the flat bones. In the skull they frequently coalesce to produce widespread irregular defects usually likened to a map and described as the 'geographical skull', both tables often suffering extensive osteolysis (Fig. 7.39). Lesions in the mandible and maxilla begin round the tooth roots, so that the teeth, which are never affected, remain dense and appear to 'float in air' (Fig. 7.35). Several vertebrae may be completely or partially collapsed and extensive lesions may develop in the scapulae, ribs and pelvis. Osteolytic pelvic lesions or vertebral collapse in a child are suggestive of this disease. The long bones are by no means exempt, but their involvement is less common (Fig. 7.40).

If observed in a relatively early stage, sclerotic reaction round the sharply defined margins of these lesions will be conspicuous by its absence. When healing, which is often attributed to radiotherapy, does occur the lesions fill in by sclerosis in the same way as eosinophil granulomas. Such healing, however, is frequently spontaneous and it is common to find that all the lesions in the skeleton tend to be at the same stage of destruction or repair. However, new lesions may appear after the original ones have begun to heal, emphasizing again the wide spectrum of radiological change in histiocytosis.

The lungs show a fine nodular infiltration in the acute phase. With healing, these fibrose and persist as linear strands of increased density, but the presence of pulmonary changes in histiocytosis always increases the gravity of the prognosis (Fig. 7.41).

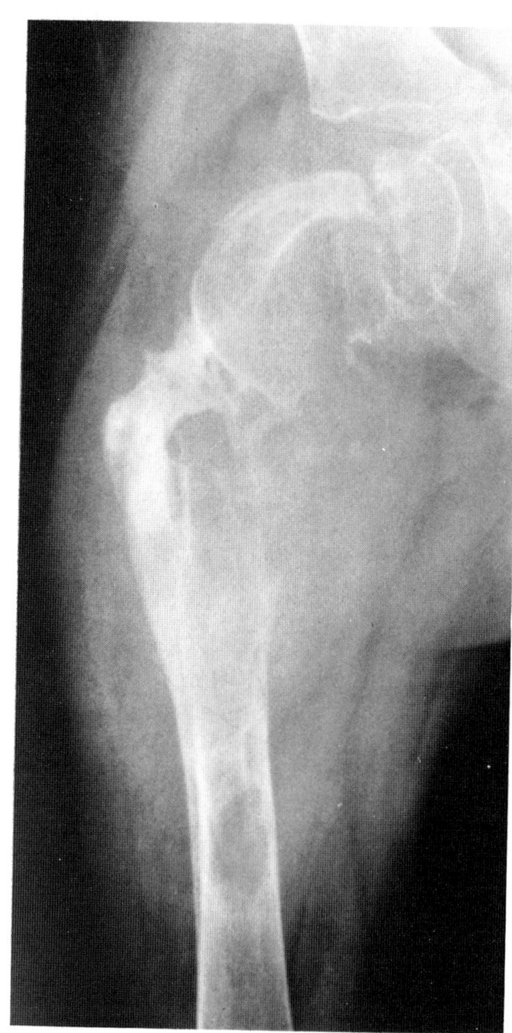

Fig. 7.40 Histiocytosis. Hand–Schüller–Christian type. Very extensive radiolucencies are present both in the metaphysis and diaphysis of this child's femur. A healed pathological fracture is present. Histiocytosis should always be considered in the differential diagnosis of bizarre bone lesions.

LETTERER–SIWE DISEASE

This is an acute or sub-acute disseminated form of the disease, occurring very rarely in infants below the age of 2 years and presenting a much more severe clinical picture. It is characterized by a pyrexia, with a rash and mouth sores, bleeding gums, respiratory symptoms and failure to thrive. Particular involvement of the extraskeletal tissues occurs with enlargement of the liver, spleen and lymph nodes. The disease usually ends fatally, often in a few months and at the most in 2 years. In those cases with a rapidly fatal outcome, skeletal lesions are unlikely to be demonstrated radiologically, apparently having insufficient time to develop. Nevertheless, histological change may be present in the bone marrow, with widespread masses of histiocytes and eosinophilic infiltration, comparable with the early histological picture of the benign eosinophil granuloma. Only in the rare cases that survive do fibrosis and cholesterol-containing foam cells become apparent.

Radiological changes. Bone lesions, when they occur, are indistinguishable from those of Hand–Schüller–Christian disease, but tend to be even more widely spread, both in

Fig. 7.41 Histiocytosis. Adult pulmonary involvement (male aged 20). **A.** A localized view from a chest X-ray demonstrates a coarse interstitial pulmonary fibrosis. Note also a pathological fracture of the left fourth rib due to a bony deposit. **B.** A CT scan demonstrates clearly peripheral interstitial pulmonary fibrosis with focal emphysema. (L 374, W 400.)

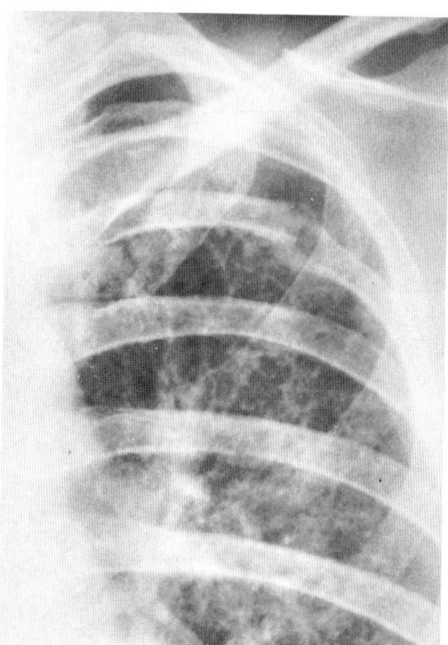

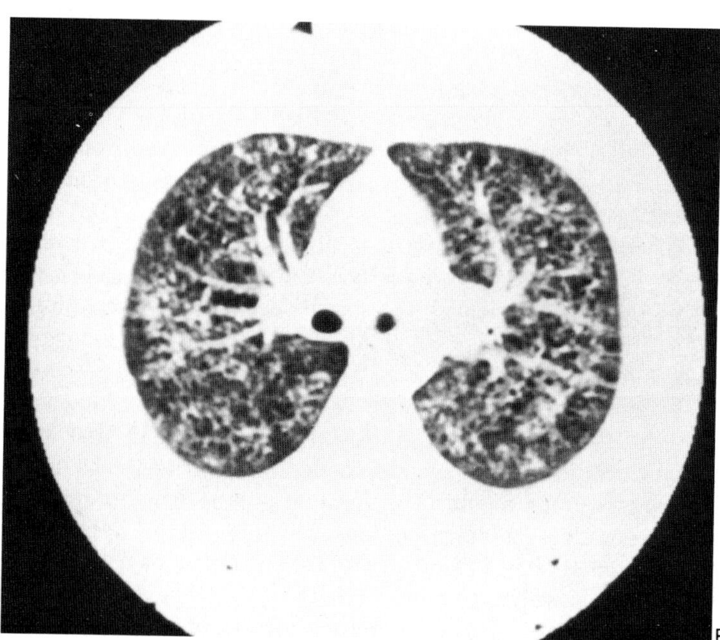

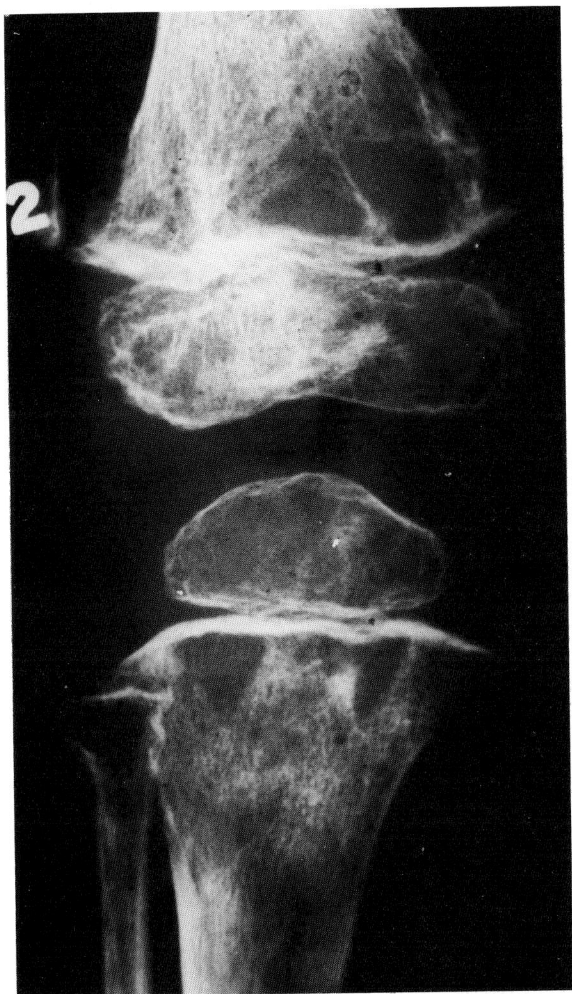

Fig. 7.42 Histiocytosis. Letterer–Siwe type. Massive destructive lesions are present throughout the skeleton, but affecting particularly the metadiaphyseal areas of the long bones. A similar appearance could be produced by metastases from a neuroblastoma or the advanced stages of leukaemia.

the flat bones and even more in the metadiaphyseal areas of the long bones (Fig. 7.42). They show no trace of the sclerotic reaction round their sharply-defined, punched-out margins. Diffuse pulmonary infiltration is common. This may closely resemble miliary tuberculosis and is a variety of honeycomb lung.

In summary, *histiocytosis* is a disease primarily of childhood, although exceptionally, its more benign manifestations may be observed in early adult life. The older the child, and the more the lesions are confined to the skeleton rather than other tissues, the better the prognosis. It must be appreciated that the benign eosinophil granuloma may deteriorate to a chronic, multifocal form of the spectrum, and that, conversely, a change to this same chronic form may be the salvation of a small number of those patients afflicted with the most aggressive form, Letterer–Siwe disease.

STORAGE DISORDERS OF THE LYMPHORETICULAR SYSTEM

A number of conditions have been described in which the lymphoreticular system is the site of abnormal deposition of lipoproteins, usually as a result of inborn errors of metabolism. The commonest of these rare disorders are Gaucher's disease and Niemann–Pick disease.

GAUCHER'S DISEASE

Young Jewish females are particularly susceptible to this hereditary conditions caused by deficiency of B-glucosadase. It is not confined by any means to this ethnic group or sex. Although manifestations of the condition commonly become apparent in the later years of childhood and in early adult life, the disease may be so chronic, and of such insidious onset, that it may be recognized for the first time only in middle age or even later life. In infancy the rapidly fatal course of this systemic disease is characterized by gross neurological changes and pulmonary infiltration.

In the juvenile and young adult variety the principal complaint is of weakness and fatigue with progressive dementia. On clinical examination splenic enlargement is detected in 95% of cases. Bone pain may be present, sometimes sufficiently severe to permit clinical confusion with osteomyelitis. It is in the chronic form of the disease that characteristic and often diagnostic bone changes may be expected. Histological examination reveals numerous large histiocytes within which an abnormal lipoprotein, *kerasin*, is present. These cells are disseminated throughout the marrow of the haematopoietic skeleton, in addition to the spleen and liver.

Radiological changes. Diffuse infiltration of the bone marrow is likely to cause widespread and irregular medullary radiolucency. Only when collections of the abnormal histiocytes occur, do destructive medullary lesions become visible, but even before this, *abnormal modelling* of the long bones may be evident. Expansion of the distal ends of the femora begins with a loss of the normal concavity of the medial sides. Eventually this justifies the classical description of 'flask-shaped', on the analogy of the contour of the Erlenmeyer flask (Fig. 7.43). This feature is, however, not diagnostic of Gaucher's disease and may be seen in other conditions including haemolytic anaemias (thalassaemia), leukaemia, osteopetrosis and lead poisoning. Other bones, notably the tibia and humerus, may be similarly affected. *Destructive lesions*, due to conglomerations of abnormal cells, present as osteolytic areas, which may cause localized endosteal cortical erosions, with sharply defined, scalloped borders. As these larger lesions increase in size and coalesce, the areas of bone abnormality may become exceedingly widespread, both in the individual bone and in the

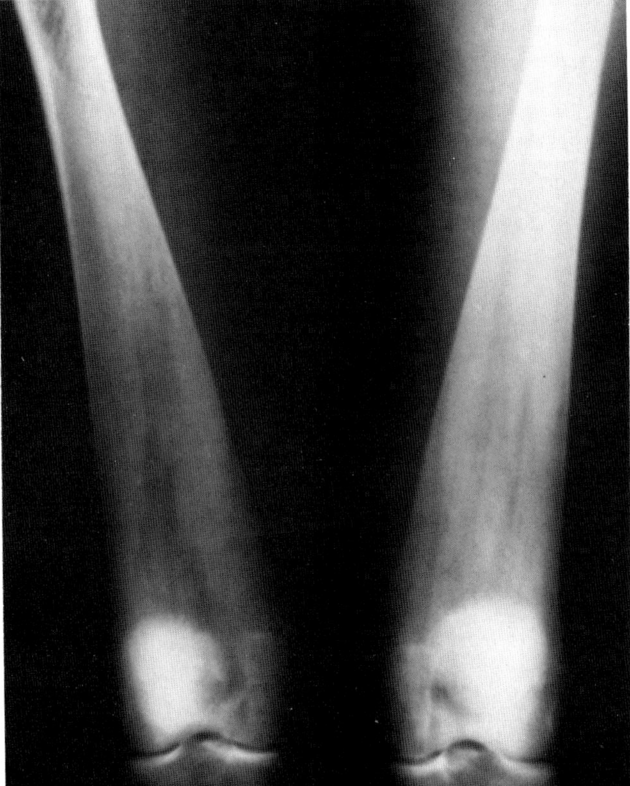

Fig. 7.43 Gaucher's disease (female aged 20). Abnormal modelling of the distal ends of the femora has resulted in typical flask-shaped appearance. An osteolytic lesion with a coarse trabecular pattern is present in the right femur.

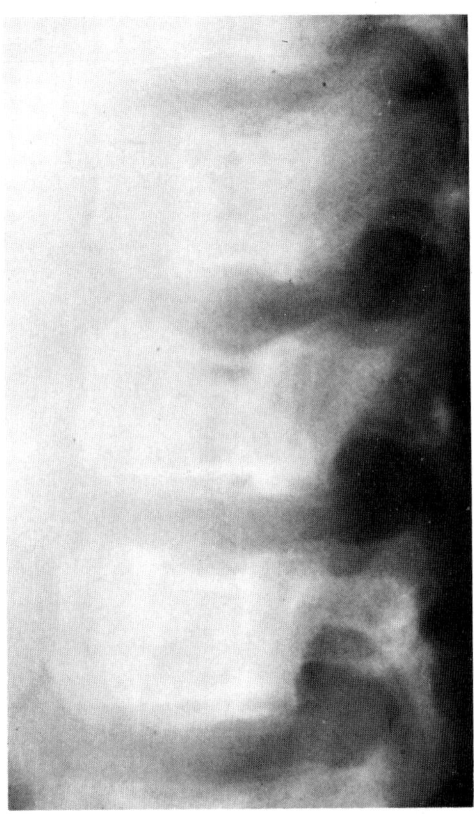

Fig. 7.44 Gaucher's disease. Infarctions in vertebral bodies have produced the 'bone within a bone' appearance throughout the lumbar spine in this child.

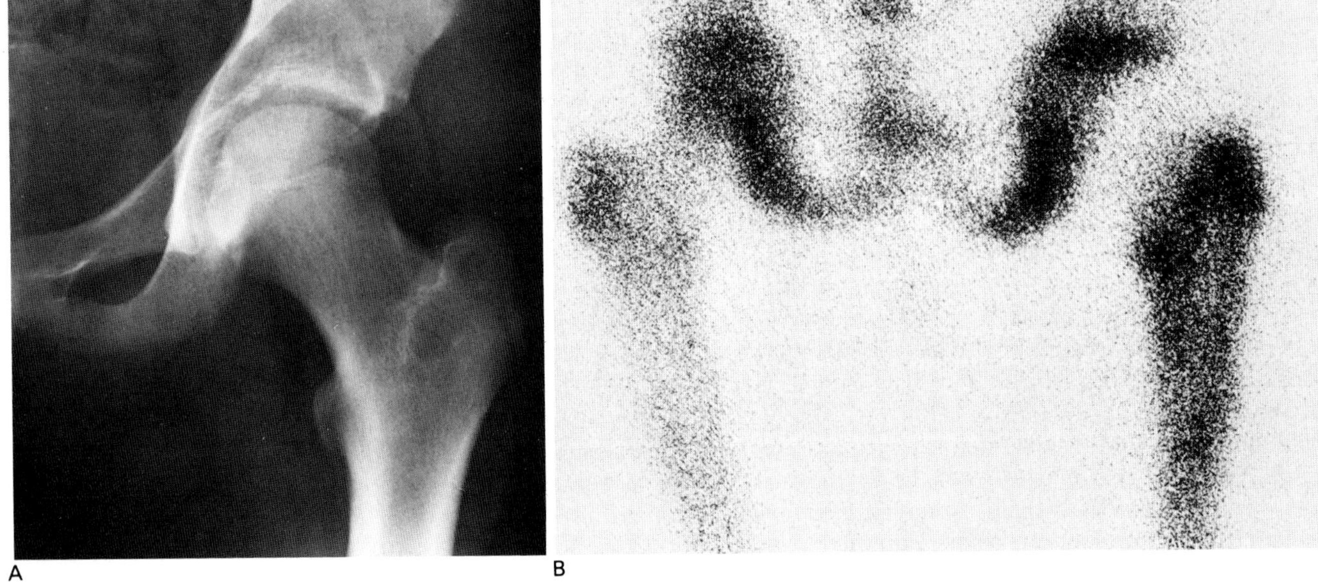

Fig. 7.45 Gaucher's disease — acute bone infarction. **A**. A radiograph of a 13-year-old girl, with known Gaucher's disease, presenting with acute hip pain of 12 hours' duration. Slight endosteal sclerosis is shown in the inferior pubic ramus and an area of ill-defined radiolucency in the intertrochanteric region. **B**. The delayed phase of a bone scan reveals the femoral head and neck to be markedly photon-deficient consistent with acute infarction. Abnormally increased activity is present also at site of previous disease.

keleton as a whole. *Infarction* of bone is not uncommon (Fig. 7.44). The femoral and humeral heads, especially the former, are often involved in this way. In a child such infarction may simulate Perthes' disease. In an adult the destructive changes in the femoral head that develop cannot be differentiated from avascular necrosis of other origin. Bone scintigraphy may be helpful in the assessment of acute bone pain in order to detect early infarction (Fig. 7.45). Subsequent disruption of articular surfaces promotes secondary osteoarthritis (Fig. 7.46).

Pathological fractures may follow relatively minor trauma. While fractures may occur through any affected bone, compression of a vertebral body is the usual lesion. As in many other conditions these compression fractures are most likely to be found in the lower dorsal or lumbar regions, the areas of greatest stress. Frank zones of osteolysis in the spine are rare in Gaucher's disease, but generalized osteoporosis is common. Pathological fractures also occur in the femoral neck causing coxa vara, and in sites where no concomitant radiological abnormality can be identified. In all such cases extensive radiological survey of the skeleton is indicated to establish or exclude the presence of characteristic pathological lesions.

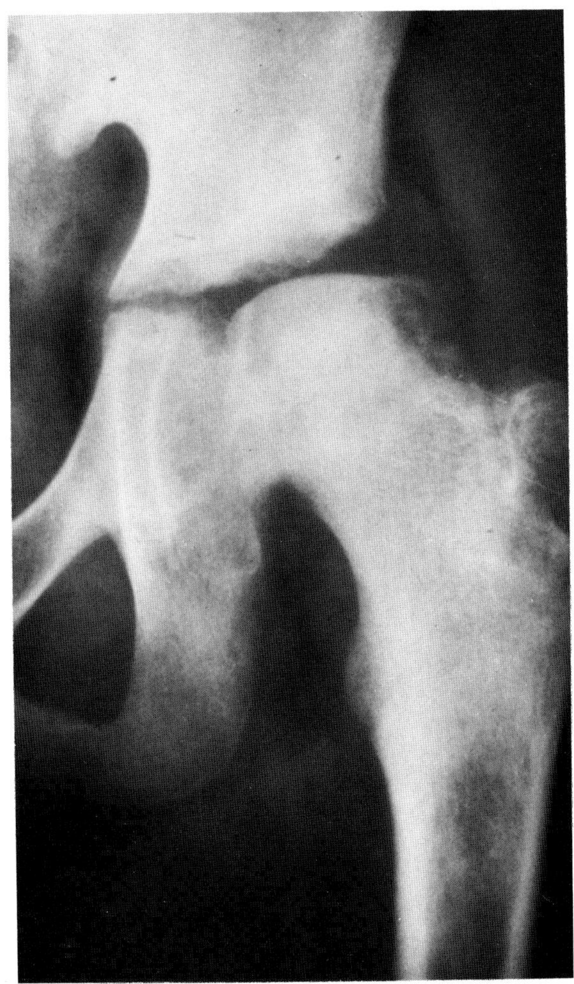

Fig. 7.46 Gaucher's disease. This adolescent has considerable deformity of the femoral head and acetabulum secondary to episodes of infarction. Evidence of degenerative arthritis is present already.

Usually bone trabeculae are destroyed, but in the chronic form of the disease a state of equilibrium may be reached which is characterized by *sclerotic reaction* within the bone. This may be due to actual thickening of the trabeculae that remain, or to osseous metaplasia. A coarse network of dense medullary strands results which may give the appearance of a honeycomb, not unlike that observed on rare occasions in multiple myelomatosis. In addition, endosteal thickening may develop, as in the later stages of sickle cell disease and myelosclerosis, the appearances again being suggestive of 'a bone within a bone'. On the outer surface, diffuse periosteal reactions may develop, usually overlying an intact cortex.

As a result of these reactive changes in the later stages of the disease, the radiological picture may be confusing. It is particularly important for differentiation from *chronic osteomyelitis* to be made, as misguided surgical intervention sometimes has been followed by chronic and resistant infection with persistent discharging sinuses.

Unlike some of the other diseases in this group, notably the chronic haemolytic anaemias, the distribution of these lesions tends to be of a peripheral rather than a central pattern. The chronic form of the disease may cause characteristic changes in the first decade; the diffuse medullary osteoporosis and abnormality of modelling in the distal ends of the femora are likely to be the first radiological manifestations. The changes may be widespread and may resemble thalassaemia, except that the bones of the hands and feet are usually completely or relatively exempt.

In the adult, the long tubular bones are usually the site of lesions, destructive processes in the pelvis and thoracic cage rarely being evident. Nevertheless involvement of the axial skeleton does occur, as shown by the frequency of spinal osteoporosis and occasional vertebral collapse, which may be apparent even in the absence of other radiological evidence of this disease. No characteristic lesions are recognized in the skull, but diffuse osteoporosis has been reported. Frank cystic areas of destruction have been noted round the tooth roots in the mandible.

In the radiological assessment of any skeletal abnormality, appreciation of associated abnormalities of soft tissue is of the utmost importance. In this instance the combination of the changes described above, with a patient with an appropriate ethnic background and with *splenomegaly* provides a strong diagnostic triad. Enlargement of the spleen, and often the liver, is almost constant in this disease. Pulmonary involvement is unusual, but an appearance suggestive of interstitial fibrosis may be observed, particularly in young children, even in the absence of skeletal involvement.

NIEMANN-PICK DISEASE

This rare disorder of the lymphoreticular system, of a type similar to Gaucher's disease, has, in its classical form, a predilection for Jewish females under the age of 2 years. The abnormal lipoprotein in the 'foam cells' in this instance is *sphingomyelin*. Osseous changes, in comparison to Gaucher's disease are less severe. Nevertheless, careful study may disclose generalized osteoporosis, minor coarsening of the trabeculae and minor modelling abnormalities. Overt areas of osteolysis do occur, but are unusual and may resemble the lesions of histiocytosis. On the other hand interstitial pulmonary infiltration, causing a 'honeycomb' lung appearance and hepatosplenomegaly, are common in classical cases, for which the prognosis is grave. Other types of the condition have been recognized in older children.

DISORDERS OF THE COAGULATION MECHANISM

HAEMOPHILIA AND ITS VARIANTS

The normal process of blood coagulation, which terminates in the formation of a network of fibrin, to arrest the passage of blood cells, depends on a number of factors. Many of these have been recognized relatively recently and their individual deficiencies have led to descriptions of several disease entities within the haemophiliac group.

From the radiological aspect the most important of these disorders are classic **haemophilia,** due to deficiency of Factor VIII and the even rarer **Christmas disease,** due to deficiency of Factor IX. These hereditary diseases primarily affect males being an X-linked, usually recessive disorder. The degree of affliction is related to the level of deficiency.

The bleeding tendency is usually observed during the first year of life and may affect any tissue system. Christmas disease is usually less severe. The actual bleeding is considered to result from trauma, possibly very slight, rather than being spontaneous. Bleeding into the joint spaces is characteristic. Such episodes commonly become more frequent during the later years of childhood and adolescence. In adult life the patient, having become aware of his peculiar disability, is less likely to suffer. Milder forms of the disease may cause formation of large, soft tissue haematomas without significant joint involvement. This is true of one other bleeding disorder, **von Willebrand's disease,** which affects both sexes equally and is transmitted in an autosomal dominant manner. If, however, the Factor VIII level is low, bleeding into joints can occur in this condition.

Radiological changes in the skeleton are caused by bleeding into joints, within bony structures and beneath the periosteum. Frequent repetition of such episodes, particularly at an early age, increases their severity.

Intra-articular haemorrhage. In the early stages of the disease, the soft tissue distension of a joint due to a haemarthrosis cannot be distinguished radiologically from a frank traumatic or inflammatory synovial effusion. The traumatic episode responsible for it, however, may have been so slight as almost to escape notice. Frequent repetition of haemorrhagic incidents results in synovial thickening and articular erosions. Initially these erosions tend to be marginal in distribution. At the same time the bony structures in the vicinity of an affected joint are likely to become porotic, partly through disuse, but even more through persistent hyperaemia associated with organization of the haemarthroses. This latter factor, as with hyperaemia of any other cause, commonly causes enlargement of the growing epiphyses (Fig. 7.47). Such epiphyses may also become abnormal in shape and often fuse prematurely. Differentiation from a chronic inflammatory synovitis, particularly one of tuberculous aetiology, is of importance and may present some radiological difficulty. The trabecular pattern of the bone becomes coarse and often has a lattice appearance. In later life secondary degenerative changes develop prematurely (Fig. 7.48).

The knee, being the joint predominantly subject to traumatic stresses and strains, is affected almost invariably, involvement being frequently bilateral. The intercondylar notch becomes wide and deep. The patella may develop an unusually rectangular shape and its proximal articular surface is a common site of an erosion.

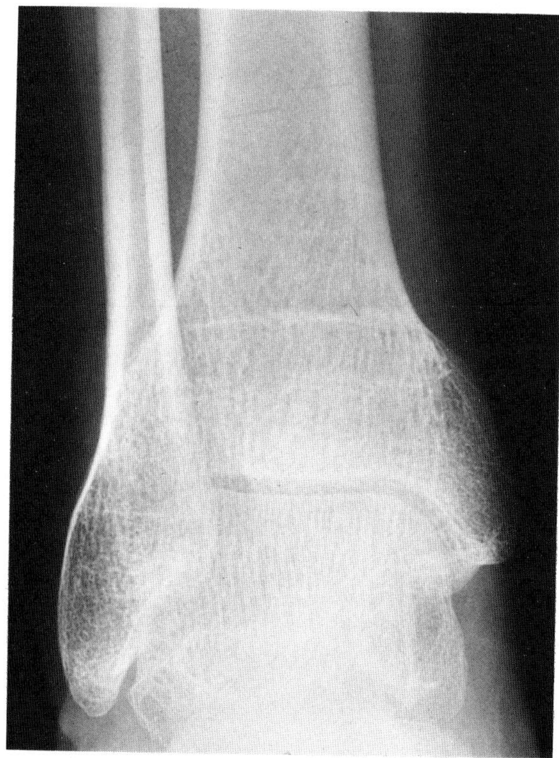

Fig. 7.47 Haemophilia. The former epiphyses are disproportionately large, presenting a 'squared' appearance. Hyaline cartilage thickness at the ankle joint is reduced.

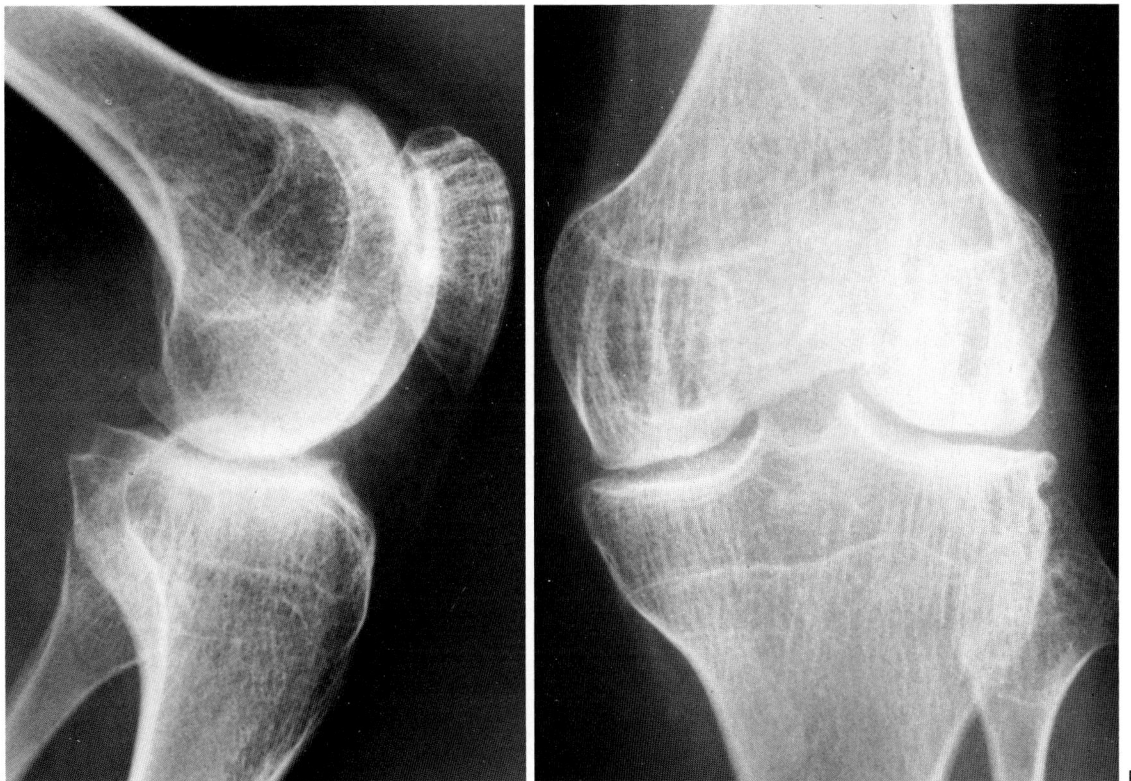

Fig. 7.48 A and **B**. Haemophilia. Typical appearances in an adult patient subject to recurrent haemarthroses since childhood. As well as the enlarged, squared appearance of the former epiphyses, hyaline cartilage width is reduced, and osteophytes are present due to secondary osteoarthritis. Areas of radiolucency within medullary bone probably represent old intraosseous haemorrhages.

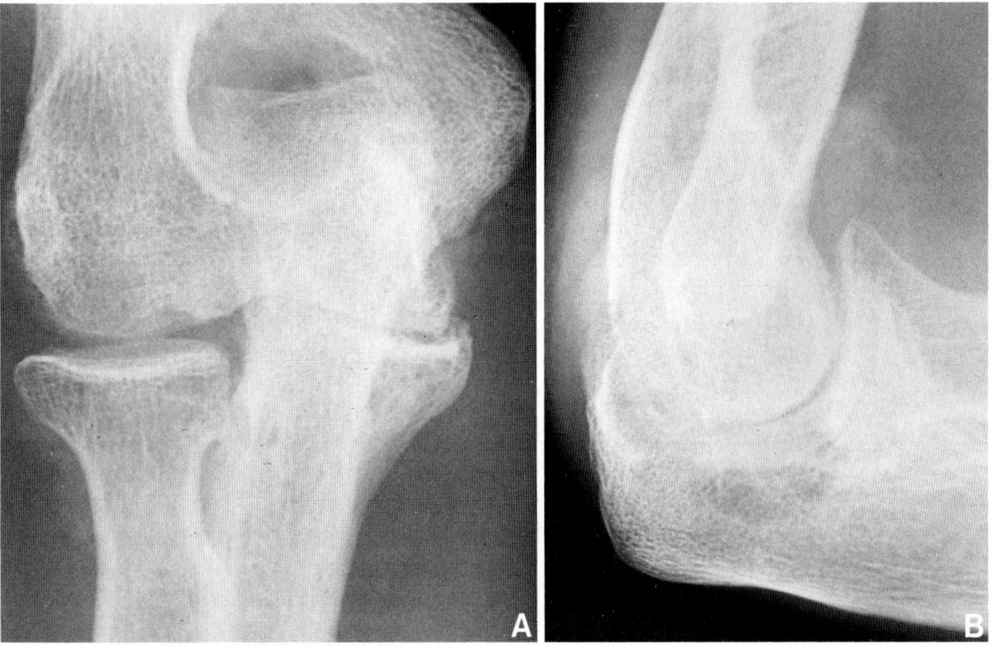

Fig. 7.49 Haemophilia. Repeated intra-articular haemorrhages have caused overgrowth of the epiphyses, particularly the head of the radius. The joint capsule is distended and the synovium is amorphously dense due to the deposition of haemosiderin from recurrent haemarthroses. A subarticular cyst is present in the olecranon fossa, and degenerative changes, in the form of hyaline cartilage thinning and osteophyte formation, are present.

The elbows and ankles also are affected commonly. A characteristic abnormality in the former joint is an enlarged and deformed radial head. The shoulders and wrists are less frequently involved. Bleeding into the hip is unusual, but when this does occur avascular necrosis of the femoral head causes an appearance comparable to Perthes' disease. Growth lines in diaphyses adjacent to affected joints commonly mark previous haemorrhagic episodes. Distended joint capsules, particularly those of the elbows, may become radiologically dense by deposition within them of haemosiderin (Fig. 7.49).

Intra-osseous haemorrhage. Juxta-articular cystic lesions may be observed in the later stages of the disease, with a peculiar predilection for the proximal humeral epiphyses and the olecranon processes. While many are comparable to the post-traumatic subarticular cysts of degenerative joint disease, the fact that some of these cysts are remote from the articular surfaces has led to the belief that they may be caused by haemorrhage within the bone itself.

Subperiosteal haemorrhage. The recognition of large osteolytic lesions in this disease, although still relatively rare, has become more frequent in recent years. These lesions are known as *haemophiliac pseudotumours* and occur in about 1 or 2% of severely affected patients. They have been observed especially in the iliac wings and in the shafts of the long bones of the lower limb, although other bones, including the calcaneus, have been involved (Fig. 7.50). These destructive lesions have been attributed to bleeding below the periosteum and often are accompanied by large swellings, sometimes relatively painless, of the soft tissues. Relation to a former traumatic incident occasionally may be established. Absorption of the underlying cortex and medulla with elevation of the periosteal margins results in an appearance which may be highly suggestive of a malignant bone tumour. Calcification is not uncommon within the space occupying lesions. A diagnostic clue, however, may be provided by evidence in an adjacent joint of a haemophiliac arthropathy. Failure to appreciate the nature of this entity, nevertheless, has resulted in iatrogenic disasters by unnecessary amputation.

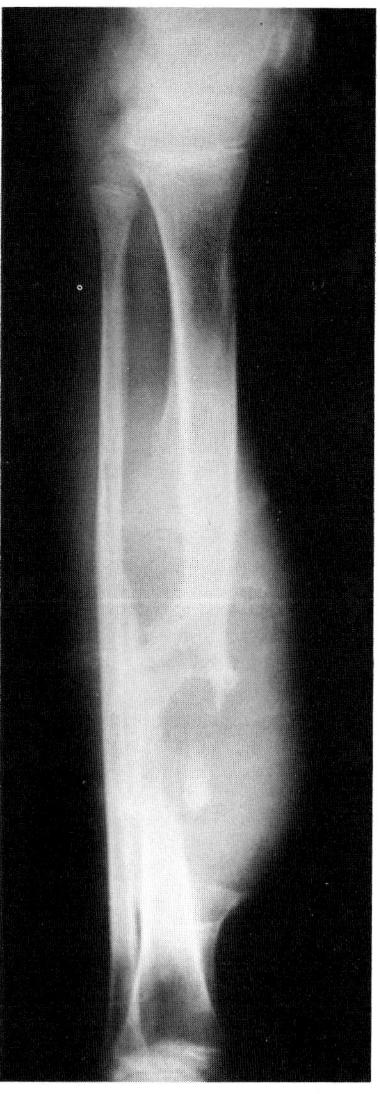

Fig. 7.50 Haemophiliac pseudotumour. A huge destructive lesion in the tibia, with relatively well-defined margins, is associated with some periosteal reaction. Although an initial impression may be of a malignant tumour changes of haemophilic arthropathy can be seen in the knee and ankle.

The diagnosis of haemophilia is likely to be made clinically, but the radiologist must be aware of its skeletal manifestations, including not only the typical arthropathies and bone cysts, but also and importantly the rare haemophiliac pseudotumours.

REFERENCES AND SUGGESTIONS FOR FURTHER READING (chapters 5–7)

Dahlin, D. C. (1978) *Bone Tumors*, 3rd edn. Springfield: C. C. Thomas

Edeiken, J. (1981) *Roentgen Diagnosis of Diseases of Bone*. 3rd edn. Baltimore: Williams & Wilkins.

Resnick, D., Niwayama, G. (1981) *Diagnosis of Bone and Joint Disorders*. Philadelphia: W. B. Saunders.

Murray, R. O., Jacobson, H. G (1977) *The Radiology of Skeletal Disorders*, 2nd edn. Edinburgh: Churchill Livingstone.

Wilner, D. (1982) *Radiology of Bone Tumors and Allied Disorders*. Philadelphia: W. B. Saunders.

Yaghmai, I. (1979) *Angiography of Bone and Soft Tissue Lesions*. Berlin: Springer-Verlag.

Osteoid osteoma

Omojola, M., Cockshott, W. P., Beatty, E. G. (1981) Osteoid osteoma: an evaluation of diagnostic modalities. *Clinical Radiology*, **32**, 199–204.

Osteoblastoma

Marsh, B. W., Bonfiglio, M., Brady, L. P., Enneking, W. F. (1975)

Benign osteoblastoma: Range of manifestations. *Journal of Bone and Joint Surgery*, **57A**, 1–9.

Osteosarcoma
Dahlin, D. C. (1967) Osteogenic sarcoma. A study of 600 cases. *Journal of Bone and Joint Surgery*, **49A**, 101–110.

Parosteal osteosarcoma
Lorentzon, R., Larsson, S. E., Boquist, L. (1980) Parosteal (juxtacortical) osteosarcoma. *Journal of Bone and Joint Surgery*, **62B**, 86–92.

Chondroblastoma
Nolan, D., Middlemiss, J. H. (1975) Chondroblastoma of bone. *Clinical Radiology*, **26**, 343–350.

Chondromyxoidfibroma
Beggs, I. G., Stoker, D. J. (1982) Chondromyxoid fibroma of bone. *Clinical Radiology*, **33**, 671–679.

Chondrosarcoma
Barnes, R., Catto M. (1966) Chondrosarcoma of bone. *Journal of Bone & Joint Surgery*, **48B**, 729–764.

Mesenchymal chondrosarcoma
Salvador, A. H., Beabout, J. W., Dahlin, D. C. (1971) Mesenchymal Chondrosarcoma. Observations on 30 new cases. *Cancer*, **28**, 605–615.

Radiation sarcoma
Smith, J. (1982) Radiation-induced sarcoma of bone: Clinical and radiographic findings in 43 patients irradiated for soft tissue neoplasms. *Clinical Radiology*, **33**, 205–221.

Non-ossifying fibroma
Maudsley, R. H. (1956) Non-osteogenic fibroma of bone (fibrous metaphyseal defect). *Journal of Bone and Joint Surgery*, **38B**, 714–733.

Desmoplastic fibroma
Rabhan, W. N., Rossi, J. (1968) Desmoplastic fibroma of bone. *Journal of Bone and Joint Surgery*, **50A**, 487–502.

Fibrosarcoma
Larsson, S. E., Lorentzon, R., Boquist, L. (1976) Fibrosarcoma of Bone. *Journal of Bone and Joint Surgery*, **58B**, 412–417.

Malignant fibrous histiocytoma
Feldman, F., Norman, D. (1972) Intra- and extra-osseous malignant histiocytoma (malignant fibrous xanthoma). *Radiology*, **104**, 497–508.

Giant cell tumour
Jacobs, P. (1972) The diagnosis of osteoclastoma (giant cell tumour): a radiological and pathological correlation. *British Journal of Radiology*, **45**, 121–136.

Solitary bone cyst
Lodwick, G. S. (1958). Juvenile unicameral bone cyst. *American Journal of Roentgenology*, **83**, 495–504.

Ewing's tumour
Dahlin, D. C., Coventry, M. B., Scanlon, P. W. (1961) Ewing's sarcoma: a critical analysis of 165 cases. *Journal of Bone and Joint Surgery*, **43A**, 185–192.

Adamantinoma
Huvos, A. G., Marcove, R. C. (1975) Adamantinoma of long bones. A clinicopathological study of fourteen cases with vascular origin suggested. *Journal of Bone and Joint Surgery*, **57A**, 148–154.

Vascular tumours
Unni, K. K., Ivins, J. C., Beabout, J. W., Dahlin, D. C. (1971) Haemangioma, haemangiopericytoma and haemangioendothelioma (angiosarcoma) of bone. *Cancer*, **27**, 1403–1414.

Haemangiomatosis
Halliday, D. R., Dahlin, D. C., Pugh, D. G., Young, H. H. (1964) Massive osteolysis and angiomatosis. *Radiology*, **82**, 637–644.

Cystic angiomatosis
Schajowicz, F., Aiello, C. L., Francone, M. V., Giannini, R. E. (1978) Cystic angiomatosis (hamartous haemolymphangiomatosis) of bone. A clinicopathological study of three cases. *Journal of Bone and Joint Surgery*, **60B**, 100–106.

Aneurysmal bone cyst
Bonakdarpour, A., Levy, W. M., Aegerter, E. (1978) Primary and secondary aneurysmal bone cyst: a radiological study of 75 cases. *Radiology*, **126**, 75–83.

Neurofibromatosis
Meszaros, W. T. (1966) Neurofibromatosis. *American Journal of Roentgenology*, **98**, 557–569.

Parosteal lipoma
Jacobs, P. (1972) Parosteal lipoma with hyperostoses. *Clinical Radiology*, **23**, 196–198.

Macrodystrophia lipomatosa
Goldman, A. B., Kaye, K. J. (1977) Macrodystrophia lipomatosa: radiographic diagnosis. *American Journal of Roentgenology*, **128**, 101–105.

Chordoma
Firooznia, H., Pinto, R. S., Lin, J. P., Baruch, H. H., Zausner, J. (1976). Chordoma: radiologic evaluation of 20 cases. *American Journal of Roentgenology*, **127**, 797–805.

Chronic anaemias
Minagi, H., Steinbach, H. L. (1966) Roentgen appearance of anomalies associated with hypoplastic anaemias and congenital hypoplasia anaemia (erythrogenesis imperfecta). *American Journal of Roentgenology*, **97**, 100–109.
Moseley, J. E. (1974) Skeletal changes in the anaemias. *Seminars in Roentgenology*, **9**, 169–182.

Thalassaemia (Cooley's anaemia)
Middlemiss, J. H., Raper, A. B. (1966). Skeletal changes in the haemoglobinopathies. *Journal of Bone and Joint Surgery*, **48B**, 693–702.

Sickle cell disease
Bohrer, S. P. (1970) Acute long bone diaphyseal infarcts in sickle cell disease. *British Journal of Radiology*, **43**, 685–697.

Leukaemia
Ngan, H., James, K. W., McCready, V. R., Macdonald, J. S. (1966) Bone changes in adult acute leukaemia. *British Journal of Radiology*, **41**, 66–69.
Simmons, C. R., Harle, T. S., Singleton, E. B. (1968) The osseous manifestations of leukaemia in children. *Radiological Clinics of North America*, **6**, 115–130.

Myeloid metaplasia and mastocytosis
Barer, M., Peterson, L. F., Dahlin, D. C., Winkelmann, R. K., Stewart, J. R. (1968) Mastocytosis with osseous lesions resembling metastatic lesions in bones. *Journal of Bone and Joint Surgery*, **50A**, 142–152.
Pettigrew, J. D., Ward, H. P. (1969) Correlation of radiologic, histologic and clinical findings in angogenic myeloid metaplasia. *Radiology*, **93**, 541–548.

Hodgkin's disease
Granger, W., Whitaker, R. (1967) Hodgkin's disease in bone with special reference to periosteal reaction. *British Journal of Radiology*, **40**, 939–948.

Non-Hodgkin's lymphoma
Pear, B. L. (1974) Skeletal manifestations of the lymphomas and leukaemias. *Seminars in Roentgenology*, **9**, 229–240.
Ivins, J. C., Dahlin, D. C. (1953) Reticulum cell sarcoma of bone. *Journal of Bone and Joint Surgery*, **35A**, 835–842.
Ngan, H., Preston, B. (1975) Non-Hodgkin's lymphoma presenting with osseous lesions. *Clinical Radiology*, **26**, 351–356.

Whittaker, L. R. (1973) Burkitt's lymphomas. *Clinical Radiology*, **24**, 339–346.

Multiple myelomatosis

Meszaros, W. T. (1974) The many facets of multiple myeloma. *Seminars in Roentgenology*, **9**, 219–228.

Murray, J. A. (1975) Multiple myeloma. *Current Practice in Orthopaedic Surgery*, **6**, 145–170.

Histiocytosis

Schajowicz, F., Sluttitel, J. (1973) Eosinophilic granuloma of bone and its relationship to Hand-Schuller-Christian and Letterer-Siwe Syndromes. *Journal of Bone and Joint Surgery*, **55B**, 545–565.

Takahashi, T., Martel, W., Oberman, H. A. (1966) The variable roentgenographic appearance of idiopathic histiocytosis. *Clinical Radiology*, **17**, 48–53.

Gaucher's disease and Niemann-Pick disease

Greenfield, G. B. (1970) Bone changes in chronic adult Gaucher's disease. *American Journal of Roentgenology, Radium Therapy and Nuclear Medicine*, **110**, 800–807.

Lachman, R., Crocker, A., Schulman, I., Strand, R. (1973) Radiological findings in Niemann-Pick disease. *Radiology*, **108**, 659–664.

Haemophilia

Stoker, D. J., Murray, R. O. (1974) Skeletal changes in haemophilia and other bleeding disorders. *Seminars in Roentgenology*, **9**, 185–193.

CHAPTER 8

SKELETAL DISORDERS OF METABOLIC AND ENDOCRINE ORIGIN

In this chapter emphasis will be laid on radiological appearances. Nevertheless, it is important that the radiologist should also have some knowledge of the clinical, biochemical and histological features of these disorders. X-ray examination has considerable limitations in the early diagnosis of many of the diseases discussed below, and it is essential that the radiologist should appreciate such shortcomings and improve his diagnostic accuracy by relating his findings to those of the biochemist and perhaps the histopathologist.

The radiologist may suspect the possibility of metabolic bone disease by the observation of diffuse or multiple change on fortuitous radiographic examination; further investigation is required to establish the presence of generalized disease.

Routine examination in suspected *metabolic disease* should include films of the following regions:

A. PA chest (if possible, using a 43 × 35 cm film with its long axis horizontally to include the shoulders)
B. AP of abdomen for renal areas, when indicated
C. Lateral thoracic and lumbar spine
D. AP pelvis
E. AP knees
F. PA hands.

An aluminium step-wedge or some other reference system, for example, a bone phantom, will provide a simple densitometric method.

In *endocrine disease*, in addition to the density of bone, assessment of its size and maturity may be required.

The films considered to be most useful will vary with the disease, but radiographs of the skull, including the pituitary fossa and teeth, chest, pelvis, knees, forearm and hands, are commonly required. Assessment of skeletal age may be achieved by the use of recognized standard films, usually of the hands (Pyle, et al 1971). In certain instances, other areas are more valuable, for example, the iliac crest apophyses in late adolescence. It cannot be overemphasized that the published standards have a wide standard deviation and are usually based on a single racial group. They therefore cannot be used universally without careful consideration of their limitations.

The bony skeleton has several functions. Firstly, it has a supportive and protective role. It is normally fashioned under metabolic and endocrine influences, whilst growing and remodelling in response to gravity and muscle stress. Secondly, it serves as a depository of calcium and phosphorus which are required for the normal function of all tissues. The bones and teeth contain approximately 99% of the calcium and 80% of the phosphorus in the body.

The organic matrix of bone is known as osteoid and nearly 90% of this matrix is collagen, a protein of great tensile strength. The structure and density of the skeleton therefore depends on the supply of protein, minerals, vitamins, etc., the normal balance of endocrine function and the normal stresses of pressure and traction in everyday life.

Bone is a living tissue which is constantly being remodelled, resorbed and repaired, even in the adult. Growth and remodelling in the child proceeds at a much faster pace. It therefore follows that any disturbance in the availability of the basic substances necessary for bone formation will affect the X-ray appearance in due course. The problem is that the standard radiographic examination is not sensitive enough to demonstrate the early and minor changes of bone loss in the adult. In the growing child, reduction in mineralization of osteoid is demonstrated best at the sites of maximal growth, for example the wrists and knees.

Despite the limitations of X-ray examination in this group of diseases, there are still many diagnostic features which the radiologist can recognize on the X-ray film in metabolic bone disease. To demonstrate these requires a high-quality radiographic technique and careful attention to detail in the radiologist's observations. In the early stages of many metabolic bone diseases, the use of a magnifying lens, or a magnification radiographic technique, is also valuable (Fig. 8.1).

RADIOLOGICAL ASSESSMENT OF BONE DENSITY

The density of bone varies widely with a number of factors

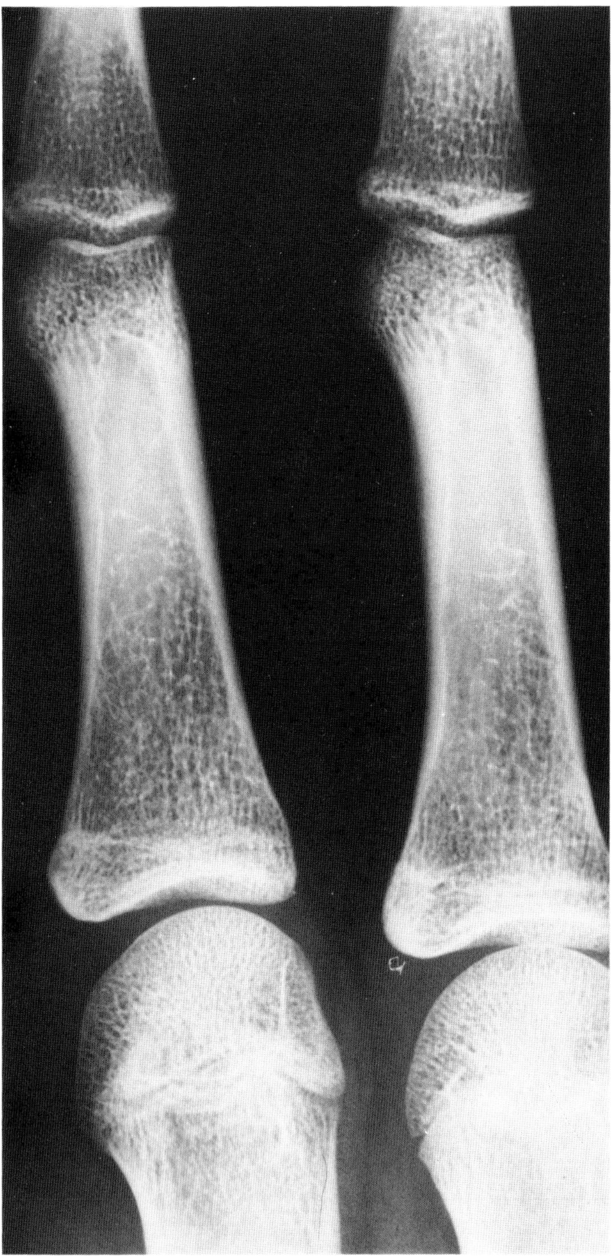

Fig. 8.1 Magnification. Definition of bone structure is improved by this technique, in this case a normal hand using a microfocus X-ray tube.

including age, sex, race and physical activity. Although the effect of a metabolic or endocrine disease is generalized, its radiological signs may vary from one part of the skeleton to another, either in its primary effect or its complications.

Nevertheless there is some value in the radiological assessment of bone density, particularly in a longitudinal study or the assessment of the effect of treatment.

No simple, effective method is available, but various approaches to the problem have been made.

1. **Radiographic densitometry.** The optical density of the image of a bone on an X-ray film is best assessed by the inclusion of an aluminium step-wedge, whereby the radiographic and soft tissue variations can be minimized. A refinement of this technique is to immerse the part to be examined in a water-bath. The use of a grid in this or any other densitometric technique is inadvisable. An extension of this principle employs the rapid decrease in attenuation coefficient of bone mineral with increasing energy of the incident beam. Comparison of films obtained at 62 and 250 kVp and subtraction of the soft tissue density obviates the need for a water-bath.

2. **X-ray spectrophotometry.** This method measures the attenuation of two energies of radiation in a highly collimated dual beam. It may be applied to almost any bone in the body, mainly representative of either cortical or medullary bone.

3. **Photon absorptiometry.** Measurement of absorption by the bone of a monochromatic, low-energy photon beam is made by a scintillation counter. The method has the great merit of eliminating unnecessary radiation and can be used to compare with a known standard. It involves the use of elaborate equipment, but appears to give reliable and reproducible results.

4. **Radiogrammetry.** This term embraces all the techniques of measurement of the thickness of cortical bone and is especially valuable in serial studies. Various bones have been studied: radius, humerus, clavicle and particularly the right second metacarpal (Fig. 8.2). Various indices of measurement have been suggested, but the simplest (total midshaft width − total medullary width at the same level) seems also to be the most satisfactory. Its great advantage lies in its use of inexpensive apparatus.

5. **Total-body neutron activation analysis (TBNAA).** This technique is at present in an experimental stage and estimates total body calcium rather than skeletal calcium.

6. **CT scanning.** As a result of its ability to define small volumes of bone and measure their density, the CT scanner is being used increasingly for quantitative analysis of bone mineral in metabolic disorders. Although largely investigative at present, this is a growth area with encouraging initial results. It seems to provide for the first time a precise, sensitive method for measurement of the vertebral spongiosa.

Nomenclature

The radiologist should avoid the use of terms which denote a disorder of bone in his description of radiographic appearances. It is particularly reprehensible to use the term *osteoporosis* for all conditions where a general reduction in bone density occurs. The term *osteopenia* has proved valuable as it includes all conditions where the mass of calcified bone is reduced, whether that bone is normal in quality or not. It should be remembered that the radiologist *observes* a generalized reduction in the optical density of bone; he may *deduce*, or give it as his opinion that this is due to osteoporosis, osteomalacia, hyperparathyroidism etc.

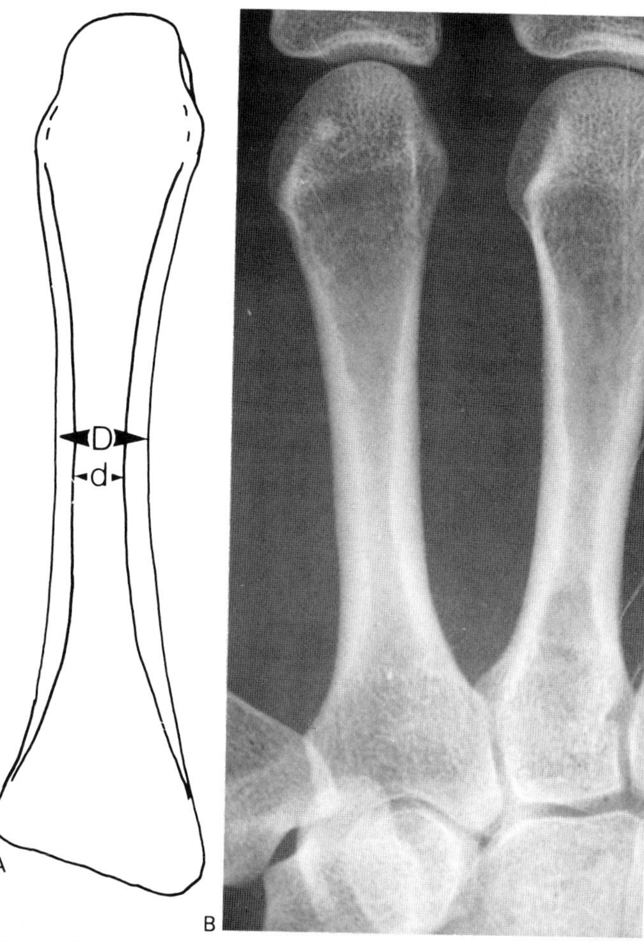

Fig. 8.2 A. and **B**. Cortical thickness. Measurement of the cortical thickness, particularly of the right second metacarpal shaft, has been used widely in assessing bone mass. The measurement D−d = total thickness of cortical bone and is probably the most satisfactory of the simple indices that have been proposed (Patterson, C. R., 1974).

Table 8.1 Classification of metabolic bone disease (after Reifenstein, 1957)

TOO LITTLE CALCIFIED BONE	
A. *Too little bone formed*:	
Too little matrix	Osteoporosis
Too little calcification of matrix	Osteomalacia or rickets
B. *Too much bone resorbed*:	Hyperparathyroid bone disease (osteitis fibrosa)
TOO MUCH CALCIFIED BONE	
A. *Too much bone formed*:	
Too much matrix	Poisonings Excessive stress Compensatory repair
Too much calcification of matrix	No such disorder described
B. *Too little bone resorbed*:	Osteosclerosis, e.g. osteopetrosis

A simplified classification of metabolic bone disease is shown in Table 8.1.

QUALITATIVE ASSESSMENT OF BONE STRUCTURE

As a result of the need for the early recognition of subtle changes in metabolic bone disease, a variety of techniques have been employed, particularly in examination of the hands.

1. **Optical or radiographic magnification.** Magnification may provide diagnostic information not available on orthodox examination. A tube with a focal spot of 50 μm and magnification of 4 to 6 times has been employed. It is likely that limits of film quality for this technique have probably been reached.

The radiologist, without the refinement of a micro-focus X-ray tube, can achieve films of the hand of acceptable quality by employing fine-grain industrial or mammographic film and optical magnification.

2. **Xeroradiography**. This electrostatic imaging system is most commonly used for mammography and other soft tissue radiography. It has advantages of better resolution and greater latitude. It has been employed in patients with metabolic bone disease, but probably without a discernible advantage.

The most effective methods for assessing bone density are sophisticated and expensive. In metabolic bone disorders the general radiologist should be content to provide X-ray films of the hand of good quality and include an aluminium step-wedge if he finds this helpful. Such films may be examined with a magnifying lens and, if necessary, cortical bone thickness can be measured (Fig. 8.2).

BIOCHEMICAL FINDINGS IN BONE DISEASE

These are of considerable diagnostic importance in both endocrine and metabolic disease. A summary of the main changes are listed in Table 8.2.

RADIONUCLIDE IMAGING IN METABOLIC BONE DISEASE

Bone scanning is a very sensitive, but *non-specific* method of identifying skeletal disease. If the disease is focal, e.g. in Paget's disease, and the diagnosis is established, scanning can serve a useful purpose in demonstrating the extent and response of the disease. In osteoporosis, the scan rarely suggests a metabolic disease, but can identify acute fractures in osteoporotic patients; it is likely to underestimate the overall extent of vertebral fractures in such patients.

In osteomalacia, primary hyperparathyroidism and renal osteodystrophy the scan is likely to suggest a metabolic bone disease by the presence of some or all of the following

Table 8.2 Biochemical values in metabolic bone disease

	Plasma calcium (fasting)	Plasma phosphorus (fasting)	Alkaline phosphatase	Urinary calcium	Plasma urea
Normal adults*	2.2–2.6 mmol/l (8.8–10.4 mg/dl)	0.80–1.5 mmol/l (2.5–4.8 mg/dl)	20–100 iv/l (3–13 KA units/100 ml)	*Males* 3.75–7.5 mmol/24 hours (150–300 mg/24 hours) *Females* 2.5–6.25 mmol (100–250 mg)	2.5–8.4 mmol/l (15–50 mg/dl)
Normal children	2.2–2.6 mmol/l (8.8–10.4 mg/dl)	1.15–2.30 mmol/l (3.5–7.0 mg/dl)	35–140 iv/l (5–20 KA units/dl) (higher at puberty)	as above but often low	2.5–8.4 mmol/l (15–50 mg/dl)
Osteoporosis	Normal	Normal	Normal	Normal	Normal
(in active phase and transiently with fractures alkaline phosphatase and urinary calcium may be raised)					
Vitamin D deficiency, rickets and osteomalacia	Low or normal	Low or normal (raised in renal failure)	Raised	Low	Normal (raised in renal failure)
Familial hypophosphataemia	Normal	Low or very low	Normal or raised	Normal	Normal
Primary hyperparathyroidism	Raised	Low normal or low	Raised in patients with bone disease	High normal or raised	Normal unless renal damage secondary to hypercalcaemia
Hyperparathyroidism secondary to glomerular failure	Normal or low	Raised	Raised	Low	Raised
Hyperparathyroidism secondary to gastrointestinal disease	Normal or low	Normal or low	Raised	Low	Normal
'Tertiary' hyperparathyroidism	Raised	Low in malabsorption (raised in renal failure)	Normal or raised	Normal or raised	Normal in malabsorption (raised in renal failure)
Myelomatosis	Normal or raised	Normal	Usually normal	Normal or raised	Normal unless secondary renal damage

*a. Biochemical ranges vary between laboratories and the figures quoted here must therefore be regarded only as a general guide.
b. Nearly half the serum calcium is protein-bound and most laboratories report serum calcium 'corrected' to the serum albumin level. This results in a narrower range of normal values.

features — increased uptake by the axial skeleton, long bones, wrists and costo-chondral junctions; prominent calvaria and mandible; a 'tie' sternum; faint or absent renal images. Positive scans may be expected in most cases of renal osteodystrophy and over 50% of patients with a biochemical diagnosis of hyperparathyroidism or osteomalacia; this is a greater percentage diagnosis of metabolic disease than is obtained radiographically. In osteomalacia, Looser's zones are identified slightly more often by the scan than the radiograph and, of course, the scan offers a quicker, cheaper record of such lesions, with less ionizing radiation to the patient.

SKELETAL CHANGES IN DEFICIENCY OR EXCESS OF VITAMINS

Metabolism of vitamin D

In recent years considerable progress has been made in the understanding of the mode of action and metabolism of vitamin D.

Vitamin D is derived from the diet as vitamin D_3 (cholecalciferol) and vitamin D_2 (ergocalciferol). Bile salts are necessary for its absorption in micelle form and osteomalacia due to biliary obstruction can be cured by physiological amounts of cholecalciferol given parenterally. The main source of the vitamin is through the action of sunlight; ultraviolet light converts 7-dehydrocholesterol to cholecalciferol in the skin. After absorption, this is hydroxylated in the liver to 25-hydroxycholecalciferol (25-HCC). Further hydroxylation takes place in the kidney to form 1,25 dihydroxycholecalciferol (1,25 DHCC), the active hormonal form of vitamin D. Such hydroxylation is confined to the kidney and is related to renal mass, not excretory function. Both 25-HCC and 1,25 DHCC probably have an enterohepatic circulation, which may be disturbed in some cases of malabsorption, resulting in hypocalcaemia and osteomalacia, previously thought to be the direct result of malabsorption of vitamin D.

1,25 DHCC acts on several target organs:

A. The intestine, where it initiates synthesis of a calcium-binding protein in the mucosa, thus promoting active absorption of calcium and phosphorus. It is 12 times more active in this respect than vitamin D.

B. In the kidney it stimulates production of a relatively inert metabolite, 24,25 DHCC, and thereby limits its own production by a feedback mechanism.

C. Receptors exist in the breast, placenta, pituitary and elsewhere, probably reflecting the increased demand for calcium during growth, pregnancy and lactation.

A diagram summarizing present knowledge of vitamin D metabolism is provided in Figure 8.3.

Calcitonin, a hormone produced in man, by C-cells, principally within the thyroid gland, is released in response to hypercalcaemia, amongst other stimuli. It inhibits bone resorption and, in this respect, is antagonistic to parathormone. Elevated levels of 1,25 DHCC meet the requirements of growth, pregnancy and lactation by enhancing absorption from the gut. The unwanted effect of bone resorption is counteracted by increased secretion of calcitonin. Its place in normal bone metabolism is incompletely understood but, when used in the treatment of Paget's disease it reduces the excessive bone turnover.

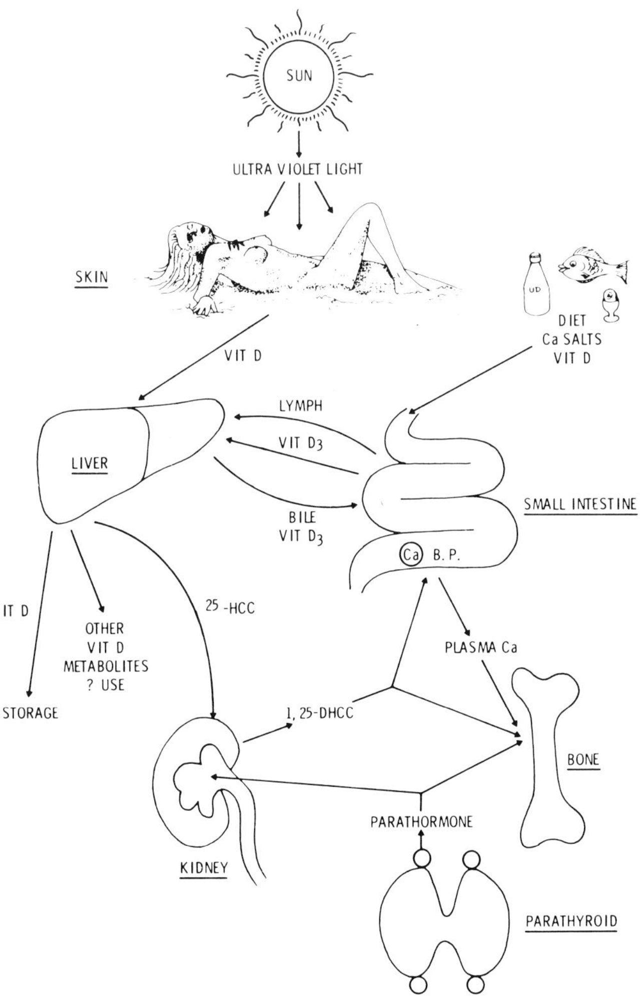

Fig. 8.3 Calcium and vitamin D metabolism. This simplified diagram illustrates the metabolic pathways in calcium metabolism. (25–HCC = 25 hydroxycholecalciferol 1,25–DHCC = 1,25 dihydroxycholecalciferol.

VITAMIN D DEFICIENCY: RICKETS AND OSTEOMALACIA

Rickets in children and osteomalacia in adults are the bone disorders caused by lack of vitamin D. The biochemical and histological abnormalities are identical in the two conditions, which differ only in the age of onset. Vitamin D lack can result from a deficient diet, failure to absorb the vitamin or defective metabolism. All these disorders have in common the defective production of 1,25-DHCC. The definitive definition of rickets and osteomalacia is based on histological criteria (Fig. 8.4), although in the majority of cases an initial diagnosis is made on biochemical and radiological grounds without resorting to bone biopsy.

Nutritional deficiency of vitamin D only occurs where patients have *both* a deficient diet *and* lack of adequate exposure to ultraviolet light. Two groups of patients are particularly vulnerable:

Coloured immigrants (particularly Asians) who by nature of their previous diet often with a high phytate content, have low stores of vitamin D and who come to live in Northern Europe. Such high dietary content of phytate may contribute by reducing the intestinal calcium content. A low exposure to ultraviolet light occurs as a result of their pigmented skins, the northern latitude and, in the case of women particularly, dark swathed clothing and often social isolation.

The middle-aged and elderly, particularly those living in poor areas of large cities for similar reasons of diet and lack of sunshine, but sometimes with other factors superimposed.

Dietary rickets and osteomalacia are therefore still seen in certain groups in developed countries, in addition to a wider incidence in India, Africa and South America. In North America, and to a lesser extent Northern Europe,

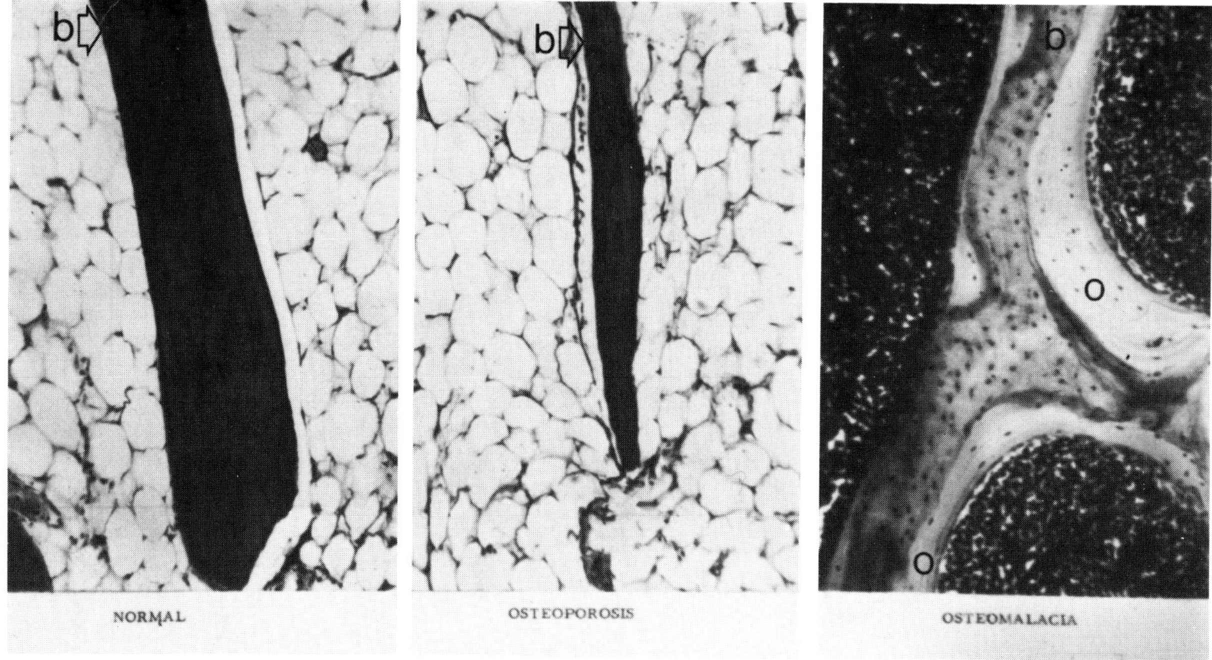

Fig. 8.4 Histology of osteoporosis and osteomalacia. The histology of osteoporosis shown in this section resembles that of normal bone except that the bony trabecula (b) is thinner in osteoporosis, i.e. bone is reduced in quantity. In osteomalacia, stained to show uncalcified bone, the osteoid (o) covers the entire bony trabecula to a considerable depth. In normal bone osteoid covers a minority of the trabecular surface.

fortification of food with vitamin D has almost eliminated the disorders in the general population.

Malabsorption syndromes of any type can result in osteomalacia or rickets (Fig. 8.5). In addition, the small bowel in coeliac disease may show 'resistance' to the action of vitamin D on calcium transport.

Osteomalacia occurs in a very small minority of patients after partial gastrectomy and responds to vitamin D. Its occurrence in obstructive jaundice has already been mentioned; it is rare and sometimes combined with osteoporosis. Rickets also may occur in neonates as a result of hepatitis and biliary atresia or obstruction.

Renal tubular disorders associated with phosphorus depletion and/or acidosis produce skeletal abnormalities radiologically and histologically identical with osteomalacia and rickets. Certain authorities exclude these disorders from the group when no evidence of a defect in vitamin D metabolism is shown. For the purpose of this book they are included and, indeed, failure of renal synthesis of 1,25-DHCC is a finding in many of these disorders.

Prolonged therapy with anticonvulsants produces osteomalacia or rickets by induction of hepatic enzymes which degrade vitamin D to less active metabolites. Such an effect is greater in those, for example Coloured immigrants, whose vitamin D intake is already low (Fig. 8.6). Treatment consists of increasing the oral intake of vitamin D. A similar mechanism may operate in the osteomalacia reported following the administration of the sedative glutethimide and the anti-tuberculosis agent rifampicin.

Poisoning by excessive consumption of aluminium hydroxide leading to phosphate deficiency, magnesium sulphate excess or cadmium intoxication, may occur. Cadmium poisoning leading to tubular damage has resulted from inhalation of fumes and ingestion of dust of cadmium oxide in the manufacture of alkaline batteries. The painful 'itai-itai' (translation 'ouch!-ouch!') disease produced osteomalacia in people drinking cadmium-polluted water in Japan.

RICKETS

Although rickets and osteomalacia are accepted as synonymous terms, it is convenient to preserve the two names as the radiological features of vitamin D deficiency differ in the immature and mature skeleton. In the first 6 months of life, rickets can present with tetany or convulsions. Later, the child will show swollen, tender joints. An abnormal waddling gait may be as much the result of bone pain as associated hypotonia.

Radiological features

These are due to non-calcification of recently formed osteoid and to the effects of stress on the weakened bone. They are, therefore, most obvious at the more rapidly growing metaphyseal regions, for example wrists and knees, and in the subperiosteal regions of florid cases.

The earliest radiological sign is narrowing or loss of the 'zone of provisional calcification' which borders the meta-

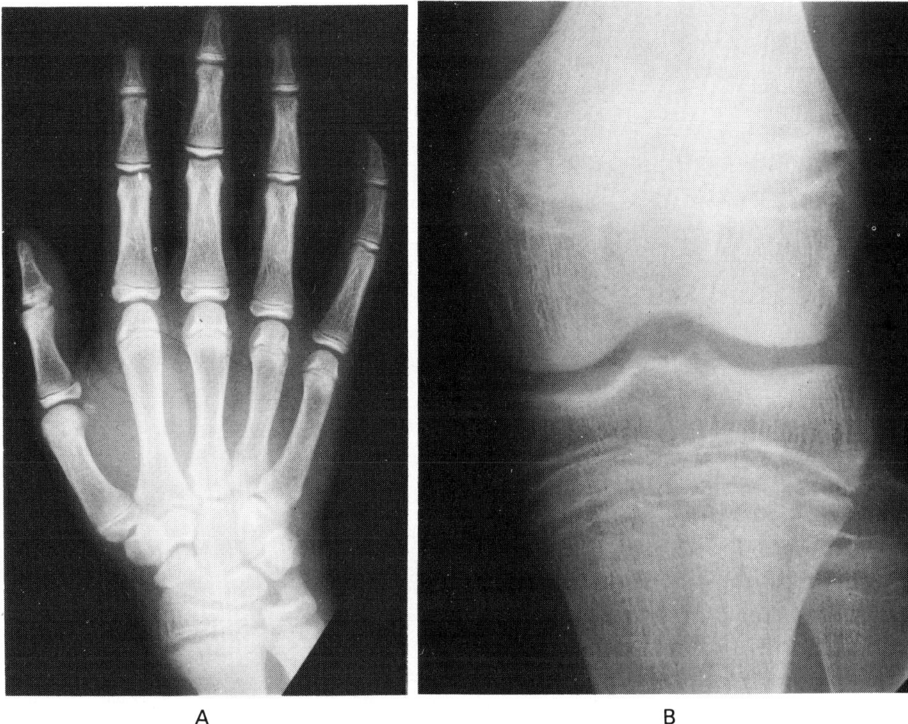

Fig. 8.5 A. and **B**. Rickets. This 23-year-old man developed steatorrhoea due to gluten sensitivity. Epiphyseal fusion is grossly delayed, with wide distal 'growth plates' of the radius and ulna. The phalanges exhibit the early cortical erosions of secondary hyperparathyroidism. The knees show alternating lucent and dense bands, indicating the periodicity of the process.

physeal margin of the growth plate. Subsequently, this metaphyseal margin becomes indistinct and frayed in appearance, followed by an increase in the apparent width of the growth plate, due to the presence of much uncalcified metaphyseal bone. Splaying and cupping of the visible metaphyseal bony margin (Fig. 8.6) results from the stress of weight-bearing and may be quite striking in the wrists if the child reverts to crawling. X-ray examination will also reveal swelling of the metaphyses due to piling up of osteoid which cannot be modelled normally by osteoclastic activity. Similar change takes place in the subperiosteal layer, where newly formed osteoid fails to calcify, but is more subtle and may show only as a less distinct cortical margin than normal. Changes also take place within the less rapidly growing parts of the skeleton, but are less obvious. All unfused growth plates are not growing at a similar rate; growth, and hence rachitic change, occurs maximally at the wrist, 0–6 years, at the knee, 5–10 years, and at the iliac crests, 14–18 years. It has to be remembered, in addition, that chronic rickets is also associated with delay in maturation and epiphyseal fusion. A generalized reduction in bone density may supervene in time and the clarity of the trabecular pattern is lost, although this is rarely a diagnostic feature. Fractures occur in long-standing cases; Looser's zones are demonstrated less often than in osteomalacia.

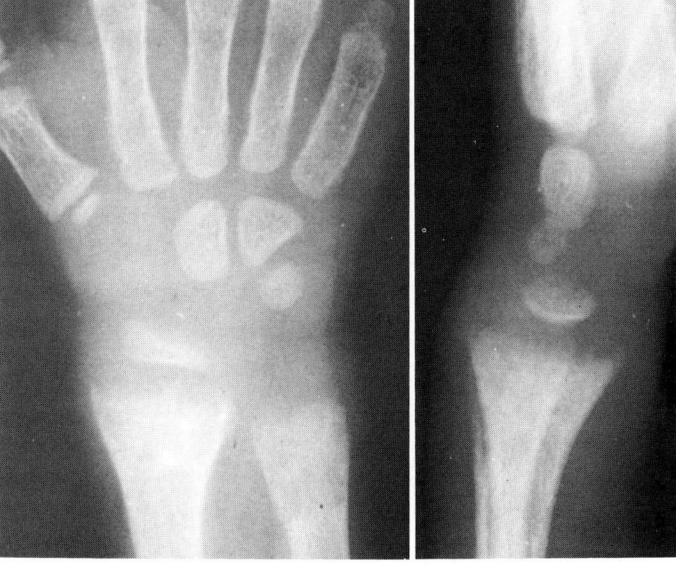

Fig. 8.6 Phenytoin rickets. Deficient metaphyseal mineralization with irregular cupped bony margins is typical of rickets of any aetiology. The wrists appear swollen. This West Indian child was under treatment with Phenytoin and other anti-convulsant drugs.

Epiphyseal changes follow the same pattern, with reduced peripheral mineralization and hazy cortical margins, in contrast to the sharp thin cortices in scurvy. Within 2 to 3 weeks of adequate therapy, radiological evidence of healing is seen and total recalcification is usually complete in 2 months. Initially, the dense line of provisional calcification appears, bordering the growth plate and separate from the bony metaphysis. Further mineralization of the osteoid unites this with the metaphysis. In the epiphysis and shafts a return of density occurs first in the subperiosteal layer (Fig. 8.7). Initially new woven bone is formed and, at this stage, the absence of modelling is striking. Osteoclastic and osteoblastic activity subsequently restores the normal architecture of lamellar bone.

When vitamin D ingestion has been intermittent or when treatment is inadequate, the process of calcification and repair is irregular and patchy sclerosis of the metaphysis is seen, sometimes with alternating sclerotic and lucent bands (Fig. 8.5B). In severe malnutrition (rickets may be associated with scurvy and protein deficiency) bone growth may be so retarded that little osteoid forms. In long-standing cases or in familial hypophosphataemia (vitamin D resistant rickets), curvature of the bones occurs due to multiple infractions with intermittent attempts at healing. The child is small and stunted. Thoracic kyphosis may be present with a deep narrow ('pigeon') chest. A Harrison's sulcus may appear on the lower thorax at the site of the rib attachments of the diaphragm. Enlargement of the anterior metaphyses of the ribs produces a rachitic 'rosary'; this term is essentially a descriptive clinical one, matched radiologically by the widened anterior ends of the ribs. The skull is bossed. Appendicular skeletal deformities mainly affect the lower limbs (Fig. 8.8). Characteristic lateral bowing of the legs may be present from the age of 2 or 3 years, with associated varus deformity of the hips and knees. When the onset of rickets is later in childhood, genu valgum may occur.

Localized stress changes dictate the appearances at growth plates close to weight-bearing joints, e.g. the knees. When the lower limbs are bowed, the growth plates become widened medially; with knock-knees, the stress is applied laterally and widening of the plate occurs on this side of the limb.

The completion of modelling and replacement of bone may take several years and, in the intervening period, many children show coarse trabeculation and growth arrest lines in the affected metaphyseal regions.

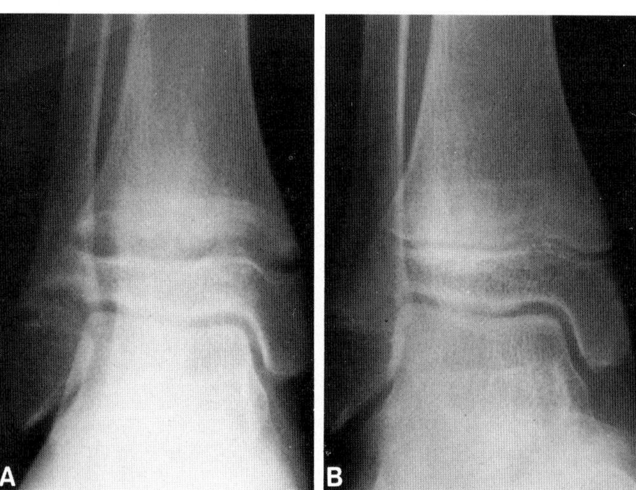

Fig. 8.7 Healing of rickets. The influence of vitamin D therapy is shown in this patient. **A**. Established rickets with loss of the zone of provisional calcification at the metaphysis which is irregular. **B**. After treatment, the growth plate is now of normal depth and its bony margins are reconstituted. Altered density at the metaphysis will disappear in time during the remodelling process.

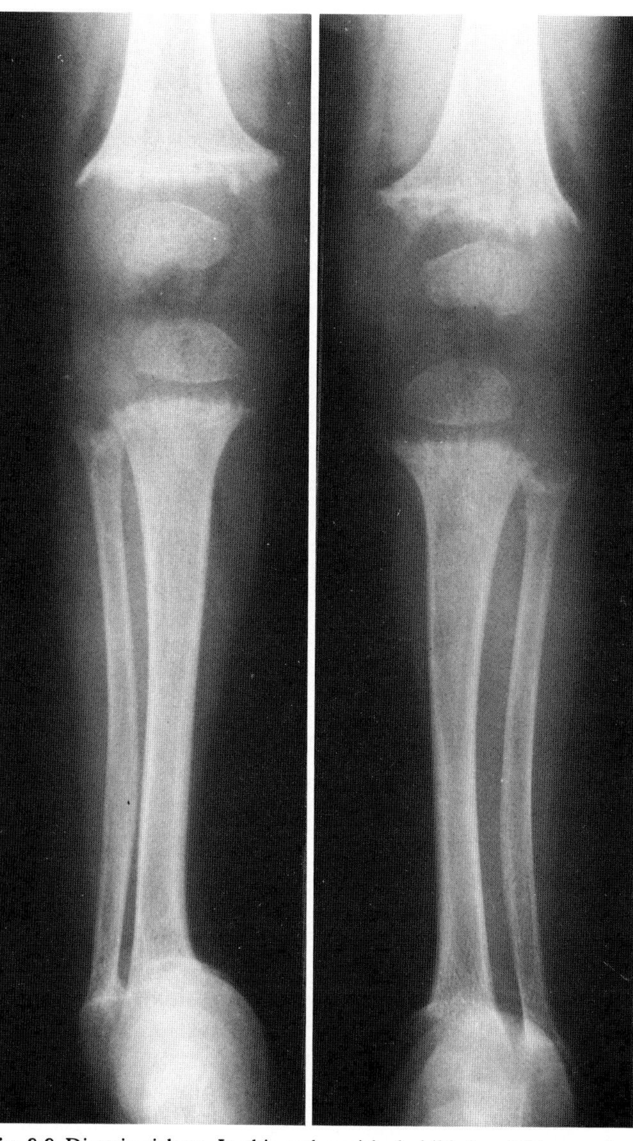

Fig. 8.8 Dietetic rickets. In this malnourished child, in addition to the characteristic metaphyseal changes, generalized osteopenia is evident. The bowing of the legs is S-shaped, varus deformity in the distal tibial shaft correcting the tendency to valgus deformity more proximally.

Pre-term infants

Rickets is common in pre-term infants of very low birthweight. The pathogenesis is uncertain, but it may be severe enough to cause spontaneous fractures and respiratory difficulty. Infants of under 34 weeks gestation require vitamin D supplements of at least 1000 iu per day in their first 2 months; rickets may occur despite this if calcium and phosphorus intake is inadequate.

Renal tubular rickets

A number of renal tubular disorders, when presenting first in childhood, may be associated with the radiological picture of rickets.

Familial hypophosphataemia

This is the commonest of the disorders previously known as vitamin D resistant rickets. It is usually inherited in a dominant sex-linked manner; females pass the disease on to half their sons and half their daughters, whilst affected males pass the disease to none of their sons and all of their daughters. Penetrance is incomplete. Radiographically, the appearances simulate dietetic rickets, but deformity of the pelvis and spine is not seen. Similar changes occur in cystinosis (Fanconi syndrome). Metaphyseal chondrodysplasia (Schmid type), transmitted as an autosomal dominant, sometimes shows some resemblance radiologically and must be distinguished.

Mild cases may present in adult life with bones of normal density, but show hyperostotic changes in the spine and sacro-iliac joints mimicking ankylosing spondylitis. Hyperostotic narrowing of the lumbar spinal canal is reported. Radio-ulnar synostosis may occur.

Acquired forms of hypophosphataemic rickets or osteomalacia

This group of uncommon disorders includes those patients with simply a high renal phosphate clearance.

Hypophosphataemia leading to rickets or osteomalacia has been described in association with tumours of bone or soft tissue. Resolution of the metabolic bone disease often occurs following ablation of such tumours, which are commonly of fibrous tissue origin or haemangiopericytomas. A similar association has been observed occasionally with more generalized diseases — fibrous dysplasia and neurofibromatosis, where surgical cure cannot unfortunately be contemplated.

Renal tubular acidosis

Probably not a single disorder; affected children show retarded growth and adults reduced height. Radiological features are nephrocalcinosis, nephrolithiasis and osteomalacia (Fig. 8.9). Symptomatic bone disease is uncommon but, in the absence of vitamin D excess, the combination of nephrocalcinosis and osteomalacia is almost diagnostic of

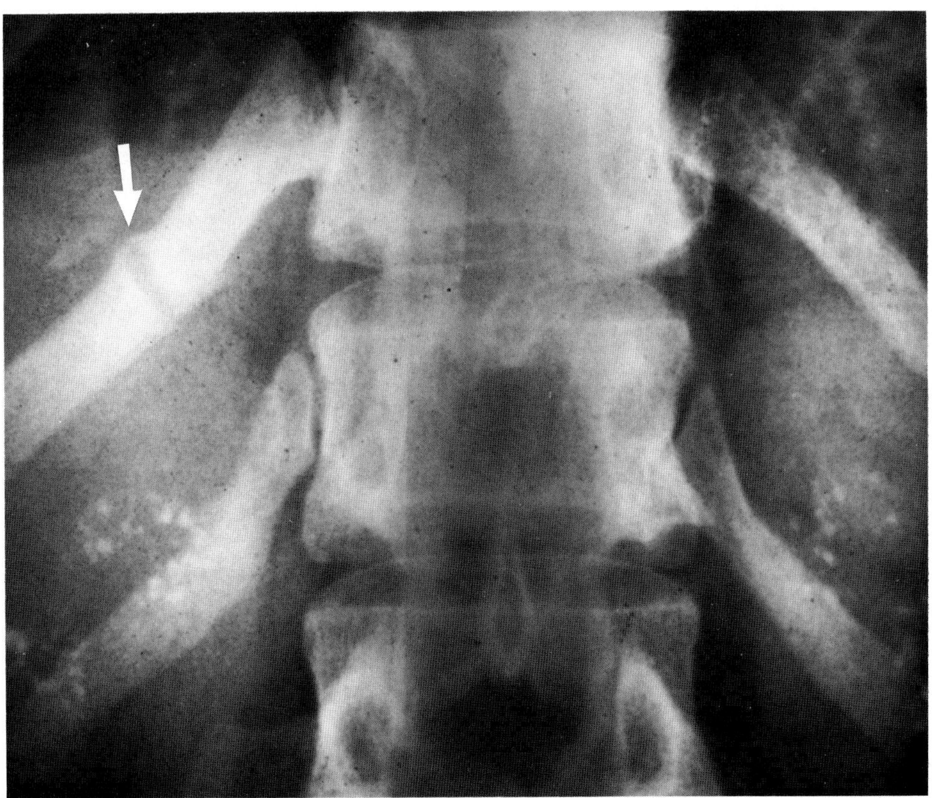

Fig. 8.9 Renal tubular acidosis. The combination of nephrocalcinosis and osteomalacia (Looser's zone (↓) in the right 11th rib) is characteristic, although symptomatic bone disease affects only a minority of patients.

renal tubular acidosis. Hyperparathyroid bone disease is very rare in this disorder, in the absence of renal failure.

DIFFERENTIAL DIAGNOSIS OF CAUSE OF RICKETS

Rachitic changes are essentially similar from all causes but it is sometimes possible to suggest a cause from the radiographic appearances. In the majority of cases of hypophosphataemic rickets, the changes at the knee are greater than at the wrist; the radial growth plate may even appear normal. Even if this differential involvement is not striking, in this disease, short, ill-modelled limb bones may be found particularly in girls.

Similarly, although theoretically, secondary hyperparathyroidism can occur in any form of rickets, it is commonest in those patients with renal osteodystrophy.

Lower limb deformity (bow legs or knock-knees) occurs predominantly in familial hypophosphataemic and nutritional rickets, as such patients are ambulatory. Children with Fanconi's syndrome, renal tubular acidosis and renal osteodystrophy are often chronically ill so that they do not subject their limbs to weight-bearing stresses.

OSTEOMALACIA

This term is confined to the bone changes of vitamin D deficiency in the mature skeleton. Very little evidence exists to suggest that a low calcium intake alone ever causes osteomalacia in otherwise healthy people, although it contributes to the clinical problem in the face of vitamin D deficiency, disease of the small bowel or any other cause of osteomalacia. Bone pain is prominent in the disorder as is myopathic weakness.

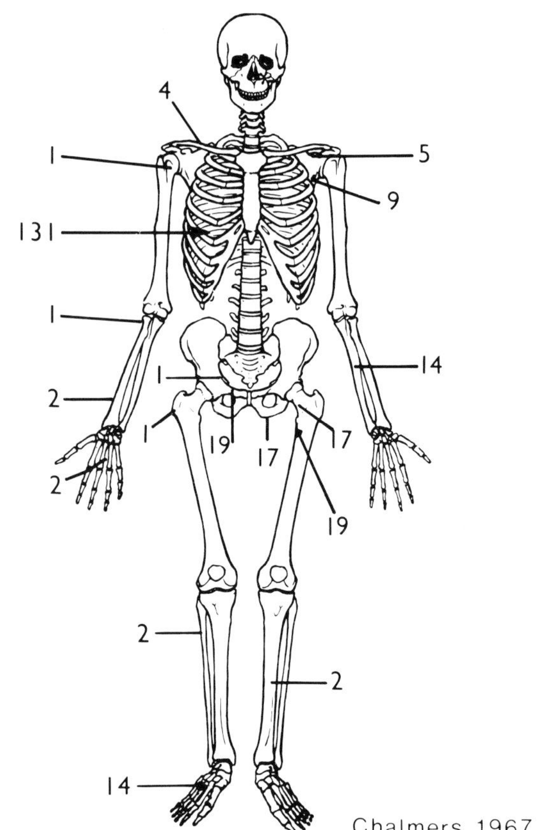

Fig. 8.10 Looser's zones in osteomalacia. Sites of incidence in a group of middle-aged and elderly patients with dietetic osteomalacia.

Radiological features

Early. Although patients with osteomalacia, as a group, possess bones with less calcium content than normal, this may not be recognizable by serial radiography or densitometry. If reduced bone density is detected, it is unlikely to be distinguishable from the other forms of osteopenia, although more likely than osteoporosis to affect the appendicular skeleton. The radiological hall-mark of osteomalacia is the *Looser's zone* (*pseudo-fracture*). This is a narrow (2–3 mm wide) radiolucency which transects one or both cortical margins of a bone. It may lie perpendicularly or obliquely to the line of the cortex. The degree of clarity with which a Looser's zone is seen depends upon its age. Initially it is poorly demarcated, then increases in width before becoming relatively prominent with slight sclerosis of its margins. It is generally accepted that these zones are regions where stress infractions have been repaired by osteoid in the absence of normal mineralization of the bone. This may not be the whole story, as some Looser's zones occur commonly in sites where stress fractures are rarely shown. A helpful feature is the tendency for Looser's zones to occur symmetrically in particular sites (Fig. 8.10). These include the lower ribs, the pubic rami, the neck and medial cortex of the proximal shaft of the femur, the axillary border of the scapula and certain long bones, particularly of the forearm and leg (Fig. 8.11). Looser's zones may progress to complete fractures and the radiologist should suspect the diagnosis in a middle-aged or elderly female presenting with bilateral symmetrical fractures of the femoral necks (Fig. 8.12). As in rickets, bone pain is experienced by most patients with osteomalacia. It is not unusual, however, to find a number of unsuspected and sometimes healed rib fractures in a patient presenting with the condition (Fig. 8.13). Following treatment, undisplaced Looser's zones generally disappear without trace.

Late. The typical appearance of untreated osteomalacia resembles that of 'late' rickets, although the deformity and stunting of growth is less. The bones are small and overall density is reduced with thin cortices and sparse trabecular bone. As osteoporosis is predominantly a disorder of the elderly, thinning of the upper cortex of the clavicles to below 2 mm, without erosion of their outer ends, should suggest osteomalacia on the chest film of a patient under 45 years of age. The vertebral bodies are reduced in density and biconcave ('cod fish' vertebrae) (Fig. 8.13). The inter-

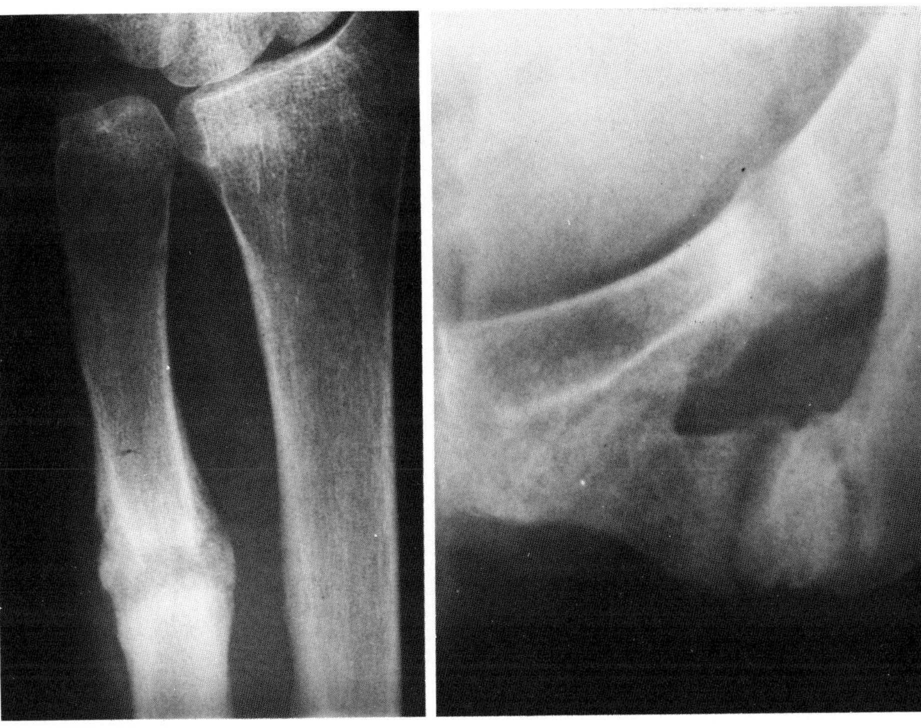

Fig. 8.11 Osteomalacia. Looser's zones in (**A**) the distal third of the ulnar shaft; (**B**) the ischio-pubic rami. Healing is occurring.
Looser's zones may heal with or without adequate treatment.

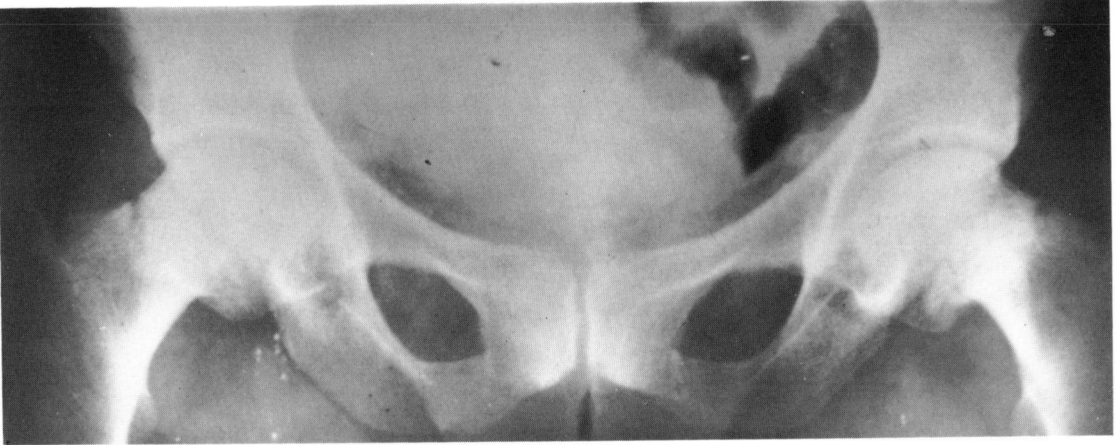

Fig. 8.12 Osteomalacia. Patient with carcinoma of the cervix and a long history of diarrhoea who presented with bilateral fractures of the femoral necks. The osteomalacia proved to be secondary to gluten enteropathy.

vertebral discs are large and biconvex in comparison and this appearance may be the more striking. Wedging of the vertebral bodies due to compression fracture is seen (Fig. 8.13), but is less common than in osteoporosis. The shape of the pelvic brim tends to be triradiate. True protrusio acetabuli is rare. Coxa vara results from bowing of the femoral neck; the clavicles and various limb bones may also be bowed. If the disease is still active, Looser's zones will be apparent. Treatment produces rapid relief of the clinical symptoms, especially bone pain and those due to the myopathy. Radiological healing occurs, but deformities persist.

Blood chemistry

Almost all patients with vitamin D deficient osteomalacia have a high serum alkaline phosphatase (ALP) in association with often a low serum phosphorus and sometimes a low serum calcium. The radiologist's contribution to the diagnosis lies mainly in the demonstration of Looser's zones. However, they are not shown radiographically in all patients with osteomalacia, thus emphasizing the need for estimation of the serum ALP and for the use of radionuclide bone scans in suspect patients. A few patients with osteomalacia due to malabsorption have a normal serum ALP. In hypophosphataemic osteomalacia (the adult form

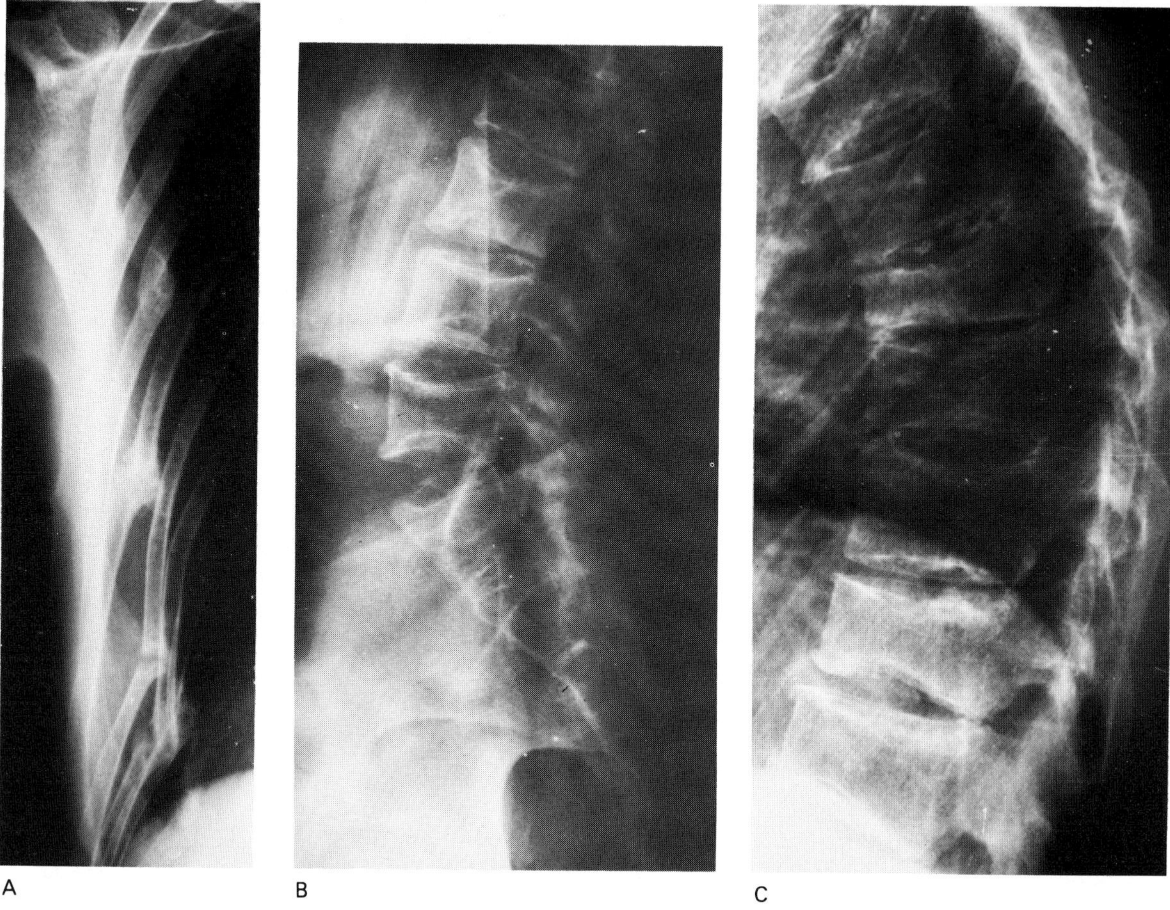

Fig. 8.13 Osteomalacia. In this patient numerous rib fractures (**A**) in various stages of development and healing are evident with at least one Looser's zone. Whilst vertebral collapse in the lumbar region has resulted in biconcavity of the vertebral bodies (**B**), in the thoracic spine, wedging predominates (**C**).

of familial hypophosphataemia) the serum ALP is often elevated, but its level is not always related to the severity of the bone disease.

Histopathology (Fig. 8.4)

In both osteomalacia and rickets the characteristic feature is failure of ossification of new bone. The histological diagnosis is made on the presence of *excess* osteoid and for this an *uncalcified* bone section is required. In addition to the presence of excess osteoid of abnormal thickness covering all trabeculae, the absence of a normal 'calcification front' may be evident with special staining techniques.

HYPOPHOSPHATASIA

This rare disorder is inherited as an autosomal recessive trait and is characterized by a low or very low serum alkaline phosphatase, an abnormal bone formation resembling rickets or osteomalacia and an increased urinary excretion of phosphoethanolamine. Several clinical forms are recognized. The early appearance of the disease is a sign of severity and the neonatal variety has a lethal outcome. Mild and asymptomatic forms are found.

Radiological changes in bone are characteristic with bowing of long bones, reduced bone density and distorted metaphyseal ossification. Although resembling rickets, the extent of uncalcified metaphyseal bone is usually much greater and initial ossification more irregular. Islands of non-ossified tissue are projected into the metaphyses (Fig. 8.14). Deformities of the distal phalanges and S-shaped tibiae are present. The major complications are fractures, craniostenosis and nephrocalcinosis. No specific therapy is known, but the effect of vitamin D is deleterious. Heterozygotes tend to show diminution of serum alkaline phosphatase levels and many excrete phosphoethanolamine in the urine.

AXIAL OSTEOMALACIA AND FIBROGENESIS IMPERFECTA OSSIUM

A brief account of each of these rare disorders is appropriate. Axial osteomalacia, as its name implies, is charac-

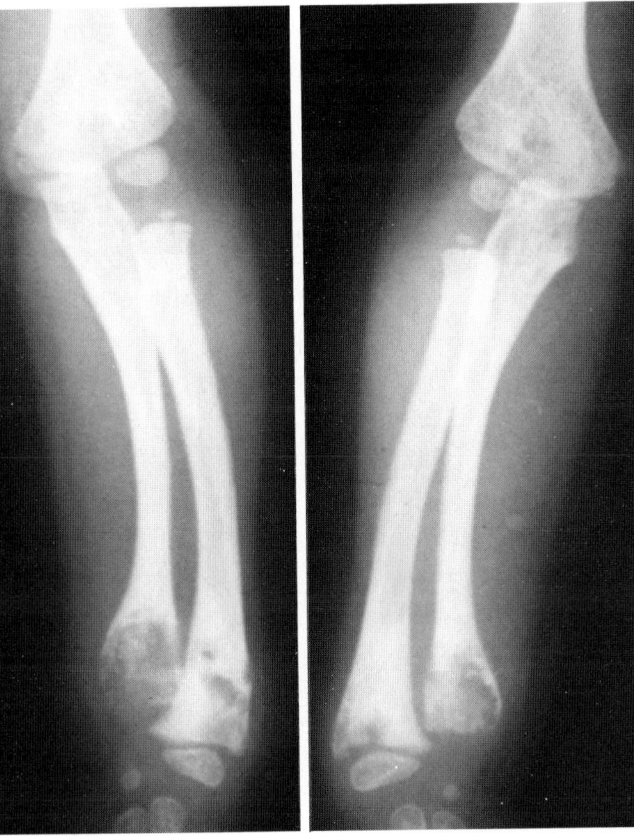

Fig. 8.14 Hypophosphatasia. In this child metaphyseal ossification is delayed in the ulnae whilst the distal radii contains islands of non-ossified tissue.

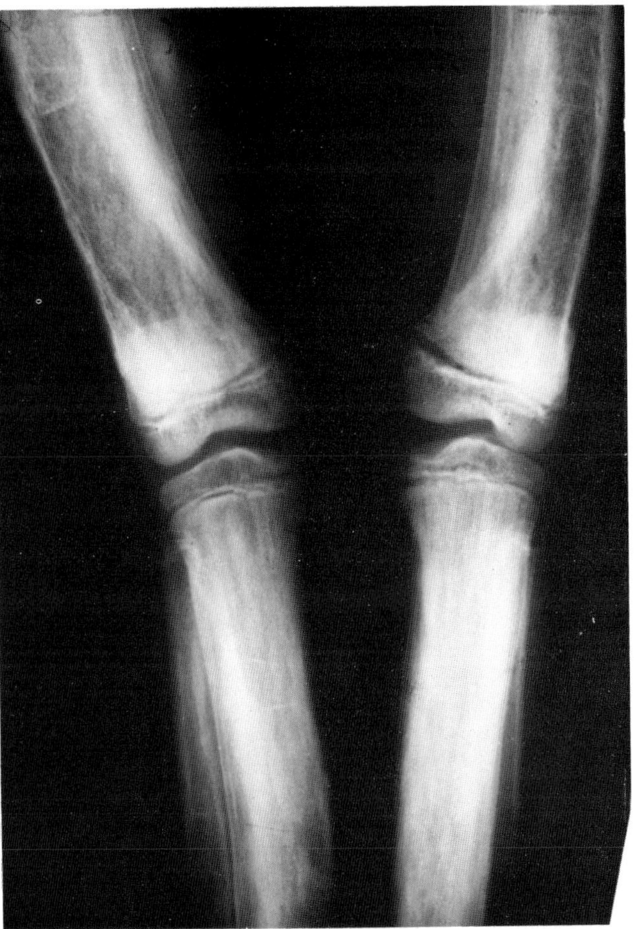

Fig. 8.15 Familial hyperphosphatasaemia. The radiological appearances in this child are diagnostic. The bones are widened with loss of differentiation of cortex and medulla. A coarse trabecular pattern and bowing are also evident. These features resemble those of Paget's disease.

terized by coarsening of the trabecular pattern of the vertebrae, ribs and pelvis. Symptoms are mild and the prognosis is good. The serum ALP is often in the normal range but the histology is that of osteomalacia.

Fibrogenesis imperfecta ossium, first described in 1950, shows a similar radiological pattern in the axial skeleton, but the limb bones are also affected with trabecular coarsening at the ends of the bones. The patients are middle-aged and have multiple fractures. Serum ALP is elevated; histologically, wide 'osteoid seams' are evident but examination with the polarizing microscope shows the collagen fibres to be grossly abnormal and deficient.

FAMILIAL HYPERPHOSPHATASAEMIA

This extremely rare syndrome was first described in 1956. It shows autosomal recessive inheritance and presents between the third and eighteenth month of life, with progressive enlargement of the head and bowing of the limbs. All patients show elevation of the serum acid and alkaline phosphatase levels.

Radiological features are characteristic, with thickening of the skull vault and patches of increased density. The long bones are widened and of cylindrical shape with loss of modelling (Fig. 8.15). The medulla is widened at the expense of the cortex, which is thin and shows microfractures. The disease is differentiated from Paget's disease by the age of onset and the general symmetrical involvement of bone. It should *not* be called juvenile Paget's disease, since we do not know the aetiology of either disorder.

DEFICIENCY OF VITAMIN C

Scurvy

About 90% of the matrix of mature bone consists of collagen. Vitamin C (ascorbic acid) is necessary for the hydroxylation of proline to form hydroxyproline, which with hydroxylysine is almost unique to collagen. Lack of dietary vitamin C therefore results in deficient formation of bone matrix — scurvy. This disorder is a form of osteoporosis and in the adult cannot be differentiated radiologically from other forms. Scurvy is rare before the age of 6 months because the newborn infant normally possesses an adequate stock of vitamin C; it is also rare in breast-fed infants. The occasional report of scurvy in Western medical literature relates to children fed on sterilized cow's milk with no fruit or vitamin supplements, or to total aversion to fruit in the older child.

Infants and young children present with irritability and limb pains, sometimes progressing to pseudoparalysis, and a characteristic radiological appearance.

Bone density is generally reduced, the bone cortex is thin and the trabeculae sparse. The zone of provisional calcification at the growing metaphysis is dense and sharp, but on its diaphyseal side the bone shows a lucent band due to deficient ossification. This weakened zone fractures easily and marginal metaphyseal infractions in various stages of healing protrude to form lateral spurs (Pelkan). The epiphyses are small and show finely pencilled dense margins, producing a ring or 'halo' appearance (Wimburger's sign) (Fig. 8.16).

Deficiency of vitamin C also results in capillary fragility, bruising and subperiosteal haemorrhages. In children, these cause stripping of the loosely attached periosteum and quite extensive formation of periosteal new bone, especially following treatment (Fig. 8.17). The new bone so formed becomes resorbed completely. Soft tissue oedema may be observed in association with subperiosteal haemorrhage.

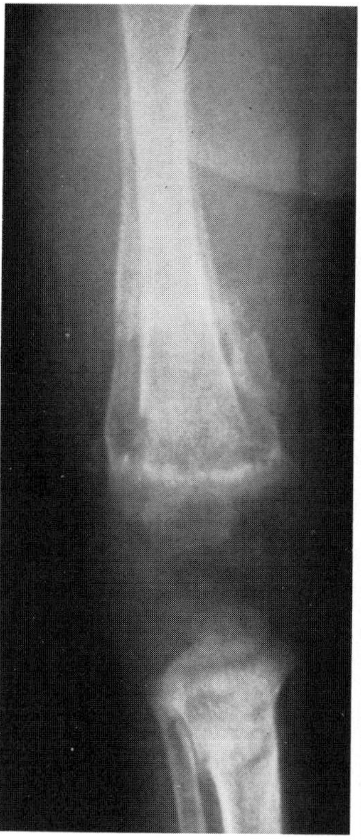
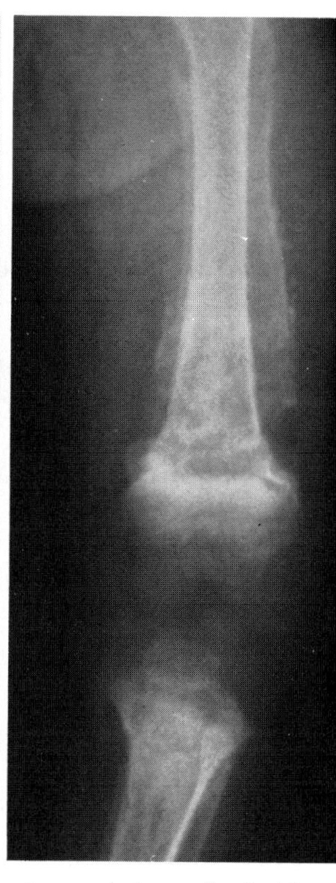

Fig. 8.17 Severe scurvy. Generalized osteoporosis is associated with a fracture of the right tibial shaft. Metaphyseal fractures are also present and a shell of subperiosteal bone marks the site of haemorrhage.

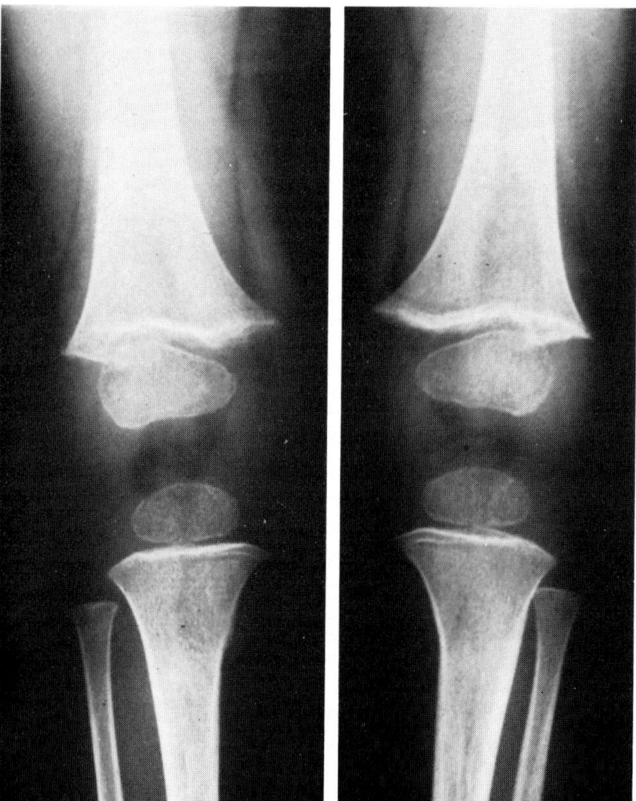

Fig. 8.16 Scurvy. A 10-month-old child with painful limbs shows the changes of early scurvy. Dense white lines at the metaphyseal margins contrast with a general reduction in bone density. Sharp spurs are present at the femoral metaphyseal margins and the epiphyses exhibit a 'halo' appearance.

Healing elsewhere is rapid and the zones of provisional calcification may be incorporated, leaving dense bands in the shafts of long bones resembling growth arrest lines and 'ghost' ring densities of the epiphyseal centres. In scurvy occurring in the older child, vertebral collapse more suggestive of adult osteoporosis may occur. Radiographic evidence of bone disease, apart from generalized osteoporosis, is rare in adults, but periosteal reaction, particularly in the legs, may be observed secondary to haemorrhage.

Scurvy may sometimes mimic, or be mimicked by, certain features of unrecognized skeletal trauma (battered child syndrome). The latter condition is recognized by the normal bone density, the presence of normally ossified cortices and metaphyses and fractures in various stages of healing.

HYPERVITAMINOSES

Vitamin A poisoning

Chronic hypervitaminosis A is uncommon and results from overdosage in prophylaxis, misconceived medication or in

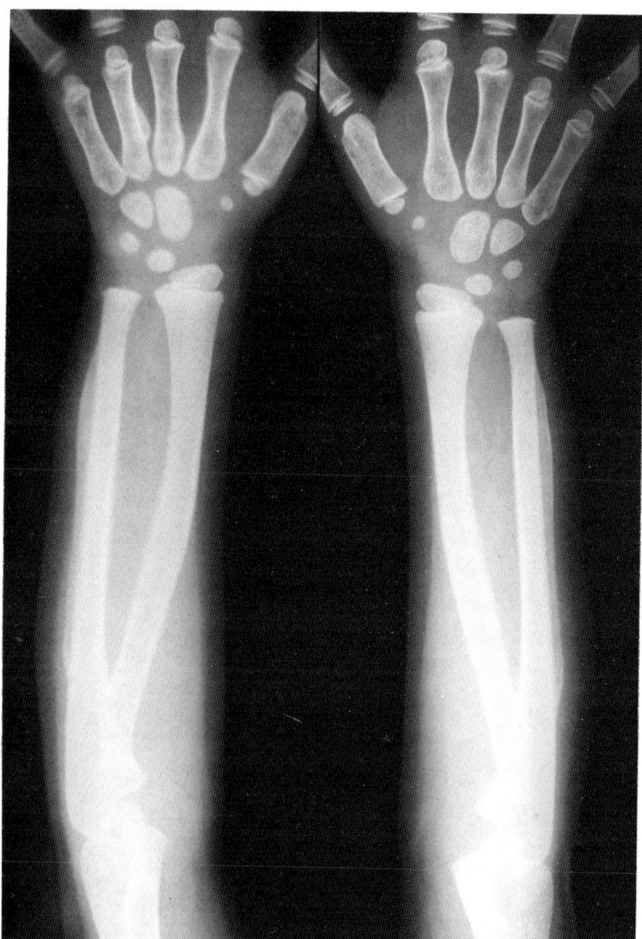

Fig. 8.18 Vitamin A poisoning. Organizing periosteal reactions of both ulnae are present in this child as the only skeletal abnormality.

hyperalimentation in infants. Hypercalcaemia may occur in children, but is rare in adults. Tender swellings, especially in the limbs, are associated with underlying periosteal new bone formation (Fig. 8.18). Following withdrawal of the medication, such hyperostoses become assimilated and remodelled. *Radiologically*, the disorder simulates infantile cortical hyperostosis, which is usually apparent by 4 months of age whereas, in most cases, hypervitaminosis A is not recognized in the first year of life.

Vitamin D poisoning

At one time vitamin D was advocated in the treatment of a wide variety of diseases and this resulted in many cases of vitamin D poisoning. Today vitamin D is used in large doses mainly in the treatment of hypoparathyroidism and hypophosphataemic rickets. The doses employed may approach the toxic range. The symptoms are generally those of hypercalcaemia — fatigue, weakness, thirst and polyuria, anorexia, nausea and vomiting, abdominal pain.

Radiologically, in children dense metaphyseal lines, simulating those of lead poisoning, may be found and growth may be retarded. Generalized osteosclerosis is occasionally found at all ages. The principal finding is of metastatic calcification, either confined to the kidney or extensively involving arterial walls, periarticular tissues and other subcutaneous regions.

OSTEOPOROSIS

Osteoporosis is not a single disease, but a heterogenous group of disorders of bone which have one factor in common — a reduction in bone mass, below the limits of normal. The bone that remains is normally mineralized and apparently normal in its microstructure (Fig. 8.4). Osteoporosis is the commonest disorder in metabolic bone disease, yet despite extensive research, considerable controversy still exists over the aetiology of even the common varieties. The major causes of osteoporosis are shown in Table 8.3.

Table 8.3 Classification of generalized osteoporosis

Immobilization
Localized
Generalized
Combined with hyperaemia (e.g. in arthritides)
Prolonged space flight
Hypogonadal
Post-menopausal
Eunuchoidal
Gonadal dysgenesis
Senile
Excess of catabolic agents
Adrenal corticosteroids
spontaneous — Cushing's syndrome
iatrogenic
Thyroid hormones
thyrotoxicosis
Cytotoxic chemotherapy
Miscellaneous
Hepatic osteoporosis
Heparin osteoporosis
Juvenile osteoporosis
Scurvy
'Idiopathic' osteoporosis

One initial problem lies in the concept of *normal* bone loss. With aging, an overall loss of bone occurs, but great individual variation exists; some subjects even increase their bone mass. It is possible, however to accept the concept of an age-related bone loss which is physiological. This bone loss starts a decade earlier in women than men and once begun it tends to progress in linear fashion. Such physiological bone loss should not be confused with the common accelerated osteoporosis of post-menopausal females, although the two processes overlap. Significant loss of bone in males is uncommon before the age of 65 years but, in females, bone loss may be rapid and severe after the age of 50. The osteoporosis correlates well with loss of

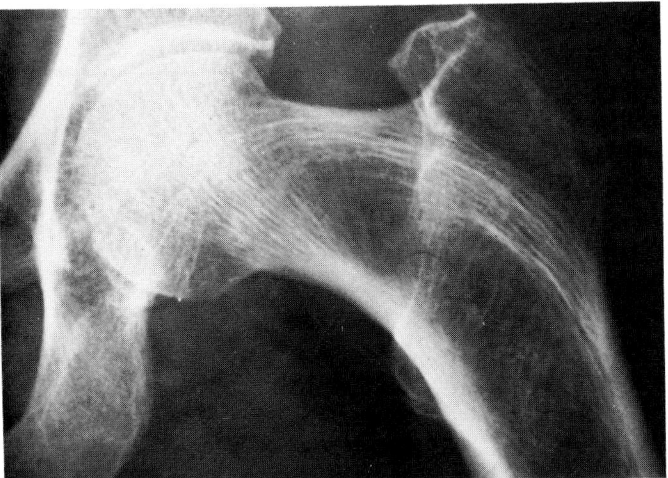

Fig. 8.19 Osteoporosis. In this patient, resorption of the secondary trabeculae has left the primary trabeculae to delineate the lines of stress within the femoral necks.

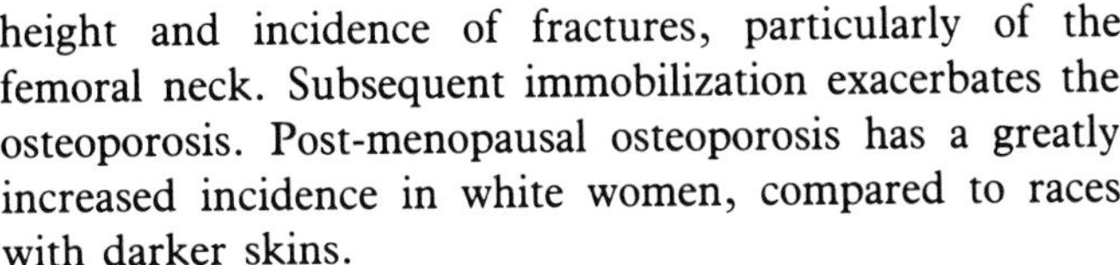

height and incidence of fractures, particularly of the femoral neck. Subsequent immobilization exacerbates the osteoporosis. Post-menopausal osteoporosis has a greatly increased incidence in white women, compared to races with darker skins.

In addition to the presumption that post-menopausal osteoporosis may be related to reduced ovarian endocrine function, evidence has been presented that it relates to oestrogen levels and can be prevented by the continued administration of oestrogen. Once osteoporosis is established, oestrogen therapy will usually not affect the radiographic density.

Radiologically the earliest change in osteoporosis is usually in the axial skeleton. Secondary trabeculae in the lower thoracic and lumbar vertebrae are resorbed, with resultant loss of density. Mean vertebral height in the osteoporotic subject is less than in the normal, even in the absence of an identifiable fracture. It is, however, not a sensitive indicator of spinal osteoporosis and does not always correlate with fractures of the femoral neck. Trabecular loss in the proximal femur and calcaneus makes the remaining primary trabeculae appear more prominent and demonstrates the lines of stress within the bone (Fig. 8.19). This observation has been used in the proximal femur as a method of identifying those patients who are at risk from compression fractures of the vertebrae. Once secondary trabeculae have been removed, they rarely reform. Restoration of a positive calcium balance and osteoblastic activity leads to appositional bone formation on the primary trabeculae and the characteristic coarse pattern of chronic osteoporosis (Fig. 8.20). Generalized reduction in bone density is difficult to assess without recourse to some of the techniques outlined earlier in this chapter. Removal of much trabecular bone and perhaps a loss of 40% of total

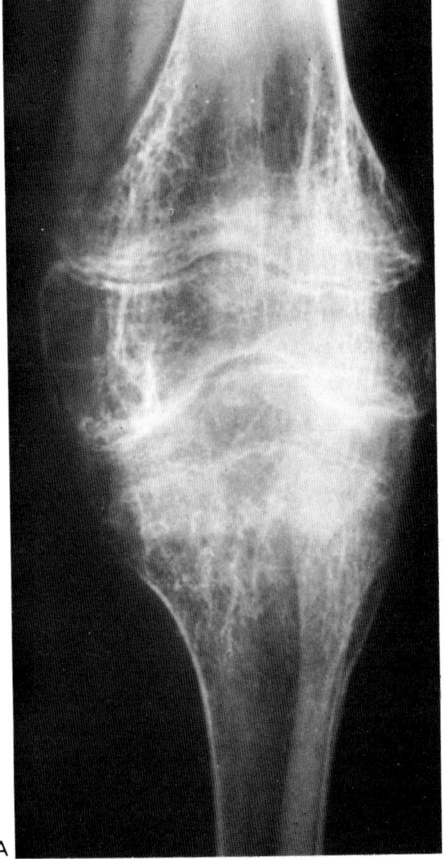

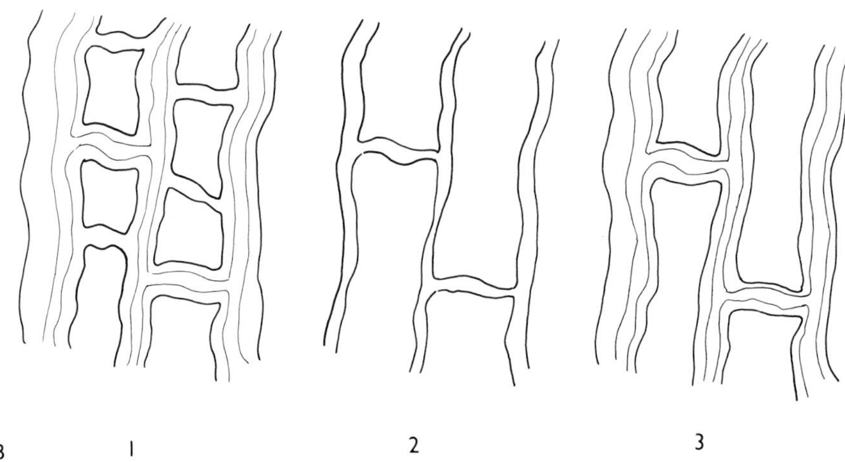

Fig. 8.20 Chronic osteoporosis. **A**. Long-standing periarticular osteoporosis in this child with Still's disease has resulted in sparse but coarse trabeculation in the medulla. **B**. Diagram to show that when normal bone (1) is involved by osteoporosis, the secondary trabeculae are resorbed (2). Re-ossification leads to the laying down of bone on the remaining primary trabeculae (3) and coarsening of the pattern of the spongiosa.

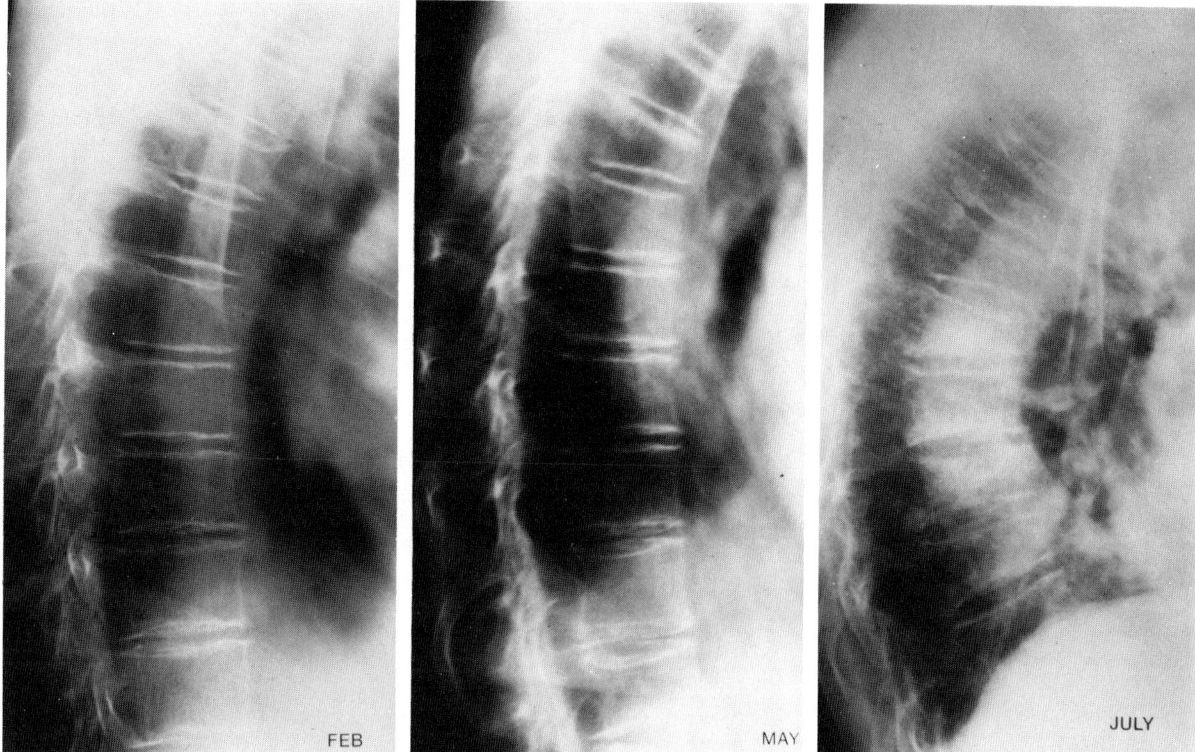

Fig. 8.21 Post-menopausal osteoporosis. Serial films in this patient show the progressive development of kyphosis as a result of anterior wedging of the thoracic vertebral bodies, during the course of 6 months.

bone mass may not be identified on routine X-ray examination. As the vertebrae become more brittle, anterior wedging occurs, due particularly to compression of the superior vertebral plates, with supervening dorsal kyphosis (Fig. 8.21). Biconcavity of vertebral bodies may also occur, as in osteomalacia, but the two types of deformity generally coexist in osteoporosis. Complications mainly comprise fractures of which those of the vertebrae, femoral necks and distal radius are most common. General cortical thinning occurs, yet despite this the cortex is clear and sharp, due mainly to loss of the adjoining trabecular bone. Bone loss in osteoporosis results because resorption exceeds bone formation, primarily due to reduced osteoblastic activity. Cortical resorption occurs mainly on the medullary surface, although osteocytic resorption of bone occurs within the cortex. A correlation between osteoporosis and the presence of calcification of the aorta has been noted, but is unexplained.

Whilst osteoporosis is a common radiological finding in the middle-aged and elderly, the radiologist must be alert to the possibility that other conditions may present with a similar appearance. These include curable conditions such as Cushing's disease and treatable conditions such as myelomatosis, which may present no identifiable focal lesions and only generalized osteopenia.

Idiopathic juvenile osteoporosis

This is a rare disease, affecting both sexes, originally reported in the 8 to 15 year age group, but seen in some cases under the age of 5 years. Patients present with bone pain, backache or limp. Fractures, particularly at the metaphyses of long bones, occur with minimal trauma and, radiologically, multiple collapsed vertebrae are shown; changes in the skull are minimal. The diagnosis is made by exclusion of such conditions as leukaemia, lymphoma and hypercorticosteroid states. It differs from osteogenesis imperfecta by the absence of a family history, blue sclerae and dental changes. Spontaneous recovery is the rule, but may take as long as five years.

Hepatic osteoporosis

Bone disease in biliary obstruction may be osteomalacia, osteoporosis or a combination of the two. In primary biliary cirrhosis, osteoporosis predominates. Osteoporosis has also been observed in alcoholics, not all of whom have hepatic cirrhosis.

Heparin osteoporosis

Long-term therapy with heparin may cause serious loss of bone with spontaneous fractures. Heparin therapy of this duration is now used rarely.

THE SKELETAL EFFECTS OF ENDOCRINE DISEASE

The endocrine system exerts considerable control over the growth and maturation of the skeleton as a whole and several hormones have direct actions on bone, notably growth hormone, the thyroid hormones, parathormone, calcitonin and the gluco-corticosteroids. Endocrine disease may therefore produce a variety of responses by bone.

THE PITUITARY

Pituitary insufficiency

Apart from the retardation in growth and maturation in children, no specific features are found. The untreated skeleton is small, but normally proportioned with slender bones, unfused growth plates and skull sutures. Epiphyseal closure is delayed, sometimes until the fifth decade.

Gigantism

The converse applies, with overgrowth of bones when an eosinophil adenoma arises in childhood. Ultimately, in addition to over-production of growth hormone, a deficiency of the other pituitary trophic hormones occurs. Thus, not only is growth accelerated, but continues for an unusually long time, resulting in a very tall individual. Later, acromegalic features are superimposed on those of gigantism.

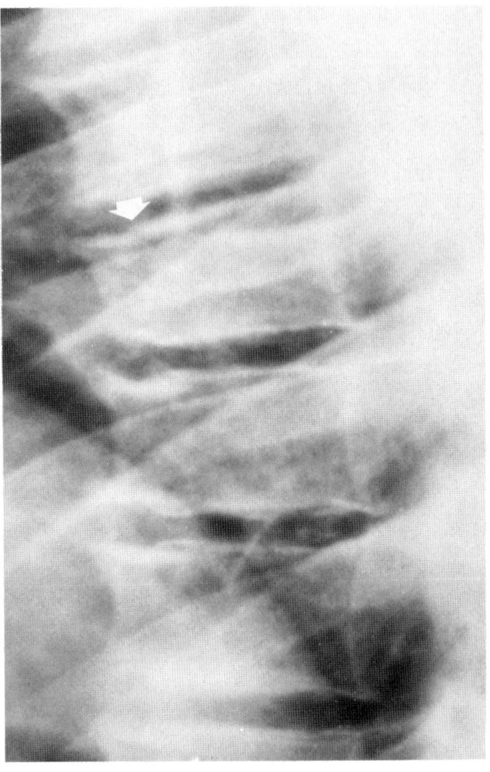

Fig. 8.22 Thoracic spine in acromegaly. The vertebral bodies appear flat as a result of the laying down of appositional new bone, mainly anteriorly. The original margin of the vertebral border can be identified (arrow).

Acromegaly

This condition results from the effect of excess growth hormone on the mature skeleton. Because the growth plates are closed, new bone formation is appositional and affects particularly the skull, spine and extremities.

The skull vault is thickened and the sinuses and mastoid air cells are greatly enlarged. The pituitary fossa is enlarged by the adenoma in nearly every case, but tomography may be required to demonstrate the floor of the fossa which may be depressed asymmetrically. The mandible is hypergnathic, with an increased angle. In the spine, kyphosis is common. The deposition of new bone anteriorly and laterally on the vertebral body is apparent and it may be possible to discern the underlying original shape of the vertebral body (Fig. 8.22). Posterior scalloping may be present and osteophyte formation is common. In association with the kyphosis, an increase in the sagittal diameter of the chest occurs. Although the total width of the long bones is increased, the cortical thickness is often unaltered. No evidence exists for acromegaly being a cause of true osteoporosis. Characteristic changes are present in the hands and feet. Bone overgrowth enlarges the bases of the phalanges and the terminal tufts, which become shaped like arrow-heads. Muscle attachments are prominent and widening of joint spaces, particularly those of the metacarpophalangeal joints, due to growth of articular cartilage, is shown. Typical 'hooks' are present on the heads of the metacarpals (Fig. 8.23). The hands and feet are large overall, due to enlargement of all tissues. A diagnostic feature is the thickness of the heel-pad measured from the X-ray film (Fig. 8.24). In the absence of injury or other cause for soft tissue swelling, it is rare for the normal heel-pad to exceed 21.5 mm in females and 23 mm in males. However, even with a precisely defined method of measurement it is not possible to separate completely normal subjects from acromegalic patients (Kho et al, 1970). Enlargement of the viscera, particularly the heart, liver and kidneys may be evident. Calcification within the pinna of the ear is sometimes present. In addition to an increased depth of articular cartilage, joints may show premature degenerative disease as a result of bony overgrowth producing incongruity of the opposing articular surfaces. This is particularly evident in the shoulders (Fig. 8.25), hips and knees. Premature osteophytosis with preservation or increase of the cartilage space is almost diagnostic. Extension of subchondral cortical bone into the articular cartilage is sometimes observed. Although an associated crystal arthropathy has been proposed, chondrocalcinosis is uncommon.

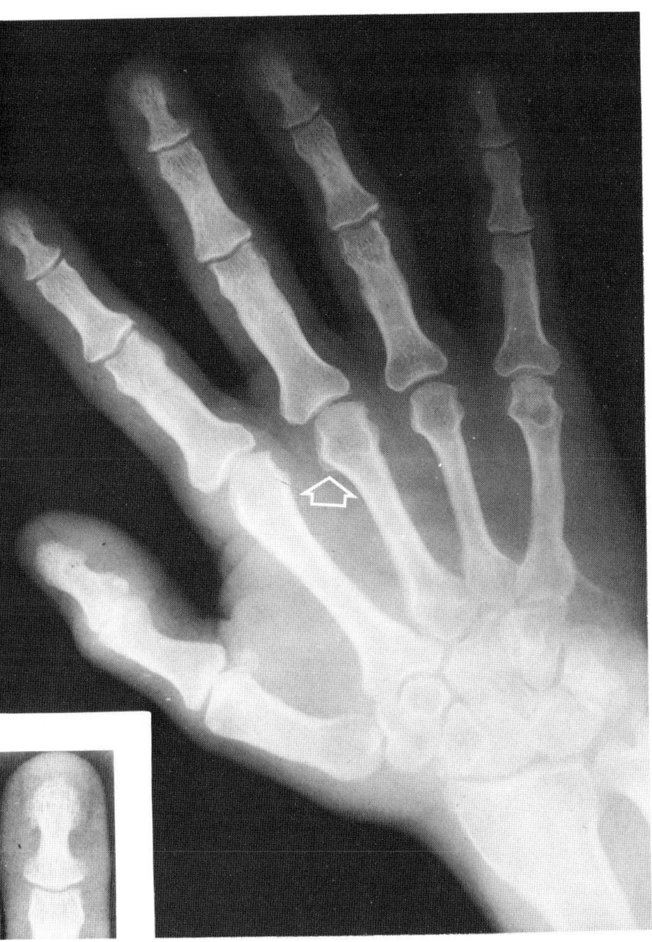

Fig. 8.23 The hand in acromegaly. The fingers are broad as a result of soft tissue enlargement and broadening of the terminal tufts. An early 'hook' is present on a metacarpal head (arrow) and the metacarpophalangeal cartilage spaces are widened.

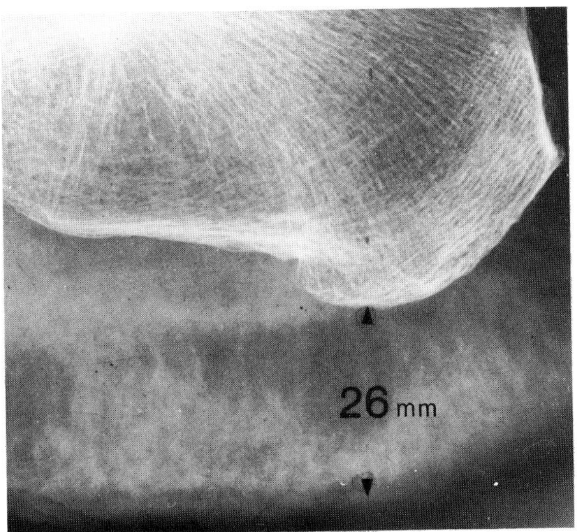

Fig. 8.24 Heel pad thickness in acromegaly. The heel pad is measured perpendicularly to the superior calcaneal line by the method of Kho *et al.* (1970).

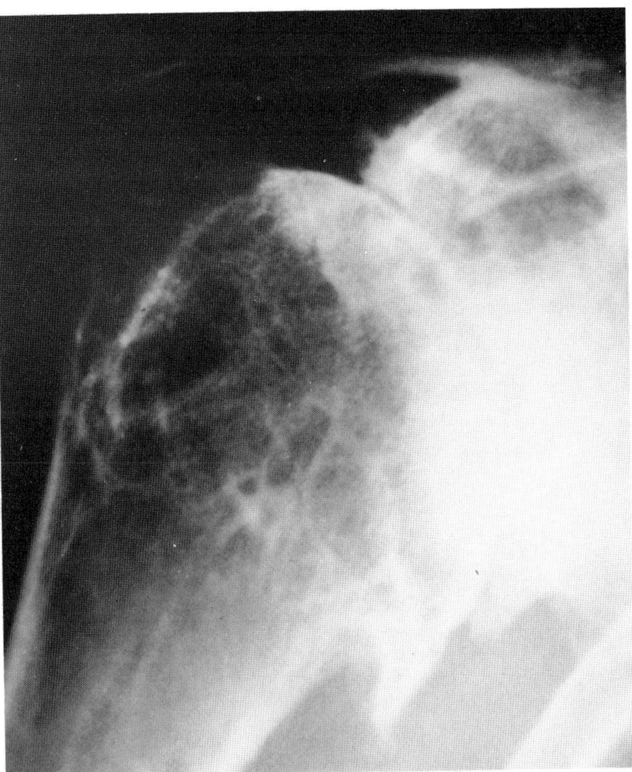

Fig. 8.25 Degenerative joint disease in acromegaly. Narrowing of the joint space is associated with subarticular sclerosis and osteophyte formation. Osteoarthrosis of the shoulder joint is uncommon in the absence of a clear predisposing cause.

THE THYROID

Hypothryoidism

Characteristic findings in the skeleton of patients with *cretinism* and *juvenile myxoedema* may lead to the radiologist being the first to make the diagnosis. Ossification centres are delayed in their appearance, although eventually they appear in normal sequence (Fig. 8.26). Once they do ossify, their growth is retarded. They are commonly multicentric and irregularly ossified. These changes are bilateral and symmetrical. Such changes in the hips must be differentiated from bilateral Perthes' disease and multiple epiphyseal dysplasia (Fig. 8.27). Epiphyseal and sutural closure is delayed. The skull has a short base and development of vascular markings and diploic differentiation are delayed. In the infant and young child, the sella is immature and 'bowl' like; in the older child, rebound hypertrophy of the pituitary causes a relatively large round 'cherry' sella. The paranasal sinuses are poorly developed. A kyphosis at the thoraco-lumbar junction is usually associated with a hypoplastic or 'bullet' vertebral body, usually the first or second lumbar. This is probably due to the stress effect of sitting on the vertebrae of a hypotonic child. All the long bones are shorter than normal, the pelvis is often narrow with coxa vara deformities. The incidence of slipped femoral capital epiphysis is increased. The most marked skeletal changes are seen in adult cretin dwarfs (Fig. 8.28).

Following prompt replacement therapy in early infancy, the bone changes return to normal and, more importantly, so does intellectual progress.

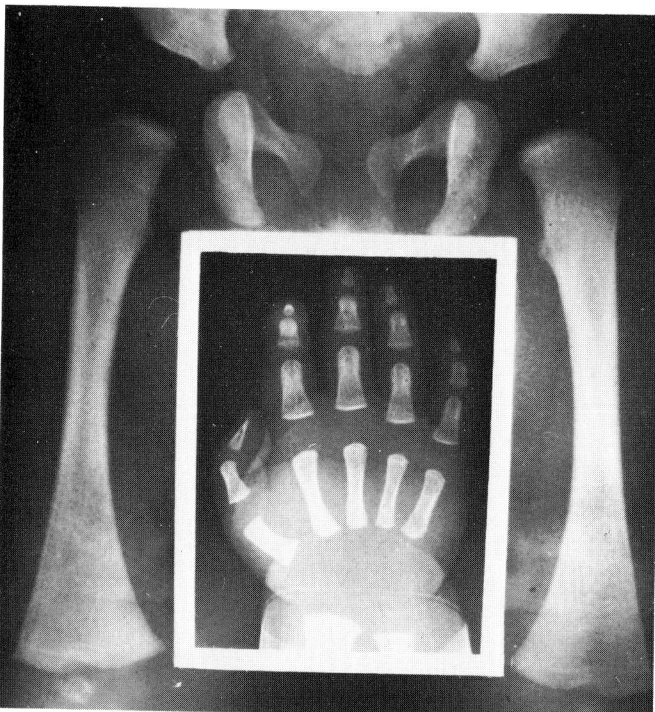

Fig. 8.27 Hypothyroidism. In this child the epiphyses of the proximal femur show multiple ossification centres. In the differential diagnosis, symmetrical involvement in Perthes' disease is rare and multiple epiphyseal dysplasia can usually be confirmed by the radiographic appearance of other epiphyses.

Hyperthyroidism

Skeletal changes are rarely symptomatic. The principa radiographic finding in adults is a generalized loss of bon (osteoporosis) associated with intracortical striations. Ove half the patients show cortical bone thickness.

Thyroid acropachy is a rare, late manifestation. It is mor common in males and nearly always affects patients treate by thyroid ablation who may have been euthyroid or hypothyroid for years. The extremities are swollen an clubbed. Exophthalmos and pretibial myxoedema are al most always present. A quite distinct periosteal new bon formation is found in the extremities, particularly th hands. A spiculated or feathery appearance affects mainly the metacarpals of the thumb, index and little fingers, bu also the phalanges (Fig. 8.29). It must be distinguished

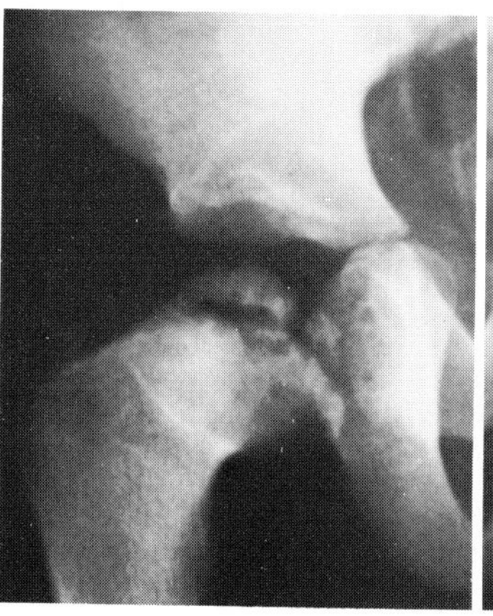

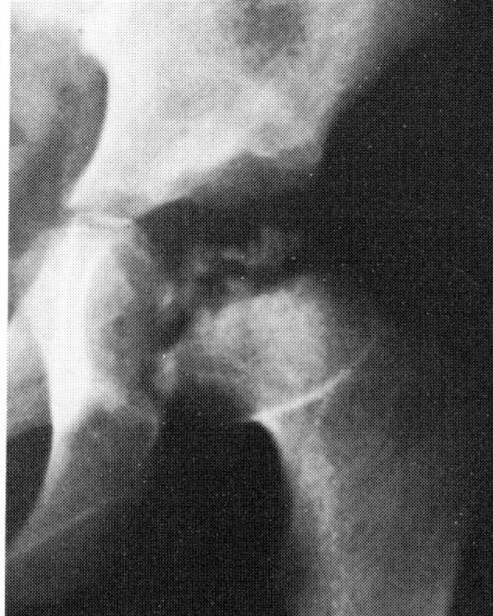

Fig. 8.26 Cretinism. Marked skeletal retardation was present in this 12-month-old child. Note that the carpal and proximal femoral centres have not yet appeared.

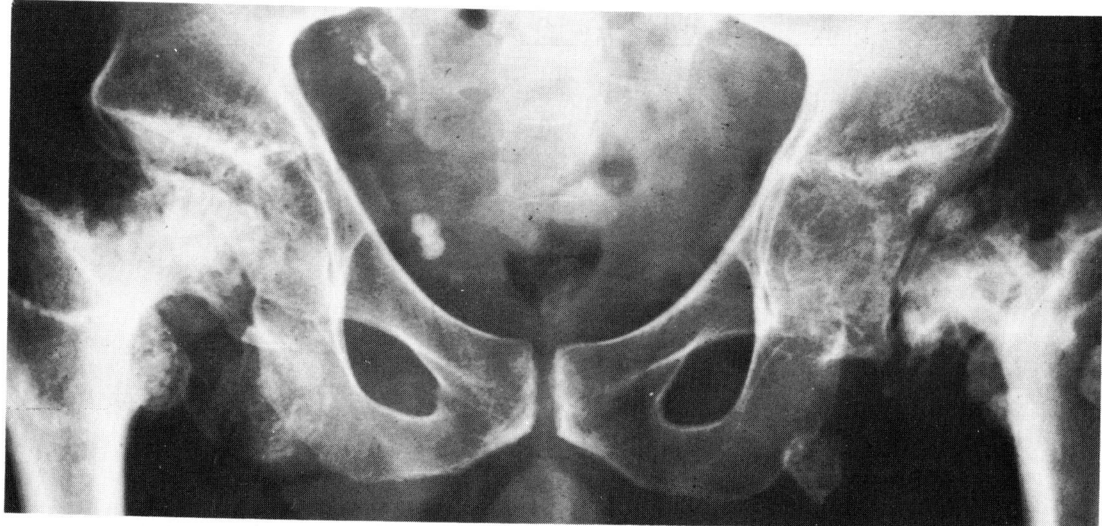

Fig. 8.28 Adult cretinism. This 39-year-old man received no therapy until 4 years before this film was obtained. Coxa vara is present whilst the femoral heads are deformed and irregularly ossified in the absence of thyroid hormone during development.

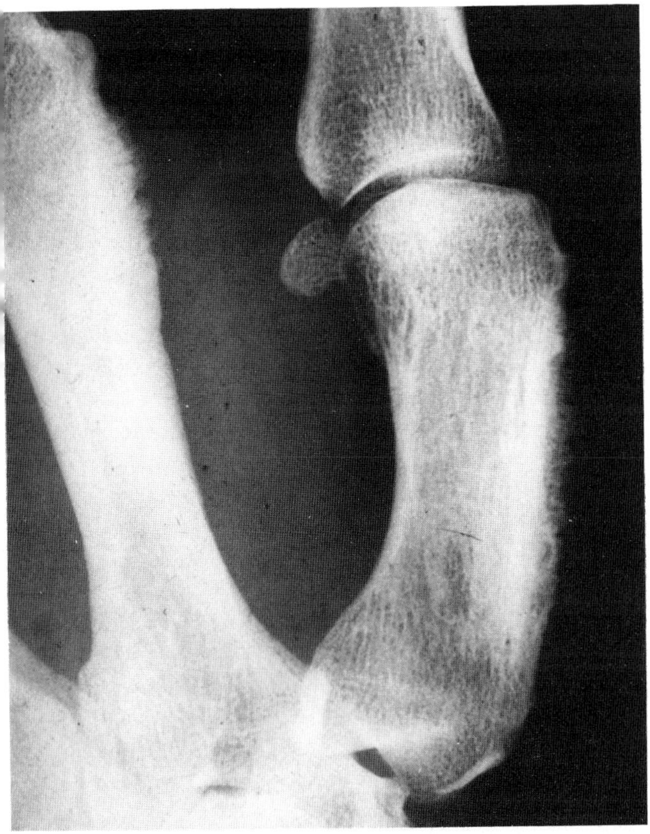

Fig. 8.29 Thyroid acropachy. A characteristic feathery periosteal reaction affects the radial aspect of the metacarpal shafts.

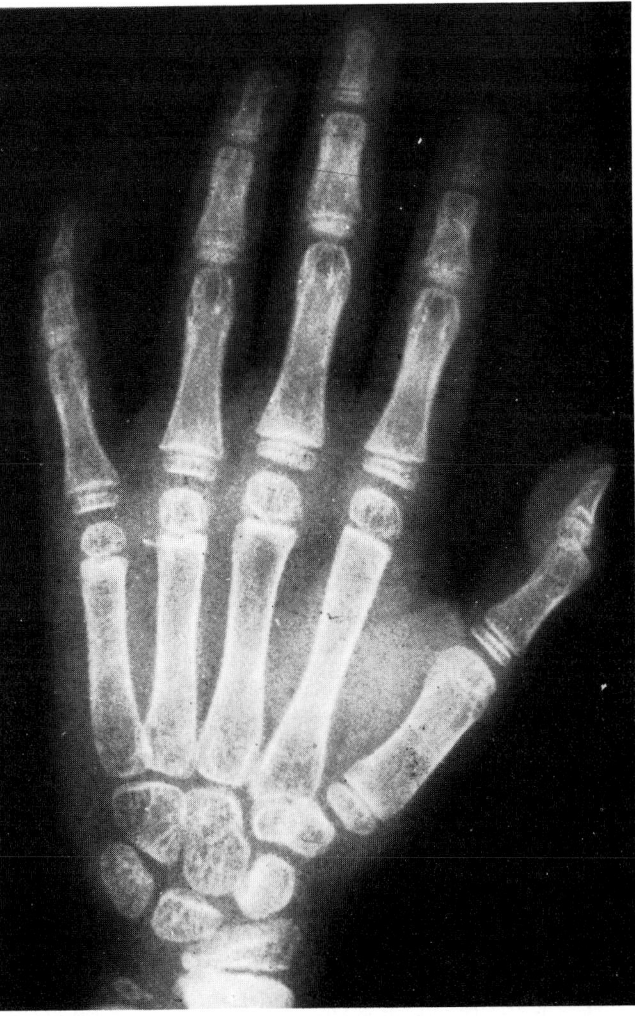

Fig. 8.30 Hyperthyroidism in a child of 3 years. The rare appearance of this disorder in childhood has resulted in premature ossification of the carpal centres. Evidence of osteoporosis is also present.

from hypertrophic osteoarthropathy which shows more dense wavy new bone and is not often confined to the bones of the hands and feet.

In the rarely occurring hyperthyroidism of childhood, the most obvious radiological feature is the precocious appearance of the ossification centres, which are otherwise normal (Fig. 8.30).

THE PARATHYROID GLANDS: HYPERPARATHYROIDISM

PRIMARY HYPERPARATHYROIDISM

Excessive production of parathormone resulting from a disorder of one or more of the parathyroid glands causes a metabolic disturbance characterized by an elevated plasma calcium level. The depression of the plasma phosphate and elevation of urinary calcium are rarely as reliable or constant features. Urinary phosphate determinations are most helpful in occult hyperparathyroidism when combined with calcium infusion or phosphate deprivation. Serum alkaline phosphatase is raised only when bone disease occurs. Hypercalcaemia is the most valuable single diagnostic feature and results from (1) increased intestinal absorption of calcium; (2) increased bone turnover, particularly resorption; (3) increased tubular reabsorption of calcium. Clinical features may therefore relate to the hypercalcaemia itself with lassitude, weakness, thirst, polyuria, anorexia and nausea; or to bone or renal complications. Symptoms of psychiatric and pancreatic disorder may be found. The true incidence of primary hyperparathyroidism (HPT) is not known, but the introduction of biochemical screening using the autoanalyser has revealed many unsuspected patients. It is more common in women, particularly after the menopause. The disorder may be found at all ages from birth to old age, but the greatest incidence occurs between 20 and 60 years. A familial incidence has been described in some cases. HPT may form part of either type of multiple endocrine neoplasia. The main parathyroid lesions are adenoma, accounting for three quarters of the cases, hyperplasia and carcinoma.

Hyperparathyroidism is rare in infancy. Histologically and radiologically it is indistinguishable from the equally uncommon intrauterine hyperparathyroidism found in neonates born to mothers with poorly controlled hypoparathyroidism; this, however, tends to improve spontaneously as the secondary parathyroid hyperplasia regresses. Both disorders may result in increased incidence of fractures at birth.

Bone changes (osteitis fibrosa)

Unlike osteomalacia, bone pain is not a common feature of HPT. Advanced bone disease is now rarely seen. It used to be said that radiological evidence of bone disease was present in one-quarter of cases, but with the increase in asymptomatic patients, this proportion is now reduced to about 10%.

Radiographic evidence of *osteopenia* is also uncommon, although absorptiometric methods reveal decreased mineral values in 50% of patients. Nevertheless, in advanced cases bone density is reduced, with loss of the normal fine trabecular pattern and sometimes a 'ground-glass' appearance. In the lateral radiograph of the skull, this featureless appearance may be exaggerated by erosion of the margins o the vascular grooves which makes these markings les distinct.

Subperiosteal erosion of the cortex is almost pathognomonic of bone disease in HPT. First the sharp margi of cortical bone is lost with progression and local destruction leaving a spiculated or 'lace-like' appearance of th thinned cortex. Definition between the cortex and the medulla is lost. This osteoclastic activity is progressing in th whole skeleton, but may be demonstrated only in th hands, where fine-detail radiography is possible. Such cortical erosion is most common on the radial aspect of th middle phalanges (Fig. 8.31A & B). Erosion of the terminal tufts of the phalanges is further evidence of this process (Fig. 8.31B). Other involved areas include the latera and sometimes the medial ends of the clavicles, medial as-

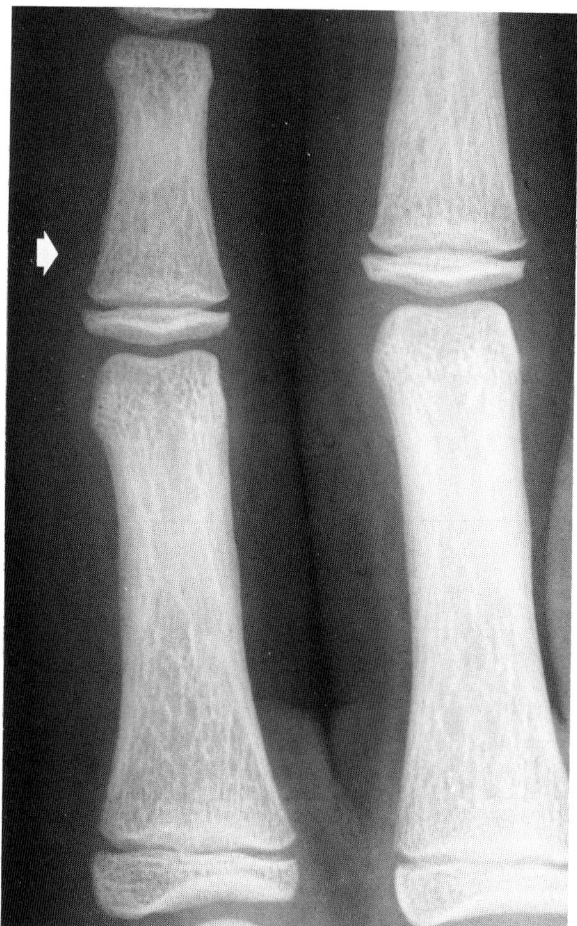

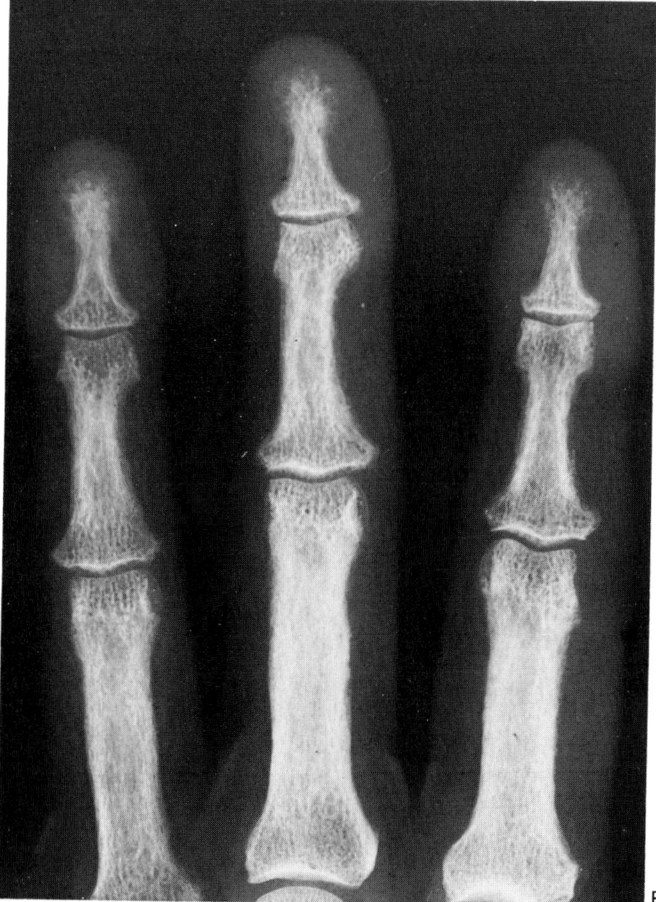

Fig. 8.31 Hyperparathyroidism. **A**. The hand of this child has been recorded by a magnification technique. The arrow indicates the site of the earliest changes of cortical erosion in this disorder — the proximal metaphyseal region of the middle phalanx on the radial aspects. **B**. In this adult patient erosive change is present in the subperiosteal bone of the phalangeal shafts, particularly on their radial aspects. The terminal tufts are eroded, in addition to more generalized change in bone architecture due to increased osteoclastic activity.

ect of the proximal tibia, pubic symphysis, ischial tuberoities and the medial aspect of the neck of the femur. n most of these sites a predominantly metaphyseal location preferred. When other bones show cortical erosion, the ands are almost inevitably affected. Disappearance of the amina dura around the teeth may occur in HPT. It is, owever, not a specific sign and occurs in both local and eneralized conditions, including osteomalacia, osteoporsis, myelomatosis and Paget's disease. The radiographic ppearance of osteoclasis progresses from small surface iregularities to deeper pits which coalesce to produce extenive, ill-defined scalloping of the cortex. With such rogress, other bones become involved and the changes are rossly abnormal. However, stress must be laid on the imortance of diagnosing the early subtle lesion with good adiographic technique and some form of magnification. When HPT occurs in the immature skeleton, a much grosser appearance of metaphyseal destruction may be apparent. This is particularly marked in the femoral and humeral necks. Displacement, with varus deformity, may occur through such an eroded area.

Diffuse cortical change. In addition to the surface changes, multiple oval or cigar-shaped lucencies, measuring 2–5 mm in length, may perforate the cortex (Fig. 8.32). These represent deeper osteoclasis in the Haversian canals or possibly osteocytic resorption; such cortical striation is a reflection of rapid turnover and is found in other states, e.g. normal childhood, osteomalacia and acute osteoporosis, particularly the reflex sympathetic dystrophy syndrome. Ultimately, a 'basket-work' appearance may result, which merges with the medullary trabeculae. Such lytic changes in the skull are the cause of the so-called 'pepper-pot' skull (Fig. 8.33). As a reactive change in the long-standing case some thickening of trabeculae may occur. Osteosclerosis, either localized or diffuse, is extremely rare, in contradistinction to secondary HPT.

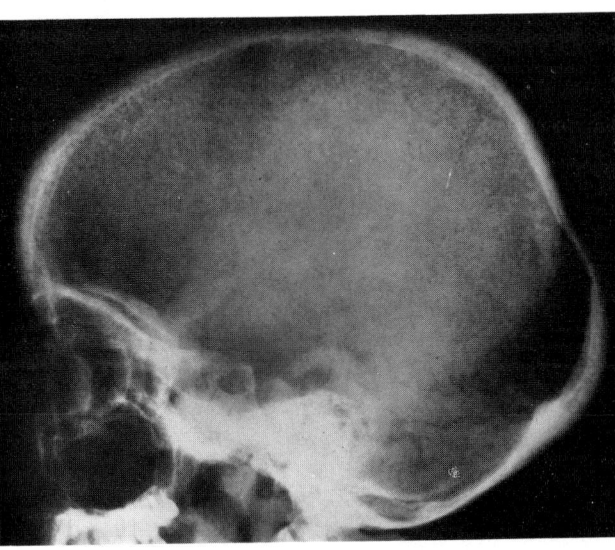

Fig. 8.33 Hyperparathyroidism. Generalized reduction in bone density derives from many small osteoclastic lucencies throughout the vault (the 'pepper-pot' skull). The vascular markings are poorly defined.

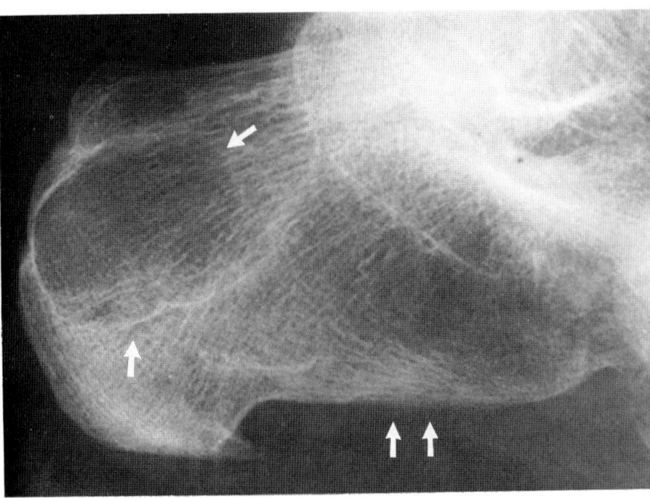

Fig. 8.32 Hyperparathyroidism. This radiograph of the calcaneus shows most of the features of hyperparathyroid bone disease — osteopenia, cortical striation (↑ ↑) cortical erosion and, in the posterosuperior part of the bone, increased lysis (↑) which proved to be due to the presence of a brown tumour.

Formation of brown tumours. These are locally destructive areas of intense osteoclastic activity. They should not be called cysts, which they rarely are, nor osteoclastomas, a term which has links with giant cell tumour of bone and is best avoided. They may occur anywhere in the skeleton and may expand the bone, with or without cortical destruction. They are often well-defined and multilocular and, when solitary, may mimic several varieties of benign tumours or cysts of bone (Figs. 8.32 & 8.34). In this circumstance, presentation may be the result of pathological fracture. When they are multiple, less confusion should occur. After removal of the parathyroid tumour, several responses are possible. Some bone tumours slowly fill in and revert to a normal bony structure; others become hyperostotic, almost resembling ivory osteomas. Uncommonly, a third group remain unchanged for years. These are usually those that have been the site of destructive central haemorrhage and therefore remain cystic.

Soft tissue calcification is common in the secondary form of HPT in both periarticular and vascular locations, but may occasionally occur to a significant degree in the primary disease.

Joint disorders

Joints may be involved in a variety of ways in HPT. Firstly, marginal erosions occur in relation to joints as a result of osteoclastic activity. Weakening of the subarticular bone may, in addition, lead to infraction with struc-

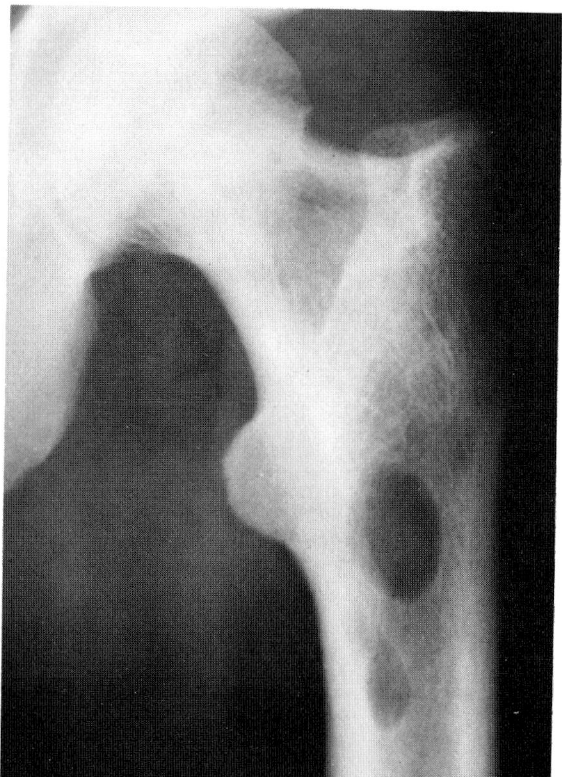

Fig. 8.34 Primary hyperparathyroidism. The well-defined lytic lesions in the proximal femoral shaft are brown tumours. The clarity of the margins of two of the lesions indicates cortical involvement. No other obvious features of hyperparathyroid bone disease are present in the film.

tural collapse. This appearance may mimic rheumatoid arthritis. Secondly, chondrocalcinosis may occur (Fig. 8.35). Such intra-articular deposition of crystals of calcium pyrophosphate dihydrate may lead to episodes of pseudo-gout. Thirdly, true gout may result from hyperuricaemia.

Renal lesions

Renal tubular dysfunction results from the direct effect of parathormone on the kidney and is corrected by parathyroidectomy. Renal calculi have been reported in as many as 50% of patients. Such calculi are often small and result in the patient presenting with renal colic. Most stones are formed of calcium oxalate and/or apatite mixtures, but a minority are uric acid stones.

Nephrocalcinosis

This is less common. The term depends upon radiological evidence; calcification is sometimes difficult to demonstrate and may be undetected unless tomography is employed. Deposition of calcium is generally in the region of the renal pyramids, but forms no diagnostic pattern. Uraemia is a major cause of death in untreated HPT.

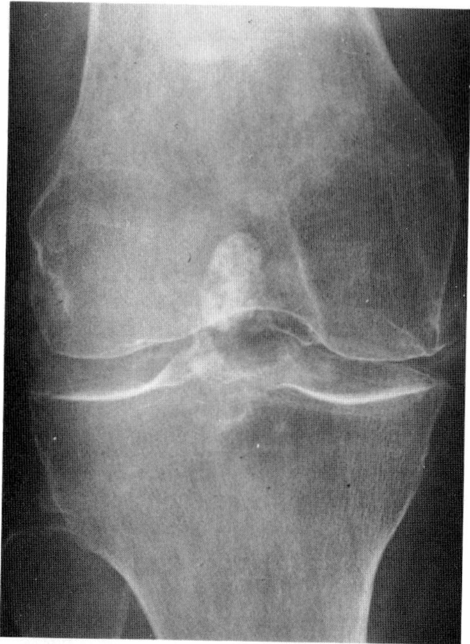

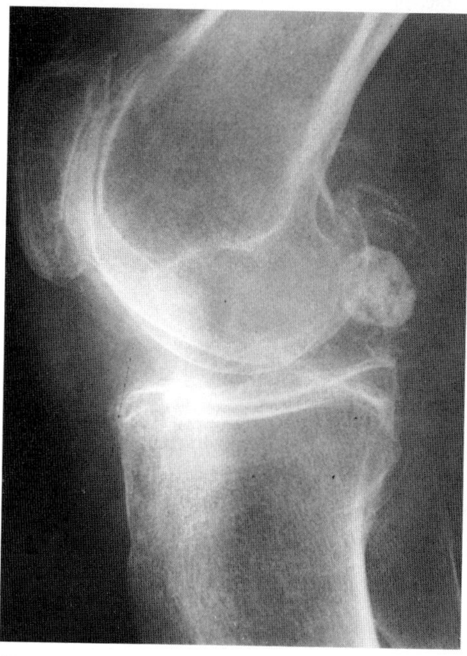

Fig. 8.35 Hyperparathyroidism. In addition to chondrocalcinosis, this patient shows calcification of the joint capsule or synovium.

Other findings

Parathyroid tumours may occasionally indent the upper oesophagus on a barium swallow. Parathyroid adenomata may calcify. Cardiomegaly is generally the sequel of complicating hypertension. An increased incidence of peptic ulcer in HPT is likely.

SECONDARY HYPERPARATHYROIDISM

Hyperplasia of all the parathyroid glands occurs in reonse to persistent hypocalcaemia of any cause. Secondary PT is found in many patients with rickets, osteomalacia renal failure. HPT is part of the picture of uraemic osodystrophy which will be discussed later.

Long-standing osteomalacia is a less common cause of condary HPT and often shows only as subperiosteal eroons superimposed on the established changes of osteoalacia. Diffuse changes similar to primary HPT do occur, ut brown tumours are uncommon. Arterial calcification common and ectopic soft tissue calcification is seen, ough less often than in HPT associated with renal disase. Bone sclerosis may occur, just as in the secondary yperparathyroidism of uraemic osteodystrophy.

'TERTIARY' HYPERPARATHYROIDISM'

his term is employed to describe patients with secondary IPT who develop an autonomous parathyroid adenoma. t may follow osteomalacia or renal failure and is characerized by hypercalcaemia. The HPT fails to respond to reatment of the underlying disorder and where possible arathyroidectomy should be performed.

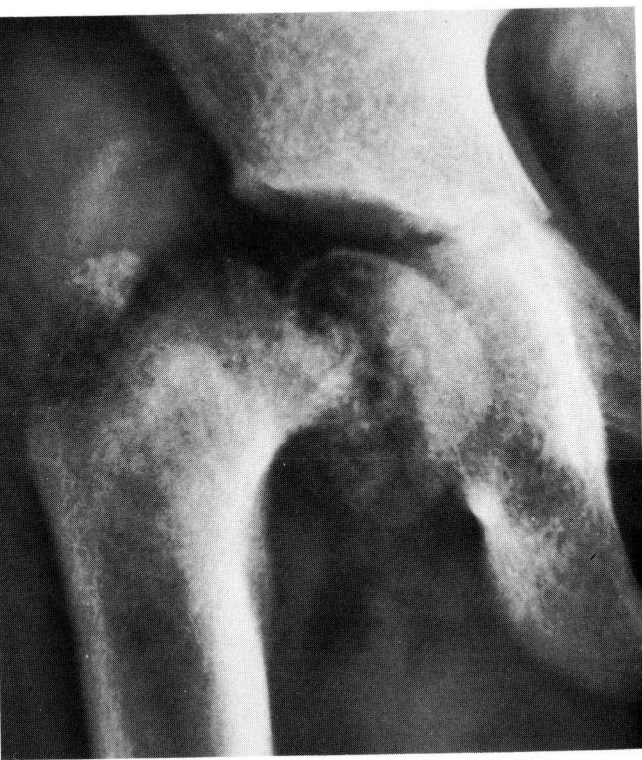

Fig. 8.36 Uraemic osteodystrophy in childhood. In this child with chronic renal failure the combination of rickets and secondary hyperparathyroidism affects the skeleton. The femoral metaphysis is irregular and the capital epiphysis shows considerable displacement. The metaphyseal appearance has been likened to a 'rotting fence post'.

URAEMIC OSTEODYSTROPHY
(Renal glomerular osteodystrophy)

This entity requires separate mention because it consists of (1) osteomalacia or rickets; (2) bone changes of secondary hyperparathyroidism; and (3) osteosclerosis. Few paients present with symptoms due to the bone disease. The most prevalent cause is bilateral *chronic pyelonephritis*, often associated with vesico-ureteric reflux. *Chronic glomerulonephritis* is a less common finding. In both conditions, endstage renal disease is evidenced by small contracted kidneys. Rarely, polycystic disease is the primary lesion. Nephrocalcinosis is rare, but renal calculi may be associated with the pyelonephritis.

Children. The skull, pelvis, scapulae, vertebrae and metaphyses of tubular bones, consisting primarily of cancellous bone, show an increase in bone mass and often osteosclerosis. This change relates to the duration of the uraemia and at first the bone density may be radiologically normal or reduced. Vertebral sclerosis may be confined to the upper and lower thirds of each body producing the transverse bands of a 'rugger-jersey' spine. Metastatic calcification is less common than in adults. Metaphyseal changes resemble those of vitamin D dependent rickets, with poorly mineralized metaphyseal spongiosa. To this is added to cortical erosion of HPT, producing the 'rotting fence post' appearance of the femoral necks (Fig. 8.36). Shearing stresses may result in epiphyseal separation. The apparent epiphyseal plate is less wide than in untreated vitamin D dependent rickets, however, and the metaphysis less cupped, but with poorly orientated spongiosa. Growth and skeletal maturation are delayed.

Biopsy reveals predominant osteomalacia in one quarter, hyperparathyroidism in one quarter and a mixed pattern in the remaining half. The type of bone disease on biopsy often does not correlate well with the radiographic appearances. Nevertheless, children with abnormal radiographs always show abnormal biochemistry.

Adults. The changes of HPT are the most prominent with subperiosteal resorption most easily detected in the phalanges (Fig. 8.31). Metastatic calcification is observed (Fig. 8.37) in arterial walls, articular cartilage and periarticular regions. Radiographic evidence of visceral calcification is rare, apart from in the kidneys. Osteosclerosis produces the 'rugger-jersey' spine (Fig. 8.38) and increased density causing some obliteration of the medullary cavity of the long bones. The residual changes of osteomalacia are mainly those of Looser's zones, although the general bone changes must be an inextricable mixture of the two conditions.

Although the basic factors leading to osteosclerosis are uncertain, a number of possible contributory causes have to be considered:

1. Elevation of the serum phosphate level leads to a raised calcium/phosphate product. In the presence of ex-

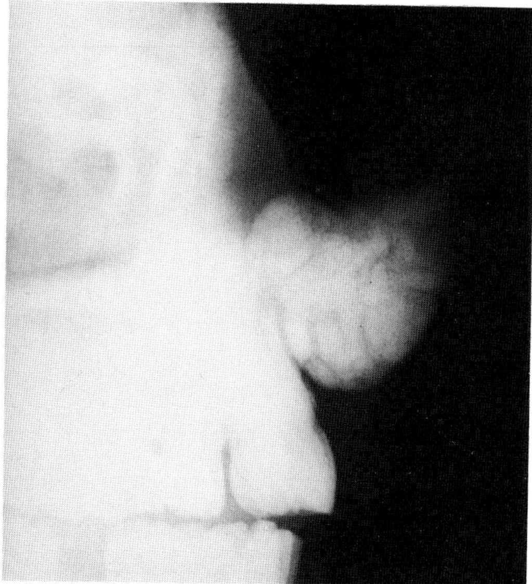

Fig. 8.37 Metastatic calcification in secondary hyperparathyroidism (uraemic osteodystrophy). Calcium salts have been deposited, rather unusually, in the soft tissues above the upper lip.

cess osteoid (osteomalacia), regional increases in mineralized bone may therefore be expected.

2. Excess of parathyroid hormone (rather than any calcitonin effect) can produce osteosclerosis under experimental conditions, probably due to a direct effect on bone.

3. Periosteal osteogenesis may contribute in a minority of patients.

4. Osteosclerosis tends to increase *pari passu* with the severity of osteitis fibroma. Hæmodialysis has resulted in increasing survival of patients with osteodystrophy and hence more osteosclerosis is observed nowadays.

HAEMODIALYSIS AND RENAL TRANSPLANTATION

Haemodialysis has no effect on the abnormal vitamin D metabolism of azotaemia. Hence, one would expect little change in the appearance of the bone lesions. Indeed, a progressive symptomatic bone disease has been recognized in some dialysis patients at some centres. These patients develop bone pain, fractures and progressive rarefaction (Fig. 8.39). The cause is unknown, but it is not universal and may be related to local conditions, for example, some contaminant of local tap water. Metastatic calcification does not usually change on dialysis and may increase (Fig. 8.40).

Successful renal transplantation does correct the biochemical abnormalities, although sometimes only after a delay of some months.

Changes in the bone and soft tissue in patients on chronic haemodialysis or following renal transplantation may reflect the persistence of uraemic osteodystrophy or additional features. These latter include osteonecrosis, osteomyelitis and certain connective tissue complications. Osteonecrosis is usually attributable to treatment with corticosteroids and occurs in between 4 and 28% of transplanted patients. The most common site is the femoral head (Fig. 8.41); others include the distal femoral condyles, both ends of the humerus, the talus, cuboid and other carpal and tarsal bones. Osteomyelitis and septic arthritis are also thought to relate to steroids and immunosuppressive agents; the infecting organisms comprise common bacteria, including *Mycobacterium tuberculosis*, as well as opportunist organisms.

OXALOSIS

Primary hyperoxaluria is a rare metabolic disorder inherited as an autosomal recessive trait. It is characterized by

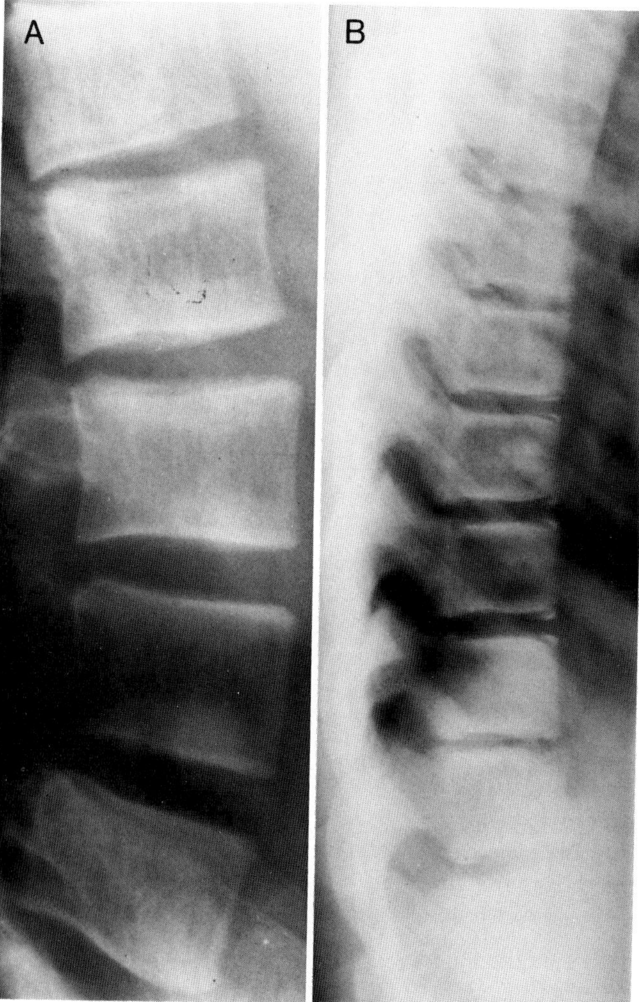

Fig. 8.38 Spine in renal osteodystrophy. **A.** Affected adult showing typical 'rugger-jersey' change of increased density of cancellous bone nearest the vertebral end-plates. **B.** Similar changes in a child with additional density on either side of Hahn's clefts.

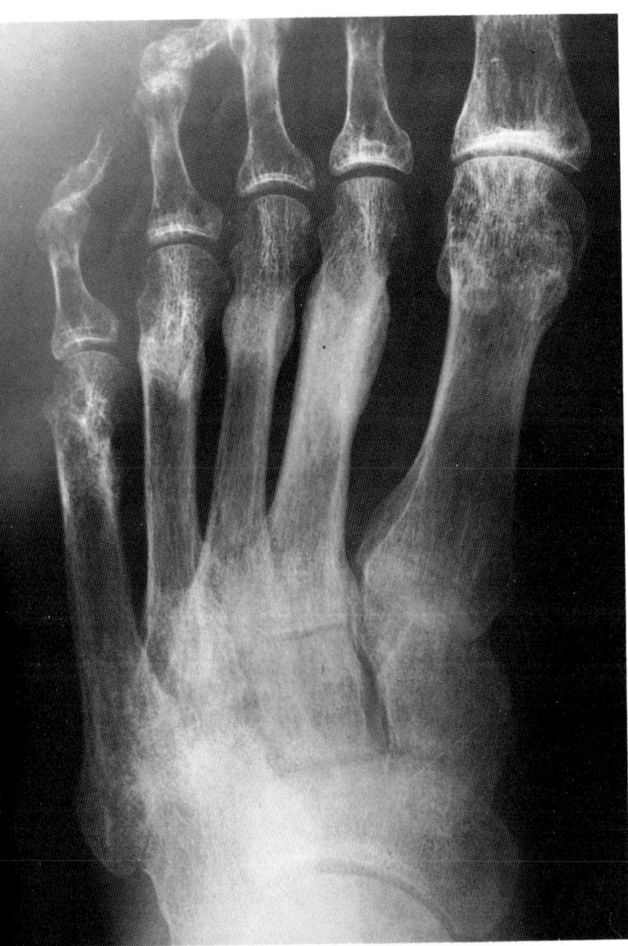

Fig. 8.39 'Dialysis bone disease'. In this patient on long-term haemodialysis, a general reduction in bone density is shown. Multiple fractures of the metatarsals are present in various stages of healing.

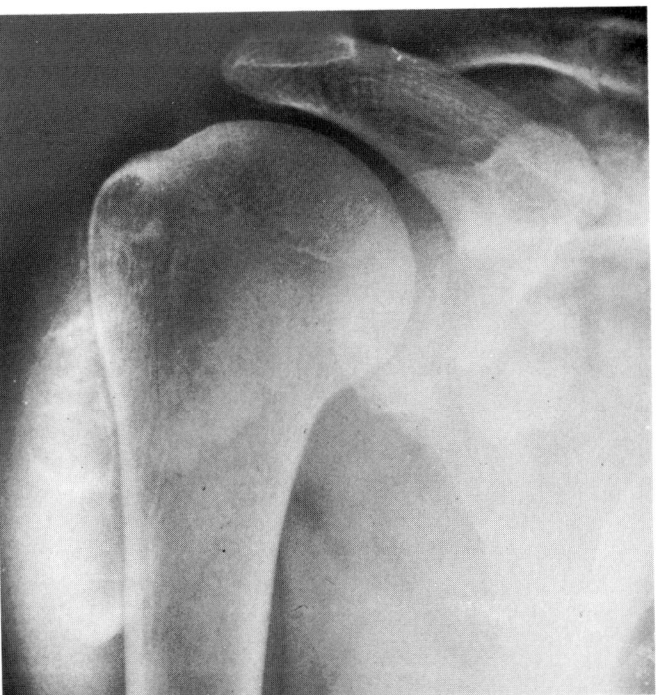

Fig. 8.40 Soft tissue calcification in uraemia. Massive calcification is present in the soft tissues around the shoulder joint. Such calcification may occur without dialysis therapy, but this 25-year-old patient had been receiving regular haemodialysis in the 18 months since bilateral nephrectomy. Fracture of the clavicle occurred spontaneously.

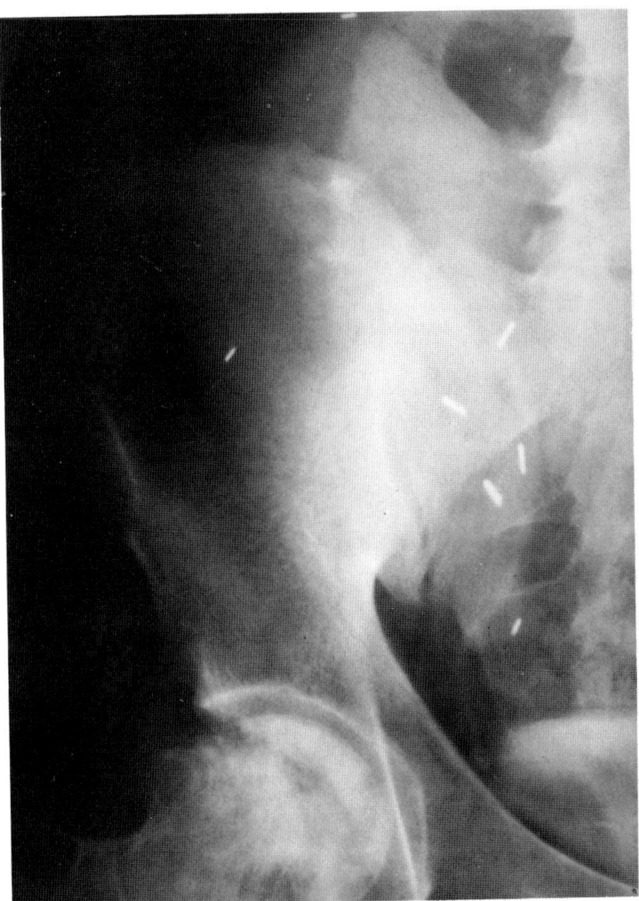

Fig. 8.41 Osteonecrosis in femoral head following renal transplantation. Operative clips and a nephrographic image of the transplanted kidney are observed in this urographic examination. Osteosclerosis and early structural collapse of the femoral head indicate avascular necrosis following immuno-suppressive therapy.

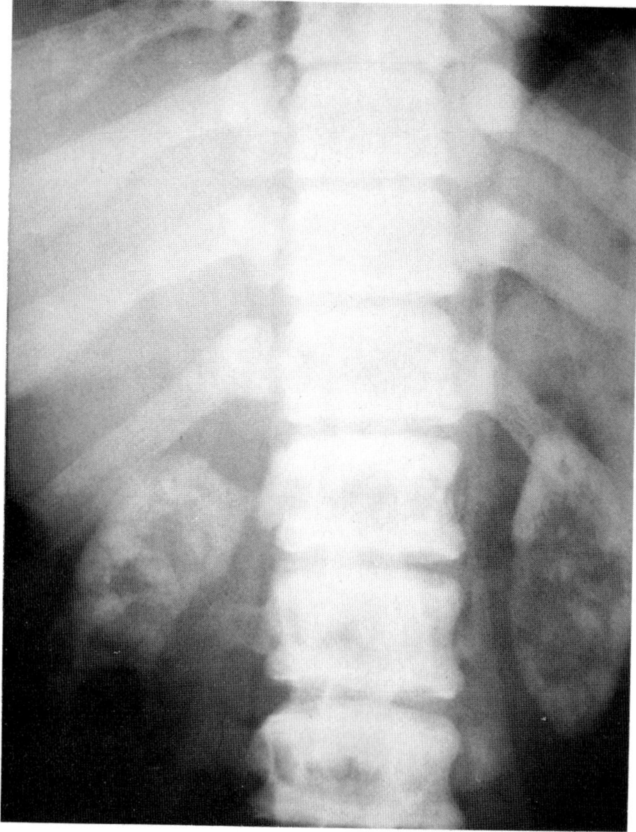

Fig. 8.42 Oxalosis. Classical changes in this rare disorder are shown by the presence of small calcified renal outlines and density of the bones, especially close to the vertebral end-plates and the heads of the ribs.

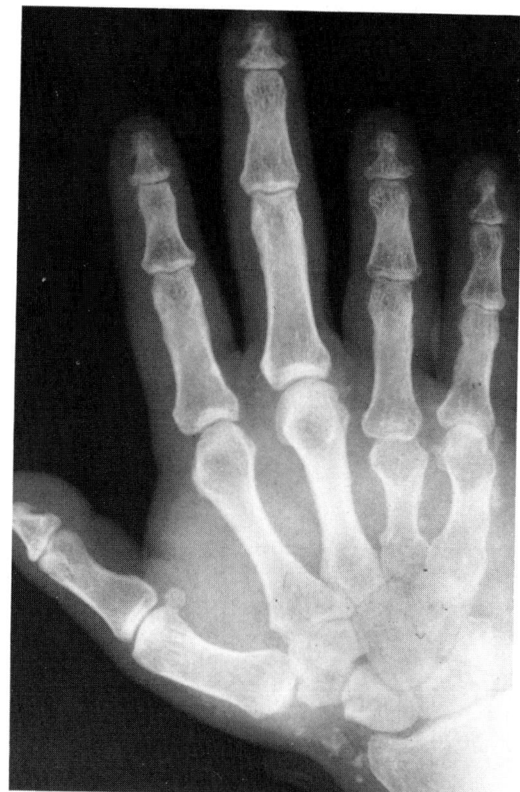

Fig. 8.43 Pseudohypoparathyroidism (PHPT). In this disorder shortening of one or more metacarpals or metatarsals is common and may be associated with phalangeal shortening. Such changes may occur in many other conditions and the diagnosis of PHPT is established principally by biochemical means.

recurrent urinary calculi and progressive renal failure. The continuous deposition of calcium oxalate in the soft tissues and bone (oxalosis) may occur in those who survive through dialysis treatment (Fig. 8.42).

HYPOPARATHYROIDISM, PSEUDO-HYPOPARATHYROIDISM AND PSEUDO-PSEUDO-HYPOPARATHYROIDISM

HYPOPARATHYROIDISM

This is an uncommon disorder which may follow thyroid surgery, ^{131}I therapy or be idiopathic, either of autoimmune or familial aetiology. The skeleton is usually normal. The main radiological feature of idiopathic hypoparathyroidism is calcification of the basal ganglia (Ch. 58) and, occasionally, in the cerebrum and cerebellum. Discrete ectopic calcification may occur in periarticular and subcutaneous regions, for example of the scalp.

The serum calcium is always low (under 1.8 mmol/l). A phosphate diuresis follows the administration of parathormone.

PSEUDO-HYPOPARATHYROIDISM

In this disorder of dominant inheritance, the chemical changes in the blood are similar to those of idiopathic hypoparathryoidism with hypocalcaemia and hyperphosphataemia, but do not respond to parathormone. The principal radiological findings are short stature, with short metacarpals, metatarsals and phalanges, affecting particularly the fourth and fifth metacarpals (Fig. 8.43). The teeth may show hypoplasia and defects in the enamel. Calcification may be present in the basal ganglia, cerebellum and skin. The children have characteristic moon faces. Deformities due to chronic tetany have been reported. Secondary hyperparathyroidism is a well-recognized feature of this disorder.

PSEUDO-PSEUDO-HYPOPARATHYROIDISM

This presents the same skeletal syndrome, but with normal blood chemistry. Whilst idiopathic brachydactyly might be a better name, the similarity does suggest some genetic link with the preceding disorder.

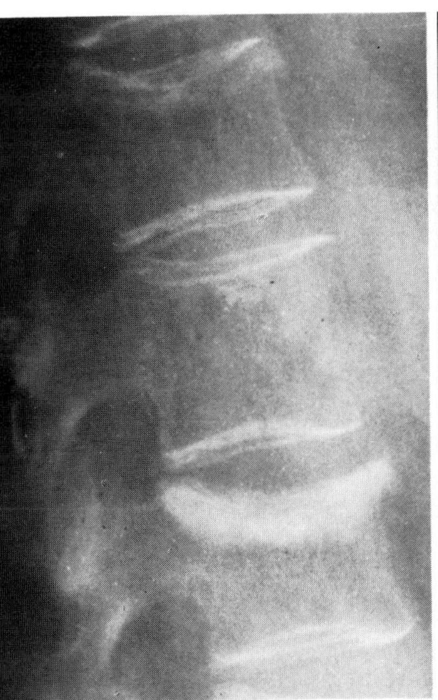

Fig. 8.44

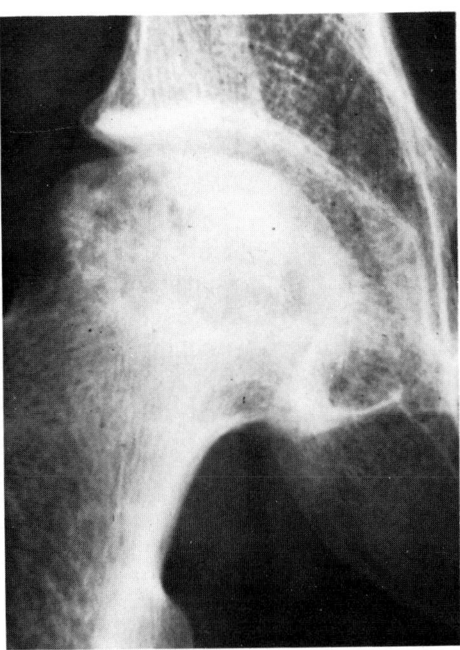

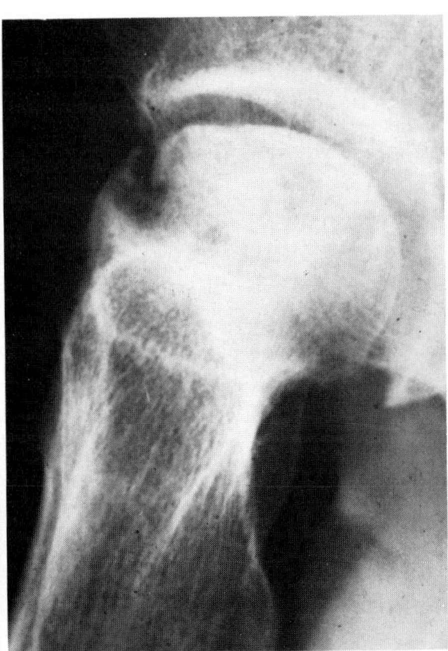

Fig. 8.45

Fig. 8.44 Cushing's syndrome. Generalized reduction in bone density simulates post-menopausal osteoporosis in this patient. The compression fracture of the superior border of the body of L4 has characteristically produced dense callus. This feature is almost, but not entirely, pathognomonic of glucocorticosteroid excess.

Fig. 8.45 Osteonecrosis due to steroids. Aseptic necrosis with structural failure of the subarticular bone has occurred in this patient receiving systemic steroid therapy. Subsequent damage to the other side of the joint will inevitably lead to arthropathy.

GLUCOCORTICOID EXCESS (*Cushing's syndrome*)

Excessive action by glucocorticosteroids may result from:

A. A tumour of the adrenal cortex
B. Adrenal hyperplasia as a result of excessive production of corticotrophin by the anterior pituitary
C. Therapy with corticosteroids or corticotrophin
D. Ectopic production of corticotrophin-like peptides by non-endocrine tumours, for example, carcinoma of the bronchus.

If prolonged, any of these disorders may produce disturbances of calcium metabolism and skeletal change. Iatrogenic prescription is at present the commonest cause of the syndrome. Corticosteroids are catabolic and, in excess, result in osteoporosis. This is most marked in the axial skeleton, where vertebral collapse occurs frequently. The vertebral bodies are wedged or biconcave and often show marginal density below the collapsed vertebral plate, due to the formation of florid immature callus (Fig. 8.44). This appearance is an important diagnostic clue to the aetiology of this osteoporosis. Rib fractures are common, multiple and often painless. Here too, callus formation may be excessive. Bone changes of osteoporosis in the appendicular skeleton are not striking. Ischaemic necrosis of the femoral heads is a frequent complication of corticosteroid excess (Fig. 8.45). It leads to structural failure and secondary arthritic change. Its mechanism is unknown, but it is not related to osteoporosis *per se*. Other joints, for example, the knee and shoulder, are affected much less frequently.

The administration of corticosteroids to children tends to retard growth and development. As they may control disorders which do the same, for example, juvenile rheumatoid arthritis, the balance may be a fine one, in respect of ultimate development. Characteristically, pain sense is partially or completely suppressed so that arthropathy or multiple fractures may be revealed as incidental findings. Similarly, infections of bones and joints may supervene and spread silently in the absence of normal pain sense. Widespread infection makes a significant contribution to morbidity and mortality in Cushing's syndrome.

TOXIC CHANGES IN BONE

A number of ingested materials may be incorporated into the skeleton and cause radiographic changes.

Lead poisoning

This condition is found mainly in children who ingest lead-containing paint flaking from old buildings or woodwork.

Lead has now vanished from currently available household paints. Nevertheless, lead-containing paint can be found covering older articles and in the deeper layers of repainted furniture. The habit is a form of *pica*, often associated with boredom, being commoner in children who are neglected and left without playthings. An abdominal X-ray will often show multiple dense flakes of paint within the intestine (Fig. 8.46). Other sources include contamination of water supplied via lead pipes and inhalation of lead when old batteries are burned. The amount of lead in the atmosphere derived from combustion of petrol is not known to produce radiographic change in the skeleton. In the growing skeleton lead is deposited in the growing metaphyseal regions, especially at the wrist, knee and ankle (Fig. 8.46). A mild general osteosclerosis is occasionally seen. Modelling deformities occur, for example, flask-shaped femora due to interference with osteoclastic activity. Although some of the density is due to lead itself ($Z = 92$) it is mostly due to reactive change. The differential diagnosis lies between normal metaphyseal density, other metallic poisoning and healed rickets. The bone changes are insignificant beside the damage caused by lead encephalopathy, which may be prevented by removal of the toxic cause. Increased intracranial pressure may be revealed by widened skull sutures.

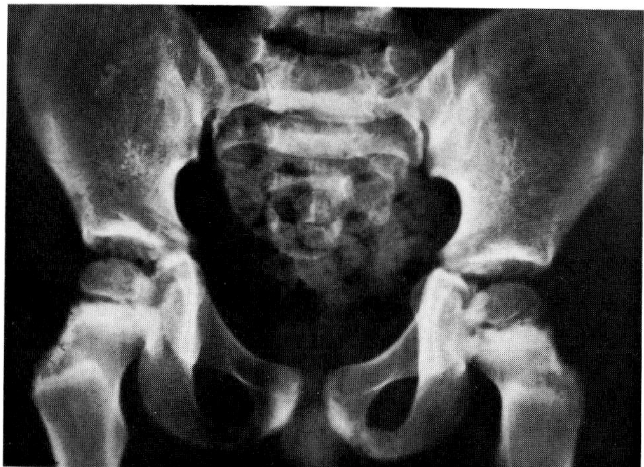

Fig. 8.46 Lead poisoning. Increased metaphyseal density of the femora and probably the iliac crests is due to lead deposition. The radio-opacities overlying the right iliac wing indicate pica for lead-containing paint.

Other metallic poisonings

These are less common.

Bismuth taken in large quantities for the treatment of congenital syphilis of past generations produced similar skeletal changes to those due to lead. The banning of dangerous yellow *phosphorus* has eliminated the osteonecrosis of 'phossy jaw'. Substitution of the sesquisulphide in safety matches only rarely results in its deposition in bone with metaphyseal sclerosis when match heads are eaten as a form of pica.

Miscellaneous poisons

The hazards of radium poisoning due to the painting of luminous dials is of historical interest only. Changes include bone necrosis, osteoporosis, mixed focal sclerosis and lucency and, in the long term, sarcomatous change. Another recognized industrial poison is *vinyl chloride*. At risk are those who clean tanks following the polymerization process in the manufacture of plastics (PVC). They inhale the monomer dust and may develop Raynaud's phenomenon, limb pains and erosions of bone, particularly in the fingers, with characteristic lucencies of the central portion of the terminal phalanges (Fig. 8.47). Sacro-iliitis occasionally occurs. The erosions heal rapidly after withdrawal of the toxic material. The occurrence of haemangiosarcoma of the liver following exposure to this toxic agent is mentioned elsewhere. Elimination of the hazards should result in disappearance of these complications.

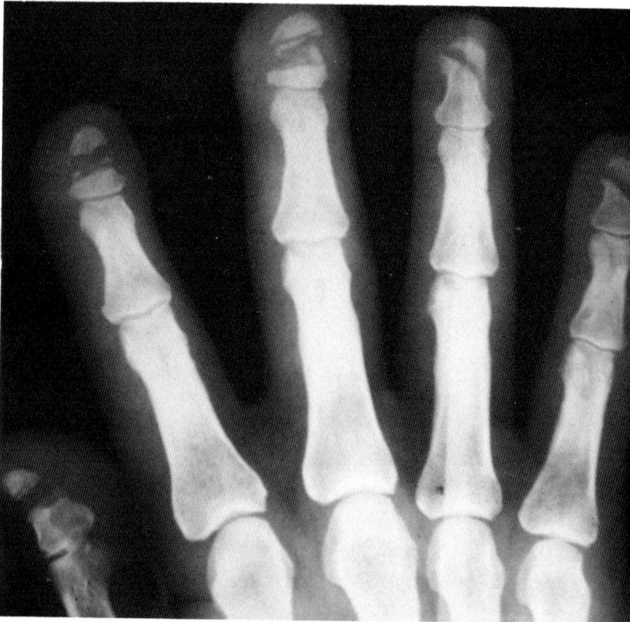

Fig. 8.47 Vinyl chloride poisoning. Inhalation or ingestion of vinyl chloride may produce this characteristic resorption of the central portions of the terminal phalanges.

Fluorosis

Chronic fluoride poisoning is almost always endemic, due to the subject living in an area where the drinking water has a high fluoride content, sometimes exceeding 10 parts per million. Such areas include parts of the Indian subcontinent, countries bordering the Persian Gulf and China.

Fluorine is inhaled or ingested otherwise in aluminium melting and other industries, habitual inhalation of fluorinated hydrocarbons, and in wine drinkers where fluorine is used as a preservative.

Fluorosis is manifested by mottled dental enamel and diffuse osteosclerosis of the skeleton. Sclerosis is not due to the density of the deposited fluoride (Z = 9), but to the osteoblastic response it provokes. Many adults in endemic areas are asymptomatic all their lives, despite radiographic evidence of osteosclerosis. In fact, a small amount of fluoride incorporated within the hydroxyapatite crystal improves its stability and protects against caries and age-related loss. Endemic fluorosis in children is rare, but may occur before the age of 10 in areas with an exceptionally high fluoride content and be associated with crippling stiffness and pain. In addition to a generalized increase in density, the affected bones show thickening of the cortex at the expense of the medullary cavity. Ossification takes place at ligamentous and musculotendinous attachments. This gives rise to a characteristic 'fringed' appearance which may be diagnostic (Fig. 8.48). Ossification in the intraosseous membranes of paired bones may lead to synostosis.

MISCELLANEOUS METABOLIC DISORDERS

Ochronosis (alkaptonuria)

This is a rare hereditary disorder of amino-acid (tyrosine) metabolism which results in the excessive production of derivatives of homogentisic acid. These are excreted in the urine and rarely are deposited in the tissues. The radiological features mainly reflect changes in the joints due to premature degenerative disease in response to pigment deposition in articular cartilage. The axial skeleton shows reduced bone density with generalized calcification of the narrowed intervertebral discs and kyphoscoliosis (Fig. 8.49). Ankylosis often follows. Extensive degenerative change affects the major synovial joints, for example, knees, shoulders and hips (Fig. 8.50). The diagnosis is confirmed by identification of homogentisic acid in the urine.

Hepatolenticular degeneration (Wilson's disease)

This rare disease of autosomal recessive inheritance is a disorder of copper metabolism primarily presenting with neurological abnormalities in adolescence, but bone changes also occur. These consist of rickets or osteomalacia

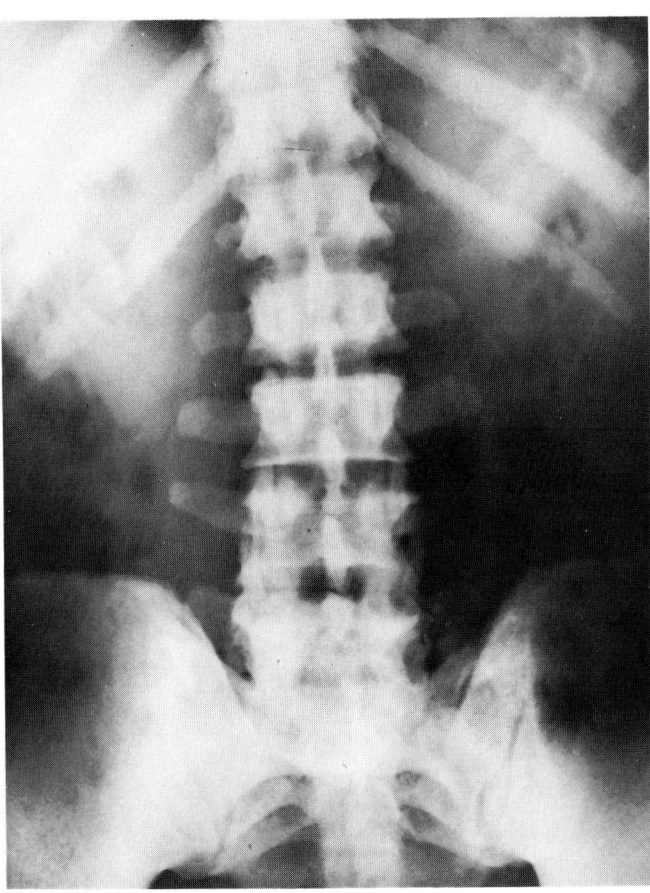

Fig. 8.48 Fluorosis. In this condition a generalized and non-specific skeletal sclerosis may be associated with a more diagnostic irregularity of bone margins shown here in the lower ribs.

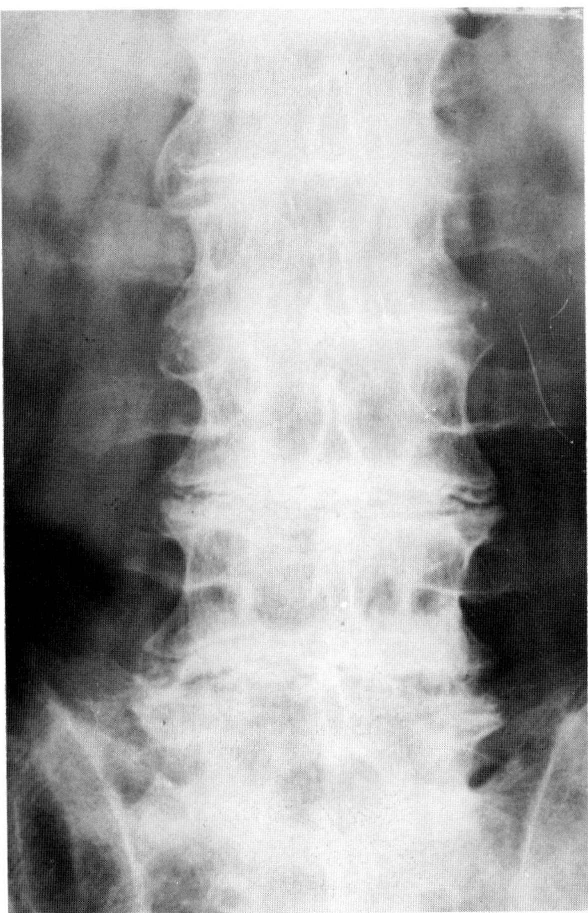

Fig. 8.49 Ochronosis. The intervertebral disc spaces are generally narrowed and calcified. Such widespread change is uncommon in uncomplicated degenerative spondylosis.

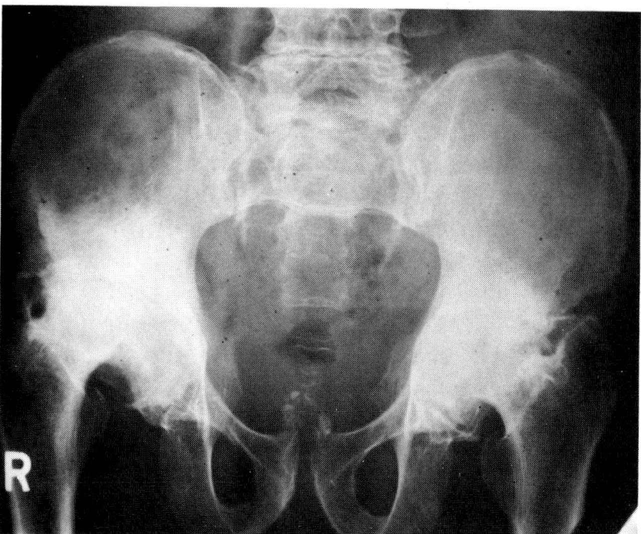

Fig. 8.50 Ochronosis. Gross narrowing of the joint spaces of both hips is associated with other evidence of severe degenerative disease. The intervertebral disc spaces are calcified and narrowed.

and joint abnormalities. Involvement of the peripheral joints predominates, especially wrists, hands, knees and hips. Fine irregularities of the subchondral bone may lead to a 'fringed' appearance which is diagnostic. Chondrocalcinosis is sometimes observed. Premature osteoarthrosis occurs in those who survive.

Copper deficiency in infants

Copper deficiency is rare in man. It is reported as an anaemia responsive to copper supplements in malnourished infants, in chronic malabsorption and in long term parenteral nutrition in infants. Radiographic changes include reduction in bone density, cortical thinning, metaphyseal irregularity and delay in ossification. In contrast to rickets, the zone of provisional calcification is preserved.

Haemochromatosis

This is a rare disease of iron metabolism where haemosiderin is deposited in the tissues. Osteopenia occurs, in common with other causes of iron-overload. A destructive arthropathy may occur in association with chondrocalci-

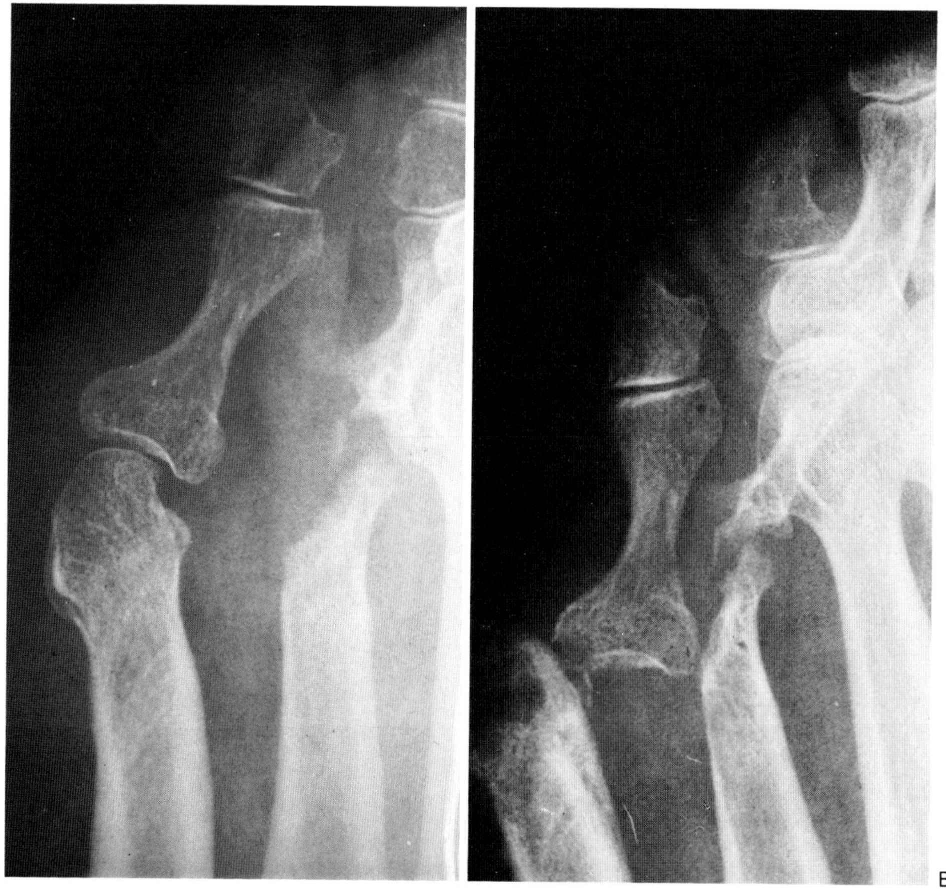

Fig. 8.51 A. and **B.** Diabetic foot. Progressive changes affect the lateral side of the foot in two films taken at a year's interval. By the time of the second film, soft tissue swelling is less but a destructive arthropathy has involved the metatarso-phalangeal joint of the little toe with dislocation. Such change was associated with the development of a penetrating ulcer.

nosis. A helpful sign in the differential diagnosis is the predominance of the involvement of the metacarpophalangeal joints of the index and middle fingers.

Calcium pyrophosphate dihydrate deposition disease (pyrophosphate arthropathy, pseudo-gout)

This disease, of unknown aetiology, is one of the major causes of chondrocalcinosis. Clinically, it may present with an acute episode of joint pain, but differs from gout in that the blood chemistry is normal and para-articular erosions do not occur. Often joint symptoms are insidious and chronic. The disorder results from the deposition of calcium pyrophosphate crystals in cartilage and synovial fluid, from where they may be aspirated and identified under polarized light. Calcification occurs in both hyaline and fibrocartilage. Although the knee is most commonly involved, the wrist, hip and shoulder joints, pubic symphysis and spine may be affected. Differentiation from other causes of chondrocalcinosis is essential.

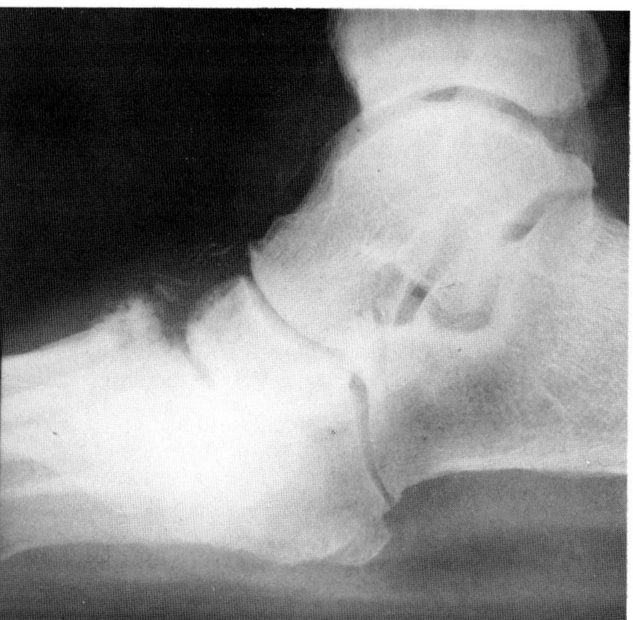

Fig. 8.52 Diabetic foot. Classical neuropathic changes are demonstrated at tarso-metatarsal joints with disorganisation of the joints, sclerosis of the subarticular bone and fragmentation.

Homocystinuria

This disorder is due to deficient activity of the enzyme cysthathionine synthetase, which converts homocysteine to cystathionin and cysteine; blood and urinary homocystine therefore increases. Two different molecular defects account for this biochemical abnormality and clinical picture. One form is vitamin dependent and responds to pharmacological doses of pyridoxine, the other is pyridoxine resistant and necessitates a perpetual low methionine diet. In the former group, treated children will have normal skeletal development. Skeletal changes include osteoporosis, scoliosis, sternal deformities, valgus deformity at the knees and hips, enlarged epiphyses and arachnodactyly. Though having many features in common with Marfan's syndrome, it differs in its autosomal recessive inheritance, mental retardation, osteoporosis, normal or reduced joint mobility and a high incidence of vascular thrombosis.

Diabetes mellitus

The deficient production of insulin does not result in bone disease. However, some complications of diabetes merit consideration. Premature degenerative change leads to increased and often widespread vascular calcification, which is particularly suggestive of diabetes below the age of 40. In males, calcification of the *vas deferens* is almost pathognomonic of the disease and may occur as early as the third decade. The diabetic foot is probably a combination of vascular, infective and neuropathic changes and affects as many as one in two chronic diabetics. In diabetes, neurotrophic change results in phalangeal resorption (Fig. 8.51), whilst a Charcot-type of neuropathic change most often affects the metatarsophalangeal, tarsometatarsal and intertarsal joints (Fig. 8.52). Overall, osteopenia is more common than the bone sclerosis associated with neuropathy, but the two processes frequently co-exist. An increased incidence of idiopathic skeletal hyperostosis is found in diabetics.

REFERENCES AND SUGGESTIONS FOR FURTHER READING

Metabolic bone disease: general

Doyle, F. H (1975) Current concepts in metabolic bone disease. In Lodge, T., Steiner, R. (eds) *Recent Advances in Radiology*, ch. 3. Edinburgh: Churchill Livingstone.

Fogelman, I., Carr, D. (1980) A comparison of bone scanning and radiology in the evaluation of patients with metabolic bone disease. *Clinical Radiology*, **31**, 321–326.

Jackson, W. P U. (1967) *Calcium Metabolism and Bone Disease*. London: Arnold.

Murray, R. O., Jacobson, H. G (1977) *The Radiology of Skeletal Disorders*, 2nd edn. Edinburgh: Churchill Livingstone.

Paterson, C. R. (1974) *Metabolic Disorders of Bone*. Oxford: Blackwell.

Pyle, S. I., Waterhouse, A. M., Greulich, W. W. (1971) *A Radiographic Standard of References for the Growing Hand and Wrist*. Chicago: Year Book Medical Publishers.

Reifenstein, E. C. Jr. (1975) Definitions, terminology and classification of metabolic bone disorders. *Clinical Orthopedics*, **9**, 30–45.

Resnick, D., Niwayama, G. (1981) *Diagnosis of Bone and Joint Disorders with Emphasis on Articular Abnormalities*. Philadelphia: W. B. Saunders.

Shapiro, R. (1962) Metabolic bone disease — a basic review. *Clinical Radiology*, **13**, 238–251.

Assessment of bone density and morphology

Dequeker, J., Johnston, C. C. Jr. (eds) (1982) *Non-invasive Bone Measurements: Methodological Problems*. Oxford, Washington D.C.: I.R.L. Press.

Exton-Smith, E. A, Millard, P. H., Payne, P. R., Wheeler, E. F. (1969) Method for measuring quantity of bone. *Lancet*, **2**, 1153–1154.

Genant, H. K. et al. (1980) Computed tomography of the musculoskeletal system. *Journal of Bone and Joint Surgery*, **62-A**, 1088–1011.

Genant, H. K., Cann, C. E. (1981) Vertebral mineral determination using quantitative computed tomography. In: DeLuca, H. F. (ed.) *et al. Osteoporosis: Recent Advances in Pathogenesis and Treatment*, pp. 37–47. Baltimore: University Park Press.

Omnell, K. A. (1957) Quantitative roentgenographic studies on changes in mineral content of bone in vivo. *Acta Radiologica* (Suppl.), **148**, 7–86.

Papworth, M. P. (1972) The physical measurement of bone mineral in humans. I. Measurement by diagnostic radiography. *Australasian Radiology*, **16**, 320–324.

Direct radiographic magnification

Doi, K., Genant, H., Rossman, K. (1975) Effect of film graininess and geometric unsharpness on image quality in fine detail skeletal radiography. *Investigative Radiology*, **10**, 35–42.

Genant, H., Doi, K., Mall, J. C (1975) Optical versus radiographic magnification for fine detail skeletal radiography. *Investigative Radiology*, **10**, 160–172.

Meema, H. E. (1973) The combined use of morphometric and microradioscopic methods in the diagnosis of metabolic bone disease. *Radiologie*, **13**, 11–16.

Xeroradiography

Roach, J. F. (1970) Xeroradiography. *Radiological Clinics of North America*, **8**, 271–275.

Vitamin D, osteomalacia and rickets

Callenbach, J. C., Sheenan, M. B., Abramson, S. J., Hall, R. T. (1981) Etiologic factors in rickets of very low-birth-weight infants. *Journal of Pediatrics*, **98**, 800–805.

Chalmers, J., Conacher, W. D. H., Gardner, D. L., Scott, P. J. (1967) Osteomalacia — a common disease in elderly women. *Journal of Bone and Joint Surgery*, **49-B**, 403–423.

Goel, K. M., *et al.* (1976) Florid and subclinical rickets among immigrant children in Glasgow. *Lancet*, **1**, 1141–1145.

Pitt, M. J., Haussler, M. R. (1977) Vitamin D: Biochemistry and clinical applications. *Skeletal Radiology*, **1**, 191–208.

Steinbach, H. L., Noetzli, M. (1964) Roentgen appearance of the skeleton in osteomalacia and rickets. *American Journal of Roentgenology*, **91**, 955–972.

Swischuk, L. E., Hayden, C. K. Jr. (1979) Rickets: A roentgenographic scheme for diagnosis. *Pediatric Radiology*, **8**, 203–208.

Yendt, E. R. (1970) Vitamin D. Part II in International encyclopaedia of pharmacology and therapeutics. Section 51, Vol. 1: Ramussen, H. (ed.) *Parathyroid Hormone, Thyrocalcitonin and Related Drugs*, pp. 139–195. Oxford: Pergamon.

Hypophosphatasia

Kozlowski, K. *et al.* (1976) Hypophosphatasia. Review of 25 cases. *Pediatric Radiology*, **5**, 103–117.

Familial hyperphosphatasaemia

Caffey, J. (1972) Familial hyperphosphatasaemia with ateliosis and hypermetabolism of growing membranous bone. *Bulletin of the Hospital for Joint Diseases*, **33**, 81–110.

Scurvy

McCann, P. (1962) The incidence and value of radiological signs in scurvy. *British Journal of Radiology*, **35**, 683–686.

Idiopathic hypercalcaemia of infancy

Dupont, B. (1970) Idiopathic hypercalcaemia of infancy. The elfin face syndrome. *Danish Medical Bulletin*, **17**, 33–46.

Vitamin A poisoning

Caffey, J. (1951) Chronic poisoning due to excess of vitamin A. *American Journal of Roentgenology*, **65**, 12–26.

Osteoporosis

Gordon, G. S., Vaughan, C. (1976) *Clinical Management of the Osteoporoses*. Aylesbury: H. M. & M. Publishers.

Houang, M. T. D., Brenton, D. P., Renton, P., Shaw, D. G. (1978) Idiopathic juvenile osteoporosis. *Skeletal Radiology*, **3**, 17–23.

Pogrund, H. *et al.* (1981) Determination of osteoporosis in patients with fractured femoral neck using the Singh index. *Clinical Orthopedics*, **156**, 189–195.

Singh, M., Riggs, B. L., Beabout, J. W., Jowsey, J. (1972) Femoral trabecular-pattern index for evaluation of spinal osteoporosis. *Annals of Internal Medicine*, 77, 63–67.

Acromegaly

Lang, E. K., Bessler, W. T. (1961) Roentgenologic features of acromegaly. *American Journal of Roentgenology*, **86**, 321–328.

Kho, K. M., Wright, A. D., Doyle, F. H. (1970) Heel pad thickness in acromegaly. *British Journal of Radiology*, **43**, 119–125.

Thyroid

Meema, H. E., Schatz, D. L. (1970) Simple radiologic demonstration of cortical bone loss in thyrotoxicosis. *Radiology*, **97**, 9–15.

Hyperparathyroidism

Genant, H. K. *et al.* (1973) Primary hyperparathyroidism. *Radiology*, **109**, 513–524.

Jensen, P. S., Kliger, A. S. (1977) Early radiographic manifestations of secondary hyperparathyroidism associated with renal disease. *Radiology*, **125**, 645–652.

Pyrah, L. N., Hodgkinson, A., Anderson, C. K. (1966) Primary hyperparathyroidism. *British Journal of Surgery*, **53**, 245–316.

Uraemic osteodystrophy

Shapiro, R. (1972) Radiologic aspects of renal osteodystrophy. *Radiologic Clinics of North America*, **10**, 557–568.

Mehls, O. *et al.* (1973) Roentgenological signs in the skeleton of uremic children. *Pediatric Radiology*, **1**, 183–190.

Resnick, D. (1978) Abnormalities of bone and soft tissue following renal transplantation. *Seminars in Roentgenology*, **13**, 329–340.

Oxalosis

Brancaccio, D. *et al.* (1981) Bone changes in end-stage oxalosis. *American Journal of Roentgenology*, **139**, 935–939.

Hypoparathyroidism and pseudo-hypoparathyroidism

Taybi, H., Keele, D. (1962) Hypoparathyroidism: a review of the literature and report of two cases. *American Journal of Roentgenology*, **88**, 432–442.

Steinbach, H. L., Young, D. A. (1966) The roentgen appearances of pseudohypoparathyroidism and pseudo-pseudohypoparathyroidism. *American Journal of Roentgenology*, **97**, 49–66.

Adrenal hypercorticism

Murray, R. O. (1961) Steroids and the skeleton. *Radiology*, **77**, 729–743.

Toxic effects on bone

Betts, P. R., Watson, S. M., Astley, R. (1973) A suggested role of radiology in lead poisoning. *Annales de Radiologie*, **16**, 183–187.

Harris, D. K., Adams, W. G. F. (1967) Acro-osteolysis occurring in polymerization of vinyl chloride. *British Medical Journal*, **3**, 712–714.

Kilmar, S. P., Kemp Harper, R. A. (1963) Fluorosis in Aden. *British Journal of Radiology*, **36**, 497–502.

Miscellaneous

Ward, P. R., Engelbrecht, P. J. (1963) Alkaptonuria and ochronosis. *Clinical Radiology*, **14**, 170–174.

Ross, P., Wood. B. (1970) Osteoarthropathy in idiopathic hemochromatosis. *American Journal of Roentgenology*, **109**, 575–580.

Grunebaum, M., Horodinceanu, C., Steinherz, R. (1980) The radiographic manifestations of bone changes in copper deficiency. *Pediatric Radiology*, **9**, 101–104.

Resnick, D., Niwayama, G., Goergen, T. G., *et al.* (1977) Clinical, radiographic and pathologic abnormalities in calcium pyrophosphate dihydrate deposition disease (CPPD): Pseudogout. *Radiology*, **122**, 1–16.

Rosenor, V. M., Mitchell, R. C. (1959) Skeletal changes in Wilson's disease (hepatolenticular degeneration). *British Journal of Radiology*, **32**, 805–809.

Brenton, D. F., *et al.* (1972) Homocystinuria and Marfan's syndrome. *Journal of Bone and Joint Surgery*, **54-B**, 277–298.

Thomas, P. S. P., Carson, N. A. J. (1978) Homocystinuria. The evolution of skeletal changes in relation to treatment. *Annales de Radiologie*, **21**, 95–104.

Kellett, M. A. (1967) The radiologic features of diabetes mellitus. *Radiological Clinics of North America*, 5, 239–248.

Geoffroy, J., Hoeffel, J. C., Pointel, J. P., *et al.* (1979) The feet in diabetes: Roentgenographic observation in 1501 cases. *Diagnostic Imaging*, **48**, 286–293.

CHAPTER 9

SKELETAL TRAUMA — GENERAL CONSIDERATIONS

The diagnosis of traumatic lesions of the skeleton forms a major portion of the work of most radiological departments being, in many cases, complementary to frank clinical evidence of a fracture. However, it should be appreciated that on occasion radiological changes of an unusual nature may be traumatic in origin. Some skill then may be required in their differentiation from such conditions as infections and neoplasms. Since most traumatic lesions show a strong tendency to spontaneous healing, recognition of a purely traumatic origin may be of considerable value in management and prognosis, in the avoidance of unnecessary biopsy and in reassurance of the patient. The radiologist should be prepared, when necessary, to support his radiological opinion by confirmatory clinical examination and it should be remembered that failure to observe and record even an unimportant fracture may result in legal proceedings.

The patient with a suspected skeletal injury must be investigated methodically. Two projections are the minimal radiographic requirement, since one may fail to demonstrate a fracture (Fig. 9.1). Standard positioning permits the student to develop a confident knowledge of normal radiological appearances, whilst sometimes supplementary projections and techniques may be of value. Radiographs of the normal counterpart of the opposite side of the body provide an eminently satisfactory control; such examinations are never to be regarded as routine, and are only obtained to resolve a problem in paediatric trauma, e.g. epiphyseal displacement at the elbow. Certain undisplaced fractures may be invisible immediately after injury and only subsequent bone resorption along their margins or the development of callus formation after an interval of 10–20 days may permit the diagnosis to be established (Fig. 9.2). The use of fluoroscopy for the routine examination and reduction of fractures is no longer justified.

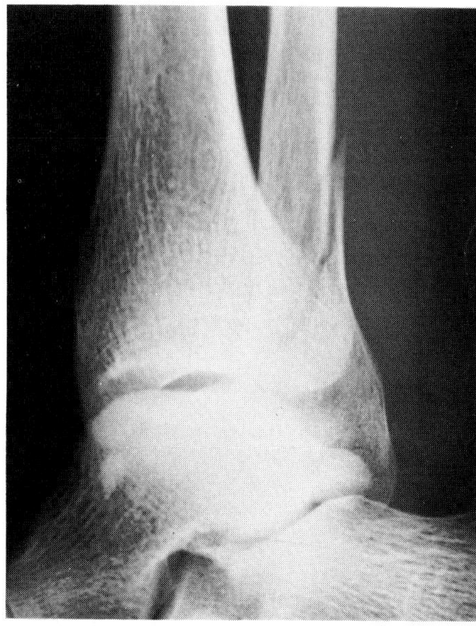

Fig. 9.1 One view alone is not enough in the examination of fractures. This fibular fracture was visible only in the oblique projection. In this area even two views may be inadequate.

GENERAL PRINCIPLES

Radiological examination permits assessment of:

1. **Presence of a fracture,** and whether this has occurred through normal or pathological bone. Variation from normal anatomical contours, a break in cortical continuity, disturbance of normal joint relationships or the presence of a line of increased density from overriding bone fragments, each may provide the first clue to diagnosis.
2. **Type and position of fracture,** showing whether it is simple or comminuted, whether a dislocation or subluxation is also present, or, in children, whether displacement of an epiphysis has occurred (Fig. 9.3). It is often possible to deduce the mechanical forces involved in its production. The examination is repeated as a routine procedure after manipulative or open reduction to check the degree of restoration of anatomical position.

Flake fractures at the attachments of tendons and ligaments may indicate considerable soft-tissue damage. Differentiation must be made from accessory ossicles, which always have clearly defined, smooth cortical margins.

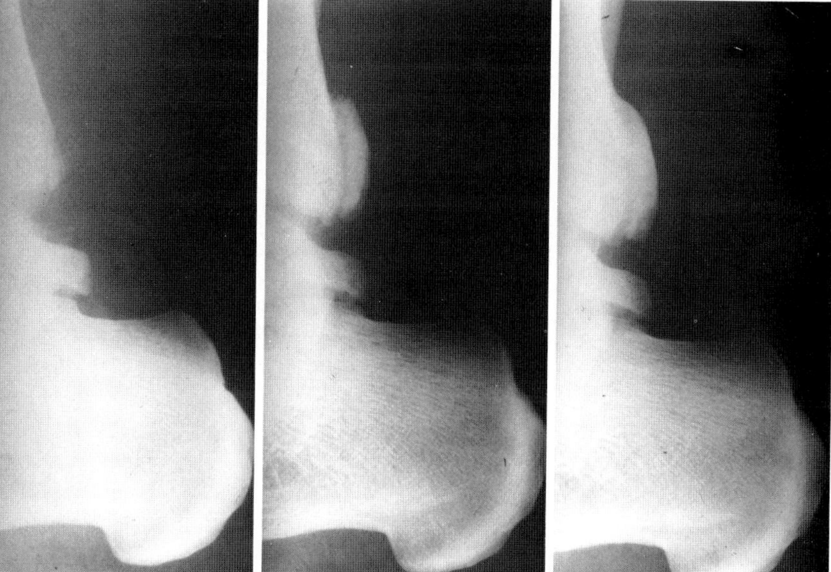

Fig. 9.2 Post-traumatic hyperostosis. A marginal cortical fracture of the posterior malleolus is shown on serial radiographs to form a plaque of periosteal new bone which then becomes organized. Such periosteal reaction may occur in the absence of fracture due to avulsion of the posterior tibio-fibular ligament.

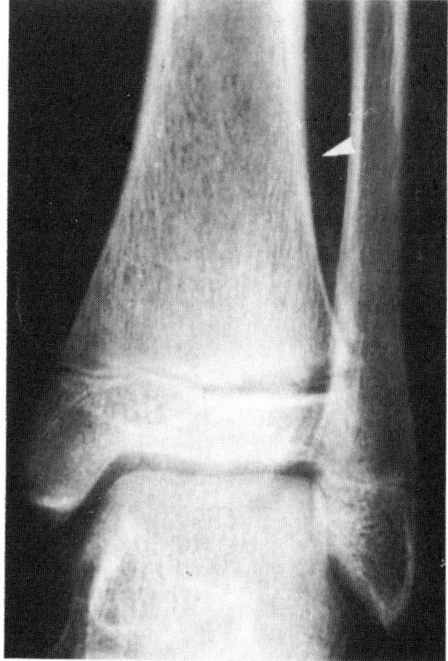

Fig. 9.3 Mild traumatic separation of the distal tibial epiphysis caused by adduction strain a few days before. Periosteal reaction is visible on the lateral side of the distal end of the tibia (arrow).

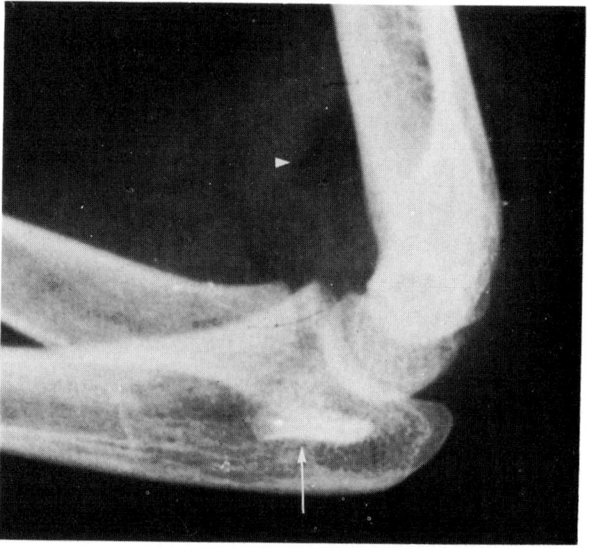

Fig. 9.4 Separation of the epiphysis for the head of the radius (↑). An effusion within the intact joint capsule has displaced the lucent fat pads which normally lie in close apposition to the humerus (▶).

3. **Associated soft-tissue shadows.** Provided the joint capsule remains intact, its distension by an *effusion* may be evident. Effusions of the elbow joint displace the pads of fat lying on the anterior and posterior aspects of the capsule so that they become evident as displaced translucent areas (Fig. 9.4). In such cases, particular care should be taken before a fracture is excluded. The presence of *free fat within a synovial compartment* is presumptive evidence of bone injury and may be observed in the shoulder and knee when a fluid level results from fat floating on top of synovial fluid. This feature is demonstrated only when the exposure is made with a horizontal beam (Fig. 9.5). Haemorrhage from bone injuries assumes importance with fractures of the dorsal spine, when the resulting *haematomata* may resemble paravertebral abscesses (Fig. 9.6). The introduction of air from the atmosphere into the soft tissues may result from compound fractures or from puncture of the lungs by a rib fracture, producing the linear translucencies of *surgical emphysema*.

The physiological *vacuum phenomenon* — a translucency due to gas within a joint — may be evident in radiographs of a joint under stress, as in the shoulders of infants suspended by the arms. It is produced often in the knee when films are obtained with abduction or adduction

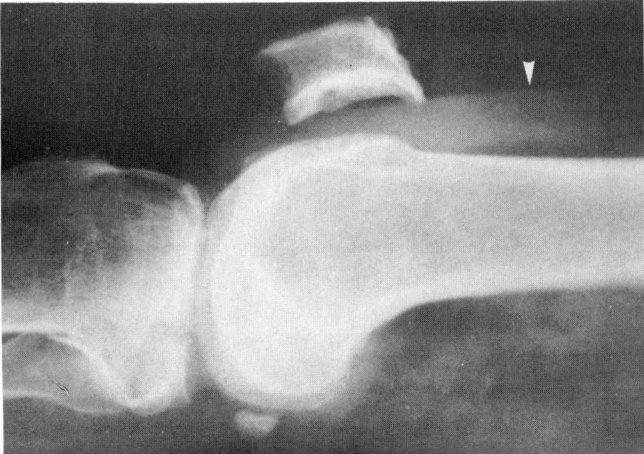

Fig. 9.5 Fat-fluid level. This depression fracture of the posterior portion of the lateral tibial condyle was caused by a fall from a height. The film was obtained with the patient supine, using a horizontal beam. The fluid level (arrow) shown in the distended capsule is due to the presence of free fat within the joint and provides presumptive evidence of a bone injury.

stress. This phenomenon is not observed when an intra-articular effusion is present. Similar translucencies may be visible in degenerate intervertebral discs. They appear to have no special pathological significance.

4. **Age and healing of fractures.** The repair of a fracture passes through the following stages:

a. A *haematoma* forms between the bone ends and, especially in children, may elevate the adjacent periosteum.

b. *Granulation tissue* is formed on the fracture surfaces. With absorption of the haematoma this tissue provides the first continuity between the fragments.

c. *Callus* (essentially immature osteoid tissue) is formed on both the periosteal and endosteal surfaces of the bone. It acts as a natural splint which first becomes calcified and then undergoes osseous modification, such woven bone being resorbed as the original fracture surfaces develop firm bony union.

The corresponding radiological signs in a recent fracture are sharply-defined margins without bone resorption plus soft-tissue swelling due to oedema and haemorrhage. As repair progresses, after 10–14 days, definition of the fracture line becomes less precise, as a result of localized bone resorption and hyperaemia associated with the

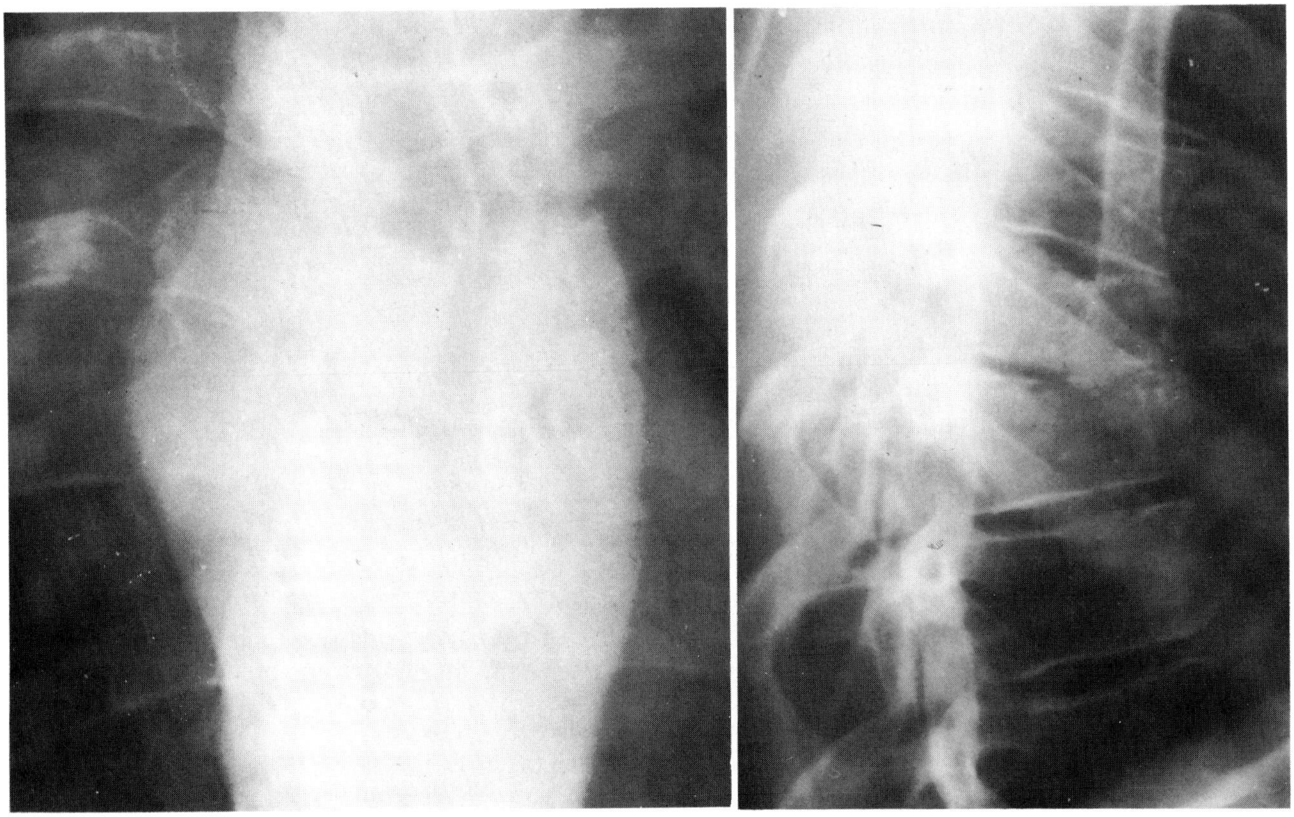

A B

Fig. 9.6 A. and **B**. Compression fractures of the vertebral bodies of T7, 8 and 9 with large bilateral haematomata. The latter took many months to absorb, still being visible after the fractures had consolidated.

formation of granulation tissue. Thus, when no displacement of the fragments has occurred, the fracture is easier to identify several days after the injury. By this time the associated soft tissue swelling has regressed and after another two or three weeks it should have resolved completely. During this further stage, formation of periosteal and endosteal callus becomes visible, first as irregular mottled calcification around the fracture, then increasing in density and quantity. A characteristic bony texture ultimately develops. This reparative bone tissue then undergoes organization with the peripheral margins, becoming smooth and clearly defined. In some regions such as the skull and the neck of the femur, where periosteal function is less active, callus formation may not be evident. The development of a continuous trabecular pattern across the fracture line provides the final radiological criterion of sound union (Fig. 9.7).

In a healthy adult, the whole process from injury to consolidation takes about four months for a single fracture of a large tubular bone such as the femur — longer in the case of multiple fractures (Fig. 9.8). The healing process is functionally adequate in about two months for a bone like the humerus, in which prolonged protection from weight-bearing is not required. Oblique fractures tend to heal more quickly than transverse fractures, since they present greater areas for repair. Healing is slower in the elderly and quicker in children. Some degree of disuse osteoporosis almost always accompanies immobilization and is likely to be especially prominent in the bones distal to a fracture in a limb. This osteoporosis is due to hyperaemia and a physiological impairment of osteoblastic function in the absence of active use. Even in young adults, such loss of density is most prominent in former metaphyseal areas, where an increase of vascular supply may persist for many years after epiphyseal fusion (Fig. 9.9).

The presence of abundant callus which is beginning to organize is usually found to coincide with clinical union; the final process of consolidation by bone only develops later. Provided that the position of the bone ends has remained constant in serial films, particularly if accompanied by a surrounding sheath of organizing callus, it is usually justifiable to permit a return to limited active use, even though the original fracture remains visible. Union must, however, be regarded as inadequate when clinical examination reveals any suggestion of movement at the fracture site. Excessive callus formation may be observed with minimal but persistent movement at the fracture site due to incomplete immobilization in a plaster cast which has become loose as soft tissue swelling has regressed. A similar phenomenon has been observed in patients with persistent

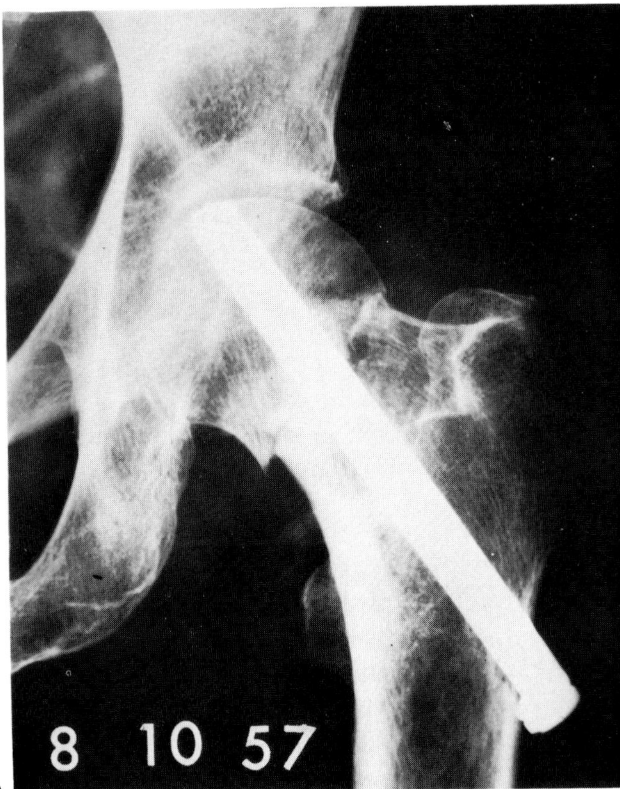

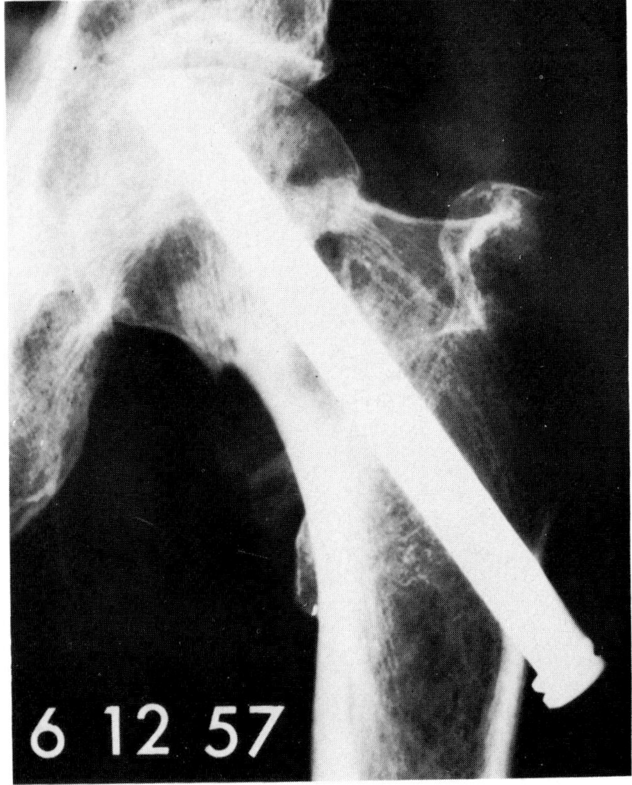

Fig. 9.7 Development of bone union. **A.** This transcervical fracture of the femoral neck was immobilized in good position with a Smith-Petersen nail. **B.** 2 months later, trabeculation crossing the fracture line constituted radiological evidence of union. The periosteum in this intracapsular region is bound down by Sharpey's fibres, so that callus formation is usually absent or minimal.

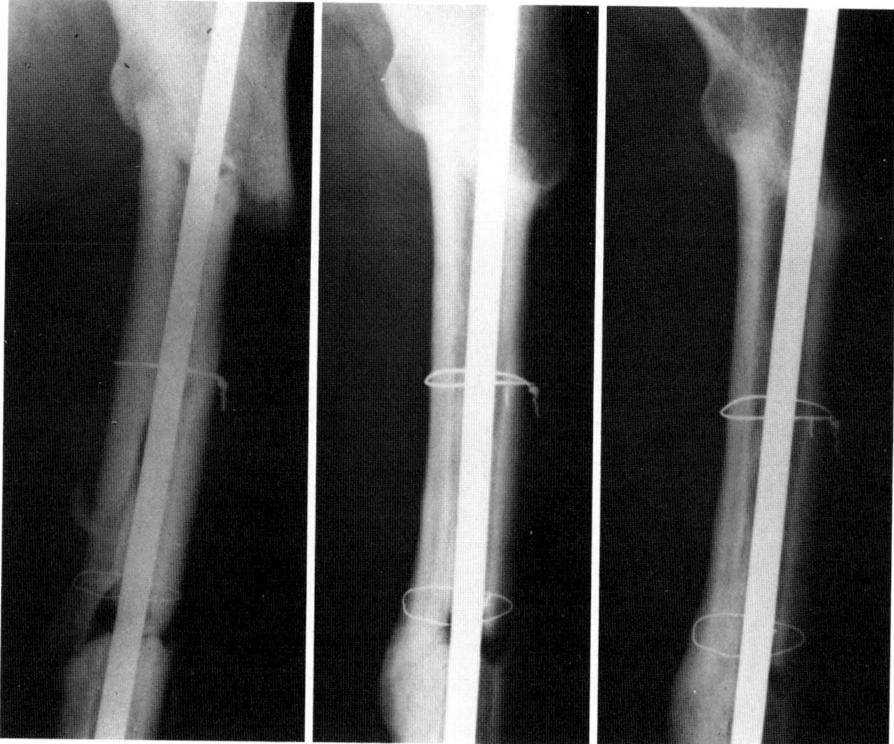

Fig. 9.8

Fig. 9.8 Development of bone union. These comminuted fractures in a 24-year-old male were immobilized with a Kuntschner nail. A protective caliper was required for a further 15 months.

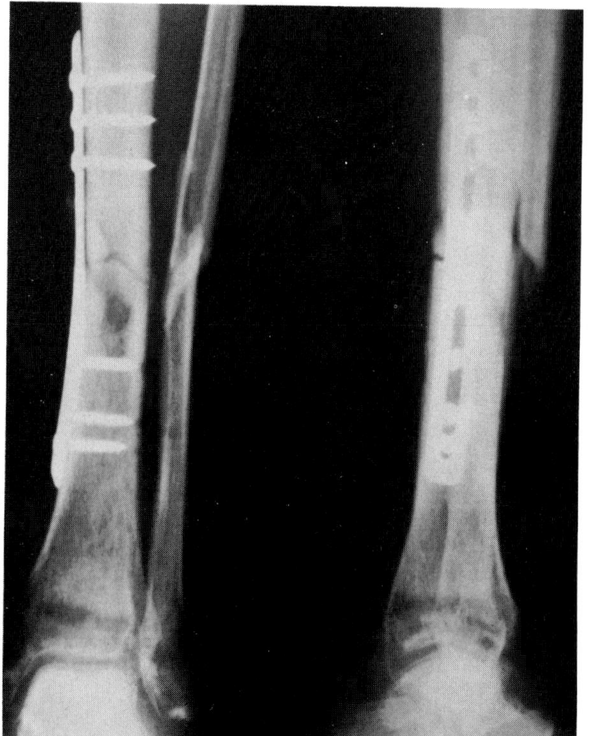

Fig. 9.9

Fig. 9.9 Malunion after open reduction. This comminuted fracture of the tibia was immobilized in a plaster which obscured all bony points of reference. The fracture united with 30 degrees external rotation of the distal fragments. This could have been deduced from the anteroposterior film taken through plaster, which showed the interval between the proximal fragments of the tibia and fibula to be much greater than that between the distal fragments. The lateral view also showed posterior displacement of the distal fragment of the fibula. Note the use of a slotted plate to allow satisfactory impaction of the fracture; round holed plates may be responsible for some residual distraction and delay in healing. Disuse atrophy is particularly evident in former metaphyseal areas, which are still highly vascular in a young adult.

tremor in Parkinson's disease. Similarly, hyperplastic callus commonly occurs around fractures in osteogenesis imperfecta.

COMPLICATIONS OF FRACTURE

1. **Delayed union** is usually due to some form of interference with the healing process. This may be purely *mechanical* and associated with distraction of the fracture fragments, possibly by the application of excessive traction, or inadequate internal fixation. Healing tends to be slower in the *elderly* owing to physiological diminution in osteoblastic activity. Such activity is also impaired by *vitamin C deficiency* so that insufficient osteoid tissue is formed. In

vitamin D deficiency, by contrast, calcification of the formed osteoid tissue is incomplete. The presence of *infection* delays union. Most, but not all, *pathological* fractures are slow to unite. Finally, union is sometimes inexplicably delayed despite good reduction and immobilization.

2. **Non-union** commonly results from *incomplete immobilization*. It may also be due to *interposition of soft tissue*. Bone absorption round the fracture margins is followed by their becoming sclerosed and irregular with an obvious intervening translucency. Surrounding callus may form and organize, but the fracture line is seen to persist through this natural splint. Once this characteristic radiological appearance has developed, the state of non-union may be regarded as being established. Fractures of the tibia and scaphoid are particularly subject to this complication (Fig. 9.10). *Infection* also inhibits union, usually with the development of osteomyelitis. Much irregular bone destruction and a sclerotic reaction may develop and be accompanied by the formation of one or more sequestra.

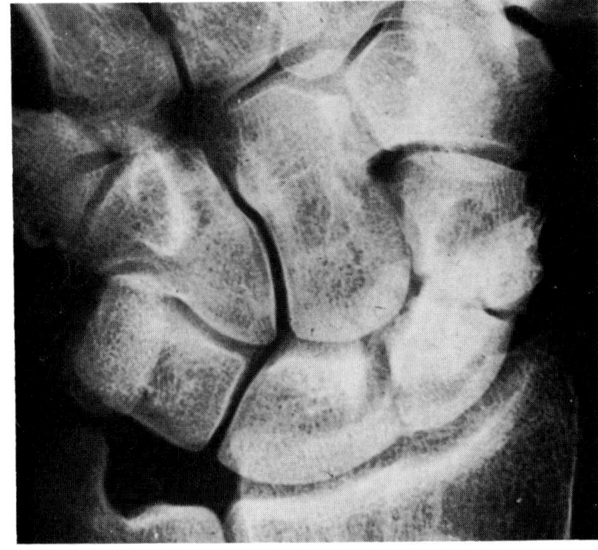

Fig. 9.10 Non-union. The sclerosed margins of this fracture of the waist of the scaphoid indicate that it will never unite spontaneously. Without early and adequate immobilization, this complication is relatively common, particularly when significant damage is sustained by the intercarpal ligaments. Deformity in the articular surface predisposes towards subsequent degenerative joint disease. Cystic degeneration is present in the distal portion of the bone.

3. **Malunion,** due to incomplete reduction, results in residual deformity (Fig. 9.9). In adults, when the plane of a weight-bearing joint such as the ankle is altered, the resultant abnormal stresses predispose to the development of premature degenerative joint disease (Fig. 9.11). Similar degenerative change is likely to occur when a step deformity in an articular surface cannot be corrected.

4. **Avascular necrosis.** Deprivation of blood supply to a segment of bone, as with any other tissue, causes cell death. The most common cause is an injury, resulting in *post-traumatic necrosis*. Less frequent causes, such as physical agents and infarction in generalized disorders, are discussed later in this chapter as *systemic necrosis*.

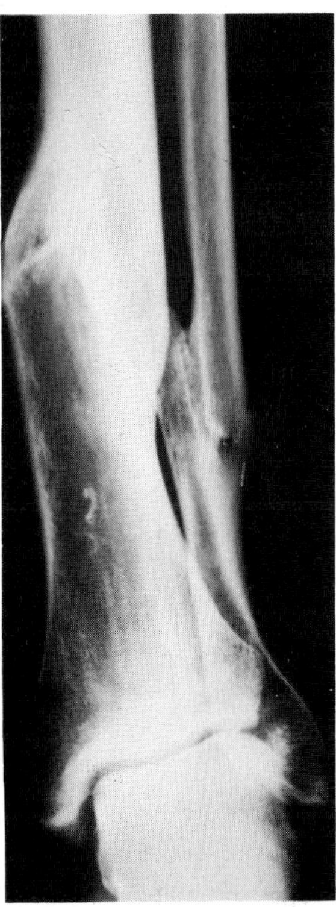

Fig. 9.11 Malunion. Although these fractures of the tibia and fibula have united soundly, the residual valgus tilt of the ankle provides an unwelcome disability and makes this joint particularly susceptible to premature degenerative change.

Because of the local vascular anatomy avascular necrosis is liable to affect especially

1. the head of the femur in subcapital fractures of the femoral neck;
2. the proximal pole of the scaphoid and
3. the body of the talus.

The initial stages of avascular necrosis cause no radiological abnormality, but in due course the dead, weakened structure is liable to collapse and crumble. Much controversy has been aroused by the appearance of an apparent fairly uniform increase of density in the affected bone fragment. This density usually develops after an interval from the time of injury varying from two months in children to two years or even longer in elderly adults. To some degree such increase may be relative, owing to the osteoporosis of disuse which develops in surrounding bones. True increase of density, however, for long regarded as the primary manifestation of bone necrosis, now is recognized to be due to revascularization and repair.

Histological studies of femoral heads removed after subcapital fractures of the femoral neck, prior to insertion of a prosthesis, have been most informative. In the early stages of cell death the bone structure appears radiologically normal and the development of increased density corresponds to the process of revascularization; a thin layer of calcifying osteoid tissue is laid down on the scaffolding provided by the necrotic trabeculae (Fig. 9.12). In these elderly individuals, translucent cystic areas correspond to

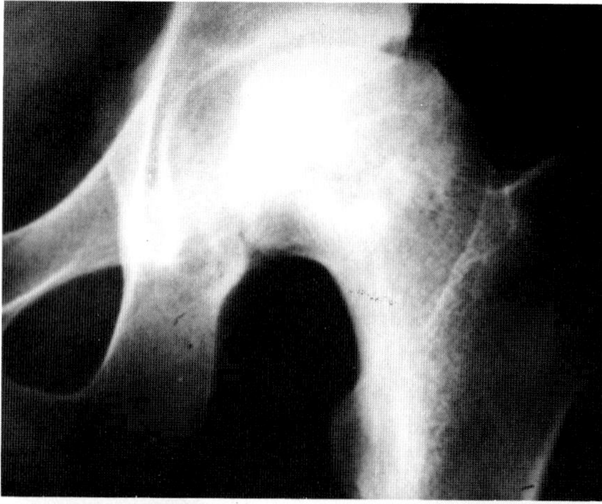

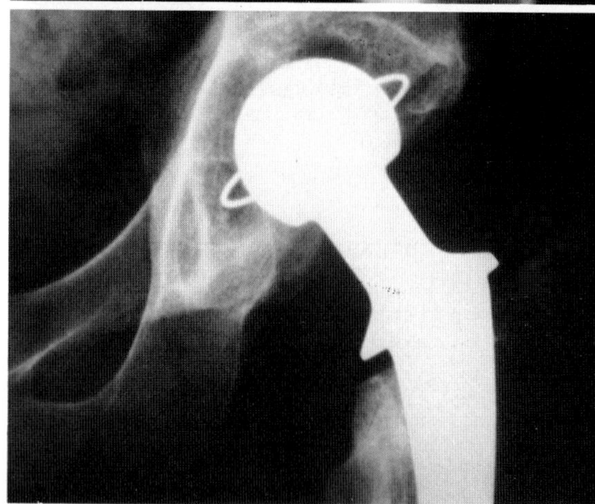

Fig. 9.12 Avascular necrosis following renal transplantation. The changes of avascular necrosis in the femoral head consist of central lucency with surrounding sclerosis; secondary degenerative joint disease is already apparent. The lower film shows the appearance following arthroplasty.

zones of absorption of fragmented trabeculae by revascularizing tissues. The degree of repair is often insufficient to prevent the crumbling and collapse which is so often a late sequel of ischaemic necrosis. Nevertheless it does appear, especially in younger patients with adequate protection, that this process can be successful and permit reconstruction of the dead trabeculae and replacement with normal viable bone.

On occasion, the radiological changes of avascular necrosis may be greatly delayed, depending on the time taken for revascularizing tissue to invade the necrotic structure. Although the initial radiograph after an injury in such cases may have failed to demonstrate a fracture, subsequent developments indicate strongly that traumatic disturbance of the blood supply had in fact occurred.

5. **Traumatic subperiosteal ossification** may develop in an acute form after injury to a bone which need not necessarily be sufficiently severe to cause a fracture. It is due to ossification within a subperiosteal haematoma. The callus and new bone are derived from the stripped periosteal cells. Initially a mass of diffuse and irregular density develops adjacent to, but usually separate from, the site of injury. The soft tissues on the anterior aspect of the femur are commonly affected in this way after a direct blow. The new bone eventually organizes and tends to leave a permanent flat periosteal elevation resembling a sessile exostosis (Figs. 9.2 and 9.13). Confusion with an osteosarcoma should not arise where an adequate history is available. Serial studies show the ossification in a haematoma in soft tissues to develop far more quickly than a neoplasm. Ultimately, of course, these lesions either regress completely or leave a focus of residual ossification. Ossification of the same type or calcification may follow avulsion of ligamentous attachments — as for example at the superior pole of the patella and the medial collateral ligament of the knee, the latter being known as the *Pellegrini–Stieda lesion* (Fig. 9.14). A comparable condition may also arise as a result of repeated low-grade trauma, the most typical example being the formation of a 'rider's bone' in the adductor muscles of the thigh.

Such lesions have been described as *myositis ossificans* — a misnomer.

6. **Sudeck's atrophy** (painful post-traumatic osteoporosis). A relatively rare complication of traumatic lesions of the extremities is the development of a particularly severe form of disuse osteoporosis known as *Sudeck's atrophy*. It is confined almost entirely to the bony structures distal to the point of injury. These bones develop a patchy osteoporotic mottling, often to an extreme degree, with cortical thinning, but with remarkable clarity of the articular margins (Fig. 9.15). The condition may follow relatively trivial trauma, possibly even without bone damage. It differs from an ordinary severe disuse osteoporosis only by the clinical presence of swelling of the soft tissue, smooth, rather shiny skin and severe pain and immobility. Its aetiology remains obscure.

During recent years attention has been drawn, mainly by French authors, to the entity of *transient osteoporosis*, which is believed to be a type of Sudeck's atrophy, but in which a frank history of trauma is exceptional. The condition mainly affects the hip or the knee and causes severe pain and disability. Subarticular demineralization is the usual presenting radiological abnormality but involvement of a larger area, for example, of a femoral condyle, may simulate a lesion such as a giant-cell tumour. Bone scanning shows localized increased uptake. Biopsy reveals

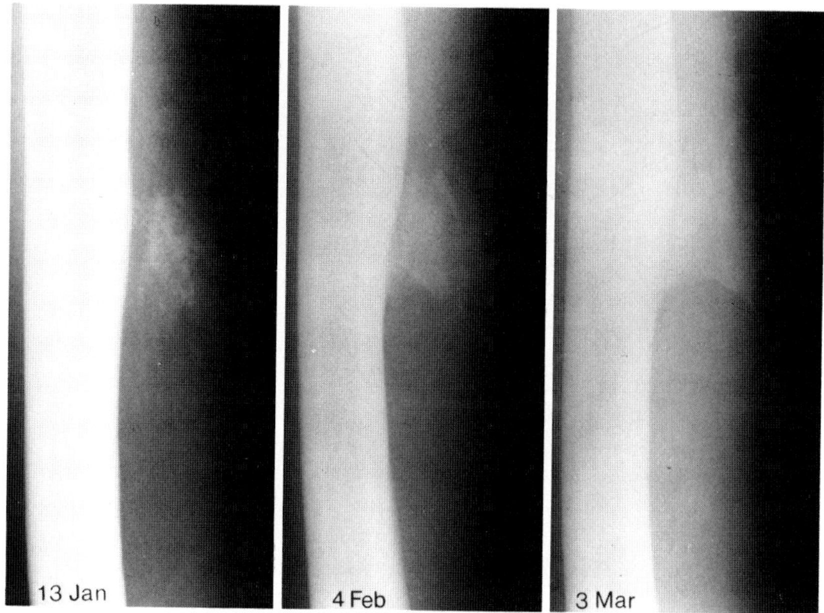

Fig. 9.13 Ossifying haematoma. The ossification in the soft tissues of the arm in this young adult followed a blow during a football match. Serial films show the soft tissue bone is maturing and becoming attached to the underlying cortex, thereby resembling an exostosis. A malignant bone-forming tumour would not exhibit such benign characteristics and, indeed, might be expected to erode the underlying bone.

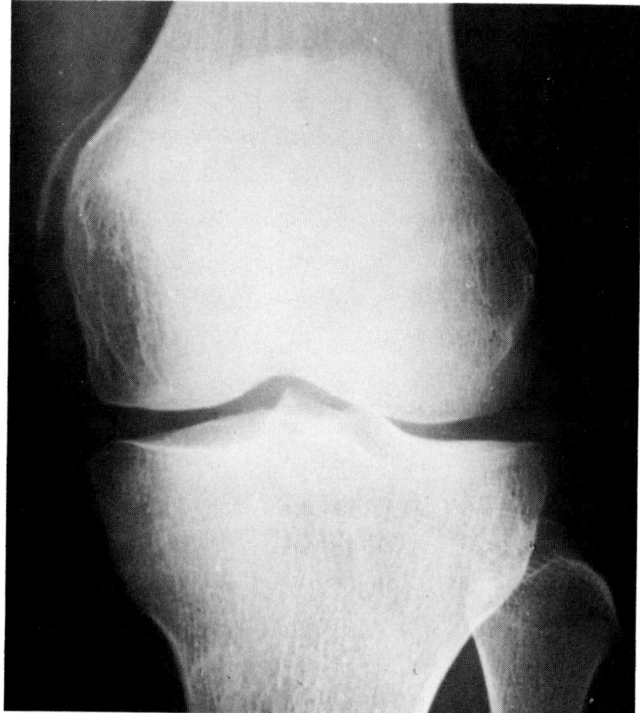

Fig. 9.14 Pellegrini–Stieda lesion. Post-traumatic calcification is shown in relation to the medial femoral condyle following a tear of the medial collateral ligament.

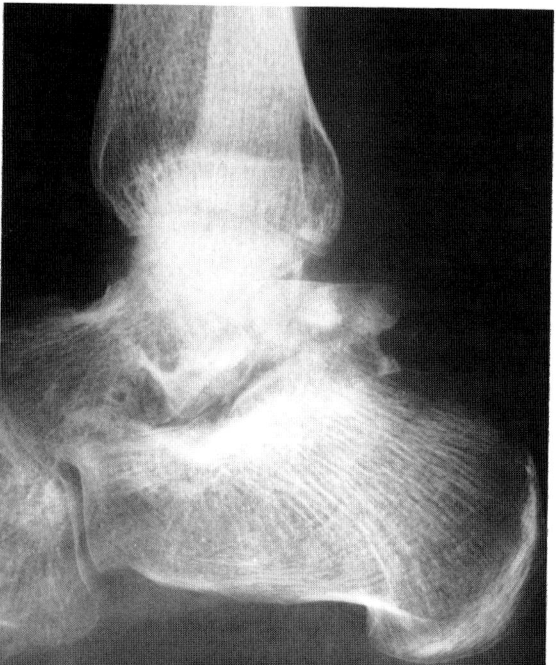

Fig. 9.15 Sudeck's atrophy. Loss of bone density affects mainly the cancellous bone in the subarticular regions of the ankle and hind foot. These appearances are non-specific and it is only the association with severe painful symptoms that merits the name of Sudeck's atrophy. Such cases form part of the reflex sympathetic dystrophy syndrome.

only osteoporosis. Symptoms resolve spontaneously in four to eight months with restoration of a normal radiological appearance.

7. **Traumatic arterio-venous pseudo-aneurysms** may develop after vascular injuries, often in association with fractures. The aneurysms form in the soft tissue intervening between an artery and a vein and, by pressure erosion, produce large osseous defects with smooth, clearly defined and slightly sclerosed margins (Fig. 9.16). A bruit may be detected clinically and should lead to radiological confirmation by arteriography. The development of these lesions, which are uncommon, is analogous to the pressure erosion of the anterior aspects of the lower thoracic vertebrae which sometimes result from direct contact with a pulsating aortic aneurysm.

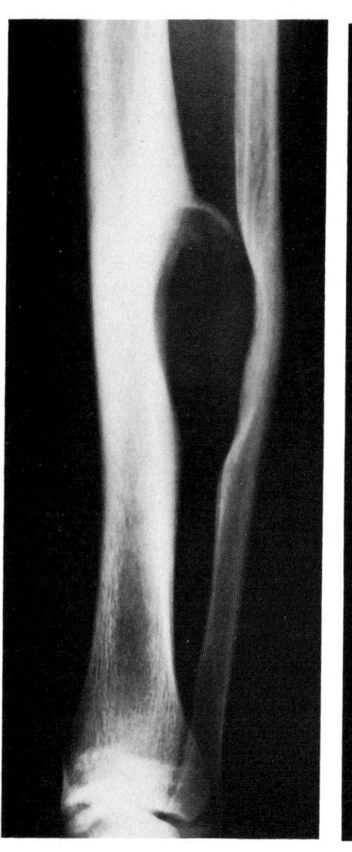

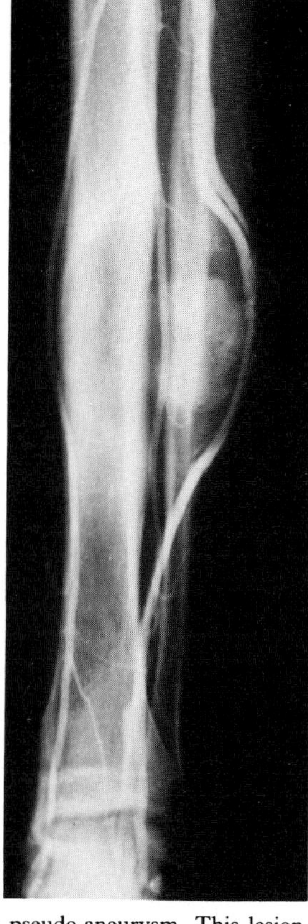

Fig. 9.16 Post-traumatic arterio-venous pseudo-aneurysm. This lesion was found a few years after a stab injury. Slow growth of the aneurysm has deformed the tibia and fibula. The margins of the bony destruction are smooth and corticated. Arteriography confirms the diagnosis, showing early venous filling.

INTERNAL FIXATION OF FRACTURES

Open reduction and immobilization of fractures is indicated:

1. when satisfactory position cannot be achieved by manipulation;
2. when good position after manipulation cannot be maintained;
3. when the fracture is of a type in which union is slow and
4. when established non-union has taken place.

Autogenous bone grafts are usually taken from the iliac crest, from a rib, or from the tibia. They may be cut into a specific shape for either onlay or inlay application or be broken up into bone chips. Only the peripheral cells of the graft survive transplantation. The remainder become necrotic, but provide a scaffold for the formation of new bone in the healing process. Fracture of the weakened donor site is not unknown, especially in the tibia. In some cases specially prepared exogenous grafts derived from a bone bank or from animals are used with varying success.

Metallic implants have been employed successfully for many years, usually permitting early active movement with a consequent reduction in the time of healing and restoration of normal function. Ideally, such implants must be free from tissue reaction, corrosion and mechanical failure. Fractures vary greatly in type and bones in their size, texture and strength. An impressive array of devices for internal fixation is available; these can be classified roughly into:

a. screws, of differing types for either engaging cortical bone or holding firm in cancellous bone;
b. plates and screws for bridging fractures. Blade plates may be employed in fractures close to joints;
c. intramedullary nails and screws, with features to prevent axial rotation;
d. circlage wires, usually of metal, are sometimes employed in the accurate alignment of spiral fractures, e.g. in the tibia.

Suitable metals employed for implants are:

1. certain stainless steels,
2. alloys of chromium, cobalt and molybdenum (e.g. Vitallium),
3. Titanium

Displaced subcapital fractures of the femoral neck in the elderly are treated by excision of the femoral head and replacement by metallic prostheses of various types (Fig. 9.12). The prolonged periods of recumbency required by conservative treatment in the past are no longer necessary.

The introduction of high density polythene and other materials has enabled effective replacement of the acetabulum as well as the femoral head in suitable patients. In fractures of long tubular bones intramedullary nails are frequently employed for internal fixation. In the development of metal implant techniques it has been necessary to overcome the following disadvantages.

1. **Electrolytic destruction.** Although now of decided historical interest only, the use of metals such as steel and bronze produced marked electrolytic corrosion of the implant and destruction of adjacent bone, to such a degree that a bone tumour or infection might be suspected. Research in biomedical engineering has so advanced the quality of the materials now used that the incidence of disruption or major corrosion has been greatly reduced.

2. **Inadequate immobilization.** The implant must have the physical strength for its intended purpose and be designed so that it will stay in position. Plating of femoral fractures has been replaced largely by the use of intramedullary nails (Fig. 9.8). Delayed union with minimal movement round a fracture usually causes resorption of bone around the whole of the implant, with some reactive marginal sclerosis. This sometimes happens with pin fixation of a femoral neck fracture. The pin then becomes loose and tends to extrude.

3. **Residual distraction** of a fracture of a long bone tends to delay healing and is liable to occur with the use of round-holed plates. Slotted plates permit adequate fixation in the long axis and allow the fracture surfaces to impact firmly together. This complication is less common with intramedullary nailing, but may still occur (Fig. 9.17).

4. **Infection** must be avoided by scrupulous aseptic technique. Infection should be suspected by the radiologist when bone resorption is visible round an implant, especially if this is localized. Infections associated with compound fractures must be controlled by antibiotic therapy before the insertion of an implant is considered. Radionuclide scans are helpful at an early stage, again if increased uptake is localized or if change is observed on serial scans. The use of gallium in addition to technetium radionuclide scans has given promising results.

TRAUMATIC LESIONS OF THE SKELETON IN CHILDREN

Fractures in children differ from those of adults because children are subject to different types of trauma and because their skeletons are in a phase of active growth.

Fractures of the lower arm and forearm are much more common than in adults. Together they account for nearly half the total of fractures in children. Another fifth of chil-

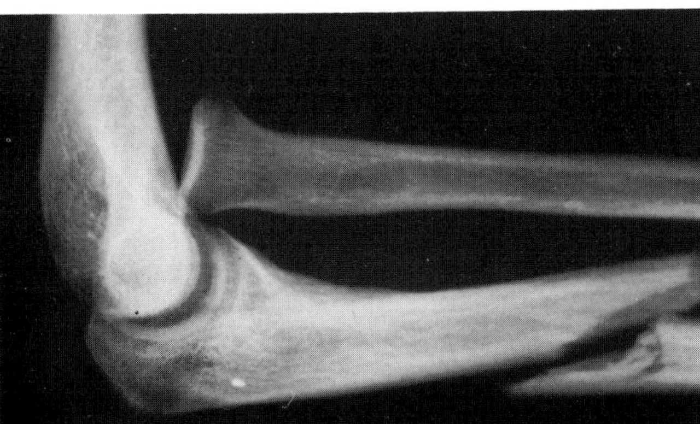

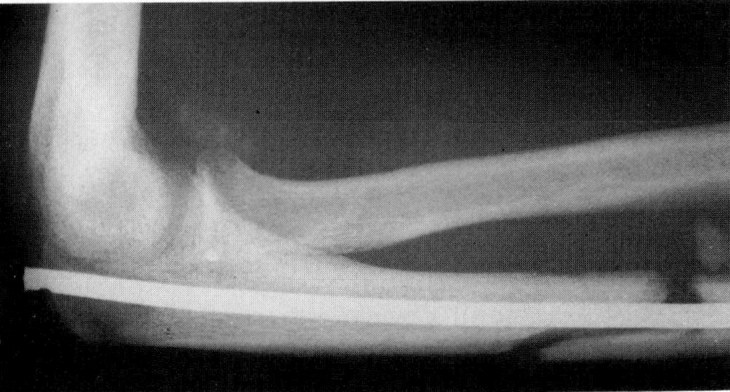

Fig. 9.17 A Monteggia fracture-dislocation showing the characteristic overlap of the ulnar fragments with the common anterior dislocation of the radial head. The residual distraction of the ulnar fracture, following intramedullary nailing, delayed healing. Note also post-traumatic new bone formation in the soft tissues anterior to the reduced radial head in the later film.

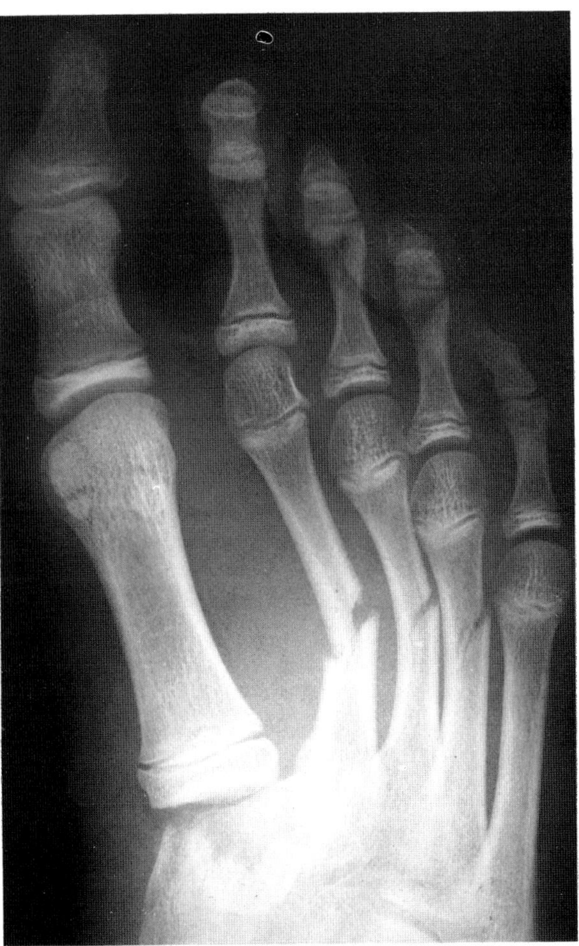

Fig. 9.18 In this child the three central metatarsals are fractured. The second metatarsal shows a complete fracture but the fractures of the shafts of the third and fourth metatarsals are incomplete on their medial sides — greenstick fractures.

dren's fractures involve the leg. Such fractures nearly always occur in the shafts of long bones, the joint surfaces being affected only rarely.

Many of these fractures are incomplete, and may show the characteristic cortical wrinkle (Fig. 10.21) or the classical 'greenstick' type of fracture (Fig. 9.18). Such fractures unite rapidly in continuity. Of more recent interest is the rarer plastic bowing fracture, most often involving the ulna, radius or fibula without visible radiographic evidence of fracture. Accurate reduction of complete fractures may result in a temporary increase in length. With fractures of the femur and tibia, reduction in good alignment with slight overlap of the fragments is often considered desirable, in order to avoid a transient inequality of leg length.

Remodelling. Active growth allows the juvenile skeleton to heal much more quickly than the adult, and callus formation usually develops rapidly within a few days. Moreover, children have a remarkable ability to correct deformities of alignment by remodelling during the remaining years of growth (Fig. 9.19). This corrective power diminishes progressively as age advances. It is more effective with small-angle fractures and with those which are situated near the ends rather than those in the middle of the shafts of long bones. Compressed vertebral bodies are also capable of almost complete reconstruction (Fig. 9.20). Remodelling, however, cannot correct residual deformities

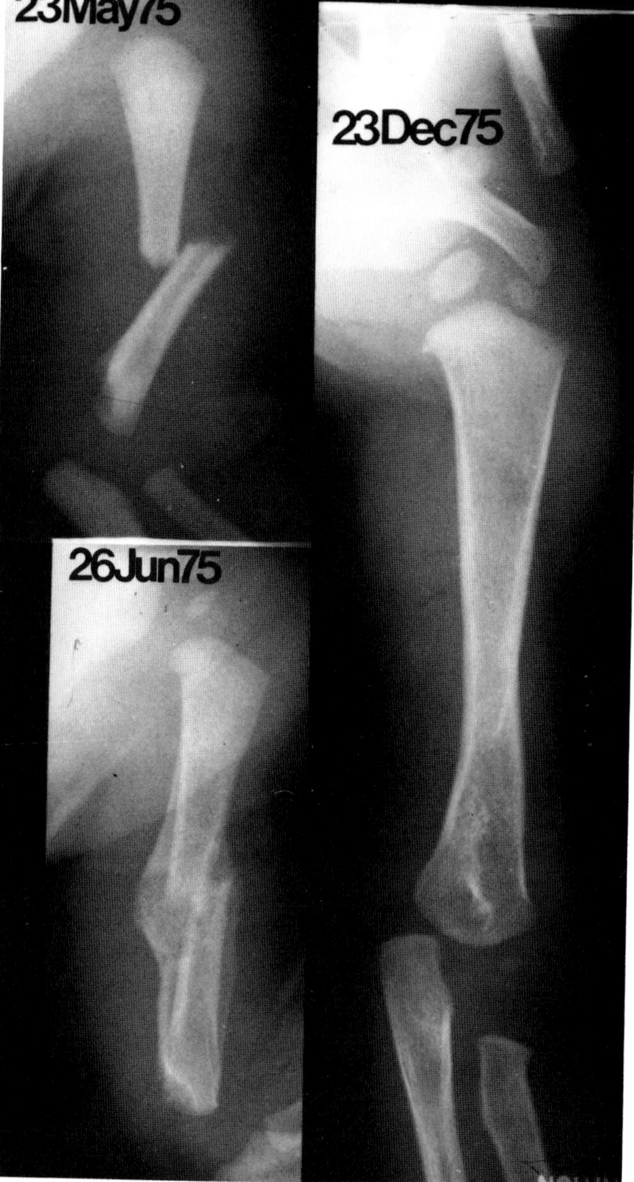

Fig. 9.19

Fig. 9.19 In this child the fracture of the midshaft of the humerus has united despite the less than satisfactory alignment. In under 9 months, remodelling of the excess callus has left a relatively normally shaped bone.

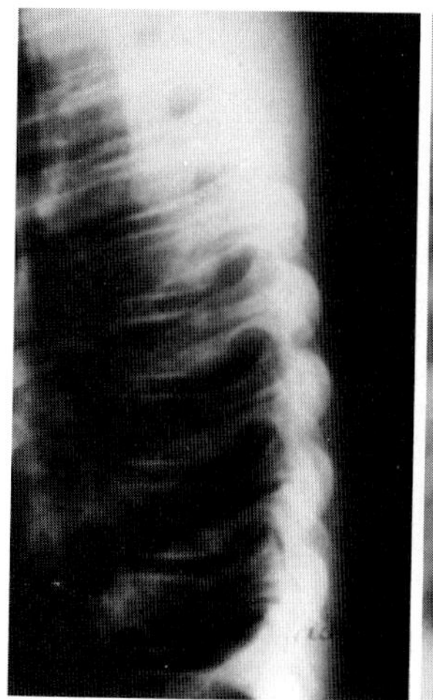
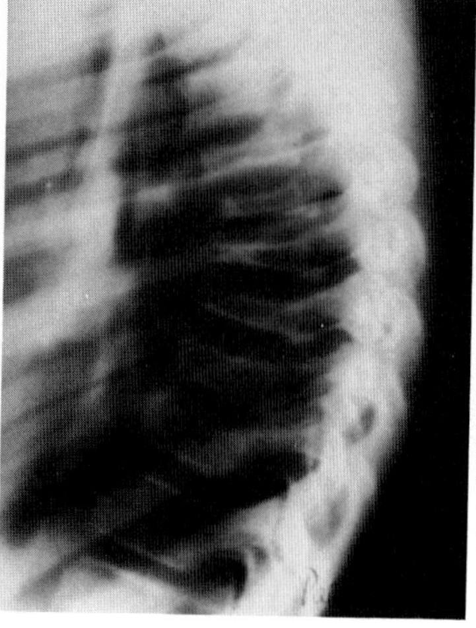
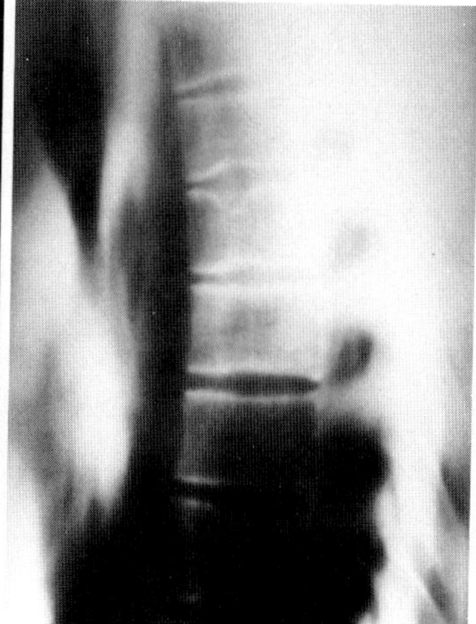

Fig. 9.20

Fig. 9.20 Compression fractures of the dorsal spine due to muscle spasm in tetanus. This 9-year-old boy was knocked over by a car and suffered multiple abrasions. The initial X-ray showed no abnormality, but severe compression fractures resulted from subsequent muscle spasm. In the third film, obtained 9 years later, almost complete vertebral reconstruction has taken place. Two residual Schmorl's nodes are seen in this tomogram.

f rotation. Similarly, coxa vara following a fracture of the roximal end of the femur, and facial bone deformities annot be corrected.

EPIPHYSEAL FRACTURE-SEPARATIONS

Iowever fortunate this excellent corrective mechanism nay be, an added danger for the growing child is that of piphyseal separation. This lesion is not uncommon ecause the growth plate offers a site of relative weakness. uvenile injuries of this type are usually accompanied by letachment of a portion of the metaphysis from the side owards which the epiphysis is displaced. Spontaneous eduction may take place before radiography is undertaken o that, if the metaphyseal fragment is small or absent, dentification of this severe traumatic lesion may be difficult. The elbow joint is a common site for such injuries, and it is often advisable to obtain radiographs of the other elbow for comparison. The injured epiphyseal plate is likely to be wider than its counterpart.

These injuries of the growth plate have been classified by Salter and Harris. Type I: Separation of the whole epiphysis. Type II: Separation of the epiphysis with a peripheral metaphyseal fragment. Type III: Partial separation of the epiphysis. Type IV: Partial separation of the epiphysis with an adjacent metaphyseal fragment. Type V: Compression injury involving the growth plate with little or no initial radiological abnormality, yet an increased risk of premature fusion (Figs 9.21–9.24).

Premature epiphyseal fusion of the injured growth plate constitutes the major danger of these lesions. In the arm this may produce only a cosmetic deformity (Fig. 9.24), but in the leg any consequent inequality of length may cause considerable disability. Early weight-bearing must therefore be avoided. Even if frank premature fusion does not occur, some impairment of growth may cause slight shortening. Should premature fusion of an epiphysis be incomplete, abnormalities such as tibia recurvatum may occur and ultimately may require corrective osteotomy.

Surgical measures to correct inequality include:

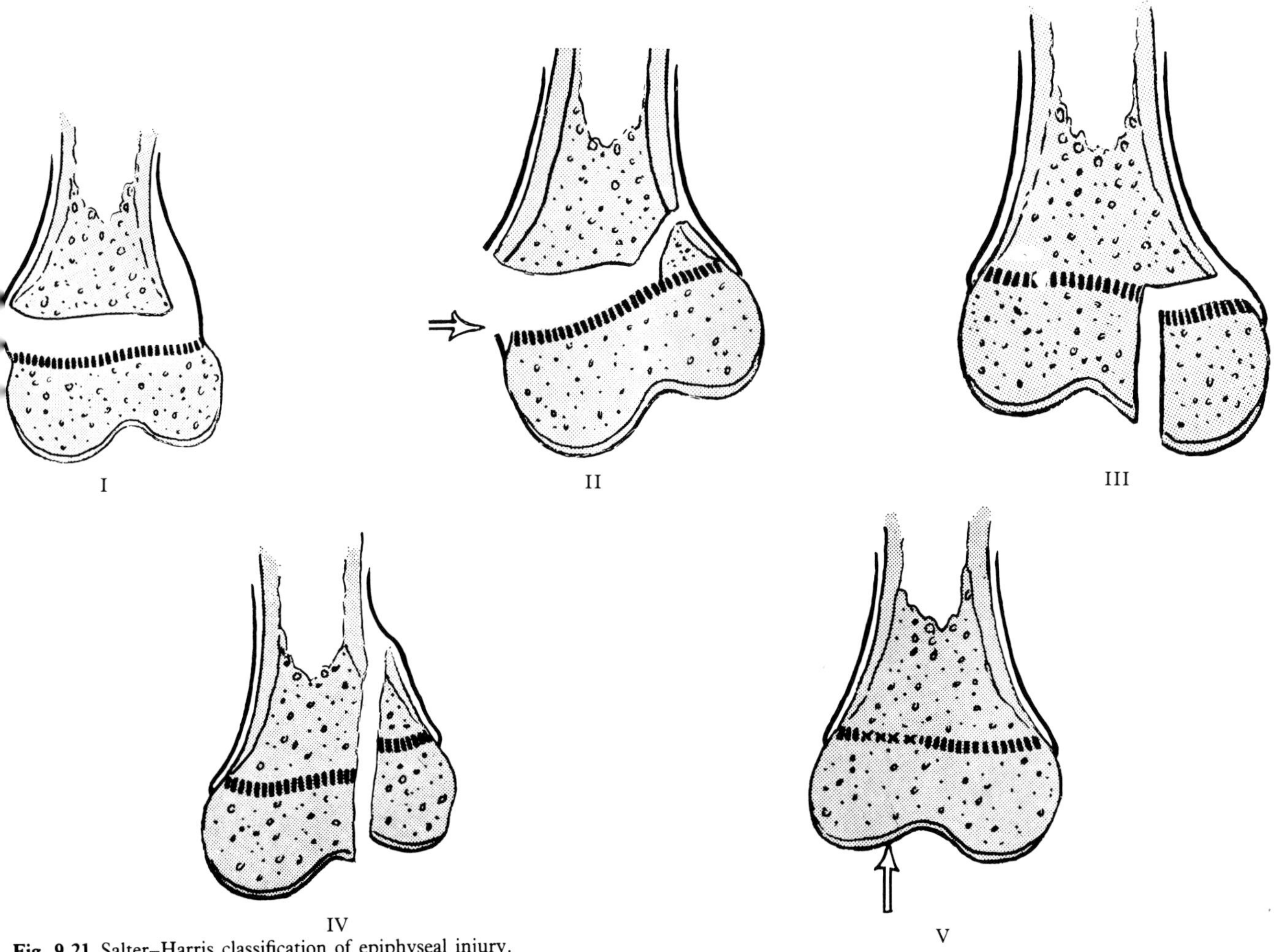

Fig. 9.21 Salter–Harris classification of epiphyseal injury.

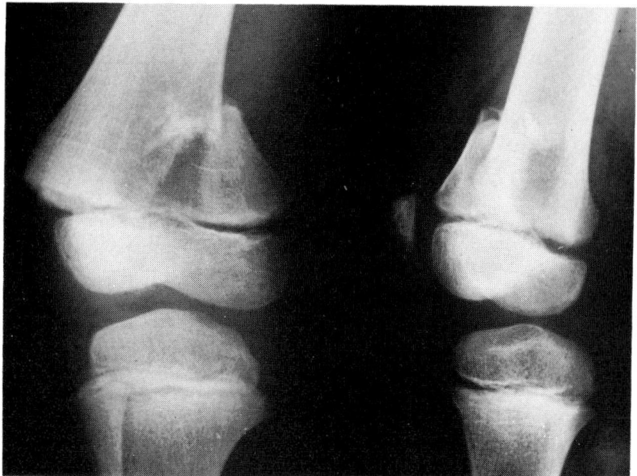

Fig. 9.22 Fracture-separation of the distal femoral epiphysis in an anteromedial direction, carrying with it a large fragment of the femoral metaphysis — the relatively common Salter–Harris Type II injury.

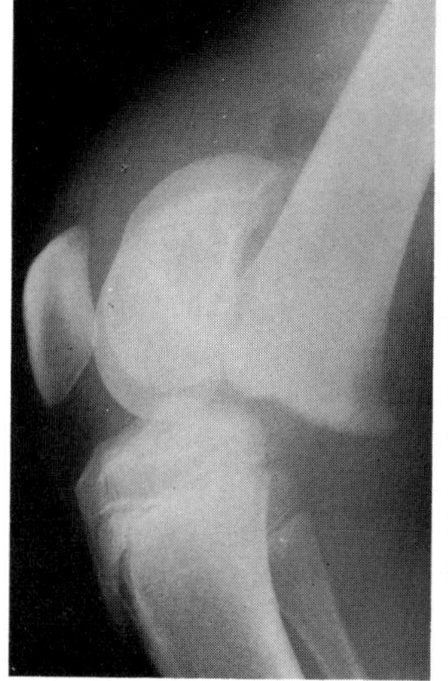

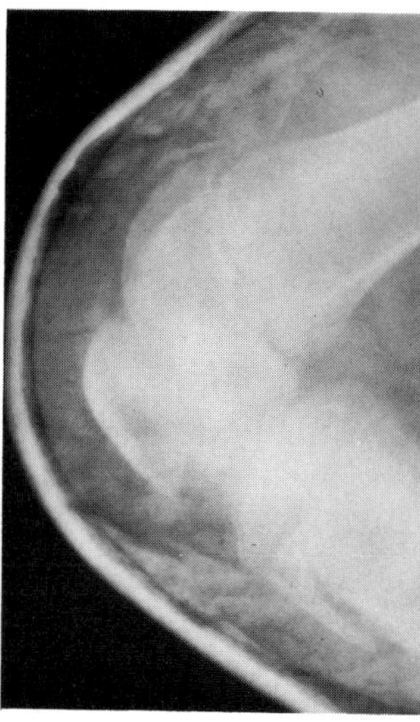

Fig. 9.23 Post-traumatic displacement of the distal femoral epiphysis in this 12-year-old boy was unaccompanied by separation of a metaphyseal fragment — the rare Salter–Harris Type I. Following reduction, no other bone injury could be identified. Such injuries carry a high risk of premature fusion at the growth plate.

1. resection of a central segment of the normal femur; 2. fusion of the growth plates around the normal knee (epiphysiodesis) or impairment of their growth by the insertion of metallic staples; 3. Lengthening the short femur or tibia by the more time-consuming and unpredictable procedure of performing central osteotomies and applying prolonged distraction. By the last method about 6 cm increase in length is usually obtained, but the treatment requires at least a year.

SLIPPED FEMORAL CAPITAL EPIPHYSIS (SFCE)
(*Epiphysiolysis, adolescent coxa vara*)

Slipped epiphysis is a disorder of adolescence (Figs 9.25–9.30). Its specific aetiology is not known but it usually coincides with the growth spurt of puberty; hence its onset is earlier in girls (mean age 11.5 years) than in boys (mean age 14 years). Boys are affected more often than girls but the previously recorded preponderance of 3 : 1 is probably now less, perhaps on account of increased athletic participation by girls in recent decades. A history of specific injury is rarely obtained, but repeated low-grade trauma may well be a causative factor. Some authors have proposed a constitutional cause and the incidence is greater in both overweight and asthenic children. Bilateral involvement probably occurs in 20–40% of cases, though some authorities claim an incidence of over 90%.

Patients usually present with a limp with or without pain in the hip or knee. The diagnosis is suspected clinically by the limitation of internal rotation of the hip, but a firm diagnosis requires adequate radiological examination.

Early diagnosis is essential, as in the majority of cases initial management is directed at internal fixation of the femoral epiphysis without attempting to correct the

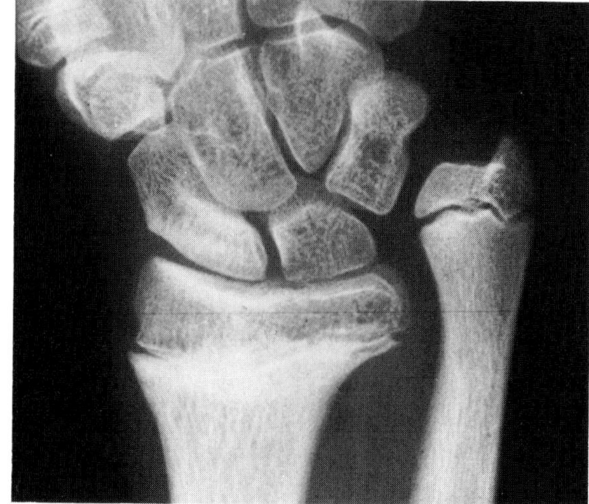

Fig. 9.24 Premature fusion of the distal radial epiphysis, following a fracture-separation 7 years before, with relative overgrowth of the ulna.

deformity, as such interference increases the incidence of chondrolysis and therefore premature degenerative joint disease. Early diagnosis depends on a high index of suspicion by the general practitioner leading to orthopaedic confirmation and adequate radiological examination.

The **radiological appearance** is that of displacement of the epiphysis in relation to the metaphysis, almost always in a predominantly posterior direction. Displacement occurs in two stages:

1. A slow posterior migration. This results in coxa vara following remodelling and is best recorded by use of Bill-

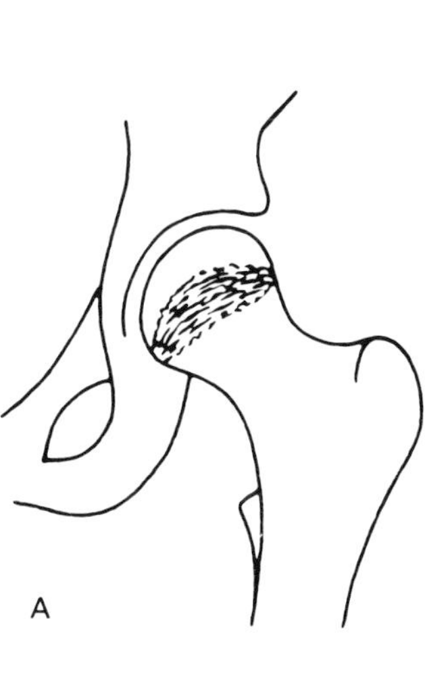

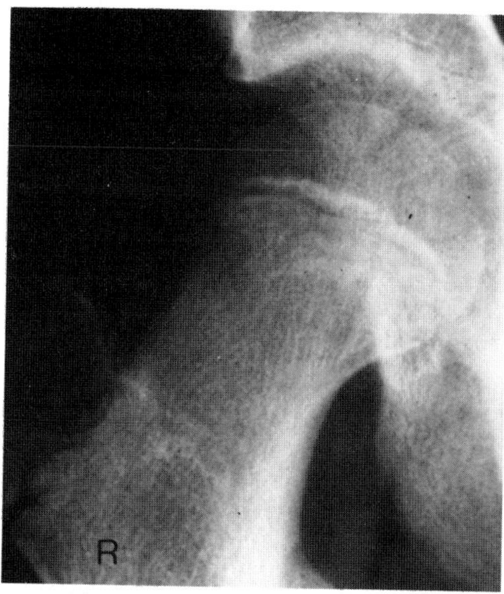

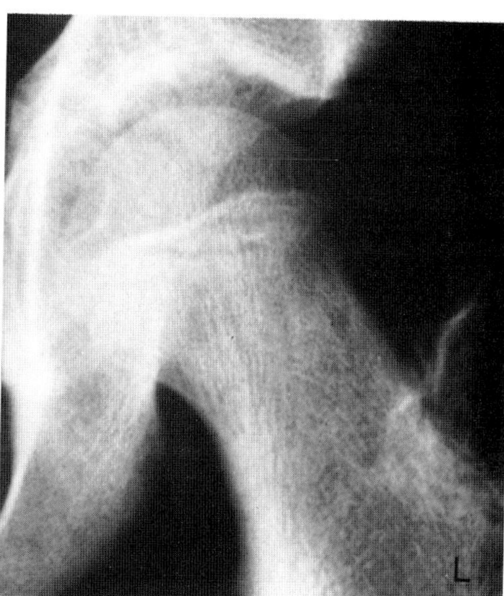

Fig. 9.25 Slipped epiphysis. **A**. Changes in the metaphyseal appearance are diagramatically shown. **B**. In this child, the interdigitating lucent lines of the metaphysis of the normal left femur are clear. In the affected right femur, clarity of the lines is lost and the overlying posteriorly slipped epiphysis has caused some increased density of the metaphysis.

ings views. These should be obtained when monitoring the other hip in following up a slipped epiphysis; in 20–40% of patients the slip is bilateral. The views are also valuable in late cases to determine the extent of the deformity prior to corrective osteotomy.

2. A more rapid, sometimes episodic, fracture-separation, which produces other radiographic appearances.

The most useful diagnostic signs on the anteroposterior radiograph are:

a. *Blurring of the metaphysis* (Fig. 9.25) due to trauma to its margins by the fracture-separation and to superimposition of the posteriorly displaced epiphysis.

b. *Displacement of the femoral metaphysis* from the acetabulum (Fig. 9.26). The medial third of the metaphysis no longer overlaps the posterior margin of the acetabulum.

c. *Increased width of the growth plate* (Fig. 9.27), most useful in unilateral slipped epiphysis.

d. *Prolongation of superior neck line* (Fig. 9.28). A straight line drawn along the superior margin of the femoral neck usually transects part of the epiphysis. If it fails to do so, or transects a smaller segment than in the other femur, a slipped epiphysis is to be suspected.

e. *Reduction of epiphyseal height* (Fig. 9.29). This is certainly abnormal when reduced by 2 mm or more as compared with the other normal side, or when a 2 mm reduction occurs on serial films.

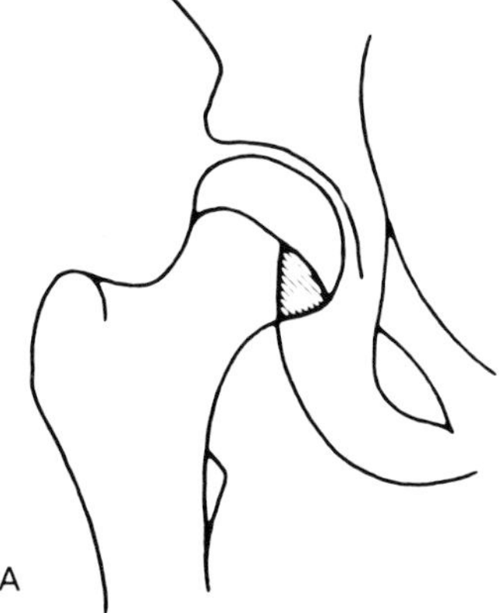

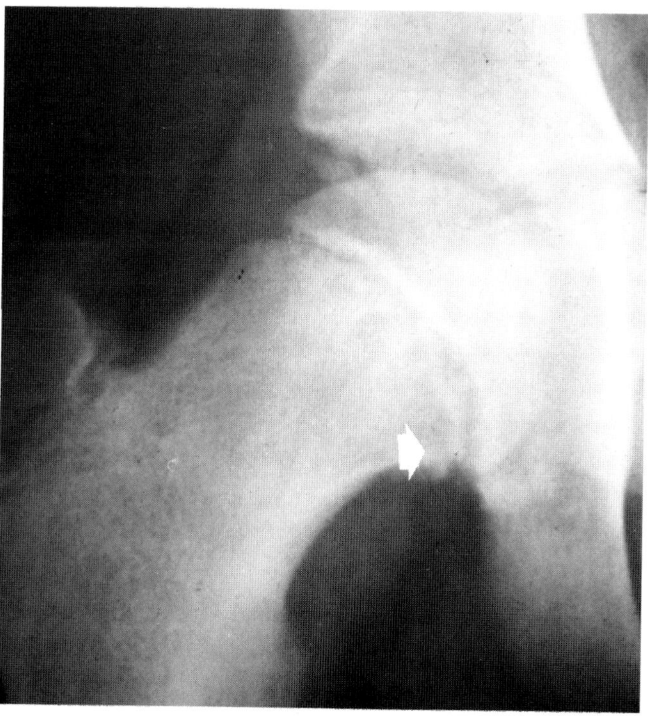

Fig. 9.26 Slipped epiphysis. **A**. The diagram of a normal hip shows that the posterior acetabular wall overlaps the medial third of the femoral metaphysis. **B**. In the radiograph the metaphysis lies completely clear of the acetabulum (➧).

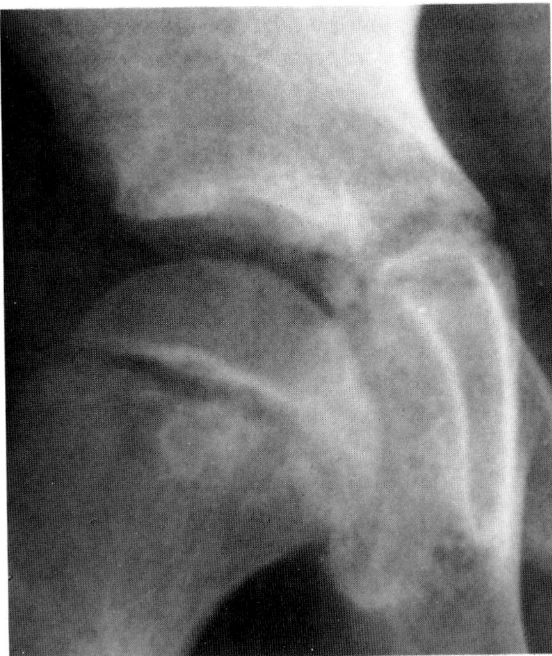

Fig. 9.27 Slipped epiphysis. The growth plate is abnormally wide as a result of the slip. Irregularity of the metaphysis is also present.

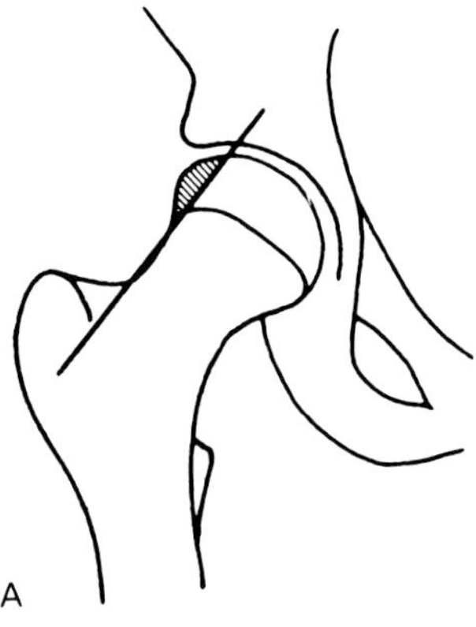

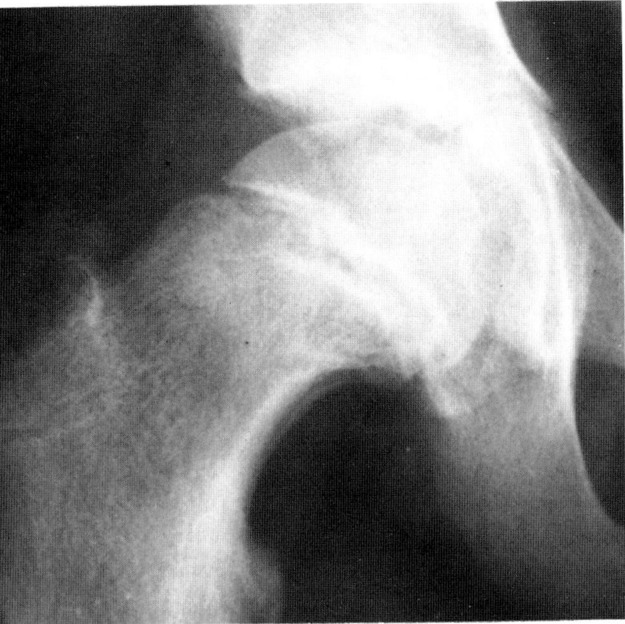

Fig. 9.28 Slipped epiphysis. **A**. A line drawn along the superior femoral neck line cuts a significant part of the epiphysis in the normal subject. **B**. The medial element of the slip has resulted in a situation where a line drawn along the superior part of the femoral neck would not cut the epiphysis at any point.

These signs on anteroposterior radiographs are valuable in *suspecting* the presence of a slipped femoral epiphysis. The abnormality is *confirmed* on a lateral film (Fig. 9.30). In at least 10% of cases no abnormality will be apparent on the AP radiograph and both AP and frog lateral projections are therefore always necessary in adolescent patients with a painful hip or limp.

Because of the high incidence of bilateral slip, it is essential that all such patients are kept under clinical surveillance until natural fusion occurs at the femoral growth plates. An acute slip can occur quite rapidly, within the space of a month, but frequent radiographic examination is not acceptable.

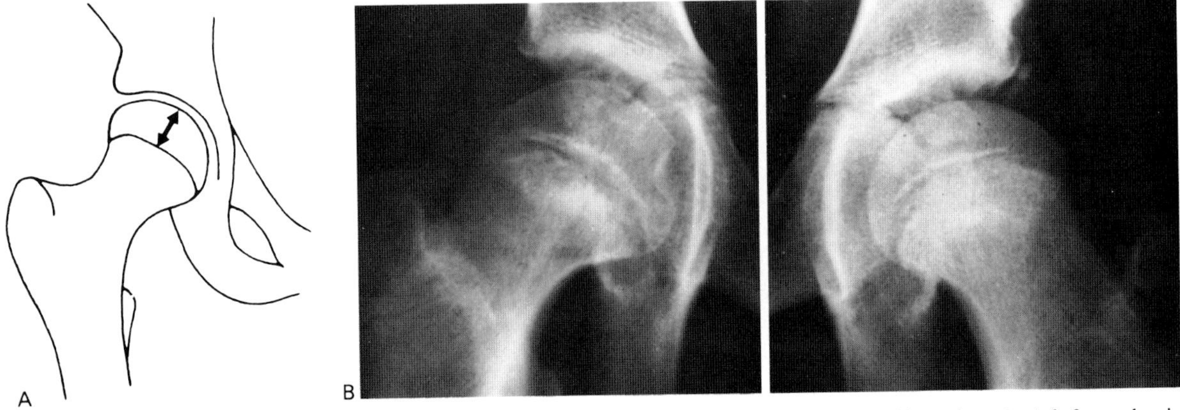

Fig. 9.29 Slipped epiphysis. **A**. Diagram showing the method of measurement of epiphyseal height. **B**. In this patient the left femoral epiphysis is smaller than the right, even though the patient has bilateral slipped epiphyses. The slip on the left is much greater and the height of the epiphysis was 3 mm less than that on the other side.

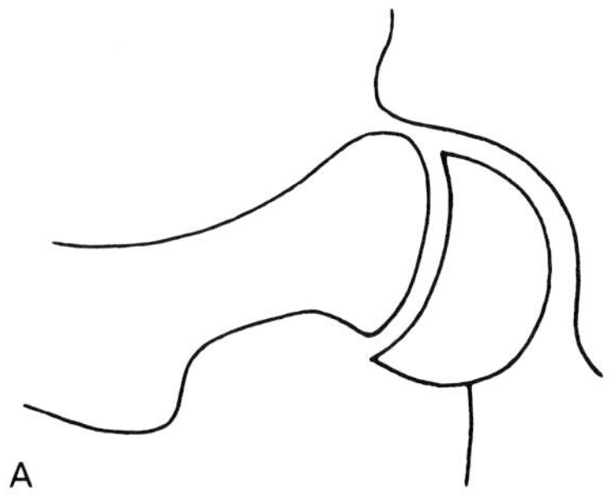

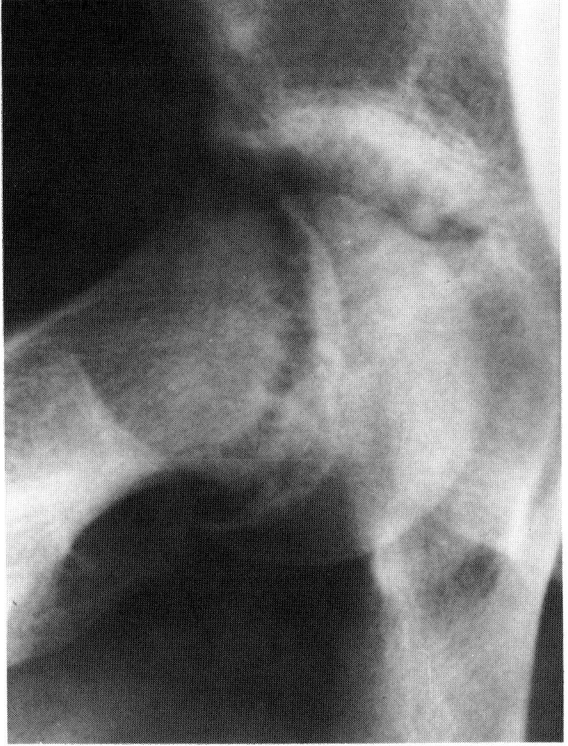

Fig. 9.30 Slipped epiphysis. **A**. Diagram of an early epiphyseal slip in the lateral projection. **B**. Radiograph showing a similar appearance with posterior slip.

Appropriate management consists of obtaining baseline Billing views of the normal hip, keeping the patient under frequent orthopaedic surveillance and repeating the radiographic examination at any sign of change.

Following epiphyseal slip with or without internal fixation, premature fusion may be expected. Fusion in an unacceptably deformed position may require osteotomy, often triplane, to improve function and hopefully to reduce the chance of secondary osteoarthrosis. It is well known that a minor slip of the femoral capital epiphysis may remain asymptomatic and undetected during the growth period and takes its toll in middle life.

An unusual late complication, responsible for persistent pain and stiffness, is *necrosis of the articular cartilage* (chondrolysis; Waldenström's disease), causing narrowing of the joint space, irregularity of the articular surfaces, disuse osteoporosis and, ultimately, osteoarthrosis. Very rarely, the slip may take place in the reverse direction or laterally.

Radiological recognition of the early slipped epiphysis is most important. All too often minor degrees of asymmetry, which always require explanation, are not appreciated. The displacement progresses insidiously, only to become overt months later, with great increase in difficulty of surgical management.

In a significant minority of cases no limp or pain in the hip is present; it will appreciated that radiological examination of the hips is mandatory in an adolescent patient with unexplained pain in the knee.

TRAUMATIC CORTICAL HYPEROSTOSIS; SUBPERIOSTEAL HAEMATOMA

Trauma may result in elevation of the periosteum by haematoma in the absence of a frank fracture. The initial radiograph may reveal no bony abnormality and only after an interval is the injury to the bone revealed by the presence of appositional new bone.

In children and, particularly, infants the periosteum is only loosely attached by incomplete Sharpey's fibres. As a consequence, it is easily stripped from the underlying cortex by the formation of a haematoma. A special example of this type of injury is the so-called *cephalhaematoma* of the skull sometimes observed in neonates after forceps delivery.

Under certain circumstances, in young infants, a history of trauma may be suppressed by the parents or guardians. The affected areas may be tender and swollen but external bruising may be absent. Radiographic examination, in this situation, may reveal periosteal reaction due to subperiosteal haematomata in the absence of fracture; such lesions are produced by gripping or twisting movements to the limbs by the guilty adult and are part of the spectrum of non-accidental injury to children (Fig. 9.31). Such haematomata are essentially similar to those in scurvy (q.v.), where capillary fragility is an important factor.

Traumatic cortical hyperostosis must not be confused with the rare disease of unknown origin *infantile cortical hyperostosis*.

The natural history of periosteal hyperostosis is for incorporation of the bone into the cortex. The degree of remodelling depends on the age of the patient — the younger the patient, the more likely is it that the new bone so formed will be totally resorbed.

NON-ACCIDENTAL INJURY; THE BATTERED CHILD SYNDROME

First described in 1946 by Caffey, the incidence, or at least its recognition, has increased considerably in the past 20 years. Caffey reported the association of multiple fractures

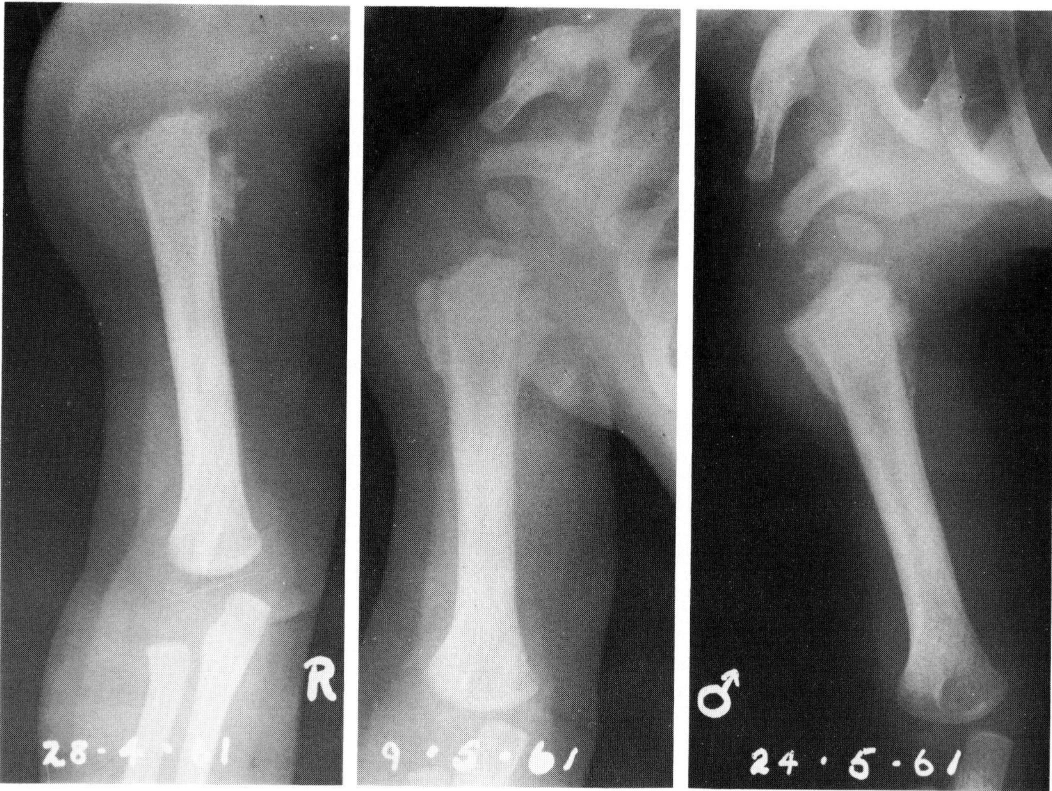

Fig. 9.31 Traumatic cortical hyperostosis. This 6-month-old male was brought to hospital because he was unwilling to use his right arm. The subperiosteal haematomata round the upper end of the humerus and detachment of a bone fragment from the metaphysis indicated a traumatic origin, despite the absence of such history. Subsequent progress of the lesion confirmed this conclusion. The culprit was eventually found to be a 6-year-old brother who had been swinging him round by the arms. That this game had been in progress for some time is shown by the healed fracture of the right clavicle. Very similar lesions were found in the left arm of this patient, and in both arms of a female twin.

of the long bones in children suffering from chronic subdural haematomas. Such injuries were 'either not observed or were denied when observed' by the parent or guardian. The children are usually under school age and frequently under the age of 2 years. It is now accepted that these injuries are inflicted by adults in charge of the children.

The essential feature of the syndrome is evidence of repeated injury. *Clinical* manifestations include multiple bruises or burns of varying age, inconsistencies in the history given by the parent or guardian and often a withdrawn child exhibiting the signs of social and intellectual neglect. The possibility of trauma is often not mentioned by the parent.

The **radiographic characteristic of** the disorder is the presence of multiple fractures at different stages of healing, and either of unusual type or incompatible with the declared form of injury. Particularly common are marginal metaphyseal fractures with or without epiphyseal displacement and exuberant subperiosteal ossification (Fig. 9.31). Such injuries often result from vigorous shaking of a child which is being gripped by a limb or limbs. Skull fracture or diastasis is common and fractures rarely found in accidental trauma, in flat bones, ribs and spine, are observed (Fig. 9.32).

Although suspicion that undeclared skeletal trauma has been sustained by a child may be aroused by clinical and social information, the radiologist has a duty to communicate the possibility of the diagnosis when the findings are suggestive. Such notification should be given verbally to the clinician in the first instance. Some skeletal injuries are almost diagnostic, some are suggestive, whilst child abuse can occur without evidence of skeletal damage. Many children subjected to battering die of a subsequent assault. A radiographic skeletal survey is indicated when non-accidental injury is suspected; this should include the skull, AP and lateral projections of the whole trunk and AP views of the whole length of all extremities.

Differential diagnosis: 1. Birth injury: infants born by breech delivery are prone to epiphyseal/metaphyseal fractures, especially of the lower extremities. Radiographic evidence of such a fracture would not be present after the twelfth day of life; 2. Meningomyelocoele and rarer causes of neurosensory defect such as congenital indifference to pain; 3. Osteogenesis imperfecta; 4. Congenital syphilis; 5. Scurvy; 6. Infantile cortical hyperostosis.

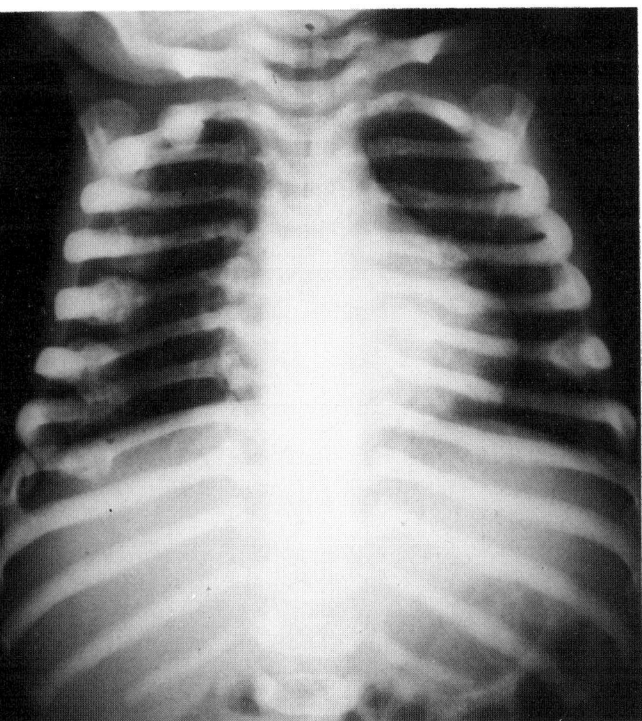

Fig. 9.32 Non-accidental injury. The radiograph shows multiple rib fractures at different stages of healing, probably the result of repeated compression injuries to the thorax. The child was admitted with a recent skull fracture.

The combination of clinical and radiographic features will generally differentiate such disorders from non-accidental injury.

It is important to remember that illness and child abuse are not separated in a distinct manner. Children leaving hospital after in-patient therapy show a greater incidence of subsequent non-accidental injury.

SPECIAL TYPES OF SKELETAL TRAUMA

MUSCLE SPASM

Violent muscle spasm may exert sufficient force to cause fractures. These are well recognized as a complication of epileptic fits, when crush injuries of the vertebral bodies and even fractures of the femoral necks may ensue. Vertebral compression fractures in the thoracic region also occur in *tetanus*, during the stage of opisthotonus, more frequently than is appreciated (Fig. 9.20). Anterior wedging of the vertebral bodies takes place during tonic hyperextension of the spine because it is physiologically impossible to obliterate the normal dorsal kyphos even in the gross degrees of hyperextension achieved by acrobats.

In children such fractures may undergo virtually complete reconstruction during the subsequent years of growth (Figs 9.19 and 9.20). Similar injuries occurred with *electro-convulsive therapy*, prior to the routine prophylactic use of curare-like drugs and in accidental *electric shock*. Involuntary *reflex spasm* may cause transverse fractures of the patella and violent voluntary effort may detach fragments of bone from the origins of muscles or the insertions of tendons. Such trauma due to resisted muscular pull is not uncommon at the pelvic and scapular origins of major limb muscles.

CHRONIC TRAUMA

a. **Stress or fatigue fractures.** The description of the cause of these lesions by Brandt, quoted by Golding, cannot be bettered: 'rhythmically repeated, subthreshold, mechanical insults which only by summation lead to structural changes and severance of continuity'. These fractures have been observed in many bones, in each of which their sites tend to be characteristic. The constant or repeated stress from which they result is very often some form of athletic or occupational activity. They may occur in the absence of any unusual precipitating factor, especially when periods of prolonged bed rest have caused the skeleton to develop disuse osteoporosis. These lesions are often productive of pain before radiological evidence of their presence becomes evident. However they are usually detectable even at this early stage by radionuclide scanning.

The radiograph may show a hairline translucency of a crack fracture, usually running transversely across the bone. By the time radiographic examination is undertaken some evidence of callus formation in relation to the injury almost always has become evident. When visible the cortical element of the fracture is a fine lucent line, while the medullary fracture shows only the density of callus formation. The fracture line, indeed, may never be identified, even with tomography, and the diagnosis may depend on the recognition of callus formation, particularly at one of the sites where these lesions typically develop. Confusion with new bone formation by a tumour should not arise, but if any doubt exists, serial examinations will show progressive maturation of the repair process. Such errors have been made in the past and may have been responsible for some apparent cures of 'malignant bone tumours'. The comparable error is to biopsy a stress fracture and for the immature osteoid of the callus to be confused with an osteosarcoma. Biopsy should be avoided in such circumstances as repeat radiographic examinations after 2–3 weeks will usually show maturation and such a delay will not affect the prognosis of osteosarcoma significantly. Furthermore, in several documented cases, biopsy has led to the stress lesion being converted to a complete fracture.

March fractures of the *metatarsal* necks, especially the second, are much the most common stress fractures (Fig. 9.33). The name is descriptive of the cause. The proximal third of the *tibia* not infrequently is affected in children (Fig. 9.34). In adults the lesion is more common in the middle or distal part of the tibial shaft, affecting long distance runners and male ballet dancers (Fig. 9.35). The distal *fibular* fracture of this type is associated with long distance running and that of the proximal shaft with repeated jumping from a height, as in training for para-

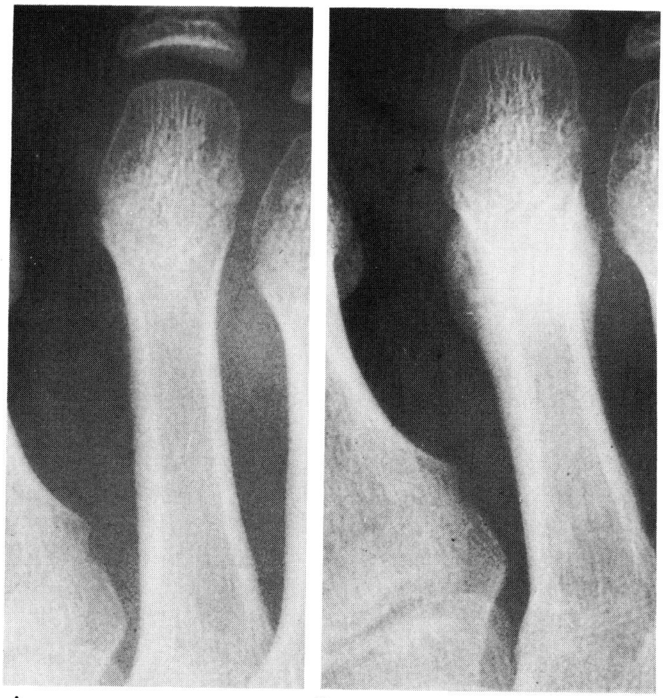

A B

Fig. 9.33 Stress fracture of second metatarsal. Following a cross-country run this 12-year-old boy presented with pain in the right forefoot of one week's duration. **A**. The initial film showed minimal periosteal reaction on the neck of the second metatarsal. **B**. The diagnosis of a stress fracture was confirmed by the examination three weeks later which showed much organized callus surrounding the lesion.

chute jumping. Other bones sometimes involved incluc the *lower ribs* in the mid-axillary line from chron coughing; the *first rib*, from carrying a heavy pack; th *femur* (Fig. 9.36); the *calcaneus* and the *clavicle*. This li is by no means exhaustive.

Spondylolisthesis is a forward slip of one lumbar vertebr on another. Normally, this movement is prevented b resistance to forward thrust by the integrity of the anteri part of the neural arch, comprising the pedicle, the pa interarticularis and the inferior articular process. The la

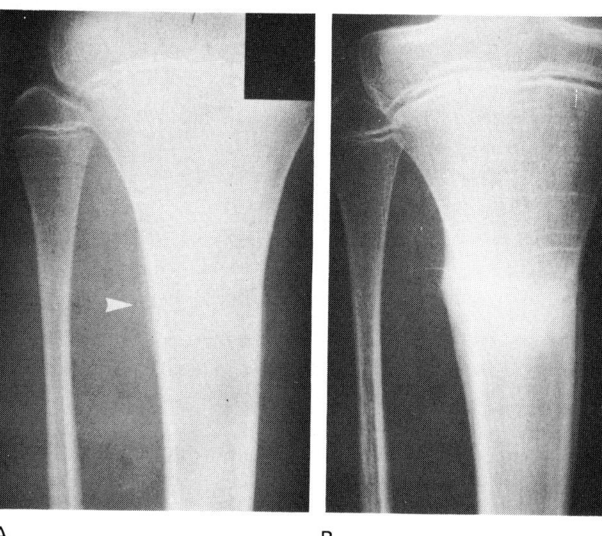

A B

Fig. 9.34 Stress fracture of tibia. **A**. Minimal periosteal reaction is shown on the tibial shaft. The fracture line itself is not evident. **B**. 6 weeks later the periosteal reaction has increased and sclerosis has developed round the fracture line. Such appearances must not be mistaken for tumours.

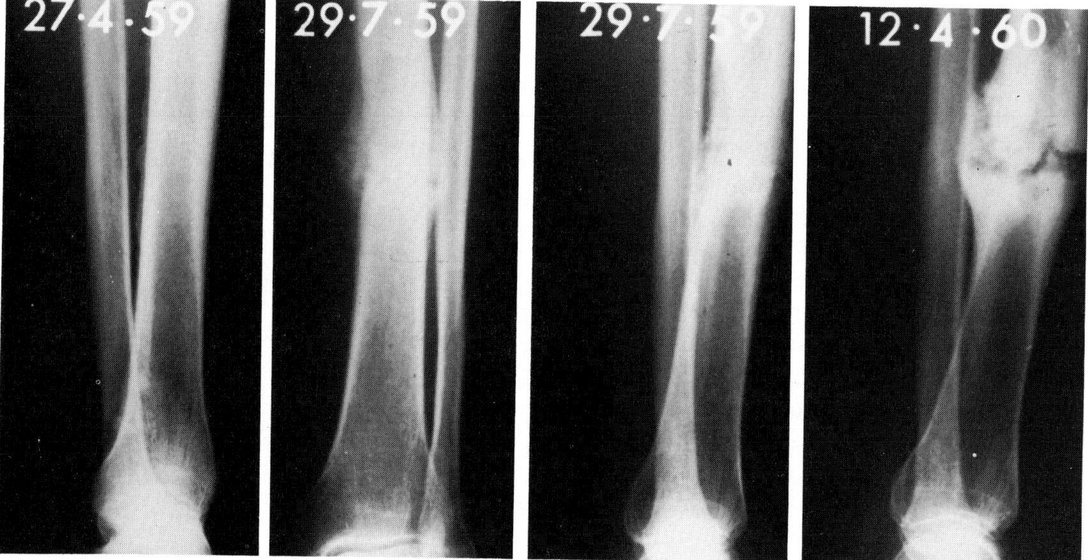

Fig. 9.35 Stress fracture of the midshaft of the tibia in a 58-year-old man. Following the second examination, surgical exploration was undertaken in the belief that the lesion was due to infection. Non-union followed, as indicated by the sclerotic margins of the ununited fracture. This man's work involved repeated jumping from a height, so that an occupational background was suspected.

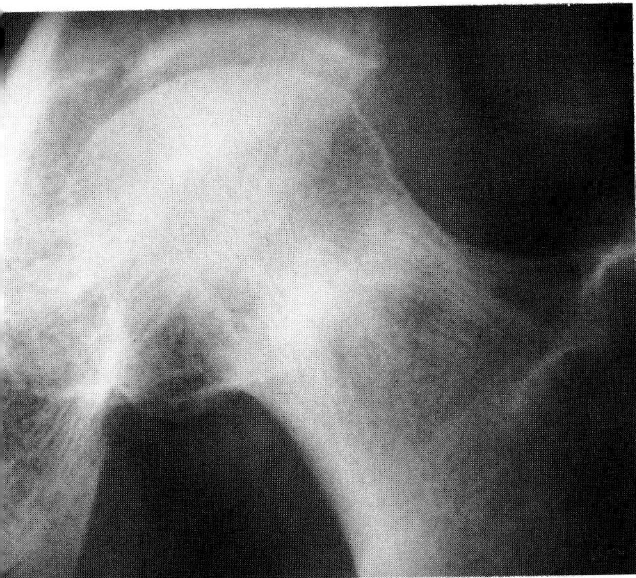

ig. 9.36 Stress fracture of femoral neck. Increased density in the edulla in the subcapital region of the neck shows a linear direction nd indicates the presence of callus within the cancellous bone. Such actures usually present as low-grade pain in the hip unrelated to any pecific injury.

is held in position by the superior articular process of the vertebra below, with the posterior intervertebral joint lying between. In the oblique projection the shape of the neural arch may be compared to the silhouette of a Scots terrier (Fig. 9.37), the transverse process representing the nose, the superior articular process representing the ear and the inferior articular process the front leg. A defect ofthe pars interarticularis breaks the 'neck' of the dog. The majority of these lesions are attributable to stress fractures of one or both sides of the neural arch through the relatively weak pars interarticularis (Fig. 9.38). Such fractures are difficult

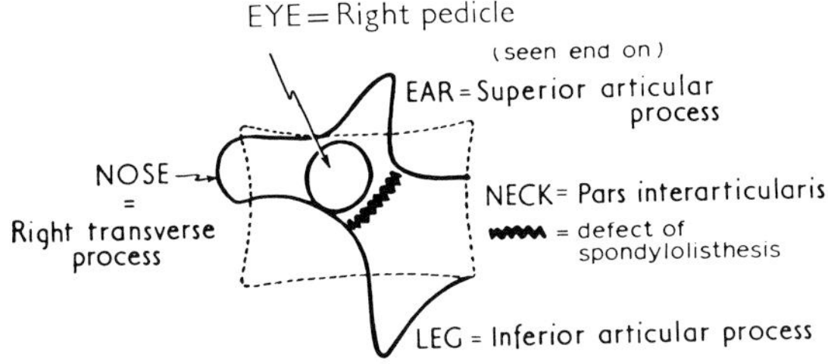

Fig. 9.37 Diagram of oblique projection of neural arch of a lumbar vertebra presenting an appearance comparable to a Scots terrier dog. The defect in the pars interarticularis in spondylolysis corresponds with a collar around the neck of the dog.

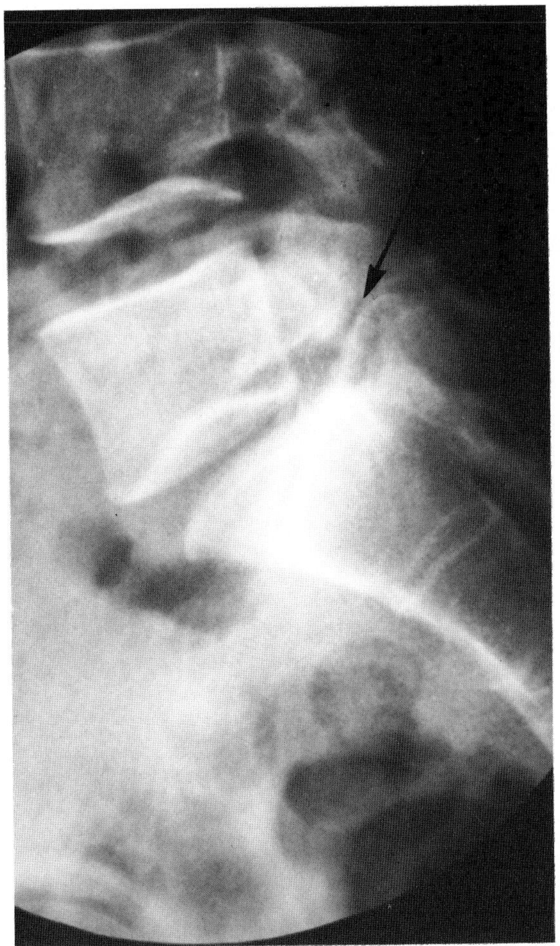

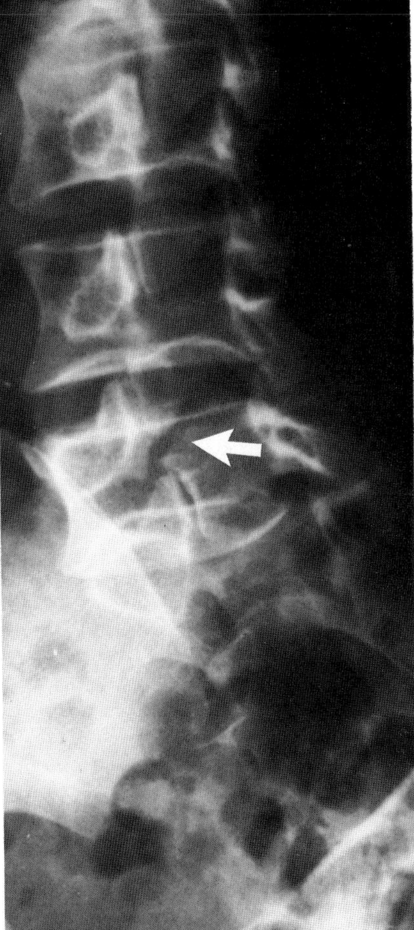

Fig. 9.38 Acute spondylolisthesis. This middle-aged patient suffered severe pain in the lower part of his back during heavy lifting. **A**. The lateral projection shows a forward slip of L5 on S1 of about 20%. The defect in the pars interarticularis is visible (arrow). **B**. In the oblique view the right pars shows a fracture with sharp margins (arrow), indicating that it is recent. The patient was found to have an old resorbed pars defect on the left side at the same level.

to detect in their early stages and are likely to be visible only in oblique projections. Owing to the distraction caused by the forward thrust, non-union is common, leaving a residual defect with sclerosed margins (Fig. 9.39A and B), or a gap resulting from bony resorption. Even when union does occur, the pars interarticularis may be elongated. The slipping of the vertebral bodies is demonstrated best in the lateral projection. Almost always the upper vertebra slips forwards and in the extreme case it may be completely in front of a line through the anterior margin of the lower vertebral body. Such gross disturbance is confined largely to the lumbo-sacral level. Owing to the associated lordosis, in the anteroposterior view, the fift lumbar vertebral body presents a semi-axial projection an is superimposed on the sacrum, presenting the 'bow-lin of Brailsford (Fig. 9.39C). By obtaining a 30 degre cephalad-angled AP radiograph, in lesser degrees of spor dylolisthesis, the defect in the pars interarticularis may b revealed. The presence of a pars interarticularis defe without forward slipping of the vertebra is known a *spondylolysis*.

Although about half the cases of spondylolisthesis can b attributed to these stress fractures of the neural arch, th remainder of these abnormalities are divided almost equall

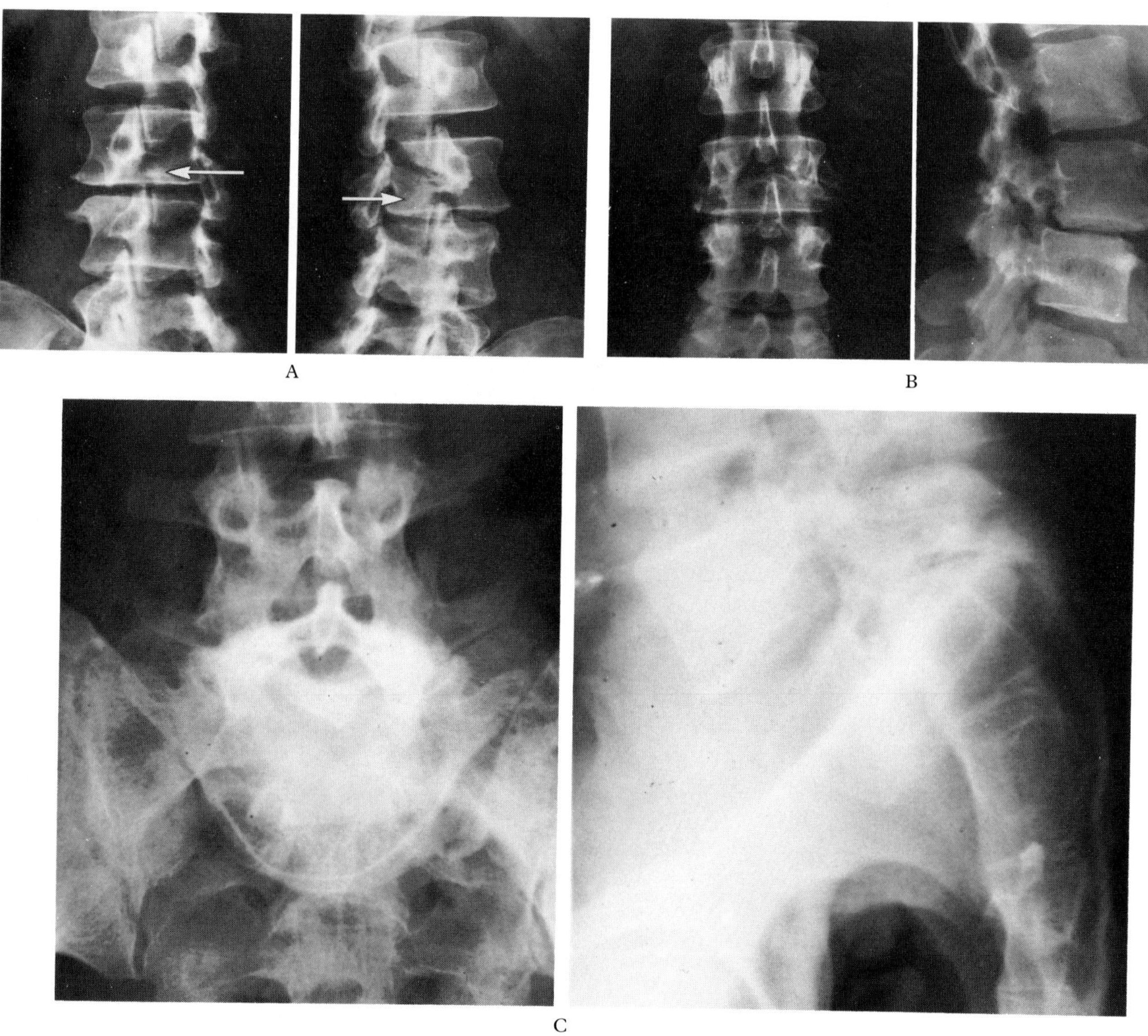

Fig. 9.39 A. and **B.** Spondylolisthesis. This 47-year-old female ballet dancer had complained of periodic attacks of back pain since the age of 18. L3 is displaced forwards in relation to the body of L4. Bilateral pars interarticularis defects are present and are demonstrated best in the oblique projections with marginal sclerosis. They were attributable to old ununited stress fractures. Narrowing of this intervertebral disc space indicated degenerative change in the L3–L4 intervertebral disc with some secondary degenerative change. A traction spur (arrow) is present (see text), an abnormality usually indicative of spinal instability. **C.** Gross lumbo-sacral spondylolisthesis. In the anteroposterior view the fifth lumbar vertebral body is projected through its vertical diameter, so that its anterior surface presents the classical 'bow-line' appearance.

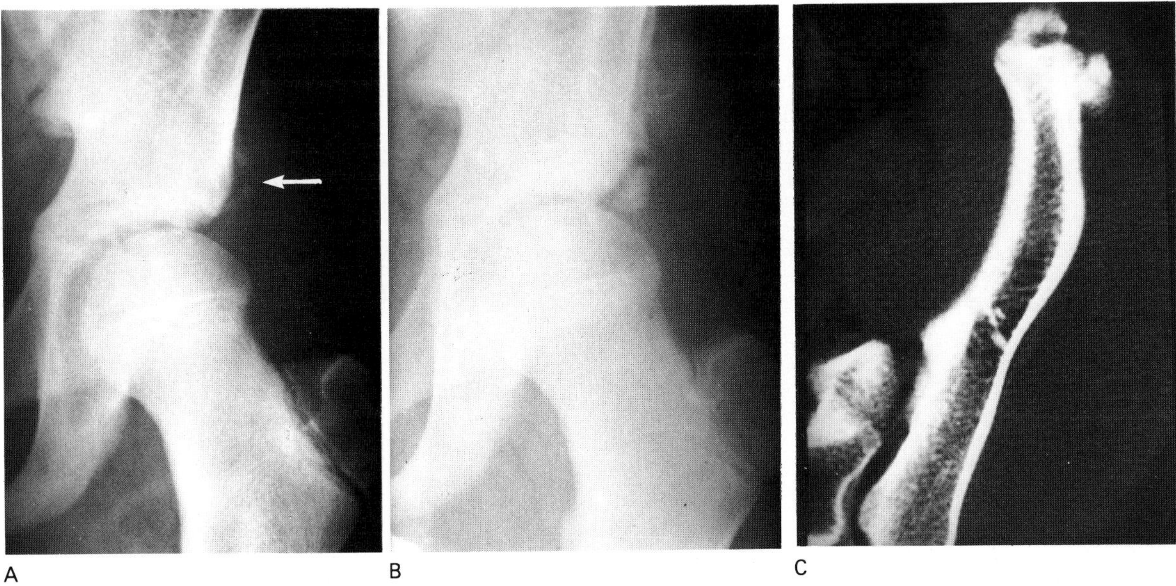

ig. 9.40 Avulsion injury of origin of rectus femoris in a child complaining of pain in left hip. **A**. On the early film a small amount of periosteal one is evident adjoining the acetabular margin (←). **B**. Some 48 days later this bone has increased in amount in a somewhat florid way causing ie surgeon to be concerned about the possible presence of a tumour. **C**. CT scan of the anterior inferior iliac spine showing the new bone rmation but excluding a neoplastic cause in the absence of bone destruction and soft tissue extension. (Courtesy of Dr R. Mitchell, Northwick ark Hospital.)

nto those resulting from degenerative changes in the osterior intervertebral joints and those associated with ongenital hypoplasia of articular processes. Acute and athological fractures of a pars interarticularis are distinctly ncommon.

The degree of spondylolisthesis is best recorded by bserving the percentage movement of one vertebral body n that below. Large slips are found in developmental and pondylotic forms; degenerative change in the apophyseal oints rarely produces spondylolisthesis in excess of 20%.

b. **Acute and chronic avulsion injuries**. Some of the lesions described under the heading of osteochondritis (see Ch. 3) are accepted generally as being attributable to chronic or repeated trauma. For example, the irregularities of the tibial tuberosity and the lower pole of the patella, referred to respectively as Osgood-Schlatter's disease and Sinding–Larsen disease, result from chronic strain on ligamentous attachments to growing bone.

Avulsion injuries are especially common around the hip. Such lesions are incurred often in the growing skeleton as a result of athletic activity. A frequent site to be affected is the anterior inferior iliac spine (Fig. 9.40), from which originates the straight head of rectus femoris, the muscle mainly employed in kicking a football. The formation of an irregular tuft of new bone provides the diagnostic feature of skeletal asymmetry (a feature *always* demanding an explanation) and sometimes may account for chronic hip pain and a limp in children, especially boys. Similar irregularities may be observed to correspond with the origin of the adductor muscles on the ischial apophysis and the insertion of the psoas major muscle on the lesser trochanter. Around the shoulder the repeated action of throwing a ball may provoke a similar reaction on the inferior aspect of the neck of the glenoid, the origin of the triceps muscle (Fig. 10.7).

Brief mention may be here of another cause of chronic groin pain, *instability of the symphysis pubis*, demonstrated by comparison of films obtained with weight-bearing on each leg in turn. Such a state may be suggested by widening of the fibrocartilage and irregularity and sclerosis of the margins of the pubic bones (Fig. 9.41). The condition is not infrequently observed in professional athletes and in women as a result of prolonged parturitional stress. Coincidental stress changes elsewhere in the pelvic ring at one or other sacro-iliac joint may be found.

The term 'osteochondritis', although still in common use, should no longer be employed to describe these different entities which share the common factor of chronic stress. (The condition of post-traumatic necrosis is therefore considered below.)

c. **Post-traumatic necrosis.** The term osteochondritis has long been used, again inaccurately, to describe the radiographic appearances of death of a single bone, such as the lunate, or of a growing epiphyseal centre, such as the head of the second metatarsal (see Ch. 3). These particular entities are also known as Kienböck's and Freiberg's diseases respectively, but many eponyms exist for similar lesions in other parts of the skeleton. Kienböck's disease, incidentally, appears frequently to be attributable to occupational stresses in manual workers. A further example is the so-called 'adult osteochondritis' of the navicular, with the occurrence of flattening, density and

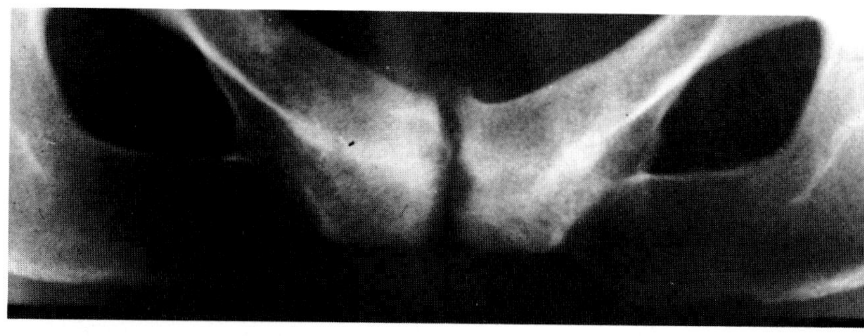

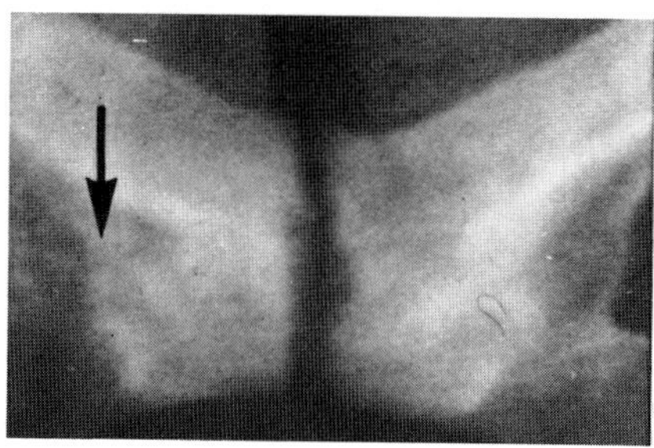

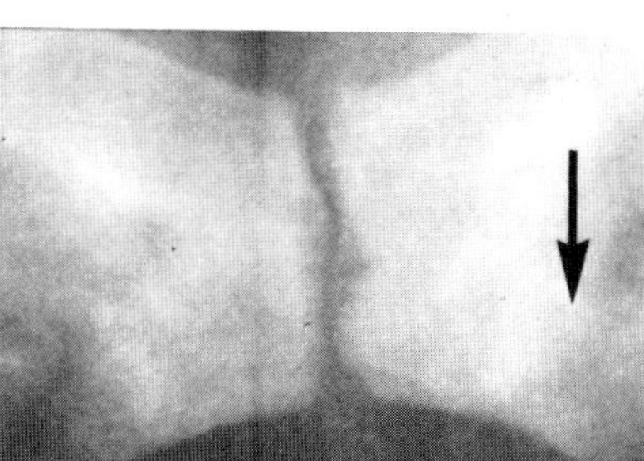

Fig. 9.41 Instability at pubic symphysis. The bony margins of the symphysis are irregular and sclerotic, suggesting trauma leading to chronic instability. The lower figures show radiographs obtained during weight-bearing on each leg in turn (arrows). Even the minor displacement shown here, which amounted to only a few mm, indicates significant instability at this site.

fragmentation which are characteristic of avascular necrosis.

Although a definite history of trauma is occasionally obtained from patients affected by this condition, the majority are quite unaware of any specific injury. The essential abnormality is deprivation of vascular supply, usually as a result of chronic stress, producing the changes of avascular necrosis as described in Chapter 3. For example, many workers have suspected that the avascular necrosis of the femoral head observed in Perthes' disease is post-traumatic. To a large extent this theory is supported by the work of Kemp and Boldero, who have shown that the condition may follow a traumatic effusion into the hip joint, with radiological evidence of widening of the joint space, again providing asymmetry. Such a discrepancy is often the only radiological abnormality to be found in the 'irritable hip syndrome' in children, which is occasionally followed by frank necrosis of the femoral head. These workers attributed the deprivation of vascular supply to be due to blockage of the *venous* drainage system as a result of the formation of granulation tissue within the medial compartment of the joint. Accumulations of pus within a hip joint affected by septic arthritis or blood in a haemophiliac may precipitate similar necrosis of the capital epiphysis.

The fundamental fact must be repeated that alteration in the radiological appearances of necrotic bone only takes place during the phase of revascularization and attempted repair.

Radionuclide scanning will show lack of photon activity in areas of vascular deprivation in bone, before any radiographic abnormality becomes apparent. During the later stage of revascularization, when increased density is evident radiographically, increased uptake can be expected on the radionuclide scan.

The theory that 'osteochondritis dissecans' has a traumatic origin has likewise been substantiated. These lesions of articular surfaces are now regarded as being caused by chronic stress. Specific athletic acitivites may be associated with specific lesions, affection of the proximal articular surface of the talus, for example, being a complication of

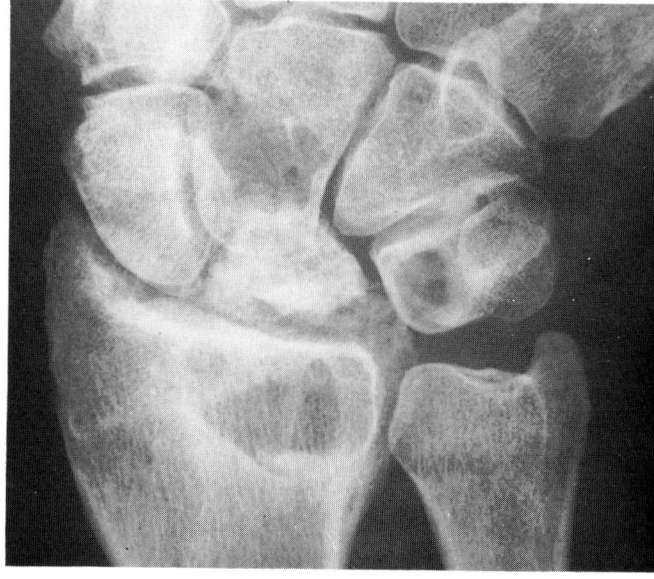

Fig. 9.42 Vibration syndrome. Fragmentation and flattening of the lunate due to avascular necrosis is typical of Kienböck's disease, accompanied by extensive cystic changes in the surrounding bones. These abnormalities occurred in a compressed air drill worker who had been exposed to this repeated trauma for many years.

high-jumping. The bilateral lesions sometimes observed in the femoral condyles may be associated with abnormal stresses related to walking and running with a mild knock-knee deformity.

d. **The vibration syndrome ('driller's disease').** Degenerative cystic changes may develop in the bones of the hand and wrist following the constant use of vibrating tools for five or more years, often associated with the occupational 'dead hand' syndrome. These radiological changes are more common in the guiding hand than the driving hand. They are more likely to develop when the frequency of impulse is greater than 2500 per minute (Fig. 9.42).

A similar appearance, however, may be observed in the bones of the hands and wrists of heavy manual workers, so that definitive radiological diagnosis of this condition is difficult.

OTHER CAUSES OF AVASCULAR NECROSIS

a. **Ionizing radiation.** Penetration of bone by radiation has a tendency to injure the tissue; if the dose is sufficient, cell death results. The incidence of osteonecrosis has been progressively reduced with the introduction of higher kilovoltage techniques. Spontaneous fracture may occur in the devitalized bone, and subsequent attempts at repair, as discussed previously, may result in the development of areas of increased density. It is important that these should not be interpreted as osteoblastic metastases and subjected to still more radiation. Such errors have occurred with avascular necrosis in the pelvis following irradiation for carcinoma of the cervix. Therapeutic radiation involving the region of a growing epiphysis can result in premature fusion.

b. **Thermal effects.** *Frostbite* may be followed by intense osteoporosis of terminal phalanges after about 10 days and the development of avascular necrosis, bone resorption without new bone formation, and premature fusion of epiphyses in children. Secondary ulceration and sepsis predispose to osteomyelitis. Some severe *burns* have been followed by avascular necrosis of bone.

c. **Dysbaric osteonecrosis (caisson disease).** Over-rapid decompression from high atmospheric pressures in tunnel workers and deep-sea divers is believed to result in the liberation of nitrogen bubbles in the blood stream which are responsible for the painful condition known as 'the bends'. These bubbles may block capillaries and cause avascular necrosis in bone. Irregular areas of increased bone density may be found, indicative of earlier medullary infarctions (see Ch. 3). Although usually without symptoms, the most common regions to show radiographic change are the shafts of long bones, often in the lower limbs. More important in terms of sequelae are infarctions in the medulla, at the ends of long bones, just deep to the subarticular cortex. The commonest site for such changes is the humeral head; the femoral head is next most commonly affected. The earliest radiographic signs constitute subtle densities, which may progress to linear lucencies in the subarticular bone. Structural collapse or dissecting lesions may follow (Fig. 9.43). It should be remembered that similar infarctions of articular surfaces occur in Gaucher's disease, sickle-cell disease (see Ch. 7) and chronic alcoholism with pancreatitis.

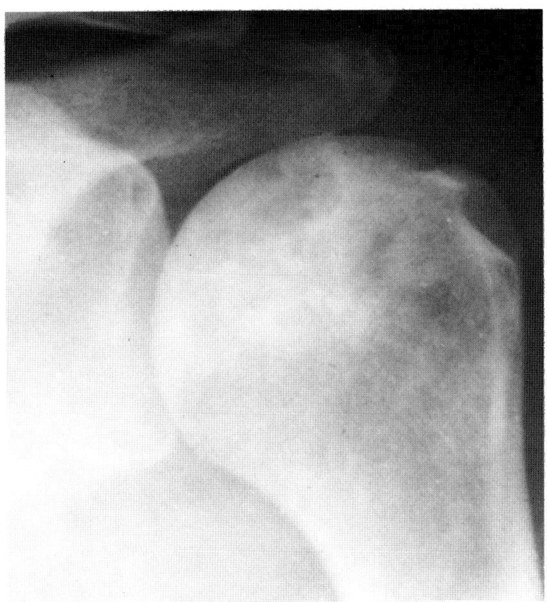

Fig. 9.43 Dysbaric osteonecrosis. Sclerosis is present in the medulla of the humeral head, indicating repair of the infarct. Some lucency in the subarticular bone is associated with evidence of early structural collapse.

SKELETAL LESIONS OCCURRING WITH DIMINUTION OF PAIN SENSE (NEUROPATHIC)

The reflex action of muscular contraction in response to painful stimuli is of inestimable value in the protection of bones and joints from damage. Repeated trauma in the absence of normal pain and proprioceptive sensation is responsible for the severe arthropathies known as Charcot joints. These were described in 1868 by the great French neurologist, whose name they bear, long before the advent of radiology. This eponym has become almost synonymous with the lesions of neurosyphilis, but it is evident that some of Charcot's original cases were caused by syringomyelia. As both diseases have declined in incidence during recent years, other causes of neuropathic changes have been recognized increasingly. It should be appreciated that such joints need not necessarily be painless, as a diminution of pain sense just sufficient to destroy the protective reflexes may be responsible for their production. Similarly, the occurrence of relatively painless fractures, though less common, must be recognized. Fixation of these joints and fractures by operative measures is frequently unsuccessful,

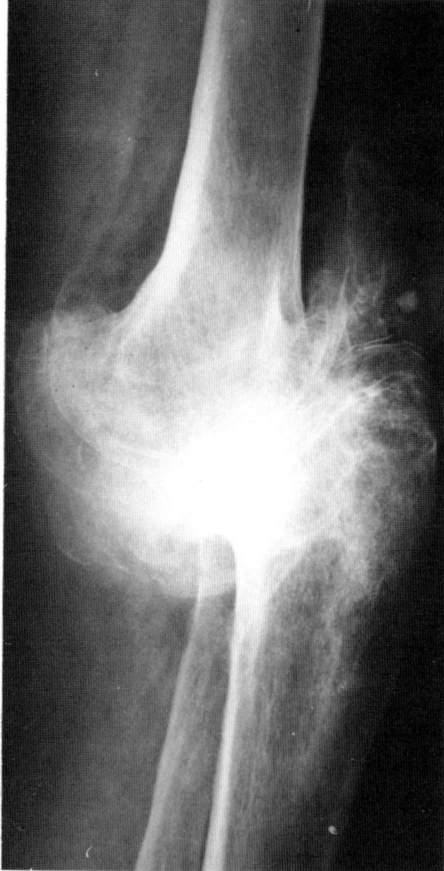

Fig. 9.44

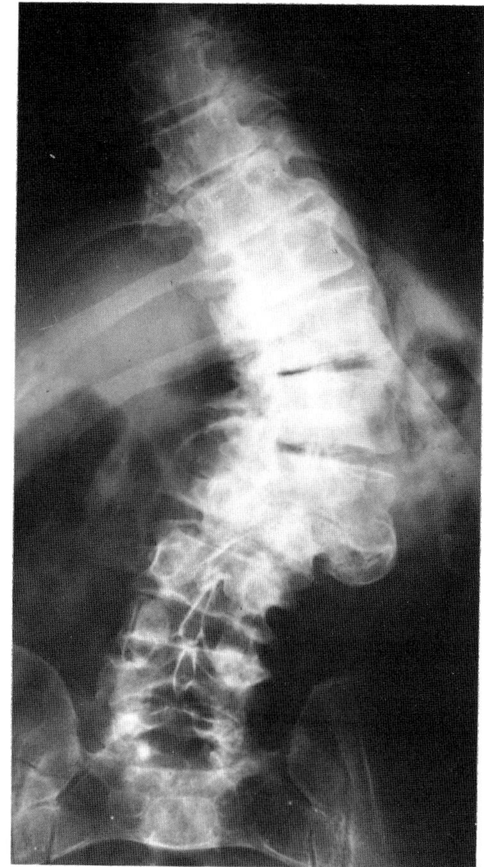

Fig. 9.45

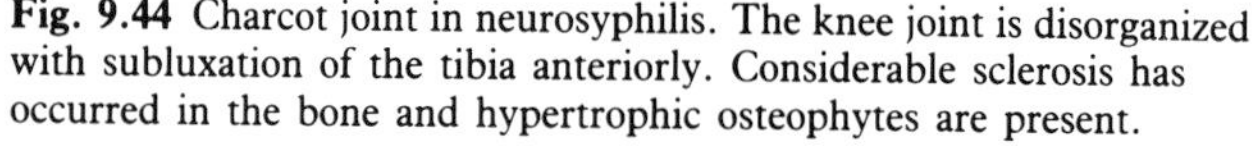

Fig. 9.44 Charcot joint in neurosyphilis. The knee joint is disorganized with subluxation of the tibia anteriorly. Considerable sclerosis has occurred in the bone and hypertrophic osteophytes are present.

Fig. 9.45 Charcot spine. This patient was noted to have a painless prominence in the lumbar region caused by the kyphoscoliosis shown here on X-ray examination. Although narrowing of the disc spaces and osteophyte formation simulates degenerative spondylosis, the lateral subluxation in the upper lumbar region is typical of a neuropathic spine (the 'tumbling bricks' appearance).

Fig. 9.46 Syringomyelia. Among the neuropathic changes observe the straight margin of the defect which almost simulates surgical intervention. Marginal sclerosis is a prominent feature.

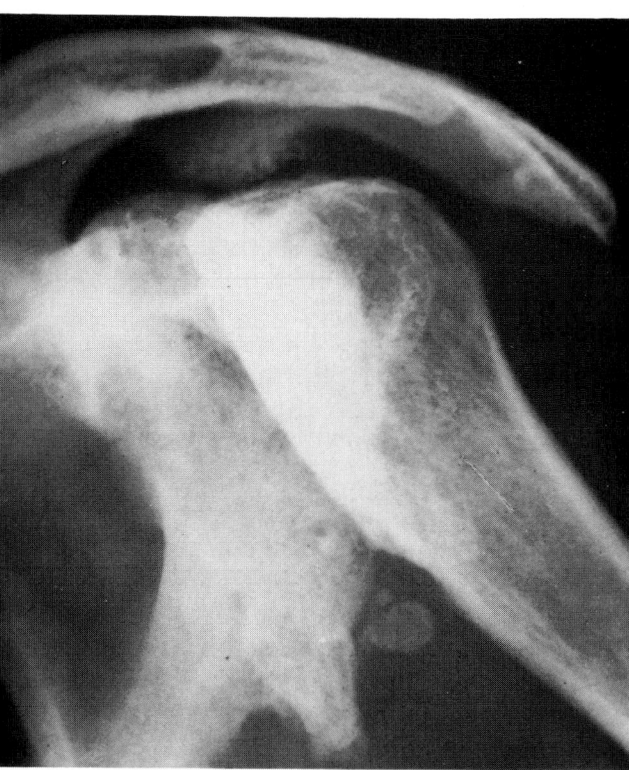

Fig. 9.46

and if fixation is achieved, similar changes may develop proximally or distally to the original lesion. The following causes should be considered:

a. **Neurosyphilis**. Disintegration of joint surfaces may produce most bizarre clinical findings with painless hypermobility and deformity. Instability, swelling and deformity are the common complaints. Serial radiological examinations show progressive destruction with multiple loose fragments of bone (Fig. 9.44). These may be ground down into myriads of minute bone particles, so that the radiological appearance may suggest amorphous calcification.

'he margin of the area of destruction may be so straight nd clearly defined as to suggest previous surgical intervention. Dislocation and derangement of the affected joints s frequent. An important diagnostic feature, common to nost neuropathic lesions in the absence of complicating nfection, is preservation of normal bone density, or even n actual increase of periarticular sclerosis. The lower imbs are more commonly affected than the upper, the nee being particularly susceptible; small joints are relaively exempt. Involvement of the lumbar spine may lead o considerable deformity, including scoliosis, and cause oss of height. The appearance in the frontal view has been ikened to 'tumbling bricks' (Fig. 9.45). Spinal changes all ppear to be neurosyphilitic in origin. The progression rom an initial and apparently trivial or unnoticed injury o gross disorganization may take less than a year. These esions are essentially traumatic and must not be confused vith syphilitic osteitis. The main radiological differential liagnosis is severe degenerative joint disease.

b. **Syringomyelia.** In this condition pressure on the racts in the cervical portion of the spinal cord by a syrinx s responsible for loss of pain sense in the upper limbs. The houlder, and to a lesser extent, elbow and wrist are the ites of predilection; radiological appearances are identical o those of neurosyphilis (Fig. 9.46). Again, the small oints are rarely affected.

c. **Congenital indifference to pain (congenital asymbolia).** A number of cases of this rare neurological disorder ave been reported. Affected children are able, without pain, to undertake physical feats such as jumping from a height, which are quite impossible for their normal contemporaries. As a result, they suffer from neuropathies and painless fractures, especially of the lower limbs (Fig. 9.47). The skin is usually extensively scarred from numerous abrasions and burns. These, though frequently infected, remain painless. Even the lesions of a complicating osteomyelitis may attract attention only through associated pyrexia.

d. **Spina bifida** is sometimes accompanied by complete or partial loss of pain sense in a lower limb, often in the ankle and foot, thus precipitating similar neuropathic changes. If these are found in a child, either this condition or congenital indifference to pain should be suspected, since neurosyphilitic lesions are unknown at this age. As with other neuropathic conditions, trophic ulcers on the feet may develop with secondary bone infection.

Neuropathic fractures in children are productive of a quite abnormal amount of reparative callus. The first

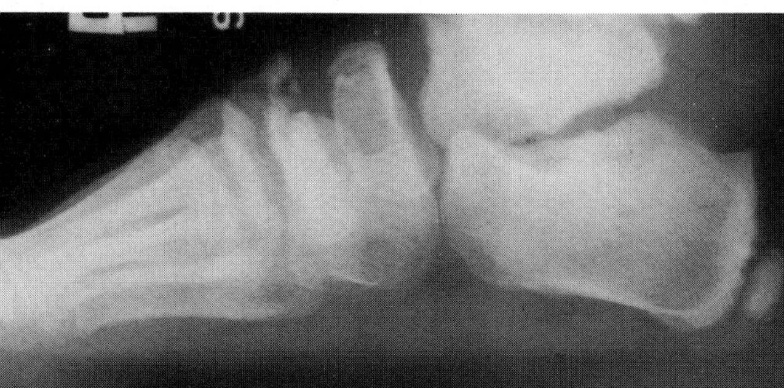

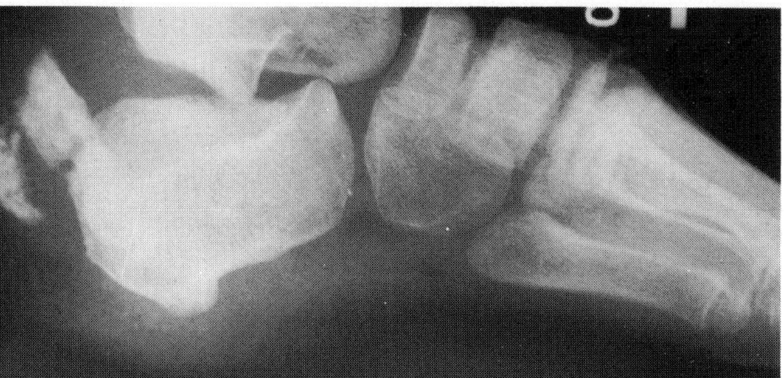

'ig. **9.47** Congenital absence of pain sense. These neuropathic joint hanges and fractures caused deformity without pain in the feet of this '-year-old girl who had delighted in showing that she could jump lown from a much greater height than her contemporaries.

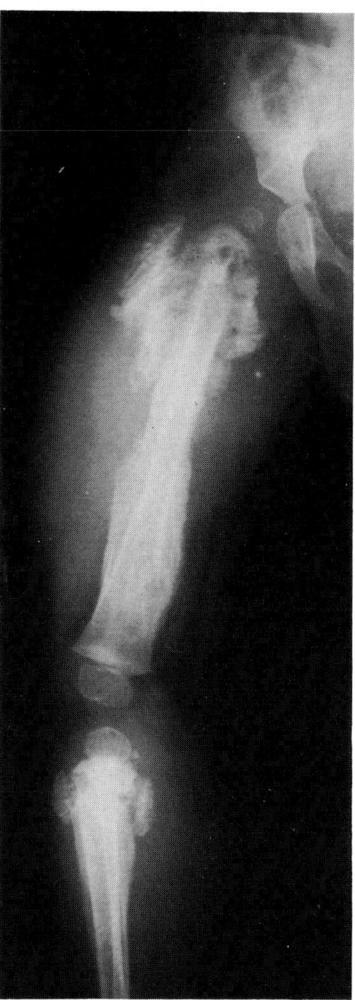

Fig. 9.48 Neuropathic fractures in the paralysed limb of a child. Note the large amount of reparative callus. Such lesions are often discovered only incidentally.

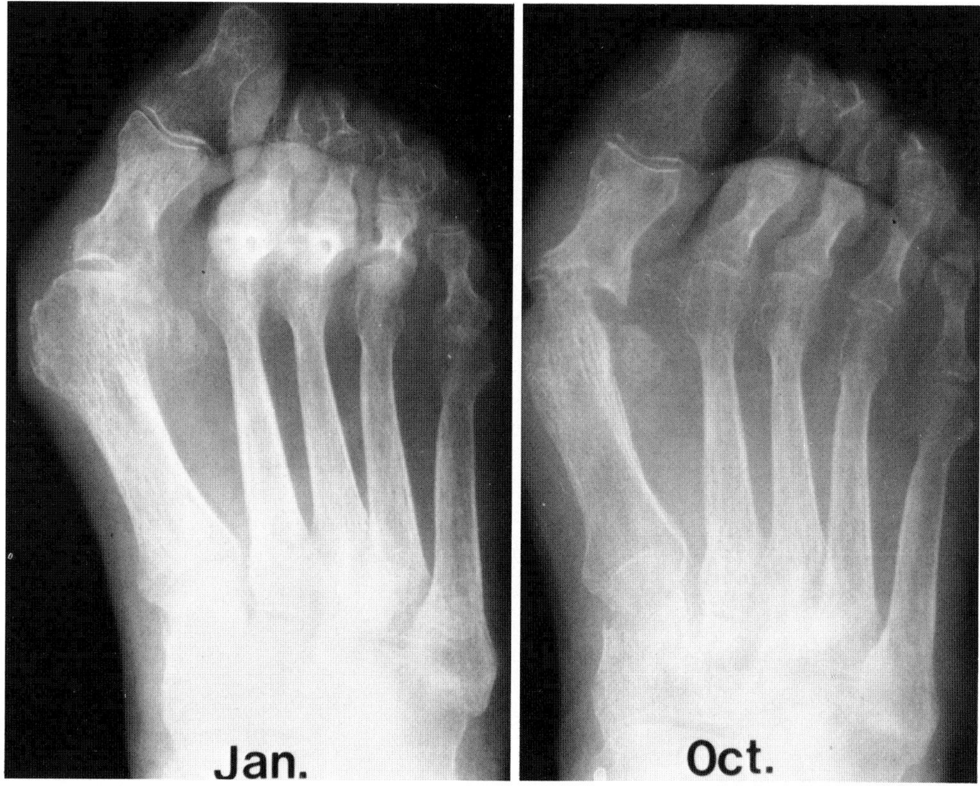

Fig. 9.49 Diabetic foot. Periarticular osteoporosis is present but erosive change involves the head of the first metatarsal and progress is shown on the serial films. The predilection for osteomyelitis and infective arthritis of the first metatarsophalangeal joint is almost always due to an associate penetrating ulcer on the sole of the foot.

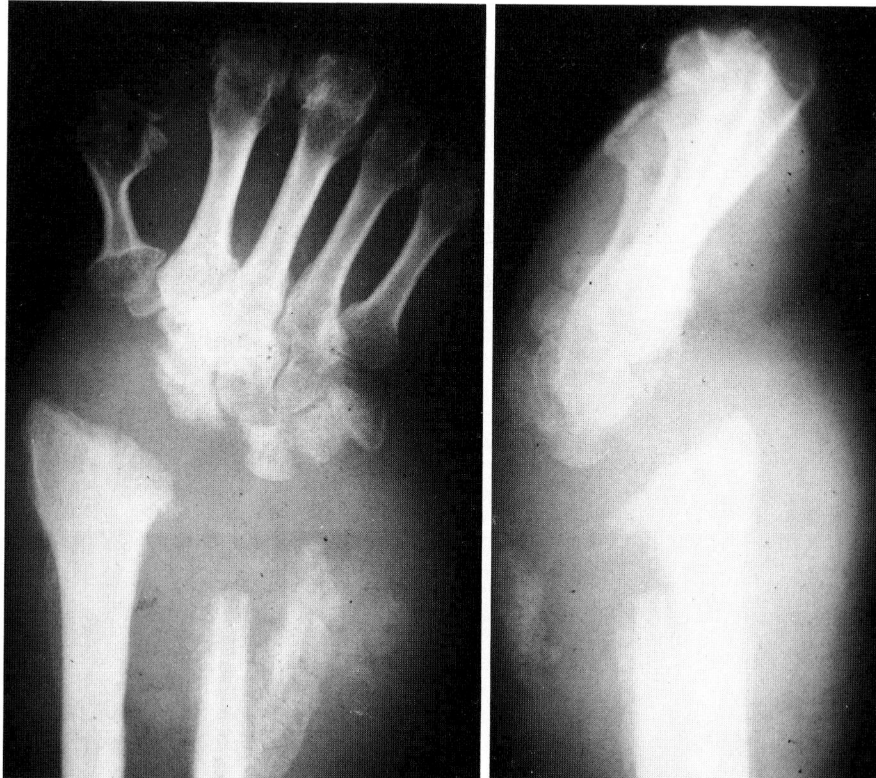

Fig. 9.50 Leprosy. Destructive change is present in the wrist and carpus without loss of bone density, confirming the neuropathic nature of the disorder. The large soft tissue swelling reflects secondary infection which in this patient was painless.

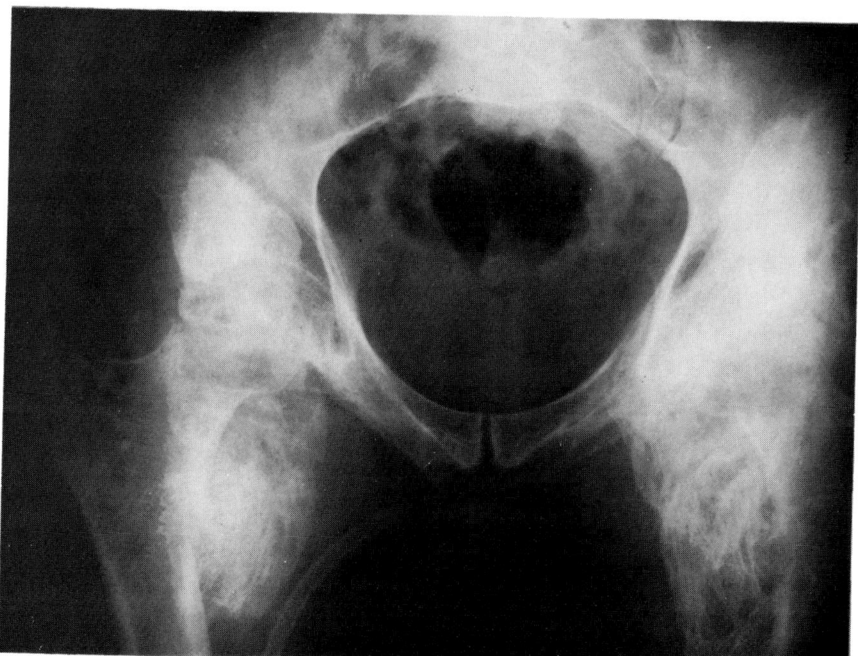

Fig. 9.51 Myositis ossificans associated with paraplegia. Very extensive soft tissue ossification is visible round both hip joints.

indication of such a lesion may be the clinical observation of a large bony mass, which may even be suspected of representing a bone tumour (Fig. 9.48). Fractures of this type presumably result from inadvertent damage in children; they are not observed in adults.

e. **Diabetic neuropathy.** The changes essentially affect the small joints of the feet and it has been suggested that this is due to loss of peripheral pain sense through vascular starvation of sensory nerves (Fig. 9.49). Neuropathies have developed without the formation of trophic ulcers, so that they cannot be attributed to infection, although the subsequent development of this complication is common. Arterial calcification is a frequent finding. The combination of neuropathy, vascular insufficiency and infection results in the final disability of the diabetic foot.

f. **Leprosy.** Impaired pain sensation in this condition causes neuropathic changes in the hands and feet. In the former, the interphalangeal joints and, in the latter, the metatarso-phalangeal joints are especially prone to this development, each corresponding to the zones of maximum movement (Fig. 9.50). (See Ch. 3). Disintegration of tarsal bones may occur and neurotrophic changes leading to the 'sucked barley sugar' appearance of phalanges and metatarsals.

7. **Paralytic conditions,** such as poliomyelitis, are sometimes complicated by fractures in a paralysed limb. These result from the vulnerability of the hypoplastic bone to stress. They are not truly neuropathic as no sensory deficit exists. Adults, however, do occasionally develop neuropathic changes in a paralysed limb and a further radiological complication which must be considered in paraplegic patients is the appearance of extensive soft tissue ossification, usually described as myositis ossificans (Fig. 9.51) (See Ch. 55).

REFERENCES AND SUGGESTIONS FOR FURTHER READING

See end of Chapter 10.

CHAPTER 10

SKELETAL TRAUMA — REGIONAL

It is not possible in the space available to describe the many varieties of fractures that may affect the skeleton and for detailed consideration the reader is referred to textbooks specifically devoted to these subjects. In this chapter we can draw attention only to common injuries and to those in which correct radiological interpretation is of particular importance.

THE SHOULDER AND ARM

The clavicle may be fractured during the passage of the fetus through the birth canal. This is the commonest of such birth injuries and occurs at the junction of the middle and distal thirds of the bone.

The common fracture in later life follows a fall on the outstretched arm. The fragments often overlap considerably and their anatomical relationship may be demonstrated by a supero-inferior view obtained with the patient leaning forward over the film. Accurate reduction is desirable to avoid a residual cosmetic defect. Dislocation or subluxation of the acromio-clavicular joint (Fig. 10.1) may follow similar trauma or a fall on to the point of the shoulder. Although increased width of the joint space may be demonstrated by an erect film of both shoulders with heavy weights in the patient's hands, the examination is often unrewarding. This is mainly due to the patient lifting the weights rather than letting his arms hang down and to the overall inadequacy of the stress employed. Very rarely, dislocations of the sterno-clavicular joints occur. Clinical suspicion of such a deformity often requires tomography for confirmation.

Post-traumatic osteolysis of the clavicle may follow such injuries or affect those undertaking repetitive occupational movements at the shoulder. Essentially this is a post-traumatic arthritis in which the resorption of the outer end of the clavicle is an occasional complication in a few patients.

The shoulder is a frequent site of injury. Frank *dislocations* occur, most usually in an anterior direction, so that the head of the humerus lies in a *subcoracoid* location (Fig. 10.2A and B). The characteristic deformity makes the diagnosis apparent clinically. The articular surfaces of the humeral head and the glenoid fossa should normally be parallel to each other. A *posterior* dislocation is relatively rare. These injuries are usually associated with severe muscle spasm, such as occurs with electric shocks and epilepsy, but also occur in contact sports. Although no instantly recognizable clinical deformity is present, dislocation should be suspected by the almost complete loss of external rotation. It is important that a true antero-posterior projection of the shoulder joint is taken, i.e. with the patient rotated at least 30 degrees to the affected side. With the glenoid articulation in profile therefore, any loss of parallelism or overlap by the humeral head must indicate it is dislocated (Fig. 10.3). The humeral head may through its abnormal rotation present an abnormally circular 'light bulb' appearance, again with loss of the normal parallel relationship of the gleno-humeral surfaces

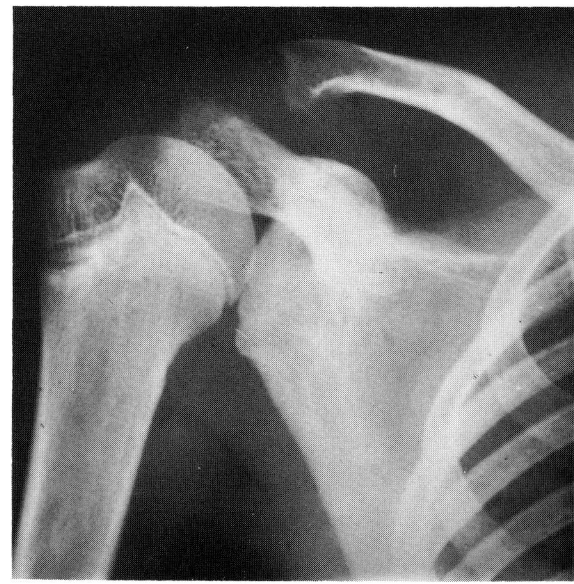

Fig. 10.1 Dislocation of the acromio-clavicular joint following a fall on the point of the shoulder. The deformity is accentuated by examination in the erect position with weights being carried in both hands.

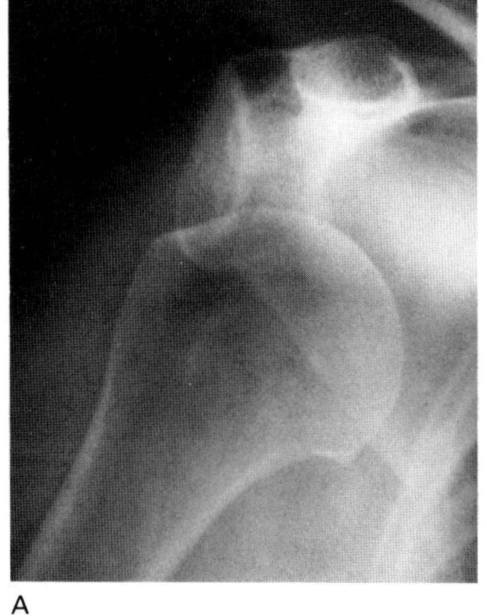

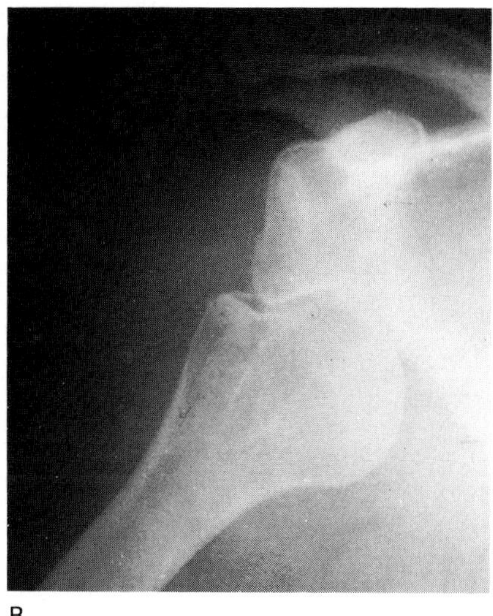

Fig. 10.2 Subcoracoid (anterior) dislocation of the shoulder. **A**. The humeral head is displaced forward, medially and inferiorly to lie in the subscapular fossa. **B**. Luxio erecta: the humeral head has lodged below the glenoid fossa, so that the humerus is abducted. This is a rarer type of injury. The pressure defect on the outer part of the humeral head caused by the inferior rim of the glenoid fossa illustrates clearly the mechanism whereby a recurrent dislocation defect is produced.

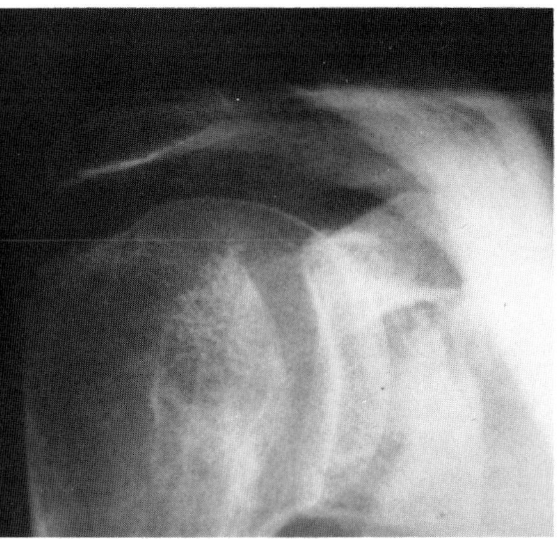

Fig. 10.3 Posterior dislocation of the humerus. The glenoid process is seen in profile yet is overlapped by the humeral head, which must therefore be dislocated. In an anterior dislocation the humeral head would be depressed, so the dislocation must be posterior even without a confirmatory additional projection. The patient was an epileptic.

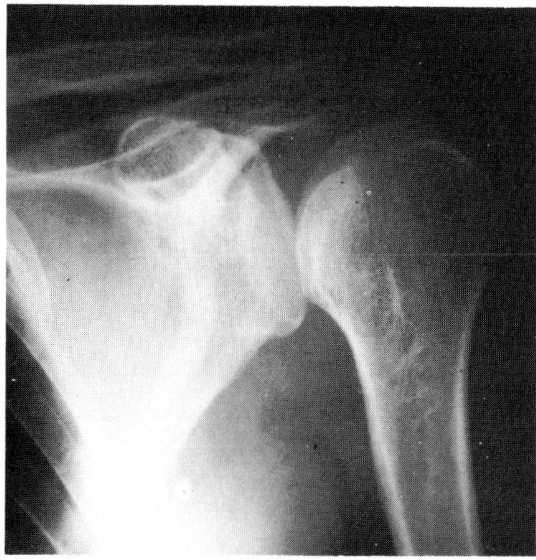

Fig. 10.4 Posterior dislocation of the shoulder. Note the circular appearance of the humeral head and the lack of parallelism between this and the glenoid fossa. The injury followed a severe electric shock causing muscle spasm, which had also precipitated compression fractures of the fifth and sixth thoracic vertebral bodies in this patient. (Courtesy of Dr J. L. Boldero).

(Fig. 10.4). In addition, as in all cases of shoulder injury, an *axial view* should be taken, with the X-ray beam centred on the axilla from below to a film held horizontally above the joint.

Thus, posterior dislocation presents the problem of non-reduction; when the dislocation is recognized and reduced, it usually remains stable, having been caused by unusual force. In anterior dislocation, the main complication is recurrence of the dislocation, made possible by either capsular damage or detachment of part of the glenoid labrum (the 'Bankart' lesion). During the course of dislocation, the humeral head often sustains a compression fracture on its posterolateral aspect against the hard edge of the glenoid labrum (Fig. 10.5). Such a defect does not necessarily indicate recurrent dislocation as it can occur after a single episode; its identification is however valuable when other evidence to support the diagnosis or direction of a previous dislocation is missing. Such a defect was recognized by anatomists in the late eighteenth century and radiologically in 1898. When the abnormality is large, the term 'hatchet' defect is usefully descriptive. Although it can be visualized sometimes on the axial view and on 60 degrees internal rotation, it is shown most consistently by means of the Stryker projection (Fig. 10.6).

The rotator cuff is the name applied to the expansion of the conjoined tendons of the supraspinatus, infraspinatus, teres minor and subscapularis muscles just before their insertion into the greater tuberosity of the humerus.

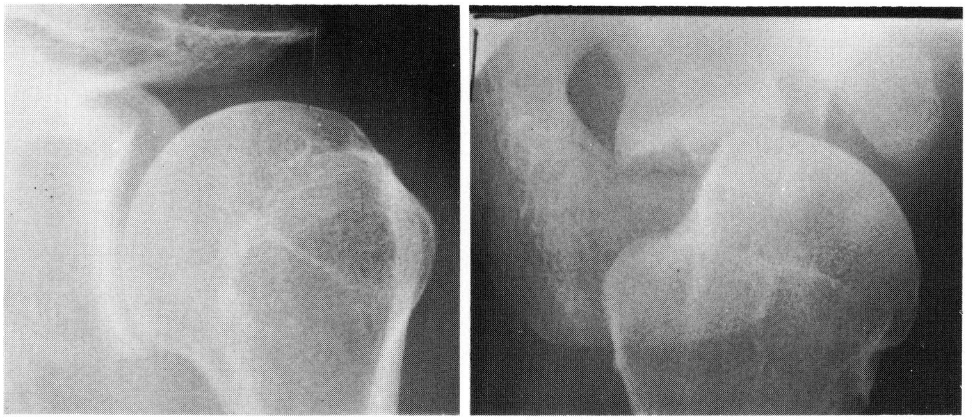

Fig. 10.5 A. and **B.** Recurrent anterior dislocation of the shoulder. The characteristic 'hatchet' defect is well shown in the axial projection. A large defect of this nature is even clearly visualized in the AP projection. It is however rarely possible to identify small defects on a simple frontal projection; in addition to the axial view, a film in 60 degrees internal rotation or a Stryker view may be required.

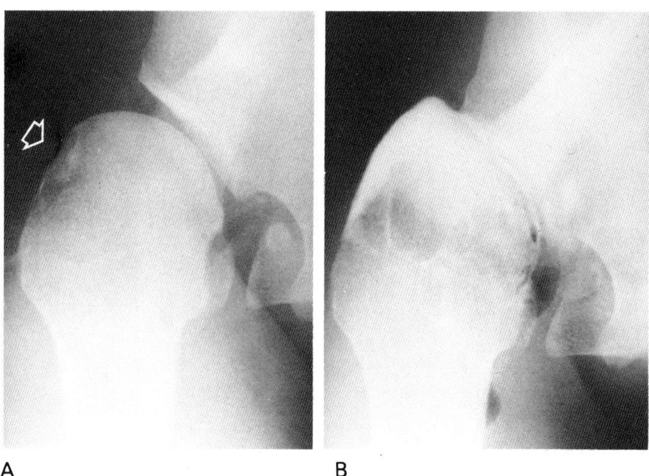

Fig. 10.6 A. and **B.** Recurrent anterior dislocation (Stryker projection). This offers the best and most consistent opportunity to demonstrate the defect, particularly if it is small (arrow). **A.** Plain radiograph; **B.** During double contrast arthrography. As the patient is supine and the defect posterior, it fills with the positive contrast medium.

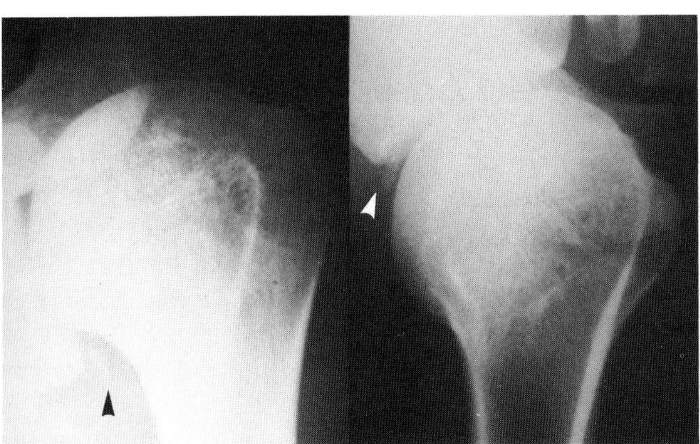

Fig. 10.7 Avulsion fracture of glenoid. A young footballer involved in a collision with two other players sustained an anterior dislocation of the shoulder. The bony fragment revealed on a subsequent examination was the avulsed bony origin of the long head of the triceps.

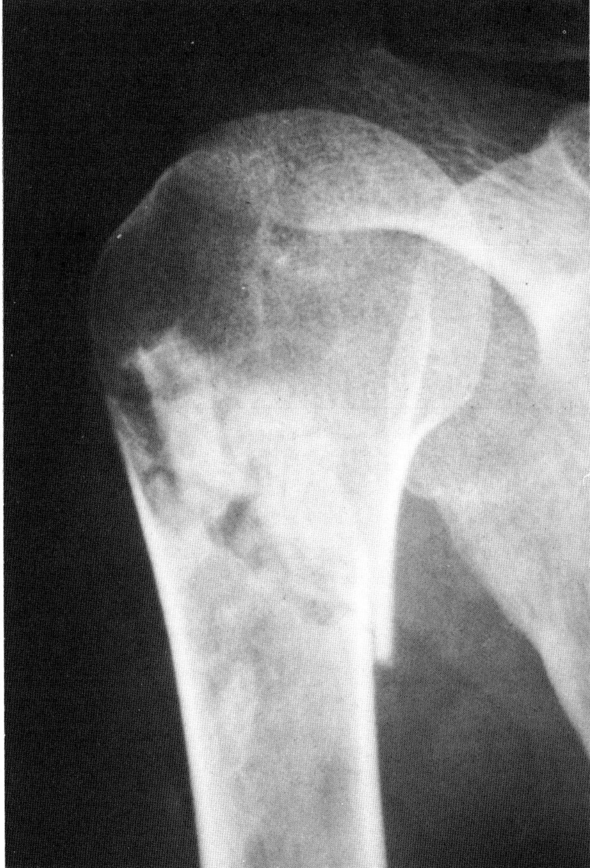

Fig. 10.8 Fracture of surgical neck of humerus. This fracture shows comminution of its margins; it united in satisfactory position with conservative management.

Tears of the rotator cuff are often sustained in fractures and dislocations at the shoulder joint. More commonly, patients present with a painful arc of abduction due to a chronic tear of the rotator cuff in the absence of bony injury; such tears may be confirmed by shoulder arthrography.

The scapula. Being protected by its site and covering by muscles, the scapula is rarely injured without severe trauma. Four-fifths of such injuries involve the body or neck and their radiological demonstration is simple; a tangential projection should always supplement the frontal view.

Fracture of the coracoid process or the glenoid rim may accompany anterior dislocation of the humerus and injuries of this type may require axial or angled views for their demonstration. It is less well recognized that fractures of the margins and processes of the scapula may result from avulsion or resisted stress at muscle attachments (Fig. 10.7).

The proximal humerus. The common site of fracture is the surgical neck. The patient is usually a female in middle life who has fallen on her outstretched hand. Associated fissure fractures of the greater tuberosity are common. Such fractures are often impacted, but anteroposterior and lateral projections are required to exclude displacement (Fig. 10.8). More extensive fractures are described by the Neer classification as one, two, three of four-part fractures. The numbers relate to the number of fragments and their degree of angulation or displacement (Neer, 1970).

The humeral shaft. Such fractures are relatively

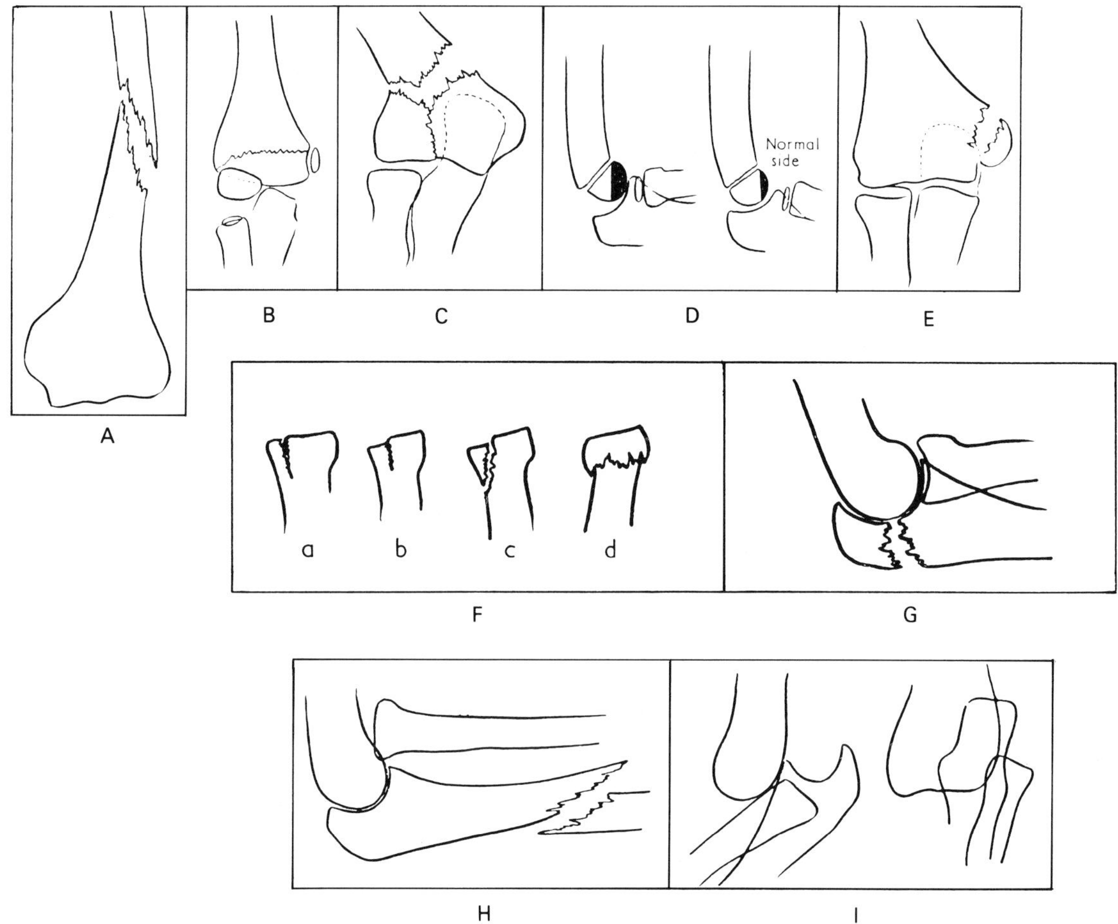

Fig. 10.9 Injuries round the elbow joint. **A.** *Spiral fracture of distal humeral shaft.* This fracture is often associated with damage to the radial nerve. **B.** *Supracondylar fracture of humerus* in a child. **C.** *Supracondylar fracture of humerus* in an adult. Observe the extension of the fracture line downwards to involve the articular surface. **D.** *Forward displacement of the distal humeral epiphysis in a child.* The degree of displacement is shown by comparison of the shaded areas in the normal and abnormal sides. In children it is always advisable to compare the radiographs of the suspected injury with those of its normal counterpart. **E.** *Avulsion fracture of medial epicondyle of humerus.* This point is the weak link in the extensor system of the forearm and, in children especially, it is possible for the detached fragment to be trapped within the joint. In such injuries the relationship of the head of the radius to the capitulum always must be assessed consciously, to avoid failure to recognize subluxation. **F.** *Types of fracture of radial head*: (a) Vertical crack in the outer third; (b) a similar lesion with depression of the lateral fragment; and (c) with detachment of this fragment; (d) a transverse fracture of the radial neck with impaction and some disturbance of alignment. **G.** *Fracture of olecranon process of ulna.* **H.** *Monteggia fracture-dislocation.* Overlap of the oblique ulnar fracture with an intact radius has resulted in forward dislocation of the radial head. Posterior dislocation of the radial head with this injury is considerably less common. **I.** *Postero-lateral dislocation of the elbow.* These injuries are often complicated by separation of the tip of the coronoid process of the ulna.

common but heal satisfactorily, usually without complication. Damage to the radial nerve affects less than one in six patients. The injury is usually a fall or a motor accident, but torsion fractures, as in throwing sports or arm wrestling, are described.

Fractures round the elbow joint (Fig. 10.9)

The distal humerus. The supracondylar fracture accounts for 60% of all fractures about the elbow in children. The fracture is transverse and results from a fall on the outstretched hand. The distal fragment is displaced anteriorly and rotated to a varying degree. The fracture line may be difficult to identify and the frontal view is usually less than satisfactory owing to the limitation of extension. The lateral projection will usually reveal a haemarthrosis displacing one or both fat pads (Fig. 10.10) and a line drawn along the anterior cortex of the humerus does not traverse the middle third of the capitulum (Fig. 10.11). The normal *carrying angle* at the elbow is of the order of 170 degrees, but greater in females than males. A cubitus varus deformity may occur following a supracondylar fracture and lead to difficulty in carrying or throwing. An increased carrying angle, cubitus valgus, may lead later to symptoms from pressure on the ulnar nerve.

A fracture of the lateral condyle is the second commonest injury to the elbow in childhood. It is usually an oblique fracture-separation involving the joint surface.

Fractures of the distal humerus in adults rarely present diagnostic problems; they are transverse, T or Y-shaped, involving the articular surface in the majority of cases.

The medial epicondyle in children is an apophysis that gives origin to the common flexor muscles. Avulsion can occur as a result of valgus stress during a fall. The epicondyle is displaced distally and can become trapped within the temporarily widened joint space (Fig. 10.12). Rarely, paralysis of the posteriorly located ulnar nerve accompanies this injury. The radiologist has a responsibility to diagnose epicondylar entrapment by identifying the avulsed fragment within the joint and noting the absence of the epicondylar centre from its normal position.

A working familiarity with the normal development of

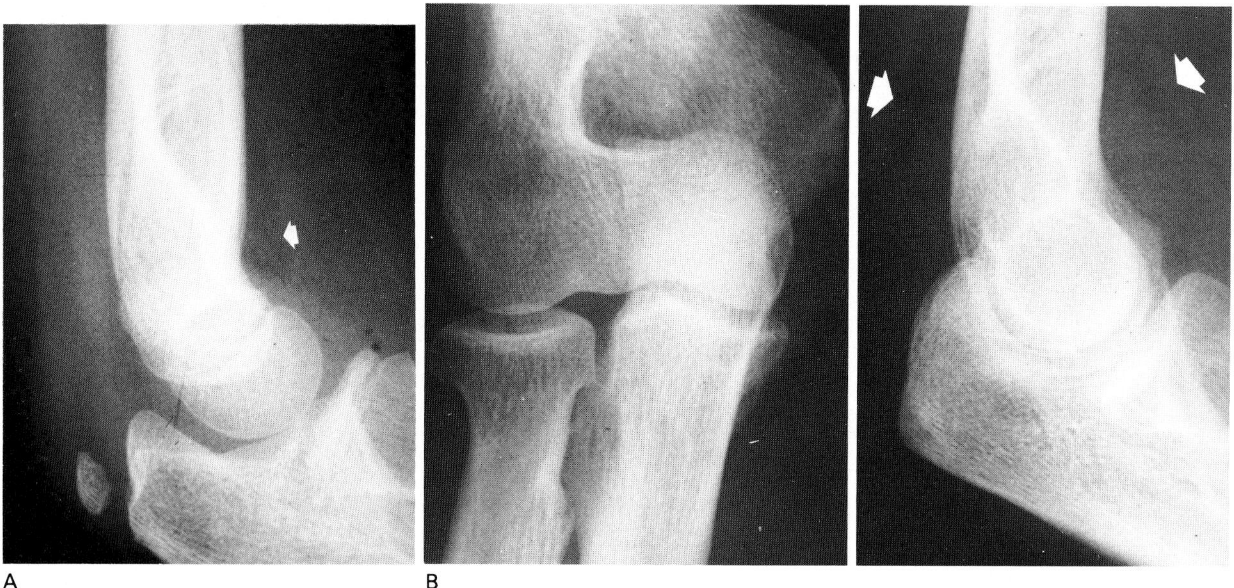

Fig. 10.10 Post-traumatic effusion of the elbow joint. **A.** Lateral projection of a child's normal elbow. The posterior fat pad is not visible. The anterior fat pad (arrow) is seen in a normal location, applied to the cortex of the distal part of the shaft of the humerus. **B.** An undisplaced fracture of the radial head is demonstrated on the AP film. In the lateral projection, an associated haemarthrosis has displaced the anterior fat pad anteriorly.

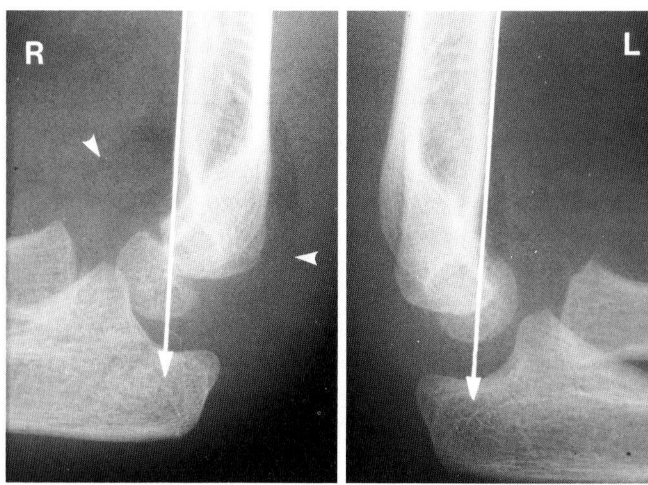

Fig. 10.11 Supracondylar fracture of humerus. The left humerus is normal; the line extending from the anterior cortex of the shaft passes through the middle third of the capitellum. A haemarthrosis of the right elbow joint displaces both fat pads and a similar line cuts the posterior third of the capitellum, indicating the anterior displacement of the fragment.

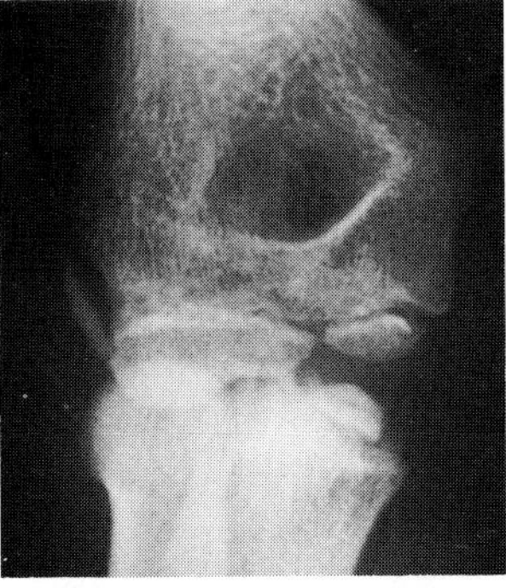
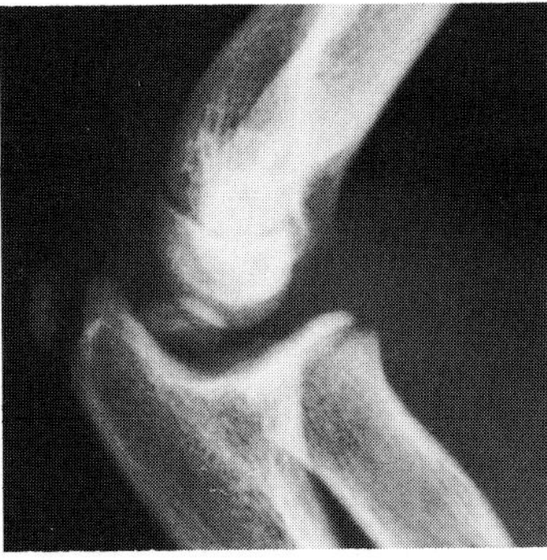

Fig. 10.12 Avulsion of medial epicondyle of the humerus. The centre for the lateral epicondyle has ossified in this child, therefore the medial epicondyle also should have appeared. It is not in its normal location but lies within the medial compartment of the elbow joint.

the ossification centres around the elbow is essential; this will indicate that, as the medial epicondyle ossifies before the lateral, the absence of the medial centre while the lateral one is in correct position should suggest that the medial epicondyle is displaced. Table 10.1 gives a mnemonic, helpful in recalling the order in which ossification takes place.

Table 10.1 Mnemonic — to recall the order in which ossification takes place.

		Rough age of first ossification
Can	Capitellum	1
Radiology	Radius	5
Make	Medial epicondyle	7
Trauma	Trochlear	10
Less	Lateral epicondyle	11
Obscure	Olecranon	11

(**NB** Ossification varies widely with the individual and its gender. Such figures as are given here owe less to complete accuracy than to the aid to memory of a rhythmical scan!)

Fracture of the capitellum may be associated with fracture of the radial head. A shearing force, however, can result in the intra-articular displacement of a segment of the capitellum which thereby becomes an osteochondral loose body (Fig. 10.13).

The head and neck of the radius. Fracture of the radial head is the commonest elbow injury in adults (Fig. 10.9F). About half of such fractures are undisplaced; the fracture involves the joint surface and is vertical (Figs. 10.10B and 10.14). A fracture should be suspected in the presence of radiographic evidence of a joint effusion. Because the elbow joint consists of more than one articulation, two standard views may prove inadequate and need to be supplemented by oblique or pronated projections.

The equivalent injury in the child or adolescent is an epiphyseal fracture-separation (Fig. 9.4) (mostly Salter–Harris II). Purely metaphyseal fractures of the radial neck are also observed in children.

The proximal end of the ulna. Fractures of the olecranon are less common than those of the radial head and neck; they result from a direct injury such as a fall on to the point of the elbow or indirectly from a fall in the outstretched hand. The common injury is a transverse fracture across the deepest part of the olecranon notch (Fig. 10.9G). Separation may occur as a result of the pull of the triceps muscle. Fractures of the coronoid process may complicate elbow dislocations.

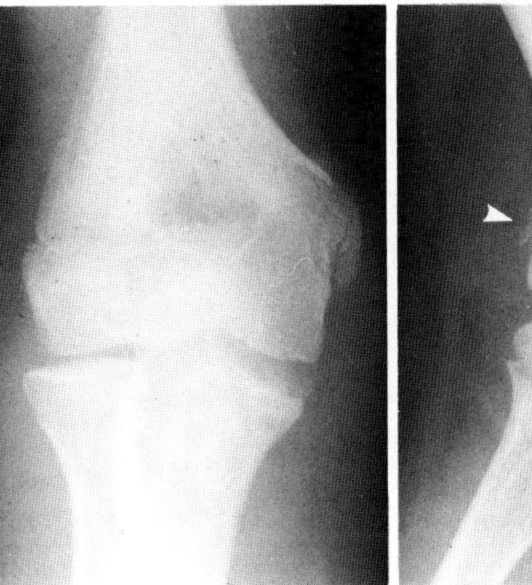
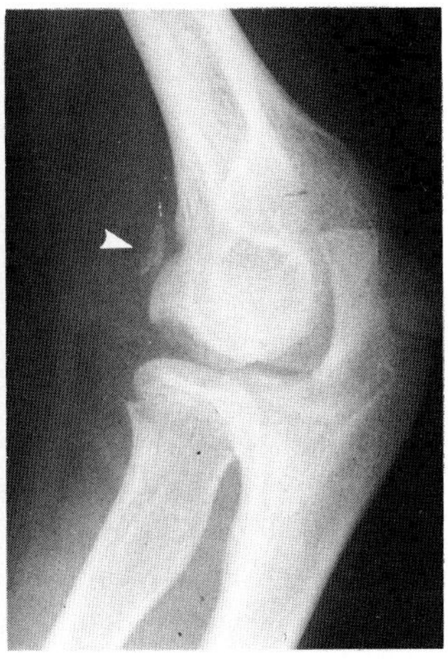

Fig. 10.13 Osteochondral fracture of the capitellum. This child complained of recurrent pain and stiffness of the elbow. The defect of the surface of the capitellum is seen best in the oblique view with the detached partially-ossified fragment lying within the synovial cavity above it (arrow). The loose body was removed at operation.

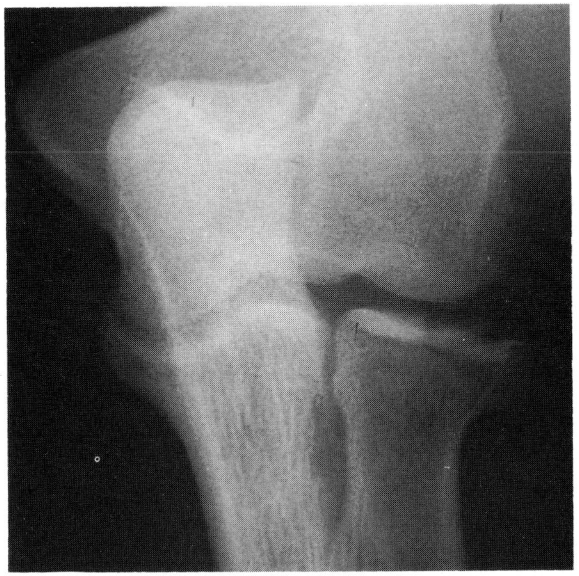

Fig. 10.14 Vertical fracture of head of radius. This typical injury resulted from a fall on the outstretched arm.

Dislocations at the elbow. Almost 90% of elbow dislocations are posterior or posterolateral; their radiographic demonstration is usually easy, but associated fractures should be sought and identified on post-reduction views. The severe soft tissue injury required to dislocate the elbow is sometimes complicated by the formation of heterotopic bone (myositis ossificans).

Isolated *dislocation of the head of the radius* is uncommon and should not be diagnosed before an associated fracture of the ulnar shaft is excluded. The combination of these two injuries is the *Monteggia* fracture-dislocation (Figs. 9.17 and 10.15).

Most radial dislocations are anterior in situation. Confirmation of dislocation or subluxation is achieved by showing that an axial radial line does not pass through the centre of the capitulum. In the normal subject such a transection occurs, whatever the radiographic projection (Fig. 10.16).

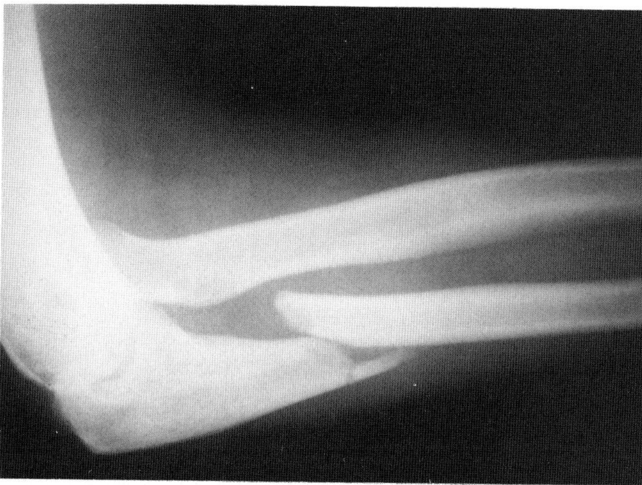

Fig. 10.15 Monteggia fracture-dislocation. The ulna is fractured obliquely in its proximal third with some shortening. The radial head is dislocated anteriorly, thus accommodating the ulnar shortening without fracture of the radius.

Fractures of the shafts of the forearm bones. These are quite common. Usually both bones are fractured during a fall, but the shaft of a single bone may fracture as a result of a direct blow, such as the *parry* fracture of the ulna, when the arm is raised to protect the face. In all cases, radiographic examination of the forearm bones should include both the elbow and wrist. When a single forearm bone is fractured in a fall an associated dislocation can be expected. The commoner *Monteggia* fracture-dislocation combines an ulnar fracture, usually of the proximal one-third of the shaft with a dislocation of the radial head, usually anteriorly (Fig. 10.15). The *Galeazzi* fracture-dislocation is characterized by an oblique displaced fracture of the radial shaft in its distal third and disruption of the distal radio-ulnar joint (Fig. 10.17).

Fractures of the distal radius and ulna. One of the commonest sites for fracture. Many are designated by eponyms.

Colles' fracture usually affects the older person, particularly females, and is caused by a fall on the outstretched hand. This is essentially a rotational fracture but the radiologist can usually recognize and quantify only impaction and posterior angulation; the element of supination is almost impossible to evaluate. Radiographic appearances are obvious (Fig. 10.18) and the ulnar styloid is fractured incidentally in over 50% of cases. It is important to remember that the normal radial articular surface in the lateral projection is angulated 10–15 degrees in a palmar direction. A post-reduction position that does not restore at least a neutral position will restrict the patient's grip function in the future and can only be accepted in an elderly subject with limited physical expectations.

Smith's fracture (reversed Colles' fracture) is less frequent and resembles a Colles' fracture in the frontal

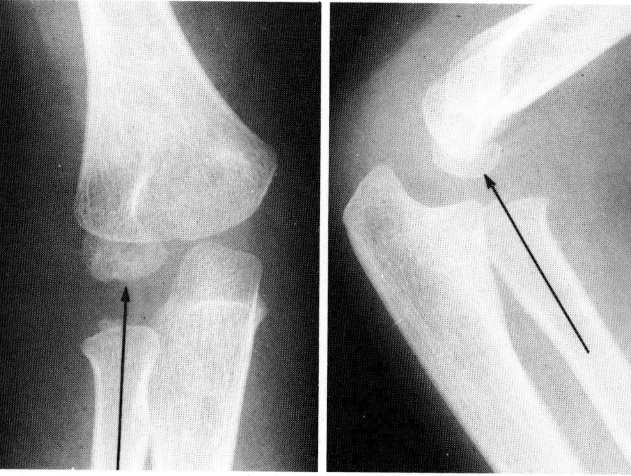

Fig. 10.16 Normal elbow. An axial line through the radius will always transect the centre of the capitellum. If it does not, either the radius or the capitellum is displaced.

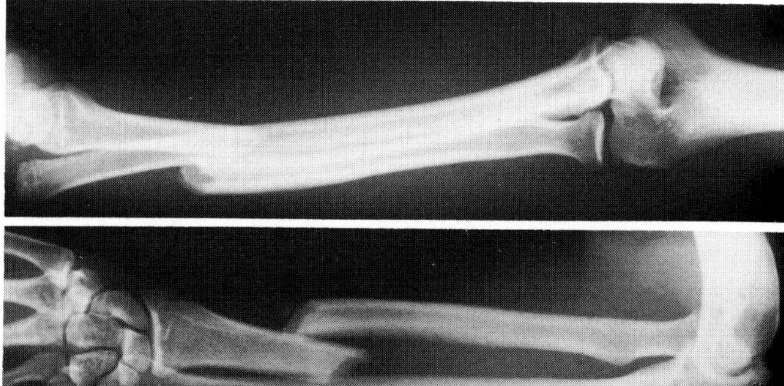

Fig. 10.17 Galeazzi fracture-dislocation. The radial shaft is fractured with overlap due to the rupture of the distal ligaments and dislocation of the radio-ulnar joint.

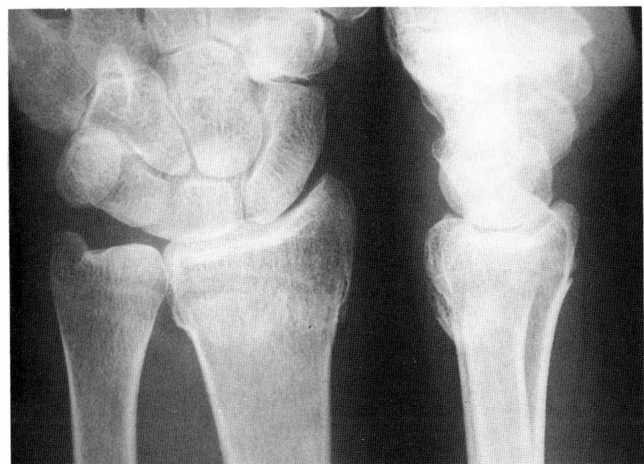

Fig. 10.18 Colles' fracture. In this patient only minor displacement is present, characterized by reversal of the normal palmar angulation of the distal radial surface. Minor impaction is also evident.

projection. The lateral projection shows an oblique fracture with forward displacement and angulation (Fig. 10.19). This is an unstable fracture which often requires internal fixation.

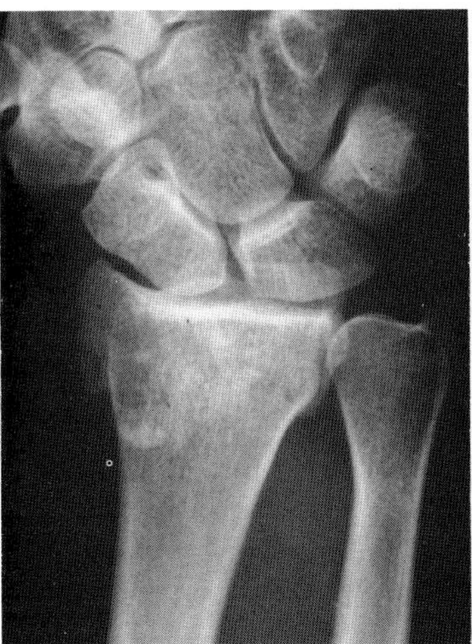

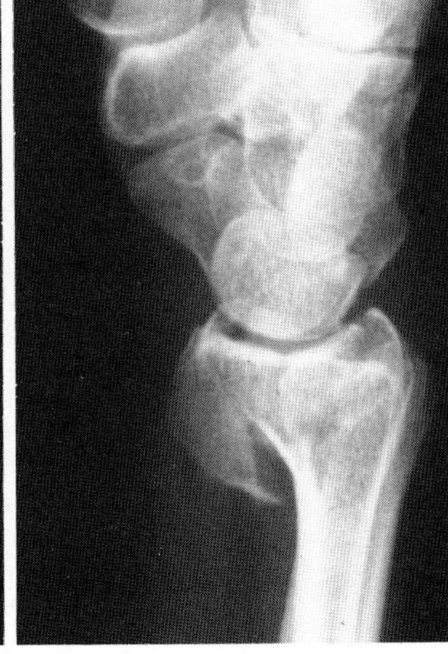

Fig. 10.19 Smith's fracture. The obliquity of the fracture makes it potentially unstable. The comminution and involvement of the radial articular surface shows some elements of the reversed Barton's fracture.

Barton's fracture is a marginal posterior fracture passing through the radial articular surface. When the fracture line separates the anterior radial rim it is usually termed a *reverse Barton's fracture*.

These fractures are illustrated diagramatically in Figure 10.20.

Fractures of the distal radius and ulna are common in **children and adolescents.** Between the ages of 5 and 10 years most involve the shafts 2–4 cm proximal to the distal radial growth plate. Usually these are of the 'wrinkle' or 'torus' type (torus = the protruding semicircular moulding at the base of a classical column) (Fig. 10.21). True greenstick and complete fractures are less common. Typically the distal fragment is angulated dorsally as in Colles' fracture.

Similar falls may result in separation of the distal radial metaphysis (Fig. 10.22). These tend to affect children over the age of 10 years and are usually Salter-Harris Type II. Premature fusion may result (Fig. 9.24).

Fractures of the carpus. Any carpal bone may be injured, but the commonest fracture involves the scaphoid following a fall on the outstretched hand (Fig. 10.23). Adequate radiographic examination requires at least four views — postero-anterior, lateral, 45-degree pronated oblique, and postero-anterior in ulnar deviation. Because the carpal bones are mostly cancellous in structure, hairline fractures sometimes escape identification. With clinical signs of a fracture, good practice demands the application of a plaster cast and repeating the X-ray examination in 10–14 days. By that time, resorption at the fracture margins will ensure the fracture is more apparent. An alternative management would be to undertake radionuclide scanning (Fig. 10.24); a normal result would tend to exclude fracture, but such studies are often not readily available to accident patients. Some 70% of scaphoid fractures involve the waist of the bone and 20% the distal pole. The least common site, the proximal pole, is involved in only 10% but accounts for most cases of delayed union and post-traumatic osteonecrosis, as the blood supply enters the bone in its middle third. Associated injuries include fractures of the radial styloid, capitate and triquetrum and perilunate dislocations.

Non-union of a fracture of the waist of the scaphoid may occur (Fig. 9.10). Such an occurrence suggests that some displacement of the bony margins must have occurred, probably in association with damage to the intercarpal ligaments.

The *triquetrum* is the second commonest carpal bone to be injured, but usually only by a marginal avulsion fracture of its dorsal surface, demonstrated on the lateral radiograph of the wrist. Fractures of the other carpal bones are unusual, but include certain occupational and sporting injuries such as the fracture of the hook of the hamate in golfers and those using racquets.

Carpal dislocations. Essentially the radiologist has to distinguish between lunate and perilunate dislocations. In dislocation of the *lunate* the bone is invariably displaced anteriorly with rupture of the capitolunate and the radiolunate ligaments. The lunate pivots on the intact attachment of the palmar radiolunate ligament and in the frontal projection presents a triangular rather than a quadrilateral contour (Figs 10.20 and 10.25). The key to the diagnosis lies in the lateral projection, however, where the lunate is

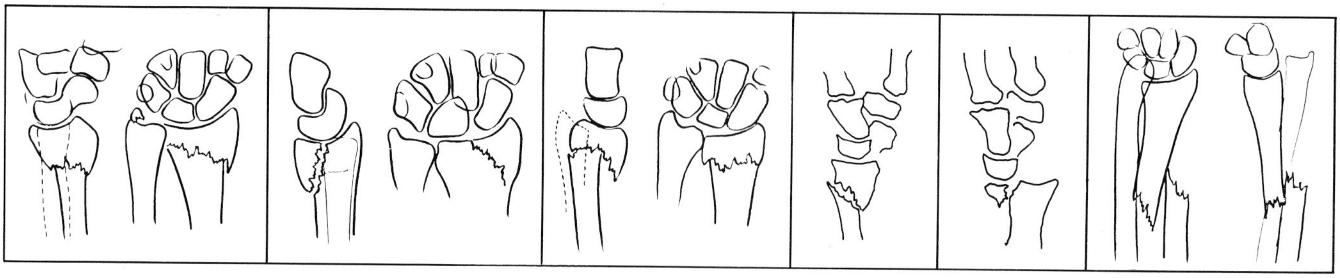

A B C D E F

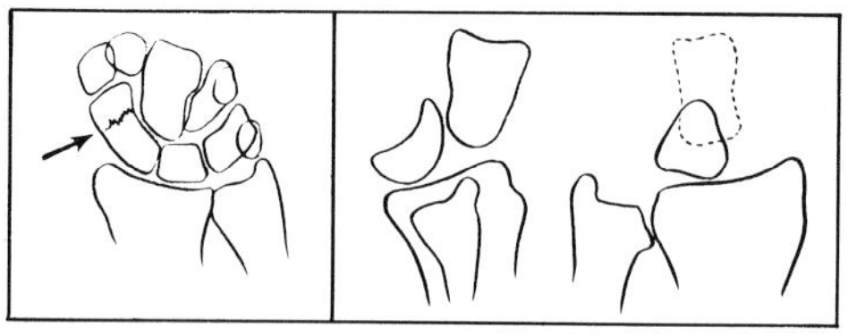

G H

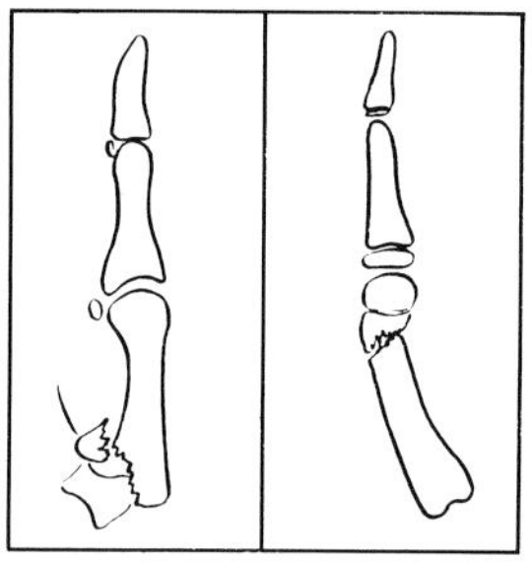

J K

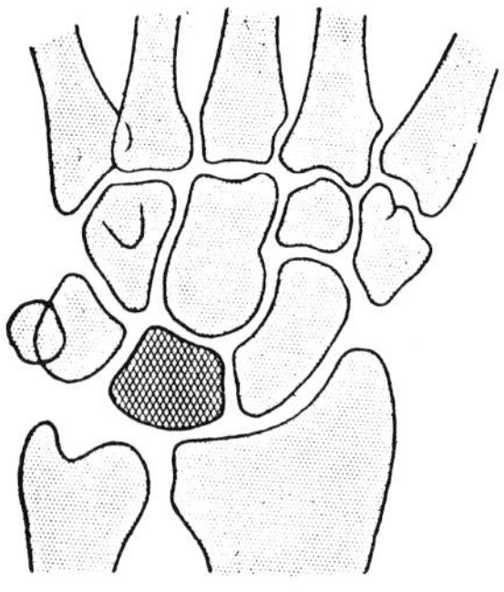

Dislocation of the lunate.

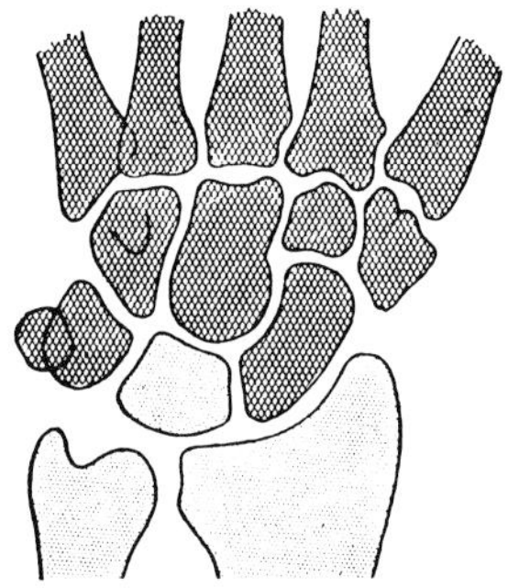

Perilunar dislocation of the carpus.

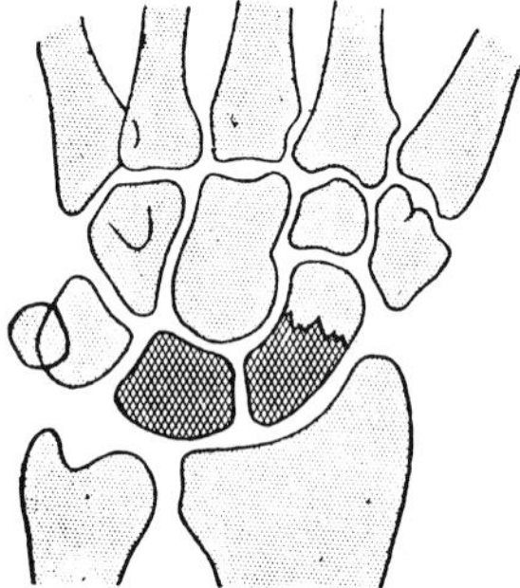

Dislocation of the lunate and half scaphoid.

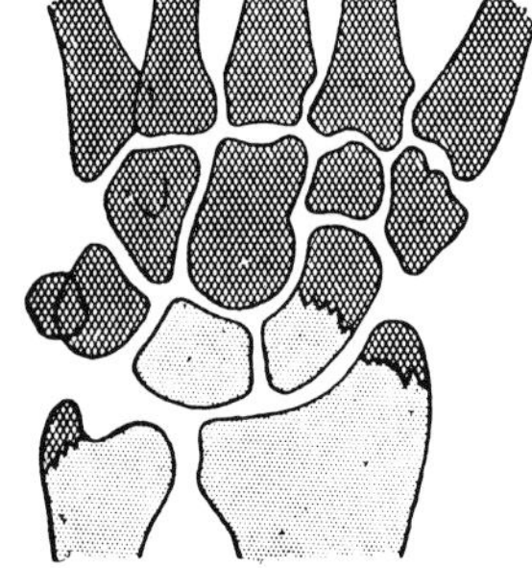

Trans-scapho-perilunar dislocation.

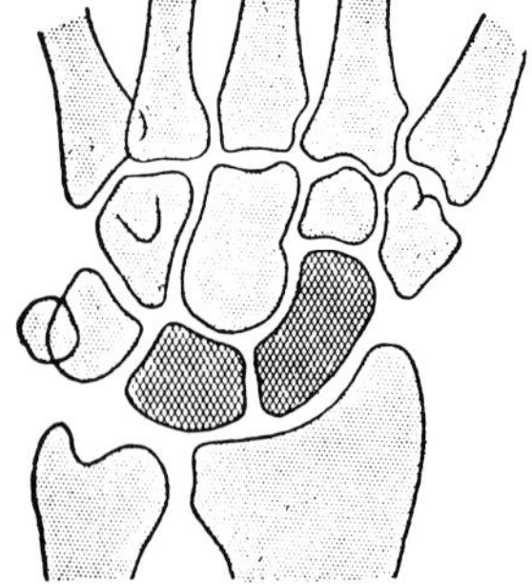

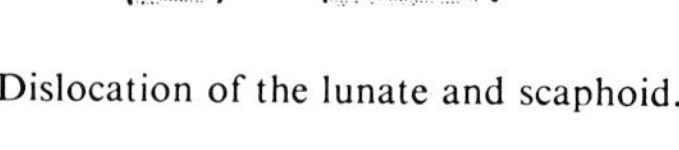

Dislocation of the lunate and scaphoid.

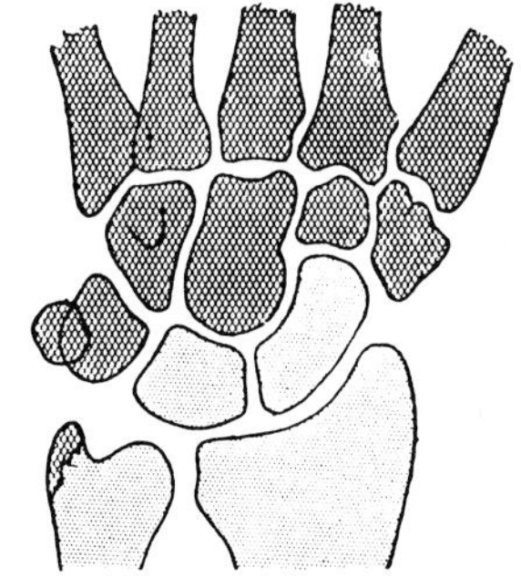

Peri-scapho-lunar dislocation.

I

Fig. 10.20 Injuries round the wrist. **A**. *Colles' fracture*. The distal fragment of the radius is tilted dorsally. The radial styloid process is depressed. The ulnar styloid process has been avulsed. **B**. *Colles' fracture* with separation of radial styloid process. This fracture involves the articular surface of the radius. Note the associated dorsal subluxation of the carpus. **C**. *Smith's fracture*. The distal fragment of the radius is displaced forwards and impacted. **D**. *Smith's fracture*. In this variety the obliquity and lack of impaction leads to shortening and deformity; internal fixation may be required. **E**. *Barton's fracture*. The marginal posterior radial fracture involves the articular surface. For the carpus to be displaced posteriorly, as shown here, the anterior radiocarpal ligament complex must also be disrupted. **F**. *Galeazzi fracture-dislocation*. The oblique fracture of the radial shaft shows overlap of the fragment. Owing to the ulna remaining intact, the distal radio-ulnar joint has been dislocated. **G**. *Fracture of the scaphoid*. A transverse hairline crack is frequently seen in the waist of the bone. It may be visible only on oblique projections. **H**. *Dislocation of lunate*. The base of the capitate has been displaced dorsally out of its normal cup on the articular surface of the lunate, which is tilted forwards. Note that in the anteroposterior view the bone thus assumes a triangular appearance. **I**. Classification of dislocation of the carpus. The dislocated bones are shown in dark shading and the undisplaced bones in plain shading. Note that in each pair the dislocation on the left is the counterpart of that on the right. It is quite simple. (*Courtesy of the late Sir Reginald Watson-Jones*). **J**. *Bennett's fracture-dislocation of the base of the first metacarpal*. The fracture has permitted the major fragment to displace proximally over the saddle-shaped trapezium. **K**. *Greenstick fracture of the neck of the fifth metacarpal*, with slight angulation. This is a very common injury in adolescence.

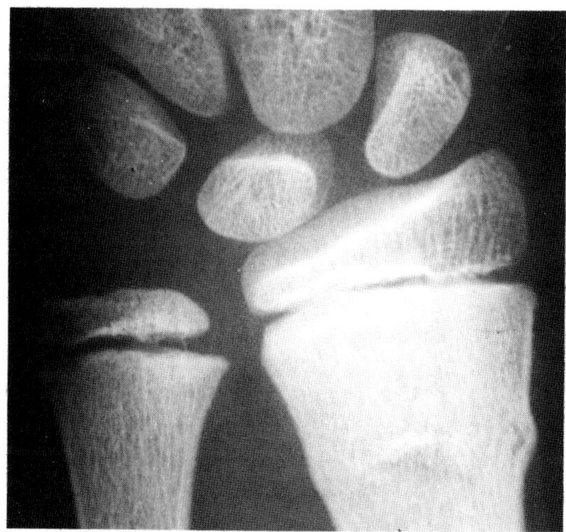

Fig. 10.21 'Torus' fracture of distal radial shaft. Such fractures are common in children and require only immobilization to achieve an excellent result. They are not 'greenstick' fractures but complete fractures within an almost intact periosteum.

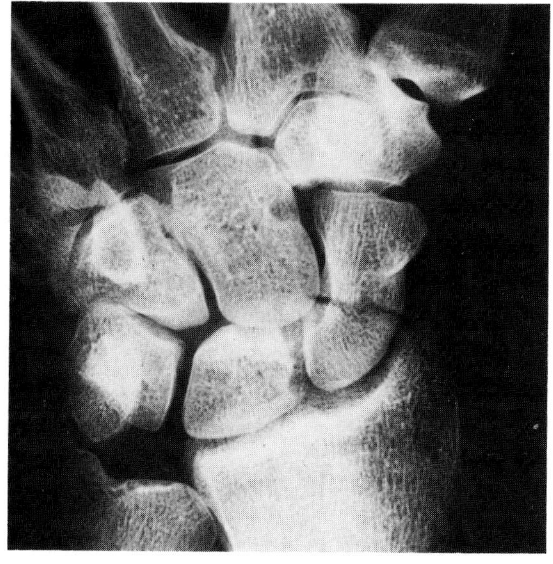

Fig. 10.23 Fracture of the waist of the scaphoid. This recent fracture is virtually undisplaced. Many scaphoid fractures are much less obvious.

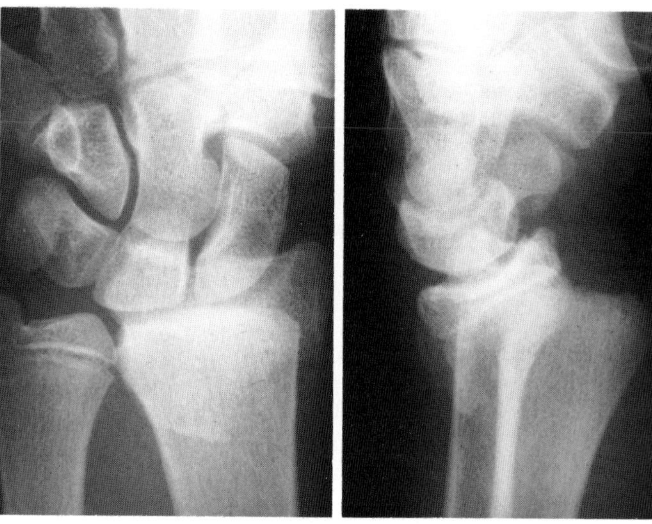

Fig. 10.22 Posterior fracture-separation of distal radial epiphysis. Equivalent to the adult Colles' fracture, the small retained posterior metaphyseal fragment indicates that this is a Salter–Harris Type II lesion.

demonstrably articulating neither with the radius nor the capitate (Fig. 10.25).

Conversely, in the more common *perilunate* dislocation of the carpus, the lunate retains its normal anatomical relationship with the radius, but the remainder of the carpus is dislocated posteriorly (Fig. 10.26). In the majority of perilunate dislocations, the scaphoid is also fractured. Occasionally, the carpal bones occupy an intermediate position with the lunate tilted but not dislocated; such indeterminate appearances have been referred to as dorsal midcarpal dislocations. In all such carpal dislo-

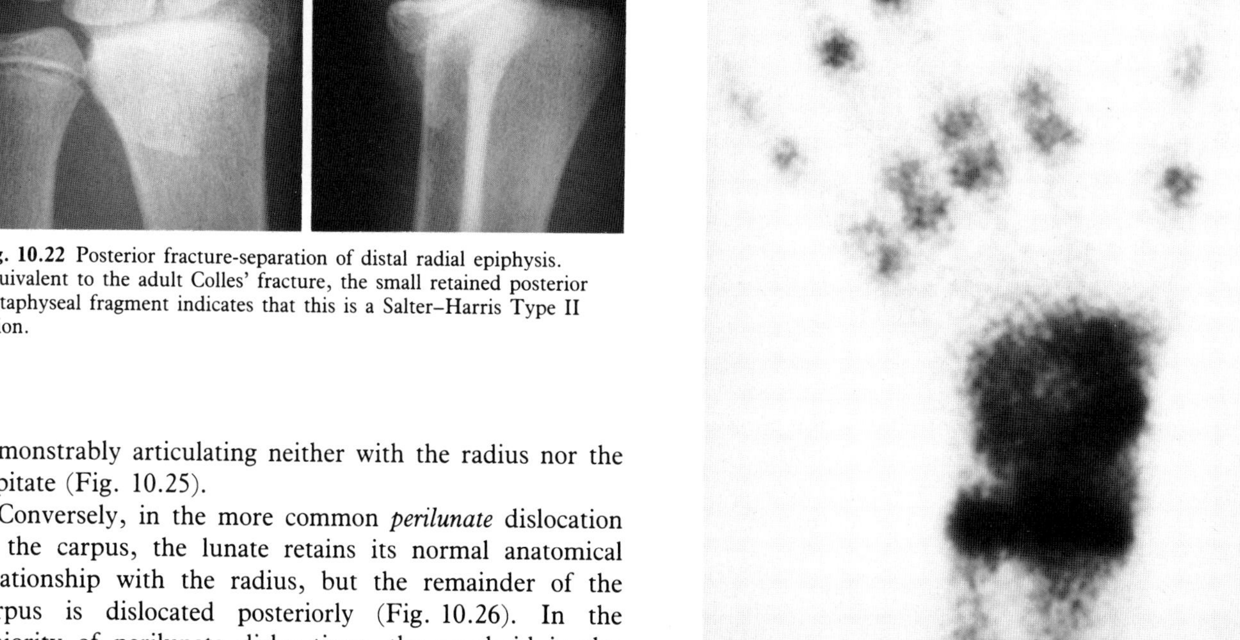

Fig. 10.24 Radionuclide bone scan in scaphoid fracture. Although generalized increase in uptake is evident at the wrist and carpus in this immature patient, activity is greatest over the scaphoid and at the radial and ulnar growth plates. A later scan would be expected to show a reduction in the blood pool activity.

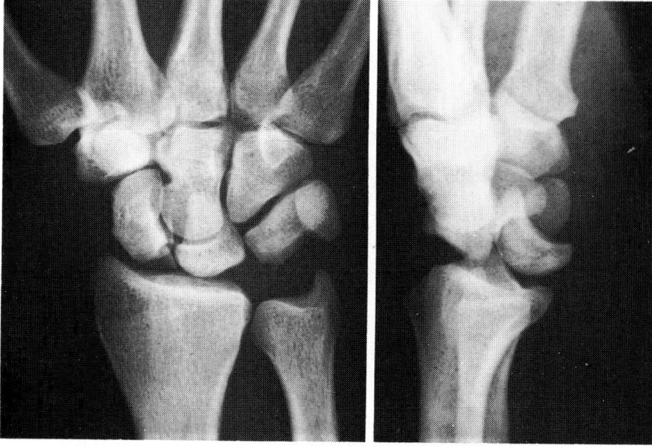

Fig. 10.25 In the anteroposterior projection the lunate bone appears to be triangular instead of quadrilateral in shape and the lateral projection shows clearly that it is displaced forwards. The distal concavity no longer contains the base of the capitate. Because this appearance is perhaps intermediate between a lunate and a perilunate dislocation, nowadays it is better referred to as a dorsal midcarpal dislocation. A chip fracture of the proximal scaphoid is also present.

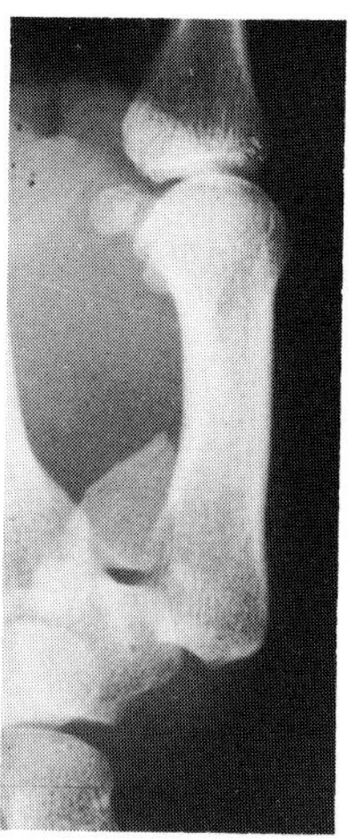

Fig. 10.27 Bennett's fracture-dislocation. The articular surface of the base of the first metacarpal is involved and the main portion of the bone is displaced proximally in relation to the trapezium.

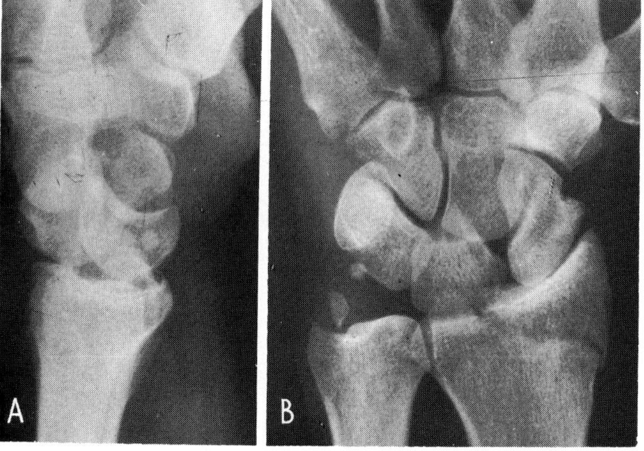

Fig. 10.26 Perilunar dislocation of the carpus. With the exception of the lunate, the whole of the carpus has been dislocated dorsally in relation to the radius. Both the radial and ulnar styloid processes have been fractured. Note loss of articulation between lunate and adjacent carpal bones.

cations displacement indicates rupture of the appropriate carpo-radial and intercarpal ligaments.

Lesser magnitudes of dislocation are observed in the carpus. These include the rotational dislocation of the scaphoid with widening of the scapho-lunate joint space and dorsal or palmar instability, in which dislocation of the radio-lunato-capitate axes is demonstrable in the lateral projection.

The hand. Fractures of the hand are common and often without specific radiographic features. The *mallet finger* deformity results from avulsion of the long extensor insertion at the base of the terminal phalanx. The radiologist should be aware that such avulsion is only associated with an identifiable fragment of bone from the phalanx in about one-quarter of cases. The metacarpal bone of the thumb is fractured proximally in almost 80% of cases. The most important of these injuries to recognize is *Bennett's fracture*, in fact, a fracture-dislocation. An oblique fracture of the base of the first metacarpal allows dorsal subluxation or dislocation of the remainder of the bone (Fig. 10.27). Recognition of this unstable injury is important as open reduction or percutaneous pin fixation is usually required.

THE PELVIS AND LOWER LIMB

THE PELVIS

This large bony ring is generally damaged in severe trauma such as motor vehicle accidents when unstable fractures result from breaking of the ring in at least two places (Fig. 10.28). Associated visceral damage and considerable internal haemorrhage are common. When one fracture is found in the pelvic ring, a search should be made for an associated break in the opposite arc. It is unusual for a sacro-iliac joint to be dislocated, but disruption of the pubic symphysis is relatively common. Stable fractures are more common and consist of unilateral fractures of the ischiopubic rami, isolated fractures of the sacrum or ilium and avulsion injuries.

Unilateral fracture of a ramus is the most common pelvic fracture. A straddle injury may result in fracture of the superior and inferior public rami on both sides.

Pathological fractures of these areas often complicate osteomalacia, and this condition should be suspected when symmetrical fractures occur with inadequate trauma.

Stress fractures of the pubic rami occur in runners and in the elderly, when they may be mistaken for metastases

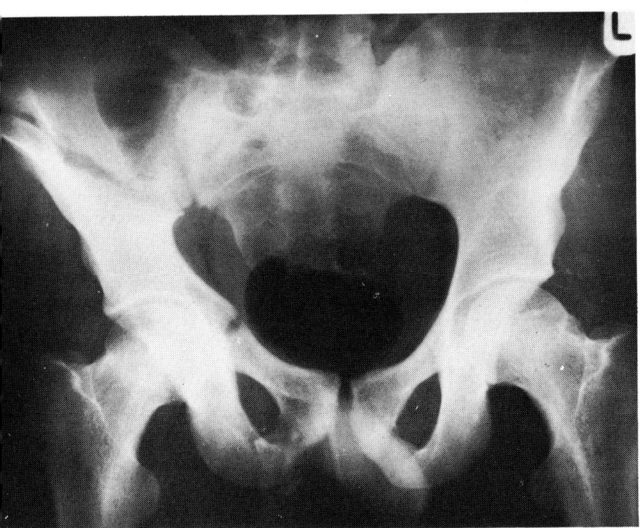

Fig. 10.28 Multiple fractures of the right innominate bone. Note that the obturator ring is broken in two places (both superior and inferior pubic rami).

(Fig. 10.29). Stress lesions of the pubic symphysis have been discussed above.

Isolated fractures of the sacrum usually result from the direct trauma of falling heavily on the buttocks. They are usually transverse and often difficult to visualize on routine radiographic views; an anteroposterior projection with the beam angled 30 degrees in a cephalad direction is usually needed. Failing this, as in other pelvic fractures, CT will demonstrate the fracture clearly (see below).

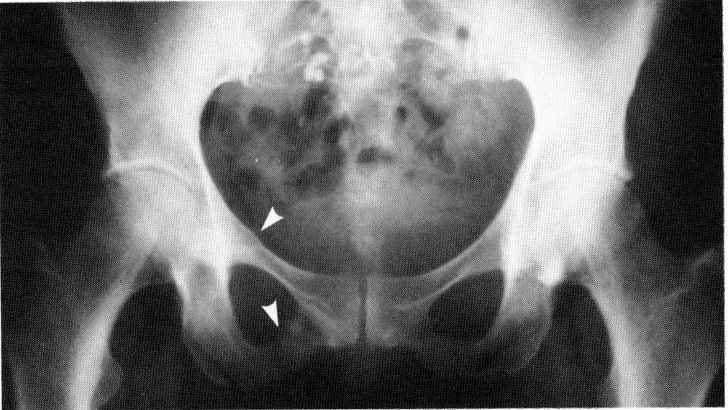

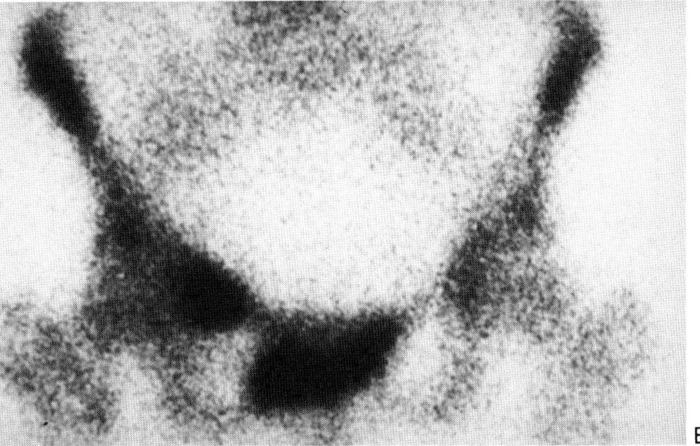

Fig. 10.29 Fractures of ischio-pubic rami. **A.** The healing stress fractures of the right inferior pubic and superior ischio-pubic rami are easily identified (arrows). **B.** The radionuclide bone scan confirms activity at these sites.

THE HIP AND FEMUR (Fig. 10.30A–I)

Fractures of the femoral neck are especially common in the elderly, particularly the elderly female, stressing the importance of osteoporosis in their aetiology. Intracapsular fractures are mostly subcapital (Figs. 9.7 and 10.31), but fractures also occur uncommonly in the middle third and base of the femoral neck. The line of a subcapital fracture is surprisingly constant, forming a short spiral, so that an anteromedial spike of femoral neck is detached with the head. Such fractures may be impacted, often in a valgus position, or displaced. Displaced fractures are usually associated with external rotation of the main part of the femur so that apparent shortening of the neck is evident on the frontal radiograph. With such intracapsular fractures the capacity for formation of periosteal callus does not exist. Most fractures are immobilized by some variety of nail or transcervical pin. Because of the possibility of non-union with avascular necrosis (Fig. 9.12), many surgical authorities favour early prosthetic replacement of *displaced* fractures. The average incidence of radiologically demonstrable avascular necrosis following a subcapital fracture is 25% with few cases in impacted undisplaced fractures and many more when displacement has occurred.

Stress fractures occur in two major groups — younger patients with athletic or occupational stresses and the elderly osteoporotic subject; fractures in the latter group are sometimes referred to as fatigue fractures. Fractures in other disorders, although similar in appearance, are pathological fractures. Most stress fractures are found either subcapitally or on the medial aspect of the base of the femoral neck. Early changes may show only an ill-defined band of linear density in the medulla (Fig. 9.36). Early stress fractures are often difficult or impossible to demonstrate radiographically; a suggestive history should lead to a radionuclide bone scan which will show increased uptake at the site of stress injury (see below). Symmetrical fractures of both femoral necks in the elderly should raise the possibility of osteomalacia.

The equivalent childhood injury to fracture of the femoral neck is a post-traumatic epiphyseal separation, usually Salter–Harris Type I (fig. 10.32). These are fortunately rare as they carry a high incidence of avascular necrosis and/or premature fusion or non-union.

Intertrochanteric fractures are common in the elderly, but without predominance in females. Separation of one or both trochanters is common. Because the blood supply is excellent, good results can be anticipated with treatment by internal fixation and early ambulation.

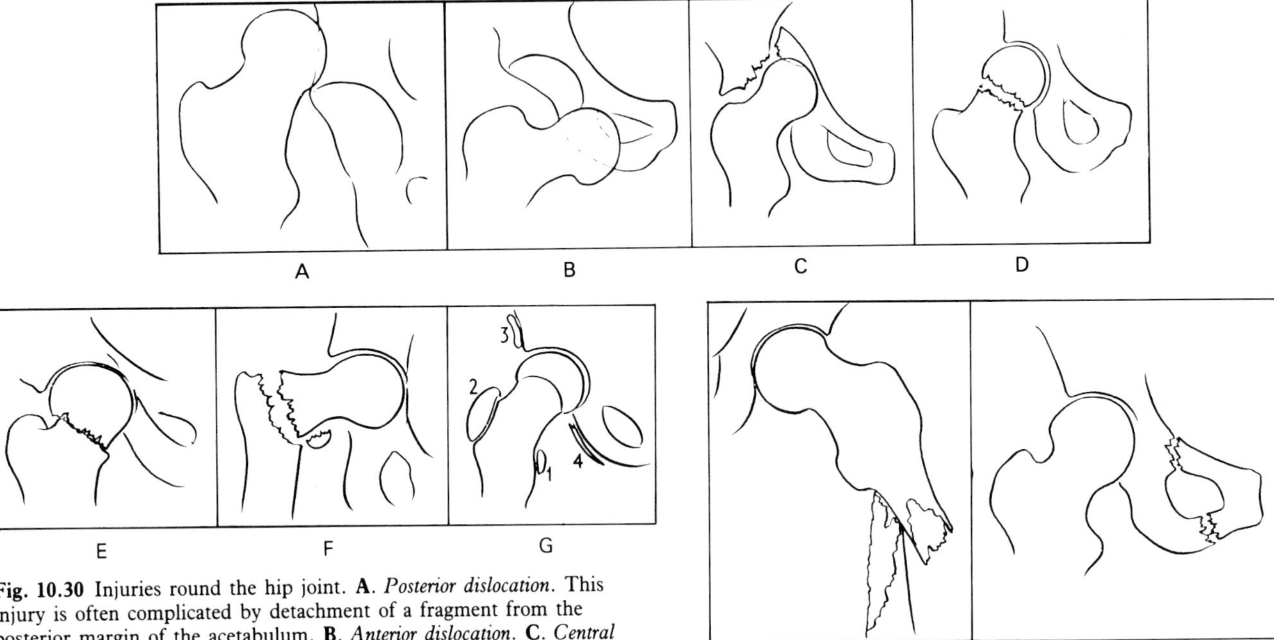

Fig. 10.30 Injuries round the hip joint. **A**. *Posterior dislocation*. This injury is often complicated by detachment of a fragment from the posterior margin of the acetabulum. **B**. *Anterior dislocation*. **C**. *Central dislocation* with an associated fracture of the acetabulum.
D. *Transcervical adduction fracture of femoral neck*. Approximately half the fractures of the femoral neck occur at this site. The remainder occur approximately equally in the subcapital and basal areas.
E. *Impacted abduction type fracture of femoral neck*. The position is acceptable, but internal splinting is usually undertaken.
F. *Intertrochanteric fracture of femur*. The lesser trochanter is characteristically separated. **G**. *Sites of avulsion lesions in childhood and adolescence*: (1) Lesser trochanter — common; (2) Greater trochanter — rare; (3) Anterior inferior iliac spine — very common; (4) Ischial apophysis — common. **H**. *Subtrochanteric fracture of femoral shaft*.
I. *Fractures of the obturator ring*. As with other bony rings, two fractures may be expected.

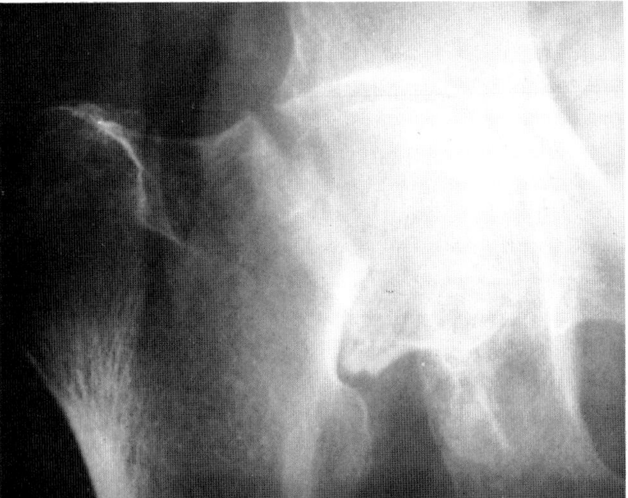

Fig. 10.31 Subcapital fracture of femoral neck. The fracture is displaced with varus deformity. The characteristic inferior extension of the fracture line into the femoral neck is well shown. Because of the displacement, prosthetic replacement was undertaken.

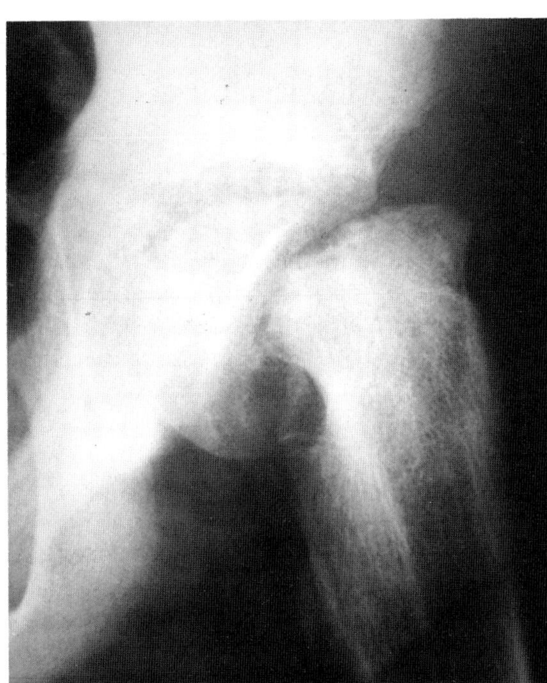

Fig. 10.32 Epiphyseal fracture-separation. The displacement at the growth plate followed a severe injury and the lesion should not therefore be termed a slipped epiphysis. The injury was complicated by osteonecrosis of the entire femoral capital epiphysis and premature fusion.

Dislocations and fracture-dislocations of the hip. Dislocation of the hip is relatively rare and the majority of cases occur in motor vehicle accidents. Most dislocations are *posterior*. With the hip flexed and adducted a severe impact against the dashboard will cause posterior dislocation without fracture of the posterior wall of the acetabulum (Fig. 10.33); this fracture is stable when reduced. With the thigh in a neutral or abducted position, the posterior wall of the acetabulum will be detached, leaving an unstable femoral head. The demonstration of the fracture of the acetabular wall requires supplementary oblique views; CT has proved of inestimable value in the demonstration of this and other acetabular injuries.

Anterior dislocations are uncommon, easily recognised radiographically and usually result from a forced abduction in flexion (Fig. 10.34).

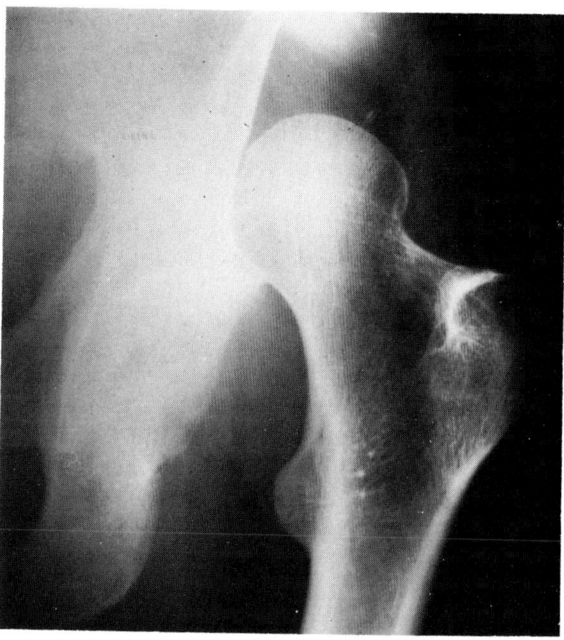

Fig. 10.33 Posterior dislocation of the hip. The acetabulum is intact.

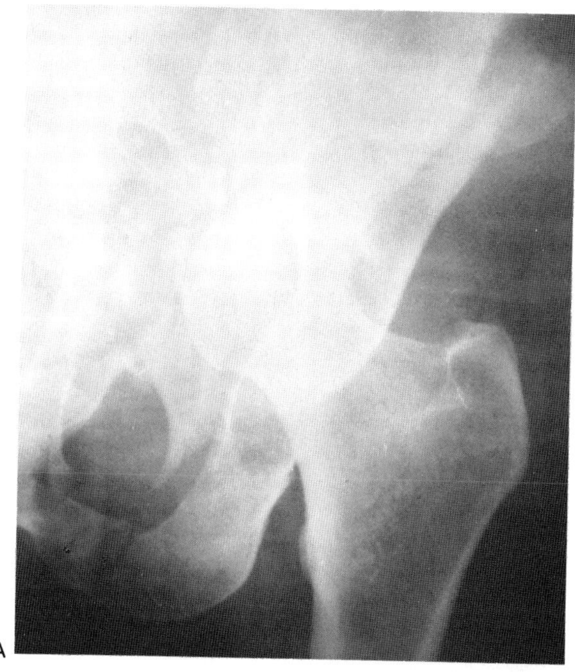

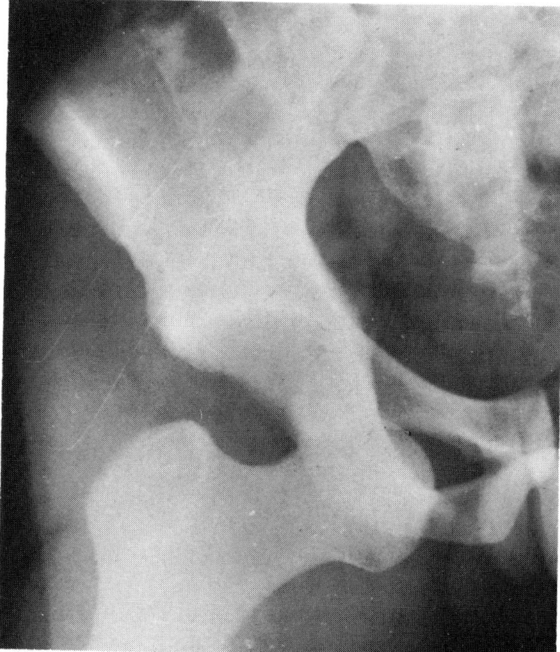

Fig. 10.34 Anterior dislocation of the hip, resulting from overabduction.

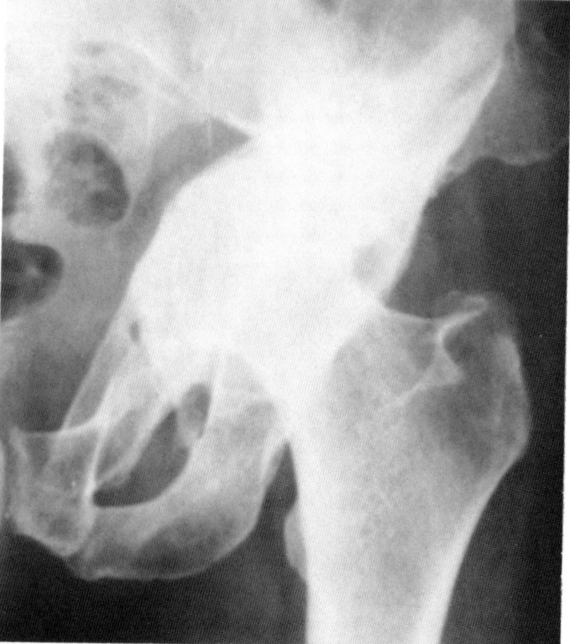

Fig. 10.35 Central dislocation of the femoral head. **A**. Early, in association with an extensive oblique iliac fractures. **B**. Following union, showing a residual protrusio acetabuli deformity.

Acetabular fractures are fractures of the pelvis but are considered separately here. Apart from fracture of the posterior rim associated with posterior dislocation, fractures may be central (Fig. 10.35), sometimes associated with central dislocation of the femoral head, or involve the anterior (ilio-pubic) or posterior (ischio-pubic) columns. Demonstration of these fracture lines is best achieved by internal and external oblique (Judet) views (Fig. 10.36). CT has proved so valuable in this pelvic region that it should be employed whenever possible in such circumstances (see below).

Fractures of the *femoral shaft* usually indicate severe violence. Commonly transverse or oblique in the mid shaft (Fig. 9.8), treatment is directed to correction of shortening

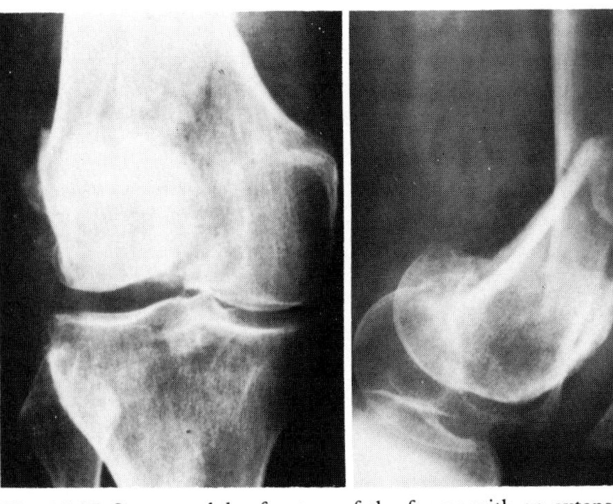

Fig. 10.37 Supracondylar fracture of the femur with an extension reaching to the intercondylar notch and a resultant step deformity of the lateral femoral condyle. The patella was also fractured.

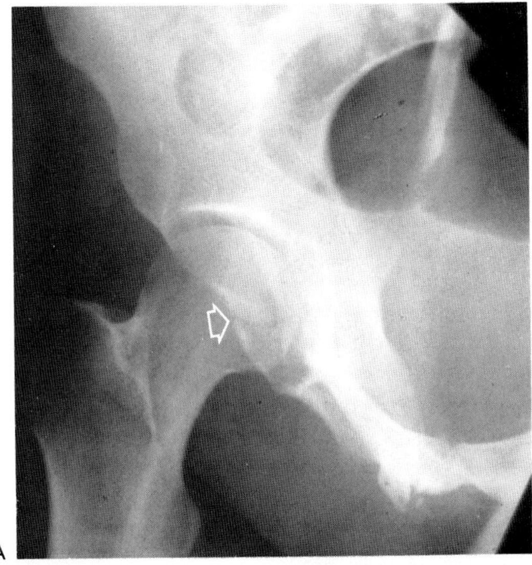

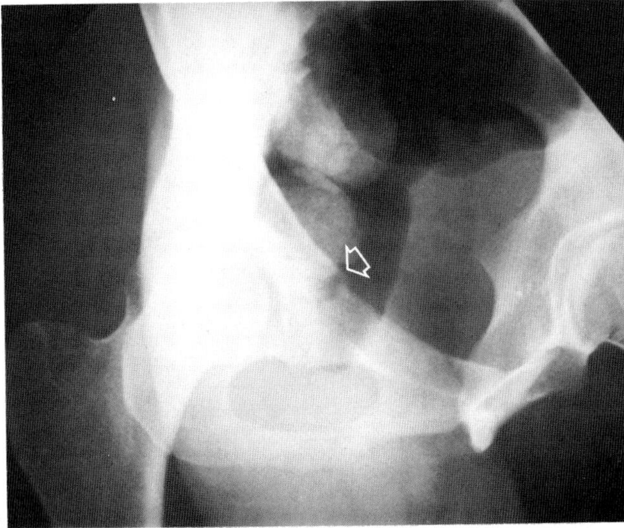

Fig. 10.36 A. and **B.** Judet views in fracture of the pelvic wall. The two oblique views demonstrate respectively the passage of the fracture line through the posterior and anterior pillars. When readily available to accident cases, CT has replaced such special views which require sometimes painful movement by the patient.

and fixation with an intramedullary nail. Supracondylar fractures of the femur often show posterior angulation of the distal fragment (Fig. 10.37). Such fractures may be comminuted and extension into the knee joint may occur.

THE KNEE AND LEG (Fig. 10.38)

Fractures of the femoral condyles may either extend from supracondylar fractures or result from impaction forces which often fragment and separate the condyles; such fractures are, of course, intra-articular (Fig. 10.308A). The **patella** may be fragmented by a direct blow or break transversely, with or without separation. Vertical fractures are less common and difficult to detect without an axial (skyline) view (Fig. 10.39). Misinterpretation of the accessory ossification centre of a bipartite patella as a fracture should not occur. The centre is larger than the segment of the patella it replaces, always occupies the superolateral quadrant, and the adjoining margins of the two bones are corticated.

Avulsion fractures of the superior or inferior poles are identifiable on the lateral projection.

Dislocation of the patella is almost always in a lateral direction. Similarly, *recurrent or habitual dislocation of the patella* is usually in a lateral direction and associated with hypoplasia of the lateral femoral condyle with a shallow frontal groove. An osteochondral fracture of the medial margin of the patella may be observed in the skyline projection.

Ligamentous injuries are rarely accompanied by visible radiographic evidence of avulsion of their bony attachments. Occasionally the tibial attachment of a cruciate ligament is identified as an apparent loose fragment with incomplete cortication of its margin. Such fragments often remain in the intercondylar region (Fig. 10.40). The region

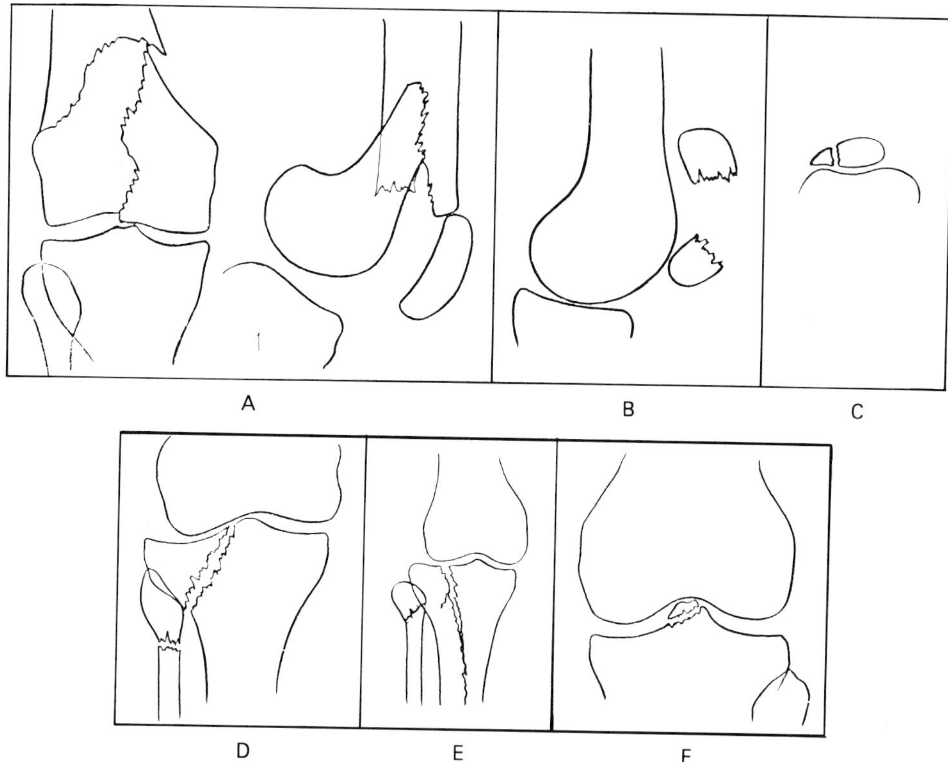

Fig. 10.38 *Injuries of the knee and leg.* (**A**) *Supracondylar fracture of the femur* with extension to involve the articular surface. (**B**) *Transverse fracture of the patella* with wide separation of fragments. (**C**) *Vertical fracture of the patella* visible only in the axial projection. (**D**) *Fracture of the lateral condyle of the tibia and neck of fibula.* This injury has resulted from forced abduction with impact of the surface of the lateral femoral condyle upon the tibia. Involvement of the articular surface is minimal and this injury carries a good prognosis. (**E**) *A more severe fracture of the lateral tibial condyle* with a crack running downwards into the tibial shaft. This has been caused by complete rupture of the internal lateral ligament and the cruciate ligaments so that the lateral margin of the femur has impacted upon the surface of the lateral tibial condyle to produce the injury. The articular surface is involved. The neck of the fibula is also fractured. (**F**) *Avulsion injury* to extra-synovial intercondylar region of tibia.

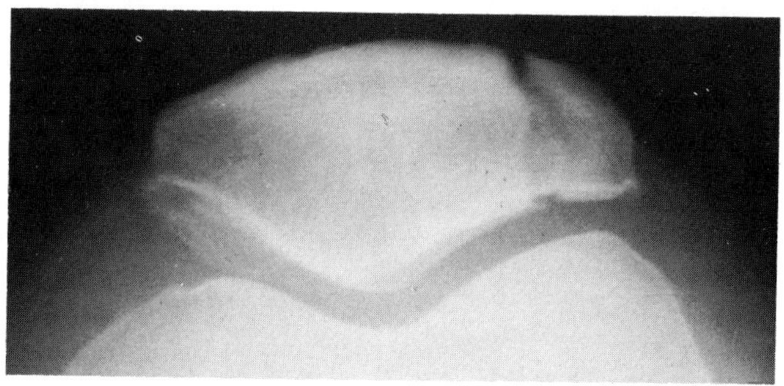

Fig. 10.39 Vertical fracture of the patella. Some of these lesions are only visible in the axial view.

from which the bony fragment is derived is identified only rarely on the radiograph. Effusions are diagnosed most accurately in the lateral projection when fluid causing capsular distension separates the normal fat planes. In accident cases the lateral view should be obtained with a horizontal beam. The presence of a fat–fluid interface (Fig. 9.5) indicates free fat from the bone marrow has entered the joint; in the absence of gross femoral disruption, this usually indicates a fracture of the tibial plateau as patellar fractures almost never produce this sign.

Fractures of the tibial plateau are common but can be difficult to detect (Fig. 10.41). The radiologist must determine the degree of depression, if any, of the fragment and remember that the patient's ultimate disability may relate as much to the associated ligamentous disruption as to the fracture. Clinical suspicion of soft-tissue damage within the joint, e.g. to the menisci or cruciate ligaments can be confirmed by arthrography or arthroscopy later in the patient's management. Such fractures are the result of valgus force on the knee causing compression of the tibial plateau which is weaker than the femoral condyle. Although classically called the 'bumper' fracture (Fig. 10.42), the majority affect middle-aged women following falls with a rotational element. Most consist of a compression or shearing fracture of the lateral tibial condyle or a combination of the two.

The shafts of the tibia and fibula are commonly fractured. Indirect injury leads to spiral or oblique fractures, while the superficial position of the bones anteriorly makes compound fractures relatively common following direct

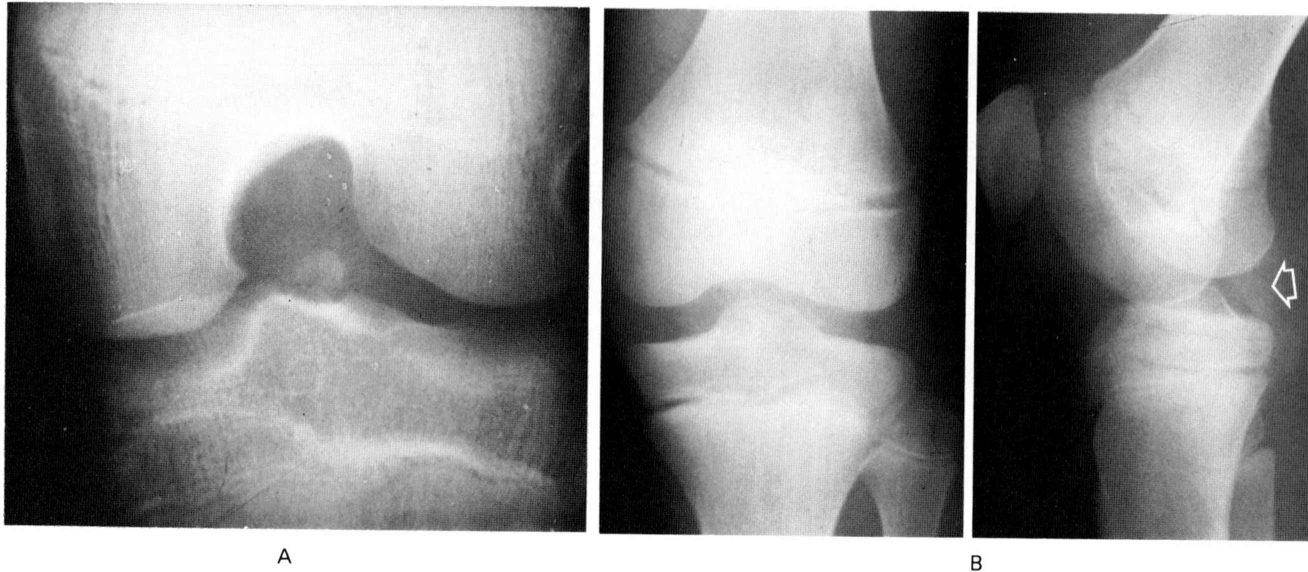

Fig. 10.40 A. In this intercondylar view a bony fragment is shown close to the tibial crest. At exploration it proved to be the proximal attachment of the anterior cruciate ligament to the medial aspect of the lateral femoral condyle. **B.** Avulsion of tibial attachment of posterior cruciate ligament. The ligament is attached to the posterior margin of the tibial plateau. The detached bony fragment is visible (arrow) and was reattached at operation.

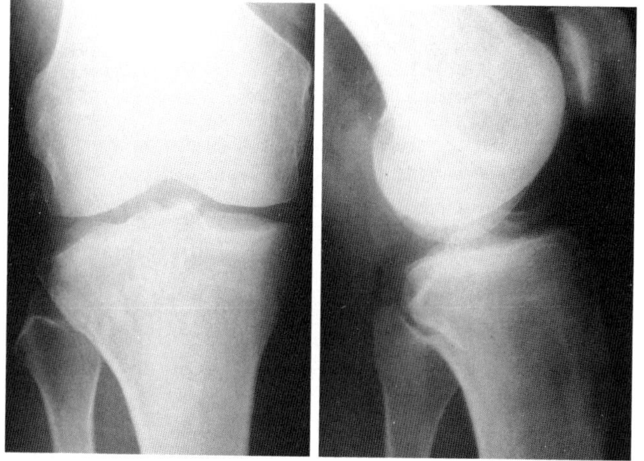

Fig. 10.41 Fracture of lateral tibial condyle. A valgus injury has resulted in depression of the lateral half of the tibial plateau. A horizontal fracture of the fibular shaft has been sustained in its proximal third (not shown).

injury. The whole length of both bones should be included on both projections because: (a) the two bones are often not fractured at the same level. Any shortening at a tibial fracture site must indicate a fibular fracture or its dislocation at one or other tibio-fibular joint; (b) Particularly after reduction, a residual external rotation deformity may be present (Fig. 9.9). In such cases the distal fibular fragment is displaced posteriorly and the space between the distal shafts of the bones, in the anteroposterior view, narrows compared to the proximal shafts.

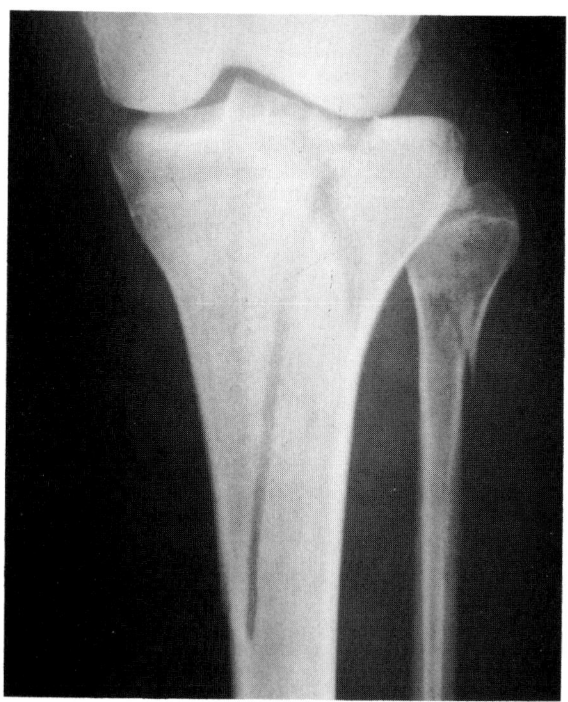

Fig. 10.42 'Bumper' fracture of the tibia. The injury has resulted from the impaction of the lateral condyle of the femur on the lateral condyle of the tibia. This has suffered a depression type vertical fracture with a corresponding fracture of the neck of the fibula.

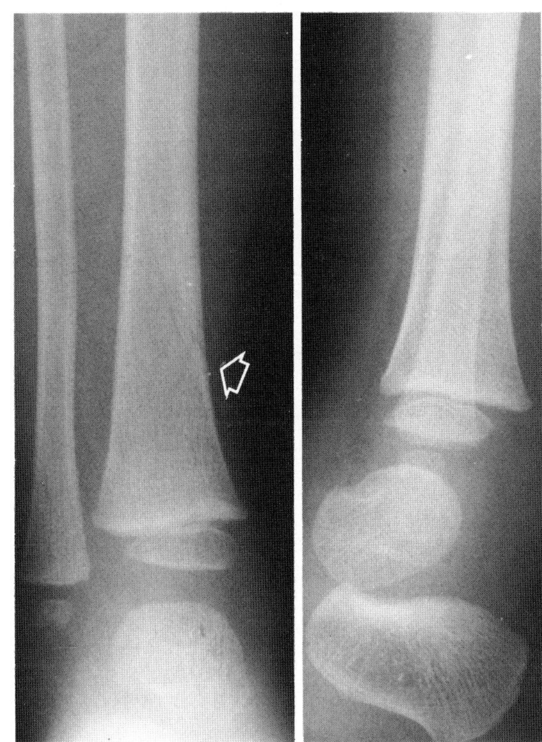

g. **10.43** Spiral 'toddler's' fracture of tibia. The undisplaced fracture ie is identified in the anteroposterior, but not the lateral, projection.

Fractures of the leg in children commonly consist of ›iral fractures of the tibia without fracture of the fibula. nder the age of 2, the 'toddler's fracture' is an undislaced spiral fracture which is identifiable on the anteroosterior or the lateral projection, but rarely in both views ⁽ig. 10.43). Such children often present with a refusal to ear weight following one of the many falls to which chilren of this age are prone.

Stress fractures affect long distance runners, ballet ancers and those indulging in other acrobatic sports. The ommonest location is the proximal half of the shaft of the bia, less often the midshaft of the tibia or the fibula. A ansverse band of increased density is often found; periosal callus is minimal or absent, but chronic stress leads to ie formation of appositional new bone to a variable degree Figs. 9.33 and 9.34).

THE ANKLE AND FOOT (Fig. 10.44)

Fracture-dislocations of the ankle (Pott's fracture). orces applied at the ankle result in a variety of bony and gamentous injuries. Many combinations of injury to the iedial and lateral joint margins result in instability, so the erm fracture-dislocation is appropriate.

The medial malleolus may fracture transversely in assocition with an oblique or spiral fracture of the fibula in its distal shaft (a bimalleolar fracture). The fibular fracture line extends proximally from anterior to posterior (Fig. 9.1). This fracture-dislocation is caused by *external rotation* stress and is the commonest of such injuries (Fig. 10.45). Posterior displacement of the talus may result in an additional fracture of the posterior tibial margin, resulting in a trimalleolar or third degree fracture-dislocation (Fig. 10.46). The less common *adduction* or *inversion* results in an oblique or almost vertical fracture of the medial malleolus associated with rupture of the lateral collateral ligament or a transverse fracture through the lateral malleolus. The radiologist should always assess the position of the talus in the ankle mortice. Any asymmetry needs explanation. If bimalleolar fractures are not present, movement can result if tibio-fibular separation occurs, either by rupture of the distal tibio-fibular ligament or avulsion of its tibial attachment. Fractures of the fibular shaft may occur more proximally than could be demonstrated on a standard radiograph of the ankle. Any unexplained asymmetry must lead to the demonstration of the entire fibula. The combination of a posterior malleolar fracture with an oblique fracture of the proximal shaft of the fibula is termed a *Maisonneuve fracture.*

The lateral ligament is more commonly ruptured due to the frequency of inversion injury. Instability due to such ligamentous injury is eatablished by X-ray examination of both ankles in an anteroposterior projection in forced inversion (Fig. 10.47). Sometimes local or general anaesthesia is required and this is especially the case in tears of the distal tibio-fibular ligament. A simple avulsion fracture of the tip of either malleolus has the same significance as a severe sprain of the ligament. Radiographic confirmation of anteroposterior instability can also be demonstrated by stress views.

Fractures of the *talus* are either avulsions or fractures of the neck, less commonly the body, following forced dorsiflexion of the foot. About half of such fractures are associated with dislocation at the ankle or the subtalar joint, and avascular necrosis of the body of the talus is not an infrequent complication.

Osteochondral fractures of the dome of the talus usually are a consequence of a severe inversion injury.

Fractures of the **calcaneus** should always be suspected after a fall from a height and radiography of both feet should be undertaken in these circumstances. Both lateral and axial views are obligatory. Compression fractures result in displacement and Böhler's angle is useful in evaluation of such injuries. The angle is formed at the junction of two lines drawn on the lateral projection of the foot — from the superior posterior margin of the tuberosity through the tip of the posterior facet and through the tip of the posterior facet to the superior margin of the anterior process. The normal angle measures 20–40 degrees and is reduced by many compression injuries. It should be remembered that the type of force causing such injuries

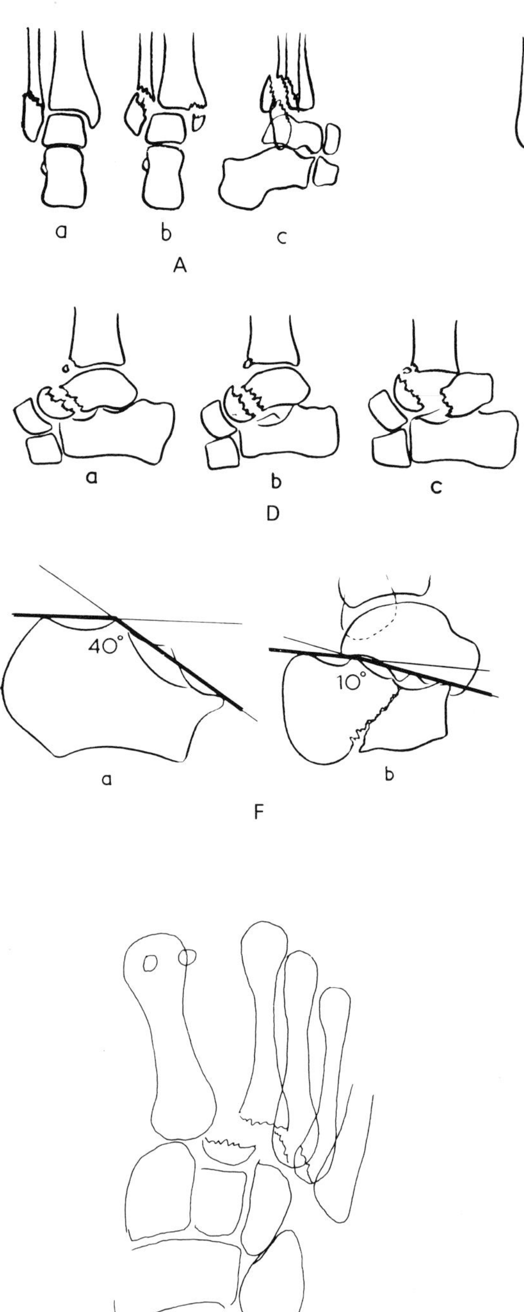

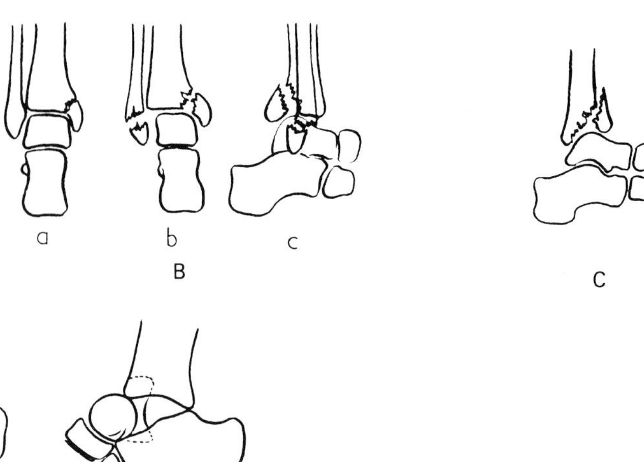

Fig. 10.44 Injuries round the ankle joint and foot. **A**. *Pott's fracture abduction–external rotation type*: (a) First degree — simple oblique fracture of fibula; (b) Second degree — the fibular fracture is accompanied by a transverse fracture of the medial malleolus and lateral subluxation of the talus within the ankle mortice; (c) Third degree. In addition to the fibular fracture, the posterior malleolus o the tibia has been fractured and displaced upwards and the talus ha subluxated backwards within the ankle mortice. **B**. *Pott's fracture — adduction type*: (a) First degree — vertical fracture of medial malleol (b) The fracture of the medial malleolus is accompanied by a transv fracture of the lateral malleolus and medial subluxation of the talus within the ankle mortice; (c) Third degree. The talus is dislocated backwards. The posterior malleolus of the tibia is fractured and the is a transverse fracture of the lateral malleolus. **C**. *Pott's fracture — unusual vertical compression type* with separation of the anterior part the distal end of the tibia and forward subluxation of the talus with the ankle mortice. (*After Wilson, J. N. (ed.) Watson-Jones Fractures Joint Injuries*, Edinburgh; Churchill Livingstone). **D**. *Examples of dorsiflexion injuries to the talus*. In each, the anterior margin of the ti has been fractured by impingement of the talus upon it in a positio extreme dorsiflexion. (a) Fracture of the neck of the talus; (b) Fract of the neck of the talus combined with some forward subluxation o the body of the talus; (c) A large fragment of the body of the talus been dislocation backwards. **E**. *Total dislocation of the talus*. This is plantar flexion injury. (After W. D. Coltart, *Journal of Bone & Join Surgery*, 52, 545, 1952). **F**. *Fracture of the calcaneus*. The normal an formed between the subtalar joint and the upper margin of the tuberosity of the calcaneus should be about 40°. Diminution of this angle should arouse suspicion of a fracture, but this may only be clearly shown in the axial projection. (a) Normal Böhler's angle measurement; (b) Increased angle with fracture of body of calcaneus **G**. *Lisfranc tarso-metatarsal fracture-dislocation*. In this example the fo lateral metatarsals are separated from the first metatarsal opening a between the first and second metatarsals. Note that the base of the second metatarsal is usually fractured in this injury.

also predisposes to fractures in the thoracolumbar spine in 10% of cases and that the patient may not, at first, complain of backache.

Many other injuries may be encountered in the foot. These include fracture of the navicular process of the calcaneus which is identifiable, in most cases, only an oblique projection. Important fractures vary fr the common avulsion fracture of the base of the metatarsal, where the fracture line is coronal and caus by the pull of the peroneus brevis tendon (Fig. 10.48),

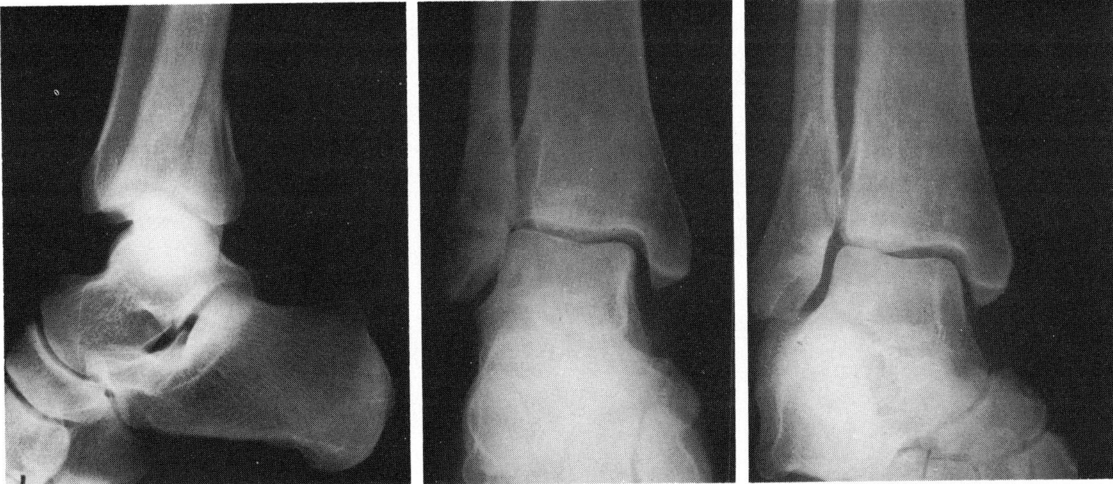

ig. 10.45 Abduction-external rotation type of Pott's fracture. The fracture of the distal end of the fibula is best shown with slight internal ›tation. The talus is subluxated backwards and laterally within the ankle mortice and the posterior malleolus of the tibia has been fractured, ausing a slight step deformity.

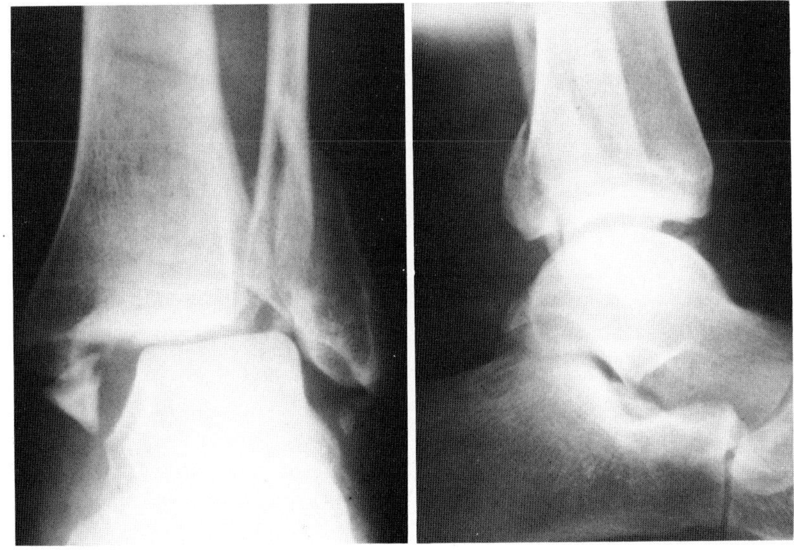

Fig. 10.46 Trimalleolar or third degree fracture-lislocation of the ankle. The posterior malleolus is hown to be fractured. This is an unstable dislocation, he talus being displaced laterally in the ankle nortice.

the rare tarso-metatarsal fracture-dislocation. This latter injury, essentially a dorsal displacement sustained during the course of a fall, is dignified by the name of *Lisfranc*. The force almost inevitably fractures the base of the 2nd metatarsal which is inset between the medial and lateral cuneiform bones (Fig. 10.44).

Brief mention should be made of the occasional fracture of a sesamoid bone of the great toe, usually that on the medial side. A bipartite medial sesamoid bone is found in about 10% of patients and differentiation from a fracture is similar to the process in respect of the patella (see p. 306). Oblique or axial views may be necessary for the clear demonstration of a sesamoid fracture.

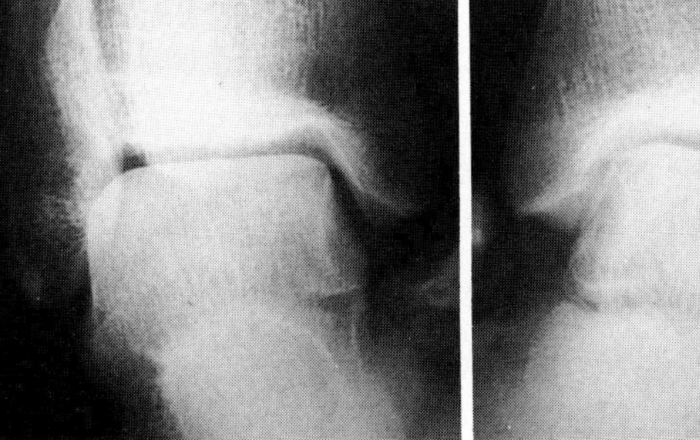

Fig. 10.47 Tear of external lateral ligament. An anteroposterior film in full forced inversion shows abnormal tilt of the left talus within the ankle mortice. Since some degree of tilt may take place physiologically, comparison with the normal ankle is essential.

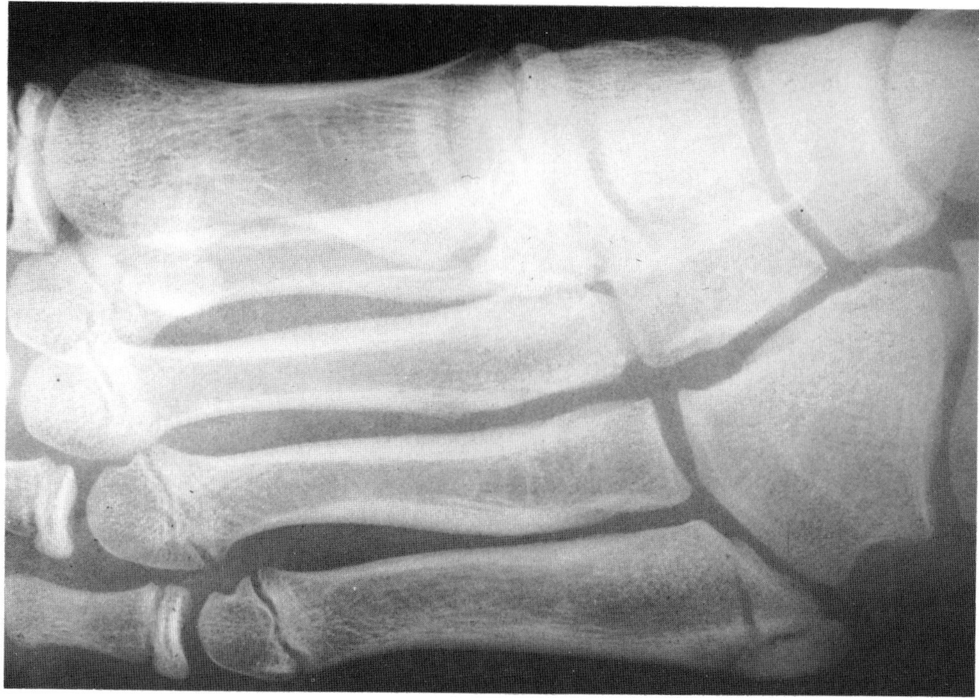

Fig. 10.48 Fracture of the base of the fifth metatarsal. This relatively common fracture is transverse and has to be distinguished in the young from the normal axially aligned apophyseal growth plate. In this child both the fracture and the growth plate coexist.

THE SKULL

In head injury, prevention of further damage to brain tissue is of the first importance. The purpose of radiological examination of the skull is to detect and to evaluate direct evidence of cranial injury and therefore indirect evidence to the cranial contents. Thus, although severe brain damage can occur in the absence of a skull fracture, the presence of a fracture indicates a significant and often deforming injury to the cranium. Much over-emphasis of the value of skull radiography has been made by accident units and compounded by the legal profession. Numerous radiologically orientated papers stressing the absence of logic in many requests for X-ray examination of the skull have failed to alter the pattern of requests. A few hospitals have instituted policies employing criteria producing a high yield of abnormal skull radiographs. Such criteria include:

a. Unconsciousness at time of presentation
b. Documented evidence of deterioration in level of consciousness or mental state
c. Clinical evidence of skull fracture, e.g. depression of skull surface
d. Discharge of fluid or blood from nose or ear
e. Bilateral orbital ecchymoses
f. Unexplained focal neurological signs

In one analysis of patients without high yield criteria, abnormal skull X-rays were found in only 5% and in none did the finding contribute to patient care in a period of 4 weeks. It must be stressed that radiographic examination of the skull in no way absolves the clinician from a full neurological examination. Films taken of a restless unco-operative patient may not be adequate for diagnostic purposes and it can be advantageous to delay X-ray examination until resuscitative measures are established.

Something like 80% of skull fractures are *linear*. These have to be distinguished from vessel markings. Fractures are more lucent, may be short or long, do not usually branch, and are more likely to angulate than follow a smooth curve (Fig. 10.49). Sometimes the fracture line through the outer and inner tables of the skull is not superimposed and the fracture may appear to widen at some point. It is often quite difficult to differentiate some vascular grooves from fractures; in general, arterial vascular grooves which are found in characteristic locations, have thin sclerotic margins and branch. Venous grooves are more wide and tortuous.

Linear fractures of the calvaria may extend into the skull base where they can be very difficult to demonstrate; here clinical evidence of a basal fracture is all-important. In such cases the lateral projection obtained using a horizontal beam may show a fluid level due to the presence of blood in the sphenoid sinus. Linear fractures of the vault heal readily in children except in the case of the 'growing' fracture which may presage a leptomeningeal cyst due to the

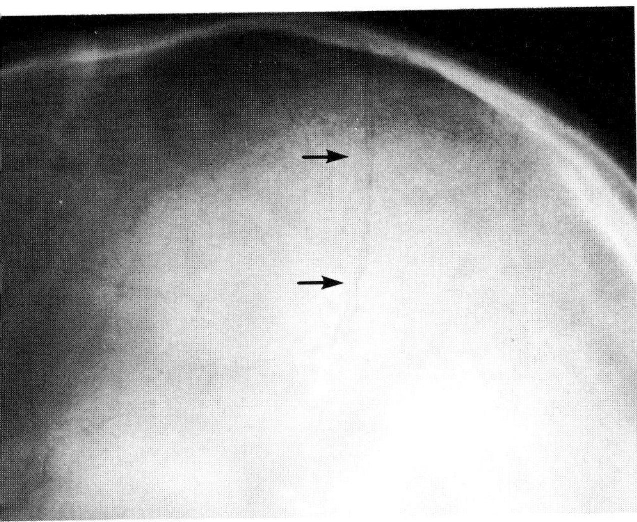

Fig. 10.49 Linear fracture of skull vault. The straightness, clarity and intermittent 'tram-lining' of the linear lucency show it to be a fracture of the parietal bone and not a vascular groove.

entrapment of the arachnoid mater in the fracture line. Pulsation within such cysts causes progressive erosion of bone (see Ch. 57).

Fractures involving the middle ear, sphenoid and ethmoid sinuses are usually difficult to demonstrate; those of the frontal sinuses are usually easy to see. All are essentially compound fractures and may be accompanied by cerebrospinal fluid otorrhoea or rhinorrhoea.

Depressed fractures are usually associated with brain damage and overlap of the fragments often provides an irregular line of double density on the radiograph. Accurate tangential views provide conclusive evidence of depression.

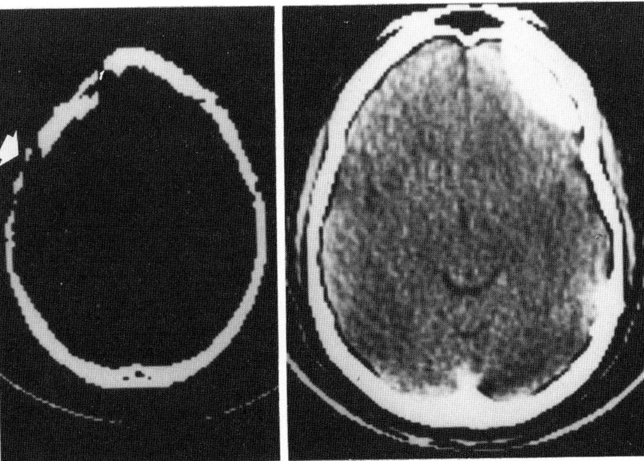

Fig. 10.50 Extradural haematoma (CT scan). The defect on the left scan (arrow) was at the site of a vault fracture. The patient nevertheless shows a frontal extradural haematoma on the opposite side with oedema of the underlying brain and slight displacement of the ventricular system. (Courtesy of Dr G. Hart, Consultant Radiologist, Atkinson Morley's Hospital, London.)

Most *foreign bodies* within the cranium result from gunshot wounds. Metallic and bone fragments are carried deep to the entry wound and must be localized.

Indirect evidence of intracranial injury is provided by lateral shift of the calcified pineal in excess of 2 mm.

The use of computed tomography however has proved invaluable in the assessment of head injuries, particularly in respect of depressed fractures and intracranial haemorrhage (Fig. 10.50). The use to which the investigation is put depends upon its accessibility to the individual patient; in certain cases it could be the primary investigation and precede plain film examination. CT is an essential method for identifying intracranial haematoma in a case of head injury. The combination of skull fracture and any impairment of consciousness makes a haematoma likely to be present in one patient in four, whereas if neither of these two features is present the risk is only 1 in 6000.

FACIAL BONES

The face is a primary target for injury in automobile accidents, particularly when a full lap and diagonal seat belt is not worn by the driver or front-seat passenger. Other injuries to the face are mostly the result of fights or assaults. Clinical assessment is hampered by swelling, but the presence of extensive bruising of the face and periorbital regions makes an underlying fracture very probable. Full assessment is necessary even if other more life-threatening injuries are present; the need to preserve an airway, to prevent ocular complications and residual deformity of the jaws are all of great importance.

The architecture of the face is designed to resist injury. Areas of strength include the body of the zygoma, the frontal process of the maxilla and the alveolar ridge of the maxilla. Unfortunately, this leads to the concept that areas of weakness exist; such lines of weakness were defined by LeFort in 1901 and led to the three major fractures of the facial skeleton bearing his name (Fig. 10.51).

The LeFort 1 fracture is a low transverse line separating the alveolar process from the rest of the maxilla.

The LeFort 2 (pyramidal) fracture separates the central portion of the face and often displaces it posteriorly. The fracture line passes obliquely through the ethmoids, the inferior orbital rim, the maxillary antra and the pterygoid plates.

The LeFort 3 fracture is a high transverse fracture separating the whole facial skeleton from the skull.

Demonstration of facial fractures requires a full series of routine projections consisting of occipito-frontal (or reverse), occipitomental (or reverse) (Fig. 10.52) and lateral views. Supplementary projections, such as submentovertical and obliques, are obtained if appropriate and if the patient's other injuries permit.

The nasal bones are not protected from direct frontal injury. Fractures are identified easily in lateral views.

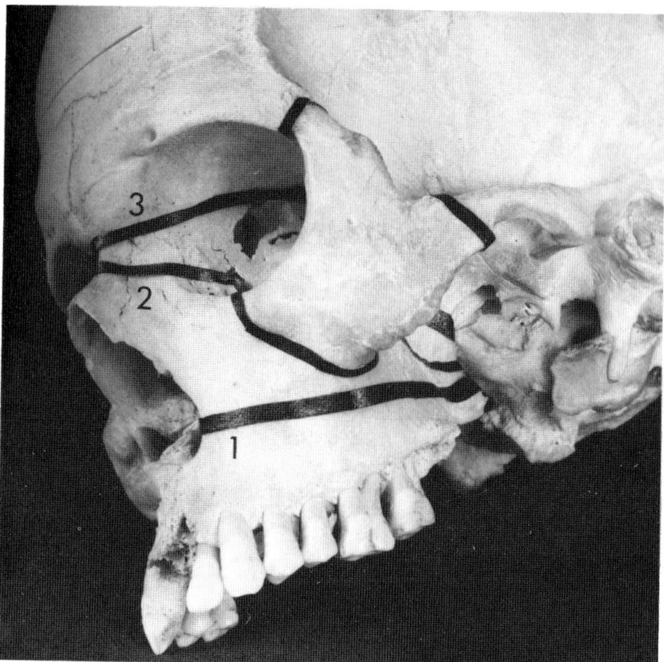

Fig. 10.51 Facial fracture lines. The lines of the common facial fractures are marked on the skull. (1) The low transverse fracture; (2) Pyramidal fracture and (3) high transverse fracture. The numbers also relate to the Le Fort lines of weakness.

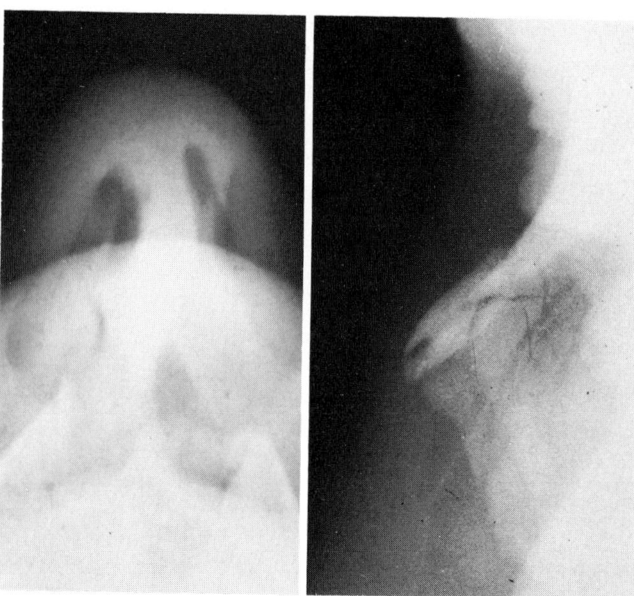

Fig. 10.53 Fracture of the nasal bones. Displacement is evident also in the axial view.

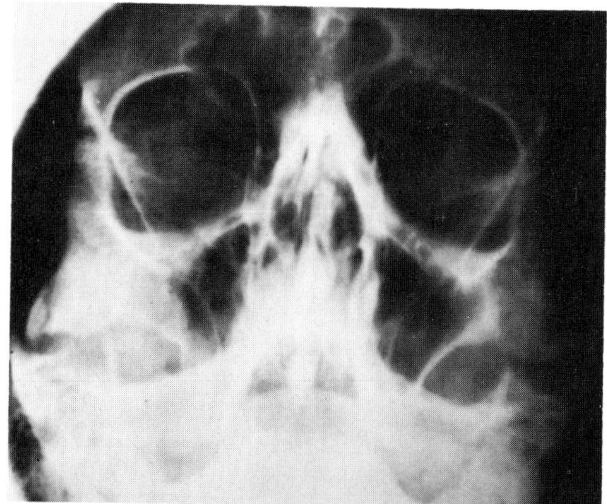

Fig. 10.52 Fracture of right zygoma. The occipito-mental view shows the bony ring to have been damaged in two places with separation of the right zygomatico-frontal synchondrosis and slight depression of the floor of the right orbit.

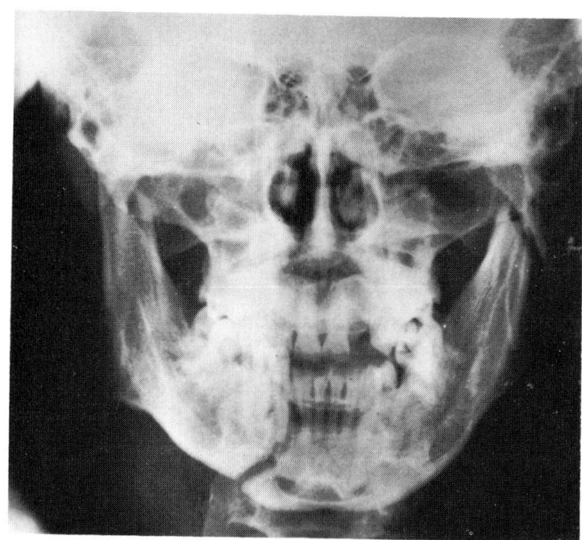

Fig. 10.54 Fractures of the mandible following direct injury. As with other bony rings, fractures in two places are common. Fractures involve the right canine region and the neck of the left condyle.

Lateral displacement is shown best in an axial view with an occlusal film held in the mouth, although the nasal bones may be obscured when the forehead is protuberant (Fig. 10.53). Fractures of the **mandible** are most common at the point of greatest weakness, which corresponds with the canine tooth. They are virtually always compound into the mouth and accurate reduction is necessary to avoid subsequent malocclusion of the teeth. As this bone is essentially a bony ring, the presence of a second fracture must always be excluded. This is especially liable to affect the neck of the condyle on the opposite side to the main injury (Fig. 10.54).

THE SPINE (Fig. 10.55)

Most spinal injuries are due to indirect force; the commonest result from hyperflexion and cause *anterior compression* of one or more vertebral bodies. Such lesions are common in the thoracic and thoraco-lumbar regions, especially in the osteoporotic bones of the elderly. They usually heal spontaneously and may only be revealed years later as an incidental finding. Wedging therefore usually persists except in children where considerable vertebral reconstruction may occur. Acute compression of a thoracic vertebral body may be accompanied by a haematoma resembling a small paravertebral abscess (Fig. 9.6).

The radiologist must appreciate the presence of many spinal ligaments (Fig. 10.55A) and understand that severe ligamentous damage may be sustained in achieving a minor fracture or displacement of bone.

Radiographic assessment of injuries to the spine seeks the answer to two questions. (1) Is a fracture or dislocation

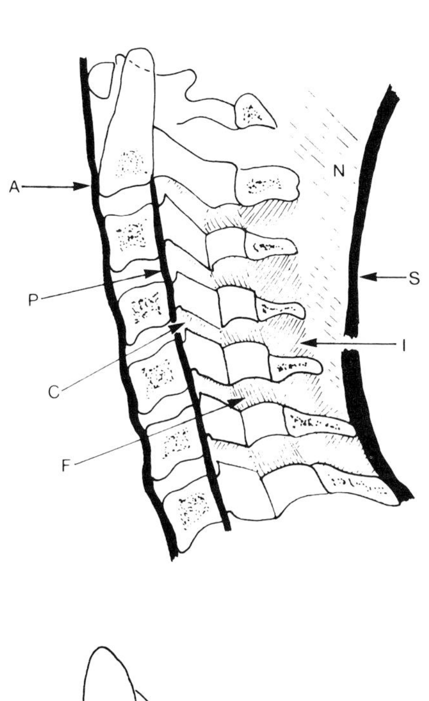

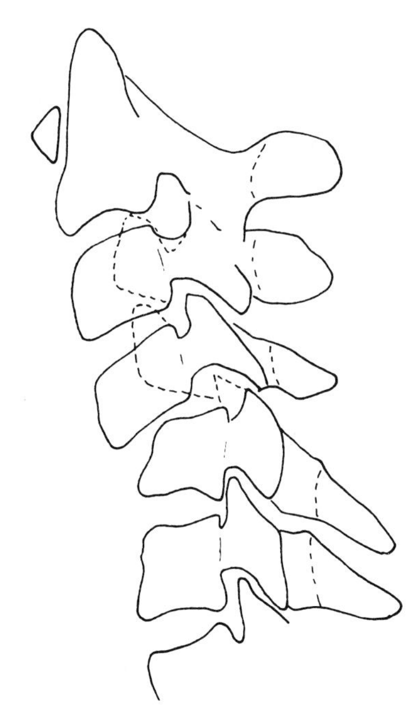

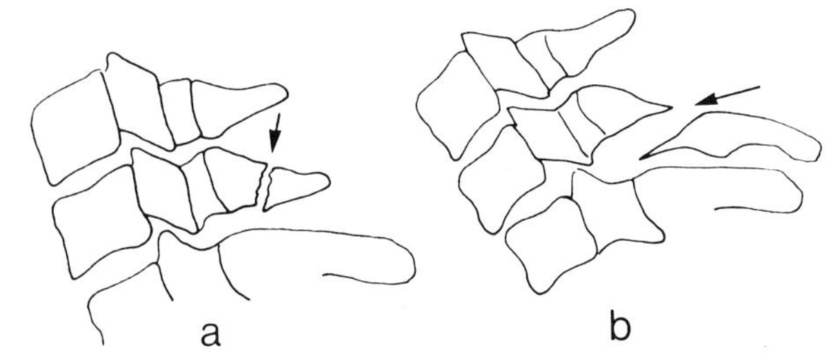

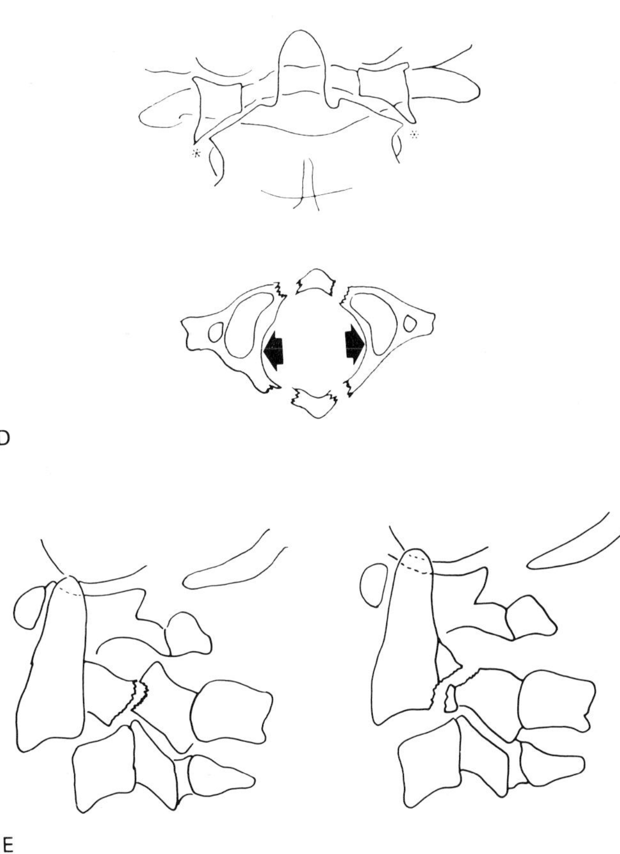

Fig. 10.55 Cervical spinal injuries. **A.** Normal ligamentous anatomy. A = anterior longitudinal ligament, P = posterior longitudinal ligament, the anterior margin of the spinal canal, C = capsular ligaments of apophyseal joints, F = ligamenta flava, I = interspinous ligaments, N = ligamentum nuchae, S = supraspinous ligament. **B.** Flexion-rotation injury with interlocked facets. Note the rotational element at C3 and C4 where the articular processes are no longer superimposed but show a 'bow-tie' appearance. **C.** Fractures involving spinous process. (a) Near vertical 'clay-shoveller's' fracture — caused by avulsion, and stable. (b) Horizontal fracture which is part of a severe hyperextension injury causing extensive damage to the posterior ligament complex. **D.** Jefferson fracture. Extension of the margins of C1 beyond the borders of C2 must indicate fracture of the ring of the atlas in at least two places. **E.** Two varieties of hangman's fracture of C2 involving the arch in the region of the pedicle and the facet joint respectively.

demonstrated? (2) Is the lesion stable or unstable? Nowhere is this more important than in the cervical spine. Radiographic examination here must include a lateral view of all seven vertebrae. This is sometimes difficult in an injured patient as the soft tissue of the shoulder obscures the lower vertebral bodies. As fractures of C6 and C7 are relatively common, attempts have to be made to depress the shoulders whilst a horizontal beam lateral view is obtained. Failing this, oblique or 'swimmer's' views can be useful. Well-penetrated films employing a high kV, even at the expense of film quality, are helpful and often essential at the cervico-thoracic junction (Fig. 10.56). In the final event, if efforts are unsuccessful, traction may have to be applied and further radiographic attempts made when the initial spasm has passed. CT scans, when available, can provide valuable information to supplement the plain films. CT is particularly valuable in the C1–C2 region (Fig. 10.57) and in hyperflexion injury lower in the cervical spine.

The main objective of management in assessing the stability of a cervical fracture-dislocation is the prevention of further neural damage.

Dislocation or subluxation of the posterior interve tebral joints occurs most commonly in the cervical region a prolonged skull traction may be required for reductio The commonest injury is of the hyperflexion ty occasioned by a rapid braking force, such as occurs in collision (Fig. 10.58). The general use of the term 'whipla injury' should be avoided as this is an injury sustain by the passenger in a car struck from behind; it consis of *hyperextension* followed by *flexion* and usually causes severe ligamentous strain without bony injury on radi graphic examination.

While, in hyperflexion injuries, some disturbance in tl bony relationships is usually identified, it is possible for r radiographic abnormality to be noted in the presence (a complete quadriplegia, the original dislocation havir undergone spontaneous reduction.

Likewise, cord damage is not inevitable and man unreduced lesions show no neurological damage an proceed to spontaneous fusion.

Important diagnostic signs of a hyperflexion injur

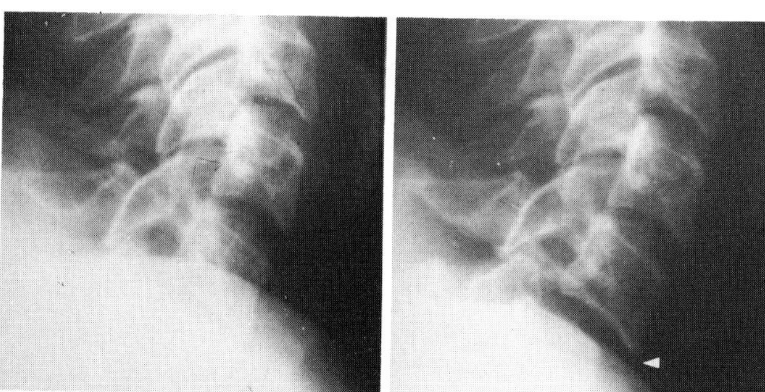

Fig. 10.56 Fracture-dislocation at C6–C7 level. The film on the left was obtained with inadequate penetration at 70 kV and failed to demonstrate the seventh cervical vertebra. The only diagnostic clue to the diagnosis was subluxation of the posterior intervertebral joints. A more penetrated projection at 100 kV demonstrates clearly the fracture-dislocation. Observe widening of the angle between the spinous processes and disruption of the smooth line on the posterior side of the neural canal.

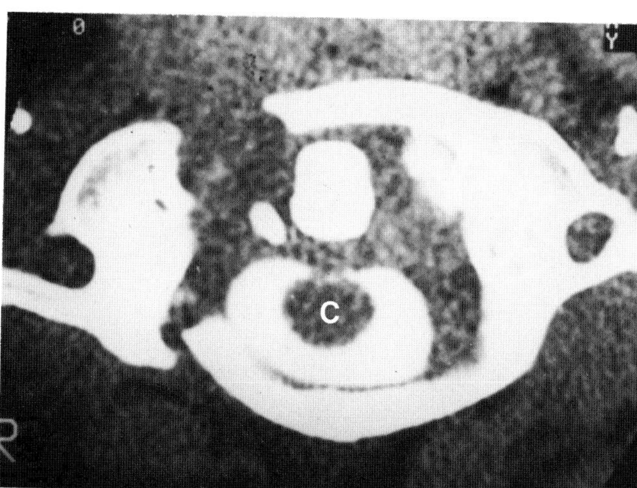

Fig. 10.57 CT scan of 'Jefferson' fracture of atlas. The right side of the arch of C1 is fractured in two places. Contrast medium has been injected into the subarachnoid space to demonstrate the spinal cord (C). (Courtesy of Dr David Sutton.)

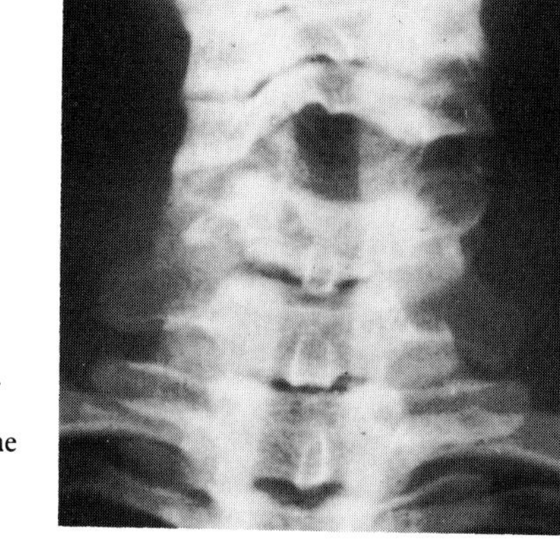

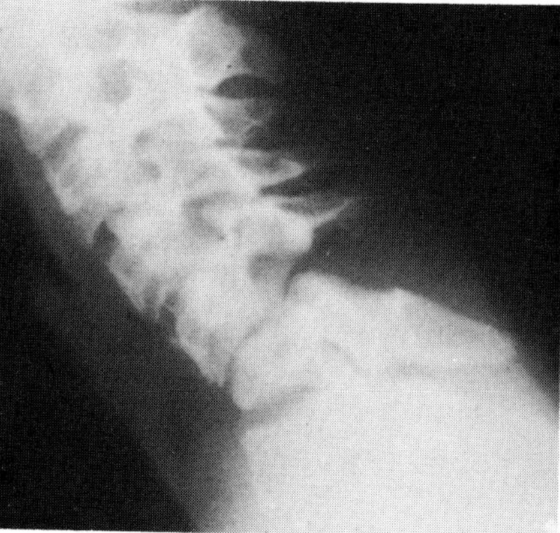

Fig. 10.58 Hyperflexion fracture-dislocation with secondary instability following a road traffic accident. The body of C5 is dislocated forwards in relation to the body of C6, with slight wedging of the latter. The synovial articular surfaces and spinous processes are widely separated.

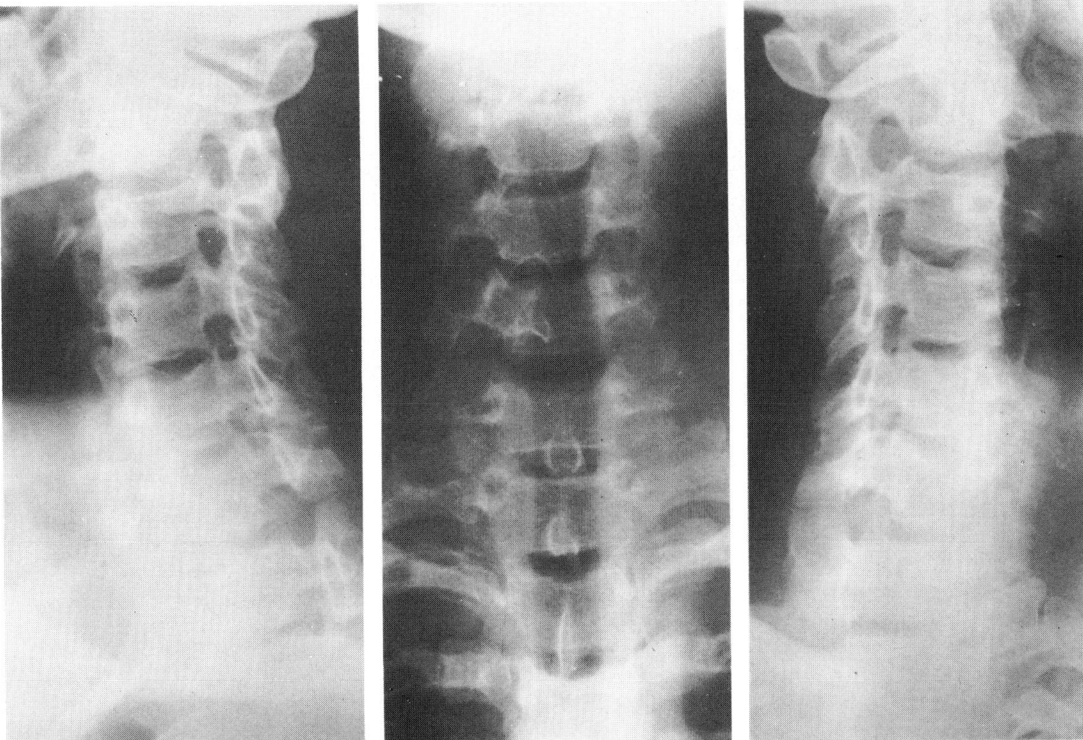

Fig. 10.59 Dislocation of cervical spine. (Male aged 20). This young man fell while inebriated and developed paraplegic signs which resolved with traction. Both the posterior intervertebral joints at the C6–C7 level are dislocated, the articular facets being 'locked'. The displacement on the left side is the more severe, with relative enlargement of this exit foramen and disruption of alignment of the spinal canal. The discrepancy between the degree of involvement of these joints has caused an element of rotation, which can be deduced in the frontal view from malalignment of the spinous processes above and below the widened C6–C7 space.

include (1) loss of the smooth posterior line of the vertebral bodies, the anterior wall of the spinal canal. When, in the presence of apophyseal dislocation, a vertebral body is displaced forwards by more than half its anteroposterior diameter, both facet joints must be dislocated (Fig. 10.55B); (2) Hyperflexion injury leads to loss of the normal cervical lordosis and increased separation of the spinous processes at the affected level (Fig. 10.58); (3) Malalignment of the spinous processes in the frontal projection indicates asymmetrical subluxation (Fig. 10.59) or, more commonly, unilateral dislocation.

Hyperextension injuries are often associated with extensive disruption of the paraspinal ligaments (Fig. 10.55A) and often severe neurological damage. Plain radiographic evidence of such a catastrophic injury may be confined to a small marginal 'tear-drop' fracture of the anterior margin of a vertebral body. It is emphasized that the clinical state of such a patient can never be judged from inspection of the radiograph.

Isolated fractures of the vertebral appendages may result from direct trauma or violent muscular stress, such as in fractures of the lumbar transverse processes. Fractures of the pars interarticularis may occur in acute trauma but are much more commonly the result of chronic stress. The *clay-shoveller's* fracture is a stress fracture of the spinous process of a lower cervical vertebra in the coronal plane (Fig. 10.60A). It must not be confused with a horizontal fracture of the spinous process which is part of a severe hyperflexion disruption of the posterior elements (Figs 10.6B and 10.55C).

Certain vertebral injuries require individual consideration:

1. **Fracture of the atlas (Jefferson fracture).** This rare injury is due to transmission of force through the occipital condyles, and is caused often by impact of the head on the bottom of a swimming bath after a dive or by a heavy blow on the vertex. Separation of the fragments may be shown with an anteroposterior view through the open mouth, when the lateral masses of the atlas overlap those of the axis, indicating that the arch of the atlas is broken in at least two places (Figs 10.61, 10.55D and 10.57). Spinal cord compression is responsible for an immediate mortality of 10%, but the remainder have a remarkably good prognosis and usually suffer only slight residual disability.

2. **Dislocation of the atlas**. Atlanto-occipital dislocations are usually fatal. Atlanto-axial dislocation is the most common dislocation in this region. In anterior and rotatory dislocations the lateral view shows a disturbance of the relationship of the anterior arch to the odontoid process,

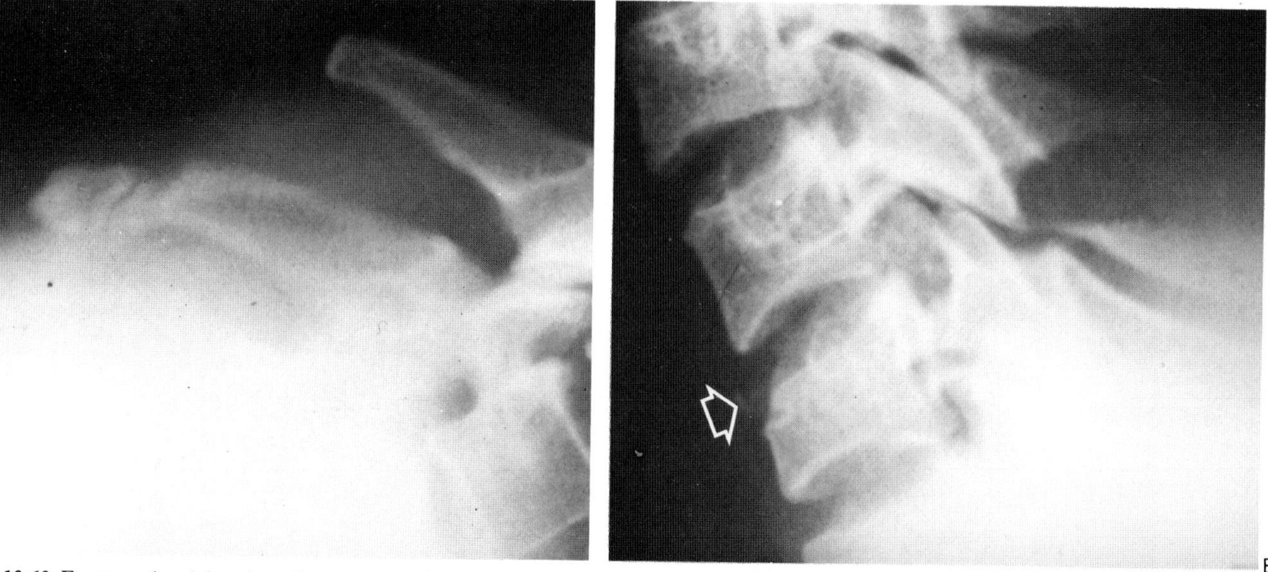

Fig. 10.60 Fractures involving the spinous process (see also Fig. 10.55 C). **A**. Clay-shoveller's fracture — an isolated avulsion fracture. **B**. Horizontal fracture as part of a severe hyperflexion injury. The separation of the two parts of the process indicates the severe ligamentous damage. The anterior tear-drop fracture (arrow) shows that the adjoining vertebra has impinged at some time.

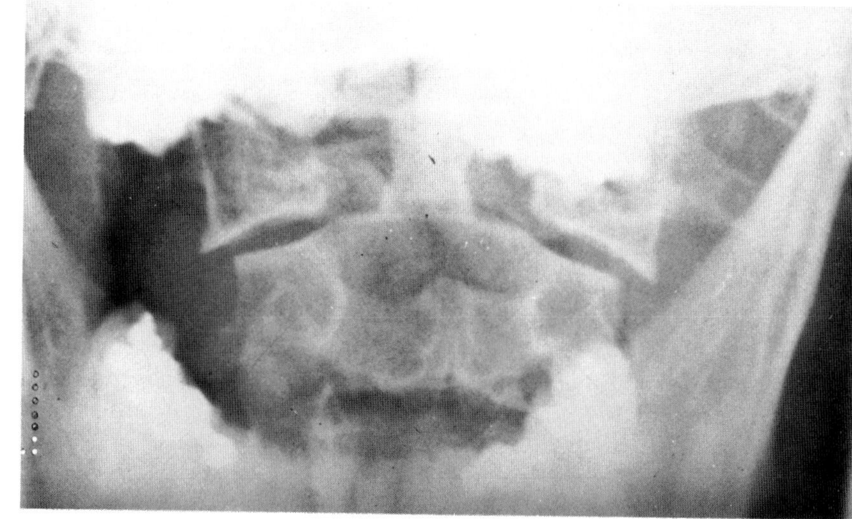

Fig. 10.61 Jefferson fracture of atlas. In the open-mouth projection the lateral masses of the atlas extend beyond those of the axis, indicating that the arch of C1 must be fractured in several places.

the space between these structures becoming abnormally wide. Rotation is usually associated with a variable degree of torticollis, making radiography difficult and radiographs difficult to interpret. Tomography may be required, but even CT fails to resolve the spatial relationships in some cases. Dislocations are often associated with a fracture of the odontoid process (Fig. 10.62). The forward type of atlantal dislocation has been recognized to occur spontaneously in children with throat infections and has been attributed to laxity of the transverse atlantal ligament associated with hyperaemia. Such spontaneous dislocations with adjacent inflammatory lesions are not confined to this joint.

3. **Fracture of the axis.** The odontoid process is the homologue of a vertebral body. It develops from separate ossific centres which very rarely may fail to develop or fail to fuse. Fractures usually occur at the base of the odontoid process, with displacement rarely exceeding a few millimetres in either a forward or backward direction (Fig. 10.62), but it is especially important to recognize those which are undisplaced in order that adequate protection may be provided. Fractures are visualized best in the anteroposterior open-mouth projection, but have to be distinguished from the mach effect produced by the anterior or posterior arch of the atlas, or air in the buccal cavity. The prognosis is considerably better with this injury

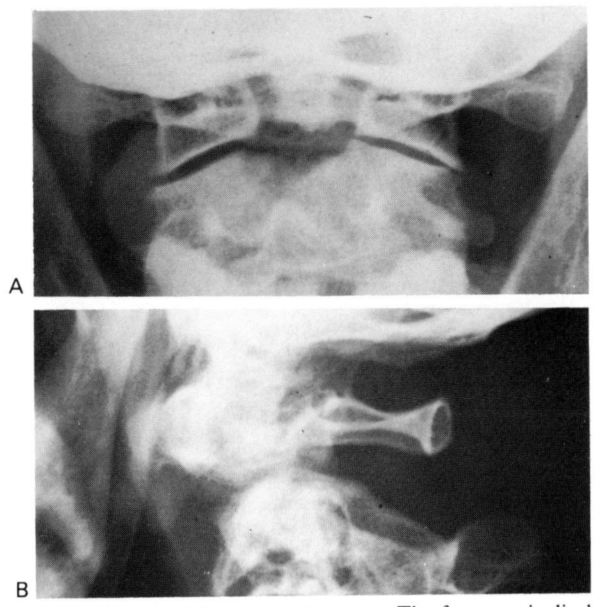

Fig. 10.62 Fracture of the odontoid process. The fragment is displaced forwards with an associated dislocation of the atlas.

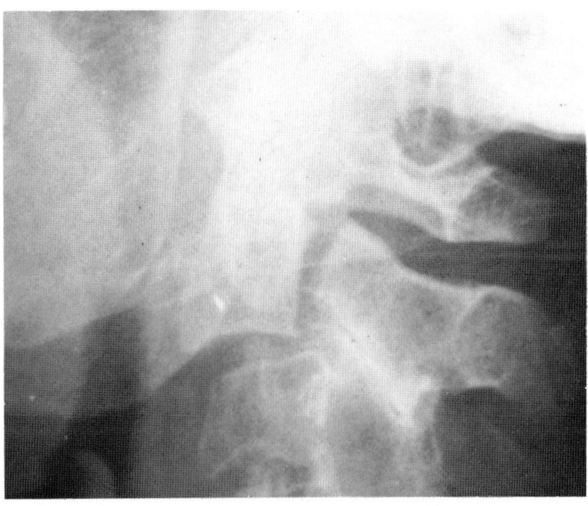

Fig. 10.63 Hangman's fracture of axis. The bilateral fractures of the pedicles are seen best in the lateral projection. The body of the axis lies slightly anterior to C3; this is an *unstable* fracture.

than it is with a rupture of the transverse ligament of the atlas, which crosses immediately behind the odontoid process. The latter injury permits dislocation of the atlas and may result in fatal cord compression.

Instability at the atlanto-axial level, demonstrated by comparison of lateral films in flexion and extension, is sometimes observed with absence of the odontoid process. Such absence has long been regarded as a congenital variant, but verified cases have been reported of this appearance following a fracture in childhood with necrosis and absorption of the fragment.

The most common cause of atlanto-axial instability, however, is rheumatoid arthritis. Identification of such instability is paramount prior to general anaesthesia and intubation of affected patients.

Fracture of the axis on one or other side of the junction of the pedicle and body constitutes a *'hangman's fracture'* (Figs. 10.55E and 10.63), although it usually results from a traffic accident or a non-judicial fall.

4. **'Chance' or 'lap-strap' fractures** are the result of acute flexion injuries of the lower thoracic or lumbar spine incurred in road accidents while wearing a single lap strap without restraint of the upper part of the torso by a diagonal strap. Marked angular kyphosis is demonstrated with a fracture traversing both the apical vertebral body and its appendages (Fig. 10.64).

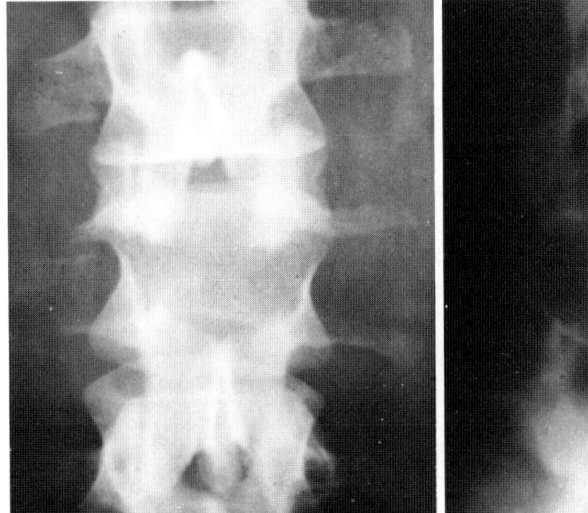

Fig. 10.64 'Chance' or 'lap-strap' fracture of L2. The fracture is due to a hyperflexion injury with disruption of the posterior ligament complex and involvement of the posterior arch and the margin of the vertebral body in this case. In the anteroposterior radiograph, the 'empty' appearance of the vertebra results from separation of the fractured arch by the persistent kyphosis.

DISC LESIONS

While it is clear that many of these spinal injuries also cause damage to the intervertebral discs, a localized disc lesion is relatively rarely attributable to a fracture. The nucleus pulposus is a gelatinous fluid collection lying between the cartilaginous end-plates of the vertebral bodies, and is contained peripherally by the tough anulus fibrosus. Either sudden or chronic trauma may cause annular rupture with or without protrusion of the incompressible fluid centre of this shock-absorber system through its fibrous wall. Should protrusion occur in a posterior or postero-lateral direction to encroach on the neural canal, cord or nerve root, pressure may result with consequent segmental root pain and secondary muscle spasm. The lesions are most common in men of middle age when the weight load of the skeleton has been increased by obesity and the muscle tone has been diminished by a sedentary life. In younger individuals, no abnormality may be visible in the radiograph, the disc spaces being of normal height. Abnormal reduction in height of an inter vertebral space indicates a previous disc lesion. Evidence of chronic disc derangement is provided by malalignment of the vertebral bodies recognized most easily by a slight step deformity between their posterior borders. The upper body may show a little backward slip in relation to the lower. Comparison of lateral views in flexion and extension may exhibit localized limitation of movement due to muscle spasm at the affected level. On the other hand, such views may reveal instability at the affected level. Instability should be suspected when a small spur of bone is evident on the anterior aspect of a vertebral body at a point slightly removed from the articular margin. These abnormalities have been described by Macnab as 'traction spurs' and correspond to the attachments of the anterior longitudinal ligament. They are not to be confused with osteophytes, which are direct outgrowths from the margin of the articular cartilage. Osteophytes appear to represent a physiological response to a disordered joint mechanism, in an attempt to limit movement and thus reduce painful symptoms. Traction spurs, as their name implies, reflect the stresses on the spinal ligaments following the irregular movements of vertebrae in relation to an abnormal, often degenerate, disc.

As age advances, the affected disc space narrows progressively and degenerative spondylosis develops. This alteration of anatomical relationship also predisposes to the development of degenerative osteoarthritis in the associated apophyseal joints. The lesions are most frequently found at the lumbo-sacral and L4–L5 levels, the latter being especially liable to occur with the common sacralization of the fifth lumbar vertebra. Spontaneous disc herniation in the dorsal area is unusual but tends to produce cord compression at an early stage because of the relatively narrow spinal canal.

Degenerative changes in the cervical discs are exceedingly common in the elderly and especially between C5 and C7. Acute cervical disc prolapse is uncommon, but may occur after trauma. Radiation of pain to the arms in the middle-aged may be associated with secondary osteophytic encroachment on the intervertebral foramina demonstrated most clearly in oblique projections.

Myelography is of considerable value in assessing the type and position of disc protrusions and, in particular displacement or compression of nerve roots.

Discography, the direct injection of radio-opaque medium into the nucleus pulposus, may reveal extensive rupture and displacement of a nucleus pulposus when plain films have shown no abnormality. Its major use is in the lumbar spine to establish the presence of normal discs adjoining a site of proposed surgical fusion.

Computed tomography, employing the new generation machines, has been shown to have a comparable accuracy to water-soluble myelography in the demonstration of disc disease. Its value in spinal stenosis and degenerative disease of the apophyseal joints is even greater, but its value in direct delineation of nerve root involvement has yet to be established.

Magnetic resonance imaging at the present time is not widely available and has yet to secure its place. Although the discs and ligaments are visualized better than with CT, the poor definition of bone is a limiting factor in anatomical definition.

THE THORACIC CAGE

Fractures of the ribs are common in adults and result from direct trauma. Their demonstration may be of importance medico-legally, but the greatest value of radiological examination is in excluding complications. These include *pneumothorax, surgical emphysema*, the presence of *fluid (usually blood) in the pleural space* or *collapse of underlying lung tissue* (see Ch. 19). The rib fractures themselves are largely splinted by the intercostal muscles.

The presence of multiple old healed rib fractures, unassociated with a history of serious trauma, should suggest such conditions as alcoholism, steroid therapy or osteomalacia.

Fractures of the **sternum** usually result from direct impact on a steering wheel in road accidents. These are commonest at the junction of the body and manubrium and are best shown with lateral views.

ISOTOPES AND CT

In traumatic conditions radiography remains the most useful, accessible and cheap method of imaging in the management of the patient. Nevertheless, two scanning techniques — radionuclide scanning and computed tomography — because of their differing mechanisms, are complementary both to orthodox radiography and to each other.

RADIONUCLIDE SCANNING (scintigraphy)

Radionuclide imaging reflects the activity or rate of turnover of bone thereby providing dynamic information relating to its blood supply and metabolism; it is therefore valuable in demonstrating the reactive changes in bone following trauma. The technique carries a high sensitivity and low specificity, so is best employed to localize a lesion whilst other techniques identify the cause. As the dose is similar whether single or multiple lesions are present, it should not generally be used for serial studies, e.g. to monitor fracture healing, where radiography would be more appropriate.

In most cases of trauma, radionuclide scans are unnecessary, although fractures older than 3 days are identifiable in 95% of cases. In the first 5 days following injury, increased activity due to soft tissue trauma and hyperaemia may be difficult to differentiate from fracture and an unequivocal result cannot always be expected. In trauma, positive scans may be found, in the absence of fracture, in stress sclerosis (Fig. 10.65) and subperiosteal haematoma. The bone scan offers its greatest value in locating fractures in bones with a mainly cancellous structure, such as the scaphoid or vertebral body, where radiographic demonstration of the fracture line may be difficult. A scan cannot differentiate between a fracture through normal and abnormal bone.

Activity may persist for a variable period after apparent healing of the fracture; fractures under 6 months of age however show a greater activity than older lesions. Activity persisting for over 18 months is generally associated with incomplete fractures or malunion. Radionuclide bone scanning may be of use in the evaluation of non-accidental injury in childhood in that fractures and periosteal reactions may be identified prior to radiographic evidence of their presence. In other circumstances, unsuspected fractures may be revealed (Fig. 66).

COMPUTED TOMOGRAPHY (CT)

The value of CT in trauma to the head is already proven to be unique and cost-effective. Similarly, information of incomparable value has been provided in injury to the soft tissues within the thorax and abdomen.

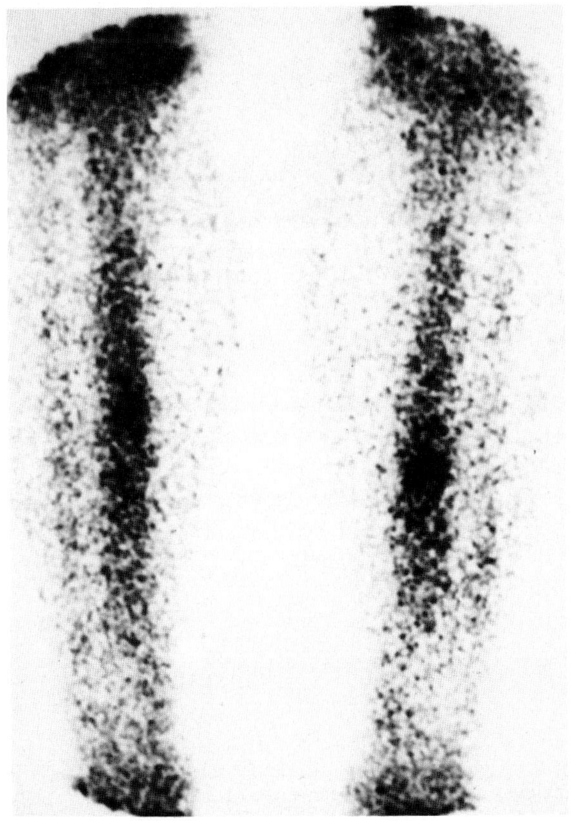

Fig. 10.65 Radionuclide scan of legs of a ballet dancer showing increased uptake in association with stress fractures of the tibiae. Such activity may precede radiographic evidence of fracture by as much as three weeks.

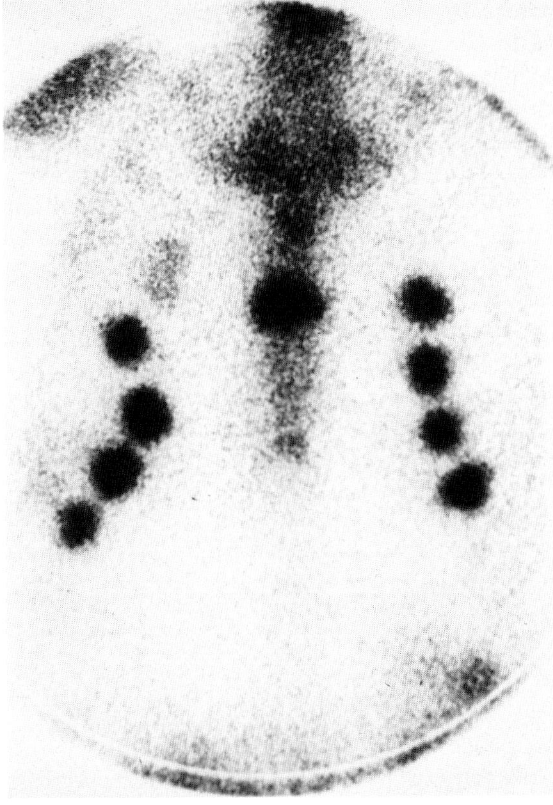

Fig. 10.66 Radionuclide scan of a patient resuscitated by external cardiac massage showing uptake in multiple anterior rib fractures.

Injury to bone was initially not given priority in CT scanning because of the excellent detail provided by radiography and the relative inaccessibility of CT to many Accident Departments. It is now obvious that CT can offer much valuable information in trauma, particularly in the axial skeleton. In contrast to the several disadvantages of CT — cost and availability — it has the advantage that seriously injured patients, who are sufficiently unencumbered by splints etc. to be able to enter the CT port, can be scanned without the further movement that might be required by special radiographic projections.

Spinal trauma. In evaluation of injuries to the *cervical* region, CT will show the presence of multiple fractures in the vertebral arch, such as in the Jefferson fracture of C1 (Fig. 10.57). Further information, helpful in the management of hyperflexion injuries lower in the cervical spine, may be afforded, but odontoid fractures, being in the plane of the scan, generally can only be shown well with sagittal reconstruction. In the *thoracolumbar* spine, anatomical detail is again provided in areas where conventional radiography is difficult. In particular, encroachment on the spinal canal and cord by fracture fragments can be uniquely shown by this form of imaging (Fig. 10.67).

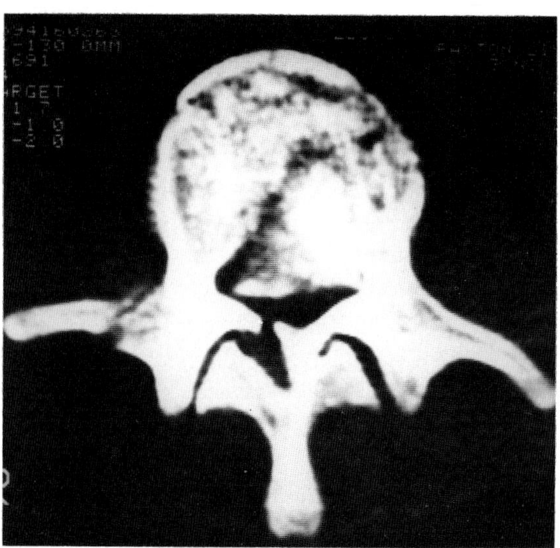

Fig. 10.67 CT of fractured lumbar vertebra. Observe the displacement of a fragment of the body posteriorly to encroach on the spinal canal. (Courtesy of Professor J. Best, Edinburgh.)

Pelvic and acetabular fractures, The complex anatomy of the bony pelvis often provides limitations to conventional radiography. The acetabulum is supported by two columns of bone, the anterior and posterior pillars. Demonstration of fractures requires special views with rotation of the patient (Judet views, q.v.). CT has been shown to be of great value in the demonstration of fragments which the surgeon can then locate and remove before they cause irreparable damage to the joint or other structures, such as blood vessels. Postoperative CT enables the surgeon to confirm his achievements in this region. The orientation of the sacrum makes its demonstration difficult by radiography and here too CT will establish the spatial relationships of the fracture fragments (Fig. 10.68). Needless to say, the great value of the technique in demonstration of the soft tissues can result in the identification of large haematomata within the pelvic cavity.

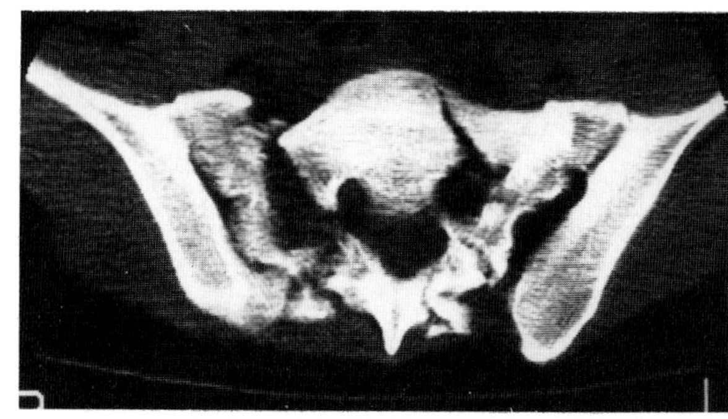

Fig. 10.68 CT of comminuted fracture of sacrum due to lateral compression of the pelvis. Note splaying of left sacroiliac joint posteriorly. (Courtesy of Professor J. Best, Edinburgh.)

The appendicular skeleton. The contribution here is less significant as conventional radiography is usually adequate or better. CT will probably prove to have value in injuries of less accessible (sternoclavicular) and complex (knee, ankle) joints. It may provide information through a plaster cast, denied to radiography, and in the soft tissues, e.g. in a compartment syndrome; the information may again be unequalled by other imaging modalities.

REFERENCES AND SUGGESTIONS FOR FURTHER READING (Chapters 9 & 10)

General

Grech, P. (1981) *Casualty Radiology*. London: Chapman & Hall.

Harris, J. H., Jr., Harris, W. H. (1975) *The Radiology of Emergency Medicine*. Baltimore: Williams & Wilkins Co.

Murray, R. O., Jacobson, H. G (1977) *The Radiology of Skeletal Disorders*, 2nd edn. Edinburgh: Churchill Livingstone.

Ozonoff, M. B. (1979) *Pediatric Orthopaedic Radiology*. Philadelphia: W. B. Saunders Co.

Rogers, L. F. (1982) *Radiology of Skeletal Trauma*. New York, Edinburgh: Churchill Livingstone.

Wilson, J. N. (ed.) (1976) *Watson Jones Fractures and Joint Injuries*. 5th edn. Edinburgh: Churchill Livingstone.

Specific Conditions

Aichroth, P. (1974) Osteochondritis dissecans of the knee. *Journal of Bone and Joint Surgery*, **53B**, 440–447.

Bloomberg, T. J., Nuttall, J., Stoker, D. J. (1978) Radiology in early slipped femoral capital epiphysis. *Clinical Radiology*, **29**, 657–667.

Caffey, J. (1972) The parent-infant traumatic stress syndrome (Caffey-Kempe syndrome) (battered baby syndrome). The First Annual Neuhauser Presidential Address to the Society for Pediatric Radiology. *American Journal of Roentgenology*, **114**, 217–229.

Crowe, J. E., Swischuk, L. E. (1977) Acute bowing fractures of the forearm in children. A frequently missed injury. *American Journal of Roentgenology*, **128**, 981–984.

Dolan, K. D., Jacoby, C. G. (1978) Facial fractures. *Seminars in Roentgenology*, **13**, 37–51.

Greaney, R. B., Gerber, F. H., Laughlin, R. L. *et al.* (1983) Distribution and natural history of stress fractures in U.S. marine recruits. *Radiology*, **146**, 339–346.

Harris, J. H. Jr. (1978) *The Radiology of Acute Cervical Spine Trauma.* Baltimore: Williams & Wilkins Co.

Harris, N. H., Murray, R. O. (1974) Lesions of the symphysis in athletes. *British Medical Journal*, **4**, 211–214.

Johnson, J. T. H. (1967) Neuropathic fractures and joint injuries. Pathogenesis and rationale of prevention and treatment. *Journal of Bone and Joint Surgery*, **49A**, 1–30.

Keen, J. S., Goletz, T. H., Lilleas, T., *et al.* (1982) Diagnosis of vertebral fractures. A comparison of conventional radiography, conventional tomography and computed axial tomography. *Journal of Bone and Joint Surgery*, **64A**, 586–594.

Lequesne, M. *et al.* (1977) Partial transient osteoporosis. *Skeletal Radiology*, **2**, 1–8.

Neer, C. S. (1970) Displaced proximal humeral fractures. *Journal of Bone and Joint Surgery*, **52A**, 1077–1089.

Nelson, S. W. (1966) Some important diagnostic and technical fundamentals in the radiology of trauma, with particular emphasis on skeletal trauma. *Radiological Clinics of North America*, **4**, 241–259.

Newman, P. H. (1963) The aetiology of spondylolisthesis. *Journal of Bone and Joint Surgery*, **45B**, 39–59.

Reckling, F. W. (1982) Unstable fracture-dislocations of the forearm (Monteggia and Galeazzi lesions). *Journal of Bone and Joint Surgery*, **64A**, 857–863.

Ryan, M. D., Taylor, T. K. F. (1982) Odontoid fractures. *Journal of Bone and Joint Surgery*, **64B**, 416–421.

Salter, R. B., Harris, W. R. (1963) Injuries involving the epiphyseal plate. *Journal of Bone and Joint Surgery*, **45A**, 587–622.

Walker, R. H., Burton, D. S. (1982) Computerized tomography in assessment of acetabular fractures. *Journal of Trauma*, **22**, 227–234.

Warrick, C. K. (1965) Posterior dislocation of the shoulder joint. *British Journal of Radiology*, **38**, 758–761.

PART 2

THE CHEST

CHAPTER 11

THE NORMAL CHEST: METHODS OF INVESTIGATION AND DIFFERENTIAL DIAGNOSIS

THE NORMAL CHEST: METHODS OF INVESTIGATION

1. Plain films: PA, lateral,
   AP, decubitus, supine, oblique, inspiratory, expiratory, lordotic, apical, penetrated, magnified.
2. Tomography
3. Fluoroscopy
4. Isotope studies
5. CAT scanning
6. Fine needle biopsy
7. Bronchography
8. Ultrasound
9. Pulmonary angiography
10. Bronchial arteriography
11. Diagnostic pneumothorax
12. Barium swallow
13. Lymphangiography
14. MRI.

The *plain chest film* is the most frequently requested radiological examination. Because of the inherent contrast of the tissues of the thorax, visualization of the lung fields is excellent. A routine examination should include PA and lateral films. Comparison with old films is valuable and should never be omitted. Current plain films are mandatory before proceeding to more complex diagnostic procedures.

Tomography is the investigation of choice for assessing the peripheral lung mass and the abnormal hilum, although high kVp chest films have reduced the need for tomography in many cases.

CAT scanning has developed a place in the evaluation of the hilum. It is also of great value for pleural and chest wall lesions, and for staging malignancy. It is particularly valuable in assessing mediastinal masses and aneurysms (see Ch. 12).

Radio-isotope scans excel in the diagnosis of pulmonary embolus, and also in excluding this diagnosis; only rarely, such as when embolectomy is contemplated, does angiography become necessary.

Ultrasound has a small part to play in locating and confirming the presence of pleural fluid. *Bronchography* remains the best investigation for demonstrating bronchiectasis, but its use has otherwise declined.

Fine needle biopsy of peripheral pulmonary lesions has gained wide popularity. It should only be considered when non-invasive techniques have failed to establish a definite diagnosis. This technique is invaluable when a positive result is obtained. A negative result is of little diagnostic assistance.

MRI has so far proved of most value in elucidating mediastinal and vascular lesions. As yet it appears less useful for intrapulmonary lesions.

Most of the techniques listed are discussed in detail below.

PLAIN FILMS

The PA view. By definition the patient faces the film chin up with shoulders rotated forwards to displace the scapulae from the lung fields. Exposure is made on full inspiration for optimum visualization of the bases, centring at T5. The breasts should be compressed against the film to prevent them obscuring the lung bases.

There is no general consensus regarding the kilovoltage used for chest radiography. High kVp, low kVp or intermediate kVp techniques are used with various film-screen combinations, grids or air gap techniques.

Using a low kVp (60–80 kV) produces a high contrast film (Fig. 11.1). For larger patients a grid is needed to reduce scatter. A FFD of six feet reduces magnification and produces a sharper image.

With high kilovoltages of 120–150 kVp the films are of lower contrast (Fig. 11. 2) with increased visualisation of the hidden areas of the lung fields due to better penetration of overlying structures. The bones and pulmonary calcification are less well seen. Pulmonary markings are better demonstrated. A grid or air gap is necessary to reduce scatter and improve contrast. An air gap of 15–25 cm between patient and film necessitates an increased FFD of 8 feet to reduce magnification.

An automatic exposure system and dedicated automatic chest unit are desirable in a busy department.

The lateral view. A high kVp or normal kVp technique may be used with or without a grid. For sharpness the side of interest is nearest the film. With shoulders parallel to the film the arms are elevated, or displaced back if the anterior mediastinum is of interest.

Lesions obscured on the PA view are often clearly demonstrated on the lateral view; in contrast, clearcut lesions on the PA view may have an insignificant appearance on the lateral film because the lung fields are superimposed. This is particularly so with a large pleural effusion (Fig. 11.3). Anterior mediastinal masses, encysted pleural fluid (Fig. 11.4), lobar collapse and posterior basal consolidation are well demonstrated.

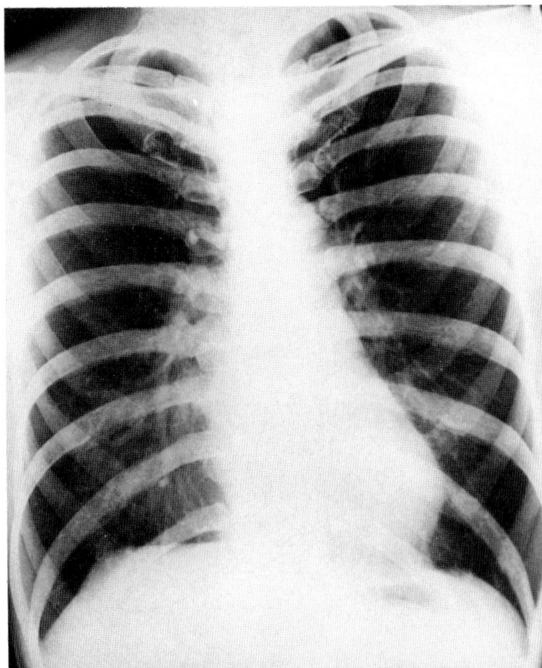

Fig. 11.1 Radiograph taken at 60 kVp.

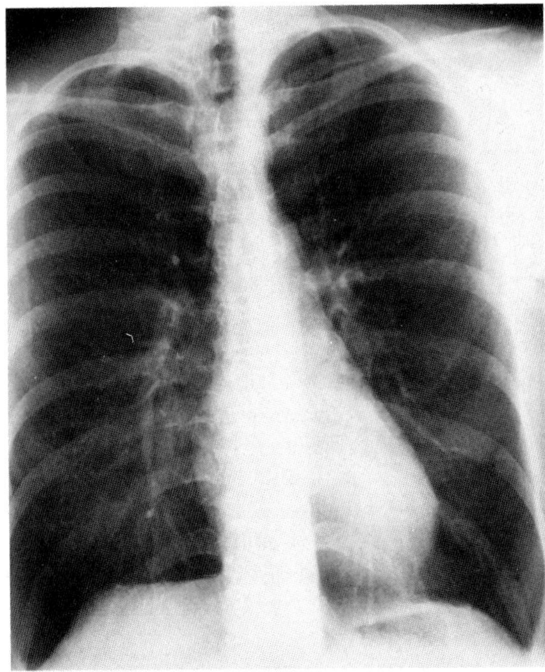

Fig. 11.2 Radiograph of same patient taken at 140 kVp. Note the improved visualization of the main airways, vascular structures and the area behind the heart including the spine.

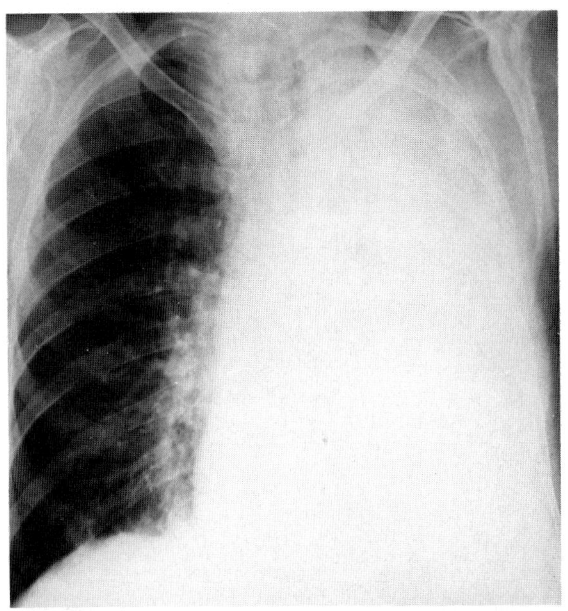

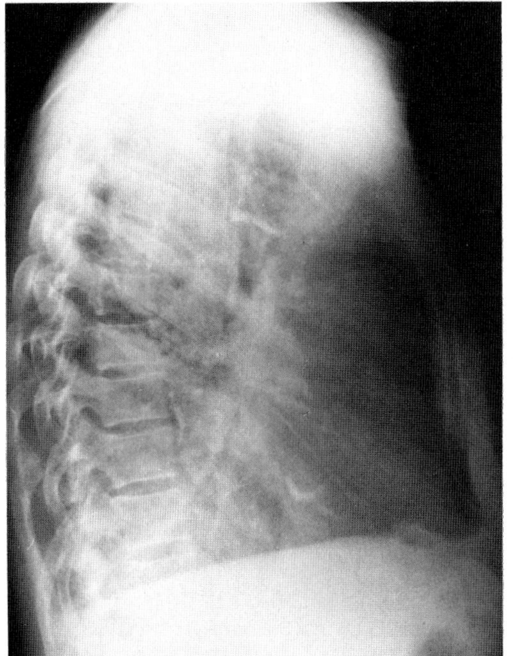

Fig. 11.3 (**A**) Collapse and consolidation of the left lung. (**B**) Lateral film. The appearances are less dramatic than on the PA film. Only the right hemidiaphragm is visible. The radiolucency of the lower vertebrae is decreased.

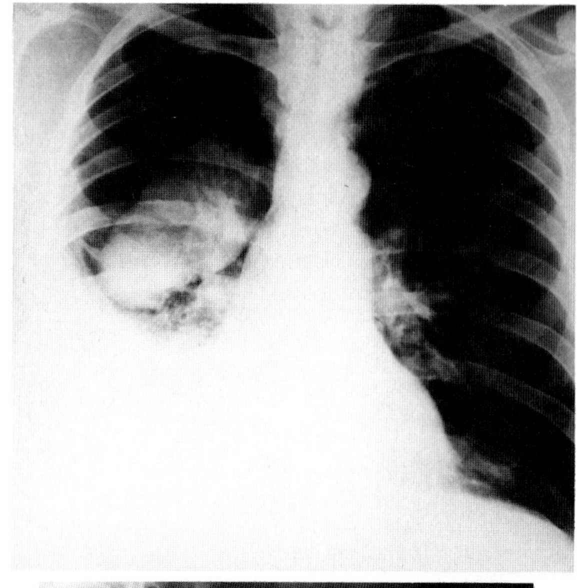

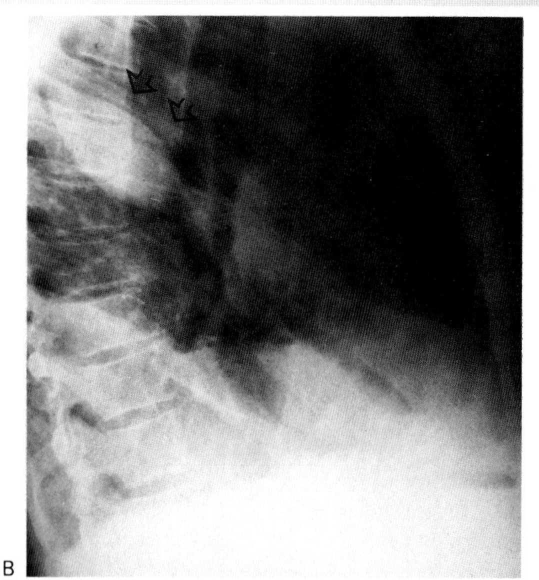

Fig. 11.4 Encysted pleural fluid. (**A**) PA film. A large right pleural effusion and a large mass above. (**B**) Lateral film. Loculated fluid is demonstrated high in the oblique fissure.

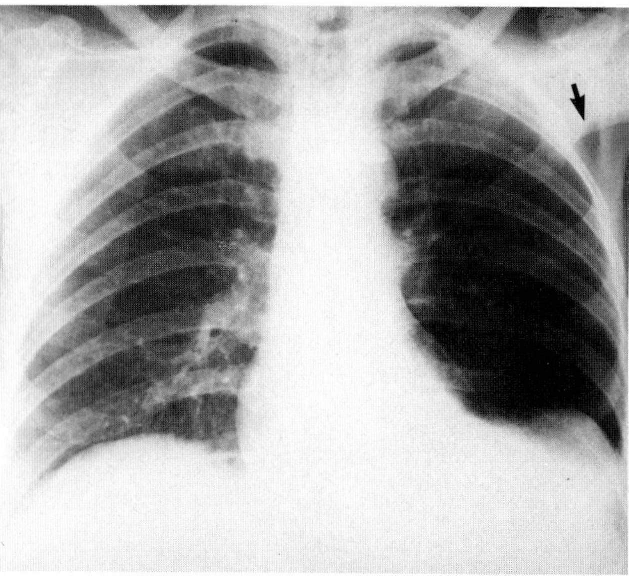

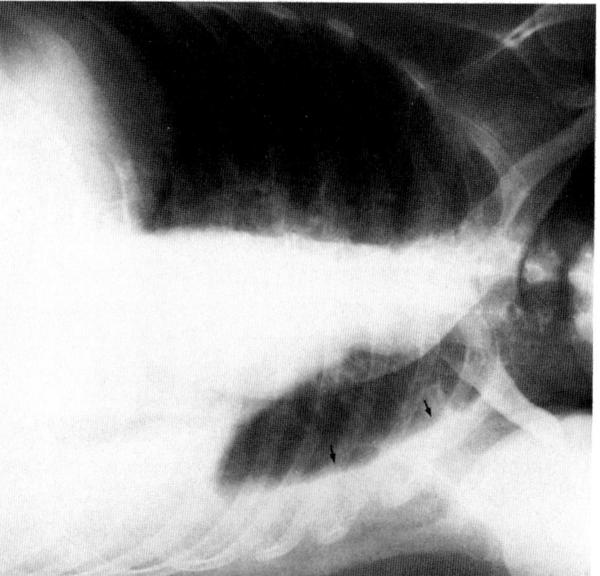

Fig. 11.5 Subpulmonary pleural fluid. (**A**) Erect PA radiograph. There is apparent elevation of the left hemidiaphragm. Increased translucency of the left lung is due to a left mastectomy. Note the abnormal axillary fold (arrow). (**B**) Left lateral decubitus film (with horizontal beam.) Pleural fluid has moved to the most dependent part of the left lung (arrows).

Other views. Additional plain films may assist with certain diagnostic problems. To show the hidden areas of the PA film, rib destruction, cavitation, calcification, an air bronchogram and the main airways, a *penetrated film* should be obtained. The retrocardiac area and posterior costophrenic angles are demonstrated on oblique views. In the AP position the ribs are projected over different areas of the lung and the posterior chest well shown. Good visualization of the apices requires projecting the clavicles up, as in the *apical view* with the tube angled up 50–60 degrees, or down, as in the *lordotic view* with the patient in a lordotic PA position. In the lordotic view a middle lobe collapse shows clearly as a well-defined triangular structure.

A subpulmonary effusion is often difficult to distinguish from an elevated diaphragm or consolidation. In the *supine* and *decubitus* (Fig. 11.5) *positions* free fluid becomes displaced; on the supine projection this results in the hemithorax becoming opaque. The decubitus film shows fluid levels particularly well.

Paired *inspiratory* and *expiratory* films demonstrate air trapping and diaphragm movement. Small pneumothoraces and interstitial shadowing may be more apparent on an expiratory film.

VIEWING THE PA FILM

Before a diagnosis can be made an abnormality, if present,

must be identified. Knowledge of the normal appearances of a chest radiograph is essential. Also the radiologist must develop a routine which ensures that no areas of the radiograph fail to be scrutinized. A suggested scheme is as follows, examining each point in turn.

Request form	Name, age, sex, date. Clinical information.
1. Technical	Centring, position, markers. Degree of inspiration.
2. Trachea	Position, outline.
3. Heart and mediastinum	Size, shape, displacement.
4. Diaphragms	Outline, shape, relative position.
5. Pleura	Position of horizontal fissure. Costophrenic and cardiophrenic angles.
6. Lung fields	Local or generalized abnormality. Compare the two sides for lung markings and translucency.
7. Hidden Areas	Apices. Diaphragms. Mediastinum, hila. Bones.
8. Hila	Density, position, shape.
9. Below diaphragm	Gas shadow, calcification.
10. Soft tissues	Mastectomy, densities etc.
11. Bones	Destruction etc.

Some radiologists prefer initially to view the film without studying the clinical information. Comparison with previous chest radiographs is essential.

1. Technical

Centring. If the film is well centred the medial ends of the clavicle are equidistant from the vertebral spinous processes at the T4–T5 level. Small degrees of rotation distort the mediastinal borders, and the lung nearest the film appears less translucent. Thoracic deformities, especially scoliosis, negate the value of conventional centring.

Penetration. The vertebral bodies should be just visible through the cardiac shadow. Underpenetration increases the likelihood of missing an abnormality overlaid by another structure. Overpenetration results in loss of low density lesions such as early tuberculous shadowing, although a bright light may reveal the abnormality.

Degree of inspiration. On full inspiration the anterior ends of the sixth ribs or posterior ends of the tenth ribs are above the diaphragms; variation occurs with patient build. Pulmonary diseases such as SLE and fibrosing alveolitis are associated with reduced pulmonary compliance, which may result in reduced pulmonary inflation and therefore elevated diaphragms. On expiration the heart seems larger and basal shadowing may occur from crowding of normal vessels.

2. The trachea

The trachea should be examined for narrowing, displacement and intraluminal lesions. It is mid-line in its upper part, then deviates slightly to the right around the aortic knuckle. On expiration tracheal deviation to the right may be quite marked. Also shortening occurs on expiration; an endotracheal tube situated just above the carina on an inspiratory film may occlude the main bronchus on expiration.

Calibre is even. Translucency decreases caudally. On the right the tracheal margin can be traced down to the right main bronchus. This border is known as the *right paratracheal stripe*. It is present on 60% of films. Normally it measures less than 5 mm. Widening occurs with tracheal malignancy, mediastinal tumours, mediastinitis and pleural effusions. The left paratracheal line is rarely visualized.

The *azygos vein* lies in the angle between the right main bronchus and trachea. Enlargement occurs in the supine position but also with portal hypertension, IVC and SVC obstruction, right-sided cardiac failure and constrictive pericarditis.

On inspiration the carinal angle of 60–75 degrees widens. Pathological causes of widening include an enlarged left atrium (Fig. 11.6) and enlarged carinal lymph nodes.

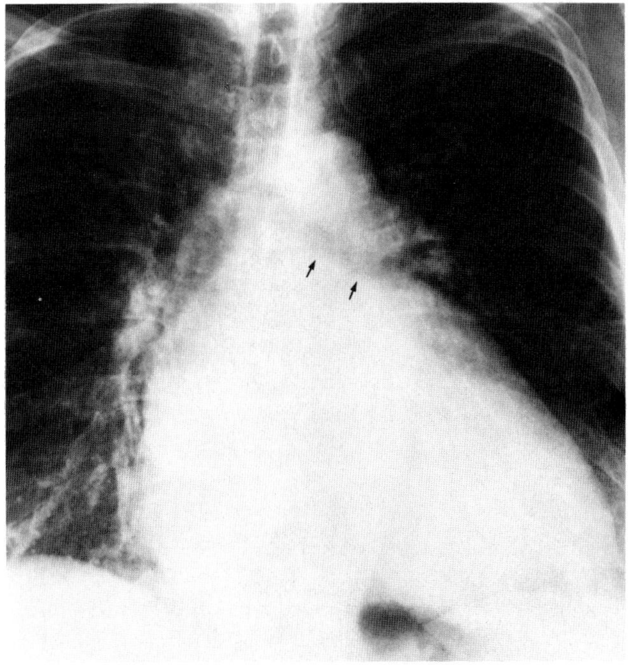

Fig. 11.6 Elevated left main bronchus (arrows) and widened carina. Patient with mitral valve disease and an enlarged left atrium.

3. Mediastinum and heart

The central dense shadow seen on the PA chest film comprises the mediastinum, heart, spine and sternum. With good centring two thirds of the cardiac shadow lies to the left of the midline and one third to the right, although this is quite variable. The transverse cardiac diameter and cardiothoracic ratio are assessed. Measurements in isolation are of less value than when measurements of previous examinations are available. An increase of 1.5 cm in the transverse diameter is significant. However, apparent cardiac enlargement occurs with a short FFD, on expiration, in the supine and AP projections and when the diaphragms are elevated.

All borders of the heart and mediastinum are clearly defined except where the heart sits on the left hemidiaphragm. The right superior mediastinal shadow is formed by the SVC and innominate vessels; a dilated aorta may contribute to this border. It is sharper than the left which is formed by the subclavian artery above the aortic knuckle.

In babies and young children the normal *thymus* is a triangular sail shaped structure with well-defined borders projecting from one or both sides of the mediastinum (Fig. 11.7). Both borders may be wavy, the 'wave sign of Mulvey', from indentation by costal cartilages. The right border is straighter than the left which may be rounded. Thymic size decreases on inspiration and in response to stress and illness. It is absent in di George's syndrome. Enlargement may occur following recovery from an illness. Large thymuses are more common in boys.

Adjacent to the vertebral bodies run the *paraspinal lines*, usually 1 or 2 mm wide. Enlargement occurs due to osteophytes, a tortuous aorta, obesity, vertebral and adjacent soft tissue masses, and a dilated azygos system.

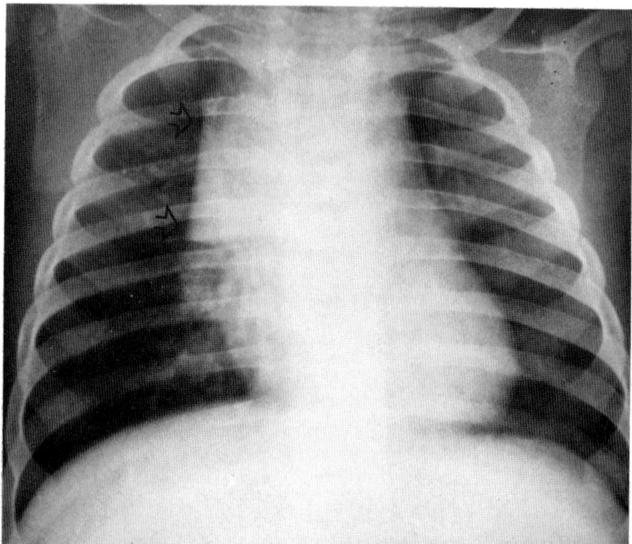

Fig. 11.7 Normal thymus in a child, projecting to the right of the mediastinum (arrows).

A search should be made for abnormal densities, fluid levels, mediastinal emphysema and calcification. Spinal abnormalities may accompany mediastinal masses; for example, hemivertebrae with neuroenteric cysts.

4. The diaphragm

In most patients the right hemidiaphragm is higher than the left. This is due to the heart depressing the left side and not to the liver pushing up the right hemidiaphragm; in dextrocardia with normal abdominal situs the right side is lowest. The hemidiaphragms may lie at the same level and in a small percentage of the population the left side is the higher; this is more likely to occur if the stomach or splenic flexure are distended with gas. A difference greater than 3 cm is significant.

On inspiration the domes of the diaphragms are at the level of the sixth rib anteriorly and at or below the tenth rib posteriorly.

Both domes have gentle curves which steepen towards the posterior angles. The upper borders are clearly seen except on the left side where the heart is in contact with the diaphragm. On occasions *fat pads* in the cardiophrenic angles cause some loss of diaphragmatic definition. Otherwise loss of outline indicates that adjacent tissue has become non-air containing, for example with consolidation.

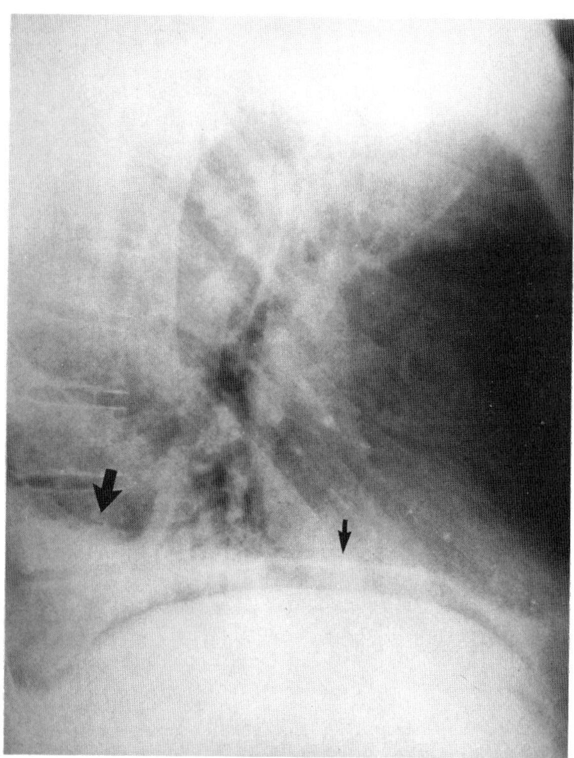

Fig. 11.8 Pneumoperitoneum after laparotomy. The thin right cupola (small arrow) is outlined by the adjacent aerated lung and the free abdominal gas. Posterior consolidation (large arrow) obscures the outline of the diaphragm superiorly.

Only the superior surface is seen unless free intraperitoneal gas is present to outline the undersurface (Fig. 11.8).

Congenital variations and other lesions of the diaphragm will be considered later.

5. The fissures

The main fissures. Visualization of the fissures occurs when the X-ray beam is tangential. In the PA view only the horizontal fissure is seen. It runs from the hilum to the region of the sixth rib in the axillary line.

It may be straight or have a slightly downward curve. Often this fissure is incomplete. Occasionally a double appearance occurs.

All fissures are clearly seen on the lateral film. The horizontal fissure runs anteriorly and often slightly downwards. Both oblique fissures commence posteriorly at the level of T4 or T5, passing through the hilum. The left is steeper and finishes 5 cm behind the anterior costophrenic angle, whereas the right ends just behind the angle.

Accessory fissures. (a) The *azygos* fissure is comma shaped with a triangular base peripherally and nearly always right sided (Fig. 11.9). It occurs in the apex of the lung and consists of paired folds of parietal and visceral pleura plus the azygos vein which has failed to migrate normally. Enlargement occurs in the supine position. At post-mortem the incidence is 1% but radiologically it is 0.4%. If left sided, the fissure contains the hemiazygos vein.

b. *The superior accessory* fissure separates the apical from the basal segments of the lower lobes. Commoner on the right it occurs in 5% of the population. On the PA film it resembles a horizontal fissure. The lateral film shows it running posteriorly from the hilum.

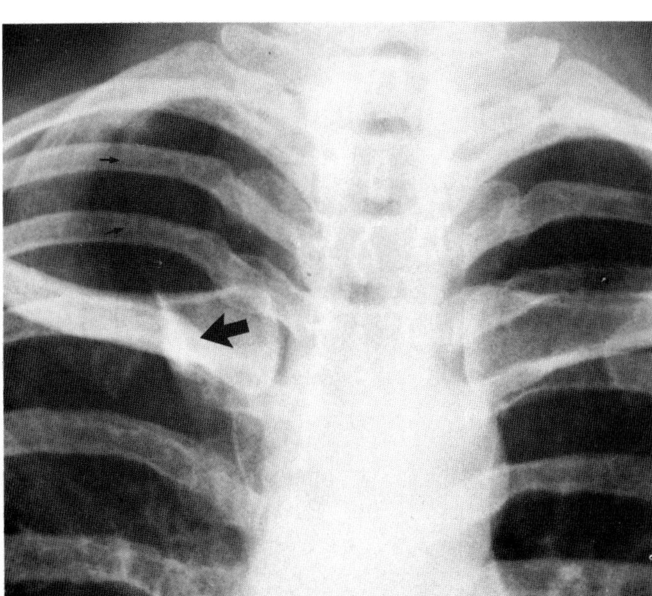

Fig. 11.9 Azygos fissure. The azygos vein is seen to lie at the lower end of the fissure (large arrow).

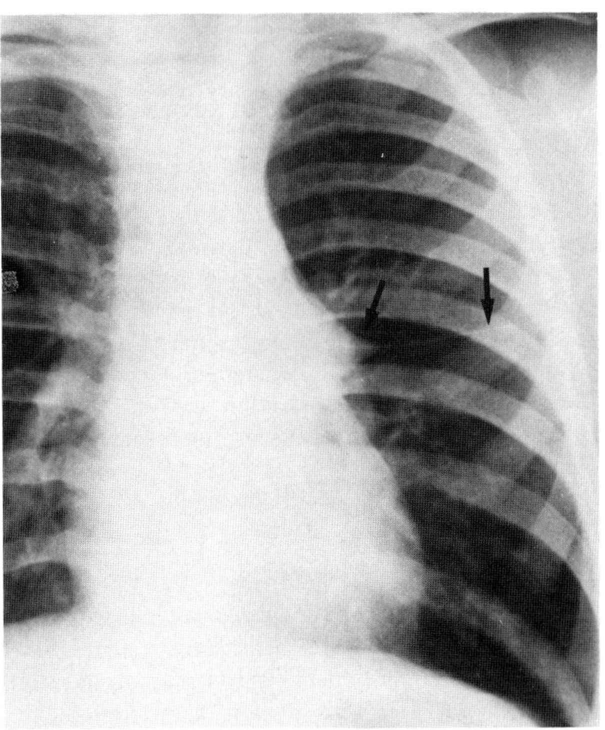

Fig. 11.10 Left-sided horizontal fissure.

c. The *inferior accessory* fissure appears as an oblique line running up from the cardiophrenic angles. It separates the medial basal from the other basal segments. Commoner on the right its incidence is 5%.

d. The *left sided horizontal* fissure, (Fig. 11.10) separates the lingula from the other upper lobe segments.

The angles. The normal costophrenic angles are acute and well defined. When the diaphragms are flat these angles are obliterated. Not infrequently the cardiophrenic angles contain low density ill-defined shadows caused by fat pads.

6. The lung fields

By comparing the lung fields, areas of abnormal translucency or of decreased or increased lung markings are easier to detect. The upper and lower zone vessels are compared for size.

An abnormal shadow should be closely studied to ensure that it is not a combination shadow formed by superimposed normal structures such as vessels and costal cartilage. The extent and location of the shadow is determined. Any specific features such as calcification are noted. A general survey to look for other lesions and displaced landmarks is made.

7. **The hidden areas**

The apices. On the PA film both apices are partially obscured by ribs, costal cartilages, clavicles and soft tissues. Visualization is very limited on the lateral view.

Mediastinum and hila. Central lesions may be obscured by these structures, or appear as a superimposed density. The abnormality is usually detectable on the lateral film.

Diaphragms. Because of the downward curve of the posterior diaphragm, the posterior and lateral basal segments of the lower lobes and the posterior sulcus are partially obscured. Visualisation is further diminished if the film is not taken on full inspiration.

Bones. A pulmonary lesion at any site may be hidden by bone or costal cartilage. Determining whether a density is pulmonary or bony may be difficult; AP, expiratory and oblique films are helpful in this situation.

8. **The hilum**

Normally the left hilum is 0.5–2.0 cm higher than the right. They should be of equal density and similar size with concave lateral borders. This concavity occurs where the upper lobe veins meet the pulmonary arteries. Unfortunately there is a wide normal range for the size and appearance of the hila. Any shadow which is not obviously vascular must be regarded with a high degree of suspicion and merits further investigation; old films for comparison are very helpful.

Of all the structures in the hilum only the pulmonary arteries and upper lobe veins significantly contribute to the hilar shadows on a plain radiograph. Normal lymph nodes are not seen. The air within the lumen of the proximal bronchi is apparent but bronchial walls are only demonstrated if seen end on; the upper lobe bronchus frequently appears as a ring shadow adjacent to the upper outer hilum (Fig. 11.11). Occasionally bronchial narrowing or occlusion may be shown.

The pulmonary vessels. The left pulmonary artery lies above the left main bronchus before passing posteriorly, whereas on the right side the artery is anterior to the bronchus, so that the left hilum is higher. Size is very variable. The maximum diameter of the normal descending branch of the right pulmonary artery is between 10 and 16 mm in males (9 and 15 mm in females).

The upper lobe veins are lateral to the arteries, which are separated from the mediastinum by approximately 1 cm of lung tissue. The lower lobe vessels are larger than those in the upper lobes in the erect position, where perfusion and aeration of the upper zones is reduced. This is not, however, the case in young children. In the supine position the vessels equalize. In the right paracardiac region the lower lobe vessels are always prominent.

Most of the normal shadows in the peripheral lung fields are vascular. Distribution within the lung fields should be similar. Local areas of decreased vascularity may be due to bullae or compensatory emphysema.

Pulmonary arteries and veins have different characteristics. The arteries, accompanying the bronchi, lie posterosuperiorly. The veins have fewer branches, are straighter, less well defined and larger. They do not follow the bronchi but drain via the interlobular septa, eventually forming superior and basal veins which converge on the left atrium. This confluence of veins may appear as a rounded

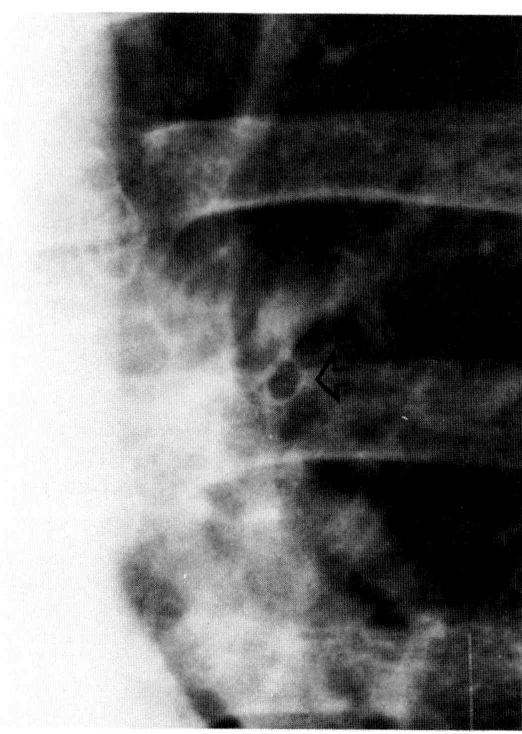

Fig. 11.11 Upper lobe bronchus seen end on appears as a ring shadow.

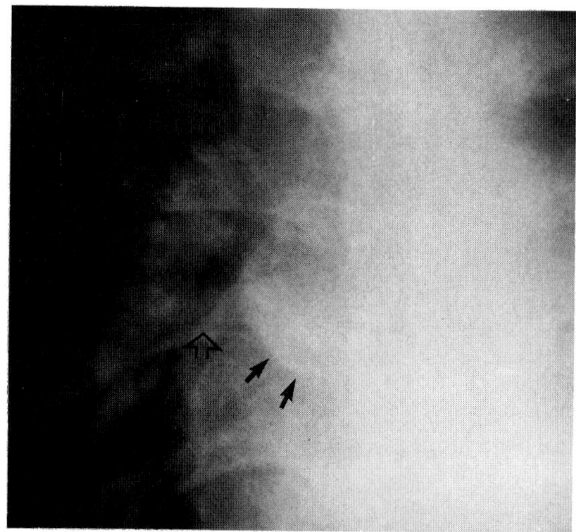

Fig. 11.12 Confluence of pulmonary veins (small arrows). A large vein is seen draining into this (open arrow).

structure to the right of mid-line superimposed on the heart, sometimes simulating a large left atrium (Fig. 11.12).

The bronchial vessels. Normally these are not seen on a chest film. The arteries arise from the ventral surface of the descending aorta at the T5–T6 level. Anatomy is very variable. Usually there are two branches on the left and one on the right which often shares a common origin with an intercostal artery. After entering the hila, the bronchial arteries accompany the bronchi. The veins drain mainly into the pulmonary veins and to a lesser extent into the azygos system.

Enlarged bronchial arteries appear as multiple small nodules around the hilum and as short lines in the proximal lung fields. Occasionally enlarged arteries may indent the oesophagus. Enlarged bronchial arteries may be general as in cyanotic heart disease, or local with local pulmonary lesions.

Causes of enlarged bronchial arteries

1. General enlargement	e.g. cyanotic congenital heart disease (pulmonary atresia, severe Fallot's tetralogy)
2. Local enlargement,	e.g. bronchiectasis, primary carcinoma.

The pulmonary segments and bronchi. The pulmonary segments (Figs 11.13 and 11.4) are served by segmental bronchi and arteries but unlike the lobes are not separated by pleura. Normal bronchi are not visualized in the peripheral lung fields.

The right main bronchus is shorter, steeper and wider than the left, bifurcating earlier, the upper lobe bronchus arising after 2.5 cm. On the left the upper lobe bronchus arises after 5 cm. The bronchi divide between 6 and 20 times before becoming bronchioles. Terminal bronchioles

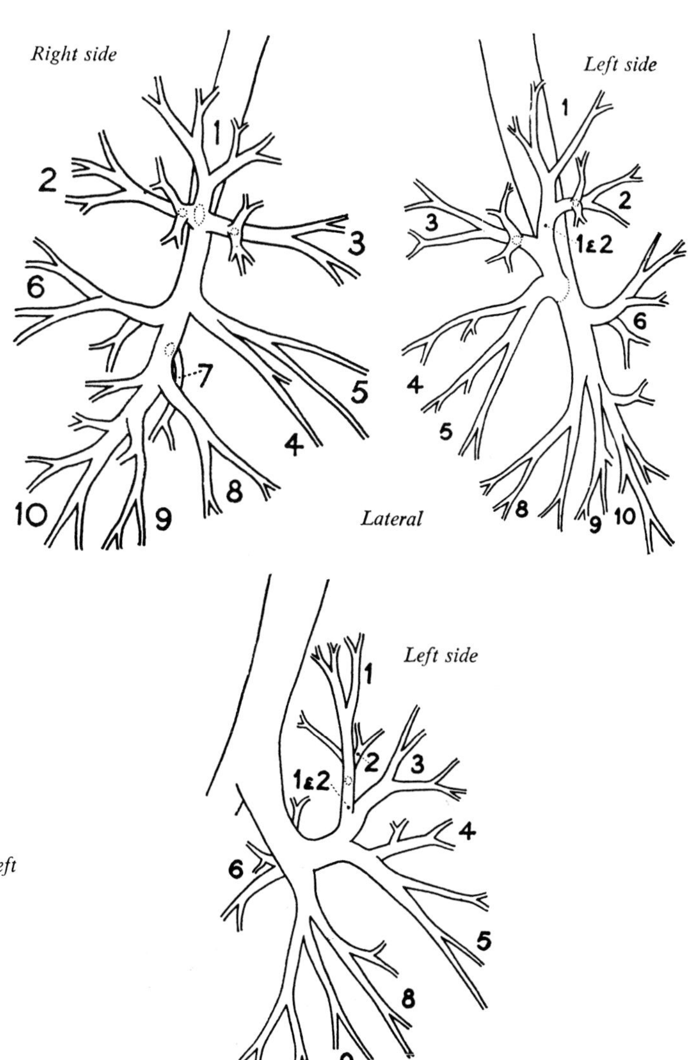

Fig. 11.13 Diagram illustrating the anatomy of the main bronchi and segmental divisions. Nomenclature approved by the Thoracic Society. (Reproduced by kind permission of the Editors of *Thorax*.)

UPPER LOBE
1. Apical bronchus
2. Posterior bronchus
3. Anterior bronchus

Right	*Left*
MIDDLE LOBE	LINGULA
4. Lateral bronchus	4. Superior bronchus
5. Medial bronchus	5. Inferior bronchus

LOWER LOBE

Right	*Left*
6. Apical bronchus	
7. Medial basal (cardiac)	6. Apical bronchus
8. Anterior basal bronchus	8. Anterior basal bronchus
9. Lateral basal bronchus	9. Lateral basal bronchus
10. Posterior basal bronchus	10. Posterior basal bronchus

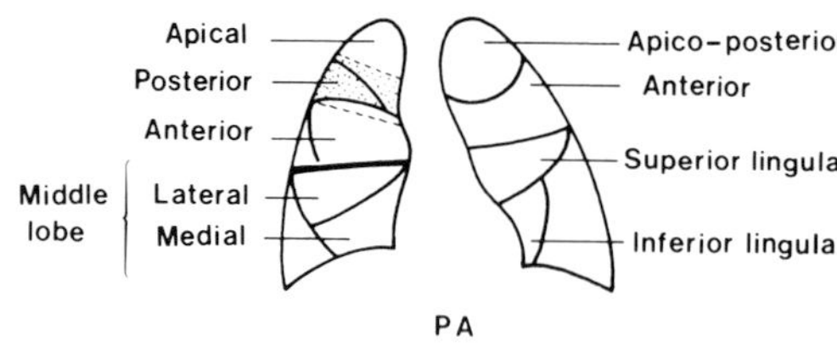

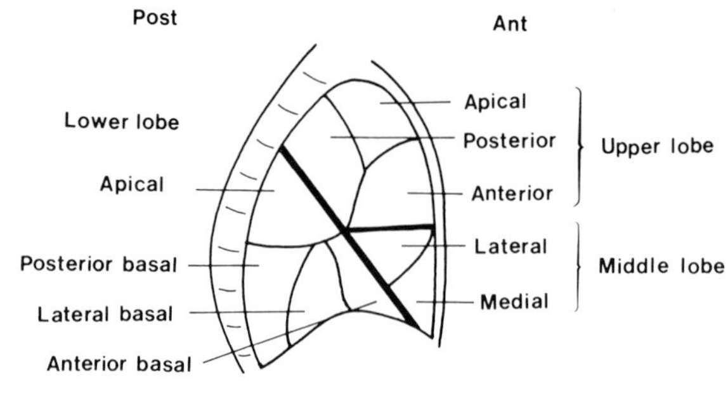

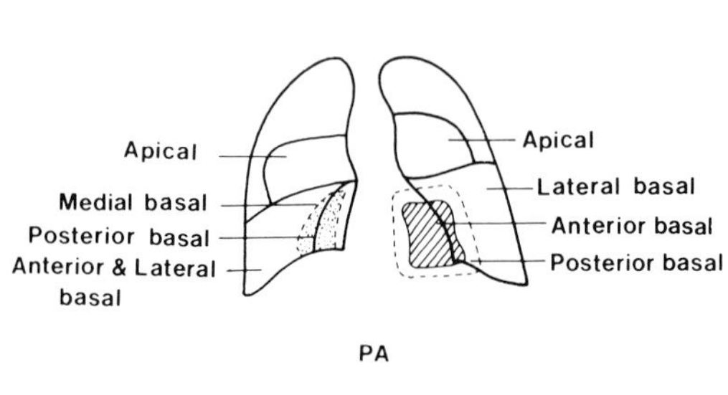

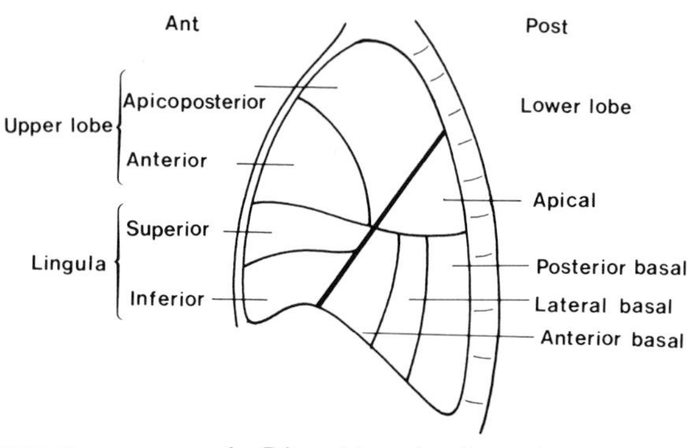

Fig. 11.14 Diagrams illustrating the approximate positions of the pulmonary segments as seen on the PA and lateral radiographs.

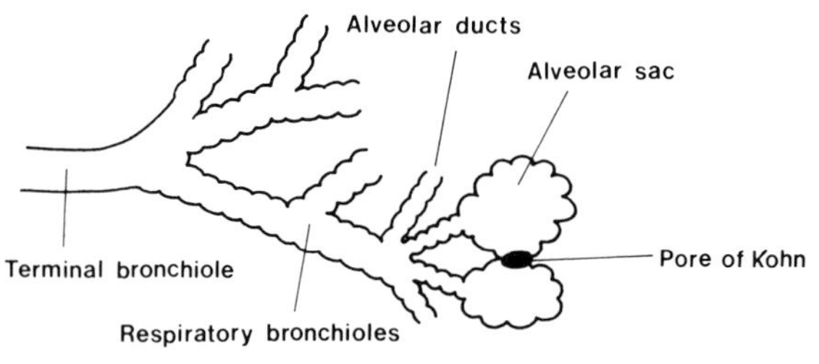

Fig. 11.15 A diagrammatic representation of the acinus.

are 0.2 mm in diameter. Each receives two or three respiratory bronchioles which connect with between two and 11 alveolar ducts. Each duct receives between two and six alveolar sacs which are connnected to alveoli. The *acinus*, which is generally considered to be the functioning lung unit, is that portion of the lung arising from the terminal bronchiole (Fig. 11.15). When filled with fluid it is seen on a radiograph as a 5–6 mm shadow, and this comprises the basic unit seen in alveolar (acinar) shadowing.

The primary lobule arises from the last respiratory bronchiole. The secondary lobule is between 1 and 2.5 cm in size and is the smallest discrete unit of lung tissue surrounded by connective tissue septa. When thickened these septa become Kerley B lines (Fig. 11.16).

Other connections exist between the air spaces, allowing collateral air drift. The pores of Kohn, 3–13 μm in size, connect the alveoli. The canals of Lambert (30 μm) exist between bronchioles and alveoli.

The lymphatic system. Lymphatics remove interstitial fluid and foreign particles. They run in the interlobular septa, are connected with the subpleural lymphatics and drain via the deep lymphatics to the hilum. Normal lymphatics are not seen. Thickening of the lymphatics and surrounding connective tissue results in the well-described Kerley B lines, which may be transient or persistent. The lymphatics themselves only contribute a small percentage towards the thickness of these lines, which are mainly formed by thickened connective tissue.

Table 11.1 Kerley lines

A lines: Thin non-branching lines radiating from the hilum. May represent interlobular septa or anastomotic lymphatics.

B lines: Transverse thin lines of 1–3 cm
Seen at the bases, lying perpendicular to the pleura
Formed by thickened interlobular septa

C lines: A spider's web appearance

Cause of Kerley B lines:

Pulmonary oedema	Scleroderma
Mitral valve disease	Alveolar cell carcinoma
Pneumoconiosis	Lymphoma
Lymphangitis carcinomatosa	Lymphatic obstruction
Interstitial fibrosis	Lymphangiectasia
Sarcoidosis	Idiopathic (in the elderly)

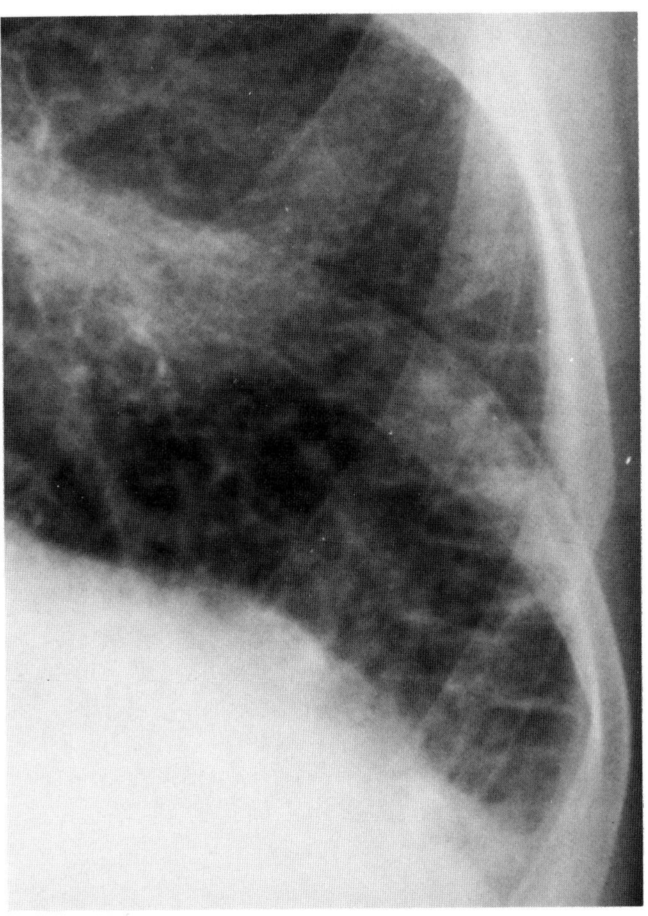

Fig. 11.16 Kerley B lines. Thickened interlobular septa in a patient with mitral valve disease.

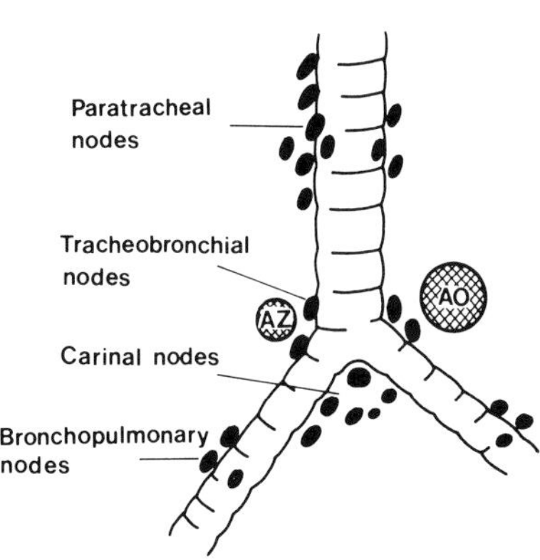

Fig. 11.17 The middle mediastinal nodes.

The lymph nodes. The intrapulmonary lymphatics drain directly to the bronchopulmonary nodes; therefore this group is the first to be involved by a peripheral tumour. The node groups and drainage have been well described (Fig. 11.17). There are extensive intercommunications between the groups, but on occasions the pattern of nodal involvement can suggest the likely site of a primary tumour. Mediastinal lymph nodes may be involved by disease both above and below the diaphragm.

A. *The anterior mediastinal* nodes, in the region of the aortic arch, drain the thymus and right heart.
B. *The intrapulmonary* nodes lie along the main bronchi.
C. *The middle mediastinal* nodes drain the lungs, bronchi, left heart, lower trachea and visceral pleura. They are divided into four groups.
   i. Bronchopulmonary (hilar) nodes which drain into groups ii and iii. When enlarged they appear as lobulated hilar masses.
   ii. Carinal nodes
   iii. Tracheobronchial nodes which lie adjacent to the azygos vein on the right side and are near the recurrent laryngeal nerve on the left side.
   iv. Paratracheal nodes are more numerous on the right side. A significant amount of drainage occurs from the left to the right group.
D. *The posterior mediastinal* nodes drain the posterior diaphragm and lower oesophagus. They are situated around the lower descending aorta and oesophagus.
E. *The parietal* nodes consist of anterior and posterior groups, situated behind the sternum and posteriorly in the intercostal region, draining the soft tissues and parietal pleura.

9. **Below the diaphragm**

A pneumoperitoneum is frequently more obvious on an erect chest film than an abdominal film, and is most obvious in an erect lateral film. A search should be made for other abnormal gas shadows, such as dilated loops, abscesses, displaced gastric bubble and intramural gas. Interposition of bowel between liver and diaphragm, Chilaiditi's syndrome (Fig. 11.18), is a common and often transient occurrence; the obvious bowel pattern distinguishes it from free intraperitoneal gas. However subdiaphragmatic fat may be difficult to distinguish from free gas on a single film.

Calcified hepatic tumours, granulomas and gallstones may be demonstrated.

10. **Soft tissues**

A general survey of the soft tissues includes the chest wall, shoulders and lower neck. Comparison of the two sides is helpful.

It is important to confirm the presence or absence of breast shadows (Fig. 11.19). The breasts may partially obscure the lung bases. Nipple shadows are variable in position, may be asymmetrical and not infrequently only one shadow is seen; care must be taken to avoid misinterpretation as a neoplasm or vice versa. The nipple shadows tend to be better defined laterally than medially. Inspiratory and expiratory films with metal nipple markers are often helpful.

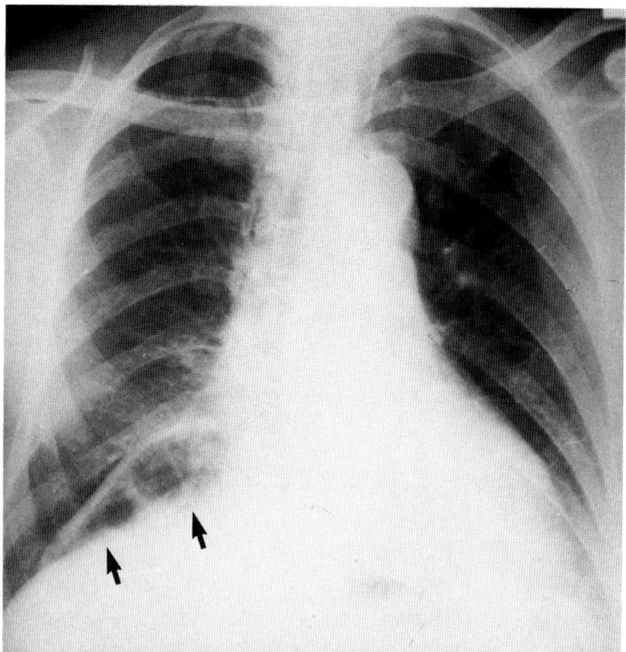

Fig. 11.18 Chilaiditi's syndrome. Interposition of colon between liver and diaphragm. Note the colonic haustral pattern.

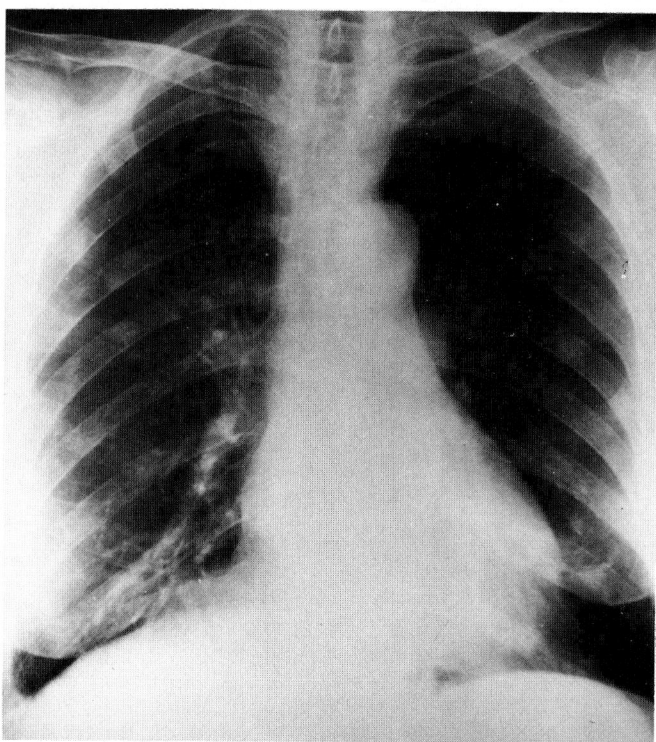

Fig. 11.19 Gynaecomastia in a male patient treated with stilboestrol for carcinoma of the prostate. Note the sclerotic rib metastases.

The anterior axillary fold is seen as a curvilinear shadow extending from the axilla onto the chest, frequently causing ill-defined shadowing which must be differentiated from consolidation.

At the apices the sternocleidomastoid muscles curve down and slightly outwards, and may simulate an apical cavity or bulla. The floor of the supraclavicular fossa often resembles a fluid level.

Peripherally in the subpleural area at the bases or near the apices slight thickening may be due to subcostal muscles or fat and should not be diagnosed as pleural fluid.

Companion shadows are 2–3 mm in thickness running parallel to the upper border of the clavicles and inferior borders of the upper ribs. They are formed by the soft tissues adjacent to the bone.

Abnormalities of the soft tissues will be discussed later.

11. **The bones**

A survey should be made of all the bones demonstrated on a chest film. Not infrequently a normal bony structure or a lesion may be difficult to distinguish from a pulmonary lesion. Identification of a bone abnormality in association with pulmonary disease may help to narrow the differential diagnosis.

The sternum. The number, shape, position and growth rate of the ossification centres is extremely variable. Usually there are single centres in the manubrium and xiphoid, with three or four centres in the body. Parasternal ossicles can be confused with a lung nodule. Slight patient rotation can result in apparent mediastinal widening in part due to the sternal shadow, and in the infant the ossification centres may cause confusion.

The clavicles. The rhomboid fossa is an irregular notch with a well-corticated margin lying up to 3 cm from the medial end of the clavicle inferiorly; it should not be mistaken for a destructive process. The medial epiphyses fuse late and are another source of confusion with a lung nodule. Superior companion shadows are usually present.

The scapulae. On the lateral film the inferior angle of the scapula simulates a pulmonary mass. The spine of the scapula may cast a linear shadow which appears pleural in aetiology on a PA film.

The ribs. Companion shadows are frequently present on the upper ribs. Pathological rib notching, as seen in aortic coarctation, should not be confused with the normal notch present on the inferior surface just lateral to the tubercle. The contours of the ribs must be evaluated for destruction; the inferior borders of the middle and lower ribs are usually indistinct however.

To decide whether a nodule is intrapulmonary or bony, inspiratory, expiratory, lateral and oblique films are helpful.

On the PA film the first *costal cartilage*, which usually calcifies early and is often very dense, obscures part of the upper zone. On the lateral film the anterior end of a cartilage seen behind the sternum should not be interpreted as a pulmonary node. Costal cartilage calcification is very rare before the age of 20. Central homogenous or spotty calcification occurs in females whereas in men it is usually in the cartilage edge.

The spine. Routine evaluation for destruction of vertebral bodies, disc spaces and scoliosis is necessary. A scoliosis often results in apparent mediastinal widening. The transverse processes may look like a pulmonary mass.

In the neonate the vertebral bodies have a sandwich appearance due to large venous sinuses. Residual grooves may persist in adults.

EXAMINING THE LATERAL FILM

A routine similar to that for the PA film should be used. The posterior basal segments of the lower lobes are particularly well seen. Kerley B lines are frequently well demonstrated anteriorly.

Important observations are (Fig. 11.20):

1. The clear spaces
2. Vertebral translucency
3. Diaphragm outlines

1. **The clear spaces**. There are two clear spaces which are areas of increased translucency corresponding to the sites where both lungs meet; they are the retrosternal and retrocardiac areas. Loss of translucency indicates local pathology. Obliteration of the retrosternal space occurs with anterior mediastinal masses such as a thymoma (Fig. 11.21). Normally this space measures less than 3 cm at its widest point.

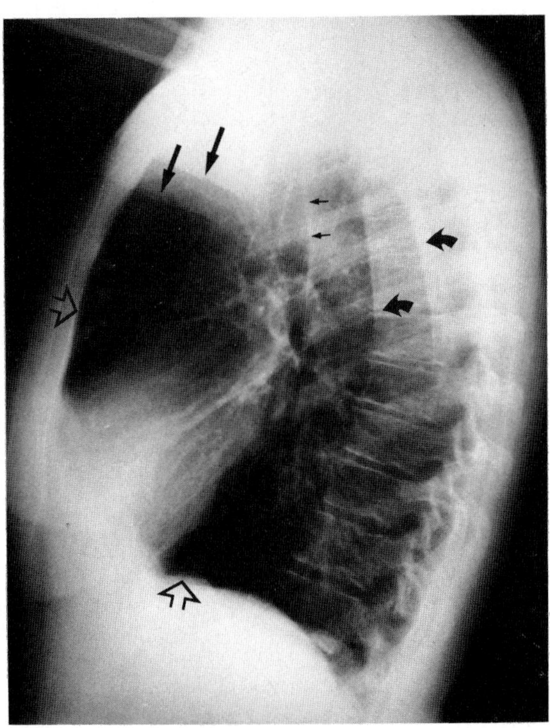

Fig. 11.20 Normal lateral film. Note the retrosternal and retrocardiac clear spaces (open arrows) and the increased translucency of the lower vertebrae. The axillary folds (large arrows) and scapulae (curved arrows) overlie the lung fields. The tracheal translucency is well seen. (small arrows).

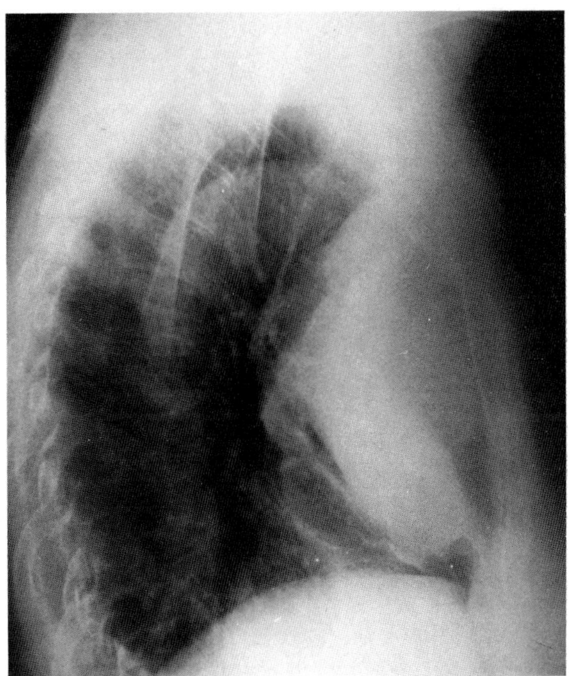

Fig. 11.21 Thymoma. Obliteration of the retrosternal space.

2. **Vertebral translucency.** The vertebral bodies become progressively more translucent caudally. Loss of this translucency may be the only sign of posterior basal consolidation.

3. **Diaphragm outline**. Both diaphragms are visible throughout their length except the left anteriorly where it merges with the heart. Loss of outline occurs with pleural effusions and consolidation (Fig. 11.22). The posterior costophrenic angles are acute; small amounts of pleural fluid may be detected by blunting of these angles.

4. **Other features**. Displacement and thickening of the fissures should be noted. Loculated interlobar effusions are particularly well shown. The left oblique fissure is steeper than the right, terminating 5 cm behind the anterior cardiophrenic angle.

The trachea passes down in a slightly posterior direction to the D6 or D7 level. It is partly overlapped by the scapulae and axillary folds. Anterior to the carina is the right pulmonary artery. The left pulmonary artery is superior and posterior. The veins are inferior. Their confluence creates a bulge on the posterior cardiac border.

The normal posterior tracheal wall measures less than 5 mm. Actually this includes both tracheal and oesophageal walls and widening may occur with disease of both these structures. Shadowing, frequently present in the region of

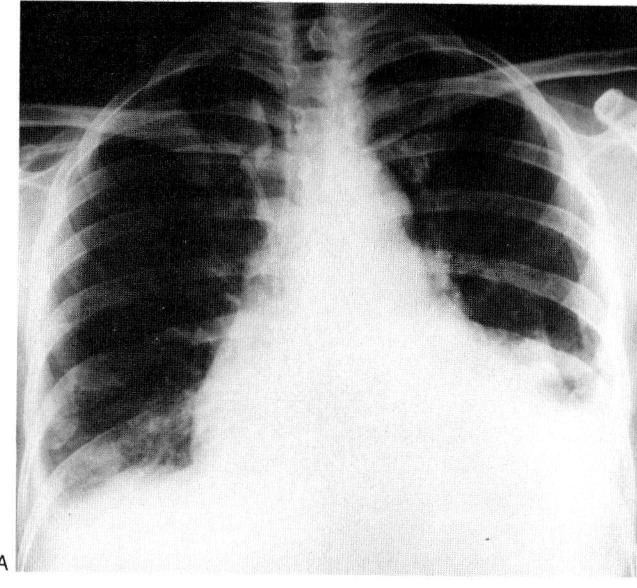

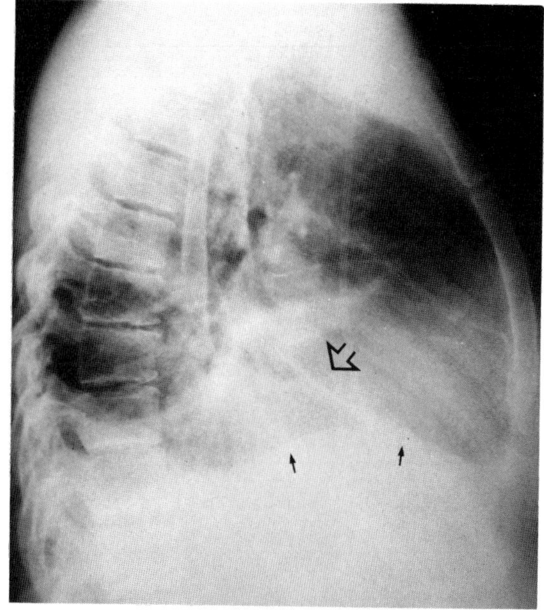

Fig. 11.22 (**A**) PA film. A moderate-sized left pleural effusion and a small right effusion. (**B**) Lateral film. There is loss of translucency of the lower vertebrae, thickening of the oblique fissure (open arrow) and absence of the left hemidiaphragm, with loss of the right hemidiaphragm posteriorly.

the anterior cardiophrenic angle, is thought to be created by mediastinal fat plus the interface between the two lungs.

The soft tissues and bones must be surveyed. The scapulae and their inferior angles often cast confusing shadows. The sternum is well shown.

INTERPRETATION OF THE ABNORMAL FILM: HELPFUL RADIOLOGICAL SIGNS: DIFFERENTIAL DIAGNOSIS

THE SILHOUETTE SIGN

Described by Felson the silhouette sign permits localization of a lesion on a PA film by studying the mediastinal and diaphragmatic outlines. These outlines are visualized because the adjacent alveoli are aerated. If the air is displaced, the adjacent borders are obliterated and the lesion localized, provided the film is adequately penetrated. Conversely if the border is retained and the abnormality is superimposed, the lesion must be either anterior or posterior. In 8–10% of normal people a short segment of the right heart border is obliterated by a fat pad or pulmonary vessels and should not be interpreted as middle lobe disease.

Obliteration of these borders may be due to adjacent pleural or mediastinal lesions. In addition, lesions of the right middle lobe (Figs 11.23 and 11.24) or lingula affect the right and left cardiac borders. Loss of aortic outline on the right occurs with disease of the anterior segment of the upper lobe, or the middle lobe. Obliteration of the aortic knuckle is a feature of disease in the apicoposterior segment of the upper lobe (Fig. 11.25).

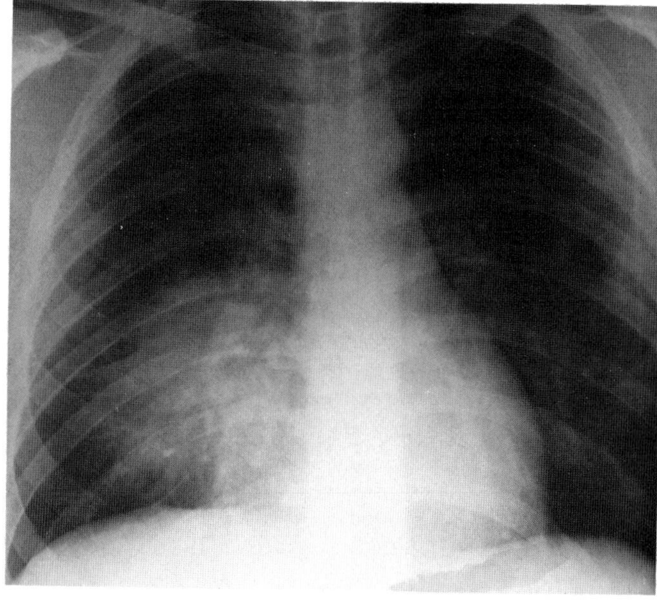

Fig. 11.23 Right middle lobe consolidation, demonstrating the silhouette sign with loss of outline of the right heart border.

Using the same principle, a well-defined mass seen above the clavicles is always posterior. An anterior mass is in contact with soft tissues, not aerated lung, and is ill-defined. This constitutes the cervicothoracic sign.

The 'hilum overlay' sign helps distinguish a large heart from a mediastinal mass. With the latter the hilum is seen through the mass, whereas with the former the hilum is displaced so that only its lateral border is visible.

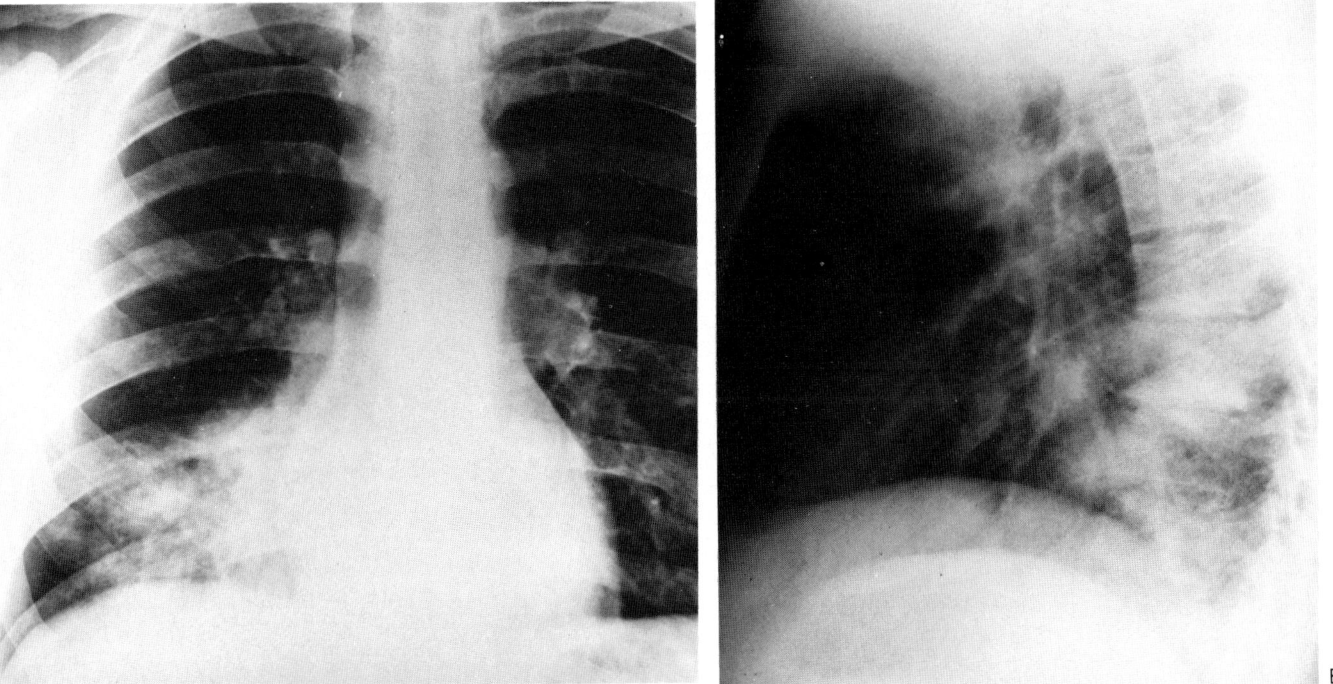

Fig. 11.24 Right lower lobe consolidation. (**A**) Shadowing at the right base but the cardiac border remains visible. (**B**) Lateral film. Consolidation in the posterior basal segment of the lower lobe with obliteration of the outline of the diaphragm posteriorly and loss of translucency of the lower vertebrae.

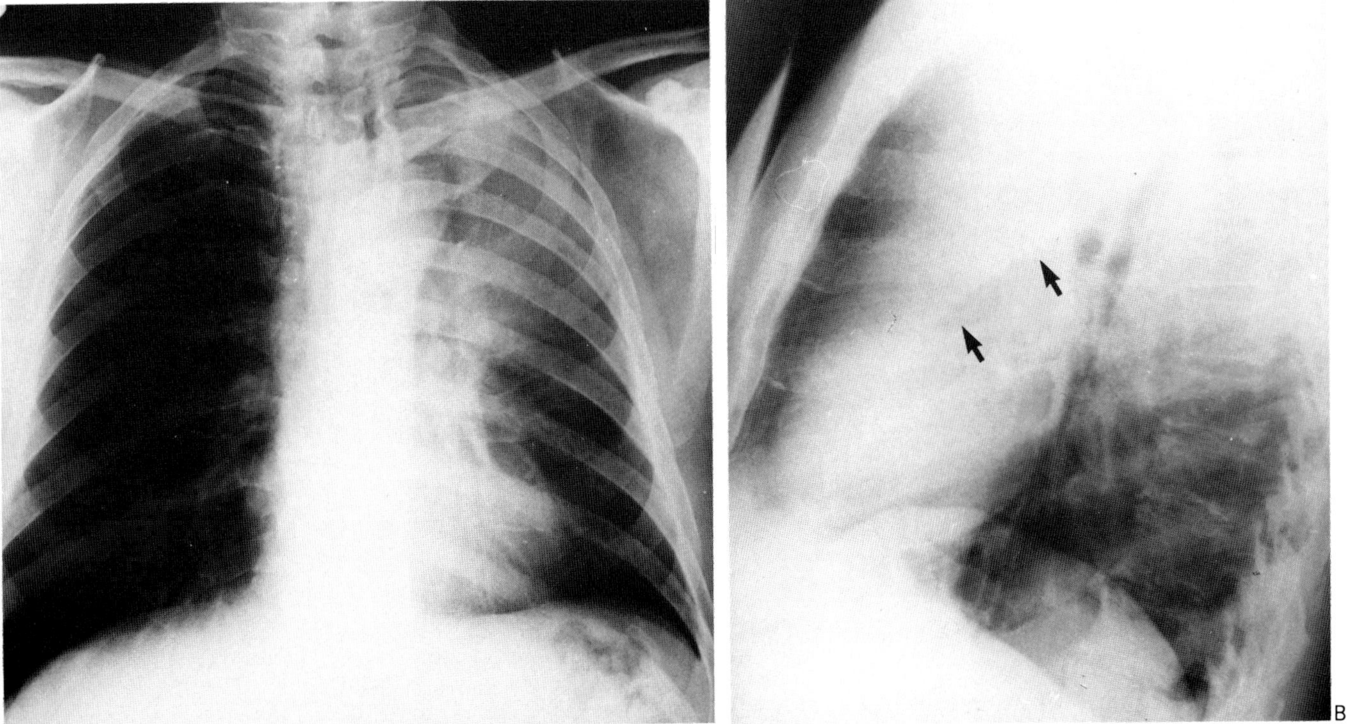

Fig. 11.25 Left upper lobe collapse. A carcinoma was present at the hilum. (**A**) Shadowing in the upper zone with loss of outline of the upper cardiac border and aortic knuckle. There is tracheal deviation. (**B**) Anterior displacement of the collapsed lobe and greater fissure.

THE AIR BRONCHOGRAM

Originally described by Fleischner, and named by Felson, the air bronchogram is an important sign that shadowing is intrapulmonary. The bronchus, if air filled and not fluid filled, becomes visible when air is displaced from the surrounding parenchyma. An air bronchogram does not occur within pleural fluid or a solid tumour. It may be present in consolidation distal to a malignancy if the bronchus remains patent (Fig. 11.26). It commonly occurs in alveolar shadowing but has been described accompanying interstitial disease.

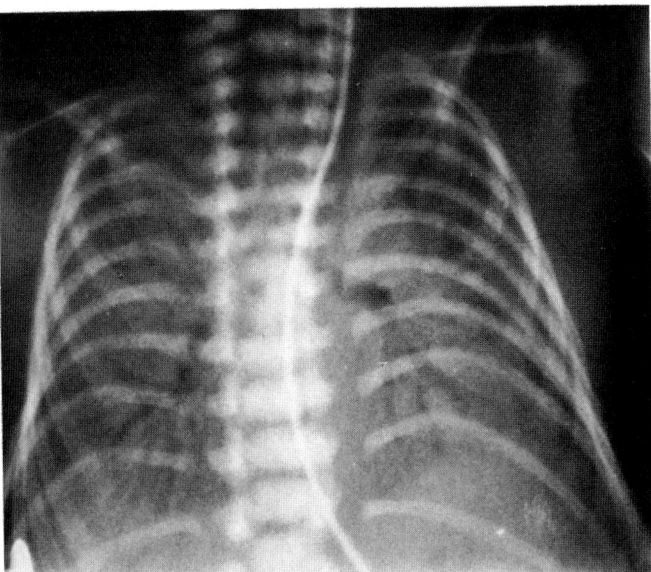

Fig. 11.27 Hyaline membrane disease. Extensive homogenous consolidation with a prominent air bronchogram.

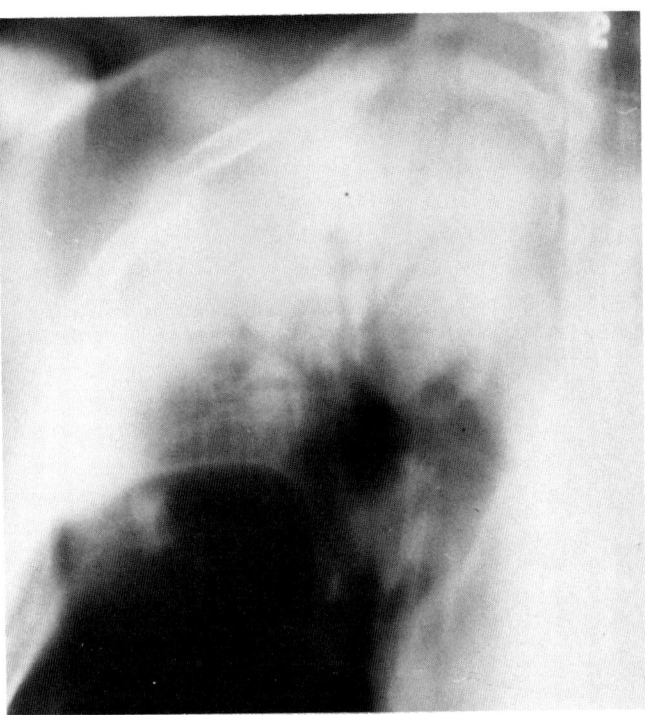

Fig. 11.26 Air bronchogram. An air bronchogram is clearly seen in the consolidated right upper lobe. A proximal carcinoma was present, although it is unusual for an air bronchogram to occur in the presence of a neoplasm.

Table 11.2 Causes of an air bronchogram

Common:	Consolidation Pulmonary oedema Hyaline membrane disease (Fig. 11.27)	*Others*:	Lymphoma Sarcoidosis Alveolar proteinosis Alveolar cell carcinoma Adult respiratory distress syndrome

ALVEOLAR SHADOWING (ACINAR SHADOWING)

The division of pulmonary shadowing into alveolar and interstitial is convenient but strictly incorrect; most disease processes involve both interstitium and acinus on histological examination. When the acinus is fluid filled it forms

Table 11.3 Causes of alveolar shadowing

1. **Pulmonary oedema**
   a) *Cardiac*
   b) *Non-cardiac*:
   Fluid overload, hypoalbuminaemia, shock lung, fat embolus, drowning, hanging, high altitude, aspiration (Mendelsohn's syndrome), blast injury, uraemia, oxygentoxicity, inhalation of noxious gases, heroin overdose, malaria, drugs (e.g. nitrofurantoin), raised intracranial pressure.
2. **Pneumonia**
   Localized, e.g. pneumococcus
   Generalized, e.g. pneumocystis, parasites, fungi
3. **Neonatal**
   Hyaline membrane disease
   Aspiration
4. **Alveolar blood**
   Pulmonary haematoma
   Goodpasture's syndrome
   Pulmonary infarction
5. **Tumours**
   Lymphoma
   Alveolar cell carcinoma
   Leukaemia
6. **Miscellaneous**
   Alveolar proteinosis
   Desquamative pneumonitis
   Radiation pneumonitis
   Loeffler's syndrome
   Eosinophilic infiltration
   Mineral oil aspiration and ingestion
   Sarcoidosis
   Polyarteritis nodosa
   Drugs

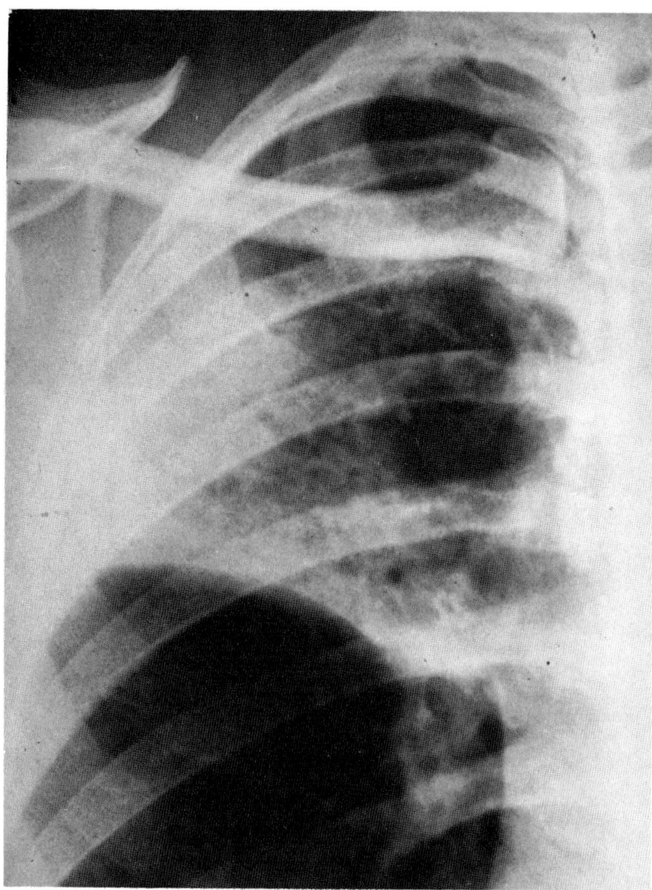

Fig. 11.28 Right upper lobe consolidation. Upper bowing of the horizontal fissure indicates some collapse. There is an acinar pattern with some confluence.

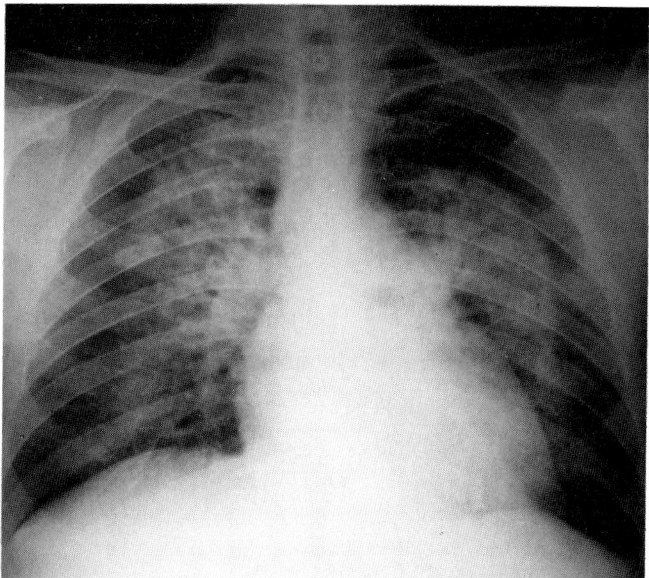

Fig. 11.29 Acute intra-alveolar pulmonary oedema with a batswing distribution.

a 7 mm shadow. These rapidly coalesce into fluffy, ill-defined cotton wool shadows, homogenous or patchy but well-defined adjacent to the fissures (Fig. 11.28). The air bronchogram and silhouette sign are characteristic features. Vascular markings are lost. During resolution a mottled appearance may occur.

Alveolar shadowing may have a bat's-wing distribution (Fig. 11.29), when homogenous shadows spread from the hila with a peripheral translucent rim. Commonly due to cardiac failure, when clearing quickly occurs after treatment, it may also be seen with pneumocystic infection, alveolar proteinosis and noncardiac causes of pulmonary oedema. Occasionally oedema is unilateral or peripheral.

Infections are usually localized; if generalized shadowing is present it may well be due to an opportunistic infection.

INTERSTITIAL SHADOWING

Thickening of the parenchymal perivascular tissues, that is interstitial lung disease, may appear radiologically as reticular, nodular, reticulonodular or ground glass shadowing; most diseases, however, have a reticulonodular pattern. Correlation between radiographic changes and the severity of respiratory disease is often poor; a normal film may accompany gross interstitial disease.

Unlike alveolar shadowing, interstitial shadowing is not homogenous. Kerley lines and honeycomb shadowing may be present. The bronchi remain patent so that lobar collapse is not a feature; loss of volume may occur as a result of fibrosis. Care is needed to avoid mistaking normal vascular markings for interstitial disease. Normal vessels are not seen in the peripheral 1.5 cm of the lung fields and, unlike interstitial shadows, vessels taper and branch. Diffuse interstitial shadowing (Fig. 11.30) occurs in a large number of disease processes. Certain features may help to narrow the differential diagnosis.

A. **A history** of industrial dust exposure, occupation, pigeon racing and disease processes such as rheumatoid arthritis is very helpful.

B. **Miliary** nodules (Fig. 11.31) are discrete, usually 2–3 mm in size, and occur in only a few diseases, most frequently tuberculosis. Pneumoconiosis, apart from asbestosis, and sarcoidosis initially spare the bases; haemosiderosis is predominantly midzone. Dense miliary shadows indicate the presence of calcium or metals, although assessing density can be difficult being dependent on radiographic factors (Fig. 11.32).

C. **Large nodules** are usually metastases. Alveolar disease processes such as infections may have a nodular appearance, but these tend to be less well-defined, changing from day to day and resolve after treatment. Pulmonary infarcts take longer to resolve.

Table 11.4 Causes of miliary shadowing (0.5–3.0 mm)

Soft tissue density	Tuberculosis Sarcoidosis Pneumoconiosis Metastases Hyaline membrane disease Histoplasmosis	High density	Alveolar microlithiasis Calcification: Tuberculosis Chicken pox Dust inhalation: Tin Barium etc. After lymphography Ectopic bone (mitral valve disease) Haemosiderosis

Table 11.5 Causes of larger nodular shadows (interstitial and others)

Malignancy: metastases, lymphoma, alveolar cell carcinoma
Tuberculosis
Sarcoidosis
Pneumoconiosis
Haemosiderosis
Pulmonary infarcts, fat emboli
Collagen diseases: Rheumatoid arthritis
Wegener's granuloma etc.
Allergic lung disease: Drugs, extrinsic allergic alveolitis
Alveolar shadowing: Infections, pulmonary haemorrhage
Pulmonary oedema (any cause)
Hyaline membrane disease
Artefacts: Skin nodules, e.g. neurofibromatosis
Clothing, hair
Pleural: Tumours, loculated effusions

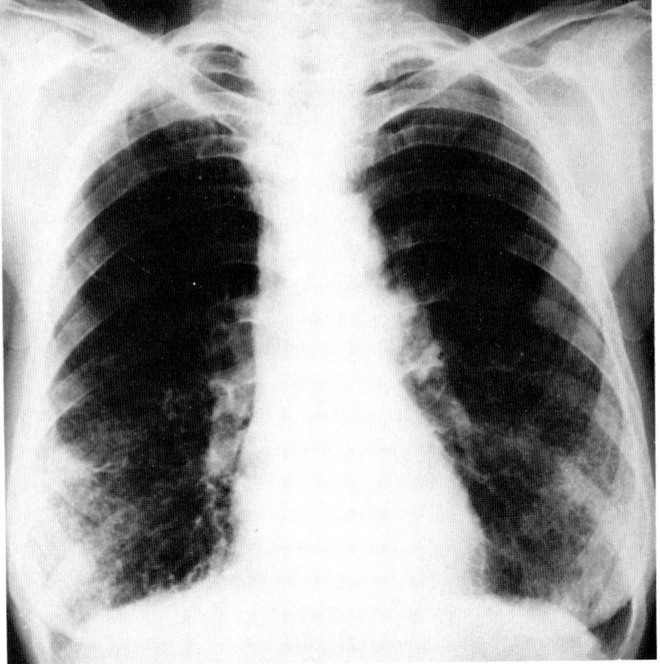

Fig. 11.30 Fibrosing alveolitis. Reticulo-nodular shadowing maximal in the lower zones.

Table 11.6 Causes of diffuse interstitial shadowing

Infections	Bacterial — tuberculosis, mycoplasma etc. Viral Fungal Protozoan — pneumocystis Parasites
Cardiac	Left heart failure Haemosiderosis Obstructed total anomalous pulmonary venous drainage
Neoplastic	Lymphangitis carcinomatosa Lymphoma Leukaemia
Collagen diseases	SLE Polyarteritis nodosa Scleroderma Rheumatoid arthritis
Drugs	Busulphan Methotrexate Bleomycin
Dust disease	
Honeycomb shadowing	
Miscellaneous	
Fibrosing alveolitis Extrinsic allergic alveolitis Sarcoidosis Amyloidosis Hepatic cirrhosis Bronchiectasis Oil emboli Chronic lipoid pneumonia Chronic interstitial pneumonia Desquamative pneumonitis	Gaucher's disease Histiocytosis X Tuberose sclerosis Neurofibromatosis Pulmonary myomatosis Congenital adenomatoid malformation

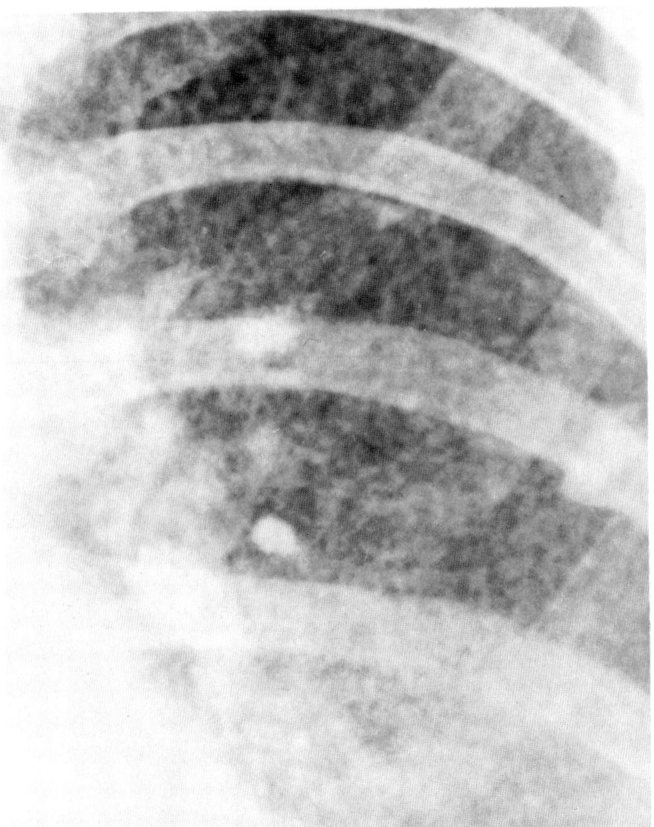

Fig. 11.31 Miliary tuberculosis. Widespread fine nodular shadowing without confluence.

D. **A linear** pattern is often present. A search must be made for Kerley lines. A coarse linear pattern may occur with the development of fibrosis. Associated displacement of structures may be seen. Fibrosis occurs in a large number of conditions such as tuberculosis, sarcoidosis, pneumoconiosis and fibrosing alveolitis (Fig. 11.33).

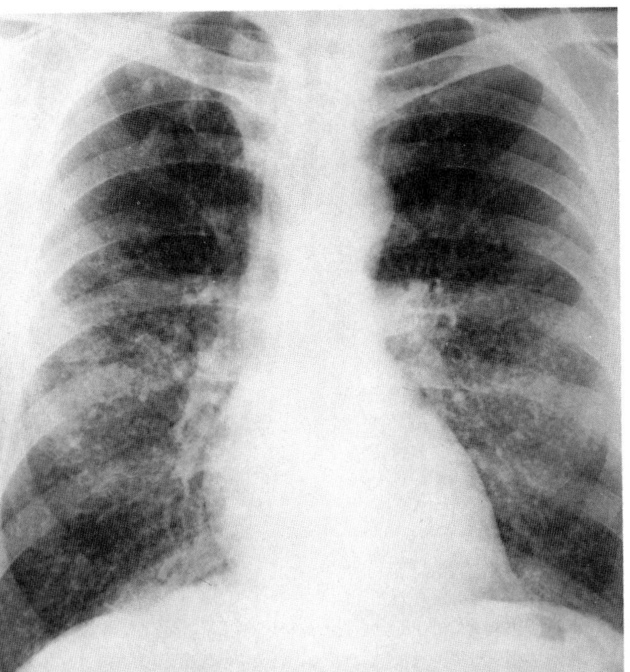

Fig. 11.32 Siderosis. Extensive dense miliary shadowing in an iron foundry worker.

HONEYCOMB SHADOWING

The parenchymal destruction which may occur with interstitial lung disease can result in the formation of thin-walled cysts. When these cysts are between 5 mm and 10 mm in size, the term honeycomb shadowing is used. It is associated with an increased risk of pneumothorax.

Honeycomb shadowing is a particular feature of histiocytosis X. Fibrosing alveolitis frequently has a small honeycomb pattern with cysts smaller than 3 mm. The larger pattern may develop.

Table 11.7 Causes of honeycomb shadowing

Common:	Histiocytosis X	Rare:	Tuberose sclerosis
	Scleroderma		Amyloidosis
	Rheumatoid lung		Gaucher's disease
	Idiopathic interstitial fibrosis		Chronic lipoid pneumonia
	Pneumoconiosis		Chronic interstitial fungal infections
	Sarcoidosis		Pulmonary myomatosis
			Biliary cirrhosis

Similar appearance: Bronchiectasis (and cystic fibrosis)

THE SINGLE PULMONARY NODULE

The commonest solitary pulmonary nodules are primary tumours, metastases and granulomata. Soft tissue masses, artefacts and extrapleural masses may appear as intrapul-

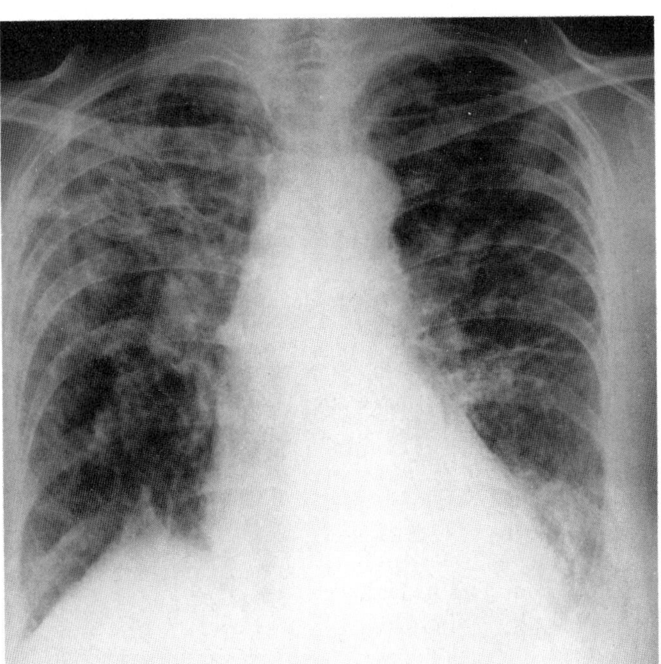

Fig. 11.33 Sarcoidosis. Fibrosis mainly affecting the upper zones with elevation of the hila and tenting of the right hemidiaphragm. A 55-year-old female with a long history of sarcoidosis.

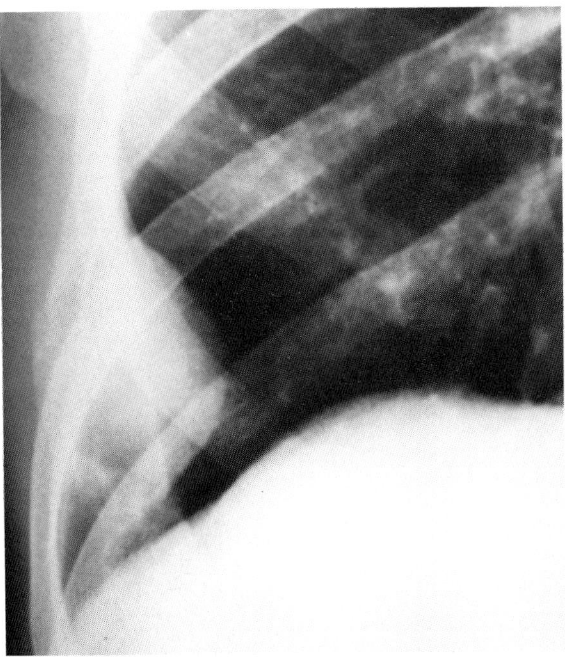

Fig. 11.34 Reticulum cell sarcoma of right lower rib with an extrapleural mass.

monary lesions on the PA view, but a lateral film usually helps distinguish them from parenchymal masses. Extrapleural (Fig. 11.34) and mediastinal masses characteristically form obtuse angles with the lung edge, whereas an intrapulmonary lesion forms an acute angle.

A search should be made for associated abnormalities such as bone destruction, pleural effusions, collapse, septal lines and enlarged lymph nodes. Previous films are necessary to assess the rate of growth. Malignant tumours may enlarge intermittently, but no growth over a period of two years implies that a nodule is benign. When the diagnosis is in doubt and if the mass is accessible, a fine needle biopsy is indicated if other non-invasive investigations have been unsuccessful.

Infective processes may appear rounded, but some change in appearance occurs on follow up films after treatment. Frequently a carcinoma develops within the upper zone and has an irregular spiculated or notched outline. Calcification suggests that a lesion is benign, although carcinomas can arise coincidentally at the site of an old calcified tuberculous focus. Hamartomas often develop popcorn calcification. Calcified metastases are rare and the primary tumour is usually an osteogenic sarcoma or chondrosarcoma (Fig. 11.35).

Granulomas frequently calcify, are usually well defined and frequently lobulated. Metastases are often well defined but may have an irregular outline. Arteriovenous malformations characteristically have associated dilated arteries and veins, usually well seen on tomography.

Table 11.8 Causes of a solitary pulmonary nodule

Malignant tumours:	Primary, secondary, lymphoma, plasmacytoma
Benign tumours:	Hamartoma, adenoma, arteriovenous malformation
Granuloma:	Tuberculosis, histoplasmosis, paraffinoma, fungi, parasites
Infections:	Pneumonia, abscesses, hydatid, amoebic abscess
Pulmonary infarct	
Pulmonary haematoma	
Collagen diseases:	Rheumatoid arthritis, Wegener's granulomatosis
Sarcoidosis	
Sequestrated segment	
Retention cyst	
Impacted mucus	
Amyloid	
Intrapulmonary lymph node	
Pleural:	Fibroma, tumour, Loculated fluid
Non-pulmonary	e.g. skin lesions

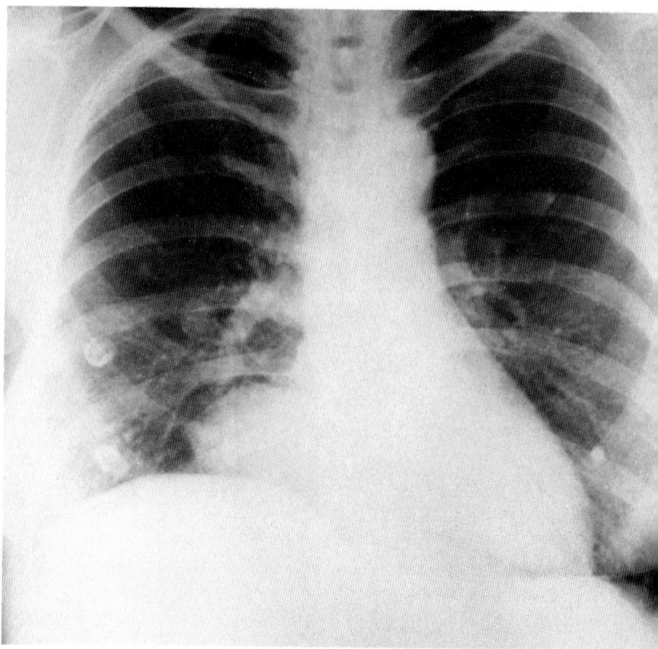

Fig. 11.35 Multiple calcified metastases from a chondrosarcoma of the right tenth rib.

Very large masses are most often a primary carcinoma, a cannonball metastasis or a pleural fibroma.

CAVITATION

A cavity is a translucency within the lung parenchyma surrounded by a complete wall. Particular features of importance are the site of the cavity, its outline, wall thickness, the presence of a fluid level, contents of the cavity, satellite lesions and the appearance of the surrounding lung tissue. Tomography is often necessary. Only films taken with a horizontal beam will demonstrate a fluid level.

The common cavitating lesions are tuberculous, staphylococcal infections (Fig. 11.36) and carcinoma. Cavitation may occur within a tumour or in the lung distal to the mass.

The site. Tuberculous cavities are usually upper zone, in the posterior segments of the upper lobes or apical segments of the lower lobes. Abscesses which are due to aspiration are most often right sided and lower zone, although site is related to which part of the lung was dependent at the time.

Amoebic abscesses are nearly always in the right lower lobe, infection extending directly from the liver. Sequestrated segments are mainly left sided. Pulmonary infarcts are most common in the lower zones.

The wall of the cavity. The majority of cavitating malignant tumours are squamous cell carcinomas. Usually the wall is thick and irregular with eccentric cavitation; rarely a squamous carcinoma may form a thin walled cavity.

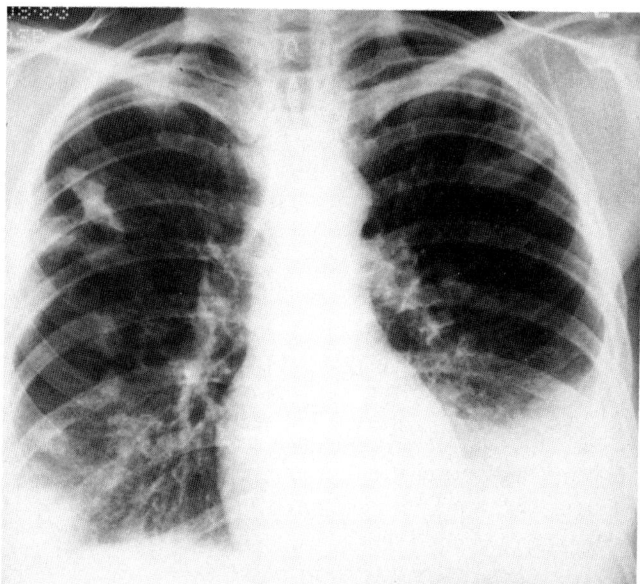

Fig. 11.36 Staphylococcal abscesses. Multiple cavitating abscesses in a young male heroin addict. Bilateral effusions also present.

Cavitating metastases are not common but are usually thick-walled, as are infective abscesses and Wegener's granulomas.

The common thin-walled lesions are pneumatoceles and bullae (Fig. 11. 37), although these are not cavities in the true meaning of the word. Chronic tuberculous cavities are often thin-walled whereas acute cavities tend to be thick-walled; adjacent changes of fibrosis or acute infection are usually present.

Table 11.9 Cavitating pulmonary lesions

Infections:	*Staphylococcus, klebsiella.* tuberculosis, histoplasmosis. amoebic, hydatid. paragonimiasis fungal
Malignant:	Primary, secondary, lymphoma
Abscess:	Aspiration
Pulmonary infarct Pulmonary haematoma	
Pneumoconiosis:	PMF Caplan's syndrome
Collagen diseases:	Rheumatoid nodules, Wegener's granuloma
Developmental:	Sequestrated segments, bronchogenic cysts
Cystic bronchiectasis	
Sarcoidosis	
Bullae, pneumatocele	
Common causes of multiple cavities	
Abscesses Lymphoma Metastases Rheumatoid nodules Wegener's granuloma Coccidiodomycosis	

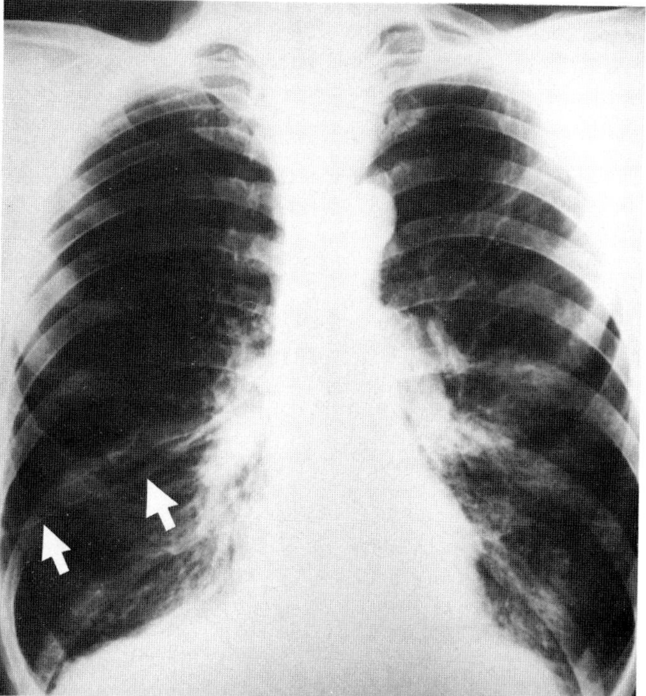

Fig. 11.37 Bullous emphysema. Curvilinear shadows in the right middle zone (arrows) with a lack of vascular markings in the upper zone due to the presence of bullae.

Satellite lesions are a common feature of benign lesions, usually tuberculous.

Fluid levels and the meniscus sign. Fluid levels are

Table 11.10 Fluid levels on a chest radiograph

Intrapulmonary	
Hydropneumothorax:	Trauma, surgery Bronchopleural fistula*
Oesophageal:	Pharyngeal pouch, diverticulae Obstruction (tumour, achalasia) Oesophagectomy (bowel interposition)
Mediastinal:	Infections Oesophageal perforation (endoscopy, trauma)
Pneumopericardium:	Diagnostic aspiration, surgery Trauma
Chest wall:	Plombage with lucite balls (Fig. 11.39) Fractures Infections
Diaphragm:	Hernias, eventration rupture

*A bronchopleural fistula should be considered if a hydropneumothorax persists or enlarges after chest surgery.

common in primary tumours; irregular masses of blood clot or necrotic tumour may be seen within the cavity.

Cavitating metastases and tuberculous cavities contain fluid infrequently.

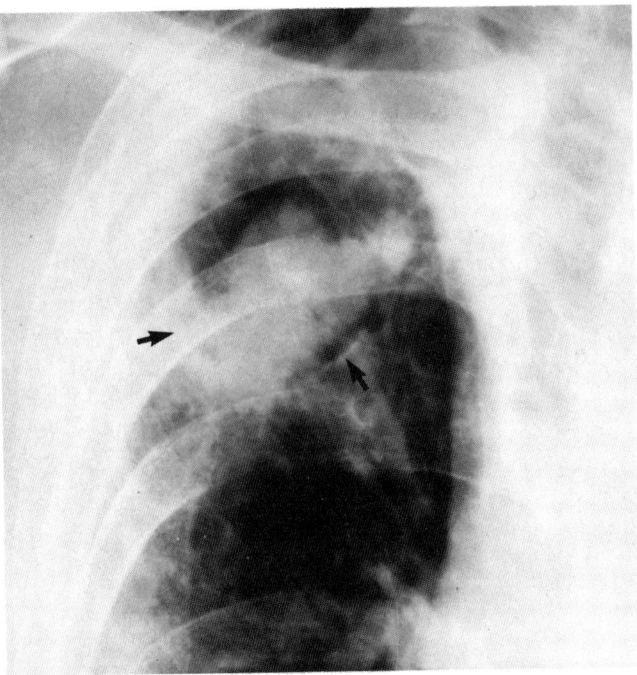

Fig. 11.38 Aspergillus mycetoma. A large mycetoma within an old tuberculous cavity in a fibrotic upper lobe. The mycetoma is surrounded by a halo of air.

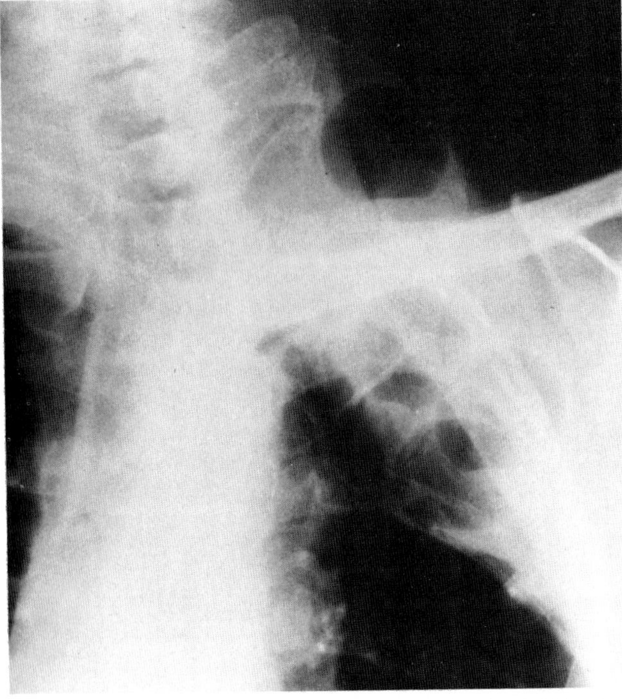

Fig. 11.39 Apical plombage. Hollow lucite spheres with fluid levels which have formed because of leakage of the walls of the spheres.

An aspergilloma (Fig. 11.38) within a cavity gives rise to the meniscus sign of a crescentic air shadow above the fungus ball. Movement occurs with change in patient position. When an hydatid cyst ruptures the daughter cysts floating within the cavity appear like a waterlily, hence the waterlily sign. Other lesions which may be seen within a cavity include inspissated pus, cavernoliths or blood clot. Blood clot may occur in cavitating neoplasms, tuberculosis and pulmonary infarcts.

CALCIFICATION

Calcification is most easily recognized on tomography and with low kVp films. In the elderly calcification of tracheal and bronchial cartilage is a common occurrence. Calcification in the walls of the bronchioles, osteopathia racemosa, is of no significance.

Table 11.11 Calcification on the chest radiograph

Intrapulmonary:	Granuloma infections — Tuberculosis, histoplasmosis, chicken pox, coccidioidomycosis, actinomycosis, hydatid cyst
	Abscess — Chronic
	Tumours — Metastases (osteogenic sarcoma, chondrosarcoma) cystadenocarcinoma arteriovenous malformation hamartoma, carcinoid.
	Haematoma
	Infarct
	Mitral valve disease
	Broncholith — tuberculosis
	Alveolar microlithiasis
	Idiopathic
	Rare — Metabolic (hypercalcaemia) Silicosis Sarcoidosis Rheumatoid arthritis Amyloid Osteopathia racemosa
Lymph nodes:	Tuberculosis, histoplasmosis
	Sarcoidosis
	Silicosis
	Lymphoma after irradiation
Pleural:	Tuberculosis
	Asbestosis, talcosis,
	Haemothorax, empyema
Mediastinal:	Cardiac, vascular
	Tumours, e.g. thymus, thyroid, dermoid
Pulmonary artery:	Pulmonary hypertension
	Aneurysm
	Thrombus
Chest wall:	Costal cartilage; bone
	Breasts, e.g. tumours, fat necrosis
	Soft tissues, e.g. parasites

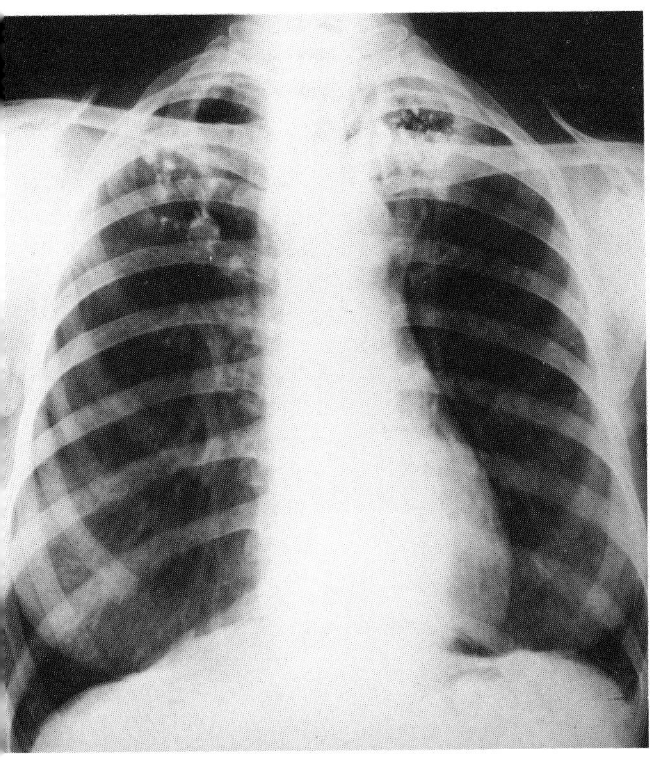

Fig. 11.40 Pulmonary tuberculosis. Numerous calcified foci in both upper zones with left upper lobe fibrosis.

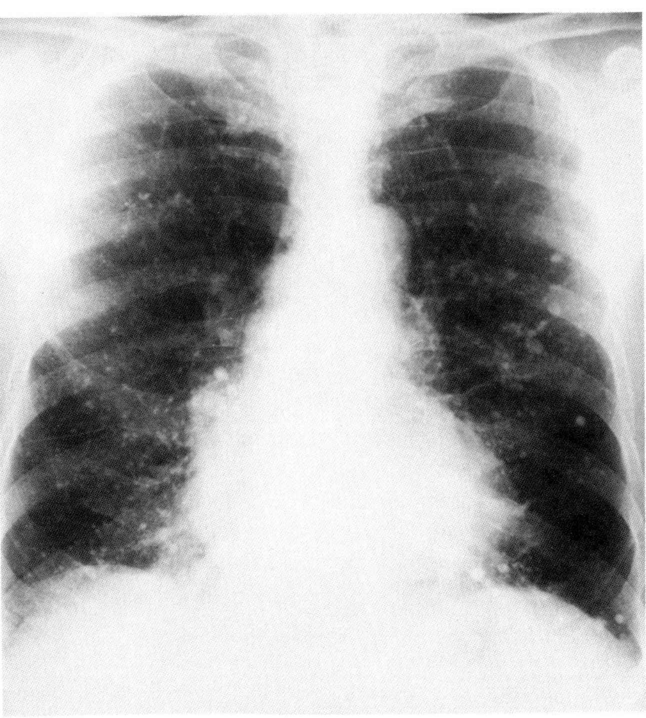

Fig. 11.41 Chickenpox. Widespread small calcified opacities following a previous chickenpox pneumonia.

By far the commonest cause of intrapulmonary calcification is *tuberculosis* (Fig. 11.40) The foci are usually upper zone, scattered and variable in size. *Chicken pox foci* (Fig. 11.41) are smaller (1–3 mm), regular sized and widely distributed. Characteristically the foci of *histoplasmosis* are surrounded by small haloes.

Alveolar microlithiasis appears as tiny sand-like densities in the mid and lower zones, due to calcium phosphate deposits in the alveoli. *Hamartomas* often have popcorn calcification. Occasionally *phleboliths* are present in arteriovenous malformations. Rarely a fine rim of calcification forms in the wall of an *hydatid cyst*.

Pleural plaques may contain irregular areas of calcification. In asbestosis the plaques may appear as thin linear deposits on the parietal diaphragmatic surfaces (Fig. 11.42).

Calcification of the lymph nodes occurs in a number of conditions (Table 11.11). An eggshell pattern is characteristic of *sarcoidosis* and *silicosis*. Very rarely calcified intrapulmonary nodes are present in these conditions.

LINEAR AND BAND SHADOWS

There are many disease processes which may result in linear shadows within the lung fields. Causes which must be considered include the following:

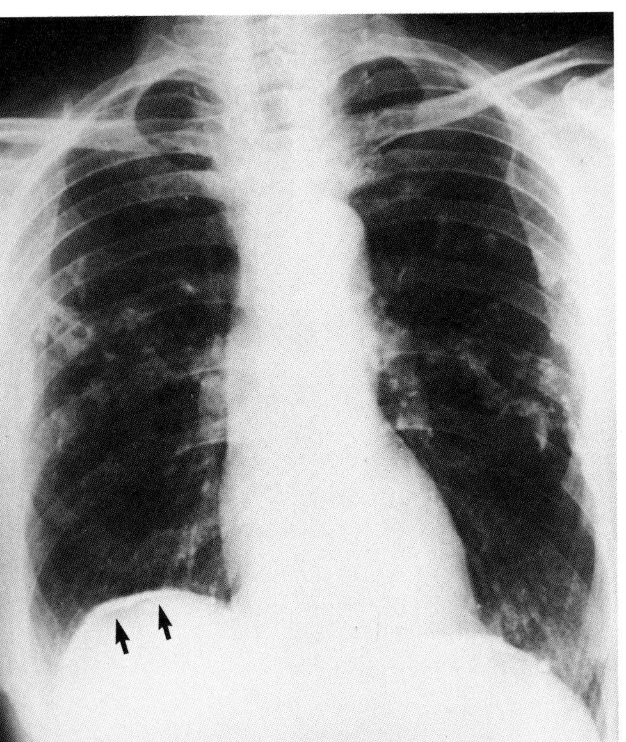

Fig. 11.42 Asbestos exposure. Extensive irregular bilateral calcified pleural plaques including the right dome of the diaphragm (arrows). Previous employment involved working with asbestos.

Pulmonary infarcts	The fissures
Sentinel lines	Curvilinear shadows (Bullae, pneumatoceles)
Kerley lines	Bronchial wall thickening
Plate atelectasis	Mucus filled bronchi
Pulmonary and pleural scars	Artefacts
Resolving infection	

Pulmonary infarcts are very variable in appearance. Frequently they form irregular thick wedge-shaped lines with the base adjacent to the pleura. They are often basal and peripheral. Adjacent diaphragm splinting and a pleural reaction may occur. Resolution tends to be slow, in contrast to infections which often resolve fairly rapidly.

Originally described by Fleischner, *plate atelectasis* is commonly seen on post-operative films and is thought to develop as a result of underventilation. They lie at the bases, running parallel to the diaphragms, are several centimetres long and between 1 mm and 3 mm thick. Resolution is rapid.

Mucus filled bronchi, or bronchoceles, form branching tubular structures seen peripherally or near the hilum. Bronchial obstruction due to malignancy, a tuberculous stenosis or a benign intrabronchial mass, and bronchiectasis are the usual causes.

Sentinel lines are also thought to represent mucus filled bronchi. Most frequently they are left sided and associated with a left lower lobe collapse. These coarse lines ar curved upwards and lie peripherally in contact with th pleura. They probably develop as a result of kinking of th bronchi adjacent to the collapse.

Kerley B lines lie in a similar position but are shorter Unilateral Kerley lines are usually an indication c lymphangitis carcinomatosa but may occur in early cardia failure.

The normal and accessory *fissures* have been described Thickening of the fissures is frequently seen in cardia failure. Bulging fissures indicate lobar expansion (Fig. 11.43). They may be a feature of an abscess, acut infections such as *Klebsiella* and *Staphylococcus*, tubercu losis and large tumours.

Old pleural and pulmonary scars do not change in appear ance on serial films. Pulmonary scarring is a common en result of infarction. Associated pleural thickening an tenting are often present. Pleural scars extend to th pleural surface.

Curvilinear shadows indicate the presence of bullae pneumatoceles (Fig. 11.44) or cystic bronchiectasis Vascular markings from unaffected adjacent lung may b superimposed.

Thickened bronchial walls cast thin parallel shadows which are called tramline shadows. When seen end o these bronchi appear as ring shadows. They are a commo finding in bronchiectasis.

A
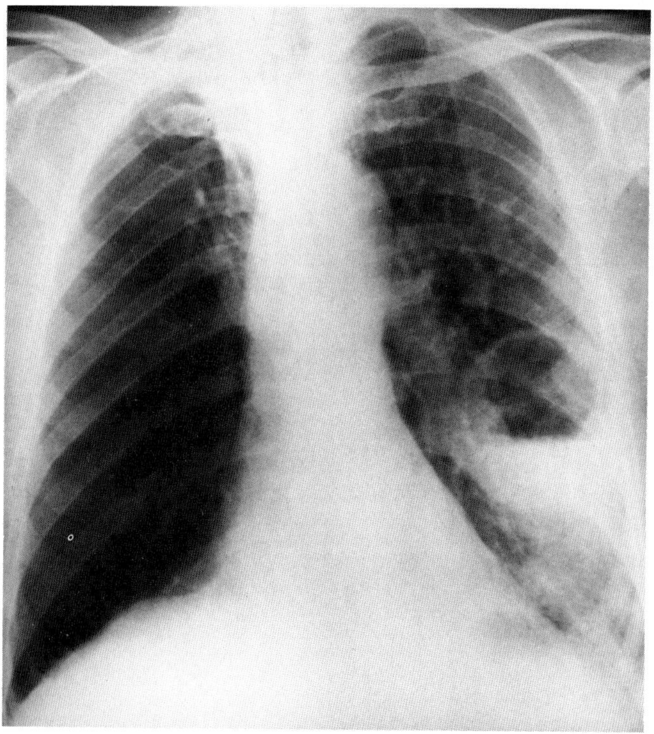

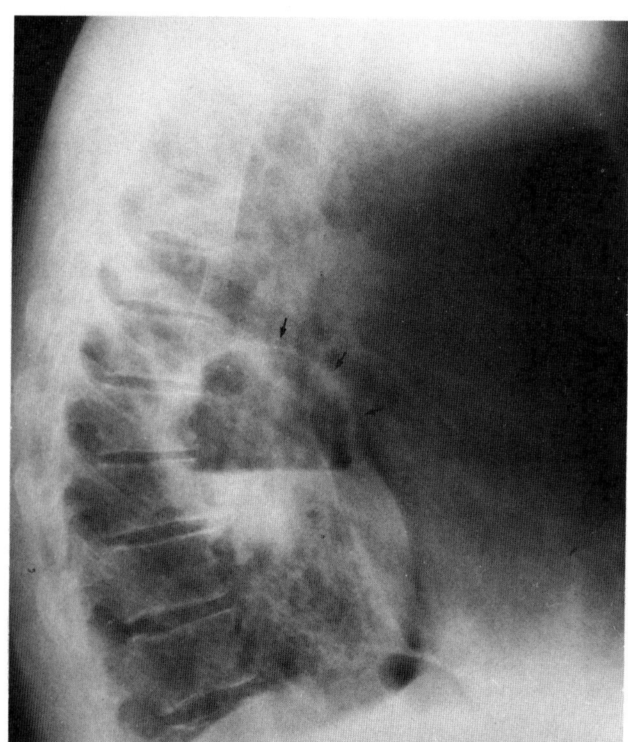
B

Fig. 11.43 (**A**) A large lung abscess with a fluid level distal to a hilar carcinoma. There is an old right upper lobe collapse with compensatory emphysema. (**B**) Note bulging of the oblique fissure adjacent to the abscess.

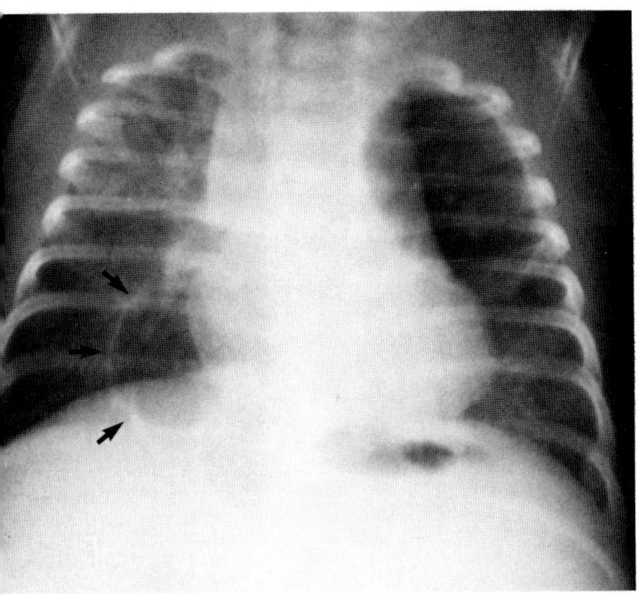

Fig. 11.44 Pneumatocele. Child with a staphylococcal pneumonia. Consolidation in the right upper lobe and a pneumatocele adjacent to the right heart border.

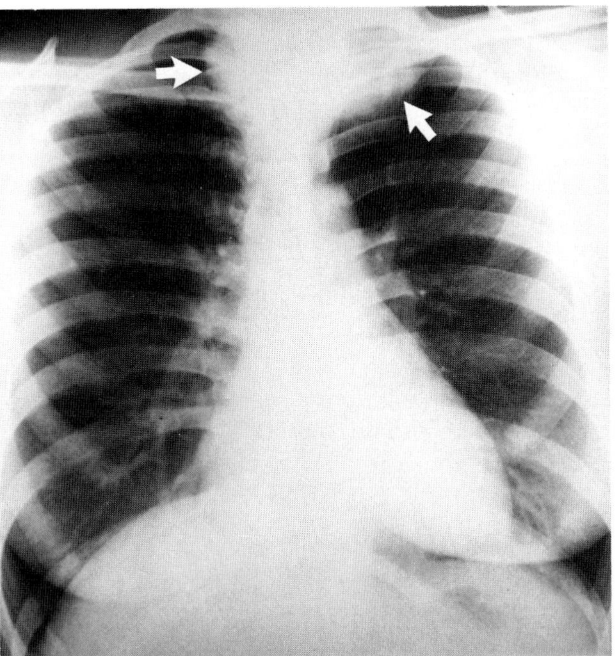

Fig. 11.46 A female patient with her hair in a plait overlying the upper mediastinum and simulating mediastinal widening.

APICAL SHADOWING

Most shadows seen in the apices are *pleural caps*. These crescentic shaped shadows may be unilateral or bilateral, when they are usually asymmetrical. Their significance is doubtful; they may represent old pleural thickening. It is important that they should not be misdiagnosed especially when a *Pancoast tumour* is present (Fig. 11.45). If there is any doubt about rib erosion, penetrated films and tomography should be obtained.

The apices are frequently the site of *tuberculosis*. Assessing activity is difficult when changes of previous infection, such as upper zone fibrosis, pleural thickening and calcification, are present. Previous films for comparison are invaluable.

Table 11.12 Common causes of apical shadows

Pleural caps	Pancoast tumour
Pleural fluid	Infections
Bullae	Pneumothorax
Soft tissue, e.g.	companion shadows, hair (Fig. 11.46) sternocleidomastoids

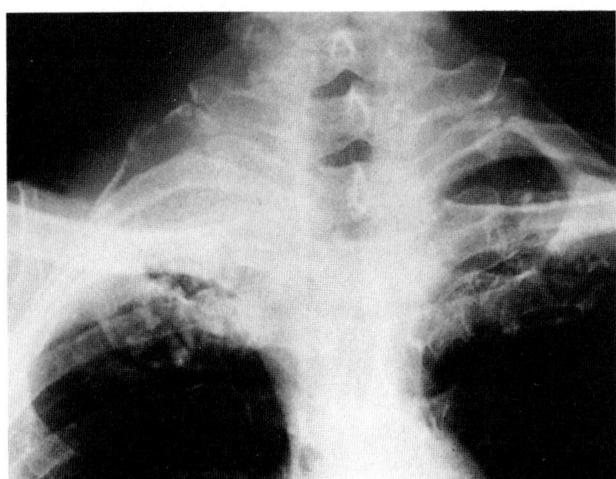

Fig. 11.45 Pancoast tumour. There is apical shadowing on the right side simulating pleural thickening. Note destruction of the first rib.

SIGNS OF LOSS OF VOLUME

With a significant loss of lung volume structures are displaced towards the collapse (Fig. 11.47) or fibrosis. These additional signs of loss of volume are important for parenchymal changes are not always apparent on a PA radiograph.

Within the collapse, crowding together of the vascular markings may be apparent, with the vessels in the normal adjacent lobes showing separation as a result of compensatory emphysema; this also results in increased transradiancy. The fissures may be bowed or displaced (Fig. 11.48). As a result of displacement the hilum changes shape, often appearing smaller with upward rotation. Herniation of the contralateral lung is shown by displacement of the anterior mediastinal line. With major collapse the diaphragm becomes elevated, although there are numerous other causes for this. With upper lobe fibrosis tracheal displacement is angular whereas with collapse it is smooth. Ipsilateral rib crowding is a late feature, more apparent in children.

Fig. 11.47 Pulmonary agenesis. The right lung is absent. The heart and mediastinum are displaced to the right. Note herniation of the left lung across the midline (arrows). The rib spaces are narrowed on the right.

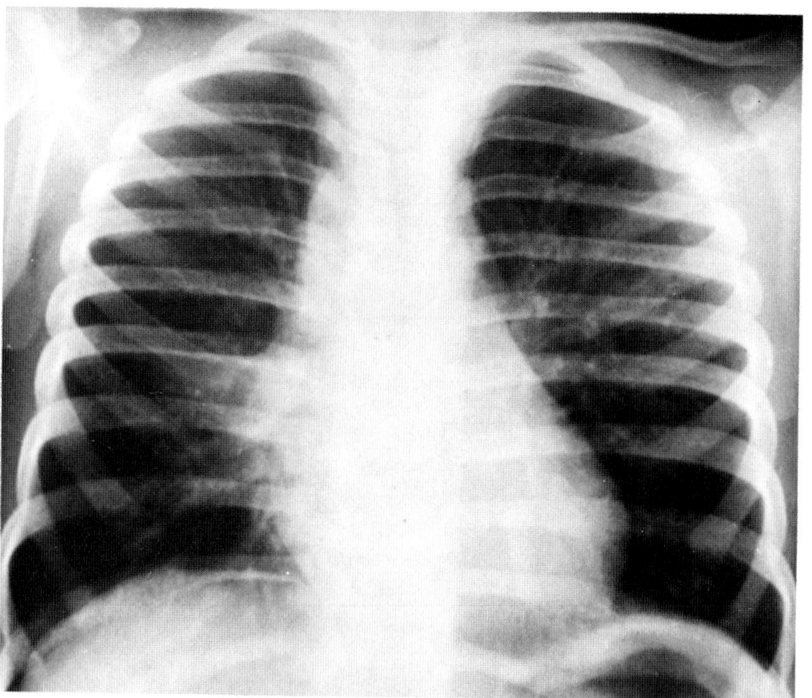

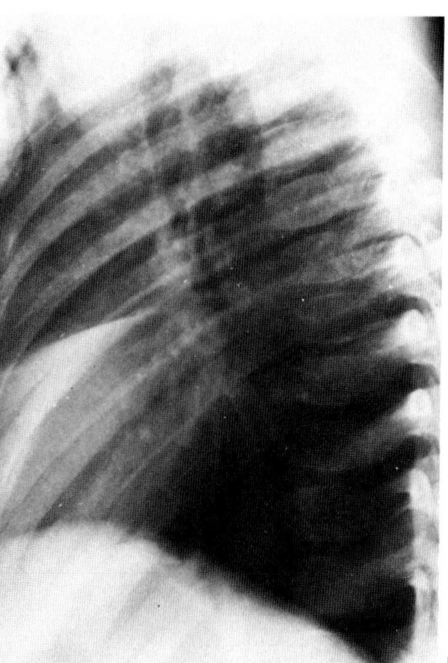

Fig. 11.48 Right middle lobe collapse. (**A**) Loss of definition of the right heart border with adjacent shadowing. (**B**) Lobar collapse with displacement of the fissures.

HILAR ENLARGEMENT

Unfortunately the pulmonary hilum has a very variable appearance. It is often extremely difficult to decide whether enlargement is due to a mass or to a prominent pulmonary artery; the arteries can often be identified and distinguished from mass lesions by tracing the branch vessels arising from them. However, tomography is frequently necessary.

Enlarged lymph nodes are lobulated and the adjacent bronchi may be slightly narrowed. Enlargement is usually bilateral in sarcoidosis, whereas in lymphoma it tends to be asymmetrical (Fig. 11.49). Tuberculous lymphadenopathy, without an identifiable peripheral pulmonary lesion, is uncommon in the Asian population. In the presence of malignancy an enlarged hilum may be due to the primary tumour itself or to lymph node involvement by a peripheral tumour.

able 11.13 Causes of hilar enlargement

nilateral	
pparent:	Rotation, scoliosis A small contralateral hilum
ormal:	Young women
ymph nodes:	Tuberculosis, lymphoma carcinoma Fungi, histoplasmosis
umours:	Benign, malignant
ulmonary artery:	Aneurysm, poststenotic dilatation pulmonary embolus
uperimposed anterior or osterior mass	
ericardial defect	
ilateral	
xpiratory film	
odes:	Lymphoma, sarcoidosis Carcinoma Glandular fever, whooping cough Tuberculosis, histoplasmosis, fungi pneumoconiosis
ulmonary artery:	Pulmonary hypertension Congenital heart disease
)rugs	

'able 11.14 Causes of a small hilum

Jnilateral
pparent — rotation, scoliosis
Jormal — especially left
.obar collapse
Iypoplasia
AcCleod's syndrome
Jnilateral pulmonary embolus

ilateral
Cyanotic congenital heart disease,
e.g. Fallot's tetralogy)
Central pulmonary embolus

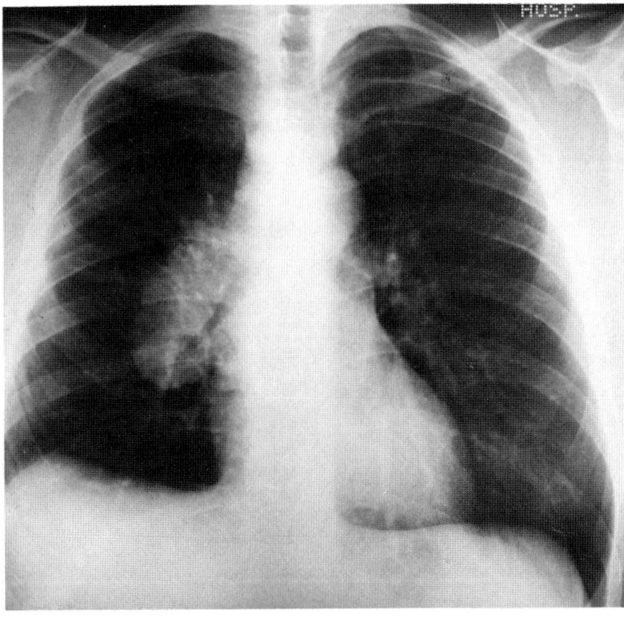

Fig. 11.49 A young male patient with Hodgkin's disease. An enlarged lobulated right hilum typical of glandular enlargement.

UNILATERAL INCREASED TRANSRADIANCY

Comparison of the lung fields should reveal any local or general abnormality of transradiancy. Increased transradiancy may be accompanied by signs of obstructive or compensatory emphysema such as separation of the vascular markings, splaying of the ribs, mediastinal displacement and depression of the diaphragm.

Rotation or scoliosis are the commonest causes of increased transradiancy. With rotation to the left, the left side becomes more radiolucent. Mastectomy is another important cause, and an abnormal axillary fold will be seen if a radical mastectomy has been performed.

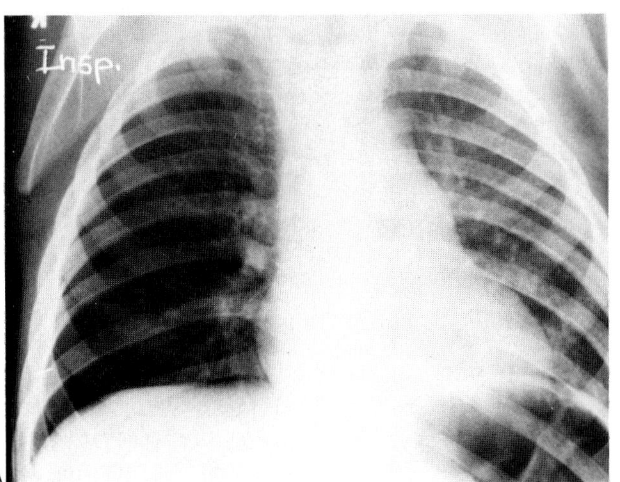

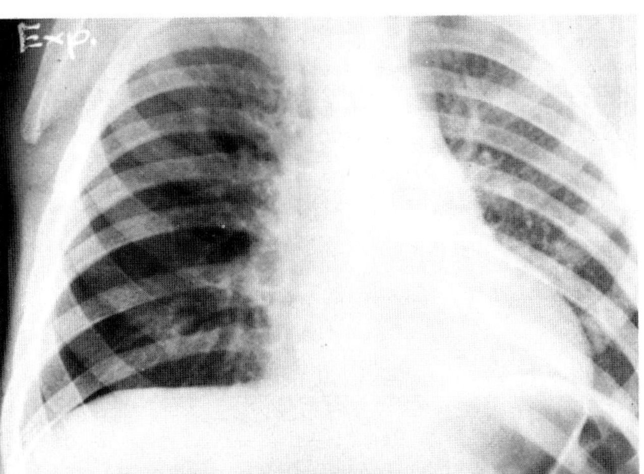

Fig. 11.50 Obstructive emphysema. Child inhaled a peanut. (**A**) Inspiratory film shows a hypertransradiant right lung. (**B**) Expiratory film. There is air trapping on the right side with further shift of the mediastinum to the left.

With conditions such as McCleod's syndrome, congenital lobar emphysema and inhaled foreign body, obstructive emphysema (Fig. 11.50) can be demonstrated on an expiratory film. The mediastinum moves away from the affected side and the ipsilateral diaphragm remains depressed. A small pulmonary artery occurs in McCleod's syndrome, congenital absence and arterial hypoplasia.

Signs of previous surgery or pulmonary collapse may be apparent.

Table 11.15 Causes of unilateral hypertransradiancy

Normal	Contralateral lung is of increased density, e.g. pleural effusion, thickening; consolidation
Technical	Rotation, scoliosis
Soft tissue	Mastectomy, congenital absence of pectoralis major Poliomyelitis
Compensatory emphysema	Lobar collapse, lobectomy
Obstructive emphysema	Foreign body, tumour McCleod's syndrome Congenital lobar emphysema
Bullous emphysema	
Vascular	Absent or hypoplastic pulmonary artery Obstruction of pulmonary artery (tumour, embolus) McCleod's syndrome
Pneumothorax	

THE OPAQUE HEMITHORAX

All the causes of unilateral hypertransradiancy are also responsible for apparent contralateral increased density. When a hemithorax is opaque, penetrated and lateral films are indicated. Signs of collapse, fluid levels, mediastinal displacement and rib abnormalities are important. Pulmonary agenesis is most frequently left sided with associated hypoplastic ribs.

Table 11.16 Causes of an opaque hemithorax

Technical	Rotation, scoliosis
Pleural	Large effusion, hydrothorax Thickening, mesothelioma
Surgical	Pneumonectomy, thoracoplasty
Congenital	Pulmonary agenesis
Mediastinal	Gross cardiomegaly, tumours
Pulmonary	Collapse, consolidation, fibrosis
Diaphragmatic hernias	

THE CHEST FILM OF THE ELDERLY PERSON

With age the thorax changes shape and the AP diameter increases. A kyphosis develops, frequently resulting in the patients chin overlying the apices. Often only an AP film in the sitting position can be obtained, usually with a poor degree of inspiration so that the lung bases are not clearly seen.

Bone demineralization increases. Vertebral body compression and rib fractures occur. The bony margins become irregular. Calcification of the costal cartilage and vascular structures is prominent. Not infrequently there is calcification of the cartilagenous rings of the trachea and bronchi.

The major blood vessels become unfolded. On a lateral film the aorta is visualized throughout its length. Unfolding of the subclavian and innominate vessels result in widening of the superior mediastinum. Prominence of the hilar vessels is partly due to the presence of chronic obstructive airways disease. The peripheral vessels become more obvious as well.

Changes of previous pathology such as linear scars, pleural thickening, tenting of the diaphragm and calcified foci are apparent. Blunting of the costophrenic angles is often seen. With age the diaphragms tend to be flatter.

LIMITATIONS OF THE PLAIN CHEST FILM

It should be remembered that chest radiography has limitations in the diagnosis of certain disease processes.

First the radiologist may fail to spot a lesion. Felson has reported that 20–30% of the significant information on a plain film may be overlooked by a trained radiologist.

Secondly the disease process can fail to appear as a visible abnormality on the film. This occurs when the lesions are small as with miliary shadowing, metastases and fine interstitial shadowing. Such abnormalities are identified earlier on CT scans. Both chronic obstructive airways disease and extensive bronchiectasis can be associated with a normal film; inflamed bronchi are not usually seen. Small pulmonary emboli without infarction can rarely be diagnosed without a radioisotope scan.

Finally, the shadow patterns themselves are rarely specific to a particular disease process. For example both pulmonary infarcts and pneumonia cause consolidation with identical appearances.

OTHER METHODS OF INVESTIGATION

TOMOGRAPHY

Indications. Tomography is performed:

1. To improve visualization of a lesion.
2. To locate the site of a mass, especially prior to biopsy.
3. For evaluation of the hilum and proximal airways.
4. To demonstrate a suspected lesion, e.g. metastases.
5. For evaluation of the mediastinum and chest wall adjacent to a lung mass.

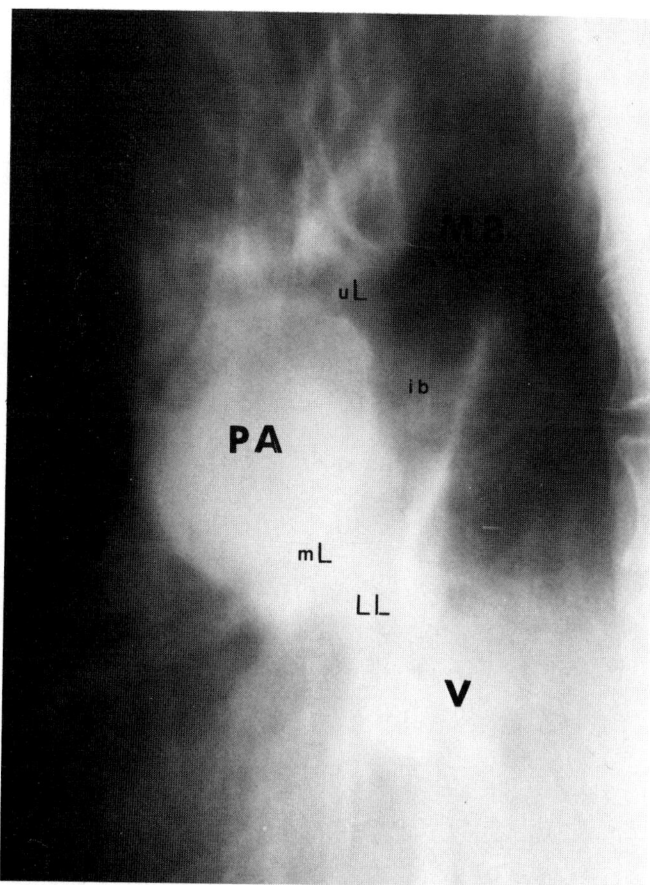

Fig. 11.51 Right posterior oblique (55°) tomogram of right hilum. PA = Pulmonary artery. V = Pulmonary vein. MB = Main bronchus. uL = upper lobe bronchus. ib = Intermediate bronchus. mL = Middle lobe bronchus. LL = Lower lobe brochus.

Technique. Tomography must never be performed in the absence of a recent chest film and should be closely supervised by a radiologist. Particular attention must be paid to radiographic technique. Care is needed to ensure that the area of interest has been included on those cuts taken. Linear tomography is usually adequate although more complex movements may be used. Cuts at 1 cm intervals are necessary; on occasions closer cuts at the level of an abnormality are indicated.

AP tomography, supplemented occasionally with lateral tomography, is satisfactory for peripheral lesions. The hilum is best visualized in the 55° posterior oblique position with the side of interest dependent (Fig. 11.51). On this view the bronchi are projected in profile. A penetrated AP view demonstrates the carina and should be obtained routinely.

The peripheral mass The main reason for performing tomography of a mass is to determine whether there are any features which indicate whether it is benign or malignant. Features of diagnostic importance include calcification, cavitation, outline, bronchial narrowing and the presence of an air bronchogram (Fig. 11.52).

The hilum. On plain films the normal hilum has a very variable appearance and assessment is difficult. Hilar tomograms are not easy to interpret. It is helpful to remember that normal sized lymph nodes are not usually seen, and if they are enlarged are well defined. Also

Fig. 11.52 Oat cell carcinoma. (**A**) Peripheral mass adjacent to the ribs. (**B**) Oblique tomogram shows an irregular mass with thin strands extending into the surrounding lung.

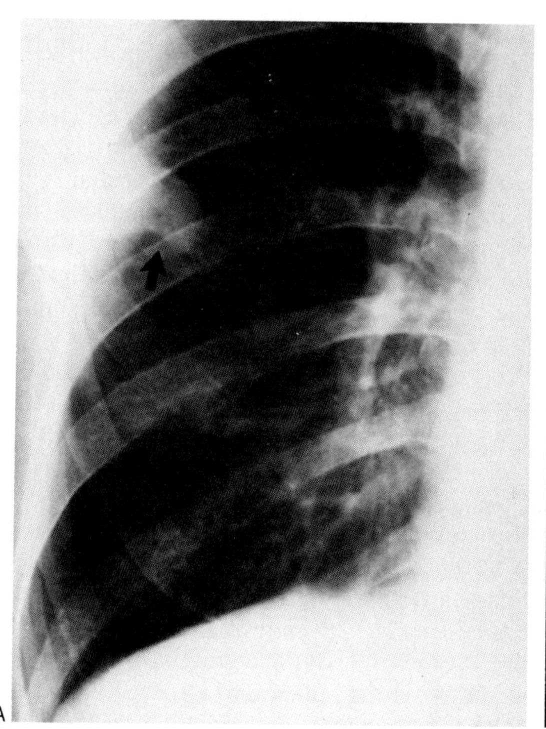

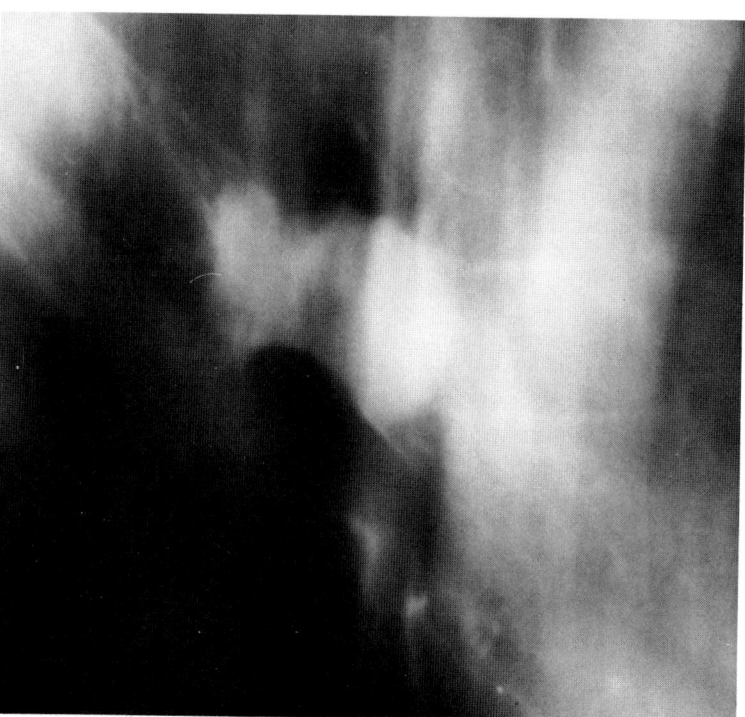

pulmonary vessels branch and taper, and this helps to distinguish them from hilar masses. If a mass is identified the adjacent bronchi must be examined for narrowing or occlusion.

FLUOROSCOPY

Fluoroscopy is of value for assessing diaphragm movement, and also for demonstrating mediastinal shift when obstructive emphysema is suspected. It is frequently helpful with young children when the radiograph is not diagnostic because of movement and poor inspiration.

Occasionally it can be used for locating the site of a mass by rotating the patient and noting movement of the lesion with respect to the sternum or spine. Pulsation is a misleading sign. Frequently pulsation is transmitted from adjacent vascular structures and the mass in question is not vascular. Masses of vascular origin change size with the Valsalva manoeuvre and on change of patient position. If there is doubt about whether a mass is intrapulmonary or mediastinal, screening whilst the patient breathes deeply shows a pulmonary lesion to be mobile whereas a mediastinal lesion fails to move with respiration.

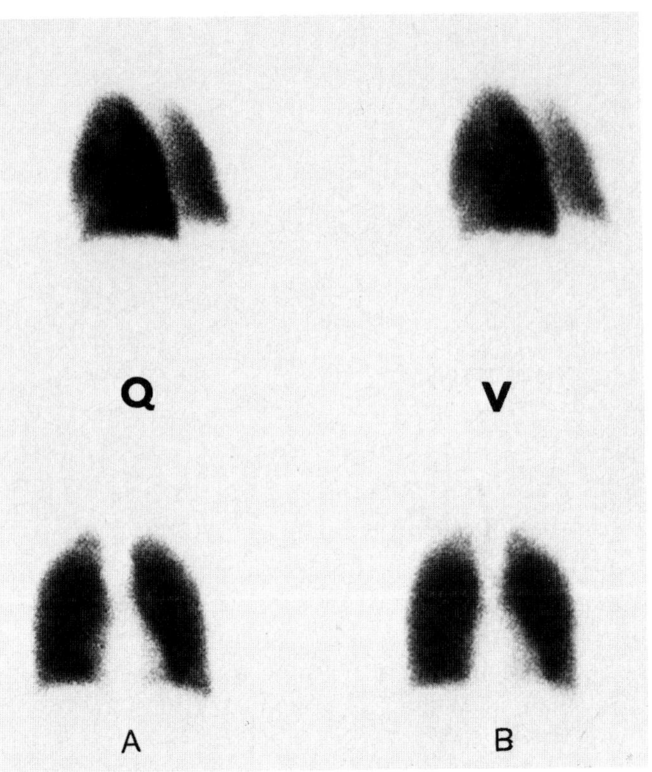

Fig. 11.53 Normal radio-isotope scans. (**A**) Perfusion lung scan (Q) using ^{99}Tc^{m}-labelled macroaggregates. (**B**) Ventilation scan (V) using ^{133}Xe. Note the isotope within the trachea.

RADIO-ISOTOPE SCANNING

Isotope scanning of the lungs is of most value in the diagnosis of pulmonary embolism, when a normal perfusion scan virtually excludes the diagnosis. Unfortunately the major drawback of this technique alone is its lack of specificity so that occasionally interpretation must be guarded. A report must always be made in the light of a current chest film and a ventilation scan if available.

Main indications

a. Diagnosis of pulmonary embolus
b. Evaluation of emphysema
c. To determine the extent of parenchymal disease and malignancy
d. Monitoring the effect of therapy.

Perfusion scans. ^{99}Tc^{m} labelled albumin microspheres or macroaggregates are injected intravenously. Caution is necessary with patients suffering from pulmonary hypertension and right to left shunts. 0.1% of the pulmonary capillaries are occluded for a few hours until phagocytosis occurs. The perfusion pattern of the lungs is dependent upon patient position. Anterior, posterior and both oblique views are taken (Fig. 11.53).

Decreased areas of perfusion occur if there is arterial occlusion. Similar perfusion defects may be seen with emphysema, consolidation, pulmonary collapse and after irradiation, although all of this group will have abnormal ventilation scans as well. Perfusion defects are also seen with fibrosis, although in a small percentage of cases ventilation appears normal.

Conditions where perfusion is abnormal and ventilation normal include vasculitis and pulmonary artery compression as well as embolism. Perfusion scans are helpful when congenital abnormalities such as pulmonary artery agenesis and hypoplastic lung are suspected.

Ventilation scans. Ventilation defects are nearly always associated with corresponding perfusion defects. Exceptions include asthma, inhaled foreign bodies and some cases of carcinoma of the lung, when perfusion scans are normal. ^{133}Xe with a half life of 5.7 days is commonly used; ^{81}Kr^{m} is also widely available and has a half life of 13 seconds. The views taken are as those described for the perfusion scan (Fig. 11.53).

With ^{133}Xe, scanning after a single inhalation of isotope reveals areas of underventilation. Washout scans after rebreathing an air-isotope mixture demonstrates air trapping and is of use in assessing bullous emphysema, and in confirming the presence of obstructive emphysema.

With ^{81}Kr^{m}, scanning is performed during tidal respiration. Due to its better physical characteristics it more accurately demonstrates regional pulmonary ventilation, and can be used concurrently with perfusion imaging.

Pulmonary embolus. Multiple segmental perfusion defects (Fig. 11.54) in the presence of a normal ventilation scan and chest radiograph are virtually diagnostic of

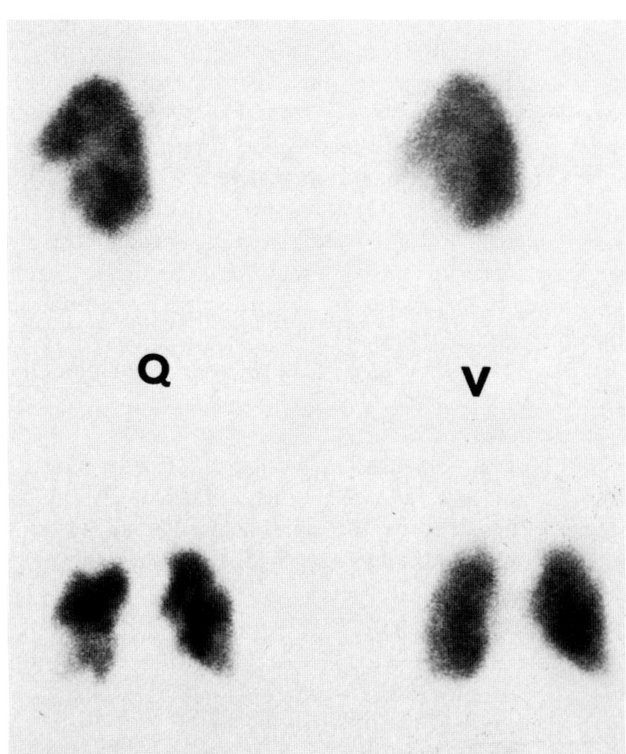

Fig. 11.54 Multiple pulmonary emboli. The perfusion (Q) scan shows multiple large defects in both lungs. There are no defects on the ventilation (V) scan. This V/Q mismatch is characteristic of pulmonary embolism.

pulmonary emboli. A normal perfusion scan excludes pulmonary emboli in vessels larger than 1 mm. A saddle embolus may give an apparently normal perfusion scan by causing symmetrically reduced perfusion in both lungs, or perfusion may be normal.

Gallium-67 citrate imaging. Gallium can demonstrate the extent of an inflammatory process with greater accuracy and earlier than on a chest film. It is also of value in assessing the degree of activity of a disease process and in demonstrating response to treatment. Apart from inflammation, uptake is also increased in abnormal nodes and tumours, but not all secondaries. Thus gallium may be used for assessing the activity and extent of pulmonary sarcoidosis, tuberculosis, interstitial fibrosis, drug pneumonitis and pneumocystis infection. Pulmonary infarcts fail to take up the isotope unless they become infected; this lack of uptake helps to differentiate infection from infarction.

CT SCANNING

CT scanning is developing a rapidly expanding list of applications in the evaluation of pulmonary and chest wall pathology.

Lesions such as metastases, interstitial fibrosis and pleural abnormalities are identifiable earlier than on conventional films and the staging of malignancy has become more accurate. Increasing use is being made of CT guided needle biopsy.

Unfortunately, due to the partial volume effect it is often difficult to determine whether calcification is present within a small pulmonary nodule. Although the CT number does tend to be slightly higher in the presence of calcification, there is considerable overlap with that of the noncalcified lesion so that differentiating between metastases and granulomata may be difficult or impossible without biopsy.

Technique. Supine scanning on suspended inspiration is routine. Prone and decubitus scans may be necessary to demonstrate free fluid and posterior metastases. Window settings of 1000 HU width and –250 to –500 HU level are optimal for the lung fields; settings should be adjusted to view other areas.

Normal appearances (Fig. 11.55). The pulmonary vessels appear as linear densities radiating from the hilum

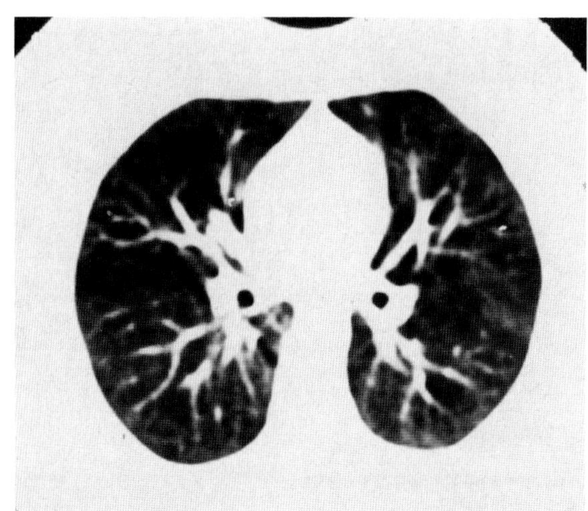

Fig. 11.55 Normal CT scan at level of the hila. Window settings L-700 W 425.

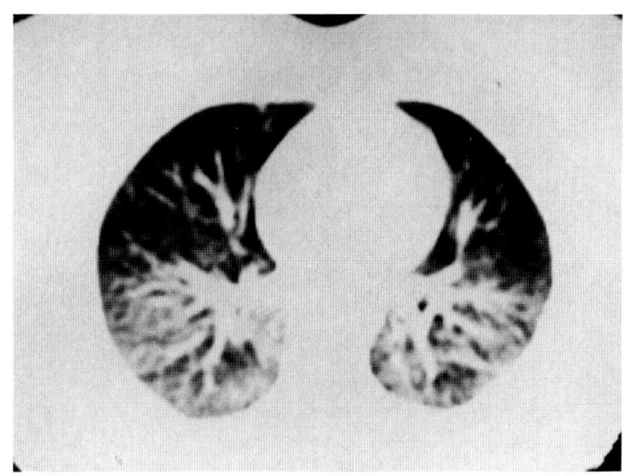

Fig. 11.56 Normal CT scan taken on expiration. Note the increased density of the gravity dependent lung posteriorly. L-700 W425.

and extending almost to the periphery. In the supine position the vessels are strikingly prominent at the bases posteriorly because of the effect of gravity (Fig. 11.56). This gravity dependent perfusion effect is reduced on inspiration and may be eliminated by the presence of emphysema or interstitial fibrosis. Often a vessel is seen to suddenly cut off; this is because it has passed out of the plane of the tomographic cut and does not indicate an occlusion.

Anteriorly in the upper zones both the internal mammary arteries and first ribs may simulate superficial pulmonary nodules. All the ribs are poorly demonstrated because of their oblique lie. Neither the fissures nor the diaphragm are well seen, the diaphragm merging imperceptibly with the upper abdominal organs and heart.

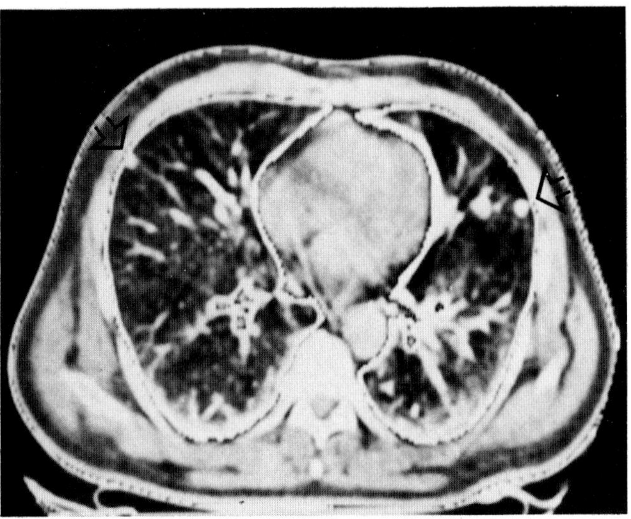

Fig. 11.57 Metastases from a squamous cell carcinoma of the axilla. Note the subpleural position of the metastases (arrows).

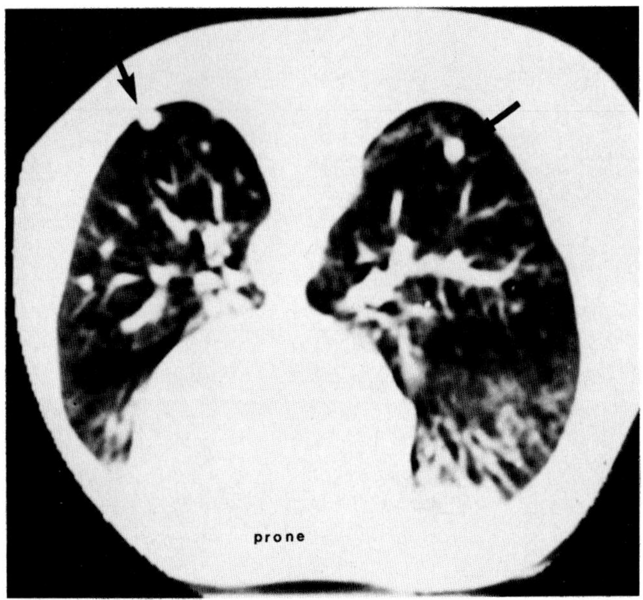

Fig. 11.58 Prone scan of the same patient shows improved visualization of the lung bases where several metastases are present peripherally.

Metastases. Nodules of 3 mm may be demonstrated (Fig. 11.57). Metastases tend to be subpleural and must not be confused with blood vessels, which can be followed through adjacent cuts. In the prone position the vessels change in size and the posterior lung bases are better visualized because the anterior lung becomes gravity dependent; therefore posterior metastases may become apparent. (Fig. 11.58)

Bullae. These show as areas of reduced attenuation, and do not contain vessels, although displaced vessels are present around them.

The pleura. Plaques and calcification secondary to asbestos exposure are seen early, particularly in the posterior sulcus and on the diaphragms. Pleural fluid and tumours are well seen and may be distinguished from each other. Lung which is obscured by an effusion on a plain film is clearly visualized.

LUNG BIOPSY

When non-invasive techniques have failed to establish a definite diagnosis, a lung biopsy is indicated.

Techniques

a. With an **open biopsy** obtained at surgery an adequate specimen is obtained, but this procedure does entail the risks associated with anaesthesia and thoracotomy.

b. With **fibre-optic biopsy** using a fibre-optic bronchoscope, a central lesion can be biopsied; brushings, washings and bacteriological samples may be taken. The success rate is high and the complication rate low.

c. **Catheter biopsy** can also be used for central masses. A French 7 or 8 catheter is guided under screen control into the relevant bronchus, having been inserted via the cricothyroid membrane.

d. **Percutaneous fine needle biopsy**. The main indication for this technique is to determine the nature of a peripheral mass; it does have a use for obtaining bacteriological specimens as well.

The procedure is contraindicated if the patient is on anticoagulants, has a bleeding diathesis or if the mass is thought to be vascular. It is inadvisable in patients with bullae or in those who have had a pneumonectomy. Patient co-operation is needed and uncontrolled coughing is a contraindication. Because of the risk of anaphylaxis, biopsy is inadvisable if the mass is thought to be a hydatid cyst.

The site of the lesion should be determined on plain films, tomograms and screening, preferably biplane. Patient position is adjusted so that the shortest route to the mass is chosen for the passage of the needle. The site of puncture is marked and anaesthetized. A long narrow auge (18–22) needle is inserted during suspended respir-ion. Some resistance is usually felt on entering the mass. creening while slightly obliquing the patient should onfirm that the needle is correctly positioned. Ideally the iopsy is taken from the periphery of the mass, where the uccess rate for positive biopsy is higher. Suction is applied vith a syringe; the needle is manipulated to and fro within he mass and then withdrawn. The advice of the cytologist hould be sought to obtain the best slides.

Immediately after the biopsy, inspiratory and expiratory lms should be obtained, with repeat films after three ours. Bed rest is indicated.

omplications reported include:

. Pneumothorax — 10–20% of cases. Most are shallow and resolve spontaneously.
. Haemoptysis — 5% of cases; usually transient
. Haemothorax
. Empyema
. Subcutaneous emphysema
. Transplanting malignant cells.

Using fine needle biopsy the dangers of the latter four omplications are extremely low.

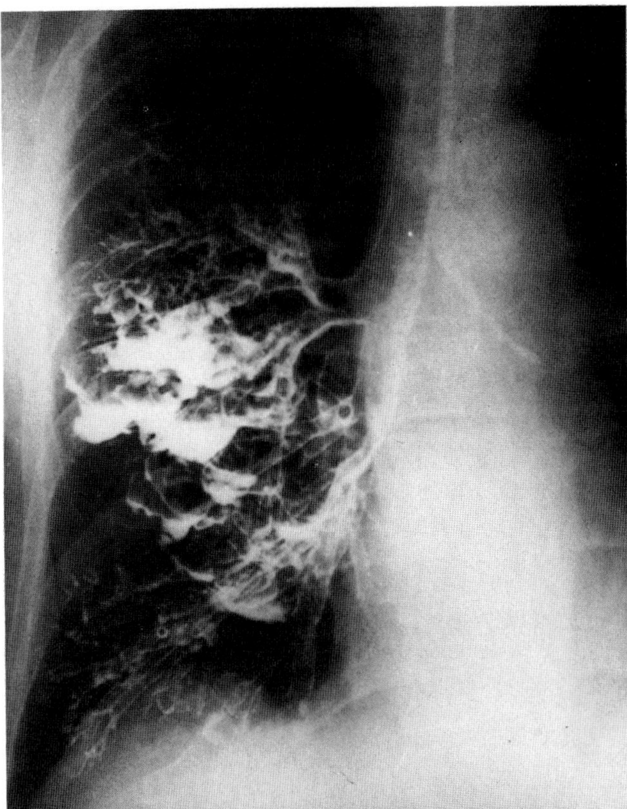

Fig. 11.59 Bronchogram. Patient with cystic bronchiectasis. The majority of the bronchi outlined with contrast are dilated.

BRONCHOGRAPHY

ronchography remains the definitive investigation for the iagnosis of bronchiectasis (Fig. 11.59) and for demon-trating the extent of the disease. With the introduction of ibre-optic bronchoscopy, biopsy techniques and CT scan-ning, its other uses have declined. Occasionally bron-chography is indicated to investigate haemoptysis when all ther investigations are negative. It is helpful for demon-strating congenital abnormalities such as sequestration and ulmonary agenesis and rarely may be used to elucidate the nature of a pulmonary lesion by assessing bronchial distor-tion and displacement.

Severely impaired pulmonary function is a contraindi-cation and partial impairment necessitates only a limited examination. Massive haemoptysis, recent pneumonia, active tuberculosis and a history of allergy are other recog-nized contraindications.

The technique is well described elsewhere. Approaches include a cricothyroid puncture, nasal or transoral drip, and tracheal intubation under local or general anaesthesia. Bronchography by contrast inhalation has failed to become widely accepted. Good physiotherapy before and after the procedure, and atropine to reduce the secretions, are essen-tial. Films taken include AP, lateral and obliques and, if necessary, tomograms. Delayed films demonstrate distal filling. Cinebronchography has its exponents.

On examining the films all the bronchi should be identi-fied. A search must be made for bronchial narrowing or occlusion, intraluminal filling defects and dilated mucous glands. The latter commonly occur with bronchitis and bronchiectasis.

ULTRASOUND

The acoustic mismatch between the chest wall and adjacent aerated lung results in virtually total reflection of the ultra-sonic beam so that ultrasound can only be used for inves-tigating superficial lesions. It is most valuable for diagnosing a pleural effusion, differentiating an effusion from a mass or a subphrenic collection, and in locating the site of fluid prior to a diagnostic tap. Diaphragm movement can be studied as well.

A real time sector scanner with a 3.5 or 5.0 mHz trans-ducer is preferable. On supine scanning the right diaphragm and surrounding areas are clearly visualised through the liver (Fig. 11.60). However, on the left side visualization is hampered by intervening bowel. By filling the stomach with fluid to act as an acoustic window, and then obliquing the patient, visualization can be improved.

In the supine position free pleural fluid appears as a triangular anechoic area, with a well-defined posterior wall, in the posterior costophrenic angle (Fig. 11.61). Internal echoes may be due to blood or pus, and septa indicating

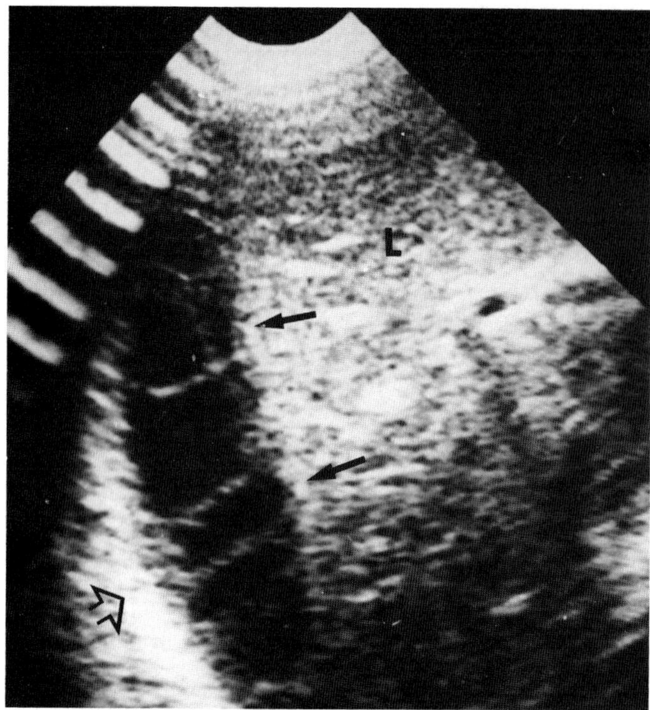

Fig. 11.60 Ultrasound of subphrenic abscess. There is a transonic area (arrows) between the liver (L) and diaphragm (open arrow). Strands crossing this area indicate loculation.

loculation may be seen. Frequently an empyema has a thick wall.

PULMONARY ANGIOGRAPHY

Main indications:

a. Diagnosis of pulmonary embolism
b. Evaluation of pulmonary hypertension
c. Diagnosis of vascular lesions, e.g. arteriovenous malformations, pulmonary hypoplasia, pulmonary artery aneurysms
d. Diagnosis of left atrial myxoma.

The newer imaging techniques have resulted in a marked decline in the number of occasions when pulmonary angiography is necessary. Left atrial myxomas are now usually diagnosed using echocardiography. In the majority of cases pulmonary embolus is excluded by a normal perfusion radioisotope scan. However for a definitive diagnosis of embolism, particularly if surgery is anticipated, angiography is performed (Fig. 11.62).

The right heart may be approached via the femoral vein or the basilic vein after cutdown. In the case of a suspected pulmonary embolus the femoral approach should be preceded by an ascending phlebogram to exclude the presence of iliac or femoral vein thrombus, which could be dislodged by catheterisation.

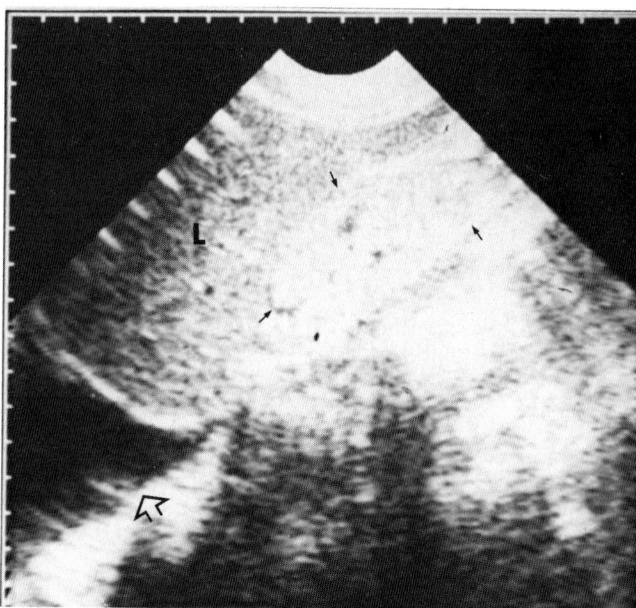

Fig. 11.61 Ultrasound of a pleural effusion. A patient in renal failure with acute glomerulonephritis. There is a moderate sized effusion (open arrow) seen as a transonic area in the posterior sulcus above the diaphragm. Note the highly echogenic kidney (small arrows).

All procedures require ECG monitoring and pressure studies, including right heart and pulmonary wedge pressures. A fairly rapid injection of a large bolus of contrast (50–60 ml at 20–25 ml/s) is required for good visualiz-

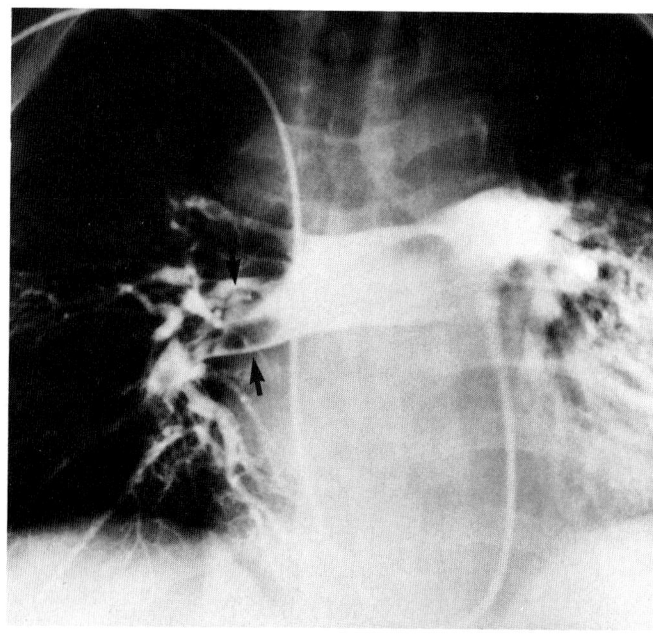

Fig. 11.62 Pulmonary angiogram. A 55-year-old male, 4 days after a thoracotomy developed a DVT and pulmonary embolism. There are large thrombi (arrows) in the main arteries and peripheral perfusion is poor.

tion of the pulmonary vessels, although caution is needed when pulmonary hypertension is present.

BRONCHIAL ARTERIOGRAPHY

Arteriography followed by embolization of bronchial and intercostal branches is a recognized treatment for life threatening or recurrent severe haemoptysis when surgery is contraindicated. Its value is limited for investigating the nature of pulmonary abnormalities. Malignant and inflammatory lesions often have a similar vascular pattern.

The anatomy of the bronchial arteries is very variable and not infrequently spinal branches arise from the intercostal arteries or intercostal-bronchial trunks. This is an absolute contraindication to embolization because of the risk of spinal cord infarction.

DIAGNOSTIC PNEUMOTHORAX

Although rarely performed nowadays, a diagnostic pneumothorax may be used to distinguish a pleural from a pulmonary lesion. A mass within the lung or visceral pleura moves with the lung and becomes displaced from the chest wall, whereas a parietal pleural or chest wall mass is unchanged in position.

BARIUM SWALLOW

CT scanning has almost replaced the barium swallow as a method of diagnosing the non-oesophageal mediastinal mass by displacement or obstruction of the oesophagus. However a barium swallow is necessary to demonstrate lesions such as an hiatus hernia, achalasia and scleroderma, all of which may be associated with pulmonary changes.

LYMPHANGIOGRAPHY

Chylous reflux resulting in the formation of a chylothorax may be demonstrated by conventional lymphangiography.

THE CHEST WALL

THE BONES

The sternum. *Developmental abnormalities* such as perforation, fissures and agenesis are rare. Agenesis is associated with an increased incidence of congenital heart disease. Other sternal lesions associated with congenital heart disease include pigeon chest and depressed sternum, which are found with atrial septal defects, and premature obliteration of the ossification centres, associated with ventricular septal defects. Double ossification centres have an increased incidence in Down's syndrome whereas delayed epiphyseal fusion is a feature of cretinism.

In the presence of a *depressed sternum* the anterior ribs are more vertical and the posterior ribs more horizontal than normal (Fig. 11.63). The heart is displaced to the left and appears enlarged with a straight left border and an indistinct right border. The lower thoracic spine is clearly

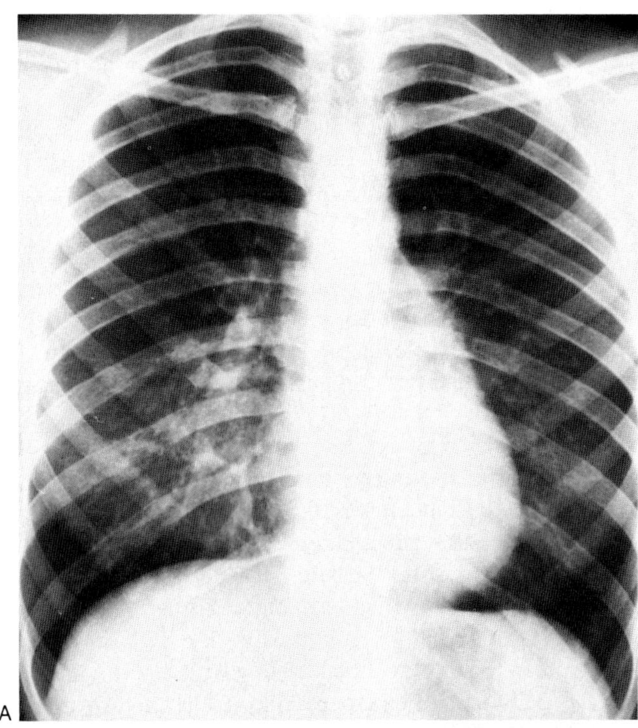

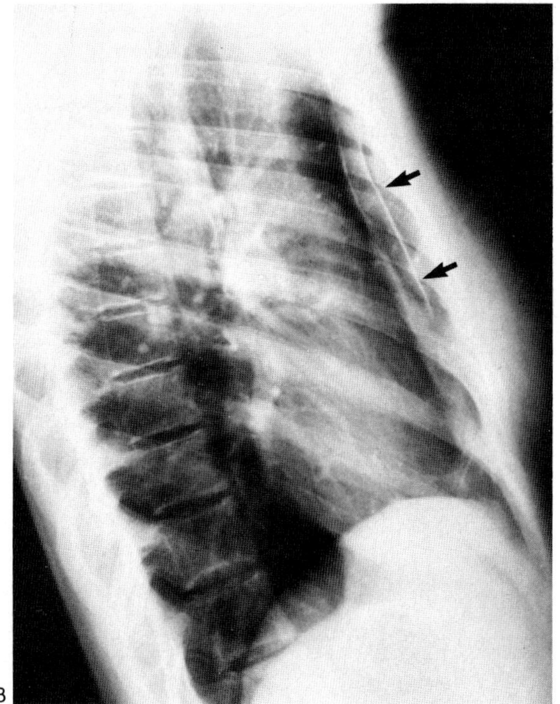

Fig. 11.63 Pectus excavatum (depressed sternum). (**A**) Prominent shadowing adjacent to the right heart border. The heart is displaced to the left and has a straight left border. (**B**) Note the posteriorly displaced sternum (arrows).

visualized. Ill-defined shadowing is seen in the right cardiophrenic region and must not be confused with middle lobe consolidation or collapse.

Erosion of the sternum may occur due to adjacent anterior mediastinal lymphadenopathy, aortic aneurysms and mediastinal tumours or as a result of an infective process.

Primary *tumours* are rare and are usually cartilagenous. The sternum may be the site for metastases, lymphoma and myeloma.

Fractures of the sternum may be associated with injury of the thoracic spine, especially as a result of a steering wheel injury, when the sternum and ribs become separated.

The clavicles. Duplication of the clavicle and a pseudarthrosis of the middle third are rare abnormalities. Absence or defective development of the outer end of the bone is a feature of cleidocranial dysostosis. The clavicles are small in patients with progeria and may actually disappear completely.

Erosion of the outer ends of the clavicles occurs with rheumatoid arthritis, infections and hyperparathyroidism. Erosion of the medial ends is also seen with infections and rheumatoid arthritis but is more difficult to demonstrate.

The clavicle may be the site of metastases, myeloma, giant cell tumours, Ewing's sarcoma, eosinophilic granuloma (Fig. 11.64) and Paget's disease.

Fractures are common, often healing with mal-union, and they are easily missed on a chest film if the fracture affects the middle third of the bone which is often foreshortened and poorly seen.

The scapulae. Sprengel's shoulder is associated with Klippel Feil syndrome and congenital heart diseases; rib and vertebral anomalies are often present as well. Fractures are easily missed. Both primary and secondary tumours and Paget's disease may occur within the scapula.

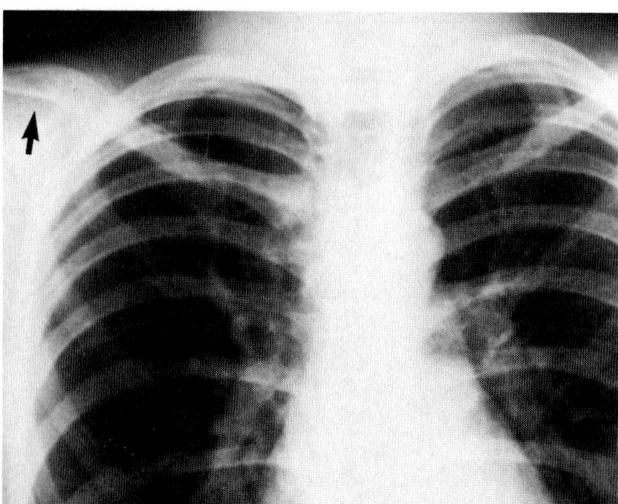

Fig. 11.64 Eosinophilic granuloma of the right clavicle. Asymptomatic. An expanding lytic lesion. Biopsy confirmed the diagnosis.

The Ribs. *Rib notching* may occur on the superior or inferior surface and be unilateral or bilateral.

Superior notching (Fig. 11.65) may be a normal occurrence in old age, but has been recorded in patients with rheumatoid arthritis, SLE, hyperparathyroidism, neurofibromatosis and in polio victims.

Inferior notching (Fig. 11.66) develops as a result of hypertrophy of the intercostal arteries and veins or with neurogenic tumours. When the aorta is obstructed, blood flow through the intercostal arteries is reversed.

With coarctation notching of the first and second ribs does not develop, because the arteries arise proximally, and the middle ribs are usually affected. Notching of the lower ribs may be seen with a blocked abdominal aorta. If a coarctation is preductal notching does not occur.

Congenital anomalies of the ribs are common. They may be bifid or hypoplastic and bridging between ribs may occur. Hypoplastic first ribs must be distinguished from cervical ribs (Fig. 11.67); the latter arise from C7, the transverse processes of which point caudally whereas

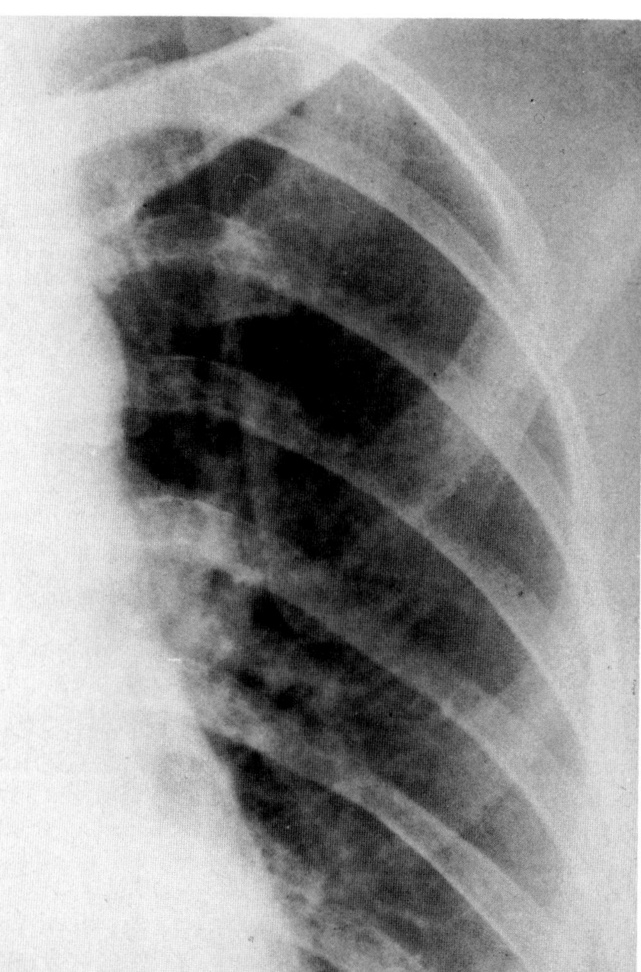

Fig. 11.65 Superior rib notching in a patient with a long history of paralysis following poliomyelitis.

hypoplastic ribs arise from D1, the transverse processes of which are cranially inclined.

Eleven pairs of ribs are often present in patients with *Down's syndrome*.

An *intrathoracic rib* is uncommon. It appears as a ribbon-

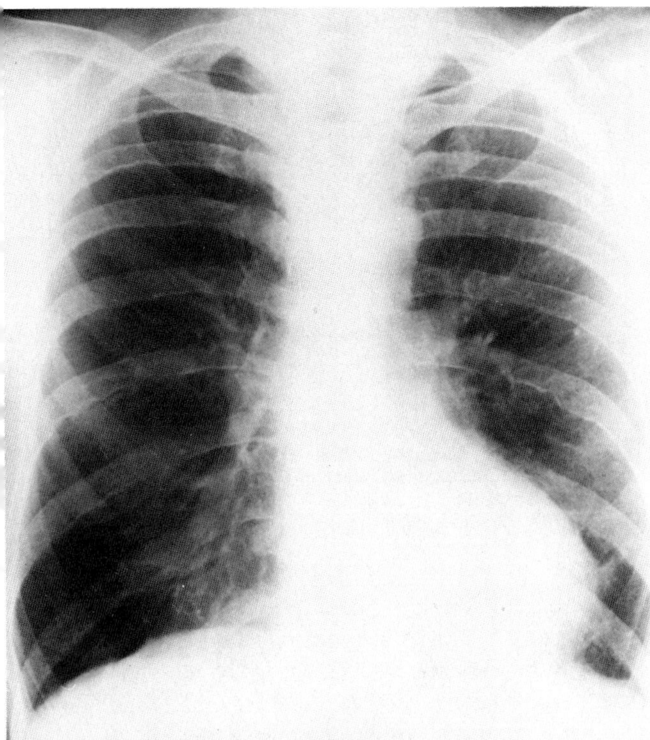

Fig. 11.66 Inferior rib notching. An elderly male who presented with hypertension. Coarctation of the aorta with rib notching most prominent in the fourth to eighth ribs.

Table 11.17 Causes of inferior rib notching

Aortic	Coarctation; occlusion
Subclavian	Takayashu disease Blalock–Taussig operation (unilateral)
Reduced pulmonary flow	Pulmonary atresia, pulmonary stenosis Fallot's tetralogy Truncus Type IV
Venous	SVC, IVC obstruction
Shunts	Pulmonary or intercostal arteriovenous fistula Intercostal-pulmonary fistula
Others	Hyperparathyroidism Neurogenic tumours Idiopathic
Unilateral notching	Blalock–Taussig operation Subclavian artery block Coarctation involving the left subclavian artery Coarctation with an anomalous right subclavian artery

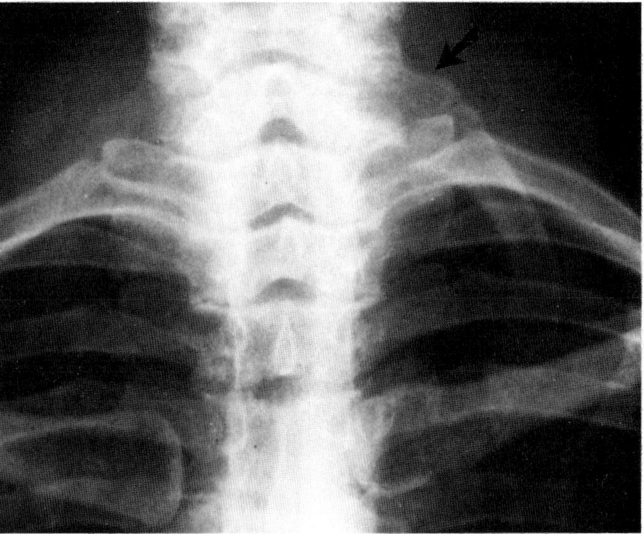

Fig. 11.67 Cervical ribs. Note the downward direction of the transverse process of C7 (arrow).

like shadow near to the spine attached at one or both ends of the posterior part of a rib.

In *Tietze's syndrome* the anterior ends of the ribs are invariably normal but occasionally they may be enlarged and have a spotty appearance.

Absence, irregularity, partial amputation or displacement may be the result of *previous surgery* (Fig. 11.68). *Localized rib displacement* may be accompanied by pressure erosion and is characteristic of a soft tissue mass such as a neurofibroma or lipoma.

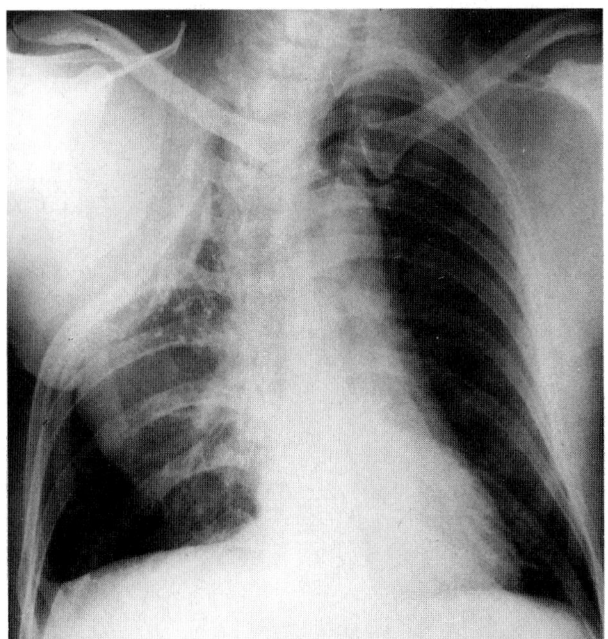

Fig. 11.68 Right thoracoplasty for tuberculosis. Removal of the upper ribs with collapse of the upper lobe.

Crowding of the ribs is a sign of major pulmonary collapse but also frequently accompanies a scoliosis. The ribs tend to have a horizontal lie in conditions resulting in hyperinflation.

Fractures are common, although often difficult to spot on a routine chest film. An associated extrapleural haematoma, pneumothorax or surgical emphysema may occur. The usual site for *cough fractures* is in the sixth to ninth ribs in the axillary line. *Stress fractures* are usually seen in the first ribs.

Pathological fractures indicate a local rib lesion or are due to generalized diminution of bone mass as occurs in senile osteoporosis, myeloma, steroid therapy, Cushing's syndrome and other endocrine disorders, and diffuse metastases. Those occurring in Cushing's syndrome develop abundant callus.

The *Looser's zones* of osteomalacia represent areas of uncalcified osteoid and the resulting rib deformities may give the thorax a shape like a bell.

Sclerosis of the ribs may be seen in generalized disorders such as osteopetrosis, myelofibrosis, fluorosis and metastases, or with localized lesions such as Paget's disease (Fig. 11.69) when the affected rib is enlarged. *Post-irradiation necrosis* is frequently seen associated with a mastectomy; un-united rib fractures, bony sclerosis and an abnormal trabecular pattern may occur with soft tissue calcification.

Localized *expansion* of the rib occurs in fibrous dysplasia and Gaucher's disease, and with benign tumours including eosinophilic granuloma, haemangiomata, chondromata,

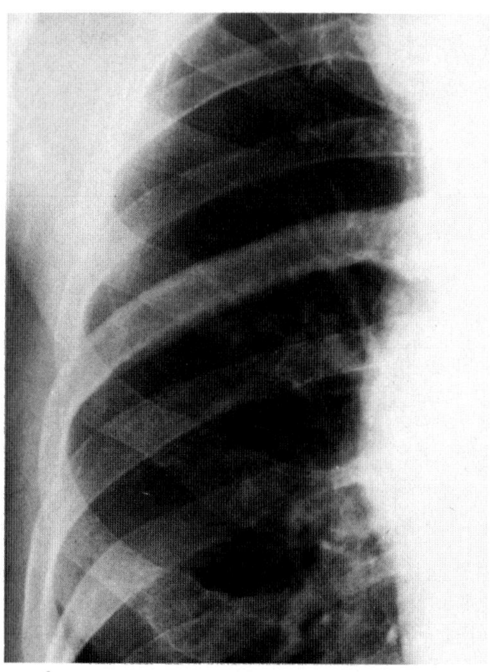

Fig. 11.69 Paget's disease. An enlarged sixth rib with a coarse trabecular pattern and of increased density.

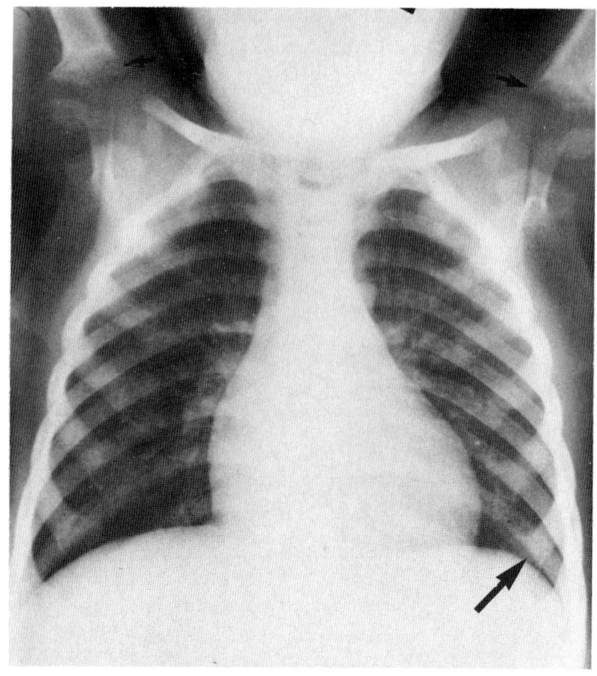

Fig. 11.70 Rickets. Enlargement and cupping of the anterior ends of the ribs. Note the metaphyseal changes in the humeri.

brown tumours of hyperparathyroidism and aneurysmal bone cyst. In Hurler's syndrome there is generalized expansion of the ribs, sparing the proximal ends. In thalassaemia expansion is most marked proximally and is associated with abnormal trabeculation. Widening of the rib ends occurs with scurvy and rickets (Fig. 11.70).

Rib destruction may be the result of a primary lesion or due to involvement by an adjacent infection or tumour of the lung, pleura or soft tissues. An extrapleural mass is often associated.

The rare actinomycosis infection is usually associated with a wavy periostitis of the rib. Many malignant processes including lymphoma, myeloma and metastases commonly affect the ribs.

The thoracic spine. A survey of the spine should be made to check for abnormal curvature or alignment, destruction of the bone or intervertebral discs, abnormal sclerosis, congenital lesions and paravertebral soft tissue masses.

Butterfly vertebrae and other anomalies may be seen. Scoliosis and Klippel Feil syndrome are associated with an increased incidence of congenital heart disease. With a severe scoliosis, when the curve exceeds 60°, cardiorespiratory complications are common in adults.

In the *straight back syndrome* the normal thoracic kyphosis is reduced so that the sternum and spine are virtually parallel, resulting in compression of the mediastinum. Characteristically on the PA film the heart appears to be enlarged, displaced to the left and with a prominent left atrial appendage and aorta. On auscultation there is an ejection systolic murmur with accentuation on expiration.

Anterior erosion of the vertebral bodies with sparing of the disc spaces can develop as a result of aneurysms of the descending aorta, vascular tumours, gross enlargement of the left atrium and neurofibromatosis. In the latter posterior scalloping of the vertebral bodies and an enlarged intervertebral foramen may also be seen.

Destruction of a pedicle is characteristic of a metastasis. Collapse of a vertebral body may be due to a local lesion or a generalized disease such as osteoporosis. The presence of disc destruction is always highly suggestive of an infective process. Calcification of the discs is not uncommon. It is often idiopathic or post traumatic but may occur in ankylosing spondylitis and ochronosis.

The single dense, or ivory, vertebra is the classical appearance of lymphoma, but may be seen with other conditions such as Paget's disease and metastases.

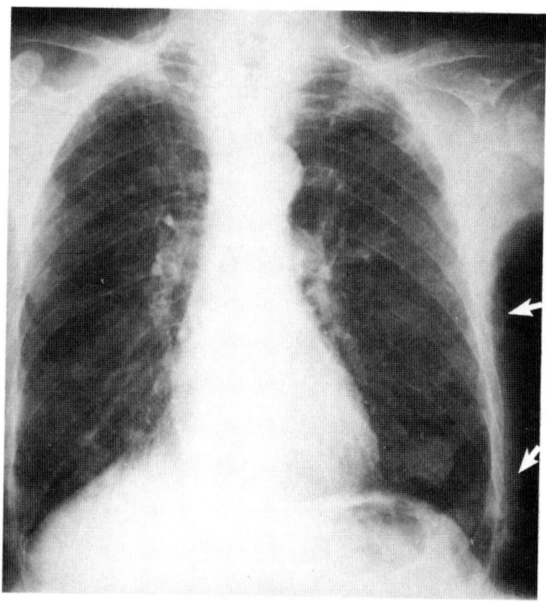

Fig. 11.72 Neurofibromatosis. Multiple soft-tissue lesions, those overlying the lung fields simulating intrapulmonary nodules.

THE SOFT TISSUES

Artefacts. Overlying hair plaits, hair fasteners, buttons, jewellery and clothing may cast confusing shadows which can simulate pulmonary pathology such as a tuberculous infection (Fig. 11.71).

Tracing the edges of the lesion to its extremity will show if it extends beyond the lung fields.

Skin lesions. Soft tissue tumours including naevi and lipomas can mimic intrapulmonary nodules. Pedunculated lesions have well-defined edges because they are surrounded by air and lung markings should be seen through the lesion. The patient must be examined, although a lateral film should confirm that a lesion is extrapulmonary. Multiple nodules occur in neurofibromatosis (Fig. 11.72).

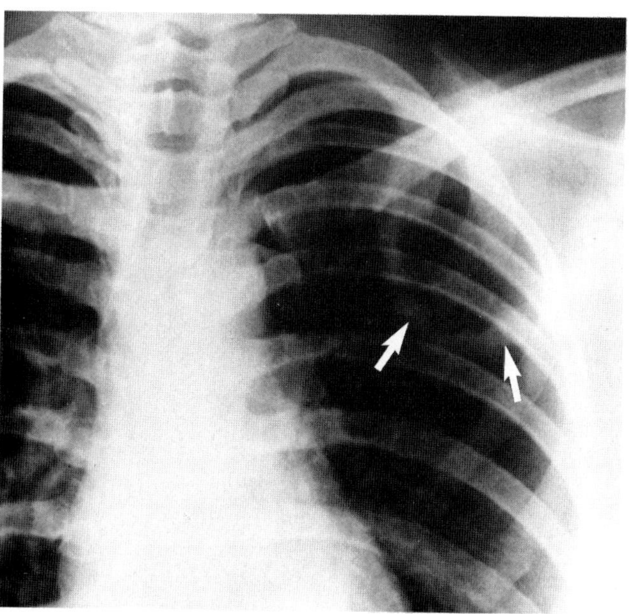

Fig. 11.71 Hair overlying the left upper zone forms a curvilinear shadow simulating a cavity.

In the presence of a soft tissue mass the adjacent bone and lung must be assessed. Occasionally gas may occur within an abscess.

The breast. Mastectomy is probably the commonest cause of a translucent hemithorax. With a radical mastectomy the normal downward curve of the axillary fold is replaced by a dense ascending line, as a result of abscence of pectoralis major (Fig. 11.73). This may also occur as a congenital abnormality, or after amputation of an arm. An absent pectoralis major, associated with syndactyly, is known as *Poland's syndrome*.

A simple mastectomy is associated with normal axillary folds. Accompanying changes of bone necrosis and soft tissue calcification due to irradiation may be present.

Surgical emphysema. Surgical emphysema is often present with a pneumothorax (Fig. 11.74) and pneumomediastinum. After surgery an increase in the extent of the emphysema on serial films suggests that a bronchopleural fistula has developed. Similar appearances may be seen with a tension pneumothorax.

Densities. Calcified nodes and the lesions of cysticercosis may be superimposed on the lung fields. After lymphangiography contrast may be seen in the thoracic duct especially in the left upper zone where the duct drains into the innominate vein; within the lungs transient miliary shadows due to oil emboli may occur. Occasionally after myelography the residual Myodil tracks along the intercostal nerves to give a bizarre appearance.

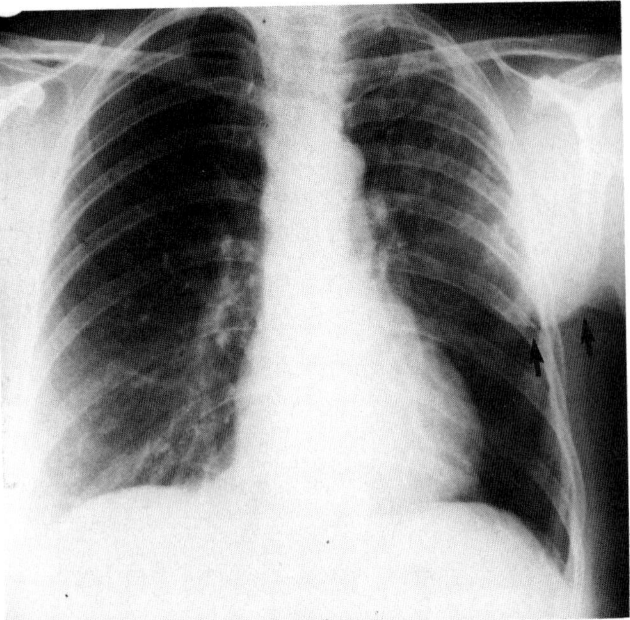

Fig. 11.73 Left mastectomy. Note the abnormal left axillary fold passing cranially (arrows). The left lung is hypertransradiant at its base. Note radiation necrosis of the upper ribs and soft tissue calcification.

THE DIAPHRAGM

The normal appearances of the diaphragm have already been described.

Normal variants

1. *Scalloping* (Fig. 11.75). This variant appears as short curves of diaphragm, convex upwards and mostly seen on the right side.

2. *Muscle slips* (Fig. 11.75). Most commonly seen in patients with emphysema and those who are tall and thin, these appear as small curved lines concave upwards. They are usually right sided.

3. *Diaphragmatic humps and dromedary diaphragms* (Fig. 11.75). Both these variants are probably mild forms of eventration. They occur anteriorly and are usually right-sided. On the PA film the hump appears as a shadow in the right cardiophrenic angle which must be differentiated from a fat pad, lipoma, pericardial cyst and Morgagni hernia; it contains liver but is not a true hernia because there is no defect in the diaphragm. On the lateral film it overlies the heart and must not be confused with middle lobe consolidation.

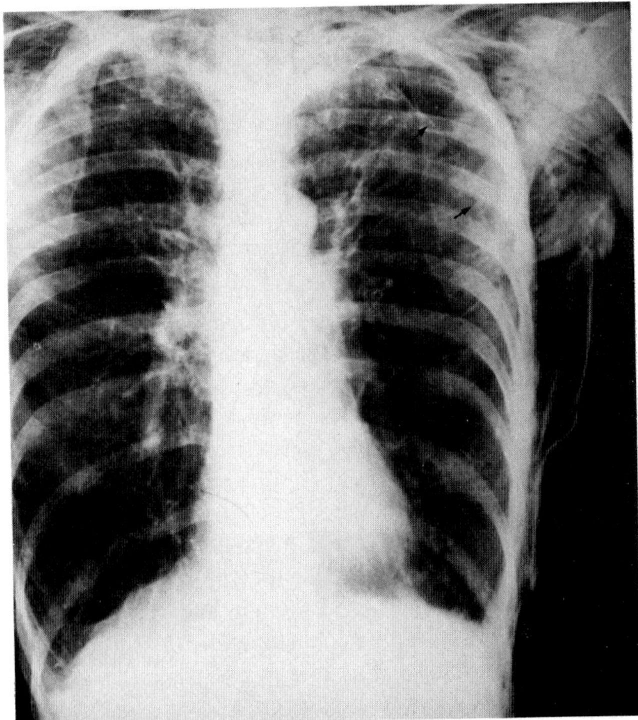

Fig. 11.74 Surgical emphysema following a small left pneumothorax (arrows) in a man with chronic obstructive airways disease.

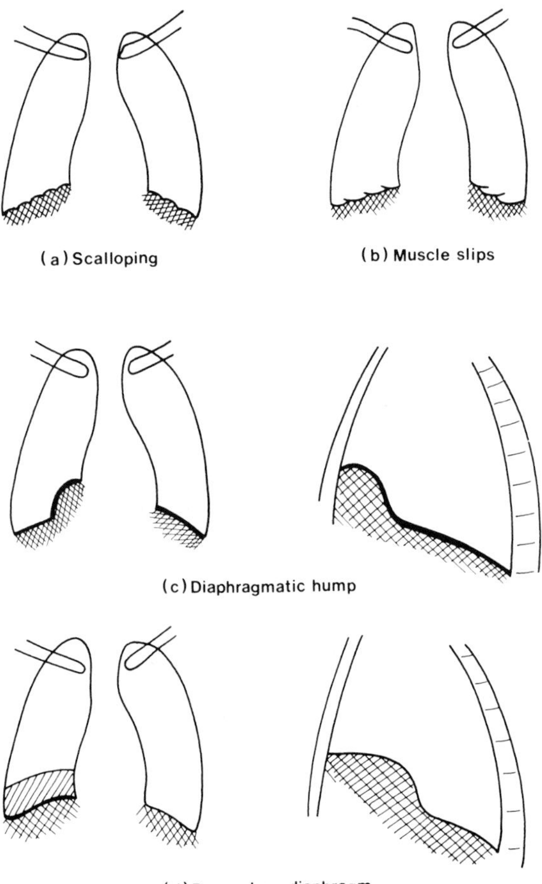

Fig. 11.75 Diagrams to show the normal variants of the diaphragm.

The dromedary diaphragm is a more severe form of the diaphragmatic hump and appears as a double contour on the PA view.

4. *Eventration* (Fig. 11.76). This is nearly always left sided, the hemidiaphragm being considerably elevated with characteristically marked mediastinal displacement to the right, a feature rarely seen with diaphragmatic paralysis.

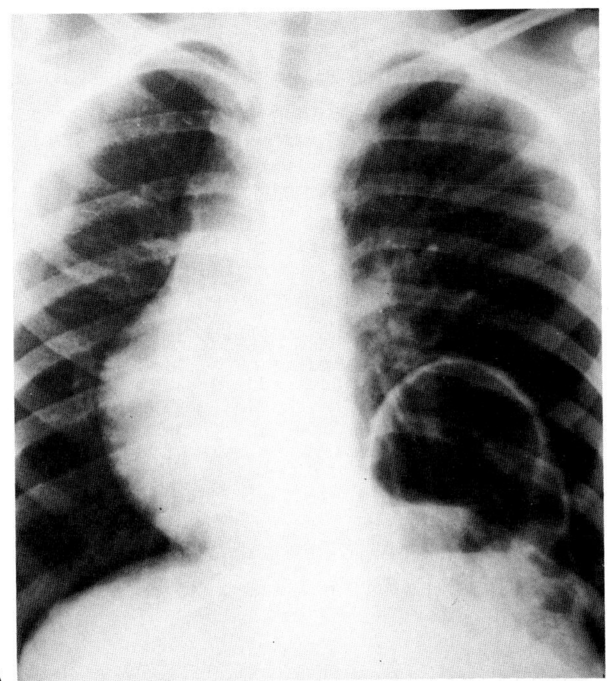

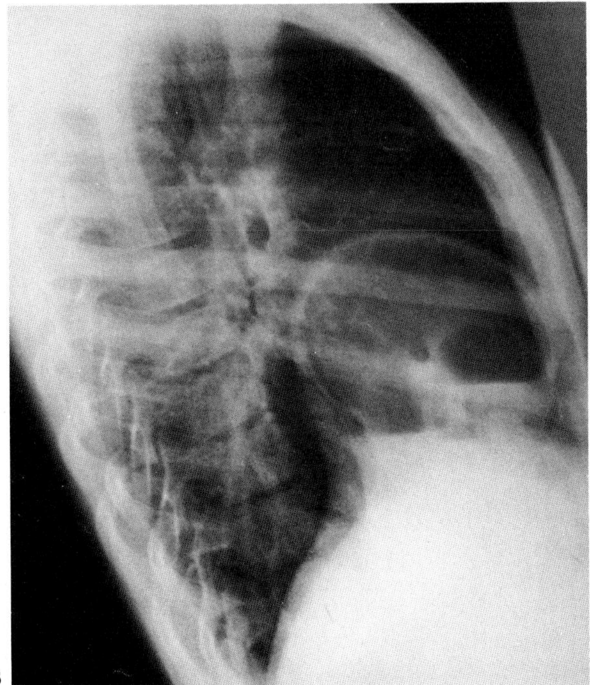

Fig. 11.76 Eventration. (**A**) The left cupola is elevated and the heart displaced to the right. (**B**) The lateral film shows the elevated left cupola with a distended stomach and a normal right cupola.

On fluoroscopy, movement is reduced, absent or paradoxical. The muscle is thin and weak. A partial gastric volvulus with rotation along its long axis so that the greater curve is uppermost may be associated. On occasions eventration may ressemble absence or rupture of the diaphragm and must also be distinguished from paralysis.

5. *Accessory diaphragm*. This is a rare condition which is asymptomatic and usually right sided. The hemithorax is partitioned by the accessory diaphragm which runs parallel to the oblique fissure and resembles a thickened fissure. The blood supply is often anomalous.

Diaphragm movement

Respiratory excursion is easily assessed on fluoroscopy. Normally the left diaphragm moves more than the right, excursion being between 3 and 6 cm. Paradoxical movement occurs when the pressure exerted by the abdomen exceeds that of the weak diaphragm so that it moves upwards on inspiration or sniffing. Paradoxical movement, known to occur in a small percentage of normal subjects, may be demonstrated with diaphragmatic paralysis, subdiaphragmatic infection and eventration.

The elevated diaphragm

The causes are listed in Tables 11.18 and 11.19.

Table 11.18 Causes of unilateral elevation of the diaphragm

Paralysis:	Surgery and trauma Idiopathic Neoplastic. Diabetes mellitus Infections. Herpes zoster. Tb glands
Congenital:	Eventration and humps
Pulmonary:	Lower lobe collapse, pulmonary hypoplasia Pulmonary embolus, basal pneumonia
Pleural:	Thickening, pleurisy Subpulmonary effusion
Bony:	Scoliosis, rib fractures
Subdiaphragmatic:	Gas distended viscus Subphrenic abscess, pancreatitis Abdominal mass, hepatomegaly Splenomegaly

Table 11.19 Causes of bilateral elevation of the diaphragm

Reduced pulmonary compliance, e.g. SLE, fibrosing alveolitis	
Technical:	Supine film. Expiratory film
Subdiaphragmatic:	Ascites, obesity Pregnancy

Frequently no cause can be found to explain elevation of a hemidiaphragm. The clinical history is important. It is essential to exclude the presence of an active lesion, especially malignancy, by carefully surveying the lung fields, hila and the mediastinum. Eventration is usually associated with marked cardiac displacement. Pleural thickening is often fairly obvious. Tenting of the diaphragm, with loss of definition, obliteration or blunting of the costophrenic angles and thickening of the fissures may be accompanying features. Subpulmonary fluid can appear as an elevated diaphragm. It usually has a straighter surface and will shift with change of patient position if it is not loculated; decubitus, supine films and ultrasound are helpful. If the fluid is loculated it may be impossible to differentiate from an elevated diaphragm on plain films, although ultrasound should clearly distinguish between them.

Splinting of the diaphragm may be seen with upper abdominal inflammatory processes and pneumonia. Elevation frequently occurs with a pulmonary embolus.

It may be difficult to decide whether diaphragm elevation is due to paralysis or to pressure from below by an abdominal mass. Locating the position of the liver edge on an abdominal film may then be helpful. If the liver edge is displaced down towards the pelvis it is likely that there is a mass between the liver and diaphragm, whereas a high liver edge is consistent with paralysis. On the left side the position of the stomach bubble may be studied using the same principle. Depressed diaphragms are a feature of pulmonary hyperinflation.

Subphrenic abscess

A subphrenic abscess is usually associated with recent abdominal surgery or sepsis. It is commoner on the right side and fortunately it is easier to diagnose a right-sided abscess than one which is left-sided. Although ultrasound is now the investigation of choice, plain films, including a chest film, contrast studies and CT scans are also helpful.

Plain film signs of a subphrenic abscess. On the chest radiograph there may be ipsilateral basal pulmonary shadowing or atelectasis and a pleural effusion. The diaphragm is frequently elevated with decreased or paradoxical movement. Beneath the diaphragm abnormal gas shadows formed by gas within the abscess may be identified (Fig. 11.77). Depression of the gastric fundus and the liver edge may occur. Films taken with a horizontal beam, (i.e. erect and decubitus positions) increase the likelihood of visualizing the abscess cavity.

The thickness of the diaphragm

On the left side the gastric bubble within the fundus is well applied to the lower surface of the diaphragm in the erect position. Together the stomach wall and diaphragm form a linear density which measures between 5 and 8 mm in thickness.

If this measurement is greater than 8 mm several pathological conditions must be considered although it may be a normal variation. Tumours of the diaphragm, stomach and pleura, subpulmonary fluid and diaphragmatic humps may be responsible. Abdominal lesions include subphrenic abscess, an enlarged liver and spleen and other masses.

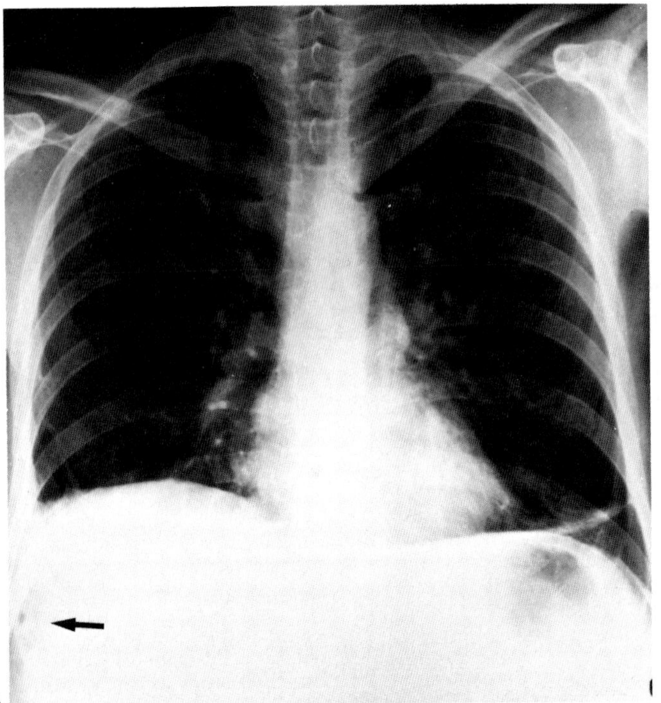

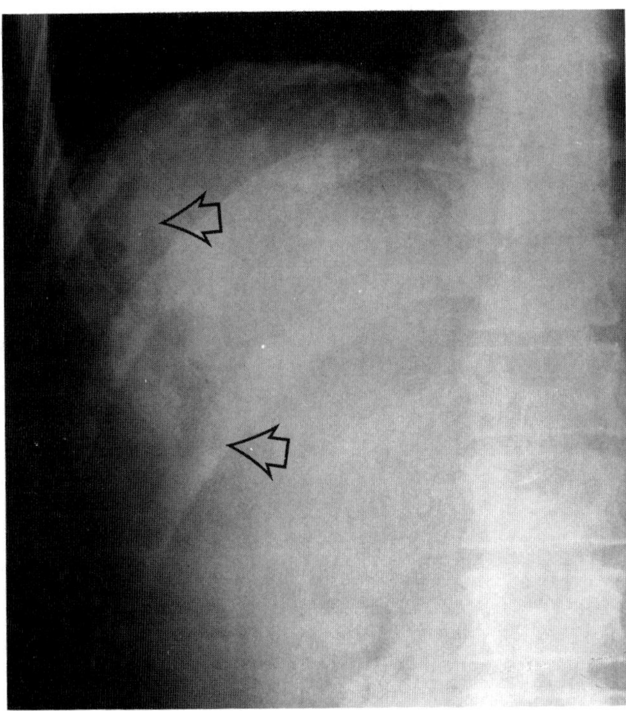

Fig. 11.77 Subphrenic abscess. A male patient with Crohn's disease developed a pyrexia and right shoulder tip pain a few days after laparotomy. (**A**) Abnormal gas shadows are just visible below the right cupola (arrow). There is blunting of the right costophrenic angle. (**B**) Gas shadows within the abscess are clearly seen (open arrows) in penetrated film of abdomen.

Tumours of the diaphragm

These are rare, and benign tumours include lipomas, fibromas, neurofibromas and cysts. Sarcomas are often associated with a pleural effusion. Tumours may appear smooth or lobulated and must be differentiated from intrapulmonary masses, diaphragmatic humps and hernias, and liver tumours.

Hernias of the diaphragm

The classical appearance of a *hiatus hernia*, with a fluid level superimposed on the cardiac shadow, is well known (Fig. 11.78). A *Bochdalek hernia* occurs in the posterolateral part of the diaphragm and is frequently congenital. It may present at birth as neonatal respiratory distress. This hernia is most commonly left sided and may contain omentum, fat, spleen or kidney. The *Morgagni* hernia is uncommon. It is usually right sided, and anterior, appearing as an homogenous shadow in the cardiophrenic angle. The hernia contains fat, or occasionally bowel, and is asymptomatic.

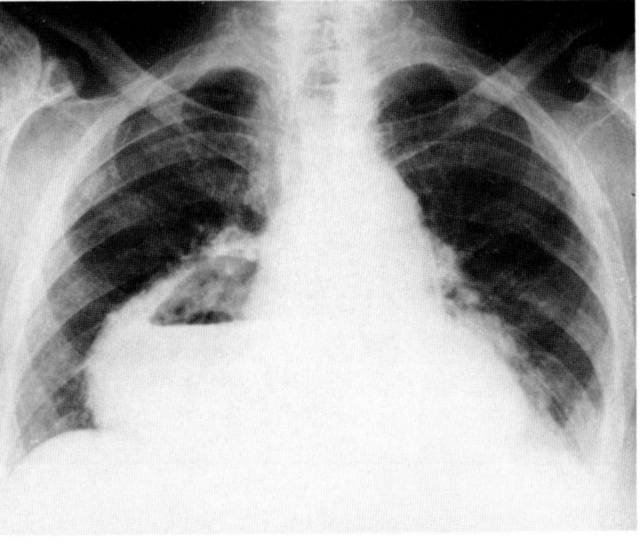

Fig. 11.78 Hiatus hernia. An elderly asymptomatic patient. A large fluid level superimposed on the cardiac shadow. A typical appearance of a hiatus hernia.

Rupture of the diaphragm

Rupture usually occurs as a result of trauma but may be idiopathic or related to previous diaphragmatic surgery. Some 90% of cases are left sided. Frequently the stomach herniates through the diaphragm resulting in gastric obstruction, which may give an appearance that can be confused with a pneumothorax or eventration, although the distended stomach rarely abuts all the borders of the thoracic cage. It is essential that these conditions are differentiated and oral contrast or passage of a nasogastric tube should give the answer. Colon, spleen and kidney may herniate through the defect but this is less common. If there is no herniation of abdominal contents, the diaphragm may appear to be normal on a plain film, or may be elevated with an abnormal outline.

REFERENCES AND SUGGESTIONS FOR FURTHER READING

Boone, M. L., Swenson, B. E., Felson, B. (1964) Rib notching: Its many causes. *American Journal of Roentgenology*, **91**, 1075–1088.

Campbell, J. A. (1963) The diaphragm in roentgenology of the chest. *Radiologic Clinics of North America*, **1**, 394–410.

Felson, B. (1967) The roentgen diagnosis of disseminated pulmonary alveolar diseases. *Seminars in Radiology*, **2**, 3–21.

Felson, B. (1973) *Chest Roentgenology*. Philadelphia: W. B. Saunders.

Felson, B. (1979) A new look at pattern recognition of diffuse pulmonary disease. *American Journal of Roentgenology*, **133**, 183–189.

Fleischner, F. G. (1941) Linear shadows in the lung. *American Journal of Roentgenology*, **46**, 610–618.

Freeman, L. M., Blaufox, M. D. (1980) Radionuclide studies of the lung. *Seminars in nuclear medicine*, **X**, 198–310.

Fraser R. G., Pare J. A. P. (1978) Diagnosis of diseases of the chest. Vol. 1. 2nd edn. Philadelphia: W. B. Saunders.

Heitzman, E. R. (1981) Computed tomography of the thorax: Current perspectives. (Fleischner Lecture) *American Journal of Roentgenology*, **136**, 3–12.

Keats, T. E. (1979) *An atlas of normal roentgen variants that may simulate disease*. 2nd edn, pp. 427–500, Chicago: Year Book Medical Publishers.

Kerr, I. H. (1984) Interstitial lung disease: The role of the radiologist. *Clinical Radiology*, **35**, 1–7.

Lalli, A. F., McCormack, L. J., Zelch M. et al (1978) Aspiration biopsies of chest lesions. *Radiology*, **127**, 35–40.

McCleod, R. A., Brown, L. R., Miller, W. E. & DeRemee, R. A. (1976) Evaluation of the pulmonary hila by tomography. *Radiologic Clinics of North America*, **14**, 51–84.

Miller, W. E., Crowe, J. K., Muhm, J. R. (1976) The evaluation of pulmonary parenchymal abnormalities by tomography. *Radiologic Clinics of North America*, **14**, 85–104.

Milne, E. N. C. (1973) Correlation of physiologic findings with chest radiology. *Radiologic Clinics of North America*, **11**, 17–47.

Reed, J. C., Madewell J. E. (1975) The air bronchogram in interstitial disease of the lungs. *Radiology*, **116**, 1–9.

Simon, G. (1975) The anterior view chest radiograph — criteria for normality derived from a basic analysis of the shadows. *Clinical Radiology*, **26**, 429–437.

Simon, G. (1978) Principles of chest X-ray diagnosis, 4th edn. London: Butterworths.

Strickland, B. (1976) Sentinel lines — an unusual sign of lower lobe contraction. *Thorax*, **31**, 517–521.

Trapnell, D. (1973) The differential diagnosis of linear shadows in chest radiographs. *Radiologic Clinics of North America*, **11**, 77–92.

CHAPTER 12

THE MEDIASTINUM

Mediastinal lesions are usually first demonstrated radiologically on a chest radiograph, which may show either a round or oval mass, widening of the mediastinum or a pneumomediastinum. However a small tumour in the anterior mediastinum behind the sternum or a small paravertebral mass in the posterior mediastinum behind the heart may in fact be present, even though the chest radiograph appears to be normal.

The frequency of different mediastinal mass lesions in one series of over 1000 patients was as follows:

1. Neurogenic tumours 20%
2. Thymic tumours 20%
3. Benign cysts 20%
4. Lymph node mass 15%
5. Teratodermoid tumours 10%
6. Thyroid tumours 5%
7. Mesenchymal tumours 5%
8. Miscellaneous masses 5%

Another large series of nearly 800 patients showed a completely different incidence of 65% for lymph node masses, 10% for vascular abnormalities and 25% for all other mediastinal tumours. Most of these large series have a surgical bias and therefore exclude some mediastinal lesions such as hiatus hernia, aortic aneurysms and neoplastic or inflammatory causes of lymph node enlargement. This makes them unhelpful to the radiologist when considering the possible differential diagnosis of the mediastinal abnormality on the chest radiograph. The commonest lesions at X-ray are lymph node masses, vascular abnormalities and hiatus hernias in adult patients and the normal thymus gland in infants and children. The typical sites for the common and rare mediastinal masses are shown in Figure 12.1 and Table 12.1.

Table 12.1 The anatomical location of mediastinal masses

Position in mediastinum	Common lesions	Rare lesions
Anterior division	1. Tortuous innominate artery Lymph node enlargement Retrosternal goitre Fat deposition	Aneurysm of innominate artery Parathyroid adenoma Lymphangioma
	2. Lymph node enlargement Aneurysm of ascending aorta Thymoma Teratodermoid tumour	Sternal mass Lipoma Haemangioma
	3. Epicardial fat pad Diaphragmatic hump Pleuropericardial cyst	Morgagni hernia
Middle division	4. Lymph node enlargement Aneurysm of aortic arch Enlarged pulmonary artery Dilatation of superior vena cava Bronchogenic cyst	Tracheal lesion Cardiac tumour
Posterior division	5. Neurogenic tumour Pharyngo-oesophageal pouch	
	6. Hiatus hernia Aneurysm of descending aorta Oesophageal dilatation Dilatation of azygos vein	Neuroenteric cyst Pancreatic pseudocyst Sequestrated lung segment
	7. Neurogenic tumour Paravertebral mass	Bochdalek hernia Extramedullary haemopoiesis

ANATOMY

The mediastinum is situated between the lungs in the centre of the thorax. It extends from the thoracic inlet above to the central tendon of the diaphragm below with the sternum anteriorly, the thoracic spine posteriorly and the parietal pleura laterally.

The anatomical location of a mass lesion within the

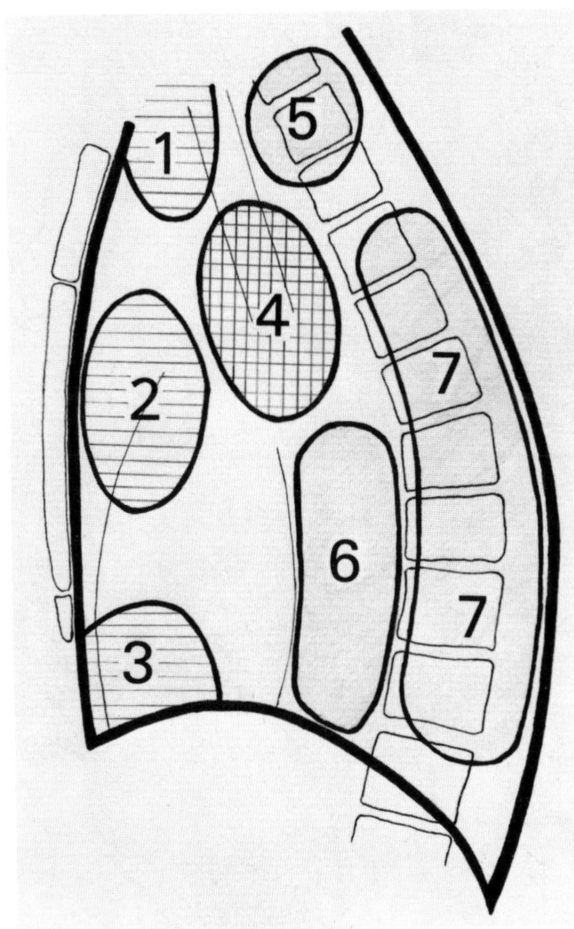

Fig. 12.1 Diagram illustrating the typical sites of the common and rare mediastinal masses listed in Table 12.1.

mediastinum affects its differential diagnosis and therefore from a radiological point of view the mediastinum is best divided into three divisions, which all extend from the root of the neck to the diaphragm. The *anterior* division lies in front of the anterior pericardium and trachea, the *middle* division within the pericardial cavity but including the trachea, and the *posterior* division lies behind the posterior pericardium and trachea. Some normal structures such as the thoracic aorta and the mediastinal lymph nodes are present in all these divisions and some very large mass lesions can involve adjacent divisions of the mediastinum. This can make the diagnosis of a mass lesion difficult, because its site of origin is obscure.

All the anatomical structures in the mediastinum are surrounded by fatty connective tissue and therefore the larger structures such as the aorta, vena cavae, pulmonary arteries and trachea are easily demonstrated by computerized tomography (CT) in the normal adult patient (Figs 12.2 and 65.92).

The trachea is a thin-walled air containing structure, lying in front of the thoracic spine in the mid-line, and terminating below in the right and left main bronchi. The oesophagus also often contains air and lies behind the trachea just to the left of the mid-line.

Contrast enhancement of the blood pool at CT highlights the vascular structures, particularly when used in conjunction with a first pass technique — dynamic CT. The innominate veins lie behind the sternum and unite to form the superior vena cava on the right. The innominate artery, the left common carotid artery and the left subclavian artery arising from the arch of the aorta are situated between the innominate veins and the trachea with the arch of the aorta extending backwards to the left of the midline, above the tracheal bifurcation. The horizontal part of the azygos vein lies in the right tracheo-bronchial angle and extends forwards from the right of the midline to join the superior vena cava.

In front of the tracheal bifurcation the main pulmonary artery lies to the left of the midline with the ascending aorta and superior vena cava on the right. The superior vena cava lies behind the ascending aorta. The left pulmonary artery passes over the left main bronchus and the right pulmonary artery is situated behind the superior vena cava but in front of the right main bronchus. The descending aorta lies behind the tracheal bifurcation on the left.

The right and left pulmonary veins drain into the left atrium below the tracheal bifurcation and the superior vena cava drains into the right atrium. At the same level the ascending aorta and main pulmonary artery arise from the left and right ventricles with the main pulmonary artery in front of the ascending aorta. The inferior vena cava drains into the right atrium just above the diaphragm with the descending aorta and oesophagus lying in front of the thoracic spine just to the left of the mid-line.

In children and young adult patients the normal thymus gland can nearly always be demonstrated by CT, and with the third and fourth generation scanners the involuting thymus gland can often be identified in adult patients and occasionally even in elderly patients. The thymus lies below the left innominate vein in front of either the main pulmonary artery or ascending aorta and usually appears as either an arrow-head structure or two separate eliptical lobes pointing towards the sternum. Occasionally only one of these lobes can be identified by CT. Up to the age of 20 years the attenuation value of the gland is similar to that of soft tissue, but above the age of 40 years it falls as fatty involution occurs and the gland decreases in size.

In obese patients there is an excess of mediastinal fat and this allows the smaller structures such as the vertical part of the azygos vein, the thoracic duct and even the normal sized mediastinal lymph nodes to be identified.

CT also demonstrates the right sided azygo-oesophageal recess behind the right main bronchus and the left sided aorto-pulmonary window between the left pulmonary artery and the aortic arch. An abnormal mass lesion

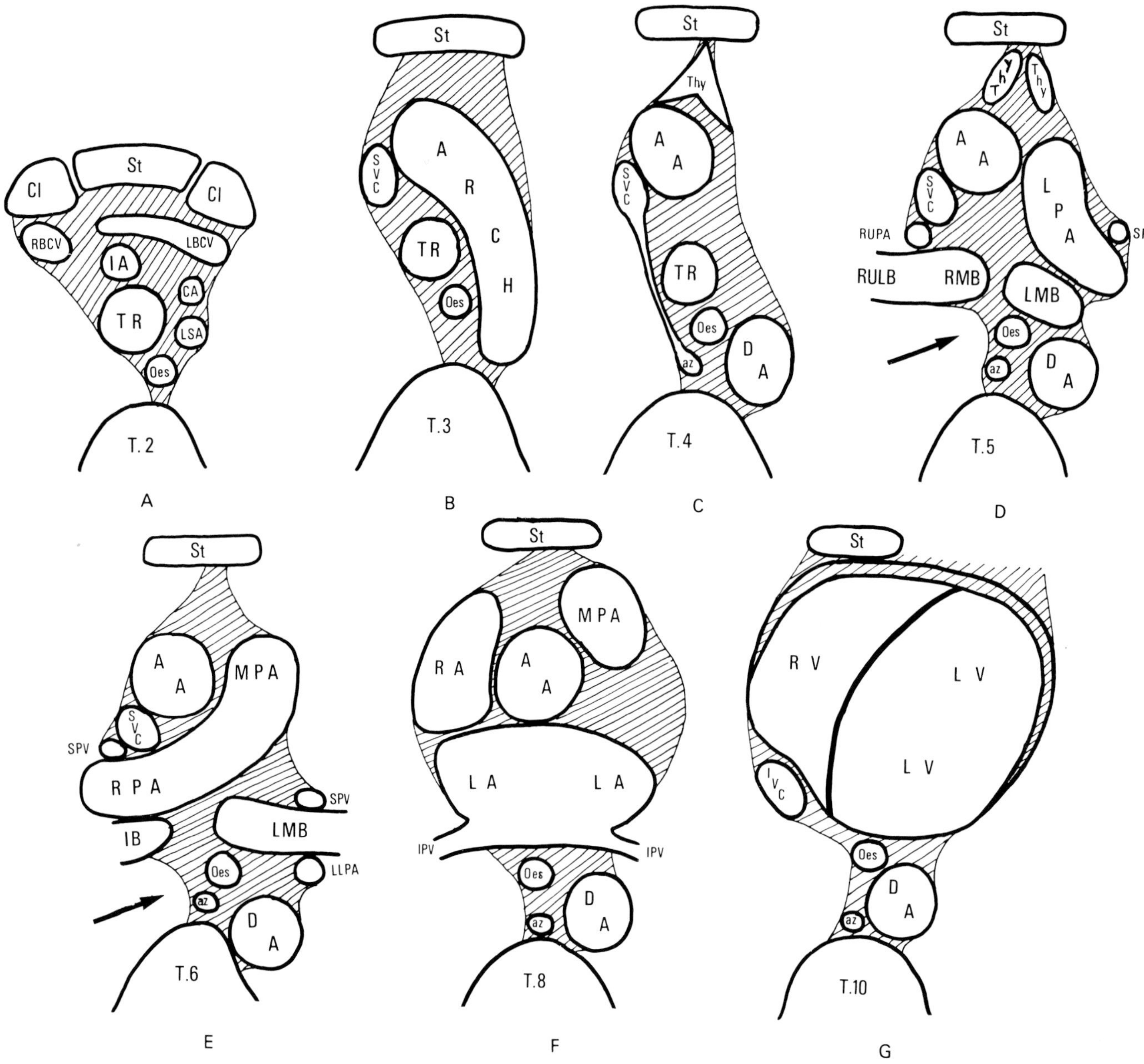

Fig. 12.2 Diagrams illustrating normal mediastinal anatomy at various levels through the thorax and features which can be identified by CT. (**A**) Above the aortic arch through the sternoclavicular joints. (**B**) Arch of aorta. (**C**) Below the aortic arch through the aorto-pulmonary window. (**D**) Left pulmonary artery. (**E**) Main and right pulmonary arteries. (**F**) Left and right atria. (**G**) Left and right ventricles. Key: Arch = arch of aorta; AA = ascending aorta; DA = descending aorta; IA = innominate artery; CA = left common carotid artery; LSA = left subclavian artery; MPA = main pulmonary artery; RPA = right pulmonary artery; LPA = left pulmonary artery; RUPA = right upper lobe pulmonary artery; LLPA = left lower lobe pulmonary artery; SPV = superior pulmonary vein; IPV = inferior pulmonary vein; SVC = superior vena cava; IVC = inferior vena cava; az. = azygos vein; RBCV & LBCV = right and left brachiocephalic or innominate veins; TR = trachea; RMB = right main bronchus; LMB = left main bronchus; IB = intermediate bronchus; RULB = right upper lobe bronchus; LV = left ventricle; RV = right ventricle; LA = left atrium; RA = right atrium; Oes = oesophagus; St = sternum; Cl = clavicle; Thy = thymus gland; → = azygo-oesophageal recess. (Compare Fig. 65.92.)

in either of these sites is very easy to detect as they are normally occupied by air filled lung and mediastinal fat respectively. The way the various mediastinal lines (e.g. the paraspinal, para-aortic, paratracheal, para-oesophageal, pericardial and anterior and posterior pulmonary junctional lines) are produced on a chest radiograph becomes apparent when viewing the mediastinum with CT. Normal mediastinal anatomy at various critical levels through the thorax is illustrated diagrammatically in Figure 12.2. These diagrams should be compared with the CT sections in Chapter 65 (Fig. 65.92).

RADIOLOGICAL INVESTIGATION

Patients with mediastinal lesions may present with an

asymptomatic incidental radiological abnormality on a chest radiograph or with clinical symptoms and signs suggestive of intra-thoracic pathology. The clinical presentation may be quite unhelpful with symptoms such as chest pain, cough and weight loss, but more specific symptoms such as dysphagia or stridor are useful in localizing the mediastinal lesion to a particular anatomical site. Occasionally there is a very specific clinical problem and the best example of this is the patient who presents with myasthenia gravis. About 15% of patients with this auto-immune neurological condition turn out to have a thymoma on investigation.

The various radiological methods of investigating the mediastinum include:

1. Standard high kV chest radiography
2. Computerized tomography
3. Conventional mediastinal tomography
4. Barium studies
5. Arteriography and venography
6. Isotope scan
7. Ultrasound
8. Urography
9. Myelography
10. Needle biopsy

The roles of nuclear magnetic resonance imaging (MRI), digital chest radiography and digital subtraction angiography in the investigation of the mediastinum are at present still being evaluated (Figs 12.3–12.5).

The chest radiograph may be the only radiological investigation necessary to confirm the cause of a mediastinal mass lesion (e.g. a hiatus hernia or bilateral hilar lymphadenopathy due to sarcoidosis). However this is often not so and with ideal radiological working facilities the next investigation should be a CT scan, which can confirm such diagnoses as aortic aneurysm or fat deposition. The other more traditional radiological investigations, such as conventional mediastinal tomography, barium studies and arteriography can be used instead of CT and of course need to be used in many hospitals where this imaging facility is not available. Even with CT a histological diagnosis cannot necessarily be made as there are many mediastinal lesions which appear as round or oval masses of soft tissue density such as neurogenic tumours or bronchogenic cysts. The presence of calcification within the mass may not be diagnostic (e.g. a thyroid tumour or a thymoma) although the presence of fat usually is (e.g. a teratodermoid tumour).

Investigations such as an *isotope scan*, *ultrasound*, *urography* and *myelography* are occasionally used to confirm the diagnosis of a mediastinal lesion (e.g. echocardiography for a pleuropericardial cyst). Myelography with non-ionic water soluble contrast medium may be used in conjunction with CT. Fine needle aspiration biopsy of mediastinal masses can be used to produce a cytological diagnosis in about 80% of cases. This procedure is done under either fluoroscopic or CT guided control using a 22 gauge short bevelled 15 cm long needle. Complications such as slight haemoptysis and minor pneumothorax occur in about 15% of patients, with a major pneumothorax in only 3% of cases. This technique can be used instead of a diagnostic surgical procedure but in about 20% of

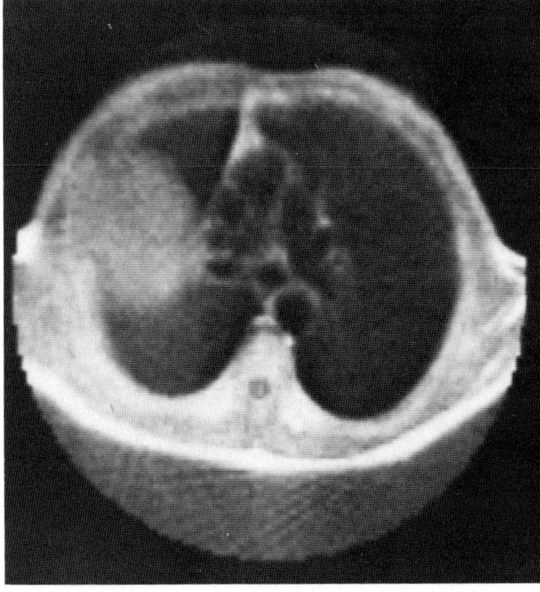

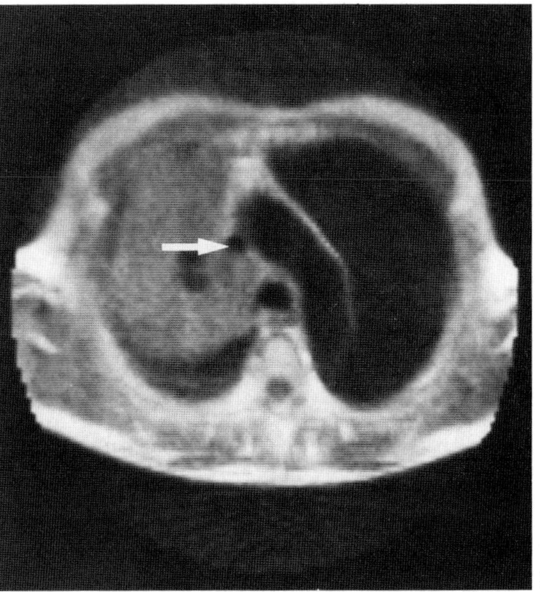

Fig. 12.3 Carcinoma of the bronchus. Steady state free precession (SSFP) MRI scans in two patients with bronchial carcinomas. Scan A below the level of the aortic arch shows the smaller tumour in the right lung without mediastinal involvement. Scan B at the level of the aortic arch shows the larger cavitating tumour in the right lung involving the mediastinum and compressing the superior vena cava (→). In the scans a high signal (white) is produced by fat and a low signal (black) is produced by air and flowing blood. (Courtesy of Professor B. S. Worthington.)

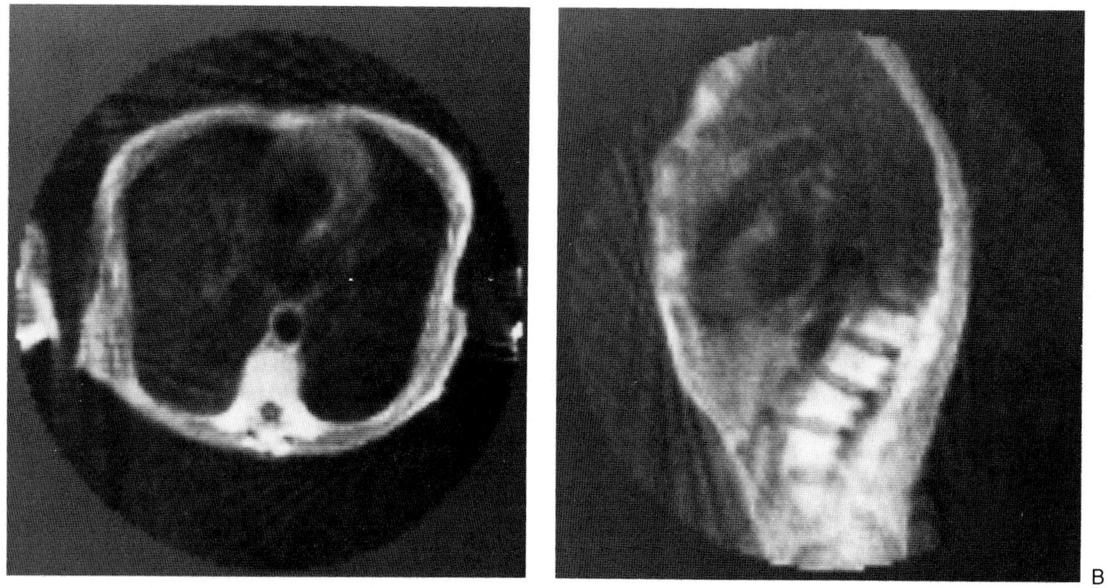

Fig. 12.4 Anterior mediastinal mass. Axial view (**A**) below the level of the aortic arch and sagittal view (**B**) near the midline show an anterior mediastinal mass around the main pulmonary artery and ascending aorta. Diagnosis not confirmed by surgery but thought to be either a dermoid tumour or a thymoma in this elderly asymptomatic female patient. (Courtesy of Professor B. S. Worthington.)

patients a specific cytological diagnosis cannot be made because of the limitations of cytology in the diagnosis of various tumours, such as lymphomas.

Of the newer techniques magnetic resonance imaging (MRI) is probably the most exciting and it could prove to be superior to CT in the assessment of the mediastinum (Figs 12.4 and 12.5). This is because with MRI the images can be displayed in any plane with equal resolution, whereas with CT the axial plane is generally superior to the reconstructed views in the sagittal or coronal planes; also, as flowing blood produces no signal in MRI, the heart and great vessels can be easily distinguished from a solid or cystic mass lesion, without the need for contrast media, which is usually required in CT imaging. The scan times for MRI are still rather long (e.g. 2–4 minutes per slice) in comparison to CT and at present there is much research into both cardiac and respiratory gating to reduce movement artefact (see Ch. 68). At present CT can still be

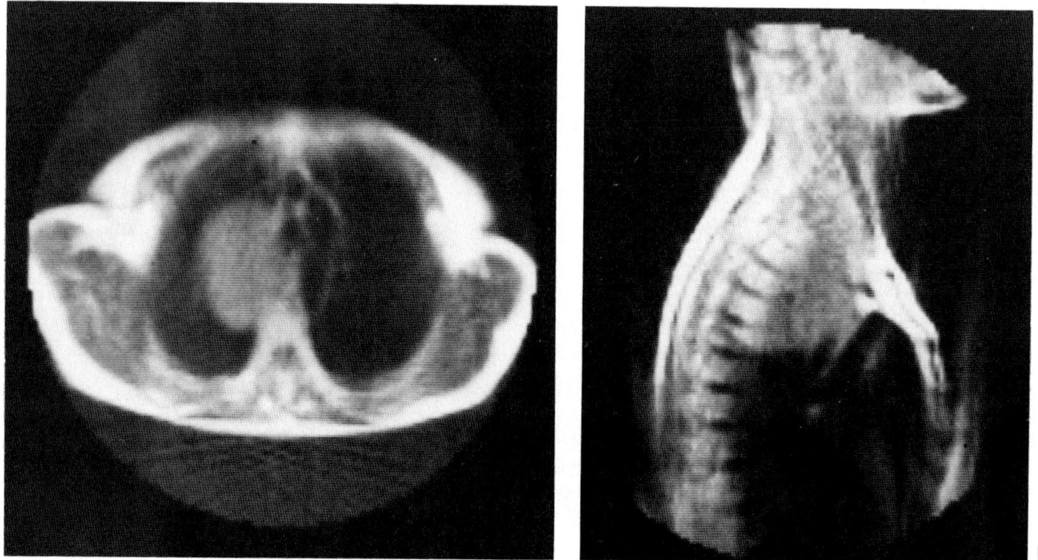

Fig. 12.5 Posterior mediastinal mass. Axial view (**A**) at the level of the aortic arch and sagittal view (**B**) at the midline show a posterior mediastinal mass extending into the middle mediastinum with forward displacement of the trachea. Diagnosis of a neurofibroma confirmed by surgery in this female patient (Courtesy of Professor B. S. Worthington.)

egarded as the best single radiological investigation for the nediastinum and its uses include:

1. The investigation of an obvious mediastinal mass on a chest radiograph.
2. The investigation of suspected mediastinal disease when the chest radiograph is normal (e.g. a thymoma in a patient with myasthenia gravis).
3. The investigation of the widened mediastinum on a chest radiograph (e.g. fatty deposition in an obese patient).
4. The investigation of the abnormal hilum on a chest radiograph.
5. The investigation of the extent of malignant disease (e.g. mediastinal lymph node involvement in a patient with a carcinoma of the bronchus).
6. The investigation of a suspected vascular abnormality.

Table 12.2 The causes of calcification in a mediastinal mass

Anterior mediastinum:	Aneurysm of ascending aorta Retrosternal goitre Thymoma Teratodermoid tumour Lymphoma after radiotherapy Haemangioma
Middle mediastinum:	Lymph node enlargement: Tuberculosis Histoplasmosis Lymphoma after radiotherapy Sarcoidosis Silicosis Aneurysm of aortic arch Bronchogenic cyst
Posterior mediastinum:	Aneurysm of descending aorta Neurogenic tumour: Neuroblastoma Neurofibrosarcoma Ganglioneuroma Abscess Haematoma Leiomyoma of oesophagus

ANTERIOR MEDIASTINAL MASSES

THYROID TUMOUR

Less than 5% of enlarged thyroid glands in the neck extend into the mediastinum to produce a retrosternal goitre. Enlargement can be due to non-toxic enlargement of the gland, thyrotoxicosis, carcinoma of the thyroid gland and Hashimoto's disease. An intrathoracic goitre also occasionally develops in a heterotopic thyroid gland in the anterior mediastinum.

A retrosternal goitre can present either as an anterior mediastinal mass on a chest radiograph of an asymptomatic adult female patient, or with a soft tissue swelling that moves on swallowing in the root of the neck. The goitre can also produce dysphagia, but stridor, vocal cord paralysis or a superior vena caval compression syndrome indicate the development of malignancy.

A retrosternal goitre appears as an oval soft tissue mass, in the superior part of the anterior mediastinum, which extends down from the neck. The outline is well defined in the mediastinum but fades off into the neck due to its anterior location (a mass situated posteriorly in the thoracic inlet has a sharply defined upper and lower margin due to the posterior position of the lung apices). The soft tissue mass more commonly projects to the right side of the mediastinum with displacement and compression of the trachea to the left (Fig. 12.6). However about 20% of thyroid goitres are retrotracheal producing displacement of the oesophagus posteriorly and the trachea anteriorly. The soft tissue mass may also contain central nodular, linear or crescentic patterns of calcification (Fig. 12.7). This is of course not a diagnostic radiological sign because calcification also occurs in thymic tumours, teratodermoid tumours, aneurysms and enlarged lymph nodes as shown in Table 12.2. Rapid increase in the size of the mass indicates internal haemorrhage into a cyst.

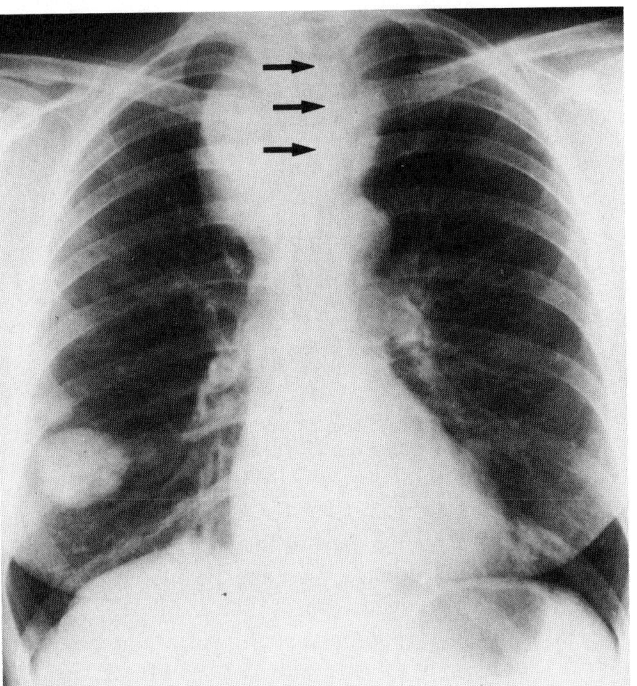

Fig. 12.6 Carcinoma of the thyroid. 53-year-old female presenting with a painful goitre and dysphagia. PA film shows an oval mass in the superior part of the anterior mediastinum with displacement of the trachea (→) to the left and multiple pulmonary metastases.

The diagnosis is confirmed if necessary by an *isotope scan*, using either $^{99}Tc^{m}$-sodium pertechnetate or ^{123}I-sodium iodide, which shows an area of increased isotope activity extending below the sternal notch.

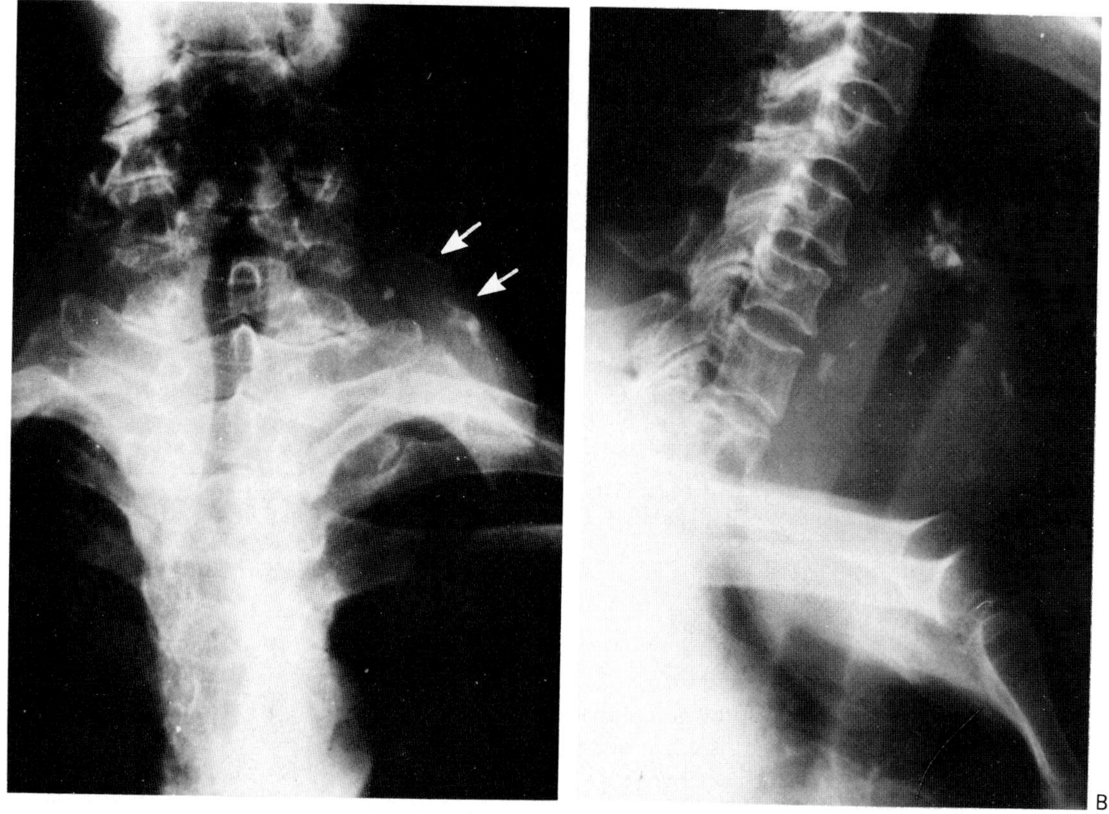

Fig. 12.7 Thyroid adenoma. 68-year-old male presenting with a goitre. AP (**A**) and lateral films (**B**) show a large mass, which contains calcification (arrows), in the root of the neck. There is slight retrosternal extension of the cervical goitre, which is compressing the trachea and also extending behind it.

THYMIC TUMOUR

The normal thymus gland is the commonest cause of a mediastinal abnormality on a chest radiograph in infants. It produces a triangular soft tissue mass, which projects to one side, often the right, of the anterior mediastinum (hence the sail sign). The normal thymus gland becomes more prominent on an expiratory or slightly rotated film, but may disappear radiologically in the presence of a severe neonatal infection or after the use of corticosteroids. The complete absence of the normal thymus gland occurs in immune deficiency disease involving the T-lymphocytes, such as Di George's syndrome. With the increasing availability of CT, the normal thymus gland can now be identified in children, adult and elderly patients. It usually appears as a triangular mass of soft-tissue attenuation within the fat of the anterior mediastinum at the level of the origins of the great vessels arising from the heart.

The commonest of the thymic tumours in the mediastinum are the benign and malignant thymoma, but this group of tumours also includes hyperplasia of the gland, thymic cysts, thymolipomas and carcinoid tumours.

Some 25% of thymomas may eventually prove locally malignant, but frank secondaries, most usually by seeding round the pleura, are less common. Other malignant tumours such as malignant lymphoma and malignant germ cell tumours can also arise in the thymus. Finally there is a significant incidence of non thymic malignancy in patients with benign thymoma.

A thymoma usually presents as an anterior mediastinal mass on a chest radiograph in an asymptomatic adult patient, but can also present with myasthenia gravis. In fact about 15% of patients with myasthenia have a thymic tumour and about 10% of patients with a thymoma have myasthenia gravis. It is most important to look for a thymoma in patients with myasthenia, because surgical removal of the tumour may partially reduce or completely abolish the effects of this auto-immune neurological condition. A thymic tumour can also occur in patients with endocrine or immunological diseases such as Cushing's syndrome, thyrotoxicosis, hypo- and agammaglobulinaemia.

A thymoma appears as a round or oval soft tissue mass, which projects to one side of the anterior mediastinum when large but may be undetectable on the PA film if small. However the outline is well defined on lateral tomography (Fig. 12.8). The soft tissue mass may also contain a peripheral rim or central nodules of calcification. A very large soft tissue mass with less radiographic density than expected for its size and which alters in shape on respiration is usually due to a thymolipoma. Thymic cysts may also occur. The presence of pleural metastases indi-

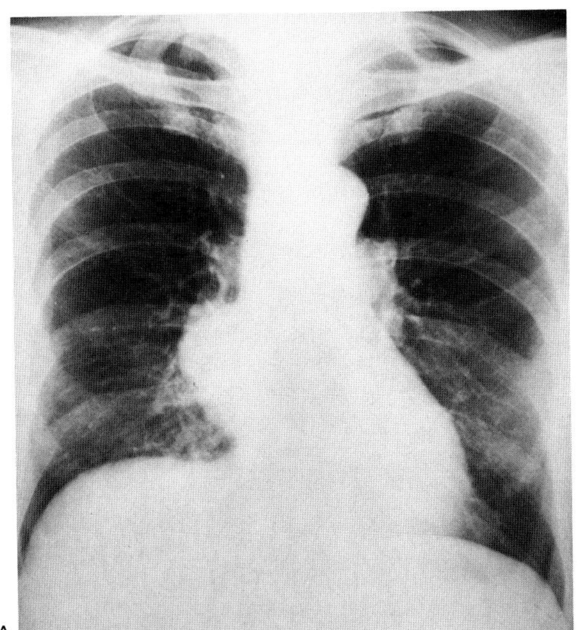

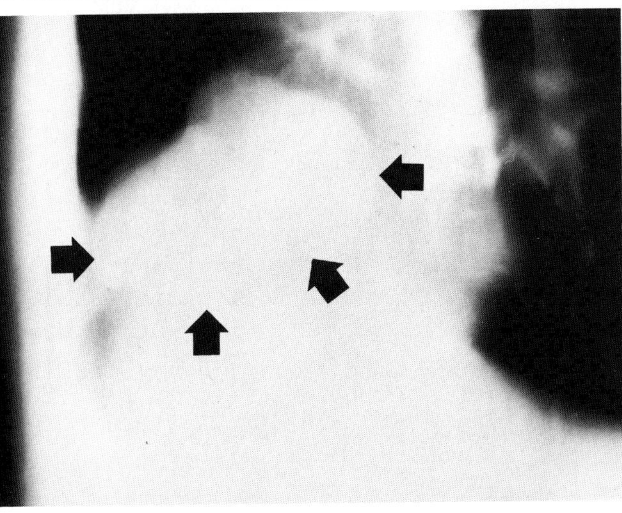

Fig. 12.8 Thymoma. 58-year-old male with a long history of myasthenia gravis, but no evidence of a thymoma on initial investigation several years before. PA film (**A**) and lateral tomogram (**B**) (arrows) now show a lobulated mass in the anterior mediastinum projecting to the right of the heart. Diagnosis confirmed by needle biopsy.

cates a malignant thymoma, as these tumours tend to seed around the pleura (Fig. 12.9).

The diagnosis is confirmed by CT, which shows a solid mass of soft tissue attenuation, which occasionally contains calcium or cyst fluid (Fig. 12.9). Direct needle puncture of a thymoma with aspiration biopsy is occasionally performed under CT or fluoroscopic guidance to confirm the diagnosis in patients with myasthenia gravis. CT is far more sensitive than conventional X-rays in defining thymic tumours and there should be no hesitation in proceeding to CT where simple X-rays have proved negative or equivocal in suspected cases.

TERATODERMOID TUMOURS

The commonest of the **germ cell tumours** in the mediastinum are the *dermoid cyst* and the *benign* and *malignant teratoma*. This group of tumours also includes *choriocarcinomas, embryonal cell carcinomas, endodermal sinus tumours* and *seminomas*. These tumours are all thought to arise from primitive germ cell rests in the urogenital ridge. The dermoid cyst consists mainly of ectodermal tissues, whereas the solid teratoma usually contains tissues of ectodermal, mesodermal and endodermal origin. About 70% of teratodermoid tumours are benign.

A teratodermoid tumour usually presents as an anterior mediastinal mass on a chest radiograph in an asymptomatic young adult patient. The tumour can also produce dyspnoea, cough and chest pain and may become infected to form an abscess. This can rupture into the mediastinum, the pleural cavity or the bronchial tree, producing the diagnostic symptom of trichoptysis, if there is hair in the cyst.

A benign dermoid cyst appears as a round or oval soft tissue mass, which usually projects to only one side of the anterior mediastinum. The outline is well defined but becomes irregular in very large tumours due to peripheral atelectasis in the surrounding compressed lung (Fig. 12.10). The soft tissue mass may also contain a peripheral rim or central nodules of calcification, a fat–fluid level or a rudimentary tooth, which is of course a diagnostic radiological sign. Rapid increase in the size of the mass indicates either internal haemorrhage or the development of malignancy. An air–fluid level is present after rupture of an infected cyst into the bronchial tree. A malignant teratoma appears as a lobulated soft tissue mass, which projects on both sides of the anterior mediastinum.

The diagnosis is confirmed by CT, which shows a solid mass of variable attenuation which contains soft tissue, cyst fluid, calcium, bone or fat. Rarely a terato-dermoid tumour may occur in the posterior mediastinum.

FAT DEPOSITION

The excessive deposition of fat in the mediastinum usually presents with widening of the superior part of the mediastinum and large epicardial fat pads in an asymptomatic obese adult patient. This can also occur in patients with Cushing's syndrome and in patients receiving long term high dose corticosteroid treatment. Steroids cause mobilization of body fat with its subsequent redistribution in the anterior mediastinum and cardiophrenic angles. This widening of the mediastinum can be difficult to differentiate from both mediastinal lymphadenopathy and a dissecting aortic aneurysm. The diagnosis is easily confirmed by CT, which shows an excessive amount of mediastinal fat (Fig. 12.11).

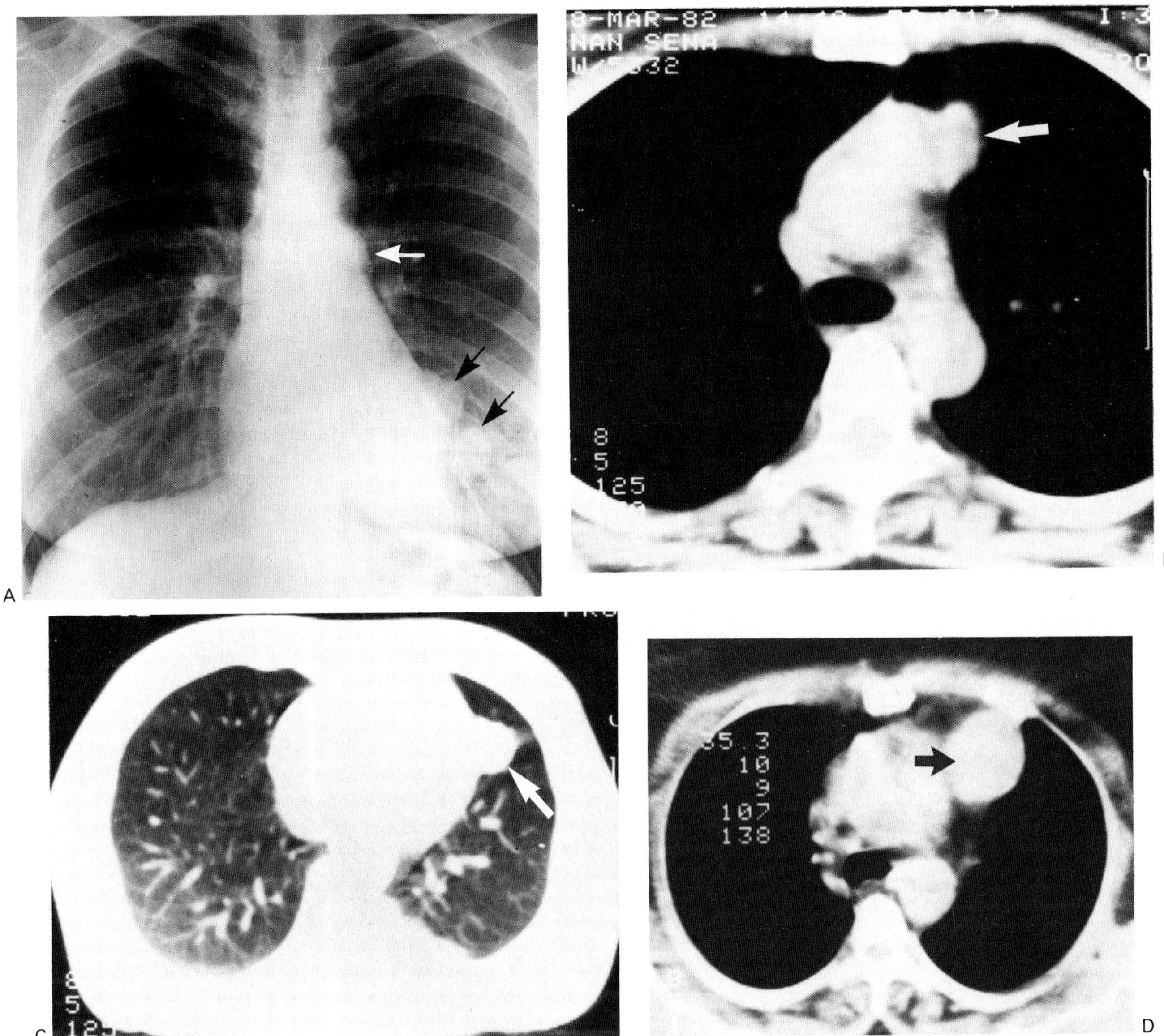

Fig. 12.9 (**A–C**) Malignant thymoma. 45-year-old female with myasthenia gravis (**A**) PA film shows small opacity overlying pulmonary artery (←) and two rounded opacities at left heart border (←). The latter were pleural deposits adjacent to the heart. (**B**) CT shows the mass to the left of the ascending aorta (←) (W512 L +36). (**C**) CT shows one of the metastases adjacent to the heart (←) (W836 L-700) (*Courtesy of Dr David Sutton*). (**D**) Thymoma. 37-year-old female presenting with myasthenia gravis. CT scan (L + 40, W 512) at the level of the tracheal bifurcation shows a round soft tissue mass (→), 4 cm in size, in the anterior mediastinum projecting to the left of the heart.

PLEUROPERICARDIAL CYST

A pleuro-pericardial cyst usually presents as an anterior (or middle) mediastinal mass on a chest radiograph in an asymptomatic adult patient. About 75% of pleuro-pericardial cysts occur in the right anterior cardiophrenic angle (Fig. 12.12). The cysts have thin walls, lined by mesothelial cells and contain clear fluid (hence their name of 'spring-water cysts'). They appear as a round, oval or triangular soft tissue mass, in the anterior or middle mediastinum and can alter in shape on respiration. The differential diagnosis of a soft tissue lesion in the right anterior cardiophrenic angle includes an *epicardial fat pad*, *a partial eventration* of the right hemidiaphragm, *right middle lobe* or *pleural pathology*, a *Morgagni hernia* and a *right atrial* or *pericardial tumour*.

The diagnosis is confirmed by either *ultrasound*, which shows a transonic mass adjacent to the pericardium, or *CT*, which shows a thin walled cyst containing fluid of low attenuation (0–10 HU) (Fig. 12.12). Direct *needle puncture* of a pleuropericardial cyst with aspiration of its fluid contents is occasionally performed under CT or ultrasonic guidance.

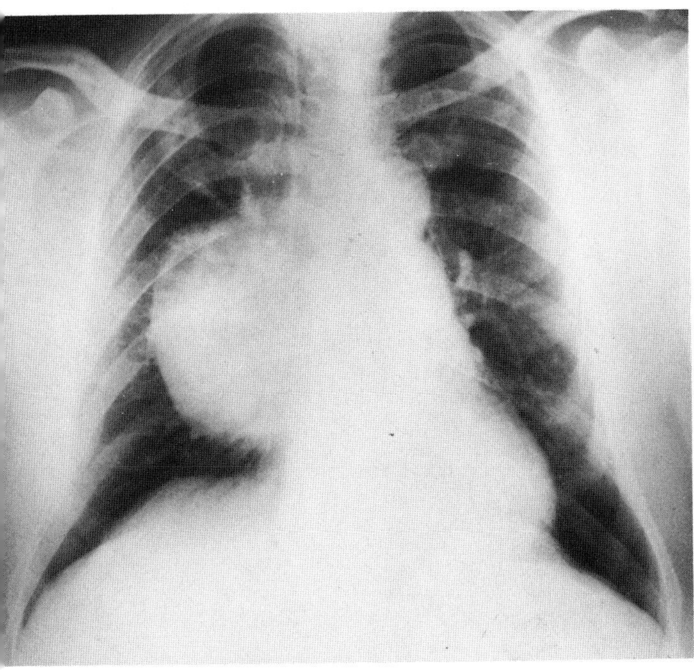

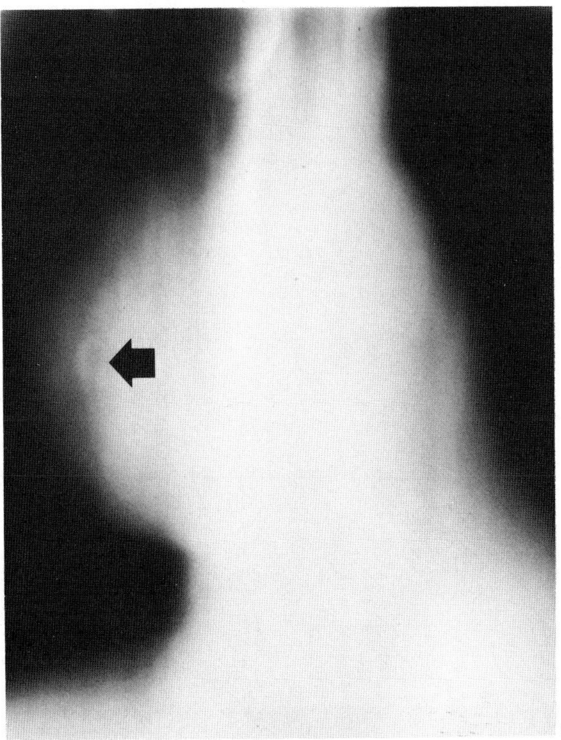

Fig. 12.10 Benign teratoma. 65-year-old male presenting with chest pain. PA film (**A**) and AP tomogram (**B**) show a large round mass, which contains calcification (←), in the anterior mediastinum overlying the right hilum. Diagnosis confirmed by surgery.

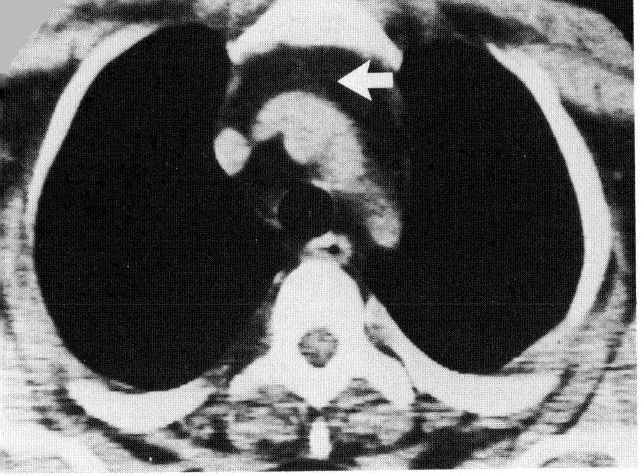

Fig. 12.11 Fat deposition. 43-year-old male presenting with chest pain and a widened mediastinum on a chest film. CT scan (L + 40, W 512) above the tracheal bifurcation shows excess deposition of fat throughout the mediastinum, particularly anteriorly (←).

MORGAGNI HERNIA

The foramen of Morgagni is a persistent developmental defect in the diaphragm anteriorly, between the septum transversum and the right and left costal origins of the diaphragm. A hernia through the foramen of Morgagni usually presents as an anterior mediastinal mass on a chest radiograph in an asymptomatic adult patient. The hernia can also produce retrosternal chest pain, epigastric discomfort and dyspnoea, but strangulation of the contents of the hernial sac is rare.

More than 90% of Morgagni hernias are situated in the right anterior cardiophrenic angle, due to the protective effect of the pericardium on the left. The smaller hernias contain omentum, which appears as a round or oval soft tissue mass, but with less radiographic density than expected for its size. This can be difficult to differentiate from an *epicardial fat pad*, a *pleuropericardial cyst* or *right middle lobe pathology*, although occasionally the properitoneal fat line can be seen continuing upwards from the anterior abdominal wall around the hernial sac on a lateral chest film. The larger hernias usually contain transverse colon, which appears as a soft tissue mass containing either gas or an air–fluid level, but they can also contain liver, stomach or small intestine.

The diagnosis is confirmed by a barium meal and follow through or a barium enema, which shows either upward tenting of the transverse colon towards the hernia or a loop of transverse colon above the diaphragm and within the chest.

PARATHYROID ADENOMA

An adenoma in an ectopic parathyroid gland in the chest usually presents with hypercalcaemia in an adult patient with hyperparathyroidism. It is a rare tumour that occurs in the superior part of the anterior mediastinum. The

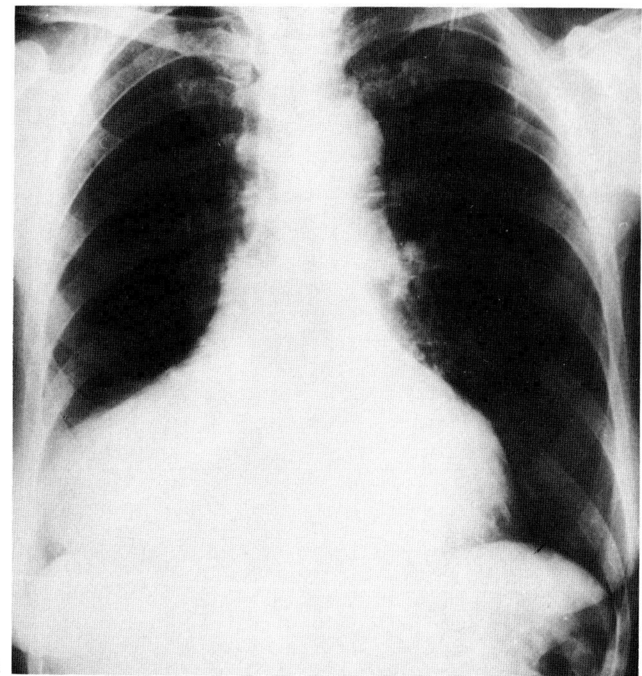

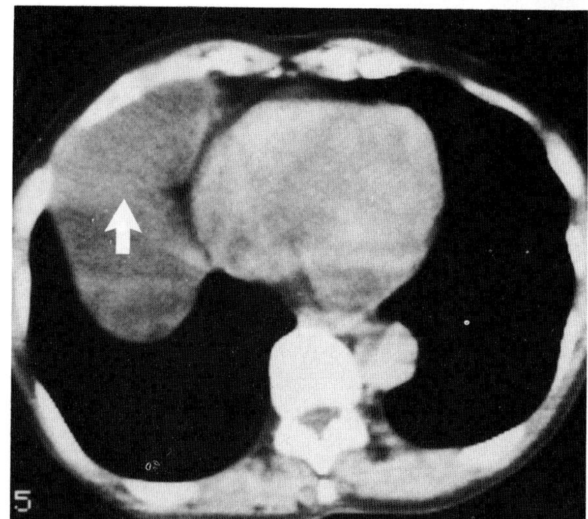

Fig. 12.12 Pleuro-pericardial cyst. 72-year-old female presenting with dyspnoea. PA film (**A**) shows a large oval mass in the right cardiophrenic angle and CT scan (L + 40, W 512) (**B**) below the tracheal bifurcation shows an oval mass ($\uparrow$), 10 cm in size, separate from the heart in the anterior and middle mediastinum. The density of the mass (Average: + 9 HU) is typical of cyst fluid.

mediastinum appears normal on the chest radiograph, although there may be evidence of nephrocalcinosis or renal calculi on an abdominal film and hyperparathyroid bone disease on a skeletal survey. The diagnosis is confirmed by an *isotope scan*, using ^{201}Tl-thallium chloride, with computerized subtraction of the thyroid image using ^{99m}Tc-sodium pertechnetate, to leave the parathyroid image, which shows an area of increased isotope activity in the anterior mediastinum (Fig. 12.13).

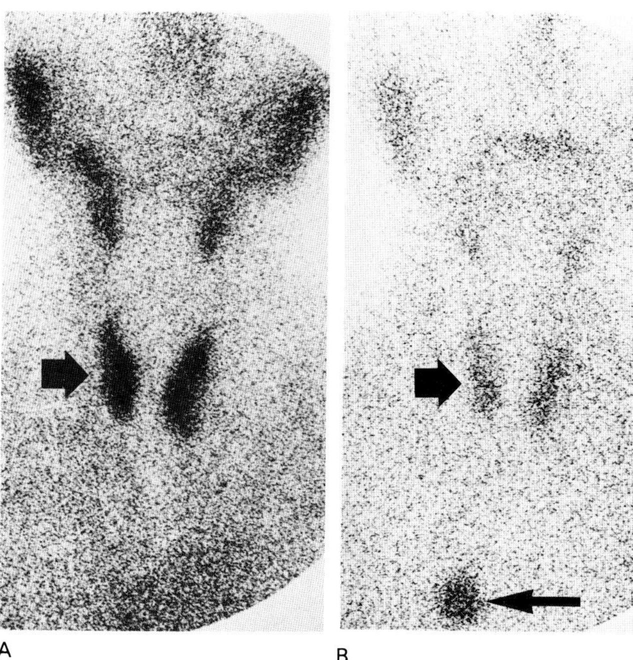

Fig. 12.13 Parathyroid adenoma. 64-year-old female presenting with hypercalcaemia. Isotope scans using ^{99}Tc^{m} (**A**) and ^{201}Tl (**B**) show isotope activity in the salivary glands and thyroid gland ($\rightarrow$), and in the parathyroid adenoma in the mediastinum ($\leftarrow$). The latter is shown only on the thallium scan even without computerized subtraction of scan **A** from scan **B**.

LYMPHANGIOMA

A lymphangioma or cystic hygroma usually presents as a soft tissue swelling that trans-illuminates in the root of the neck in children. It is a rare mesenchymal tumour that occurs in the superior part of the anterior mediastinum and it appears as an oval soft tissue mass, which extends up into the neck and can alter in shape on respiration, but does not displace the trachea. A chylothorax may also occur. The diagnosis is confirmed by CT.

LIPOMA

A lipoma usually presents as an incidental mediastinal lesion on a chest radiograph in an asymptomatic adult patient. It is also a rare mesenchymal tumour, which occurs in the anterior (or posterior) mediastinum. It appears as a round or oval soft tissue mass with less radiographic density than expected for its size, and which can alter in shape on respiration (Fig. 12.14). Malignant degeneration into a liposarcoma may also occur. The diagnosis is confirmed by CT, which shows a solid mass of tissue of fatty attenuation (−50 to −100 HU) (Fig. 12.14).

OTHER RARE ANTERIOR MEDIASTINAL MASSES

Apart from lymphangioma, lipoma and liposarcoma other tumours of mesenchymal origin can also occur

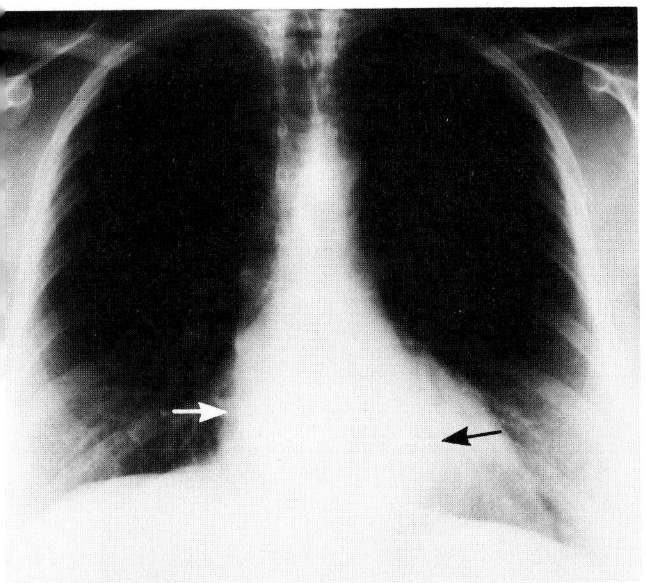

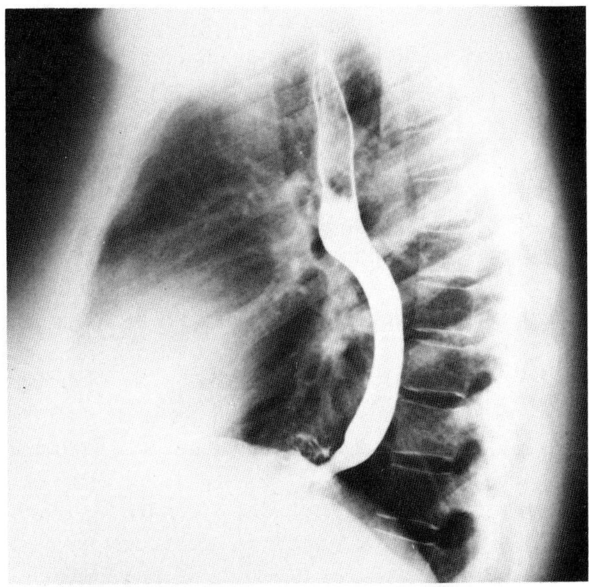

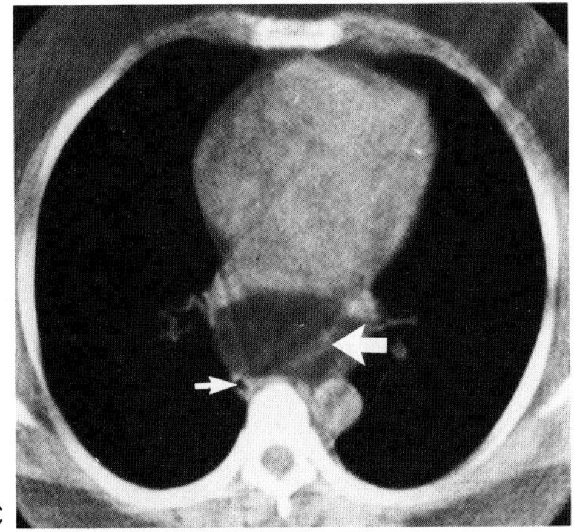

Fig. 12.14 Lipoma. Asymptomatic 42-year-old female. PA film (**A**) and barium swallow (**B**) show an oval mass, with less density than expected for its size, particularly in the lateral view, behind the heart. CT scan (L–150, W 800) (**C**) below the tracheal bifurcation shows an oval mass of fat density, (←), 8 cm in size, in the posterior mediastinum with displacement of the oesophagus (→) to the right. (*Plain films courtesy of Dr P. Ho and CT scan courtesy of Dr T.J. Bloomberg.*)

in the mediastinum and these include *fibroma*, *fibrosarcoma*, *haemangioma*, *haemangiopericytoma* and *haemangioendothelioma*. About 50% of mesenchymal tumours are malignant.

The small benign tumours are usually asymptomatic, whereas the large benign tumours and the malignant tumours tend to produce symptoms such as retrosternal chest pain, back pain or dysphagia depending upon their anatomical location. They appear as widening of the mediastinum or a round or oval soft tissue mass in the anterior (or posterior) mediastinum. The presence of phleboliths is of course diagnostic of a haemangioma.

A *plasmacytoma* of the sternum and an *osteochondroma* or a *chondrosarcoma* of a rib may also result in a tumour mass that involves the anterior mediastinum.

MIDDLE MEDIASTINAL MASSES

LYMPH NODE ENLARGEMENT

Lymph nodes occur in the anterior, middle and posterior mediastinum but are found predominantly in its middle division, where the paratracheal, tracheobronchial, bronchopulmonary (hilar) and subcarinal groups are situated. Enlargement of lymph node groups usually presents as a middle mediastinal mass on a chest radiograph in an asymptomatic adult patient, but can also present with generalized lymphadenopathy or cough, dyspnoea and weight loss. There are many causes of enlargement of the mediastinal lymph node groups and these include metastatic disease, lymphoma, leukaemia, sarcoidosis, tuberculosis, histoplasmosis and other infections and granulomas.

Metastatic disease can produce enlargement of any of the lymph node groups within the mediastinum. The primary tumour is usually intrathoracic, such as a bronchial or oesophageal carcinoma, but may occasionally be extrathoracic in origin — breast carcinoma, renal carcinoma, adrenal tumours, testicular tumours and tumours of the pharynx and larynx. Pulmonary metastases or lymphangitis carcinomatosa are also frequently present with these tumours when there is mediastinal lymphadenopathy. A bronchial carcinoma situated either peripherally or centrally in the lung metastasizes early to the mediastinal lymph nodes producing either a unilateral hilar mass with an irregular outline (due to surrounding infiltration, atelectasis or consolidation) or widening of the superior part of the middle mediastinum due to a superior vena caval compression syndrome. A bronchial carcinoma is the commonest primary tumour to metastasize to the mediastinal lymph nodes. A carcinoma of the breast may involve the lymph nodes of the internal mammary chain in the anterior mediastinum and an oesophageal carcinoma may involve the posterior mediastinal lymph nodes. A renal carcinoma or an adrenal neuroblastoma can metastasize to the hilar lymph nodes, usually on the right, whereas a testicular teratoma or seminoma usually metastasizes to the paratracheal lymph nodes.

Hodgkin's disease, the **non-Hodgkin's lymphomas** and the **lymphatic leukaemias** usually involve the paratracheal and tracheobronchial lymph nodes producing an asymmetrical bilateral widening of the superior part of the middle mediastinum. Involvement of the subcarinal lymph nodes splays the carina and a unilateral or bilateral hilar mass can also occur. The lymphomas, particularly Hodgkin's disease, also frequently involve the anterior mediastinum producing a lobulated soft tissue mass due to indentation by the anterior ribs (Fig. 12.15). Parenchymal lung disease may also occur and lymph node calcification occasionally develops in Hodgkin's disease after irradiation.

Radiotherapy to the mediastinum produces a reduction in the size of lymph node masses in radio-responsive metastatic diseases, such as lymphoma and seminoma during treatment, but may also produce a chronic mediastinitis with fibrosis extending into the lungs. This is quite characteristic and appears as a straight line, widening the mediastinum on both sides and corresponding to the treatment field (Fig. 12.16). This mediastinal fibrosis may also develop at lower therapy doses in patients who are also receiving cytotoxic chemotherapy, particularly cyclophosphamide.

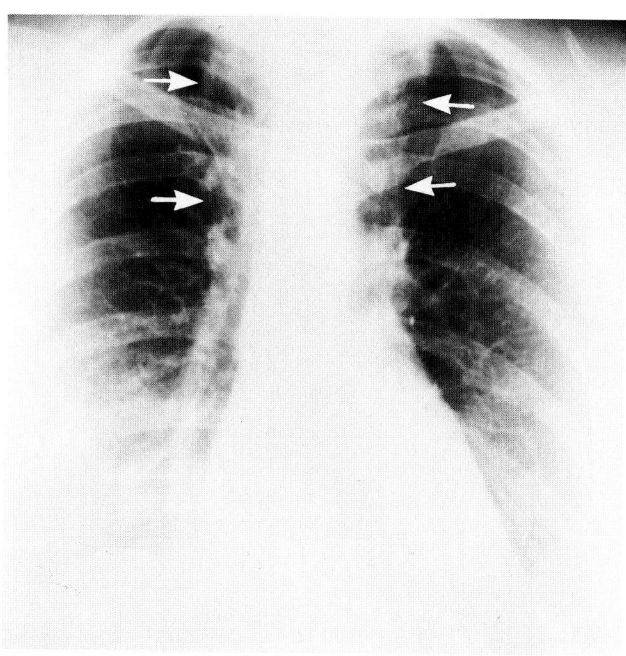

Fig. 12.16 Radiotherapy to the mediastinum. Asymptomatic 40-year-old female with Hodgkin's disease in remission treated with mediastinal radiotherapy several years ago. PA film shows widening of the superior part of the mediastinum due to radiation fibrosis extending into the lungs (arrows).

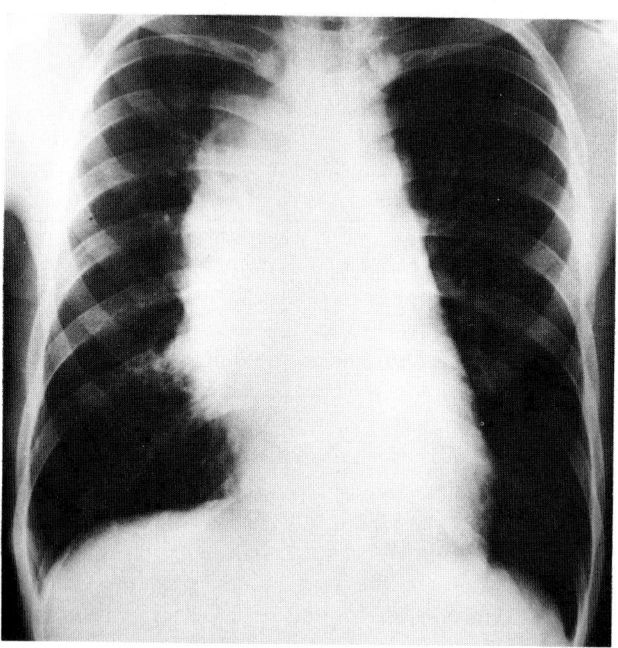

Fig. 12.15 Hodgkin's disease. 18-year-old male presenting with cervical lymphadenopathy. PA film shows asymmetrical lobulated widening of the mediastinum, due to involvement of the middle and anterior mediastinal lymph nodes, particularly on the right.

Sarcoidosis typically causes enlargement of the bronchopulmonary lymph nodes producing bilateral lobulated hilar masses with well-defined outlines. Sarcoid granulomata also frequently involve the tracheobronchial, right paratracheal and left aorto-pulmonary lymph nodes. Parenchymal lung disease commonly develops and peripheral calcification occasionally occurs in the lymph nodes (hence the sign of 'egg shell' calcification).

A **primary tuberculous infection** of the lung in children or young adult patients produces an area of consolidation in one of the lobes with a small pleural effusion and a unilateral hilar mass. Calcification may develop in both the primary Ghon focus and the mediastinal lymph nodes as healing occurs. Tuberculosis can also produce a unilateral paratracheal mass of lymph nodes without obvious pulmonary or pleural involvement (Fig. 12.17). This type of infection occurs in the adult immigrant population and in patients who are immunosuppressed by cytotoxic drugs.

In the USA, **fungal infections** such as *histoplasmosis*, *coccidioidomycosis* and *blastomycosis* may produce enlargement of the hilar or paratracheal lymph nodes and calcification may also develop in the lymph nodes in healing histoplasmosis. The only fungus in this country which causes unilateral hilar lymphadenopathy is *actinomycosis* and this can be difficult to differentiate from a bronchial carcinoma.

There are many other inflammatory causes of unilateral : bilateral hilar lymphadenopathy and these include *infec-ous mononucleosis* or glandular fever, *measles*, *whooping ɔugh*, *mycoplasma infection*, *adenoviruses* and a *pyogenic lung bscess*. Peripheral or egg shell type of calcification may :cur in the hilar nodes in patients with *silicosis* and atients with *cystic fibrosis* may have enlarged hilar shadows due to enlarged lymph nodes or cor pulmonale. Finally *Castleman's giant mediastinal lymph node hyperplasia* may also produce a large middle mediastinal mass.

The diagnosis of mediastinal lymph node enlargement is usually apparent on the chest radiographs, but can be confirmed by CT with enhancement of the blood pool to differentiate the lymph nodes from the vascular structures (Fig. 12.18).

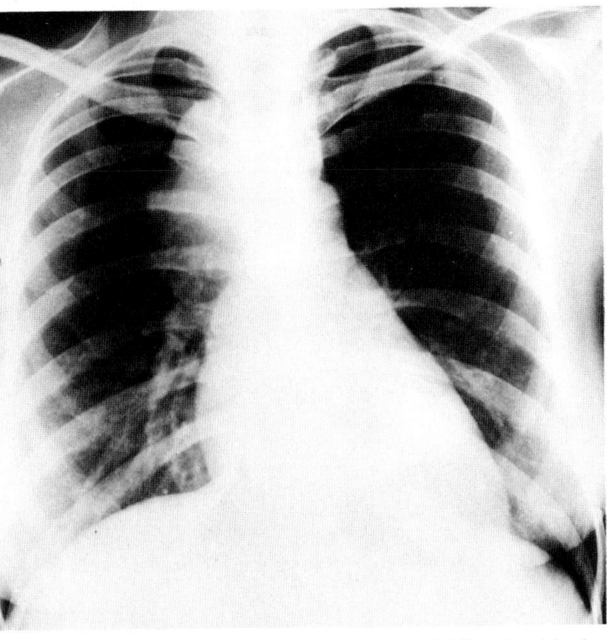

Fig. 12.17 Tuberculosis. Asymptomatic 29-year-old female with chronic renal disease treated with immunosuppressive drugs. PA film shows a right paratracheal mass of enlarged lymph nodes in the middle mediastinum.

AORTIC ANEURYSM AND VASCULAR ANOMALIES

The thoracic aorta passes through all the anatomical divisions of the mediastinum and the great vessels arising from it lie in the superior part of the mediastinum. Abnormalities of the aorta and great vessels usually present as a mediastinal mass or widening of the mediastinum on a chest radiograph in an asymptomatic elderly patient. (e.g. an unfolded aorta, a tortuous innominate artery or an aortic aneurysm). Aortic aneurysms can also produce chest pain radiating into the back (e.g. a dissecting aortic aneurysm), aortic incompetence (e.g. an aneurysm of the ascending aorta), hoarseness due to involvement of the left recurrent laryngeal nerve (e.g. an aneurysm of the arch of the aorta) and dysphagia (e.g. an aneurysm of the descending aorta). There are many causes of aneurysms of the thoracic aorta and these include atherosclerosis, hypertension, blunt chest trauma, syphilitic aortitis, a mycotic origin and congenital anomalies such as coarctation of the aorta and Marfan's syndrome.

Aortic aneurysms produce either widening of the mediastinum or a round or oval soft tissue mass in any part of the

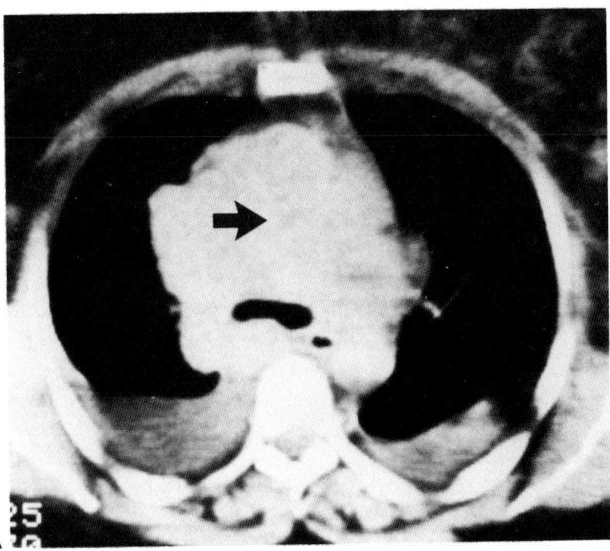

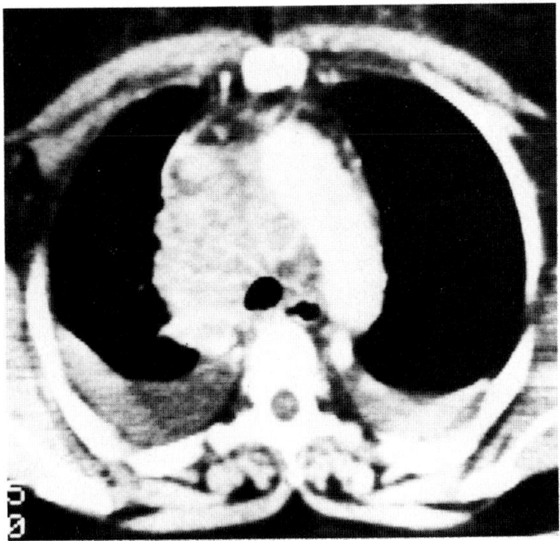

Fig. 12.18 (**A**) Carcinoma of the bronchus. 55-year-old female presenting with superior vena caval compression syndrome. CT scan (L + 40, W 512) at the level of the tracheal bifurcation shows extensive mediastinal tumour with loss of the normal fat planes between the large vascular structures, (→) due to involvement of the middle and posterior mediastinal lymph nodes and also bilateral pleural effusions. Enhancement of the the blood pool would demonstrate the vascular structures within the tumour mass. (**B**) Non-Hodgkin's lymphoma. CT scan (L + 45, W 512) following contrast enhancement. The aortic arch is well shown, but the superior vena cava is compressed.

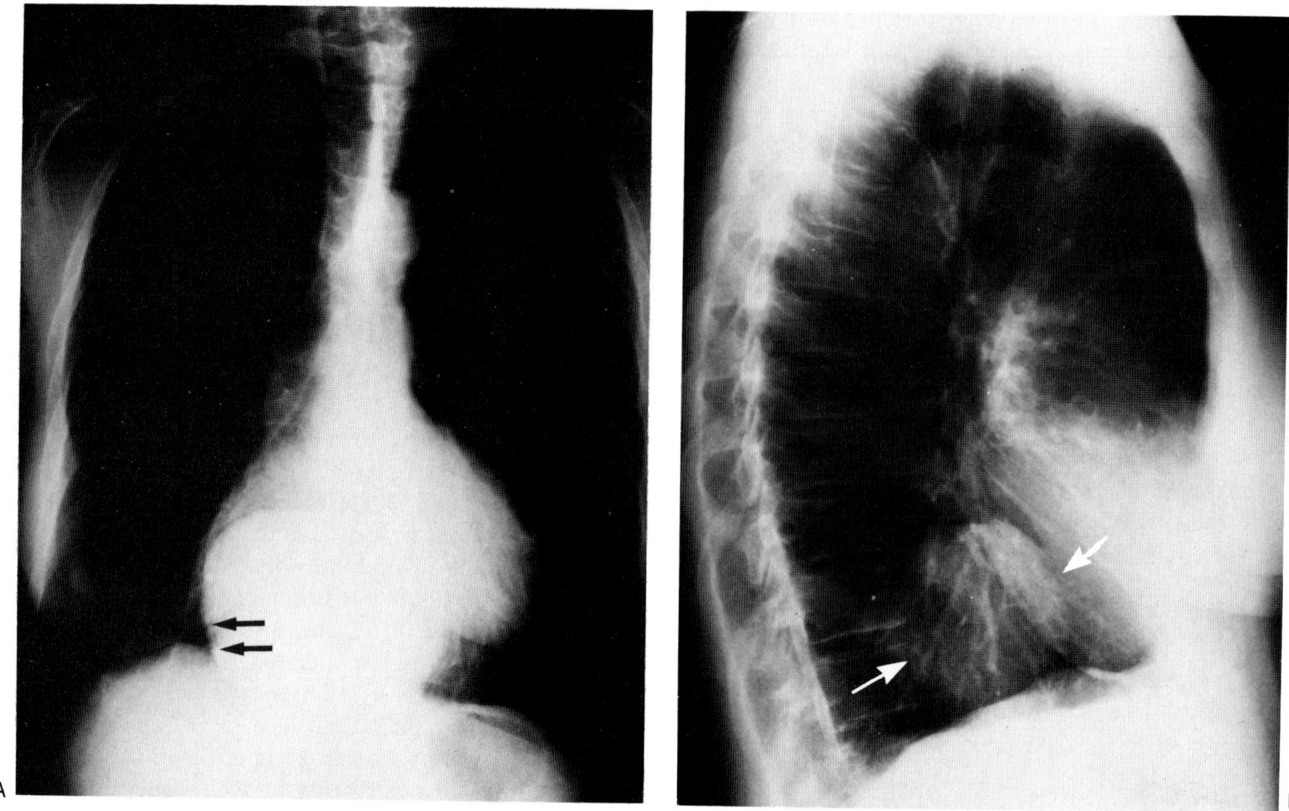

Fig. 12.19 Aneurysm of descending aorta. 69-year-old female presenting with haematemesis from a benign gastric ulcer. PA (**A**) and lateral films (**B**) show a large round mass, which has some peripheral calcification in its wall (arrows), in the posterior mediastinum behind the heart. Diagnosis confirmed by ultrasound using the liver as a window into the mediastinum.

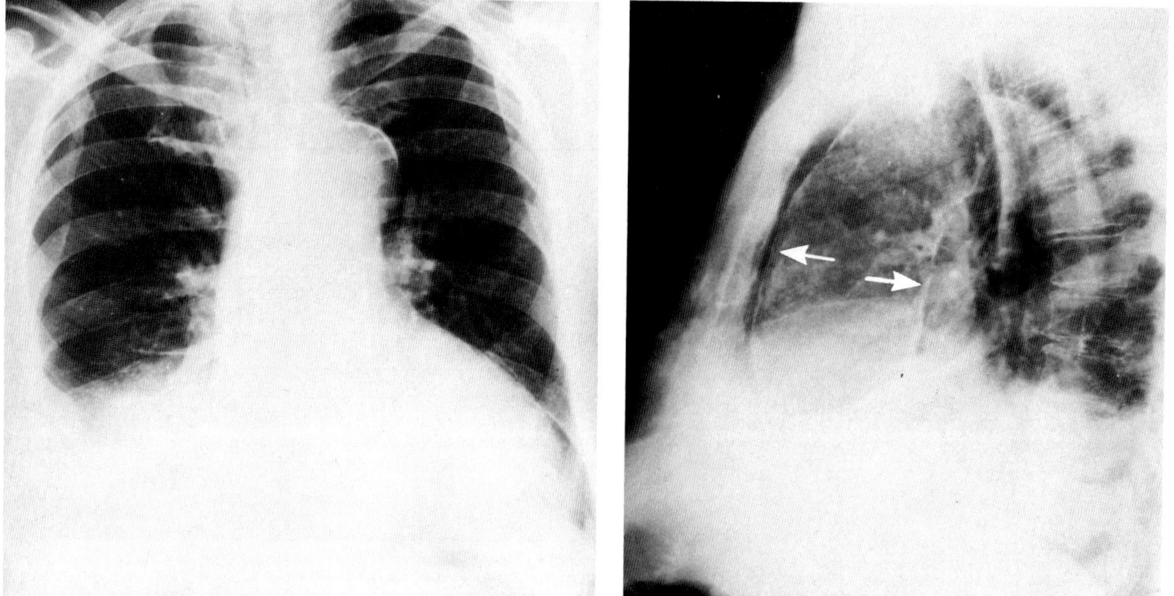

Fig. 12.20 Aneurysm of ascending aorta. 73-year-old male presenting with right lower lobe pneumonia. PA (**A**) and lateral films (**B**) show pneumonic consolidation in the right lower lobe and curvilinear calcification in the wall of an aneurysm of the ascending aorta (arrows), due to syphilitic aortitis.

mediastinum with a well-defined outline and sometimes a peripheral rim of calcification (Fig. 12.19). Curvilinear calcification in an ascending aortic aneurysm can be due to either syphilitic aortitis or rarely atherosclerosis (Fig. 12.20). On fluoroscopy aortic aneurysms appear as pulsatile masses but this is not a diagnostic radiological sign because any mass lesion adjacent to the aorta transmits its pulsation. Aortic aneurysms may also involve adjacent bones producing a pressure erosion defect of the sternum or anterior scalloping of one or two vertebral bodies.

The diagnosis may be confirmed by thoracic aortography or digital subtraction angiography but preferably by CT; this shows a dilated aorta containing a central lumen of blood of high attenuation, due to enhancement of the blood pool with water soluble contrast medium (80–100 HU) and a peripheral layer of clot of lower attenuation on the wall of the aorta, which may contain calcification. The subintimal flap and false lumen of a *dissecting aortic aneurysm* can also be demonstrated by CT (Fig. 12.21).

A *tortuous innominate artery* occurs in about 20% of elderly patients with hypertension and produces widening of the superior part of the mediastinum on the right without displacement of the trachea to the left. However a true aneurysm of the innominate or subclavian arteries is rare as a cause of a mass in the superior part of the mediastinum. Another common abnormality is a *tortuous aneurysmal descending thoracic aorta*, which produces widening of the mediastinum on the left, often at the level of the left hilum. The hilar vessels can be seen

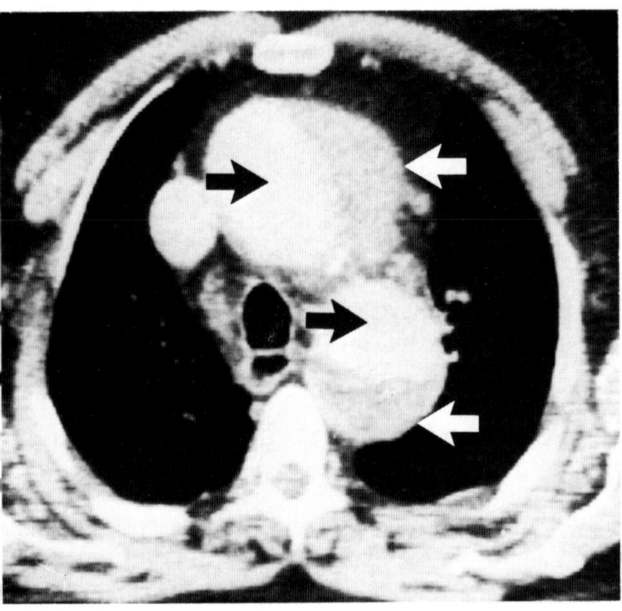

Fig. 12.21 Dissecting aneurysm of aorta (De Bakey type 1). 60-year-old male presenting with chest pain and a widened mediastinum on a chest film. CT scan (L + 40, W 512) above the tracheal bifurcation shows dilatation of the ascending and descending aorta with enhancement of the blood in the true lumen (→), but not the false lumen which contains clot (←).

through this apparent hilar mass indicating that the descending thoracic aorta lies posterior to the hilum. *Dilatation of the main pulmonary artery* can also produce an apparent left hilar mass through which the hilar vessels can again be seen, but in this case the main pulmonary artery lies anterior to the hilum. Enlargement of the main pulmonary artery can be due to many causes and these include primary or secondary pulmonary arterial hypertension, the post-stenotic dilatation of pulmonary valve stenosis and a pulmonary artery aneurysm.

A *right sided aortic arch* and other congenital anomalies of the aorta can also produce an abnormal mediastinal configuration. A truncus arteriosus and Fallot's tetralogy may occur in association with a right-sided aortic arch.

DILATATION OF MEDIASTINAL VEINS

The superior vena cava lies in the middle mediastinum and the azygos vein lies in the posterior mediastinum. Dilatation of the veins in the mediastinum usually presents with cough, dyspnoea and swelling of the ankles in an adult patient.

Dilatation of the superior vena cava is produced by a raised central venous pressure, which occurs in congestive cardiac failure, tricuspid valve disease, constrictive pericarditis, a cardiomyopathy, a right atrial tumour, partial anomalous pulmonary venous drainage (to a right sided superior vena cava) and a mediastinal tumour with a superior vena caval compression syndrome. A dilated superior vena cava produces widening of the superior part of the middle mediastinum on the right.

A raised central venous pressure also results in dilatation of the azygos vein. This also occurs in portal hypertension, complete occlusion of the superior or inferior vena cava and azygos continuation of the inferior vena cava. A dilated azygos vein produces an oval soft tissue mass in the right tracheobronchial angle. This can be difficult to differentiate from an enlarged lymph node although the azygos vein alters in size with a change in posture or during the Valsalva manoeuvre.

Total anomalous pulmonary venous drainage (to a right or left sided superior vena cava) or an isolated left sided superior vena cava produce an abnormally wide mediastinal configuration, whereas complete transposition of the great vessels produces an unusually narrow mediastinal configuration.

The diagnosis of dilatation of the mediastinal veins is confirmed by vena cavography, digital subtraction angiography or CT in some cases.

BRONCHOGENIC CYST

A bronchogenic cyst usually presents as a middle (or posterior) mediastinal mass on a chest radiograph in an asymptomatic child or young adult patient. The cyst can also produce stridor in children and cough, dyspnoea and chest pain in adults. Infection with rupture into the bronchial tree is rare. The majority of bronchogenic cysts occur around the carina in the *paratracheal, tracheobronchial* or *subcarinal* regions. The cysts have thin walls lined by ciliated columnar epithelium of respiratory origin and contain mucoid material. They appear as a round or oval soft tissue mass in the middle mediastinum frequently on the right near the carina (Fig. 12.22) and can alter in shape on respiration. Rapid increase in the size of the mass indicates internal haemorrhage. An air–fluid level is present after rupture of an infected cyst into the bronchial tree.

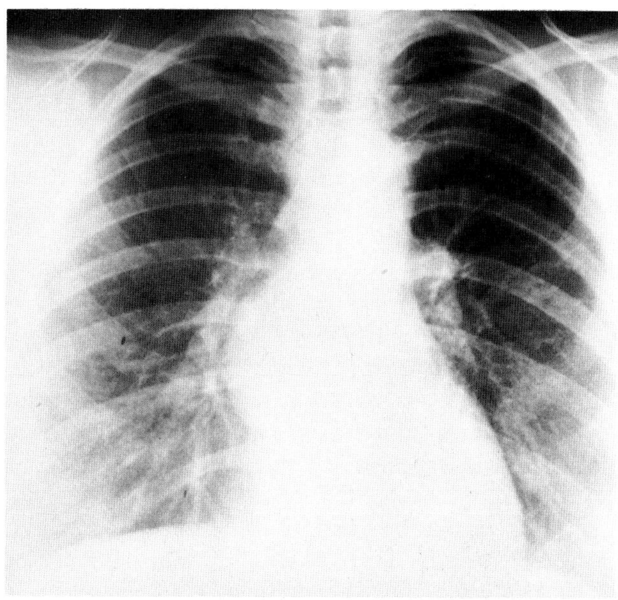

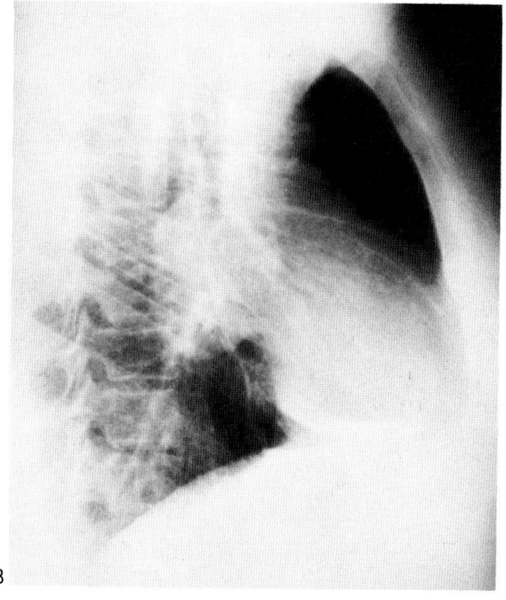

Fig. 12.22 Bronchogenic cyst. Asymptomatic 21-year-old female. PA (**A**) and lateral films (**B**) show an oval mass in the middle mediastinum below the carina on the right. Diagnosis confirmed by surgery.

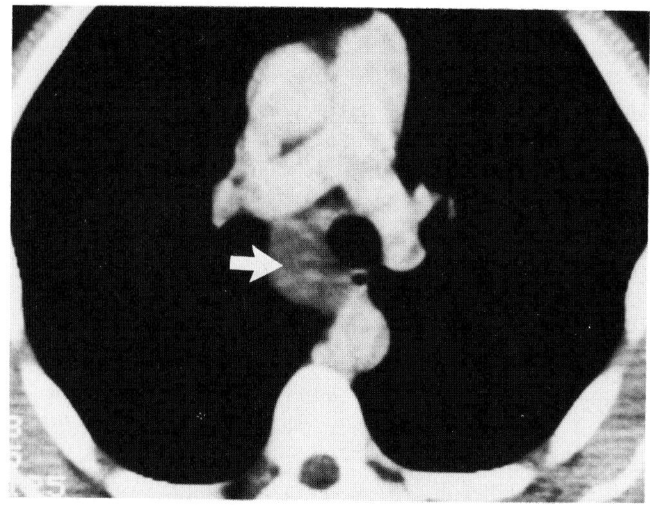

Fig. 12.23 Bronchogenic cyst. 25-year-old male presenting with a cough. CT scan (L + 40, W 512) at the level of the tracheal bifurcation shows a round mass (→), 3 cm in size, in the middle mediastinum with enhancement of the blood pool. The density of the mass (average + 45 HU) is typical of mucoid material.

The diagnosis is suggested by CT, which shows a mass of soft tissue attenuation (10–50 HU) (Fig. 12.23), but is usually confirmed at surgery. A pericardial defect may occur in association with a bronchogenic cyst.

RARE MIDDLE MEDIASTINAL LESIONS

A **tracheal tumour**, such as a *carcinoma*, a *cylindroma* or a *plasmacytoma* usually presents with cough, haemoptysis and dyspnoea or stridor in an adult patient. They are rare tumours, which occur in the middle mediastinum and although the mediastinum may appear normal on the initial inspection of the chest radiograph there is narrowing of the tracheal lumen by a small soft tissue mass on review of the films. The diagnosis is confirmed by conventional tomography.

Tracheobronchomegaly or the Mounier-Kuhn syndrome and *tracheomalacia* may produce widening of the superior part of the mediastinum due to dilatation of the trachea.

POSTERIOR MEDIASTINAL MASSES

NEUROGENIC TUMOURS

The commonest of the **neurogenic tumours** in the mediastinum in adults are the *neurofibroma* and the *neurilemmoma* (or Schwannoma), which develop from the peripheral intercostal nerves; the *ganglioneuroma* and the *neuroblastoma*, which arise in the thoracic sympathetic ganglia, are the commonest of the neurogenic tumours in the mediastinum in children. This group of tumours also includes *neurofibrosarcomas, phaeochromocytomas* and *chemodectomas*, which occur in paraganglionic nerve tissue. About 30% of neurogenic tumours are malignant.

A neurogenic tumour usually presents as a posterior mediastinal mass on a chest radiograph in an asymptomatic child or young adult patient. The tumours can also produce back pain and may extend through an intervertebral foramen into the spinal canal (hence their name of 'dumb-bell' tumours) to produce a spinal cord compression syndrome. A neurofibroma or neurofibrosarcoma in the mediastinum may be part of the generalized neurofibromatosis of Von Recklinghausen's disease, but it should be remembered that a mediastinal mass in this neurocutaneous disease can also be caused by a lateral thoracic meningocoele.

A neurogenic tumour appears as a round or oval soft tissue mass with a well-defined outline in the paravertebral gutter which projects to only one side of the posterior mediastinum. A ganglioneuroma may appear as a rather elongated soft tissue mass, in comparison to the more circular appearance of the neurofibroma, due to its extensive mediastinal origin (Fig. 12.24). A neuroblastoma may contain central spicules or a peripheral rim of calcification. This can also occur in neurofibrosarcomas and ganglioneuromas. However calcification is generally not a feature of the benign neurogenic tumours and does not occur in the mediastinal lymph node metastases from an adrenal neuroblastoma.

Neurogenic tumours may also involve the posterior ribs or adjacent thoracic vertebrae. The benign tumours can produce splaying of several posterior ribs, a localized pressure erosion defect of one or two vertebral bodies and of course rib notching. On the other hand a bony destructive process indicates a malignant tumour. Enlargement of an intervertebral foramen is diagnostic of a dumb-bell shaped neurogenic tumour, usually a neurofibroma (Fig. 12.25). Rapid increase in the size of the mass or a pleural effusion indicates malignant degeneration.

The diagnosis is confirmed by CT, which shows a solid mass of soft tissue attenuation which may contain calcium and involve the adjacent bones. Intraspinal extension may also be demonstrated by enhancement of the CSF with non-ionic water soluble contrast medium in the spinal canal. Rarely a neurogenic tumour may occur in the anterior or middle mediastinum.

HIATUS HERNIA

A fixed or irreducible hiatus hernia is one of the commonest causes of a mediastinal mass and usually presents as a posterior mediastinal mass on a chest radiograph in an asymptomatic elderly patient. The hernia can also produce dyspnoea, retrosternal chest pain and epigastric discomfort, but incarceration of the stomach is rare.

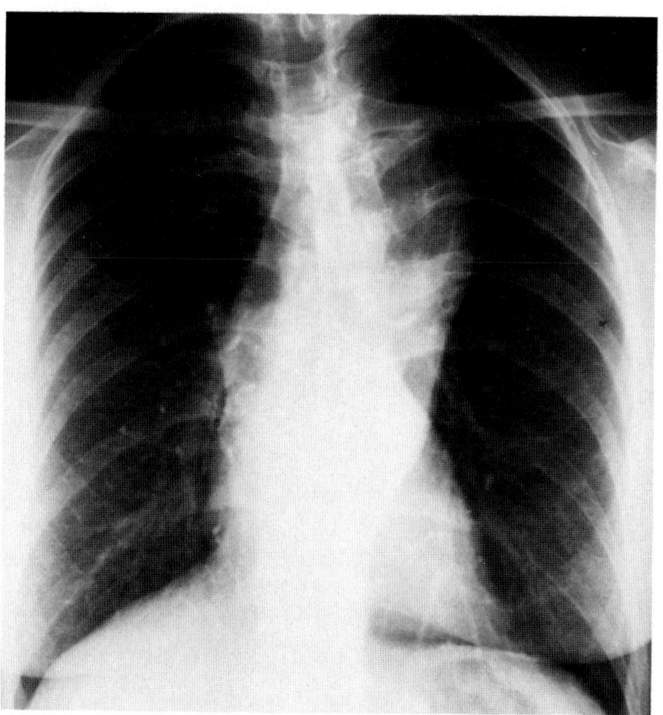

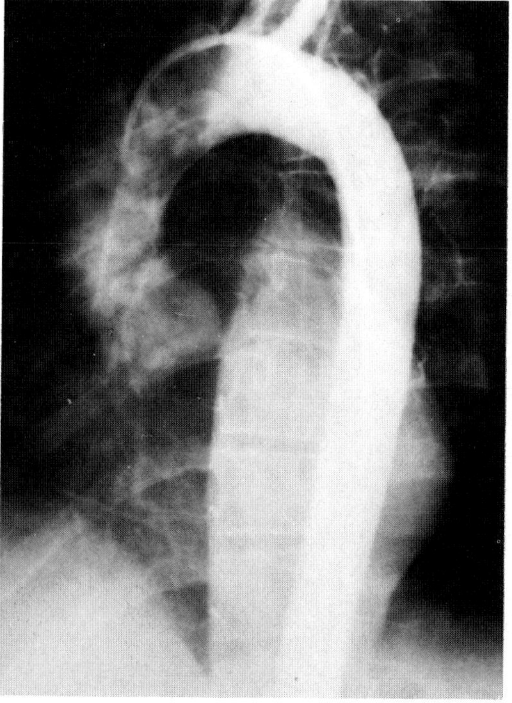

Fig. 12.24 Ganglioneuroma. 44-year-old female presenting with chest pain. PA film (**A**) shows an elongated mass in the posterior mediastinum with loss of the normal outline of the arch of the aorta and a scoliosis of the dorsal spine convex to the left. Arch aortogram (**B**) was normal, but a myelogram (not illustrated) showed intraspinal extension of the tumour.

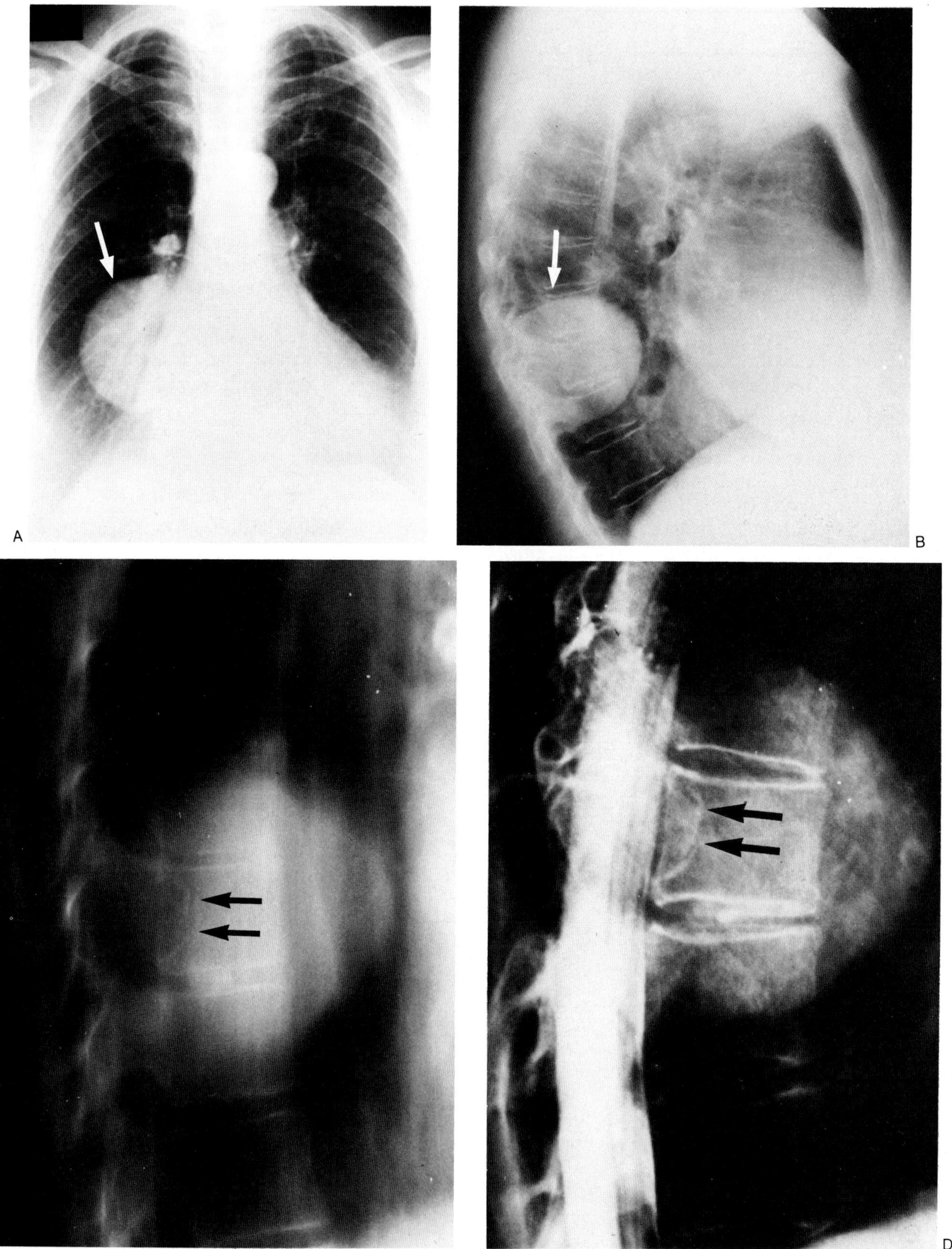

Fig. 12.25 Neurofibroma. Asymptomatic 57-year-old female. PA (**A**) and lateral films (**B**) show a round mass in the posterior mediastinum behind the heart on the right. The lateral tomogram (**C**) shows enlargement of the intervertebral foramen (←), but the myelogram (**D**) does not show significant intraspinal extension of the tumour.

A hiatus hernia appears as a round soft tissue mass ntaining an air–fluid level directly behind the heart, hich lies to the left of the midline in the posterior mediasnum in about 70% of cases. The larger hernias can also ntain liver, omentum and small intestine.

The diagnosis is easily confirmed by a penetrated PA film, lateral film or a barium meal, which shows the stomach bove the diaphragm within the chest.

OESOPHAGEAL LESIONS

esions of the oesophagus usually present with dysphagia an adult patient, but can also produce an aspiration neumonitis, due to spill of the oesophageal contents into e trachea and main bronchi.

A *pharyngo-oesophageal pouch* or Zenker's diverticulum produced by herniation of the pharyngo-oesophageal ucosa through Killihan's dehiscence, usually on the left, etween the muscle fibres of the inferior constrictor uscle. The mediastinum appears normal on a chest radioraph when the pouch is small, but a large pouch appears s a round soft tissue mass in the superior part of the osterior mediastinum, which contains an air-fluid level. he soft tissue mass lies in the midline and displaces the achea forwards.

A *carcinoma* and even a *leiomyoma* of the oesophagus may e large enough to produce a soft tissue mass in the osterior mediastinum and a large *diverticulum* of the lower oesophagus occasionally produces a soft tissue mass behind the heart.

There are several causes of a dilated or *mega-oesophagus* and these include *achalasia* of the cardia, a *benign oesophageal stricture, a carcinoma* of the oesophagus, *presbyoesophagus, systemic sclerosis* and South American trypanosomiasis or *Chagas' disease*. The oesophagus dilates proximal to the long standing obstruction or due to the degeneration of Auerbach's plexus in its wall. A mega-oesophagus produces widening of the posterior mediastinum behind the heart on the right, extending from the thoracic inlet to the diaphragm (Fig. 12.26), sometimes with bowing around the azygos vein. There is often an air–fluid level in the superior part of the posterior mediastinum with the non-homogeneous mottled appearance of food particles mixed with air beneath it, and no air in the fundus of the stomach. There may also be patchy pneumonic consolidation, bronchiectasis or even occasionally pulmonary fibrosis in both lower lobes, due to the recurrent aspiration pneumonitis.

The diagnosis of all oesophageal lesions is confirmed by a barium swallow, which can also be useful in the investigation of other posterior mediastinal masses. The dilated oesophagus is also easily confirmed by CT (Fig. 12.27).

Oesophageal lesions are discussed in more detail in Chapter 29.

PARAVERTEBRAL LESIONS

Neurogenic tumours causing paravertebral masses have been discussed above. Other paravertebral lesions of the dorsal spine usually present with back pain in an adult patient. There are several common causes of a paraver-

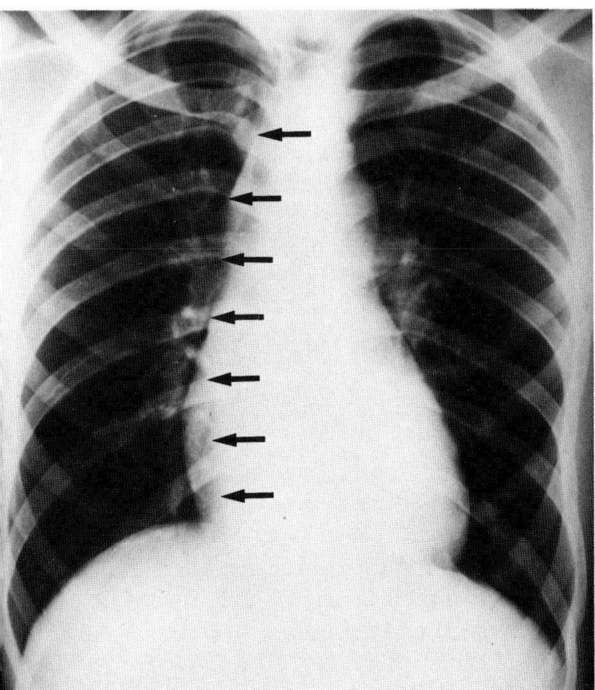

ig. 12.26 Achalasia of the cardia. 19-year-old male presenting with aemoptysis. PA film shows a dilated oesophagus (arrows) behind the eart on the right with absence of air in the gastric fundus. Diagnosis onfirmed by barium swallow.

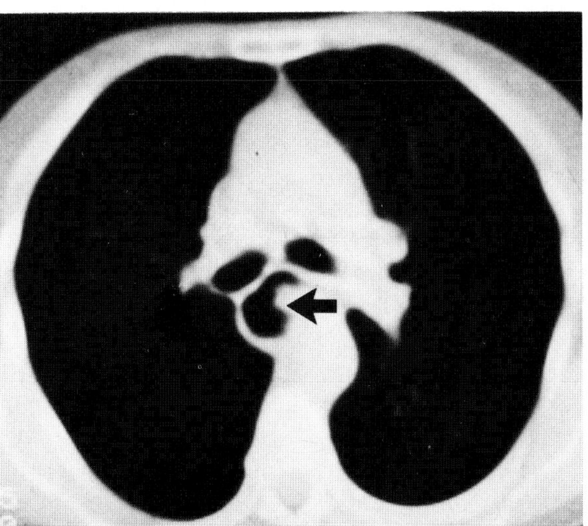

Fig. 12.27 Carcinoma of the oesophagus. 62-year-old male presenting with dysphagia. CT scan (L, O, W 2000) at the level of the tracheal bifurcation shows dilatation of the oesophagus with tumour projecting into the air-filled lumen (←).

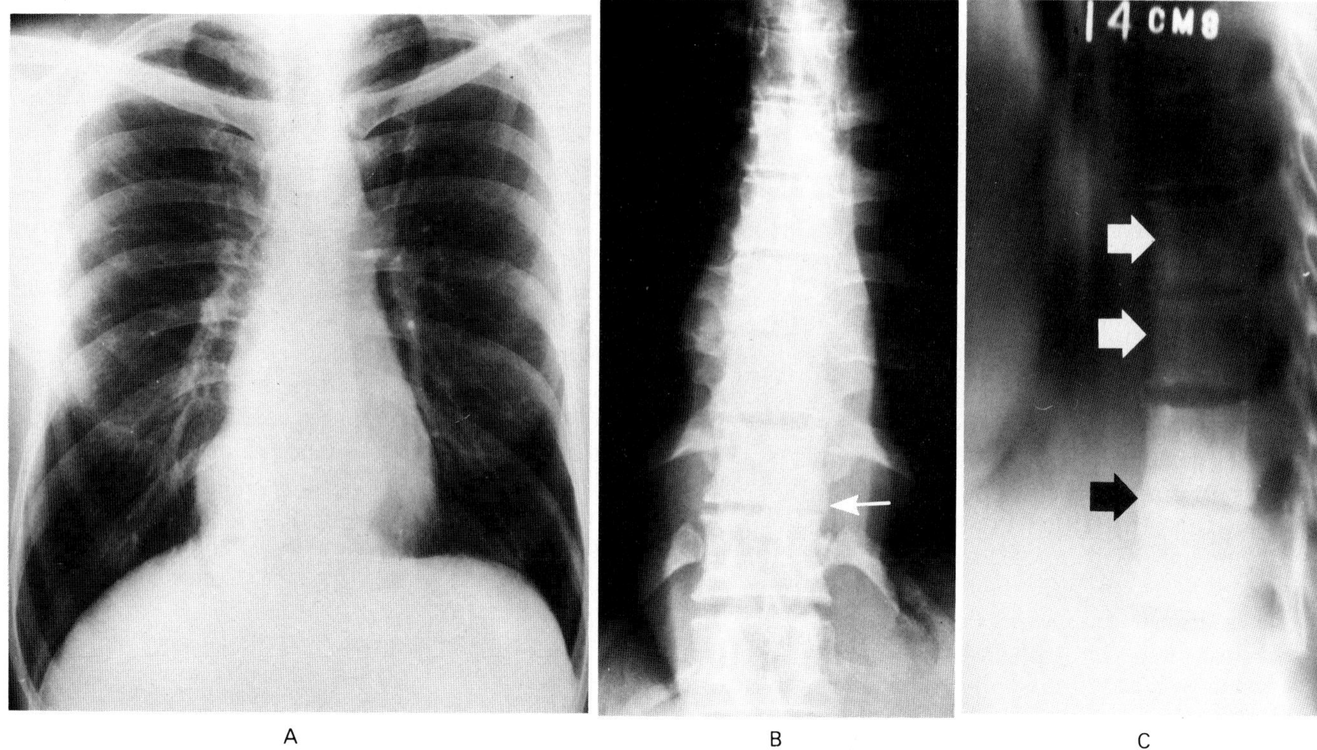

Fig. 12.28 Tuberculous paravertebral mass. 37-year-old male presenting with back pain. PA film (**A**), penetrated PA film (**B**) and lateral tomogram (**C**) show a paravertebral mass in the posterior mediastinum behind the heart with loss of intervertebral disc space at the D10–D11 level (←) and erosion of the anterior surfaces of the vertebral bodies above this (→). Diagnosis confirmed by surgery.

tebral mass and these include a traumatic wedge compression fracture of a vertebral body with haematoma formation, a pyogenic or tuberculous paraspinal abscess, multiple myeloma, disseminated lymphoma and metastatic carcinoma with paraspinal extension. Extramedullary haemopoietic tissue can also produce paravertebral masses (see p. 197).

A paravertebral mass appears as an elongated or lobulated soft tissue shadow with a well-defined outline which usually projects on both sides of the posterior mediastinum (Fig. 12.28). Paravertebral masses also usually involve the adjacent thoracic vertebrae or intervertebral disc spaces. This allows the radiologist to differentiate between the inflammatory lesions, which usually involve and narrow the intervertebral disc space as well as producing bone destruction, and the neoplastic lesions, which only produce bone destruction.

The diagnosis is confirmed by a penetrated PA film, a lateral film or conventional tomography. Direct needle puncture of a paravertebral mass with aspiration biopsy can also be performed under CT or fluoroscopic guidance to confirm the diagnosis.

BOCHDALEK HERNIA

The foramen of Bochdalek is a persistent developmental defect in the diaphragm posteriorly produced by a failur of the pleuroperitoneal canal membrane to fuse with th dorsal oesophageal mesentery medially and the body wal laterally. A hernia through the foramen of Bochdalek ca present either as a posterior mediastinal mass on a ches radiograph in an asymptomatic adult patient or with acut respiratory distress in the neonatal period. Strangulatio of the herniating bowel is rare.

About 90% of Bochdalek hernias occur in the left hemi diaphragm, because of the protective effect of the live on the right. The smaller hernias usually contain retro peritoneal fat, kidney or spleen which appears as a sof tissue mass in the posterior costo-phrenic angle. Th smaller hernias can also contain the splenic flexure of th colon (Fig. 12.29).

The larger hernias contain jejunum, ileum and colo which appears as multiple ring shadows in the chest due t the airfilled loops of bowel. They may displace the hear and mediastinum into the contralateral hemithorax. Ther is also absence of aerated lung in the affected hemithora due to the associated compressed hypoplastic lung abov the loops of bowel. The larger hernias can also contai liver.

The diagnosis is confirmed by a barium meal and follov through, which shows loops of small intestine and colo within the hemithorax. An isotope scan, ultrasound o

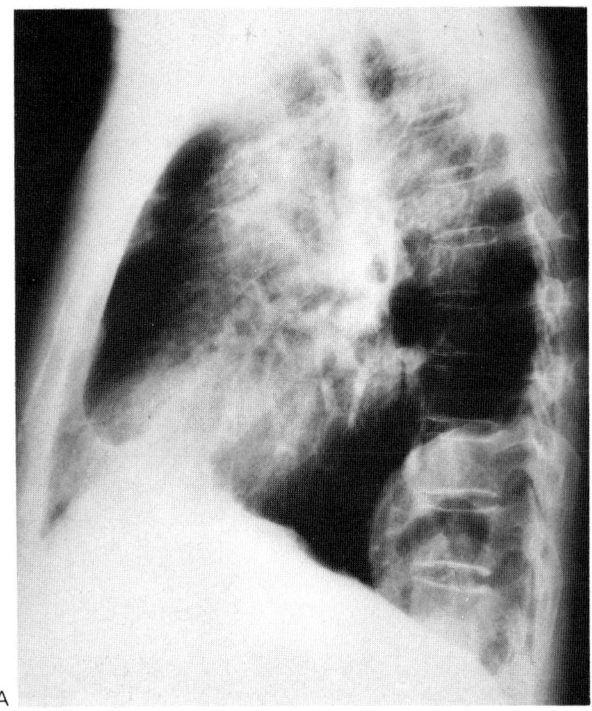

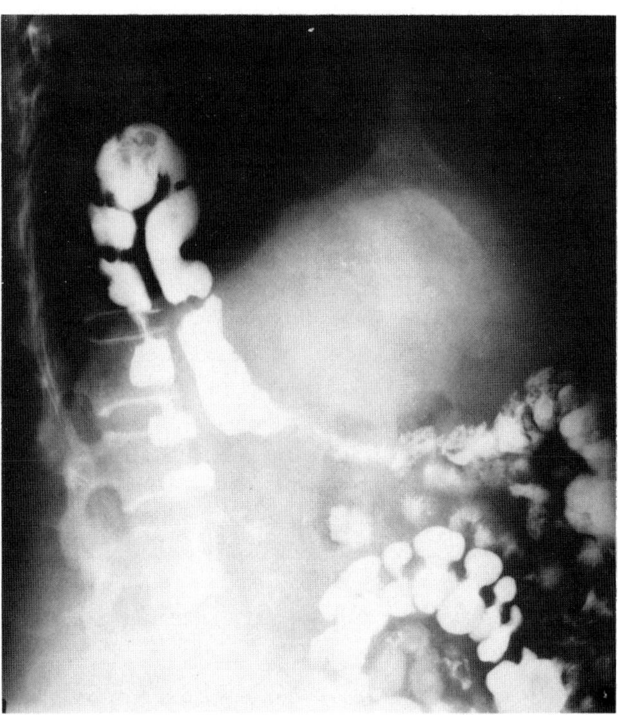

Fig. 12.29 Bochdalek hernia. Asymptomatic 65-year-old male. Lateral film (**A**) shows an oval mass, which contains a loop of bowel, in the left posterior costo-phrenic angle. Barium meal and follow through (**B**) showed the splenic flexure of the colon within the hernia.

intravenous urography can also confirm the diagnosis by showing liver, spleen or kidney above the diaphragm. Thirteen pairs of ribs may occur in association with a Bochdalek hernia.

NEUROENTERIC CYSTS

The developmental anomalies, produced by partial or complete persistence of the neurenteric canal or its incomplete resorption, include *gastro-intestinal reduplications, enteric cysts, neuroenteric cysts, anterior meningocoeles* and *cysts of the cord.*

A neuroenteric cyst usually presents with respiratory distress or feeding difficulties in infants, whereas an anterior meningocoele is usually asymptomatic. An enteric cyst may produce chest pain in children or young adult patients if peptic ulceration occurs within it. Infection with rupture into the oesophagus is rare. These rare developmental cysts are closely related not only to the oesophagus, to which there may be fibrous attachments, but also to the thoracic spine, in which there may be congenital bony abnormalities such as block vertebra, hemivertebra and butterfly vertebra (hence the split notochord syndrome). The cysts have thin walls lined by stratified squamous epithelium or ciliated columnar epithelium of both gastrointestinal and notochordal or neural origin and contain fluid material. They appear as a round or oval soft tissue mass in the posterior mediastinum frequently on the right. An air–fluid level is present after rupture of an infected cyst into the oesophagus.

The diagnosis of a meningocoele is confirmed by myelography, which shows non-ionic water soluble contrast medium entering the meningocoele in the prone position. CT may also be diagnostic. The diagnosis of an enteric cyst is occasionally confirmed by a barium swallow, if the barium sulphate actually enters the cyst. The diagnosis of neuroenteric cysts may also be suggested by CT, which shows a mass of soft tissue attenuation, but is usually confirmed by surgery.

PANCREATIC PSEUDOCYST

A pseudocyst of the pancreas extending through the oesophageal or aortic hiatus into the chest usually presents with dyspnoea or dysphagia in a patient with acute pancreatitis. It is a rare abnormality, which occurs in the posterior mediastinum and it appears as a round or oval soft tissue mass behind the heart. A left basal pleural effusion or atelectasis in the lower lobes may also occur. The diagnosis is confirmed by CT, which shows a thin-walled cystic mass containing fluid of low attenuation (0–20 HU) extending from the abdomen into the chest through the aortic hiatus, behind the diaphragmatic crura.

EXTRAMEDULLARY HAEMOPOIESIS

Extramedullary haemopoiesis in the chest usually presents as an incidental mediastinal lesion on a chest radiograph in children or young adult patients with a chronic haemolytic anaemia, such as thalassaemia major. It is a rare abnormality, which occurs in the posterior mediastinum and it appears as a lobulated paravertebral soft tissue mass behind the heart. There may also be evidence of hepatosplenomegaly on an abdominal film (unless there has been a splenectomy) and a typically abnormal skeletal survey. The diagnosis is confirmed by a penetrated PA film. Extramedullary haemopoiesis may also occur in myelofibrosis.

OTHER RARE POSTERIOR MEDIASTINAL LESIONS

Oesophageal varices and a *cyst of the thoracic duct* may produce a soft tissue mass in the posterior mediastinum and an *osteochondroma* or a *chondrosarcoma* of a vertebra or rib may also result in a tumour mass that involves the posterior mediastinum.

OTHER MEDIASTINAL LESIONS

PNEUMOMEDIASTINUM

Air in the mediastinum presents either as an incidental radiological abnormality in an asymptomatic child or adult patient, or with chest pain, which is made worse by breathing or swallowing. The air usually tracks upwards into the root of the neck to produce surgical emphysema. There are many causes of a pneumomediastinum and these include:

1. Perforation of the oesophagus following endoscopy, dilatation of a stricture or insertion of an Atkinson or Celestin tube, or after prolonged vomiting as in the Mallory–Weiss syndrome.
2. Rupture of the trachea or main bronchi following bronchoscopy, or after blunt chest trauma.
3. After sternotomy.
4. Intermittent positive pressure ventilation, especially in neonates.
5. Asthma.
6. After prolonged coughing as in whooping cough.
7. During pregnancy, especially at the time of childbirth.
8. Pneumoperitoneum due to any cause.

Air used to be deliberately introduced into the mediastinum during a diagnostic pneumomediastinum and it also tracked into the mediastinum after diagnostic pre-sacral pneumography, but today both these procedures are obsolete.

Air in the mediastinum appears as translucent streaks of gas outlining the blood vessels and other structures, with displacement of the parietal layer of the pleura laterally. A large volume of air tracks throughout the mediastinal tissue planes and up into the neck and so can easily be identified on a PA chest radiograph (Fig. 12.30), but a small volume of air behind the sternum or behind the heart can often only be seen on the lateral film.

The presence of chest pain and fever in a patient with a pneumomediastinum indicates *acute mediastinitis* and this is usually due to perforation of the pharynx, oesophagus or trachea. In addition to the streaks of gas, the mediastinum may be widened by the oedematous mediastinal tissues which have a hazy outline and there may be a small pleural effusion. An abscess occasionally develops from

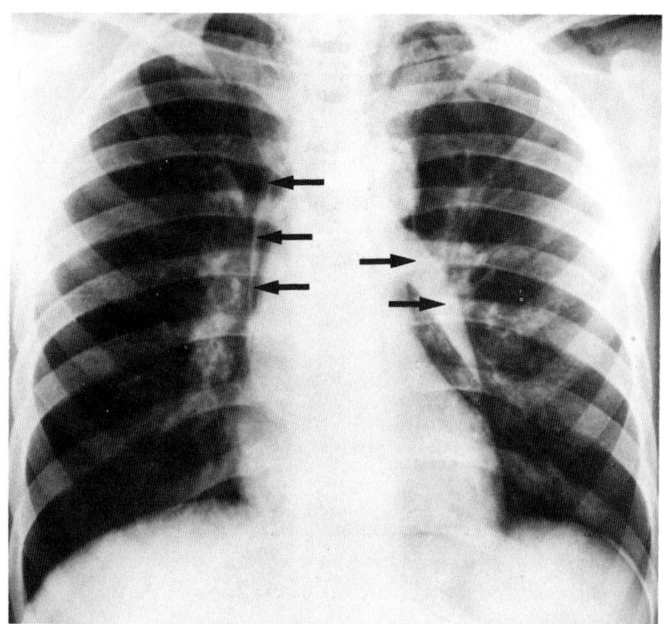

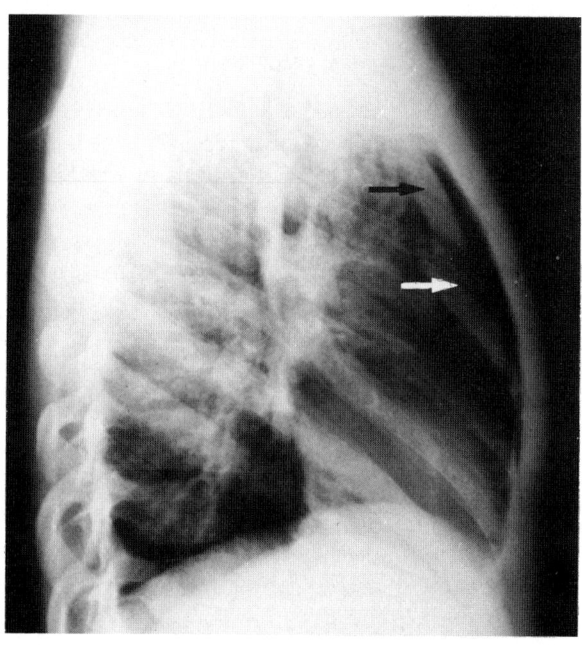

Fig. 12.30 Pneumomediastinum. 12-year-old boy with asthma. PA (**A**) and lateral films (**B**) show air in the mediastinum with displacement of the pleura (←) and demonstration of the thymus gland (→).

acute mediastinitis and appears as a round or oval soft tissue mass (Fig. 12.31), which may contain an air–fluid level, in any part of the mediastinum.

Chronic mediastinitis or *mediastinal fibrosis* usually presents with a superior vena caval compression syndrome. The commonest cause of chronic mediastinitis is radiotherapy (Fig. 12.16), but it may also be due to a chronic inflammatory condition such as tuberculosis or histoplasmosis and can be idiopathic either alone or in association with primary idiopathic retroperitoneal fibrosis. It can also occur with Riedel's thyroiditis and with drug treatment with methysergide or practolol. The mediastinum is usually widened and there may be narrowing of the trachea. The diagnosis is confirmed by superior vena cavography or digital subtraction angiography, which shows either complete occlusions or stenoses in the mediastinal veins with retrograde filling of dilated veins such as the jugular, azygos and internal mammary veins.

Apart from a pneumomediastinum and mediastinitis, the other condition that can involve any part of the mediastinum is *haemorrhage*. This is usually due to blunt or penetrating chest trauma but it may also be due to a leaking aortic aneurysm and can occur in association with bleeding disorders and anticoagulant therapy. The mediastinum is usually widened but there may be a round or oval soft tissue mass in any part of the mediastinum if a localized haematoma develops. The diagnosis can be confirmed by CT in these various situations.

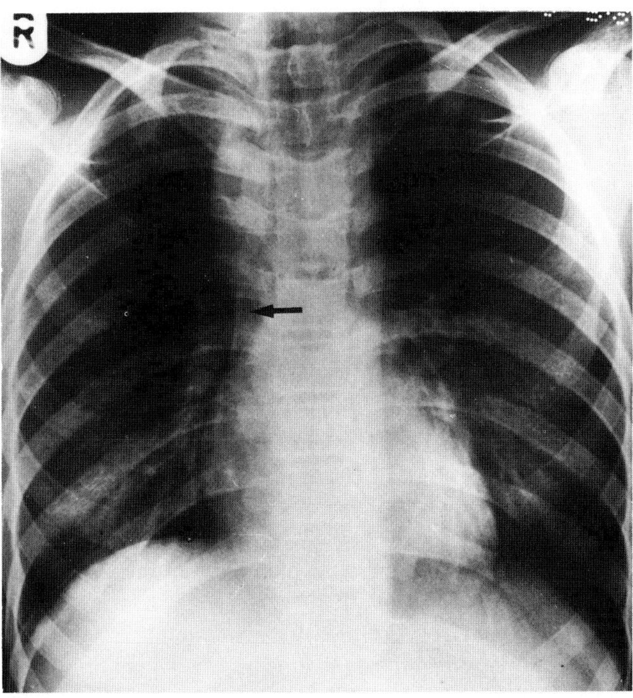

Fig. 12.31 Abscess. 15-year-old girl with a short history of pyrexia several days after a pharyngo-oesophageal tear produced by an explosion of a well known fizzy drink into her mouth as she opened the bottle with her teeth. PA film shows a right paratracheal mass in the middle mediastinum and traces of the resolving mediastinal gas (←).

REFERENCES AND SUGGESTIONS FOR FURTHER READING

Adler, O. B., Rosenberger, A., Peleg, H. (1983). Fine needle aspiration biopsy of mediastinal masses. *American Journal of Roentgenology*, **140**, 893–896.

Axel, L., Kressel, H. Y., Thickman, D., Epstein, D. M., Edelstein, W., Bottomley, P., Redington, R., Baum, S. (1983) NMR imaging of the chest at 0.12T. *American Journal of Roentgenology*, **141**, 1157–1162.

Baron, R. L., Lee, J. K. T., Sagel, S. S., Peterson, R. R. (1982) Computed tomography of the normal thymus. *American Journal of Roentgenology*, **142**, 121–125.

Baron, R. L., Levitt, R. G., Sagel, S. S., Stanley, R. J. (1981). Computed tomography in the evaluation of mediastinal widening. *Radiology*, **138**, 107–113.

Brown, L. R., Muhm, J. R., Gray, J. E. (1980). Radiographic detection of thymoma. *American Journal of Roentgenology*, **134**, 1181–1188.

Cohen, A. M., Creviston, S., Li Puma, J. P., Lieberman, J., Haaga, J. R., Alfidi, R. J. (1983). Nuclear magnetic resonance imaging of the mediastinum and hili. *American Journal of Roentgenology*, **141**, 1163–1169.

Crowe, J. K., Brown, L. R., Muhm, J. R. (1978). Computed tomography of the mediastinum. *Radiology*, **128**, 75–87.

Egan, T. J., Neiman, H. L., Herman, R. J., Malava, S. R., Sanders, J. H. (1980). Computed tomography in the diagnosis of aortic aneurysm dissection or traumatic injury. *Radiology*, **136**, 141–146.

Fraser, R. G., Breatnach, E., Barnes, G. T. (1983). Digital radiography of the chest. *Radiology*, **148**, 1–5.

Gamsu, G., Webb, W. R., Sheldon, P., Kaufman, L., Crooks, L. E., Birnberg, F. A., Goodman, P., Hinchcliffe, W. A., Hedgecock, M. (1983) Nuclear magnetic resonance imaging of the thorax. *Radiology*, **147**, 473–480.

Heitzman, E. R., Goldwin, R. L., Proto, A. V. (1977). Radiologic analysis of the mediastinum utilizing computed tomography. *Radiologic Clinics of North America*, **15**, 309–329.

Kirks, D. R., Korobkin, M. (1981). Computed tomography of the chest in infants and children: Techniques and mediastinal evaluation. *Radiologic Clinics of North America*, **19**, 409–419.

Lyons, H. A., Calvy, G. L., Sammons, B. P. (1959). The diagnosis and classification of mediastinal masses: A study of 782 cases. *Annals of Internal Medicine*, **51**, 897–932.

McLoud, T. C., Meyer, J. E. (1982) Mediastinal metastases. *Radiologic Clinics of North America*, **20**, 453–468.

Morrison, I. M. (1958). Tumours and cysts of the mediastinum. *Thorax*, **13**, 294–307.

Oudkerk, M., Overbosch, E., Dee, P. (1983). CT recognition of acute aortic dissection. *American Journal of Roentgenology*, **141**, 671–676.

Pugatch, R. D., Faling, L. J., Robbins, A. H., Spira, R. (1980) CT diagnosis of benign mediastinal abnormalities. *American Journal of Roentgenology*, **134**, 685–694.

Siegel, M. J., Sagel, S. S., Reed, K. (1982) The value of computed tomography in the diagnosis and management of paediatric mediastinal abnormalities. *Radiology*, **142**, 149–155.

Westcott, J. L. (1981) Percutaneous needle aspiration of hilar and mediastinal masses. *Radiology*, **141**, 323–329.

Wychulis, A. R., Payne, W. S., Clagett, O. T., Woolner, L. B. (1971) Surgical treatment of mediastinal tumours: A 40 year experience. *Journal of Thoracic and Cardiovascular Surgery*, **62**, 379–392.

CHAPTER 13

THE PLEURA: COLLAPSE AND CONSOLIDATION

THE PLEURA

Basic anatomy. The pleura is a serous membrane which covers the surface of the lung, and lines the inner surface of the chest wall. The visceral pleura, over the lung, and the parietal pleura, over the chest wall, are continuous at the hilum, where a fold of pleura extends inferiorly to form the inferior pulmonary ligament. The two layers of pleura are closely applied to each other, being separated by a thin layer of lubricating pleural fluid, which is normally not more than a few millilitres in volume. The parietal pleura, and the visceral pleura over the periphery of the lung are not normally visible radiographically. However, where the visceral pleura lines the interlobar fissures of the lung it is often visible, there being two layers of pleura outlined by aerated lung. The horizontal fissure of the right lung is often seen on a frontal chest film, and the oblique fissures will usually be seen on the lateral views. Some patients have one or more accessory fissures, the most common being the azygos fissure and the inferior accessory fissure of the right lower lobe. Occasionally anterior or posterior junction lines are seen in the frontal chest film, where the left and right lungs come into contact in the mediastinum.

Some physiological considerations. The normal anatomy of the lungs is maintained by a balance between different elastic forces of the chest wall and lungs. The lung has a natural tendency to collapse toward its hilum, and this is opposed by forces of similar magnitude of the chest wall to expand outwards. The visceral and parietal layers of pleura are thus kept in close apposition. If increased fluid or air collects in the pleural space the effect of the outward forces on the underlying lung is diminished, and the lung will tend to retract towards its hilum. Therefore, in an erect patient a small pleural effusion having gravitated to the base of the lung causes retraction of the lower part of the lung, but has comparatively little effect at the apex. Conversely, a small pneumothorax will collect at the apex and have little effect at the lung base. Obviously large intrapleural collections will affect the entire lung. These basic patterns may be altered by the state of the underlying lung and the presence of pleural adhesions.

Table 13.1 A summary of imaging methods useful in pleural disease

1. Standard PA and lateral projections. This is the starting point for investigation of pleural disease. High kV technique may provide all the necessary information.
2. Expiratory film. This may show a shallow pneumothorax that is not apparent on the standard PA film.
3. Penetrated grid film. This may show an air bronchogram in what appears as a homogenous opacity on a standard film, and differentiate consolidation from diffuse pleural shadowing.
4. Apical lordotic projection. This may clarify the extent of apical pleural shadowing, and help confirm or exclude a mass.
5. Conventional tomography. This may be helpful to evaluate apical pleural shadowing and the adjacent bones.
6. Lateral decubitus projection and horizontal beam. With the patient lying on the affected side, a small free pleural effusion will layer out against the chest wall, and can be differentiated from pleural thickening. It may also demonstrate the presence of a sub-pulmonary effusion. With the patient lying on the normal side a small pneumothorax may be more easily seen against the chest wall of the upper side. This may be especially useful in young children.
7. Supine AP projection with vertical beam. This may be used to demonstrate a sub-pulmonary effusion, which, if free, will flow over the posterior chest wall, producing veiling of the lung, but showing the true level of the diaphragm.
8. Fluoroscopy. This is helpul in determining the best tangential projections to demonstrate loculated effusions, and pleural plaques and calcification.
9. CT. Most sensitive method for detecting and assessing pleural effusions, pleural plaques and pleural tumours. It can also differentiate between pleural and parenchymal opacities, and is useful to assess lung that is obscured by surrounding pleural thickening or fluid.
10. Ultrasound. This may be useful to differentiate between pleural thickening and loculated pleural fluid, and is particularly useful in the aspiration of loculated fluid.
11. Percutaneous needle biopsy. Not strictly an imaging technique, but is part of the radiologist's diagnostic armamentarium. Localized pleural thickening or loculated pleural fluid may be sampled, usually using fluoroscopy, but ultrasonic or CT guidance can be used.
12. Diagnostic pneumothorax. This has been used to differentiate between pleural and peripheral lung opacities, but has been superseded by CT

Fibrotic, emphysematous or consolidated lung may not be able to retract, and adhesions may prevent the usual distribution of air or fluid.

DISEASES OF THE PLEURA

Pleural fluid

Fluid which accumulates in the pleural space may be transudate, exudate, pus, blood or chyle. Radiographically they produce similar shadows and are, therefore, indistinguishable. However, there may be clinical data to point to the aetiology, or the chest film may show other abnormalities, such as evidence of heart failure or trauma, which indicate the cause. Sometimes the definitive diagnosis is only made after thoracentesis or pleural biopsy, or not infrequently remains obscure.

a. **Transudates**. Transudates contain less than 3 g/dl of protein, and are usually clear or faintly yellow, watery fluids. A pleural transudate may be called a hydrothorax. They are often bilateral. The commonest cause is *cardiac failure*, when the effusion usually accumulates first on the right, before becoming bilateral. Other causes are *hypoproteinaemia* (especially the nephrotic syndrome, hepatic cirrhosis and anaemia), *constrictive pericarditis, Meig's syndrome* and *myxoedema*.

b. **Exudates** contain in excess of 3 g/dl of protein, and vary from amber, slightly cloudy fluid, which often clots on standing, to frank pus. A purulent pleural effusion is termed an empyema. The commonest causes of pleural exudate are *bacterial pneumonia, pulmonary tuberculosis, carcinoma of the lung, metastatic malignancy* and *pulmonary infarction*. Less common causes are *subphrenic infection, connective tissue disorders* (especially systemic lupus erythematosus and rheumatoid disease) and *non-bacterial pneumonias*. Unusual causes include post-myocardial infarction syndrome, acute pancreatitis and primary neoplasia of the pleura.

c. **Haemothorax**. Bleeding into the pleural space is almost always secondary to open or closed *trauma* to the chest. Rarely it is due to *haemophilia*. The effusions associated with pulmonary infarction and carcinoma of the lung are frequently blood-stained, but rarely pure blood.

d. **Chylothorax.** Chyle is a milky fluid high in neutral fat and fatty acids. Chylothorax may develop secondary to damage or obstruction of the thoracic lymphatic vessels. The commonest cause is chest *trauma*, usually surgical. Other causes include carcinoma of the lung, lymphoma and filariasis. Lymphangiomyomatosis is a rare cause.

Radiological appearances of pleural fluid

Free fluid. Pleural fluid not surprisingly casts a shadow of water or soft tissue density on the chest radiograph. In the absence of pleural adhesions, the position and morphology of this shadow will depend upon the amount of fluid, the state of the underlying lung and the position of the patient. The most dependent recess of the pleura is the posterior costophrenic angle. A *small effusion* will, therefore, tend to collect posteriorly, and in most patients 1–2 dl of fluid are required to fill in this recess before fluid will be seen above the dome of the diaphragm on the frontal view (Fig. 13.1). Small effusions may thus be seen earlier on a lateral film than on a frontal film, but it is possible to identify effusions of only a few millilitres using decubitus views with a horizontal beam (Fig. 13.2), ultrasound (Fig. 13.2D) or CT (Fig. 13.23). As more fluid accumulates the costophrenic angle on the frontal view fills in, and with increasing fluid a homogenous opacity spread upwards obscuring the lung base. Typically this opacity has a fairly well-defined, concave upper edge, is higher laterally than medially and obscures the diaphragmatic shadow (Fig. 13.3). Frequently fluid will track into the pleural fissures (Fig. 13.4). If the film is sufficiently penetrated, pulmonary vessels in the lung masked by the effusion will be seen. A *massive effusion* may cause complete radio-opacity of a hemithorax. The underlying lung will have retracted towards its hilum, and the space occupying effect of the effusion will push the mediastinum towards the opposite side (Fig. 13.5). In the presence of a massive effusion, lack of displacement of the mediastinum suggests that the underlying lung is completely collapsed, and this is likely to be due to carcinoma of the bronchus. In the presence of pleural disease the ipsilateral hemidiaphragm

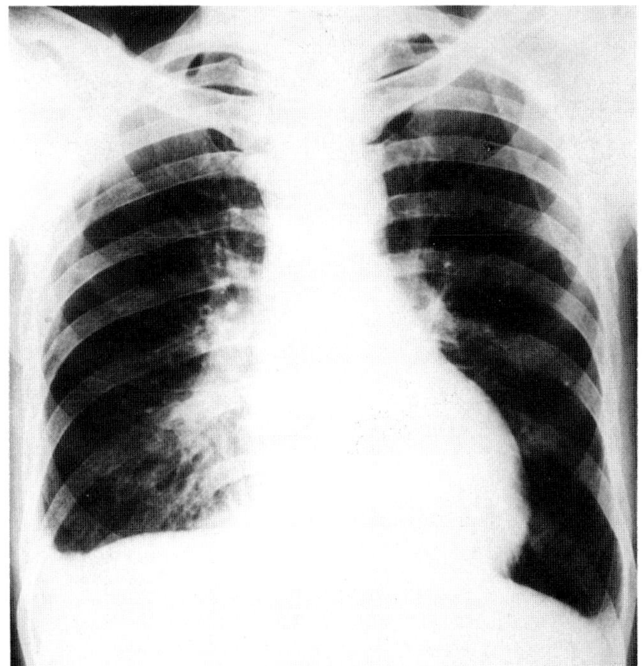

Fig. 13.1 Small bilateral pleural effusions. Male aged 58 years with ischaemic heart disease. The left costophrenic angle is blunted by a small effusion. The right pleural effusion is larger, and fluid is beginning to extend up the chest wall.

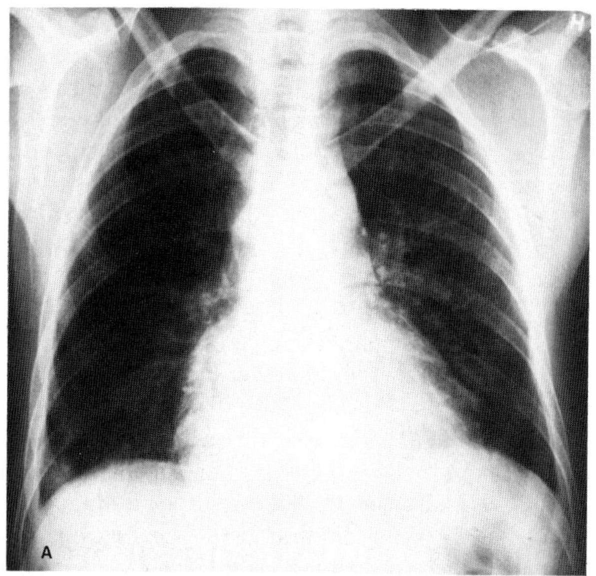

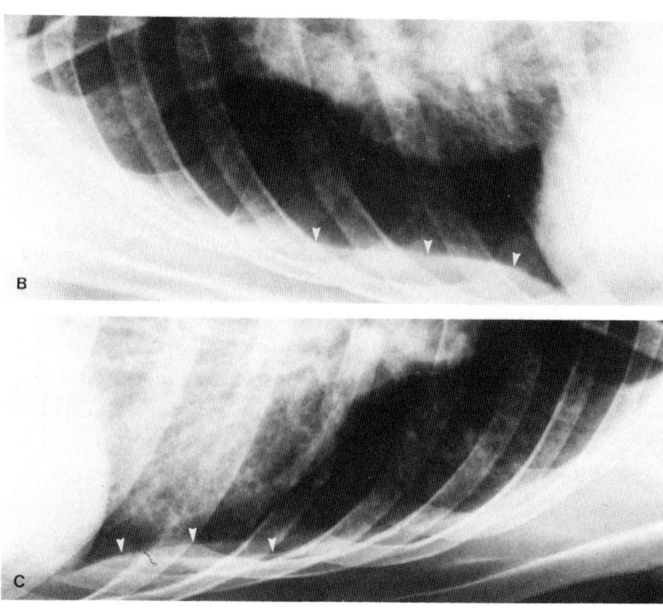

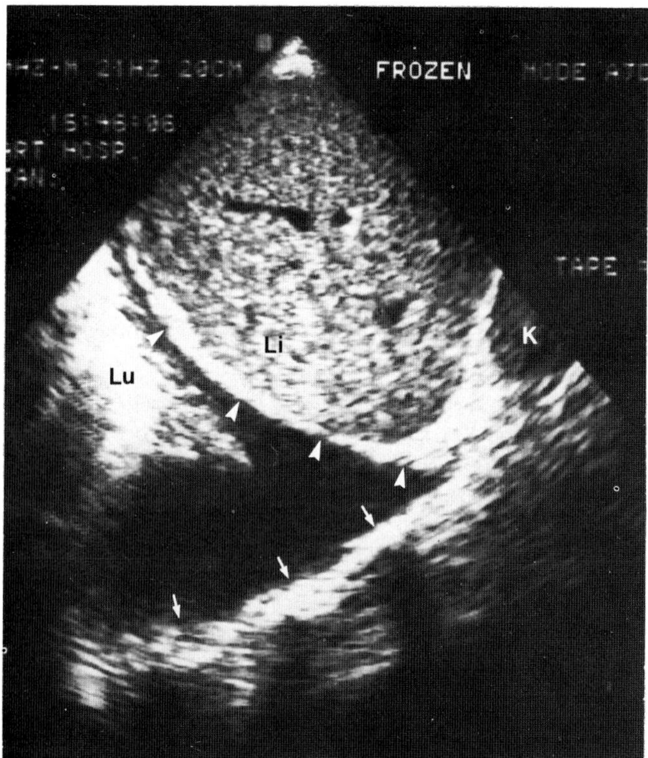

Fig. 13.2 Small bilateral pleural effusions. Male aged 34 years. Renal transplant patient with cytomegalovirus pneumonia. The effusions probably relate to renal failure rather than the pneumonia. (**A**) PA film shows subtle filling in of both costo-phrenic angles. (**B** and **C**) Horizontal ray right and left lateral decubitus films shown obvious free pleural effusions collecting along the dependent lateral costal margins (arrowheads). (**D**) Pleural effusion: ultrasonic demonstration. Male aged 47 years with ischaemic heart disease. Liver scan performed for hepatomegaly; no evidence of pleural effusion clinically or on chest radiograph. Patient scanned supine. Sagittal section through liver (Li) and right kidney (K) demonstrates base of right lung (Lu) floating in echo-free effusion above diaphragm (arrowheads) and posterior chest wall (arrows).

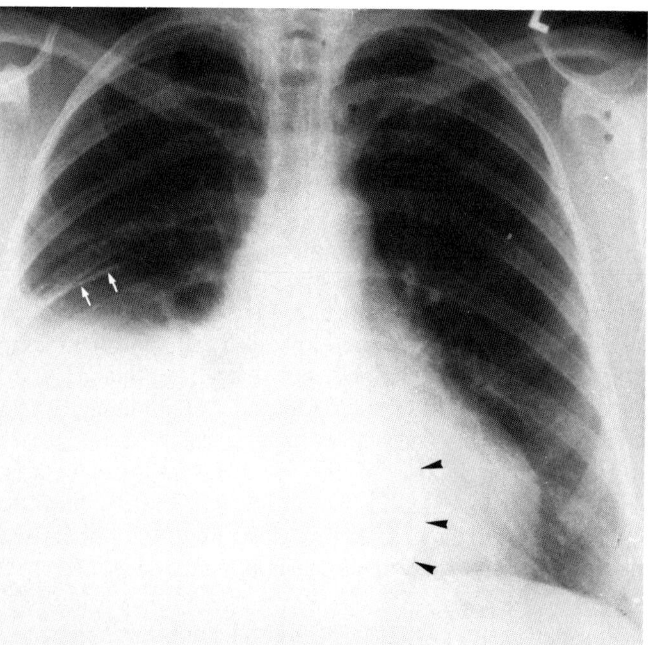

Fig. 13.3 Moderate size pleural effusion. Female aged 56 years. Effusions of unknown aetiology. PA film demonstrates typical pleural opacity with concave upper border, slightly higher laterally, and obscuring the diaphragm and underlying lung. Fluid is extending into the fissure (arrows), and also into the azygo-oesophageal recess producing a retro-cardiac opacity (arrowheads).

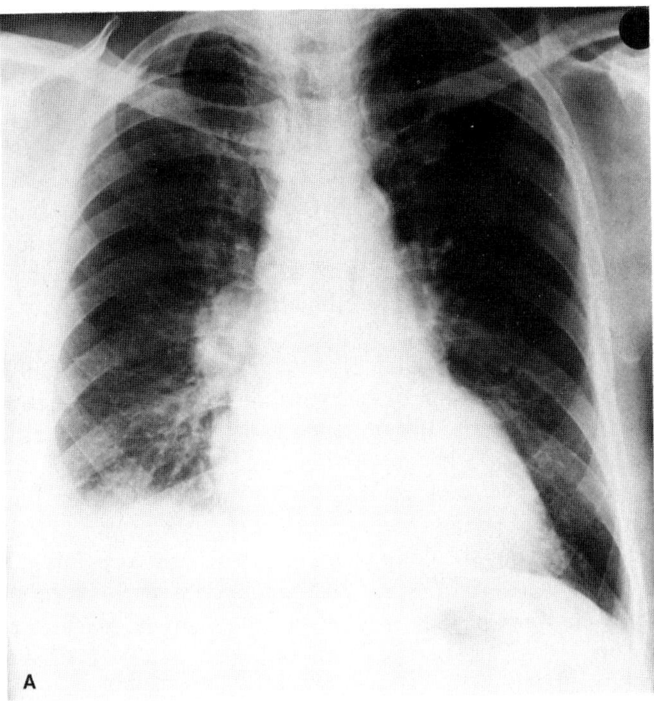

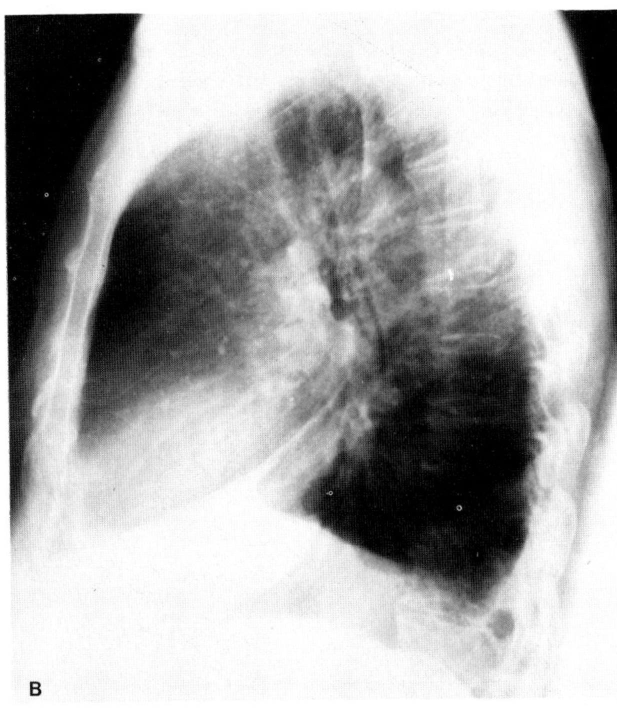

Fig. 13.4 Small pleural effusion. Male aged 72 with ischaemic heart disease. (**A**) PA film shows hazy contour of right hemidiaphragm and filled-in costophrenic angle. (**B**) Lateral film shows hazy contour of right hemidiaphragm posteriorly, and fluid extending into right oblique fissure. The contour of the left hemidiaphragm is clearly seen in both projections.

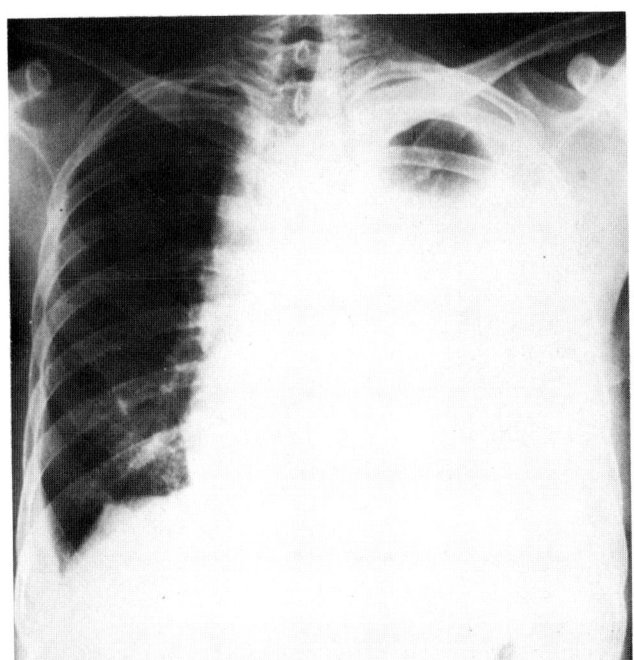

Fig. 13.5 Large pleural effusion. Male aged 28 years with well-differentiated lymphocytic lymphoma. PA films shows a large left pleural effusion extending over apex of lung and pushing mediastinum to the right. A small right pleural effusion is also present, and right paratracheal shadowing represents lymphadenopathy.

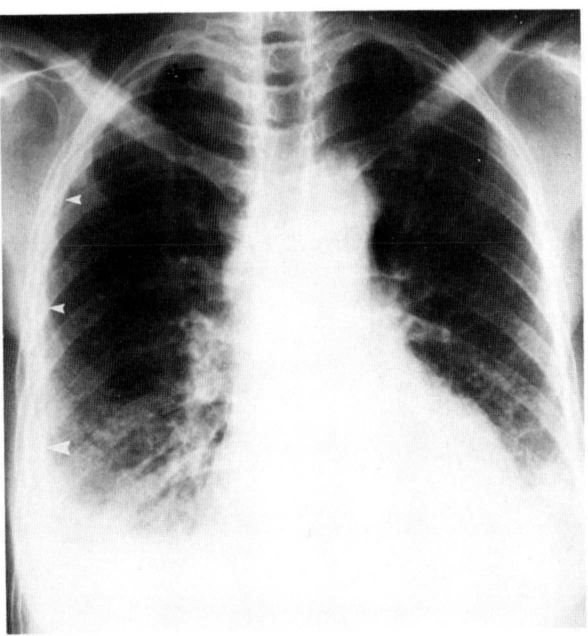

Fig. 13.6 Lamellar pleural effusion. Female aged 60 years with Sjögren's syndrome. Erect PA film shows small bilateral pleural effusions and bilateral basal interstitial lung disease. The right pleural effusion extends up the lateral costal margin (arrowheads).

is usually elevated. However, the weight of a large effusion may cause inversion of the diaphragm, and this sign is probably best demonstrated by ultrasound.

Atypical distribution of pleural fluid is quite common. *Lamellar effusions* are shallow collections between the chest wall and lung surface (Fig. 13.6), sometimes sparing the costophrenic angle. They occur most often in children and patients with heart disease. Occasionally quite large effusions accumulate between the diaphragm and under surface of the lung, mimicking elevation of that hemidiaphragm. This is the so-called *sub-pulmonary pleural effusion*. The contour of the 'diaphragm' is altered, its apex being more lateral than usual, and there may be some blunting of the costophrenic angle or tracking of fluid into fissures (Fig. 13.7). On the left side increased distance between the gastric air-bubble and lung base may be apparent. A sub-pulmonary effusion in a free pleural space will move with changes of posture, as can be demonstrated by horizontal beam lateral decubitus or supine films. A large right pleural effusion may collect in the *azygo-oesophageal recess* and mimic a retro-cardiac mass (Fig. 13.3). The reasons for atypical distribution of pleural fluid are often unclear, but it may be associated with abnormality of the underlying lung.

Loculated fluid. The pleural space may be partially obliterated by pleural disease causing fusion of the parietal and visceral layers. Encapsulated and free pleural fluid can be distinguished by gravitational methods. Encapsulated fluid, however, may be difficult to differentiate from an extrapleural opacity, parenchymal lung disease or mediastinal mass, but there are some useful diagnostic points.

An encysted effusion is often associated with free pleural fluid or other pleural shadowing, and may extend into a fissure (Fig. 13.8). Loculated effusions tend to have comparatively little depth, but considerable width, rather like a bi-convex lens. Their appearance, therefore, depends on whether they are viewed '*en face*', in profile or obliquely. Fluoroscopy is often helpful in determining the best projection for radiographic demonstration. Extrapleural opacities tend to have a much sharper outline, with tapered, sometimes concave edges where they meet the chest wall. Parenchymal lesions may show an air bronchogram. The differentiation between pleural thickening or mass and loculated pleural fluid may be difficult on plain

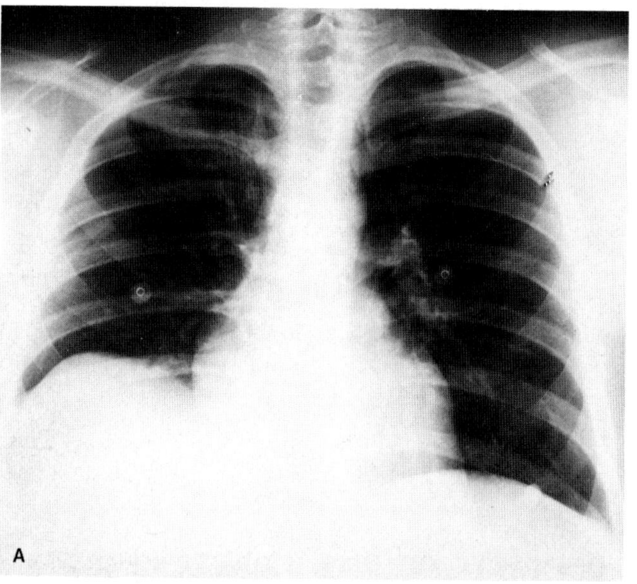

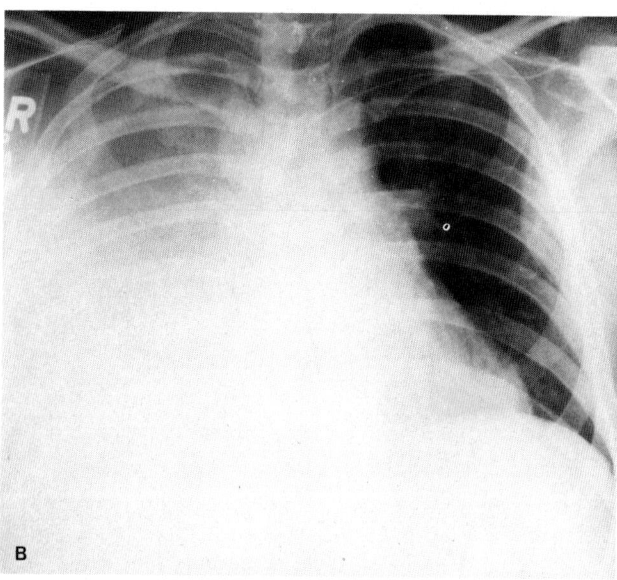

Fig. 13.7 Sub-pulmonary pleural effusion. Male aged 21 years with portal fibrosis. (**A**) Erect PA film shows apparent elevation of right hemi-diaphragm with apex more lateral than usual, and blunting of costophrenic angle. (**B**) Supine film demonstrates shift of pleural fluid from below lung to collection posteriorly and laterally veiling entire right lung.

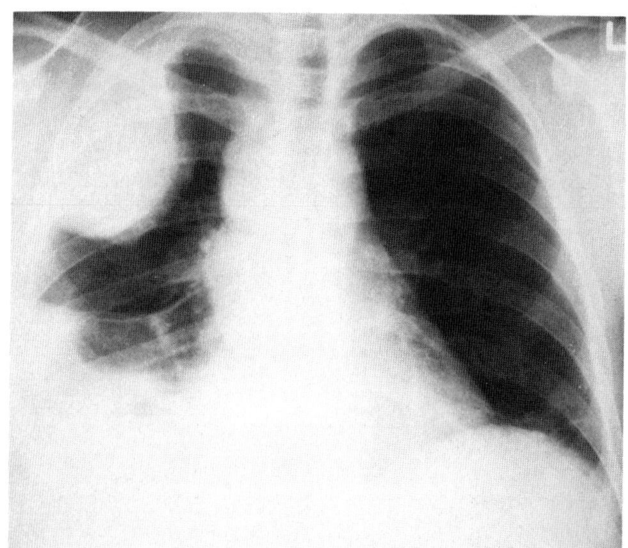

Fig. 13.8 Loculated pleural effusion. Male aged 19 years with non-Hodgkin's lymphoma. Erect PA film shows well-circumscribed, convex opacity adjacent to right upper costal margin, and extending around apex of lung. Right paratracheal shadowing is partly due to lymph node enlargement, and partly due to loculated pleural fluid. Pleural fluid is also present at the right base extending into the horizontal fissure.

films. Ultrasound is particularly useful in this context (Fig. 13.24), especially if aspiration of fluid is planned. Loculated fluid is anechoic, whereas pleural thickening and masses have internal echoes.

Loculated effusions occur most commonly along the chest wall, usually posteriorly or laterally. Since the advent of antibiotics their incidence has dropped. When viewed *en face* these effusions produce a radio-opacity of relatively low density. Loculated mediastinal effusions can be difficult to distinguish from a mediastinal mass, and in this location CT is particularly useful.

Fluid may become loculated in one or more of the interlobar fissures. This is an uncommon occurrence and is most often seen in heart failure. The appearances depend upon which fissure is affected and the quantity of fluid. Fluid collecting in the *horizontal fissure* produces a lenticular, oval or round shadow, with well-demarcated edges. Fluid extending into the adjacent parts of the fissure may make it appear thickened. In both frontal and lateral projections the shadow appears rounded. Loculated fluid in an *oblique fissure* may be less well defined on a frontal

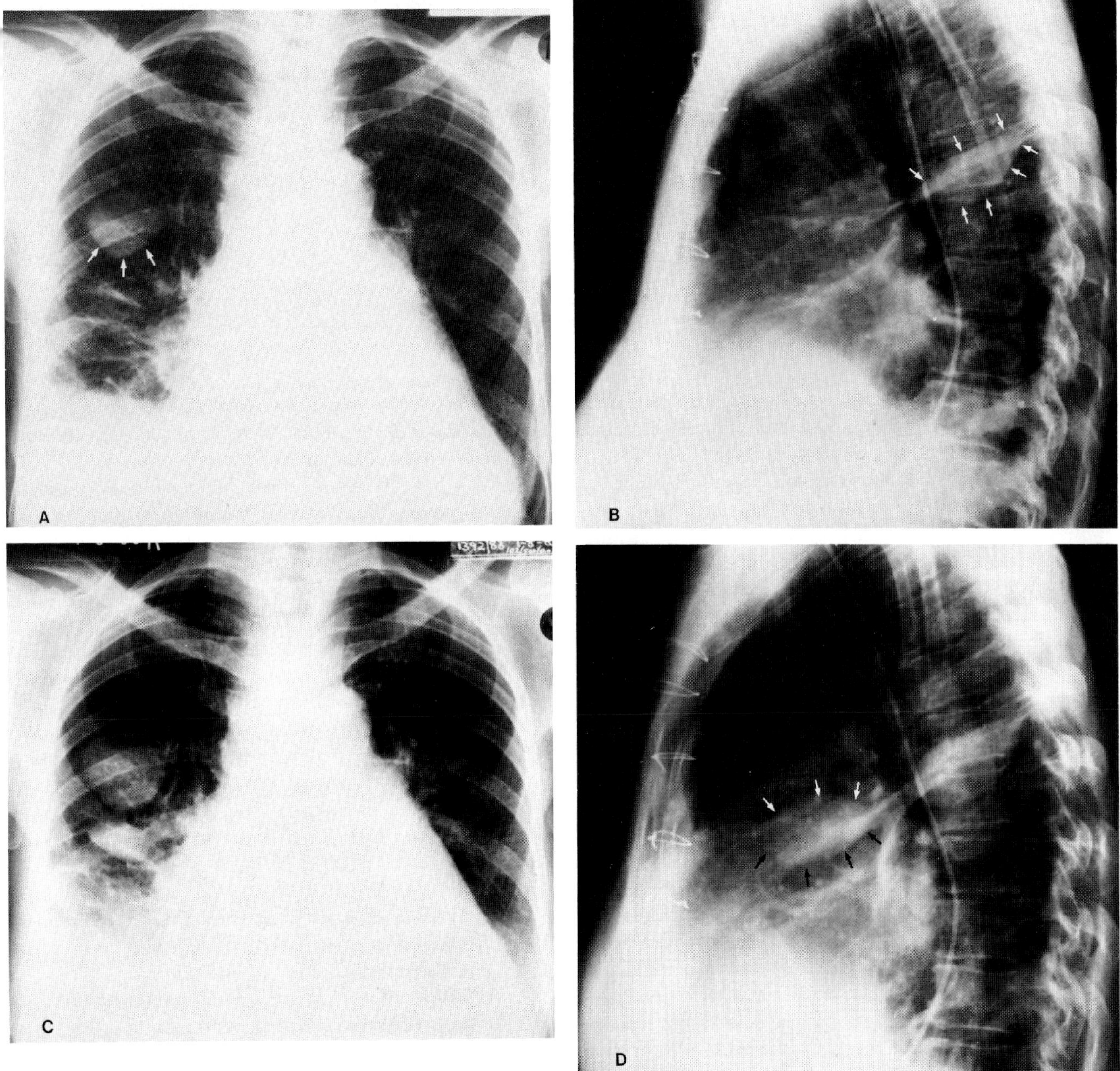

Fig. 13.9 Loculated interlobar pleural effusions. Female aged 60 years. Post-replacement of aortic root. (**A**) 19 days post-operatively a right mid zone opacity appears (arrows), with a sharp lower margin and an indistinct upper margin. The right costophrenic angle has also filled in. (**B**) Lateral projection demonstrates typical lenticular configuration of fluid loculated in the oblique fissure (arrows). (**C**) 7 days later a second round opacity has appeared below the first. This opacity is well circumscribed. (**D**) Lateral projection confirms that this is fluid loculated in the horizontal fissure (arrows).

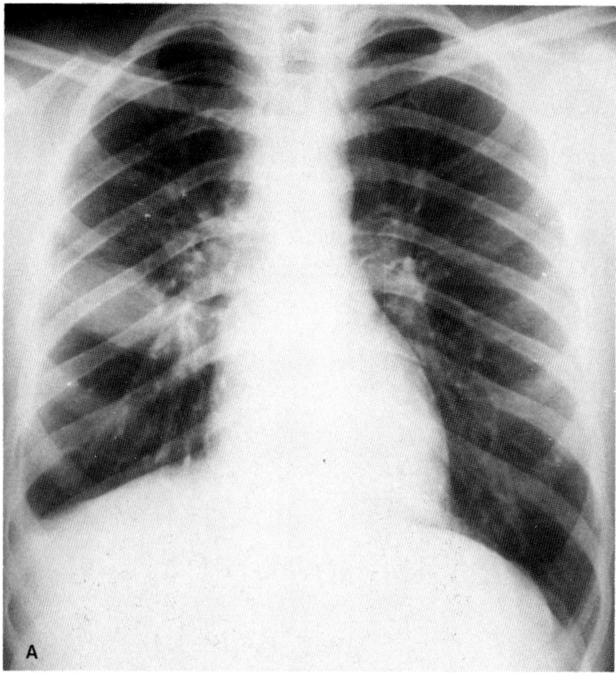

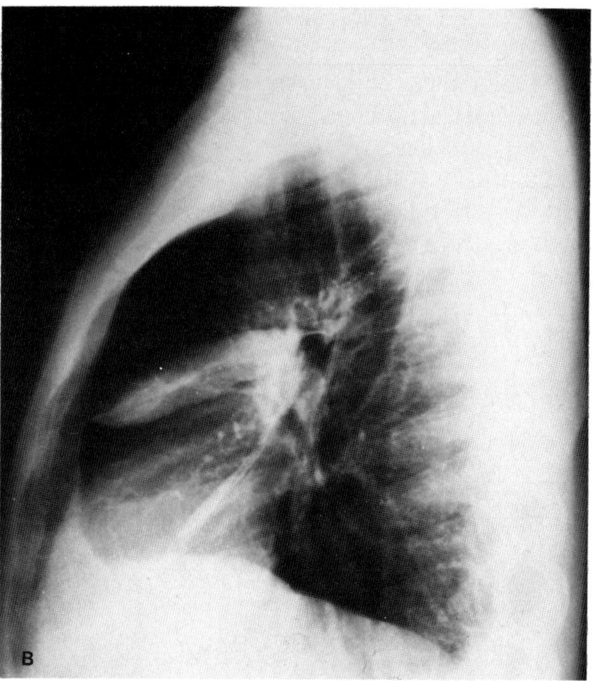

Fig. 13.10 Loculated interlobar effusion. Male aged 32 years on treatment for pulmonary tuberculosis. (**A**) PA film shows blunted right costophrenic angle, and fairly well-circumscribed right mid zone opacity. (**B**) Lateral projection shows typical lenticular configuration of fluid loculated in the horizontal fissure, and also fluid extending into oblique fissure.

radiograph, but a lateral film is usually diagnostic since the fissure is seen tangentially, and the typical lenticular configuration of the effusion is demonstrated (Fig. 13.9).

Loculated interlobar effusions can appear rounded on two views. Following treatment they may disappear rapidly, and are hence known as 'pseudo-' or 'vanishing' tumours. They may recur in subsequent episodes of heart failure. Interlobar fluid may mimic right middle lobe consolidation, but its lenticular shape and extension into the fissure are usually characteristic, and obscuration of the right heart border is very unusual (Fig. 13.10).

Pneumothorax

Pneumothorax is the presence of air in the pleural cavity. Air enters this cavity through a defect in either the parietal or the visceral pleura. Such defects are the result of lung pathology, trauma or deliberate introduction of air, respectively giving rise to *spontaneous, traumatic* or *artificial* pneumothoraces. If pleural adhesions are present the pneumothorax may be localized, otherwise it is generalized. If air can move freely in and out of the pleural space during respiration it is an *open* pneumothorax; if no movement of air occurs it is *closed*, and if air enters the pleural space on inspiration, but does not leave on expiration it is *valvular*. As intrapleural pressure increases in a valvular pneumothorax a *tension pneumothorax* develops.

Aetiology

Spontaneous pneumothorax is the commonest type, and typically occurs in young adult males, due to *rupture of a congenital pleural bleb*. Such blebs are usually in the lung apex and may be bilateral.

In older patients chronic bronchitis and emphysema are common factors. Rarer causes include bronchial asthma, rupture of a tension cyst in staphylococcal pneumonia, rupture of a sub-pleural tuberculous focus, rupture of a sub-pleural tension cyst in carcinoma of the bronchus, and rupture of a cavitating sub-pleural metastasis. Other associations include many of the causes of interstitial pulmonary fibrosis (cystic fibrosis, histiocytosis, tuberous sclerosis, sarcoidosis and some of the pneumoconioses).

Traumatic pneumothorax may be the result of a penetrating chest wound, closed chest trauma (particularly rupture of a bronchus in a road accident), rib fracture, pleural aspiration or biopsy, lung biopsy, bronchoscopy, oesophagoscopy, and positive pressure ventilation. The pleura may also be violated during mediastinal surgery and nephrectomy.

Artifical pneumothorax as treatment for pulmonary tuberculosis is now of historical interest only, as is diagnostic pneumothorax.

Radiological appearances. A small pneumothorax in a free pleural space in an erect patient collects at the apex. The lung apex retracts towards the hilum and on a frontal chest film the sharp white line of the visceral pleura will be visible, separated from the chest wall by the radiolucent pleural space, which is devoid of lung markings (Fig. 13.11). The affected lung usually remains aerated; its

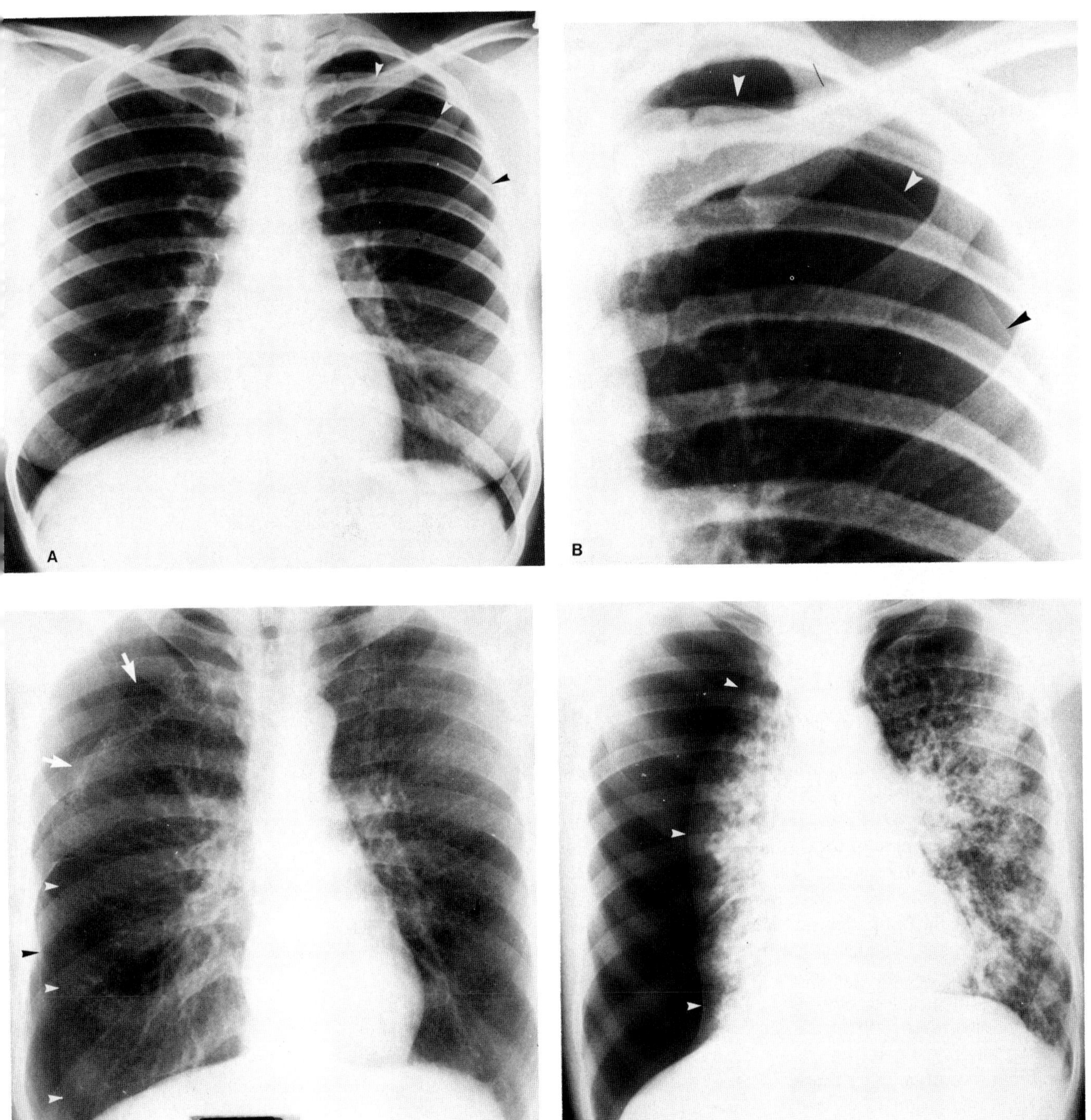

Fig. 13.11 Spontaneous pneumothoraces. (**A** and **B**) Female aged 22 years. PA film shows apical pneumothorax. The visceral pleura (arrowheads) separates aerated lung from the radiolucent pleural space. (**C**) Male aged 25 years. PA film shows a moderate pneumothorax affecting the whole lung (arrowheads), secondary to rupture of an apical bulla (arrows). (**D**) Male aged 16 years with cystic fibrosis. PA film shows diffuse nodular and ring shadows in the lungs, left hilar enlargement and a large right pneumothorax (arrowheads).

perfusion is reduced in proportion to its ventilation, and, therefore, its radiodensity remains normal. A small pneumothorax may easily go unseen, and it may be necessary to examine the film with a bright light. An expiratory film will make a closed pneumothorax easier to see since on full expiration the lung volume is at its smallest, while the volume of pleural air is unchanged. A lateral decubitus film with the affected side uppermost is sometimes helpful, as the pleural air can be seen along the lateral chest wall. This view is particularly useful in infants, since small pneumo-

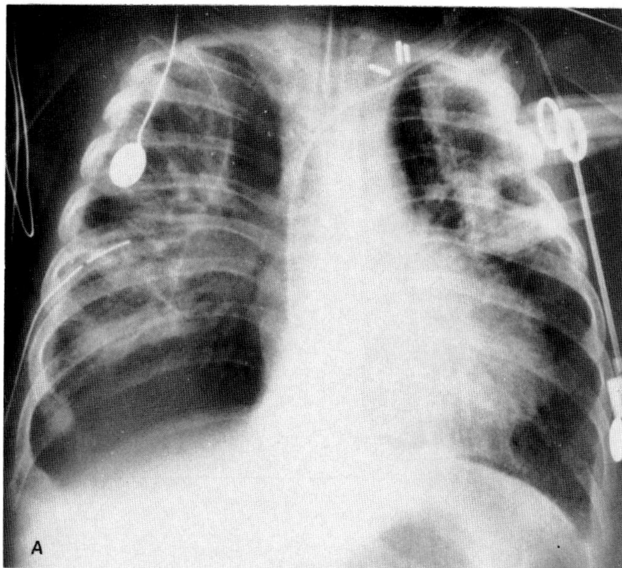

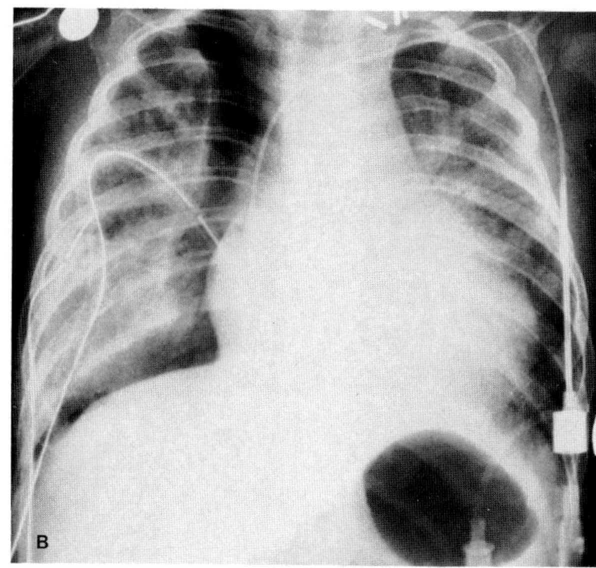

Fig. 13.12 Medial tension pneumothorax. Female aged 1 year on ventilator following closure of patent ductus arteriosus and resection of coarctation of aorta. (**A**) Supine AP film demonstrates a right pneumothorax, the intra-pleural air collecting anteriorly and medially, and the lung collapsing posteriorly and laterally. The pleural tube is situated laterally, and is, therefore, not decompressing the pneumothorax. The right hemidiaphragm is depressed, and the mediastinum is displaced to the left, indicating a tension pneumothorax. (**B**) Following insertion of another pleural tube more medially, the pneumothorax is smaller, and the right hemidiaphragm and mediastinum have returned to their normal positions.

thoraces are difficult to see in supine AP films, as the air tends to collect anteriorly and medially (Fig. 13.12).

A large pneumothorax may lead to complete relaxation and retraction of the lung, with some mediastinal shift towards the normal side, which increases on expiration.

Tension pneumothorax (Figs. 13.12 and 13.13) may lead to massive displacement of the mediastinum, kinking of the great veins and acute cardiac and respiratory embarrassment. Radiologically the ipsilateral lung may be squashed against the mediastinum, or herniate across the midline, and the ipsilateral hemidiaphragm may be depressed. On fluoroscopy the mediastinal shift to the contralateral side is greatest in inspiration, an observation that distinguishes a tension pneumothorax from a large pneumothorax not under strain.

Complications of pneumothorax. Pleural adhesions may limit the distribution of a pneumothorax and result in a loculated or *encysted pneumothorax*. The usual appearance is an ovoid air collection adjacent to the chest wall, and it may be radiographically indistinguishable from a thin-walled sub-pleural pulmonary cavity, cyst or bulla. *Pleural adhesions* are occasionally seen as line shadows stretching between the two pleural layers, preventing relaxation of the underlying lung (Fig. 13.13). Rupture of an adhesion may produce a haemopneumothorax, or discharge of an underlying infected sub-pleural lesion, leading to a pyopneumothorax. *Collapse* or *consolidation* of a lobe or lung in association with a pneumothorax are important complications which may delay re-expansion of the lung.

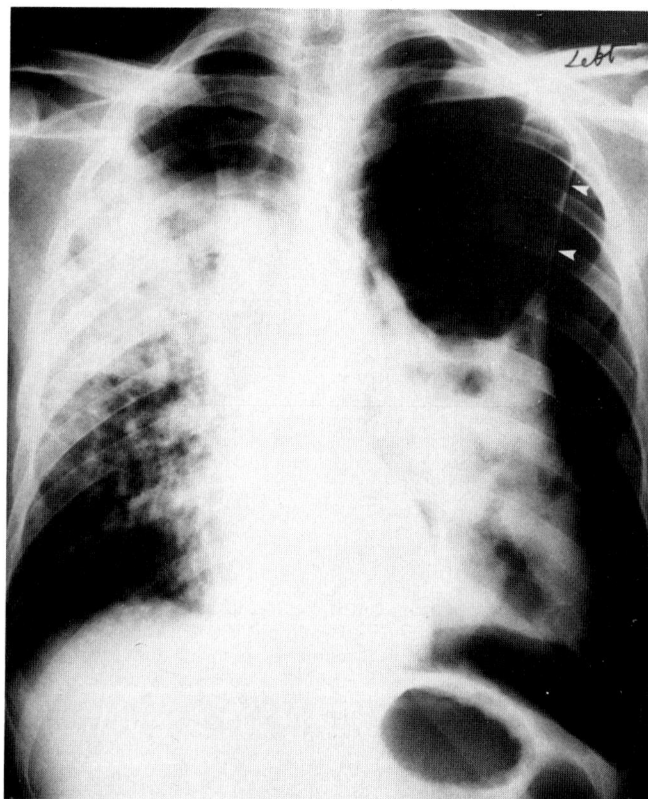

Fig. 13.13 Tension pneumothorax and pleural adhesion. Elderly male with spontaneous pneumothorax secondary to extensive cavitating pulmonary tuberculosis. The left lung is prevented from collapsing completely by the extensive consolidation, and by tethering of an adhesion (arrowheads). The mediastinum is displaced to the right.

Since the normal pleural space contains a small volume of fluid, blunting of the costophrenic angle by a short fluid level is commonly seen in a pneumothorax (Fig. 13.14). In a small pneumothorax this fluid level may be the most obvious radiological sign. A larger fluid collection usually signifies a complication and represents exudate, pus or blood, depending on the aetiology of the pneumothorax.

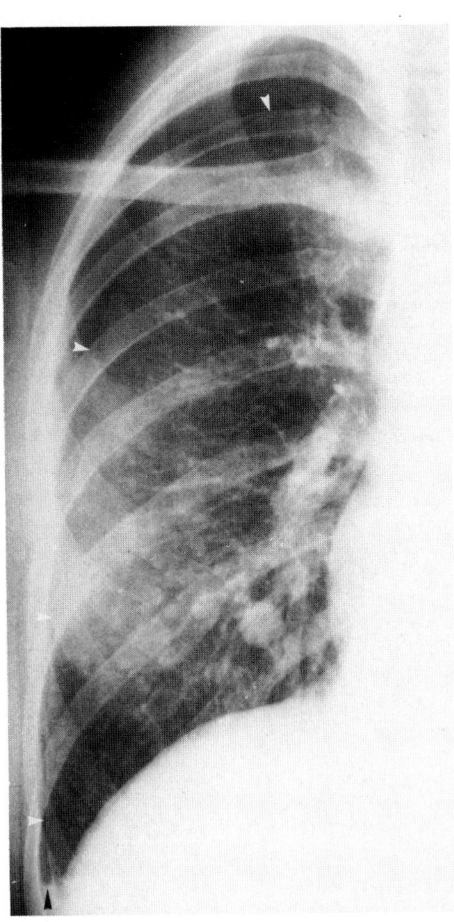

Fig. 13.14 Shallow hydropneumothorax. Male aged 18 years. Spontaneous pneumothorax probably due to rupture of sub-pleural cavitating metastatic osteogenic sarcoma. The primary tumour was in the right scapula, which has been removed, and pulmonary metastases are seen in the right lower zone. The visceral pleura is faintly seen (white arrowheads) and a short fluid level (black arrowhead) is present just above the right costo-phrenic angle.

The usual radiological appearance of a *hydropneumothorax* is that of a pneumothorax containing a horizontal fluid level which separates opaque fluid below, from lucent air above. This demonstration requires a horizontal beam film (Fig. 13.15), so that if the patient is not fit enough for an upright film a lateral decubitus film or 'shoot through' lateral film may be indicated.

If a pneumothorax becomes chronic, *thickening* of the visceral or parietal pleura may occur. The former may prevent re-expansion of the lung, and surgical decortication may be necessary if respiratory function is significantly impaired. Rarely *fibrin bodies* may develop in a chronic pneumothorax. These are small round or ovoid opacities which sometimes calcify; they may be mobile within the pleural space, and are sometimes referred to as 'pleural mice'.

Bronchopleural fistula

Bronchopleural fistula is a communication between the airway and the pleural space. It is most frequently a complication of complete or partial *pneumonectomy*, and is discussed under post-operative complications. Other causes include *carcinoma of the bronchus* and *ruptured lung abscess*. The radiological appearance is that of a hydro- or pyo-pneumothorax.

Pleural thickening

Blunting of a costophrenic angle is a frequent incidental finding on a chest X-ray. It is due to localized pleural thickening and usually results from a previous episode of pleuritis, although a previous history of chest disease is often lacking. In the asymptomatic patient and in the absence of other radiological abnormality it is of no other significance. It may mimic a small pleural effusion, and if a previous film is not available for comparison a lateral decubitus film will exclude free pleural fluid. Localized pleural thickening extending into the inferior end of an oblique fissure may produce so-called tenting of the diaphragm, and is of similar significance. This latter appearance may also result from basal intrapulmonary scarring, due to previous pulmonary infection or infarction.

Bilateral apical pleural thickening is also a fairly common finding. It is more frequent in elderly patients, and is not due to tuberculosis. Its aetiology is uncertain, but ischaemia is probably a factor. Such apical shadowing is usually symmetrical (Fig. 13.16). Asymmetric or *unilateral apical pleural thickening*, however, may be of pathological significance, especially if associated with pain. If asymmetric, apical pleural shadowing may represent a Pancoast tumour, and it is important to visualize the adjacent ribs and spine (Fig. 13.17). Penetrated films and tomography may be indicated, since evidence of bone involvement will almost certainly indicate a carcinoma.

More extensive *unilateral pleural thickening* is usually the result of a previous thoracotomy or pleural effusion. Empyema or haemothorax are especially likely to resolve with *pleural fibrosis*. Chronic pneumothorax is a rarer cause. These causes of pleural fibrosis all involve the visceral layer and the thickened pleura may calcify. If the entire lung is surrounded by fibrotic pleura, this is termed a fibrothorax. The pleural peel may be a few centimetres thick, and may cause reduced ventilation of the surrounded lung, and subsequent decrease in volume of that hemithorax. If the

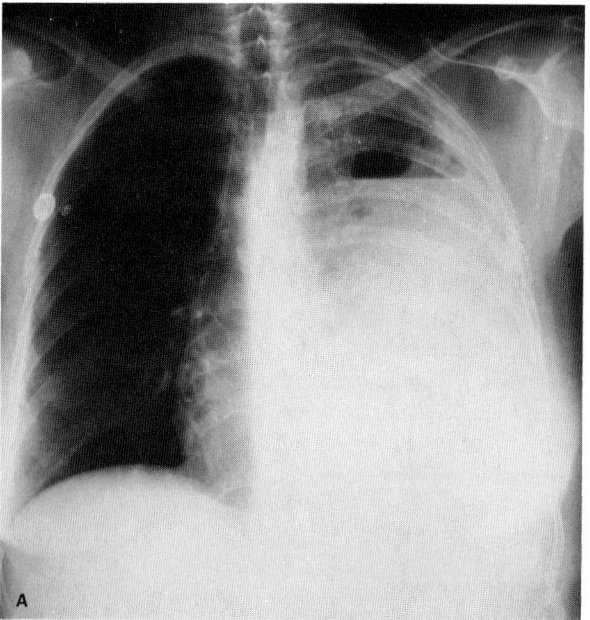

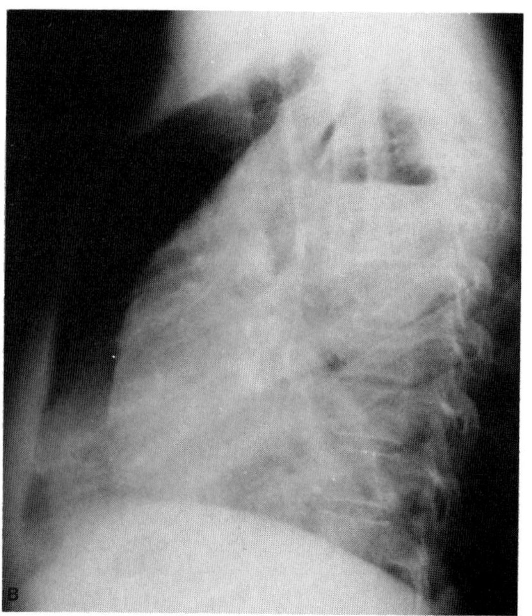

Fig. 13.15 Loculated pyo-pneumothorax. Female aged 45 years, following gunshot wound to chest. (**A**) Erect PA film shows a fluid level in the left upper zone, and pleural thickening over the apex. (**B**) Lateral film shows that the fluid level is situated posteriorly. The differential diagnosis lies between a pyo-pneumothorax and a lung abscess. (**C**) Horizontal ray left lateral decubitus film demonstrates a long fluid level (arrowheads) which can only be in the pleural cavity. Some smaller loculated collections are also seen

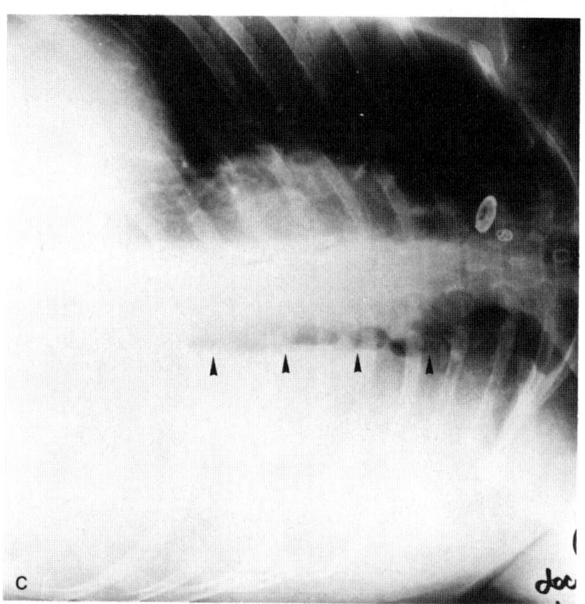

chest X-ray shows that the vascularity of the affected lung is decreased relative to the other lung, then significant ventilatory restriction is likely, and surgical decortication may be necessary.

Bilateral pleural plaques are a common manifestation of asbestos exposure, and occasionally more diffuse pleural thickening is seen (Fig. 13.18).

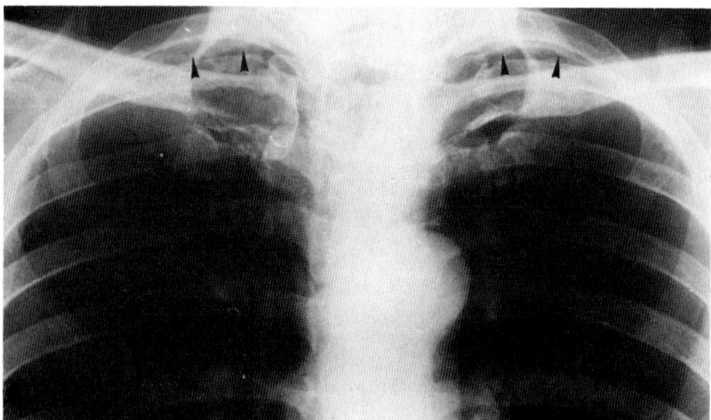

Fig. 13.16 Bilateral apical pleural thickening. An incidental finding in a 67-year-old man with ischaemic heart disease. The apical pleural shadowing (arrowheads) is symmetrical, although the edge is better seen on the left.

Pleural calcification

Pleural calcification has the same causes as pleural thickening. Unilateral pleural calcification is, therefore, likely to be the result of previous empyema, haemothorax or pleurisy, and bilateral calcification occurs after asbestos exposure and in some other pneumoconioses, or occasionally after bilateral effusions. As with the incidental finding of pleural thickening, pleural calcification may be discovered in a patient who is not aware of previous or current chest disease.

The calcification associated with previous pleurisy, empyema or haemothorax occurs in the visceral pleura, and

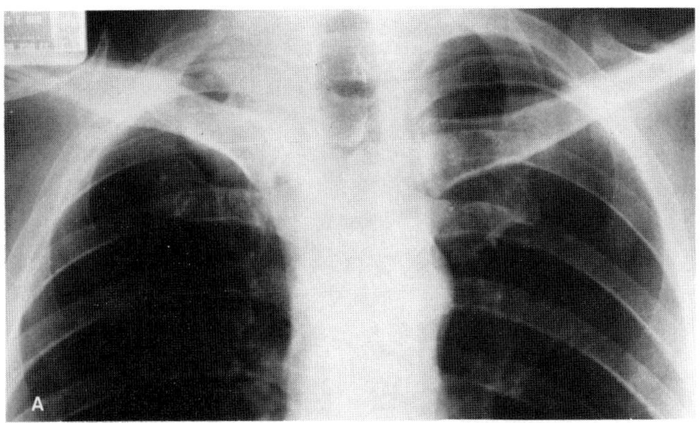

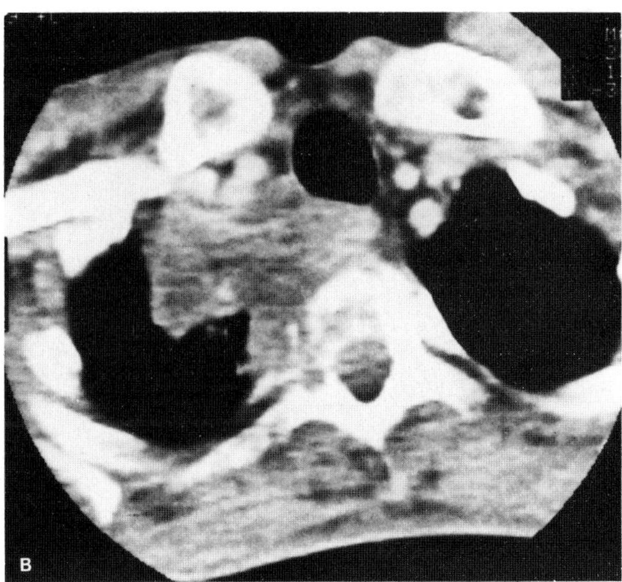

Fig. 13.17 Unilateral apical pleural thickening. Male aged 46 years with pain in right side of neck and right arm. (**A**) Dense pleural shadowing is present at the right apex. The left apex is clear. A dorsal spine film (not shown) demonstrated absence of the right pedicle of T3. (**B**) CT demonstrates a right apical mass infiltrating the third thoracic vertebra. Histology: anaplastic carcinoma.

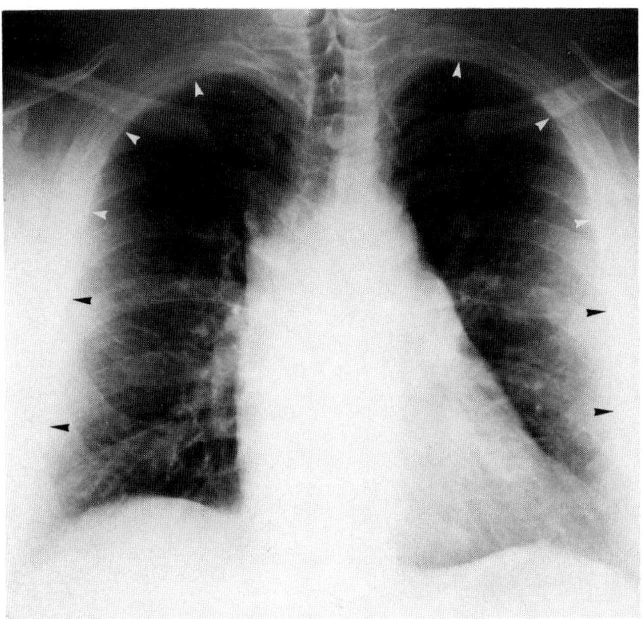

Fig. 13.18 Diffuse pleural thickening. Male aged 60 years, with history of asbestos exposure when working as a Post Office engineer and in gas works. The patient was an asymptomatic tuberculosis contact. Both lungs are surrounded by pleural thickening (arrowheads).

associated pleural thickening is almost always present, and separates the calcium from the ribs. The calcium may be in a continuous sheet or in discrete plaques, usually producing dense, coarse, irregular shadows, often sharply demarcated laterally (Fig. 13.19). If a plaque is viewed *en face* it may cast a less well-defined shadow and mimic a pulmonary infiltrate. However, a lateral view will often demonstrate the calcified plaque over the anterior or posterior pleura, but it may be necessary to fluoroscope the patient to obtain the best tangential projection for demonstration of the plaque.

The calcification associated with asbestos exposure is usually more delicate and bilateral (Fig. 13.20). It is frequently visible over the diaphragm (Fig. 13.21) and adjacent to the axillae. Tangential views show it to be situated immediately deep to the ribs, and it is in fact located in the parietal pleura (Fig. 13.22). The most sensitive method for demonstrating a pleural plaque is CT (Fig. 13.23), and ultrasound can be helpful in differentiating a plaque from loculated fluid.

Pleural tumours

Primary neoplasms of the pleura are rare. Benign tumours of the pleura include local mesothelioma (or fibroma) and lipoma. The commonest malignant disease of the pleura is metastatic (Fig. 13.24), the most frequent primary tumours being of the bronchus and breast. Primary malignancy of the pleura (malignant mesothelioma) is usually associated with asbestos exposure.

Pleural fibromas usually present with finger clubbing and joint pains due to hypertrophic osteoarthropathy, but may be an incidental finding on a chest X-ray. The radiographic appearance is of a well-defined lobulated mass adjacent to the chest wall, mediastinum, diaphragm or a pleural fissure (Fig. 13.25). The mass may be small or occupy most of the hemi-thorax (Fig. 13.26). In the presence of osteoarthropathy the diagnosis is almost certain, but if necessary percutaneous needle biopsy is probably the investigation of choice.

Sub-pleural lipomas appear as well-defined rounded masses. They may change shape with respiration being soft tumours, and if large enough may erode adjacent ribs.

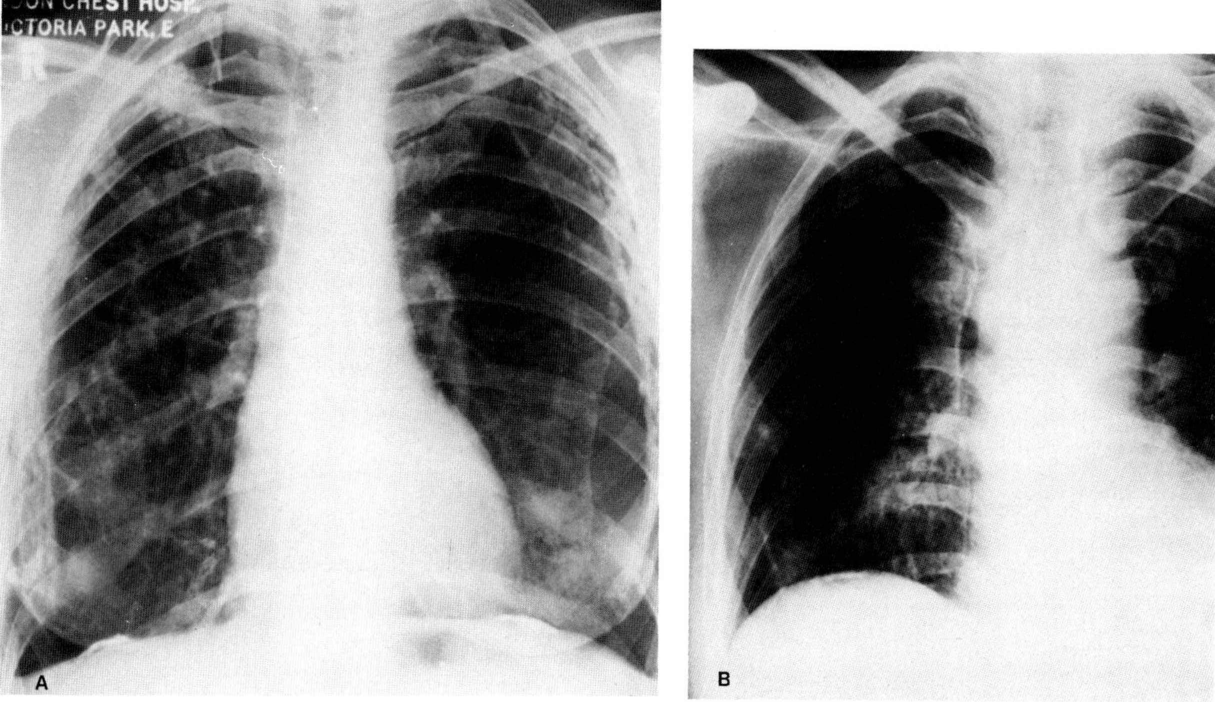

Fig. 13.19 Pleural calcification. (**A**) Middle-aged woman with history of recurrent episodes of pleurisy, presumed to be tuberculous. Extensive plaques of pleural calcification surround both lungs. (**B**) Male aged 40 years with no history of thoracic illness. Extensive pleural calcification is present around the right lung.

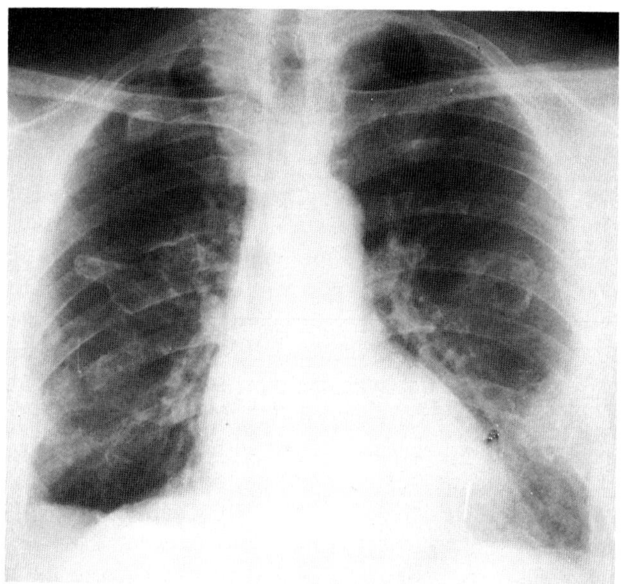

Fig. 13.20 Bilateral calcified pleural plaques due to asbestos exposure. Male aged 48 years with ischaemic heart disease — incidental finding. Pleural thickening is present in the periphery of both mid and lower zones, and calcified pleural plaques are seen *en face* in both lung fields.

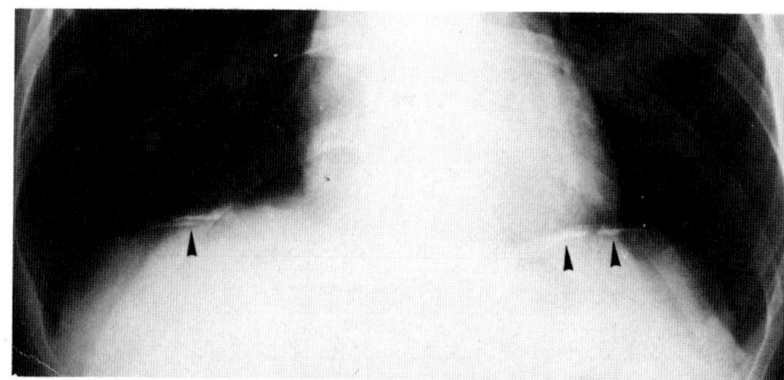

Fig. 13.21 Bilateral calcified pleural plaques due to asbestos exposure. Male age 50 years. TB contact — incidental finding. Pleural calcification is present over both domes of the diaphragm (arrowheads). The lungs appear normal

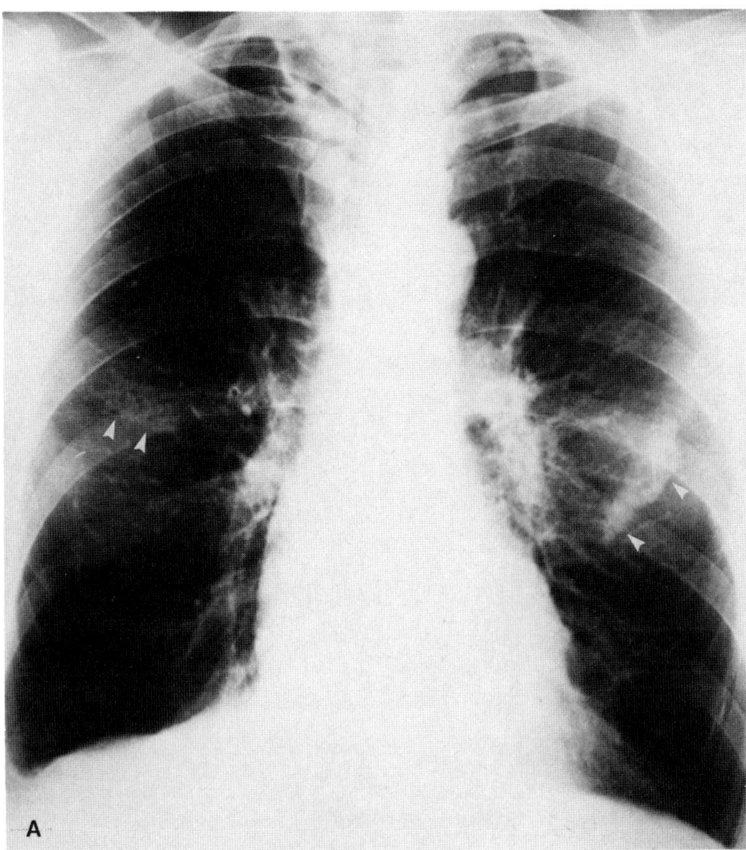

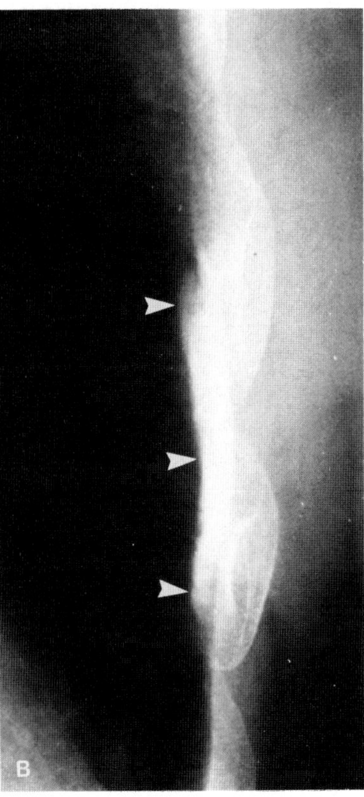

. **13.22** Pleural calcification due to asbestos exposure. Male aged 51 years with chronic obstructive airways disease. (**A**) The lungs are perinflated. Calcified pleural plaques are present in both mid zones (arrowheads). (**B**) An oblique film, aided by fluoroscopy, shows the left-ed plaque tangentially (arrowheads); it is situated in the parietal pleura, immediately deep to the ribs.

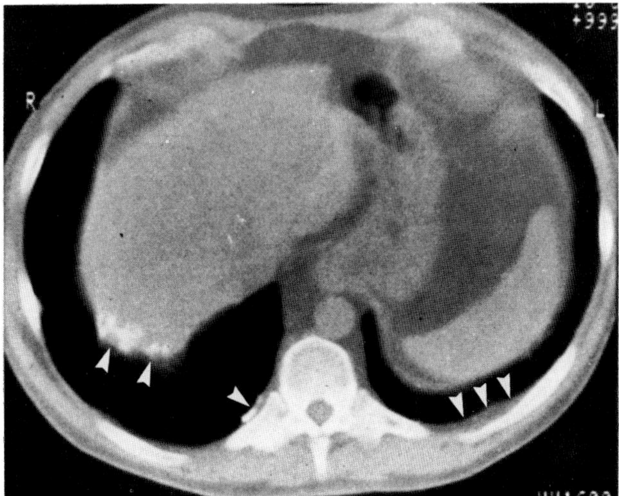

Fig. 13.23 CT demonstration of three pleural abnormalities not apparent on the PA chest film. Male aged 54 years with history of asbestos exposure. (A) A small calcified pleural plaque is present in the right paraspinal gutter (single arrowhead). (B) Pleural calcification is present over the right hemidiaphragm (two arrowheads). (C) A small left pleural effusion (three arrowheads) is present.

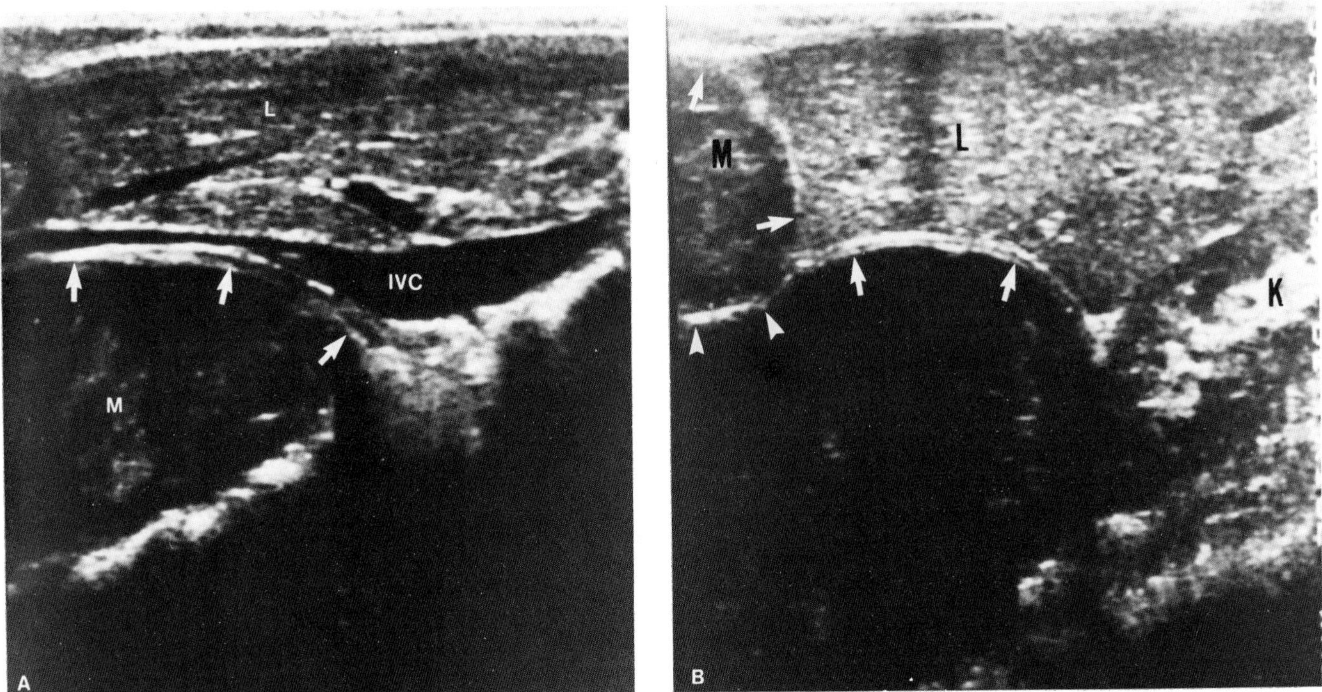

Fig. 13.24 Pleural metastases from a sarcoma. Female aged 14 years. The right hemithorax was opaque on the chest radiograph (not shown), thought to be due to a large pleural effusion. Ultrasound demonstrates pleural masses. (**A**) Sagittal scan through liver (L) and inferior vena cava (IVC). A pleural mass (M) with a few internal echoes lies adjacent to the diaphragm (arrows). (**B**) Sagittal scan through liver and right kidney (K) demonstrates eversion of the diaphragm (arrows) by pleural fluid and a mass. An interface (arrowheads) is seen between the mass and pleural fluid. (*Courtesy of Dr W. Lees.*)

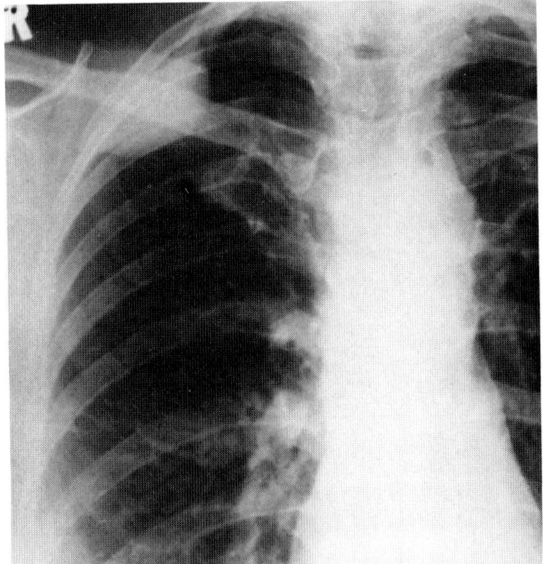

Fig. 13.25 Pleural fibroma or benign mesothelioma. Female aged 48 years. Incidental finding in patient with past history of left apical tuberculosis. A sharply demarcated peripheral upper zone opacity is present, making an obtuse angle with adjacent chest wall, and without other pleural abnormality. It was removed. Histology: benign fibrous mesothelioma.

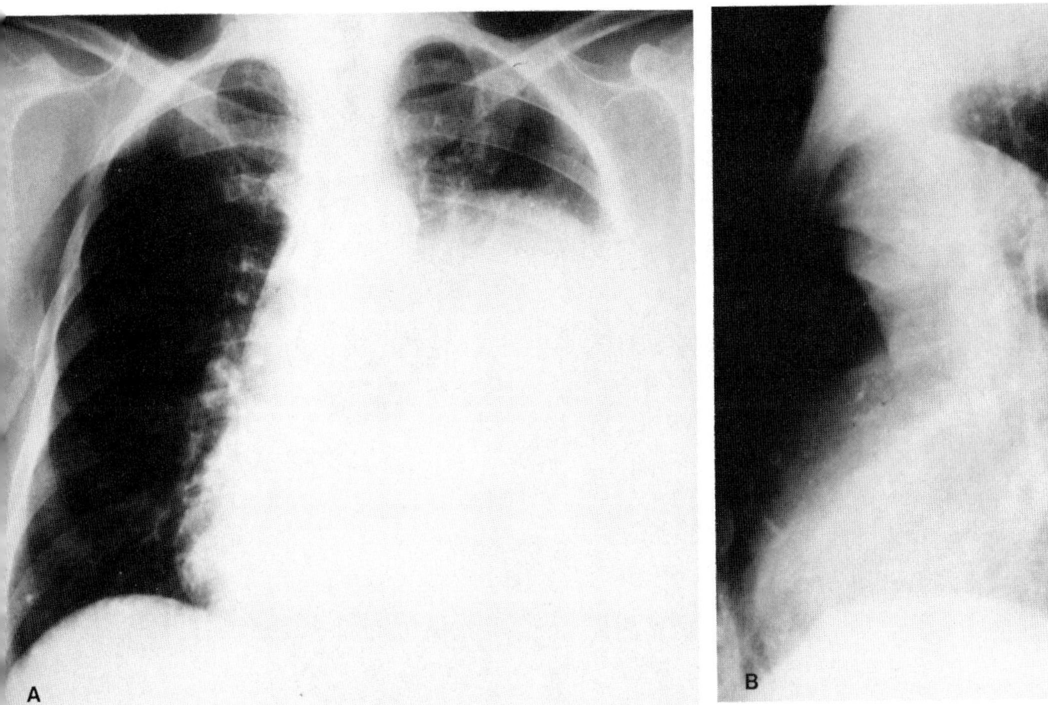

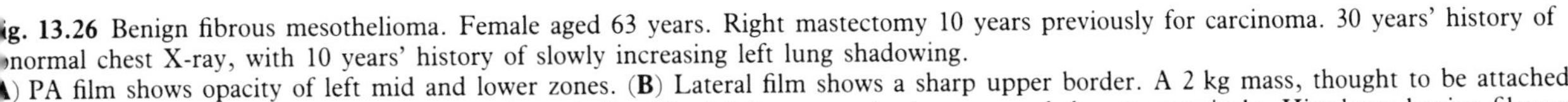

Fig. 13.26 Benign fibrous mesothelioma. Female aged 63 years. Right mastectomy 10 years previously for carcinoma. 30 years' history of abnormal chest X-ray, with 10 years' history of slowly increasing left lung shadowing.
(**A**) PA film shows opacity of left mid and lower zones. (**B**) Lateral film shows a sharp upper border. A 2 kg mass, thought to be attached to the phrenic nerve by a narrow stalk, was removed surgically. The left lung completely re-expanded post-operatively. Histology: benign fibrous mesothelioma.

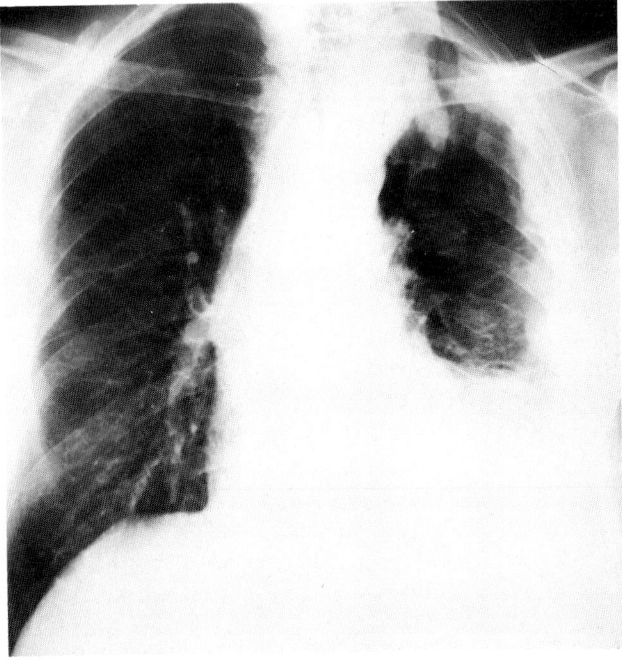

Fig. 13.27 Malignant mesothelioma of the pleura. Irregular, nodular pleural thickening surrounds the left lung. Percutaneous biopsy revealed malignant mesothelioma of mixed epithelial and fibroblastic pattern.

Malignant mesothelioma is usually due to prolonged exposure to asbestos dust, particularly crocidolite. The usual appearance is nodular pleural thickening around all or part of a lung (Fig. 13.27). A haemorrhagic pleural effusion may be present, but the lung changes of asbestosis may be absent. The effusion may obscure the pleural masses. Often the mediastinum is central, despite the presence of a large effusion, and this is thought to result from volume loss of the underlying lung secondary to either ventilatory restriction by the surrounding tumour, or bronchial stenosis by tumour compression at the hilum. Rib involvement may occur with malignant mesothelioma, but the presence of a pleural mass and adjacent rib destruction is more likely to be due to metastatic bone tumour, or possibly a primary bone tumour.

The extent of malignant mesothelioma is best assessed by CT (Fig. 13.28). CT may also help differentiate between malignant mesothelioma and benign pleural plaques. Nodular extension into fissures, pleural effusion and volume loss of the ipsilateral lung all suggest malignancy. A tissue diagnosis may be obtained by percutaneous needle biopsy.

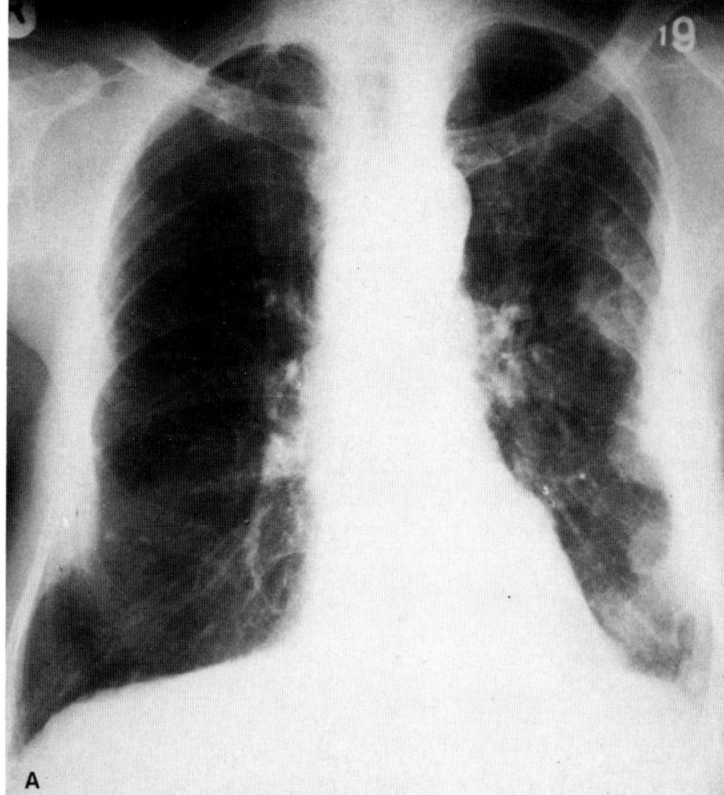

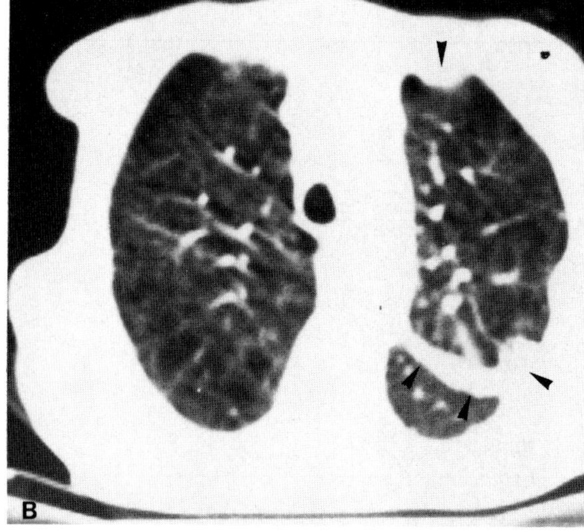

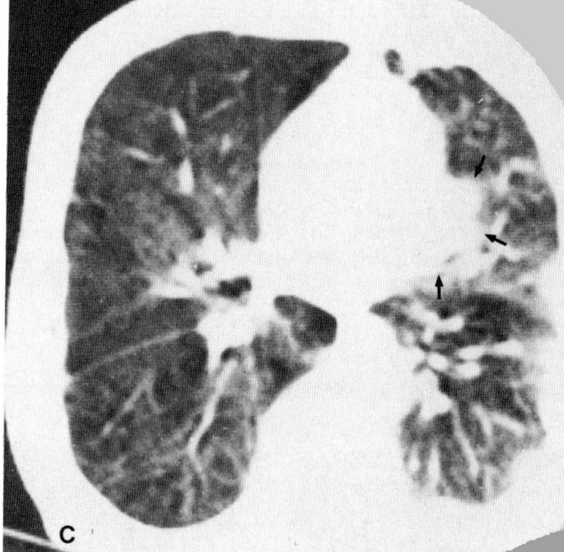

Fig. 13.28 Malignant mesothelioma. History of carcinoma of colon 14 years previously. Presents with abnormal chest radiograph (**A**) which shows lobulated left pleural opacities. (**B** and **C**) CT demonstrates reduced volume of left lung, peripheral pleural masses with extension into the oblique fissure (arrowheads), and masses adjacent to the left heart border (arrows) not seen on the chest radiograph. Percutaneous biopsy: malignant mesothelioma. (*Courtesy of Dr B. Strickland.*)

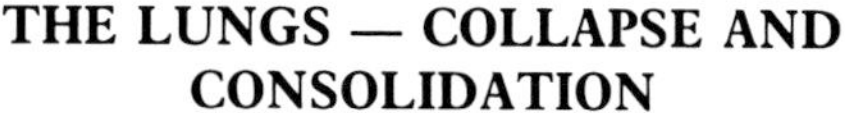

THE LUNGS — COLLAPSE AND CONSOLIDATION

COLLAPSE

Partial or complete loss of volume of a lung is referred to as collapse or atelectasis. Current usage has made these terms synonymous, and they imply a diminished volume of air in the lung with associated reduction of lung volume. This contrasts with consolidation, in which a diminished volume of air in the lung is associated with normal lung volume. Fraser and Paré describe four different mechanisms which may cause pulmonary collapse.

Mechanisms of collapse

1. *Relaxation or passive collapse.* This is the mechanism whereby the lung tends to retract towards its hilum, when air or increased fluid collects in the pleural space. It is discussed under diseases of the pleura.

2. *Cicatrization collapse.* As discussed in the section on the pleura, normal lung expansion depends upon a balance between outward forces of the chest wall and opposite elastic forces of the lung. When the lung is abnormally stiff this balance is disturbed, lung compliance is decreased and the volume of the affected lung is reduced. This occurs with pulmonary fibrosis.

3. *Adhesive collapse.* The surface tension of the alveoli is decreased by surfactant. If this mechanism is disturbed, as in the respiratory distress syndrome, collapse of alveoli occurs, although the central airways remain patent.

4. *Resorption collapse.* In acute bronchial obstruction the gases in the alveoli are steadily taken up by the blood in the pulmonary capillaries, and are not replenished, causing alveolar collapse. The degree of collapse may be modified by collateral air drift if the obstruction is distal to the main bronchus, and also by infection and accumulation of secretions. If the obstruction becomes chronic, subsequent resorption of intra-alveolar secretions and exudate may

result in complete collapse. This is the usual mechanism of collapse seen in carcinoma of the bronchus.

Radiological signs of collapse

The radiographic appearance in pulmonary collapse depends upon the mechanism of collapse, the degree of collapse, the presence or absence of consolidation, the pre-existing state of the lung and the state of the pleura. Signs of collapse may be considered as direct or indirect. Indirect signs are the results of compensatory changes which occur in response to the volume loss.

Direct signs of collapse

1. *Displacement of interlobar fissures.* This is the most reliable sign, and the degree of displacement will depend on the extent of the collapse.
2. *Loss of aeration.* Increased density of a collapsed area of lung may not become apparent until collapse is almost complete. However, if the collapsed lung is adjacent to the mediastinum or diaphragm, obscuration of the adjacent structures may indicate loss of aeration.
3. *Vascular and bronchial signs.* If a lobe is partially collapsed crowding of its vessels may be visible; if an air bronchogram is visible, the bronchi may appear crowded.

Indirect signs of collapse

1. *Elevation of the hemidiaphragm.* This sign may be seen in lower lobe collapse, but is rare in collapse of the other lobes.
2. *Mediastinal displacement.* In upper lobe collapse the trachea is often displaced towards the affected side, and in lower lobe collapse the heart may be displaced.
3. *Hilar displacement.* The hilum may be elevated in upper lobe collapse, and depressed in lower lobe collapse.
4. *Compensatory hyperinflation.* The normal part of the lung may become hyperinflated, and it may appear hypertransradiant with its vessels more widely spaced than in the corresponding area of the contralateral lung. If there is considerable collapse of a lung, compensatory hyperinflation of the contralateral lung may occur, with herniation across the midline.

Patterns of collapse

An air bronchogram is almost never seen in resorption collapse, but is usual in passive and adhesive collapse, and may be seen in cicatrization collapse if fibrosis is particularly dense.

Pre-existing lung disease, such as fibrosis, and pleural adhesions may alter the expected displacement of anatomic landmarks in lung collapse. There also tends to be a reciprocal relationship between the compensatory signs, e.g. in lower lobe collapse, if hemidiaphragmatic elevation is marked, hilar depression will be diminished.

Complete collapse of a lung

Complete collapse of a lung, in the absence of pneumothorax or large pleural effusion or extensive consolidation, causes opacification of the hemithorax, displacement of the mediastinum to the affected side and elevation of the diaphragm. Compensatory hyperinflation of the contralateral lung occurs, often with herniation across the midline (Fig. 13.29). Herniation most often occurs in the retrosternal space, anterior to the ascending aorta, but may occur posterior to the heart or under the aortic arch.

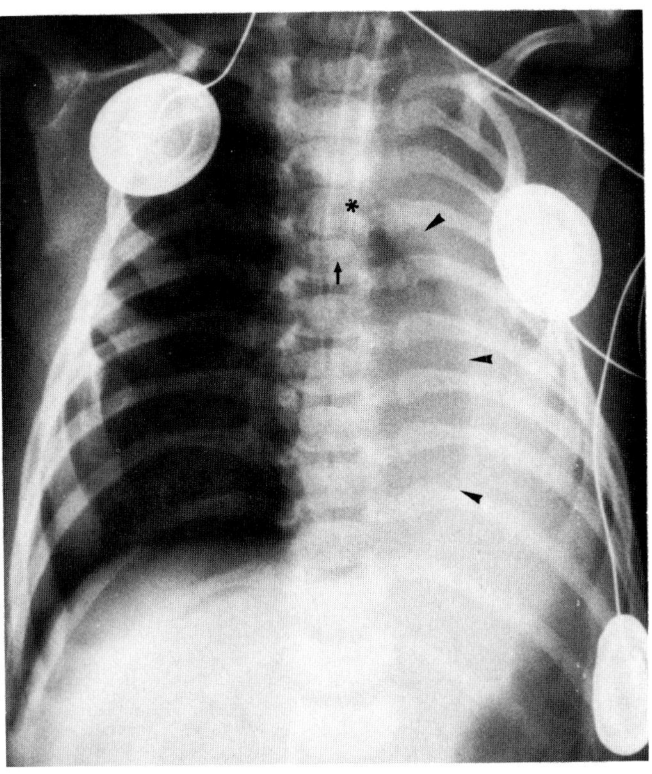

Fig. 13.29 Complete collapse of the left lung. A newborn child with complex cyanotic heart disease. The tip of the endotracheal tube (arrow) is beyond the carina (asterisk) and down the right bronchus, causing collapse of the left lung, and compensatory hyperinflation of the right lung, which has herniated across the mid-line (arrowheads).

Lobar collapse

The following descriptions describe collapse of individual lobes, uncomplicated by pre-existing pulmonary or pleural disease. The line drawings (Figs. 13.30, 13.32, 13.34, 13.36 and 13.39) represent the alteration in position of the fissures as seen in the frontal and lateral projections, resulting from increasing degrees of collapse. Only the fissures are represented. The indirect signs of collapse are not indicated.

Right upper lobe collapse (Figs. 13.30 & 13.31) The normal horizontal fissure is usually at the level of the right fourth

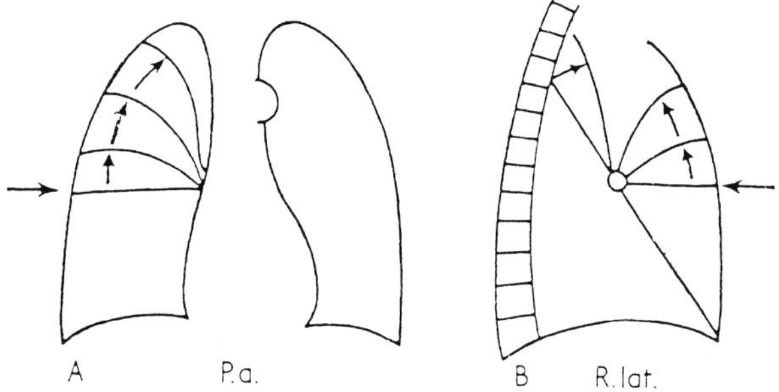

Fig. 13.30 Right upper lobe collapse. (**A**) PA projection. Note how lesser fissure is drawn upwards, and often curved, towards the apex and mediastinum. (**B**) Right lateral view. Lesser fissure also displaced upwards. Note some forward displacement of greater fissure above the hilum.

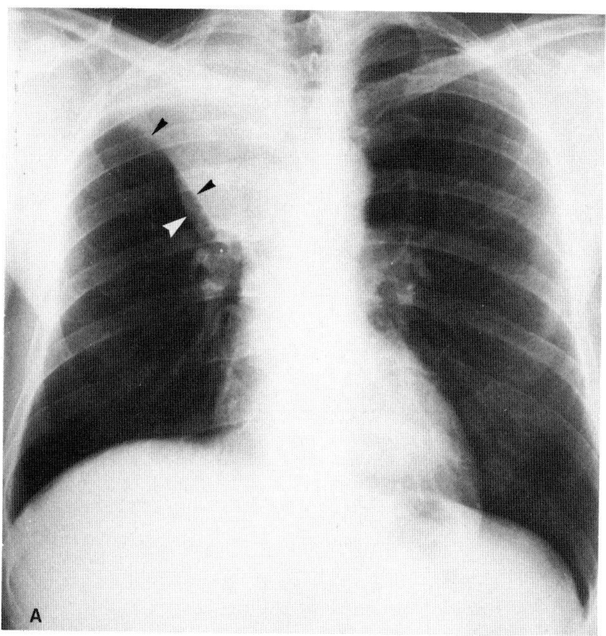

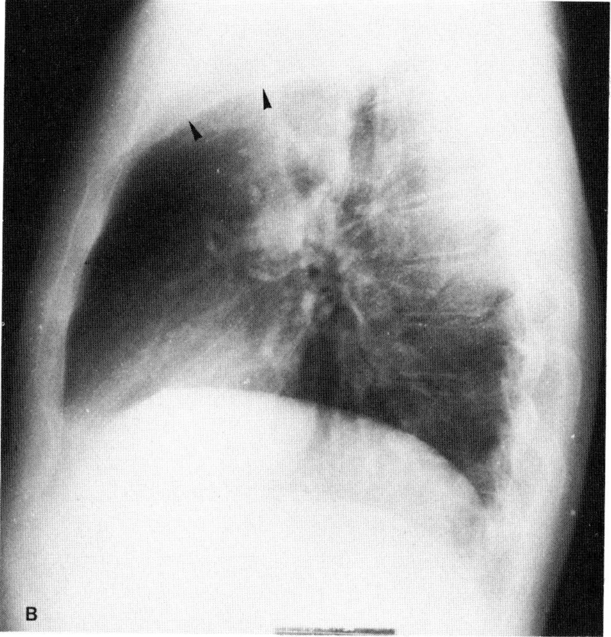

Fig. 13.31 Right upper lobe collapse. Male aged 54 years with squamous carcinoma of right upper lobe. (**A**) PA film shows a mass (white arrowhead) above the right hilum, and elevation of the horizontal fissure (black arrowheads). There is compensatory hyperinflation of the right lower lobe. (**B**) Lateral film shows anterior displacement of part of oblique fissure (arrowheads).

rib anteriorly. As the right upper lobe collapses the horizontal fissure pivots about the hilum, its lateral end moving upwards and medially towards the superior mediastinum, and its anterior end moves upwards towards the apex. The upper half of the oblique fissure moves anteriorly. The two fissures become concave superiorly. In severe collapse the lobe may be flattened against the superior mediastinum, and may obscure the upper pole of the hilum. The hilum is elevated, and its lower pole may be prominent. Deviation of the trachea to the right is usual, and compensatory hyperinflation of the right middle and lower lobes may be apparent.

Right middle lobe collapse (Figs. 13.32 and 13.33). In right middle lobe collapse the horizontal fissure and lower half of the oblique fissure move towards one another. This ca best be seen in the lateral projection. The horizontal fissu tends to be more mobile, and, therefore, usually show greater displacement. Signs of right middle lobe collaps are often subtle on the frontal projection, since the horizontal fissure may not be visible, and increased opaci does not become apparent until collapse is almo complete. However, obscuration of the right heart bord is often present, and may be the only clue in this projection. The lordotic AP projection brings the displace fissure into the line of the X-ray beam, and may elegant demonstrate right middle lobe collapse. Since the volum of this lobe is relatively small, indirect signs of volume lo are rarely present.

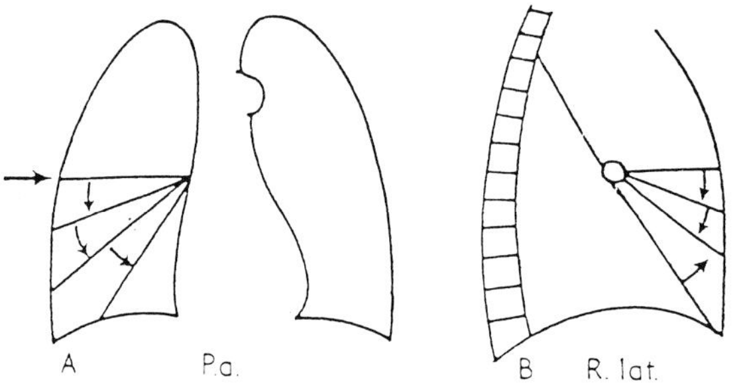

Fig. 13.32 Right middle lobe collapse. In both projections the lesser fissure is drawn downwards. In the PA view the fissure finally merges with the mediastinum and disappears. Note in the lateral view that the lower part of the greater fissure may be displaced forwards.

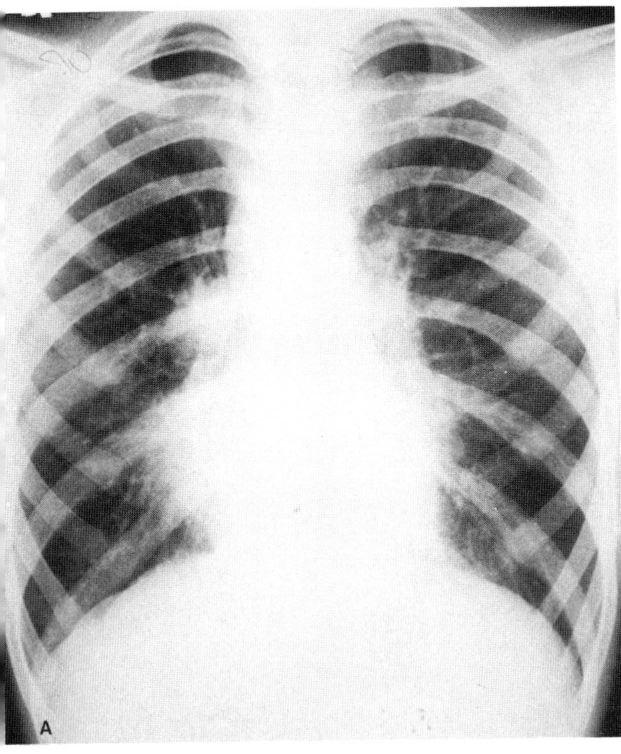

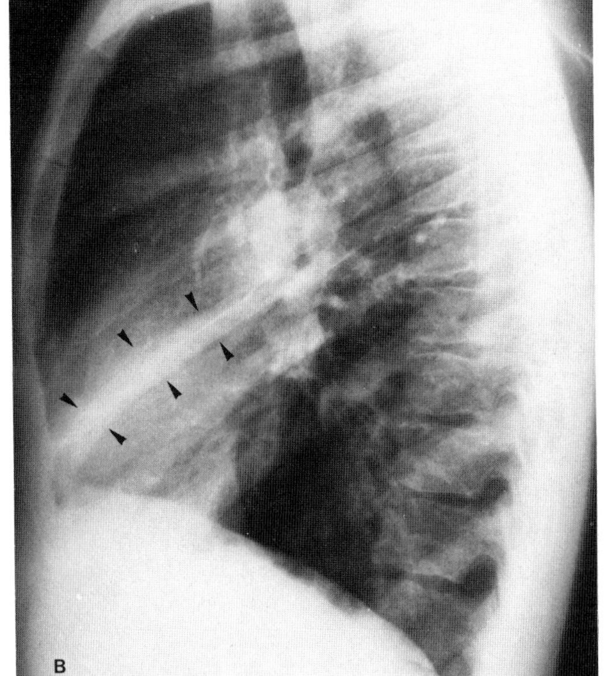

ig. 13.33 Right middle lobe collapse. (A) PA film shows obscuration right heart border, indicating loss of aeration of part of right middle be. (B) Lateral film shows complete collapse of right middle lobe rrowheads) as a thin opacity between the displaced horizontal and blique fissures. (C) Lordotic film brings the collapsed wedge of tissue to profile — an elegant but unnecessary demonstration in this case.

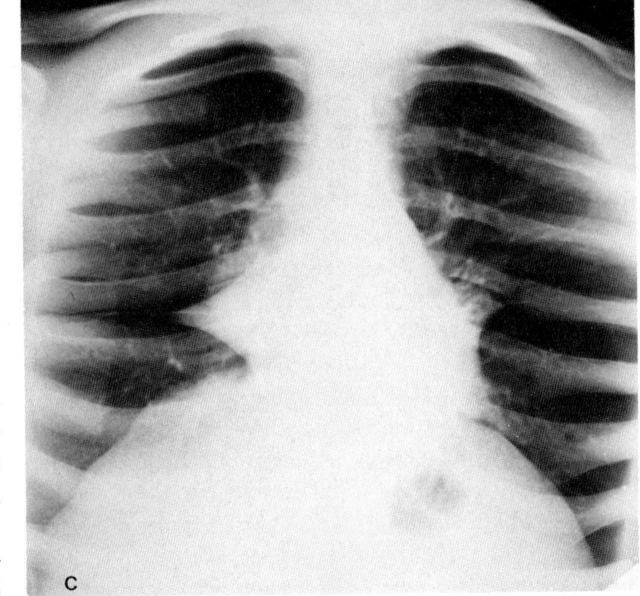

Lower lobe collapse (Figs. 13.34–13.37). The normal oblique issures extend from the level of the fourth thoracic ertebra posteriorly to the diaphragm, close to the ternum, anteriorly. The position of these fissures on the ateral projection is the best index of lower lobe volumes. When a lower lobe collapses its oblique fissure moves posteriorly but maintains its normal slope. In addition to posterior movement, the collapsing lower lobe causes nedial displacement of the oblique fissure, which may then become visible in places on the frontal projection.

Right lower lobe collapse causes depression of the horizontal fissure, which may be apparent on the frontal projection. Increased opacity of a collapsed lower lobe is usually visible on the frontal projection. A completely

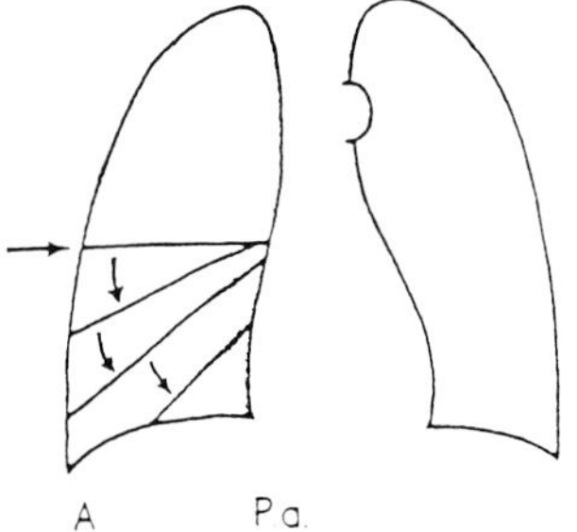

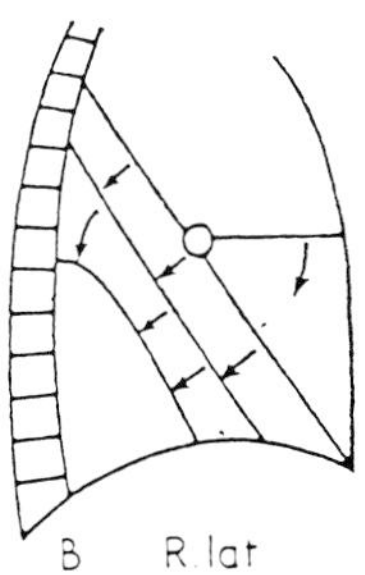

Fig. 13.34 Right lower lobe collapse. In the PA projection the greater fissure is not visible until the collapse is fairly complete. The lesser fissure is displaced downwards as in collapse of middle lobe. The degree of displacement seen may be greater in collapse of the lower lobe than of the middle lobe, as the middle lobe tends to retract towards the hilum and the fissure may disappear. In the lateral view, the oblique fissure moves backwards, tending to retain its obliquity. The upper part of the oblique fissure may curve backwards and downwards, so becoming visible in the PA projection.

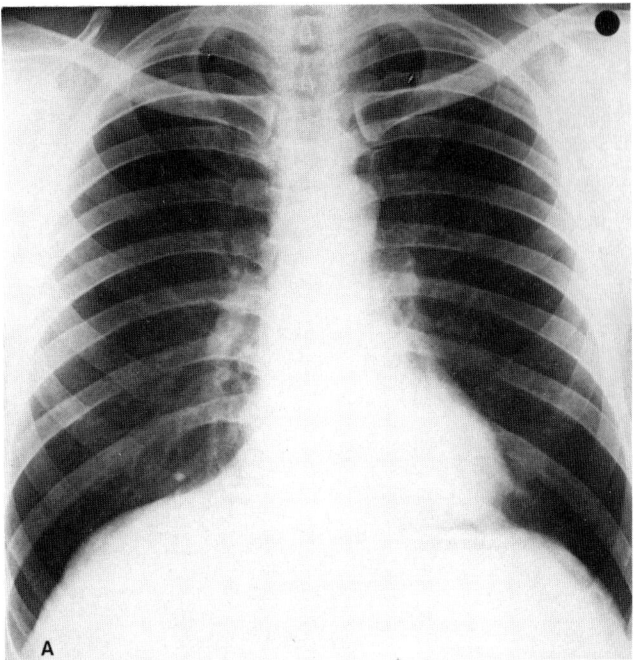

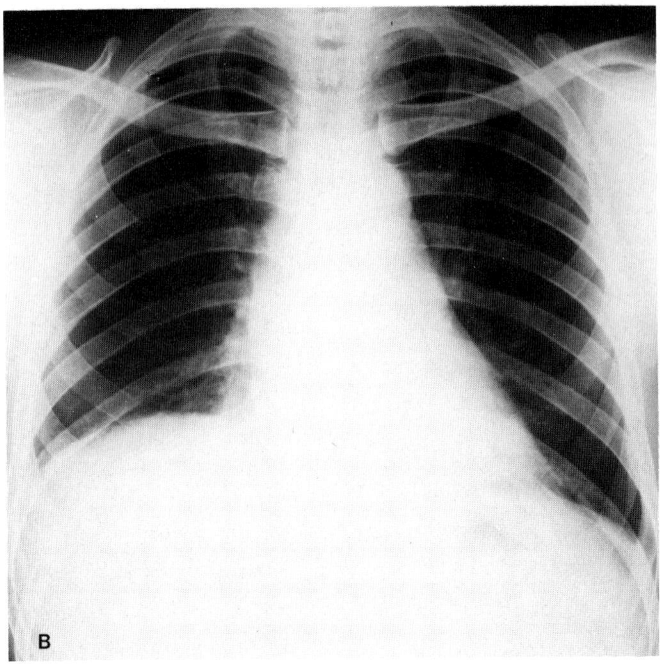

Fig. 13.35 Right lower lobe collapse. Male aged 49 years with ischaemic heart disease. (**A**) Normal pre-operative film. (**B**) Following coronary artery bypass surgery the right lower lobe has collapsed with depression and medial rotation of the hilum, elevation of the right hemidiaphragm and hyperinflation of the right upper lobe.

collapsed lower lobe may be of such small volume that it flattens and merges with the mediastinum, producing a thin, wedge-shaped shadow. On the left this shadow may be obscured by the heart, and a penetrated view with a grid may be required for its visualization. If complete left lower lobe collapse is still in doubt a right oblique film may demonstrate the wedge of tissue between spine and diaphragm. Mediastinal structures and parts of the diaphragm adjacent to the non-aerated lobe are obscured.

The hilum is usually depressed and rotated medially, and upper lobe hyperinflation is evident, but diaphragmatic elevation is not usual.

Lingular collapse (Fig. 13.38). The lingula is often involved in collapse of the left upper lobe, but it may collapse individually, when the radiological features are similar to right middle lobe collapse. However, the absence of a horizontal fissure on the left makes anterior displacement of the lower half of the oblique fissure and increased opacity anterior to it important signs. On the frontal projection the left heart border becomes obscured.

Left upper lobe collapse (Figs. 13.38–13.40). The pattern of upper lobe collapse is different in the two lungs. Left upper lobe collapse is apparent on the lateral projection as anterior displacement of the entire oblique fissure, which becomes orientated almost parallel to the anterior chest wall. With increasing collapse the upper lobe retracts posteriorly and loses contact with the anterior chest wall.

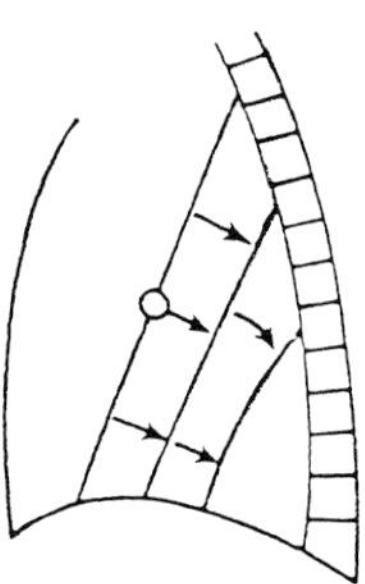

Fig. 13.36 Left lower lobe collapse. No fissure is visible in the PA projection. The lateral view shows that the greater fissure is displaced posteriorly as in collapse of the right lower lobe. The upper part of the fissure may also be drawn downwards as well as backwards.

The space between the collapsed lobe and the sternum becomes occupied by either hyperinflated left lower lobe or herniated right upper lobe. With complete collapse, the left upper lobe may lose contact with the chest wall and diaphragm and retract medially against the mediastinum. On a lateral film, therefore, left upper lobe collapse appears as an elongated opacity extending from the apex and reaching, or almost reaching the diaphragm; it is anterior to the hilum and is bounded by displaced oblique fissure posteriorly, and by hyperinflated lower lobe anteriorly.

A collapsed left upper lobe does not produce a sharp outline on the frontal view. An ill-defined hazy opacity is

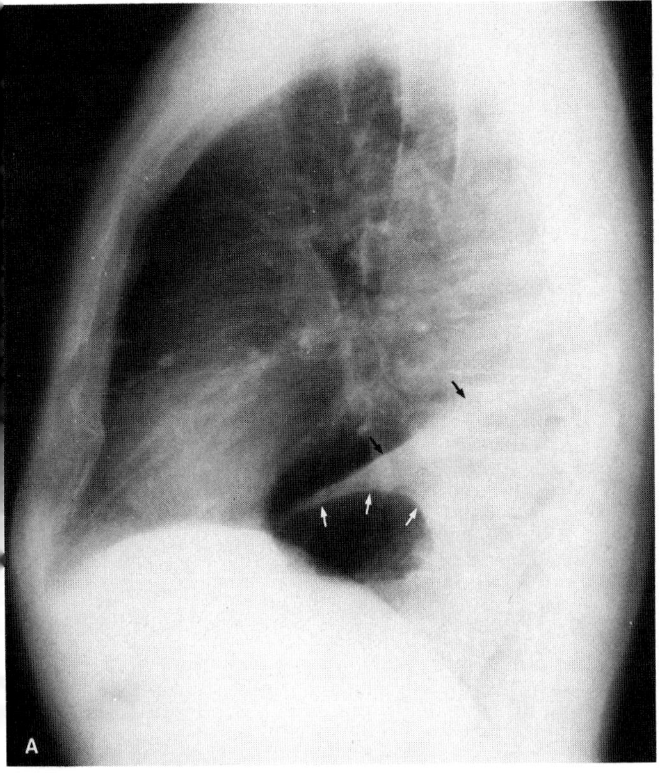

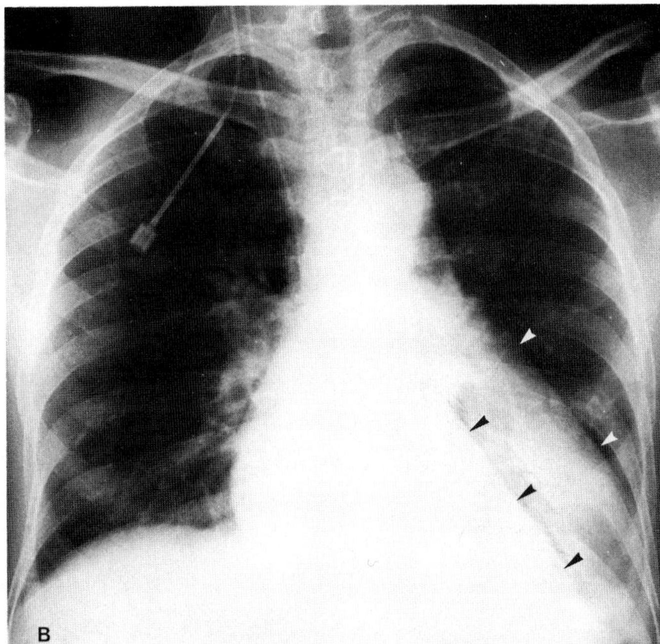

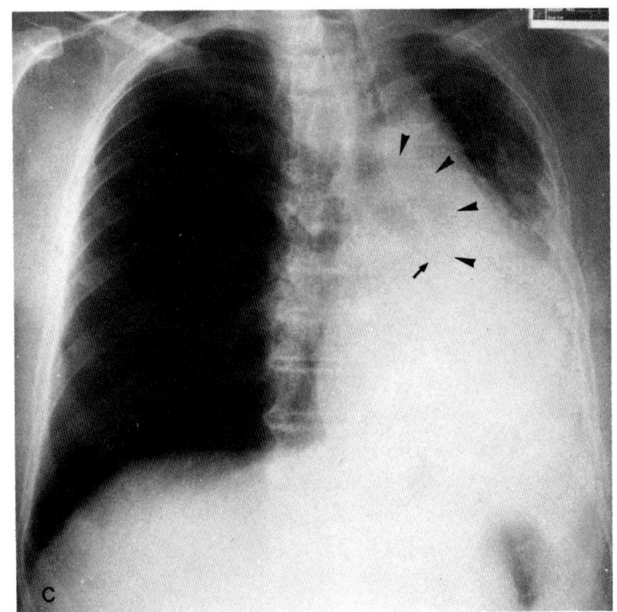

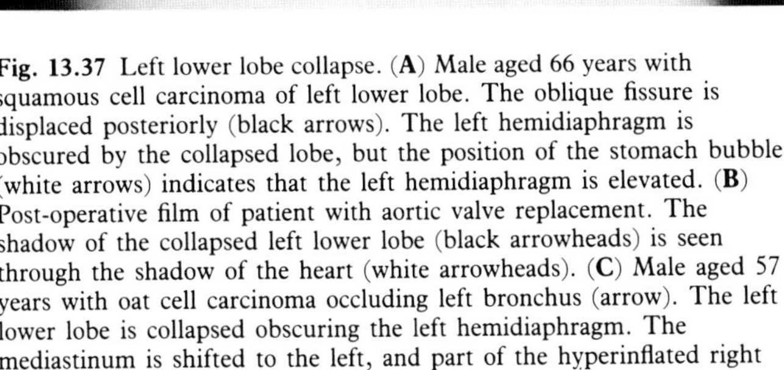

Fig. 13.37 Left lower lobe collapse. (**A**) Male aged 66 years with squamous cell carcinoma of left lower lobe. The oblique fissure is displaced posteriorly (black arrows). The left hemidiaphragm is obscured by the collapsed lobe, but the position of the stomach bubble (white arrows) indicates that the left hemidiaphragm is elevated. (**B**) Post-operative film of patient with aortic valve replacement. The shadow of the collapsed left lower lobe (black arrowheads) is seen through the shadow of the heart (white arrowheads). (**C**) Male aged 57 years with oat cell carcinoma occluding left bronchus (arrow). The left lower lobe is collapsed obscuring the left hemidiaphragm. The mediastinum is shifted to the left, and part of the hyperinflated right lung has herniated across the mid-line (arrowheads).

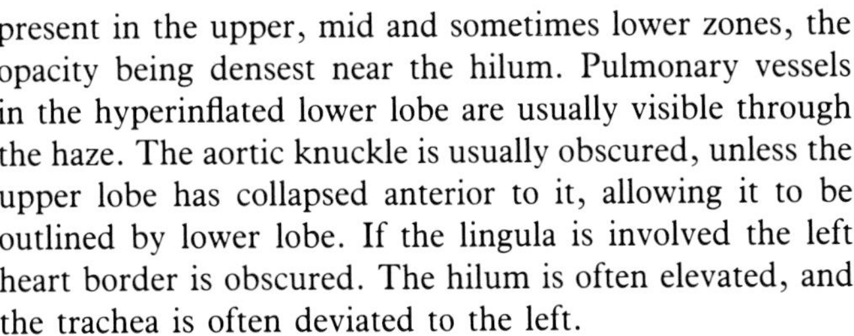

present in the upper, mid and sometimes lower zones, the opacity being densest near the hilum. Pulmonary vessels in the hyperinflated lower lobe are usually visible through the haze. The aortic knuckle is usually obscured, unless the upper lobe has collapsed anterior to it, allowing it to be outlined by lower lobe. If the lingula is involved the left heart border is obscured. The hilum is often elevated, and the trachea is often deviated to the left.

Rounded atelectasis (Fig. 13.41). This is a rare form of collapse, but is mentioned because it may be misdiagnosed as a pulmonary mass. It appears as a homogeneous mass, of up to 5 cm. diameter, with ill-defined edges. It is always pleural-based, and associated with chronic pleural thickening. Vascular shadows may be seen to radiate from part of the opacity, mimicking a comet's tail. The appearance is caused by peripheral lung tissue folding in on itself. It may be related to asbestos exposure, but is probably not of any other pathological significance.

CONSOLIDATION

Functionally the pulmonary airways can be divided into two groups. The proximal airways function purely as a conducting network; the airways distal to the terminal bronchioles are also conducting structures, but more important, are the site of gaseous exchange. These terminal airways are termed acini, an acinus comprising respiratory

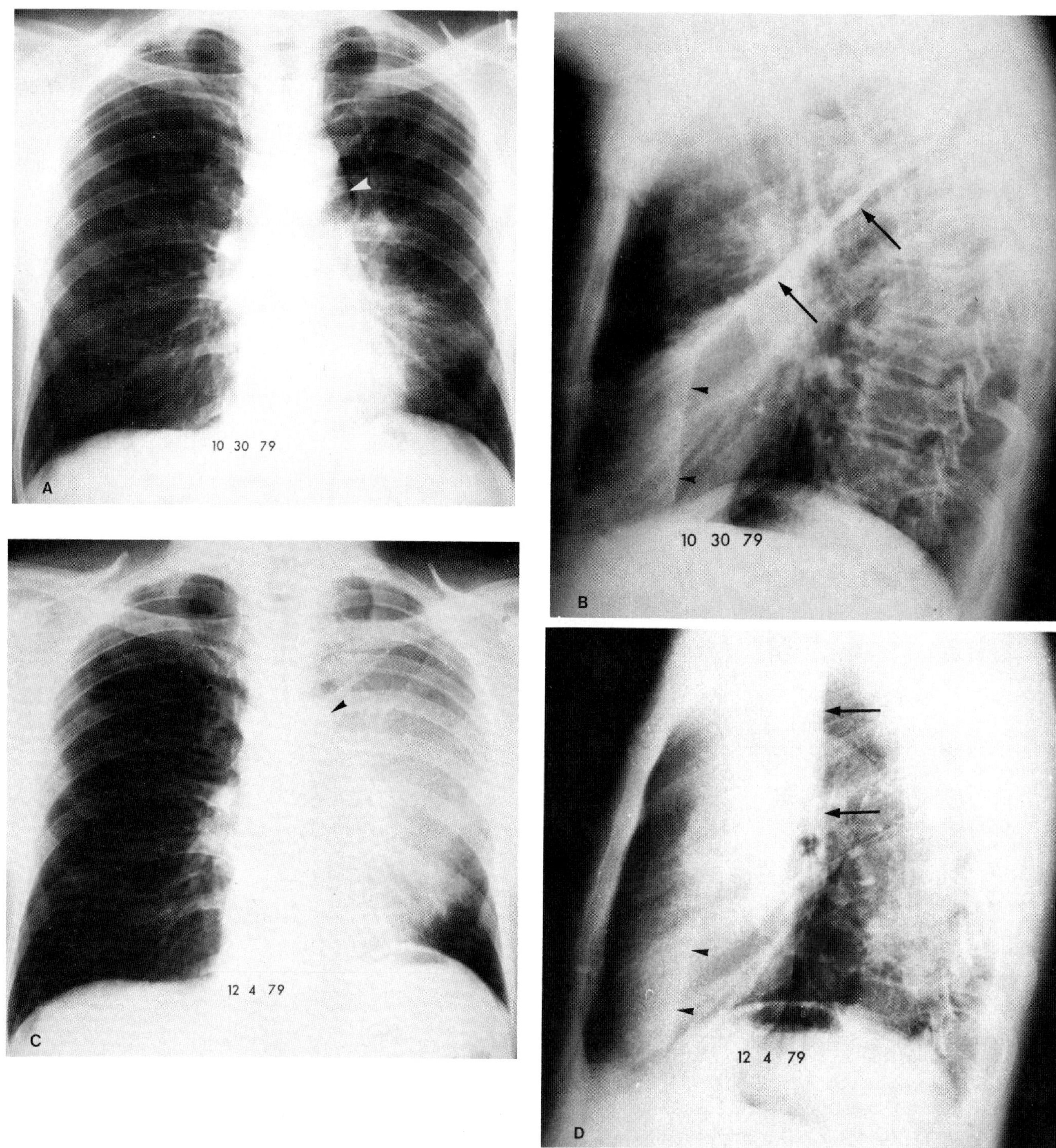

Fig. 13.38 Lingular and left upper lobe collapse. Adult male with carcinoma at left hilum. (**A**) PA film shows hazy left heart border indicating loss of aeration of lingula. A mass is present in the aortico-pulmonary window (arrowheads). (**B**) Lateral film shows collapse-consolidation of lingula, with anterior displacement of lower part of oblique fissure (arrowheads). The upper part of the oblique fissure (arrows) is thickened, but in normal position. (**C**) 5 weeks later the left upper lobe has collapsed. A hazy opacity covers most of the left hemithorax. Vessels in the hyperinflated left lower lobe can just be seen through the haze, and the aortic knuckle is obscured (arrowhead). (**D**) Lateral film shows that the oblique fissure is now displaced anteriorly (arrows).

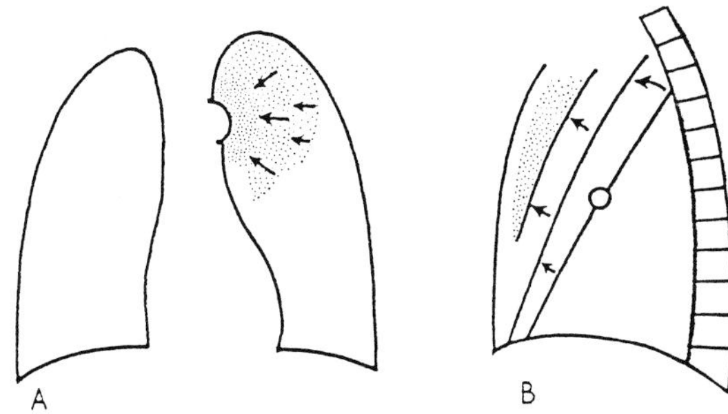

Fig. 13.39 Left upper lobe collapse. (**A**) The greater fissure does not become visible in the PA projection. When the degree of collapse is fairly complete the lobe shows a uniform loss of translucency (this may be due to accompanying consolidation), which increases in density as the degree of collapse increases. Vessel markings seen through this opacity are those in the overexpanded lower lobe. (**B**) In the lateral view, initially the fissure moves bodily forward, the lingula remaining in contact with the diaphragm. With increasing collapse the lingula retracts upwards; and the bulk of the upper lobe moves posteriorly, and becomes separated from the sternum by aerated lung. This is usually overexpanded lower lobe, though occasionally a portion of the right lung may herniate across the mid-line.

bronchioles, alveolar ducts, alveolar sacs and alveoli arising from a terminal bronchiole. Consolidation implies replacement of air in one or more acini by fluid or solid material, but does not imply a particular pathology or aetiology. The smallest unit of consolidated lung is a single acinus, which casts a shadow approximately 7 mm. in diameter. Communications between the terminal airways allow fluid to spread between adjacent acini, so that larger confluent areas of consolidation are generally visible and are frequently not confined to a single segment.

The commonest cause of consolidation is acute inflammatory exudate associated with pneumonia. Other causes include *cardiogenic pulmonary oedema, non-cardiogenic pulmonary oedema, haemorrhage* and *aspiration. Neoplasms* such as alveolar cell carcinoma and lymphoma can produce consolidation, and *alveolar proteinosis* is a rare cause. In an individual patient consolidation may be due to more than one basic aetiology. For example a patient with major head trauma may be particularly susceptible to infection, aspiration and non-cardiogenic pulmonary oedema.

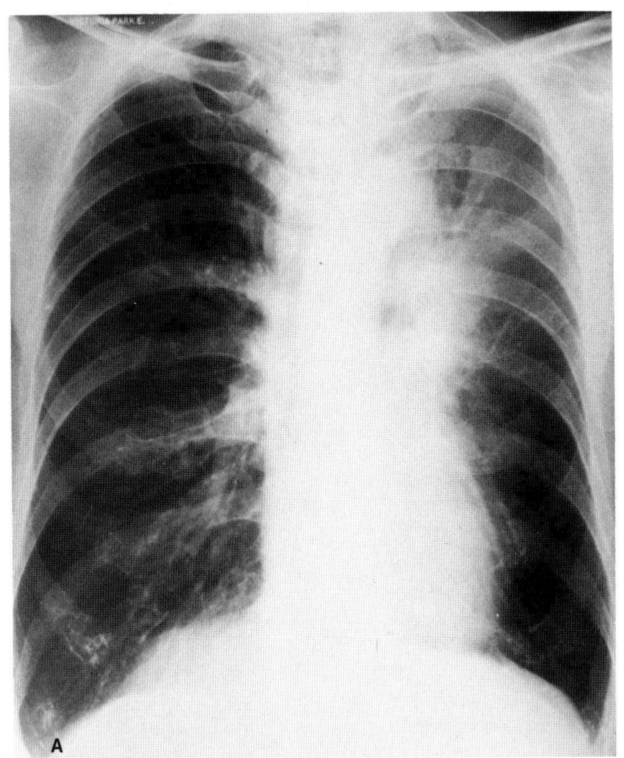

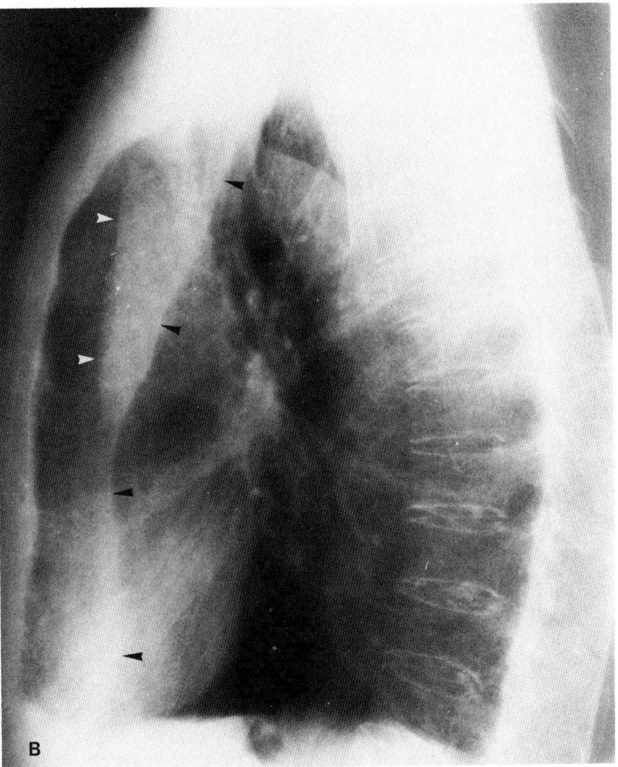

Fig. 13.40 Left upper lobe collapse, due to squamous cell carcinoma. (**A**) PA film shows typical upper zone haze, through which are seen the elevated and enlarged left hilum, and vessels of the hyperinflated lower lobe. The contour of the aortic knuckle is indistinct, but the decending aorta is sharply outlined. (**B**) Lateral film shows the collapsed left upper lobe between the anteriorly displaced oblique fissure (black arrows) and part of the hyperinflated lower lobe.

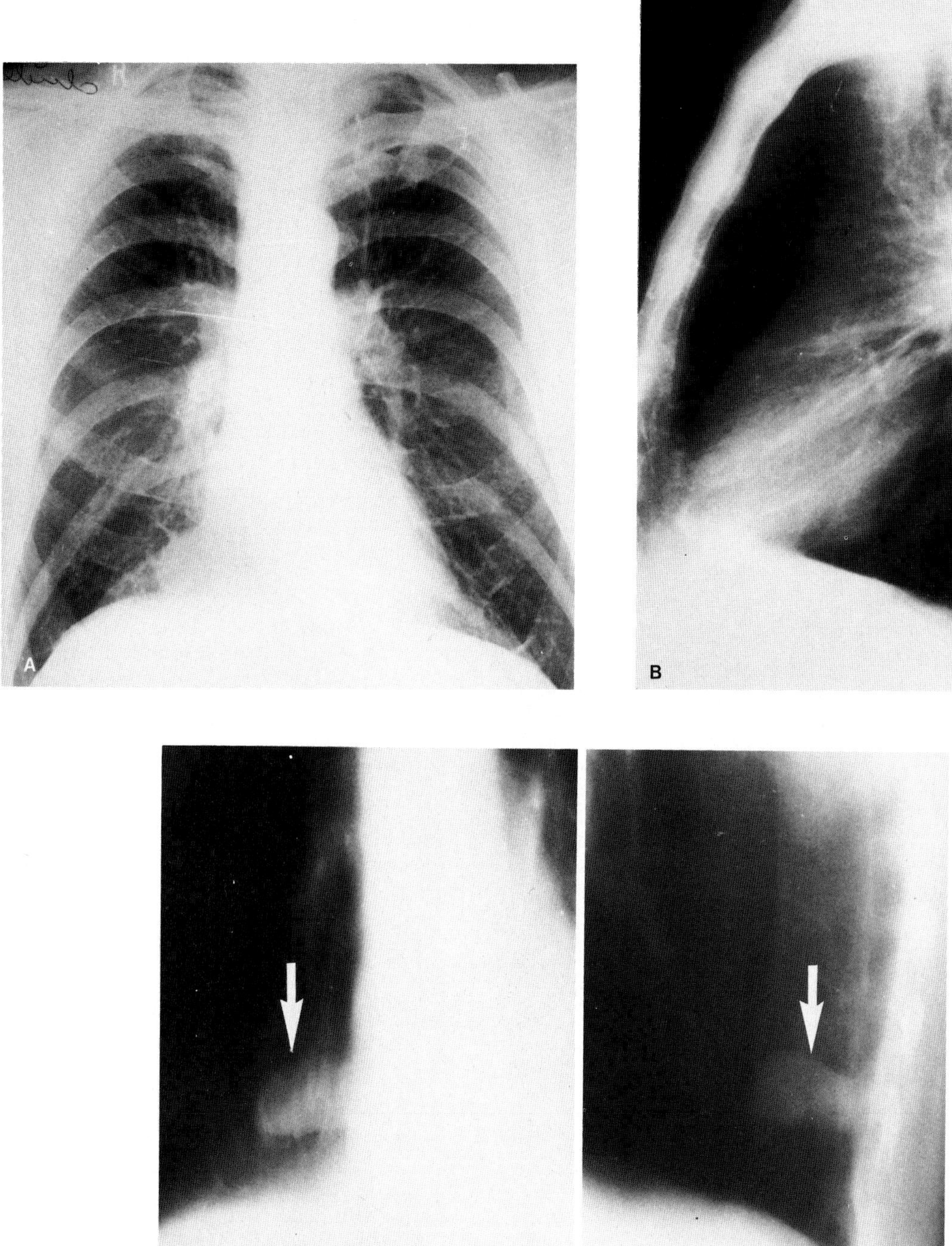

Fig. 13.41 Rounded atelectasis. (**A**) PA film shows a round opacity overlying the right cardiophrenic angle. (**B**) Lateral film shows a posterior pleural-based mass and (**C** and **D**) tomography confirms a pleural-based mass with associated pleural thickening. Following a negative percutaneous needle biopsy a thoracotomy was performed and revealed normal lung.

When consolidation is associated with a patent conducting airway an *air bronchogram* (Fig. 13.44) is often visible. This sign is produced by the radiographic contrast between the column of air in the airway and the surrounding opaque acini. If consolidation is secondary to bronchial obstruction, however, the air in the conducting airway is resorbed, and replaced by fluid, and the affected area is of uniform density.

The volume of purely consolidated lung is similar to normal lung since air is replaced by a similar volume of fluid or solid. However, collapse and consolidation are often associated with one another. When consolidation is due to

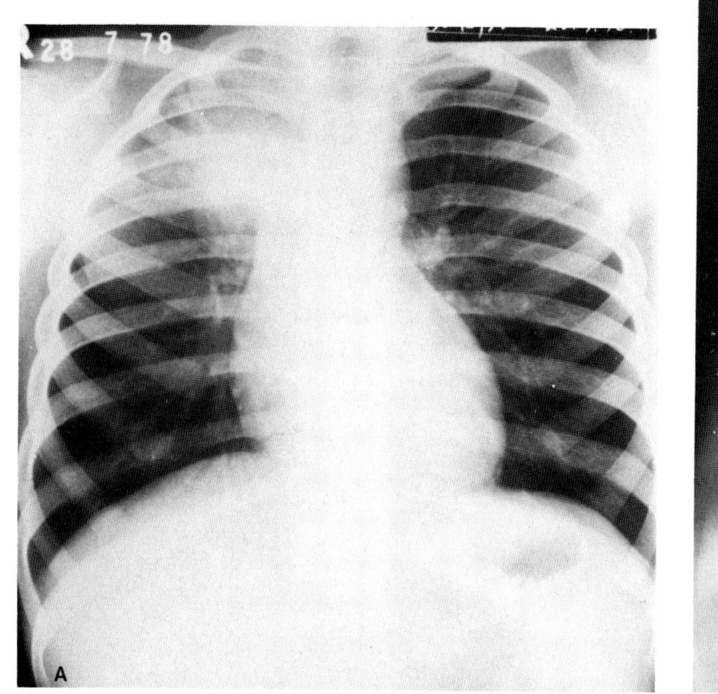

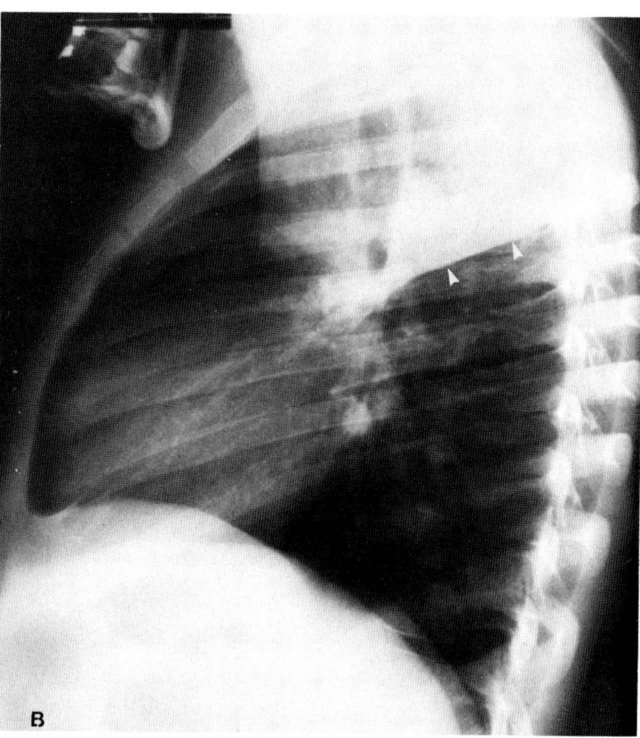

Fig. 13.42 Right upper lobe consolidation. Male aged 6 years with aortic valve disease. (**A**) Opacity in the right upper zone obscures the upper mediastinum. (**B**) Lateral film shows consolidation anterior to the upper part of the oblique fissure (arrowheads), mostly in the posterior segment of the right upper lobe.

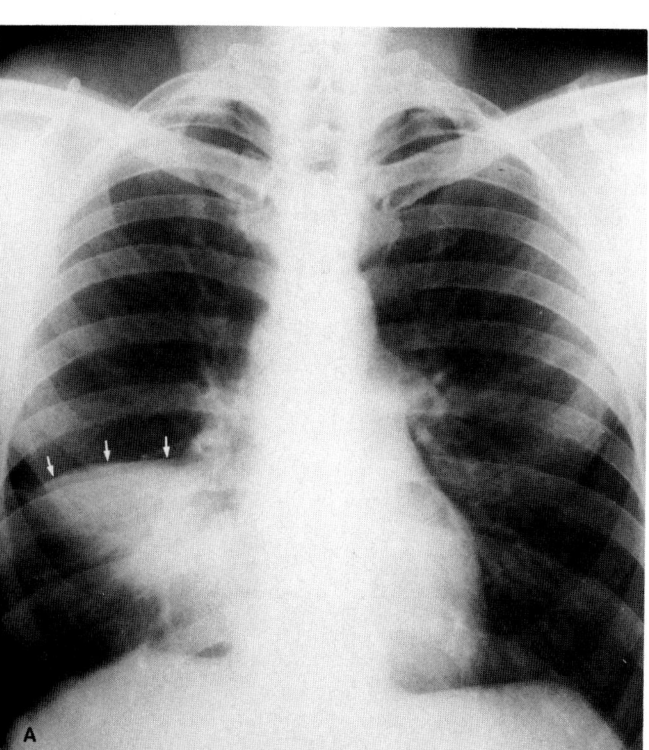

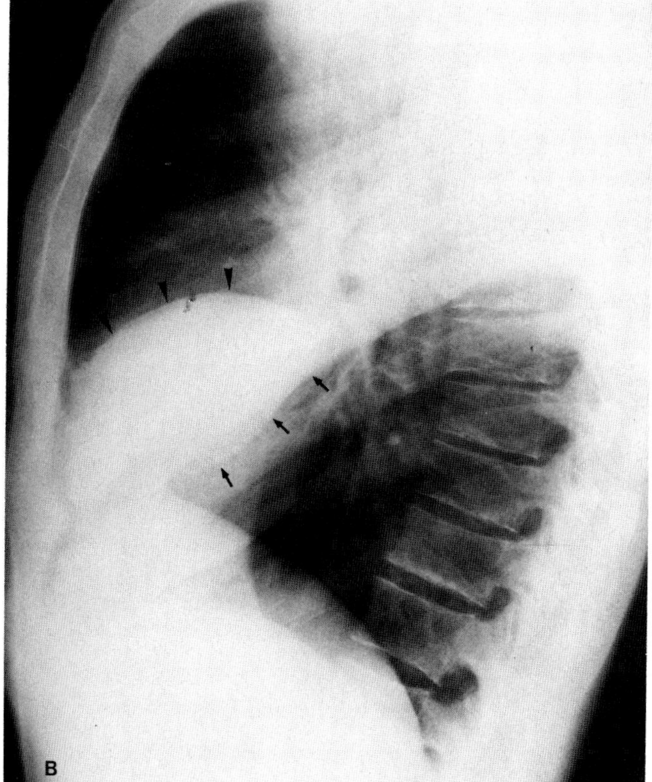

Fig. 13.43 Right middle lobe consolidation. Male aged 37 years with squamous cell carcinoma of right middle lobe. (**A**) PA film shows homogeneous opacity limited by horizontal fissure (arrows) and obscuring right heart border. (**B**) Lateral film shows consolidation bounded by horizontal fissure (arrowheads) and lower half of oblique fissure (arrows).

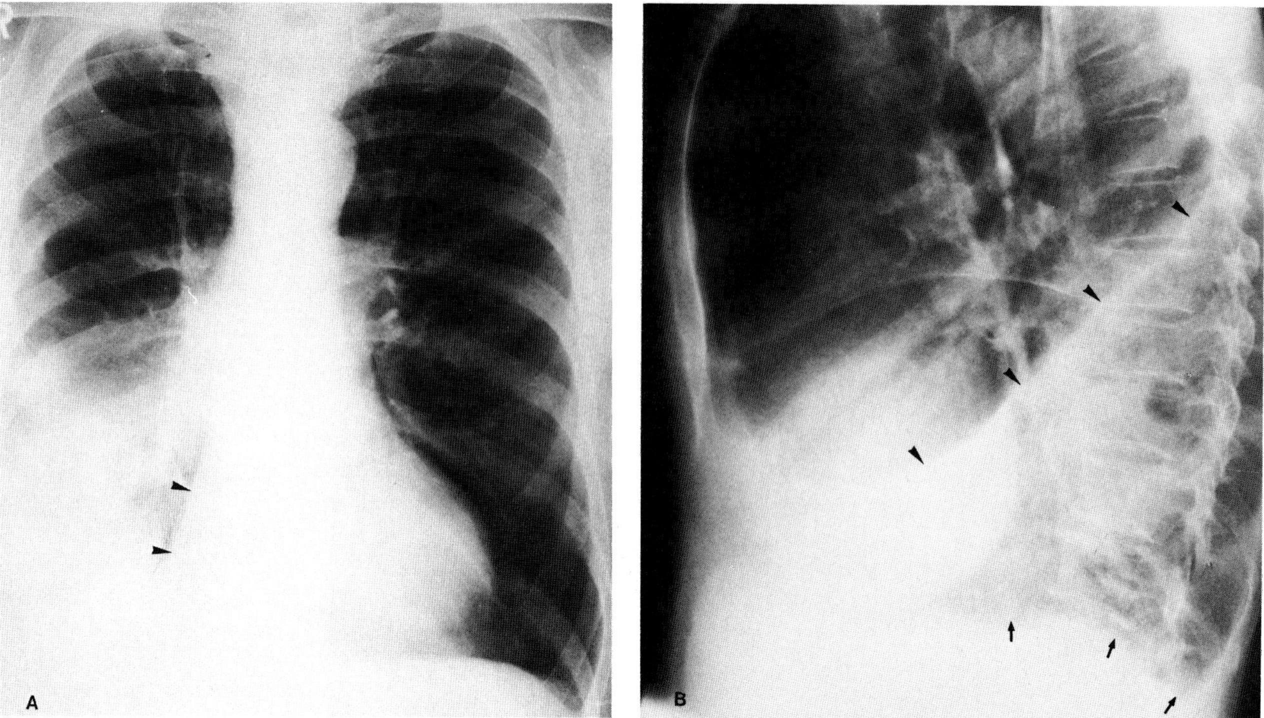

Fig. 13.44 Right lower lobe consolidation. Aerobacter aerogenes pneumonia in a chronic bronchitic. (**A**) PA film shows right lower zone shadowing obscuring the diaphragm, but not the right heart border (arrowheads). (**B**) Lateral film shows shadowing with air bronchogram, limited by oblique fissure anteriorly (arrowheads). The left hemidiaphragm is visible (arrows) but the right is obscured.

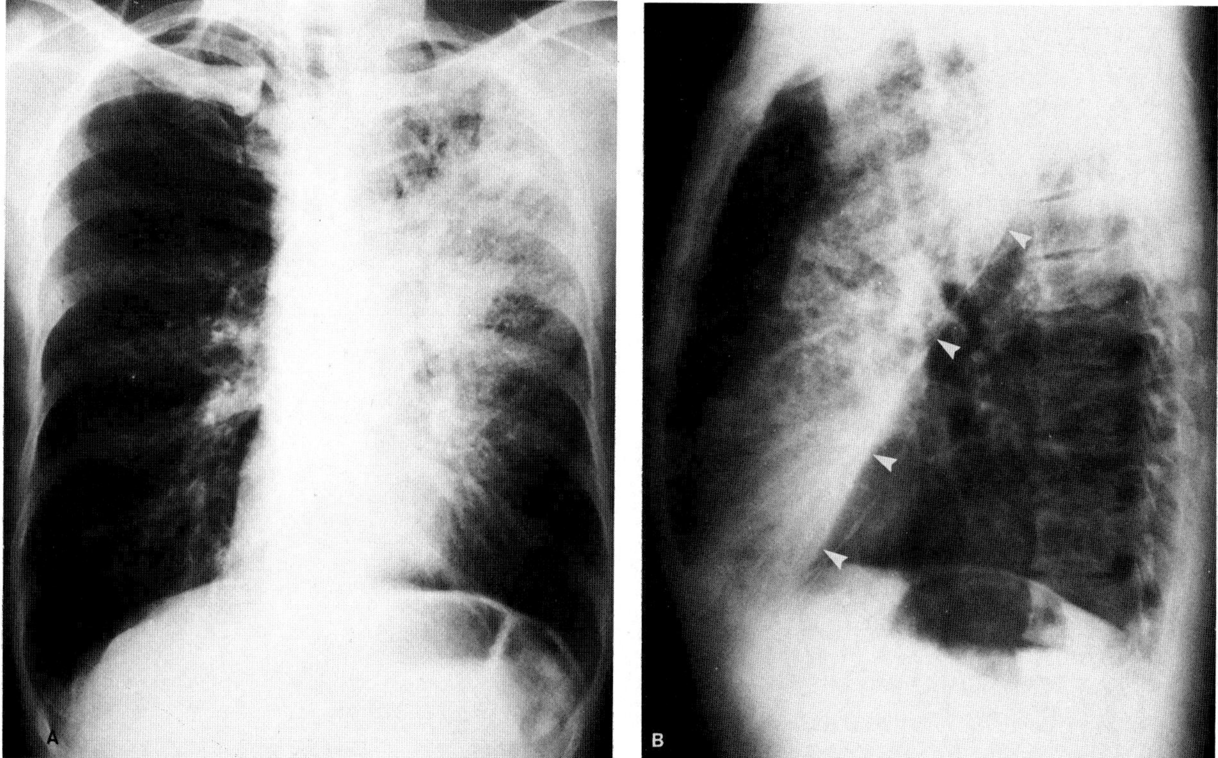

Fig. 13.45 Left upper lobe and lingular consolidation. Male aged 70 years with left upper lobe carcinoma. (**A**) Patchy consolidation obscures the left heart border and aortic knuckle. (**B**) The consolidation is bounded posteriorly by the oblique fissure (arrowheads).

uid its distribution is influenced by gravity, so that in cute pneumonitis consolidation is often denser and more learly demarcated inferiorly by a pleural surface, and is ess dense and more indistinct superiorly.

obar consolidation

Consolidation of a complete lobe produces a homogenous pacity, possibly containing an air bronchogram, delinated by the chest wall, mediastinum or diaphragm and the ppropriate interlobar fissure or fissures. Parts of the iaphragm and mediastinum adjacent to the non-aerated ung are obscured.

Right upper lobe consolidation (Fig. 13.42) is confined by the horizontal fissure inferiorly, and the upper half of the oblique fissure posteriorly, and may obscure the right upper mediastinum.

Right middle lobe consolidation (Fig. 13.43) is limited by the horizontal fissure above, and the lower half of the oblique fissure posteriorly, and may obscure the right heart border.

Lower lobe consolidation (Fig. 13.44) is limited by the oblique fissure anteriorly, and may obscure the diaphragm.

Left upper lobe and lingular consolidation (Fig. 13.45) are limited by the oblique fissure posteriorly. Lingular consolidation may obscure the left heart border, and consolidation of the upper lobe may obscure the aortic knuckle.

REFERENCES AND SUGGESTIONS FOR FURTHER READING

General

elson, B. (1973) *Chest Roentgenology*. Philadelphia: W. B. Saunders Co.

raser, R. G., Pare, J. A. P. (1977–79) *Diagnosis of Diseases of the Chest*, 2nd ed. Philadelphia: W. B. Saunders Co.

imon, G. (1978) *Principles of Chest X-ray Diagnosis*, 4th ed. London: Butterworths.

he pleura

lexander, E., Clark R. A., Colley D. P. & Mitchell S. E. (1981) CT of malignant pleural mesothelioma. *American Journal of Roentgenology*, **137**: 287–291.

lbelda, S. M., Epstein, D. M., Gefter, W. B. & Miller, W. T. (1982) Pleural thickening: Its Significance and relationship to asbestos dust exposure. *American Review of Respiratory Disease*, **126**: 621–624.

ustin, J. H. M., Carsen, G. M. (1977) Radiologic Diagnosis of Pleural Effusions In: *Current Concepts in Radiology*, **3**: 261–281, St. Louis: C. V. Mosby.

lack, L. F. (1972) The pleural space and pleural fluid. *Mayo Clinic Proceedings*, **47**: 493–506.

leischner, F. G. (1963) Atypical arrangement of free pleural effusion. *Radiologic Clinics of North America*, **1**: 347–362.

aensler, E. A., Kaplan A. J. (1971) Asbestos pleural effusion. *Annals of Internal Medicine*, **74**: 178–191.

Ieller, R. M., Janower, M. E., Weber, A. L. (1970) The radiological manifestations of malignant pleural mesothelioma. *American Journal of Roentgenology*, **108**: 53–59.

Iillerdal, G. (1983) Malignant mesothelioma 1982: Review of 4710 published cases. *British Journal of Diseases of the Chest*, **71**: 321–343.

ipscomb, D. J., Flower, C. D. R., Hadfield, J. W. (1981) Ultrasound of the pleura: an assessment of its clinical value. *Clinical Radiology*, **32**: 289–290.

AcLeod, T. C., Isler, R. J., Novelline, R. A. Putman, C. E. Simeone, J. & Stark, P. (1981) The apical cap. *American Journal of Roentgenology*, **137**: 299–306.

Aoskowitz, P. S, Griscom, N. T. (1976) The medial pneumothorax. *Radiology*, **120**: 143–147.

Raasch, B. N., Carsky, E. W., Lane, E. J., Callaghan, J. P. O. & Heitzman, E. R. (1982) Pleural Effusion: Explanation of some typical appearances. *American Journal of Roentgenology*, **139**: 899–904.

argent, E. N., Gordonson, J., Jacobson, G., Birnbaum, W. & Shaub, M. (1978) Bilateral pleural thickening: a manifestation of asbestos dust exposure. *American Journal of Roentgenology*, **131**: 579–585.

Stark, D. D., Federle, M. P., Goodman, P. C., Podrasky, A. E. & Webb, W. R., (1983) Differentiating lung abscess and empyema: Radiography and computed tomography. *American Journal of Roentgenology*, **141**: 163–167.

Williford M. E., Hidalgo H., Putman, C. E., Korobkin, M. & Ram, P. C. (1983) Computed tomography of pleural disease. *American Journal of Roentgenology*, **140**: 909–914.

Woodring, J. H. (1984) Recognition of pleural effusion on supine radiographs: How much fluid is required? *American Journal of Roentgenology*, **142**: 59–64.

Wright, F. W. (1976) Spontaneous pneumothorax and pulmonary malignant disease — a syndrome sometimes associated with cavitating tumours. *Clinical Radiology*, **27**: 211–222.

Collapse and consolidation

Krause, G. R., Lubert, M. (1958) Gross anatomico-spatial changes occuring in lobar collapse; a demonstration by means of three-dimensional plastic models. *American Journal of Roentgenology*, **79**, 258.

Proto A. V., Tocino, I. (1980) Radiographic manifestations of lobar collapse. *Seminars in Roentgenology*, **15**: 117–173.

Robbins, L. L., Hale, C. H. (1945) The Roentgen appearance of lobar and segmental collapse of the lung; preliminary report. *Radiology*, **44**: 107.

Robbins, L. L., Hale C. H., Merrill, O. E. (1945) The Roentgen appearance of lobar and segmental collapse of the lung; technic of examination. *Radiology*, **44**:471.

Robbins, L. L., Hale, C. H. (1945) The Roentgen appearance of lobar and segmental collapse of the lung. III Collapse of an entire lung or the major part thereof. *Radiology*, **45**:23.

Robbins, L. L., Hale, C. H. (1945) The Roentgen appearance of lobar and segmental collapse of the lung. IV Collapse of the lower lobes. *Radiology*, **45**:120

Robbins, L. L., Hale, C. H. (1945) The Roentgen appearance of lobar and segmental collapse of the lung. V Collapse of the right middle lobe. *Radiology*, **45**:260.

Robbins, L. L., Hale, C. H. (1945) The Roentgen appearance of lobar and segmental collapse of the lung. VI Collapse of the upper lobes. *Radiology*, **45**:347.

Schneider, H. J., Felson, B., Gonzalez, L. L. (1980) Rounded atelectasis. *American Journal of Roentgenology*, **134**, 225–232.

CHAPTER 14

TUMOURS OF THE LUNG

PRIMARY MALIGNANT TUMOURS

CARCINOMA OF THE LUNG (*Bronchial or bronchogenic carcinoma*)

There is an overwhelming preponderance of carcinoma compared to other malignant primary lung tumours. It is the cause of 35,000 deaths in England and Wales annually; it is the commonest cancer in men; in women it comes after breast, colon and skin cancer but its incidence is rising. Mortality rates are also still rising in the elderly but are falling in younger people because of lower cigarette consumption in that group. Cigarette smoking is responsible for the epidemic proportions of the disease but there are other known causes and predisposing factors. These are mostly to be found in industrial processes involving nickel, arsenic, asbestos, chromium and uranium. Its association with lung scars is higher than would be expected from chance and there is an increased incidence in sufferers from fibrosing alveolitis and systemic sclerosis. It is a disease of the over-50s and is rarely considered in the differential diagnosis of lung lesions in those under the age of 40 years. Nevertheless it has been found at all ages including childhood.

Of 100 patients with carcinoma of the lung less than 10 will survive 5 years. Many will be inoperable when first seen. In general, operability is determined by absence of involvement of the mediastinum but resection rates vary widely depending on the surgeon's view of what is possible or achievable. Despite such differences 5 year survivors in reported surgical series are remarkably constant at 25%. Moreover the proportion of lobectomies to pneumonectomies does not influence the survival rate. These figures have remained unchanged over the last 30 years, the only improvement being in the operative mortality resulting from better peri-operative management. The conclusion to be drawn is that the dominant factor in survival lies in the nature of the disease process rather than in differences in timing or type of operation. Taking the group of peripheral carcinomas, 5 year survival following resection is related to tumour size, smaller lesions having a better prognosis. An exception to this rule is that, those over 6 cm in diameter have more survivors than tumours one size below indicating that peripheral tumours may be large because they are fast growing or alternatively they are slow growing with consequently less tendency to metastasize. Amongst those surviving for 5 years there is a substantial mortality rate between 5 and 10 years.

Pathology. Carcinoma of the lung is divided pathologically into the following cell types with the approximate proportions of each shown:

Squamous	50%
Adenocarcinoma, including bronchioloalveolar cell	20%
Small cell (oat cell)	20%
Large cell	10%

This does not mean that there is unanimity amongst pathologists concerning classification, merely that in the interests of comparable reporting the above is a satisfactory compromise. With rare exceptions carcinomas arise from some element of the bronchial mucosa or its metaplasia. All types are more frequent in cigarette smokers, the association being particularly strong with squamous and small cell types, less strong in adenocarcinoma and weak in bronchioloalveolar carcinoma.

Small cell carcinoma arises from the APUD system (amine precursor uptake decarboxylase) which secretes and stores 5-hydroxytryptamine and which is also the cell of origin of carcinoid tumours of the bronchus.

The distinctive feature of the *bronchioloalveolar carcinoma* is the manner of its spread over the inner surface of the terminal air spaces including alveoli, using the pulmonary architecture as a framework which initially remains intact. Primary adenocarcinomas of the alimentary tract metastasizing to the lung can produce an identical picture so that a definition of this tumour includes a rider that no primary adenocarcinoma exists elsewhere.

It is probable that *squamous carcinoma* arises in an area of bronchial mucosal metaplasia which would account for these tumours being predominantly central in position where there is greatest exposure to irritants. The *adenocarcinoma*, unrelated to metaplasia, arises anywhere along he bronchial pathway and is usually peripheral because of he greater area at risk.

The majority of carcinomas arise peripherally in the ung, that is, distal to the division into segmental bronchi, out at presentation most will have spread centripetally. Those lesions which remain peripheral have a better prognosis. There is a poor correlation between cell type and prognosis except for the general statement that prognosis is especially poor in small cell and relatively more favourable in bronchioloalveolar carcinoma.

Investigations are directed to the establishment of a diagnosis, the determination of operability and the assessment of the patient's fitness for surgery. Once a suspicion of carcinoma has been raised the prime investigations are *sputum cytology* and *bronchoscopy*.

Tomography usually contributes little more than better definition of the lesion without answering the question: 'benign or malignant?' It is useful in settling doubts concerning such features as cavitation or calcification but its main function is to determine whether hilar and mediastinal nodes are involved. *CT scanning* improves accuracy in the search for mediastinal involvement but it is not error-free and its precise place in pre-operative assessment is not yet fully evaluated. If it demonstrates normal hilar and mediastinal structures it is reliable but if it reveals an abnormal mediastinum this does not necessarily imply inoperability since enlarged nodes can be due to reactive changes. In that event recourse may then be had to *mediastinoscopy* but this too has limitations in the area which can be reached. If CT scanning is undertaken it is usual to include the adrenals which are a common site of metastatic disease.

Ventilation and perfusion *radionuclide scans* occasionally show unexpectedly large defects and then there is likely to be extensive mediastinal involvement but similar defects can result from pulmonary artery and vein occlusion. Large defects may also be found in the apparently normal lung, the first indication of serious chronic disease rendering pneumonectomy unduly hazardous.

Biopsy. An ideal biopsy is one obtained from a lesion visible at *bronchoscopy*; blind biopsy is disappointing. The fibre-optic bronchoscope has increased the area of accessible bronchial tree but small peripheral lesions still constitute a problem and it is here that *percutaneous needle biopsy* is invaluable. It is also useful for other lesions difficult of access by bronchoscopy. The determination of cell type is more reliable from bronchoscopic than from needle biopsy because of the larger specimen obtained. Nevertheless for small cell carcinoma both are reliable and this is the most important discrimination because of the implications for treatment.

Radiological appearances. The diagnosis of carcinoma of lung starts in all but exceptional cases with an abnormality on a chest radiograph. If a previous series of radiographs happens to be available it is not uncommon to find in retrospect that a lesion had been missed months or even years before. This is not surprising when the opacity is very small and of low density since only 25% of lung volume is unobstructed by the bony thorax. In a small number of cases the radiograph is still normal after the diagnosis has been established by bronchoscopy or other means.

The first indication of a central carcinoma may be a *hilar shadow* which is slightly more prominent or denser than normal (Fig. 14.1). A location within a bronchial lumen soon produces signs of obstruction — *atelectasis* or *hyperaeration* (Fig. 14.2). Collapse of individual lobes or segments each have their distinctive radiographic signs but sometimes these are not obvious. A collapsed left lower lobe may be invisible on an underexposed PA radiograph but its presence may be inferred by the redistribution of the pulmonary vessels in the overexpanded upper lobe or by one or two curved basal 'sentinel' lines due to a drawing down of bronchi by the loss of volume, the bronchi becoming visible from retained secretions. A collapsed upper lobe may paradoxically exist with a well-aerated lung apex, a circumstance often incorrectly ascribed to herniation of lung from the opposite side when it is more often due to the overexpanded apex of the lower lobe. This 'luftsichel' sign explains why the outline of the aortic knuckle is sometimes unexpectedly preserved in collapse of the left upper lobe (Figs. 14.3–6). The presence of atelectasis should always initiate a search for evidence of a hilar mass.

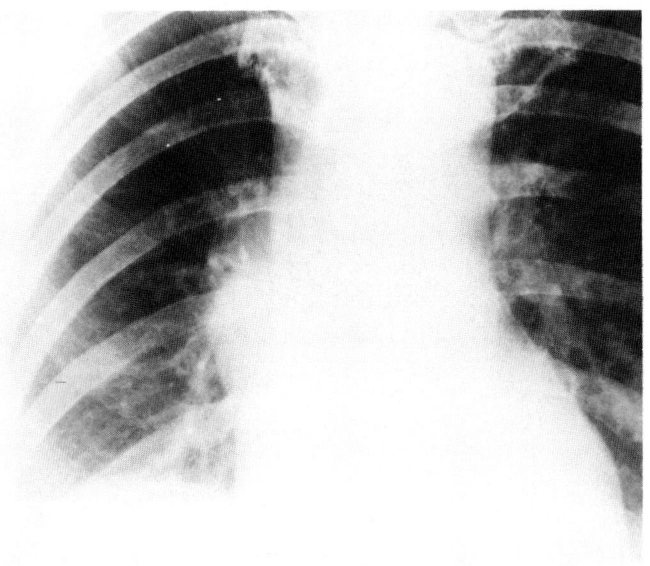

Fig. 14.1 Carcinoma of lung. Dense and enlarged right hilum.

The lung distal to a blocked lobar bronchus does not always collapse (Fig. 14.7); the air may be replaced by secretions or inflammatory exudate; microabscesses may

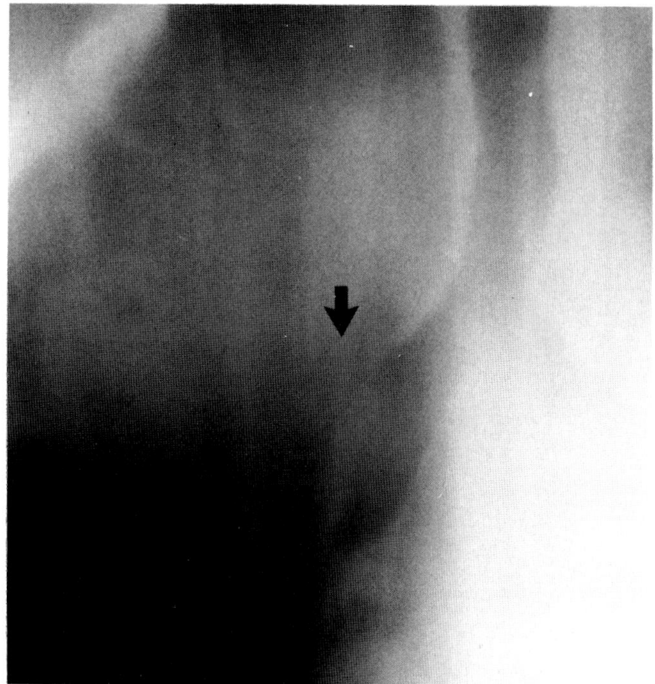

Fig. 14.2 Tomogram. Carcinoma occluding the right upper lobe bronchus.

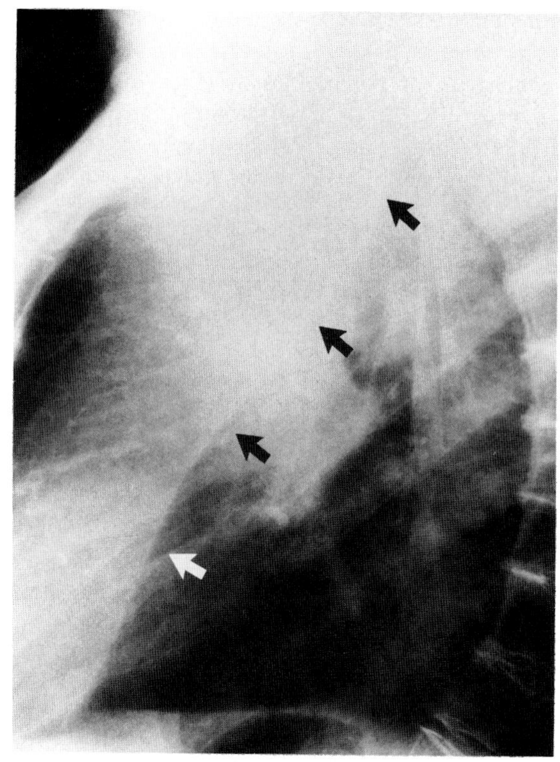

Fig. 14.4 Lateral. The collapsed lobe covers the aortic arch (arrows). The apex of the lower lobe occupies the thoracic apex.

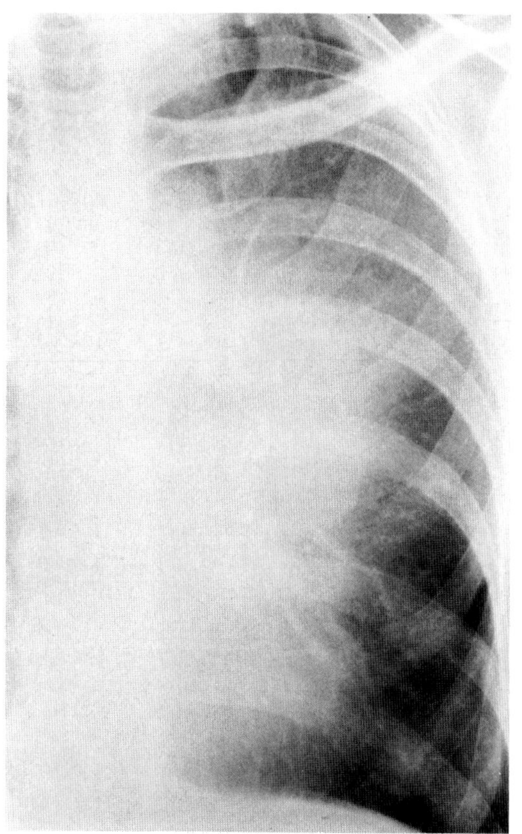

Fig. 14.3 Luftsichel sign. Collapsed left upper lobe. Aortic knuckle obscured. Aerated apex.

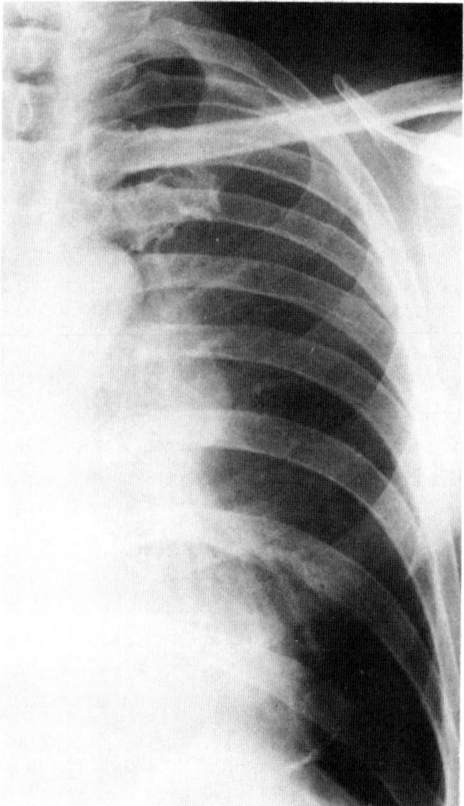

Fig. 14.5 Luftsichel sign. Collapsed left upper lobe. Aortic knuckle preserved. The apex is aerated.

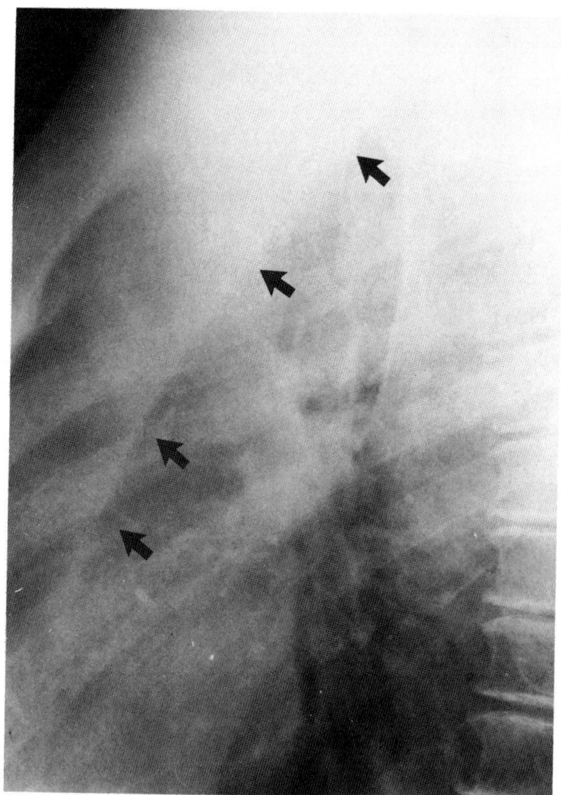

Fig. 14.6 Lateral. Aortic arch is not covered by the collapsed lobe (arrows).

form or lipid substances accumulate after release from chronic inflammatory cells. The result is a chronic fibrotic or lipoid pneumonia, hence the suspicion which attaches to a diagnosis of *unresolved pneumonia*. Air may return to an atelectatic lobe when mucosal oedema or infection subsides so that re-expansion has to be interpreted with caution in determining aetiology. *Bronchography* is now rarely used but can be useful in this situation as the appearances are always abnormal, bronchi even when patent showing irregularity, squeezing or pruning of side branches.

Accumulation of secretions within bronchi distal to a blocked segmental bronchus may result in a mucocoele which takes the form of an oval or branching opacity within aerated lung, the air reaching the segmental alveoli by collateral ventilation through the pores of Kohn (Fig. 14.8). Such collateral ventilation is inefficient and the finger-like opacities are often the centre of a *focal hyperinflation*. Regional hyperinflation can also result from a check valve bronchial obstruction.

Growth extends from the hilum along the connective tissue sheaths of bronchi and pulmonary vessels, its path revealed by dense streaks of opacity radiating from the hilar mass. As lymphatics become obstructed the flow of lymph can be reversed carrying tumour seedlings centrifugally. Lymphatic permeation of this nature results in fine

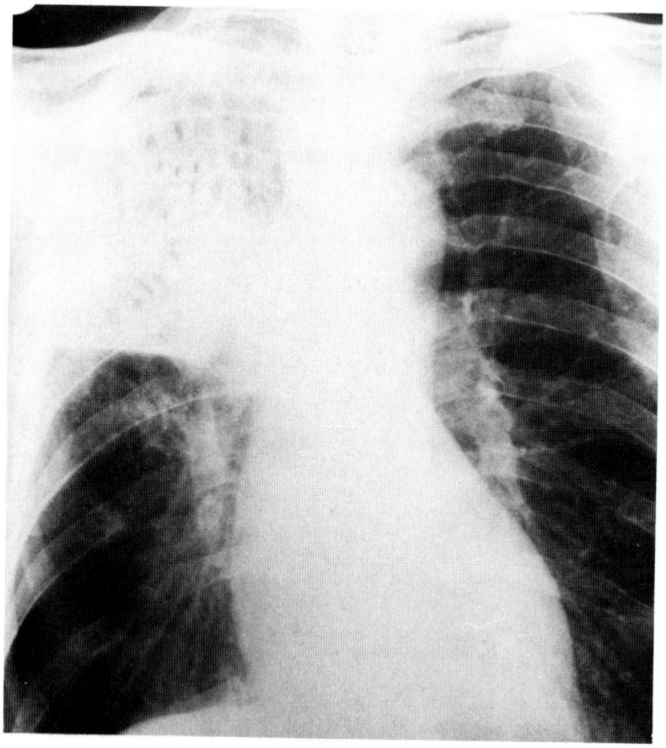

Fig. 14.7 Carcinoma of lung. Obstructive pneumonia of right upper lobe containing translucent bronchi. There was bronchiectasis distal to the tumour.

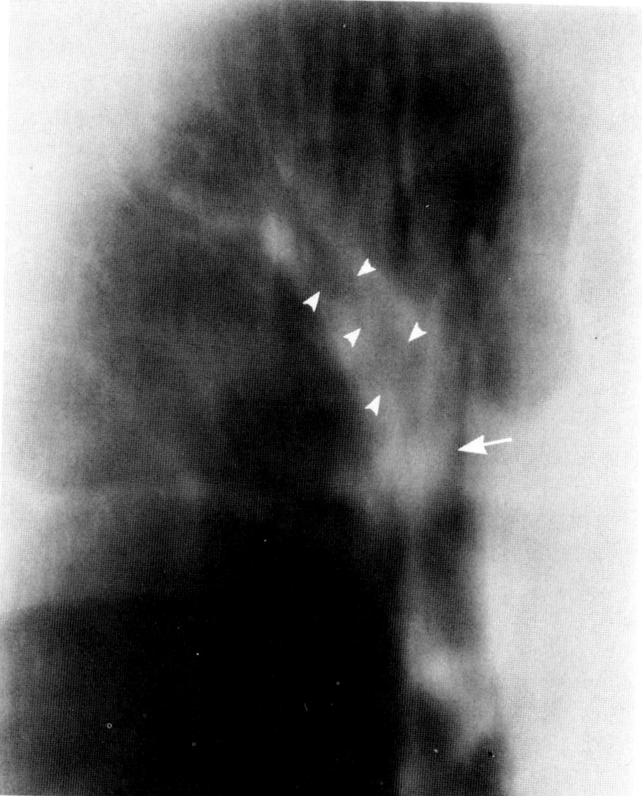

Fig. 14.8 Tomogram. Right upper lobe bronchocoele (arrowheads). The contents are relatively translucent. The obstructing lesion is visible (arrow).

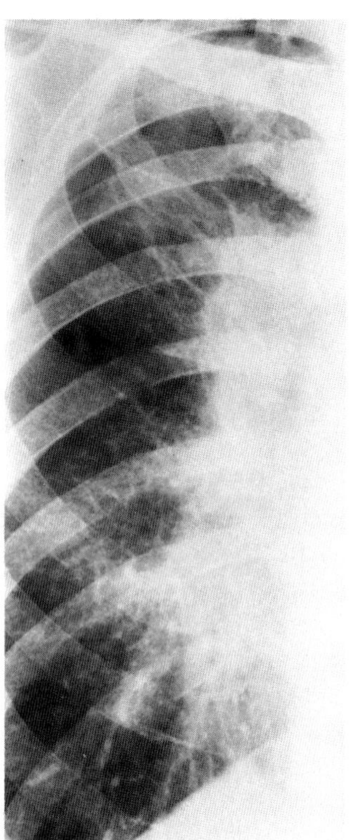

Fig. 14.9

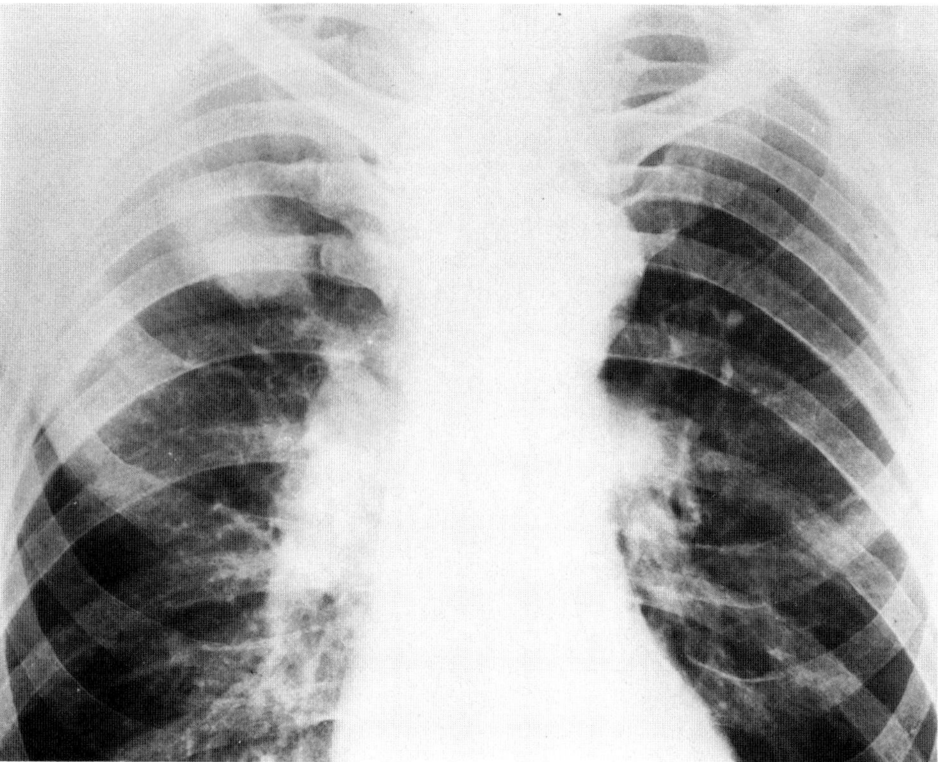

Fig. 14.10

Fig. 14.9 Centrifugal spread of carcinoma from the hilum into all lobes.

Fig. 14.10 Carcinoma in the right upper lobe with an extension into the enlarged hilum.

Fig. 14.11 Tomogram. Cavitating carcinoma. Irregular wall thickness.

linear shadows mingled with nodules of tumour. In an extreme case this leads to an appearance of *lymphangitis carcinomatosa* confined to one lung (Fig. 14.9).

An unusual form of carcinoma is one entirely confined within the mediastinum, some being genuine bronchial neoplasms. Radiographic signs may then be inconspicuous or even absent despite clinical signs of strangulation of mediastinal structures — great veins, pulmonary artery, oesophagus.

The majority of carcinomas arise at a *peripheral* site but by the time they are discovered many of them will have a band of growth extending into the hilum (Fig. 14.10). Initially they are roughly rounded in shape, growing as they do in compliant lung. A few retain this regular shape even when they achieve massive proportions but as a rule growth is attended by irregularity of outline with extensions both proximally and distally.

Cavitation is not infrequent particularly in squamous carcinomas and there are a number of possible mechanisms — infection, infarction, discharge of secretions, dissection of air into the mass (Fig. 14.11). The cavity may enlarge

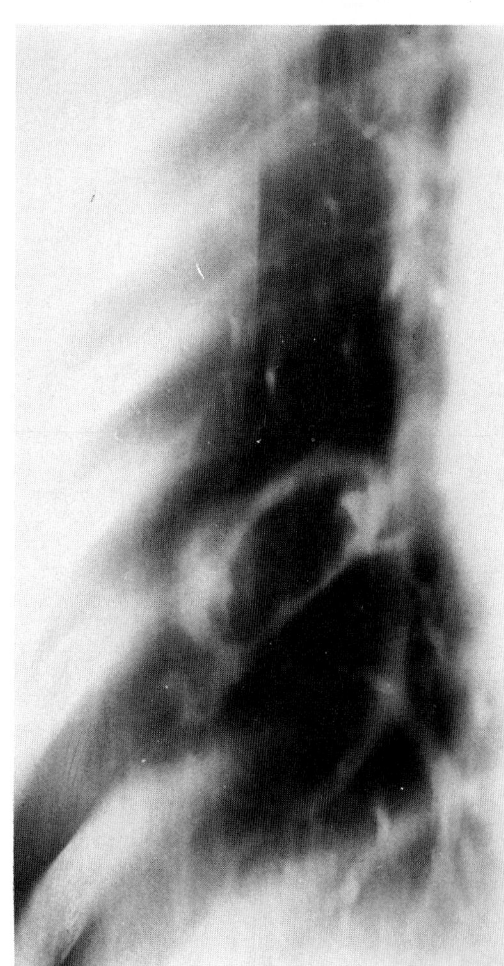

Fig. 14.11

with the growth of the tumour, necrotic debris being shed into the lumen. A needle biopsy of such a lesion may yield a pus-like material which will not be diagnostic and for this reason it is preferable to take biopsies from the growing edge rather than from the centre of a tumour. The cavities characteristically have thick irregular walls, a feature which is of use in the differential diagnosis of cavitating lung lesions. As a general rule the thicker the wall the greater the probability of malignancy. At one extreme a cavity with a uniform wall thickness of 1 mm is almost certain to be benign and conversely a wall thickness of 15 mm is almost inevitably malignant.

Rupture of such a cavity is one cause of *pneumothorax*, a rare event in primary lung neoplasms (Fig. 14.12) but rather more frequent with certain pulmonary metastases. Carcinoma of the lung metastasizes widely but those sites commonly productive of symptoms or radiographic signs are mediastinum, bone and brain. *Metastasis to lung* is usually on the ipsilateral side, the opposite lung being relatively spared. Seedling deposits close to the pleura or pericardium are likely to stimulate the formation of an *effusion* which can be difficult to control.

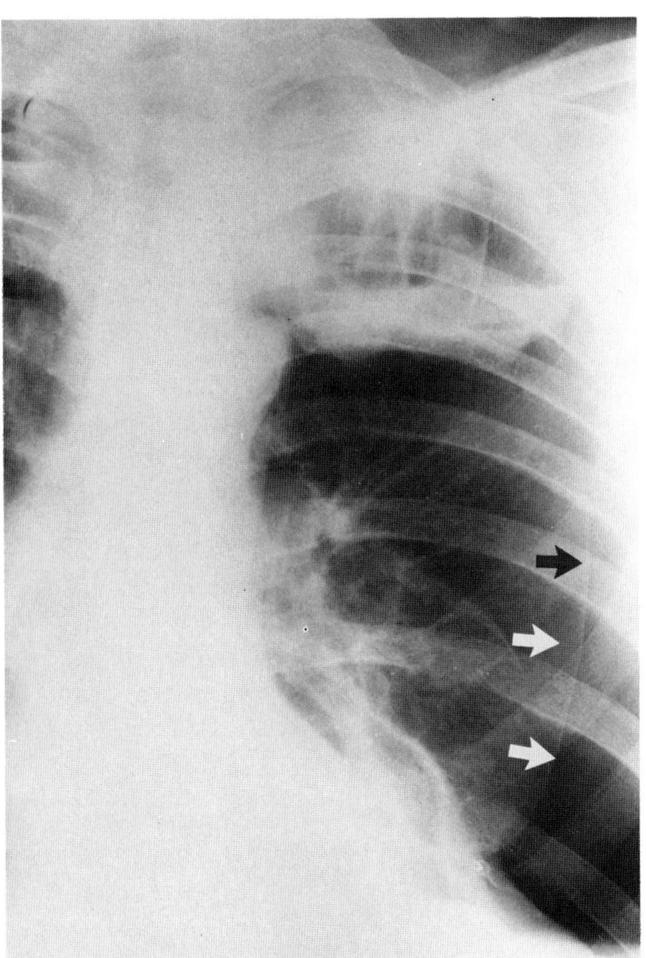

Fig. 14.12 Cavitating carcinoma with fluid content at apex. Spontaneous pneumothorax. (arrows)

A *paralysed diaphragm* due to tumour involvement of the phrenic nerve means that extension into the mediastinum has taken place and is inevitably a sign of inoperability. However, steps should be taken to try to exclude paralysis from other causes and in this respect previous chest radiographs can be invaluable. A high diaphragm may be due to a localized weakness which does not have the same significance as total paralysis and this is best assessed by fluoroscopic observation.

Hypertrophic pulmonary osteoarthropathy is most commonly caused by carcinoma of lung but it is not of itself a sign of inoperability.

The solitary lung lesion

A problem in differential diagnosis is presented by an apparently isolated single lesion. The questions that have to be answered are — 'is it a primary or secondary malignant lesion or is it benign?' There is no point in making a separate category of so-called coin lesions, the questions and management are the same irrespective of whether the lesions are strictly circular or not. In different series of such lesions the proportion of malignant primary tumours has varied between 36 and 52%. Several radiographic signs have been suggested as indicative of malignancy and conversely their absence as suggesting benignancy.

The *character of the edge*, whether irregular, spiculated or notched; a halo of emphysema; a tail of one or two lines proceeding from the lesion to the pleura. All of these have been reported as more common in malignant lesions than in benign. Unfortunately none offer sufficient discrimination on which to base management of an individual case.

Two signs have more importance — the presence of *internal calcification* and *evidence of growth*. A carcinoma may arise in a calcified scar or it may engulf a calcification during growth, but both are very rare phenomena. If it can be shown, if necessary with the aid of tomography, that there is genuine calcification present within the lesion, then this is the most reliable sign of benignancy. CT may be helpful in this respect since it is more sensitive in detecting calcification.

Growth of a lesion over a period of time has to be interpreted with caution. Carcinomas usually grow rapidly and a definite change will be noted after a few weeks but some carcinomas grow slowly at a pace matched by growth of benign lesions such as hamartomas or granulomas (Fig. 14.13). Nevertheless a lesion stable for 2 years is reliable evidence of benignancy.

In the management of these lesions there is a strong body of opinion that they should always be removed unless they are calcified or have been known to be stable for 2 years or the patient cannot stand an operation. A more conservative approach involves biopsy either percutaneously or by fibre-optic bronchoscopy with excision if the biopsy shows anything other than a benign pathology. The case for biopsy is strengthened if the patient is under 35 years old or if operation carries an extra risk.

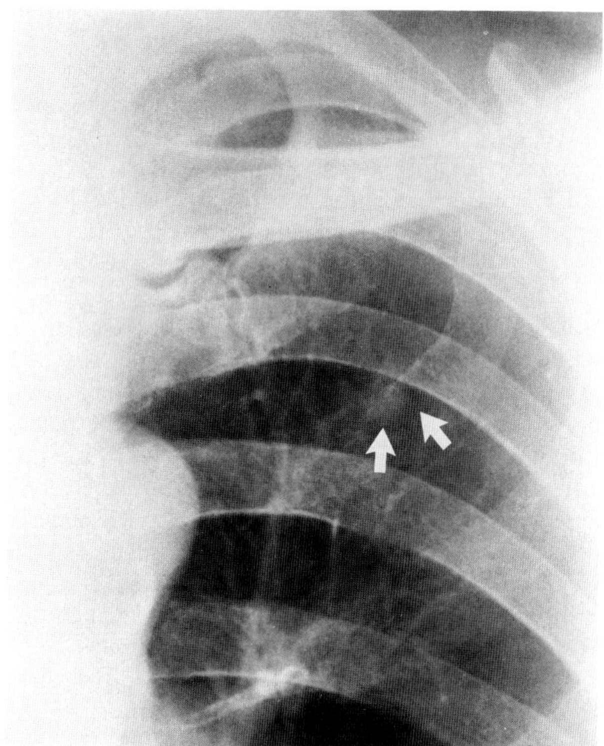

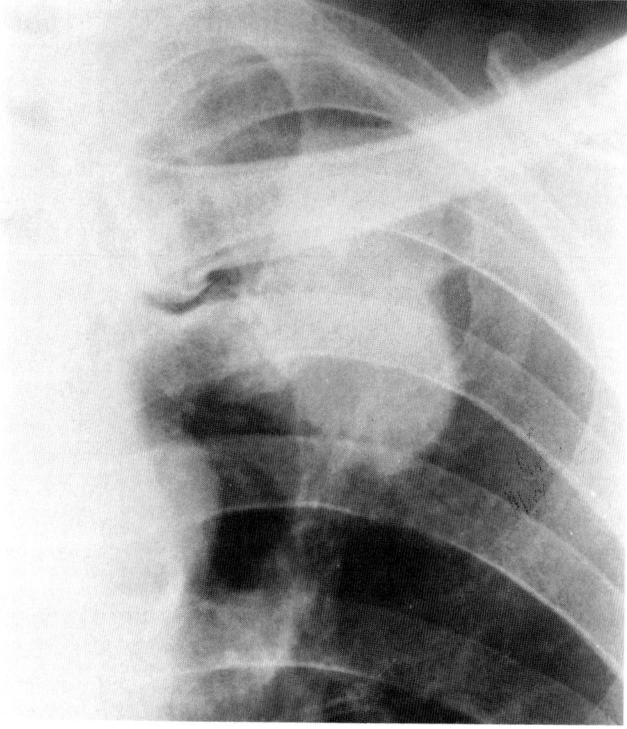

Fig. 14.13 (**A** & **B**) Carcinoma growing slowly. No treatment. Between (**A**) and (**B**) there was an interval of 3½ years.

Small cell (oat cell) carcinoma

These tumours are mostly centrally located, grow rapidly and disseminate early particularly to the bone marrow and brain (Fig. 14.14). Surgery has little to offer except for those few cases where the lesion is a peripheral nodule but even then it is not recommended if the tumour is visible at bronchoscopy. They are highly sensitive to combination chemotherapy and the thrust of research at present is to determine that combination which offers the best chance of remission (Figs. 14.15, 14.16).

Approximately 30% of small cell carcinomas secrete hormone-like substances which, if in sufficient quantity, result in corresponding endocrine or metabolic abnormalities. The substances produced are *parathormone, anti-diuretic hormone* and *corticotrophin* and the functional effects are respectively hypercalcaemia, fluid retention with hyponatraemia, Cushing's syndrome and gynaecomastia.

Other 'paramalignant' disorders seen are encephalopathy, myelopathy and myasthenia. In some instances it is

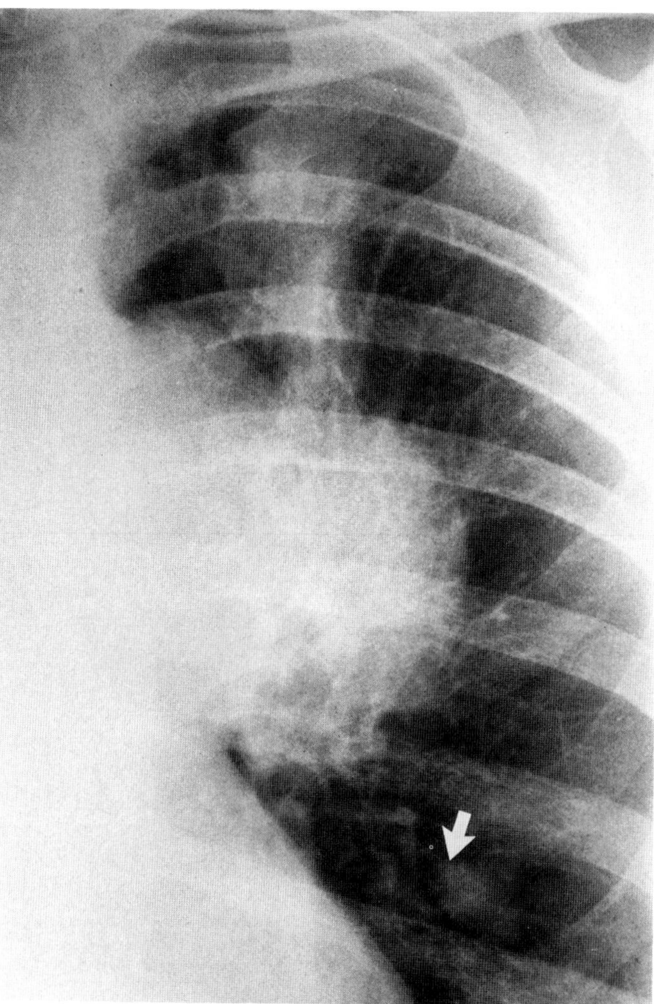

Fig. 14.14 Small cell carcinoma at left apex with an extension to the large hilum. Secondary lung deposit inferior to hilum (↓).

difficult to differentiate these syndromes from the effects of metastases. Their manifestations may appear in advance of any apparent lung neoplasm and they may remit with treatment of the primary. Other carcinoma cell types may have similar secretory properties but less frequently than the small cell type.

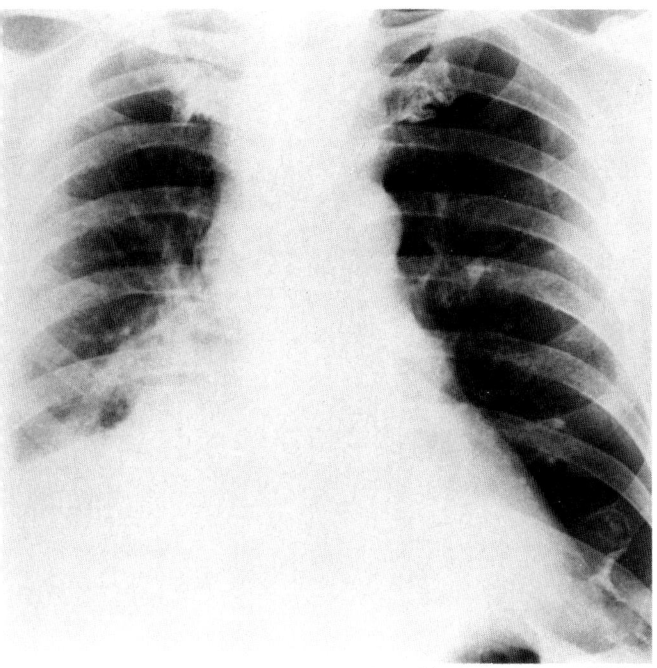

Fig. 14.15 Small cell carcinoma. Remission with chemotherapy. Right lower lobe collapse; mediastinal adenopathy.

Pancoast tumour

A carcinoma at the apex of the lung, whatever its histological type, has a propensity to invade the parietal pleura and soft tissues at the root of the neck. The term Pancoast tumour refers to the syndrome of symptoms and signs so produced which includes pain in the arm and paresis of sympathetic nerves on the same side. These tumours may be inconspicuous in the early stages, following as they do the line of the apical pleura, and be mistaken for post-inflammatory pleural thickening so common at this site. Careful search should be made for evidence of rib erosion.

Bronchioloalveolar cell carcinoma

The tumour was so-called because of the doubt surrounding the identity of the cell line from which it arises, whether from bronchioles or alveoli. Many pathologists now believe that it can arise from a number of different cell types including type 2 pneumocytes, clara cells (mucin secretors) and bronchiolar epithelium, or from a bronchiolar stem cell capable of differentiating into any of these cell lines. This places the tumour in the peripheral parts of the lung from whence it spreads into the alveolar spaces. It is not destructive of lung architecture which accounts for the relative preservation of regional lung perfusion. By definition there must be no lesion in a major bronchus or an adenocarcinoma elsewhere in the body. The cells often secrete mucin and a profuse watery sputum is characteristic. Sputum cytology may reveal adenocarcinoma cells. It is not strongly related to smoking and its incidence is roughly equal in men and women. It tends to develop in damaged lungs and there may therefore be radiographic evidence of

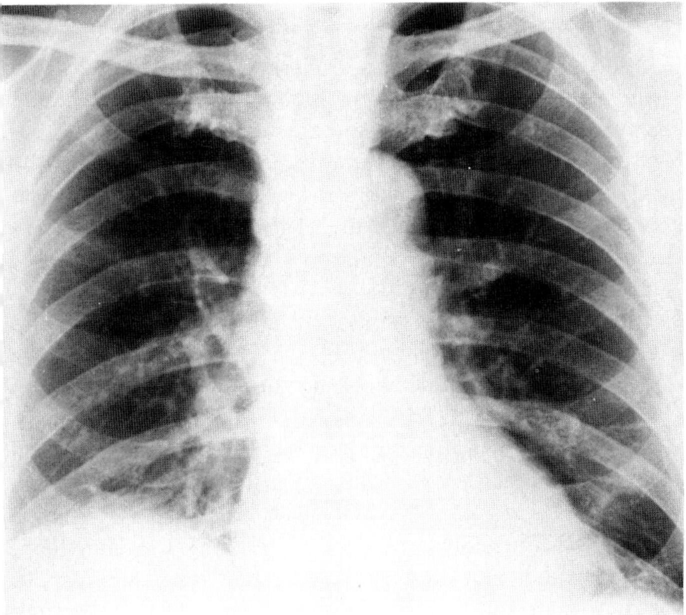

Fig. 14.16 3 years later. No sign of disease.

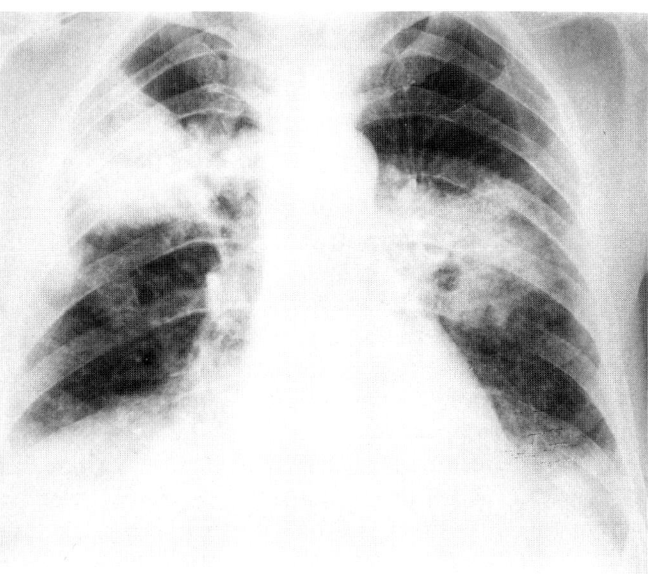

Fig. 14.17 Bronchioloalveolar carcinoma. Multiple consolidations. Small cavity lateral to the left hilum.

bronchiectasis, tuberculosis, rheumatoid pulmonary disease or systemic sclerosis.

It may be limited to a single, well-circumscribed, peripheral nodule, in which case surgical excision is likely to be curative because of the slow growth and late dissemination of this tumour. Another form of the disease is of multiple, ill-defined, variable sized nodules either confined to one lung or bilateral. The nodules coalesce as they grow and a lobar consolidation similar to pneumonia can result (Fig. 14.17). Consolidation is in part the result of airspace filling by tumour and in part by mucin. Surgery is not curative in the diffuse form and eventual spread to the opposite lung is inevitable. *CT scanning* detects spread to the opposite lung earlier than the chest radiograph. Tumour growing alongside the bronchi makes them rigid but there is no obstruction. Atelectasis does not occur and air bronchograms are visible within the lung opacity. Bronchographic abnormalities consist of absence of normal changes of calibre during the respiratory cycle, a pruned tree appearance from absence of filling of side branches and minor irregularities of the lumen. Septal lines and pleural effusion may be present. Cavitation is a rare event.

OTHER PRIMARY MALIGNANT TUMOURS OF LUNG

Most pathologists base their classification of these tumours on that proposed by a World Health Organization report in 1967. Compared to carcinoma of lung these tumours are relatively rare, are not related to cigarette smoking and in general they occur in a younger age group. Their slower rate of growth gives them a better prognosis than carcinoma. The symptoms, signs and radiographic appearances are largely determined by whether they arise within the air passages or lung.

CARCINOID

This is a tumour of slow growth and infrequent metastasis. Almost all arise within a major bronchus; a peripheral nodule is a rare exception (Fig. 14.18). It grows through the bronchial wall and the intrabronchial tumour may be the tip of an iceberg, the greater portion being extrabronchial. The cell line is the APUD system of argentaffin cells, the same as the alimentary tract carcinoids. The age group is younger than carcinoma and there is an equal incidence in men and women. The carcinoid syndrome from release of 5-hydroxytryptamine is rare but when it occurs any endocardial fibrosis is located on the left side of the heart exposed to the drainage from the tumour. The radiographic signs are those of bronchial obstruction or a smoothly circumscribed mass.

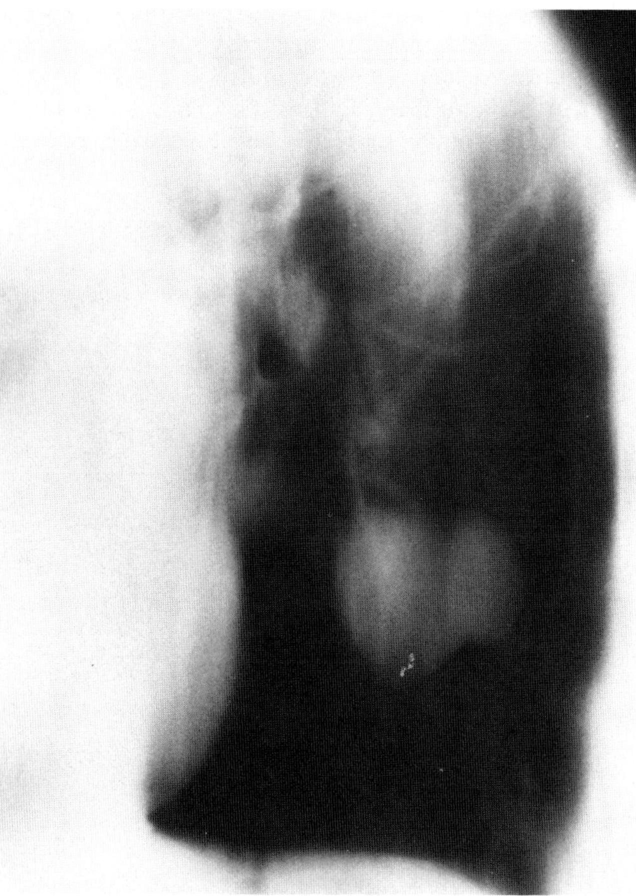

Fig. 14.18 Peripheral carcinoid. Lateral tomogram.

ADENOID CYSTIC CARCINOMA (cylindroma)

This is a carcinoma of low-grade malignancy arising from trachea, carina or main stem bronchi, locally invasive and spreading to regional hilar nodes but rarely metastasizing elsewhere (Fig. 14.19). It may extend outside or along the inside of the wall of the airway, the latter resulting in polypoid projections. Because of its site it commonly presents with obstructive symptoms particularly stridor and 'asthma'.

This tumour like others obstructing major airways can give rise to alarming symptoms while the chest radiograph remains normal. Slowly growing tumours escape detection and the patient may be labelled as asthmatic. Any asthmatic whose symptoms and signs are in any way unusual should be regarded with suspicion and any doubt settled by tomography of the major airways if necessary. These patients will usually have a characteristic flow/volume loop, a test which plots rate of flow against lung volume; obstruction in a large airway limits the rate of flow through a large part of the expiratory phase which is reflected in the flatter shape of the loop.

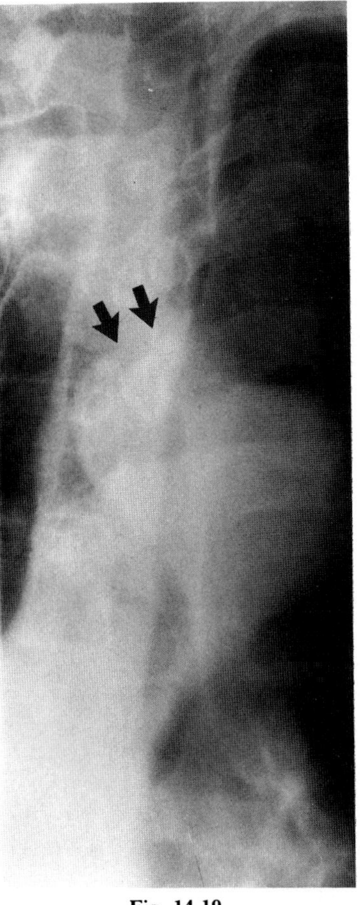

Fig. 14.19

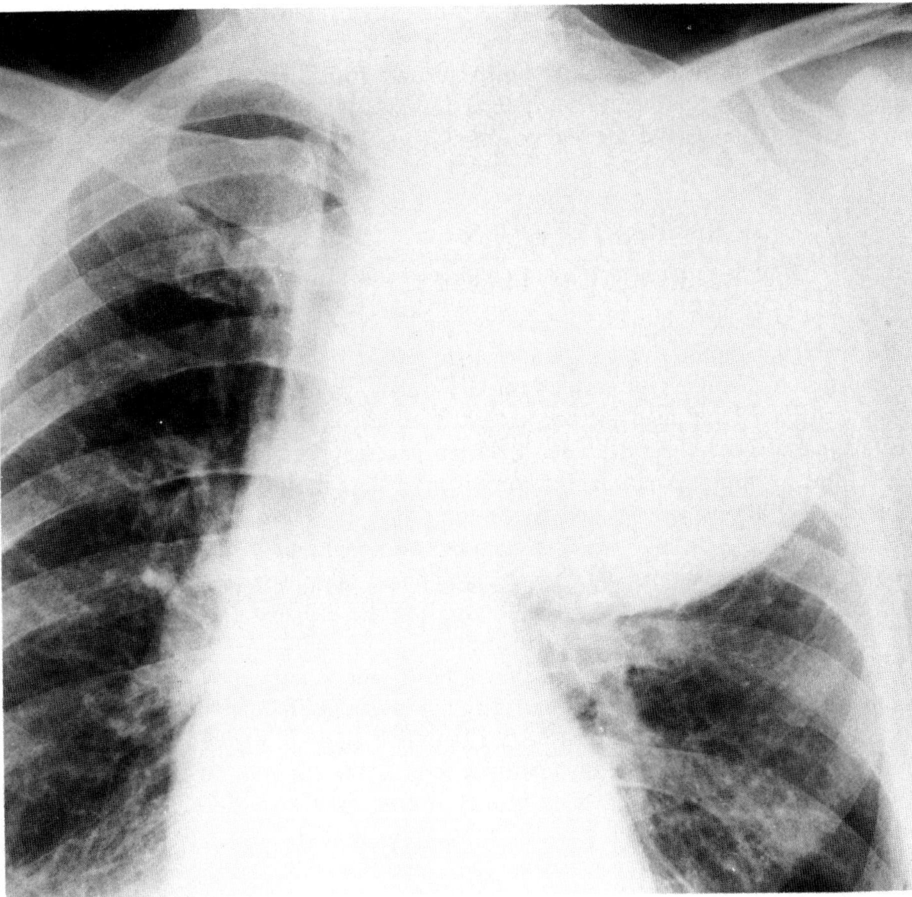

Fig. 14.20

Fig. 14.19 Adenoid cystic carcinoma of trachea. There was severe stridor and a normal chest radiograph of lung fields.

Fig. 14.20 Pulmonary blastoma. Despite the large size there is little effect on the rest of the lungs.

MUCOEPIDERMOID TUMOUR

Perhaps out of place here, this rare bronchial tumour has only exceptionally been reported as having malignant potential although it is locally invasive. A small, entirely intrabronchial sessile or polypoid tumour, found at all ages, it consists of epidermoid elements and mucus-secreting acini. The same type of tumour is found in the salivary glands.

Bronchial adenoma is an old terminology for benign intra-bronchial tumours. It is unsatisfactory on two counts; 90% of these tumours are carcinoids (which is a low-grade malignancy) and true adenomas are rare.

MIXED TUMOURS

Mixed tumours are those composed of two or more types of malignant cell. There are two lung tumours in this group:

Pulmonary blastoma. Embryonic connective tissue, muscle cells and columnar cell aggregations resembling fetal bronchioles make up this tumour. Because of its slow growth, peripheral site and absence of obstructive effects, it may become a very large round mass before discovery (Fig. 14.20). Eventually metastasis to hilar nodes and elsewhere takes place.

Carcinosarcoma. The elements of this tumour are squamous carcinoma in a sarcomatous stroma. When found in the lungs it is usually a bronchial tumour, less often peripheral; it has slow growth and the prognosis after removal is relatively good.

PRIMARY SARCOMA OF LUNG

These are rare tumours outnumbered 500 to 1 by carcinomas. Leiomyo-, rhabdomyo- and fibrosarcomas are more frequent than any others and may arise from the tracheobronchial tree, lung or pleura. As a rule they affect a younger age group than carcinomas and a number are found in children. The sex incidence is equal. Node involvement is unusual and dissemination occurs late so that prognosis after removal is relatively good especially for fibrosarcoma. The tumour may be large when discovered; depending on the site of origin, pleural lesions are likely to signal their presence by a massive effusion and bronchial lesions by obstructive signs. Peripheral lesions typically have sharply defined and regular margins.

BENIGN TUMOURS

INTRABRONCHIAL TUMOURS

Tumours arising within the bronchial tree are likely to produce striking symptoms and signs at a relatively early stage in contrast to benign pulmonary tumours which may remain undetected for long periods unless discovered incidentally on a chest radiograph. Cough, wheeze, haemoptysis, are common symptoms and the radiographic signs are those of atelectasis, bronchiectasis and air trapping.

The old term *Bronchial adenoma* included carcinoid and adenoid cystic carcinoma which are carcinomas of low-grade malignancy. True adenomas are rare and are either mucous gland adenomas (Fig. 14.21) or mucoepidermoids, the latter consisting of mixtures of mucous cells and squamous epithelium. *Papillomas* are warty tumours of the lining of the air passages and are predominantly lesions of childhood. They are frequently multiple and in the condition of *papillomatosis* the entire bronchial tree may be stuffed with tumours which have a tendency to cavitate. *Chondromas* arise from bronchial cartilage and protrude into the lumen but as in many endobronchial tumours there may be a large extrabronchial extension. *Fibromas* and *lipomas* are usually endobronchial but can be found at other sites in lung, mediastinum or in relationship to the pleura.

The *granular cell myoblastoma* is a rare polypoid bronchial tumour which was thought to derive from muscle but is now considered to have a neural origin.

PULMONARY TUMOURS

Hamartoma, leiomyoma, neurofibroma are other examples of benign tumours which can be endobronchial but they are more often found as pulmonary nodules.

Benign pulmonary tumours are characteristically sharply defined, slow growing and smoothly rounded except where they abut on a pleural surface which restrains their growth. Up to 10% of solitary pulmonary nodules are benign tumours. It may not be possible to determine whether these tumours arise from lung tissue, pleura or a small bronchus but this is not important radiologically, the critical factor being that they do not obstruct major air passages.

Hamartomas consist of mixtures of tissues normal to the organ in which they arise; in the case of the lung these are cartilage and epithelial elements. Most are under 1 cm in

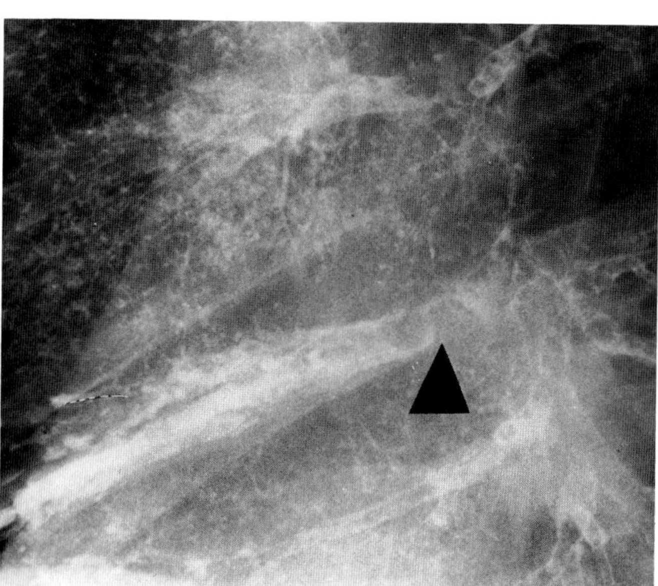

Fig. 14.21 Benign cystadenoma within the right middle lobe bronchus (large arrowhead). The lobe is collapsed (bronchogram).

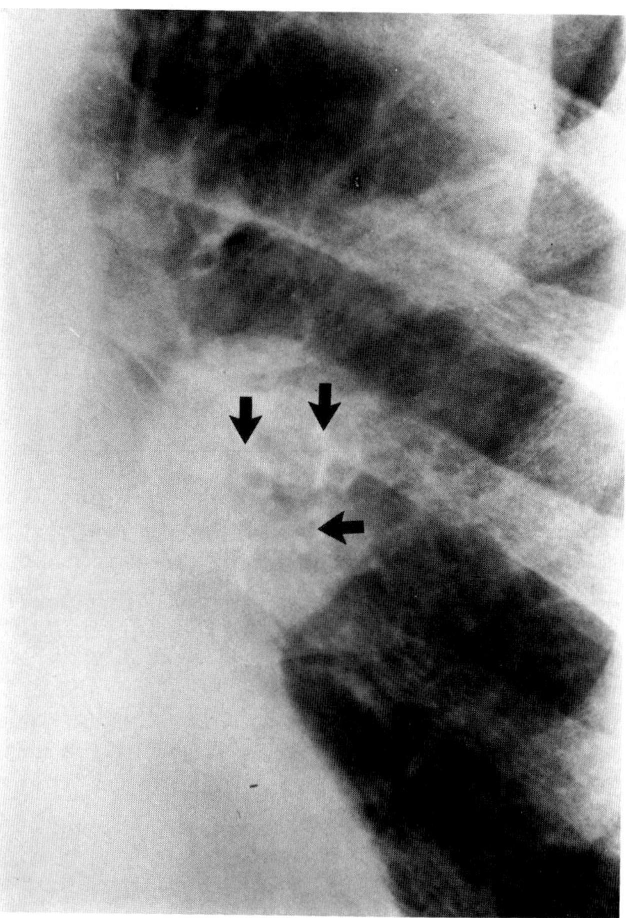

Fig. 14.22 Hamartoma. 'Popcorn' calcification is shown within the tumour (arrows).

diameter and are found incidentally at post-mortem. An average size of those found in life is about 3 cm. They grow very slowly but can reach very large size. Those discovered are usually solitary and peripheral with a sharply defined but lobulated border. The density may be inhomogenous because of fatty tissue. The cartilage element is a frequent source of calcification or ossification seen radiographically as fine stippling, coarse irregular 'popcorn' granularity or linear streaks (Fig. 14.22).

Under the general term **angioma** are lesions, arguably not true neoplasms and comprising blood-containing spaces. In the *capillary haemangioma* the spaces are of capillary size and these lesions are exemplified by the skin naevus. The spaces in the *cavernous haemangioma* are larger and their thin walls are lined by vascular endothelium. If there is a direct communication between the pulmonary artery and vein through the large spaces without the intervention of a capillary filter, the feeding artery and draining vein enlarge to accommodate what can be a considerable shunt. This is the *arteriovenous malformation or aneurysm* (Fig. 14.23). On a smaller scale the shunts are telangiectases and both types are components of the Osler-Weber-Rendu disease (*hereditary haemorrhagic telangiectasia*). *Diffuse pulmonary telangiectasia* is a rare variety and less obvious radiographically than the arteriovenous malformation, the small nodularities and exaggerated background of lung shadows being readily confused with pulmonary fibrosis. The pulmonary angiogram in diffuse telangiectasia may show enormous numbers of small vessels, but is sometimes normal.

The angiogram in arteriovenous malformation often reveals multiple lesions unsuspected on the plain radiograph together with small areas of telangiectasia. Spontaneous rupture of an angioma sometimes takes place resulting in a pulmonary haematoma. If the shunt through an arteriovenous malformation is sufficiently large there will be arterial desaturation and polycythaemia.

Neurofibromas are to be found wherever there are neural structures and therefore at any point throughout the bronchial tree. There is an association between *neurofibromatosis*, diffuse pulmonary fibrosis and phaeochromocytoma. Pneumothorax occasionally complicates thoracic neurofibromatosis (Figs. 14.24, 14.25).

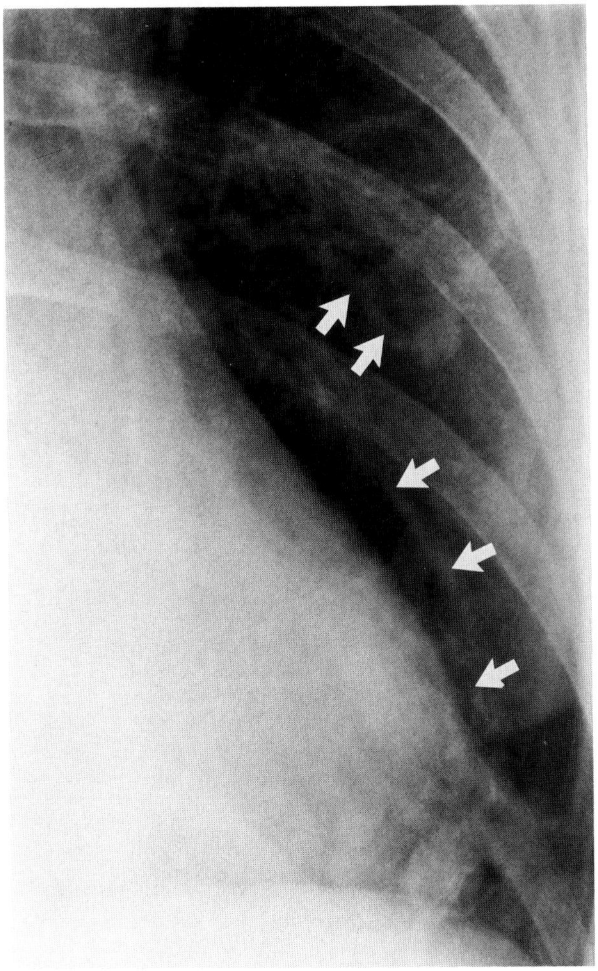

Fig. 14.23 Multiple pulmonary arteriovenous malformations. Enlarged feeding arteries (arrows).

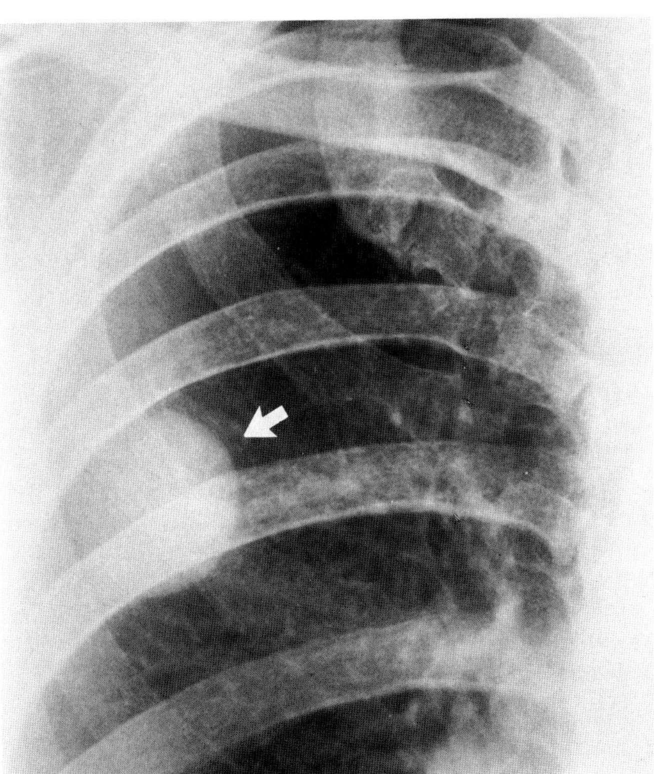

Fig. 14.24 Neurofibroma (arrow). This was intrathoracic but extrapleural.

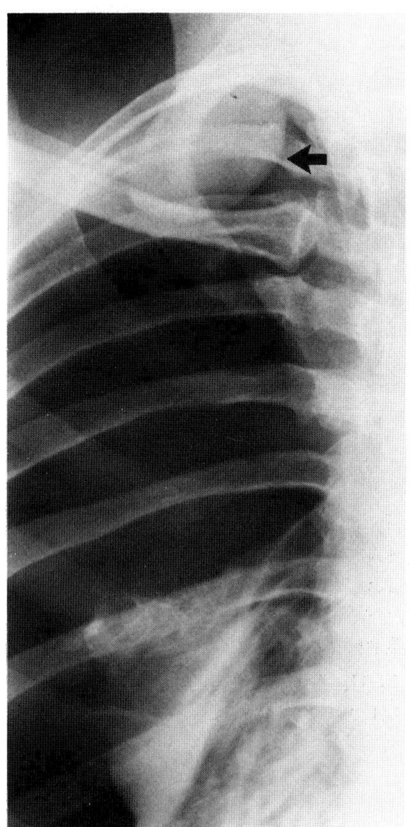

Fig. 14.25 Neurofibromatosis. Pneumothorax and an extrapleural neurofibroma (arrow).

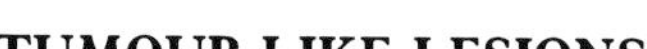

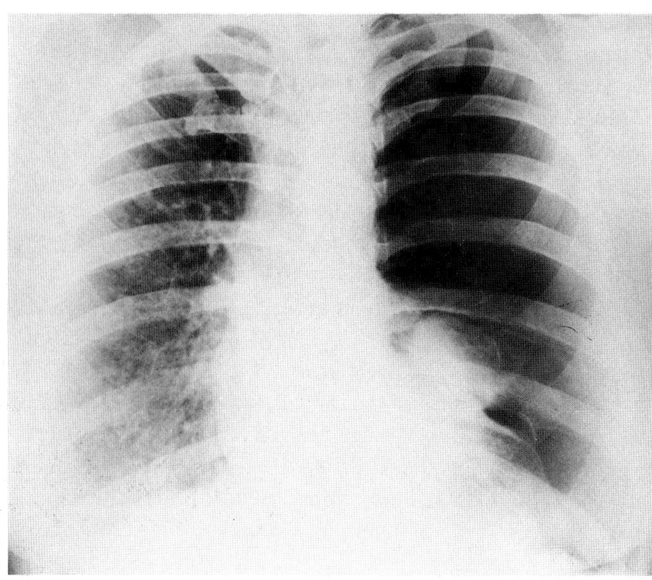

Fig. 14.26 Lymphangioleiomyomatosis. Left pneumothorax and diffuse fine reticulation in right lung.

TUMOUR-LIKE LESIONS

LYMPHANGIOMYOMATOSIS
(*Lymphangioleiomyomatosis*)

This is a rare and unusual disease of women of reproductive age, the major symptom being breathlessness but the chest radiograph may be abnormal for a considerable time before symptoms appear. Progressive respiratory insufficiency commonly leads to death within 10 years. Pathologically there is a widespread infiltration of pleura, septa and alveolar walls by proliferating muscle and lymphatics. There are obstructive effects on lymphatics, veins and small airways. Radiographically there is a fine reticulation with miliary densities distributed widely and not sparing the lung bases in contrast to eosinophil granuloma which it otherwise resembles closely (Figs. 14.26, 14.27). Other features are progressively enlarging lung volumes, small emphysematous cysts, pneumothorax, interstitial oedema, septal lines and chylous pleural effusions.

Lymphangiomyomatosis does not have a familial incidence, a point of differentiation from tuberous sclerosis which has the same pathological and radiological pulmonary manifestations.

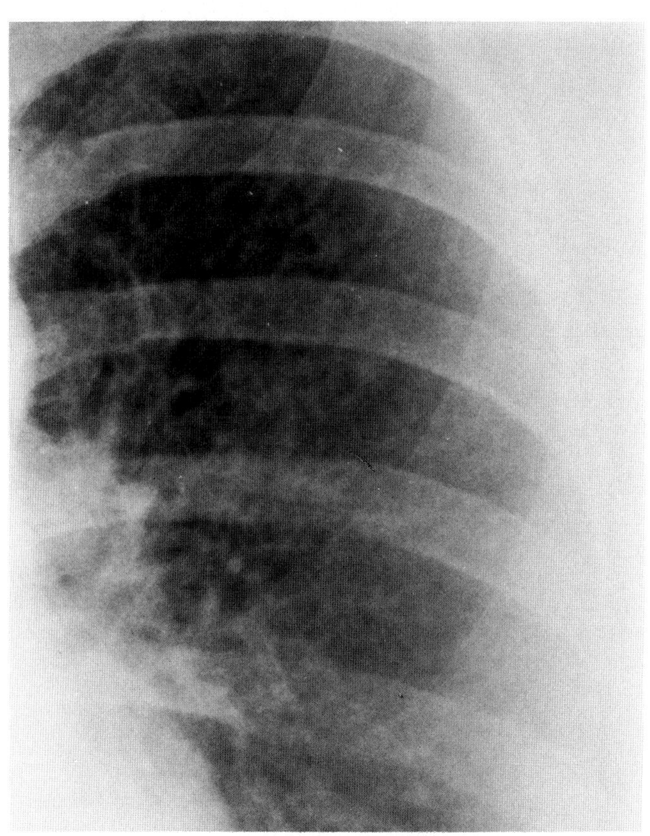

Fig. 14.27 Left lung with a reticulo-nodular pattern.

Another disease of similar pathology is *metastasising leiomyoma* from uterine leiomyomas and consequently also confined to women. The pulmonary nodules in this condition are larger, over 1 cm in diameter, and the intervening lung is normal.

PULMONARY TUBEROUS SCLEROSIS

There is a characteristic triad of epilepsy, mental retardation and adenoma sebaceum diagnostic of this genetic disorder of mesodermal tissues. Mesodermal tumours of various kinds have been found in most organs and tissues of the body but the common sites are kidney, retina, brain and bone. The lungs are rarely affected and then mostly in women. The disease may be limited to one organ in which case epilepsy and mental retardation are unusual and symptoms are delayed until adult life.

Histologically there is a diffuse leiomyomatosis in alveolar walls, small airways and vessels, in places growing into small tumours budding into the lumen. This causes bronchial obstruction and distal destruction of alveolar walls. The radiographic counterpart of these changes is a diffuse reticulation or miliary pattern progressing to honeycombing. Pneumothorax is a common complication. The prognosis is poor once symptoms appear.

ROUND ATELECTASIS (folded lung)

The radiographic appearance of this lesion is of a pleural based tumour-like mass almost always in the lower parts of the lungs. It has its origin in a sclerosing visceral pleuritis which as it contracts rolls up a portion of the underlying lung in a spiral fashion. A radiological diagnosis is possible if pulmonary vessels and bronchi can be shown to curve towards the mass as though drawn towards a vortex (Figs. 14.28, 14.29).

PLASMA CELL GRANULOMA

The histological components of this lesion are plasma cells

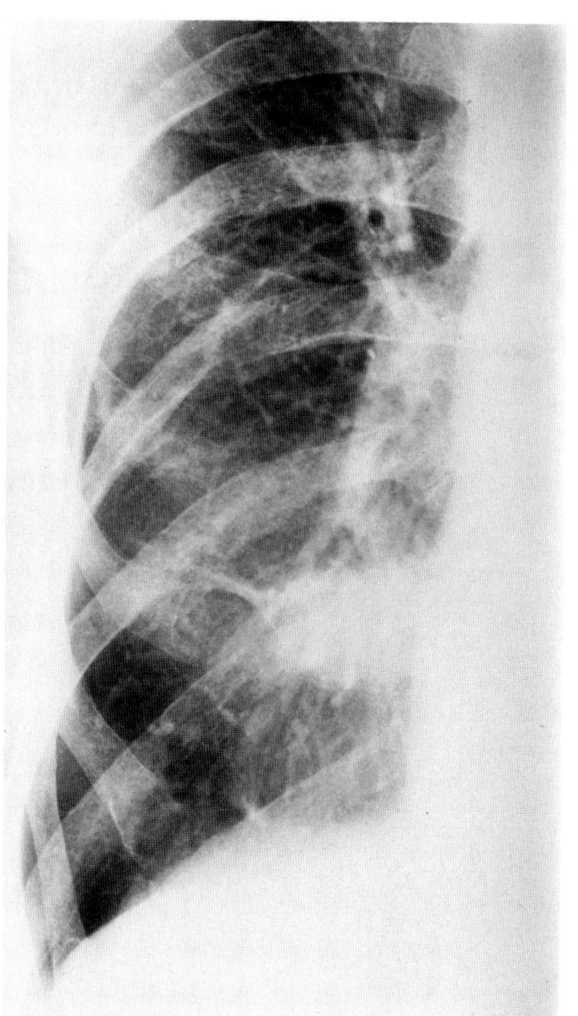

Fig. 14.28 Round atelectasis. 'Mass' at right base.

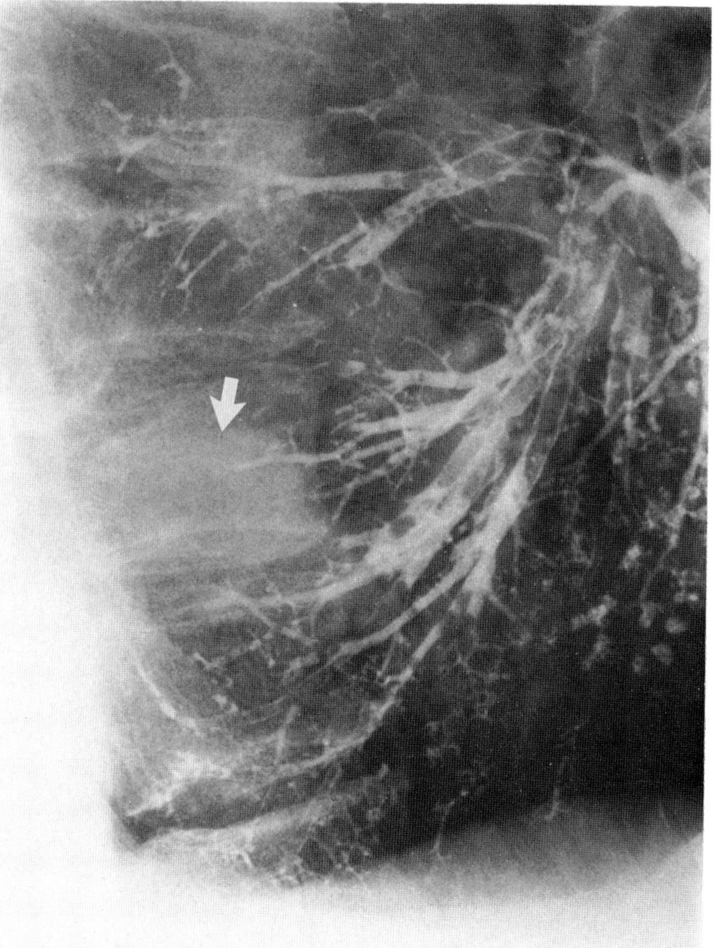

Fig. 14.29 Round atelectasis: bronchogram. Bronchi to lower lobe swept up towards the lesion (arrow).

and lymphocytes in a stroma of granulation tissue. It is now generally conceded that it is a post-inflammatory process occurring in all age groups and of equal sex distribution. When fat-laden mononuclear cells are present the terms *xanthogranuloma* or *fibroxanthoma* are sometimes applied. Usually a solitary well-circumscribed lesion, it can grow to great size but does not recur if removed. Calcification or cavitation are exceptional events. Other terms for this lesion are *histiocytoma* and *inflammatory pseudotumour*. It must not be confused with plasmacytoma which is a true tumour.

SCLEROSING HAEMANGIOMA

Although this lesion has similarities to the plasma cell granuloma above, pathologists now believe that it is possible to differentiate them on histological grounds. Nevertheless there is still dispute about their origin, whether derived from vascular endothelium or from type 2 pneumocytes. In the latter case the vascular stroma is regarded as reactive rather than neoplastic. Despite these doubts the name is retained because it is the one by which it is so commonly known. It is a sharply circumscribed lesion predominantly affecting women under the age of 50 and it has a tendency to bleed, hence the frequent symptom of haemoptysis.

METASTATIC TUMOURS

Most pulmonary metastases have their origin in malignant tumours of the genito-urinary and gastro-intestinal systems and when discovered unexpectedly a search is made for the primary site. The temptation to carry the search to absurd lengths has to be resisted. Histological examination of biopsy tissue narrows the possibilities and then the question has to be asked whether a knowledge of the primary site will affect management of that particular case.

Haematogenous metastases are tumour emboli filtered by the pulmonary vasculature. Invasion of veins by the primary tumour releases clumps of cells which pass via the cavae or vertebral venous plexus to the right heart and then to the pulmonary artery. The rare sarcoma of the pulmonary artery embolises directly into the pulmonary artery (Figs. 14.30, 14.31). Most of these tumour emboli are destroyed but those that become established behave like primary neoplasms. The tumours may remain discrete and circumscribed (Fig. 14.32) or spread through the lymphatics of the bronchovascular bundles to the hilum and mediastinum. In the latter case the lesions are irregular with intervening lung coarsened by lines and bands (Fig. 14.33). A miliary or snowstorm appearance indicates rapid growth (Fig. 14.34).

Lymphatic permeation can also take place directly from the primary, through the chest wall from breast or through the diaphragmatic crura from liver, adrenal or coeliac nodes. The mediastinum and its nodes are the first in line with this type of spread (Fig. 14.35). Mediastinal and hilar node enlargement with clear lungs is a recognized pattern of metastatic spread from renal carcinoma.

The effects on pulmonary function bear little relation to the size of individual metastases but rather to their profusion. Showers of tumour emboli in the pulmonary capillaries can cause pulmonary hypertension even when the chest radiograph is normal. Tumour cells often stimulate a fibrotic reaction in lymphatics and capillaries, a feature found in *lymphangitis carcinomatosa* which is a mixture of miliary metastases, lymphatic permeation and interstitial fibrosis (Fig. 14.36). These patients are severely dyspnoeic. Massive *pleural effusion* can add to respiratory embarrass-

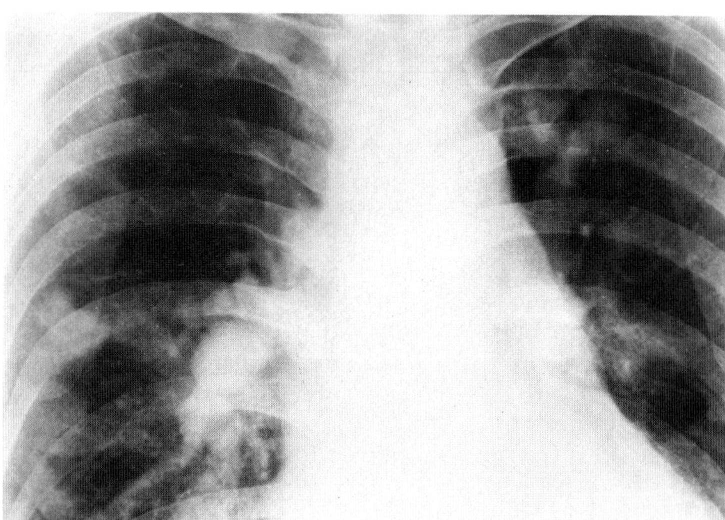

Fig. 14.30 Fibrosarcoma of pulmonary artery. Metastases growing in pulmonary artery branches.

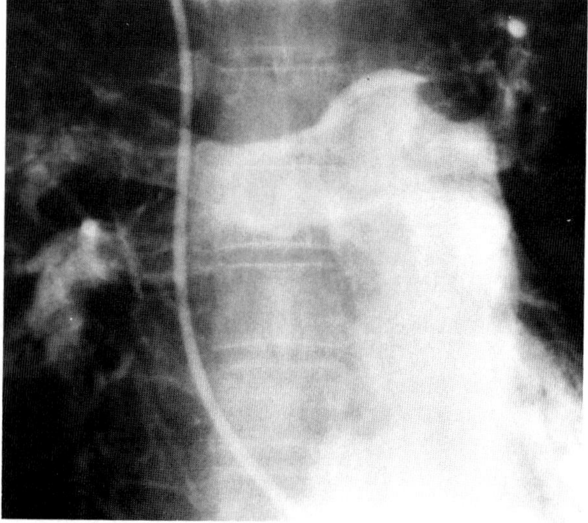

Fig. 14.31 Pulmonary angiogram. Large filling defects in pulmonary artery resembling embolus.

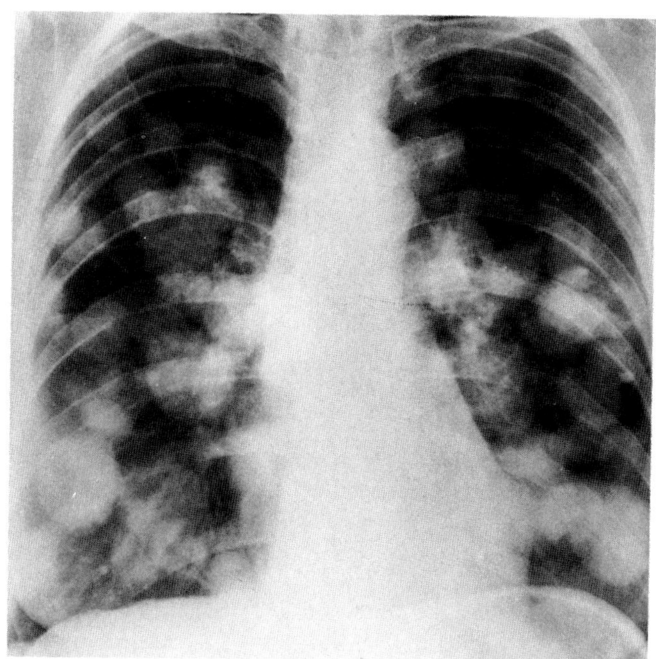

Fig. 14.32 Discrete metastases. Carcinoma of breast. The lung between lesions is normal.

ment and can be difficult to palliate. Metastases from carcinoma of thyroid may retain secretory function and can be detected by the increased uptake of ^{131}I even when the chest radiograph is normal.

At the extremes of growth rate there can be problems in the differentiation of metastases from other lesions. The sudden appearance of a profusion of lesions may seem altogether too rapid a timescale for the development of metastases and may suggest instead septicaemic abscesses (Fig. 14.37). At the other extreme is the solitary metastasis appearing many years after removal of a primary (Fig. 14.38). Multiple metastases from thyroid carcinoma can occasionally grow extremely slowly.

Calcification. Calcific densities within metastases result from a variety of pathological processes; bone formation (particularly seen in osteosarcoma), calcification in cartilage, dystrophic calcification, calcification in mucus (seen in papillary and mucinous adenocarcinoma) or following treatment.

Necrosis and cavitation is not a function of size and can occur in quite small metastases (Fig. 14.39). Cavitation always carries a risk of a *pneumothorax* (Fig. 14.40).

Fig. 14.33 Metastases with interstitial spread. The lung between nodules is abnormal. Origin unknown; the patient had both colon and breast carcinomas.

Fig. 14.34 Miliary metastases from carcinoma of stomach.

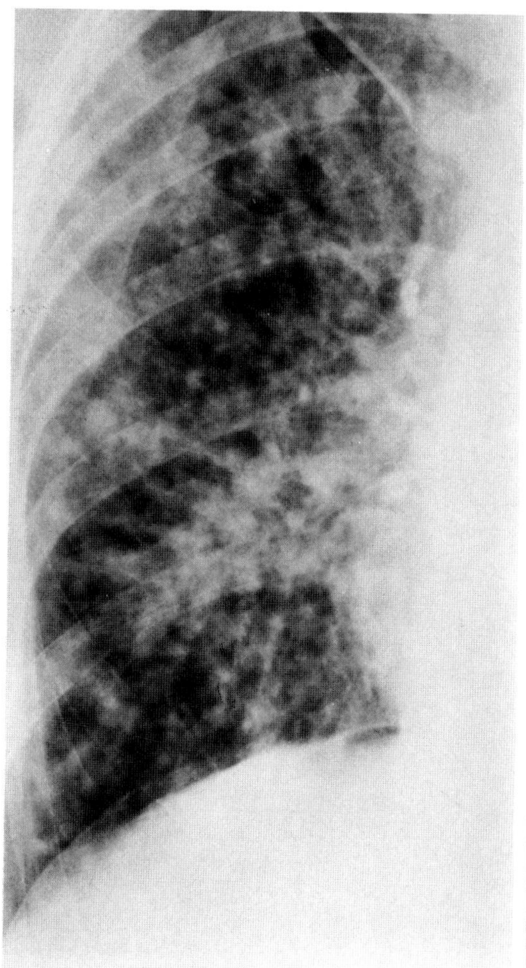

Fig. 14.33

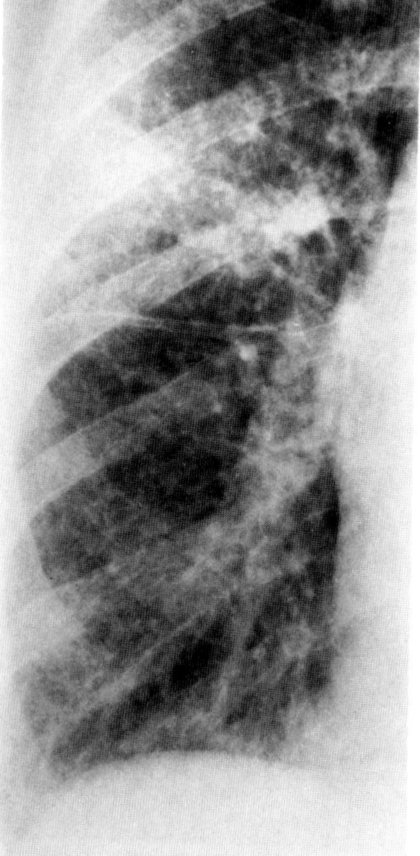

Fig. 14.34

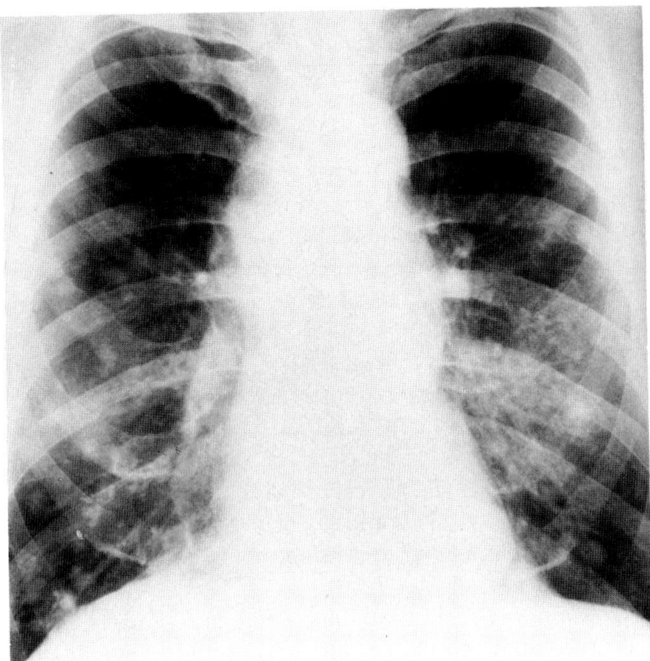

Fig. 14.35 Carcinoma of bladder. Mediastinal adenopathy and lung metastases.

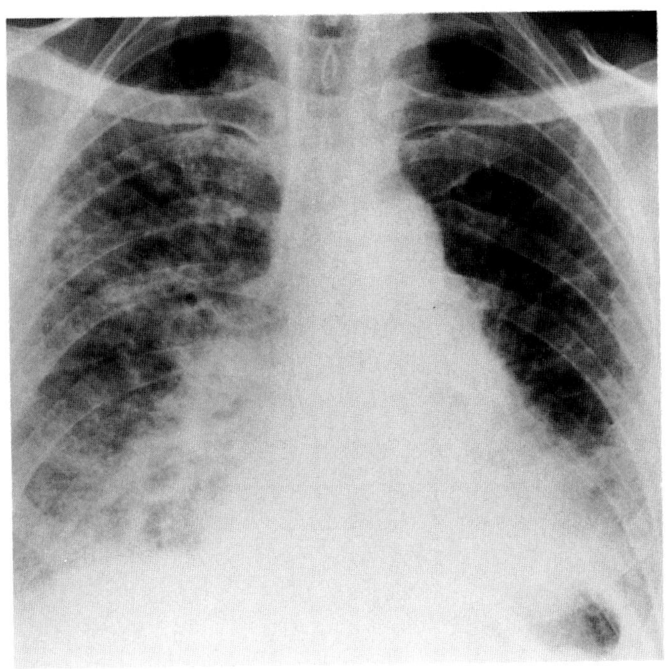

Fig. 14.36 Lymphangitis carcinomatosa.

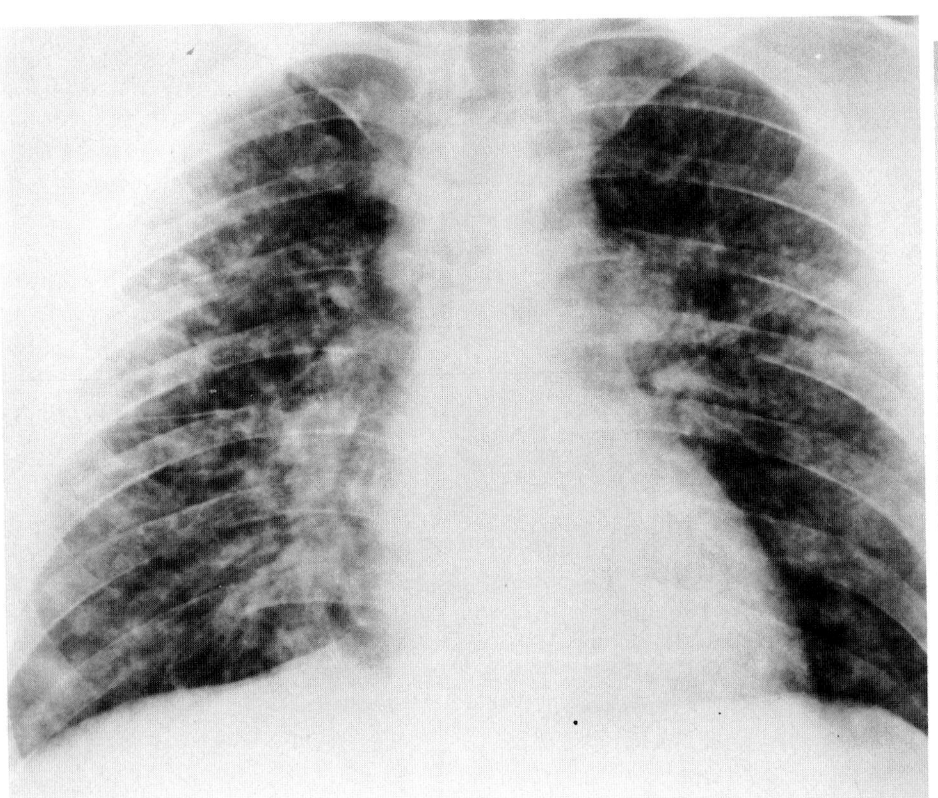

Fig. 14.37

Fig. 14.37 Metastases from malignant melanoma. Chest radiograph was normal 12 days before this.

Fig. 14.38

Fig. 14.38 Tomogram. Solitary fibrosarcoma metastasis. Fibrosarcoma removed from thigh 20 years before!

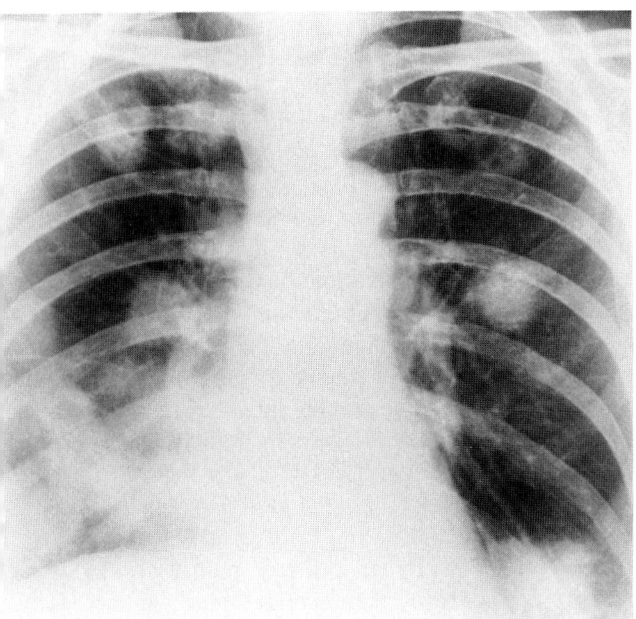

Fig. 14.39 Cavitating metastases.

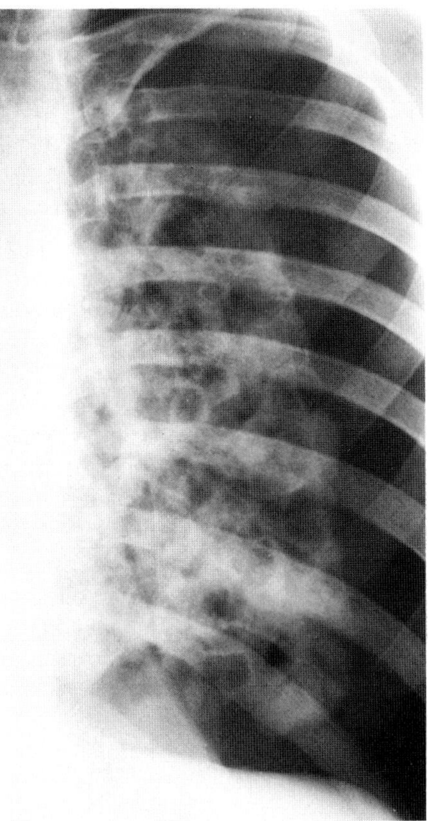

Fig. 14.40 Cavitating angiosarcoma metastases. Spontaneous pneumothorax.

Trophoblastic tumours have variable malignant potential but all are liable to embolize to the lungs where the benign varieties undergo absorption. Trophoblastic tissue is by its nature invasive and the metastases have the same characteristics. They have poor definition of their edge because they are surrounded by haemorrhage. An unusual complication sometimes follows removal of a molar pregnancy — the sudden onset of pulmonary oedema progressing into the adult respiratory distress syndrome with diffuse intravascular coagulation.

Occasionally an *endobronchial tumour* is biopsied and found to be a metastasis usually from a primary in breast, colon or renal tract. Bronchial obstruction dominates the clinical and radiographic signs, a circumstance which is otherwise rare in metastatic disease.

MALIGNANT LYMPHOMA AND LEUKAEMIA

Proliferation of lymphocytes is a feature of malignant lymphoma and also of certain benign conditions. Distinction between them on histological grounds can be difficult, compounded by the fact that some of the benign disorders eventually become transformed into malignant lymphomas.

A number of conditions predispose to the development of malignant lymphoma. These include congenital immune deficiencies (Wiskott-Aldrich syndrome, ataxia telangiectasia), auto-immune diseases (rheumatoid, systemic lupus, myasthenia gravis), occupational exposure to benzene and other solvents, organ transplantation, Sjögren's syndrome, and immunoblastic lymphadenopathy. There is also a slight excess in patients with sarcoidosis over the number expected from chance association. The drug phenytoin has an association with malignant lymphoma as well as with benign lymphoproliferative disorders. Most of the disorders which carry an increased risk have an abnormality of immune mechanisms, either immunosuppression, failure of immune surveillance or chronic subjection to antigenic stimulation. It is thought that there is a transformation by stages, first a polyclonal proliferation of lymphocytes followed by an escape of a malignant cell line.

Treatment of the malignant lymphomas is now highly effective but radiotherapy and chemotherapy are not without risk and morbidity. Treatment therefore has to be tailored to the extent and site of disease, hence the stress laid on diagnostic staging. The number and complexity of the imaging modes utilized in the staging process depends to some extent on the histological type. Centres dealing with the disease also vary in their requirements. Detailed histological classification is essential for the assessment of the efficacy of different treatment regimes under test but it has few implications as far as radiological diagnosis is concerned.

Malignant lymphoma is divided into two groups — *Hodgkin's* and *non-Hodgkin's* and each group is further subdivided on histological criteria into many varieties. Some confusion is created by the use of alternative names for the same histological type, e.g. lymphocytic lymphoma and lymphosarcoma; histiocytic lymphoma and reticulum cell sarcoma.

Hodgkin's lymphoma is a nodal disease, starting in nodes and spreading from nodes. If it starts in the thorax the *mediastinal nodes* will almost invariably be enlarged, the hilar nodes less often. The circumstance in which only the hilar nodes are enlarged is unusual but it happens sufficiently often to limit the value of site as an infallible discriminant between lymphoma and sarcoidosis. The nodes are massive and merge with each other, presenting an undulating rather than a nodular margin. If *extension into the lung* takes place it does so along interlobular, perivascular and peribronchial lymphatic channels forming deposits in the small *intrapulmonary nodes*. The latter are located at the sites of branching of the bronchovascular structures. In this way the disease can extend out to the pleura. Radiographically the sharp outline of purely central nodal disease is then replaced by a shaggy edge from a mixture of linear streaks, bands and clusters of small nodules radiating into the lungs (Figs. 14.41A and B). The individual components of this shadowing may merge into a patchy haze of progressively diminishing density as it gets further out into the lung (Figs. 14.42A & B). This pulmonary spread can take place rapidly over the course of a few days causing confusion with oedema or infection. Dense coalescent *infiltrations* may result in segmental or lobar opacities, sometimes with air bronchograms (Fig. 14.43). There may be *lung nodules*, either profuse and miliary or of larger size up to 1 cm in diameter.

Pulmonary lesions sometimes necrose with the formation of thick-walled *cavities*. An *effusion*, which may be chylous, may result from extension into the pleura and a careful search should then be made for evidence of rib erosion.

Hodgkin's disease beginning elsewhere in the body and spreading into the thorax differs from the pattern described above in that pulmonary lesions can develop without any obvious mediastinal or hilar node enlargement. This has been reported in up to 25% of cases which contrasts with the exceptional rarity of primary pulmonary Hodgkin's disease. In other respects the radiographic signs are similar.

After successful treatment the chest radiograph may not

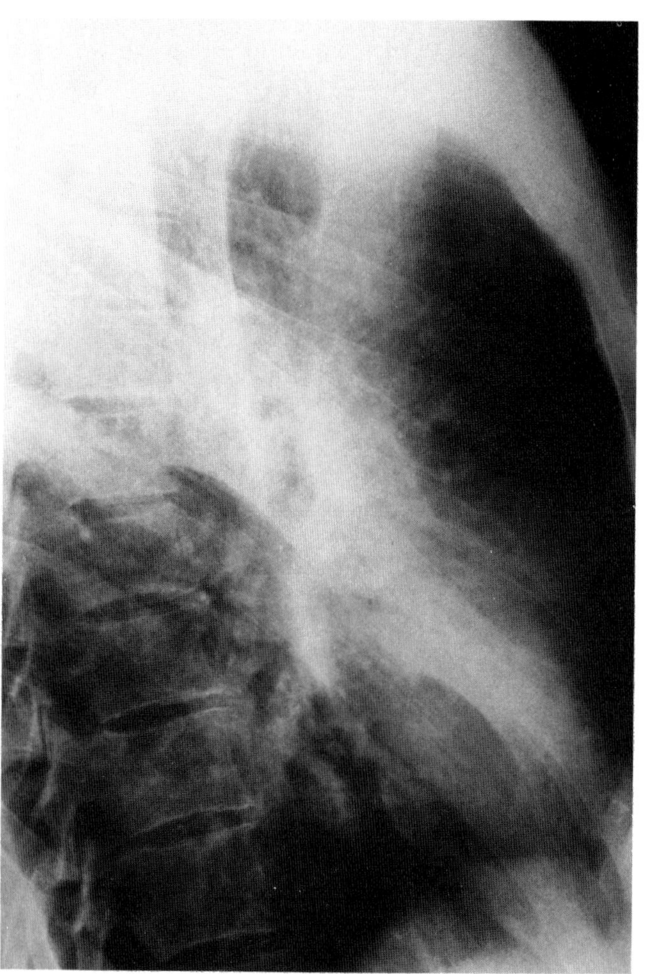

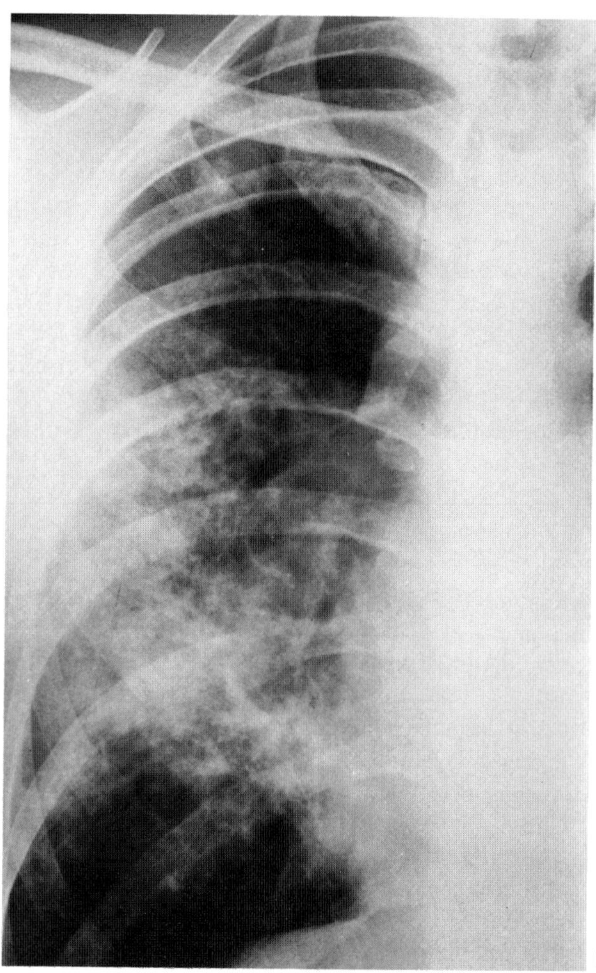

Fig. 14.41 (**A** and **B**) Hodgkin's lymphoma. Mediastinal node enlargement. Mixed nodular and interstitial pulmonary spread into upper and middle lobes.

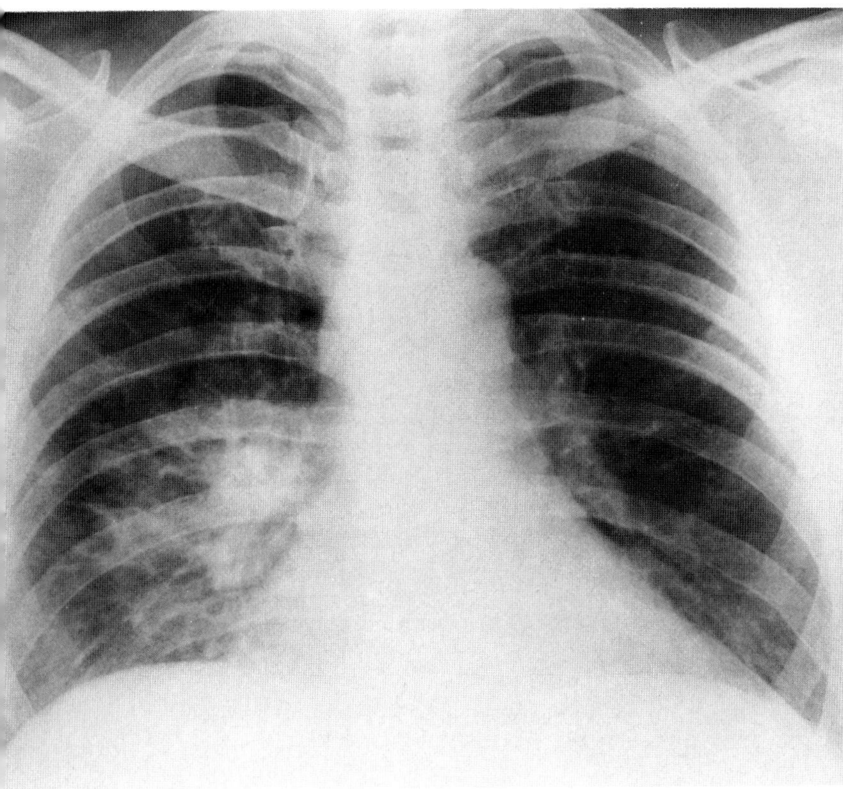

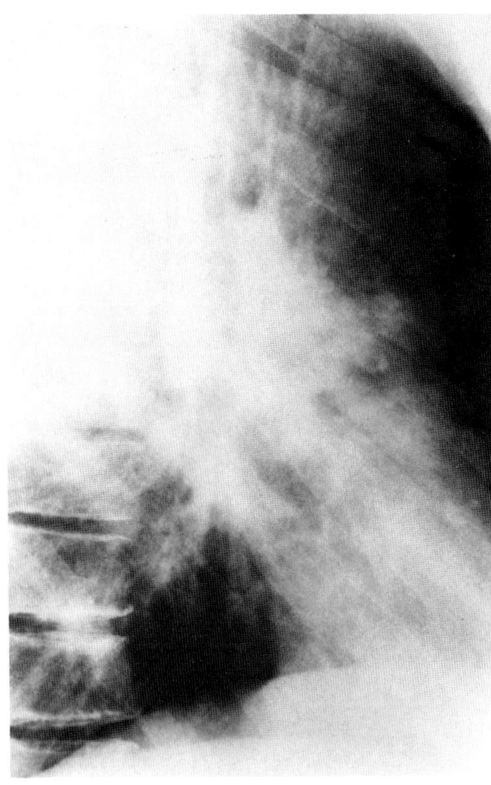

B

ig. 14.42 (**A** and **B**) Hodgkin's lymphoma. Right mediastinal and hilar node enlargement. Spreading consolidation in upper, middle and lower bes. Nodules at the edge of the consolidation and distally.

return to normal. Nodes may *calcify*, *radiation pneumonitis* appear or a residual mass of *pseudotumour* persist. To determine whether such a mass is due to pseudotumour or residual disease may require excision or biopsy. Pseudotumours consist of non-specific inflammatory reactions, fibrous tissue or amyloid.

Radiation pneumonitis is strictly confined to the volume of lung irradiated, an important point in differential diagnosis. *Recall radiation pneumonitis* is a term applied to ill-defined opacities appearing in the radiation field but only after the withdrawal of steroid therapy. It has been described as occurring up to 6 years after radiotherapy and it responds to the re-introduction of steroids.

Non-Hodgkin's lymphoma. As far as the radiographic signs are concerned the differences between Hodgkin's and non-Hodgkin's lymphoma are quantitative rather than qualitative. The disease rarely starts in the thorax and it is usually at an advanced stage when this occurs. *Mediastinal* and *hilar node masses*, radiating *perihilar streaks with small pulmonary nodules* on the lymphatic pathways, *segmental* and *lobar opacities* are all features of the disease similar to those of Hodkin's disease but *pulmonary lesions without nodal involvement* are more common (Fig. 14.44). A lobe solid with primary lymphocytic lymphoma, although rare, is not so exceptional as the equivalent in Hodgkin's disease. A *pleural plaque* or *effusion* is found in approximately 30% of patients.

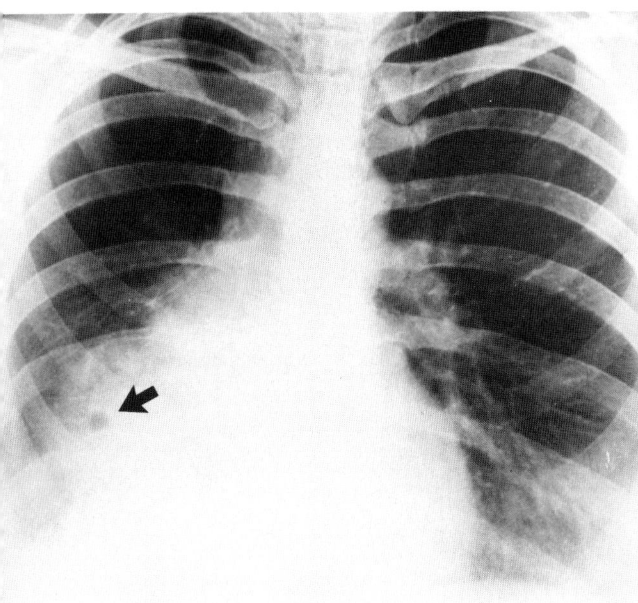

ig. 14.43 Hodgkin's lymphoma. Dense consolidation of right middle nd lower lobes with a small cavity (arrow). Mediastinal adenopathy.

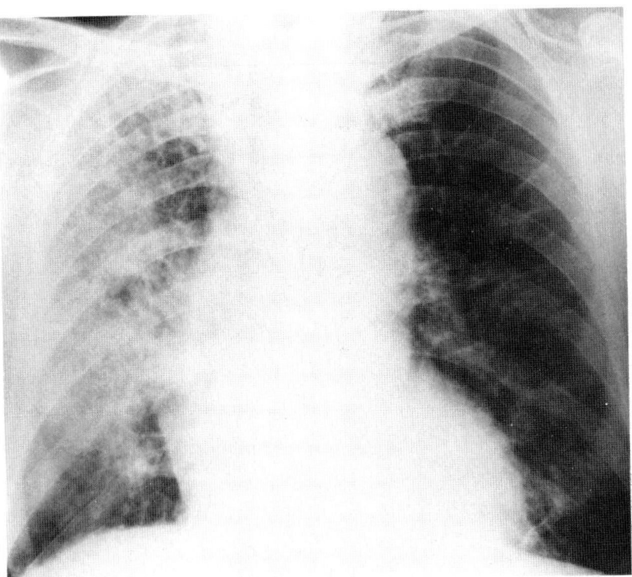

Fig. 14.44 Non-Hodgkin's lymphoma in Sjögren's syndrome. Mixed nodular and interstitial shadowing in right lung. Slow progression over 7 years. Minimal changes in left lung. No hilar or mediastinal adenopathy.

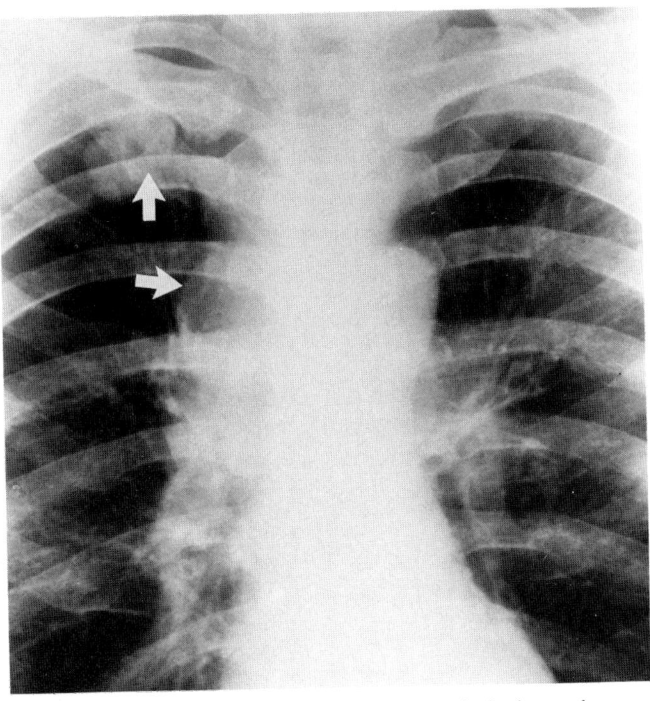

Fig. 14.45 Chronic lymphatic leukaemia. Mediastinal adenopathy. Deposit in right upper lobe (arrows).

It has been postulated that primary extra nodal malignant lymphoma belongs to a separate category of tumour derived from mucosa-associated lymphoid tissue and has a characteristic spread to histologically related tissues. An example of this spread is that which takes place in some cases of Sjögren's syndrome from the salivary glands to the lung. In this hypothesis lymphomatoid granulomatosis and pseudolymphoma are examples of primary bronchial mucosa-associated malignant lymphoma which may remain localised for long periods.

Plasmacytoma or plasmacytic lymphoma are descriptive terms for the lesions of myelomatosis and solitary tumours of this nature are identical to the disseminate form. Solitary tumours may present as pulmonary masses or obstructing endobronchial lesions.

LEUKAEMIA

In almost all cases of leukaemia that come to post-mortem there can be found microscopic infiltrations of leukaemic cells around bronchi and vessels and in alveolar walls. Macroscopic nodules from 1 mm to 2 cm in size may also be found. Nevertheless it is exceptional for these deposits to be visible on the chest radiograph, any abnormal opacity will almost certainly be the result of infection, infarction or haemorrhage. *Mediastinal* or *hilar node enlargement* is more frequent than pulmonary deposits (Fig. 14.45). Conversion of lymphoma to leukaemia is a recognized complication, particularly with lymphoblastic lymphoma and this conversion can sometimes be predicted if a mediastinal mass makes its appearance during the course of the disease. Leukaemia can also follow apparently successful treatment of lymphoma.

REFERENCES AND SUGGESTIONS FOR FURTHER READING

rnold, A. M., & Williams, C. J. (1979) Small-cell lung cancer: a curable disease? *British Journal of Diseases of the Chest*, **73**, 327–348.

lank, N., & Castellino, R. A. (1980) The intra-thoracic manifestations of the malignant lymphomas and the leukaemias. *Seminars in Roentgenology*, **15**, 227–245.

allihan, T. R., & Berard, C. W. (1980) The classification and pathology of the lymphomas and leukaemias. *Seminars in Roentgenology*, **15**, 203–218.

ho, S.-R., Henry, D. A., Beachley, M. C. & Brooks, J. W. (1981) Round (helical) atelectasis. *The British Journal of Radiology*, **54**, 643–650.

orrin, B., Liebow, A. A., & Friedman, P. J. (1975) Pulmonary lymphangiomyomatosis. *The American Journal of Pathology*, **79**, 348–382.

Lillington, G. A., & Stevens, G. M. (1976) The solitary nodule. The other side of the coin. *Chest*, **70**, 322–323.

Ray, J. F., Lawton, B. R., Magnin, G. E., Dovenbarger, W. V., Smullen, W. A., Reyes, C. N., Myers, W. O., Wenzel, F. J. & Sautter, R. D. (1976) The coin lesion story: update 1976. *Chest*, **70**, 332–336.

Seminars in Roentgenology (1977), Pulmonary neoplasms. (By various authors). No. 3. **12**, 161–246.

Wright, D. H. & Isaacson P. G. (1983) Biopsy pathology of the lympho-reticular system. London. Chapman & Hall.

CHAPTER 15

INFLAMMATORY DISEASES OF THE LUNG

Terminology. The terminology used to describe inflammatory or any other disease of the lungs is designed to satisfy clinical and pathological criteria and attempts to apply the same terms to radiographic appearances can lead to confusion. 'Infiltrate' or 'infiltration', often used to describe abnormal lung opacifications means something quite different to a pathologist. Alternatively radiographic shadows can be described in terms of their physical characteristics without any pathological overtones. Nevertheless it is difficult to completely avoid reference to such terms as 'atelectasis', 'consolidation' and 'interstitial'.

Three handicaps under which radiologists work are (1) they deal with volumes compressed into two dimensions with all the implications of superimposition; (2) terminology is imprecise and not uniform; (3) correlation between pathological and radiographic appearances is in many instances crude, particularly in the case of disseminate lung disease. Diagnosis based on purely radiographic appearances will almost always contain a large element of uncertainty but this can be reduced by a search for ancillary clues which may be clinical, pathological, radiological or statistical.

Pneumonia is an inflammatory disease of lung usually due to infection by pathogenic organisms and consolidation (the replacement of alveolar air by exudate) is assumed unless the term is qualified as in 'interstitial pneumonia'. It is seldom possible radiographically and without other evidence to differentiate inflammatory exudate from oedema fluid, blood or tumour.

Pneumonitis is a general term for any inflammatory reaction in the lung and consolidation is neither implied nor excluded. An inflammatory process that predominantly affects the alveolar wall is usually referred to as *alveolitis* in Great Britain or *interstitial pneumonitis* (*pneumonia*) in North America.

Bronchopneumonia is a multifocal bronchocentric infection based on the pulmonary lobule. The process spreads along the bronchial axis. Lesions are at first small but coalesce as they spread outwards. Their characteristic feature both pathologically and radiographically is inhomogeneity, in contrast to the homogeneity of lobar pneumonia.

Division of pneumonias into *primary* and *secondary* according to whether there is a precipitating cause is of limited help diagnostically.

ACUTE PNEUMONIA

A causative organism is only likely to be found in 50% of cases, usually because of prior treatment with antibiotics or an inability to provide a satisfactory sputum specimen. Of these organisms there will be a third each of bacterial, non-bacterial and viral.

Of the bacterial causes the *pneumococcus* (*Streptococcus pneumoniae*) in most common, with much smaller numbers of *Staphylococcus aureus*, *Haemophilus influenzae*, *Klebsiella pneumoniae* and *Legionella pneumophila*.

Of the non-bacterial causes *Mycoplasma pneumoniae* is most common. In fact it is the most common proven cause of primary pneumonia in Great Britain at the present time. Other non-bacterial causes found in small numbers are *Chlamydia psittaci* (psittacosis) and *Coxiella burnetti* (Q fever). The viruses are almost all *influenza* or *cold viruses*. Mixed infections are found in approximately 10%.

Pneumococcal pneumonia is the archetype of classical lobar pneumonia (Fig. 15.1) with homogeneous lung opacification limited by fissures. Affected lobes retain normal volume and often show air bronchograms. The onset is so acute that opacification is often at its maximum on the initial radiograph. However, consolidation is not always obvious on the radiograph and its presence may be revealed more by the silhouette sign of boundary effacement than by pulmonary opacity.

The classical appearance is now the exception rather than the rule largely because of early antibiotic treatment aborting the progression. Consolidation may not spread uniformly throughout the lobe. From the initial focus of infection a tidal wave of inflammatory oedema spreads concentrically by all available routes, not only by the air passages but also through the substance of the lung via the pores of Kohn. The opacity may therefore not conform to

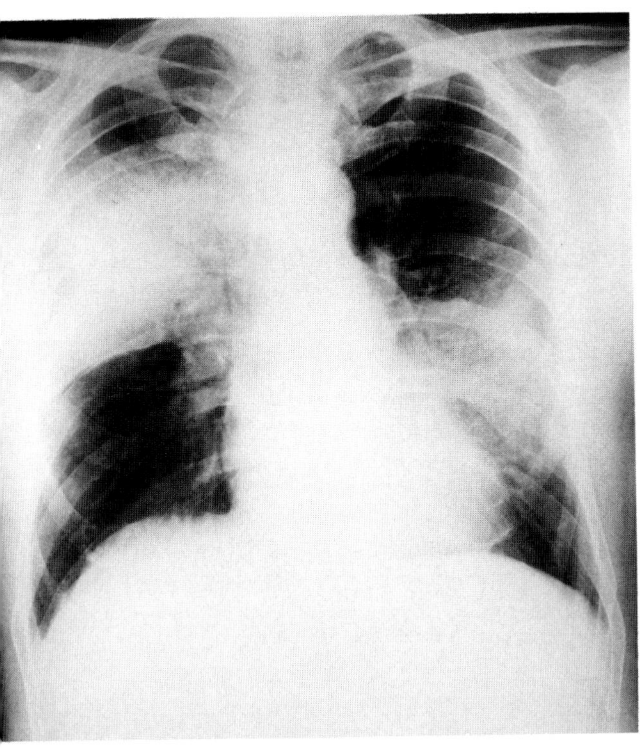

'ig. 15.1 Pneumococcal pneumonia. Lingula and right upper lobe onsolidation with sparing of apex.

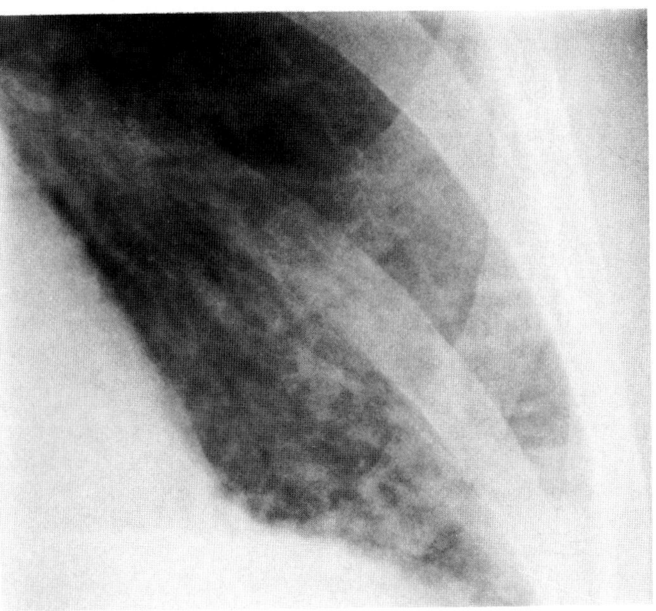

Fig. 15.2 Acute pneumonia. Oedema of interlobular septa.

egmental boundaries, it may produce rounded lesions with ll-defined margins. Kerley B lines may appear in the ffected area from a temporary overloading of lymphatics nd oedema of interlobular septa (Fig. 15.2). The distribution of the inflammatory exudate can be influenced to some degree by the effect of gravity until it becomes fixed by consolidation. Resolution is accompanied by diminution of he density of the opacity as air returns to the lobe. It is usually complete and lung architecture is restored to normal.

The complications of *empyema*, *lung abscess* or *delayed resolution* depend on such factors as host resistance and type of causative pathogen. If resolution is unduly delayed the exudate is invaded by fibroblasts and organization by *fibrosis* takes place.

There are not diagnostic features for particular pathogenic organisms but clues can sometimes be found in the radiographic pattern of pneumonia.

Staphylococcal pneumonia is usually a haematogenous dissemination and the lesions are therefore likely to be oval or round and multiple. However, this is not always the case and the staphylococcus can be a secondary invader and then the lesions will be bronchopneumonic, irregular and patchy (Fig. 15.3A, B). There is a strong tendency for colliquative necrosis to occur in the centre of staphylococcal consolidations (Fig. 15.4). As the consolidation around these *abscesses* recedes they are seen to have a thin wall. Resolution of the consolidation and resorption of the fluid contents leaves a *pneumatocoele* with a wall of hair-line thickness. These may persist for months but eventually they disappear usually leaving no trace. *Empyema* is another common complication of staphylococcal pneumonia sometimes a result of injudicious needling of a lung abscess.

Legionnaires' disease. In 1976 an explosive epidemic of severe respiratory illness occurred at an American legionnaires' convention in Philadelphia. It was a rapidly extending pneumonia complicated by shock, mental confusion, respiratory and renal failure unresponsive to the usual antibiotics with a case fatality of 16%. A previously unknown Gram-negative bacillus was eventually isolated and given the name *Legionella pneumophila*. The organism is ubiquitous in water, multiplying in water coolers, air-conditioners and showers, and infection takes place from inhalation of an aerosol mist.

It is prone to attack smokers and the debilitated. Radiographically there is spreading consolidation and although it may be confined to one lobe initially it soon extends to others and to the opposite lung (Fig. 15.5). Another characteristic feature is the slow resolution over several weeks but this is usually complete. Small *pleural effusions* are common; abscess and pneumatocoele formation rare.

Friedländer (Klebsiella) pneumonia is typically a disease of elderly debilitated men. So voluminous is the inflammatory exudate that the affected lobe may be swollen and the fissures then bulge. Although this is regarded as a helpful diagnostic sign it is in fact unusual, nor is it confined to Friedländer infections. The upper lobes are those most frequently involved and in common with other

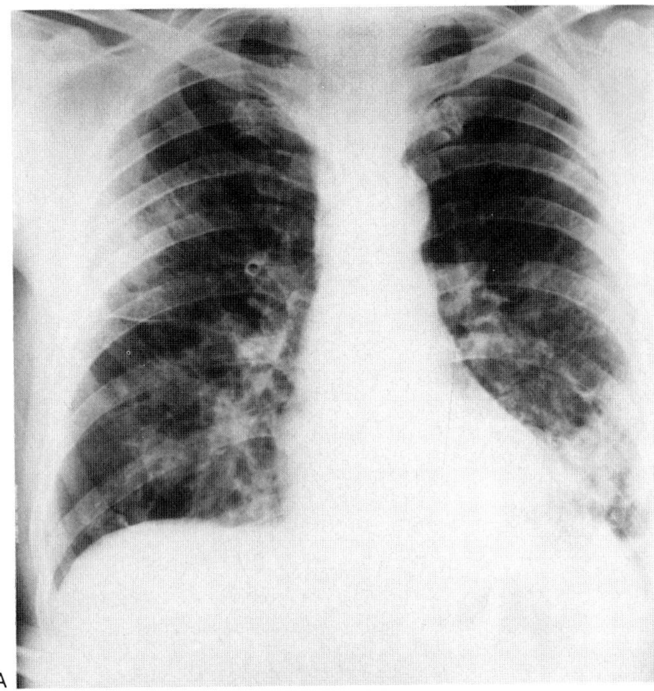

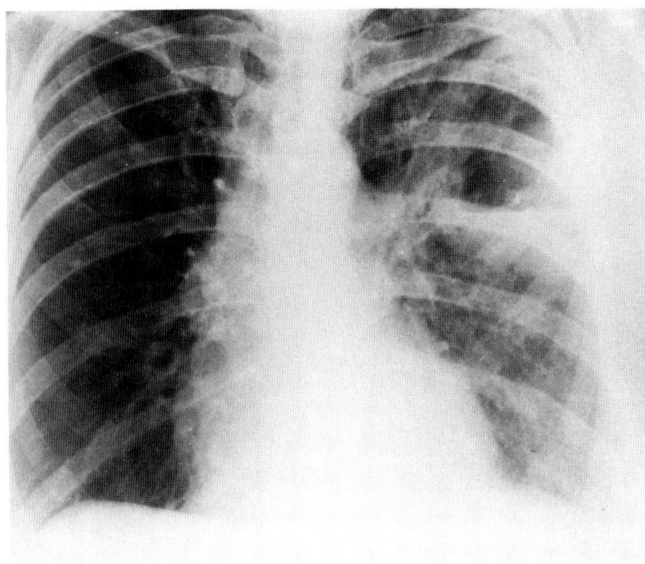

Fig. 15.4 Staphylococcal pneumonia left upper lobe with abscess formation. Influenzal illness one week before.

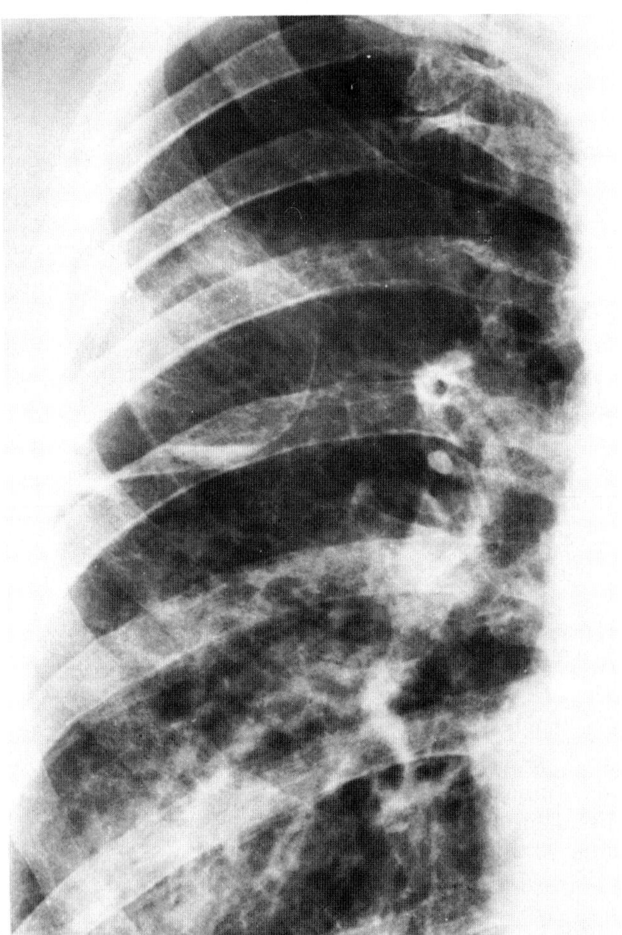

Fig. 15.3 (**A**) Staphylococcal bronchopneumonia. (**B**) A pneumatocoele has developed in the right upper lobe. The radiograph returned to normal.

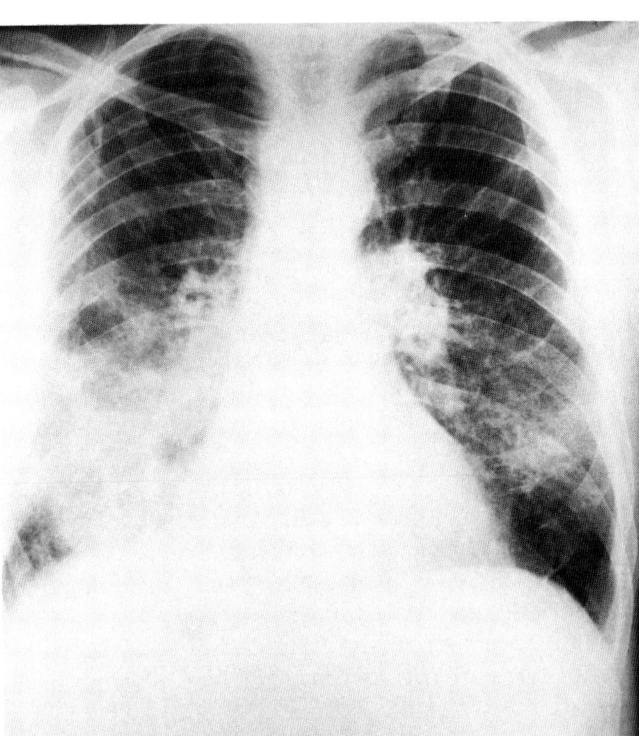

Fig. 15.5 Legionnaires' disease. Bilateral consolidations.

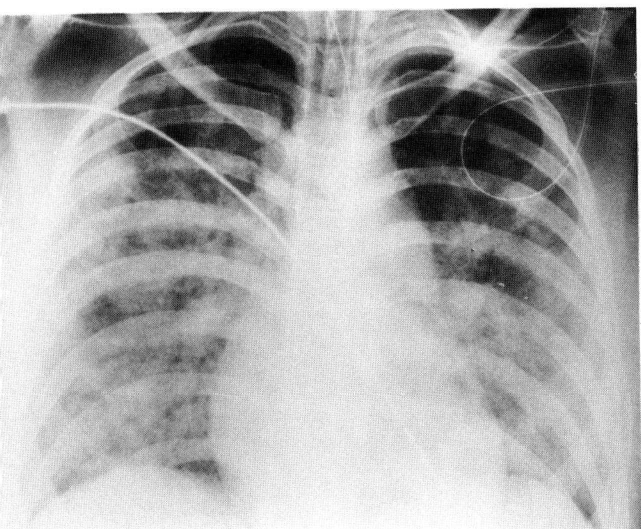

Fig. 15.6 Klebsiella (Friedländer) septicaemia. Diffuse, patchy, alveolar shadowing.

Gram-negative pneumonias there is a strong tendency to necrosis with the formation of multiple abscesses. If fibrosis takes place these cavities become permanent and by virtue of their site, mimic tuberculosis. A septicaemic infection can occur in younger patients which is radiographically indistinguishable from many other overwhelming pulmonary infections or from pulmonary oedema (Fig. 15.6).

Haemophilus influenzae is a commensal of the upper respiratory tract but since it is sometimes found in large numbers in the sputum in association with chronic lung diseases and treatment aimed at its eradication is often followed by clinical improvement it is accorded a potentially pathogenic role. It is a secondary invader found in chronic bronchitis, cystic fibrosis and debilitated states. It is also found in influenza and other virus infections. Any pulmonary opacities found in *Haemophilus* infection are disseminate and bronchopneumonic; there are no characteristic radiographic appearances (Fig. 15.7).

Pseudomonas aeruginosa is an organism widely distributed in nature and of low pathogenicity. Most infections are either acquired in hospital or occur in immunocompromised patients. Pulmonary infections follow mechanical ventilation of the lungs, inhalation therapy or the use of aerosols. It is therefore an unwelcome visitor to ITUs where the incidence of its acquisition is directly proportional to the duration of mechanical ventilation and the use of broad spectrum antibiotics. Pulmonary infection is a bronchopneumonia with a tendency to confluence and destruction of alveolar walls resulting in microabscesses which progressively enlarge. An unusual manifestation consisting of large numbers of widespread small opacities suggests a septicaemic spread.

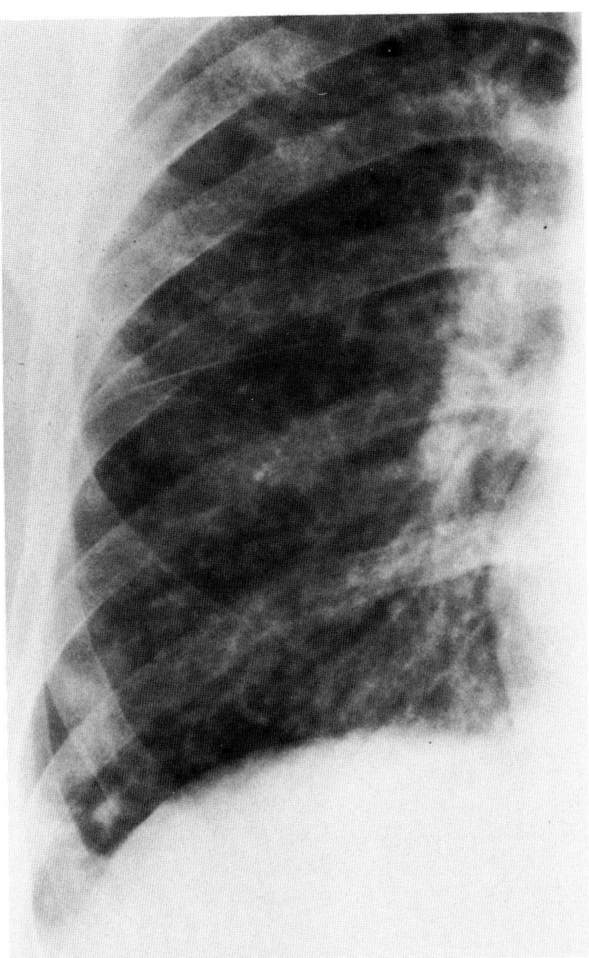

Fig. 15.7 Haemophilus infection. Widespread small opacities. Recent influenza.

Melioidosis, a disease of tropical countries of the East, is caused by *Pseudomonas pseudomallei*. It may manifest years after the patient has left an endemic area. There are two pulmonary forms, (1) septicaemic disseminate necrotizing lesions and; (2) a chronic apical pneumonia which breaks down forming a thin-walled cavity.

Tularaemia. Discovered in Tulare, California, infection with the *Francisella tularensis* is endemic amongst small mammals and is spread by ticks. Humans acquire the infection either by inoculation or inhalation. Remarkably few organisms are required to cause illness. In the bacteraemic form there are small oval pulmonary lesions and hilar adenopathy. Inhalation infection causes one or more consolidations, also with hilar adenopathy. Untreated the consolidations cavitate and fibrose and then mimic tuberculosis.

LUNG ABSCESS

Gram-negative organisms have a particular propensity to cause pulmonary infections which break down with the formation of abscesses. Three circumstances favour their development, 1) aspiration of infected material; 2) infarction by septic material; and 3) infection by anaerobic organisms. The isolation of an organism from sputum does not necessarily mean that it is the sole cause and a lack of response to treatment should lead one to suspect a mixed infection, particularly with anaerobic or microaerophilic organisms.

Commonly multiple cavities form within an area of consolidation but they only become visible when the contents are discharged and air enters. The cavities enlarge and coalesce. *Gangrene of the lung* is a rapidly spreading necrosis, the separation of the slough producing first an air crescent between itself and viable lung before falling to the bottom of the cavity. The disease has a high mortality with or without surgical resection and prognosis depends very much on finding an appropriate antibiotic.

Anaerobic and microaerophilic organisms can also be responsible for indolent pulmonary infections leading to bizarre empyemas clearing slowly over many months (Fig. 15.8).

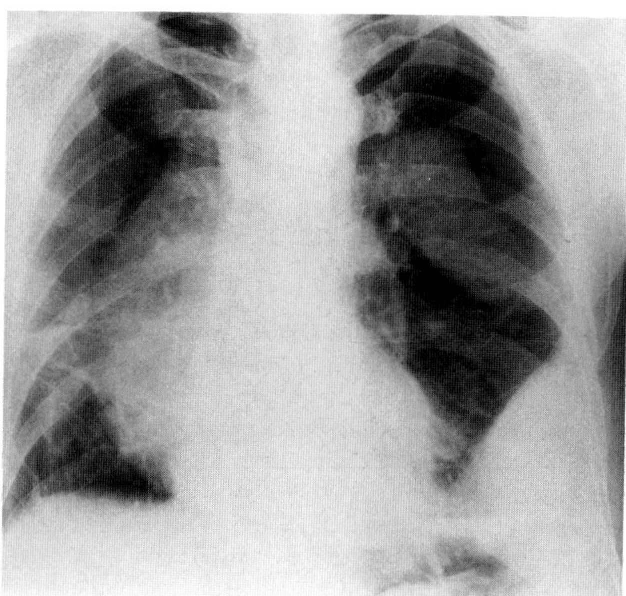

Fig. 15.8 Multiple empyemas. Aspirations sterile. Slow resolution. Probably anaerobic or microaerophilic infection.

ASPIRATION AND INHALATION

The effects of aspiration of particulate or liquid foreign material into the lungs are twofold, those due to mechanical bronchial obstruction and those due to the irritant properties of the aspirate. When the cough reflex is suppressed by stupor, alcohol or drugs, aspiration of food from the stomach during vomiting is likely to occur. The inflammatory response excited by vegetable matter intense and commonly followed by secondary infectio with commensals and anaerobic organisms. Aspiration infected material from nasal and oral sepsis is a commo cause of lung abscess. The radiological patterns are there fore those of atelectasis or suppurative bronchitis and pneu monia. Metallic or inorganic particles may excite littl

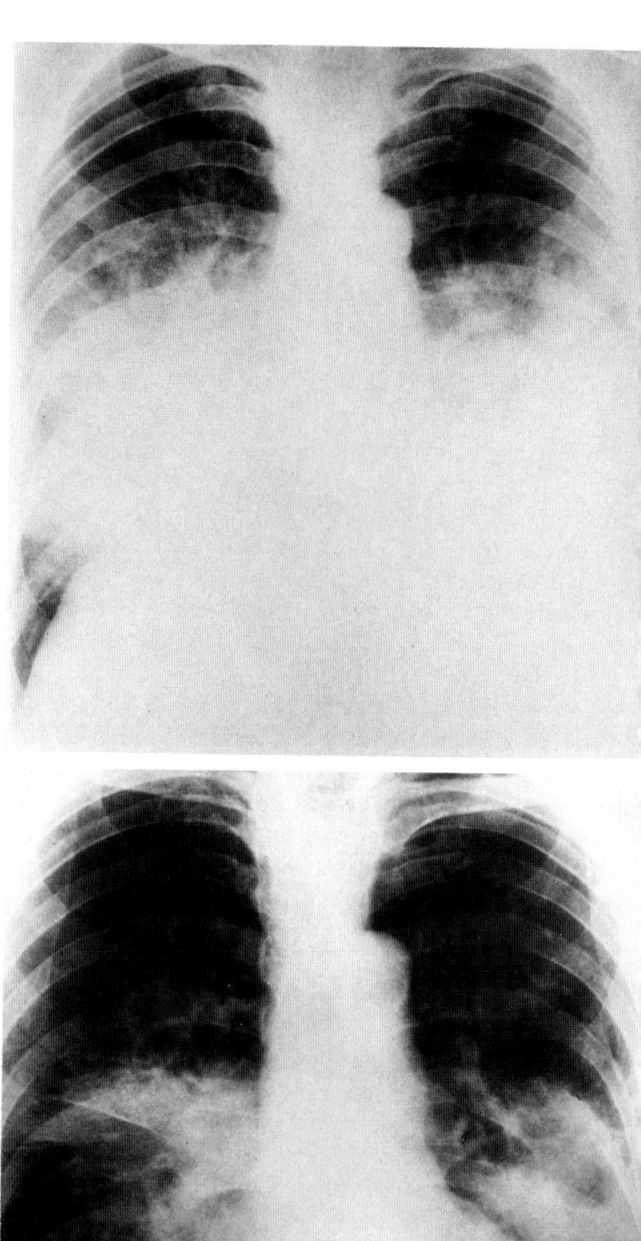

Fig. 15.9 (**A**) Lipoid pneumonia. Aspiration of liquid paraffin. (**B**) 8 years later. Significant clearance but massive residual fibrosis.

response, the mechanical effects of uncomplicated atelectasis or obstructive emphysema predominating and they may remain undetected for long periods.

Aspiration of mineral oils results in **lipoid pneumonia** (Fig. 15.9A and B). The prolonged use of liquid paraffin for constipation is the usual cause and a precipitating factor is chronic oesophageal obstruction. The oil floats to the top of any residue in the oesophagus, the optimum position for aspiration. The oil is almost inert and the reaction is indolent, granulomatous and fibrotic and any lung damage is permanent. Radiographically there are dense well-defined tumour-like masses or an extensive bilateral opacity spreading outwards from the hilar regions. Vegetable oils and animal fats such as milk induce a greater inflammatory response and the opacities are ill-defined and bronchopneumonic. Influenced by gravity the lesions of aspiration and inhalation are found predominantly in the posterior parts of the lungs. Small aspirates are common in the aged from incompetence of the closing mechanism of the larynx. These recurrent aspirations produce coarse peribronchial thickening, small patches of pneumonia and eventually fibrosis and bronchiectasis.

Mendelson's syndrome is a chemical pneumonia caused by aspiration of acid gastric contents during anaesthesia. An intense bronchospasm is rapidly followed by a flood of oedema throughout the lungs resulting in hypoxia and requiring high ventilation pressures. The radiographic appearance of massive pulmonary oedema taken together with the clinical presentation is pathognomonic (Fig. 15.10).

In cases of *near-drowning* the lungs show widespread, ill-defined alveolar opacities due to pulmonary oedema. The effects of salt water are less severe and of shorter duration than those due to hypotonic fresh water.

Inhalation of irritant gases (e.g. ammonia, chlorine, nitrogen dioxide) produces an acute focal or diffuse pulmonary oedema followed by functional derangements indicative of bronchiolar and alveolar damage. It is one cause of bronchiolitis obliterans. Widespread tubular bronchiectasis has been reported as a sequel to accidental smoke inhalation.

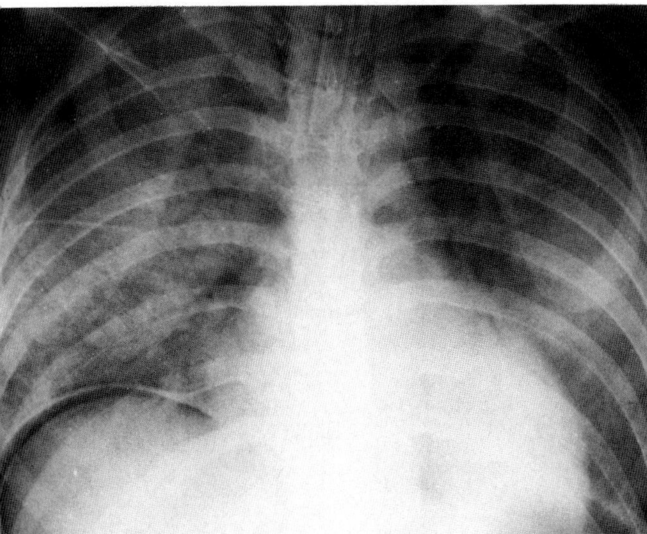

Fig. 15.10 Mendelson's syndrome. Post-operative aspiration of acid gastric contents.

IMPAIRED DEFENCE MECHANISMS

There are a number of genetically determined abnormalities, the effects of which impair the defences of the lungs against infection. Acquired immunosuppression is dealt with elsewhere.

Pulmonary cystic fibrosis

Patients are now surviving to adult life but the prognosis is still poor. The susceptibility of the lungs to infection is related to the abnormal physico-chemical properties of the bronchial mucus making it more viscous and impairing mucociliary transport. Common infecting organisms are *Staphylococcus aureus, Pseudomonas aeruginosa, Haemophilus influenzae* and *Klebsiella*. Pneumothorax occurs in 20% of cases and is difficult to manage conservatively because 50% recur and prolonged tube drainage carries a high mortality. Surgical treatment is therefore undertaken more often than would otherwise be the case. Small haemoptyses are common and on rare occasions massive haemoptyses can be life-threatening. It is in such circumstances that control by bronchial artery embolization may need to be considered.

Primary immunodeficiency disorders

These are a diverse group of *abnormalities of immunoglobulins*. The deficiencies may be selective or total and the levels reduced or absent. Adult patients are survivors from the childhood affliction and the majority have an abnormal chest radiograph, the result of recurrent bronchopulmonary infections. Thoracic manifestations include atelectasis, bronchiectasis, thymoma and lymphocytic interstitial pneumonia. These patients have an increased risk of developing lymphoid neoplasms and carcinomas.

Chronic granulomatous disease. In only rare instances do patients with this condition survive to adult life. Phagocytosis is normal but the polymorphs are incapable of destroying the ingested bacteria at a normal rate. Children suffer from recurrent pneumonias but with increasing age these become less frequent. The lungs usually show bilateral interstitial fibrosis. Other complications are bronchiectasis and granulomatous mediastinitis.

Impaired neutrophil chemotaxis. Phagocytic cells are attracted to sites of bacterial infection by chemotactic substances released by the organisms or locally produced by the host. Activated complement is one such host substance. Instances have been found of impaired neutrophil chemotactic responses which have had an adverse effect on the frequency and severity of infections.

Abscesses and skin sepsis are the common manifestations and recurrent staphylococcal pneumonias are not infrequent.

Congenital dyskinetic ciliary syndromes. The immotile cilia syndrome was the term originally applied to this group of conditions but this is too restrictive since it is now known that there can be abnormalities of synchrony as well as total immotility. It is a heterogenous mixture of structural and functional abnormalities of cilia. It is now postulated that the beating of embryonic cilia determines organ situs and if the beat is abnormal the situs will be randomly allocated and 50% will have situs inversus. Sperm tails are also cilia and males with the condition will be infertile. It also explains the curious combination of bronchiectasis, situs inversus and male infertility in Kartagener's syndrome.

The lungs suffer from the impairment of mucociliary clearance by an increased susceptibility to bronchopulmonary infections but this is only a serious problem if the infections are repeated and severe. The radiographic signs are those of bronchitis, tubular bronchiectasis, atelectasis and chronic obstructive airways disease.

Young's syndrome is a combination of obstructive azoospermia, sinusitis and chronic pulmonary infections. The latter begin in childhood and eventually most patients develop bronchiectasis. There is no structural abnormality of cilia but mucociliary transport is impaired. Spermatogenesis is normal, the infertility of these men being due to a progressive obstruction of the epididymis by inspissated secretions.

UNRESOLVED PNEUMONIA

A pneumonic consolidation which stubbornly refuses to improve over a long period presents a problem in management. It is a circumstance where excision of the lesion will have to be considered if all other diagnostic modalities have been inconclusive. Pathological examination of such lobes or lungs will usually reveal definitive or circumstantial evidence of aspiration. Proof of aspiration lies in the demonstration of identifiable particulate foreign material or extrinsic lipids. A suggestive histological pattern including foreign body giant cells is circumstantial evidence of aspiration. Only a minority are post-infective. Isolated cases will be found to be rare examples of sarcoid reaction, lymphomatoid granulomatosis, chronic eosinophil pneumonia and other miscellaneous conditions.

A few cases in which all known causes have been excluded have responded favourably to steroids and there has been relapse, sometimes in another part of the lung, when they have been withdrawn. On continuous steroid treatment the lungs become virtually normal. To distinguish this small group it has been called *cryptogenic organizing pneumonitis*.

ACTINOMYCOSIS AND NOCARDIOSIS

In the past these infections have been placed with th mycoses but the organisms concerned are now regarded a branching bacteria.

Actinomycosis

The characteristic sulphur granules found in the exudat from actinomycotic lesions consist of clumps of *Actinomyce israeli*. It is a commensal in the mouth and infection of th lung is by aspiration or direct extension from oesophagus mediastinum or elsewhere. A chronic consolidation form which with progression crosses pleural boundaries. Perihilar consolidation fanning out into the lungs may closel simulate a carcinoma. When the pleura is reached a localized encysted abscess forms which may erode a rib an break through onto the skin surface leading to drainin sinuses. An apical cavity simulating tuberculosis may form An unusual form is that of an extensive bilateral patch pneumonia.

Nocardiosis

Nocardia asteroides is a soil saprophyte of world-wide distribution and human infection is by inhalation. The lesions vary from a solitary nodule to a confluence of multiple areas of consolidation (Fig. 15.11). It is a suppurating bronchopneumonia and the consolidations can be notably dense. Multiple abscesses or a single thick-walled cavity may form. Hilar node enlargement and empyema are frequent accompaniments.

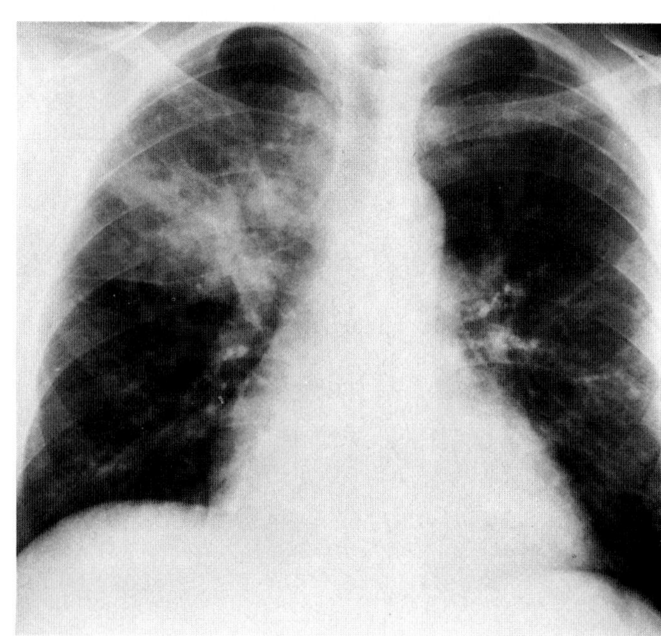

Fig. 15.11 Nocardiosis. Non-homogeneous consolidation.

CHLAMIDIAE

'he organisms responsible for the *psittacosis/lympho-*'*anuloma-venereum/trachoma* group of diseases are ɔw classified as Chlamidiae. They are obligate intra-:llular parasites but differ from viruses in having oth RNA and DNA. *Psittacosis* is acquired from sick irds — parrots, budgerigars, domestic fowl. It presents ; a lung consolidation of any size up to lobar, sometimes atchy rather than homogenous. A miliary pattern has lso been described. The hilar nodes are often enlarged. 'learing of the lesions takes place slowly over several 'eeks.

Chlamidial pneumonias are now being seen more 'equently than formerly.

MYCOPLASMA PNEUMONIA

Iycoplasma pneumoniae is an organism intermediate etween the bacteria and viruses. It is the commonest isolate from primary pneumonias in Great Britain accounting for 10–20% of cases but in only a small proportion does it cause a major respiratory illness.

Primary atypical pneumonia

This was the name given to a respiratory illness where the systemic symptoms overshadowed those due to pneumonia and the course of the disease was less dramatic but more prolonged than typical pneumonia. Primary atypical pneumonia is now known to have a number of causes including adenovirus, psittacosis and Q fever but the commonest cause is *Mycoplasma pneumoniae*.

The evolution of the pneumonia is slow so that it is possible to see a changing radiographic pattern. A fine reticulation first appears representing interstitial inflammation and this is followed by consolidation of the involved area as the alveoli become filled-in with exudate (Fig. 15.12A and B). On resolution the process is reversed. At its height there is usually a segmental or lobar consolidation but there are other possible patterns: 1) multiple irregular patches with ill-defined margins; 2) multiple well-defined small nodules; 3) rapid evolution into a fulminating fibrosing alveolitis; 4) massive bilateral bronchopneumonia with abscess formation. The last two are rare presentations. Hilar node enlargement is not uncommon but pleural effusions are rare. Resolution may take many weeks and abnormalities of pulmonary function may be detectable for up to 4 months.

Q FEVER

The 'Q' here refers to the question mark over the aetiology when first described and before it was traced to a *Rick-*

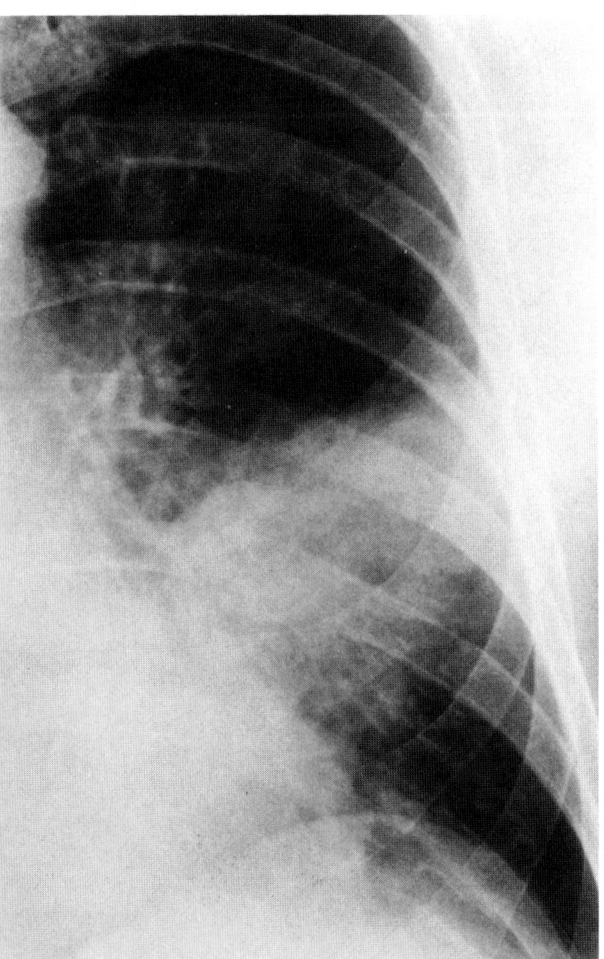

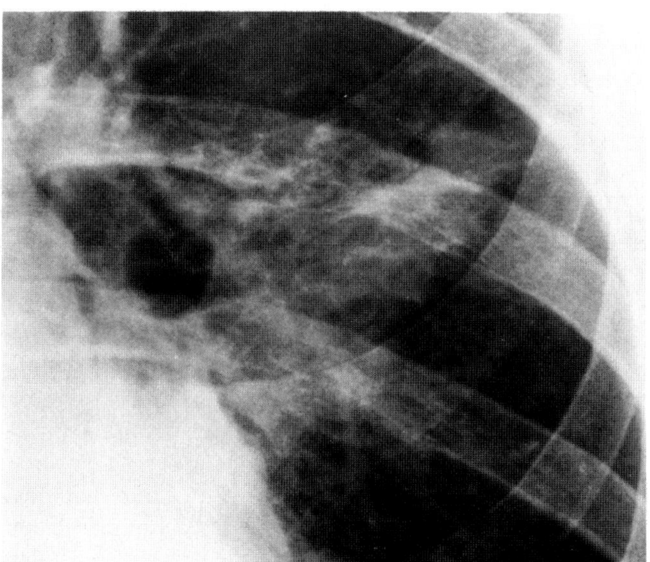

ig. 15.12 (**A**) Mycoplasma pneumonia. Linearities at the edge of the consolidation. (**B**) 2 weeks later. Reticulation becomes apparent during ɛsolution. Small bulla.

ettsia, now re-classified as *Coxiella burnetti*. The reservoirs of infection are insects and mammals, most human disease in Great Britain being acquired from contact with farm animals or their products. Most patients will have an abnormal chest radiograph at presentation. A typical appearance is of a few roughly rounded, homogeneous consolidations in both lungs. The borders of the lesions are ill-defined except at pleural surfaces. They can be quite large consolidations up to 10 cm in diameter. Alternatively it may present as a lobar consolidation. Linear streaks (plate atelectases) in association with the consolidations are also common. Nodes are not enlarged. During resolution, which averages 1 month, the ill-defined borders become sharper as the lesions shrink and become more dense. Complications include endocarditis, meningo-encephalitis and hepatitis.

ROCKY MOUNTAIN SPOTTED FEVER

The southern United States is the endemic area, as well as the Rocky Mountain regions, for this tick-born rickettsial disease. The lungs are involved as part of a bacteraemia. There is a vasculitis within the alveolar walls with spillover of haemorrhage and oedema into the alveolar spaces. Only a minority have a widespread interstitial radiographic pattern, in most there are variable numbers of alveolar opacities, an example of a predominantly interstitial histology but alveolar radiology. Pleural effusions are common. The major complication is secondary bacterial infection which has been known to lead to adult respiratory distress syndrome. The disease has a 5% mortality (Fig. 15.33).

VIRUS INFECTIONS

Characteristic features of virus pulmonary infections are described as widespread nodules, interstitial and peribronchovascular streaks radiating from the hila and mediastinal and hilar adenopathy. In contrast, bacterial infections are characterized by lobar or segmental consolidation, abscess formation and pleural effusion. In practice it is seldom possible to differentiate the two on radiographic grounds. Viral infections can present with every conceivable radiographic pattern.

The common cold

The common cold is an upper respiratory tract infection caused by many different varieties of virus — parainfluenza, rhino-, adeno-, respiratory syncytial virus. Spread of the inflammatory process into the lower respiratory tract occurs in the predisposed, asthmatics, smokers, bronchitics, so that it is not surprising to find transient small pulmonary opacities should a chest radiograph be taken. Most pulmonary complications are the result of secondary bacterial invasion analogous to the purulent sinusitis which so frequently starts from the common cold. There are however examples of virus pneumonia where the radio graph shows one or two patches of alveolar opacification with ill-defined borders (Fig. 15.13A and B). The symptoms of these virus pneumonias are often atypical of other respiratory infections.

Influenza

It is the old and sufferers from chronic debilitating disease who are most at risk of pulmonary disease during influenza infection. The influenza virus can cause pneumonia but more usual circumstance is a combination of viral and bacterial infection or bacterial secondary invasion in lun

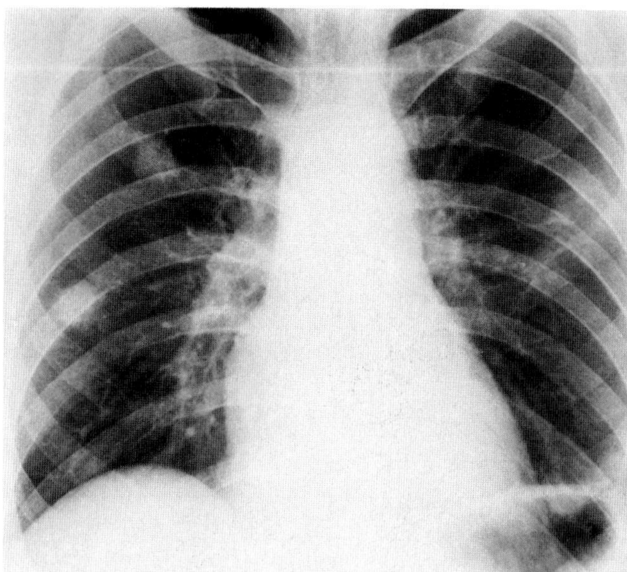

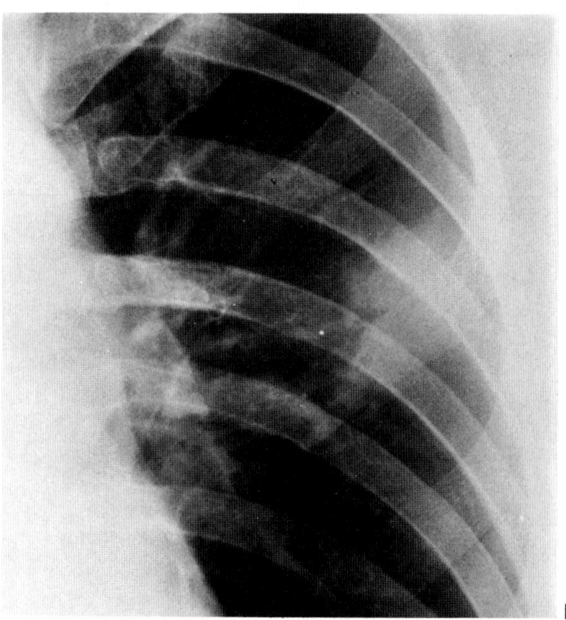

Fig. 15.13 (**A**) Adenovirus. Primary atypical pneumonia. Ill-defined edges to small patches of consolidation. Major symptoms were myositis and dysphagia. (**B**) Interval 2 weeks. The L. sided opacity becomes denser and better defined as it resolves.

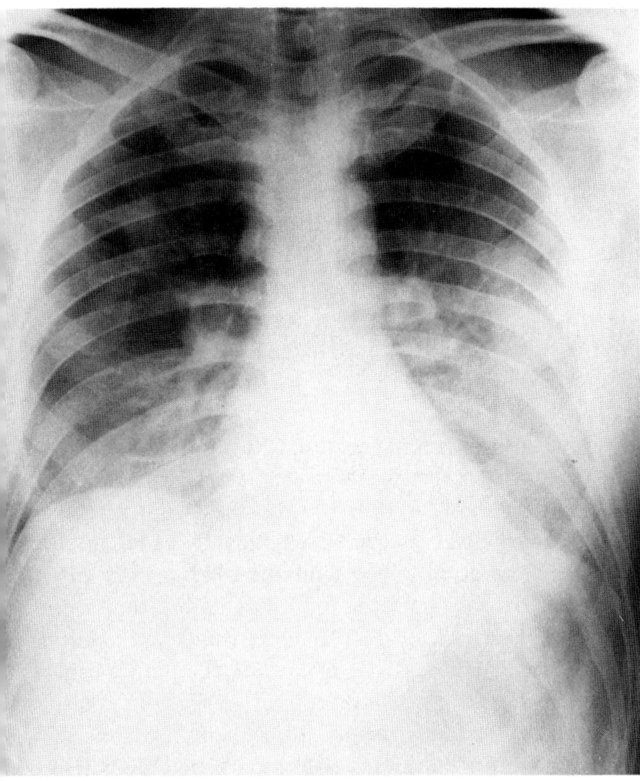

ig. 15.14 Influenza-A. Haemorrhagic consolidation at post-mortem.

lready made susceptible. Staphylococci, pneumococci and *Iaemophilus* are common secondary invaders. A distinctive ulminating virus pneumonia is seen in epidemics of the isease. It is a rapidly extending bilateral and massive onsolidation indistinguishable from non-cardiac pulmonary edema or adult respiratory distress syndrome (Fig. 15.14). Although prone to attack the debilitated it also attacks oung, previously healthy people and there is a high nortality. At post-mortem there is an intense haemorrhagic edema involving all lung structures and widespread ecrosis of pulmonary epithelium.

'aricella

Septicaemic invasion of the lungs can occur in varicella. The patients are more likely to be adults than children and he exanthem particularly severe and haemorrhagic. The ungs are studded with nodules which can be very profuse nd shifting. It is a rare complication but leaves its mark n later years by the presence of tiny calcified dots umbering from two or three up to dozens (Fig. 15.15). n Great Britain varicella is the commonest cause of these cars but not all cases give a history of unusual respiratory lisease during the original infection.

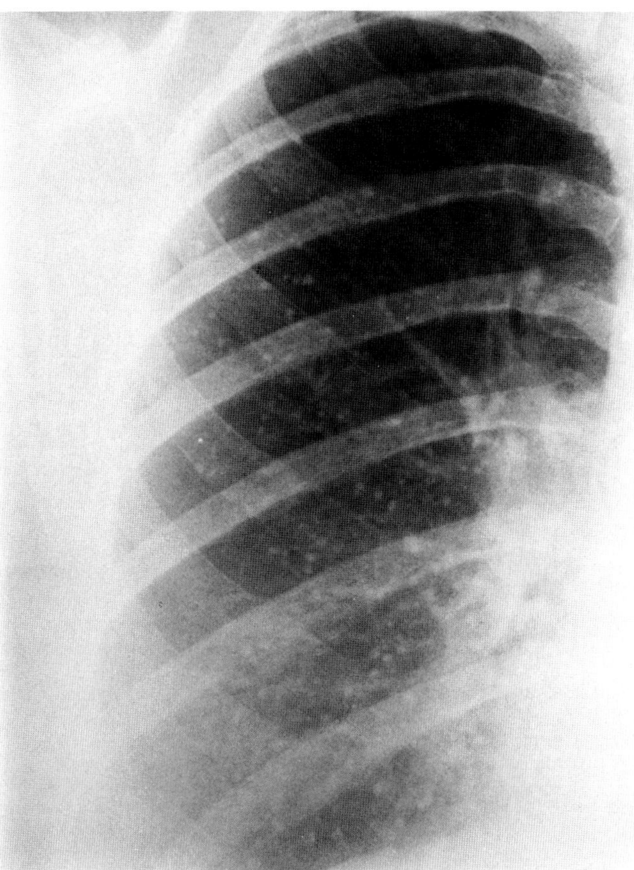

Fig. 15.15 Calcified varicella scars.

Measles giant cell pneumonia

n addition to the common secondary respiratory infections ssociated with measles there is a specific pulmonary viral infection characterized by multinucleate giant cells with cytoplasmic inclusions in the respiratory epithelium. Although a disease of childhood, it has been recorded in adults. The mediastinal and hilar nodes are commonly enlarged but other radiographic abnormalities are variable — streaky basal linearities, widespread reticulation or diffuse ill-defined opacities with a vague nodularity (Fig. 15.16). Remarkably swift resolution can take place over the course of a few days.

Infectious mononucleosis

Less than 10% have intrathoracic manifestations during the disease and node enlargement is the most frequent. The lungs may show an isolated opacity or a reticulo-nodulation.

TUBERCULOSIS

Notifications of tuberculosis in Great Britain are now of the order of 18 per 100 000 population annually. This rises to almost 400 per 100 000 amongst the immigrant population from the Indian sub-continent.

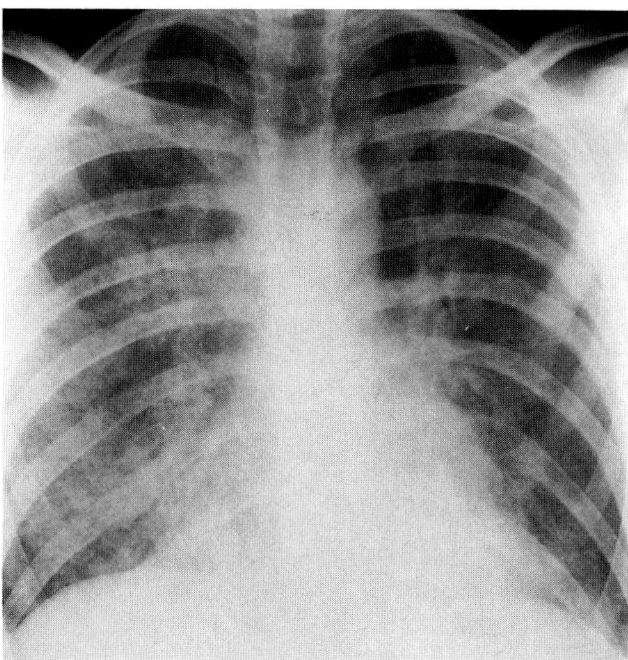

Fig. 15.16 Measles giant cell pneumonia. Extensive ill-defined opacities with a suggestion of nodularity. Patient died. There was a possible T cell deficiency.

Epidemiologically the source of tuberculosis is a patient with open pulmonary tuberculosis. Infection from inoculation of the skin, from infected milk or from the handling of pathological specimens is rare where proper measures of control are exercised. Only those patients with sputum smears positive for tubercle bacilli are infectious and after two weeks of adequate chemotherapy they can be regarded as non-infectious. Transmission is by droplet inhalation and the dose of viable organisms received is critical. Children, the immunocompromised and some immigrant groups are particularly susceptible. All these factors are reflected in the recommendations current in Great Britain concerning isolation of patients, treatment of contacts and general control measures. A chest radiograph is part of these control measures and follow-up of contacts for two years may be judged necessary.

The occupational risk of hospital personnel is, in general, minimal and only a pre-employment check which includes a chest radiograph is needed. Annual chest radiographs are not required. Those judged to be at higher risk should be offered an annual chest radiographic examination. Staff in any institution who will be in regular contact with children should have a chest radiograph as part of a pre-employment check but routine periodic radiography is not necessary.

Tuberculosis is divided into primary and post-primary stages separated by a latent interval which may stretch over decades.

PRIMARY PULMONARY TUBERCULOSIS

Organisms settle and multiply in an alveolus anywhere in the lungs but most commonly in a sub-pleural site in the well-ventilated lower lobes. The initial pulmonary lesion is the *Ghon focus* and at an early stage there is spread along lymphatics, forming tubercles on the way, into the hilar nodes. The combination of Ghon focus, lymphatic infection and hilar node involvement is the *primary complex*. Bacilli are also carried centrifugally to the pleura where they may cause a lymphocytic serous *effusion*. Healing and progression proceed simultaneously, the balance between them determined by host resistance. A fibrous capsule walls-off the lesion and calcium salts are deposited in the caseous material. From this point, if progression continues, there is little difference between lesions of primary and post-primary evolution. If the disease is not checked the caseous mass enlarges and is liquified by enzymatic digestion. Expectoration of the contents of the *cavity* disperses infection to other parts of the lungs and if this is sudden and massive an acute, diffuse *tuberculous bronchopneumonia* results. A cavity breaking through to the pleura can result in *pneumothorax*, *effusion* or *caseous empyema*.

Miliary tuberculosis results from haematogenous dissemination after erosion of a vessel by a tuberculous lesion. It is usually an early primary event but is now being seen more often in patients with post-primary tuberculosis whose defences are waning.

Involved nodes may obstruct bronchi by external compression or by discharging caseous material into the lumen. *Epituberculosis* was a term used to describe a lobar opacity in primary tuberculosis resulting from a non-caseating inflammatory exudate and attributed to a hypersensitivity reaction. This concept seems to have been abandoned. Since most epituberculosis was to be found in the right middle lobe it was probably the result of bronchial obstruction by hilar nodes.

POST-PRIMARY PULMONARY TUBERCULOSIS

This follows the primary infection after a latent interval however short or long and could conceivably be either a reactivation or reinfection. It is now generally accepted that almost all post-primary tuberculosis is due to reinfection.

The lesions usually start in the sub-apical parts of the upper lobes or in the apical segment of the lower lobes as small areas of exudative inflammation. These extend, coalesce, caseate and cavitate. Typically there is a large cavity with several smaller satellite cavities, often bilateral but more advanced on one side. Cavity walls are lined by tuberculous granulation tissue and traversed by fibrotic remnants of bronchi and vessels. A vessel which has not been totally obliterated may dilate — a Rasmussen aneurysm.

Dispersion of infection from the cavities to other parts of the lungs takes place as in the primary form and results in numerous small areas of caseous pneumonia often in the lower lobes. Massive dispersal may lead to caseation of a whole lobe.

Adhesions usually limit pleural spread but sometimes the lung becomes encased in a thick coating of caseous material, fibrosis and hyaline connective tissue. Small cavities that heal leave radiating fibrotic strands puckering the lung. Large cavities become lined by columnar or squamous epithelium and are prone to secondary infection or fungal colonization.

NON-REACTIVE TUBERCULOSIS

This is a haematogenous dissemination in the immunosuppressed. Radiographically it is miliary tuberculosis but histologically it differs in that the necrotic lesions are sharply demarcated from the surrounding lung which shows little reaction. There is also an absence of giant cell granulomas.

THE RADIOLOGY OF PULMONARY TUBERCULOSIS

Pulmonary tuberculosis has such a diversity of radiographic appearances that it is wise to include it in the differential diagnosis of virtually all pulmonary lesions.

Unusual though it is, tuberculosis can be confined to the lung bases. There is a characteristic sparing of the anterior parts of the lungs, a point of more importance in a negative rather than a positive sense. Lesions which are dominantly anterior, even though otherwise typical of tuberculosis, including cavitation, are likely to be of other aetiology.

A minimal apical lesion can easily be overlooked because of overlapping shadows of ribs and clavicle (Fig. 15.17).

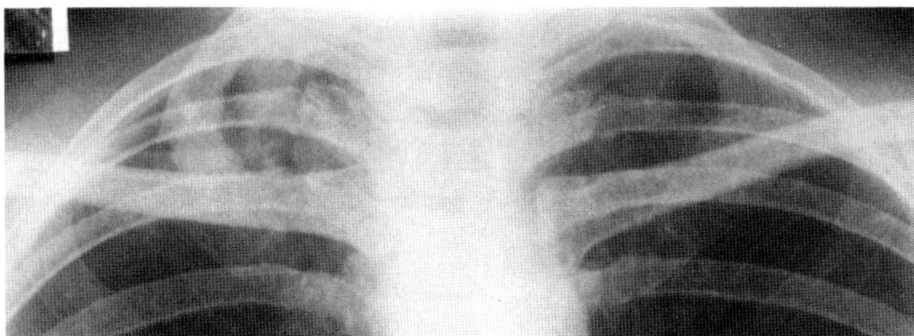

Fig. 15.17 Tuberculosis. Minimal Rt. apical lesion.

Comparison with the opposite side is then helpful, looking for asymmetries of density. The apical projection was designed to overcome this difficulty but is rarely useful and tomography is the optimum mode. The irregularity of outline and density of the lesion and the presence of small satellite shadows may give a spurious appearance of cavitation.

Until brought under control by natural healing or treatment the lesions spread at an uneven rate, reparation and destruction proceeding simultaneously. Extensive areas of lung may become involved, irregularity and patchiness being the cardinal features, homogenous opacities unusual (Fig. 15.18).

Disease activity is monitored by periodic radiographs, the appearance of new lesions or the extension of old ones indicating continued activity whereas contraction indicates

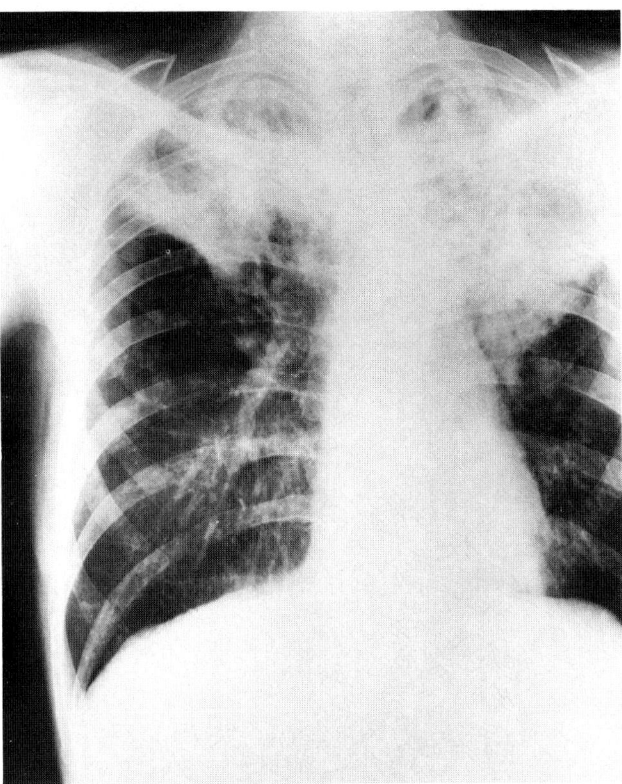

Fig. 15.18 Tuberculosis. Dense non-homogenous opacities. Contracted right upper lobe. Small lesions in other areas.

that the balance has been tilted in favour of healing. Once the radiographic signs have stabilized any subsequent change in size or density must be regarded as suspicious of reactivation, fungal colonization or complication by neoplasm.

Cavities may be thin or thick walled, central or eccentric, single or multiple (Fig. 15.19A and B). Bullae are differentiated by their hair-line walls. Acute pneumonic lesions are especially liable to rapid breakdown into multiple round cavities. Tomography is necessary both to confirm cavitation and to display its structure.

All healed lesions leave fibrotic scars very often containing calcifications. Since the upper lobes are predominantly involved the effects of fibrotic contraction are seen in the drawing over of the trachea, elevation of hilar structures and bronchovascular distortions (Fig. 15.20) Air spaces in the fibrotic areas derive from bronchiectatic cavities and emphysematous bullae as well as true cavities Atelectasis and bronchiectasis also result from endobronchial disease.

The large *pleural effusion* which may manifest early in primary tuberculosis is a reaction to sub-pleural tubercles There are few bacilli in the fluid and resolution is uncomplicated. Large caseating lesions spreading into the pleura produce a more severe *pleuritis* which is commonly confined by adhesions. Whether localized or generalized the result is a pleural space filled with tuberculous pus and caseous material which becomes grossly fibrotic. Complications which may arise from tuberculous empyema are

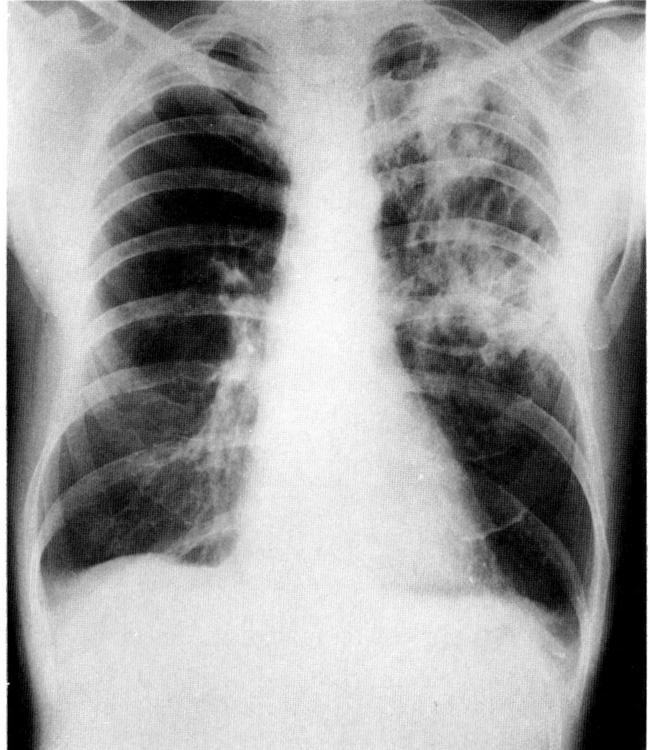

A

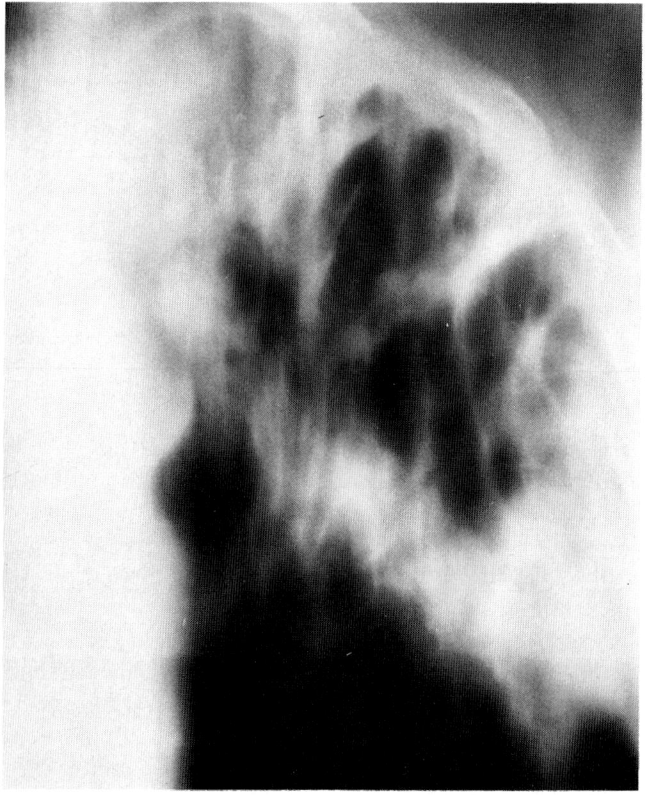

B

Fig. 15.19 (**A**) Tuberculosis. Multiloculated cavity. (**B**) Tomogram. A large part of the left upper lobe has been destroyed.

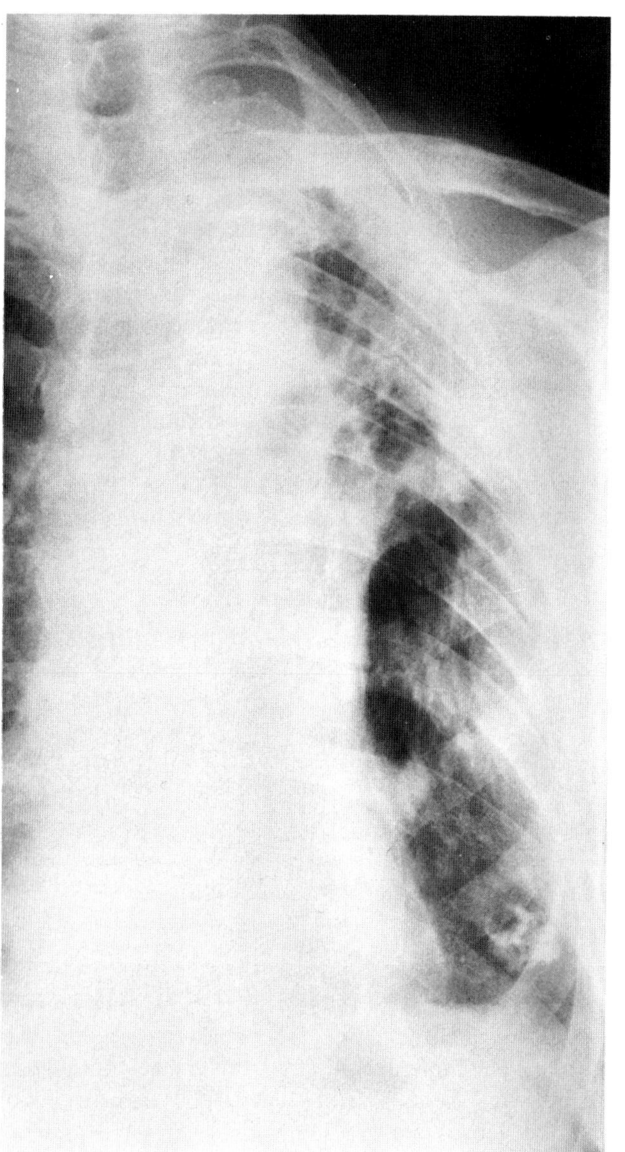

Fig. 15.20 Tuberculosis. Fibrotic shrinkage of upper lobe. Mediastinal and hilar displacement. Apex capped by thickened pleura.

osteitis of rib, chronically *discharging sinuses* to skin, *bronchopleural fistula* and *secondary infection*. These may appear after years of apparently stable pleural disease. During healing the generalized empyema develops characteristic calcific plaques on the visceral pleura (Fig. 15.21). A cap of pleural thickening commonly accompanies apical disease (Fig. 15.22).

Miliary tuberculosis can occur in the primary stage, when it is predominantly a disease of childhood, or in the post-primary stage from waning of the body's defences brought about by steroids, immunosuppression, alcoholism or any debilitating disorder. Half the cases now presenting are over the age of 60 years. Radiographically there are enormous numbers of tiny opacities 1–2 mm diameter, although superimposition may make it impossible to identify entirely discrete lesions. They are diffusely distributed throughout the lungs but there is some latitude in the profusion, size and definition of the lesions (Figs 15.23A and B). The chest radiograph may be normal or it may only show the tuberculous lesion from which the dissemination arose. Healing of miliary tuberculosis often leaves a residue of a few small grains of calcification.

Disseminate lesions of larger size than miliary and lesser profusion are found if the defences are not totally submerged. Localized dissemination also follows aspiration of infected material along bronchial pathways. A rare diffuse alveolar radiographic pattern of disease mimics pulmonary oedema.

A *tuberculoma* is a chronic, well-defined, rounded, granulomatous lesion which enters into the differential diagnosis of solitary or coin lesions. Internal calcification is then a valuable clue to its benignancy.

Considerable *enlargement of hilar* and *mediastinal nodes* may take place without any visible lesion in the lungs. If unilateral this is likely to be confused with a malignant neoplasm and if bilateral with sarcoidosis or lymphoma.

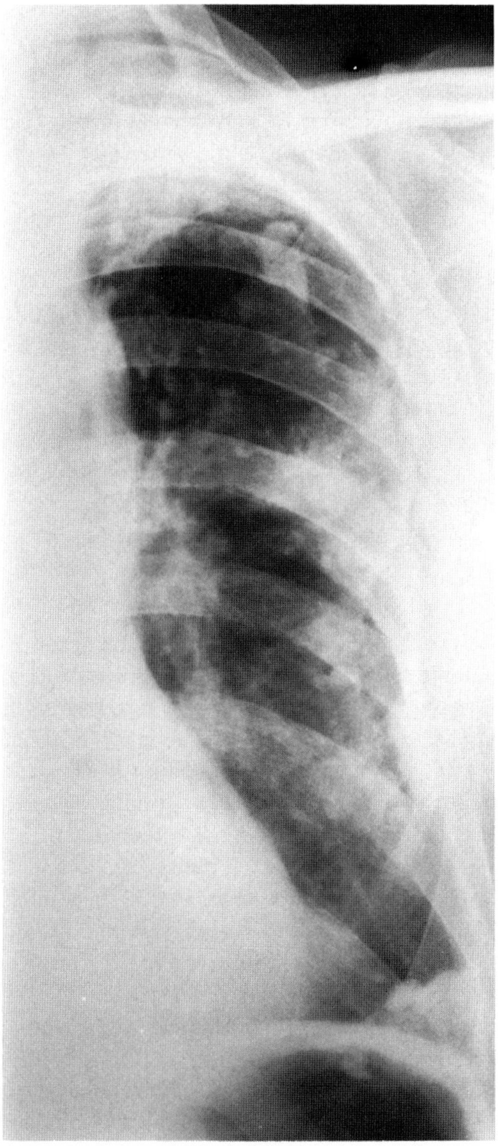

Fig. 15.21 Tuberculosis. Generalized pleural thickening. Calcified plaques on visceral pleura.

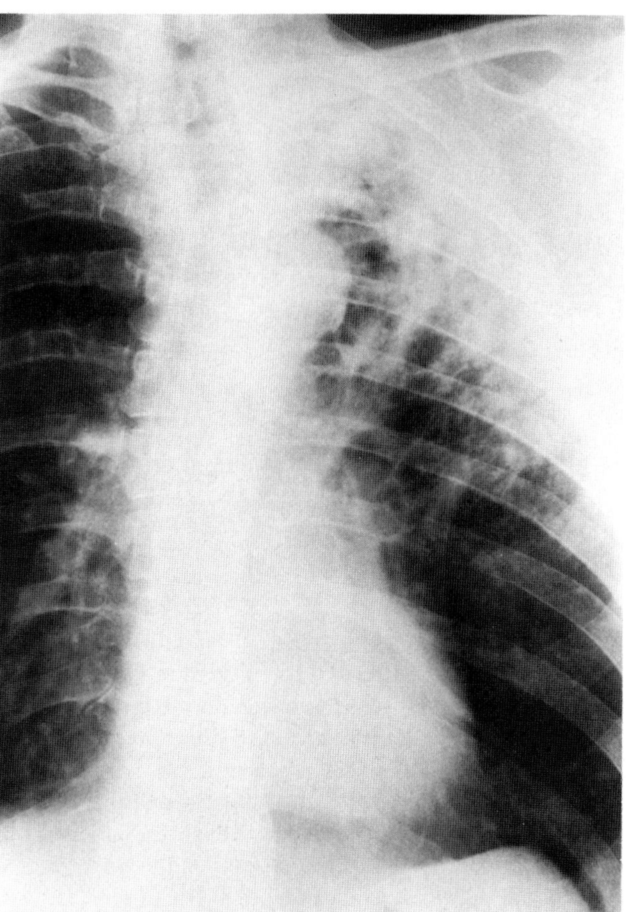

Fig. 15.22 Tuberculosis. Left upper lobe largely destroyed. Multiple small cavities. Thick pleura over apex.

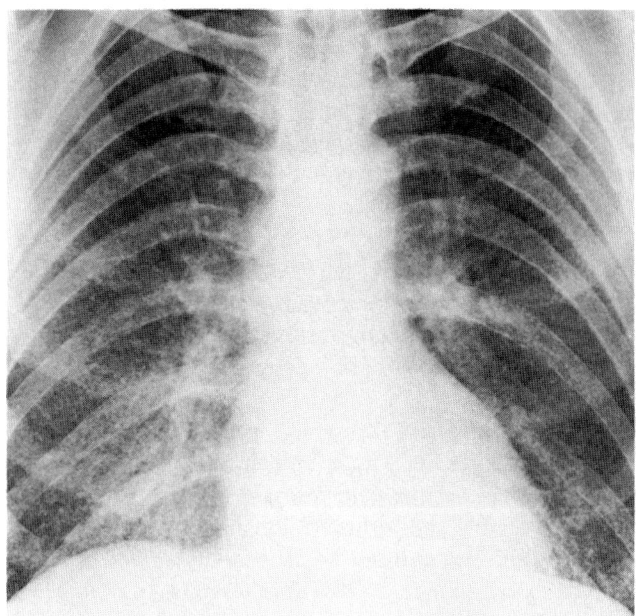
A

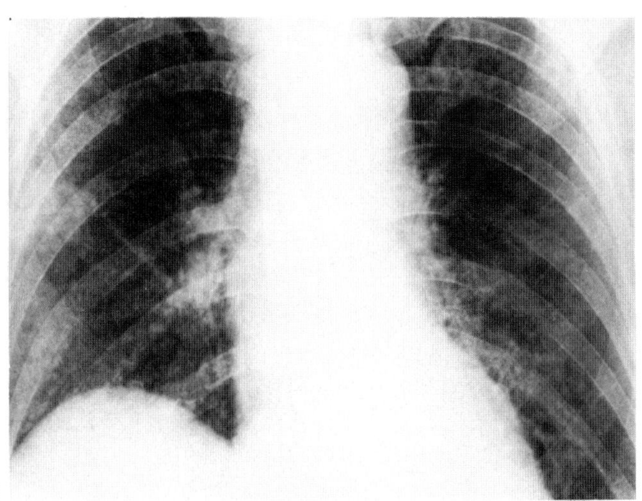
B

Fig. 15.23 (**A**) Miliary tuberculosis. Enormous numbers of lesions. Sharp definition. (**B**) Miliary tuberculosis. Lesions less profuse, less well defined and slightly larger than (A).

OTHER MYCOBACTERIAL PULMONARY INFECTIONS

There are a number of related bacilli with morphology and staining properties closely similar to the tubercle bacillus. Of these atypical mycobacteria those most frequently the cause of human disease are *M. xenopi*, *M. kansasii* and *M. battei*. Their infectivity is low but their sensitivities to drugs differs from *M. tuberculosis*. In general they cause less fibrosis, are less prone to spread but more prone to cavitate than *M. tuberculosis* infections. A common pattern is of a cluster of small opacities grouped around a central lucency. The cavities are thin-walled. Pleural disease and node enlargement are rare. These differences are not however sufficient, in an individual case, to differentiate them from *M. tuberculosis* infections.

THE MYCOSES — PULMONARY FUNGAL DISEASES

Within the family of fungi only a few cause invasive disease in humans. Outside this mainstream of fungal disease a much larger number have been reported in isolated instances as causing disease.

Refinements of taxonomy are not of much importance in the clinical context which is fortunate because exact identification can be difficult even under ideal conditions. In human disease isolation is made difficult by problems in obtaining suitable pathological material, by diversity of cultural requirements and by cross-reactivity in skin testing and antibody production.

Something more than the presence of the fungus in the environment is required before it expresses in a pathogenic role. Although the fungi of blastomycosis, cryptococcosis and histoplasmosis are present in Great Britain these diseases very rarely occur as a native infection, such few cases as are found having been acquired in endemic areas, sometimes up to 20 years previously.

The following general statements are appropriate to fungal disease: invasive disease is acquired by inhalation and the primary focus is in the lung; direct spread from animals to humans or between humans is rare; the pathology is granulomatous; dissemination through the lungs is particularly likely to occur in the immunocompromised; systemic dissemination commonly affects the central nervous system and is usually lethal.

ASPERGILLOSIS

Aspergillus fumigatus is widespread in the atmosphere and it is inevitable that man inhales the spores from time to time. It is capable of multiplying in air passages when the conditions are favourable. The pulmonary manifestations are grouped into 3 categories: (1) *Aspergilloma* — a ball of fungal hyphae growing in an old pulmonary cavity; (2) *Invasive aspergillosis* — the fungus becomes a pathogen in its own right and invades pulmonary tissue causing necrosis; (3) *Allergic bronchopulmonary aspergillosis* — asthmatics who develop transient pulmonary opacities. This is a useful classification but the boundaries of each are not rigid.

Aspergilloma. The fungus colonizes any chronic cavity or airspace except those in which tuberculosis is still active. The hyphae grow into a matted ball (a mycetoma) which lies free within the cavity. The radiographic feature is a crescent of air between the ball and the cavity wall best shown by tomography (Fig. 15.24). Since most chronic

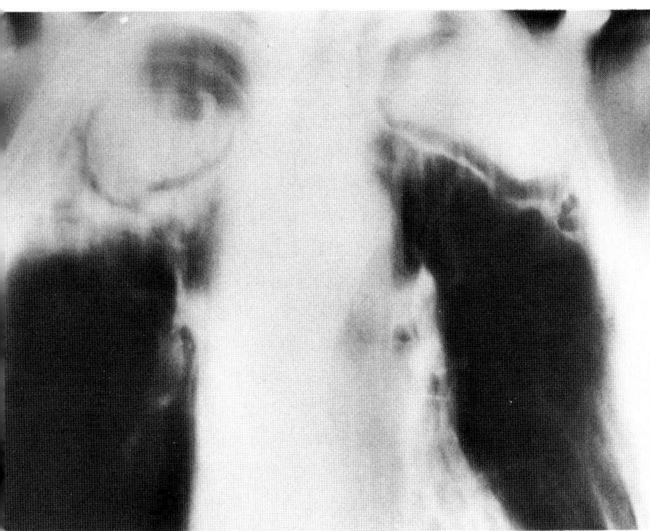

Fig. 15.24 Bilateral aspergillomas. Air crescents and fungal masses.

cavities are in the upper lobes this is where most aspergillomas will be found.

Air crescents are not always present and the diagnosis of aspergilloma should be suspected in any chronic air space which becomes opacified. Other fungi are capable of forming mycetomas and other pathologies can produce identical appearances: for example, haematoma, tumour, hydatid cyst. Rarely a mycetoma disappears on the death of the fungus but it usually returns.

Aspergilloma is an indolent condition but by no means always benign because of the tendency to bleed. Vascular granulation tissue forms in the wall of the cavity and sooner or later bleeding takes place. Small haemoptyses are frequent but occasionally a large haemoptysis can be life-threatening. Medical treatment is unsatisfactory and surgery carries a high risk from the complications of bronchopleural fistula, pneumonia, empyema and further bleeding. In these circumstances control of bleeding by embolization of bronchial and intercostal arteries has to be considered. The effects are rarely permanent but it can be repeated.

Mycetomas are also sometimes found in allergic bronchopulmonary aspergillosis. They may also become invasive, spreading through the cavity wall into normal lung. Wider dissemination is only likely to occur in the immunocompromised host.

Invasive aspergillosis. In this form the *Aspergillus* invades viable tissue and necrosis ensues. It is rarely primary and predisposing factors are chemotherapy, immunosuppression, or lung damage from other infections or radiotherapy. There is no characteristic radiographic pattern. It may take the form of a necrotising bronchopneumonia with abscess formation, organizing lobar pneumonia, widespread lesions, even a miliary spread. It can mimic an aspergilloma complete with air crescent, the differences being that it develops in apparently previously normal lung, the wall is thick and invaded by fungus and the core consists of fungus mixed with necrotic tissue (Fig. 15.25)

Allergic bronchopulmonary aspergillosis. The patient is usually an asthmatic subject who develops sensitivity to the aspergillus which has colonized the proximal bronchi. Local allergic reactions then take place resulting in two types of pathological process: 1) transient pulmonary opacities 2) bronchopulmonary damage. The transient pulmonary opacities are the same as those of other allergic reactions, an eosinophilic infiltration of alveolar walls and intra-alveolar exudate. The size varies from small nodules up to lobar dimensions. They are of low density and have ill-defined borders except at pleural boundaries (Fig. 15.26). Resolution is hastened by steroid therapy. Recurrences take place in the same or in different parts of the lungs.

The condition pursues an intermittent course over many years and the frequency of chronic changes increases with the number of acute episodes. Within areas previously the site of transient opacities the bronchi dilate and contain plugs of tough, stringy mucus mixed with small numbers of the aspergillus. Mucoid impaction is a dilated bronchus packed tightly with this material. Because of their thickened walls bronchi may be visible as tubes, rings or cavities or, if impacted, as bulbous glove-finger or branching opacities. Air may return to impacted bronchi

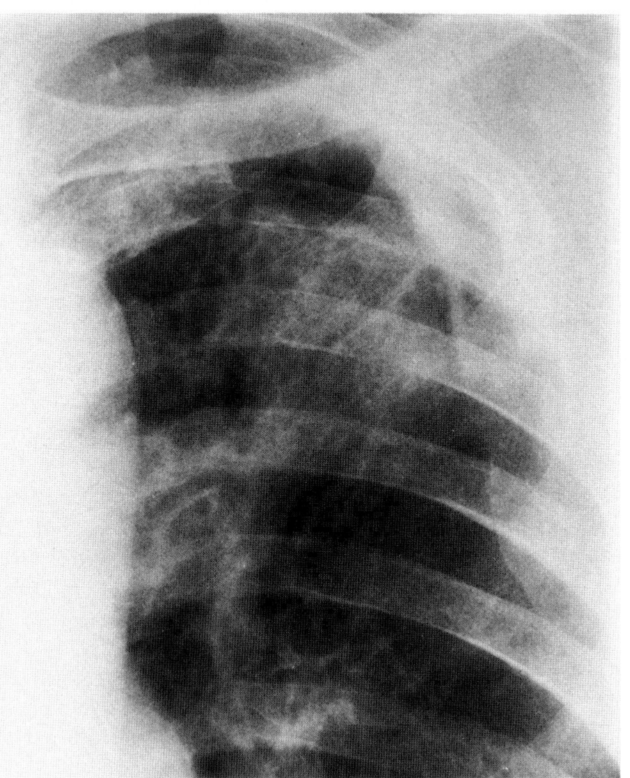

Fig. 15.25 Invasive aspergillosis. An old scarred tuberculous lesion re-opacified. Irregular borders and a tail of opacity into the hilum

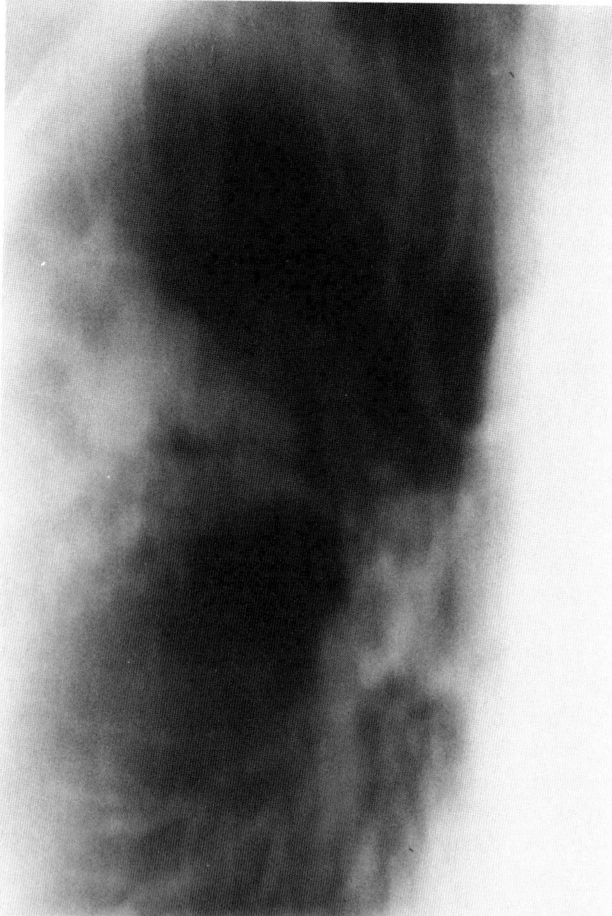

Fig. 15.26 Allergic bronchopulmonary aspergillosis. Tomogram. A wedge of opacity crossed by a patent bronchus.

if the material is coughed up. Plugging of central bronchi can lead to collapse of lobes or whole lungs. Continued damage and repair by fibrosis will lead to focal emphysema, permanent shrinkage and eventually to end-stage upper lobe fibrosis. A mycetoma may form and this is not always in the upper lobes.

If bronchography is performed a central bronchiectasis is highly characteristic, normal bronchial calibre being resumed distal to the dilatation. However, it may show only a non-specific tubular, cystic or varicose bronchiectasis.

Other fungi and moulds can produce a picture so close to that of bronchopulmonary aspergillosis both clinically and radiologically that only skin testing and precipitin reactions will be able to differentiate between them.

HISTOPLASMOSIS

Lung infection by *Histoplasma capsulatum* is usually acquired by inhalation of soil dust contaminated by bird droppings. A tiny calcified dot may be the only indication that previous infection has taken place. When many of these are scattered throughout the lungs they closely resemble the scars of miliary tuberculosis or *Varicella* pneumonia except that they tend to be rather more variable in size (Fig. 15.27 A and B).

Progression of one or more of these foci leads to larger nodules. Hilar node enlargement is common and may be the only visible manifestation. Locally progressive disease may also take the form of a consolidation, acute or chronic the latter associated with fibrosis and cavitation (Fig. 15.28). The presence of cavitation within an area of lung distorted by fibrosis is liable to be mistaken for tuberculosis. There is also a *miliary* form of diffuse lung dissemination.

An uncommon late manifestation of histoplasmosis is a *fibrosing mediastinitis* which can cause stenosis of cavae, oesophagus, trachea, bronchi or pulmonary artery. The chest radiograph will then show a widened mediastinum with large hilar shadows and opacities fanning out into the lungs. Kerley B lines may appear.

Systemic dissemination frequently gives rise to chronic ulceration of the upper air passages and destruction of the adrenal glands.

COCCIDIOIDOMYCOSIS

Some 60% of infections are asymptomatic and the commonest radiographic finding is a nodule which calcifies as it heals. Common presentations of symptomatic cases are segmental, lobar or patches of persistent consolidation together with enlarged hilar and mediastinal nodes. The adenopathy can be mistaken for sarcoidosis or lymphoma. Viable organisms persisting in healed lesions are a source of future re-activation.

Sequelae of chronic disease are fibrosis, calcification, cavitation, bronchiectasis and empyema. Cavities tend to be thin-walled but chronic apical fibro-cavitary disease can be indistinguishable from tuberculosis. There is also a miliary form of coccidioidomycosis.

It is notable that most fungal infections have a form of disease which is indistinguishable radiographically from chronic tuberculosis.

BLASTOMYCOSIS

The asymptomatic nodule, chronic pneumonia, potential for re-activation and node enlargement are indistinguishable from other fungal infections (Fig. 15.29). Cavitation is less common but when it occurs it is similar to that in coccidioidomycosis. There is no great tendency to fibrosis and healed lesions leave only small scars. Dissemination throughout the lungs can have almost any radiographic pattern (Fig. 15.30).

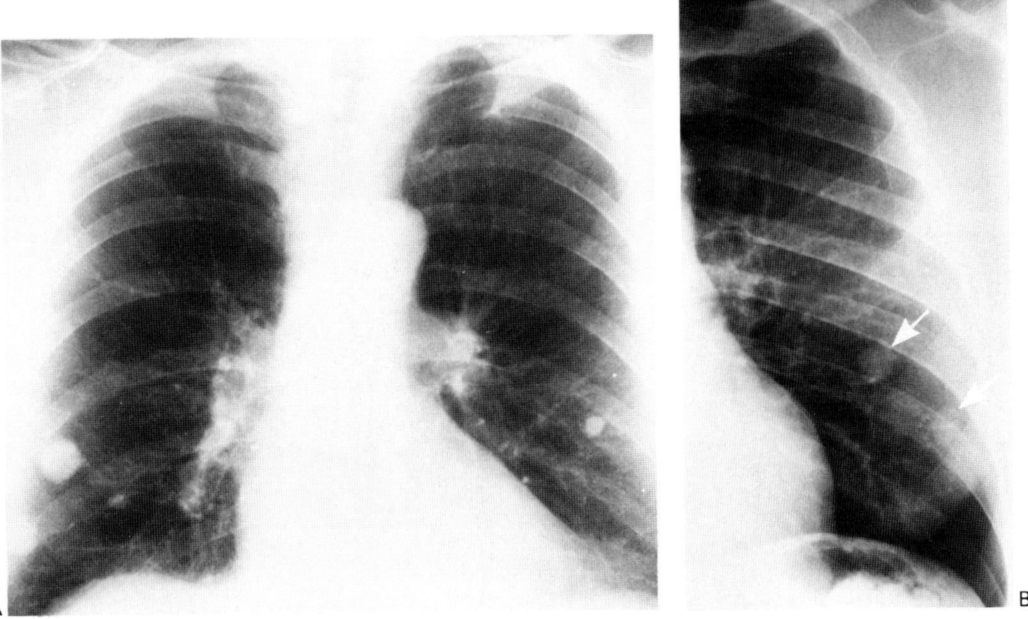

Fig. 15.27 (**A**) Histoplasmosis. Nodules with calcification. Calcified right hilar nodes. (**B**) Two small histoplasma granulomas (arrows). Tiny flecks of calcification.

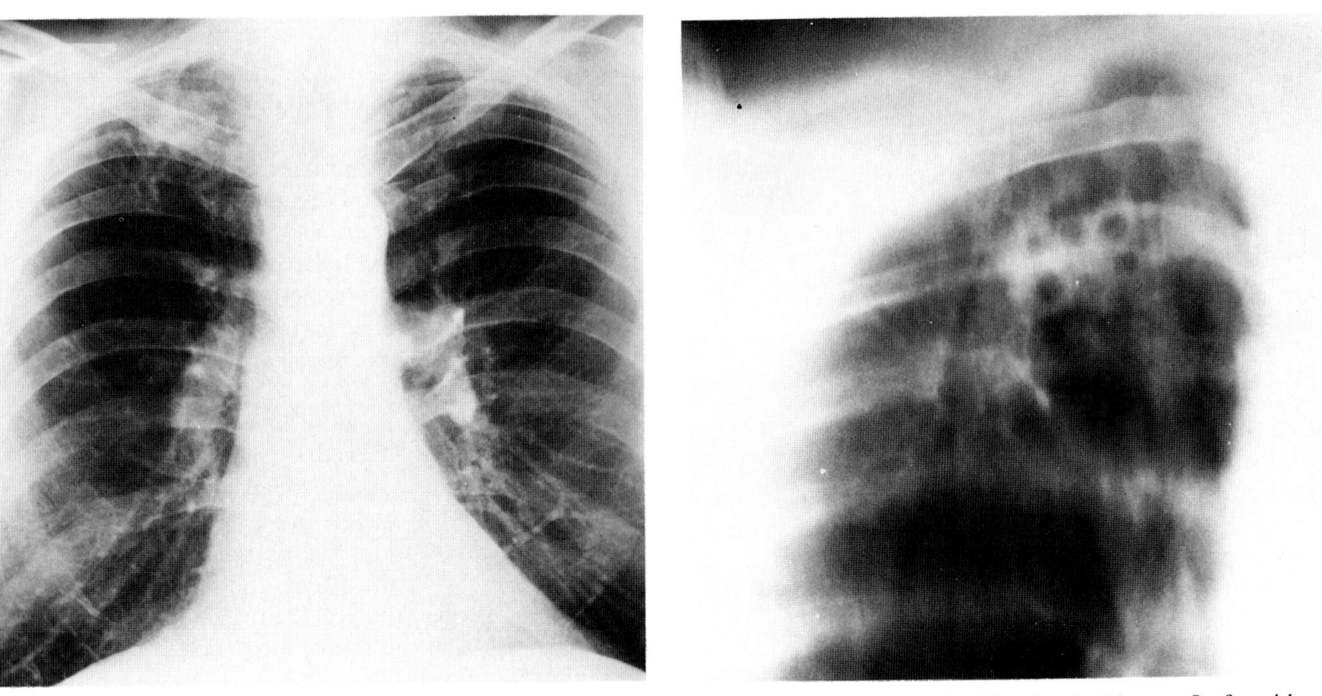

Fig. 15.28 (**A**) Histoplasmosis. Chronic disease right apex. (**B**) Tomogram. Multiple small cavities. Positive histoplasmin skin test. Confirmed by lobectomy.

CRYPTOCOCCOSIS (*Torulosis*)

Cryptococcosis neoformans is a yeast form of fungus of world-wide distribution. The reservoir for human infection is probably pigeon droppings. Lung infection is usually benign, taking the form of one or more nodules of variable size. Growth of a nodule will form a mass lesion (*toruloma*) simulating a carcinoma. Node enlargement and cavitation are rare.

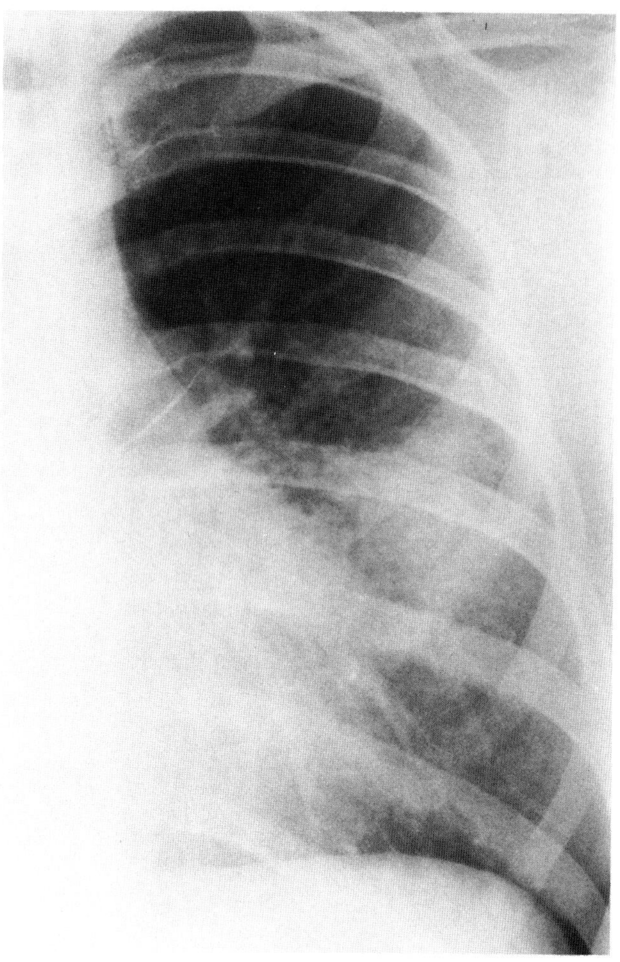

Fig. 15.29 Blastomycosis. Acute pneumonia which did not resolve. Fungus in sputum. Lingular consolidation. Resolved with treatment.

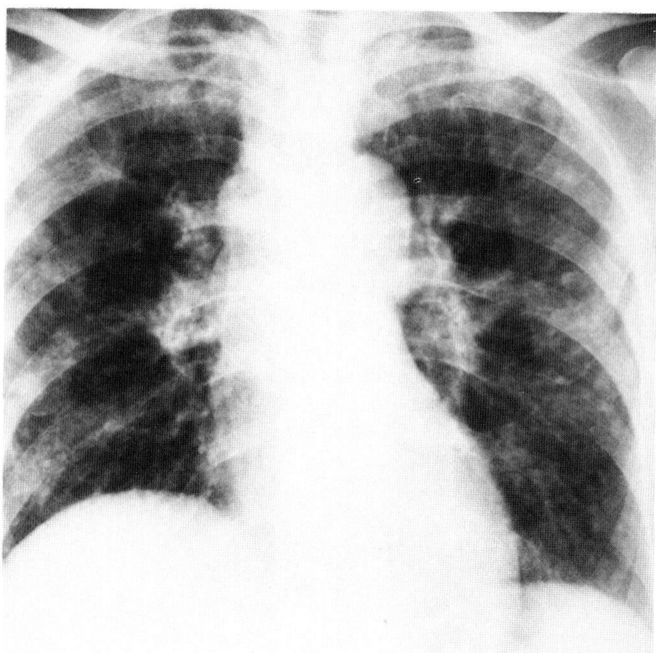

Fig. 15.30 Blastomycosis. Dissemination throughout the lungs. Multiple nodules some of which were cavitated. Mediastinal node enlargement.

CANDIDIASIS

Candida albicans is a normal mouth commensal which, when conditions are favourable, causes moniliasis (thrush), a superficial surface infection. It is rarely invasive but lung infection, when it occurs, is from haematogenous spread. The pulmonary lesion is a chronic pneumonia which breaks down with the formation of an abscess. A mycetoma may develop in the abscess which is then indistinguishable from aspergilloma.

MUCORMYCOSIS

The *Mucorales* group of fungi are best known as causes of a spreading inflammation of the face and sinuses in diabetics or the immunosuppressed. Lung infection is a rapidly progressive, dense, cavitating bronchopneumonia.

WORMS AND OTHER PARASITIC INFECTIONS

There is a common pattern running through the pulmonary manifestations of many of these diseases and the condition of **tropical pulmonary eosinophilia** can be taken as illustrative.

The endemic areas for this disease are the tropical belts of all the continents. Diagnosis is based on the symptomatology, blood eosinophilia, an abnormal chest radiograph, antibodies to filarial antigens in the blood and the striking response to specific therapy with diethylcarbamazine. Although the parasites cannot be isolated from the lungs there can be no reasonable doubt of the filarial aetiology.

Pathologically there is an eosinophilic interstitial infiltration and intra-alveolar exudate, the usual signature of a pulmonary allergic response. Patients with the disease who travel to temperate zones may be misdiagnosed as asthmatics. If the asthma has unusual features such as recurrent fever, sweating, weight loss or a high ESR, suspicion should be aroused. Untreated the disease may persist for years and can result in permanent lung damage with interstitial fibrosis.

The chest radiograph shows a subtle bilateral mid-zone haze which can readily be attributed to technical factors were it not for the accompanying loss of definition of pulmonary vessels and hila. Additionally there is a profusion of small, ill-defined, migrating nodules up to 5 mm in diameter scattered throughout the lungs, producing, in severe infestations, a snowstorm picture. Larger areas of homogenous consolidation appear transiently. There are also linear components consisting of streaks radiating from the hila and peripheral reticulations.

PARASITIC WORMS

Ascaris, *Taenia*, *Ankylostoma* and *Strongyloides* are examples of parasitic worms which lodge in or traverse the lungs at some stage of their life cycles and in so doing give rise to one or two transient and migrating opacities as a result of an allergic response. Loeffler who first described this condition believed that his original cases were due to Ascariasis. The term **Loeffler's syndrome** is now applied to almost any transient pulmonary opacities of a predominantly eosinophilic histology associated with a blood eosinophilia. The heavier the infestation the more profuse are the pulmonary lesions. *Strongyloides stercoralis* in particular is capable of causing widespread opacities and a serious pulmonary illness. Such heavy dissemination can be activated by immunosuppression.

Worms or larvae which fail to complete their migration die and a chronic granulomatous nodule will be formed. If this is removed for histological examination it is easy to miss the remains of the worm within the granuloma.

Schistosomiasis. If the eggs lodge in pulmonary arteries of less than 100 μm the lesions they cause are small granulomas like miliary tuberculosis or sarcoidosis but if they lodge in arteries of larger size the irritation causes vascular necrosis and fibrotic occlusion. The latter results in pulmonary hypertension if sufficient vessels are occluded. A third type of reaction results in diffuse interstitial fibrosis.

Paragonimiasis. The *Paragonimus* worm is endemic in the tropics and infection is acquired from eating shellfish. The worm or eggs in the lungs excite a reaction consisting of a few alveolar opacities of up to 4 cm in diameter. One or more 'bubble' cavities appear within the opacities and as the surrounding reaction subsides they are seen to have thin walls. Tuberculosis may be suspected particularly as haemoptysis is a frequent symptom.

Armillifer armillatus. This is an arachnid infestation of birds, mammals and snakes endemic in Africa and South-East Asia. Humans are infected usually from eating snakes. The larvae migrate to the lungs where they encyst, die and calcify. The radiographic appearances are pathognomonic. There are numerous thin-walled cysts less than 1 cm in diameter in a sub-pleural position containing the calcified bodies of the larvae. These appear as coils, targets and signet ring shapes.

HYDATID DISEASE

Dogs are the principal reservoir of the adult worm, *Echinococcus granulosus* and most mammals serve as intermediate host for the larvae (echinococci). The hydatid is a parasitic echinococcal cyst consisting of three layers, an adventitia formed of compressed host tissue, a middle layer of friable ectocyst and an inner germinal layer from which are produced large numbers of scolices which are the heads of developing worms. Daughter cysts are formed if the viability is threatened but in the lung the cyst is unilocular (Fig. 15.31). Smoothly spherical and of homogenous density, the cyst may grow to the size of a grapefruit. There is seldom significant reaction in the surrounding lung so that calcification is rare. Complications are those of *rupture* and *infection*.

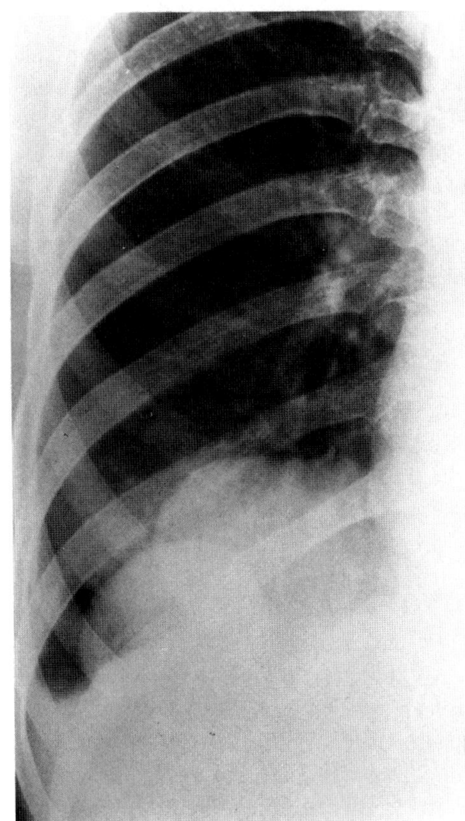

Fig. 15.31 Two hydatid cysts. Small pleural effusion.

Rupture may take place into the pleural cavity or into a bronchus. Communication with a bronchus leads to detachment of the ectocyst from the adventitia and a crescent of air separates the two. Should the cyst itself rupture the partial replacement of the fluid by air results in a fluid level.

Rupture of a *liver* hydatid into the right lung produces a characteristic combination of radiological signs. There is a basal opacity from lobar infection and atelectasis and a pleural effusion. Bronchographically there is a local bronchiectasis and the bronchial fistula into the cavity may be shown. ^{99m}Tc-labelled iminodiacetic acid scanning shows a filling defect in the hepatic uptake followed by the appearance of the radionuclide in the cyst and its progress up the bronchial tree.

The leakage of hydatid fluid into the tissues is sometimes followed by a systemic reaction. Although these reactions are uncommon, when they occur the consequences can be serious.

TOXOPLASMOSIS

Epidemiological surveys have shown a high rate of sub-clinical infection. A protozoal disease, widespread amongst mammals and birds, human acquisition is from cats or from eating infected meat. One form of presentation is in the manner of a primary atypical pneumonia with mild respiratory symptoms and mediastinal adenopathy or a pulmonary opacity.

ENTAMOEBA HISTOLYTICA

The *Entamoeba* is distributed worldwide but amoebiasis is a tropical or sub-tropical disease. The lungs can be involved by metastatic spread from the abdomen or by rupture of an hepatic amoebic abscess into the right lung base. In the latter case the radiographic signs are those of a lung abscess and bronchohepatic fistula.

IMMUNOSUPPRESSION AND PULMONARY INFECTION

Drugs are used to reduce antibody production in organ transplant recipients in order to prevent rejection and in diseases where the immune response itself is damaging as in systemic lupus. Impairment of immunological mechanisms is an unwanted side-effect of drugs used to kill malignant cells. Immunosuppression is therefore associated with administration of steroids, Azathioprine and cytotoxics. The level of suppression is proportional to the intensity of the chemotherapy. Immunological impairment is also associated with other disease states, diabetes, alcoholism, exposure to ionizing radiations and the processes of ageing.

Not only is the risk of infection increased, the tissue response is altered and potentially serious infections may give little clinical sign of their presence. For this reason periodic chest radiography is a reasonable precaution in those at risk.

The response to conventional pathogens may take a usual or an atypical form and this also applies with unusual pathogens. Certain organisms, notably *Pneumocystis carinii* and *Cytomegalovirus*, rarely if ever cause disease in the absence of immunosuppression. The organisms identified most often in these diseases are *Pneumocystis*, *Candida albicans*, *Mycobacterium tuberculosis*, *Aspergillus fumigatus* and the Herpes family of viruses.

There are many obstacles to accurate diagnosis. Infection has to be differentiated from the primary disease or a recrudescence, from the toxic effects of the drugs and from graft rejection. Mixed infections are common and the isolation of an organism does not always mean that it is the principal agent. Similarly, sero-conversion or the finding of high antibody titres is not positive proof of causation. Isolation from sputum, blood, tracheal aspiration or bronchopulmonary lavage is too variable to be reliable. Open lung biopsy is the optimum method for *Pneumocystis* but less reliable for others. Fibre-optic bronchoscopy and biopsy is useful, particularly as it is less invasive. These last two methods are not without risk of pneumothorax or bleeding and any clotting defect should be corrected beforehand. An advantage of biopsy is that it may differentiate infection from recurrence of tumour or other lesions. Unfortunately the biopsy may simply show non-specific changes of organizing pneumonia, interstitial pneumonitis or haemorrhage. Even when determined efforts are made to reach a specific diagnosis using an extensive range of tests success is elusive and in about 40% of infections no pathogen will be found.

The **radiological signs** of these infections are non-specific but the most characteristic feature is of *disseminated pulmonary lesions* with only a few showing other patterns such as lobar consolidation or isolated nodules. *Abscesses* and *cavitation* are common and their presence amongst a diffuse alveolar or interstitial shadowing, especially if there are also focal nodules, is suspicious of a mixed infection. Enlarged nodes usually imply tumour rather than infection. In leukaemia pulmonary opacities imply infection since visible deposits rarely occur. Viral infections may be accompanied by a skin rash.

Bacterial infections. An existing tuberculous lesion can be re-activated and local or miliary spread ensue. Gram-negative bacteria characteristically cause microabscesses. Nocardia has less tendency to disseminate through the lungs and a local lesion progressing rapidly to cavitation is more characteristic.

Fungal infections (Figs. 15.32–34). *Candida albicans* infections may be bronchopneumonic, *multi-nodular* or miliary. The latter may not be visible radiographically. The

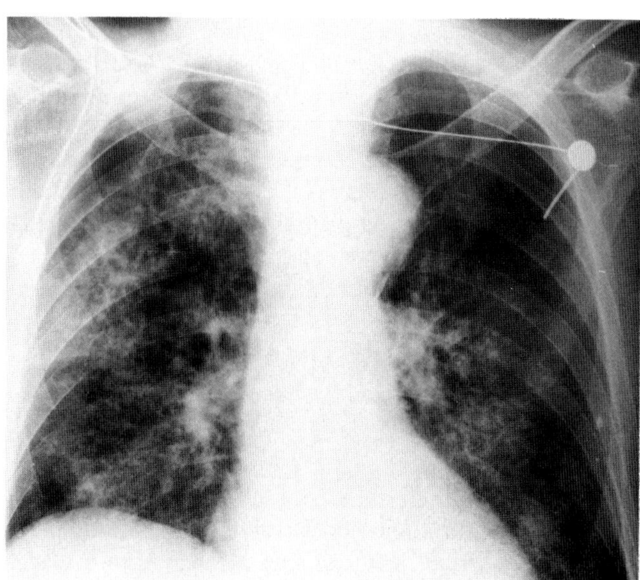

Fig. 15.32 *Candida albicans* bronchopneumonia. Mixed infection with Gram-negative organisms. Chronic alcoholic. Post-mortem confirmation.

ommon patterns in fungal infections are disseminate odules with abscesses except for histoplasmosis in which ulmonary dissemination is unusual.

Parasitic infections. In those who have lived in the opics fulminating *Entamoeba histolytica* or *Strongyloides ercoralis* pulmonary infections can occur. *Strongyloides* ay be a focal nodular or a diffuse alveolar infection.

Viral infections. These are usually of the Herpes famy consisting of Herpes simplex, Varicella/zoster and ytomegalovirus.

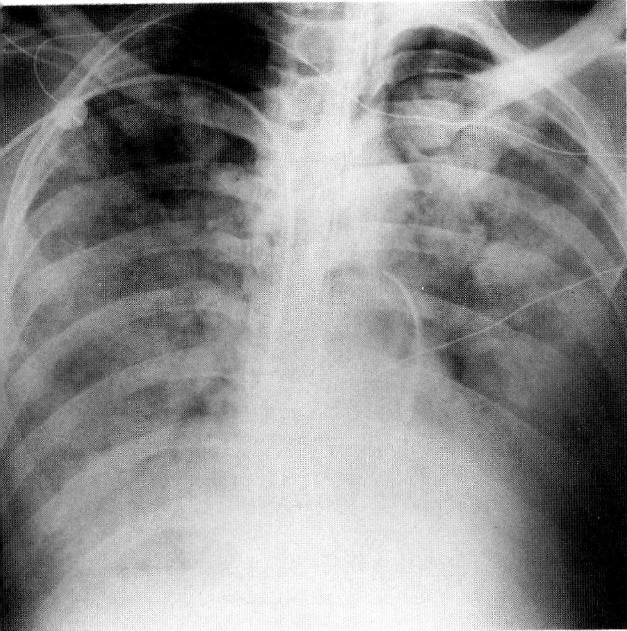

ig. 15.33 Mucormycosis. Patient an alcoholic. The fungal infection ollowed Rocky mountain spotted fever. Mixed infection with Gram egative organisms. Post-mortem confirmation.

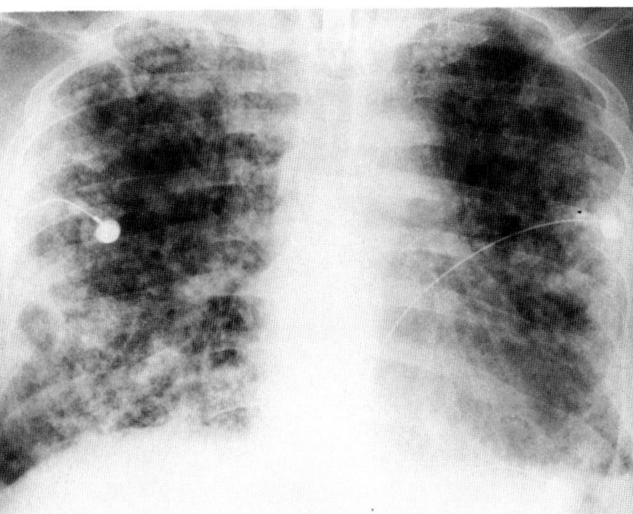

Fig. 15.34 Disseminated cryptococcosis. Mixed infection with Gram negative organisms. On steroids for systemic lupus.

Cytomegalovirus is usually acquired asymptomatically in normally immune competent people although occasionally there is an illness of infection similar to infectious mononucleosis. After primary infection the virus persists in latent form. In the immunocompromised host a reactivation of this latent infection may take place but this is not usually accompanied by clinical illness. It is a primary infection occurring in an immunocompromised host which is the cause of serious pulmonary and hepatic disease.

Diagnosis is made from the presence in cells obtained by biopsy or exfoliative cytology of characteristic 'owl eye' inclusions or from cell cultures. In the lungs it is found in pneumonic consolidation, in nodules, in wide-spread miliary lesions or in diffuse acinar perihilar opacities. Pathologically there is an interstitial infiltration and intra-alveolar exudate. The precise part which this virus plays in the pathogenesis of these lesions is uncertain because it is usually found in mixed infections.

Pneumocystis carinii infection (Fig. 15.35). This organism is worldwide in distribution but is only found in the lungs of humans and animals. Its natural habitat is not known. It is not decided whether it is protozoan or fungal but is usually classed as the former. It has not been

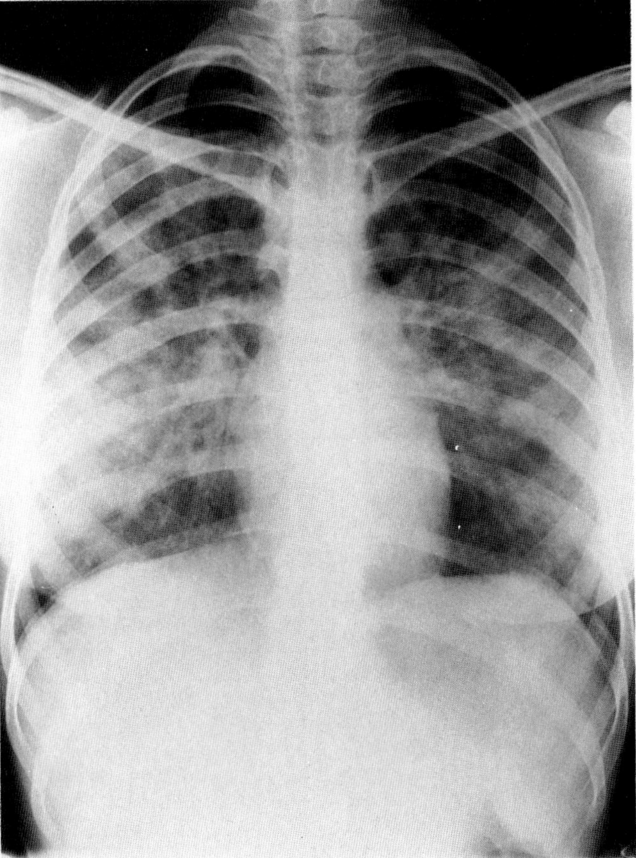

Fig. 15.35 *Pneumocystis carinii*. On cytotoxic drugs. Diffuse, patchy alveolar shadowing. Cleared on treatment.

cultured but it can be propagated in cultures of chick embryo lung cells. There is no positive evidence of transmission between humans or between animals and humans. The disease probably does not occur in otherwise healthy persons but asymptomatic infection is common as revealed by the frequency of antibodies in the population. Immune deficiency is necessary for its expression. Untreated it is almost always fatal. The pathology is that of an acute fulminating pneumonia with interstitial infiltration and intra-alveolar exudate.

Radiographically there is a diffuse bilateral pulmonary opacification, like pulmonary oedema, generally homogenous but within it there may be translucencies due to focal emphysema and air bronchograms. At a later stage many air cysts form, small at first but enlarging and some with fluid levels. Pneumothorax and pneumomediastinum are complications of the emphysema.

Open lung biopsy or bronchoalveolar lavage are the most reliable diagnostic methods. Diagnosis from sputum, needle aspiration and fibre-optic biopsy is less reliable and antibody titres are unreliable. Since invasive methods are not without risk it is sometimes better to treat on suspicion without a confirmed diagnosis.

ACQUIRED IMMUNE DEFICIENCY SYNDROM (AIDS)

This syndrome is a highly lethal combination of oppo
tunistic infections and certain rare malignancies in pe
sons who have none of the usual reasons for bein
immunosuppressed. The infections are *Pneumocystis carini*
Cytomegalovirus and *fungi*. The malignancies are *Kaposi'*
sarcoma and some *lymphoproliferative disorders*. There i
impairment of cellular immunity but humeral immunit
and phagocytosis are normal. The T-lymphocytes ar
reduced. An agent has now been identified, a human T ce
lymphotropic virus type III (HTLV-III), which seems to b
the pathogen. Whether it acts alone or in concert with othe
factors is not yet established. The population at most ris
are promiscuous homosexuals but there are a small numbe
of Haitians, Africans and haemophiliacs, the latter becaus
of their repeated exposure to blood products. It is transmit
ted sexually and by infected blood.

It is believed to have originated in Central Africa and the
spread to Haiti and North America and thence to Europe. I
is a cause of concern not only because of its high mortality
but for the epidemiological problems of control in such a
little understood condition. Once immune competence is
lost the victim becomes subject to a wide variety of othe
infections in the lungs and elsewhere.

REFERENCES AND SUGGESTIONS FOR FURTHER READING

Berkman, Y. M. (1980) Aspiration and inhalation pneumonias. *Seminars in Roentgenology*, **15**, 73–84.

Bulmer, S. R., Lamb, D., McCormack, R. J. M. & Walbaum, P. R. (1978) Aetiology of unresolved pneumonia, *Thorax*, **33**, 307–314.

Davison, A. G., Heard, B. E., McAllister, W. A. C. and Turner-Warwick, M. E. H. (1983) Cryptogenic organizing pneumonitis. *Quarterly Journal of Medicine*, **52**, 382–394.

Janower, M. L., Weiss, E. B. (1980) Mycoplasmal, viral and rickettsial pneumonias. *Seminars in Roentgenology*, **15**, 25–34.

Jewkes J., Kay. P. H., Paneth, M. & Citron, K. M. (1983) Pulmonary aspergilloma: analysis and prognosis in relation to haemoptysis and survey of treatment. *Thorax*, **38**, 572–578.

Joint Tuberculosis Committee of the British Thoracic Society (1983) Control and prevention of tuberculosis: a code of practice. *British Medical Journal*, **287**, 1118–1121.

Malo, J. L., Pepys, J., Simon, G. (1977) Studies in chronic allergic, bronchopulmonary aspergillosis. 2 — Radiological findings *Thorax*, **32**, 262–268.

Scanlon, G. T., Unger, J. D. The Radiology of bacterial and viral pneumonias (1973). *Radiologic clinics of North America*, **11**, 317–338.

Tew, J., Calenoff, L., Berlin, B. S. (1977) Bacterial and Non-bacterial pneumonia: Accuracy of radiographic diagnosis. *Radiology*, **124**, 607–612.

White, R. J., Blainey, A. D., Harrison, K. J. & Clarke, S. K. R. (1981) Causes of pneumonia presenting to a district general hospital. *Thorax*, **36**, 566–570.

CHAPTER 16

CHRONIC BRONCHITIS AND EMPHYSEMA: PNEUMOCONIOSES

CHRONIC BRONCHITIS AND EMPHYSEMA

Chronic obstruction to bronchial airflow is an abnormality that unites the group of conditions termed chronic obstructive pulmonary disease or chronic obstructive airways disease. This group is the most common form of chronic lung disease and includes chronic bronchitis, pulmonary emphysema and asthma, which are discussed in this section. Other entities in this group (cystic fibrosis and bronchiectasis) are discussed elsewhere.

Definitions

Chronic bronchitis is defined in clinical terms as 'a chronic cough without demonstrable cause, with expectoration on most days during at least three consecutive months for more than two consecutive years'.

Emphysema is defined in morphological terms as 'an increase, beyond the normal, in the size of the air spaces distal to the terminal bronchioles, with dilatation and destruction of their walls'.

Asthma is a clinical term referring to 'widespread narrowing of the bronchi, which is paroxysmal and reversible'.

Clinically a patient may have manifestations of more than one kind of chronic obstructive airways disease, and not surprisingly, therefore, the radiological and clinical pictures may be mixed.

ASTHMA

The clinical syndrome of asthma results from hyperreactivity of the larger airways to a variety of stimuli causing narrowing of the bronchi, wheezing and often dyspnoea. *Extrinsic* or atopic asthma is usually associated with a history of allergy. An important cause of extrinsic asthma is aspergillosis, and this is discussed in detail elsewhere. *Intrinsic* or non-atopic asthma may be precipitated by a variety of factors such as exercise, emotion and infection. In acute exacerbations of chronic bronchitis due to a chest infection wheezing is a common feature.

The role of radiology in asthma is limited. Most asthmatics have a normal chest X-ray during remissions. During an asthmatic attack the chest X-ray may show signs of hyperinflation (Fig. 16.1), the diaphragm being depressed and the retrosternal air-space being increased. Mediastinal emphysema may occur, presumably secondary to a rupture at terminal bronchiolar level or beyond, and occasionally this may lead to a pneumothorax. The peripheral pulmonary vessels appear normal, but if the central pulmonary arteries are enlarged irreversible pulmonary arterial hypertension is probably present. The importance of radiology is to exclude complications such as a pulmonary infection, atelectasis due to mucous plugging or pneumothorax (see Ch. 17, p. 486).

CHRONIC BRONCHITIS

The most consistent pathological finding in chronic bronchitis is hypertrophy of the mucus-secreting glands of the bronchi. Their secretions are more viscous than usual, leading to interference with the mucociliary transport mechanisms, and plugging of the small airways.

Chronic bronchitics are almost always smokers, and are usually male. Other important aetiological factors are urban atmospheric pollution, a dusty work environment and low socio-economic group. Chest infections are important precipitators of exacerbations, but are probably not a basic cause of chronic bronchitis.

The role of radiology in chronic bronchitis is to detect and assess complications of the condition, and also to detect coincidental diseases. Pulmonary emphysema is a common complication which can be assessed radiographically, as can the development of cor pulmonale. The presenting symptoms of pulmonary tuberculosis and lung cancer can be masked by chronic bronchitis, and again the chest X-ray may help.

Radiological appearances. Approximately 50% of patients with chronic bronchitis have a normal chest X-ray. In patients with a plain film abnormality the signs are due to emphysema, superimposed infection or possibly bronchiectasis.

An appearance which suggests chronic bronchitis is the so-called 'dirty chest' (Fig. 16.2). There is generalized

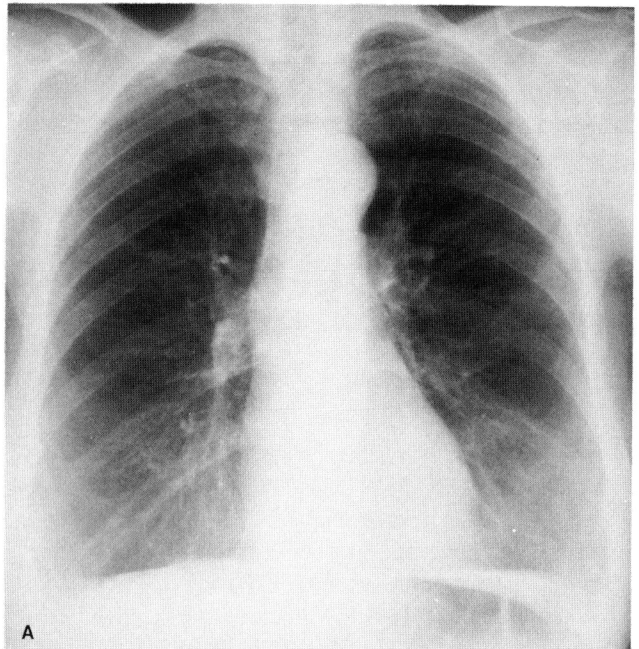

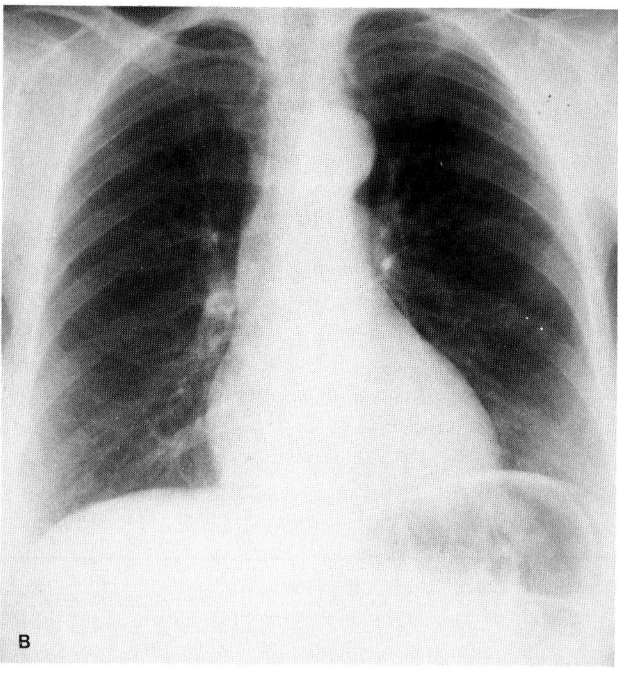

Fig. 16.1 Asthma. Female aged 64 years. (**A**) During an asthmatic attack the lungs are hyperinflated, the diaphragm being depressed and flattened. (**B**) During remission the chest radiograph is normal.

accentuation of the broncho-vascular markings. Small, poorly defined opacities may be seen anywhere in the lungs, but their perception can be extremely subjective. There is some correlation between the 'dirty chest' and the presence of perivascular and peribronchial oedema, chronic inflammation and fibrosis. If this pattern is particularly obvious, with fine linear shadows and hazy nodular opacities, the appearance may resemble interstitial fibrosis, lymphangitis carcinomatosis or bronchiectasis.

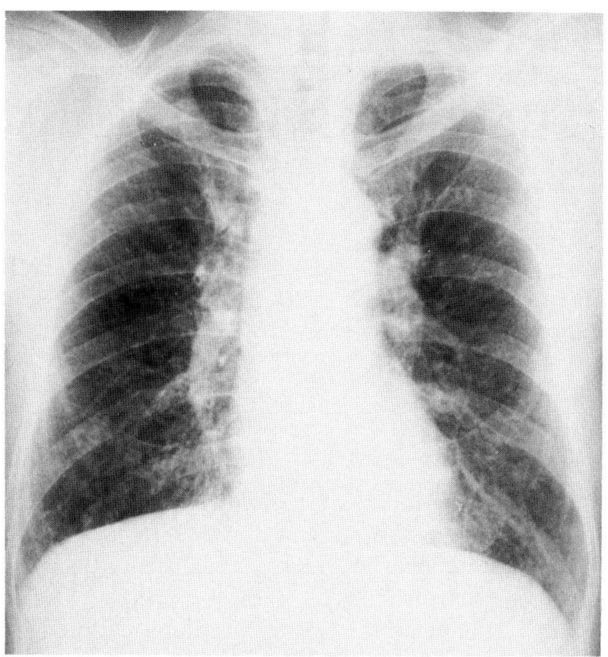

Fig. 16.2 Chronic bronchitis. Male aged 62 years. Small, poorly defined opacities are present throughout both lungs, producing the 'dirty chest'. This contrasts with the clear lungs in Figure 16.1B.

Thin tram-line or tubular shadows may also be seen, suggesting bronchiectasis, but the precise nature of these shadows is uncertain. These opacities are usually related to the hila, and may be clearly demonstrated by tomography, but again are only suggestive and not diagnostic of chronic bronchitis.

If emphysema with air-trapping is present the lungs enlarge, the diaphragm becomes flattened and the retrosternal air-space increases. The number and size of the peripheral vessels decrease, and the central pulmonary arteries may enlarge. If cor pulmonale supervenes the heart enlarges.

Bronchography is unnecessary in the diagnosis and management of chronic bronchitis, but may show a very characteristic appearance. The bronchial divisions terminate abruptly after 5–8 generations. The bronchi are often irregular and mildly dilated, and pools of contrast medium are seen in dilated terminal bronchioles. Virtually pathognomonic of chronic bronchitis is filling of dilated mucous glands best seen along the inferior margins of the main bronchi.

EMPHYSEMA

As stated above emphysema is defined in morphological terms as enlargement of the airways beyond the terminal bronchi, with dilatation and destruction of their walls. Further classification of emphysema is also based, in part, on morphology, and a basic knowledge of lung structure is, therefore, pertinent. The trachea, bronchi and terminal bronchioles are strictly conducting airways. Beyond the terminal bronchioles gas exchange takes place, so that respiratory bronchioles, alveolar ducts and alveolar sacs are both conducting and respiratory structures. The alveoli are purely respiratory in function. The *secondary pulmonary lobule* is a unit of lung structure supplied by between three and five terminal bronchioles. An acinus is the portion of lung distal to a terminal bronchiole. Therefore, a secondary pulmonary lobule comprises 3–5 acini.

Types of emphysema and associated conditions

Involvement of the secondary pulmonary lobule by emphysema may be non-selective or selective.

1. *Pan-acinar emphysema* is a non-selective process characterized by destruction of all the lung distal to the terminal bronchiole. This is sometimes termed pan-lobular emphysema. The lung may be involved locally or generally, but distribution throughout the lung is rarely uniform. It may be associated with centri-acinar emphysema, especially in chronic bronchitis, and is also seen in alpha-1-antitrypsin deficiency.

2. *Centri-acinar emphysema* is a selective process characterized by destruction and dilatation of the respiratory bronchioles. The alveolar ducts, sacs and alveoli are spared until a late stage. It is sometimes called centri-lobular emphysema. It is frequently found in association with chronic bronchitis.

3. *Focal dust emphysema* is similar to centri-acinar emphysema, except that histological evidence of inflammation is absent. It is usually the result of chronic exposure to coal dust.

4. *Paraseptal emphysema* involves the periphery of the secondary lobules, usually in the lung periphery, sometimes combined with pan- or centri-acinar emphysema, and occasionally causes bulla formation.

5. *Paracicatricial emphysema* refers to distension and destruction of terminal airspaces adjacent to fibrotic lesions, and is most frequently seen as a result of tuberculosis.

6. *Senile emphysema* or alveolar duct emphysema is probably a normal part of the aging process, and causes dilatation of the alveolar ducts. It is rarely of clinical importance or radiologically apparent.

7. *Obstructive emphysema* is strictly a misnomer, and is better termed obstructive hyperinflation since the distal airways are dilated, but not necessarily destroyed. It is discussed here for the sake of completeness. It occurs when a larger bronchus is obstructed in such a way that air enters the lung on inspiration, but is trapped on expiration. Such one-way valve obstruction may be due to an inhaled foreign body (e.g. peanuts or teeth) or due to an endobronchial or peribronchial tumour. The lung beyond the obstruction becomes hyperinflated.

8. *Compensatory emphysema* is another process that is better regarded as hyperinflation. If part or all of a lung collapses, shrinks or is removed the resulting space is occupied by displacement of the mediastinum or diaphragm, or usually more significantly by hyperinflation of the unaffected or remaining lung. This is discussed in the section on lobar collapse.

9. *A bulla* is an emphysematous space with a diameter of more than 1 cm in the distended state, and its walls are made up of compressed surrounding lung or pleura, depending on its location.

Emphysema may be classified according to the presence or absence of air-trapping at respiratory bronchiole level. Pan-acinar, obstructive and congenital lobar emphysema are associated with air-trapping and usually cause symptoms. Senile, centri-acinar, paraseptal and compensatory emphysema are not associated with air-trapping and are usually asymptomatic.

Radiological appearances

1. *Pan-acinar emphysema*

The radiographic features of pan-acinar emphysema are the results of destruction of lung tissue altering the vascular pattern, interference of ventilation decreasing lung perfusion, and air-trapping. The effects of pan-acinar emphysema are almost always apparent clinically by the time the radiographic manifestations occur, but a normal chest X-ray virtually excludes severe generalized emphysema.
The main radiographic signs are (Fig. 16.3):

a. Reduction of pulmonary vascularity peripherally
b. Hyperinflation of the lungs
c. Alteration of the cardiac shadow and central pulmonary arteries

The vascular pattern in affected areas of lung is attenuated. Involvement of the lung may be localized, or generalized, but if generalized is usually patchy. Involved areas have fewer vessels than normal, and those vessels that remain are small. Mild degrees of vascular attenuation are difficult to perceive, so it is worth comparing the size of vessels in different zones. If vessels are diminished in calibre and number in a particular zone, compared to another, that zone is likely to be emphysematous. Peripheral vascular attenuation is due to a number of factors. Perfusion of emphysematous lung is less than normal, and pulmonary blood flow is diverted to less affected areas of lung. Pulmonary vessels are displaced around emphysematous areas and bullae. Small arteries are obliterated by the primary emphysematous process, but these vessels are too small to be visualized radiographically, and this process, therefore, probably does not contribute to the oligaemic appearances, but may be a factor in increased radiolucency of affected areas. Pan-acinar emphysema has a tendency to affect the lung bases, and may cause diver-

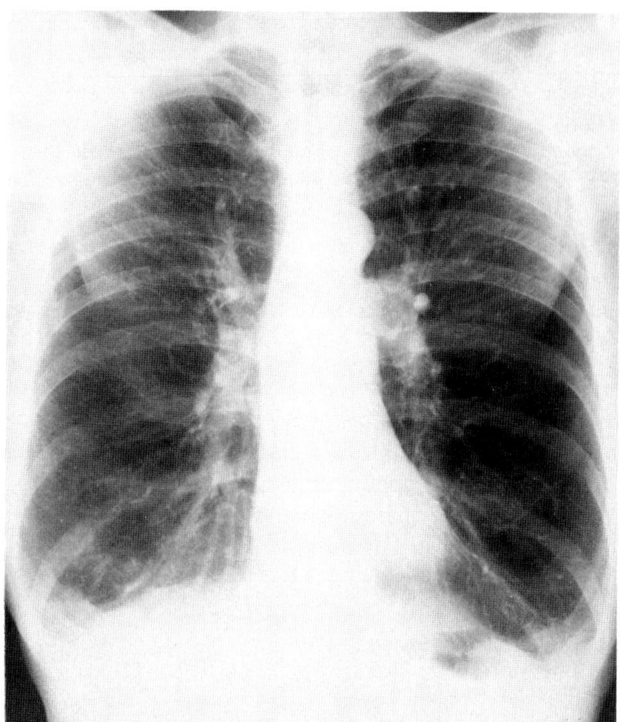

Fig. 16.3 Emphysema. Male aged 54 years. The lungs are hyperinflated, the diaphragm being low and flat. The peripheral vascular pattern is attenuated in the right mid and left mid and lower zones. The central pulmonary arteries are enlarged, indicating pulmonary arterial hypertension. The heart is elongated.

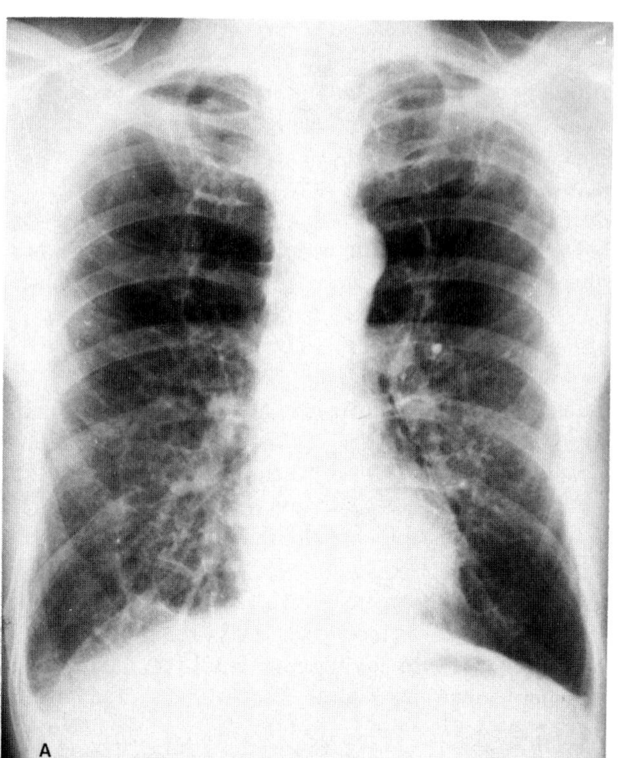

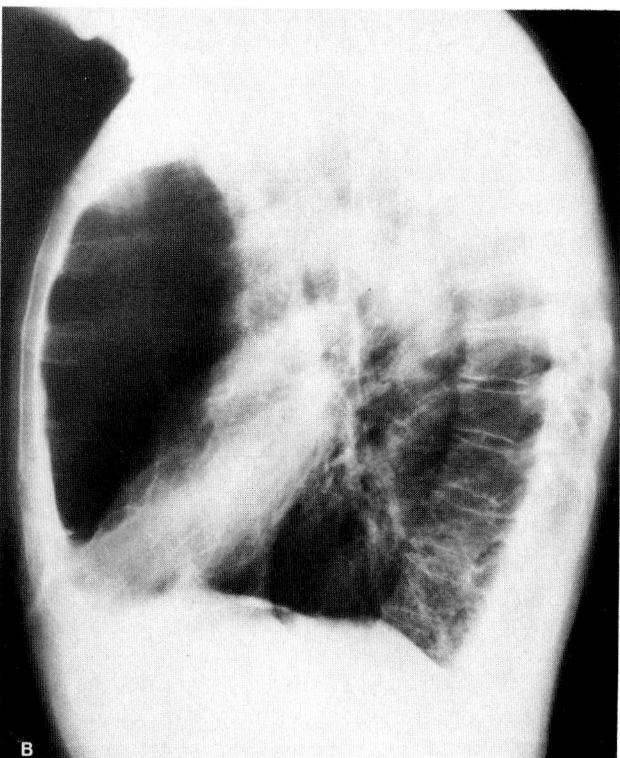

Fig. 16.4 Emphysema. Male aged 52 years. (**A**) The diaphragm is low and flat, and vascular attenuation is present in the right upper and left upper and lower zones. (**B**) Lateral film also shows increased lung volume, which is producing a barrel chest. The retro-sternal space is deeper than normal and extends more inferiorly than normal.

sion of blood flow to the upper zones, which should not be mistaken for pulmonary venous hypertension. In alpha-1-anti-trypsin deficiency the changes of emphysema tend to be basal. Air-trapping causes hyperinflation of the lungs, and may lead to flattening of the diaphragm and increased anteroposterior diameter of the thorax. Flattening of the diaphragm is often best seen on the lateral projection, the level of the diaphragm often being as low as the 11th rib posteriorly. Some normal individuals can push their diaphragm as low on full inspiration, but on expiration the diaphragm will rise 5–10 cm., whereas in emphysema excursion of the diaphragm is usually less than 3 cm. In severe emphysema the diaphragm may actually be inverted.

The 'barrel chest' is caused by bowing of the sternum, and increased thoracic kyphosis. The retrosternal air space may increase in depth, and extend inferiorly between the anterior surface of the heart and the sternum (Fig. 16.4).

The heart often appears long and narrow. This is probably due primarily to the low position of the diaphragm altering the projection of the heart. Enlargement of the central pulmonary arteries usually signifies pulmonary arterial hypertension (Fig. 16.3). If cor pulmonale develops the heart may enlarge due to right ventricular dilatation. In patients with emphysema who develop left heart failure, the signs of hyperinflation may decrease, and the level of the diaphragm will rise. This is due to pulmonary oedema increasing the compliance of the lung and thus reducing the lung volume. In these patients the distribution of oedema fluid within emphysematous lung may be bizarre.

CT scanning is at least as sensitive as the plain chest X-ray in detecting the presence and distribution of emphysema, and is probably superior (Fig. 16.7). Vascular attenuation may be detected earlier, and bullae, particularly in the lung periphery may be identified by CT when inapparent on the chest X-ray. However, chronic airways disease is such a common problem that CT cannot be regarded as a routine method of assessment, but it may help in selected cases, especially if surgical removal of a bulla is being considered.

2. *Bullous disease of the lungs*

Bullae are usually present in the lung in association with some form of emphysema, but occasionally bullae occur locally in otherwise normal lung (Fig. 16.5). They commonly occur in paraseptal emphysema, and in emphysema associated with scarring, but clinically the most important bullae are those due to pan-acinar emphysema, with or without chronic bronchitis.

Bullae appear as round or oval translucencies varying from 1 cm in diameter to occupation of almost an entire hemithorax (Fig. 16.6). They may be single or multiple, and are usually peripheral in the lung. In asymptomatic patients and in those with pulmonary scarring, bullae tend to be apical, but in chronic obstructive airways disease the bullae are found throughout the lungs (Fig. 16.7). Their walls may be visible as a smooth, curved, hair-line shadow. If the walls are not visible displacement of vessels around a radiolucent area may indicate a bullous area. Bullae may also displace fissures, and occasionally depress the hemidiaphragm or extend across the mid-line in the retrosternal space. Adjacent lung is compressed, and this is particularly important in progressive bullous emphysema, where it contributes to increasing respiratory embarrassment.

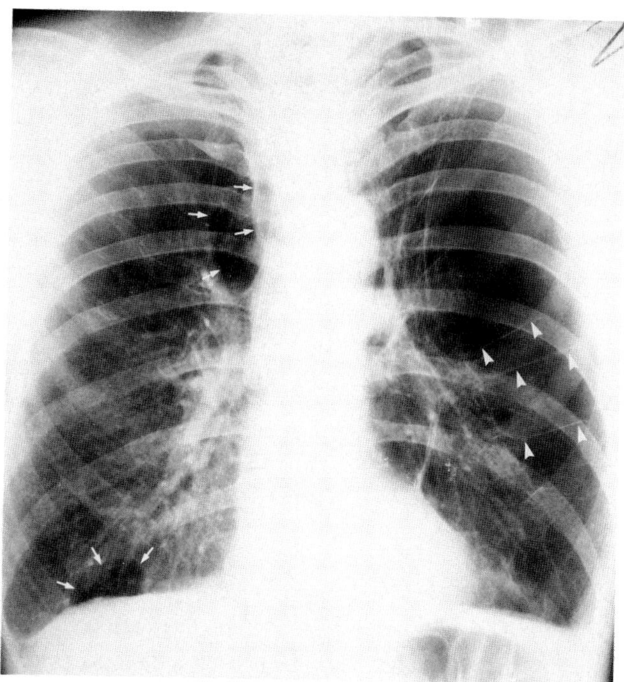

Fig. 16.6 Emphysema with bullae. Male aged 61 years. The lungs are hyperinflated. A giant bulla occupies most of the left hemithorax: compressing the left lung. Strands of lung tissue (arrowheads) are seen crossing this bulla. Small bullae (arrows) are also present in the right lung.

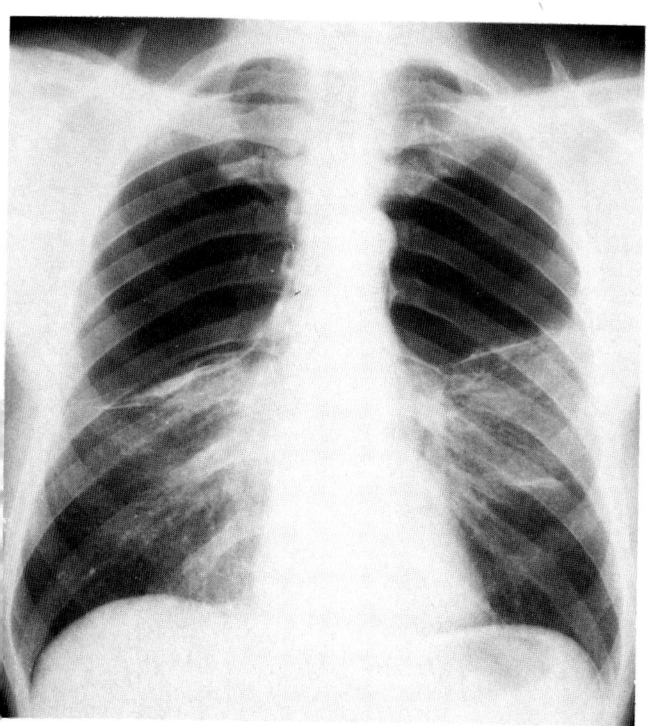

Fig. 16.5 Bilateral upper zone bullae. Male aged 35 years. 'Routine' chest X-ray — no history or symptoms of respiratory disease. Both upper zones are occupied by large bullae which are compressing the upper lobes. There is no evidence of generalized emphysema or air-trapping — the level and shape of the diaphragm are normal.

Bullae are usually air-filled but may become infected and fluid-filled. Associated inflammatory change may be present in the surrounding lung. A bulla will show a fluid level if it is partially fluid-filled, or will appear solid if completely fluid-filled (Fig. 16.8).

A giant bulla may be difficult to differentiate from a loculated pneumothorax, and tomography may be necessary to demonstrate the wall of the bulla or thin strands of lung tissue crossing it.

3. *Emphysema with chronic bronchitis*

Many patients with chronic obstructive airways disease have emphysema and chronic bronchitis. The chest X-ray may then show a combination of changes of hyperinflation, pulmonary arterial hypertension and increased broncho-vascular markings of the so-called 'dirty chest'. At one end of the clinical spectrum is the 'pink puffer' who, by major

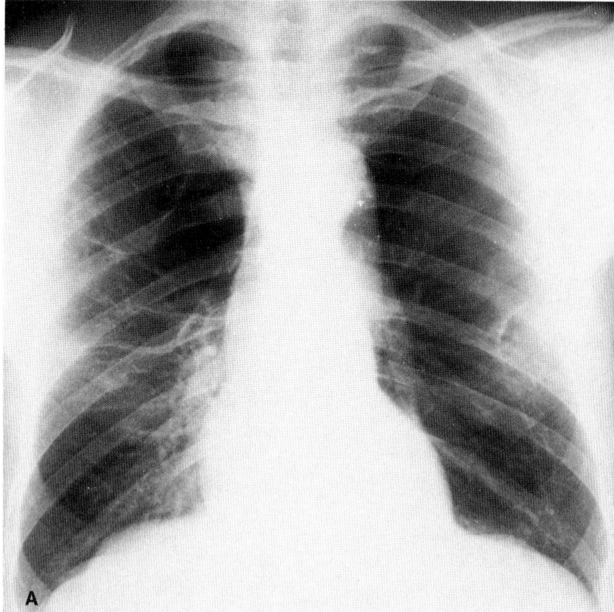

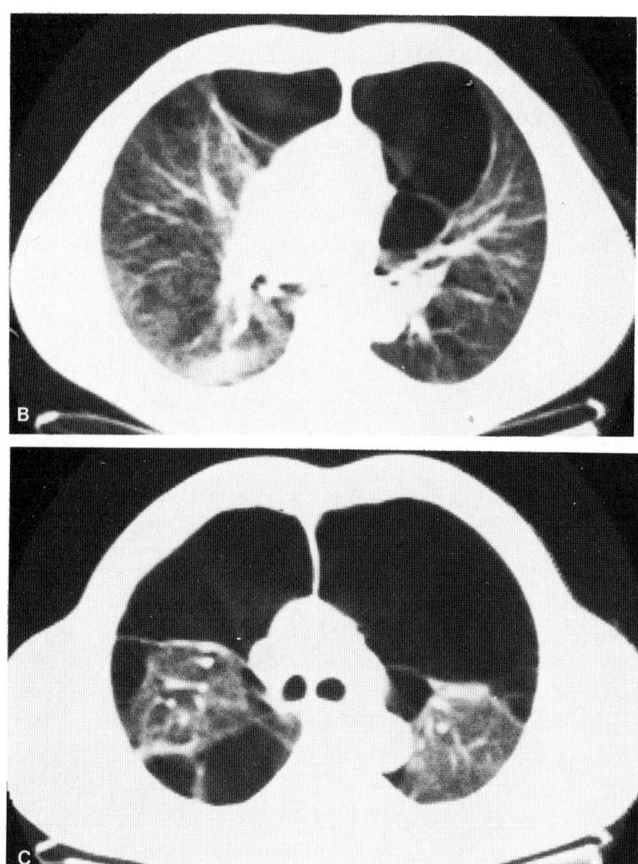

Fig. 16.7 Multiple bullae. (**A**) The chest radiograph shows bullae in both upper zones, and in the periphery of the left mid and lower zones. (**B** and **C**) CT scans demonstrate the bullae more clearly, making it easier to define their size, number and location more accurately. Comparison of expiratory and inspiratory scans makes it possible to differentiate between bullae that are ventilated and those with air-trapping. (Courtesy of Dr B. Strickland.)

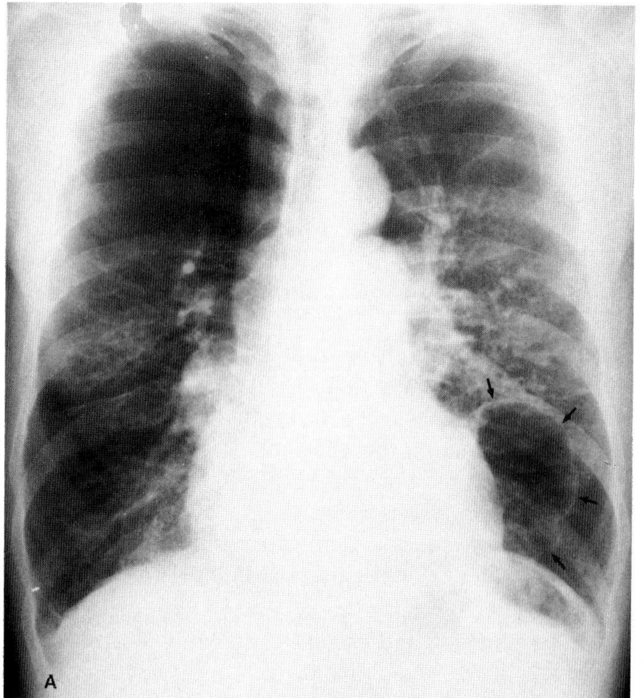

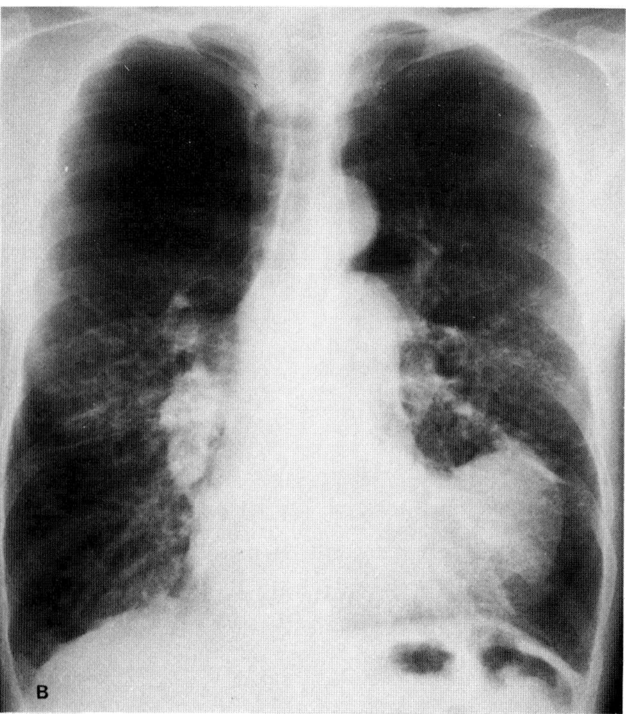

Fig. 16.8 Emphysema with infected bulla. Male aged 48 years. (**A**) The lungs are hyperinflated. The right upper zone is occupied by a large bulla, and another bulla is seen adjacent to the left heart border (arrows). The central pulmonary arteries are enlarged. (**B**) Following a chest infection the left-sided bulla has filled with fluid and appears completely opaque.

effort, ventilates sufficient alveoli to maintain normal blood gases. The lack of hypoxaemia preserves normal pulmonary artery pressure. Pink puffers tend to have predominantly pan-acinar emphysema, and the chest X-ray shows peripheral vascular attenuation and hyperinflation. This appearance may be termed the 'arterial deficiency' pattern. At the other end of the clinical spectrum is the 'blue bloater', who chronically retains carbon dioxide due to poor alveolar ventilation. The respiratory centre becomes insensitive to the persistently raised concentration of arterial carbon dioxide, and chronic cyanosis occurs. Chronic hypoxaemia causes pulmonary arteriolar constriction and in due course pulmonary arterial hypertension and cor pulmonale occur. Blue bloaters tend to have centri-acinar emphysema and less extensive panacinar emphysema. The chest X-ray shows increased bronchovascular markings, enlarged central pulmonary arteries and possibly cardiac enlargement. This appearance may be termed the 'increased markings' pattern of emphysema, and signs of hyperinflation are rarely severe. Most patients with chronic bronchitis and emphysema exhibit features between these extremes.

4. *Unilateral or lobar emphysema (Macleod's or Swyer James' Syndrome)*

This syndrome is characterized by a hypertransradiant hemithorax associated with air-trapping. It is probably the result of a childhood, viral infection causing bronchiolitis and obliteration of the small airways; the involved distal airways are ventilated by collateral air drift, and air-trapping leads to pan-acinar emphysema.

The affected lung is hypertransradiant, due to decreased perfusion, and may be smaller than normal. The ipsilateral pulmonary artery is present, but small, and the peripheral vascular pattern is attenuated. Air-trapping occurs in the affected lung, which tends to maintain its volume on expiration, resulting in displacement of the mediastinum to the normal side, and restriction of the ipsilateral hemi-diaphragm (Fig. 16.9).

Bronchography is not usually indicated, but does show a characteristic appearance. The main and segmental bronchi are normal, but the peripheral bronchi are irregularly dilated, and end abruptly after only 5–10 bifurcations, with very little peripheral bronchial filling.

The syndrome may also be illustrated by isotope scanning, when a perfusion scan will show reduced flow to the affected lung, and a ventilation scan, using xenon, will demonstrate air-trapping.

The differential diagnosis of the chest X-ray appearance includes proximal interruption of the pulmonary artery, the hypogenetic lung syndrome and pulmonary artery obstruction due to embolism. However, none of these entities exhibit air-trapping.

5. *Centri-acinar and focal dust emphysema*

These occur principally in chronic bronchitis and uncom-

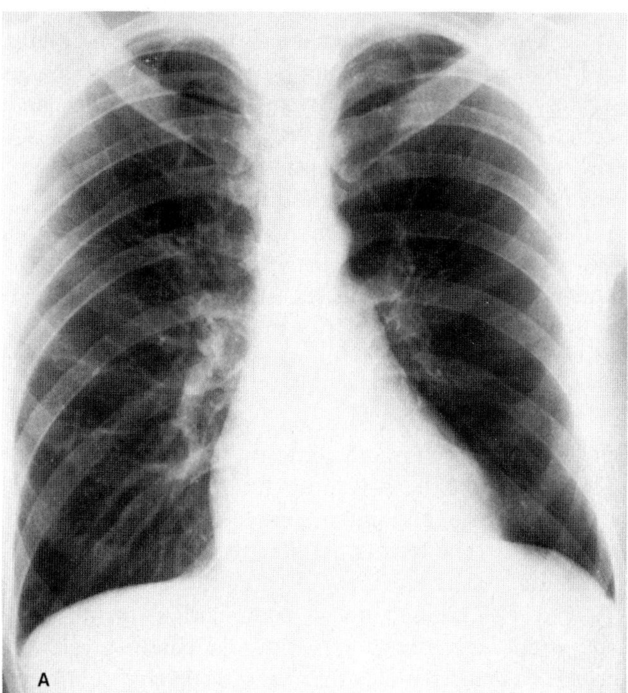

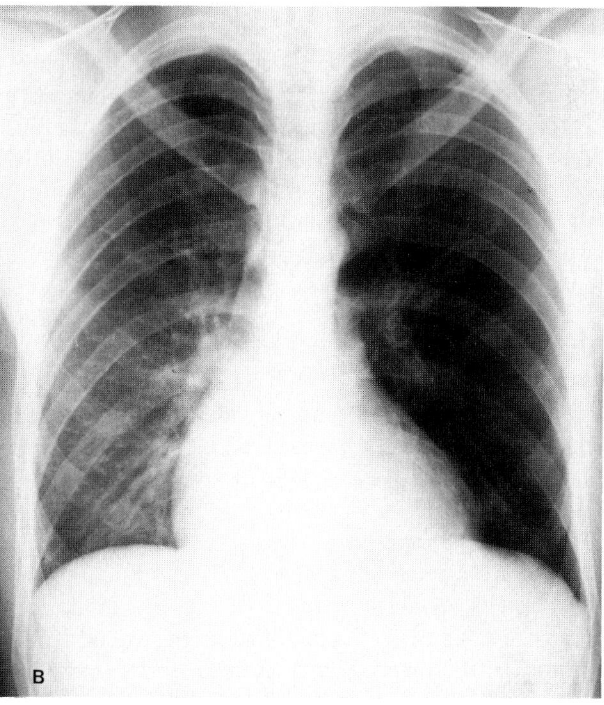

Fig. 16.9 Unilateral emphysema. Male aged 30 years. History of repeated chest infections as a child, but no current respiratory symptoms. (**A**) Inspiratory film shows normal right lung, and hypertransradiant left lung with small left pulmonary artery. (**B**) Expiratory film demonstrates displacement of mediastinum to the right and restricted movement of the left hemi-diaphragm indicating air-trapping in the left lung.

plicated coal-miners' pneumoconiosis respectively. The radiological appearance is that of the primary condition. In later stages pan-acinar and bullous emphysema may become apparent.

6. *Obstructive emphysema*
Obstructive hyperinflation may affect an entire lung, a lobe or a segment. The cause may be apparent on the chest X-ray, such as an inhaled foreign body or tooth, or a central tumour. The vascular pattern of the affected part of the lung is attenuated, and this area may appear hypertransradiant. Fluoroscopy or an expiratory film will demonstrate air-trapping in the affected area, with deviation of the mediastinum to the normal side, and restriction of the ipsilateral hemidiaphragm on expiration.

7. *Compensatory emphysema*
The radiological signs resulting from collapse or removal of all or part of a lung are discussed in the section on lobar collapse.

8. *Congenital lobar emphysema*
This is discussed in Chapter 19 (p. 529).

CRYPTOGENIC OBLITERATIVE BRONCHIOLITIS

This recently described entity presents with dyspnoea, which may be progressive and severe. The clinical picture may suggest pulmonary thromboembolic disease, but the radiographic appearance is different. The chest X-ray shows symmetrical reduction of peripheral vascularity in the mid and lower zones, and evidence of mild hyperinflation of the lungs. Bronchography shows a characteristic appearance of non-filling of the side branches of the fifth and sixth generation bronchi, abrupt termination of bronchi, and either lack of normal tapering or generalized narrowing of bronchi. The cause is unknown, but there is an association with rheumatoid disease.

A SUMMARY OF IMAGING TECHNIQUES USEFUL IN CHRONIC OBSTRUCTIVE AIRWAYS DISEASE

1. *The PA chest X-ray* may provide all the necessary information. A correctly exposed and processed film is important, since an over-exposed or over-processed film may mimic the hypertransradiant lungs of emphysema.
2. *The lateral projection* is necessary to assess AP thoracic diameter and the retrosternal space.
3. *An expiratory film or fluoroscopy* is useful to demonstrate air-trapping. In bilateral disease the excursion of both domes of the diaphragm is reduced, and with unilateral air-trapping the mediastinum is displaced to the normal side on expiration, and movement of the ipsilateral hemidiaphragm is diminished.
4. *Tomography* may be useful in detecting the presence, number, size and extent of bullae. This may be of particular importance if bullectomy is being contemplated. Tomography may also help differentiate between a large bulla and a loculated pneumothorax.
5. *CT scanning* is probably the most sensitive radiographic method of assessing the morphological changes of chronic obstructive airways disease, but its precise place in clinical management has yet to be established.
6. *Ventilation and perfusion scanning* may illustrate the physiological changes in chronic obstructive airways disease. Ventilation scanning with xenon will show areas of reduced ventilation and air-trapping, and perfusion scanning will demonstrate areas of decreased vascularity.
7. *Bronchography* may show characteristic appearances in chronic bronchitis and unilateral emphysema, or indicate the site and cause of an obstructed bronchus, but is rarely indicated clinically.

THE PNEUMOCONIOSES

Occupational disease of the chest may be due to inhalation of dusts or noxious fumes. Dusts may be inorganic or organic. In general the organic dusts cause disease by hypersensitivity reactions, and they are considered in the section on extrinsic allergic alveolitis. Noxious gases usually produce an acute inflammatory reaction, often with pulmonary oedema, which may be fatal, or may be followed by resolution, with or without subsequent pulmonary fibrosis. The pneumoconioses considered in this section are diseases due to inhalation of inorganic dusts.

Dust particles larger than 5 μm in diameter are usually deposited onto the bronchial and bronchiolar walls and are coughed up, but smaller particles may reach the alveoli. Asbestos fibres are an exception, fibres longer than 30 μm sometimes penetrating the lung parenchyma.

The diagnosis of a pneumoconiosis depends upon a history of exposure to a dust and an abnormal chest X-ray and pulmonary function tests. Occasionally a lung biopsy is necessary. The history of exposure is not necessarily one of working with a dust, but may include living near a mine or factory.

The reaction of an individual to dust exposure depends upon several factors including the nature of the dust, the concentration of particles, the duration of exposure and the individual's susceptibility. Inorganic dusts are either active or inactive. The former are fibrogenic in the lung, and the latter are relatively inert. Frequently an individual will have been exposed to a combination of dusts. The important active dusts are silica and asbestos; coal dust is usually a combination of active and inactive components.

The ILO (International Labour Office) Classification of Radiographs of the Pneumoconioses has been devised to codify the chest X-ray changes in a simple and reproducble manner. It is important in epidemiological and industrial medicine, and the interested reader is referred to the specialist publications at the end of this chapter.

SILICOSIS

Exposure to silica may occur in a variety of occupations including granite, slate and sandstone quarrying, gold mining, sandblasting, foundry work, pottery and ceramics. Exposure is usually over several years before symptoms occur, unless the exposure is overwhelming. Silica causes a fibrotic reaction in the lung, which may progress after exposure has ceased, probably due to immunological processes. Silicosis predisposes to pulmonary tuberculosis.

Radiological appearance. Simple silicosis appears as multiple, nodular shadows of fairly uniform size, usually between 2 and 5 mm. in diameter. The nodules have a fairly sharp outline, and are of uniform density (Fig. 16.10). They appear initially in the mid and upper zones, but are later found in all zones, with relative sparing of the bases. The nodules rarely calcify. Reticular shadowing may occur at any stage, and septal lines may appear. Pleural changes are rare.

Complicated silicosis is characterized by confluence of nodules (Fig. 16.11) to form homogeneous, non-segmental areas of consolidation, usually in the upper lobes. These 'massive shadows' of fibrosis migrate towards the hila, leaving peripheral areas of emphysema. When complicated silicosis develops, the possibility of tuberculosis should be considered. Cavitation of a massive shadow is usually due to ischaemic necrosis or tuberculosis.

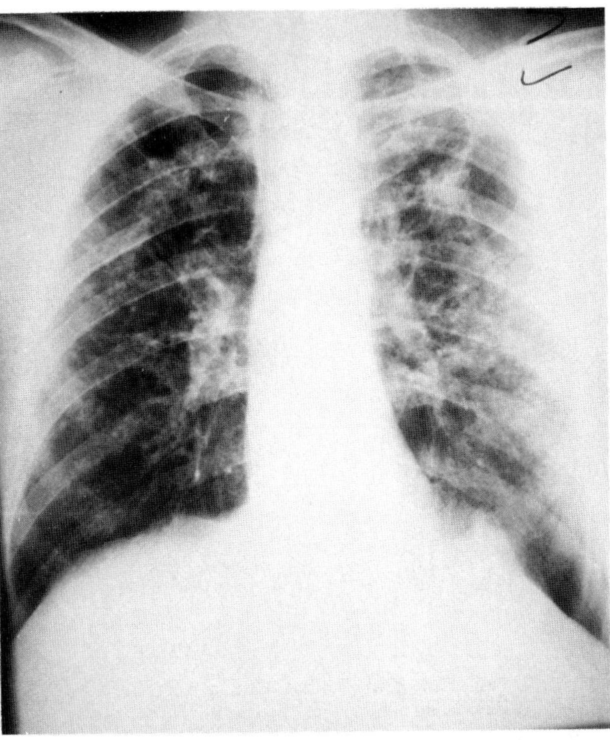

Fig. 16.11 Complicated silicosis. Roofing-felt manufacturer aged 63 years, with exposure to silica sand and talc. In addition to widespread, nodular opacities, densest in the mid and upper zones, confluent opacities are developing in the upper zones. Talc is a mixture of silica and asbestos, and sputum examination revealed asbestos bodies. Lung biopsy: mixed dust pneumoconiosis.

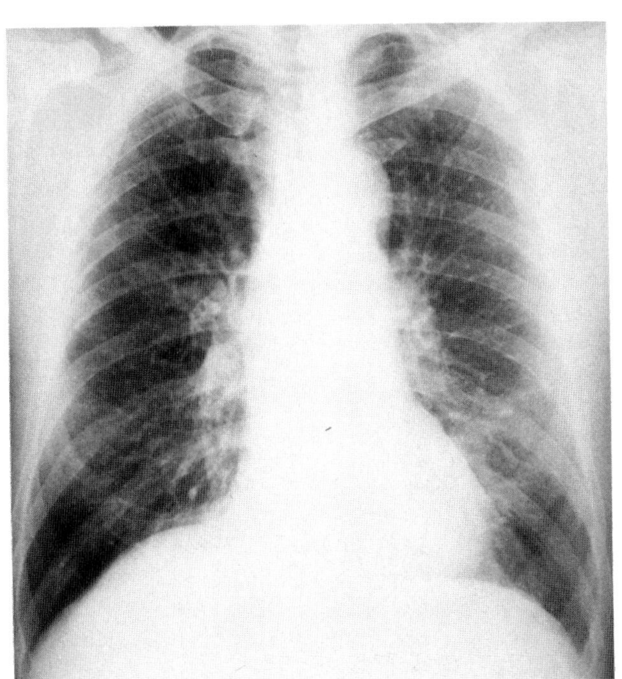

Fig. 16.10 Simple silicosis. Retired sandblaster aged 67 years. Multiple nodular opacities are present throughout both lungs, with relative sparing of the lower zones.

Hilar lymph node enlargement is common at any stage, and lymph node calcification may occur. Calcification may be diffuse throughout lymph nodes, or peripheral giving an 'egg shell' appearance (Fig. 16.12).

Extensive fibrosis may cause pulmonary arterial hypertension, and cor pulmonale may ensue.

In patients with rheumatoid disease, silicosis may be complicated by Caplan's syndrome, but, like massive fibrosis, this is commoner in coal worker's pneumoconiosis.

ASBESTOSIS

Asbestos exposure may occur in a variety of occupations. Asbestos mining and processing are obvious examples, but exposure may also occur in construction and demolition work, ship building and manufacture of some textiles. Living near such places of work also carries a risk of exposure. The duration of exposure may be very short, and the manifestation may become apparent only many years later.

The four types of asbestos that commonly cause disease are chrysolite, crocidolite, amosite and anthophyllite.

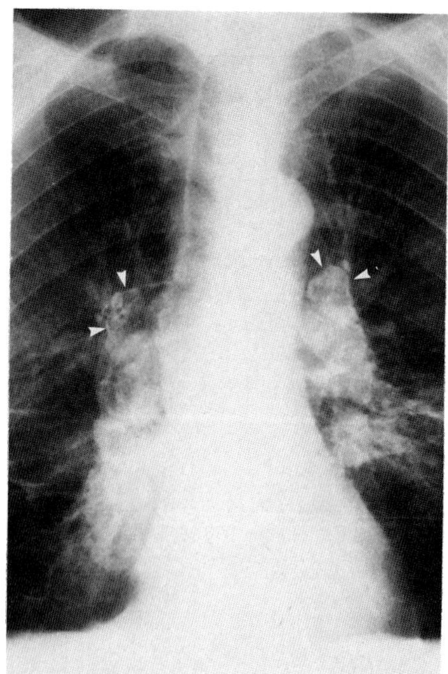

Fig. 16.12 Silicosis. Male aged 69 years. History of exposure to a variety of dusts including silica. Note bilateral hilar lymph node enlargement with 'egg-shell' calcification (arrowheads) typical of silicosis.

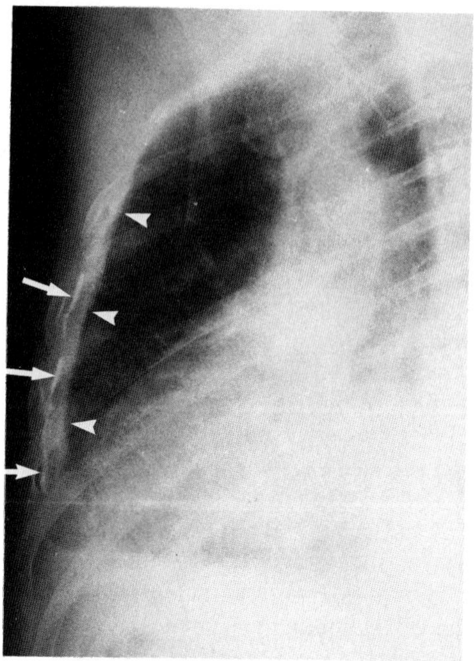

Fig. 16.13 Asbestos exposure. Retired construction worker. Oblique projection demonstrates extensive pleural thickening (arrowheads), and calcification (arrows) adjacent to ribs.

Chrysolite (or white asbestos) is the commonest, and crocidolite (or blue asbestos) is the most pathogenic.

Fibrosis is probably the result of a number of mechanisms. Direct physical irritation is almost certainly a factor in the development of pleural plaques. Asbestos is a mixture of silicates, and release of silicilic acid may be locally irritant. Lastly, a toxic effect of asbestos on macrophages leads to the release of antigens and the subsequent production of auto-antibodies. This auto-immune response is probably the cause of the fibrosing alveolitis that is a common feature. Asbestos fibres may remain in the lung for years after exposure has ceased, and this may explain the sometimes delayed development of pulmonary fibrosis.

Inhaled fibres, sometimes longer than 30 μm, may reach the alveoli and penetrate the pleura, and occasionally the diaphragm. The fibres gravitate to the lower lobes, so that changes are more severe in the lower zones, and less in the mid and upper zones.

Symptoms of asbestosis are often not apparent until 20 or 30 years after exposure. Malignant disease is an important complication. Lung cancer, usually adenocarcinoma, is relatively common, especially when asbestos exposure is combined with cigarette smoking. Compared to the non-smoker without exposure to asbestos, asbestos alone increases the likelihood of lung cancer by a factor of 5, cigarette smoking alone by a factor of 10, and the combination of asbestos and cigarettes by a factor of 50! The combination of asbestos and cigarettes also predisposes to carcinomas of the oesophagus, larynx and oropharynx. Mesothelioma of the pleura is the other malignancy closely associated with asbestos exposure, and may develop after a latent period of 20 years. Other neoplasms associated with asbestos exposure are carcinomas of the large bowel and renal tract and peritoneal mesothelioma.

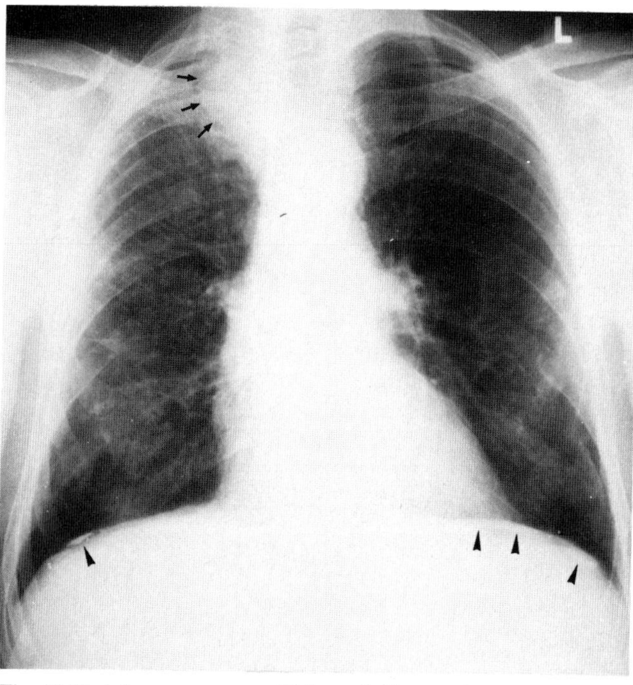

Fig. 16.14 Asbestos exposure. Male aged 60 years. Pleural shadowing in the periphery of both mid zones is due to plaques. Pleural calcification is present along both domes of the diaphragm (arrowheads). Mass at the right apex is an adenocarcinoma (arrows).

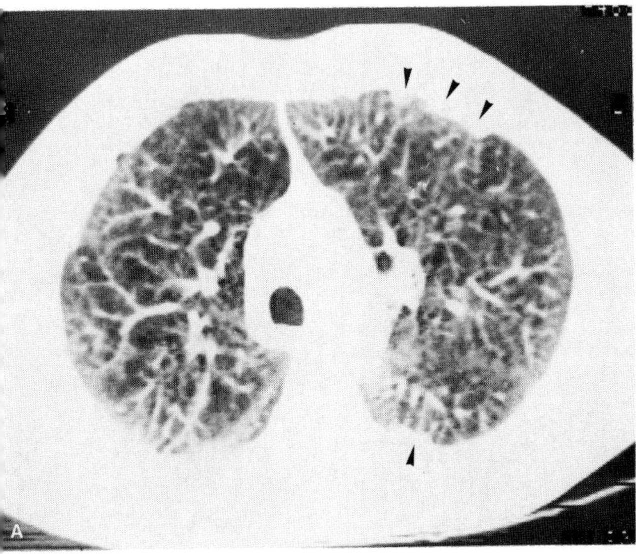

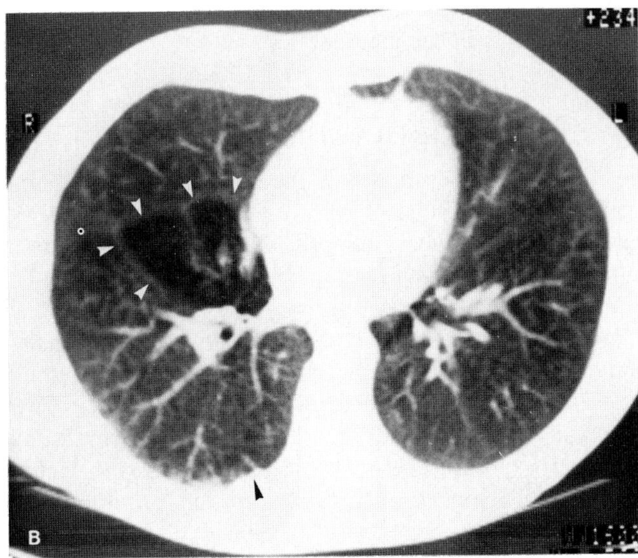

Fig. 16.15 Asbestosis. Male aged 54 years. Pipe lagger for 14 years. (**A**) CT demonstrates pleural plaques (arrowheads) and diffuse reticular and nodular shadows. (**B**) This section demonstrates further pleural plaques (black arrowhead) and bullae in the right lung (white arrowheads). The chest radiograph (not shown) demonstrated the pleural plaques, but not the lung disease.

Radiological appearance. Asbestos exposure may produce changes in the lung parenchyma and in the pleura. Pleural changes, which include plaques, calcification, diffuse thickening and effusion are seen on the chest X-ray more often than parenchymal changes.

Pleural plaques are usually bilateral, and most frequently are present peripherally in the mid zones, often adjacent to the ribs. They may be difficult to see unless viewed tangentially, so if they are suspected fluoroscopy and oblique views are helpful (Fig. 16.13). They may also be demonstrated by ultrasound and small plaques, especially close to the spine, may only be seen by CT (Fig. 13.23). Plaques are common over the diaphragm but are difficult to see unless calcified. Occasionally it may be difficult to differentiate between plaques and companion shadows. The presence of bilateral pleural plaques is almost diagnostic of asbestos exposure.

Pleural plaques frequently calcify. Calcification is, therefore, most often seen in the periphery of the mid zones and over the diaphragm (Fig. 16.14). The calcium is situated deep in the parietal pleura, just deep to the ribs or diaphragm, usually forming linear shadows, occasionally with bizarre shapes. Again tangential views (Fig. 16.13) and CT may be helpful.

Diffuse pleural thickening is an unusual manifestation (Fig. 13.18) and small pleural effusions, unrelated to malignant change, occasionally occur. Mesothelioma is discussed in the section on the pleura (Ch. 13).

Pulmonary fibrosis is usually present histologically by the time pleural calcification has developed, but may not be apparent on the chest X-ray. CT scanning is more sensitive than the chest X-ray in detecting early pulmonary fibrosis by demonstration of either nodular or linear shadows (Fig. 16.15).

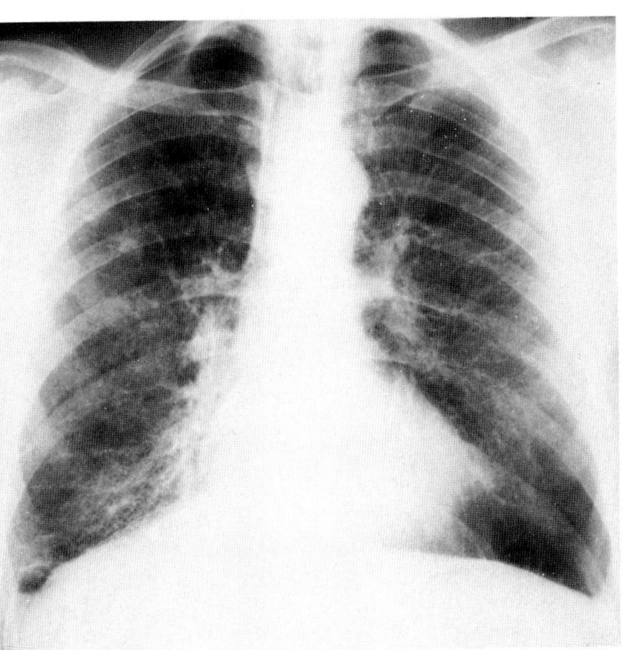

Fig. 16.16 Asbestosis. Male aged 59 years. Asbestos exposure over 25 years. Fine, reticulo-nodular shadowing is present in the mid and lower zones, best seen on the right side. Emphysematous bullae are present at the left base.

The earliest sign of pulmonary fibrosis on the chest X-ray is a fine reticular pattern in the lower zones (Fig. 16.16). This becomes coarser, leading to loss of clarity of the diaphragmatic and cardiac outlines — the so-called 'shaggy heart'. At a later stage the whole lung may be involved, but the basal preponderance persists, and emphysematous bullae may develop.

COAL-WORKER'S PNEUMOCONIOSIS

Coal dust comprises mostly carbon, but it may contain small amounts of silica. Coal-workers are susceptible to coal-worker's pneumoconiosis, silicosis, chronic bronchitis, emphysema and pulmonary tuberculosis.

Coal dust is not fibrogenic, and deposits in the lung are surrounded by areas of focal dust emphysema. The corresponding radiographic appearance is 'simple' pneumoconiosis. 'Complicated' pneumoconiosis, characterized by progressive massive fibrosis (PMF) is the result of prolonged exposure, perhaps with a complicating factor such as silica exposure, infection, or an auto-immune process with the presence of rheumatoid factor, antinuclear factor or other auto-antibodies.

Radiological appearance. The earliest signs of simple pneumoconiosis on the chest X-ray are small, faint, indistinct nodular opacities, 1–5 mm in diameter. The nodules first appear in the mid zones, with subsequent involvement of the entire lung, although the mid zone preponderance persists (Fig. 16.17). The nodules are smaller and less well-defined than those of silicosis, and may rarely calcify. Coalescence of small nodules to form opacities of 1 cm diameter or more, or the appearance of new opacities of this size signifies development of PMF (Fig. 16.18). These massive shadows are usually bilateral, and develop initially in the periphery of the upper and mid zones as round or oval shadows. They may become sausage-shaped and

Fig. 16.17 Coal-worker's pneumoconiosis. Male aged 59 years. Nodular opacities are present throughout both lungs, densest in the mid-zones. A right apical pneumothorax is also present.

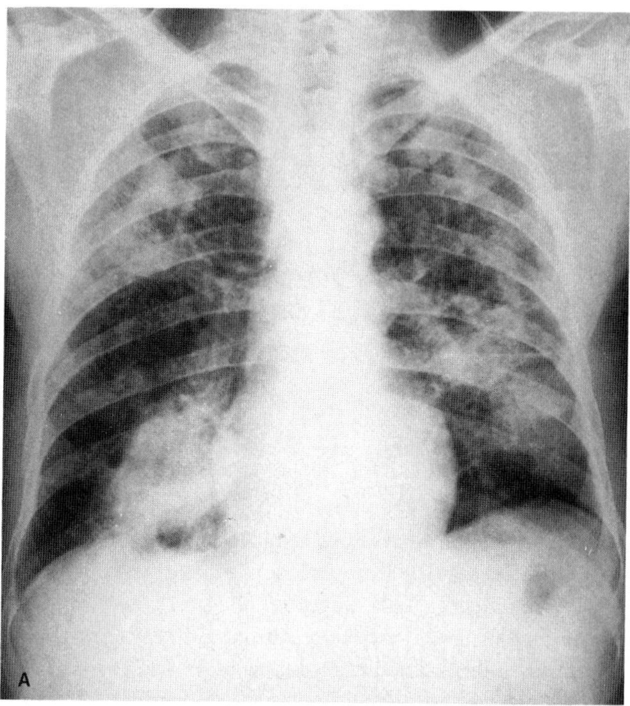

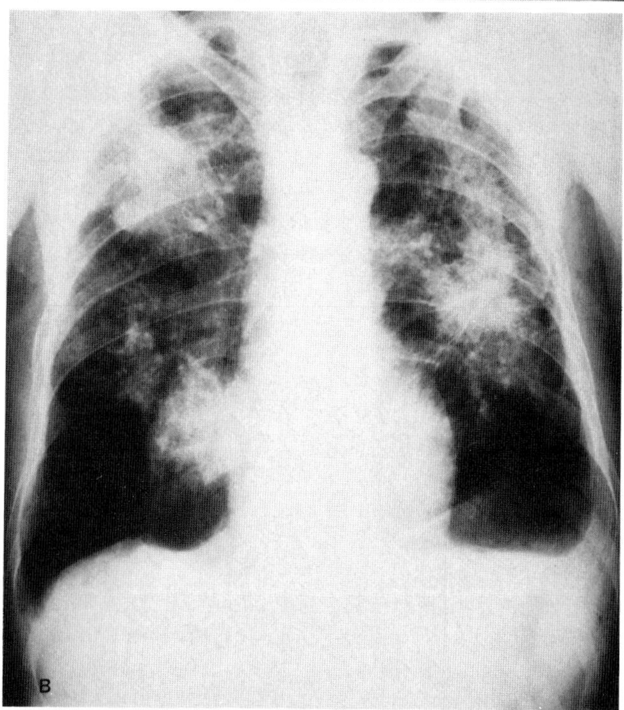

Fig. 16.18 Progressive massive fibrosis. Coal miner aged 52 years. (**A**) Nodular opacities are present throughout both lungs, and several areas of more confluent shadowing are present. (**B**) 4 years later lower zone masses have migrated centrally leaving peripheral areas of emphysema. The upper lobe opacities have enlarged.

migrate towards the hila, leaving peripheral areas of emphysema and bullae. The massive shadows may develop scattered areas of calcification, and occasionally they cavitate, and may subsequently fill with fluid.

Simple coal-worker's pneumoconiosis does not usually progress if exposure to coal dust ceases, but PMF often does.

Caplan's syndrome may occur in patients with rheumatoid disease and coal-worker's pneumoconiosis. The appearance is of multiple, round, well-defined opacities, 1–5 cm in diameter throughout the lungs, often developing rapidly, sometimes in successive crops (Fig. 16.19). These opacities represent rheumatoid nodules, and they may remain static, calcify or cavitate. The underlying changes of pneumoconiosis may not be obvious, and the appearance may then resemble pulmonary metastases.

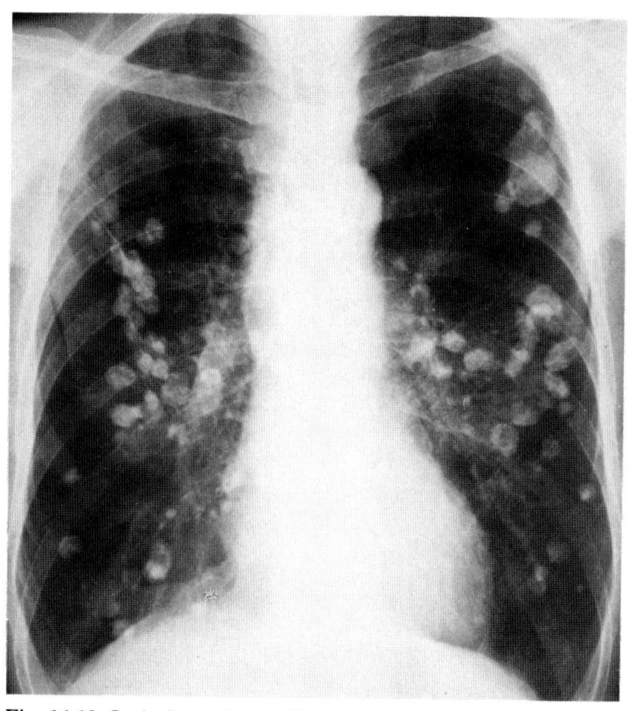

Fig. 16.19 Caplan's syndrome. Male aged 54 years. Coal worker with long-standing rheumatoid arthritis. Multiple rounded pulmonary opacities are present — some are partly calcified. Background changes of coal worker's pneumoconiosis are minimal.

BERYLLIOSIS

Chronic beryllium poisoning may produce pulmonary manifestations that resemble a pneumoconiosis, but the changes are probably due to a specific antigen–antibody reaction. Acute berylliosis is a chemical pneumonitis and the radiological appearance is that of non-cardiogenic pulmonary oedema. Chronic berylliosis is a systemic disease characterized by widespread non-caseating granulomas, which in the lung produce appearances identical to sarcoidosis. There is widespread, fine, reticular and nodular shadowing often with hilar and mediastinal lymph node enlargement, and this may be followed by widespread fibrosis (Fig. 16.20).

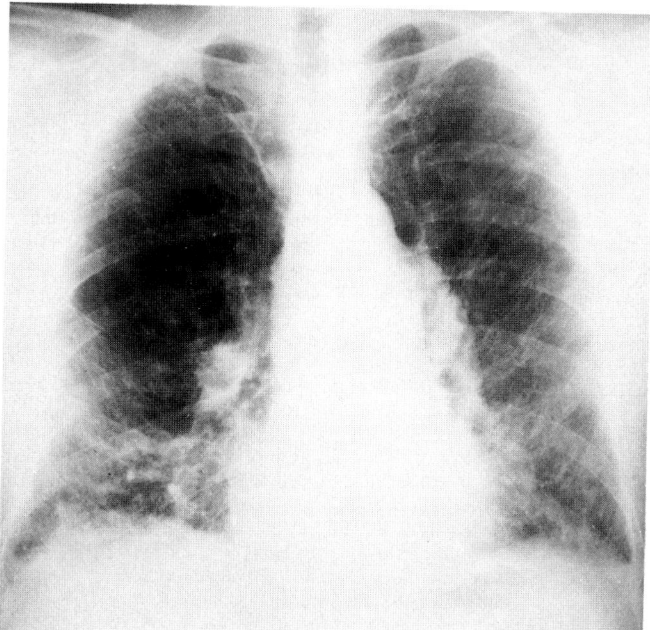

Fig. 16.20 Berylliosis. 35 years in glass blowing industry making neon lights. The chest radiograph shows diffuse reticular shadowing. The appearance is indistinguishable from end-stage sarcoidosis.

PNEUMOCONIOSES DUE TO INACTIVE DUSTS

Inactive dusts do not cause fibrosis in the lungs, but may produce changes on the chest X-ray simply by accumulating in the lungs. Symptoms are usually absent.

Siderosis is due to prolonged exposure to iron oxide dust. Widespread reticulo-nodular shadowing occurs. When exposure ceases the shadowing may regress. In silicosiderosis fibrosis may occur with a picture resembling silicosis.

Stannosis is caused by inhalation of tin oxide. Multiple, very small, very dense, discrete opacities, of 0.5–1 mm diameter are distributed throughout the lungs. Particles may collect in the interlobular lymphatics and produce dense septal lines. The opacities are denser than calcium because of the high atomic number of tin.

Barytosis results from inhalation of particulate barium sulphate, causing very dense nodulation throughout the lungs. Following cessation of exposure the shadows regress.

REFERENCES AND SUGGESTIONS FOR FURTHER READING

General

See Chapter 2.

Chronic obstructive airways disease

A report of the conclusions of a CIBA Guest Symposium: Terminology, definitions and classification of chronic pulmonary emphysema and related conditions (1959). *Thorax*, **14**, 286–299.

Anderson, A. E. Jr., Foraker, A. G. (1973) Centrilobular emphysema and panlobular emphysema: two different diseases. *Thorax*, **28**, 547–550.

Breatnach, E., Kerr, I. (1982) The radiology of cryptogenic obliterative bronchiolitis. *Clinical Radiology*, **33**, 657–661.

Carr, D. H., Pride, N. B. (1984) Computed tomography in pre-operative assessment of bullous emphysema. *Clinical Radiology*, **35**, 43–45.

Fletcher, C. M., Pride, N. B. (1984) Editorial: Definitions of emphysema, chronic bronchitis, asthma and air flow obstruction: 25 years on from the CIBA symposium. *Thorax*, **39**, 81–85.

Goddard, P. R., Nicholson, E. M., Laszlo, G., Watt, I. (1982) Computed tomography in pulmonary emphysema. *Clinical Radiology*, **33**, 379–387.

MacLeod, W. M. (1954) Abnormal transradiancy of one lung. *Thorax*, **9**, 147–153.

Morgan, M. D. L., Strickland, B. (1984) Computed tomography in the assessment of bullous lung disease. *British Journal of Diseases of the Chest*, **78**, 10–25.

Patheram, I. S., Kerr, I. H., Collins, J. V. (1981) Value of chest radiographs in severe acute asthma. *Clinical Radiology*, **32**, 281–282.

Reid, L. (1967) *The Pathology of Emphysema*. London: Lloyd-Luke.

Simon, G. (1964) Radiology and emphysema. *Clinical Radiology*, **15**, 293–306.

Swyer, P. R., James, G. C. W. (1953) A case of unilateral emphysema. *Thorax*, **8**, 133–136.

Thurlbeck, W. M., Simon, G. (1978) Radiographic appearance of the chest in emphysema. *American Journal of Roentgenology*, **130**, 429–440.

Tomashefski, J. F. (1977) Definition, differentiation and classification of COPD. *Postgraduate Medicine*, **62**, 88–97.

The Pneumoconioses

Becklake, M. R. (1976) Asbestos related diseases of the lung and other organs. Their epidemiology and implications for clinical practice. *American Review of Respiratory Disease*, **114**, 187–227.

Caplan, A. (1962) Correlation of radiological category with lung pathology in coal-workers' pneumoconiosis. *British Journal of Industrial Medicine*, **19**, 171–179.

Cunningham, C. D. B., Hugh, A. E. (1973) Pneumoconiosis in women. *Clinical Radiology*, **24**, 491–493.

Doig, A. T. (1976) Barytosis: a benign pneumoconiosis. *Thorax*, **31**, 30–39.

Epler, G. R., McLoud, T. C., Gaensler, E. A. (1982) Prevalence and incidence of benign asbestos pleural effusion in a working population. *Journal of the American Medical Association*, **247**, 617.

Greening, R. R., Helsep, J. H. (1967) The roentgenology of silicosis. *Seminars in Roentgenology*, **2**, 265–275.

Hardy, H. L. (1967) Current concepts of occupational lung disease of interest to the radiologist. *Seminars in Roentgenology*, **2**, 225–234.

Heitzman, E. R. (1973) *The Lung: Radiologic–Pathologic Correlations*. The pneumoconioses. pp. 241–258. St. Louis: The C. V. Mosby Company.

ILO/UC International Classification of Pneumoconioses (1979) Occupational Safety and Health Series. Geneva: International Labour Office.

Katz, D., Kreel, L. (1979) Computed tomography in pulmonary asbestosis. *Clinical Radiology*, **30**, 207–213.

Parkes, W. R. (1982) *Occupational Lung Disorders*. 2nd edn. London: Butterworths.

Pendergrass, E. P. (1958) Silicosis and a few of the other pneumoconioses: observations on certain aspects of the problem with emphasis on the role of the radiologist. The Caldwell Lecture 1957. *American Journal of Roentgenology*, **80**, 1–41

Rabinowitz, J. G., Efremidis, S. C., Cohen, B. et al. (1982) A comparative study of mesothelioma and asbestosis using computed tomography and conventional chest radiography. *Radiology*, **144**, 453–460.

Sander, O. A. (1976) The nonfibrogenic (benign) pneumoconioses. *Seminars in Roentgenology*, **2**, 312.

Sargent, E. N., Gordonson, J. S., Jacobson, G. (1977) Pleural plaques: a signpost of asbestos dust inhalation. *Seminars in Roentgenology*, **12**, 287–297.

CHAPTER 17

MISCELLANEOUS LUNG CONDITIONS

SARCOIDOSIS

Sarcoidosis is a multisystem disease sometimes preceded acutely by erythema nodosum or arthropathy. Although worldwide in distribution there are *racial differences* in incidence, natural history and radiographic patterns. These differences are most obvious between the Black and White races but there are also smaller variations within each group. The incidence in Black people is 12 times that in White, and the male/female ratio is 1:2 compared to 1:1 in White races. The influence of *genetic factors* is also apparent in the occasional clustering of familial cases, the excess in monozygotic compared to dizygotic twins and the fact that cases with the histocompatibility antigen HLA-B8 have less chance of developing progressive fibrosis. Genetic factors therefore can influence the natural history of the disease through the *immune response* which determines the outcome. The immune response in the lungs is distinct from the systemic immune response. The latter is reflected in a reduction in circulating lymphocytes and in T-cell proportions, an increase in gammaglobulin and anergy to tuberculin skin testing. In contrast, in the lungs there are increased proportions of lymphocytes and T-cells. The effects of the disease on function are those of impaired ventilation and alveolar gas diffusion.

There is no specific test for sarcoidosis and the diagnosis is based on a combination of symptoms, signs, histological appearances and radiographic abnormalities. Histologically there are epithelioid granulomas which do not caseate whatever size they reach. The granulomas are found in the nodes, alveolar walls and bronchial submucosa. Healing is by fibrosis which is progressive as long as the disease is active. The end result therefore lies on a scale varying from a normal chest radiograph to one with severe fibrotic lung disease. The histology is characteristic but not pathognomonic since it can be found in association with other lung diseases, particularly industrial berylliosis. Caution has to be exercised in the interpretation of biopsy material showing a sarcoid reaction as it may not be representative of the whole. The *Kveim test* is an intradermal inoculation of an extract of sarcoid tissue and if the resulting skin reaction has sarcoid histology the test is positive. Although useful, errors in the test can result from the use of a weak antigen or misinterpretation of the histology of the granuloma.

A test which would predict those cases of active pulmonary sarcoid likely to respond to steroids would be valuable. Gallium-67 uptake by the lungs, blood levels of angiotensin-converting enzyme and measurements of the cellularity of broncho-alveolar lavage fluid have all been assessed as markers of activity but without universal acceptance. Radiographic changes too do not correlate well with the inter-related triad of disease activity, functional abnormality and steroid responsiveness.

Radiological appearances. The radiographic abnormalities progress through 3 stages:

1. enlarged nodes only
2. enlarged nodes with pulmonary lesions
3. pulmonary lesions only.

The first stage is one of bilateral hilar node enlargement (Figs 17.1 and 17.2) and so characteristic is this pattern that the diagnosis is often regarded as established without recourse to biopsy. An accompanying enlargement of right paratracheal nodes is not uncommon but the diagnosis must be regarded as suspect if the nodes are solely paratracheal, if the anterior mediastinal nodes are enlarged or if the hilar involvement is unilateral. The latter may be more apparent than real and tomography may reveal contralateral nodes not appreciated on the chest radiograph. The nodes rarely calcify and do so only when there is associated pulmonary disease. Sarcoidosis is one of the causes of *egg shell calcification* of nodes.

Even in stage 1 a peripheral lung biopsy through the fibre-optic bronchoscope will show sarcoid granulomas but these are fewer in number and have less fibrosis than is found in overt pulmonary disease. Resolution of the node enlargement is the rule and recurrence is rare. There is a small group of cases in whom nodes persist for many years but even after such a long interval progression to pulmonary involvement can still occur. Progression to stage 2 occurs in from one half to two thirds of cases. If

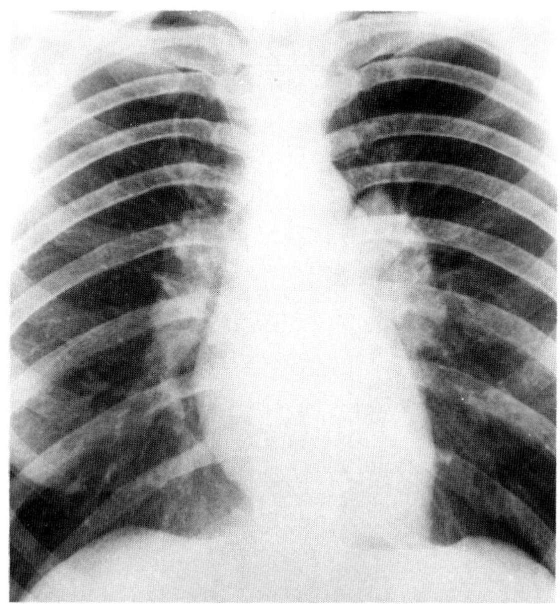

Fig. 17.1 Sarcoidosis. Bilateral hilar node enlargement.

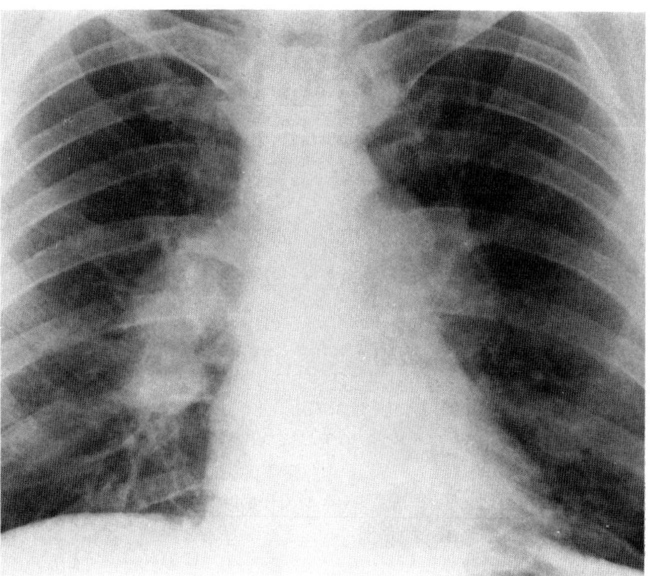

Fig. 17.2 Sarcoidosis. Hilar and tracheobronchial node enlargement. On the right the adenopathy extends to the segmental level of bronchial division.

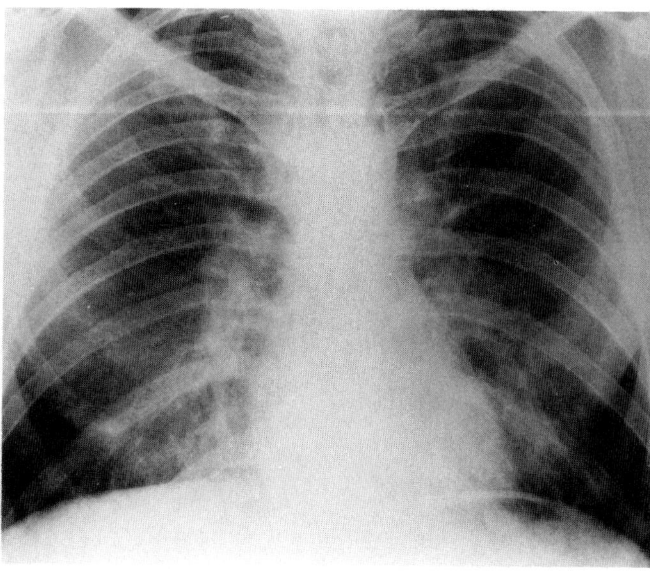

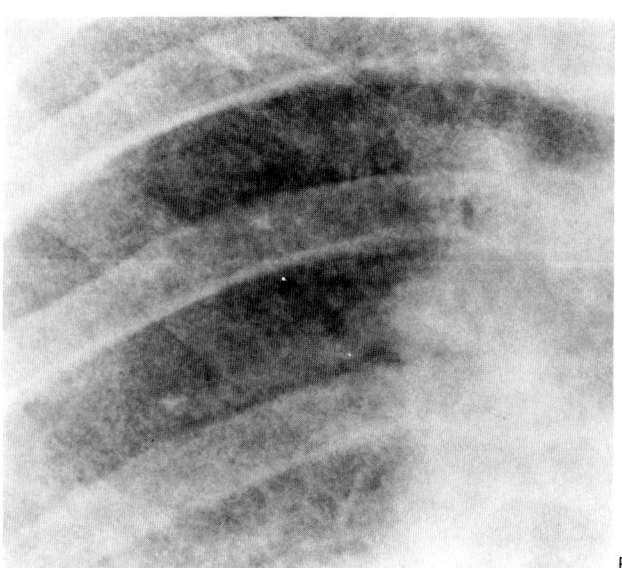

Fig. 17.3 (**A**) Sarcoidosis. Right hilar adenopathy and pulmonary disease. The latter is non-uniform. The vessels are obscured. (**B**) Close-up. Micronodulation giving a fine granular appearance.

lung disease is present on the initial chest radiograph 15–30% will develop progressive pulmonary fibrosis.

In stages 2 and 3 the pulmonary ('parenchymal') disease takes several forms, all bilateral and widespread; lobar localization is an exceptional presentation and this ultimately disseminates.

a. *small nodules*: a profuse but not uniform scattering of enormous numbers of 2–3 mm lesions fittingly described as miliary. They appear most profuse in the thicker lower parts of the lungs (Figs 17.3A and B). The overall effect may be a fine granularity or the discrete opacities may fuse into a hazy loss of translucency in which the vessels become obscured (Fig. 17.4).

b. *reticulation*: a network of fine lines or linearities radiating from the hila. There may be a few Kerley B lines from lymphatic seedlings (Fig. 17.5). The latter are not due to the effects of nodal obstruction causing lymphatic congestion; they always imply pulmonary disease.

c. *reticulo-nodular*: pure examples of nodular and reticular forms are less common than mixtures of the two (Fig. 17.6).

d. *large nodules*: these are of the order of 1 cm in diameter and the edges may be well or ill-defined (Fig. 17.7).

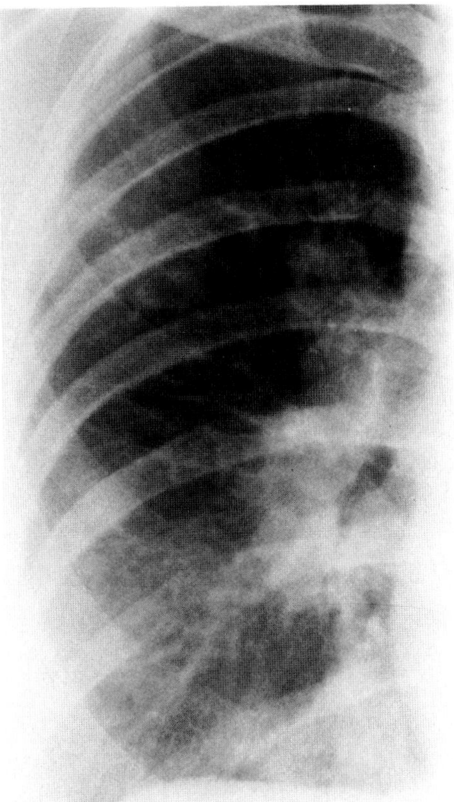

Fig. 17.4 Sarcoidosis. Hilar adenopathy. Haze or fine granularity in the lower zone and a few nodules in the upper. Vessels obscured.

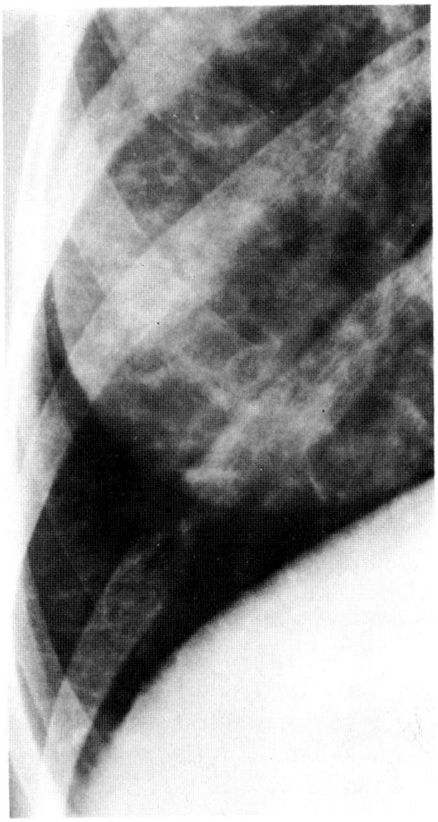

Fig. 17.5 Sarcoidosis. Basal septal lines. Reticulo-nodulation.

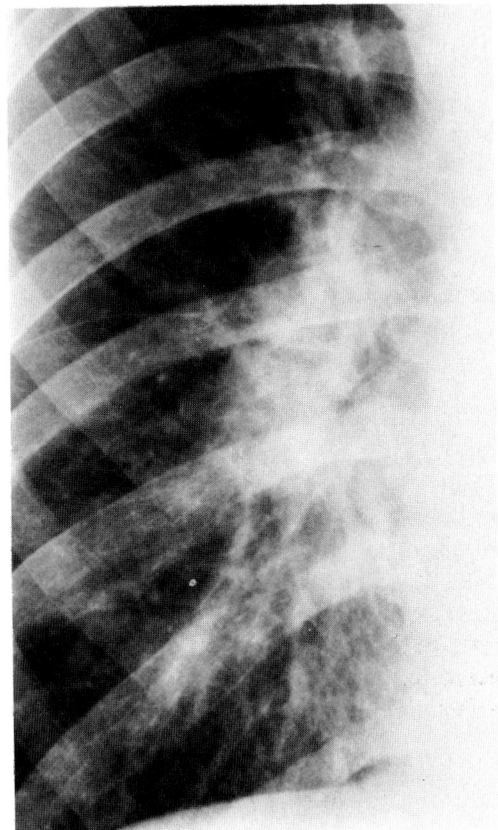

Fig. 17.6 Sarcoidosis. Hilar adenopathy and lines radiating from the hilum. Reticulo-nodulation.

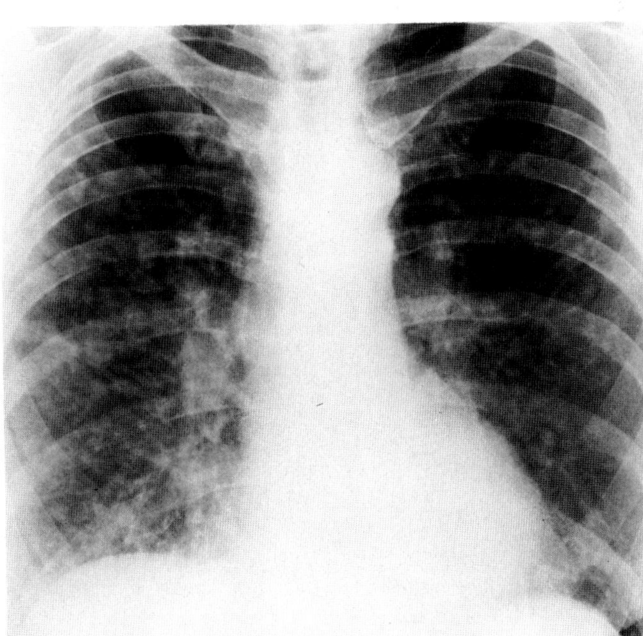

Fig. 17.7 Sarcoidosis. Larger nodules. No adenoapthy.

They may coalesce into larger opacities of segmental or lobar size and lesions such as these are prone to rapid change, either of deterioration or improvement. Ill-defined large nodules and conglomerate opacities are often described as acinar since air bronchograms may be visible within them but this is an artificial division. They encroach on, rather than grow within, the alveolar spaces. Discrete nodules of 2–3 cm size are very rarely seen in Great Britain but are found in the United States, usually in black people. Cavitation within these lesions is sometimes seen.

The pulmonary disease may regress and the chest radiograph revert to normal but it is capable of reactivation in the same areas as the original disease. Infection superimposed on sarcoid lung disease will add its own contribution to the overall radiographic appearances and it is one cause of cavitation.

e. *fibrosis*: the fibrotic sequelae lie on a scale from a few inconspicuous linear scars to a widespread interstitial fibrosis which may resemble fibrosing alveolitis. Like fibrosing alveolitis it can also lead to honeycombing, clusters of thin-walled air cysts 1 cm in diameter. Condensation and contraction of the fibrous tissue results in distortion of the pulmonary architecture, elevation of the hila, the formation of bullae and bronchiectasis (Fig. 17.8). This end-stage fibrotic disease is often predominantly apical in distribution despite the diffuse nature of the original sarcoid lesions. Bullae have thinner walls than true cavities but it is not always possible to differentiate between them (Fig. 17.9).

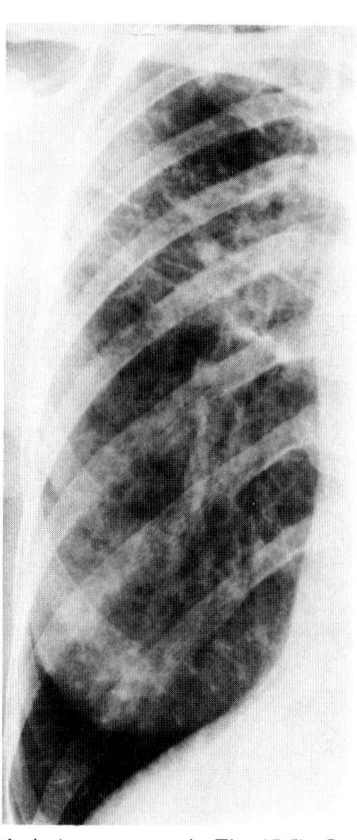

Fig. 17.8 Sarcoidosis (same case as in Fig. 17.5). Coarse reticulation. Elevation of the hilum by fibrotic contraction.

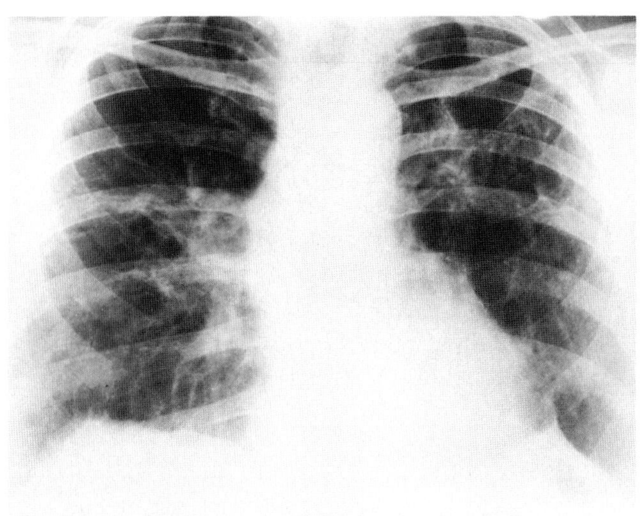

Fig. 17.9 Sarcoidosis. End-stage fibrotic disease. Apical bullae. Fibrotic contraction elevating left hilum.

Despite the fact that bronchial biopsy commonly reveals submucosal granulomas, bronchial stenosis is an unusual complication. When it occurs it is due to fibrotic strictures and not to compression by node masses or to an intraluminal granulomatous mass. It follows that stenosis is not always relieved by the resolution of hilar adenopathy.

It will usually be detected first on bronchoscopy but it requires bronchography to reveal the true extent and multiplicity of the stenoses. Atelectasis and bronchiectasis may follow the bronchial obstruction. There is a notable absence of significant pleural involvement in sarcoid pulmonary disease but pneumothorax can result from rupture of a bulla.

Necrotizing sarcoid granulomatosis is a pathological curiosity dissimilar in almost all respects from classical sarcoidosis. Discussion centres around whether it is a necrotizing angiitis with sarcoid reaction or sarcoidosis with necrosis of the granulomas and angiitis. It occupies a position between sarcoidosis and Wegener's granulomatosis. There is no other evidence of sarcoidosis such as lymphadenopathy or extrapulmonary lesions. The granulomas coalesce, necrose and occlude the lumens of bronchi and vessels. Lung architecture is destroyed. Lung distal to bronchial occlusion undergoes lipid consolidation. Although a miliary radiographic pattern has been reported the lesions are more often *solitary masses* or *large nodules* with a localized or unilateral distribution.

FIBROSING ALVEOLITIS

A widespread fibrosis involving the alveolar walls is variously called diffuse pulmonary fibrosis, diffuse interstitial fibrosis, Hamman-Rich disease or fibrosing alveolitis. As there is also a concomitant or preceding chronic inflammatory cellular infiltration the terms interstitial pneumonia or pneumonitis are also used.

There are a number of causes of alveolar injury which result in an exudation or cellular infiltration which then shows a strong tendency to progressive fibrosis. Included amongst the known causes are the inhalation of certain *industrial dusts*, *drugs*, *infections*, *radiation injury* and *oxygen toxicity*. In the end stages with severely fibrotic lungs and distorted bronchoalveolar architecture it may not be possible to trace the signs of the initiating injurious agent. In Great Britain the preferred terminology for this group of conditions is fibrosing alveolitis and if the cause is not known it is designated *cryptogenic*.

Cryptogenic fibrosing alveolitis

Although the cause is not known, and indeed there are likely to be many, the distinctive combination of symptoms, functional abnormalities, clinical signs, histology and radiographic appearances almost raise it to the status of a disease entity. The history is one of progressive exertional dyspnoea and cough with scanty sputum, finger clubbing, widespread crepitations, restricted ventilation and impaired gas exchange but little if any airways obstruction.

Histologically two patterns are recognized, one in which the cellular infiltration and fibrosis is limited to the alveolar walls, the other having additionally a filling of the alveolar spaces with mononuclear cells desquamated from the walls. They are labelled respectively *mural* (or usual interstitial pneumonitis — UIP) and *desquamative* (desquamative interstitial pneumonitis — DIP). Other distinguishing features are the variability of the histology with more intense fibrosis in the mural type whereas the desquamative has uniform histology with less fibrosis and is more responsive to steroid therapy which gives it a better prognosis. An area of dispute is whether the two types represent the two ends of a scale or are of different pathogenesis.

Progressive fibrosis leads to contraction of lung substance and destruction of architecture. Dilatation of bronchioles accounts for honeycombing. Typically there is predominant involvement of the basal parts of the lungs with a tendency to spread upwards as the disease progresses. An overgrowth of smooth muscle in the alveolar walls and interstitial tissues may be striking but is a non-specific feature of a number of fibrotic and chronic inflammatory conditions.

The course of the disease varies from a devastating progression with death in a few weeks to an indolent process spanning many years. Death is usually due to respiratory or cardiac failure. Desquamative histology has a better prognosis but it can hardly be called benign with a reported mortality of 27% and a mean survival of 12 years. Carcinoma of lung of all histological types, including the bronchioloalveolar cell, complicates the disease process in about 10% of cases.

There is no doubt that immune mechanisms play a decisive role. In over 50% of cases rheumatoid factor, nuclear, mitochondrial or smooth muscle antibodies are found in the blood and immune complexes in the blood and lungs. Immune complexes formed from antigen/antibody combination are deposited in alveolar walls and capillaries where they set in train a sequence of reactions which are locally damaging. They are found most often with a cellular histology, diminishing or disappearing in the predominantly fibrotic disease.

Diseases having an association with cryptogenic fibrosing alveolitis are generally those with an *auto-immune* pathogenesis, the connective tissue disorders rheumatoid, systemic lupus, systemic sclerosis and dermatomyositis/polymyositis being the most frequent. Other associates are Sjogren's disease, Hashimoto's thyroiditis, auto-immune haemolytic anaemia and idiopathic thrombocytopenic purpura. Cases with neurofibromatosis and an occasional familial incidence point to a possible genetic predisposition. The mural and desquamative forms do not differ in the variety of disease associates.

Radiological appearances. Characteristically the radiographic signs are basal in distribution. In the early stages the chest radiograph may be normal but some apparently normal films when reviewed later will be seen to have a subtle shadowing, not surprisingly misinterpreted as underexposure or breast shadows. *Computed tomography* shows abnormalities at an earlier stage than chest radiography. The minimal change is a triangle of ground-glass haze at the bases, more easily appreciated on the right side where it fills the cardiophrenic angle. Although bilateral it may be unequal on the two sides. The haze partially obscures pulmonary vessels and it is neither distinctly alveolar nor interstitial. With progression the changes spread upwards and out into the costophrenic angles.

Three other types of opacity may then be added to the basic pattern:

1. ill-defined and patchy
2. small (2 mm) discrete miliary (Fig. 17.10)
3. profuse, small but of irregular outline.

The latter is a reticulation and the small shadows are probably superimposition of intersecting lines (Fig. 17.11).

It might be expected that a desquamative histology would have an alveolar pattern. It has been suggested that the ill-defined patchy opacities are the radiographic counterpart of desquamative histology and miliary nodules that of the mural. However true this may be in isolated cases it is generally agreed that radiographic appearances are not a reliable discriminator of histological type in the early stages.

The subtle and fine early radiographic opacities become coarser with progression of the fibrosis. Thicker lines and

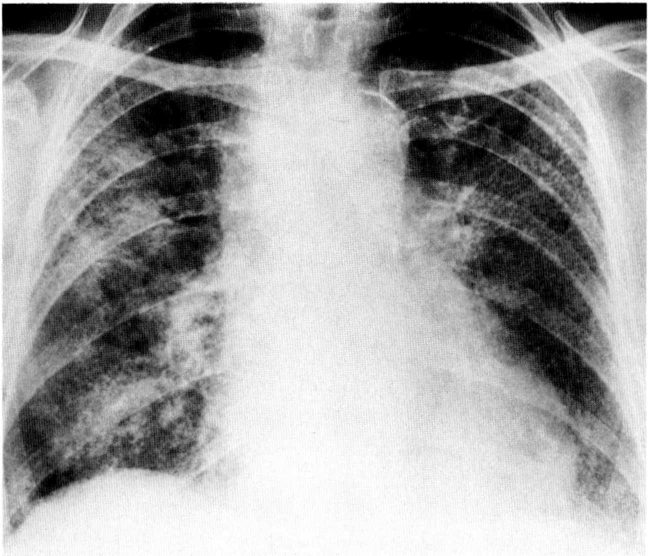

Fig. 17.10 Cryptogenic fibrosing alveolitis. Miliary opacities and a little reticulation. The apices are spared.

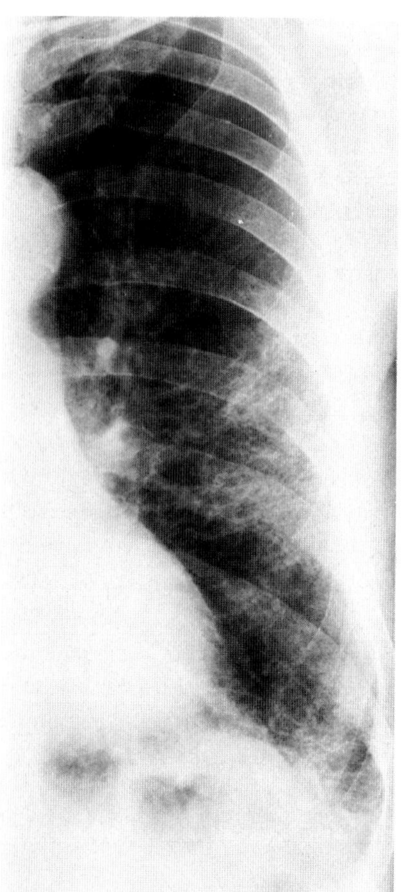

Fig. 17.11 Cryptogenic fibrosing alveolitis. Fine reticulation predominantly peripheral and sparing the apices.

denser opacities appear as the lungs shrink. Since it is the gas exchanging parts which are the site of the disease the condensation and hence the dense opacities are in the surface 'cortex' of the lungs. This is more apparent in tomographic sections than in the chest radiograph. The densities represent large volumes of condensed lung. The diaphragms rise from under-expansion of the bases.

Honeycombing is a manifestation of late stage interstitial fibrosis (Fig. 17.12). It is exceptional in the desquamative type. Hilar and mediastinal node enlargement and pleural effusions are rare. Cor pulmonale, pulmonary embolism and infections are complications which contribute to the radiographic signs.

Although bronchography is not required for primary diagnosis, the appearances are characteristic. Should it be performed for other reasons the bronchi fill right out to the pleural surface, another reflection of the condensation of alveolar spaces.

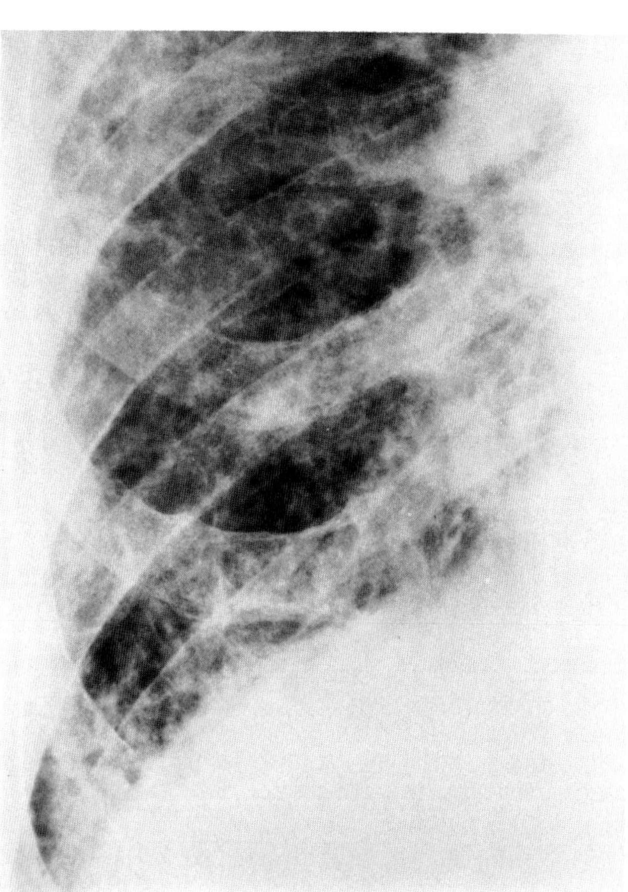

Fig. 17.12 Cryptogenic fibrosing alveolitis. Honeycombing and conglomerate fibrosis.

EXTRINSIC ALLERGIC ALVEOLITIS
(Hypersensitivity pneumonitis)

Inhaled particles of less than 10 μm size are capable of reaching the alveoli where their potential for causing damage to the gas exchanging parts of the lungs is considerable. If the particles are antigenic and the lung previously sensitized a hypersensitivity reaction ensues. Antibodies are meant to neutralize potentially harmful foreign material but sometimes the combination of antigen and antibody is itself damaging and constitutes a disease process. Extrinsic allergic alveolitis is a syndrome caused by the inhalation of dusts containing certain organisms or proteins. In *farmer's lung* the offending organism is usually *Micropolyspora faeni* from damp, mouldy hay. *Pigeon breeders* inhale dust from the dessicated droppings containing bird serum protein or from the feathers. *Mushroom growers* are affected by fungal spores from the compost used. *Air conditioning systems* may circulate fungal spores and amoebae. A similar reaction in the lungs may be induced by *drugs*, in this case blood borne, the most common examples being nitrofurantoin and salazopyrine.

Precipitating antibodies directed specifically against the antigen are found in the serum of patients but their presence only implies exposure, not necessarily disease. Some 40% of pigeon breeders have precipitins but few suffer from the disease. However the presence of precipitins to extracts of budgerigar excreta in those exposed is stronger evidence in favour of disease. The immunological reactions are predominantly type III, that is, free circulating antigen and antibody combine in the presence of complement to form complexes which are deposited in the alveolar walls. Activation of complement sets in train a sequence or reactions liberating a variety of damaging substances. The reaction is intermediate in time scale which corresponds well with the clinical presentation. Type IV reactions also play a part and here the antibody is produced and transported by lymphocytes which then aggregate at the site where the reaction takes place. The *granuloma*, a characteristic feature of type IV reactions, is the fundamental histological lesion of extrinsic allergic alveolitis.

Acute symptoms characteristically begin some six hours after exposure. The patient experiences an influenza-like illness of malaise, headache, fever, cough and dyspnoea. If the dose of antigen is small and frequently repeated acute symptoms may be absent and the presentation is then one of an insidiously progressive dyspnoea. This is a common mode of presentation of disease from budgerigars. Monday morning fever occurs in office workers in an air conditioned environment and is traceable to contamination of humidifiers.

On auscultation there are usually inspiratory crepitations but finger clubbing is rare. Lung function tests show restricted ventilation and impaired gas transfer but little airways obstruction. The best test is a bronchial challenge by the inhalation of the allergen to reproduce the symptoms and functional abnormalities. It is now rarely used but it was instrumental initially in establishing the pathogenesis of the disease.

Treatment is by removal from exposure or if that is not possible reduction of contact to a minimum. Steroids are of doubtful value. In only 50–60% of patients does the lung function return to normal and some continue to deteriorate after elimination of exposure.

The pathological lesions are *alveolar wall granulomas*, aggregates of normal constituent cells of granulation tissue — histiocytes, lymphocytes, fibroblasts, giant cells. They are widely but patchily distributed throughout the lungs, some areas being normal. After repeated attacks the acute changes give place to alveolar wall and peribronchial *fibrosis*, the granulomas then disappearing. Intra-alveolar exudate is not striking in biopsy specimens but radiographic signs of transient alveolar opacification occur in acute attacks. Bronchiolitis obliterans is common and found in 40% of specimens from farmer's lung. The pathology is similar whatever the aetiology but occasionally it is possible to identify a specific characteristic such as the fungus which causes maple bark stripper's disease or vegetable fibres in bagassosis (in cane sugar workers). In the late stages there are extensive areas of dense fibrosis representing large volumes of contracted lung in which alveolar architecture can no longer be recognized. *Honeycombing* or larger air spaces arising from dilatation of small airways or from destruction of alveolar walls then appear. These chronic changes are almost always in the upper parts of the lungs and are predominantly sub-pleural.

Radiological appearances. The chest radiograph may be initially normal but as in cryptogenic fibrosing alveolitis early changes may escape detection unless a high index of suspicion is cultivated. The minimal change consists of a widespread small nodulation with individual nodules 2 mm in diameter and having ill-defined edges in contrast to the sharp definition of lesions of similar size in miliary tubercu-

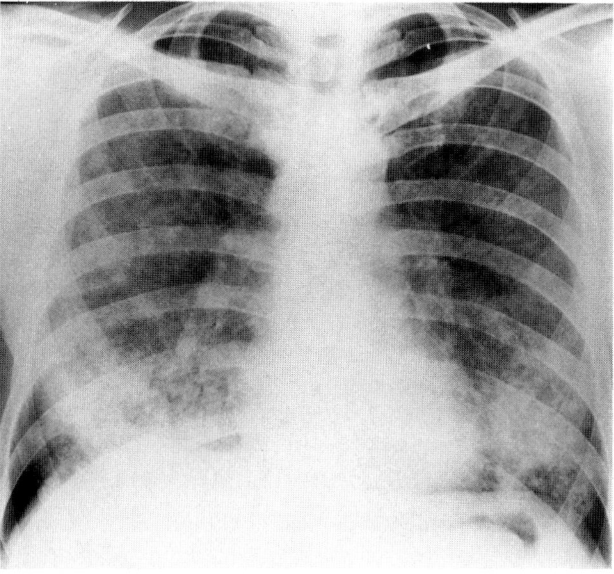

Fig. 17.13 Farmer's lung. Patchy alveolar opacification superimposed on a miliary nodulation. The costophrenic angles are clear.

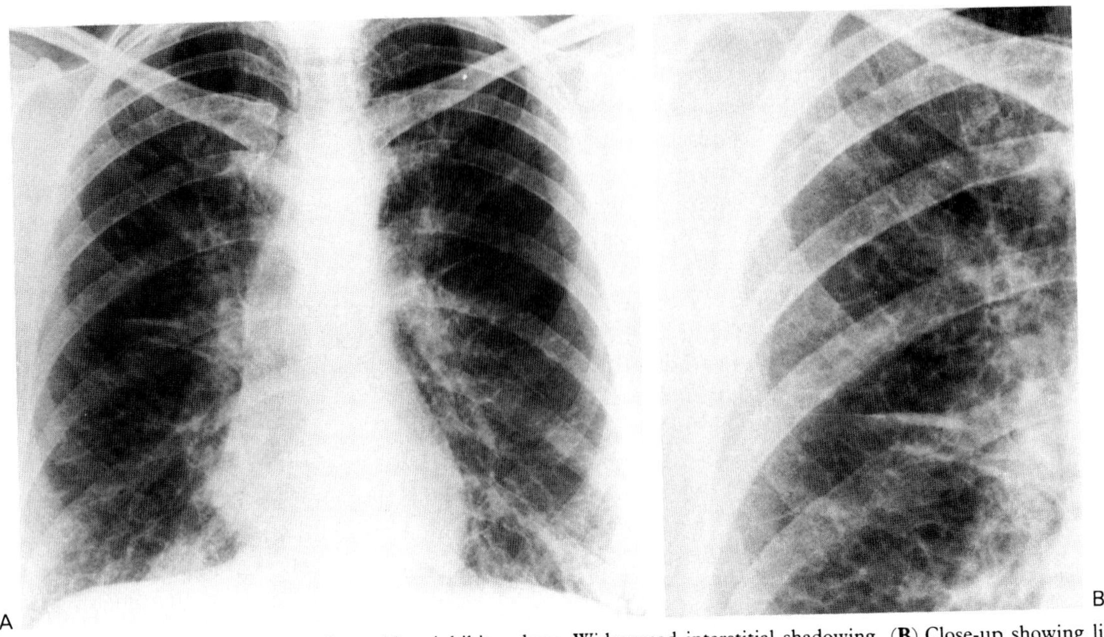

Fig. 17.14 (**A**) Allergic alveolitis due to monoamine oxidase inhibitor drug. Widespread interstitial shadowing. (**B**) Close-up showing lines from congested lymphatics. Complete resolution within 7 days.

losis (Fig. 17.13). Although widespread they may be more profuse in certain areas and typically the costophrenic angles are clear. All other radiographic changes are superimposed on this basic pattern. Patchy, ill-defined transient shadows described as 'clouding', 'mottling' or 'haze' are found in the early stages and probably represent alveolar filling during acute exacerbations. Septal lines are not uncommon (Figs 17.14A and B). The chronic stage is marked by the appearance of large dense opacities due to contraction and condensation almost always in the upper parts of the lungs. Cystic air spaces are due to bullae, bronchiectatic cavities and bronchiolar dilatations. A band of density which may be seen along the lateral chest wall, and graphically described as a 'white wall', is a condensation of subpleural alveolar spaces. Notably absent are pleural effusion, node enlargement and calcification. The sequence of radiographic changes from a diffuse abnormality to a progressive upper lobe fibrosis is highly characteristic.

Upper lobe fibrosis is a common end stage of a number of disparate diseases including extrinsic allergic alveolitis, cryptogenic fibrosing alveolitis, tuberculosis, bronchopulmonary aspergillosis, ankylosing spondylitis and many others. At this stage the natural history is the only means of differentiating between them.

PULMONARY EOSINOPHILIC CONDITIONS

Pulmonary eosinophilia is defined as the presence of transient radiographic opacities which contain eosinophils together with a blood eosinophilia. However, it is useful to consider with pulmonary eosinophilia a broader group of allied conditions some of which fall outside the simple definition.

In this broader group the brunt of the changes may fall on the peripheral pulmonary tissues or on the bronchial tree. The pulmonary element is an eosinophilic exudate and an alveolar wall granulomatous infiltration, either focal or diffuse. There is a tendency for recurrent acute attacks to lead to fibrosis.

The bronchial element consists of mucosal oedema and infiltration by eosinophils and the functional effects are more impressive than the radiological. There is smooth muscle spasm, reversible airways obstruction and the secretion of tenacious mucus. The sputum is eosinophilic and contains plugs or casts of the bronchi. There are secondary effects from infection and obstructive collapse, namely bronchiectasis and peri-bronchial fibrosis.

ASTHMA

Asthma is a state of bronchial hyper-reactivity. Stimuli ineffective in normal people produce bronchial constriction in asthmatics.

Extrinsic asthma is believed to follow inhalation of particles commonly found in the environment such as pollens, house dust and animal danders, to which the patient is allergic. The immunological response is type 1 characterized by an immediate weal on skin testing with allergens, histamine release from mast cells and attraction of eosinophils to sites of antigen/antibody reaction. The onset is in childhood and there are usually other allergic hypersensitivities such as hay fever and eczema. They have positive kin tests to a number of common allergens. These are all eatures of atopy.

Intrinsic asthma has a later onset and these patients are not atopic, the usual skin tests being negative. The onset sometimes follows a respiratory infection.

The state of heightened bronchial reactivity is also reflected in the fact that asthma may sometimes be provoked or made worse by exercise or respiratory infections. Eosinophilia in the blood is intermittent.

Radiological appearances. The chest radiograph in uncomplicated asthma is unremarkable and usually normal. During attacks the lungs are over-expanded and in severe chronic asthma this may persist. Signs of over-expansion are low diaphragms and a lung height greater than combined lung width, a reversal of normal. Bronchial wall and peribronchial thickening shows as parallel lines and once this makes its appearance it is often permanent.

Lobar or segmental collapse results from a combination of bronchial mucosal swelling and mucous plugging; rapid re-expansion is the rule. Patchy, ill-defined opacities, sometimes widespread, appear transiently but in the absence of histological verification it is not known how often these are due to eosinophilic consolidation or how often to collapse. Septal lines are sometimes seen. Rupture of alveoli results in pulmonary interstitial emphysema, mediastinal emphysema and pneumothorax.

The inter-relationship of asthma, pulmonary eosinophilia and aspergillosis are dealt with elsewhere (Ch. 15). Pulmonary eosinophilia can occur in *drug hypersensitivity* (aspirin, nitrofurantoin), after exposure to *industrial chemicals* (epoxy resins), during *parasitic infections* (Ch. 15) or the cause may be unknown.

CHRONIC EOSINOPHIL PNEUMONIA

Also known as *prolonged pulmonary eosinophilia*, the diagnosis of this unusual condition rarely presents a problem because of the highly characteristic constellation of symptoms and radiographic signs together with the blood eosinophilia, which may however be intermittent. Symptoms are often severe with fever, drenching sweats, loss of weight, dyspnoea and cough. There is a history of asthma or other atopic conditions in only one third of patients. It has been reported in identical twins. There is ventilatory restriction and impaired gas exchange with little if any airways obstruction.

Pathologically there is an alveolar exudate of eosinophils and macrophages but only mild alveolar wall infiltration. Ulcerative bronchiolitis obliterans is found in one third.

Radiological appearances. The radiographic signs have been described as pulmonary oedema in reverse, that is, ill-defined, non-segmental alveolar opacities in the peripheral parts of the lungs. This is the most distinctive pattern but central opacities are also found. They are unevenly distributed and the densities are not homogenous. Their sub-pleural position may mimic a loculated effusion but true effusions are rare. Another distinctive and almost diagnostic sign is a vertical band of shadowing roughly parallel to the chest wall but separated from it and apparently bearing no relationship to pleura, fissures, or hilum (Fig. 17.15). It is a band of sub-pleural alveolar opacification and there are two possible explanations: 1) the band is *en face* and not tangential to the X-ray beam; 2) a wide border of opaque lung clears from the periphery leaving a translucent strip between the pleura and lung still affected. It is seen most often in the stages of resolution and may recur in exacerbations of the disease.

Treatment with steroids is rapidly effective and total radiographic clearing may take no more than two or three days. Fibrotic scars are few and inconspicuous. Pulmonary function returns to normal with radiographic clearing. Relapse of symptoms and radiographic signs frequently follows reduction or withdrawal of steroids and the opacities may return in precisely the same sites, with or without the addition of fresh lesions elsewhere. They respond to the re-institution of steroids in full doses. Recurrent disease has been reported over a period of 26 years.

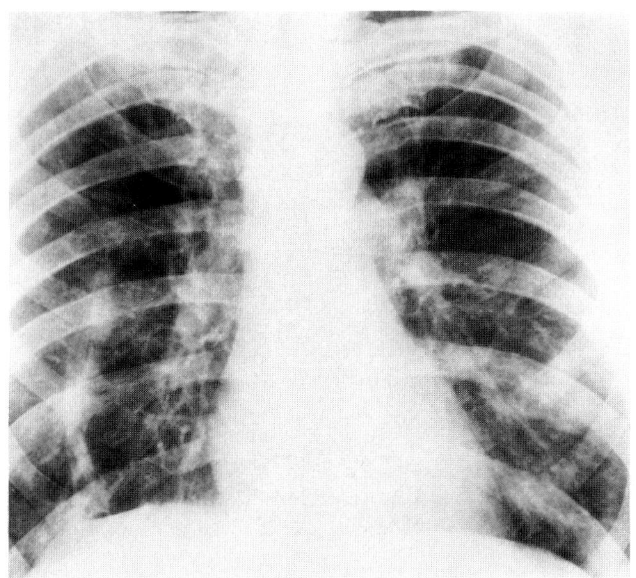

Fig. 17.15 Chronic eosinophil pneumonia. Alveolar opacities distributed peripherally. The vertical band in the right lung is characteristic.

EOSINOPHIL GRANULOMA

Eosinophil granuloma is a disease of unknown aetiology conventionally grouped with Hand–Schüller–Christian and Letterer–Siwe's diseases as histiocytosis-X disease. The pathology of eosinophil granuloma and Hand–Schüller–Christian disease is the same, the difference lying in the multi-organ distribution of the latter, especially in the cranium. Eosinophil granuloma of the lungs may or may not be associated with bone or soft tissue lesions. Isolated lung disease has a male preponderance of 5 to 1 and generally pursues a benign course which remits either spontaneously or as a result of treatment. There is no association with atopy or allergy and there is no blood eosinophilia.

There is a diffuse infiltration of alveolar walls with histiocytic granulomas, unusual in the numbers of eosinophils which they contain. The presence of Langerhans cells with granules is regarded as specific. The lesions are eventually replaced by fibrous tissue. Polypoid granulomatous lesions are also found in the bronchi.

Radiological appearances. The chest radiograph shows a fine, diffuse reticulation and sharply defined nodules 2–3 mm in size most obvious at the bases but sparing the costophrenic angles. As the lesions mature the nodules recede and the reticulation becomes more pronounced (Fig. 17.16A). An alveolar haze resembling pulmonary oedema may be seen as a transient exudative phenomenon. Honeycombing and bulla formation result from the fibrosis and the hair-line walls of these air spaces are particularly clearly seen because there are no dense fibrotic masses and the lungs are consequently well expanded (Fig. 17.16B). Bullous cysts may become very large. Pneumothorax occurs at some time in 25%. Node enlargement and pleural effusions are rare.

PULMONARY HAEMORRHAGE AND HAEMOSIDEROSIS

Under this heading will be considered those states where there is multifocal bleeding at acinar level, that is distal to the terminal bronchioles, but excluding those with a known bleeding state such as leukaemia, anticoagulation or diffuse intravascular coagulation. Haemoptysis is a common symptom but its severity does not match the large volumes of blood lost into the lungs since most of it is beyond the mucociliary clearing processes. Bleeding is severe enough to cause anaemia even at times requiring blood transfusion. Macrophages with engulfed red cells and haemosiderin fill the alveolar spaces and infiltrate the walls. These macrophages in sputum or bronchoalveolar lavage fluid are a diagnostic feature. After repeated attacks of bleeding, interstitial fibrosis is initiated but this is not sufficiently extensive to cause gross scarring or destruction of lung architecture.

A convenient classification of pulmonary haemosiderosis divides it into 5 types:

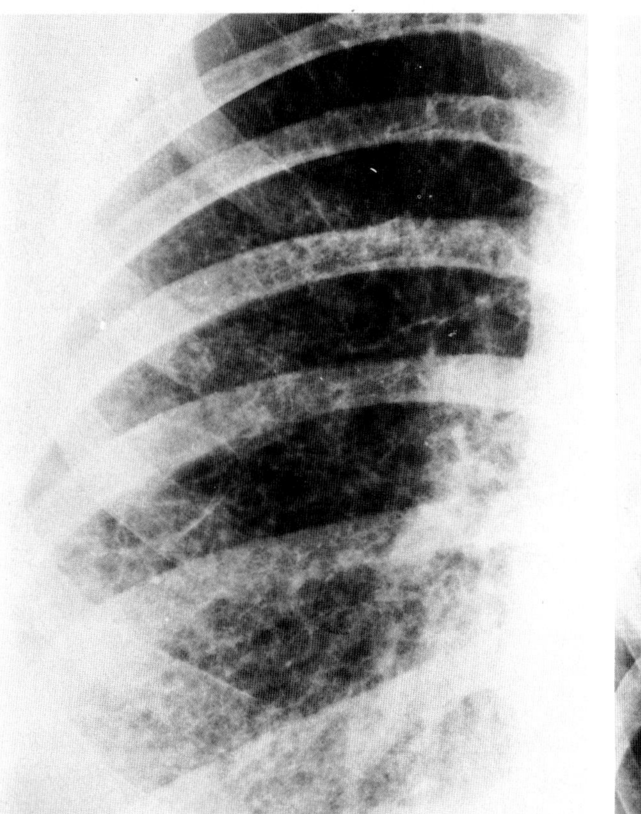

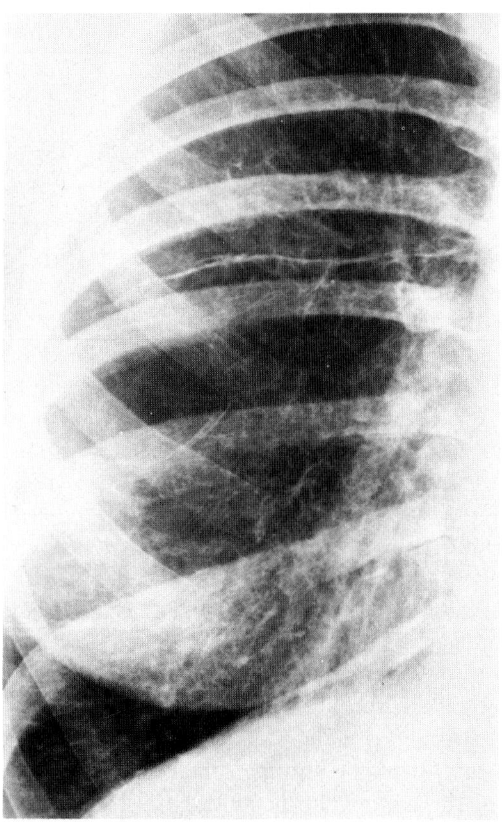

Fig. 17.16 (**A**) Eosinophil granuloma. Reticulo-nodulation. The nodulation is receding. Honeycombing and commencing bulla formation. (**B**) Later stage. The bulla has enlarged. Fine hair-line walls of other bullae visible.

1. Idiopathic
2. Associated with renal disease
3. Due to drugs (Penicillamine) or industrial chemicals (hydrocarbon fumes)
4. Part of a widespread vasculitis (Wegener's granulomatosis)
5. Miscellaneous

Idiopathic pulmonary haemosiderosis is predominantly a disease of childhood in which there are repeated episodes of haemorrhage sometimes accompanied by constitutional upset. The lungs return to normal between attacks but if these are frequently repeated permanent fibrotic changes eventually follow. The disease may remit spontaneously. The kidneys are not involved.

Pulmonary haemosiderosis with renal disease. Three sub-groups can be identified on the basis of the renal histology:

a. anti-glomerular basement membrane (GBM) antibody disease
b. immune complex renal disease
c. glomerulonephritis without either of the above.

The name *Goodpasture syndrome* should be reserved for those cases with GBM antibody. Immunofluorescence microscopy shows a linear deposit of the immunoglobulin on the glomerular capillaries sometimes with similar deposits on the alveolar capillaries. In contrast, immune complex deposits in the glomeruli are lumpy or granular. Damage to basement membranes by these deposits allows leakage to take place.

Infection, fluid overload and inhalation of toxic fumes are factors which are known to precipitate episodes of bleeding. Pulmonary function tests often indicate airways obstruction and there may be an increased uptake of *inhaled radioactive CO* by the leaked blood. The latter test is useful in differentiating haemorrhage from oedema and infection.

Treatment regimes include steroids, immunosuppression and plasmaphoresis and these are more effective in Goodpasture's syndrome than in the other types.

Miscellaneous conditions. Included in this group of pulmonary haemosiderosis are cases of heart disease which chronically elevate left atrial pressure, notably mitral stenosis. The radiographic features in the lungs are distinctive, consisting of a permanent miliary stippling from the focal nature of the bleeding.

With the exception of cardiogenic haemosiderosis noted above, the radiographic appearances of the other types are indistinguishable. Typically there are fleeting, migratory opacities with ill-defined margins, individually like pulmonary oedema (Fig. 17.17). At the edges of large confluent opacities ill-defined nodules of acinar size (6 mm) may be seen. An air bronchogram is occasionally visible within the opacities. These are characteristics of an alveolar filling process or consolidation. In severe cases both lungs can be almost totally opacified but conversely the chest radiograph may be normal in an acute attack, the decisive factor is the volume of blood lost. As the opacities resolve reticulation may become evident transiently, but a permanent reticular pattern is indicative of the evolution of interstitial fibrosis. Fibrosis only occurs after repeated episodes, usually resolution is rapid and complete. Differentiation from pulmonary infection can be difficult especially as infection is one of the precipitating factors of haemorrhage but clues to its presence are opacities which reach the apices or costo-phrenic angles, opacities limited by interlobar fissures and loss of mediastinal silhouettes. The presence of septal lines indicates fluid overload.

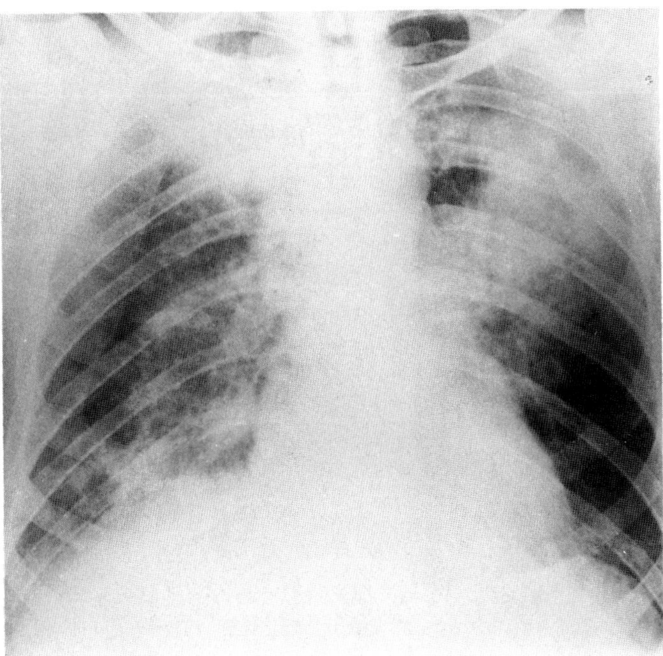

Fig. 17.17 Pulmonary haemorrhage. Goodpasture syndrome. Large alveolar opacities.

GRANULOMATOSIS WITH ANGIITIS AND LYMPHOPROLIFERATIVE DISORDERS

Wegener's granulomatosis, lymphomatoid granulomatosis and bronchocentric granulomatosis are conditions in which pulmonary angiitis is a central pathological component. These overlap with certain lymphoproliferative disorders which in turn merge with the lymphomas. Indeed, it has been suggested that some of the diseases in this group, particularly lymphomatoid granulomatosis, lymphoid interstitial pneumonia and pseudolymphoma, are in reality unusual forms of lymphoma.

WEGENER'S GRANULOMATOSIS

The essential component of Wegener's granulomatosis is

a necrotizing vasculitis, the lungs being involved as part of a widespread disease. A focal glomerulonephritis is part of the classical disease and is the most important determinant of prognosis. By *limited Wegener's granulomatosis* is meant a disease predominantly but not exclusively intrathoracic and in this form renal lesions, when present, are focal and granulomatous, not glomerulonephritic.

Symptoms referable to the upper air passages are almost always present at some time in the course of the disease, nasal obstruction, purulent discharge, sinusitis, chronic ulceration, even in some cases necrosis of nasal cartilage and bone. Cough, haemoptysis and pleurisy are usually accompanied by constitutional symptoms of malaise, weakness and fever. Rheumatoid and antinuclear factors are commonly found in the blood. Untreated the disease has a poor prognosis with an average survival of 5 months but steroids and Cyclophosphamide have transformed the outlook.

Lesions occur in any part of the respiratory tract and take the form of inflammatory necrosis in the walls of small arteries and veins leading to occlusion of the lumen. Granulation tissue containing lymphocytes, polymorphs and giant cells represents a reparative process but this also undergoes necrosis. The necrotic granulation tissue forms rubbery pulmonary masses which have a propensity to cavitate. Sometimes there is a profusion of miliary lesions. Ulceration of bronchial mucosa can result in airway narrowing and lobar collapse.

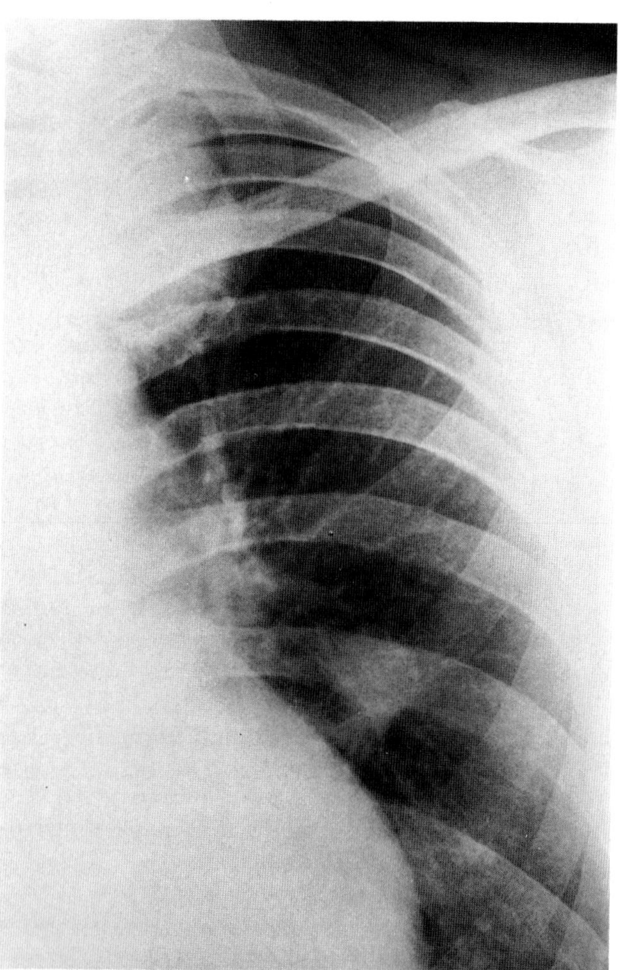

Fig. 17.18 Limited Wegener's granulomatosis. Circumscribed mass at left apex; small lesion in lingula. The large mass contained pus-like material.

Radiological appearances. Single or multiple, well-defined, round or oval pulmonary masses 1–5 cm in diameter are typical radiographic presentations (Fig. 17.18). A lobar consolidation results if the lesions extend up to the pleural fissures. Cavitating lesions may have thick or thin walls depending on how much of the necrotic material is expectorated. Multiple cavities can closely mimic tuberculosis.

A variation is a diffuse disease where the area of involved lung is still aerated but contains vaguely reticular or irregular nodular opacities.

Reactive hilar or mediastinal node enlargement can be mistaken for carcinoma especially if associated with a wedge of pulmonary consolidation or a lobe collapsed from endobronchial disease.

The lesions are not static, new ones appearing at the same time as others are resolving leaving linear scars. Relapse may occur in previously affected areas. Other frequent radiographic signs are small pleural effusions and paranasal sinus opacification. Occasional complications are pneumothorax and sub-glottic stenosis. Calcification is notably absent from the lesions.

Non-healing granuloma although of similar pathology is a separate condition characterized by gross destruction of the facial structures and responding poorly to treatment which would normally be effective in Wegener's granulomatosis. The lungs and kidneys are not involved.

LYMPHOMATOID GRANULOMATOSIS

This is a lymphoproliferative disorder with angiitis pathologically intermediate between Wegener's granulomatosis and lymphoma. Men are affected twice as frequently as women. The pulmonary disease has no distinctive clinical features but the combination with neurological symptoms and maculopapular skin lesions is suggestive of the diagnosis. Involvement of the central nervous system or peripheral nerves is found in up to one third of cases.

There are destructive lesions centred on vessels surrounded by lymphoid infiltration and granulation tissue. Neighbouring bronchioles suffer damage to their walls and obliteration of the lumen. Almost half of the patients have lesions with the same histology in the kidneys and other organs.

Radiological appearances. Bilateral pulmonary consolidations with ill-defined margins are the early signs. They have a predominantly peripheral distribution sparing the apices. With evolution the opacities become more discrete and resemble metastases. They can change rapidly, waxing and waning simultaneously in different areas. There is cavitation in 30%. In a few cases the pattern is diffuse reticulo-nodular or interstitial. Only a minority resolve, with or without residual scarring and in general the disease has a high mortality from pulmonary insufficiency, haemorrhage, secondary infection or central nervous system involvement. Hilar and mediastinal node enlargement does not occur except in the event of evolution to lymphoma which happens in approximately 10% of cases.

BRONCHOCENTRIC GRANULOMATOSIS

Bronchocentric granulomatosis is destructive, and causes granulomatous inflammation of bronchi and bronchioles. Patchily distributed shallow ulcerations of the mucosa are followed by penetration of the wall leading to destruction of cartilage in the larger bronchi. Bronchial walls are thickened and the lumen filled with masses of cheesy necrotic material. The process spreads outwards into lung tissue where the histology becomes that of an obstructive lipid pneumonia and an interstitial fibrosis. Pulmonary arteries and veins are involved incidentally by incorporation in the spreading inflammation, their lumens undergoing obliteration. There is no extrapulmonary involvement.

The disease has an equal sex incidence and the symptoms are those of chronic or recurrent pneumonia with airways obstruction. It is thought to be due to hypersensitivity to *aspergillus*. Some are asthmatics and the impacting bronchial material is then eosinophilic, otherwise it is polymorphonuclear. Steroid therapy is usually effective.

Radiological appearances. Typical radiographic presentations are a mass, a lobar consolidation or atelectasis. The opacities are frequently bilateral and migratory with the lung apex a favourite site. Less frequent presentations are small nodules or diffuse reticulo-nodulation. Reactive hilar node enlargement has been reported but is unusual.

LYMPHOID INTERSTITIAL PNEUMONIA
(*Pneumonitis*)

Areas of lung are diffusely infiltrated with mature lymphocytes within alveolar walls and in the interstitium. There is no node involvement. In places the infiltrate may form larger, round aggregates. It is a disease of slow evolution with a variable outcome, resolution, interstitial fibrosis or malignant lymphoma and it carries a 50% mortality. Frequently there is a disorder of immune globulins indicated by its association with Sjögren's syndrome, Hashimoto's thyroiditis, amyloidosis and by the presence of rheumatoid and antinuclear factors.

Radiological appearances. Radiographic reticulation is the counterpart of the interstitial histology, usually bilateral and basal, proceeding to honeycombing in those which fibrose. Added to this are coarse confluent shadows with air bronchograms suggestive of alveolar filling. This is an example of an interstitial process which, when sufficiently extensive, obliterates lung architecture and takes on the characteristics of an alveolar consolidation. There is no node or pleural involvement.

IMMUNOBLASTIC LYMPHADENOPATHY

As a cause of generalized lymphadenopathy this lies between a hyperimmune state and neoplasia. Within the enlarged nodes there is a proliferation of several types of cell but predominantly of lymphocytes and including immunoblasts containing immunoglobulins. There is also a proliferation of small blood vessels which accounts for its alternative name, angioimmunoblastic lymphadenopathy. Other features of the disorder are hepatosplenomegaly, haemolytic anaemia, polyclonal hypergammaglobulinaemia, maculopapular skin rashes and cutaneous anergy.

Radiological appearances. In the thorax the hilar and paratracheal nodes are enlarged, sometimes recurrently during the course of the disease. Pulmonary involvement is usually the result of infection and takes the form of coarse basal reticulation sometimes with an alveolar or nodular component. However, cases have been reported in which the pulmonary lesions had the same histology as the nodes. Spontaneous remission takes place in one third, but the disease is fatal in the other two thirds, from infection or renal and hepatic failure. A minority evolve into a malignant lymphoma.

SJÖGREN'S SYNDROME

Syndrome is an appropriate terminology for the constellation of signs making up this aetiologically heterogenous condition. Sjögren's syndrome is defined as dry mouth and dry eyes due to reduced exocrine gland secretions *plus* one of a number of connective tissue disorders. If the latter is missing it is called the *sicca syndrome*. Women are more often affected than men. The salivary, lachrymal and mucous glands of the mouth, nose, eyelids, pharynx, bronchial tree and stomach may all be the site of the pathological changes which consist of a massive lymphoid infiltration with eventual atrophy of the gland acini. There are minor salivary glands in the lip and this is the easiest site for a diagnostic biopsy. Although sarcoidosis may involve the salivary glands with the same functional effects it is by convention excluded from the definition of Sjögren's and sicca syndromes.

The frequency of pulmonary abnormalities has varied between 10 and 30% in different series. There are several pathogenic pathways.

1. *Infection*: reduced secretions with an increased

viscosity lowers the resistance of the air passages to infection. Recurrent pulmonary infections are common events and can lead to bronchiectasis.

2. *Direct pulmonary infiltration*: infiltrations of lymphocytes and plasma cells surround and obstruct small airways.

3. *As a manifestation of associated diseases*: by definition Sjögren's syndrome is associated with a connective tissue disorder which is usually rheumatoid arthritis or less often systemic lupus, systemic sclerosis, polyarteritis nodosa and polymyositis. Fibrosing alveolitis, lymphoid interstitial pneumonia, pseudolymphoma and malignant lymphoma also have associations with Sjögren's and sicca syndromes.

4. There is evidence pointing to a pathogenic role for *immune complex deposition* in alveolar capillaries. The sicca and pulmonary components have a predictable symptomatology but there may also be complaint of dysphagia or Raynaud's phenomenon; a few have renal tubular acidosis or primary biliary cirrhosis; there is a tendency to develop allergies to drugs. Hypergammaglobulinaemia is present in 50% of cases and there is a high incidence of organ and non-organ specific antibodies.

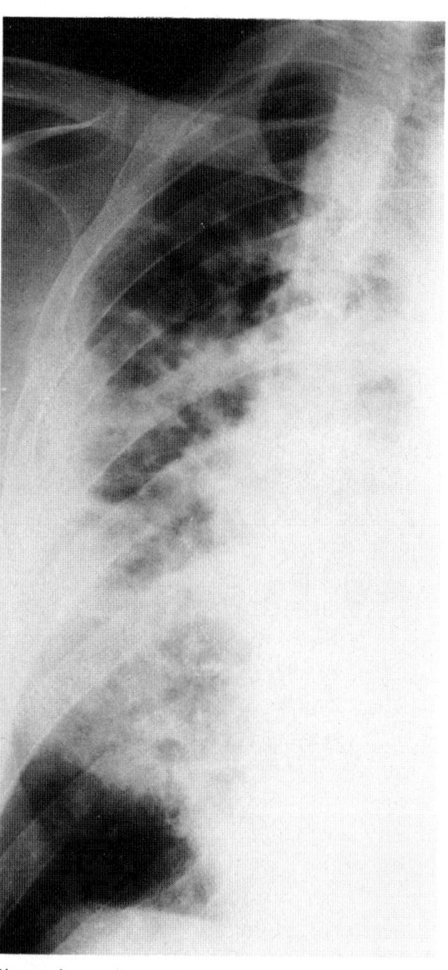

Fig. 17.19 Sjögren's syndrome. Non-Hodgkin's lymphoma. Dense conglomerate opacities mainly sub-pleural; coarse reticulation. (Same case as Fig. 14.44.)

Sialographic abnormalities although non-specific offer some diagnostic support since they are found in 50% of cases which is a much higher incidence than is found in the associated diseases uncomplicated by Sjögren's or sicca syndromes.

Radiological appearances. It is not surprising that such a heterogeneous condition has no characteristic radiographic pattern (Fig. 17.19). Infection and bronchial obstruction account for basal atelectasis, pulmonary consolidations, pleural effusion and bronchiectasis. The lymphocytic infiltrations and associated disease pathologies take a variety of forms — fine diffuse interstitial, coarse reticulonodular, diffuse alveolar; in cases with lymphocytic lymphoma multiple discrete nodules and hilar node enlargement may be found.

PSEUDOLYMPHOMA

Ambiguity surrounds the nature of this lymphoproliferative disorder, whether it should be placed with the post-inflammatory processes, the benign neoplasms or indeed whether it has any separate existence apart from the lymphomas. On the face of it the issue seems simple enough. Considering only intrathoracic lesions it is a sharply demarcated massive infiltration of the lung by well-differentiated lymphocytes and other inflammatory cells. It differs from malignant lymphoma in the maturity of the lymphocytes, by the possession of true germinal centres, a mixed cell population and an absence of Reed-Sternberg cells. Growth is slow, nodes are not involved and there is no extrathoracic spread. Bronchial walls may be invaded but the epithelium is not breached. At the periphery of the mass the infiltration is interstitial and such areas are indistinguishable from lymphoid interstitial pneumonia. However, a number progress to malignant lymphoma which poses the question whether it is a pre-malignant phase or is malignant from the beginning. Moreover, malignant lymphoma, particularly the well-differentiated lymphocytic variety, can remain limited for many years. Lymphocytic lymphoma is monoclonal whereas pseudolymphoma is polyclonal, a separation which can be made on the basis of whether the cells stain for one or more light chains. Many pseudolymphomas have had to be reclassified on the basis of this test. The drug Phenytoin has been responsible for some cases of pseudolymphoma and in these the lymph nodes may be enlarged.

Radiological appearances. On the chest radiograph the lesions either appear as round isolated opacities or as consolidations of segmental or lobar size abutting on pleural surfaces. Both types are likely to show air bronchograms. The round lesions are usually 1 to 4 cm in diameter, single or multiple with borders which shade off into the surrounding lung.

CONNECTIVE TISSUE (Collagen) DISEASES

The features common to this group of diseases are inflammation of joints, serosa, blood vessels and connective tissues. The inflammation is followed by fibrosis and the laying down of collagen. Any tissue or organ may be involved and prognosis depends on the severity in vital organs, particularly kidney, central nervous system and lung. By virtue of their rich supply of blood vessels and connective tissue the lungs are a frequent target. Criteria for entry to the group are not strict but conventionally rheumatoid arthritis, systemic lupus erythematosus (SLE), systemic sclerosis (SS), polyarteritis nodosa (PAN) and dermatomyositis/polymyositis (PMS) are regarded as founder members, with Henoch-Schönlein purpura, Goodpasture syndrome, Behçet's disease and others occupying a position on the periphery.

By re-arranging the clinical signs various sub-divisions have been created, the justification being an attempt to predict subsequent behaviour. *CREST syndrome* is a subset of SS characterized by cutaneous calcinosis, Raynaud's phenomenon, oesophageal abnormalities, sclerodactyly and telangiectasia. *Mixed connective tissue disease* consists of combined features of SLE, SS and PMS. The term *overlap syndrome* is usually applied to cases occupying the middle ground between classical PAN and allergic angiitis but it has been extended to include almost any combination so that it now lacks a precise definition.

POLYARTERITIS NODOSA

The classical form of polyarteritis nodosa affects medium sized muscular arteries in any part of the body. There is inflammation in and around the vessel followed by necrosis of the wall which is thereby weakened and gives way forming small aneurysms, the 'nodosa' of the title. Vessels are also occluded by the process. It is predominantly a male disease in the ratio 3:1. Immunological mechanisms are involved and there is immune complex deposition in vessel walls, the antigens unidentified except in those cases due to drug hypersensitivity or to the hepatitis B antigen. The protean symptomatology reflects the widespread distribution of the lesions affecting gut, skin, kidneys, heart, central nervous system, joints and muscle. Visceral angiography shows aneurysms or other arterial abnormalities in over 60% and is frequently of more diagnostic value than blind tissue biopsy.

Radiological appearances. Abnormalities in the lungs are unusual but nodules, segmental opacities, atelectases, small pleural effusions and diffuse interstitial fibrosis may be found. Opacities are usually transient except for those caused by diffuse fibrosis.

The rare disease of *relapsing polychondritis* has similarities to polyarteritis nodosa and the two conditions are sometimes found together. There is inflammation, necrosis and ultimately fibrosis of cartilage and other tissues with a high glycosaminoglycan content, which includes the aorta. The effect on the cartilage of the bronchial tree is to produce collapsible upper airways subjecting the lungs to risk of infection from impaired clearance. Fibrotic bronchial strictures may have their origin in relapsing polychondritis.

Allergic granulomatosis and angiitis (*Churg-Strauss disease*) is at one end of a scale with classical polyarteritis at the other, the middle ground being occupied by the *overlap syndrome* with features common to both. Like classical PAN, allergic granulomatosis and angiitis is a generalized necrotizing vasculitis but with certain differences. The lungs are always involved; it occurs in patients with an allergic diathesis, usually asthma; there is a blood eosinophilia; the pathology is granulomatous and eosinophils figure more prominently in the infiltrations. The differences are therefore mostly one of degree rather than of kind. It is to be suspected in asthmatics with a multisystem disorder and affects the same organs as classical

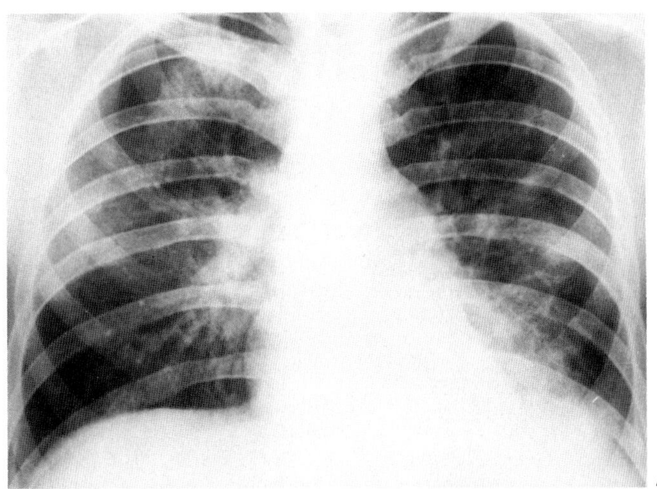

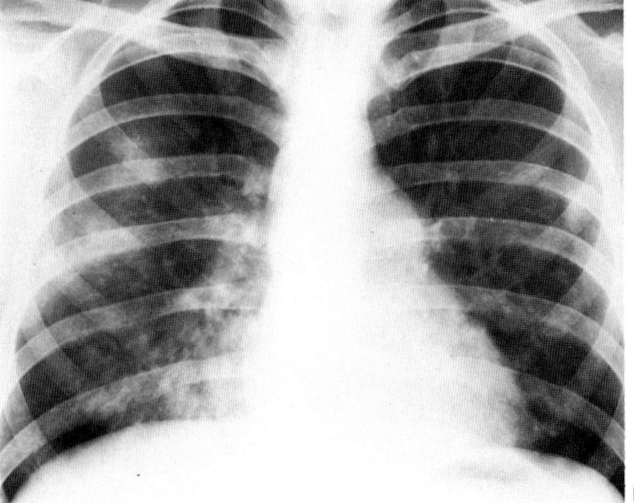

Fig. 17.20 (**A**) Henoch–Schonlein purpura. Non-segmental, migratory, alveolar opacities in all lobes. (**B**) 3 weeks later. Some lesions resolving; fresh ones have appeared at right base and right mid-zone.

PAN. Lung opacities are alveolar consolidations, sometimes massive, or a diffuse coarse reticulation and typically they wax and wane. Infarcts following pulmonary arteritis account for some of the opacities. Sometimes the presentation is acute, suggesting a precipitating insult and this *hypersensitivity vasculitis* can be induced by drugs, serum sickness or infection. Henoch–Schönlein purpura is a vasculitis of this type. These transient lung opacities are nodular, diffuse or patchy (Figs 17.20A and B).

SYSTEMIC LUPUS ERYTHEMATOSUS

Notable features of SLE are its female preponderance (F:M ratio 9:1), a butterfly facial rash, arthralgias, Raynaud's phenomenon, renal glomerulitis and nervous system involvement. The LE cell test has now been replaced by tests for *anti-nuclear antibody*, positive in 90% of cases but not an absolute requirement for diagnosis. Few patients have pulmonary symptoms or gross radiographic signs even though a majority have abnormal function tests of restrictive type. The presenting symptom may be dyspnoea without apparent cause. High diaphragms with a restricted range of sluggish movement together with basal atelectases are the result of stiff, shrunken lungs. Pathologically the alveoli have a predominantly mononuclear infiltration and hyaline membranes. Interstitial fibrosis is not a major feature and evidence of it on the chest radiograph is rarely found. Patchy pulmonary opacities are caused by pulmonary oedema, infarction or secondary infection. Infective and infarctive lesions may cavitate. There is an entity of lupus pneumonitis which is steroid responsive. Vascular thrombosis in the lungs and elsewhere is related to the presence of lupus anticoagulant, an antibody to certain clotting factors in the blood, which paradoxically increases coagulability in vivo. It is not specific to SLE and is found in other connective tissue diseases.

SYSTEMIC SCLEROSIS

The pathological abnormalities in the lungs in systemic sclerosis consist of proliferative endothelial obliteration of small arteries and an interstitial and peribronchial fibrosis. The consequences are inequalities of ventilation and perfusion, air trapping, emphysema and pulmonary hypertension. Similar pathological changes in the diaphragm and intercostal muscles adds to the respiratory dysfunction. In fact only a minority have lung disease. Radiographic changes therefore are usually inconspicuous and they are absent in the subset with CREST symptomatology (calcinosis, Raynaud's, oesophagus, sclerodactyly, telangiectasia). In the 'overlap' cases most have lung disease.

Systemic sclerosis carries an increased risk of carcinoma of the lung, particularly bronchioloalveolar cell, and at a younger age. Sjögren's syndrome also occurs with all types.

Radiological appearances. In those patients with an abnormal chest radiograph, the typical pattern is a fibrosing alveolitis, reticular or reticulo-nodular opacities spreading upwards from the bases (Figs 17.21A and B). Honeycombing may develop. Small pleural effusions are

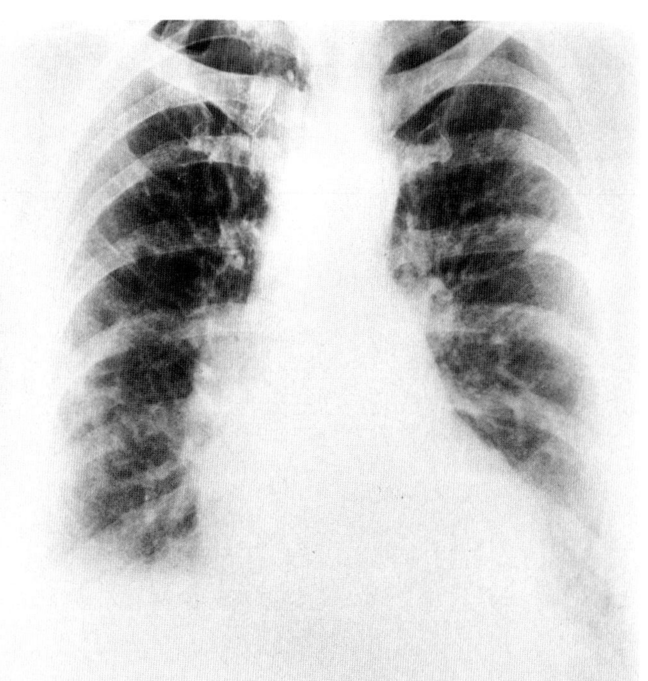

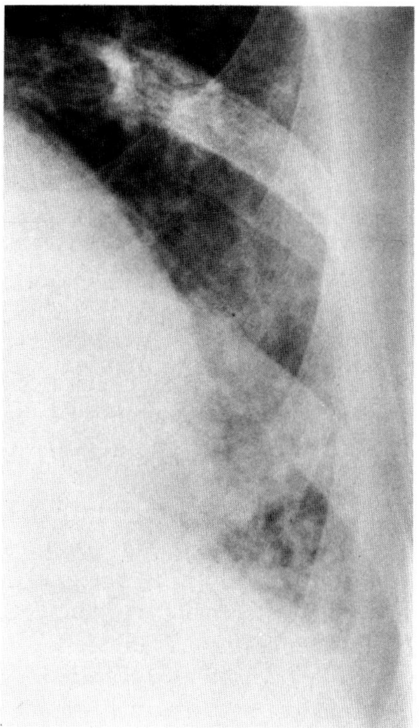

Fig. 17.21 (**A**) Systemic sclerosis. Fibrosing alveolitis spreading upwards from the bases. (**B**) Close-up. Coarse reticulation.

not uncommon and occasional findings are pneumatocoeles, pneumothorax, egg-shell calcification of hilar nodes and evidence of pulmonary hypertension. Oesophageal dysfunction can lead to aspiration pneumonitis but this is neither frequent nor important.

MIXED CONNECTIVE TISSUE DISEASE

This has features common to systemic lupus, systemic sclerosis and polymyositis, prominent amongst them being Raynaud's phenomenon, arthritis, muscle weakness and lymphadenopathy. It is steroid responsive and pursues a relatively benign course due to the absence of severe renal disease. Its immunological characteristic is a high titre of antibody to ribonuclear protein which is absent or in low titre in other connective tissue diseases. The chest radiograph is abnormal in most cases, with fibrosing alveolitis at the bases, small lung volumes and upper lobe shrinkage. A notable characteristic is a deforming erosive arthritis and acro-osteolysis.

DERMATOMYOSITIS AND POLYMYOSITIS

Lung involvement is unusual in these conditions but when present it takes the form of a basal fibrosing alveolitis. This can follow a rapidly progressive course but more often it evolves slowly with emphysema complicating the late stages.

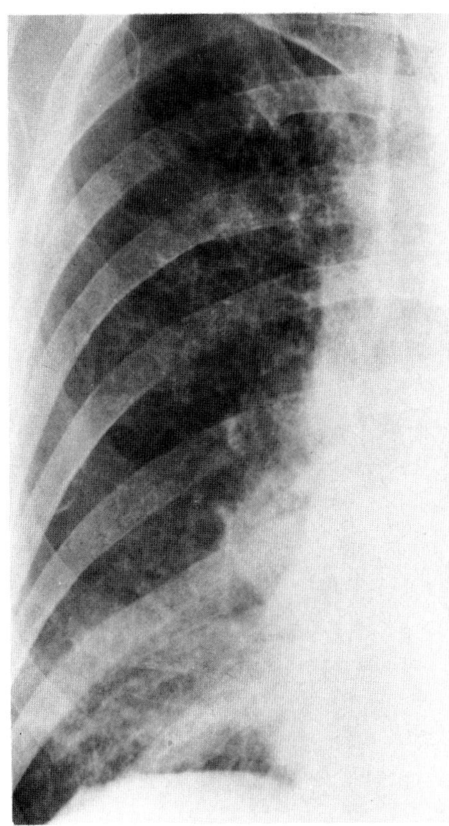

Fig. 17.22 Rheumatoid lung disease. Fibrosing alveolitis. Also a mass at right hilum. At post-mortem there was pulmonary arteritis; the mass was necrotic. The patient had received gold treatment but this bore no temporal relationship to the respiratory disease.

BEHÇET'S DISEASE

The features of this disease of unknown aetiology are ulcerations in the mouth, eye and genitalia with arthritis of large joints, thrombophlebitis and inflammatory lesions of gut. It is found most often in the Middle East and is almost exclusively a disease of men. In association with these symptoms the finding of multiple aneurysms and occlusions of pulmonary artery branches is pathognomonic. Obstruction of the cavae may also be found.

RHEUMATOID ARTHRITIS

The incidence of pleuro-pulmonary diseases directly related to rheumatoid arthritis and not just a chance association is low, no more than a few per cent. However looked at from the other direction the incidence of rheumatoid arthritis in fibrosing alveolitis is much higher than this. Intrathoracic manifestations of rheumatoid disease comprise pleural effusions, fibrosing alveolitis, rheumatoid necrobiotic lung nodules, angiitis and bronchiolitis obliterans. Occasionally these ante-date overt joint disease.

Pleural effusions are usually straw coloured exudates of moderate volume with a tendency to chronicity. The rare cholesterol effusion may remain unchanged over many years. Men are more often affected than women. Resorption of the exudate often leaves a fibrotic obliteration of the pleural space.

Cryptogenic fibrosing alveolitis and its relationship to rheumatoid disease has already been discussed but it has to be remembered that treatment with gold and penicillamine are potential causes of diffuse fibrosis (Fig. 17.22).

Rheumatoid lung nodules and subcutaneous nodules have the same histology, a necrotic centre surrounded by histiocytes, lymphocytes and fibroblasts. The nodules are round and well defined but with borders that are slightly irregular. The average diameter is 2 to 4 cm but an occasional one reaches large size. They occur in any part of the lungs and may be single or multiple but are never profuse (Fig. 17.23).

Cavitation is common and is a result of evacuation of the necrotic material (Figs 17.24A and B). The cavities may periodically fill and empty, they may become infected or rupture into the pleura in which case there will be a pneumothorax or bronchopleural fistula. Some nodules resolve leaving a scar but in general they are indolent. Large cavities have been known to close after treatment with azathioprine.

In *Caplan's syndrome* there are numerous round opacities up to 5 cm in diameter resembling metastases. It occurs on a background of simple pneumoconiosis, the two diseases modifying each other in this distinctive fashion. The solid fibrotic lesions eventually become hyalinized and may calcify. It was first described in coal miners but it is also found in asbestosis, silicosis and other industrial pneumoconioses.

Pulmonary angiitis is commonly found on histological examination of the lungs from rheumatoid patients but this does not give rise to any recognizable radiographic pattern. Isolated case reports have described acute necrotizing angiitis in association with consolidative pulmonary opacities.

Obliterative bronchiolitis is a potential cause of respiratory failure with a normal chest radiograph. It has been found in association with obstructive pneumonia and probably accounts for some large apical cavitating lesions.

Progressive upper lobe fibrosis with bullous cystic changes indistinguishable from that found in ankylosing spondylitis has also been reported.

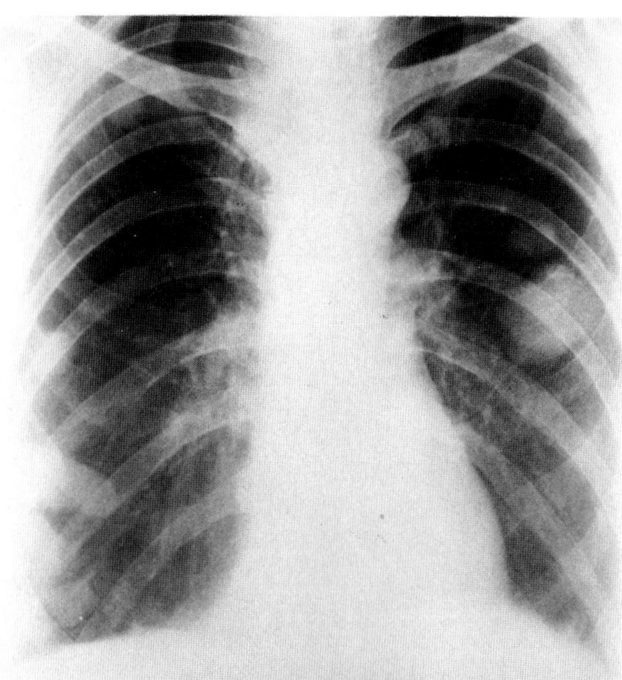

Fig. 17.23 Rheumatoid nodules. Seven can be seen. They later cavitated.

ANKYLOSING SPONDYLITIS AND PROGRESSIVE APICAL FIBROSIS

About 2% of ankylosing spondylotics of long-standing develop this complication. It begins as patchy opacities in the upper lobes with an apical cap of pleural thickening.

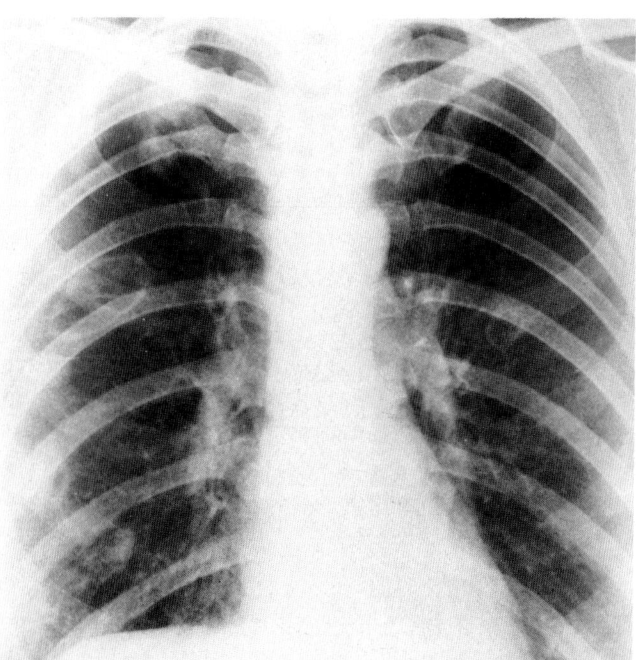

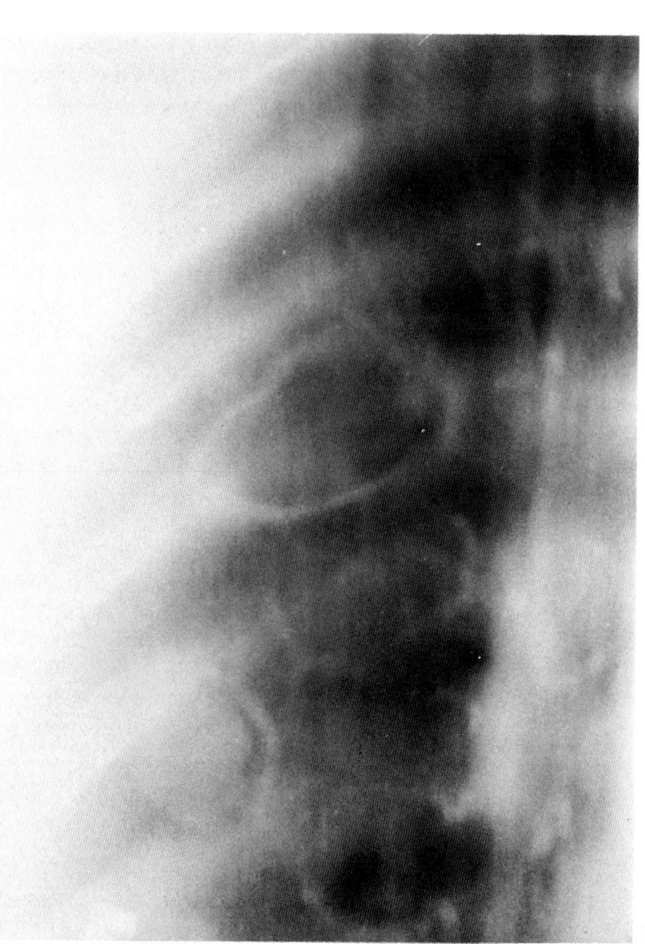

Fig. 17.24 (**A**) Cavitating rheumatoid nodules. (**B**) Tomogram. One cavity contains a central round opacity and an air crescent (compare with a mycetoma).

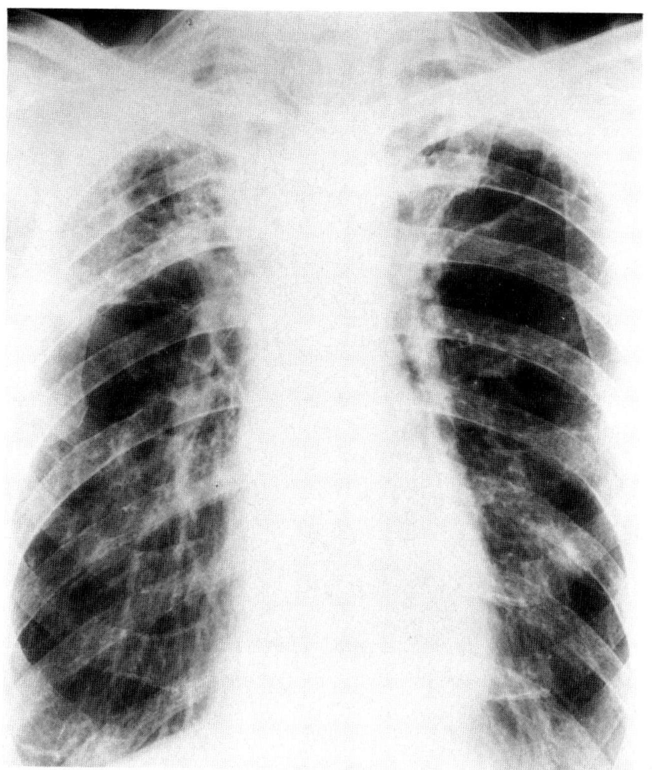

Fig. 17.25 Idiopathic progressive apical fibrosis. 9 years previously the chest radiograph was normal. The same pattern is found in many other diseases.

It may be unilateral at first but always spreads to the opposite side. The opacities enlarge and bullous air cysts appear within them at which time there may be complaint of haemoptysis. Like all chronic cavities they are susceptible to fungal colonization. Bronchi in the affected area are distorted and bronchiectatic. Pathologically the early changes are those of a patchy pneumonia with infiltration by chronic inflammatory cells and fibroblasts. There is progression to an extensive fibrosis and hyalinization destroying lung architecture.

Contracting fibro-bullous disease of this nature is not distinguishable from that caused by tuberculosis, sarcoidosis, extrinsic allergic alveolitis, pneumoconiosis, post-radiation and rheumatoid arthritis. There is also a group of idiopathic cases in which none of these causes apply (Fig. 17.25).

PULMONARY ALVEOLAR PROTEINOSIS

When this disease was first described in 1958 the pathology was characterized as 'filling of the alveoli by a PAS-positive proteinaceous material rich in lipid' which still defines the essential elements of the process. Macroscopically the lung is not uniformly affected but studded with nodules from a few millimetres up to 2 or more centimetres in diameter. The most plausible theory of causation is that it is a response to a variety of irritants including dusts and for some unknown reason there is impairment of clearance of the material so formed. This material is probably mainly formed from surfactant ingested by macrophages which then disintegrate within alveoli. Leakage of serum into alveoli also plays a part. There is a striking absence of reaction within alveolar walls unless there are complications. Men are affected three times as often as women and no age is exempt. The disease is worldwide.

Radiological appearances. Radiologically the commonest pattern is one likened to pulmonary oedema with a bilateral, fine, diffuse, radiating peri-hilar shadowing. However, the non-uniformity of the pathology may be reflected in a superimposition of patchiness taking the form either of a granularity or nodularity seen within the general opacity or at its edges (Fig. 17.26a, b). The granularity can be confused with sarcoidosis or miliary tuberculosis but the background opacity is finer than in these diseases. The irregular, coarse linearities characteristic of fibrosis or the mediastinal distortions as in chronic tuberculosis are not found unless there are infective complications but small honeycomb cysts representing distended terminal air spaces may be found at the edges of lesions and are probably the source of the occasional *pneumothorax*.

Enlargement of hilar nodes, pleural effusions and cavitation only arise with complications. There are variations to the basic 'butterfly' distribution; the opacities can be solely or predominantly unilateral or may be confined to one lung segment.

The disease may remain static over many years or it may progress. A minority resolve spontaneously, sometimes completely, at others leaving a residue of fibrosis. Recurrence after spontaneous resolution is uncommon but is now seen frequently after treatment by broncho-alveolar lavage.

Diagnosis is confirmed by *biopsy* or by the finding of the proteinaceous material in the *sputum* or *lavage fluid*. Macrophages with lamellar inclusions of lipid in the lavage fluid are also diagnostic. *Bronchoalveolar lavage* is not only diagnostic but therapeutic. Each lung in turn is filled with saline which is then repeatedly exchanged up to a total of 40 l or more. The return is at first opalescent but becomes progressively clearer. Functional improvement is immediate but radiographic clearing may be delayed and then incomplete. The procedure can be repeated as necessary.

The disease causes dyspnoea as a result of impaired gas transfer and previously carried a high mortality rate from respiratory or cardiac failure but lavage has improved the prognosis. There is an increased risk of infection not only from the usual respiratory pathogens but also from *Nocardia, Aspergillus, Cryptococcus* and other opportunistic organisms, in these circumstances likely to be disseminate. The disease is occasionally found associated with leukaemia, Hodgkin's disease and immunoglobulin deficiencies.

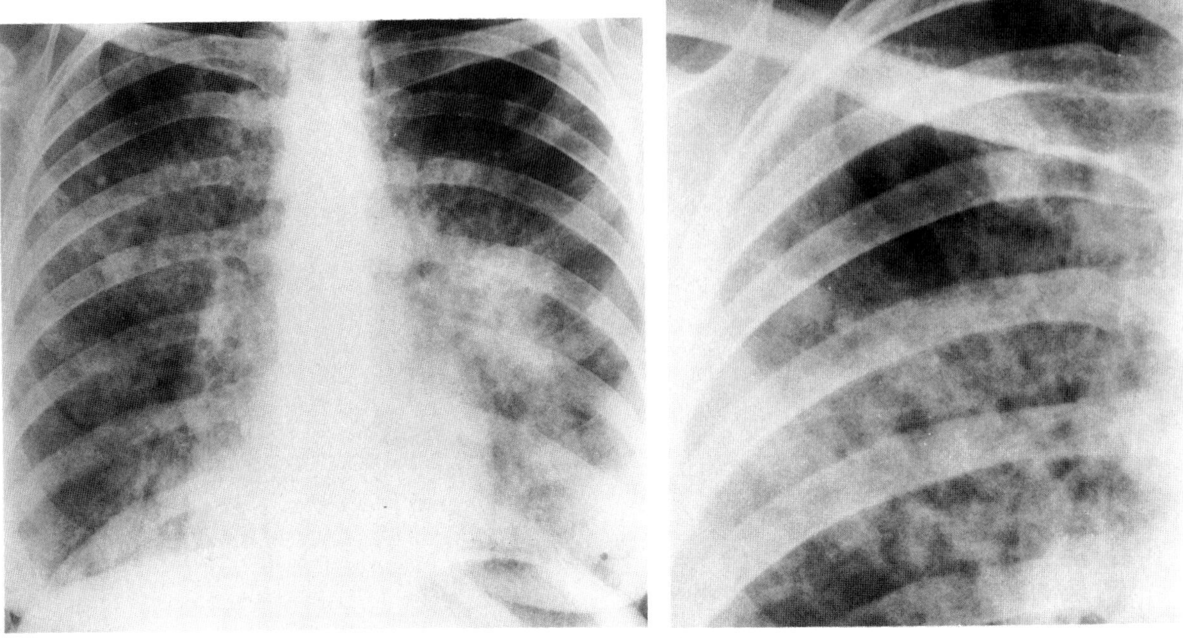

Fig. 17.26 (**A**) Pulmonary alveolar proteinosis. Central alveolar patchy densities and vague nodulation. (**B**) Close-up. Ill-defined alveolar opacities; air bronchogram visible.

AMYLOIDOSIS

Amyloid is a proteinaceous substance with specific chemical and staining properties. Amyloidosis is a group of conditions where amyloid in unusually large amounts is deposited in connective tissue, around parenchymal tissue cells and in the walls of blood vessels. The conditions are grouped into **primary** and **secondary** categories according to whether there is a prior precipitating cause. Secondary amyloidosis may arise as a complication of *chronic infection* such as tuberculosis, osteomyelitis, bronchiectasis, leprosy, but in Western countries infection now assumes less importance and the most common causes are *rheumatoid disease* and *neoplasia*. Chemical analysis and histological staining can differentiate between primary and secondary amyloid but there is a borderland represented by myeloma in which secondary amyloidosis has a chemically primary amyloid. Secondary amyloid is derived from serum (AA protein) and primary amyloid (and myeloma amyloid) from immunoglobulin light chains.

Both primary and secondary amyloidosis can occur in localized and generalized forms. Once generalized amyloidosis is established it tends to be progressive and has a poor prognosis when vital organs become involved. In 75% of the generalized disease there are amyloid deposits in the mucosa of rectal biopsy specimens. Secondary amyloid does not invoke an inflammatory response in the lungs whereas primary amyloid does so. For this reason secondary amyloidcsis in the lungs seldom causes symptoms and the chest radiograph is normal unless the initiating cause is intrapulmonary.

Further subdivision of primary pulmonary amyloidosis is based on the site involved:

Tracheo-bronchial. This may take the form of a solitary endobronchial tumour mass or polyp or it may grow down the trachea and into the bronchi in the form of nodular submucosal plaques. Radiologically the predictable effects are those of obstruction, atelectasis, distal bronchiectasis and infection. On bronchography there is a nodularity of the wall of the air passages and multiple strictures. The tumour masses may have to be removed piecemeal but they recur. Amyloid material is sometimes found in relationship to bronchial neoplasms so that caution is required in the interpretation of biopsy appearances as it may not be typical of the whole lesion.

Tracheopathia osteoplastica is a condition of cartilaginous masses lining most of the trachea and major bronchi. The masses contain amyloid deposits, calcific bodies and ossifications. It is thought in one theory to be an end stage of tracheobronchial amyloidosis.

Pulmonary (**or parenchymal**) **amyloidosis**. There are two varieties *nodular* and *alveolar septal*. In the nodular variety the lesions are discrete and solitary or multiple, sometimes in large numbers. In size they vary from one to several centimetres in diameter and they grow slowly. Approximately one third cavitate or calcify, the latter a fine stippling best appreciated on tomography. Calcification of this nature in a solitary lesion is strong evidence of amyloidosis. The second variety, alveolar septal or interstitial amyloidosis is a diffuse deposition of amyloid within alveolar walls, lobular septa and in the walls of pulmonary arterioles. Radiographically there may be a diffuse reticulation or reticulo-nodulation, a honeycomb pattern or an appearance which mimics pulmonary oedema.

Nodal. Amyloidosis may be confined to nodes (Fig. 17.27). The frequency of mediastinal and hilar node enlargement differs significantly in different reported series. It can be massive and the nodes frequently contain a coarse speckled or egg shell *calcification*.

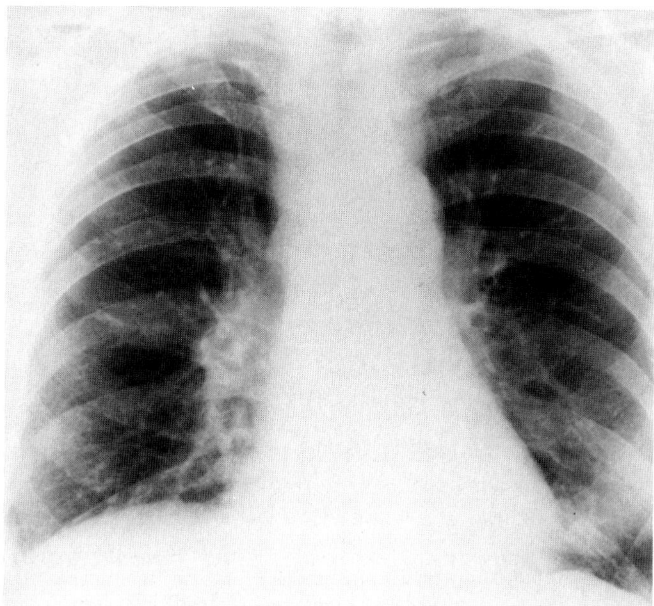

Fig. 17.27 Amyloidosis. Widening of the superior mediastinum and right hilar enlargement from adenopathy. Patient had lymphoplasmacytic lymphoma but this was not present in the mediastinal nodes which showed amyloidosis only.

Combinations of these varieties are sometimes found in the same patient. In all types the pleura is usually spared. *Cardiac amyloid* is a cause of pericardial effusion, impaired myocardial contractility and conduction defects all leading to heart failure. As the pulmonary oedema of heart failure recedes, an underlying reticulo-nodular pattern may be revealed. The combination of increasing dyspnoea with reticulo-nodular shadowing in a patient with cardiac dysfunction without obvious cause is very suggestive of myocardial amyloidosis and alveolar septal amyloidosis.

BRONCHIAL ABNORMALITIES

Bronchial abnormalities which are a part of specific diseases are considered in their respective sections.

CHRONIC BRONCHITIS

The excessive mucous secretion which is the hallmark of *chronic bronchitis* impairs the defences of the bronchial tree against infection. Sooner or later the symptoms of recurrent bronchial infection are added to those of hypersecretion and as the intervals between infections shorten the patient may have sputum which is almost continually purulent. Damage to the bronchial tree is then manifested in changes in the bronchogram — patchy non-filling of some bronchi because of retained secretions; contrast medium filling the dilated ducts of mucous glands in the epithelium of major bronchi; the epithelium is thrown into concertina folds; the even bronchial tapering is replaced by minor dilatations and narrowings; small airways dilate into small cavities. There is no sharp cut-off point between these changes and those of minor tubular bronchiectasis and bronchiolectasis; the difference is simply one of degree.

Although chronic bronchitis and chronic airways obstruction are often found together, their relationship is not a simple one of cause and effect; they are independent variables.

BRONCHIECTASIS

The incidence and severity of *bronchiectasis* has been changed substantially by improved medical management of pulmonary infections and by a reduction in the incidence of measles and whooping cough, which with their frequent complications of secondary infection, were potent initiators of bronchiectasis. The bronchial tree was permanently subjected to aspiration from pools of chronic suppuration so that surgical resection of the worst areas was no guarantee that spread to other parts would be prevented. Antibiotics have transformed the outlook so that now most at risk are those who by virtue of structural or functional abnormalities are incapable of clearing the lungs of infection. Examples of such abnormalities are *cystic fibrosis of the pancreas*, *agammaglobulinaemia* and *deficient mucociliary clearance*. In parallel with the fall in the number of surgical resections there has been a fall in the number of bronchograms performed. Diagnosis and treatment can be based on symptoms, clinical signs and non-invasive radiography so that it is no longer crucial to know the precise distribution of the bronchiectasis.

Radiological appearances. On a chest radiograph the only pathognomonic sign of bronchiectasis is a dilated, air-filled bronchus. Bronchial wall or peri-bronchial thickening has to be present before these tubes become visible (Fig. 17.28). Cavities which fill and empty, branching band shadows, grossly scarred areas of persistent collapse, are all signs suggestive but not pathognomonic of bronchiectasis. In progressive upper lobe fibrosis such as is found in tuberculosis, sarcoidosis and extrinsic allergic alveolitis,

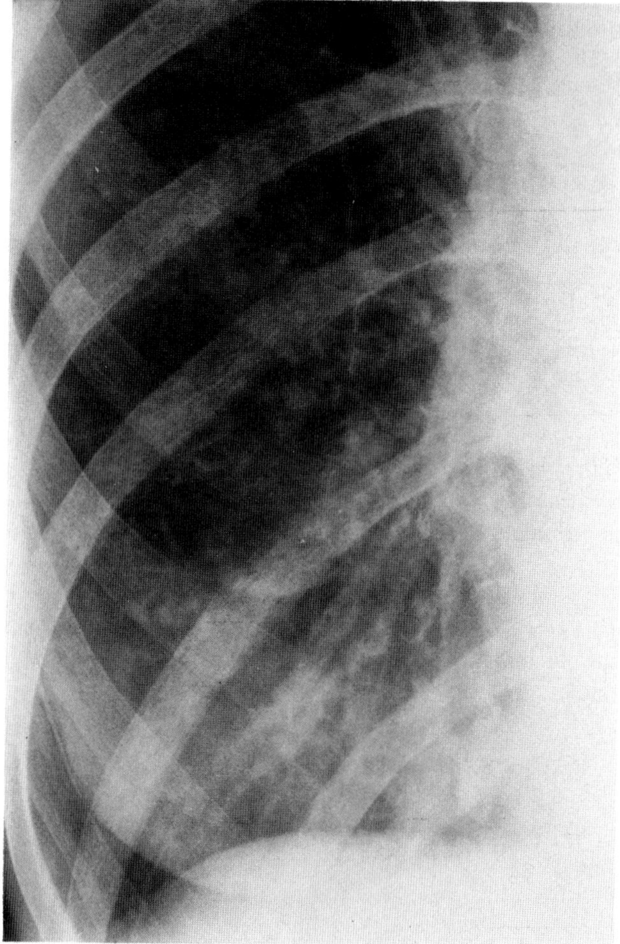

Fig. 17.28 Bronchiectasis. Thickened bronchial walls. Lumen dilated in places.

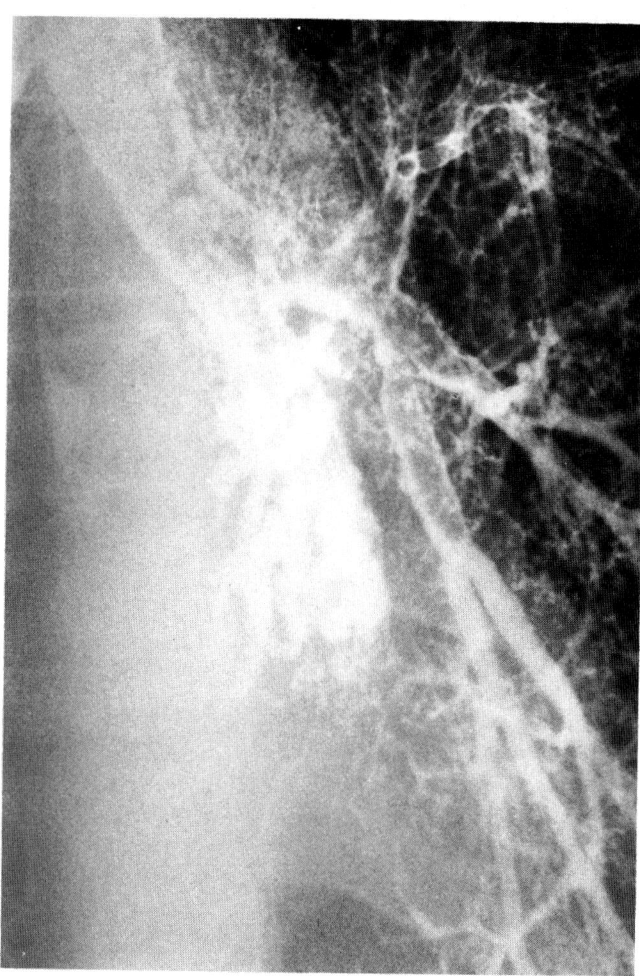

Fig. 17.29 Bronchiectasis. Diminutive left lower lobe probably from infection in infancy which arrested further growth. Dilated mucous gland ducts visible on the lingula bronchus — chronic bronchitis.

the bronchi are distorted and usually dilated. Cavities in these areas are frequently bronchiectatic in origin.

Nevertheless there are circumstances when bronchography is still required. The diagnosis may be uncertain and the chest radiograph unhelpful. The chest radiograph is occasionally normal even in the presence of quite extensive cystic bronchiectasis. Surgical resection is sometimes required for resistant infection in localized bronchiectasis and bronchography is then mandatory.

Tubular (or cylindrical) and saccular (or cystic) are descriptive terms applied to the morphology of bronchiectasis, referring respectively to dilatation along the bronchial axis or to peripheral expansions, and indicating the site of maximum damage to the airways. The side branches of the bronchial axis are spaced at first at intervals of over 1 cm but as the peripheral parts are reached the intervals reduce to 2–3 mm. The 'mm branching pattern' identifies any changes beyond as being at the bronchiolar level. Most cases of bronchiectasis however, are of mixed type but with one predominating.

A common pattern is of irregularly dilated tubes with clubbed terminations crowded together in shrunken lung (Fig. 17.29). Additional signs of chronic bronchitis are usually to be found in the large central bronchi. Saccules may remain small or enlarge to 2 to 3 cm in diameter and it is the larger which fill with greatest difficulty during bronchography. They may fill with contrast after coughing or after a delay of some hours (Figs 17.30A and B).

Allergic bronchopulmonary aspergillosis may have a unique pattern of proximal bronchiectasis with normal calibre bronchi beyond the dilatation but the common tubular bronchiectasis is more often found. Generalized bronchiectasis may be found in *alpha-1 anti-trypsin deficiency* which contrasts with the predominantly basal emphysema which is characteristic of this condition. Bronchiectasis in *cystic fibrosis* appears first in the upper lobes before spreading widely. However, bronchography is seldom required in these conditions.

BRONCHIOLITIS

Bronchiolitis is predominantly an acute infective disease of children often of viral aetiology.

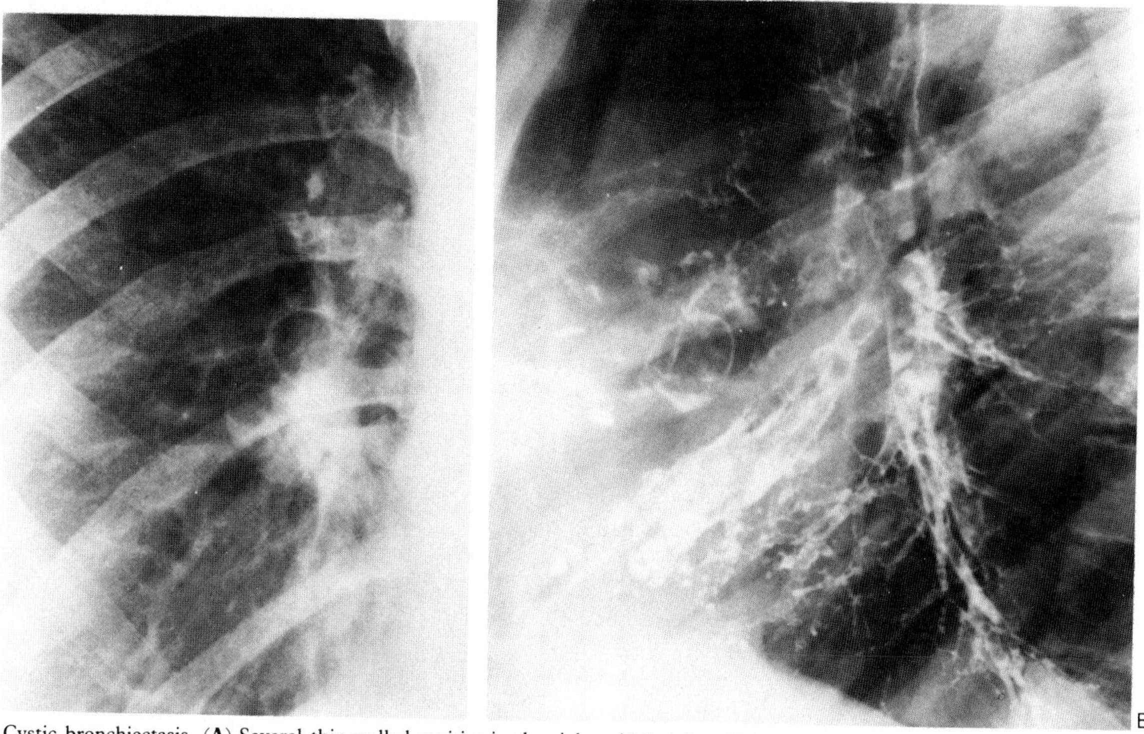

Fig. 17.30 Cystic bronchiectasis. (**A**) Several thin-walled cavities in the right middle lobe. (**B**) Bronchogram shows collapsed right middle lobe, tubular (cylindrical) bronchiectasis and sacules filling with difficulty.

Bronchiolitis obliterans has a wider spread of age incidence and aetiology. It may be caused by, or follow, viral infections or inhalation of toxic fumes; it is found in association with the lung lesions of rheumatoid arthritis, chronic eosinophil pneumonia, bronchocentric granulomatosis and allergic angiitis with granulomatosis; it is also present in 25% of farmer's lung cases; finally there is an association with bronchitis, emphysema and cigarette smoking.

After excluding cases having these known precipitating factors there remains a small number with severe, chronic, irreversible obstruction of small airways for which the terminology **cryptogenic obliterative bronchiolitis** has been proposed. The patients are almost all women with severe dyspnoea sometimes dating from a respiratory infection. Half of the patients have rheumatoid arthritis but no overt evidence of rheumatoid lung disease. Abnormalities on the chest radiograph — mild overinflation, slight reduction in vessel calibre in the lower halves of the lungs with normal central vessels — are inconspicuous but bronchographic abnormalities are more impressive with the contrast medium stopping well short of the periphery and a sparcity of side branches. There may be a generalized slight reduction in bronchial calibre. These are the changes found in unilateral lung transradiance. There are matched, non-segmental ventilation/perfusion defects on lung scanning.

BRONCHIOLECTASIS

Small peripheral saccular dilatations of the terminal and respiratory bronchioles are identified bronchographically at the level of the millimetre branching pattern (Fig. 17.31). The acinus, that is the group of alveoli distal to the terminal bronchiole, may be incorporated in the saccules which measure approximately 1 cm in diameter. Symptoms of chronic bronchitis and bronchiectasis are related to the numbers of such saccules. Bronchiolectasis has been found post mortem in patients who have had intermittent positive pressure ventilation with positive end-expiratory pressures. Patients treated identically who survived had no recognizable sequelae from which it is assumed that the condition is potentially reversible.

BRONCHOCOELE

Accumulation of mucus, pus or caseous material within distended bronchi distal to a segmental bronchus but without collapse is known as bronchocoele, bronchial mucocoele or blocked bronchiectasis. An obstructing membrane found in some cases has been interpreted as indicating a congenital origin but obstruction from any cause, including bronchial carcinoma, is capable of producing an identical appearance (Figs 17.32A and B). It is

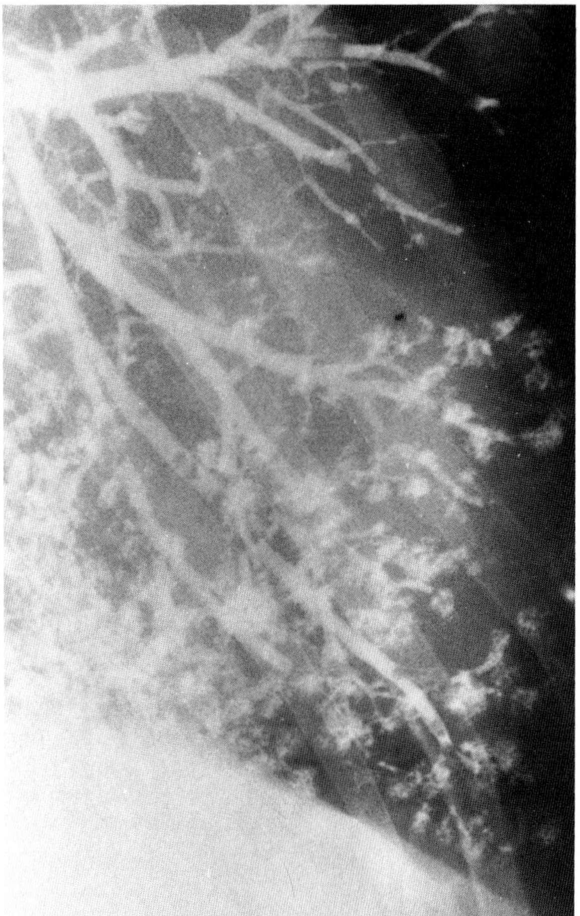

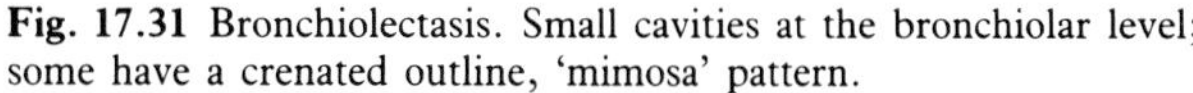

Fig. 17.31 Bronchiolectasis. Small cavities at the bronchiolar level; some have a crenated outline, 'mimosa' pattern.

relatively rare in bronchial carcinoma because of insufficient time available for its evolution before being overtaken by atelectatic changes from continued growth of the neoplasm. The characteristic appearance is a collection of oval or finger-like branching, homogenous opacities along the axis of the bronchial tree, usually in an upper lobe. The low density makes it difficult to define on the plain radiograph but it is clearly seen on tomography. The 'cyst' does not fill on bronchography, the obstruction producing a sharp cut-off in the contrast column. Aeration of the segment of lung distal to the bronchocoele is maintained by collateral air flow from adjacent segments through the pores of Kohn. For reasons which are not clear, this collateral flow is largely one way and the segment is hyperinflated. With increasing distension the bronchocoele assumes a round shape and it can then be mistaken for a

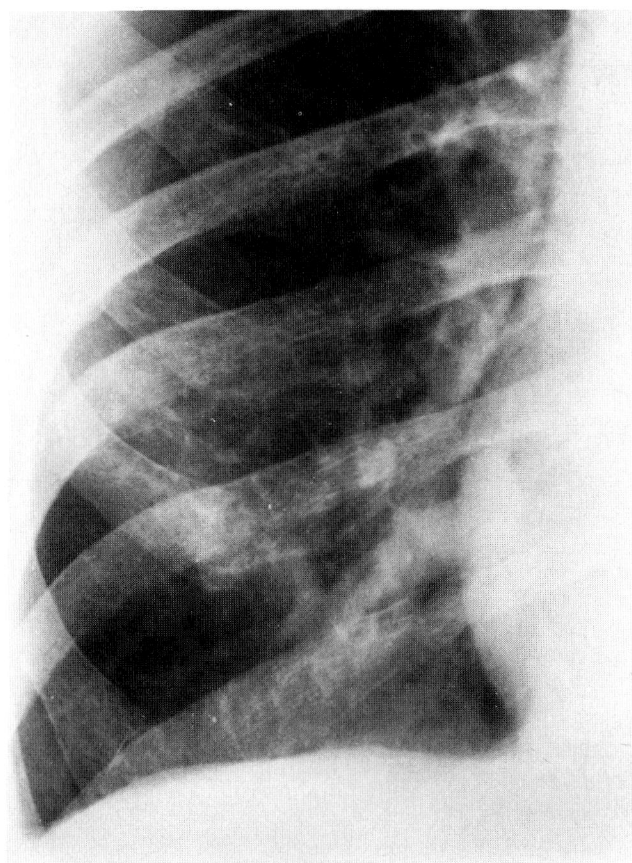

A

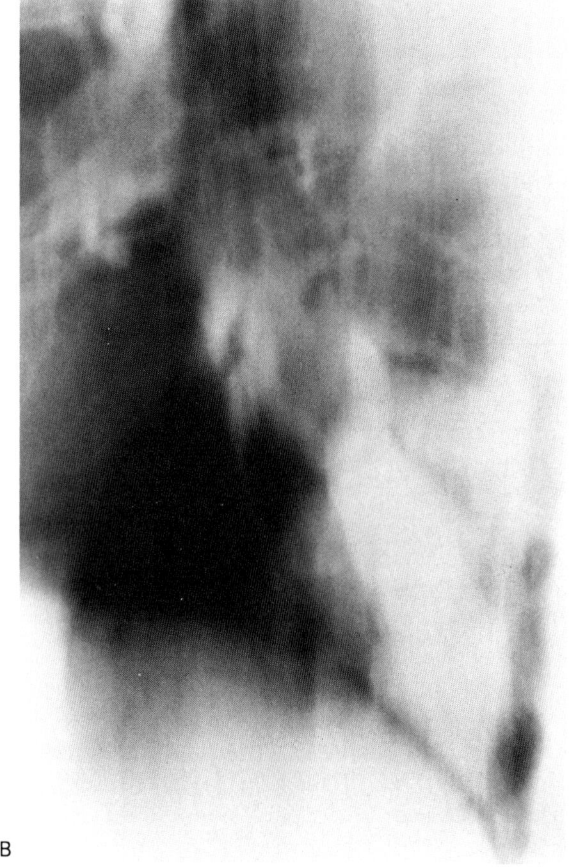

B

Fig. 17.32 (**A**) Bronchocoele due to squamous carcinoma of bronchus. (**B**) Lateral tomogram. Wide, branched bronchus. Inspissated gelatinous material was found distal to the obstructing carcinoma.

bronchogenic cyst, even to the extent of the histology since it is lined by respiratory epithelium.

BRONCHIAL MUCOID IMPACTION

Bronchial mucoid impaction has superficial similarities to bronchocoele but the aetiology and treatment of the two conditions are quite different. In the former, bronchial obstruction is caused by impaction of thick, tenacious plugs of mucus often containing a fungal mycelium. The bronchus may be dilated and may or may not fill on bronchography, depending on the tightness of the impaction. If the plugs are coughed up the obstruction is relieved. A branching opacity may be visible on the radiograph but is rarely as wide as a bronchocoele. The conditions in which it is commonly found are asthma, allergic bronchopulmonary aspergillosis and cystic fibrosis of the pancreas.

UNILATERAL LUNG TRANSRADIANCE

Increased transradiance of one lung compared to the opposite side will usually be found to be due to one of the following: 1) technical radiographic factors; 2) abnormalities of the thoracic cage. 3) pulmonary embolism; 4) compensatory or obstructive emphysema. If these causes are excluded those that remain are usually referred to eponymously as either *Macleod's* or *Swyer–James syndrome*. The vessels in the affected lung are reduced in number and calibre, a fact adequately demonstrated by *whole lung tomography* without the need for angiography. The small vessel size includes the hilum, a point of differentiation from emphysema in which these vessels are normal or enlarged (Fig. 17.33). Since the normal lung takes a larger proportion of the cardiac output its vascularity is increased.

Bronchography usually shows bronchi slightly narrower than normal with minor calibre irregularities but more importantly the contrast medium stops well short of the periphery. This is due to an absence of the effects of inspiration on the aspiration of the contrast medium peripherally. The lung is aerated but poorly ventilated with only a small change in volume between inspiration and expiration. As a consequence the mediastinum moves towards the impaired side during inspiration and diaphragmatic excursion is reduced.

There is often a history of severe respiratory infection in childhood. The condition has been observed to follow adenovirus and respiratory syncytial virus bronchiolitis but it is the site of the damage rather than the type of infection which is critical. Lung development is incomplete at birth and proliferation of newly formed alveoli continues for several years. Stunting of this growth is the cause of unilateral transradiance, the alveoli are fewer in number but larger in size. Functionally there is airways obstruction and defective gas exchange.

Although classically described as affecting one lung it may in fact be segmental or lobar or even widespread in both lungs. In the latter case the distribution is patchy, enough undamaged lung remaining to support life. Symptoms are mild, rarely more than a tendency to recurrent respiratory infections and mild dyspnoea despite the poor regional function.

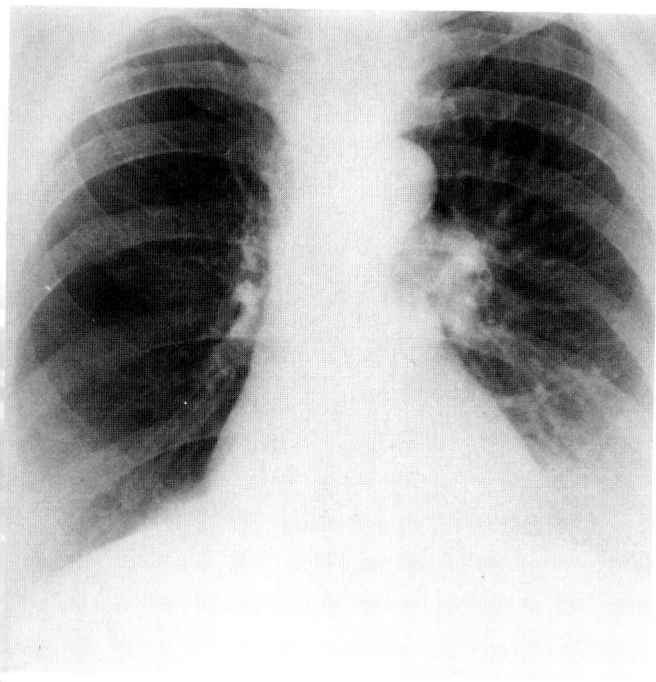

Fig. 17.33 Macleod's syndrome (unilateral lung transradiance). Small right hilum and reduced vessel calibre in right lung.

TRACHEOBRONCHOMEGALY
(*Mounier-Kuhn abnormality*)

The trachea may be as wide as the vertebral bodies and of uneven contour with bulging of the mucosa between the cartilage rings (Fig. 17.34). The dilatation may proceed no further than the main bronchi or it may be associated with a generalized bronchiectasis. The hypothesis that it results from a defect of connective tissue receives some support from its occasional association with Ehlers Danlos syndrome, a generalized connective tissue disorder.

ADULT RESPIRATORY DISTRESS SYNDROME

This condition is an *acute respiratory failure from pulmonary oedema non-cardiac in origin*. It is precipitated by a variety of insults most of which involve some form of *trauma* or *sepsis*. The list of causes is long and includes such unexpected items as miliary tuberculosis, mountain sickness, burns and major haemorrhage.

Running through these diverse situations there is a common thread of symptoms, physiological disturbances,

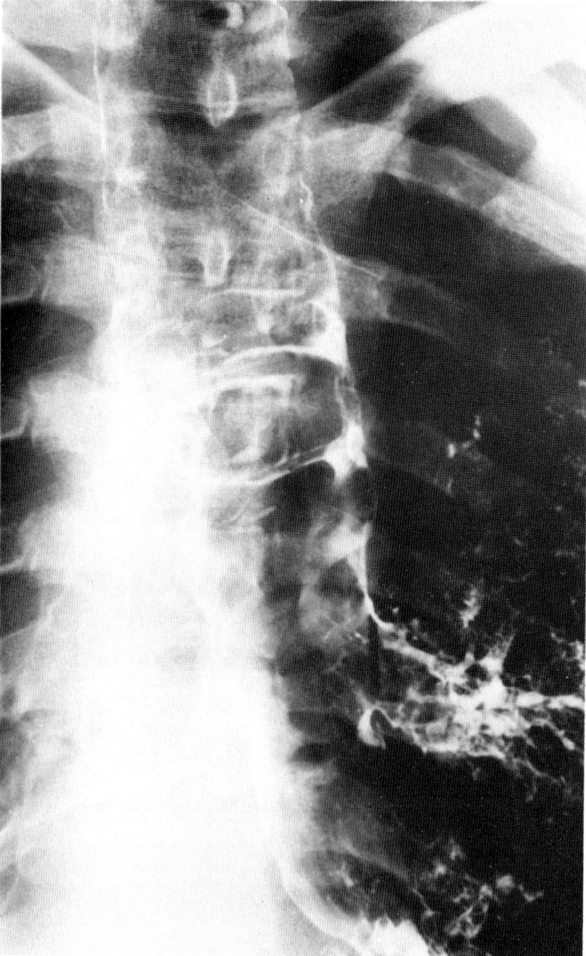

Fig. 17.34 Tracheobronchomegaly. The trachea is as wide as the vertebral bodies. The major bronchi are also wide; there was minor peripheral bronchiectasis in the lower lobes. The patient had recurrent chest infections.

pathological events and radiographic abnormalities. Following the primary insult there is a period of shock from which the patient recovers spontaneously or is resuscitated. There follows a latent interval of hours or days before respiratory distress supervenes. The patient becomes dyspnoeic, tachypnoeic, cyanosed and hypoxic. The respiratory distress is refractory and mechanical ventilation is instituted. Improvement may then follow or a deterioration requiring progressively higher ventilation pressures and oxygen concentrations. The mortality rate is approximately 40% and results from multi-organ failure, irreversible fibrotic lung disease or superadded lung infection.

This chain of events is initiated by damage to alveolar and capillary cells which allows leakage of proteinaceous oedema fluid into the alveolar walls and air spaces. The damage results from the release or activation of many injurious substances including catecholamines, serotonin, vasoactive peptides and complement. The condition is further aggravated by ischaemia, overhydration, oxygen toxicit and consumption coagulopathy. With the latter the clottin factors may be reduced to a level at which spontaneou bleeding is likely to occur.

Initially the histology is one of *haemorrhagic oedem* followed within the first week by hyperplasia of type pneumocytes and the formation of hyaline membranes Type 2 pneumocytes are the repair cells of the alveoli an anything which delays or interrupts the repair proces causes a *fibroblastic proliferation*. There is a rapid increas in lung collagen and within a few weeks the lungs ar irreversibly fibrotic and the architecture destroyed.

Radiological appearances. When the symptoms c respiratory distress first arise the chest radiograph i usually normal and this paradox will suggest massiv pulmonary embolism. A few show evidence of interstitia oedema with Kerley B lines and perivascular cuffing bu this is unusual. At 12 hours a pattern of bilateral patch alveolar opacities appears. This will suggest pulmonar oedema unrelated to heart failure because the heart size i normal. Moreover there is no pleural effusion o pulmonary vessel engorgement. Thereafter there is a rapi and massive extension of the opacities which are unaffecte by diuretics.

After the first week *complications* make their appearance Infection by Gram-negative organisms is common and wil be suggested by the presence of multiple abscess cavitie and pleural effusion. Interstitial pulmonary emphysema pneumomediastinum and pneumothorax are usuall complications of mechanical ventilation. Interstitial emphysema, producing as it does blebs of air within th pulmonary opacities, may give a spurious appearance o improvement. Segmental pulmonary angiography throug an occluding balloon catheter has been performed in th ITU using a single film technique and the results may hav prognostic significance. Those showing pruning o pulmonary artery side branches, occlusions, filling defect or early pulmonary venous filling have a poor prognosis a these changes are largely irreversible.

Examples of the adult respiratory distress syndrome ma have their own individual features relating to the nature o the initiating cause, as in 'pump' lung after cardiopulmonary by-pass, Paraquat poisoning, toxic inhalations an fat embolism (Fig. 17.35).

OXYGEN TOXICITY

Exposure to concentrations of oxygen above 50% for mor than three days is followed by signs of pulmonary damage There is increased permeability of the capillary endothelium and alveolar epithelium allowing leakage of proteinaceous fluid into the alveolar walls and air spaces. O continued exposure there follows fibroblastic proliferatio and permanent interstitial fibrosis. Radiographically th lesions are initially ill-defined alveolar opacities changin

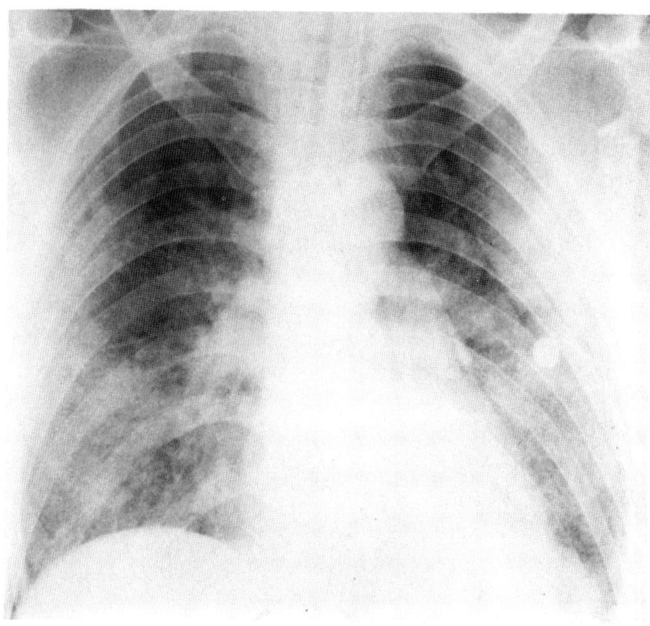

Fig. 17.35 Adult respiratory distress syndrome. Fat embolism from multiple skeletal trauma; diffuse alveolar opacities.

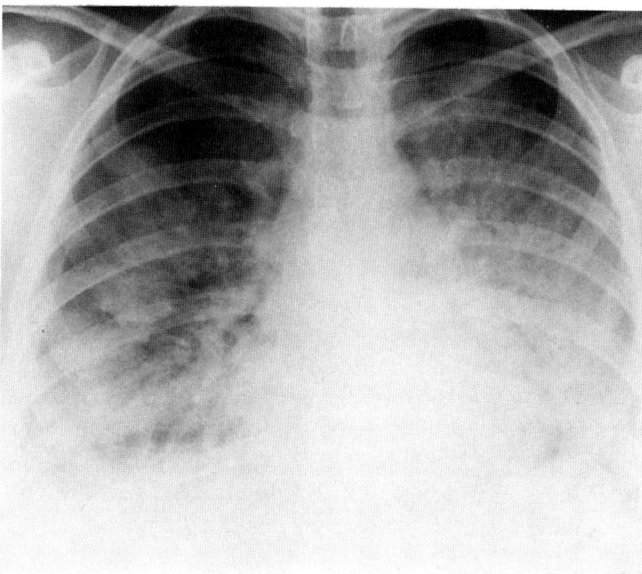

Fig. 17.36 Staphylococcal toxic shock. Extensive alveolar opacification. *Staph. aureus* phage type 3C-55 isolated from a vaginal tampon.

in the proliferative stage to coarse, linear and reticular formations.

STAPHYLOCOCCAL TOXIC SHOCK SYNDROME

This is a clearly defined syndrome caused by *Staphylococcus aureus* of certain phage types. It came into prominence when reports appeared of it affecting menstruating women using a superabsorbent type of vaginal tampon which provided an ideal environment for the growth of the organism. An exotoxin is produced and it is this which, when absorbed, causes the disease. No organisms are to be found in the blood or tissues remote from the primary site of infection. Abscesses and postoperative wound infection can also be the site of infection.

The illness has an acute onset with major systemic symptoms. Cardinal features are *hypotension*, *oliguria* and an *erythematous rash* which desquamates in the recovery stages. *Thrombocytopenia* is common and occasionally diffuse intravascular coagulation occurs. Pulmonary involvement is not invariable but when it occurs it is indistinguishable from the *adult respiratory distress syndrome* due to other causes (Fig. 17.36).

THE LUNGS IN CHRONIC RENAL FAILURE

Microscopic calcification undetected during life is often found at post-mortem in the lungs of patients who have had long-term haemodialysis. It is found in the lumen and walls of alveoli, in bronchi and vessels. If sufficiently profuse it may appear on the chest radiograph as a fine diffuse micronodulation or as 'pulmonary oedema' but only rarely is it identifiable as discrete foci of calcification. It might be suspected if the 'pulmonary oedema' is unusually dense or fails to respond to appropriate treatment. Such patients will usually also have fibrotic changes in the alveolar walls.

PULMONARY ALVEOLAR MICROLITHIASIS

Innumerable fine calculi like grains of sand form within alveoli but with surprisingly little change in other lung structures until late in the disease. There is an even distribution throughout the lungs but the shadowing is denser at the bases where the lung is thicker. The outlines of heart and vessels are obscured and the lungs may seem to be encased in a cortical shell of calcification. The only condition likely to be confused with microlithiasis is *stannosis*. Genetic factors are involved and reduced mucociliary clearance has been reported but otherwise little is known of its aetiology.

IDIOPATHIC PULMONARY OSSIFICATION

This rare condition has also been described under a variety of other names, including ossifying pneumonitis, bony metaplasia of lung and arboriform pulmonary ossification. In its usual form the delicate branching or lace-like pattern of dystrophic bone formation in the lower parts of the lungs is sufficiently distinctive to suggest the diagnosis. The cause is unknown and there are no symptoms attributable to the condition.

THE ADVERSE EFFECTS OF DRUGS ON THE LUNGS

The two types of drugs to be considered here are those which can produce reactions in all individuals and those in which idiosyncrasy or hypersensitivity are a precondition. Therapy with the first group of drugs is only justifiable in extreme circumstances since almost by definition there is a narrow margin between therapeutic and toxic dose and the research effort is directed to defining that margin or finding an effective less toxic substitute. Most of the members of this group will therefore be used in tumour chemotherapy or immunosuppression. In the second group the reaction is unexpected, albeit well recognized, and is frequently ascribed to allergy though not always correctly.

No list of drug reactions is ever complete. However thoroughly new drugs are tested in clinical trials, their introduction into widespread use will uncover unexpected reactions, hence the need for systems of surveillance.

The lungs with their large capillary bed are especially vulnerable to blood-borne injurious agents. Drugs may initiate, precipitate or potentiate asthma, common ones in this respect being *antibiotics*, *contrast media*, *aspirin* and *beta-adrenoceptor blockers*.

The gas exchanging parts of the lungs may be damaged by a direct toxic action or by processes suggestive of immunological mechanisms. In either case *fibrosis* is liable to occur following an acute inflammatory oedema, or develop insidiously. *Nitrofurantoin* is a drug which provides a model of a hypersensitivity reaction. The onset is acute with pulmonary oedema, either alveolar or interstitial and there are septal lines and pleural effusions. Eosinophilia is often present. With continued use a fibrosing alveolitis occasionally develops. Drugs with a similar exudative response include *aspirin*, *thiazide diuretics*, *sulphonamides*, *amiodarone*, *methotrexate* and *monoamine oxidase inhibitors* (Figs 17.14A and B).

Immunological mechanisms are also thought to be involved in lupus-like reactions caused by drugs such as *penicillin*, *procainamide* and *isoniazide*. The pulmonary signs are a non-specific pneumonitis, pleural effusions and pleural fibrosis.

Cytotoxic drugs such as *bleomycin*, *busulphan*, *cyclophosphamide* and *chlorambucil* are directly damaging to the lungs eliciting an intra-alveolar exudation followed by fibrous thickening of the alveolar walls. During their administration there is no interval of time after which the lungs can be considered safe from attack but after withdrawal the risk of reactions declines rapidly except in the case of cyclophosphamide where the risk can persist for months. *Radiotherapy* to the thorax potentiates the pulmonary toxicity of these drugs. Bleomycin and busulphan reactions are dose dependent. Busulphan occasionally causes pulmonary calcification or ossification. The radiographic signs are widespread reticular or reticulo-nodular opacities. An acute stage with patchy alveolar opacities is sometimes observed. The differentiation of drug reactions from recurrence or progression of the disease for which they are being given and also from opportunistic infection is clearly important and the contribution of radiology is useful but limited.

Few drug reactions feature hilar or mediastinal node enlargement, a useful point in differential diagnosis. The exception is *phenytoin* where the histology can be confused with lymphoma.

Penicillamine is unusual in the variety of its possible reactions. It can cause pulmonary eosinophilia, miliary shadows, pulmonary haemorrhage and fibrosing alveolitis.

In any diffuse lung disease the possibility that it may be due to drugs requires consideration and the appropriate enquiries should be made.

REFERENCES AND SUGGESTIONS FOR FURTHER READING

Breatnach, E. & Kerr, I. (1982) The radiology of cryptogenic obliterative bronchiolitis. *Clinical Radiology*, **33**, 657–661.

Fairfax, A. J., Haslam, P. L., Pavia, D., Sheahan, N. F., Bateman, J. R. M., Agnew, J. E., Clarke, S. W. & Turner-Warwick, M. (1981) Pulmonary disorders associated with Sjögren's syndrome. *Quarterly Journal of Medicine*, **50**, 279–295.

Davies, D., Crowther, J. S. & MacFarlane, A. (1975) Idiopathic progressive pulmonary fibrosis. *Thorax*, **30**, 316–325.

Gaensler, E. A. & Carrington, C. B. (1977) Peripheral opacities in chronic eosinophilic pneumonia: the photographic negative of pulmonary oedema. *American Journal of Roentgenology*, **128**, 1–13.

Himmelfarb, E., Wells, S. & Rabinowitz, J. G. (1972) The radiologic spectrum of cardiopulmonary amyloidosis. *Chest*, **72**,327–332.

Hunninghake, G. W. & Fauci, A. S. (1979) Pulmonary involvement in the collagen vascular diseases. *American Revue of Respiratory Disease*, **119**, 471–503.

Julsrud, P. R., Brown, L. R., Li, C–Y., Rosenow, E. C. & Crowe, J. K. (1978) Pulmonary processes of mature-appearing lymphocytes: pseudolymphoma, well-differentiated lymphocytic lymphoma and lymphocytic interstitial pneumonitis. *Radiology*, **127**, 289–296.

Liebow, A. A. (1973) Pulmonary angiitis and granulomatosis. *American Revue of Respiratory Disease*, **108**, 1–18.

MacFarlane, J. D., Dieppe, P. A., Rigden, B. G. & Clark, T. J. H. (1978) Pulmonary and pleural lesions in rheumatoid disease. *British Journal of Diseases of the Chest*, **72**: 288–300.

Scadding, J. G. (1974) Diffuse pulmonary alveolar fibrosis. *Thorax*, **29**, 271–281.

Talner, L. B., Gmelich, J. T., Liebow, A. A & Greenspan, R. H (1970) The syndrome of bronchial mucocele and regional hyperinflation of the lung. *American Journal of Roentgenology*, **110**, 675–686.

rner-Warwick, M. (1974) A perspective view on widespread pulmonary fibrosis. *British Medical Journal*, **2**, 371–376.
rner-Warwick, M., & Dewar, A. (1982) Pulmonary haemorrhage and pulmonary haemosiderosis. *Clinical Radiology*, **33**, 361–370.
Williams, D. M., Krick, J. A., & Remington, J. S. (1976) Pulmonary infection in the compromised host. *American Revue of Respiratory Disease*, **114**, 359–394.

CHAPTER 18

CHEST TRAUMA: THE POST-OPERATIVE CHEST: INTENSIVE CARE: RADIATION

CHEST TRAUMA

The thorax may be affected by direct trauma, or as a result of trauma elsewhere in the body. Direct trauma may be the result of penetrating or non-penetrating injury. The usual causes of penetrating injury are shooting, stabbing and shrapnel wounds, and are comparatively unusual except in wartime. Unfortunately, however, urban violence is on the increase, and such injuries are becoming more frequent. *Thoracic surgery* is a special category of penetrating trauma and is discussed separately. Non-penetrating injuries may be caused by falls, blows or blasts. Car accidents resulting in deceleration injuries are increasing in frequency. Trauma to other areas of the body may have thoracic complications. For example, bone fractures may cause fat emboli, and pulmonary complications are common following abdominal surgery.

Radiological techniques

The severely injured patient, the post-operative patient and the patient in the intensive care ward are a true test of the radiographer's skill. In no areas of radiography are good quality films more necessary, and in no other group of patients are good quality films more difficult to produce.

The injured patient is usually brought to the X-ray department, where, if possible, an erect PA film should be taken. A high kV technique is desirable in order to see mediastinal detail, but if this is not possible a penetrated grid radiograph should be taken. A lateral film may be useful. If the patient is severely injured it is necessary to make do with supine films. Accessory views described in the section on the pleura may be indicated. In the acute stage multiple views for rib fractures are not indicated, since it is complications of the fractures that really matter, whether or not the fractures are seen.

The post-operative and the intensive care ward patient will usually be examined with mobile X-ray equipment. An erect AP film, with the patient sitting up is preferable, but a supine film at end inspiration is better than a film taken with the patient slouched and at end expiration. The highest kV and mA possible and high speed screens will minimize motion unsharpness. Horizontal beam lateral decubitus films are often useful to assess pleural fluid, pneumothoraces and fluid levels.

Ultrasound is useful in assessing the pleura and the subphrenic areas, and a *mobile gamma camera* may be brought to the patient if pulmonary emboli are suspected.

The films of intensive care ward patients need to be examined with full clinical information, since many of the pathological processes to which these patients are susceptible produce similar radiographic manifestations. Serial films need to be evaluated for general trends, as day-to-day changes may be inapparent, and special attention needs to be given to monitoring and life support devices.

INJURIES TO THE THORACIC CAGE

Rib fractures are common, and may be single, multiple, unilateral or bilateral. Healed rib fractures are a fairly frequent incidental finding on the chest X-ray, and in the absence of a history of trauma may be associated with excessive consumption of alcohol. Acute rib fractures are often difficult to see if there is no displacement, and their presence may only be inferred by surrounding haematoma producing an extrapleural opacity. In cases of chest trauma the chest X-ray is more important in detecting a complication of rib fracture than the fracture itself. However, fracture of the first three ribs is often associated with major intrathoracic injury.

Complications of rib fracture include a flail segment, pneumothorax, haemothorax and subcutaneous emphysema. A *flail segment* is usually apparent clinically, the affected part of the chest wall being sucked in during inspiration, possibly compromising the underlying lung. The chest X-ray will show several adjacent ribs to be fractured in two places, or bilateral rib fractures.

The fractured ends of ribs may penetrate underlying pleura and lung and cause a *pneumothorax*, *haemothorax*, *haemopneumothorax* (Fig. 18.1) or *intrapulmonary haemorrhage*. Air may also escape into the chest wall and cause *subcutaneous emphysema* (Fig. 18.2).

Stress fractures of the first and second ribs are sometimes an incidental finding on the chest X-ray. *Cough*

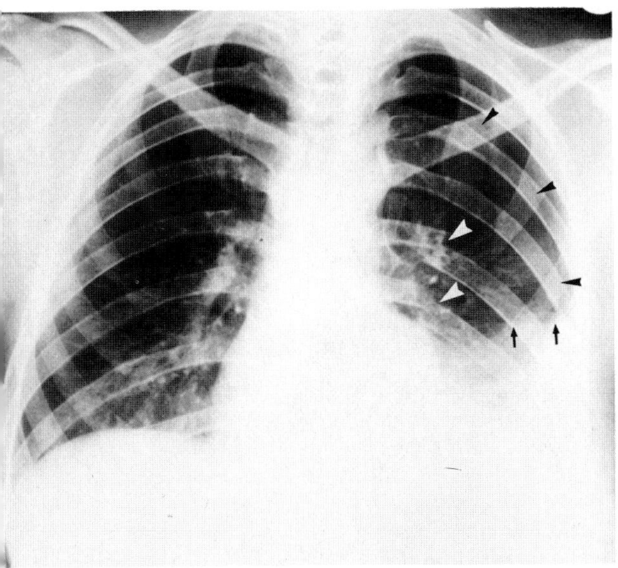

Fig. 18.1 Rib fractures and haemopneumothorax. Adult female, car accident. The left seventh and eighth ribs are fractured (white arrowheads). A pneumothorax (black arrowheads) is present, and a fluid level (arrows) is seen in the pleural space.

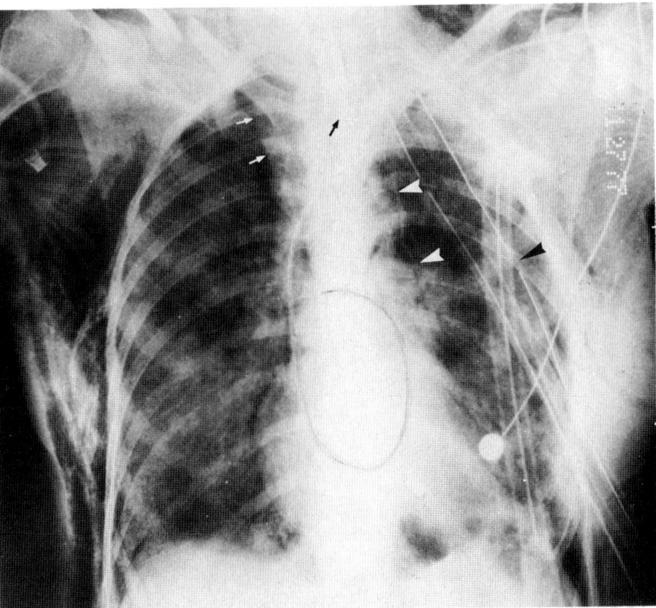

Fig. 18.2 Massive chest trauma. Adult female, car crash. Gross subcutaneous emphysema extends over the chest wall, outlining muscle planes. The right clavicle is fractured. Several ribs were fractured, but not seen on this film. Mediastinal emphysema separates pleura from the descending aorta (white arrowheads). A mediastinal haematoma is present (white arrows). Widespread lung contusion is obscured by the subcutaneous emphysema. Note tracheostomy tube (black arrow), left pleural tubes, with side-hole indicated (black arrowhead), Swan-Ganz catheter and ECG lead.

fractures usually affect the sixth to ninth ribs in the posterior axillary line, but may not be visible until callus has formed.

Fractures of the sternum usually require a lateral film or tomography for visualization.

Fractures of the thoracic spine may be associated with a para-spinal shadow which represents haematoma.

Fractures of the clavicle may be associated with injury of the subclavian vessels or brachial plexus, and posterior dislocation of the clavicle at the sternoclavicular joint may cause injury to the trachea, oesophagus, great vessels or nerves of the superior mediastinum.

Herniation of lung tissue is usually associated with obvious rib fractures, but may only be apparent on tangential views in full inspiration.

INJURIES TO THE DIAPHRAGM

Laceration of the diaphragm may result from penetrating or non-penetrating trauma to the chest or abdomen. The liver protects the right hemidiaphragm, so that the left dome is more often involved. The affected dome is not visible, and stomach, omentum, small and large bowel, spleen, kidney and pancreas may herniate into the chest (Fig. 18.3). The plain film appearance is usually characteristic, but barium swallow or enema, or rarely CT may be required for accurate assessment. *Isotope liver–spleen scan* may show a characteristic appearance of these organs in the thorax.

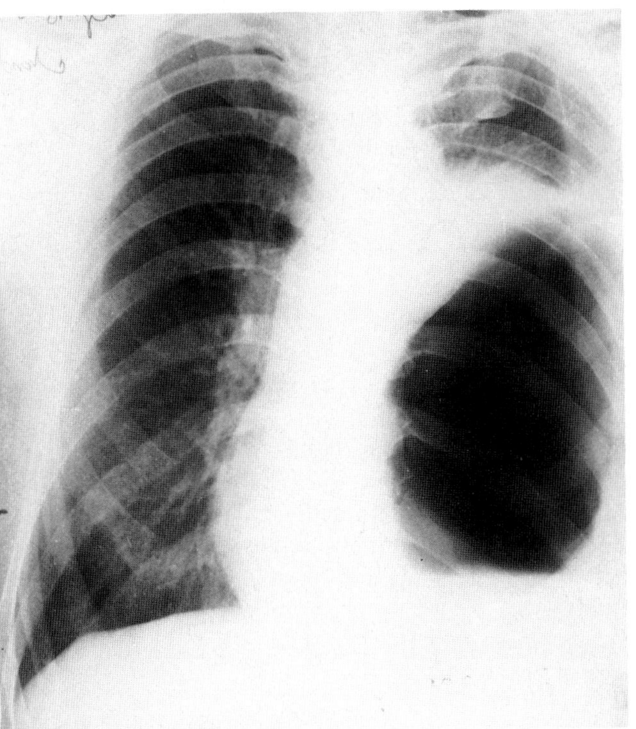

Fig. 18.3 Rupture of diaphragm. Male aged 58 years. Fell from building 13 years earlier breaking ankles and injuring chest. Presents with persistent vomiting. Chest radiograph demonstrates distended stomach in left hemithorax, confirmed by barium swallow. Thoracotomy revealed stomach herniating into left pleural cavity through 5 cm rent in left hemidiaphragm.

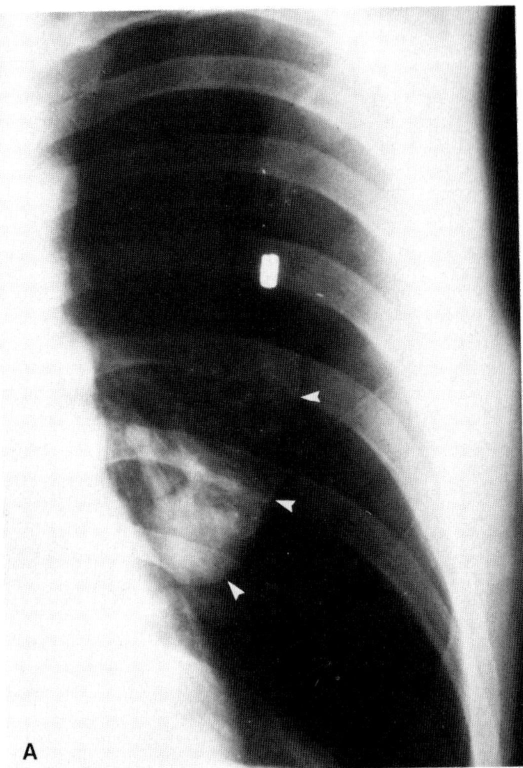

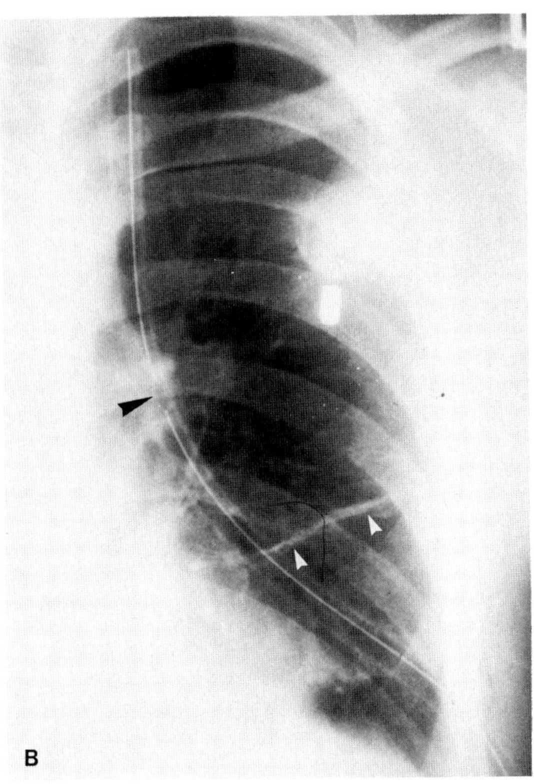

Fig. 18.4 Penetrating chest injury. Adult male, bullet wound. (**A**) Large pneumothorax (arrowheads), and bullet in chest wall. (**B**) Following insertion of pleural tube (black arrowhead) the lung re-expands revealing haematoma in bullet track. Band shadow in lower zone (white arrowheads) represents sub-segmental atelectasis.

INJURIES TO THE PLEURA

Pneumothorax, as mentioned above, may be a complication of rib fracture, and is then usually associated with a haemothorax (Fig. 18.1). If no ribs are fractured, pneumothorax is secondary to a pneumo-mediastinum or a penetrating chest injury (Fig. 18.4). Pneumothorax due to a penetrating injury is liable to develop increased pressure, resulting in a *tension pneumothorax*, which may require emergency decompression.

Haemothorax may also occur with or without rib fractures (Fig. 18.5), and is due to laceration of intercostal or pleural vessels. If a pneumothorax is also present a fluid level will be seen on a horizontal beam film (Fig. 18.1).

Pleural effusion may also result from trauma. Open injuries to the pleura are prone to infection and development of an empyema (see Fig. 13.15).

INJURIES TO THE LUNG

Pulmonary contusion is due to haemorrhagic exudation into the alveoli and interstitial spaces and appears as patchy, non-segmental consolidation (Figs. 18.5 and 18.7). Shadowing appears within the first few hours of penetrating or non-penetrating trauma, and usually shows improvement within 2 days, and clearing within 3 or 4 days (Fig. 18.6). When contusion due to a bullet wound clears, a longitudinal haematoma in the bullet track may become visible (Fig. 18.4).

Pulmonary lacerations as a result of non-penetrating trauma may appear as round, thin-walled cystic spaces. Acutely, the laceration may be obscured by pulmonary contusion, but appears as the surrounding consolidation resolves. If the laceration is filled with blood it appears as a homogeneous round opacity, and if partly blood filled it may have a fluid level. Such pulmonary haematomas or blood cysts gradually decrease in size, but may take a few months to completely resolve. Pulmonary haematomas are often multiple (Fig. 18.7).

Torsion of a lung is a rare result of severe thoracic trauma, usually to a child. The lung twists about the hilum through 180°. If unrelieved the lung may become gangrenous and appear opaque on the chest X-ray.

Atelectasis and **compensatory hyperinflation** after a chest injury may be due to aspiration of blood or mucus into the bronchi. Bronchoscopy may be indicated. Atelectasis may also occur secondary to decreased respiratory movement.

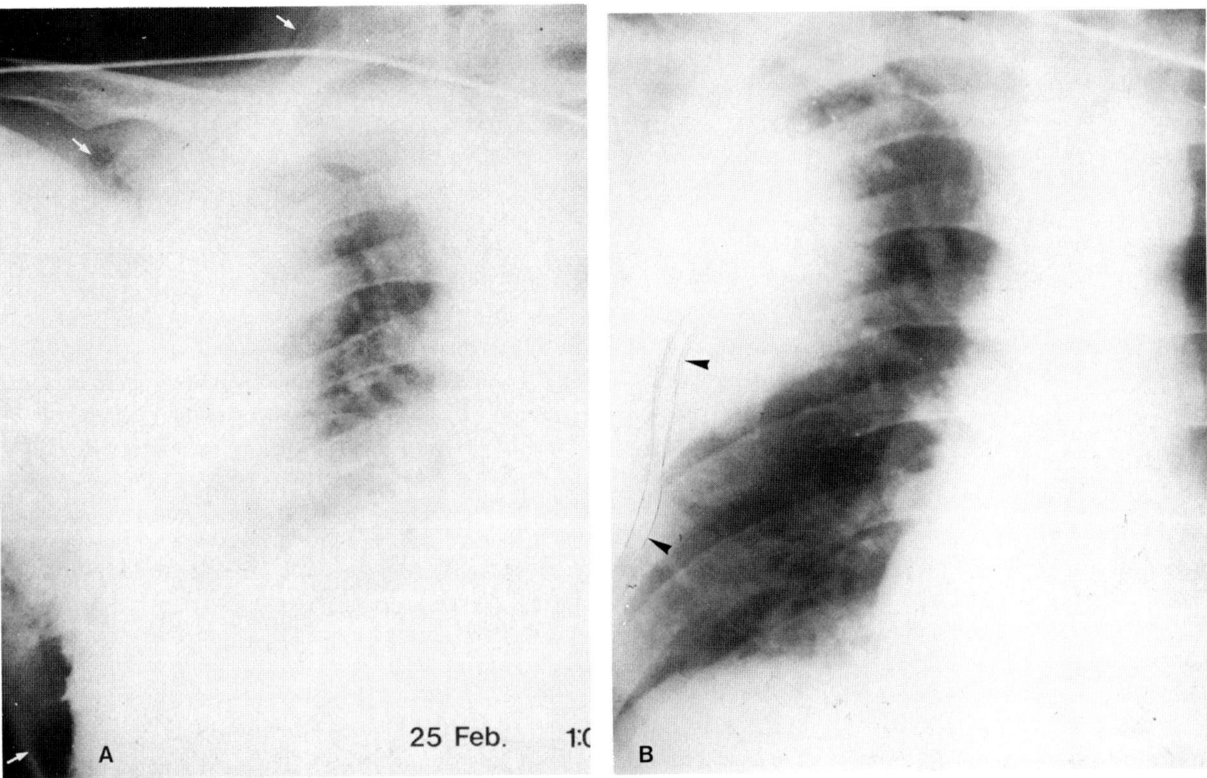

Fig. 18.5 Pulmonary contusion and haemothorax. Adult male, gun-shot injury. (**A**) Sub-cutaneous emphysema is present over chest wall (arrows), and dense shadowing extends over most of hemithorax. (**B**) Following insertion of pleural drain (arrowheads) the lower half of the shadowing, due to blood in the pleural space, has gone. The remaining opacity is pulmonary contusion. A few bullet fragments are visible above the contusion.

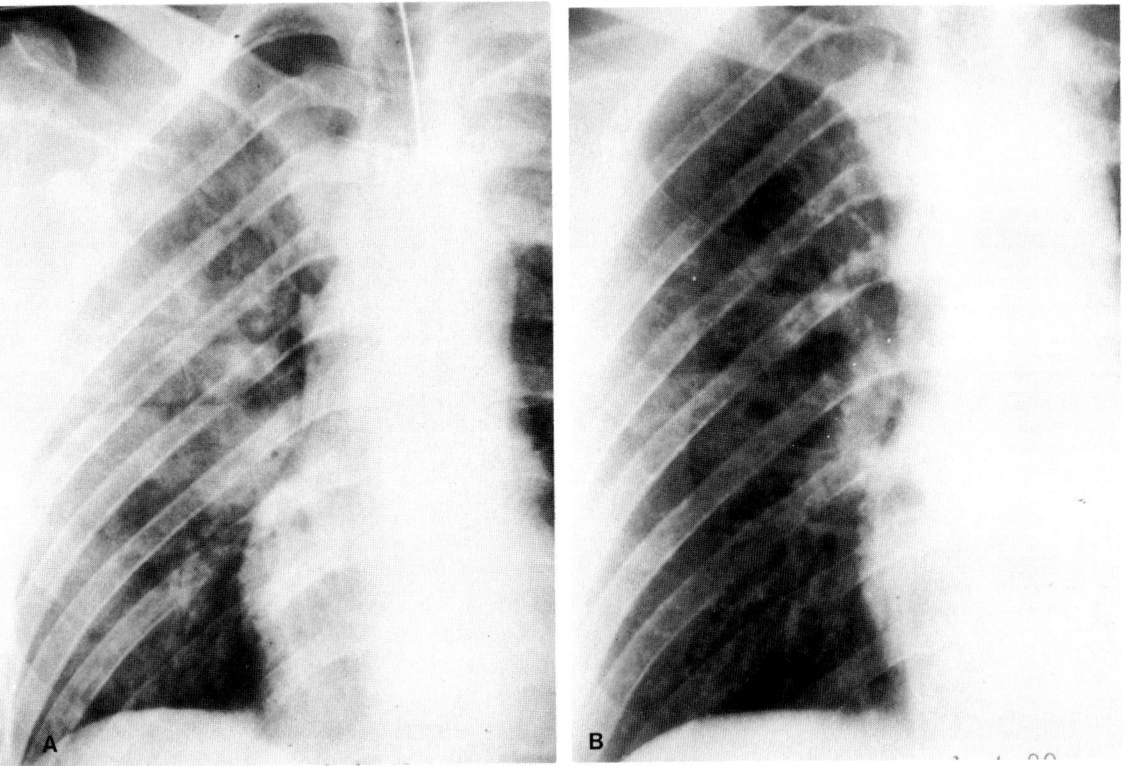

Fig. 18.6 Pulmonary contusion. Adult male, car accident. (**A**) Extensive consolidation throughout right lung. Left lung was clear. No rib fractures. (**B**) 4 days later the shadowing has resolved.

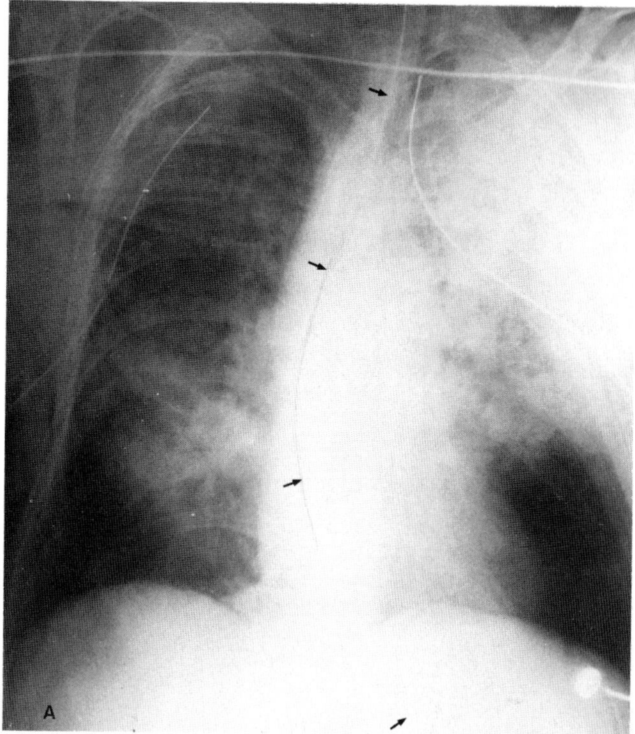

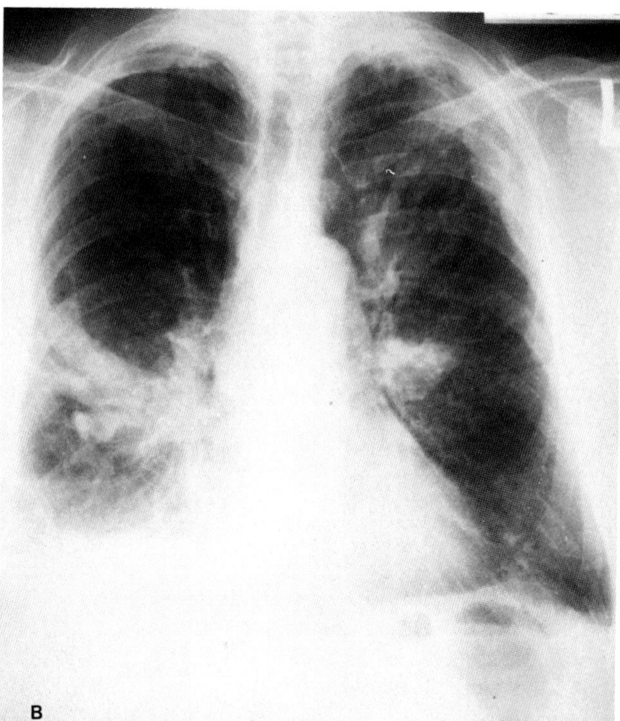

Fig. 18.7 Pulmonary contusion and haematomas. Male aged 18 years trampled on by a bull. (**A**) Extensive consolidation is present throughout both lungs, particularly in the left upper zone. Subcutaneous emphysema is seen over the right hemithorax. Bilateral pleural tubes and a naso-gastric tube (arrows) are present. (**B**) 6 days later the contusion has resolved and multiple pulmonary haematomas and some extra pleural haematomas have become visible. (**C**) One month later the haematomas are smaller.

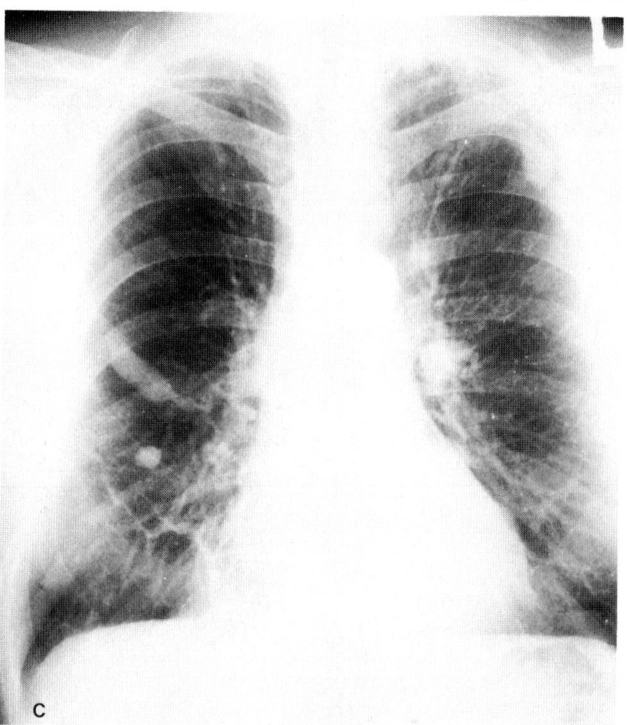

Pulmonary oedema as a manifestation of the adult respiratory distress syndrome may occur after major trauma.

Fat embolism is a rare complication of multiple fractures, due to fat globules from the bone marrow entering the systemic veins and embolising to the lungs. Poorly defined, nodular opacities appear throughout both lungs. If the patient survives the opacities resolve within a few days. The diagnosis is confirmed if fat globules are present in the sputum or urine.

INJURIES TO THE TRACHEA AND BRONCHI

Laceration or rupture of a major airway is an uncommon result of severe chest trauma, commonly in a car crash. Fracture of the first three ribs is often present, and mediastinal emphysema and pneumothorax are common (Fig. 18.8). The injury is usually in the trachea just above the carina, or in a main bronchus just distal to the carina. If the bronchial sheath is preserved there may be no immediate signs or symptoms, but tracheostenosis or bronchostenosis may occur later. Tomography may be helpful in diagnosis, but bronchoscopy is the best diagnostic method in the acute stage.

INJURIES TO THE MEDIASTINUM

Pneumomediastinum or mediastinal emphysema are terms that describe the presence of air between the tissue

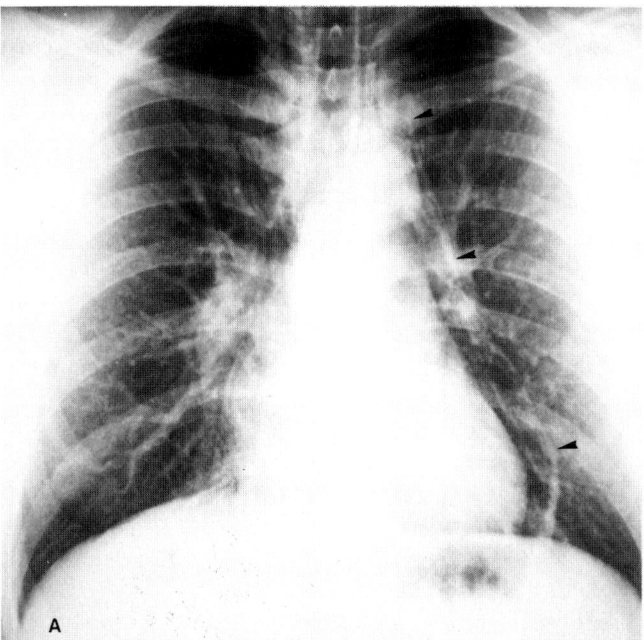

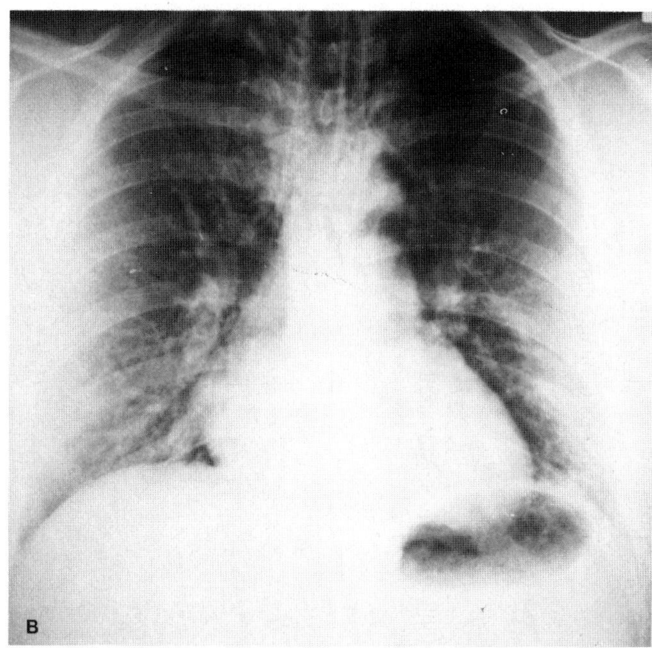

Fig. 18.8 Ruptured trachea. Adult male, deceleration injury, dyspnoea and chest pain. (**A**) Pneumomediastinum with linear lucencies in mediastinum and displacement of mediastinal pleura (arrowheads). (**B**) One hour later following a bout of coughing a left pneumothorax has developed. Bronchoscopy revealed a ruptured trachea.

planes of the mediastinum. Air may reach here as a result of interstitial pulmonary emphysema, perforation of the oesophagus, trachea or a bronchus, or from a penetrating chest injury. *Interstitial pulmonary emphysema* is a result of alveolar wall rupture due to high intra-alveolar pressure and may occur during violent coughing, asthmatic attacks, severe crush injuries, or be due to positive pressure ventilation. Air dissects centrally along the perivascular sheath to reach the mediastinum. Rarely air may dissect into the mediastinum from a pneumoperitoneum. A pneumomediastinum may extend beyond the thoracic inlet into the neck, and over the chest wall. Pneumothorax is a common complication of pneumomediastinum, but the converse never occurs.

Pneumomediastinum usually produces vertical, translucent streaks in the mediastinum. This represents gas separating and outlining the soft tissue planes and structures of the mediastinum. Gas shadows may extend up into the neck (Fig. 18.9), or dissect extrapleurally over the diaphragm, or extend into the soft tissue planes of the chest wall causing subcutaneous emphysema (Figs. 18.9 and 18.10). The mediastinal pleura may be displaced laterally, and become visible as a linear soft tissue shadow parallel to the mediastinum (Figs. 18.2, 18.8, 18.9, 18.10). If mediastinal air collects beneath the pericardium the central part of the diaphragm may be visible, producing the 'continuous diaphragm' sign (Fig. 18.10). Sometimes it may be difficult to differentiate between pneumopericardium and pneumomediastinum. In pneumopericardium gas does not extend beyond the aortic root or much beyond the main pulmonary artery (Fig. 18.14). In pneumomediastinum gas often outlines the aortic knuckle, and extends into the neck. In pneumopericar-

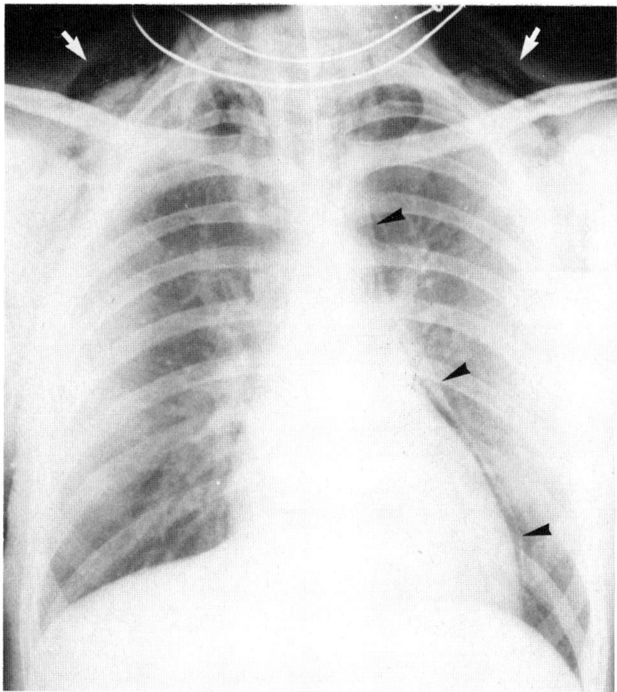

Fig. 18.9 Pneumomediastinum. Adult male, car crash. Note linear lucencies in mediastinum, extending into neck, and subcutaneous emphysema over supraclavicular fossae (arrows). The mediastinal pleura is outlined by air and displaced laterally (arrowheads).

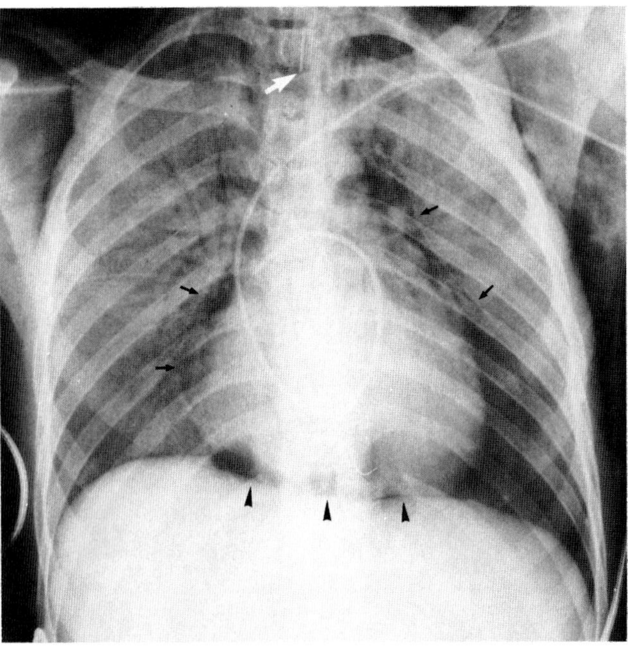

Fig. 18.10 Complications of positive pressure ventilation. Male aged 15 years. Diffuse consolidation following presumed viral pneumonia. Note endotracheal tube (white arrow) and Swan-Ganz catheter, both well positioned. Pneumomediastinum is indicated by linear lucencies in mediastinum, lateral displacement of mediastinal pleura (black arrows) and infra-pericardial air producing 'continuous diaphragm' sign (arrowheads). There is extensive bilateral subcutaneous emphysema.

dium a fluid level is often seen on horizontal beam films, and the distribution of air may alter with changes in the patient's position. The patient's position has little or no effect on a pneumomediastinum. Pneumomediastinum is relatively more common in neonates and infants and may displace the thymus or resemble a lung cyst.

Mediastinal haemorrhage may result from penetrating or non-penetrating trauma, and be due to venous or arterial bleeding. Most cases are probably unrecognized as clinical and radiographic signs are absent. Important causes include car accidents, aortic rupture and dissection, and introduction of central venous catheters. There is usually bilateral mediastinal widening (Fig. 18.11), but a localized haematoma may occur (Figs. 18.2 and 18.19).

Aortic rupture is usually the result of a car accident. Most aortic tears occur at the aortic isthmus — the site of the ligamentum arteriosum. Only 10–20% of patients survive the acute episode, but a small number may develop a chronic aneurysm at the site of the tear. The commonest acute radiographic signs are widening of the superior mediastinum, and obscuration of the aortic knuckle (Fig. 18.11). Other radiographic signs include deviation of the left main bronchus anteriorly, inferiorly and to the right, and rightward displacement of the trachea, a naso-gastric tube or the right para-spinal line. A left apical extra-pleural cap or a left haemothorax may be visible. Aortography is the definitive investigation, but CT may be diagnostic.

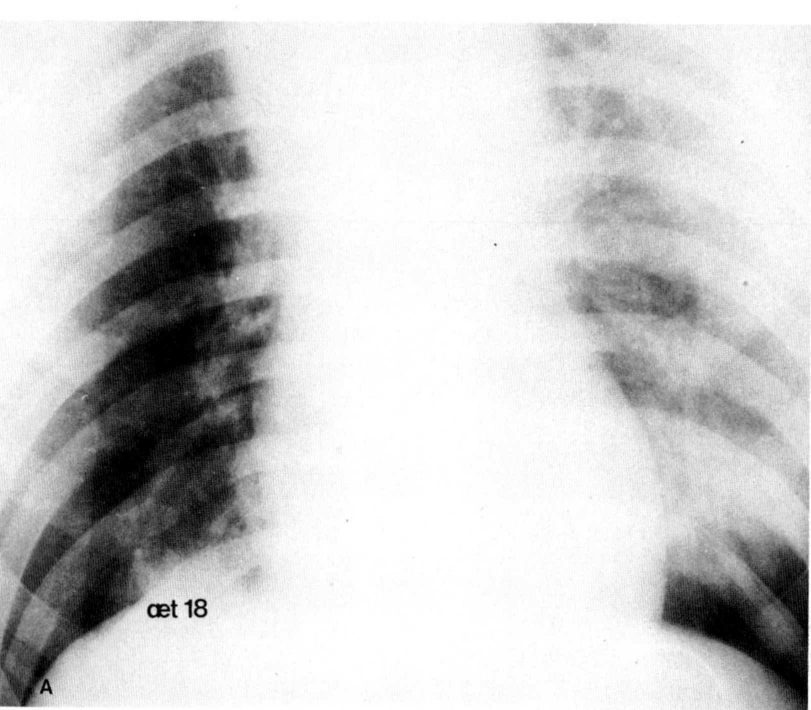

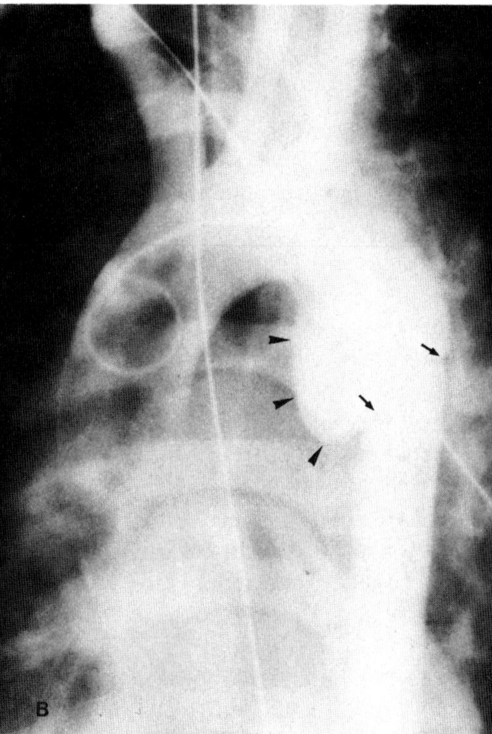

Fig. 18.11 Mediastinal haemorrhage. Male aged 18 years, car crash. (**A**) Chest radiograph shows bilateral widening of the superior mediastinum. The aorta is obscured. (**B**) Arch aortogram demonstrates aneurysm of the aortic isthmus (arrowheads) with intimal tear (arrows).

Oesophageal rupture is usually the result of instrumentation or surgery, but occasionally occurs in penetrating trauma, and is rarely spontaneous due to sudden increase of intra-oesophageal pressure (Boerhaave's syndrome). Clinically there is acute mediastinitis, and radiographically there are signs of pneumomediastinum, with or without a pneumothorax or hydropneumothorax, which is usually left sided. The diagnosis should be confirmed by a swallow using water soluble contrast medium or barium. The former is safer, and the latter radiographically superior, but carries a theoretical risk of granuloma formation in the mediastinum.

Chylothorax due to damage to the thoracic duct may become apparent hours or days after trauma. Thoracic surgery is the commonest cause.

THE POST-OPERATIVE CHEST

Intrathoracic surgery is performed most frequently for resection of all or part of a lung, or for cardiac disease. This section will discuss the usual acute changes apparent radiographically following such surgery, followed by a description of complications and late changes, and finally a description of thoracic complications of non-thoracic surgery.

THORACOTOMY

Lung resections are usually performed posterolaterally through the fourth or fifth intercostal space. Part of a rib may be resected or the ribs may simply be spread apart. Rib fractures sometimes occur, but often the surgical route is not obvious on the chest X-ray, or is marked only by some narrowing of the intercostal space, or some overlying soft tissue swelling and subcutaneous emphysema.

Following *pneumonectomy* it is important for the remaining lung to be fully ventilated, and for the mediastinum to remain close to the mid-line. Excessive mediastinal shift may compromise respiration and venous return to the heart. On the initial post-operative film the trachea should be close to the midline, the remaining lung should appear normal or slightly plethoric, and the pneumonectomy space usually contains a small amount of fluid. A drainage tube may or may not be present in the space. Over the next several days the pneumonectomy space begins to obliterate by gradual shift of the mediastinum to that side, and accumulation of fluid. The space is usually half-filled by about a week, and completely opacifies over the next 2 or 3 months (Fig. 18.12). If the mediastinum gradually moves towards the remaining lung this may indicate too rapid accumulation of fluid in the pneumonectomy space, or atelectasis in the remaining lung. A sudden shift may indicate a broncho-pleural fistula (Fig. 18.13).

Following *lobectomy* the remaining lung should expand to fill the space of the resected lobe. Immediately post-operatively pleural drains are present preventing accumulation of pleural fluid, and the mediastinum may be shifted to the side of the operation. With hyperinflation of the remaining lung the mediastinum returns to its normal position. When the drains are removed a small pleural effusion commonly occurs, but usually resolves within a few days, perhaps leaving residual pleural thickening.

With *segmental* or *subsegmental lung resections* a cut surface of lung is oversewn, and air leaks are fairly common, sometimes causing persistent pneumothorax, which may require prolonged drainage. Wire sutures or staples may be visible at the site of a bronchial stump or lesser lung resection.

Complications of thoracotomy

Post-operative spaces may persist following lobectomy and segmental or subsegmental resections. They are air spaces that correspond to the excised lung. Fluid may collect in them, but they usually resolve after a few weeks or months. If they persist and are associated with constitutional symptoms, increasing fluid and pleural thickening, an empyema or broncho-pleural fistula should be suspected.

Empyema complicating pneumonectomy, or rarely lobectomy, usually occurs a few weeks after surgery, although it may occur months or years later. Rapid accumulation of fluid may push the mediastinum to the normal side. If a fistula develops between the pneumonectomy space and a bronchus or the skin, the air–fluid level in the space will suddenly drop (Fig. 18.13). Increasing gas in the pneumonectomy space may also indicate infection by a gas-forming organism.

Broncho-pleural fistula is a communication between the bronchial tree (or lung tissue) and the pleural space. The commonest cause is a complication of *lung surgery*, but it may be the result of rupture of a *lung abscess*, erosion by a *lung cancer* or *penetrating trauma*. Broncho-pleural fistula complicating complete or partial lung resection may occur early, when it is due to faulty closure of the bronchus, but it more commonly occurs late due to infection or recurrent tumour of the bronchial stump. The usual radiographic appearance is the sudden appearance of, or increase in the amount of air in the pleural space, with a corresponding decrease in the amount of fluid in the space. A fluid level is almost always present (Fig. 18.13). If fluid enters the airways and is aspirated into the remaining lung, widespread consolidation may be seen on the chest X-ray. Sinography of the pleural space or bronchography may demonstrate the fistula.

Pleural fluid is usually seen on the chest X-ray following thoracic surgery. If the amount is excessive it may be due to bleeding or chylothorax.

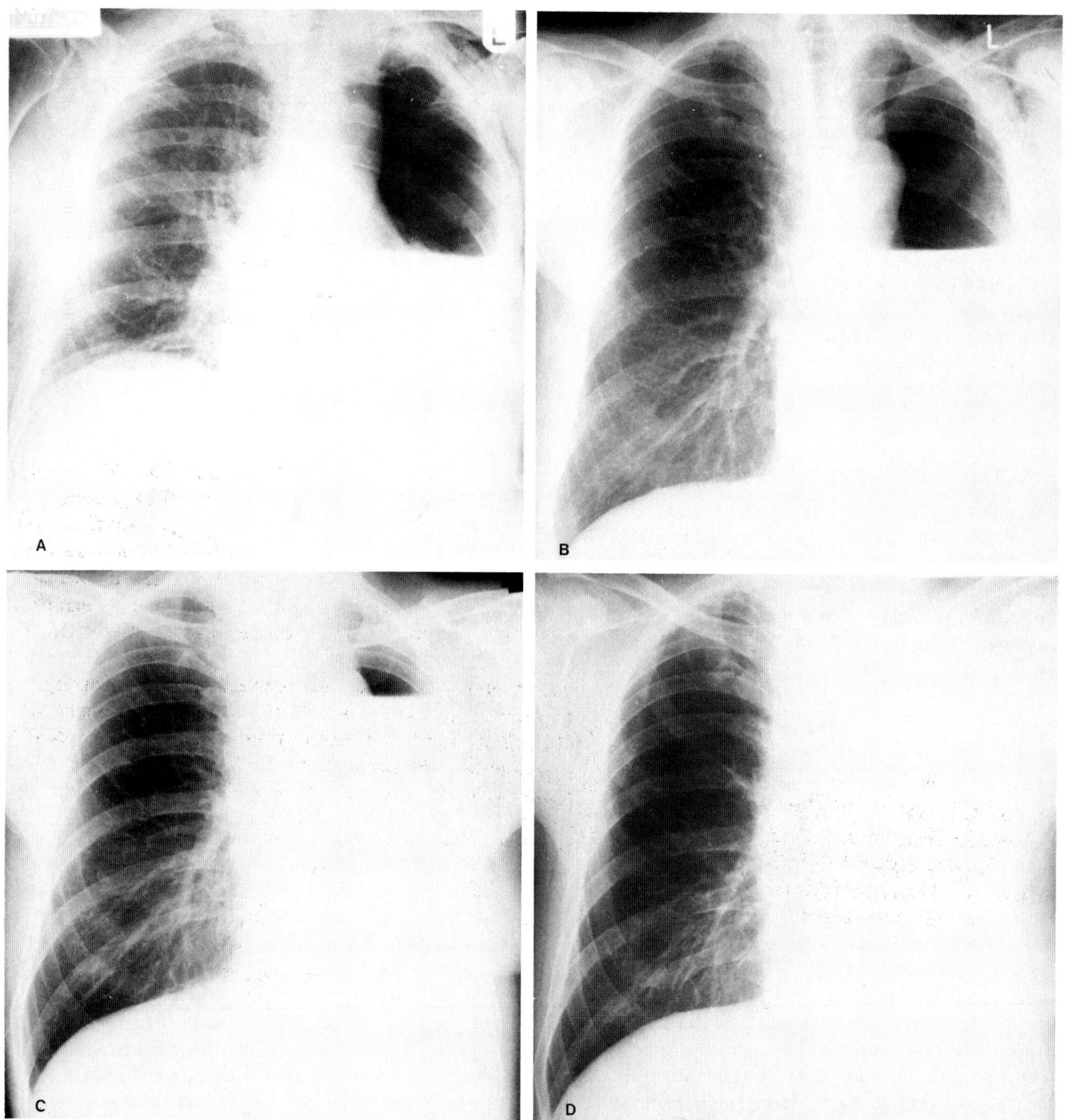

Fig. 18.12 Normal post-pneumonectomy appearances. (**A**) One day (**B**), 6 days (**C**), 5 weeks and (**D**) 8 weeks post-operatively. The pneumonectomy space is gradually obliterated by the rising fluid level, and mediastinal shift.

Diaphragmatic elevation may indicate phrenic nerve damage and is best assessed by fluoroscopy.

Other pulmonary complications of thoracic surgery include *atelectasis, aspiration pneumonia, pulmonary embolism* and *pulmonary oedema*, both cardiogenic and non-cardiogenic. These may also complicate non-thoracic surgery and are discussed below.

CARDIAC SURGERY

Most cardiac operations are performed through a *sternotomy* incision, and wire sternal sutures are often seen on the post-operative films (Figs. 18.24 and 18.25). Mitral valvotomy is now rarely performed via a *thoracotomy* incision, but this route is still used for surgery of coarctation

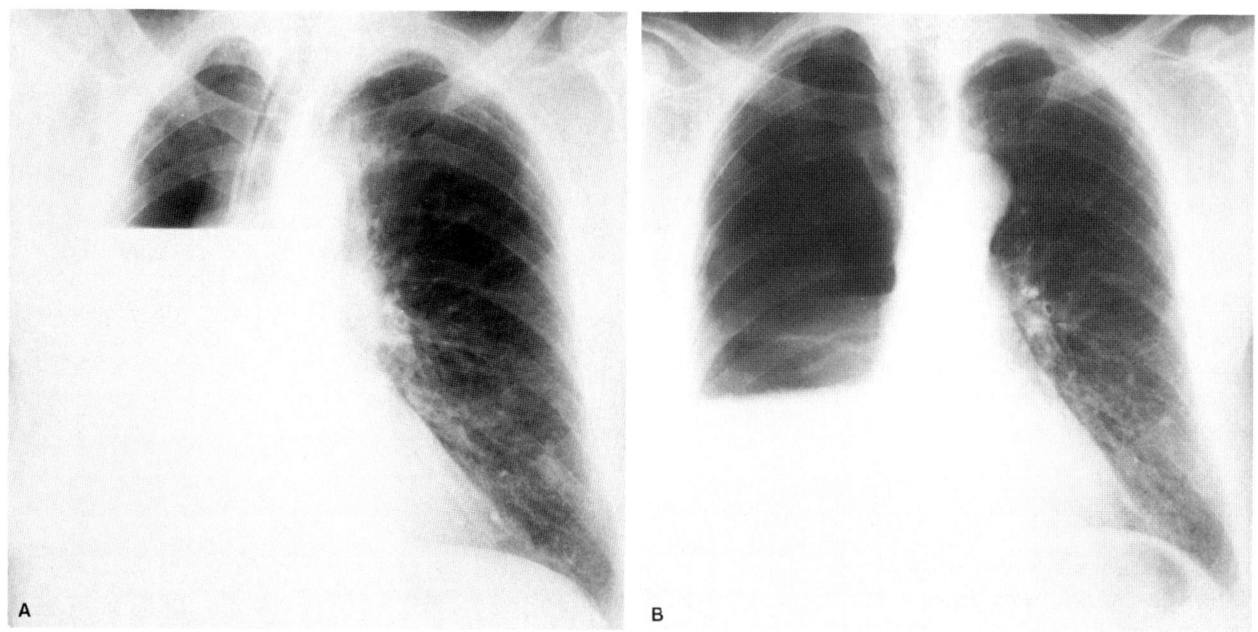

g. **18.13** Broncho-pleural fistula. (**A**) 13 days after right pneumonectomy the space is filling with fluid and the mediastinum is deviated to the right.) 2 days later after coughing up a large amount of fluid the fluid level has dropped, and the mediastinum has returned to the midline. Bronchoscopy nfirmed a right broncho-pleural fistula.

the aorta, patent ductus arteriosus, Blalock-Taussig unts and pulmonary artery banding.

Following cardiac surgery some widening of the cardio-scular silhouette is usual, and represents bleeding and dema. Marked widening of the mediastinum suggests gnificant *haemorrhage*, but the necessity for re-exploration based upon the overall clinical situation. Some air mmonly remains in the pericardium following cardiac rgery, so that the signs of *pneumopericardium* may be esent (Fig. 18.14).

Pulmonary opacities are very common following open-eart surgery, and left basal shadowing is almost invari-le, representing *atelectasis*. This shadowing usually solves over a week or two. Small *pleural effusions* are also mmon in the immediate post-operative period.

Pneumoperitoneum is sometimes seen, due to involvement the peritoneum by the sternotomy incision. It is of no athological significance.

Violation of left or right pleural space may lead to a *pneu-othorax*. Damage of a major lymphatic vessel may lead to *chylothorax* or a more localized collection — a *chyloma*. *hrenic nerve damage* may cause paresis or paralysis of a emidiaphragm.

Surgical clips or other metallic markers are sometimes sed to mark the ends of coronary artery by-pass grafts. *rosthetic heart valves* are usually visible radiographically, ut they may be difficult to see on an under-penetrated m. Their assessment fluoroscopically, angiographically or trasonographically is outside the scope of this chapter.

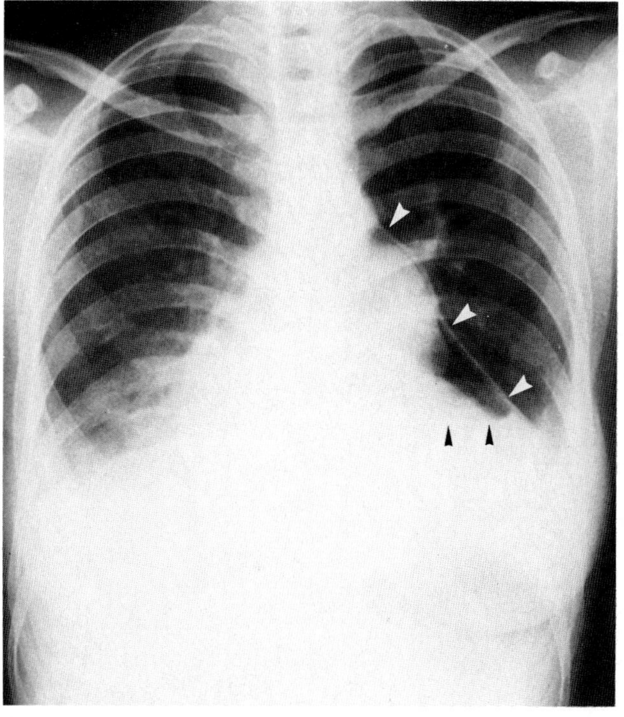

Fig. 18.14 Haemopneumopericardium. Adult female, two days after closure of atrial septal defect. The pericardium is outlined by air (white arrowheads) which does not extend as high as the aortic arch. A fluid level (black arrowheads) is present in the pericardium, and there are bilateral pleural effusions.

Sternal dehiscence may be apparent radiographically by a linear lucency appearing in the sternum and alteration in position of the sternal sutures on consecutive films. The diagnosis is usually made clinically and may be associated with osteomyelitis. A first or second rib may be fractured when the sternum is spread apart. The importance of this observation is that it may explain chest pain in the post-operative period.

The *post-pericardotomy syndrome* is probably an auto-immune phenomenon, usually occurring in the month after surgery. It presents with fever, pleurisy, and pericarditis. Pleural effusions may be visible and the cardiac silhouette may enlarge. Ultrasound will demonstrate pericardial fluid. Patchy consolidation may occur in the lung bases.

LATE APPEARANCES AFTER CHEST SURGERY

Following thoracotomy the appearance of the chest X-ray may return to normal, or evidence of surgery may persist. Resected ribs or healed rib fractures are usually obvious (Fig. 18.15). There may be irregular regeneration of a rib related to disturbed periostium. A rib space may be narrowed where a thoracotomy wound has been closed (Fig. 18.15). Rib notching may result from a Blalock-Taussig shunt between subclavian and pulmonary arteries. Pleural thickening often remains after a thoracotomy.

Re-arrangement of the remaining lung occurs after lobectomy, so that the anatomy of the fissures may be altered. Following oesophageal surgery, stomach or loops of bowel may produce unusual soft tissue opacities or fluid levels, if they have been brought up into the chest.

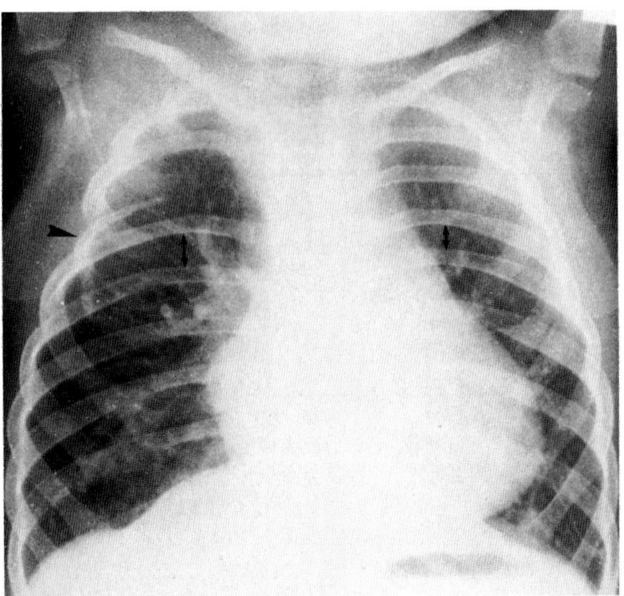

Fig. 18.15 Post-thoracotomy ribs. Right thoracotomy with partially excised, regenerating right fourth rib (arrowhead) from repair of tracheo-oesophageal fistula. Left thoracotomy, indicated by narrowed fifth intercostal space, for pulmonary artery banding for multiple ventricular septal defects.

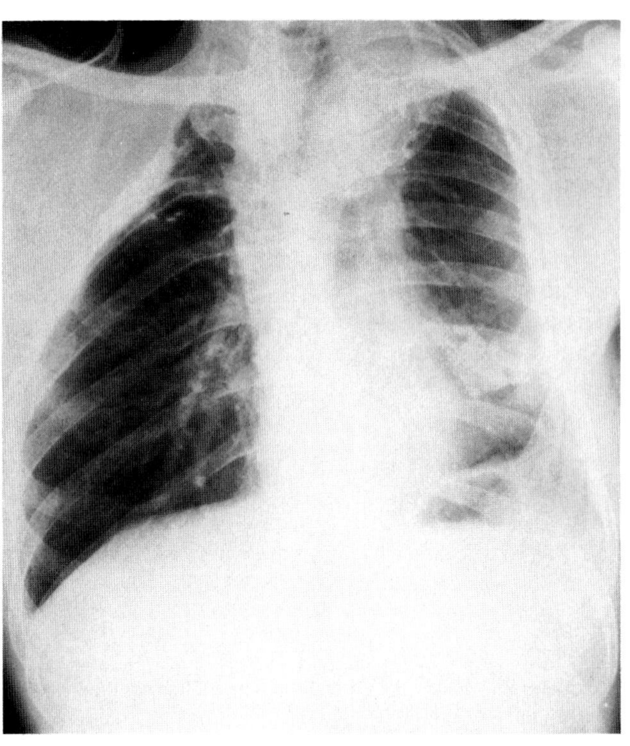

Fig. 18.16 Thoracoplasty. The first five right ribs have been removed. Left upper lobe fibrosis, bilateral apical calcification and extensive left pleural calcification are due to tuberculosis.

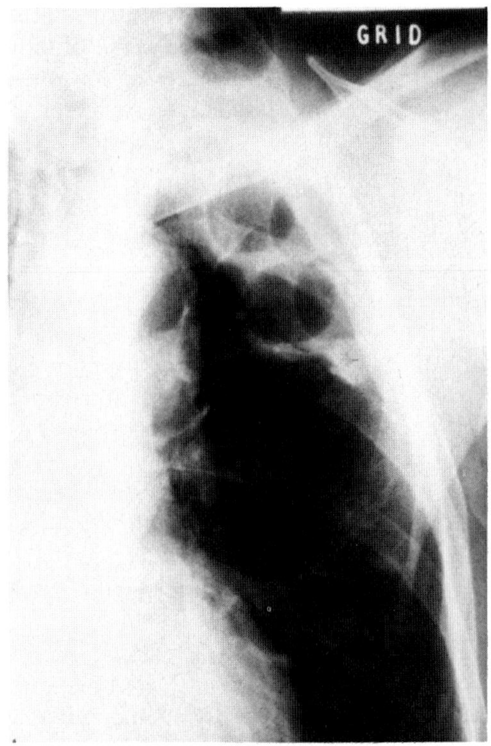

Fig. 18.17 Plombage. Several hollow balls have been inserted extra-pleurally at the left apex. The balls are slightly permeable, and the shallow fluid levels do not indicate a complication.

Surgery is now rarely performed for pulmonary tuberculosis, but many patients who have had such surgery are still alive. The object of surgery was to reduce aeration of the infected lung, usually an upper lobe. *Thoracoplasty* involved removal of the posterior parts of usually three or more ribs so that the underlying lung collapsed (Fig. 18.16). Occasionally, thoracoplasty was combined with pneumonectomy for the treatment of chronic tuberculous empyema. An alternative approach was *plombage*, which was the extrapleural insertion of some inert material to collapse the underlying lung. Solid or hollow lucite balls (Fig. 18.17) were commonly used. Other substances included crumpled cellophane packs and paraffin (Fig. 18.18).

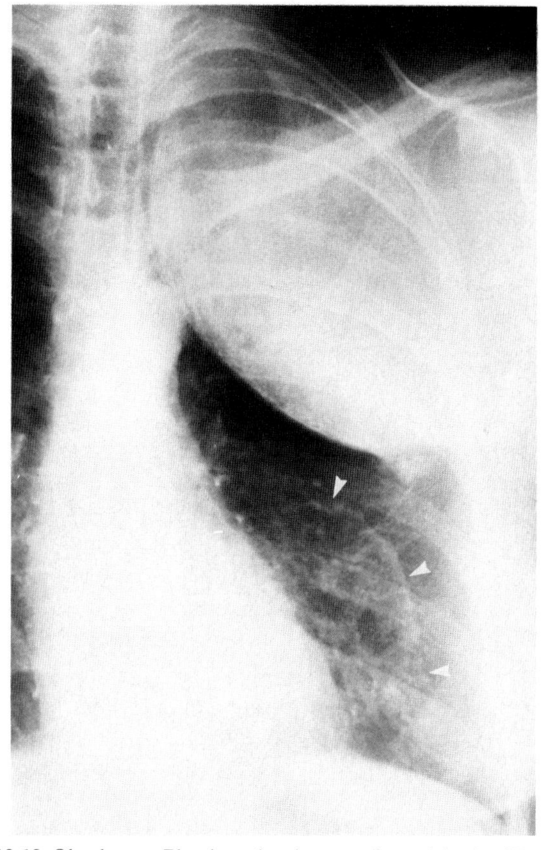

Fig. 18.18 Oleothorax. Plombage has been performed by instilling paraffin extra-pleurally through a thoracotomy with excision of the fifth rib. A thin rim of calcification has developed in the extra-pleural collection. Some paraffin has tracked inferiorly behind the lung and produced a calcified pleural plaque which is seen *en face* (arrowheads).

THORACIC COMPLICATIONS OF GENERAL SURGERY

Atelectasis is the commonest pulmonary complication of thoracic or abdominal surgery. Predisposing factors are a long anaesthetic, obesity, chronic lung disease and smoking. It is a result of retained secretions and poor ventilation. Post-operatively it is painful to breath deeply or cough. The chest X-ray usually shows elevation of the diaphragm, due to a poor inspiration. Linear, sometimes curved, opacities are frequently present in the lower zones, and probably represent a combination of subsegmental volume loss and consolidation (Fig. 18.4B). These shadows usually appear about 24 hours post-operatively and resolve within two or three days.

Pleural effusions are common immediately following abdominal surgery, and usually resolve within two weeks. They may be associated with pulmonary infarction. Effusions due to subphrenic infection usually occur later.

Pneumothorax complicating extrathoracic surgery is usually a complication of positive pressure ventilation or central venous line insertion. It may complicate nephrectomy.

Aspiration pneumonitis during anaesthesia is common, but fortunately is usually insignificant. When significant, patchy consolidation appears within a few hours, usually basally or around the hila. Clearing occurs within a few days, unless there is superinfection.

Pulmonary oedema in the post-operative period may be cardiogenic or non-cardiogenic. The latter includes fluid overload and the adult respiratory distress syndrome. If the patient is recumbent the distribution of oedema fluid may be atypical.

Pneumonia may complicate post-operative atelectasis and aspiration pneumonitis. Post-operative pneumonias, therefore, tend to be associated with bilateral basal shadowing.

Sub-phrenic abscess usually produces elevation of the hemidiaphragm, pleural effusion and basal atelectasis. Loculated gas may be seen below the diaphragm, and fluoroscopy may show splinting of the diaphragm. Subphrenic abscess can be demonstrated by CT, but the investigation of choice is ultrasound.

Pulmonary embolism may produce pulmonary shadowing, pleural effusion or elevation of the diaphragm. However, a normal chest X-ray does not exclude pulmonary embolism, and the investigation of choice is a perfusion lung scan.

THE INTENSIVELY CARED-FOR PATIENT

Patients are admitted to an intensive care ward post-operatively, following major trauma or following circulatory or respiratory failure. A number of monitoring and life-support devices may be used in their care. Radiology plays an important part in the management of these devices.

Central venous pressure (CVP) catheters are used to monitor right atrial pressure. The end of a CVP line needs to be intrathoracic, and is ideally in the superior vena cava (Fig. 18.22B). CVP lines may be introduced via an antecubital, subclavian or jugular vein. Subclavian venous

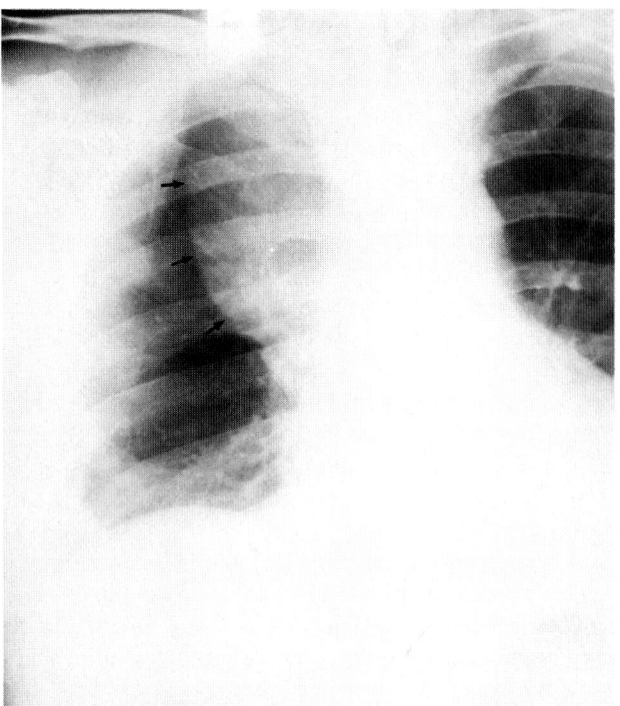

Fig. 18.19 Mediastinal haematoma. Following unsuccessfully attempted placement of a central venous line via the right subclavian vein a large extra-pleural haematoma (arrows) is present.

puncture carries a risk of pneumothorax and mediastina haematoma (Fig. 18.19). Rarely, perforation of th subclavian vein leads to fluid collecting in the mediastinur or pleura (Fig. 18.20). All catheters have a potential ris of coiling and knotting, or fracture leading to embolism.

Swan-Ganz catheters are used to measure pulmonar artery and pulmonary wedge pressures. The latter is a index of left atrial pressure. Swan-Ganz catheters ar usually introduced via an antecubital or jugular vein. A inflatable balloon at the catheter tip guides it through th right heart. Ideally the end of the catheter should be main tained 2 or 3 inches beyond the bifurcation of the mai pulmonary artery in either the right or left pulmonar artery (Fig. 18.10). When the pulmonary wedge pressur is measured the balloon is inflated, and the flow of bloo carries the catheter tip peripherally into the lung, to wedged position. After the measurement has been mad the balloon is deflated and the catheter returns to a centr position, otherwise there is a risk of pulmonary infarctior The inflation balloon is radiolucent. The balloon shoul normally be kept deflated to minimize the risk of thrombu formation.

Nasogastric tubes may not reach the stomach, or ma coil in the oesophagus (Fig. 18.21) or occasionally ar inserted into the trachea and into the right bronchu (Fig. 18.22).

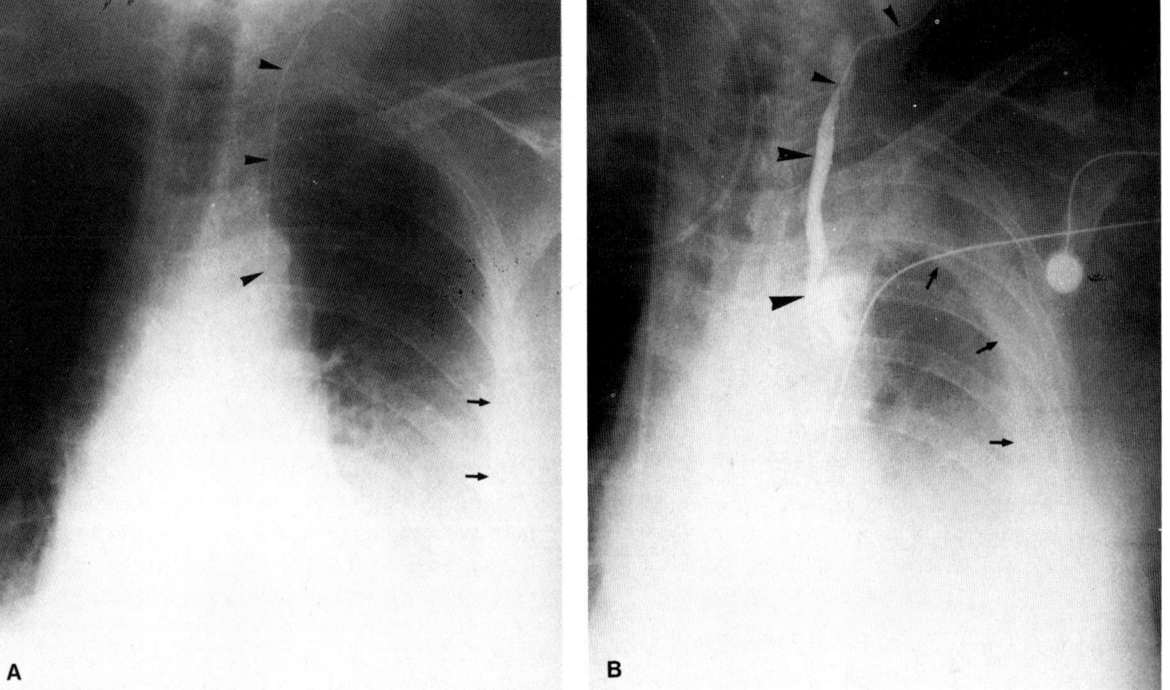

Fig. 18.20 Perforation of innominate vein. (**A**) A central venous catheter (arrowheads) has been introduced via the left jugular vein. Its tip point inferiorly, rather than to the right along the axis of the innominate vein. A pleural effusion (arrows) is present. (**B**) Next day the effusion is larger. Injection of contrast medium into the catheter (larger arrowheads) demonstrates extravasation, and communication with the pleural effusion.

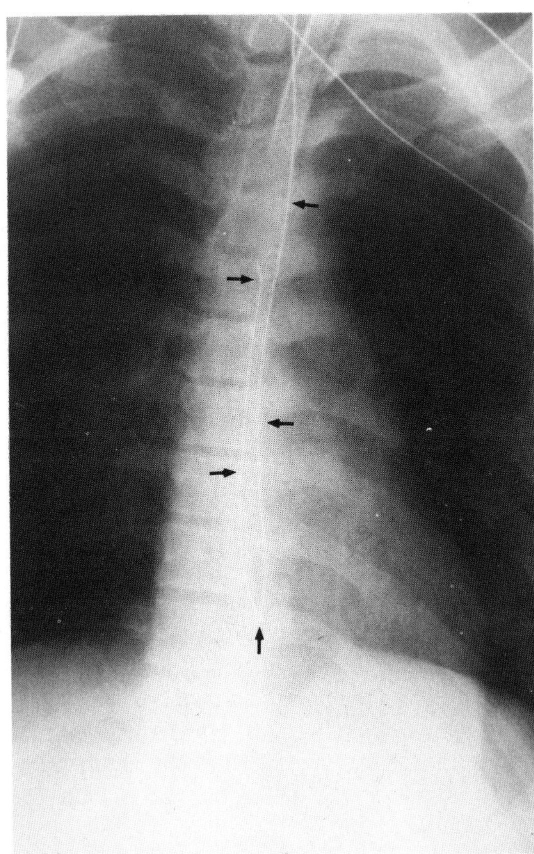

Fig. 18.21 Naso-gastric tube coiled in oesophagus. The tube does not reach the stomach, but has folded back on itself (arrows).

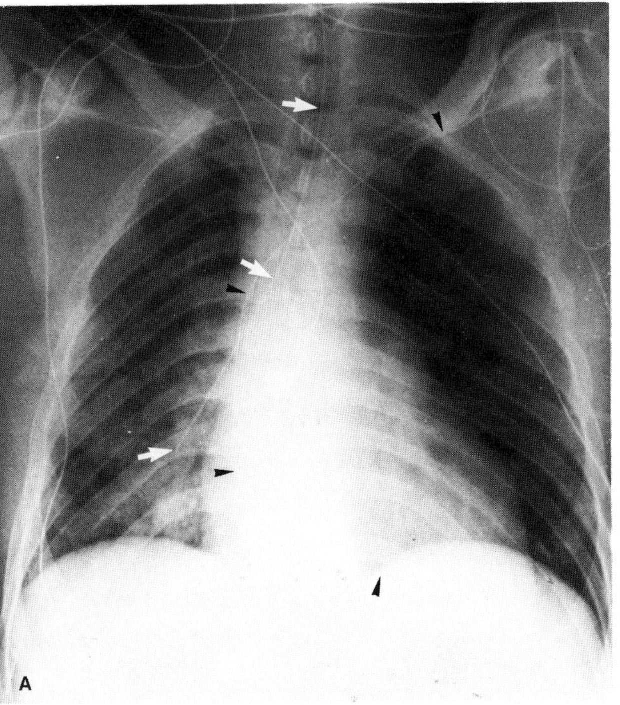

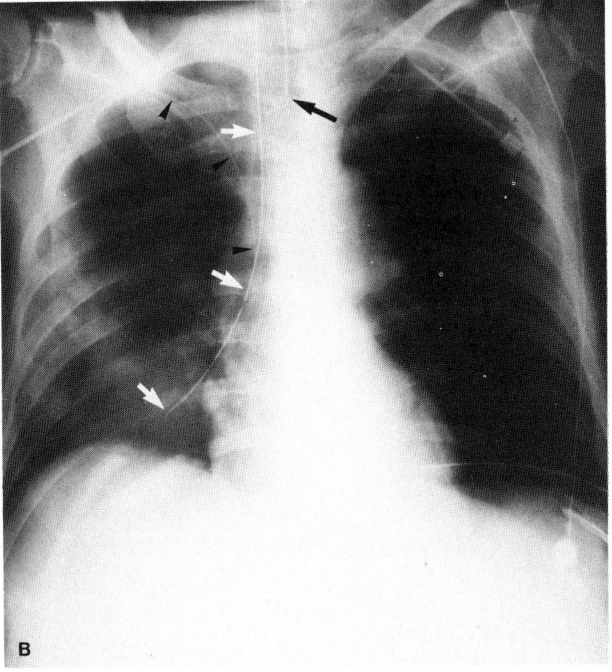

Fig. 18.22 Naso-gastric tubes in right bronchus. (**A**) The naso-gastric tube (arrows) passes down the trachea and into the right bronchus. The patient had been 'fed' via the tube, causing patchy consolidation in the right lung. A temporary pacing electrode (arrowheads) is present. (**B**) This patient with chronic renal failure developed peritonitis following peritoneal dialysis. Drains are present in the abdomen. A naso-gastric tube (white arrows) has been passed beyond an endotracheal tube (black arrow) and into the right bronchus! Two venous lines are present; the right-sided catheter (arrowheads) is well placed for central venous pressure measurements.

Endotracheal tubes are used for access to the airways for ventilation and management of secretions, and also to protect the airway. The chest X-ray is important in assessing the position of the tip of the endotracheal tube relative to the carina. Extension and flexion of the neck may make the tip of an endotracheal tube move by as much as 5 cm. With the neck in neutral position the tip of the tube should ideally be about 5–6 cm above the carina. A tube that is inserted too far usually passes into the right bronchus (Fig. 18.23), with the risk of collapse of the left lung (Fig. 13.29). If the inflated cuff of the tube dilates the trachea there is a risk of ischaemic damage to the tracheal mucosa. A late complication of an overinflated cuff is tracheostenosis.

Tracheostomy tubes are usually inserted for long-term ventilatory support. The tube tip should be situated centrally in the airways at the level of T3 (Fig. 18.2). Acute complications of tracheostomy include pneumothorax, pneumomediastinum and subcutaneous emphysema. Long-term complications include tracheal ulceration, stenosis and perforation.

Positive pressure ventilation may be complicated by interstitial emphysema, pneumomediastinum, pneumothorax and subcutaneous emphysema (Fig. 18.10).

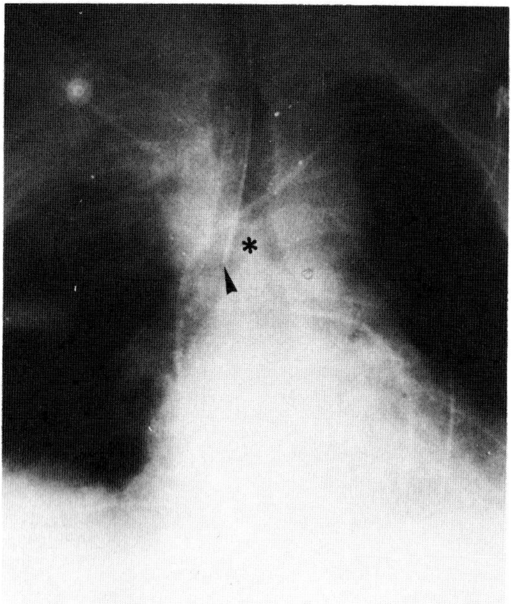

Fig. 18.23 Endotracheal tube too low. The tip of the endotracheal tube (arrowhead) is beyond the carina (asterisk) and in the right bronchus. A well-positioned Swan-Ganz catheter is present.

Pleural tubes are used to treat pleural effusions and pneumothoraces. If the patient is being nursed supine the tip of the tube should be placed anteriorly and superiorly for a pneumothorax, and posteriorly and inferiorly for an effusion. A radio-opaque line usually runs along pleural tubes, and is interrupted where there are side holes. It is important to check that all the side holes are within the thorax (Figs. 18.2 and 18.4). Tracks may remain on the chest X-ray following removal of chest tubes causing tubular or ring shadows.

Mediastinal drains are usually present following sternotomy. Apart from their position they look like pleural tubes.

Intra-aortic balloon pumps are used in patients with cardiogenic shock, often following cardiac surgery. The pump comprises a catheter, the end of which is surrounded by an elongated, inflatable balloon. It is inserted via a femoral artery and is positioned in the descending thoracic aorta. The pattern of inflation and deflation of the balloon is designed to increase coronary perfusion during diastole and to reduce the left ventricular afterload. The ideal position of the catheter tip is just distal to the origin of the left subclavian artery (Fig. 18.24). If the catheter tip is advanced too far it may occlude the left subclavian artery and if it is too proximal the balloon may occlude branches of the abdominal aorta.

Pacemakers may be permanent or temporary. Temporary epicardial wires are sometimes inserted during cardiac surgery, and may be seen as thin, almost hair-line metallic opacities overlying the heart. Temporary pacing

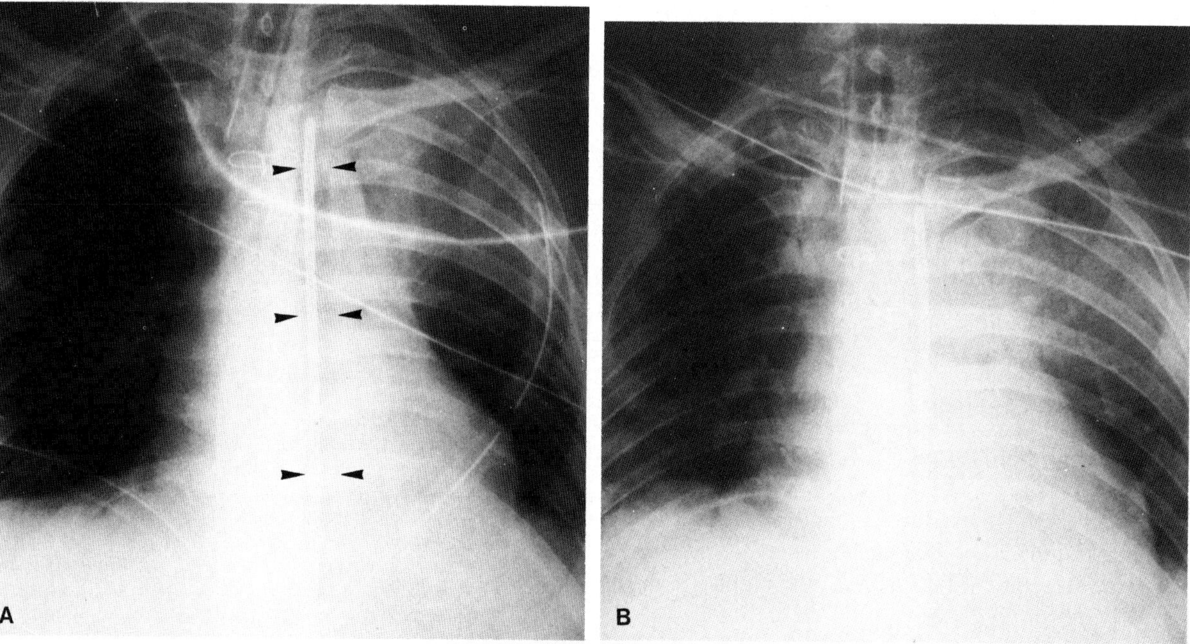

Fig. 18.24 Intra-aortic balloon pump. Post-coronary artery by-pass surgery. (**A**) Bilateral pleural and mediastinal drains and endotracheal tube are present. The pump is well sited, and its balloon is seen to be inflated (arrowheads). (**B**) The drains have been removed. When this radiograph was exposed the balloon was deflated.

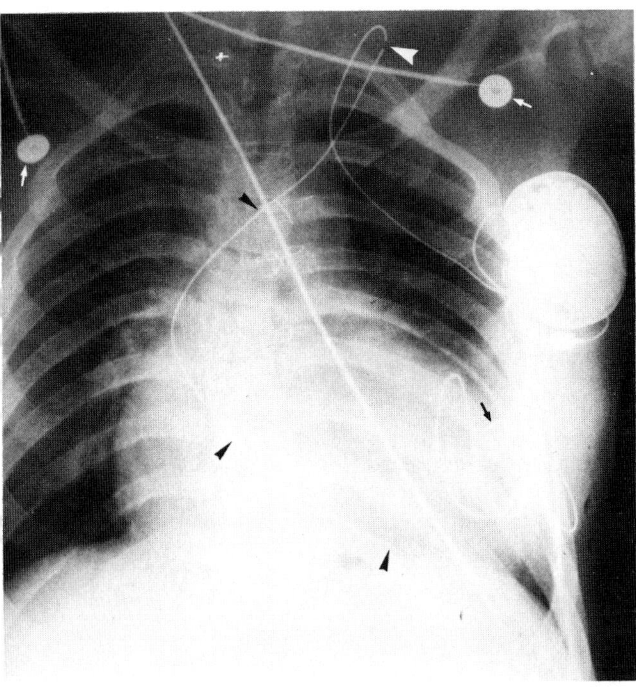

Fig. 18.25 Fractured pacing wire. Patient with surgically repaired complete atrioventricular canal. A permanent transvenous pacing system is present; the power unit is in the left axilla: the electrode (arrowheads) reaches the right ventricle by traversing the innominate vein, superior vena cava and right atrium. The electrode is fractured (white arrowhead). Note disconnected epicardial electrodes (black arrow) and ECG electrodes (white arrows).

electrodes are usually inserted transvenously via a subclavian or jugular vein (Fig. 18.22A). If a patient is not pacing properly a chest X-ray may reveal that the position of the electrode tip is unstable, or a fracture in the wire may be seen (Fig. 18.25). A full discussion of the radiology of pacemakers is outside the scope of this chapter.

RADIATION INJURY OF THE LUNG

Radiation injury of the lung usually results from treatment of a pulmonary or mediastinal neoplasm by radiotherapy. It may also be a complication of the treatment of breast cancer. The changes seen on the chest X-ray are often remarkably geometric, and correspond to the shape of the treatment portal.

The earliest pathological changes in the lung are alveolar and bronchiolar desquamation and accumulation of exudate in the alveoli. This is followed by organization and fibrosis.

The affect of radiation on the lung depends upon several factors. Healthy lung tissue is more resistant to damage than diseased lung. Previous radiotherapy and associated chemotherapy increase the likelihood of fibrosis. The total dose, the time over which it is given and the volume of lung irradiated are other factors. Radiographic changes are rare at dose rates of 2000 rad over 2–3 weeks, but are usual with doses of 6000 rad or more over 5–6 weeks.

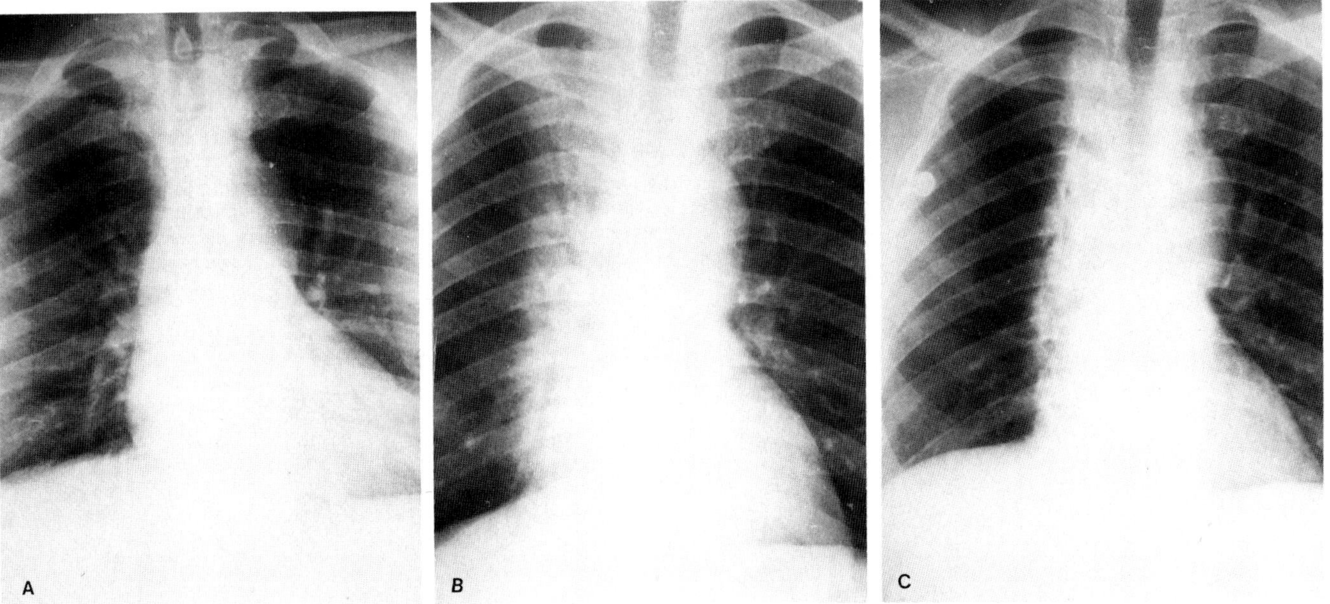

Fig. 18.26 Radiation pneumonitis. Male aged 45 years with diffuse histiocytic lymphoma, who developed upper thoracic spinal cord compression. (**A**) After surgical decompression the lungs are clear and the patient commenced radiotherapy to the spine. (**B**) 10 weeks later there is paraspinal consolidation with air bronchograms. (**C**) 14 weeks after treatment paraspinal pulmonary fibrosis has developed. The changes correspond to the shape of the treatment portal.

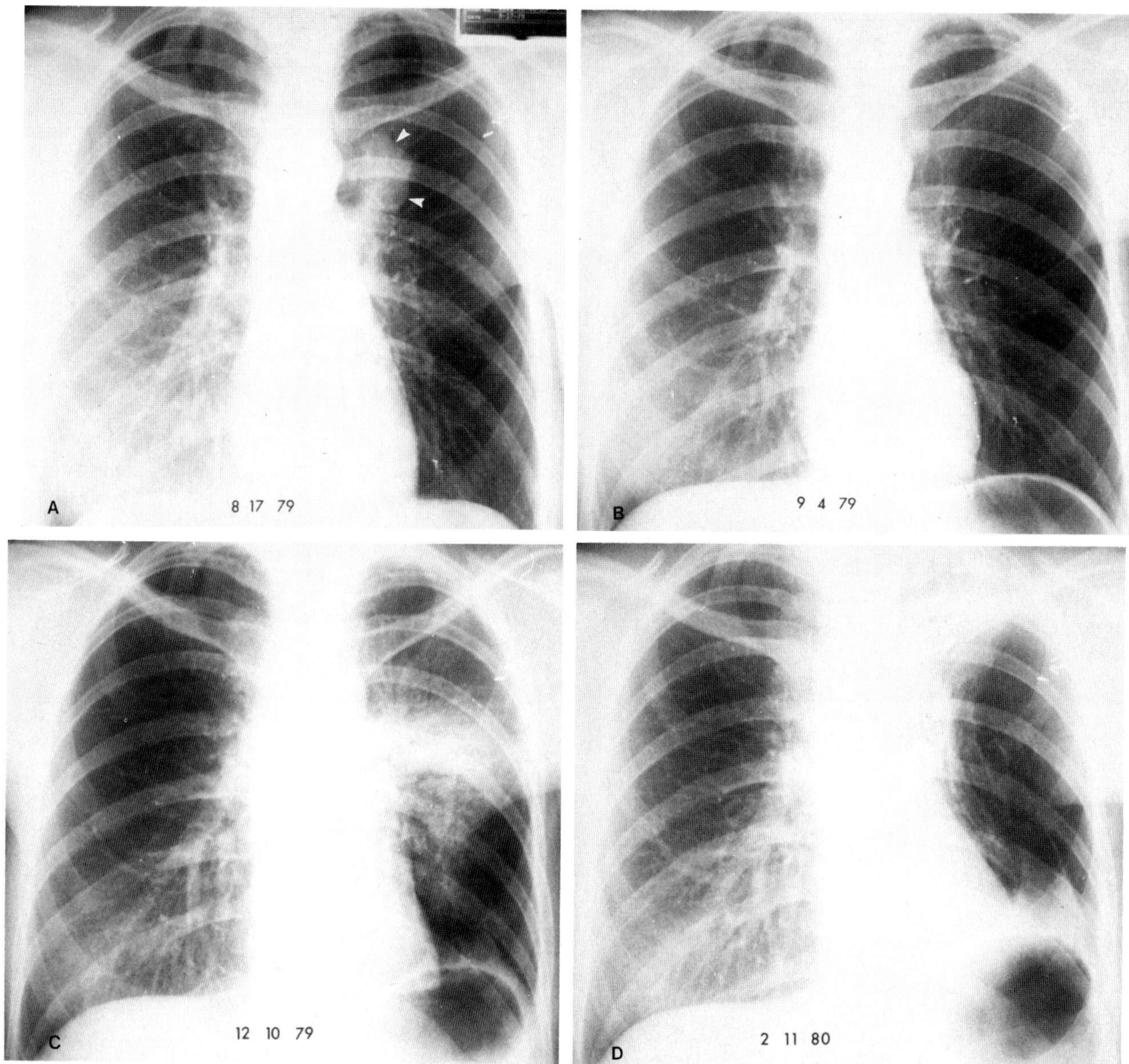

Fig. 18.27 Radiation pneumonitis. Female aged 32 years. Left mastectomy for carcinoma one year earlier; surgical clips overlie left axilla. (**A**) Medial left upper zone opacity (arrowheads) is caused by metastasis to left internal mammary lymph nodes. (**B**) 18 days later following radiotherapy the left upper zone mass has gone. (**C**) 16 weeks after treatment there is extensive consolidation in the left mid and upper zones. (**D**) 5 months after treatment there is gross left upper lobe fibrosis, the mediastinum has shifted to the left and the left hemidiaphragm is elevated. The patient remained asymptomatic throughout this time.

The radiological changes correspond to the pathology. The acute or exudative phase is not usually evident until a month or more after treatment, and may take up to 6 months to appear.

Consolidation, usually with some volume loss, occurs. It is not segmental or lobar, but corresponds to the shape of the radiation portal. An air bronchogram may be visible. The patient is usually asymptomatic, but may have a pyrexia or cough. *Fibrosis* then occurs, and is usually complete by 9–12 months (Fig. 18.26). Fibrosis, if extensive and severe enough, may cause displacement of fissures, the hila or mediastinum, and compensatory hyperinflation of the less affected lung (Fig. 18.27). Very dense fibrosis may produce an air bronchogram (Fig. 18.28).

A pleural effusion as a result of irradiation is rare, and is more likely to be due to the malignant disease being treated. Pericardial effusion may occur as a late complication of irradiation. Necrosis of ribs or a clavicle may be seen on the chest X-ray following radiotherapy.

The diagnosis of radiation pneumonitis and fibrosis is usually easy, based on the history and characteristic shape, but occasionally apical fibrosis following treatment of breast cancer may resemble tuberculosis.

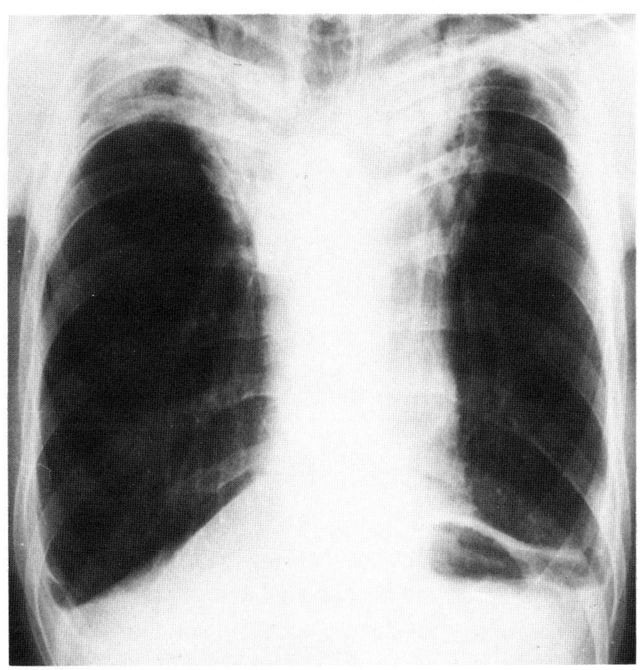

Fig. 18.28 Massive radiation fibrosis. Patient with Hodgkin's disease treated with mediastinal irradiation and chemotherapy (MOPP — Bleo). Note gross bilateral upper lobe fibrosis with extensive air bronchogram.

REFERENCES AND SUGGESTIONS FOR FURTHER READING

Trauma

Ball, T., McCrory, R., Smith, J. O. & Clements, Jr., J. L. (1982) Traumatic diaphragmatic hernia: errors in diagnosis. *American Journal of Roentgenology*, **138**, 633–637.

Cochlin, D. L. & Shaw, M. R. P. (1978) Traumatic lung cysts following minor blunt chest trauma. *Clinical Radiology*, **29**, 151–154.

Fishbone, G., Robbins, D. I., Osborn, D. J. & Grnja, V. (1973) Trauma to the thoracic aorta and great vessels. *Radiological Clinics of North America*, **11**, 543–554.

Harvey-Smith, W., Bush, W. & Northrop, C. (1980) Traumatic bronchial rupture. *American Journal of Roentgenology*, **134**, 1189–1193.

Lindsell, D. R. M., Wilson, A. G. & Maxwell, J. D. (1982) Fractures on the chest radiograph in detection of alcoholic liver disease. *British Medical Journal*, **285**, 597–599.

Parkin, G. J. S. (1973) The radiology of perforated oesophagus. *Clinical Radiology*, **24**, 324–332.

Reynolds, J. & Davis, J. T. (1966) Injuries of the chest wall, pleura, pericardium, lungs, bronchi and oesophagus. *Radiological Clinics of North America*, **4**, 383.

Sefczek, D. M., Sefczek, R. J. & Deeb, S. L. (1983) Radiographic signs of acute traumatic rupture of the thoracic aorta. *American Journal of Roentgenology*, **141**, 1259–1262.

Williams, J. R. & Stembridge, V. A. (1964) Pulmonary contusion secondary to non-penetrating chest trauma. *American Journal of Roentgenology*, **91**, 284–290.

Wiot, J. F. (1975) The radiologic manifestations of blunt chest trauma. *Journal of the American Medical Association*, **231**, 500.

The post-operative chest

Carter, A. R., Sostman, H. D., Curtis, A. M & Swett, H. A. (1983) Thoracic alterations after cardiac surgery. *American Journal of Roentgenology*, **140**, 475–481.

Goodman, L. R. (1980) Post-operative chest radiograph: I. Alterations after abdominal surgery. *American Journal of Roentgenology*, **134**, 533–541.

Goodman, L. R. (1980) Post-operative chest radiograph: II. Alterations after major intrathoracic surgery. *American Journal of Roentgenology*, **134**, 803–813.

Goodman, L. R. & Putman, C. E. (1983) *Intensive Care Radiology: Imaging of the Critically Ill*. 2nd edn. Philadelphia: W. B. Saunders.

Melamed, M., Hipona, F. A., Reynes, C. J., Barker, W. L. & Pardes, S. (1977) *The Adult Post-operative Chest*. Springfield Illinois: Charles C. Thomas.

Radiation injury of the lung

Boushy, S. F., Belgason, A. H. & Borth, L. B. (1970) The effect of radiation on the lung and bronchial tree. *American Journal of Roentgenology*, **108**, 284–292.

Freedman, G. S., Lofgren, S. B. & Kilgerman, M. M. (1974) Radiation — induced changes in pulmonary perfusion. *Radiology*, **112**, 435–437.

Gross, N. J. (1977) Pulmonary effects of radiation therapy. *Annals of Internal Medicine*, **86**, 81–92.

Libshitz, H. I. & Southard, M. E. (1974) Complications of radiation therapy: the thorax. *Seminars in Roentgenology*, **9**, 41–49.

Polansky, S. M., Ravin, C. E. & Prosnitz, L. R. (1980) Lung changes after breast irradiation. *American Journal of Roentgenology*, **139**, 101–105.

CHAPTER 19

THE CHEST IN CHILDREN

TECHNIQUES

Plain radiographs remain the basis for evaluation of the chest in childhood. In the neonate, satisfactory films can be obtained in incubators using modern mobile X-ray apparatus. The baby lies on the cassette for the film exposure. Although automatic triggering of the exposure can be made using variations of temperature at the nostril and of electrical impedance across the chest in the differing phases of respiration, an experienced radiographer will usually be able to judge the end of inspiration. An adequate inspiration will be with the right hemidiaphragm at the level of the eighth rib posteriorly. Films in expiration frequently show a sharp kink in the trachea to the right and varying degrees of opacification of the lung fields with apparent enlargement of the heart. Films are well collimated and the baby positioned as straight as possible and lordotic films avoided especially if the heart size is of particular interest. As much monitoring equipment as possible should be removed. Magnification radiography in the neonate allows better evaluation of the lung granularity in hyaline membrane disease but the construction of most incubators makes this technique difficult and its vogue has passed.

Children over 5 years old can usually cooperate sufficiently to stand for a PA film in a manner similar to adults. Below this age some form of chest stand is needed in which an assistant, preferably the mother, can hold the child in front of a cassette with a suspended protective lead apron behind which she stands. The dose to the mother with proper collimation is small and her position allows the child to be held straighter than from a position to the side. The difference between a PA and an AP projection in the small child is usually negligible. High kilovoltage techniques with added filtration and the use of a grid allow evaluation of the trachea and major bronchi which is important in stridor, mediastinal masses and to assess isomerism in congenital heart disease.

Fluoroscopy. Limitation of radiation exposure is vital in childhood but quick fluoroscopic examination of the chest can frequently prove extremely useful in the evaluation in particular of differing lung radiolucencies in suspected foreign body aspiration. With obstructive emphysema the affected lung will show little volume change in respiration and the mediastinum will swing contralaterally in expiration. Prior to the advent of computed tomography, fluoroscopy had been advocated for the detection of dubious lung metastases.

A *barium swallow* is a useful adjunct to evaluation of paediatric lung disease, especially when there is stridor or suspected mediastinal masses or vascular anomalies.

Tomography. Conventional tomography is generally poor in childhood, usually because the time of traversing the arc is relatively long for the child to be still. The indication was typically to detect metastases, especially in Wilms' tumour or osteosarcoma. Computed tomography, which is superior for this despite the larger radiation dose, has also been used to evaluate mediastinal masses. If such a mass is posterior and adjacent to the vertebral column, many advocate intrathecal water-soluble contrast medium before CT scanning.

Angiography. Angiography is infrequently used in extracardiac chest pathology. It provides valuable information however in arterio-venous malformation and pulmonary sequestrations. Digital vascular imaging has proved a less invasive technique in such cases. Embolization of bronchial arteries has been used in bronchiectatic severe haemorrhage.

Isotopes. Perfusion studies with technetium-99m macroaggregates are well established in adults but childhood combination with a ventilation scan using krypton-81m is a more useful technique especially in investigating the small lung.

Ultrasound. Ultrasound has a relatively small role. It can be particularly useful in detecting the correct site for aspiration of pleural or pericardial effusions and may show whether a mass close to the chest wall is solid or cystic.

SPECIFIC FEATURES OF THE CHEST RADIOGRAPH IN CHILDREN

The Thymus. The normal thymus is a frequent cause of widening of the superior mediastinum during the first years of life. The lateral margin frequently shows an undulation, the thymic wave, which corresponds to the indentations of the ribs on the inner surface of the thoracic cage. Particularly on the right the thymus may have a triangular 'sail-like' configuration. The thymus may involute in times of stress and a decrease in size can be induced by steroids. At times the differentiation of physiological thymus from pathology in the anterior mediastinum can be difficult. Ultrasound examination will usually differentiate cystic lesions from the homogeneous nature of normal thymic tissue. Occasionally the normal thymus can act as a significant space occupying lesion in the superior mediastinum and in such cases differentiation may be helped by computed tomography or by the exhibition of steroids.

The cardiothoracic ratio. In toddlers the cardiothoracic ratio can at times exceed 50% and care should be exercised to prevent overdiagnosis of cardiomegaly.

Kink of the trachea to the right. This is a frequent feature of a chest film taken in less than full inspiration. This is a physiological buckling and does not represent a mass lesion.

The soft tissues are frequently prominent in children and the anterior axillary fold crossing the chest wall can at times mimic a pneumothorax. Similarly skin folds can cast confusing shadows, and plaits of hair over the upper chest can mimic pulmonary infiltrations.

Pleural effusions. Whereas in adults an early sign of pleural effusion is blunting of the costophrenic angles, in childhood it is more common to see separation of the lung from the chest wall with reasonable preservation of the clarity of the costophrenic angles.

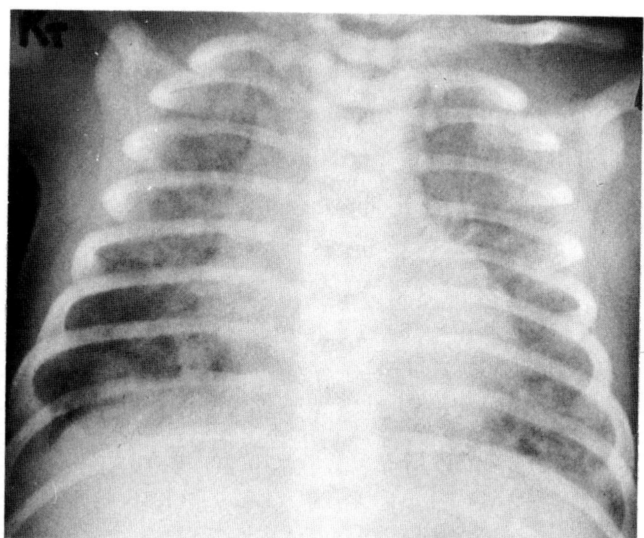

Fig. 19.1 Wet lung, or transient tachypnoea of the newborn. Patchy parenchymal shadowing in the first day of life.

THE SMALL LUNG

Discovery of a small lung on a radiograph is frequently elucidated by ventilation and perfusion radionuclide lung scans using krypton-81m and technetium-99m macroaggregates. The complete absence of isotopes in one lung in the presence of an ipsilateral opaque hemithorax with mediastinal shift to the affected side is highly suggestive of a diagnosis of pulmonary aplasia or of extreme pulmonary hypoplasia.

The complete absence of perfusion in a small lung with decreased ventilation is typical of congenital absence of the pulmonary artery. Decreased perfusion and ventilation in the presence of a small hemi-thorax may be seen in Macleod's syndrome, with post-infective maldevelopment, with aplasias of single lobes and with pulmonary hypoplasia. A segmental perfusion defect in a fully ventilated lung is associated with pulmonary sequestrations.

RESPIRATORY DISTRESS IN THE NEWBORN

Transient tachypnoea of the newborn, or wet lung disease (Fig. 19.1)

There are variable amounts of fluid in the newborn lung. This is typically quickly cleared after birth. Some babies however show a transient respiratory distress due to excess lung fluid. Predisposing conditions include prematurity, a diabetic mother and Caesarian section. The radiographs show diffuse parenchymal patchy shadowing with perihilar streakiness. The prognosis in this condition is good and there is usually progressive clearing, complete within two or three days.

Hyaline membrane disease (Fig. 19.2)

In this condition a deficiency of the pulmonary surfactant predisposes to alveolar collapse. Conditions which predispose to this include prematurity, Caesarean section and perinatal asphyxia. In mild hyaline membrane disease the radiological appearances consist of a mild granularity throughout the lung fields. As the condition becomes more severe, an air bronchogram becomes apparent. In the most severe cases the lungs are virtually opaque with loss of differentiation of the cardiac and thymic and diaphragmatic contours. Uncomplicated hyaline membrane disease is a symmetrical condition.

Bronchopulmonary dysplasia (Fig. 19.3)

Severe hyaline membrane disease is typically treated by artificial ventilation of the lungs. If ventilation needs to be prolonged especially if high pressures and high inspiratory oxygen tensions are required, damage can occur to the lungs. The hyaline membrane present in the alveoli becomes organized and fibrous tissue develops within the lungs. As a consequence, areas of the lungs become

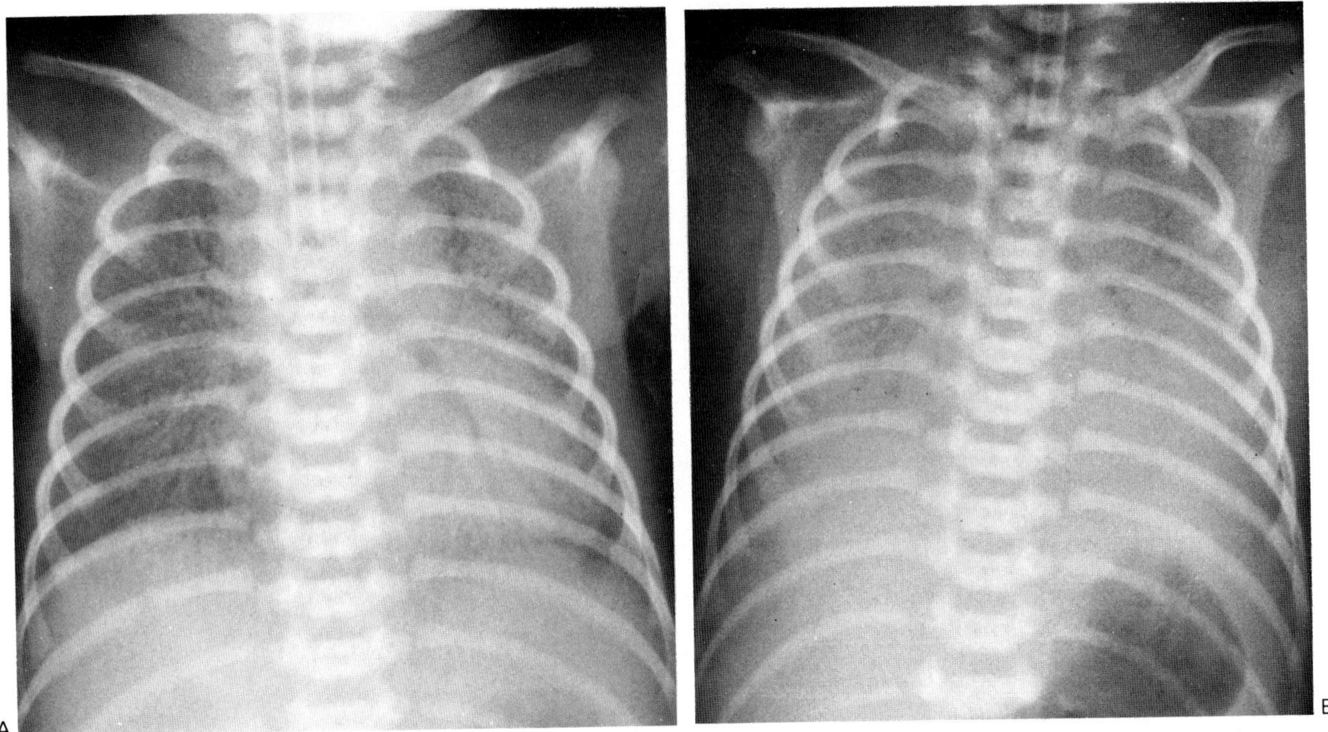

Fig. 19.2 Hyaline membrane disease. (**A**) Mild changes aged 1 day — fine reticulo-nodular shadowing with accentuation of the air bronchogram. Endotracheal tube. (**B**) More advanced changes aged 3 days — marked opacification with loss of diaphragmatic and cardiac contours.

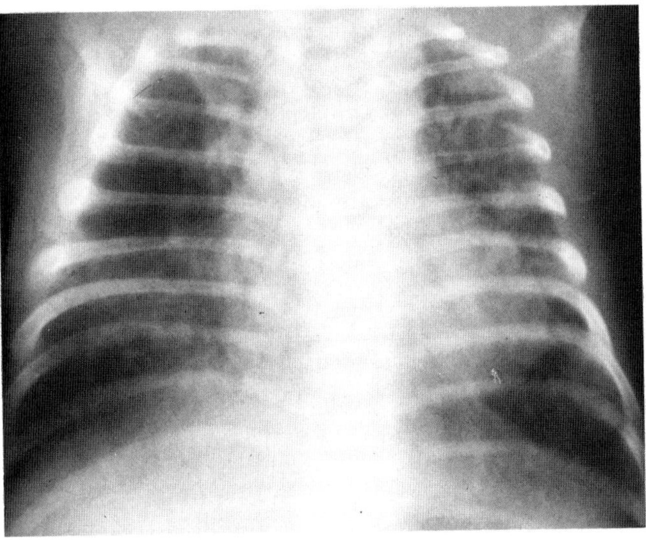

Fig. 19.3 Bronchopulmonary dysplasia. Patchy shadowing from areas of loss of volume and fibrosis, with areas of compensatory emphysema, especially in the right upper lobe.

collapsed with compensatory emphysema developing in residual aerated alveoli. This leads to a coarse reticulation and at times to variable amounts of segmental collapse and occasionally to considerable areas of localized emphysema. Whereas hyaline membrane disease, if uncomplicated, and transient tachypnoea of the newborn will quickly resolve, bronchopulmonary dysplasia can lead to severe respiratory distress lasting months and may end in respiratory failure and death.

Pulmonary interstitial emphysema (Fig. 19.4)
In this condition gas enters the interstitial tissues of the lungs and gives rise to multiple small lucencies throughout the lung fields. Some of these lucencies are due to air passing from the interstitial tissue into the relatively large lymphatics of the newborn lungs. A lung affected by interstitial emphysema is frequently larger than the contralateral one and may lead to deviation of the mediastinum. If bilateral, venous return to the heart can be impeded. Interstitial emphysema is a frequent precursor of *pneumothorax* (Fig.19.5) and pneumomediastinum.

At times the child being artificially ventilated for hyaline membrane disease will undergo marked deterioration with the appearance of a bloodstained tracheal aspirate. This is frequently due to *pulmonary haemorrhage* and is accompanied by a marked increase in the opacification of the lungs as the alveoli become filled with haemorrhagic oedema. If the child's condition stabilizes the oedema is usually quickly resorbed but such a haemorrhage can be a terminal event. It is important in the evaluation of neonatal respiratory distress to be adequately acquainted with the

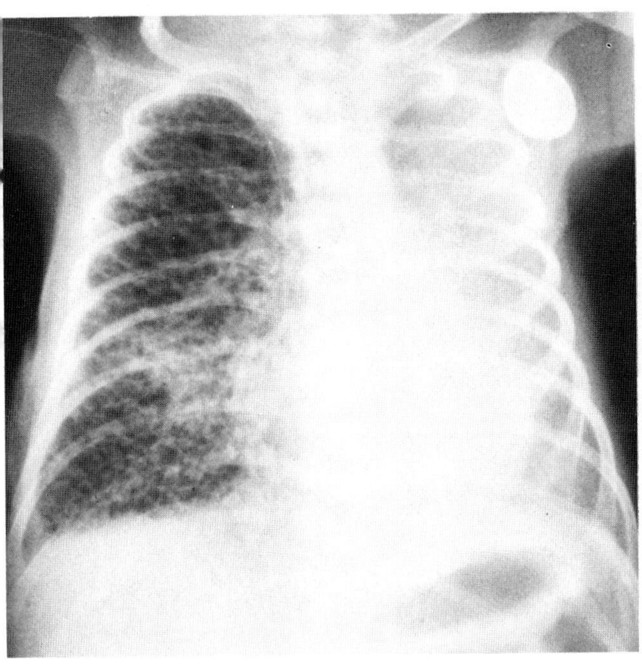

Fig. 19.4 Pulmonary interstitial emphysema. Fine reticular shadowing in the right lung with deviation of the mediastinum contralaterally. Hyaline membrane disease in the left lung.

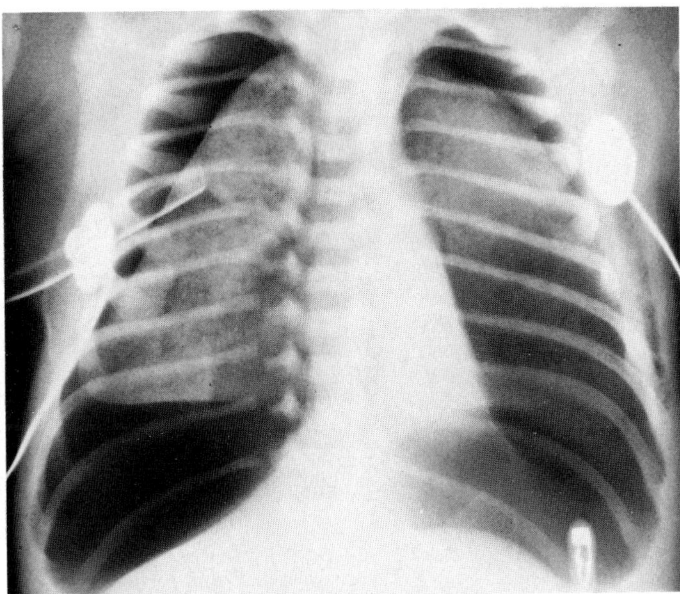

Fig. 19.5 Bilateral pneumothoraces in hyaline membrane disease. Right intercostal drain.

obstetric and maternal history. If there is a history of prolonged rupture of the membranes, patchy shadowing seen in the newborn lungs may be due to *intrauterine pneumonia*. If there has been intrauterine distress, *aspiration of meconium* can lead to respiratory embarrassment. The lungs typically show bilateral symmetrical rather coarse shadowing with frequent over-distention, complicated from time to time by pneumothorax and pneumomediastinum. Resolution of meconium aspiration can be prolonged. The *Mikity-Wilson syndrome* is essentially a radiological appearance consisting of diffuse interstitial infiltrations giving rise to a multicystic appearance. Onset is usually accompanied by apnoea and cyanosis in prematures later in the first week of life. Episodes of aspiration probably account for at least part of the syndrome and if resolution does not occur the condition can progress to bronchopulmonary dysplasia.

Pleural effusions

In the newborn these may be part of hydrops fetalis or of congestive cardiac failure. Chylothorax is the most common condition causing a large pleural effusion; this more frequently occurs in the right pleural cavity when unilateral and can lead to respiratory distress with deviation of the mediastinum. With repeated pleural aspiration the effusion usually disappears over a period of a week or two.

Congenital lobar emphysema

Gross overinflation of an upper or middle lobe in this condition leads to infantile respiratory distress with contralateral deviation of the mediastinum and compression of the other lobes of the same lung. Excision is usually necessary. A similar but less florid appearance can be produced by a persistent ductus arteriosus obstructing the left upper lobe.

Cystic adenomatoid malformation

This rare congenital cystic anomaly can lead to deviation of the mediastinum and compression of adjacent normal lung leading to neonatal distress or may present as repeated localized pneumonia. The cysts, which at times may be filled with fluid, are usually obvious.

Congenital diaphragmatic hernia (Fig. 19.6)

This is most frequently through the postero-lateral part of the diaphragm, more often on the left. The hemithorax is filled with stomach or gut and as the newborn baby swallows gas, distension leads to respiratory embarrassment with contralateral deviation of the mediastinum. Surgical correction is urgently required in an otherwise frequently fatal condition. The ipsilateral lung is usually hypoplastic. Congenital heart disease is an important association.

Pulmonary hypoplasia (Fig. 19.7)

This is a frequently lethal condition, often associated with prenatal obstructive uropathy or renal aplasia. The lungs are small and the thoracic configuration triangular. Hypoplastic lungs are seen in several skeletal dysplasias such as asphyxiating thoracic dystrophy.

At times it is difficult to differentiate whether respiratory distress is due to lung disease or due to congenital heart

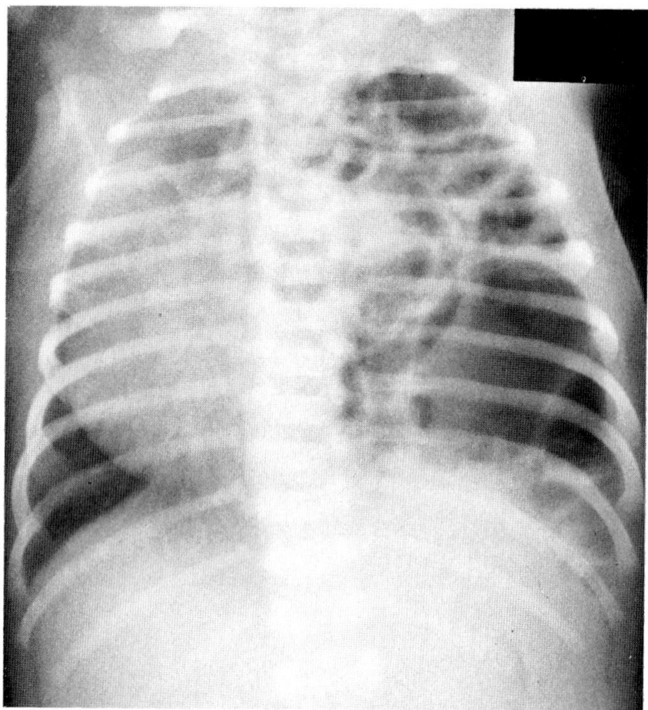

Fig. 19.6 Diaphragmatic hernia. Stomach and intestine occupy the left hemithorax with deviation of the mediastinum to the right.

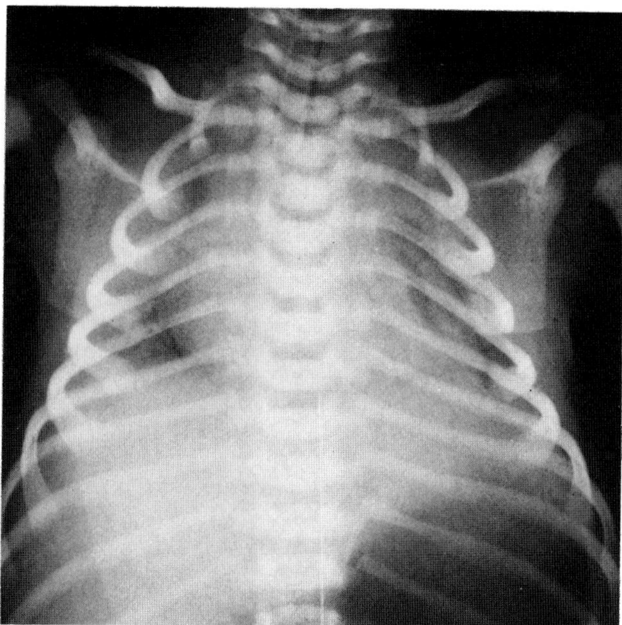

Fig. 19.7 Pulmonary hypoplasia. The rib cage shows the typical triangular configuration.

disease. However the clinical findings and the response to oxygenation and artificial ventilation will frequently allow such differentiation. The advent of real time cardiac ultrasound considerably facilitates diagnosis of structural anomalies of the neonatal heart but at times resort must be made to formal cardiac catheterization.

CONGENITAL PULMONARY SEQUESTRATION (Fig. 19.8)

This is an abnormality of development in which a portion of the lung shows separation from the normal bronchial and blood supply, though retaining some characteristics of lung tissue. They can be divided into intralobar, lying within the lung, and extralobar, in which the sequestrated segment develops enclosed in its own pleura when termed by some as an accessory lung. In intralobar sequestration there is a non-functioning portion of the lung usually lying posteriorly in the left lower lobe. The right lower lobe is the next most common situation and other lobes are rarely affected. Typically the segment is not connected with the normal bronchial tree and when communication is established it is usually in association with infection. The radiological appearances are of a soft tissue mass in the posterior part of the lower lobe usually on the left contiguous with the diaphragm. If connection has been established with the bronchial tree air-containing cystic masses with or without air–fluid levels will be seen. Bronchographic contrast medium rarely enters the lesion. The bronchial tree is spread round the mass and is typically complete in the number of its divisions. Extralobar sequestrations are much less common and usually interposed between the inferior surface of the left lower lobe and the diaphragm. They are frequently associated with other congenital anomalies and found incidentally during neonatal autopsies. Left-sided congenital diaphragmatic hernia may be associated.

Intralobar sequestrations typically derive their arterial blood supply from the aorta, usually the descending thoracic aorta, occasionally the abdominal aorta. Usually the venous drainage is via the pulmonary venous system but occasionally the inferior vena cava or azygos system. In contrast to the intralobar variety, venous drainage of extralobar sequestration is usually via the inferior vena cava, azygos or portal venous systems. The arterial supply is frequently from the abdominal aorta or one of its branches. The diagnosis of sequestrated segment should be borne in mind whenever an unusual abscess, cavity or cystic lesion is seen, particularly at the left base, and in all cases showing recurrent infection in one part of the lung.

CONGENITAL BRONCHIAL ATRESIA

The abnormality consists of an atresia of a lobar or smaller segment of bronchus and particularly affects the apical posterior segment of the bronchus of the left upper lobe. Mucous secretions inspissated within the patent airways distal to the atresia can produce an elliptical mass. Periph-

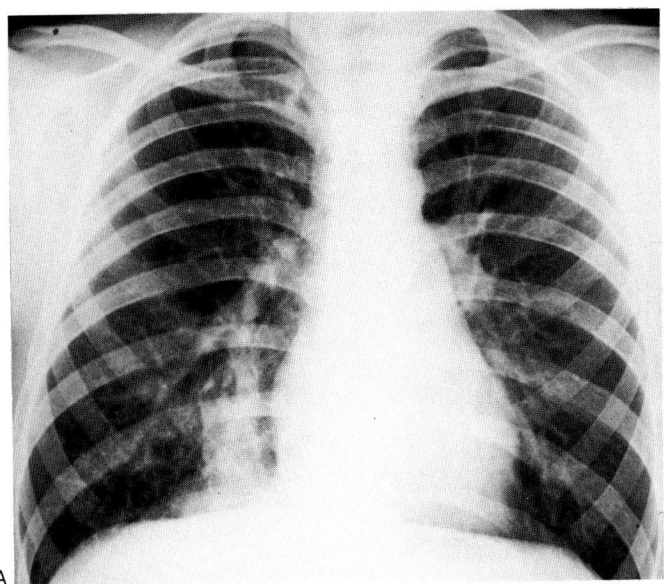

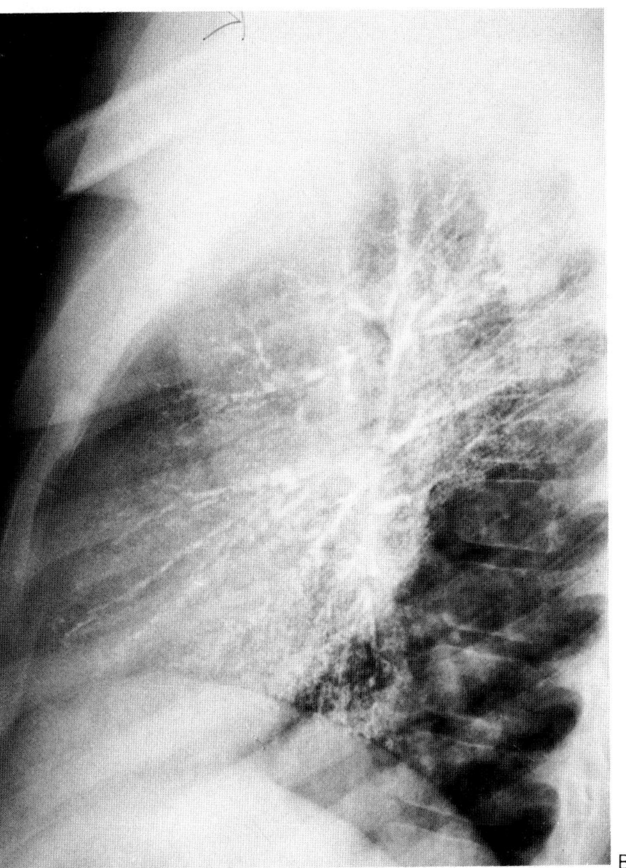

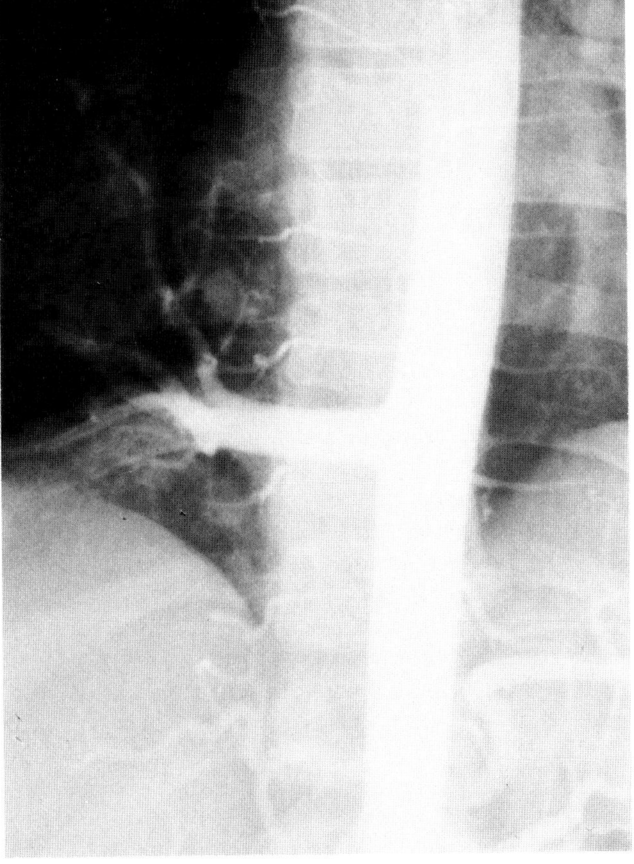

Fig. 19.8 Pulmonary sequestration. (**A**) Consolidation in the right lobe is associated with (**B**) absent bronchial filling on bronchography. (**C**) Angiography demonstrated a large feeding artery arising from the right of the descending thoracic aorta.

eral to this collateral air drift causes overinflation. Fluoroscopy will show expiratory air trapping in the involved segments and the vascular supply is diminished. Although the lesion may be associated with infection, discovery is usually on routine chest radiography.

PULMONARY ARTERIOVENOUS FISTULAE

Arteriovenous fistulae are commonly asymptomatic but some patients will show cyanosis, clubbing and polycythaemia and others will present with haemoptysis. About half of the patients with arteriovenous fistulae (Fig. 19.9) in the lungs will show such abnormal communications elsewhere in the skin and other organs (Rendu-Osler-Weber syndrome). Although the large fistulae typically present rounded homogeneous masses with enlarged serpiginous vessels radiating to the hilum, there is a high incidence of multiple lesions in the lungs and if resection is contemplated careful angiographic evaluation of both lungs should be carried out pre-operatively. Digital vascular imaging has facilitated this.

MUCOVISCIDOSIS (CYSTIC FIBROSIS OF THE PANCREAS)

Chronic suppuration in the lungs is an important feature of this condition in which many organ systems are involved. The lungs appear normal at birth but poor clearance of bronchial secretions leads to obstruction, particu-

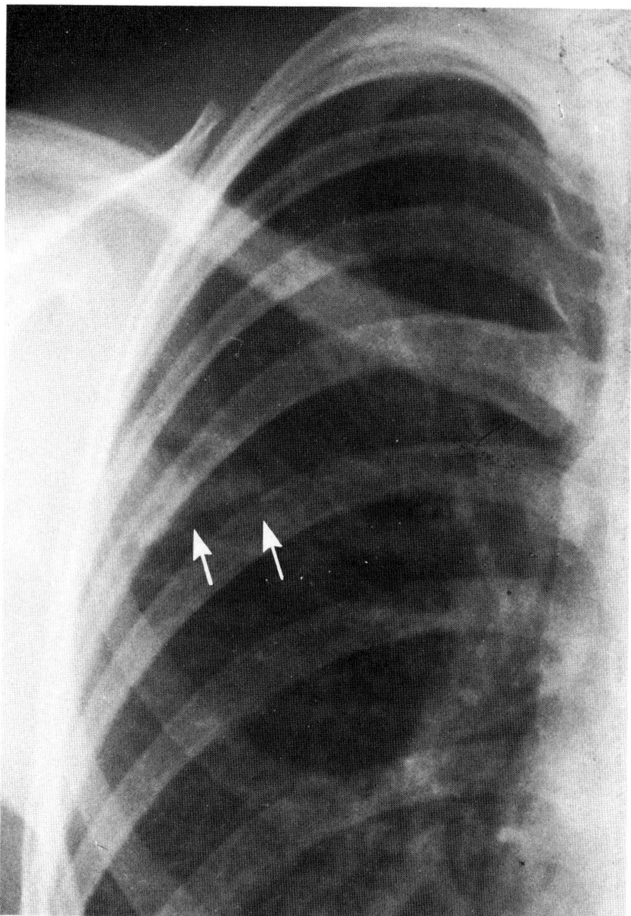

Fig. 19.9 Arterio-venous malformation. Peripheral serpiginous dilated blood vessels in the right upper lobe (arrows).

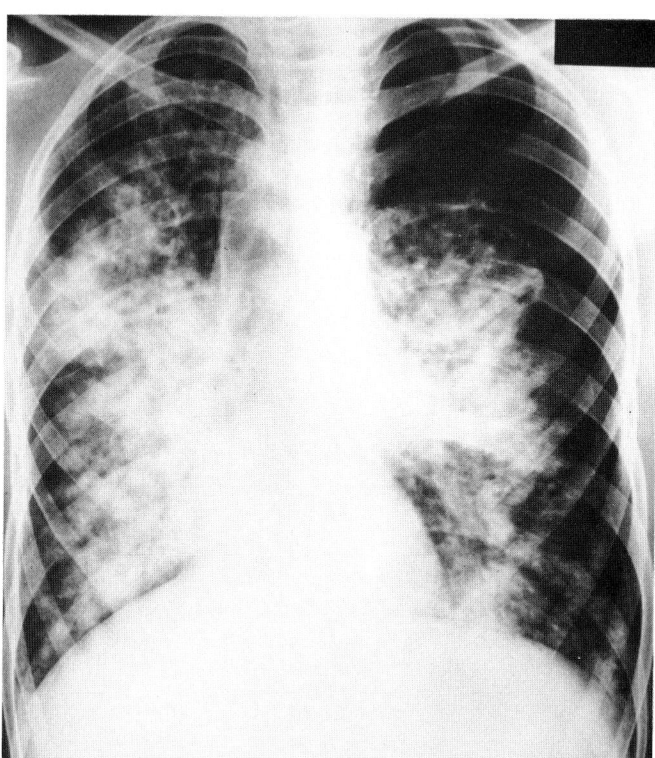

Fig. 19.10 Advanced cystic fibrosis (mucoviscidosis). Gross peribronchial shadowing with confluent pneumonic shadowing. There is a left pneumothorax with slight displacement of the mediastinum to the right.

larly of the smaller bronchi. In infancy this can lead to over-distension of the lungs resulting in flattening of the diaphragms, sternal bowing and increased dorsal kyphosis. Infiltration of the bronchial walls by lymphocytes and plasma cells is seen radiologically as peribronchial thickening particularly noticeable in bronchi seen end-on. Small discrete opacities are seen in later childhood in the periphery of the lung fields due to small peripheral abscesses. When these burst into the bronchioles they remain as small thin-walled air spaces. Segmental bronchiectasis is frequently seen consequent upon segmental collapse and consolidation. The upper lobes are more frequently involved in the bronchiectasis associated with cystic fibrosis than in other forms. Parabronchial abscesses can give rise to a more specific form of bronchiectasis with characteristic rounded shadows arising close to the medium sized bronchi with a widespread irregular distribution throughout the lung fields (Fig. 19.10). Pulmonary suppuration can lead to hilar lymph node enlargement. The hilar shadows may also be enlarged in the later stages of the disease when pulmonary hypertension arises as a complication. In later childhood peripheral areas of emphysema arise as a result of the fibrotic changes occurring more centrally. Pleural disease is an uncommon feature but pneumothorax is an important complication in the later stages of the disease and can lead to dramatic deterioration. The emphysematous changes are usually associated with a relatively narrow heart shadow but cardiac enlargement in cor pulmonale is usually a sign of a poor prognosis. Although the infections associated are usually staphylococcal, *Pseudomonas* or other Gram-negative infections, superinfection with tuberculosis and aspergillosis can occur. In the latter this may be associated with total collapse of the lung or extensive variable areas of consolidation. Repeated suppuration can lead to severe haemorrhage and bronchial artery embolization has been used to control such life-threatening episodes.

HISTIOCYTOSIS X (Fig. 19.11)

In childhood, bone and central nervous system manifestations are frequently more prominent than lung involvement. Fine wide-spread nodularity can at times resemble miliary tuberculosis but often shows a reticular pattern which may progress to 'honeycomb' lung and complicating pneumothoraces.

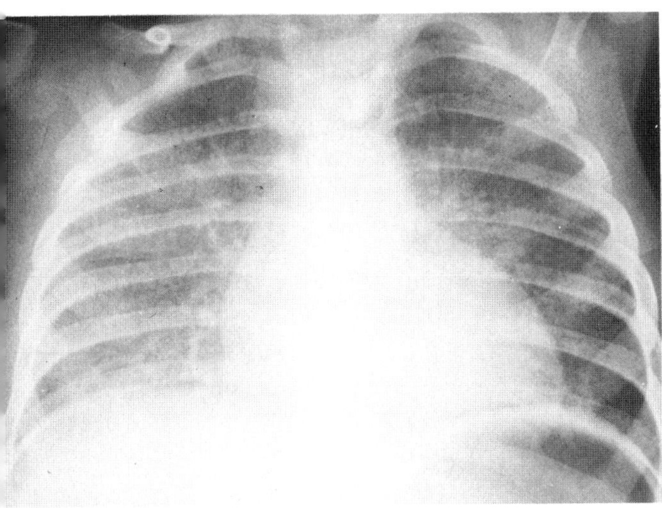

Fig. 19.11 Histiocytosis X. Fine nodularity in both lung fields.

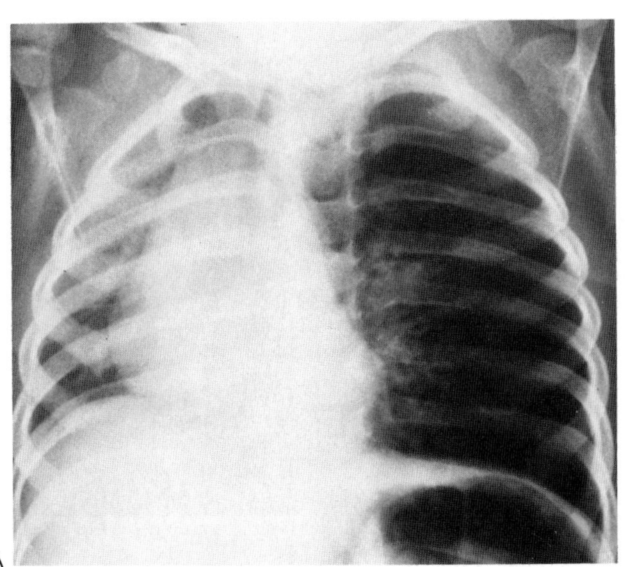

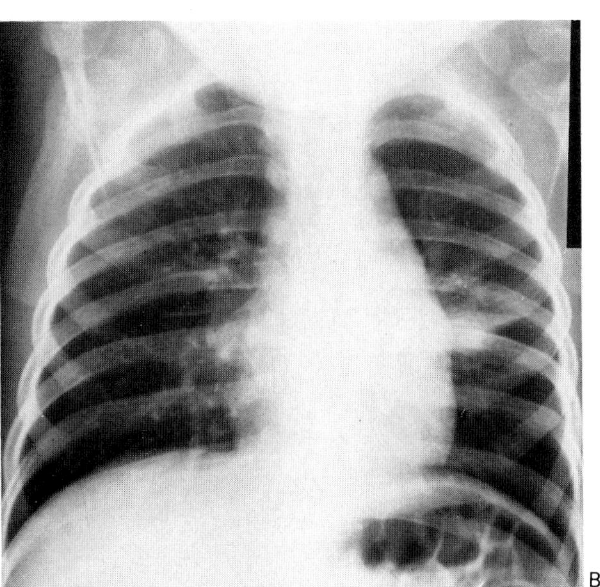

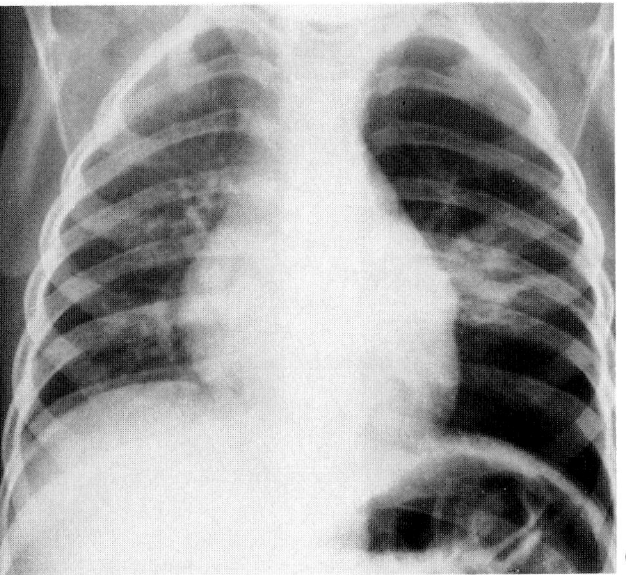

Fig. 19.12 Foreign body inhalation. (**A**) Obstructive emphysema from a foreign body in the left main bronchus. (**B** and **C**) Same child later; loss of volume in the left lung with patchy collapse in the apex of the left lower lobe; in inspiration (**B**) the mediastinum is slightly to the left; in expiration (**C**) the volume of the left lung changes little with the mediastinum swinging to the right.

BRONCHIOLITIS

This is often associated with the respiratory syncytial virus. The lungs appear overinflated with streaky peribronchiolar shadows. More confluent consolidation may complicate a frequently grave clinical condition.

INHALED FOREIGN BODIES (Fig. 19.12)

The variety of objects which children manage to aspirate is wide but peanuts are very common. There is a tendency to enter the more vertical right main bronchus. Complete obstruction will lead to peripheral collapse but partial obstruction can lead to obstructive emphysema. Films in expiration as well as inspiration supplemented if necessary by fluoroscopy will show mediastinal shift away from the obstructive emphysema on expiration. Bronchoscopy should be performed on strong clinical grounds even in the presence of normal radiography.

TRAUMA

Contusion of the lung can occur without rib fracture. Patchy resulting haemorrhagic consolidation can cavitate or resolve uneventfully.

HYDROCARBON ASPIRATION

Petrol or paraffin if accidentally swallowed frequently enter

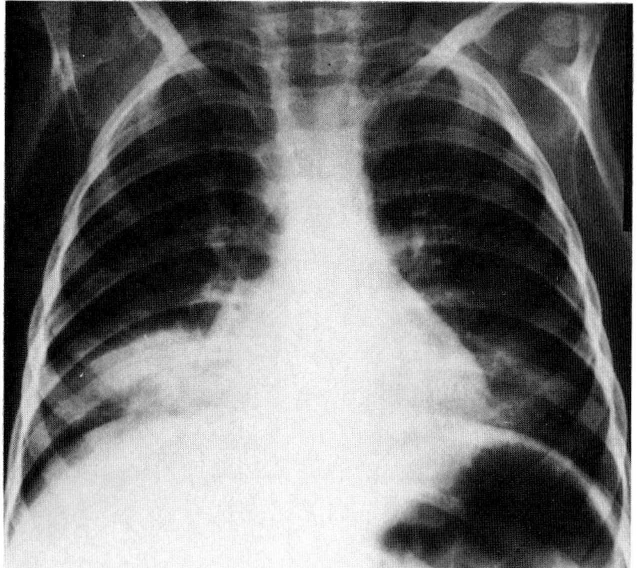

Fig. 19.13 Paraffin (kerosene) aspiration. Basal shadowing with early left basal pneumatocoele.

the trachea and may cause patchy basal lung shadowing, sometimes with delayed onset and sometimes with pneumatocoele formation (Fig. 19.13).

IMMUNE-COMPROMISE

A wide variety of common viruses, such as measles, and less common organisms such as *Pneumocystis* or cytomegalo-

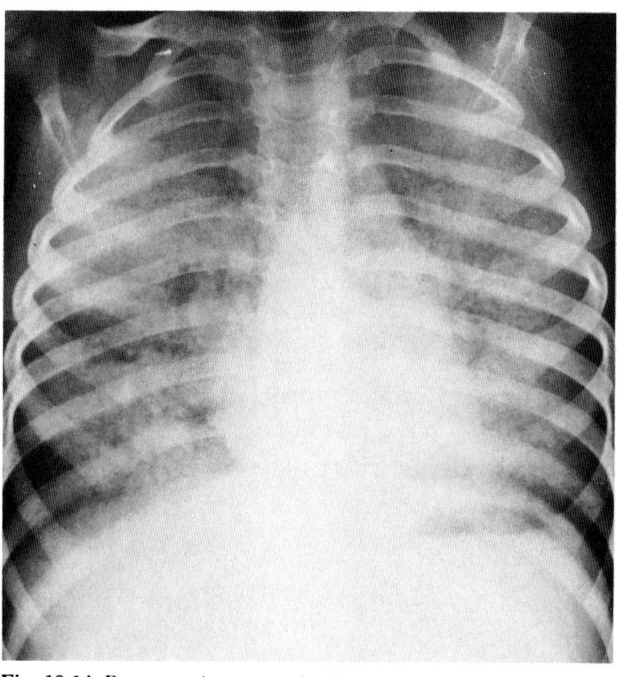

Fig. 19.14 *Pneumocystis* pneumonia. Widespread alveolar shadowing.

virus, cause extensive pulmonary shadowing in leukaemia or in children with immune deficiency or undergoing chemotherapy. Biopsy at times may be necessary to establish the diagnosis although *Pneumocystis* (Fig. 19.14) frequently has a typical appearance with gross lung opacification and an air bronchogram.

IDIOPATHIC PULMONARY HAEMOSIDEROSIS (Fig. 19.15)

This serious condition, often fatal in early adulthood starts in childhood with repeated pulmonary haemorrhages. At first it causes patchy shadowing with intervening clearing but progresses to permanent linear and reticular shadowing.

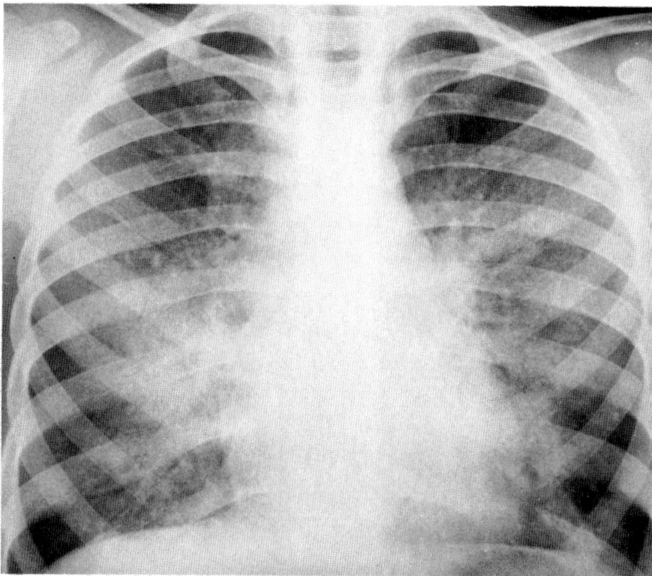

Fig. 19.15 Idiopathic pulmonary haemosiderosis. Perihilar shadowing with a reticulonodular pattern in the peripheral lung fields.

ASTHMA

Prolonged episodic bronchospasm reveals itself radiologically as over-distension of the lungs with a low flat diaphragm, sternal bowing, peribronchial shadowing seen as 'rings' end-on or 'tramlines' longitudinally and with occasional patchy shadowing.

Pneumomediastinum is most usually associated with asthma in childhood; extension results in subcutaneous emphysema particularly in the neck. Pneumothorax can at times also, but uncommonly, complicate.

TUBERCULOSIS

This is described in Chapter 15. In childhood, miliary tuberculosis is still too frequently seen (Fig. 19.16),

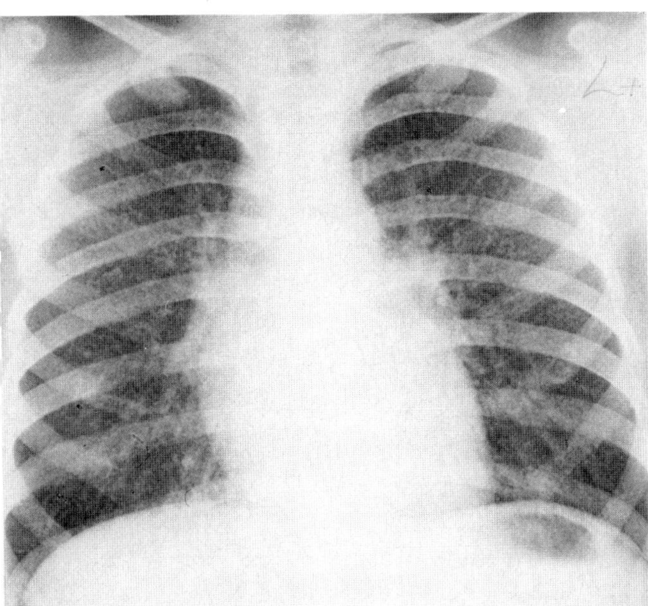

Fig. 19.16 Miliary tuberculosis. Fine nodularity throughout both lungs.

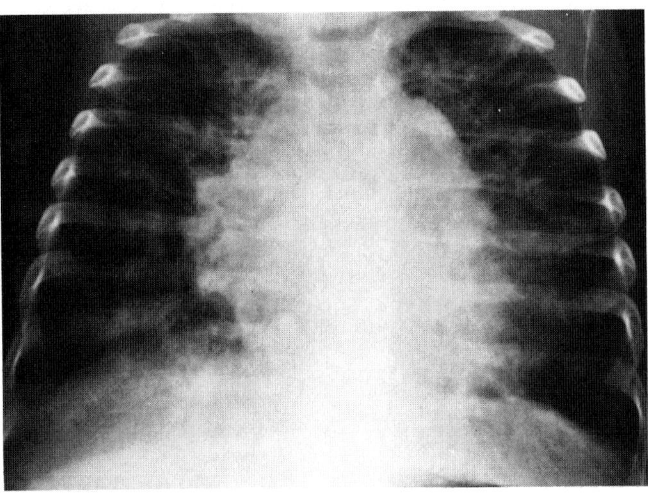

Fig. 19.17 Measles. Hilar lymph node enlargement with streaky shadowing radiating into the central lung fields.

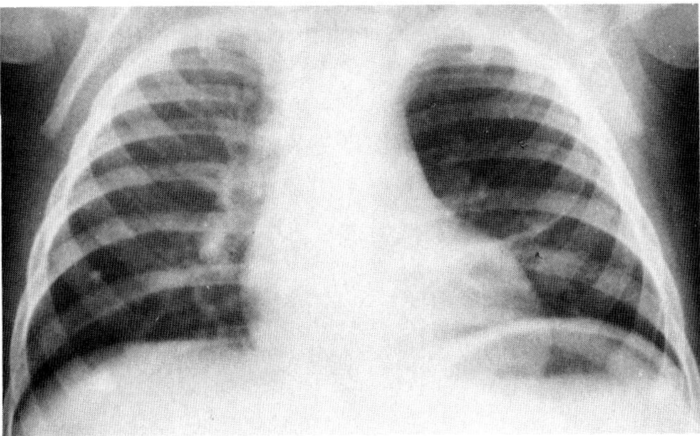

Fig. 19.18 Pneumatocoele. Previous left staphylococcal pneumonia.

especially in immigrants. A fine nodularity is evenly distributed throughout both lung fields. At times, mediastinal lymph node enlargement is also apparent.

PNEUMONIA

Many childhood pneumonias are viral (Fig. 19.17) in origin with non-specific features of patchy consolidation, overdistension and prominent hilar shadows.

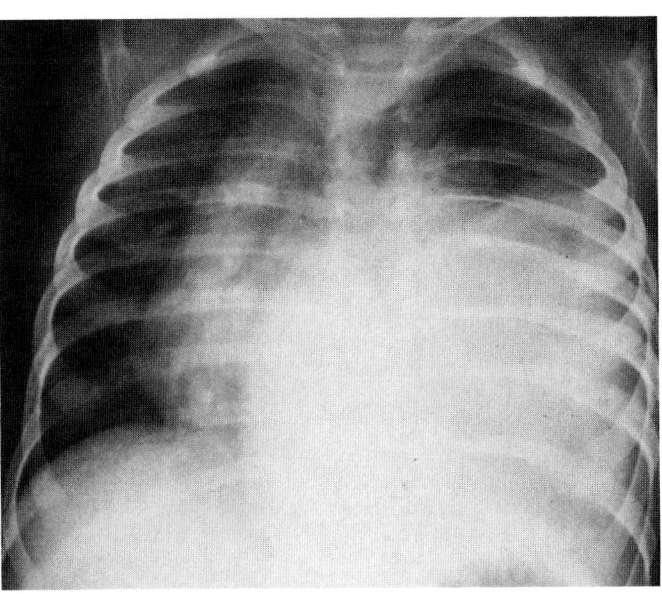

Fig. 19.19 Neuroblastoma. A large left posterior mass deviates the mediastinum to the right with thinning and separation of the adjacent posterior ends of the ribs.

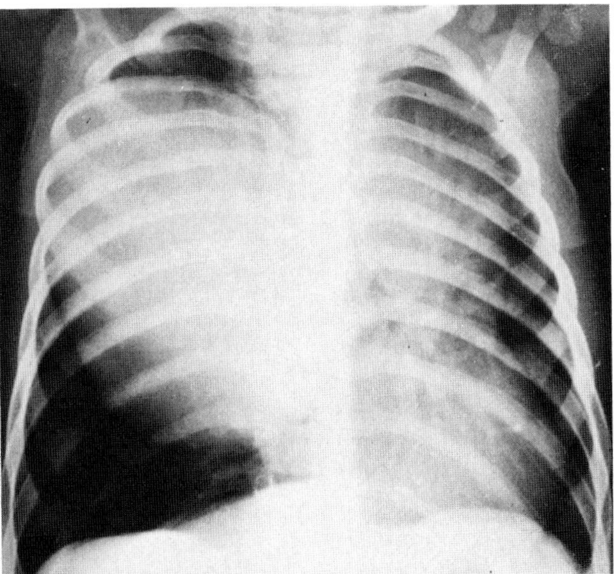

Fig. 19.20 Foregut duplication cyst with obstructive emphysema of the right lung.

Staphylococcal pneumonia, in its earlier stages non-specific in appearance, can develop highly characteristic pneumotocoeles (Fig. 19.18) showing as thin-walled radiolucencies which can rapidly enlarge and lead to pneumothorax. Their resolution is often slow with persistence long after pneumonic consolidation has resolved.

INTRATHORACIC MASSES

Neurogenic tumours such as neuroblastoma (Fig. 19.19) and ganglioneuroma are typically posterior, frequently deforming ribs. Calcification can be seen within the tumour from time to time and pleural effusions may be present.

Foregut duplication cysts (Fig. 19.20) are a common middle mediastinal mass and can cause bronchial or oesophageal compression. Vertebral anomalies are frequent. Ectopic gastric mucosa may be demonstrated by technetium-99m scanning in some of these cysts.

Cystic hygromas usually have a component in the neck as well as extension into the upper chest. Ultrasound is useful to demonstrate their characteristic massively cystic appearance.

Hilar lymph node enlargement occurs more obviously in pneumonia in childhood and is a feature of Hodgkin's disease, leukaemia and metastatic malignancies.

REFERENCES AND SUGGESTIONS FOR FURTHER READING

Avery, M. E., Fletcher, B. D., Williams, R. G. (1981) The lung and its disorders in the newborn infant, 4th edn. *Major Problems in Clinical Paediatrics*. Philadelphia: W. B. Saunders Company.

Felman, A. H. (1983) *The Pediatric Chest. Radiological, Clinical and Pathological Observations*. Springfield, Illinois: Charles C Thomas.

Griscom, N. T., Wohl, M. E. B., Kirkpatrick, J. A. (1978) Lower respiratory infections; how infants differ from adults. *Radiological Clinics of North America*. Vol XVI, pp 367–387.

Kaufmann, H. J. (ed.) (1967) *Progress in Pediatric Radiology* Vol. 1. Respiratory tract. Basel: S Karger.

Kendig, E. L., Chernick. V. (1977) *Disorders of the Respiratory Tract in Children*, 3rd edn. Philadelphia W. B. Saunders Company.

Phelan, P. D., Landau, L. I., Olinksy, A. 1982. *Respiratory Illness in Children*. 2nd edn. Oxford: Blackwell

Silverman, F. (ed.) (1985) *Caffey's Pediatric X-ray Diagnosis*. 8th edn. Chicago: Year Book.

Singleton, E. B., Wagner, M. L. (1971) *Radiologic Atlas of Pulmonary Abnormalities in Children*. Philadelphia: W. B. Saunders Company.

Swischuk, L. E. (1980) *Radiology of the Newborn and Young Infant*, 2nd edn. Baltimore: Williams and Wilkins.

Wesenberg, R. L. (1973) *The Newborn Chest*. Hagerston, Maryland: Harper and Row.

PART 3

THE HEART

CHAPTER 20

THE NORMAL HEART: METHODS OF EXAMINATION

PLAIN FILMS

The plain chest film, although it rarely provides a specific diagnosis of cardiac abnormality, is sufficiently important to be considered an integral part of the complete clinical assessment of the patient suspected of suffering from heart disease. It may indicate the nature of the functional derangement, and also its severity. To do this it should show the overall heart size, and evidence of selective chamber enlargement. It must also be of sufficient quality to enable the lung vessels to be studied. The standard cardiac series has consisted of a low KV chest film to show lung parenchyma, a penetrated PA chest to see detail within the heart, and a left lateral film with barium in the oesophagus to show left atrial size. Today, a high KV PA chest with a fine line grid represents an excellent single frontal film compromise, enabling intracardiac details and lung vessel anatomy to be seen on one film. Combined with a high quality lateral film, so that the left lower lobe bronchus may be identified, a two film cardiac study is adequate for routine purposes.

There is no place for routine oblique films in the examination of the heart. They are impossible to standardize and rarely give information which cannot be obtained more satisfactorily by other means.

FLUOROSCOPY

Image amplification fluoroscopy is easily performed but has only a limited place in the examination of the heart. Screening will show the relationship of any abnormal shadows to the heart. It is excellent for recognizing and locating intracardiac calcification, and may be of slight value in studying prosthetic valves.

Even in experienced hands it is of only limited value in the study of left ventricular aneurysm. The recognition of hilar dance in left to right shunts, and of systolic expansion of the left atrium in the diagnosis of mitral incompetence, are now of purely historical interest.

TOMOGRAPHY

Conventional tomography has virtually no place in present day cardiac radiology but *computed tomography* has been used to demonstrate pericardial effusions and thickening and also has been able to recognize tumours of the heart and dissecting aneurysms of the thoracic aorta.

ECHOCARDIOGRAPHY

Ultrasonic imaging of the heart or 'echocardiography', based on pulsed-echo techniques, allows the movements of intracardiac structures to be studied noninvasively with ease and reproducibility. The echo signal indicates the presence and location of a structure along the sound beam. Some specific details of intracardiac anatomy and pathology are much better documented by ultrasound than by X-ray imaging. There are two methods of cardiac ultrasound: one dimensional scanning is called M mode echocardiography, two dimensional scanning is variously described as the 2D echogram, cross-sectional scan or real-time scan. Pulsed Doppler can be combined with both methods to provide information about blood flow velocity and direction.

The M mode echocardiogram

The echoes reflected from different interfaces are converted electronically into spots which fall on light-sensitive paper moving at constant speed. A graph against time of the position of the reflecting structures of the heart relative to the transducer is produced. The M mode echogram requires for its interpretation the recognition of certain well-defined patterns of echo distribution and motion in closely specified beam positions which rely heavily on valve leaflet identification (Fig. 20.1). The major disadvantage is that it provides a limited 'ice-pick' view of the heart. It cannot visualize the complete left ventricular cavity, especially the apex, the right atrium and most of the leaflets of the tricuspid valve. In addition, intracardiac structures are displayed in an unfamiliar format and the spatial orientation of these structures cannot be readily appreciated.

The present indications for M mode echocardiograms are discussed individually but are summarized below:

Pericardial effusion. Quite small pericardial effusions may be detected as echo-free areas behind the left ventricle and

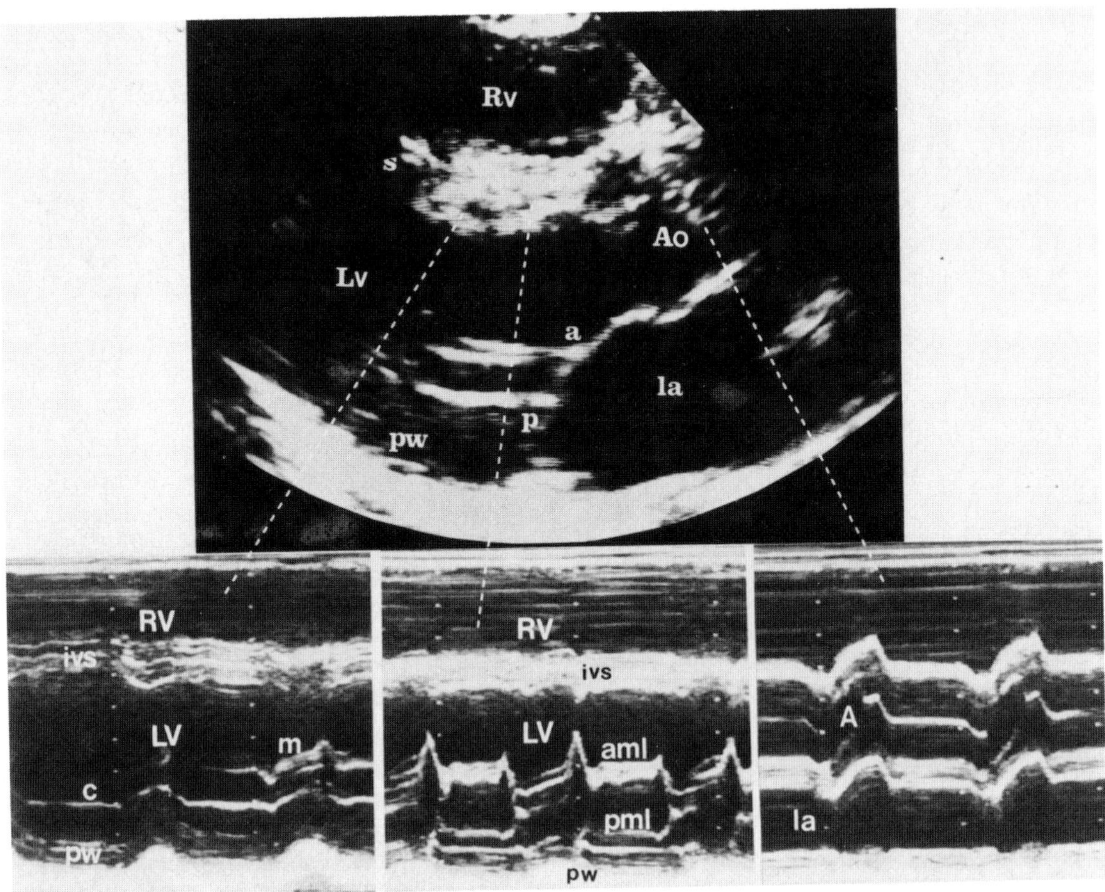

Fig. 20.1 Top. 2DE picture of a normal heart, long axis view. **Below.** M Mode pictures corresponding to the beam angles indicated on the 2DE picture, made simultaneously on a modern machine. **Left hand panel.** The beam goes through the left ventricular cavity below the level of the mitral valve. Both anterior and posterior walls of the left ventricle can be identified, together with their endocardial surfaces, and they move inwards together. Note that the cavity diameter can be measured in diastole and systole, as can the wall thickness. Without 2DE control the exact level at which the beam intersects the left ventricular cavity would be uncertain. **Middle panel.** The characteristic M shaped movement indicates that the beam is intersecting the anterior leaflet of the mitral valve. In addition the posterior leaflet of the mitral valve can be identified as moving in the opposite direction in diastole. **Right hand panel.** The box shaped opening movement of the aortic valve leaflets can be seen, which confirms that the beam is going through the aortic root. The left atrium can be identified lying behind the aorta and its long diameter can be measured.

Table of abbreviations in figures:

RV	right ventricle
LV	left ventricle
Ao, A	aorta
LA	left atrium
PW	posterior wall
a, aml	anterior leaflet mitral valve
p, pml	posterior leaflet mitral valve
c	chordae tendinae
ivs, s	interventricular septum
PA	pulmonary artery
RA	right atrium
L. ax	long axis view
S. ax	short axis view
e	endocardium
t	tricuspid valve
ias	interatrial septum
ED	end-diastole
ES	end-systole
AV	aortic valve
MV	mitral valve

in front of the right ventricle. They cannot be quantified. Difficulties may be encountered if there is a simultaneously occurring pleural effusion.

Mitral stenosis. Mitral stenosis may be recognized but its severity may not be easily estimated. Valve cusps are thickened in mitral stenosis and their movement restricted but the rate of opening is normal. Calcification cannot be distinguished from gross thickening by the echo returns. Mitral stenosis is virtually excluded if both anterior and posterior leaflets of normal thickness can be recorded simultaneously, moving in opposite directions. The thickening of the mitral valve in mitral stenosis can be distinguished from the fluttering of the anterior leaflet of the mitral valve which occurs in aortic incompetence and which may produce a similar murmur, the Austin-Flint murmur, which may cause difficulty on auscultation. A very large left atrium may be helpful in suggesting some significant degree of mitral regurgitation.

Prolapse of the mitral valve. Mid or late systolic prolapse of part of the mitral valve apparatus may be recognized but over and under diagnosis are extremely frequent.

Left atrial myxoma. M mode enchocardiography is able to detect the common prolapsing type of left atrial myxoma and to distinguish this from mitral valve disease, which it may resemble clinically. A left atrial myxoma cannot however be excluded unless the echographic recording is of the highest quality, and non-prolapsing myxomas are almost impossible to diagnose.

Aortic stenosis. The characteristic box-like opening and fine line closure of the normal aortic valve is replaced by showers of extra echoes, though usually with the same movement pattern, in calcific aortic stenosis.

Bicuspid aortic valve. A porportion of patients with bicuspid aortic valves may be recognized by restricted opening and eccentric closure of the aortic valve.

The left ventricle. A well-recorded M mode echocardiogram of the left ventricle should be able to identify the endocardial surface of both sides of the left ventricular cavity, in the region just below the main echoes of the mitral valve, and to identify the thickness of the left ventricular wall and the ventricular septum. With a good record it is possible to recognize cavity dilatation and impairment of contractility as evidence by reduced wall movement. Thus impairment of left ventricular function may be identified (when contraction remains concentric) and in addition asymmetrical thickening of the septum as opposed to the posterior wall may point to the diagnosis of hypertrophic cardiomyopathy, particularly when coupled with so-called systolic anterior movement of the mitral valve, though the latter is not specific.

Congenital heart disease. The M mode echocardiogram has virtually no place to play in the management of patients with congenital heart disease. It may show the large right ventricle and paradoxical septal movement associated with an atrial septal defect but has been entirely superseded by the 2D echogram in all other forms of congenital heart disease.

2D echogram (2DE)

By making the ultrasound beam oscillate automatically very rapidly backwards and forwards through an arc of 80 degrees, the information from a large number of M mode-scans is combined. The series of images will produce an accurate moving picture of the structures within the heart. Thus lateral as well as axial distances between structures can be appreciated, and the images obtained resemble heart structures. The 2DE allows complete visualization of all intracardiac structures. The structures shown on a 2DE depend on both the transducer position and the direction of oscillation. Two dimensional echocardiograms are effectively tomograms, showing structures in a 'slice' of the heart. The most common planes used in adult echocardiography are shown in Figs 20.2, 20.3 and 20.4.

Contrast echocardiography. Ultrasonic contrast agents rely on the injection of microbubbles of gas to produce enhancement. This is conveniently accomplished by the rapid manual injection of fluids such as 5% dextrose in water. The microbubbles are contained in the fluid or are flushed from the walls of syringes or tubing. Tricuspid regurgitation and right-to-left shunts can be directly imaged by contrast echocardiography.

Pulsed Doppler echocardiography. The application of the pulsed Doppler principles to 2DE permits blood flow information to be derived. The sample volume is positioned adjacent to the abnormal valve, or tracked along the septum to search for turbulent flow. A flow profile on

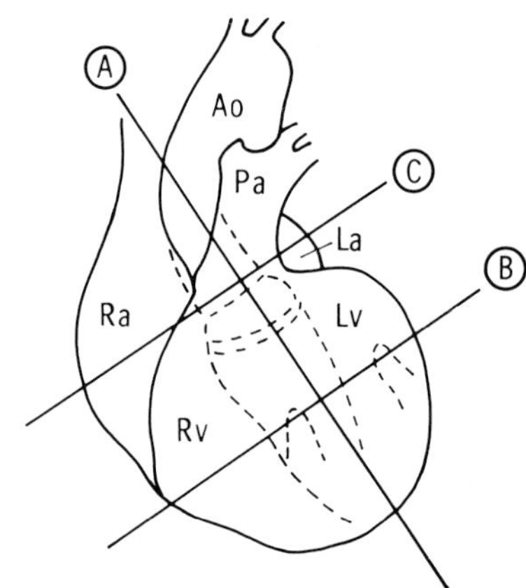

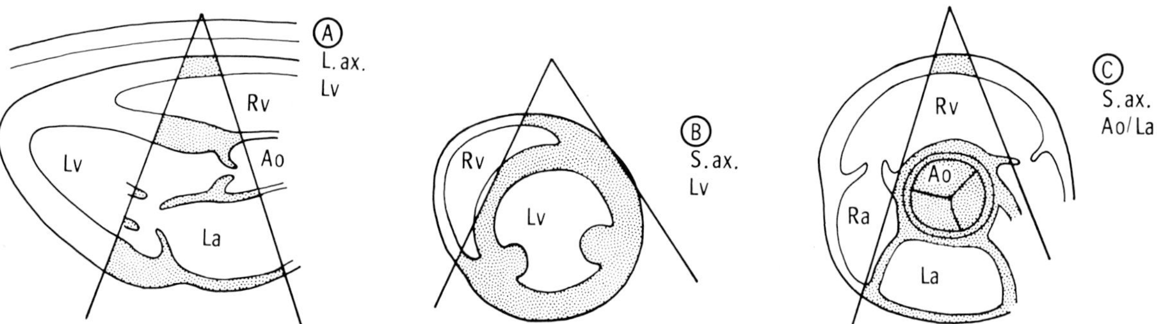

Fig. 20.2 2DE scanning of the heart. **Top left.** The heart shown diagramatically with the standard scanning planes indicated. (**A**) The long axis view. (**B**) Short axis view through the cavity of the left ventricle below the level of the mitral valve. (**C**) Short axis view more cranially than in (**B**).

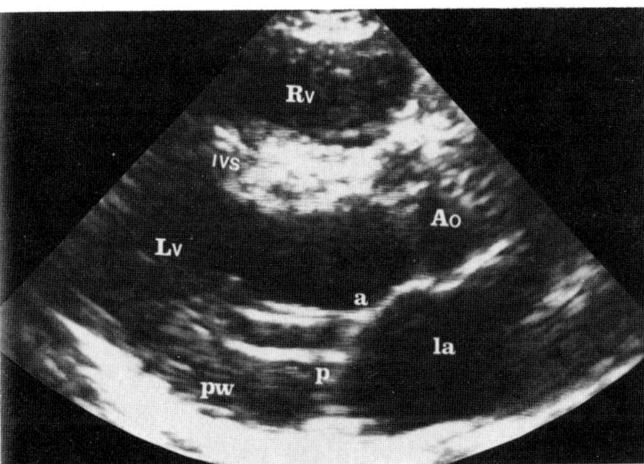

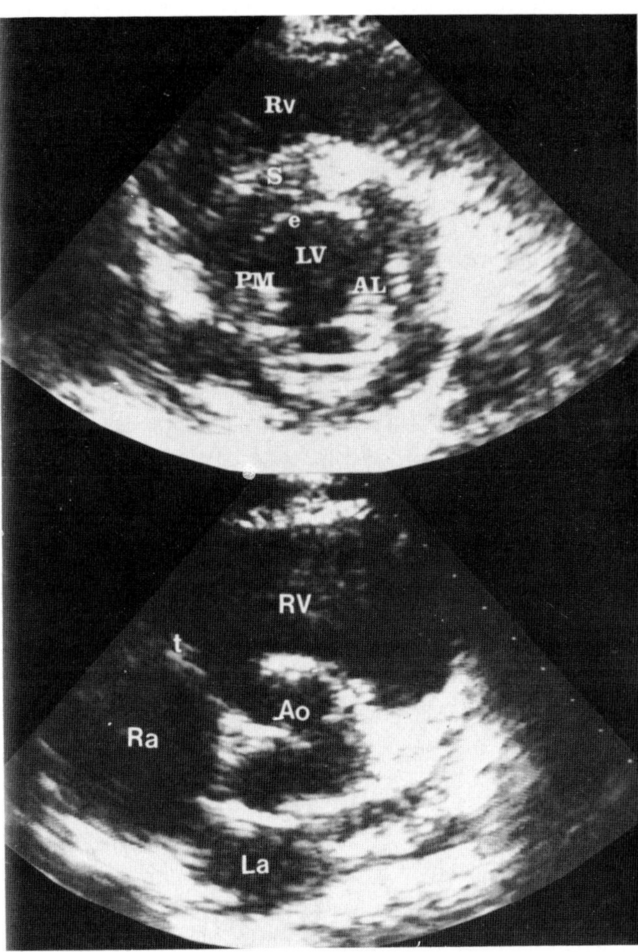

Fig. 20.3 2DE standard views corresponding to Figure 20.2. **Above.** Long axis view. This is useful for orientation of the cardiac structures and good for acquired disease of the mitral and aortic valves. It is also useful in left ventricular disease. **Top right**. A short axis cut through the left ventricle. The size and shape of the left ventricular cavity and wall thickness are demonstrated. **Below.** Short axis cut at the level of the aortic valve. As the transducer is angled cranially from the left ventricle the beam leaves the papillary muscles and intersects the mitral valve which has a characteristic 'fish-mouth' appearance. More cranial angulation intersects the aortic valve and also reveals the right ventricular outflow and in children the pulmonary valve and pulmonary artery and its bifurcation.

the direction or average flow velocity may be derived, and this provides insight into the physiological burden of valvular heart disease and intracardiac shunts.

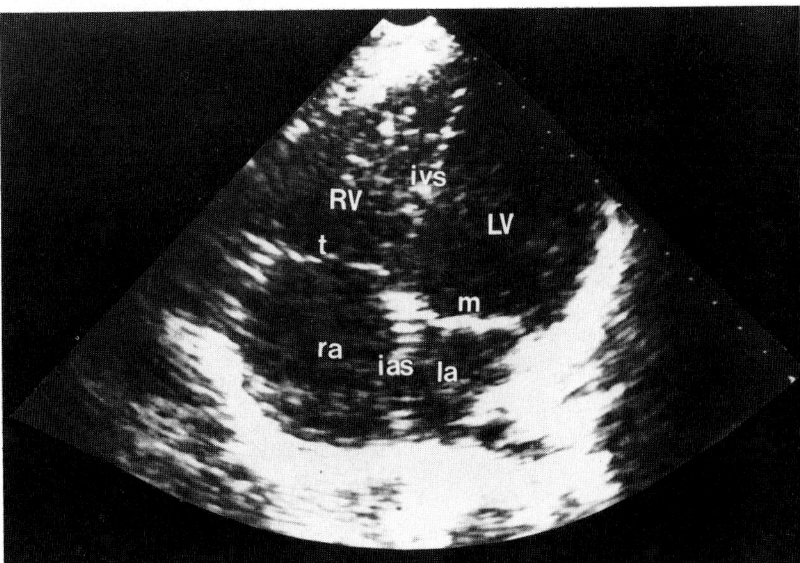

Fig. 20.4 2DE, the four chamber view. To obtain this view the transducer is rotated as well as angled so that all four chambers can be identified simultaneously together with both atrioventricular valves. This view gives one of the best demonstrations of the left ventricle and the ventricular septum and also of the atrioventricular valve. In acquired heart disease it enables structural abnormality to be seen. In congenital heart disease this view is excellent for identifying the opening of the valves into their respective ventricles. 'Drop-out' of echoes in the inter-atrial septum are common in this view, but by obtaining this view subcostally, more conclusions about the inter-atrial septum may be drawn.

ISOTOPES IN CARDIOLOGY

Isotope imaging generally is dealt with in Chapter 66 and in this section a résumé of the cardiac application is attempted. Isotopes have been used to study ventricular function and myocardial perfusion.

Ventricular function studies

Radionuclide techniques for monitoring global and regional ventricular functions fall into two major categories: 1) *First pass studies* in which the injected bolus dose is monitored during its first passage through the heart and great vessels; and 2) *Gated equilibrium studies* in which the tracer mixes with the blood pool before data collection. Both these nuclear studies can be performed at the patient's bedside using a mobile gamma camera; each technique has its own strength and weakness (Table 20.1).

Following injection the labelled radioactive tracer localizes in the heart releasing energy in the form of gamma photons which traverse overlying tissues and interact with the imaging device (single crystal or multicrystal gamma camera). A collimator permits only photons arising from specific areas of the heart to interact with the camera. The imaging device converts the gamma photon energy into an electrical signal that can be processed; an on-line computer records the information and permits the optimal visual or quantitive display of the data.

For cardiac nuclear imaging a number of heart cycles have to be averaged to provide data for accurate interpretation of structure and function. In *first pass studies* data are usually summed without regard to physiological signal; in the *gated equilibrium technique* the start of each cardiac cycle is identified from a physiological marker (the R wave of the electrocardiogram) and data from each cycle are added in the correct temporal sequence ('gated'). Gated nuclear imaging is inaccurate if the cardiac rhythm is very irregular.

First pass method. The first pass method of radionuclide angiography consists of rapidly injecting a bolus of isotope ($^{99}Tc^{m}$ pertechnetate) into the antecubital vein and obtaining images as the bolus passes through the right heart, lung fields and left heart chambers. A multidetector gamma camera with high count rate characteristics (up to 250 000 counts per second) should be used, its disadvantage being its lack of mobility. The representative cycle can be played in cine format for quantitive evaluation of wall motion; superimposed end-diastolic and end-systolic perimeters are generated to evaluate regional wall motion further (Fig. 20.5).

Table 20.1 Comparison of the two methods of radionuclide angiography

	First pass	Equilibrium
Radiopharmaceutical	Technetium-99m pertechnetate (readily available) Bolus required	Technetium-99m-labelled RBC's or HSA (preparation requires 15–20 minutes)
Camera	High count rate capabilities (multicrystal)	Conventional camera
Camera positioning	Prior to injection of agent any projection (RAO possible)	After administration of agent. LAD projection of choice
Imaging time	30 second	3–10 minutes
Measurements per injection	One measurement	Multiple repeat measurements
Advantages	1. Minimal background activity 2. Temporal separation — optimal views of chambers 3. Visualization of inferior and anterior wall motion abnormalities slightly superior 4. Analysis of lung flow possible 5. Measurement of cardiac output 6. Quantification of shunts	1. Permits repeat studies after interventions over long periods of time 2. Estimation of severity of valvar regurgitation

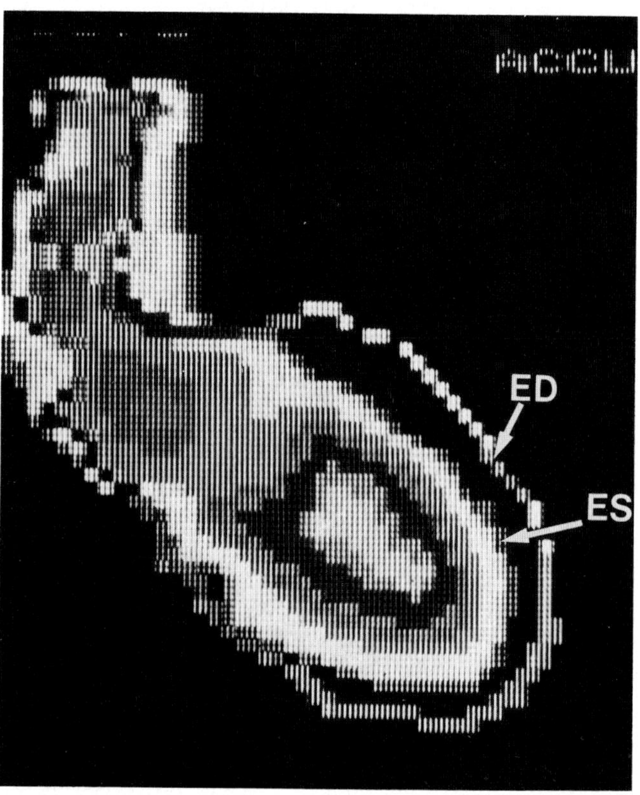

Fig. 20.5 Normal first pass isotope ventriculography. Diastole and systole can both be identified, the shape of the ventricle determined and pattern of contraction seen.

Although single crystal gamma cameras can also be used for this method, the count density obtained with them is limited and may hinder the accuracy of the values obtained. They have the advantage of mobility.

Gated equilibrium studies (Fig. 20.6). An isotope which remains fixed within the vascular space (such as $^{99}Tc^{m}$-labelled human serum albumin or red blood cells) is administered intravenously. This isotope permits the recording of data for up to four hours, thus allowing the acquisition of multiple images in various projections and also the study of the ventricular response to interventions. After equilibration, the counts are synchronized in relation to the portion of the cardiac cycle using the R wave of the electrocardiogram and the cardiac cycle is divided by the computer into a fixed number of frames. This synchronization is called 'gated' imaging. Frame durations of 40–50 ms are usually adequate. Most studies require 6–10 minutes to obtain adequate counts for data analysis. Derived data are then processed by computer to determine the variables of left ventricular contraction as with first pass data.

Non-imaging methods. A single crystal 'probe' coupled to a small processing unit is capable of producing beat to beat time/activity curves which permit the measure of ejection fraction and end-systolic and end-diastolic volumes from changes in left ventricular counts. This non-imaging device is small and readily portable. Ejection fraction may thus be measured over a long period of time if a non-diffusable indicator (such as labelled red cells) is used; the accuracy of the method is increased if electrocardiographic gating is incorporated to the system. Difficulties with the probe method arise from the correct positioning of the probe over the ventricular area of interest.

Quantitive data analysis

Ejection fraction. Semi-automatic methods for measuring cardiac ejection fraction have been in clinical use for many years. After data accumulation, the region of interest (i.e. the left ventricle) is identified and the computer generates a time/activity curve with a cyclic rise and fall in counts (Fig. 20.7). The counts are proportional

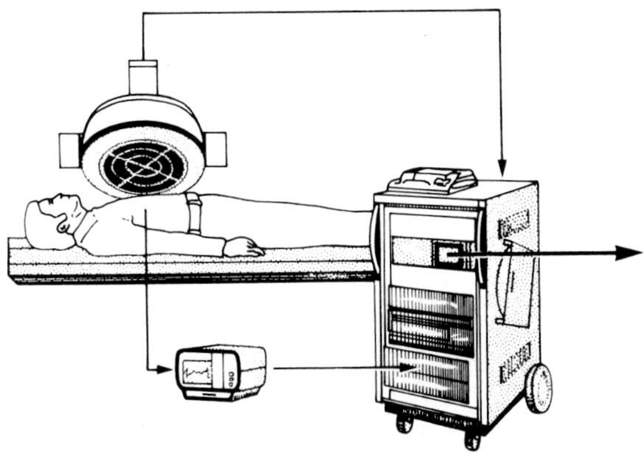

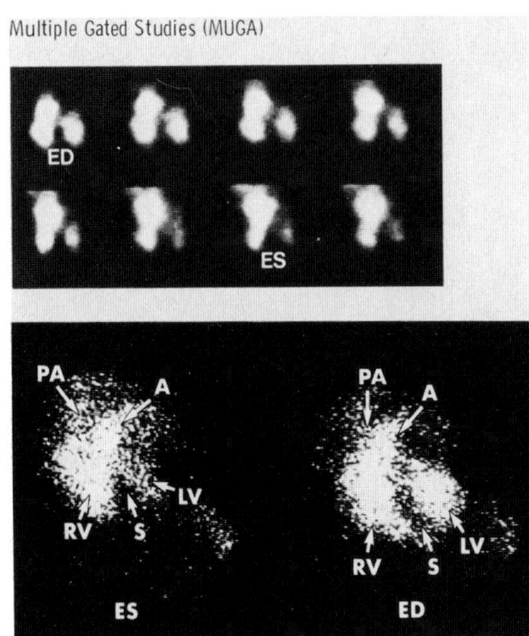

Fig. 20.6 Gated equilibrium isotope ventriculography (MUGA — multiple gated acquisition). The gamma camera is positioned in the left anterior oblique position to obtain separation of right and left ventricles; data acquisition is synchronised ('gated') by the computer to the ECG signals.

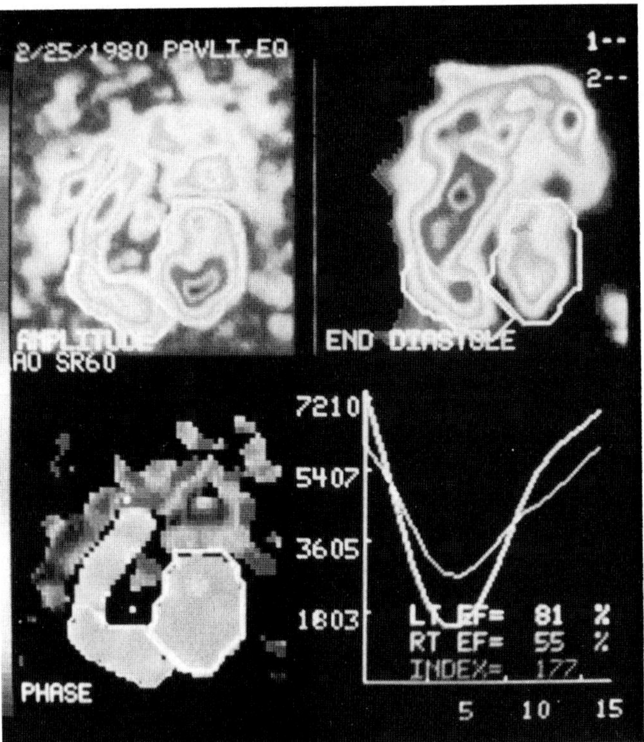

Fig. 20.7 Quantitative data analysis of the normal cardiac cycle. (Amplitude and phase image analysis) made from a gated equilibrium scan. The phase image demonstrates uniform (normal) contraction. From the time/activity curve, the ejection fraction of both ventricles (LT EF, RT EF) is calculated and expressed as a percentage.

to the volume of the chamber. The difference between peak-counts at end-diastole to trough counts at end-systole reflects the stroke counts; stroke counts divided by ED counts (after appropriate background correction) determine the ejection fraction. This time/activity curve is independent of geometric assumptions inherent in the area–length technique utilized in contrast ventriculography and echocardiography.

Regional wall motion analysis. The images are viewed in a cine film format on a continuous loop for evaluation of wall motion abnormalities; by colour coding and by recycling the images over and over again a better perception of the ventricular function is obtained. The subjective interpretation of the images is complemented by the quantitive data; normal (Figs. 20.5 and 20.6) and abnormal (Fig. 20.8) systolic wall motion in different areas of the ventricle can be assessed fairly accurately by this method. Wall motion can also be studied from display of perimetric data derived by computer analysis of the gated cardiac cycle. The cardiac cycle is divided into its various temporal frequency ccomponents, each frequency characterized by a specific *amplitude* and *phase*. The amplitude image represents the amount of contraction. The analysis of ventricular emptying and relaxation is derived from the *phase image* (Fig. 20.7), the degree of regional phase delay is generally related to the severity of contraction abnormalities and occurs in segments of the ventricle with no movement (akinetic) or in those moving paradoxically in systole (dyskinetic).

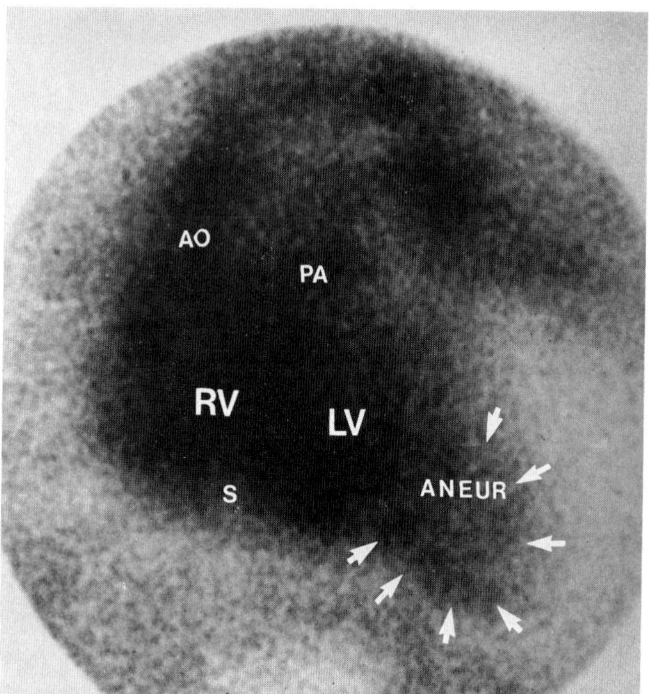

Fig. 20.8 Gated equilibrium scan in the left anterior oblique position. An apical left ventricular aneurysm has been demonstrated (arrows).

NUCLEAR TECHNIQUES FOR THE STUDY OF MYOCARDIAL PERFUSION AND INFARCT IMAGING

Assessment of myocardial perfusion

The use of thallium-201 myocardial scintigraphy for myocardial perfusion imaging has found wide acceptance in routine practice. Since thallium-201 uptake has been shown to be mainly dependent on myocardial blood flow and to a lesser degree on local cell metabolism, it can be used to assess the extent of hypoperfusion and hence ischaemic disease in the walls of the heart. Since the physical half-life of the isotope is 73 hours, transient myocardial ischaemia can be detected by comparing the uptake data at the time of exercise with those obtained 3–4 hours later at rest. The thallium is injected at maximal exercise. Ten minutes after the exercise the patient is placed beneath the detector of the gamma camera and thallium scintigrams are made successively in the left anterior oblique 45°, left anterior oblique 65° and anterior orientations (Fig. 20.9). Late imaging is performed in the same sequence after 3 to 4 hours. An area with reduced thallium uptake early after exercise may be due to either

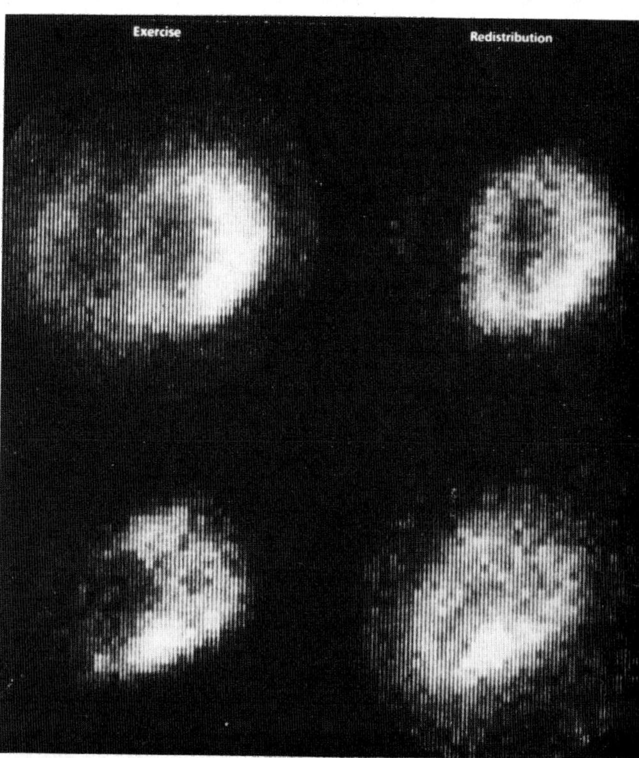

Fig. 20.9 Thallium-201 myocardial perfusion scanning. Above are the left anterior oblique views and below the lateral views of the same patient. Note the activity defect which is present in the septal aspect of the left ventricle on exercise but which fills in in the redistribution phase, seen on both views. The reversibility of the perfusion defect suggests that the myocardium is ischaemic but not necrotic. Note that the wall of the right ventricle is also demonstrated during exercise. Thallium is one of the few ways of demonstrating abnormalities of right ventricular perfusion.

ransient uptake abnormalities (ischaemia) or a previous myocardial infarction (scar). While in an acute ischaemic area the uptake defect decreases or disappears with time, (Fig. 20.9) the activity remains diminished or absent in an infarcted zone. The visual interpretation of these images depends on observer experience, image quality, ratio of myocardial to background activity, and the medium by which the images are presented. To improve the reliability of the diagnosis, computer programs have been developed for the quantitative analysis of these images. The sensitivity and specificity of exercise ^{201}Tl myocardial imaging appear to be in the range of 85–95%, a moderate but definite improvement on the exercise electrocardiogram.

Infarct imaging agents

A variety of technetium-labelled phosphates are taken up by irreversibly damaged myocardium; a positive concentration gradient is therefore achieved between infarcted and normal tissue. The main application of these radiopharmaceuticals is the serial evaluation of infarct size (usually overestimated by this method), in the differentiation between old and recent infarction (particularly in patients with bundle branch block on the ECG) and in the visualization of right ventricular infarction. The infarct may be detected as a positive focus 12 hours to one week after infarction.

ANGIOCARDIOGRAPHY

Angiocardiography is the X-ray imaging of the heart following the injection of radio-opaque contrast medium. *Selective angiocardiography*, the positioning of the contrast medium injection, through a cardiac catheter, selectively in relation to the lesion to be demonstrated, is invariably employed. With digital subtraction techniques, *non-selective (venous) angiocardiography* may well have a resurgence. Selective angiocardiography is always combined with cardiac catheterization so that intracardiac pressures and if necessary oxygen saturations can be measured. The aim is to delineate not only the types of abnormality which may be present but also their severity, so haemodynamic assessment is essential in other than coronary artery disease.

Filming is almost invariably by cine from high definition image amplifiers. 100 mm cut film may be employed in coronary arteriography as the format is large enough for direct viewing by the surgeon. 14 in. square cut film may be employed for pulmonary angiography or aortography where the large field format is particularly useful.

Selective angiocardiography requires the site of contrast injection to be chosen for the best display of the lesion suspected by clinical, echocardiographic or haemodynamic assessment. Contrast is injected downstream of *leaking valves* (cine angiography is still the best method of assessing the severity of regurgitation), upstream of *obstructions*, and in the chamber or vessel originating a *shunt*. The volume of contrast and its delivery rate is usually individually tailored to the problem to be investigated. For problems involving abnormal structure of the heart, where anatomical delineation is important, a volume of 1 ml/kg body weight should be delivered within two seconds, and the inevitable ectopic beats accepted for the sake of the high density of contrast which may be obtained. For functional cardiac studies such as left ventriculography in acquired heart disease, a slow injection should avoid ectopic beats and a low density of opacification will be accepted. Here 8–16 ml/s over 3 seconds, depending on the size and activity of the left ventricle and the quality of the X-ray equipment, will be adequate. A rate and volume controlled injector is essential.

The choice of projection will also be influenced by the problem to be studied. Projections have become more complex. The standard biplane AP and lateral series gave way to the left anterior oblique and right anterior oblique views aimed at profiling the septal and atrioventricular valve planes; these have themselves partly given way to oblique views with the addition of cranial beam angulation so that foreshortening of the profiled septum is reduced and septal and valve planes may be profiled in one view. These complex projections require ever more powerful X-ray equipment and ever more sophisticated tube suspensions.

Contrast medium

The standard ionic contrast media have pronounced effects on both the heart and the circulation. Passage of the contrast medium through the coronary circulation produces profound, though transient, changes in the ECG. These may be associated with demonstrable impairment of ventricular contraction and a rise in the left ventricular filling pressure, and associated left ventricular dilatation. The fall in blood pressure which is associated with angiocardiography is mediated in part by the impairment of ventricular contraction associated with the perfusion of the coronary arteries by the contrast and in part by the peripheral vasodilatation which the contrast medium produces. Subsequently there is an increase in cardiac output due to haemodilution. Injection of contrast medium into the pulmonary artery may be associated with a rise in pulmonary artery pressure.

The low ionic contrast media are associated with much less subjective discomfort and significantly less haemodynamic abnormality than the standard media. The non-ionic media of similar osmolarity have virtually no deleterious haemodynamic effect, their response being similar to that of normal saline. It seems likely that, in spite of their cost, these will be the agents of the future.

Angiocardiography is usually good at anatomical delineation of lesions but much less satisfactory in determining their severity and the degree of haemodynamic disturbance that they have produced. Angiocardiography can demonstrate an *obstruction* be it valvar or sub (or even supra) valvar but the severity of the obstruction must be assessed by the *pressure gradient*. This may be obtained by passing a catheter across the obstruction or by having catheters on either side. In the *right heart* the gradient across the pulmonary artery can usually be obtained by passing a catheter into the pulmonary arteries beyond the pulmonary valve and withdrawing it to the right ventricle. For tricuspid valve gradients it is customary to employ a double lumen catheter because the overall pressures are low, pressure differences are very low and balancing the pressure recording system is critical. In the *left heart* an aortic gradient may be obtained by crossing the aortic valve retrogradely to the left ventricle from the aorta or by measuring aortic and left ventricular pressures separately, the latter from a trans-septal left atrial to left ventricular catheter. Similarly mitral gradients can be obtained either using a direct left atrial pressure from a trans-septal catheter or an indirect pressure from a wedged pulmonary artery catheter, and by a catheter in the left ventricle.

When the significance of a gradient is not clear it may be necessary to measure the cardiac output (gradient depends not only on the severity of the obstruction but the flow across it) and it may be necessary to increase the cardiac output by exercise to measure a significant gradient.

The measurement of *valvar regurgitation* is difficult whatever measure is adopted. Aortic regurgitation is best assessed by cine aortography in the left anterior oblique projection and mitral regurgitation by cine left ventriculography in the right anterior oblique projection. Quantification of the appearances is not really satisfactory but gives a general guide to the severity of the condition. An attempt may be made to assess pulmonary and tricuspid incompetence by cine angiography but the significance of the findings is never clear in view of the presence of the catheter across the valve.

The number and size of *shunts* may be demonstrated by angiocardiography but the degree of shunting requires either measurements of oxygen saturation changes or other more complex methods to measure shunt volumes.

Pulmonary vascular resistance, an important measurement in the management of congenital heart disease, requires measurement not only of the pressure in the pulmonary artery and in the left atrium but also of the flow across the lungs. The present method of studying *left ventricular function*, a key factor in the surgical management of patients with acquired heart disease, consists of studying the size of the left ventricle and the proportion of its content which it ejects with each beat (ejection fraction, EF = SV/EDV*). This can be measured by measuring the volume of the ventricle on cine angiograms, based on the assumption that the left ventricle is an ellipsoid of revolution, but most radiologists base their assessment on experience. Though the ejection fraction is the best method available for measuring ventricular function it is widely influenced by factors outside the heart itself and will ultimately be replaced by a less dependent method.

*SV = Stroke Volume, EDV = End Diastolic Volume

The era of catheterization and angiocardiography in every patient with heart disease considered for surgery is already drawing to a close. Any patient with acquired heart disease in whom the number and severity of the valvular lesions can be estimated on the basis of the clinical examination and echocardiography, and in whom coronary artery disease is not suspected, can be operated on without this invasive investigation. An increasing number of patients with more complex congenital heart disease are being subjected to surgery on the basis of the clinical and 2DE examinations without angiocardiography. In some areas of anatomical delineation, particularly in the congenital abnormalities of the atrioventricular valves and their connections, 2DE is demonstrably superior to angiography. In two areas however angiocardiography is still vital. In the investigation of coronary disease there are no simple non-invasive methods available. In disorders of the pulmonary circulation associated with congenital heart disease the echocardiographer cannot easily get beyond the main pulmonary artery and to a lesser extent he has the same difficulty beyond the aortic valve; in these areas angiocardiography is still indicated.

NORMAL ANATOMY

Although the basic anatomy of the heart and its vessels is well known from the dissecting room the appearances of these structures in situ in the closed thorax may well appear unfamiliar when demonstrated by radiological methods. The normal *superior vena cava* (Fig. 20.10) forms the right border of the superior mediastinum. It is not normally visible as a discrete shadow. It may be visibly enlarged when distended as in right heart cardiac failure.

A persisting *left superior vena cava* (which usually drains to the coronary sinus and thence to the right atrium) may be recognized as a low density shadow in the left superior mediastinum (Fig. 20.11A, B).

The *inferior vena cava* is commonly recognized on good quality lateral views of the chest by its straight posterior border rising from the diaphragm to join the back of the heart in the middle of the right atrium. It may also be seen in the frontal view in the right pericardiophrenic angle (Figs 20.12A and B) and may be visibly distended in heart failure.

The *azygos vein* rises in the posterior mediastinum on the right side and passes forward to join the superior vena cava before it enters the right atrium. Occasionally the normal azygos vein may be seen as a small 'end on' shadow in the angle between the right main bronchus and the trachea.

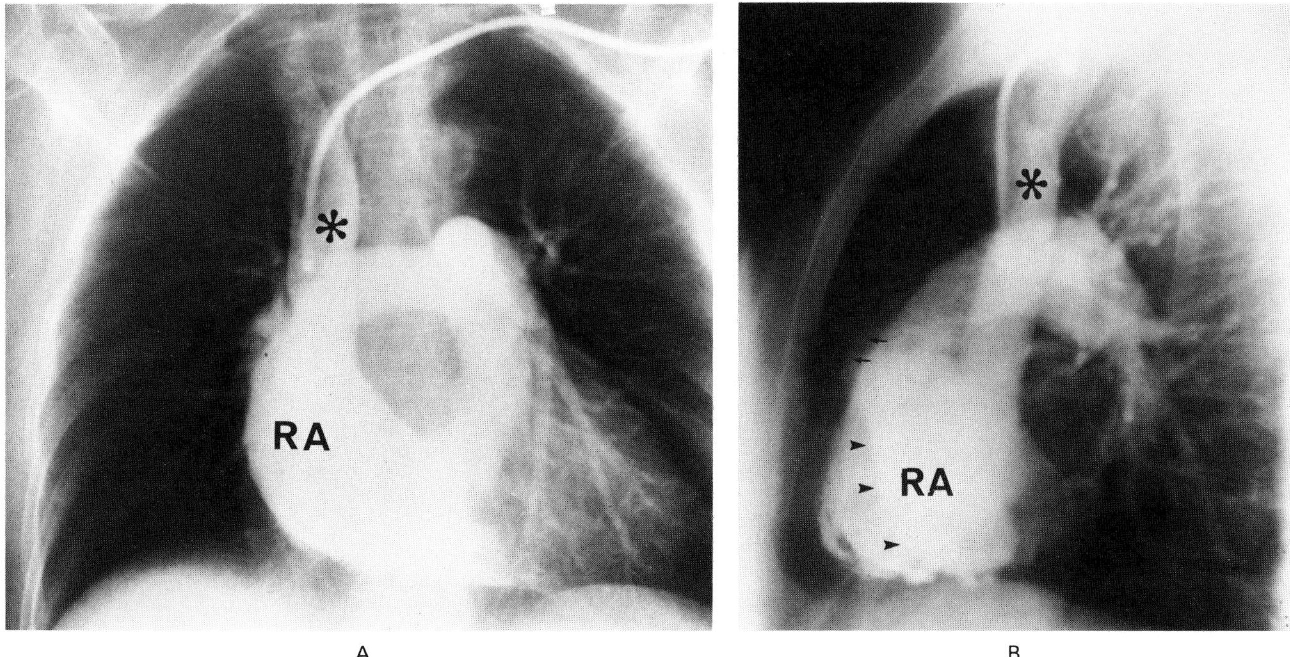

Fig. 20.10 Normal right atrial angiogram. The injection has been made from a catheter in the superior vena cava. (**A**) Frontal view. (**B**) Lateral view. * indicates the superior vena cava, arrow heads mark the front border of the right atrium in the lateral view, overlapped by the right ventricle. Arrows indicate the front border of the right atrial appendage. The superior vena cava forms the right border of the superior mediastinum and the right atrium forms the border of the heart. Only the right atrial appendage forms part of the front border in the lateral view.

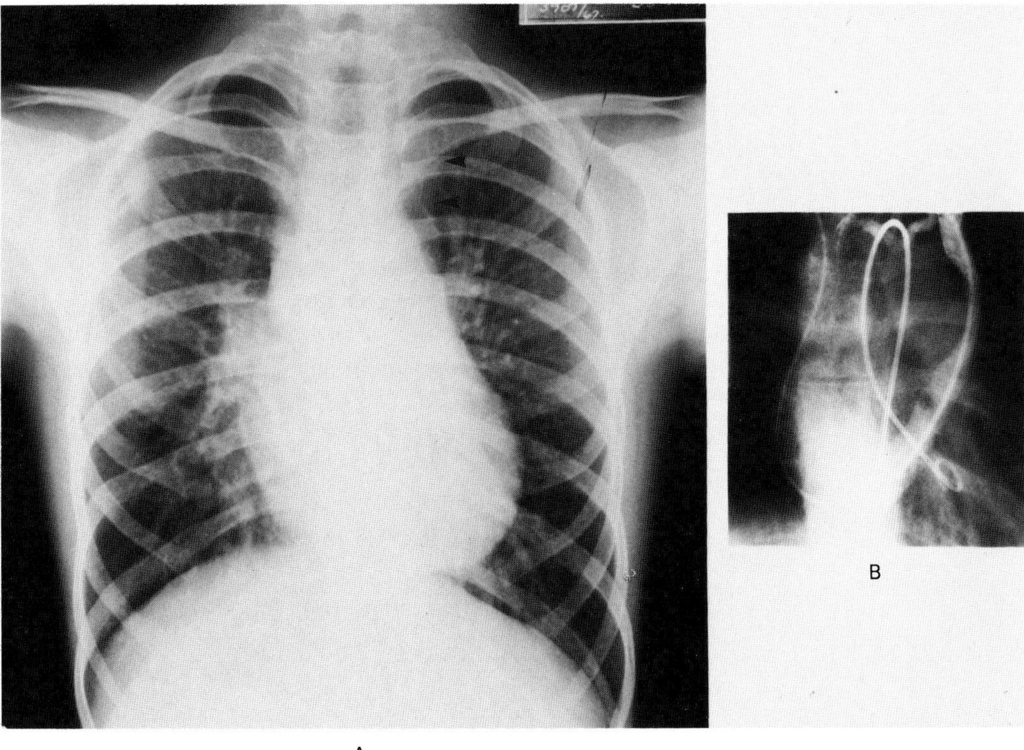

Fig. 20.11 (**A**) Persisting left superior vena cava. This appears as a low density shadow (arrowed) to the left of the superior mediastinum in the plain film (**B**) The matching angiogram shows it to descend to the left of the aortic arch.

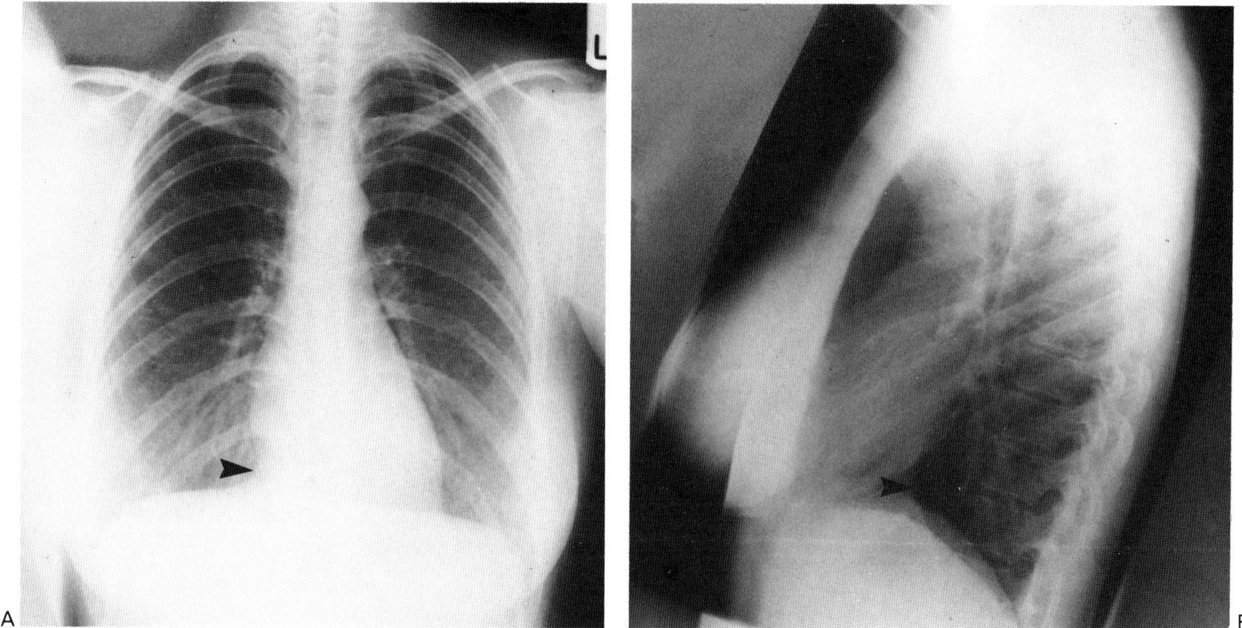

Fig. 20.12 (**A** and **B**) Normal inferior vena cava (arrowed) seen in frontal and lateral views.

When an azygos lobe is present its fissure points to the azygos vein. The azygos vein may be quite large in the absence of pathology, when it may be confused with a paramediastinal mass. Contrast studies will serve to identify the shadow as vascular. It may be pathologically enlarged when the right heart filling pressure is increased from both cardiac and non-cardiac causes as in superior vena cava or portal venous obstruction. It reaches its largest size however when there is congenital interruption of the intrahepatic part of the inferior vena cava so that the distal inferior vena cava drains directly into the azygos vein which returns all the blood from the lower half of the body (Fig. 20.13A, B). This arrangement always suggests the possibility of left isomerism or polysplenia.

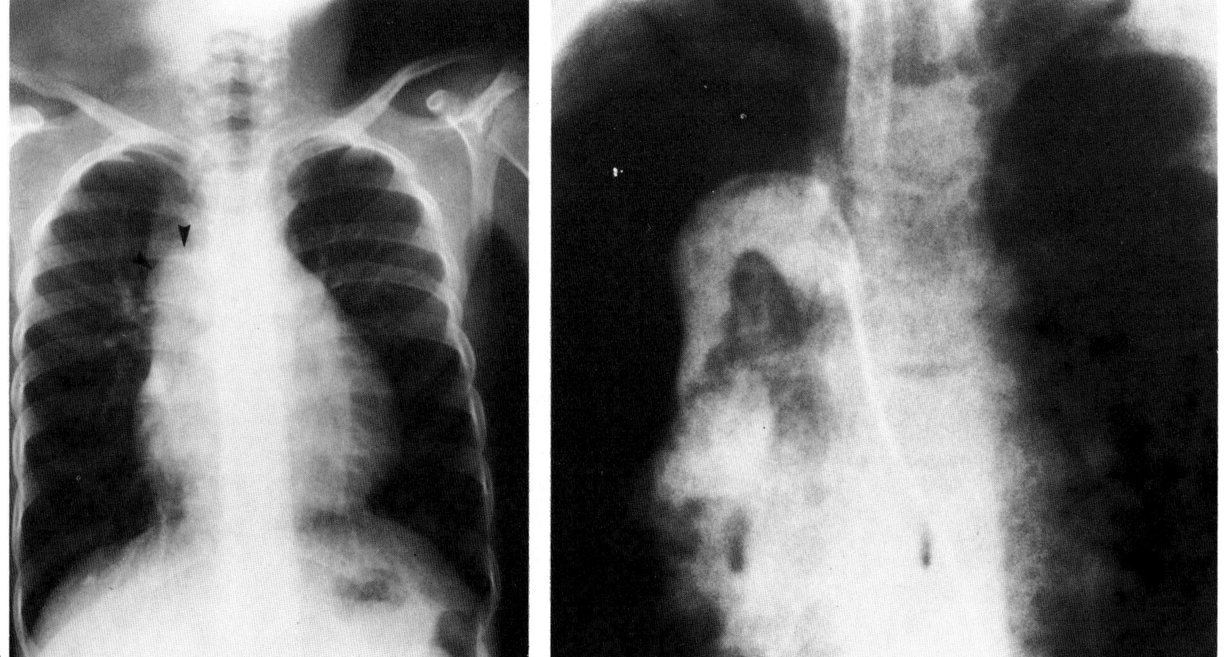

Fig. 20.13 Interruption of the inferior vena cava. (**A**) The enlarged azygos vein (arrows) may resemble the aortic arch. (**B**) Contrast studies in the same case shows the azygos continuation of the inferior vena cava arching over the right main bronchus to enter the right atrium.

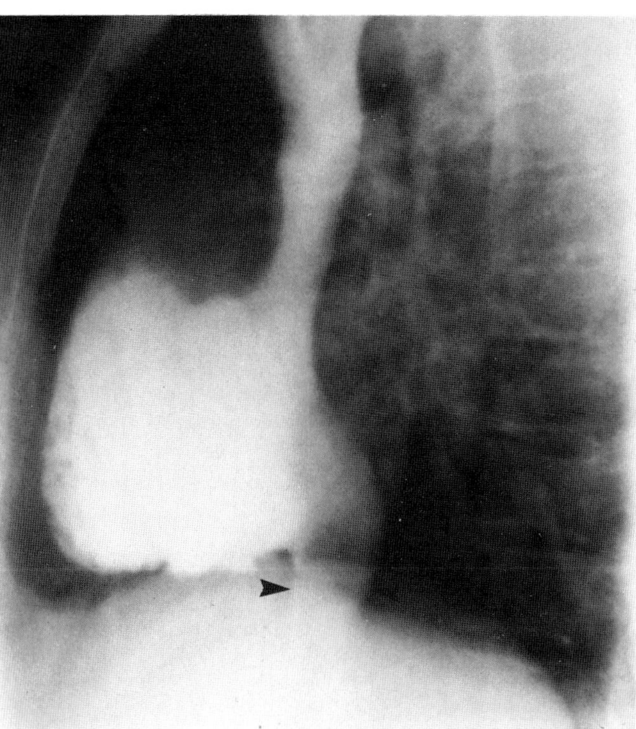

Fig. 20.14 Right atrial angiocardiogram, lateral view. Contrast has been injected into the superior vena cava and has refluxed down the inferior vena cava (arrow) showing it entering the back of the right atrium.

A left hemiazygos vein, if present, may also be enlarged for similar reasons.

The right atrium (Fig. 20.10) is a globular chamber forming the right heart border in the frontal view. Its broad based appendage passes forwards and to the left from its upper anterior aspect to sit on the front of the heart. The appendage is the only part of the right atrium seen anteriorly in the lateral view. The posterior wall of the right atrium is marked in the lateral chest film by the entrance of the inferior vena cava (Fig. 20.14).

When the right atrium is enlarged it protrudes the right heart border to the right and increases its radius of curvature, as the spherical chamber increases its diameter (Fig. 20.15A and B). A big right atrial appendage can fill in the space, seen in the lateral view, between the front of the heart and the back of the sternum.

Right atrial enlargement can occur in relation to acquired tricuspid valve disease both stenosis and incompetence, and in congenital anomalies of the tricuspid valve both stenosis and incompetence, and more particularly in Ebstein's anomaly. The right atrium can also be enlarged when it carries a high flow as in atrial septal defect.

The morphological characteristics by which the right atrium is distinguished as right, in complex congenital heart disease, are the presence of the limbus of the fossa ovalis on its septal aspect and its broad based and squat atrial appendage.

The right ventricle (Fig. 20.16) is a chamber of complex shape. In the frontal view it appears triangular.

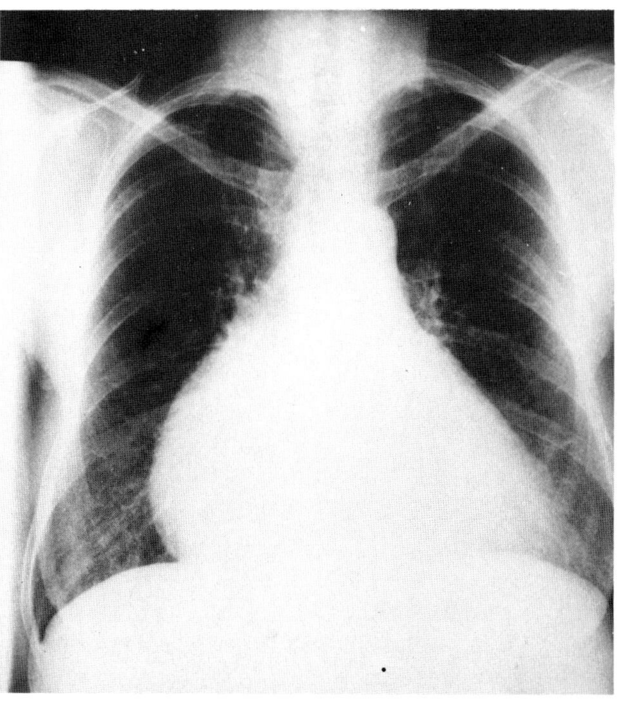

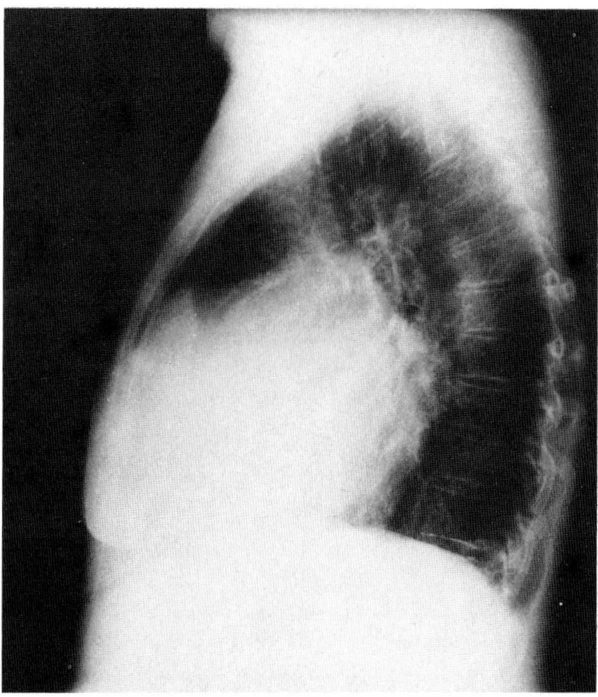

Fig. 20.15 Tricuspid stenosis. (**A**) The right heart border has bulged to the right and its radius of curvature has increased. (**B**) There is filling in of the gap between the front of the heart and the sternum in the lateral view.

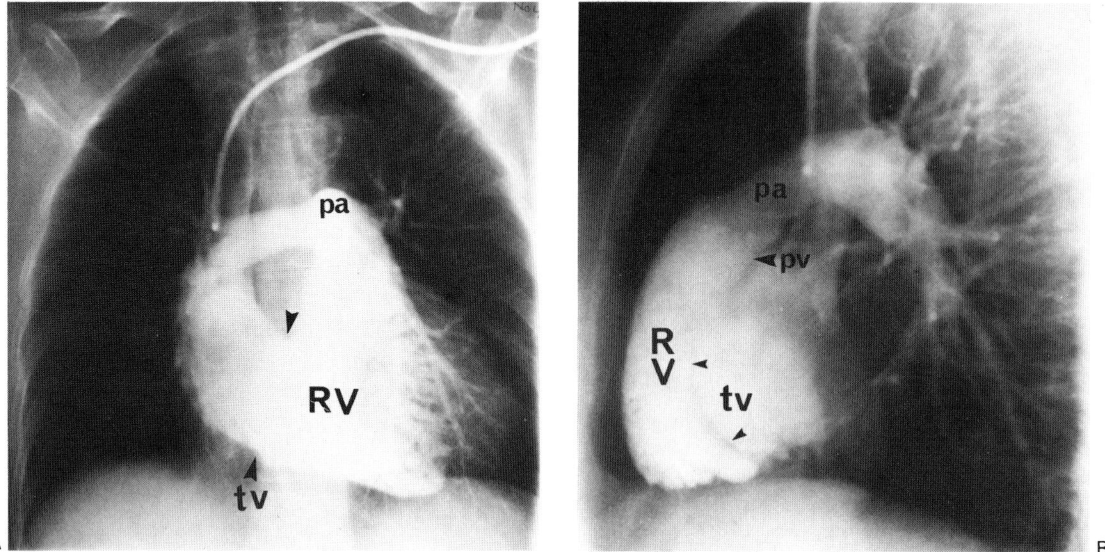

Fig. 20.16 Normal right ventricular angiocardiogram, superior vena cava injection. (**A**) Frontal view. (**B**) Lateral view. The right ventricle does not contribute to the cardiac silhouette in the frontal view except at the upper left border where its infundibulum reaches to the left border of the heart. It forms the front of the heart in the lateral view. These angiocardiograms indicate the position of the tricuspid valve, which because of its oblique lie is not seen in profile in either frontal or lateral views but its approximate position is indicated by the arrows. The pulmonary bay may be seen to be formed by the left border of the main pulmonary artery beyond the pulmonary valve and before it divides into right and left pulmonary arteries.

The triangular shape of the right ventricle in the frontal view is obvious with the pulmonary artery sitting on its infundibulum. The flat shape in the lateral view is also obvious.

The tricuspid valve enters from its right hand posterior aspect and the ventricular apex lies at the left inferior part. At the top of the right ventricle the pulmonary valve sits on the top of the muscular conus or infundibulum which separates it from the tricuspid valve. Seen from the side the right ventricle is flattened with a meniscal cross section produced by the large interventricular septum (really part of the left ventricle) bulging into the right

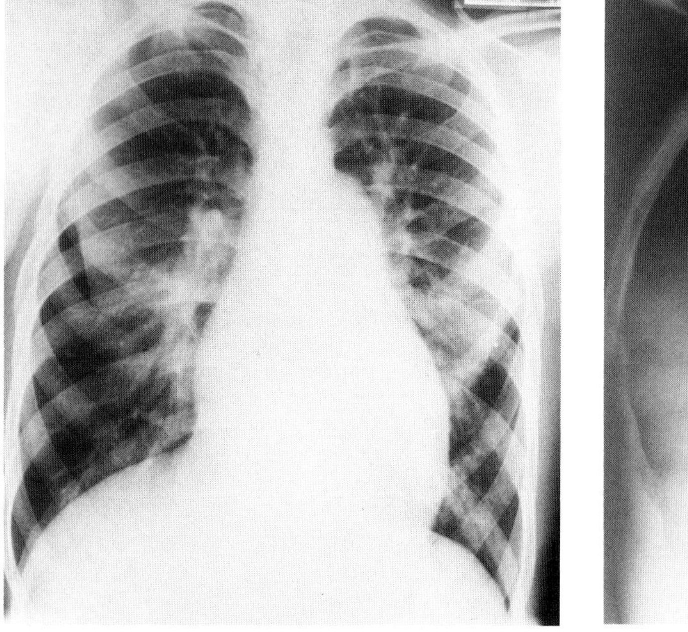

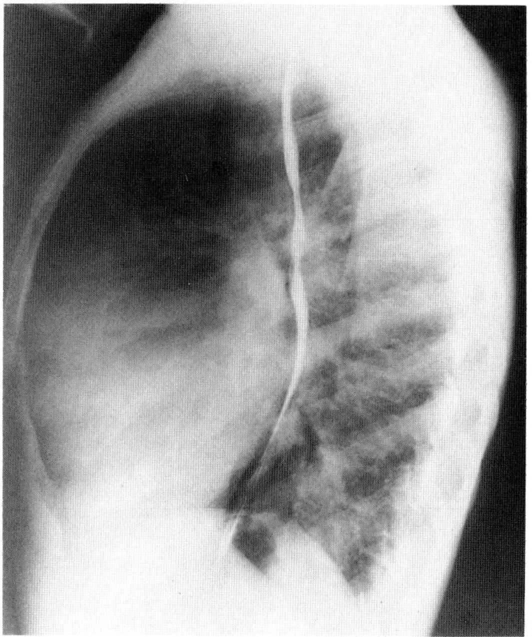

Fig. 20.17 Right ventricular enlargement due to atrial septal defect. (**A**) Frontal view. *Note* the triangular shape of the heart with an indeterminate apex and a bulge of the left mid heart border. There is also a convex pulmonary bay and pulmonary plethora (see later). (**B**) Lateral view. This shows that there is slight bulging forward of the sternum but in addition there is increased area of contact between the front of the heart and the sternum.

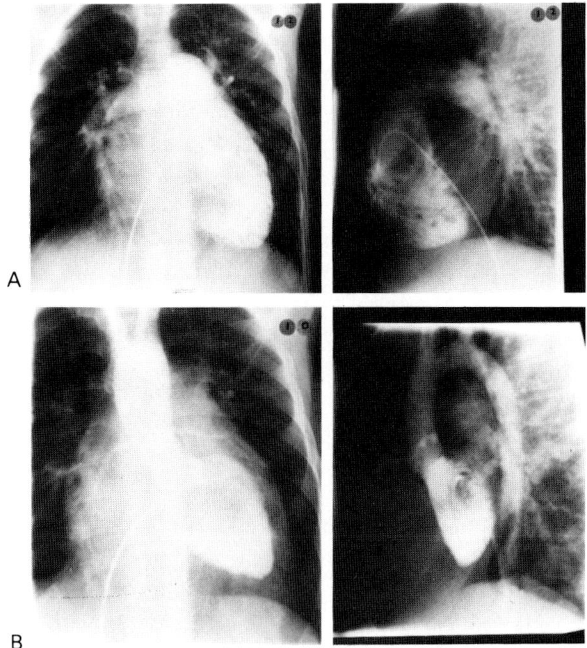

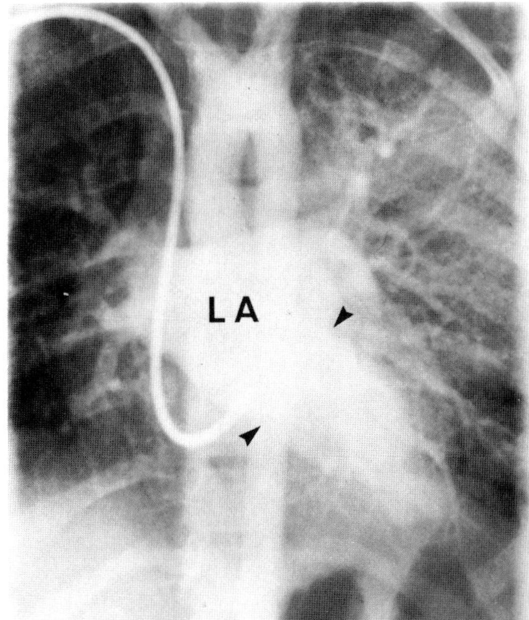

Fig. 20.18 Biventricular angiography in atrial septal defect, same patient as in Figure 20.17. (**A**) Above. Frontal and lateral right ventricular angiogram; (**B**) Below. Frontal and lateral left ventricular angiogram. Note that the left border of the heart is now formed by the markedly enlarged right ventricle which also accounts for the increased contact of the heart with the sternum in the lateral view. The left ventricle, which has been pushed back by the large right ventricle, no longer contributes to the cardiac silhouette in the frontal view.

ventricle. The right ventricle does not contribute to the cardiac outline in the frontal view but forms most of the front of the heart in the lateral view. In the normally shaped chest only the lower half of the normal heart is in contact with the sternum.

Selective enlargement imposes the triangular shape of the right ventricle on the heart in the frontal view (Figs 20.17 and 20.18). A bulge may be seen on the left heart border where the large right ventricle, usually its infundibulum, forms part of the left heart border. Alternatively the bulge may be the large right ventricle lifting up a normal left ventricle. In the lateral view selective right ventricular enlargement may be recognized by the bulging forward of the front of the heart, increasing the area of contact with the sternum. A similar filling-in may also result if the right atrial appendage is very large.

Right ventricular enlargement may occur as a result of pulmonary hypertension or pulmonary valve disease, (usually pulmonary incompetence), tricuspid valve disease or left to right shunts.

The right ventricle is characterized morphologically by its muscular conus which separates its entry from its exit valves, by its coarsely trabeculated septal aspect, and by the direct attachment of part of its valve to the septum, either by chordae tendinae or by a papillary muscle of the conus.

The left atrium (Fig. 20.19) has an oval shape when seen from the front and is flattened when seen from the side. The four pulmonary veins enter its posterior aspect, two on each side. The left atrium forms the upper posterior border of the heart, although this border cannot clearly be

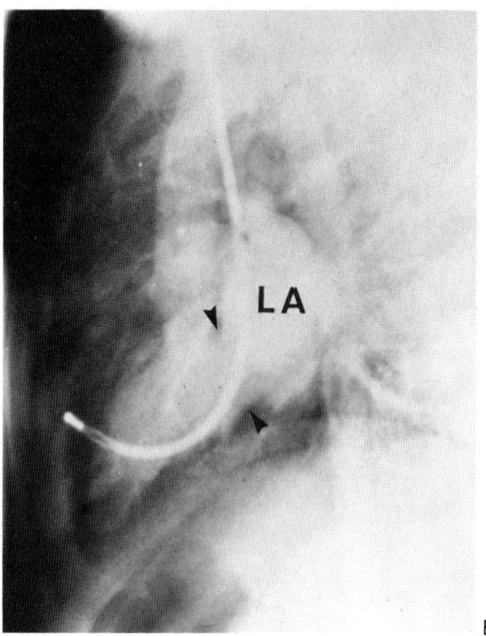

Fig. 20.19 Left atrial angiogram, follow-through angiogram. (**A**) Frontal view. (**B**) Lateral view. The left atrium forms a flattened structure, forming the upper posterior border of the heart in the lateral view, but not contributing to the cardiac silhouette in the frontal view. The arrows indicate the position of the mitral valve which is not seen in profile.

seen as it is not in contact with air-containing lung. The position of the border can be identified in good quality films as the air-containing left main bronchus lies in contact with the back of the heart; so does the oesophagus, and when this is opacified with barium it marks the back wall of the left atrium. The left atrial appendage is a narrow, finger-like, protrusion from the left upper anterior border of the left atrium, passing forward round the upper left heart border to be buried in the epicardial fat. In the normal heart, neither the body of the left atrium nor its appendage makes any significant contribution to the cardiac silhouette in the frontal view.

Left atrial enlargement (Fig. 20.20) may involve the appendage or the body or both. The enlarged appendage may be identified, first by the straightening of the normally concave left heart border, then by the appearance of a discrete bulge below the pulmonary conus and above the left ventricle. Enlargement of the left atrial body may occur to the right, where it first appears as a double shadow through the heart, progressing to form the right heart border. When gross it extends to the left. Enlargement may also occur posteriorly, displacing the left main bronchus and barium filled oesophagus backwards. As most left atrial enlargement is associated with mitral valve disease the subject is considered again in Chapter 23, but enlargement may occur in any process causing either pressure or volume load to be transmitted to the left atrium, particularly left ventricular disease. The left atrium is the most sensitive chamber for the detection of chamber enlargement.

The morphological characteristics of a left atrium are the opposite of those of the right. It lacks a limbus to the fossa ovalis and its appendage is long finger-like and narrow based.

The left ventricle (Fig. 20.21) is a carrot-shaped structure whose base is formed by the fibrous skeleton of the aortic and mitral valves. The long axis of the ventricle points from the base, downwards, forwards and to the left to the apex of the left ventricle, which in turn almost invariably forms the apex of the heart. The left ventricle forms the left border of the heart in the frontal view and the lower posterior border, below the level of the mitral valve, in the lateral view.

Left ventricular enlargement is recognized in two ways. Left ventricular hypertrophy produces a rounding of the cardiac apex. Left ventricular dilatation (Fig. 20.22A) imposes its shape on the heart in the frontal view with elongation of the cardiac apex either to the left or to the left and downwards, often combined with the rounding of the apex. Left ventricular enlargement may sometimes be identified in the lateral view when the soft tissue shadow of the left ventricle protrudes behind the line of the barium-filled oesophagus, or more than 2 cm behind the back of the

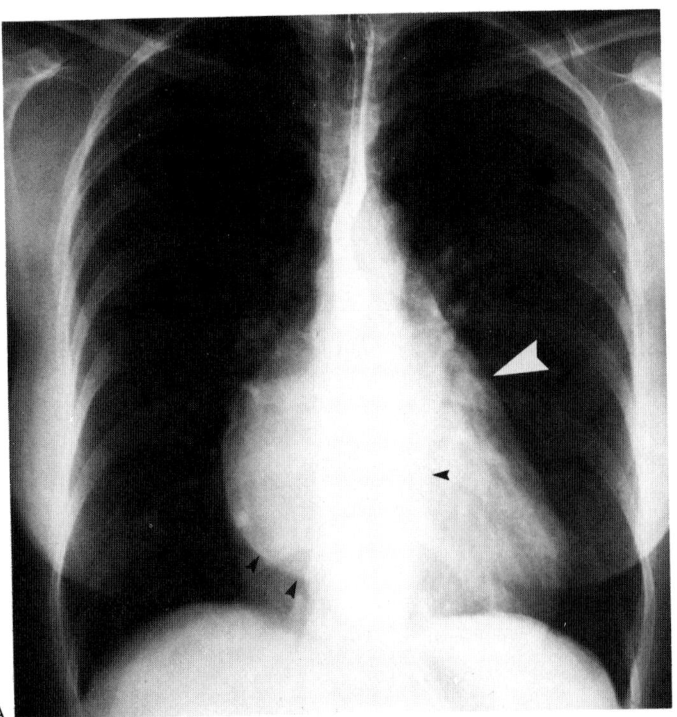

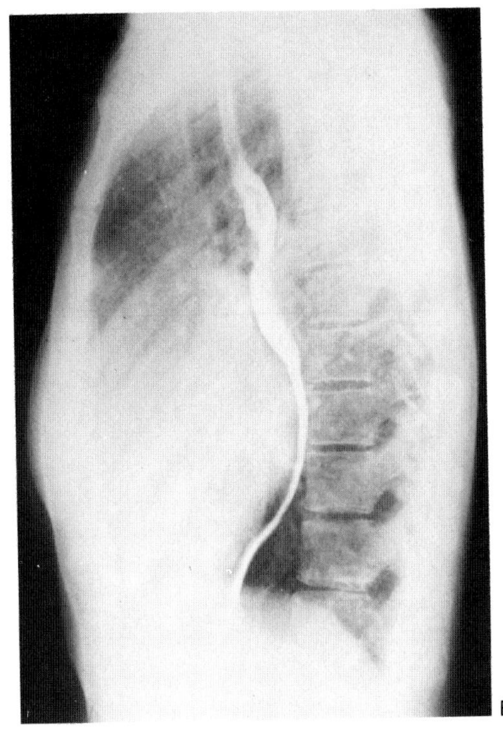

Fig. 20.20 Selective left atrial enlargement. (**A**) Frontal view. The left atrial appendage produces a localised bulge on the left heart border (white arrow) below the pulmonary bay. The double shadow (paired arrows) of the left atrium is seen through the heart shadow. The displacement of the aorta to the left is indicated by the single arrow. Note that the right atrial shadow continues below the diaphragm as it is anchored by the inferior vena cava. (**B**) Lateral view. Note the localized posterior displacement of the barium filled oesophagus which returns to its normal position at the site of the mitral valve.

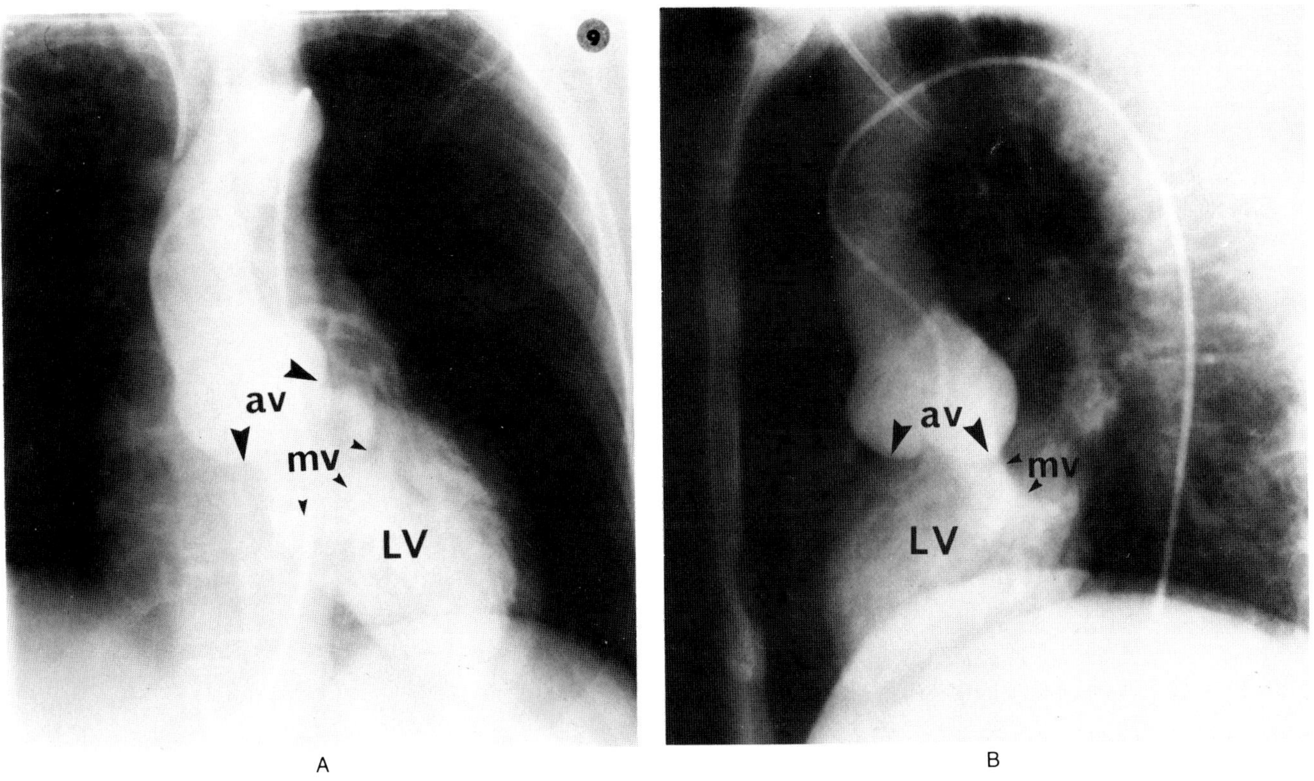

Fig. 20.21 Left ventricular angiocardiogram. (**A**) Frontal view. The left ventricle forms the left border of the cardiac silhouette and its apex forms the apex of the heart. The aortic valve lies approximately in the middle of the heart shadow. The mitral valve can be identified by the non-opaque blood entering and with contrast trapped under the posterior leaflet (small arrows). (**B**) Lateral view. The left ventricle forms the lower part of the posterior border of the heart. The aortic valve lies approximately in the middle of the heart shadow. The anterior leaflet of the mitral valve (small arrows) is suspended from the non coronary cusp of the aortic valve. The mitral valve lies obliquely and is not seen in profile in these views but its approximate position has been indicated. The aorta, beginning at the aortic valve, extends to the right of the superior mediastinum and then passes to the left of the oesophagus and trachea to reach the posterior mediastinum and turns downwards as the descending aorta. On the right the aorta is concealed by the superior vena cava and its most posterior part forms the aortic knob of the frontal chest X-ray.

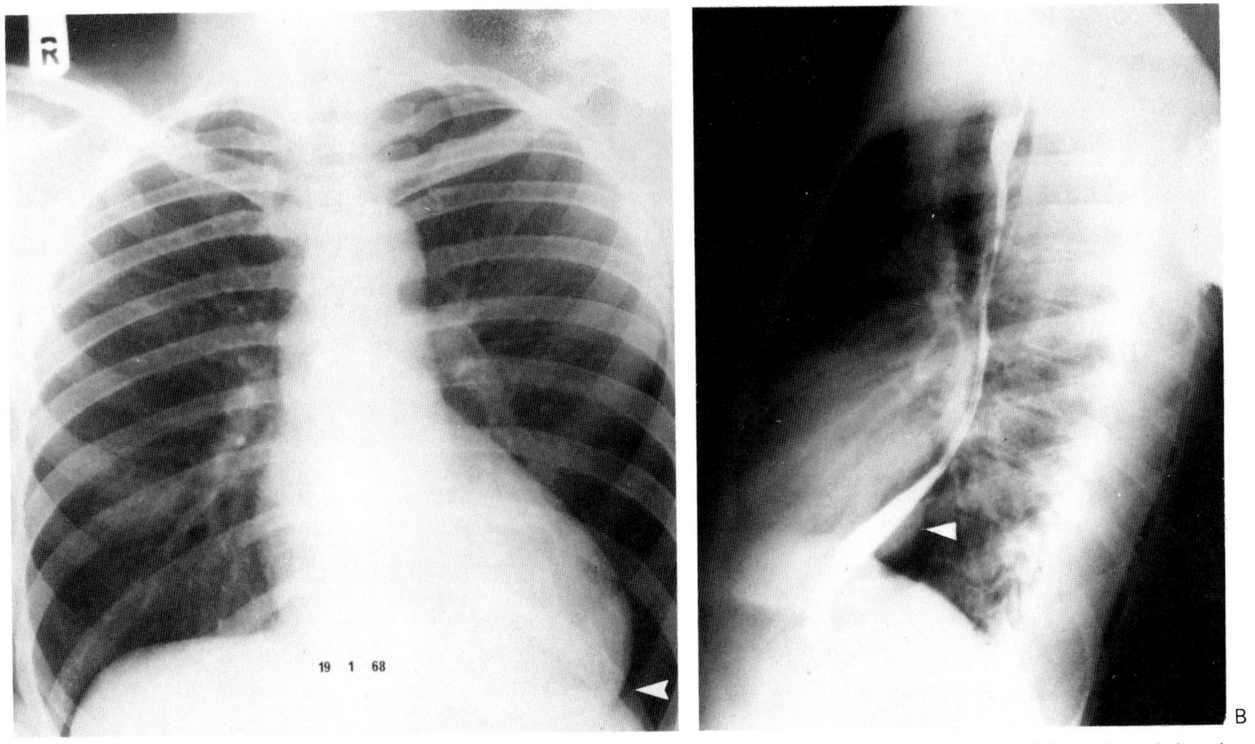

Fig. 20.22 Selective left ventricular enlargement in aortic incompetence. (**A**) Frontal view. This shows that the left ventricle has enlarged along its long axis taking the apex of the heart to the left and downwards (white arrow). (**B**) Lateral view. This shows the left ventricle extending behind the line of the barium filled oesophagus (arrow).

right atrium as indicated by the entrance of the inferior vena cava (Fig. 20.22B).

Left ventricular enlargement may occur in any pressure or volume overload of the left ventricle. Pressure overload results from hypertension, coarctation, aortic heart disease or any form of congenital aortic obstruction. Volume overload may be caused by mitral or aortic regurgitation or left to right shunt. Left ventricular enlargement may also result from diseases of heart muscle such as ischaemia or cardiomyopathy.

The morphological characteristics of the left ventricle are the lack of a muscular conus separating the entry and exit valves which are in fibrous continuity, a smooth septal aspect, and a mitral valve which is not attached directly to the ventricular septum.

The aorta (Fig. 20.21) begins at the aortic valve which lies just above the middle of the heart shadow in both frontal and lateral views. The aortic valve lies within the heart mass and does not usually cast a discrete shadow. Rarely a faint small double shadow may be seen through the heart in the frontal view, rather resembling that of the left atrium, though seen to be continuous with the ascending aorta. The normal ascending aorta does not form a discrete shadow in the right superior mediastinum, being covered by the superior vena cava. When dilated and elongated in old age or hypertension the ascending aorta bulges to the right. Only the front wall of the ascending aorta is easily identified in the lateral view, the posterior wall not being in contact with gas-containing lung is imperfectly seen. The arch of the aorta passes in front of the trachea and then backwards on the left of the trachea and oesophagus. It can usually be seen indenting the left side of the trachea, in correctly penetrated films, and also the barium-filled oesophagus. In cases of doubt those signs indicate the side of the aortic arch. The shadow of the aortic knob is formed by the most posterior part of the aortic arch. The left border of a descending aorta can usually be identified in adult patients as a straight line passing downwards and towards the midline, lying to the left of the spine and in continuity with the arch of the aorta.

The main pulmonary artery (Fig. 20.16), that part of the pulmonary artery between the pulmonary valve and the bifurcation into the right and left pulmonary arteries, forms the floor of the pulmonary bay and lies on the left between the aortic arch and the heart proper. In the normal adult the floor of the pulmonary bay tends to be straight. In children and young women a a convexity, indicating a prominent main pulmonary artery, may still be normal.

CARDIAC SIZE

The plain film is an important indicator of cardiac size. The detection of cardiac enlargement is an important aspect of its use. The customary method of assessment is the measurement of the cardiothoracic ratio (Fig. 20.23). In adult White patients this should not exceed 50% (two standard deviations above the mean), but in Coloured patients up to 55% may still be normal.

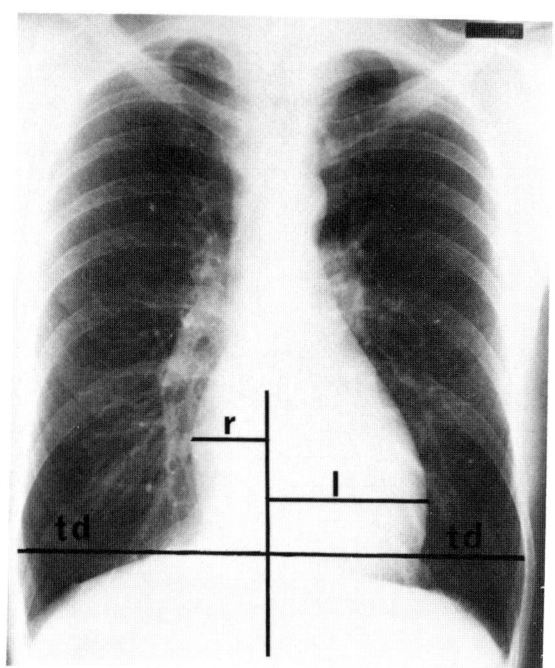

Fig. 20.23 The assessment of cardiac enlargement. The cardiac diameter should be the maximum cardiac diameter (r + 1). The transverse thoracic diameter is measured in a variety of ways. Here it is measured as the maximum internal diameter of the thorax.

The cardiothoracic ratio is increased in the elderly; this may be due to an infolding of the ribs, reducing the thoracic component of the ratio, or due to heart disease. The cardiothoracic ratio may be increased in the neonate (See p. 624).

The transverse diameter of the heart may be measured directly on radiograph taken at 6 ft. An upper limit of 16 cm for men and 15 cm for women is usual. The advantage of a single measurement is that it may be compared in serial films. A difference of 2 cm is held to be a significant change. This applies only when the heart is originally normal and physiological differences of almost that size may be encountered. In significantly enlarged hearts much less change in diameter will be significant.

The measurement of cardiac volume (Fig. 20.24), on the assumption that the heart may represent an elipsoid is not routinely performed, other than in Scandinavia.

In the *neonate*, the heart may be relatively larger compared to the thorax than in the adult, and a cardiothoracic ratio of up to 60% is not necessarily abnormal. Considerable care should be taken before diagnosing cardiomegaly radiologically as much unnecessary investigation may follow. The neonatal chest is also difficult to study radiologically as the heart shape tends to be nonspecific because of the right ventricular preponderance

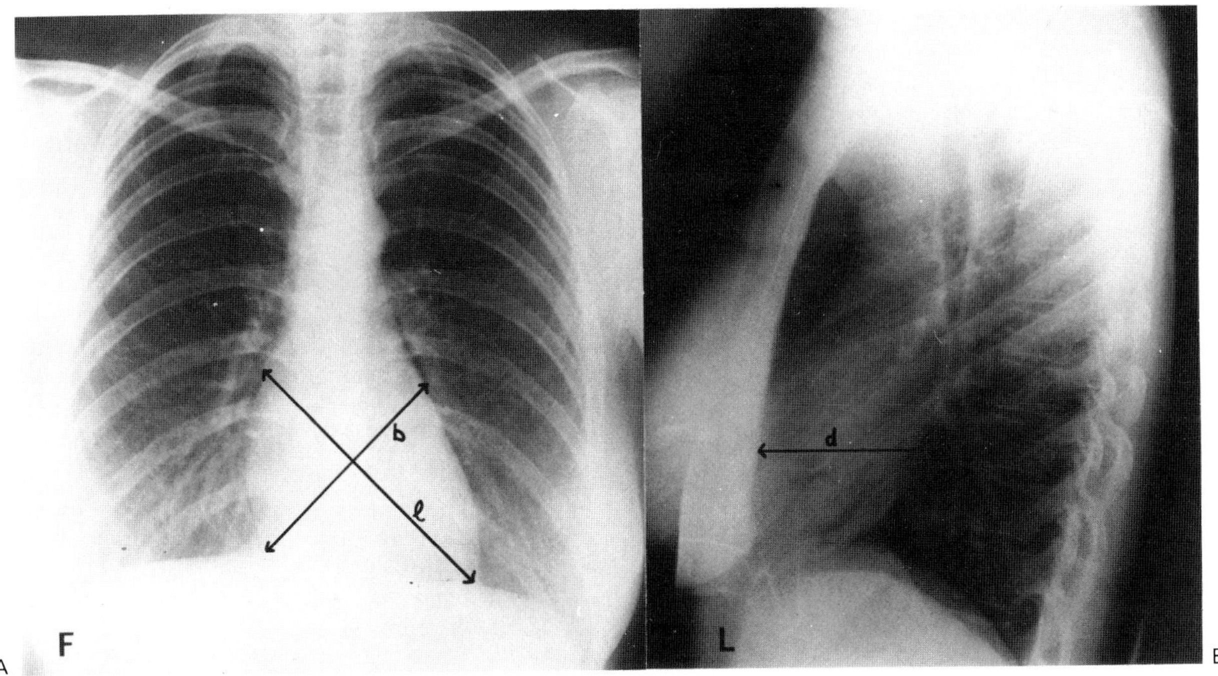

Fig. 20.24 (**A** and **B**) Measurement of cardiac volume. The volume of the heart may be measured on the assumption that the heart is an elipsoid and if its three axes can be determined its volume, $l \times b \times d \times \pi/6 \times 1/m^3$ (where m is the magnification factor) can be calculated.

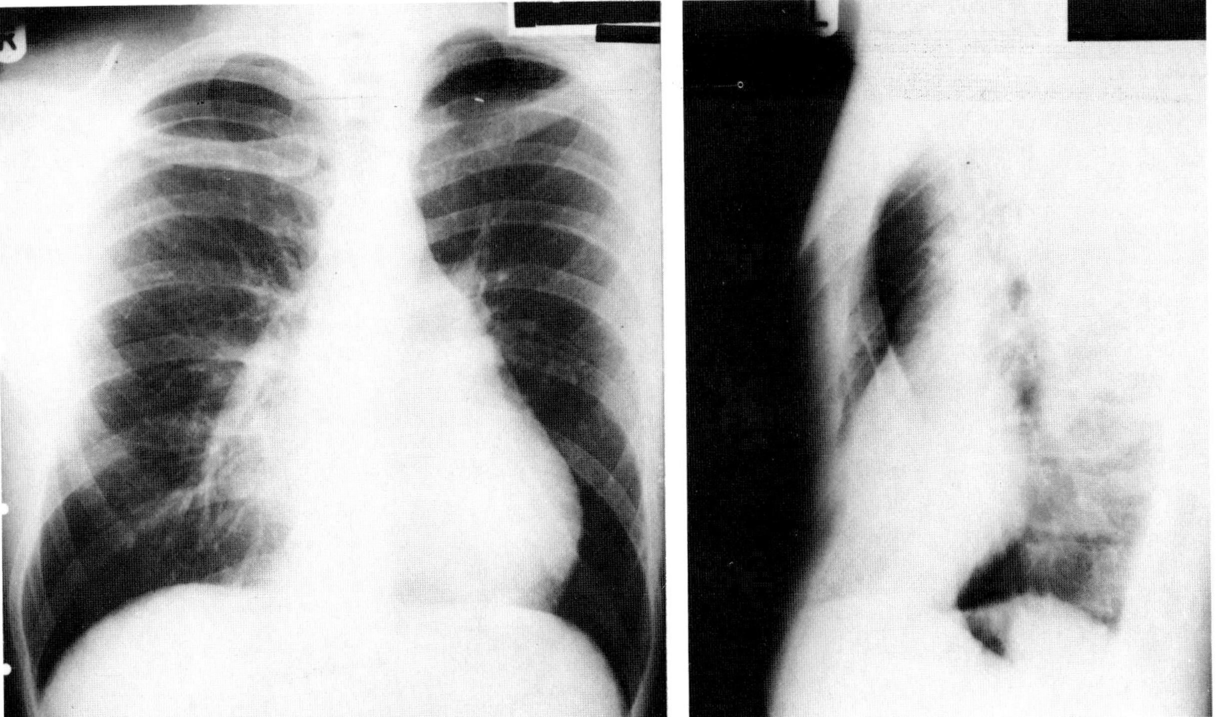

Fig. 20.25 Depressed sternum. (**A**) Frontal view. The heart is displaced to the left. Its left border is straight and there is a prominence in the position of the main pulmonary artery. There is an ill-defined shadow to the right of the vertebral column. The clue to those appearances is given by the visualization of the intervertebral discs at the level of the lower thoracic spine where normally they would disappear. (**B**) Lateral view. This demonstrates the enormous sternal depression. This patient was thought to have a normal heart.

which is present at birth. The mediastinal structures are frequently concealed by a large thymus so that identification of the side of the aortic arch and of the pulmonary bay may be difficult or impossible.

DEPRESSED STERNUM

Analysis of the size and shape of the heart may be made difficult or impossible in the presence of skeletal deformities of which depressed sternum (Fig. 20.25A, B) is the most common. The presence of odd murmurs, apparently related to the deformity, but resembling those of heart disease, may complicate the clinical examination. In the frontal view the heart shadow may appear overtly enlarged. Its left border is often straightened and the main pulmonary artery may appear prominent. The right border of the heart mav bulge to the right if the heart is compressed against the spine, but most commonly it is not seen to the right of the sternum when the heart, as is usual, is displaced to the left. The central pulmonary vessels may appear prominent, and this together with the slightly odd murmurs, may raise the possibility of an atrial septal defect. Ill-defined shadowing, often extensive, is frequently seen in the right pericardiophrenic angle which the unwary might take for a pulmonary lesion. It does not show an air bronchogram. The easy visibility of the vertebral bodies and their intervertebral discs through the heart shadow of the standard frontal film always raises the possibility that the appearances of the heart are due to depressed sternum. If downward sloping anterior ribs are present this virtually confirms the diagnosis.

The appearances on the lateral view are often rather unimpressive, varying from a slight reduction in the anteroposterior diameter of the chest from flattening of the sternum to gross sternal depression with compression of the heart against the spine. The 'straight back syndrome', whose chief radiological feature is obvious from its name, also leads to a narrowing of the anteroposterior diameter of the chest, with squashing of the heart between sternum and spine, and similar, though less marked, cardiac appearances to those of depressed sternum, in the frontal view. It may be associated with prolapse of the mitral valve.

REFERENCES AND SUGGESTIONS FOR FURTHER READING

Anderson , R. H. & Becker, A. E. (date) *Cardiac Anatomy: an Integrated Text and Colour Atlas*. Edinburgh: Churchill Livingstone.

Donaldson, R. M. & Ell, P. J. (1981) Nuclear Cardiology — a review. *British Journal of Hospital Medicine*, **25**, 111–126.

Elliott, L. P., Bargeron, L. M., Soto, B. & Bream, P. R. (1980) Axial cine-angiography in congenital heart disease. *Radiologic Clinics in North America*, **18**, 515–546.

Feigenbaum, H. (1984) *Echocardiography*, 4th edn. Philadelphia: Lea & Febiger.

Fowler, N. O. (ed.) (1983) *Non-invasive Diagnostic Methods in Cardiology*. Philadelphia: F. A. Davis.

Guthaner, D. F. & Wexler, L. (1980) New aspects of coronary arteriography. *Radiologic Clinics in North America*, **18**, 501–504.

Higgins, C. B. (ed.) (1983) *CT of the Heart and Great Vessels*. Mount Kisco, New York: Futura Publishing Co.

Netter, F. H. (1969) *The Ciba Collection of Medical Illustrations*, Vol 5, *The Heart*. London: Ciba.

Raphael, M. J. & Allwork, S. P. (1974) Angiographic anatomy of the left ventricle. *Clinical Radiology*, **25**, 95–105.

Raphael, M. J. & Allwork, S. P. (1976) Angiographic anatomy of the right heart. *Clinical Radiology*, **27**, 265–272.

Walton, S. & Ell, P. J. (1983) *Introduction to Nuclear Cardiology*. London: Current Medical Literature Ltd.

CHAPTER 21

THE PERICARDIUM

NORMAL ANATOMY

The pericardial sac consists of two layers separated by a potential space which is lubricated by a few millilitres of pericardial fluid. The parietal pericardium is a tough fibrous sac, enclosing the heart and attached to the central tendon of the diaphragm below. The visceral pericardium is closely applied to the surface of the heart. The two layers are fused next to the heart at the entry of the pulmonary veins to the left atrium posteriorly and at the entry of the inferior vena cava to the right atrium inferiorly. The two layers extend up the aorta, to fuse about half way between the aortic valve and the origin of the innominate artery; they extend along the main pulmonary artery fusing before its bifurcation, and along the superior vena cava.

Radiographic appearances. The pericardium has the same radiographic density as the heart. In spite of this it may be identified on the frontal film if there is a substantial amount of epicardial fat which produces a low density linear shadow, with a normal density shadow of the pericardium appearing as a thin white line outside it.

The *epicardial fat line* is often best identified in the lateral view and enables an estimate of the thickness of the pericardium to be made (see later).

The pericardial outline may be obscured by the pericardial fat pads which may develop in the cardiophrenic angles as ill-defined low-density triangular shadows with their vertices in the cardiophrenic angles. The outline of the heart with its pericardium is often identifiable through them. The nature of these shadows is usually obvious from the lateral view, where they have a characteristically ill-defined triangular shape with the base of the triangle abutting on the anterior chest wall. Rather similar appearances may be produced by pleural thickening over the base of the middle lobe or lingula. Only rarely do these appearances lead to difficulties in differentiation from tumours or hernias occurring in the regions of the anterior cardiophrenic angles.

Ultrasound

The parietal pericardium produces strong echoes from both M mode and sector scanning. In the absence of pericardial disease the strong echoes are continuous with the posterior wall of the left ventricle. The pericardium cannot be identified anteriorly unless it is abnormal.

CT Scanning

Using modern high speed machines the anterior and caudal part of the pericardium, where it is surrounded externally by the mediastinal fat and internally by epicardial fat, can be identified in almost all patients without the use of contrast. The normal pericardium appears as a fine line, 1–2 mm thick in front of the lower part of the right and left ventricles and right atrium. Patchy areas of apparent pericardial thickening up to a few millimetres in thickness may be identified over the right ventricle in the apparently normal patient and are thought to be movement artefacts. The normal pericardium cannot usually be identified posteriorly.

Angiocardiography

Opacification of the right atrium by contrast injection into it or the vena cava, and frontal filming, will demonstrate the combined thickness of the pericardium and the wall of the right atrium, which is normally less than 3–4 mm. Later filming, as the contrast passes through the chambers of the heart may also be helpful in detecting displacements and deformities of these chambers by pericardial disease.

Pneumopericardium

The inner aspect of the pericardium may be outlined by gas introduced during pericardiocentesis, and the thickness of the pericardium determined (see later).

DISEASES OF THE PERICARDIUM

CONGENITAL DEFECTS

These are rare and may be partial or complete, and usually involve the left side of the pericardium. Partial defects are usually asymptomatic but may produce symptoms if the left atrial appendage herniates through the defect and then

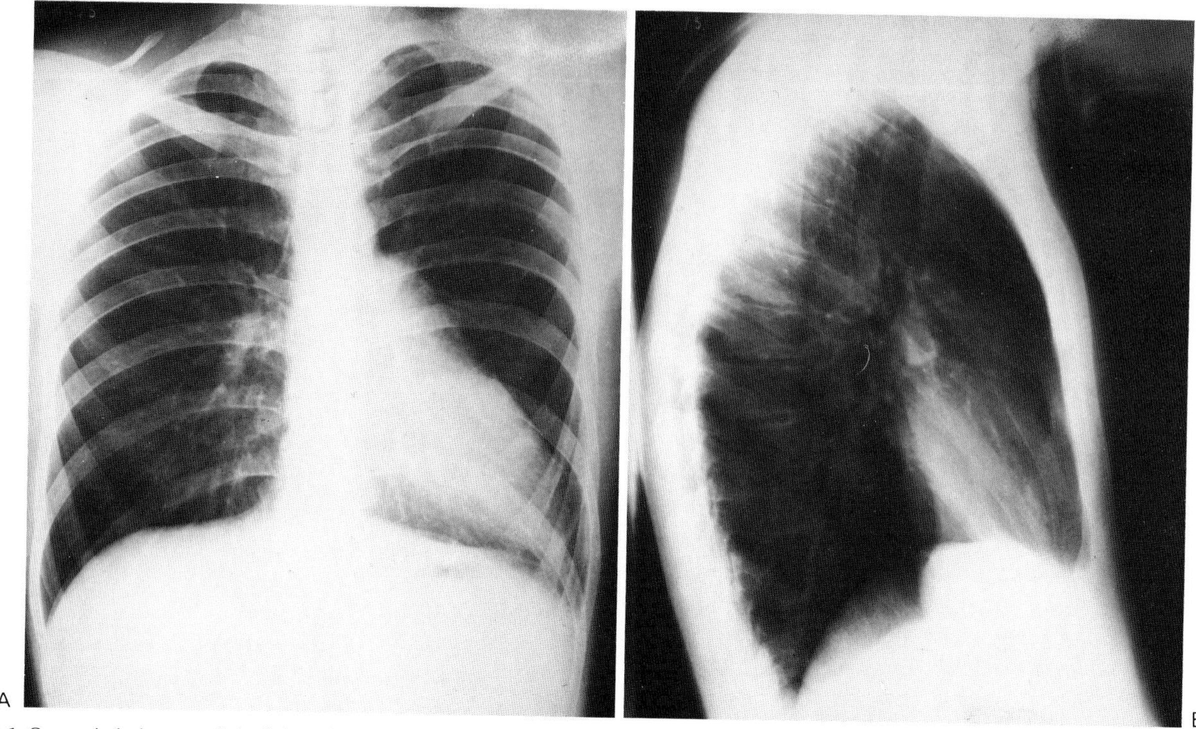

Fig. 21.1 Congenital absence of the left pericardium. (**A**) Frontal view. Note that the heart is displaced to the left and there is a prominence in the position of the main pulmonary artery. Note also that the outline of the left diaphragm is clear as far as the spine. (**B**) Lateral view. This is unremarkable.

strangulates. They may be associated with non-specific murmurs. Complete absence of the pericardium is not usually associated with specific clinical features. In both conditions, the plain films suggest the diagnosis.

In *partial defects* there is a bulge on the left heart border, usually in the position of the left atrial appendage and appearing to suggest that this structure is enlarged. However, there is no other radiological evidence of left atrial enlargement and no clinical features to suggest this, though the non-specific murmurs may be confusing. Rarely the pulmonary artery may appear enlarged if it herniates through the defect and this (Fig. 21.1), combined with non-specific murmurs, may suggest a diagnosis of pulmonary stenosis.

CT scanning reveals partial absence of the left pericardium and prominence and altered rotation of the main pulmonary artery.

Angiocardiography in the levophase of a pulmonary artery injection will confirm that the abnormal shadow is the left atrial appendage or an otherwise normal main pulmonary artery. In view of the danger of strangulation it has been suggested that the left atrial appendage should be amputated and the pericardial defect closed.

Complete defects of the left pericardium (Fig. 21.1A, B), produce a characteristic appearance with the whole heart displaced to the left with a prominent pulmonary artery shadow, perhaps a prominence of the left atrial appendage and with a slightly prominent left ventricular border. Gas containing lung may be interposed between the heart and the left diaphragm due to the absence of connection of pericardium to diaphragm.

The diagnosis is usually made with confidence from the plain film and the absence of other features of heart disease. CT scanning may demonstrate the absence of the left pericardium and the altered axis of the main pulmonary artery to the left, and thus confirm the diagnosis. If there is still doubt an artificial pneumothorax will allow gas to enter the pericardium and confirm its absence.

PERICARDIAL EFFUSION

This is the commonest abnormality of the pericardium to be encountered in routine radiological practice. The presenting features may be *pain* when the cause is inflammatory or malignant disease, or *tamponade*. The development of the latter is characterised by shortness of breath, hypotension, pulsus paradoxus, and distended neck veins, and depends on the rapidity of fluid collections; over a litre may be present without symptoms if it collects slowly, whereas 200–300 ml collecting rapidly may cause symptoms. The fluid in the indistensible pericardial sac compresses the heart and obstructs the entry of blood through the vena cavae leading to a fall in cardiac output.

The commonest disease of the pericardium, *pericarditis*, does not produce radiological abnormality unless an effusion is present.

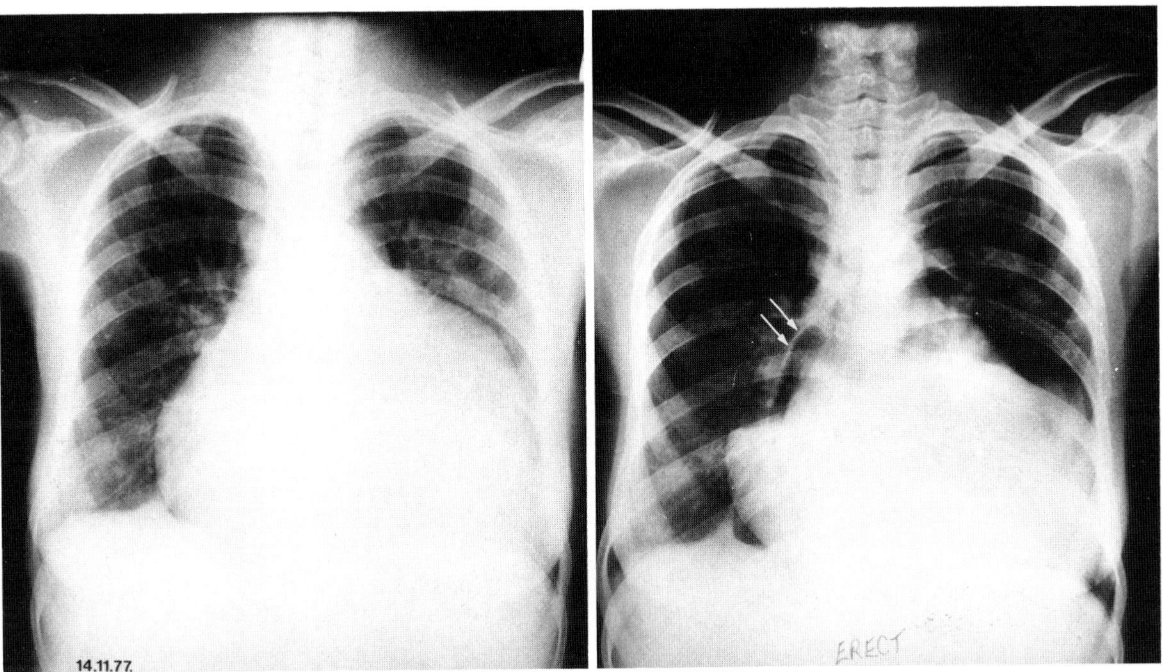

Fig. 21.2 Pericardial effusion. (**A**) Frontal view, 14.11.77. There is a large globular heart shadow with a rather localized bulge on the left upper cardiac border. The lungs are not congested. (**B**) Frontal film, 16.11.77, after aspiration and injection of carbon dioxide. The pericardium of normal thickness is outlined on its inner aspect by the carbon dioxide and on its outer aspect by the gas filled lung (arrows). Fluid levels are seen in the pericardium and a rather prominent main pulmonary artery is visible outlined by pericardial gas.

Radiological appearances. The plain film appearances depend on the amount of fluid and its distribution. If there is sufficient fluid the heart shadow will be enlarged, and in larger effusions, grossly so. It may have a globular or non-specific shape but in large effusions there is very often a rather localised bulge in the left upper cardiac border which may lead to confusion (Fig. 21.2). Although the heart shadow appears enlarged, there are no features on the film to suggest selective chamber enlargement.

The accumulation and dispersal of fluid produces rapid changes in the heart size on serial films, and when these occur they always suggest pericardial fluid as the cause.

Displacement of the epicardial fat stripe inwards, when this can be identified, also points to a pericardial effusion. This is usually better seen on the lateral view though in our experience it is rare.

Screening of the heart to show diminished pulsation and changes in shape from erect to supine posture, is of historical interest only.

The obstruction of venous return to the right heart rather than the left heart leads to a reduction in flow and pressure through the lungs so that abnormalities of the pulmonary vasculature are striking by their absence.

These features lead to one of the characteristic appearances of a pericardial effusion; a large heart with clear lungs rather than congested lungs, which usually occur in heart disease. The other feature to suggest a pericardial effusion is a rapid change in heart size over serial films.

Other investigations. Once a pericardial effusion is suspected echocardiography is the next step. *M mode echocardiography* shows separation of the posterior wall of the left ventricle from the pericardium by an echo-free space (Fg. 21.3) and if the effusion is large an echo-free space appears between the front of the right ventricular wall and the back of the sternum. The *2DE* is much easier to interpret, showing an echo-free space surrounding the heart (Fig. 21.4), and if the effusion is large the whole heart can be seen swinging in the effusion. The M mode echocardiogram is unable to detect those rare localized pericardial effusions which do not develop within the usual beam directions, though loculated effusions are well defined by 2DE (Fig. 21.4) and this technique may allow the visualization of the aspiration needle during pericardiocentesis and thus avoid penetration of the myocardium.

CT scanning is also very helpful in medium and large pericardial effusions (Fig. 21.6B), showing a continuous layer of fluid surrounding the heart. The layer may be of high or low density but this characteristic does not help in distinguishing the nature of the fluid.

Angiocardiography is now only rarely required but right atrial angiography in the AP view will show an increase in the combined thickness of the right atrial wall and the pericardium to more than 4 mm. However it does not distinguish fluid from thickening. It would also show elevation of the floor of the right ventricle due to inferior

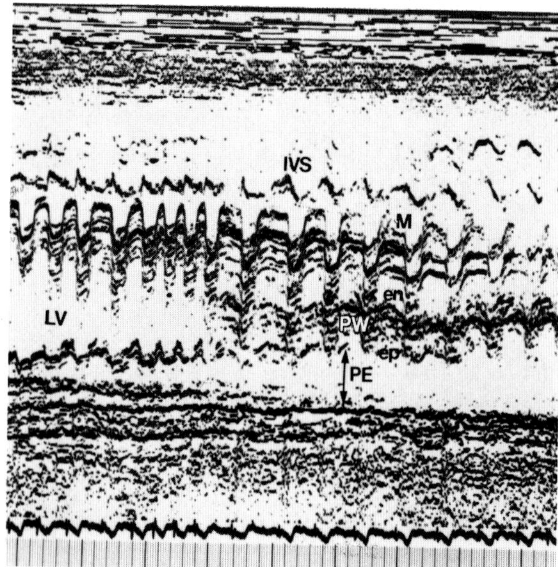

Fig. 21.3 Pericardial effusion. The M-mode echocardiogram demonstrates a separation of the posterior wall of the left ventricle (PW) marked on its outer side by the echoes of the epicardium (ep) and with a large echo-free space behind it of a pericardial effusion (PE). The transducer has been scanned from the left ventricle (LV) towards the left atrium, with the beam passing through the interventricular septum (IVS) and onto the mitral apparatus (M) and reflected off the endocardium (en).

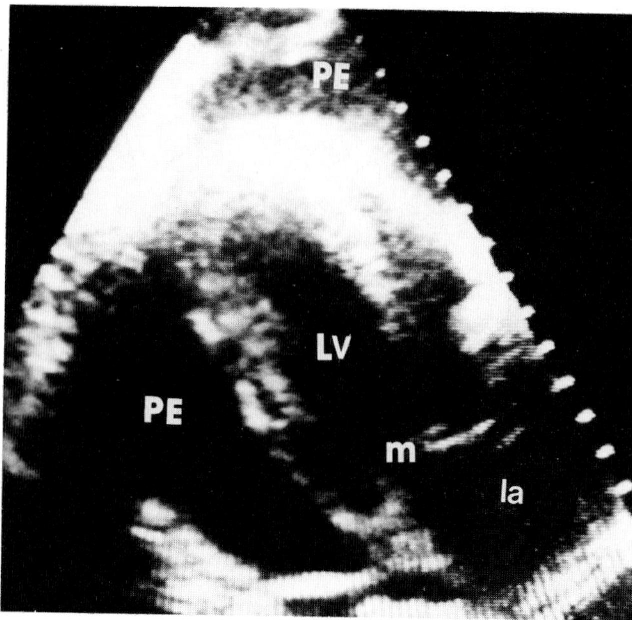

Fig. 21.4 Pericardial effusion, 2DE study. In this long axis view a large echo-free space of pericardial effusion (PE) is seen both behind and in front of the left ventricle (LV).

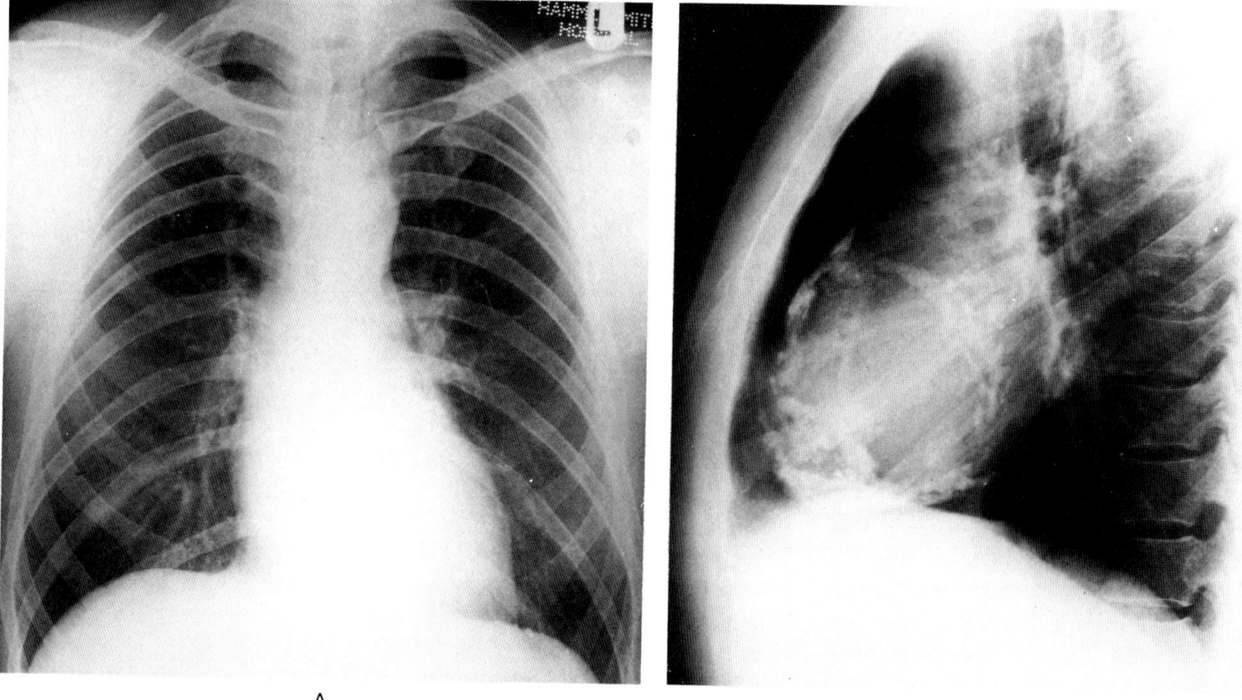

Fig. 21.5 Constrictive pericarditis. (**A**) Frontal view. In this slightly light film the heart and lungs appear normal, apart from some possible straightening of the right heart border. (**B**) Lateral view. This shows extensive pericardial calcification spreading over the front of the right ventricle and also encircling the heart in the atrio-ventricular groove. There is no calcium at the back as fluid cannot collect there.

fluid and will show any localised fluid collecting over the left ventricle.

Aspiration. The nature of the pericardial effusion may be obvious on the basis of known clinical features, otherwise fluid may be aspirated and examined. *Gas* (*or contrast*) may be introduced into the pericardium at aspiration (Fig. 21.2B), to outline the inside of the pericardium and indicate its thickness. A thin smooth pericardium suggests a transudate, a thick pericardium an infection, and localized masses on the inside of the pericardium a tumour. The heart structures are often clearly identified when there is gas in the pericardium.

A pneumo-pericardium may also result from chest or abdominal trauma or after cardiac surgery.

Aetiology. The following conditions may be associated with a pericardial effusion.

Malignant disease. Secondary malignant disease, usually from the breast, commonly produces a pericardial effusion and may lead to tamponade.

Inflammatory disease. Infections due to bacterial, tuberculous or viral aetiology may all lead to an exudative pericardial effusion.

Heart disease. A pericardial effusion may result from cardiac failure or may be associated with myocardial infarction when this is complicated by Dressler's syndrome.

Endocrine diseases. The best known of these is myxoedema which frequently has a substantial though often asymptomatic pericardial effusion.

Collagen diseases. All the collagen diseases may be associated with a pericardial effusion but in systemic lupus erythematosis it may be quite large.

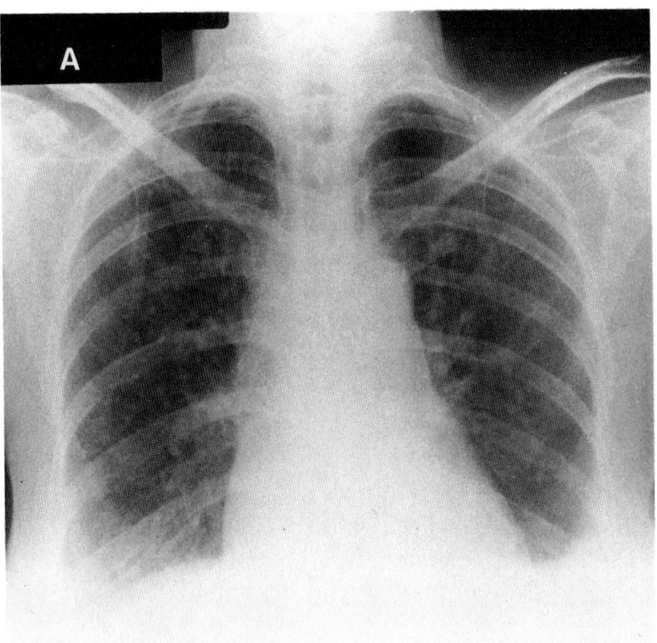

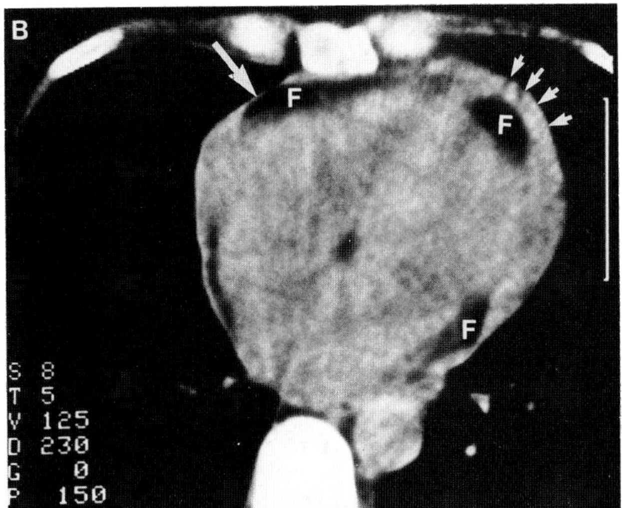

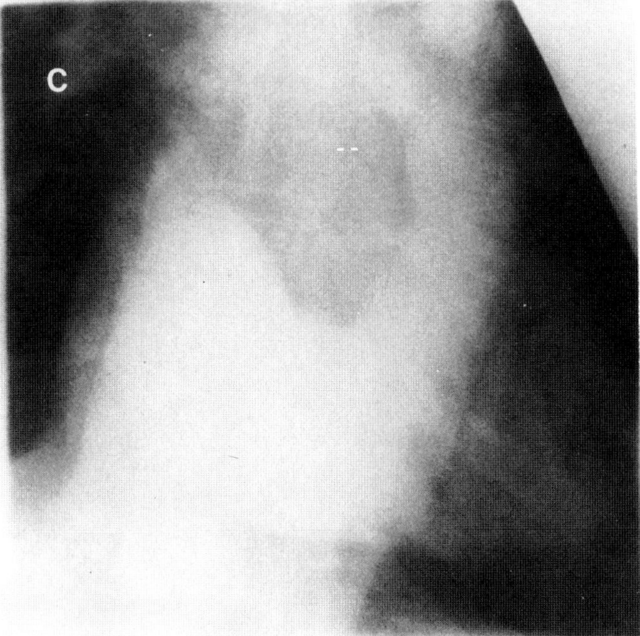

Fig. 21.6 Constrictive pericarditis. (**A**) Frontal view. The heart is normal in size with some straightening of the right heart border. There are bilateral pleural effusions larger on the left. There is also abnormal pulmonary shadowing due to active tuberculosis. This was the cause of the constriction. (**B**) CT scan of the heart without contrast, same patient Low attenuation areas of pericardial fluid (F) surround the heart. The pericardium remains of normal thickness over the right ventricle (single arrow) but is grossly thickened over the left ventricle (multiple arrows); (**C**) right atrial angiogram, same patient. The increased thickness between the opacified right atrium and the outer aspect of the cardiac shadow is clearly visible. This indicates pericardial thickening but does not necessarily indicate constriction.

Uraemia. A large pericardial effusion may be a feature of uraemia though it rarely leads to tamponade.

Haemopericardium. This may result from trauma, from rupture of the heart in the course of myocardial infarction, or be due to dissecting aneurysm leaking into the pericardium.

CONSTRICTIVE PERICARDITIS

In this condition there is impairment of filling of the chambers of the heart, almost always involving mainly the right heart, and due to thickening and hence rigidity of the pericardium. *Viral* and *tuberculous* pericarditis are the commonest causes leading to constriction but *haemopericardium* may lead to constriction as may *collagen disease* involving the pericardium.

The patient presents with oedema and may have hepatomegaly and ascites. Shortness of breath is not a feature. The diagnosis of heart disease may not be obvious as there are no murmurs and the neck veins may be so distended that pulsations are not visible, and the heart itself may not be enlarged. The diagnosis of constriction presents two problems: recognizing that the cause of symptoms is heart disease, and distinguishing constriction of the pericardium from a restrictive cardiomyopathy.

Radiological appearances. On plain film examination, the heart may be normal in size (Fig. 21.5A) or may be non-specifically enlarged. Straightening of the right heart border with smoothing out of its contour from superior to inferior vena cava may be seen. There may be pleuro-pericardial adhesions roughening the outline of the heart. About half the cases have pericardial *calcification*, seen over the front and sides of the heart but not at the back where fluid cannot collect at the insertion of the pulmonary veins into the left atrium (Fig. 21.5B). Calcification may be seen on the plain film but is often better demonstrated by fluoroscopy which is not only more sensitive but is able to locate calcification to the pericardium. Calcification also develops in the atrioventricular groove and may encircle the heart. Calcification, however, does not invariably mean constriction.

Due to constriction over the right heart the lungs are usually clear though there may be a pleural effusion. In those unusual cases where constriction in the atrio-ventricular groove obstructs left atrial emptying pulmonary oedema may develop.

Investigations. These are usually devoted to confirming the presence of constriction, and distinguishing this condition from restrictive cardiomyopathy. The *M mode echocardiogram* and the *cross-sectional scan* show normally functioning chambers with pericardial thickening and may identify pericardial calcification by the dense echoes. The *CT scan* will usually identify thickening of the pericardium and suggest a diagnosis of constrictive pericarditis. (Fig. 21.6B).

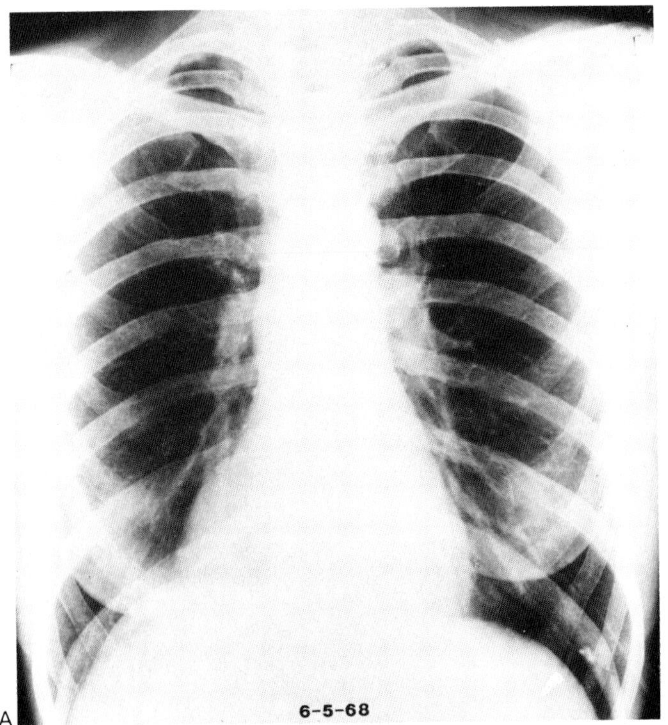

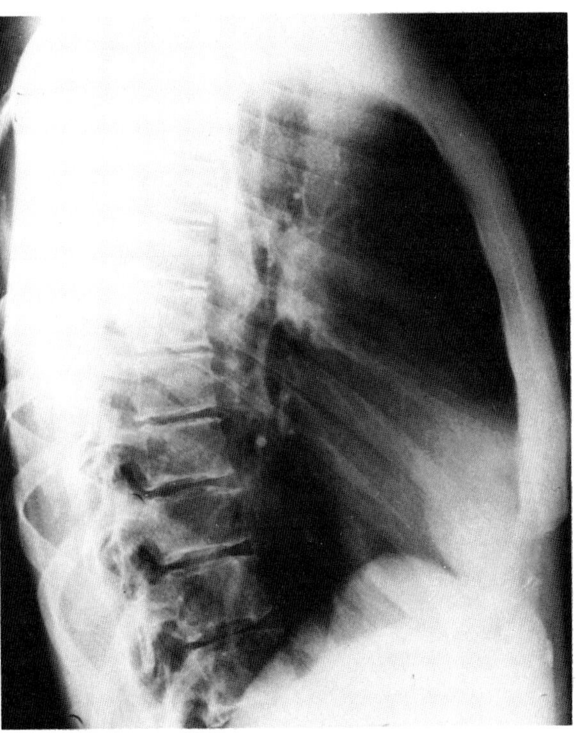

Fig. 21.7 Pericardial cyst. (**A**) Frontal chest X-ray. There is a sharply defined abnormal shadow in the right pericardiophrenic angle. (**B**) Lateral view. This is seen to lie anteriorly. This is one of the characteristic sites for a pericardial cyst.

Cardiac catheterization and angiocardiography. Right and ·ft ventricular catheterization and simultaneous pressure ·cords are required to establish a diagnosis of constriction. 7hen constriction is present the diastolic pressures in the ight and left ventricle are identical. Thickening of the ericardium can be demonstrated by a right atrial injection howing an increase in the thickness of the combined right trial wall and pericardium above the normal 4 mm Fig. 21.6C). The demonstration of thickening does not owever, inevitably point to constriction.

TUMOURS OF THE PERICARDIUM

'hese are relatively rare, the only common tumour encoun-ered is the benign *spring water cyst* (synonym *pleuro-ericardial cyst, pericardial coelomic cyst*). These cysts are nilocular and thin walled and attached to the pericardium ither intimately or by a pedicle, and are in some ways similar to pericardial diverticula, which are distinct in communicating with the pericardial cavity. They are most commonly found in the pericardiophrenic angle more often on the right than the left, though they can occur in any part of the lower half of the mediastinum. The smaller cysts may take up a rather 'tear drop' shape and lie in an elongated fashion in the lower end of the oblique fissure, though the large ones are almost always spherical. On fluoroscopy they may be seen to change shape with respiration.

The diagnosis of the majority is usually obvious on the plain radiograph when they appear as rounded sharply defined cystic shadows anteriorly in the pericardiophrenic angle (Fig. 21.7A and B). Rarely a Morgagni hernia, which may be filled only with omentum in the elderly, may cause confusion. Barium study will distinguish the two.

Secondary malignant involvement of the pericardium is common, producing a pericardial effusion and possibly tamponade. The breast is a common primary site.

REFERENCES AND SUGGESTIONS FOR FURTHER READING

Iiggins, C. B. (ed.) (1983) *CT of the Heart and Great Vessels*. Mount Kisco, New York: Futura Publishing Co.

efferson, K., Rees, S. (1980) *Clinical Cardiac Radiology*, 2nd edn. London: Butterworths.

Schiller, N. B. (1980) Echocardiography in pericardial disease. *Medical Clinics of North America*, **64**, 253.

Shabbetai et al (1979) The pericardium and cardiac function. *Progress in Cardiovascular Diseases*, **22**(**2**), 107–134.

CHAPTER 22

THE PULMONARY CIRCULATION

The pulmonary circulation begins at the pulmonary valve which sits on the infundibulum of the right ventricle. The valve cannot be identified specifically on the plain film but can be identified by 2DE. It may very rarely calcify in middle-aged patients when the valve is congenitally abnormal or the seat of bacterial endocarditis, or in the presence of pulmonary hypertension.

The *main pulmonary artery* beyond the pulmonary valve may be identified on the frontal film as its left border forms the floor of the pulmonary bay. This is the concavity of the left mediastinal shadow, below the knob-like shadow of the arch of the aorta, and above the shadow of the heart. In the normal adult the floor of the pulmonary bay is straight. In children and young women (Fig. 22.1A), a slight convexity is within normal limits.

Enlargement of the main pulmonary artery produces a convexity of the floor of the pulmonary bay. The main pulmonary artery is enlarged in *left to right shunts*, in *pulmonary hypertension* and in the *post-stenotic dilatation* of pulmonary valve stenosis; enlargement may be extreme in certain situations such as when the Eisenmenger reaction occurs in association with an atrial septal defect, and in the pulmonary hypertension associated with Bilharzia.

The main pulmonary artery divides after a variable distance into the right and left pulmonary arteries (Figs 22.1B and 22.2). The *left pulmonary artery* appears as the continuation of the main, passing backwards. It gives off the left upper lobe branches as it passes above the left main bronchus and then arches downwards as the branch to the left lower lobe before dividing into the branches to the basal segments. The left pulmonary artery and its descending branch are silhouetted against the lung and can be identified on the plain film, as forming part of the left hilum and its continuation into the left lower lobe.

The *right pulmonary artery* appears as a sharply angled branch of the main pulmonary artery and passes to the right in the mediastinum. It divides within the mediastinum and its upper lobe branch leaves the mediastinum above the right hilum to supply the upper lobe. The descending branch of the right pulmonary artery is the vessel first to be identified as it forms the lower part of the right hilum where it is outlined against the lung (Figs 22.1A and B).

In the lateral view the right and left pulmonary arteries may be distinguished. The left pulmonary artery lies above and posterior to the radiolucency of the carina 'end-on'; the right pulmonary artery in front and slightly below (Fig. 22.2).

In the lungs the arteries lie within the parenchyma roughly following the bronchial branching pattern. The short descending branches of both the right and left lower lobe arteries can usually be identified before they break up into the branches to the basal segments. The vessels to each lobe can be identified even though the branching pattern is variable. The arteries branch and taper smoothly out from the hilum and can be followed as discrete shadows to the outer third of the lung (Figs 22.1A and B).

The pulmonary arterioles, capillaries and pulmonary venules, contribute to the lung radio-opacity but cannot be identified as discrete structures.

The *pulmonary veins* form an inconstant arrangement (Fig. 22.1C). The pulmonary veins of the upper lobe collect into the superior pulmonary vein, those of the lower lobe into the basal veins which join to form the inferior pulmonary vein. The two veins on each side join the four corners of the left atrium.

The pulmonary veins may be distinguished from the arteries on the plain film (Fig. 22.3) by their course and position. The *lower lobe veins* run horizontally to reach the left atrium and are usually visible and distinguishable from the more vertically running branches of the descending branch of the pulmonary artery. *The upper lobe veins* when visible, lie lateral to the upper lobe arteries, and run vertically to pass through the hilar shadow to reach the left atrium.

The hilar shadow has a concave outer aspect, formed by the superior pulmonary vein above, and descending branch of the pulmonary artery below.

The upper lobe veins may not be visible on the erect film for two reasons. They are collapsed in the erect position as the normal left atrial pressure is inadequate to distend them, and they carry little blood as the normal pulmonary artery pressure is inadequate to perfuse the apices of the lungs. The normal upper lobe vessels in the first interspace are rarely more than 3 mm in diameter.

The diameter of the descending branch of the right pulmonary artery does not normally exceed 15 mm in women and 16 mm in men. Normally it has a rather straight outer border. A convex outer border suggests that the vessel is abnormally large, a concave outer border that it is abnormally small. These features are probably more helpful than measurements in evaluating pathology in the pulmonary circulation.

Rarely, the superior and inferior pulmonary veins may join each other, forming a confluence, before entering the left atrium. This confluence can form a descrete rounded or oval shadow on the plain film (Figs 22.4A, B), on either side, and particularly so when there is an increase in pulmonary vein pressure. This shadow may resemble a tumour but its nature is usually obvious because of its characteristic site right next to the left atrium, and once suspected can be confirmed by demonstrating its relationship to the pulmonary vein.

ABNORMALITIES OF THE PULMONARY CIRCULATION

The concept of pulmonary vascular resistance is derived by an analogy from electricity. In the lung PVR (pulmonary vascular resistance) is defined as P/F. P is the pressure across the pulmonary vascular bed between the arteries and the veins, i.e. the pressure gradient (voltage sic) in mmHg, and F is the blood flow (equivalent to current)

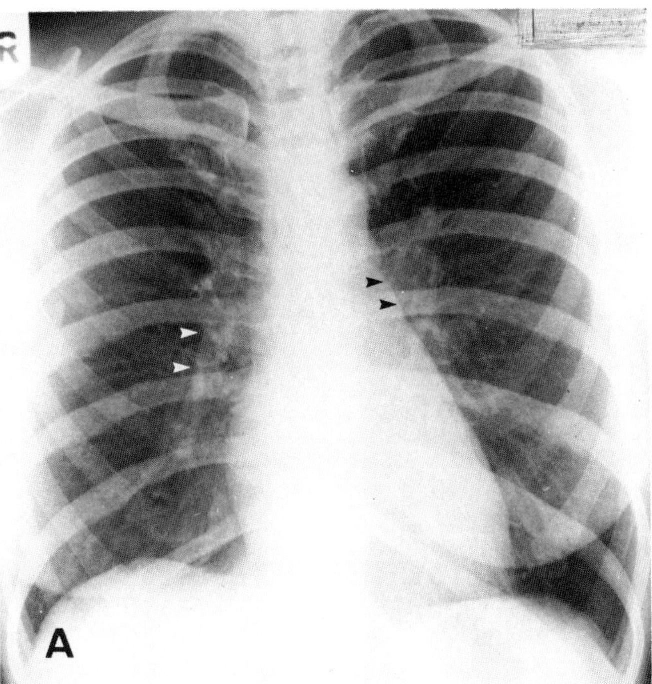

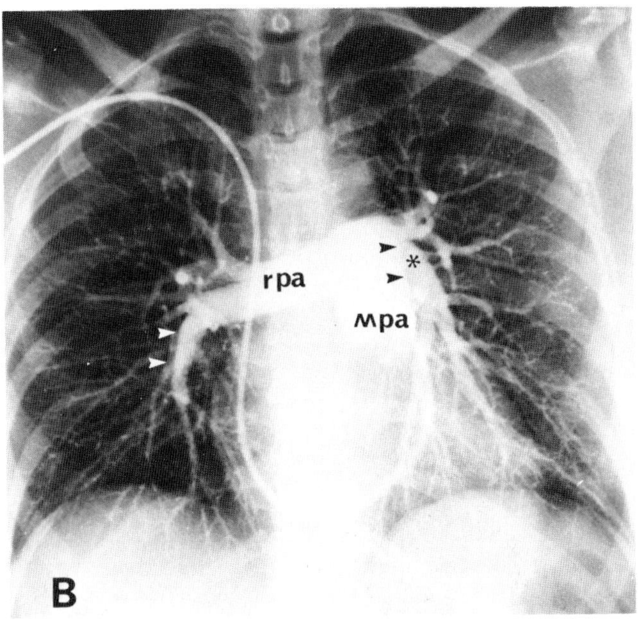

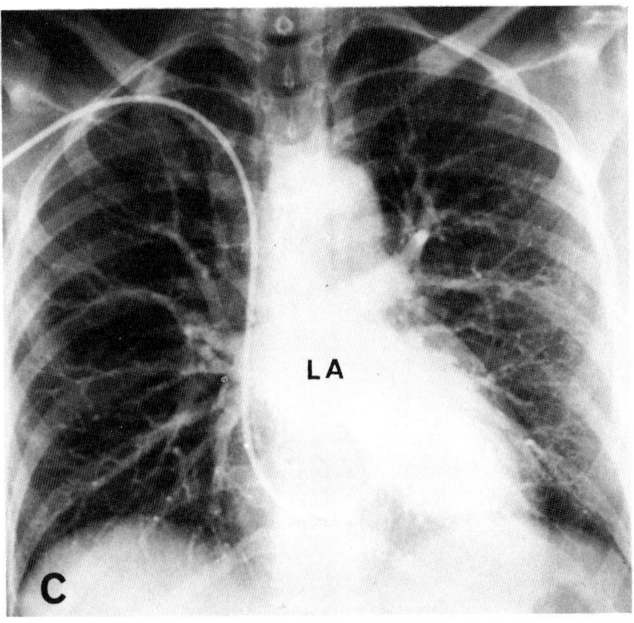

Fig. 22.1 A young woman with sudden onset of chest pain. (**A**) Frontal film. The pulmonary artery beyond the pulmonary valve produces a slight convexity of the pulmonary bay (black arrows). The normal straight outer border of the descending right pulmonary artery may also be seen (white arrows). (**B**) Pulmonary angiogram, arterial phase, same patient. The main pulmonary artery (MPA), beyond the pulmonary valve (black arrows) forms the floor of the pulmonary bay. The right pulmonary artery (RPA) appears as a branch of the main. It crosses the mediastinum and divides within it so the arteries to the right upper lobe come out from the mediastinum above the hilum. The descending branch of the right pulmonary artery can be identified (white arrows) after it leaves the mediastinum and emerges to become silhouetted against the lung. The descending branch of the left pulmonary artery (asterisk) may also be seen silhouetted against the lung as it forms the left hilar shadow. (**C**) Pulmonary angiogram, venous phase, same patient. The pulmonary veins are seen joining the left atrium. They converge to form four pulmonary veins, the superior and inferior pulmonary veins on each side, joining the four corners of the atrium.

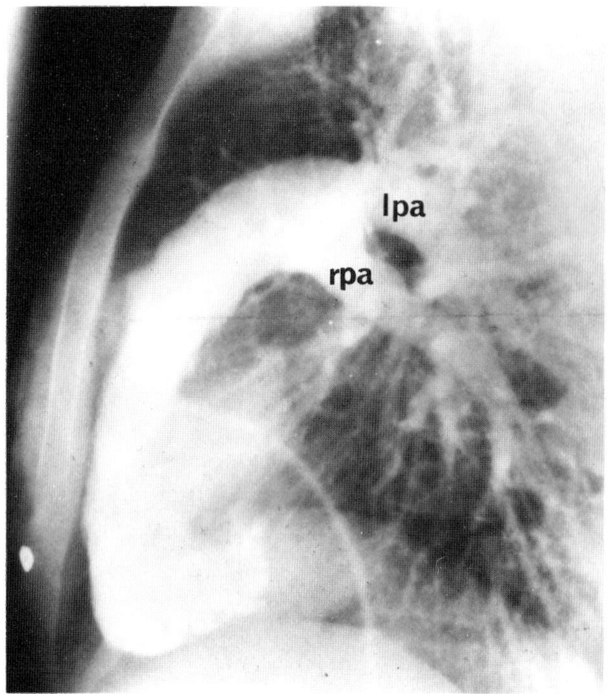

Fig. 22.2 Lateral angiogram to show the pulmonary arteries. The left pulmonary artery (LPA) lies above and behind the 'end-on' carina; the right pulmonary artery (RPA) lies below and in front.

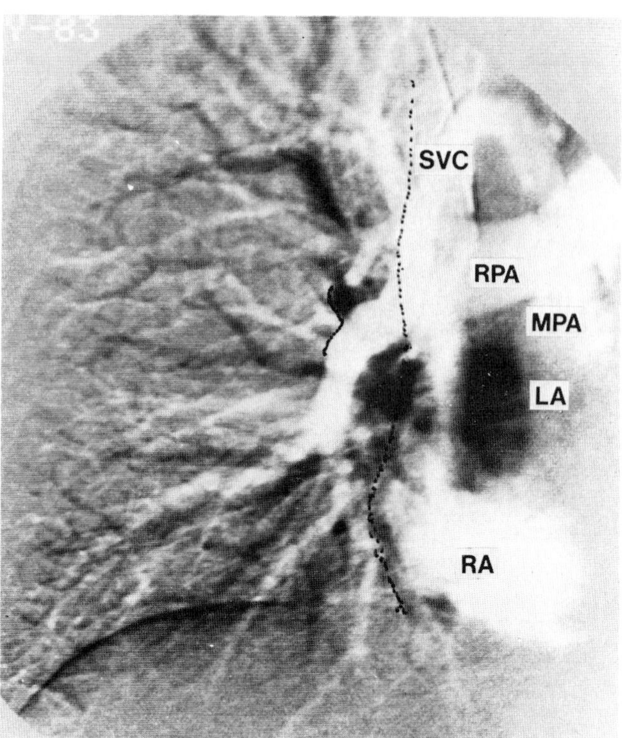

Fig. 22.3 Digital subtraction pulmonary angiogram. The use of computer techniques allows pulmonary arteries and veins to be displayed separately but simultaneously at the same study. The arterial phase appears in white, the venous phase in black, the right edge of the mediastinum has been dotted in. It is formed by the superior vena cava (SVC) above (the injection catheter, imperfectly subtracted due to movement misregistration may be seen) and the right atrium (RA) below. The concavity of the outer aspect of the right hilum has been marked in ink. It is formed by the superior pulmonary vein above, descending vertically to reach the left atrium below the hilum, and the descending branch of the right pulmonary artery below. The upper lobe artery is seen emerging from the mediastinum above the hilum and lying medial to the upper lobe pulmonary vein. The lower lobe vessels are less clearly seen due to misregistration.

through the lungs in l/min. The normal pulmonary vascular resistance is one sixth of that in the systemic circulation so that the normal pulmonary artery pressure (20/10 mmHg) is one sixth that of the systemic circulation. The pulmonary artery pressure is easy to measure, and as pulmonary venous pressure is usually small, is taken to indicate the pressure gradient, unless there is evidence of pulmonary venous hypertension.

In normal lung an increase in flow is accompanied by an increase in pulmonary artery pressure even though pulmonary vascular resistance is normal, so-called *hyperkinetic pulmonary hypertension*. When the increase in flow is reversed, pressure will fall to normal. An increase in pulmonary artery pressure may also occur if there is a rise in pressure in the pulmonary veins. This pressure will be transmitted directly back through the pulmonary vascular bed to the pulmonary artery, so called *passive pulmonary hypertension*

When a rise in pulmonary artery pressure is due to obstruction of the vessels within the lung the condition is termed pulmonary hypertension. It may be due to obstruction or destruction of the pulmonary capillary bed, to obstruction or vasoconstriction of the smaller arteries and arterioles or to obstruction of the larger arteries.

CONGENITAL HEART DISEASE

Changes in the pulmonary circulation in congenital heart disease will be fully dealt with in Chapter 25 but the general patterns of abnormality are considered briefly here. Congenital heart disease may also show abnormalities and have pulmonary changes similar to those in acquired heart disease.

Pulmonary plethora

This is the characteristic appearance of the lung vessels in the presence of increase in pulmonary flow, usually from a left to right shunt, rarely from an increase in cardiac output. The main pulmonary artery is enlarged producing a convex pulmonary bay. The pulmonary arteries and veins are increased in size and can be followed into the outer third of the lung. Upper and lower lobe flow are equilibrated. Pulmonary oedema in association with large shunts may be superimposed on the appearances of pulmonary plethora.

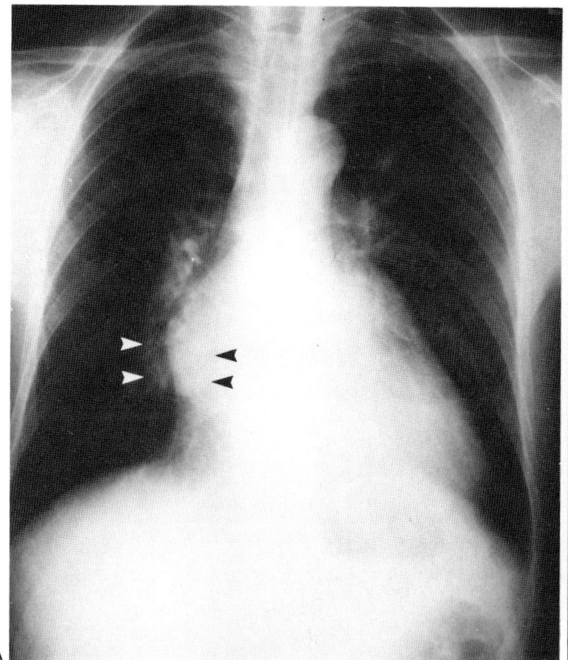

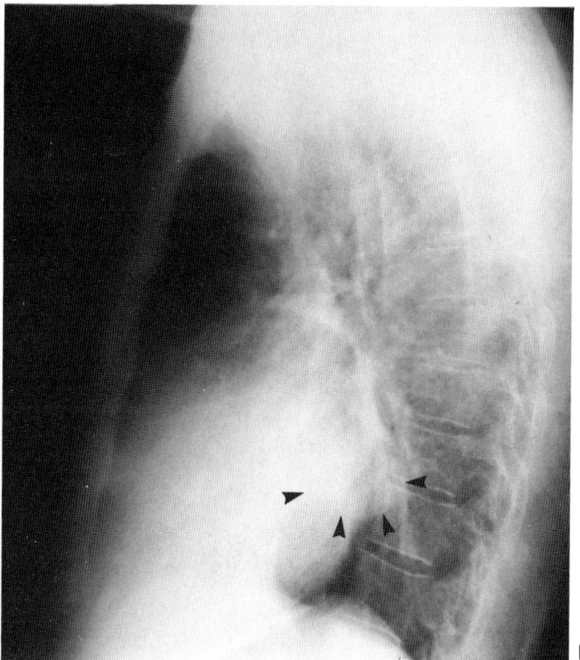

Fig. 22.4 Confluence of the pulmonary veins. In this patient with mitral valve disease there is a large sharply demarcated rounded shadow at the right corner to the left atrium (arrows). The nature of the shadow is suggested by its sharp definition and characteristic site with pulmonary veins entering it. (**A**) Frontal view. (**B**) Lateral view.

If gross pulmonary plethora is present and an enlarged pulmonary artery cannot be identified it may be normally situated but concealed by the thymus, absent as in truncus arteriosus, or misplaced in the mediastinum as in transposition of the great arteries.

In the neonate the appearances of pulmonary plethora may be mimicked by an underexposed film.

The following may produce the appearances of pulmonary plethora:

1. *Left to right shunts*
   a) Without cyanosis
      atrial shunts
      ventricular shunts
      aortopulmonary shunts
   b) With cyanosis

All the following lesions are characterized by mixing of arterial and venous blood within the heart:

transposition of the great arteries
total anomalous pulmonary venous drainage
truncus arteriosus
common atrium
single ventricle
double outlet right ventricle

2. *Increased cardiac output*
   Pregnancy
   Anaemia
   Thyrotoxicosis
   Beriberi
   Systemic arteriovenous fistulae
   Chronic liver disease
   Polycythaemia
   Paget's disease

PULMONARY ARTERY PRUNING

High pressure left to right shunts are associated with obstructive changes in the smaller pulmonary arteries and arterioles which lead to an increase in pulmonary vascular resistance and a rise in pulmonary artery pressure, ultimately to systemic levels, and hence to a reduction and then reversal of a shunt, '*the Eisenmenger reaction*'. The characteristic but not invariable appearance in this situation is of a large main, and large central pulmonary arteries which taper down rapidly to very small vessels over a few orders of branches, giving a 'pruned tree' appearance. Unless the appearances are gross the level of the increase of pulmonary vascular resistance cannot be judged by the plain film appearances.

In long-standing Eisenmenger reaction patients calcification may develop in the main and central pulmonary arteries. The Eisenmenger reaction is a common complication of large ventricular septal defects and large patent ductus arteriosus defects, but is rare in atrial septal defects. Rise in pulmonary vascular resistance may also occur in association with similar communications in transposition of the great arteries or in syndromes allied to ventricular septal defect such as double outlet right ventricle and single ventricle.

PULMONARY OLIGAEMIA

Reduced blood flow from obstruction proximal to the main pulmonary artery may lead to characteristic appearances. The main pulmonary artery is small and often displaced medially (as in the Tetralogy of Fallot) producing an empty or concave pulmonary bay. The pulmonary vessels are small and the lungs are hypertranslucent. These appearances can be mimicked in the neonate by over-exposure of the film, and are then difficult to assess, and the pulmonary bay itself may be obscured in the neonate by a large thymus.

ASYMMETRICAL PERFUSION

The plain film may demonstrate abnormal asymmetrical perfusion. There is a normal perfusion gradient from above downwards (see p. 564) and the reverse perfusion gradient of pulmonary venous hypertension is considered below. Differences in perfusion on the two sides, as evidenced by difference in the size and extent of the blood vessels on the two sides are a common feature of congenital heart disease, either as the result of revascularization surgery such as Blalock or Waterston shunt operations, or with congenital abnormalities of pulmonary flow. Localized abnormalities of perfusion, scattered throughout the lungs, are always strongly suggestive of complex pulmonary atresia (see below).

BRONCHIAL CIRCULATION

An increase in the bronchial circulation, which usually develops as a response to severe obstruction of the pulmonary circulation, leads to an enlargement of the bronchial arteries. This enlargement may be suspected by a curious spotty appearance of the lungs, spreading out from the hilum. Pulmonary oligaemia can often be seen in association with this appearance of the bronchial circulation.

PULMONARY VENOUS HYPERTENSION

Impairment of function of the valves or chambers of the left heart commonly leads to a rise in pressure in the left atrium which is transmitted back into the (valveless) pulmonary veins producing pulmonary venous hypertension. This increase in pressure leads to the distension of the normally collapsed upper lobe veins. These veins may be recognized on the erect plain film (Fig. 22.5), as enlarged and rising up towards the apex of the lung. They may enlarge alone or there may be some enlargement of the arteries which accompany them, so that the vessels above the hilum appear larger than those below. The positive identification of *upper lobe blood diversion* almost invariably indicates disorder of the left side of the heart, though basal emphysema may rarely produce similar appearances without the explanation being obvious. Rarely, local lung disease involving the upper lobes may prevent its radiological recognition. However, it is common to see the changes of pulmonary oedema (see later) indicating severe functional impairment of the left heart, without recognising upper lobe blood diversion.

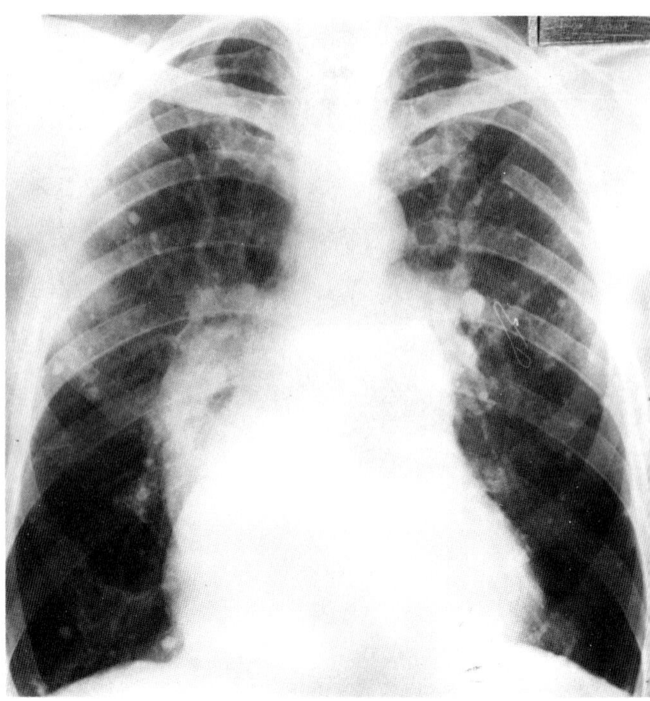

Fig. 22.5 The end result of longstanding severe pulmonary venous hypertension. There has been a closed mitral valvotomy through the left sixth rib. There is very marked upper lobe blood diversion with very large upper lobe pulmonary veins and almost no veins visible in the lower lobes. There is also severe pulmonary arterial hypertension with gross enlargement of the main and central pulmonary arteries with tapering peripherally. In addition there are the characteristic densities of pulmonary ossific nodules.

The explanation for the development of upper lobe blood diversion is not clear. It has been suggested that perivascular oedema surrounding the lower lobe veins in the erect position leads to their compression and produces the redistribution of flow to the upper lobe.

As the pulmonary venous pressure rises above 25 mmHg it exceeds the plasma osmotic pressure and enters the threshold for pulmonary oedema. This appears initially as **interstitial lines** (Figs 22.6A and B). *B lines are horizontal basal peripheral non-branching fine lines visible on the frontal* and lateral film. They are thought to be due to oedema of the interlobular septa through which the lymphatics pass. *A lines* are irregular lines mainly spreading out from the

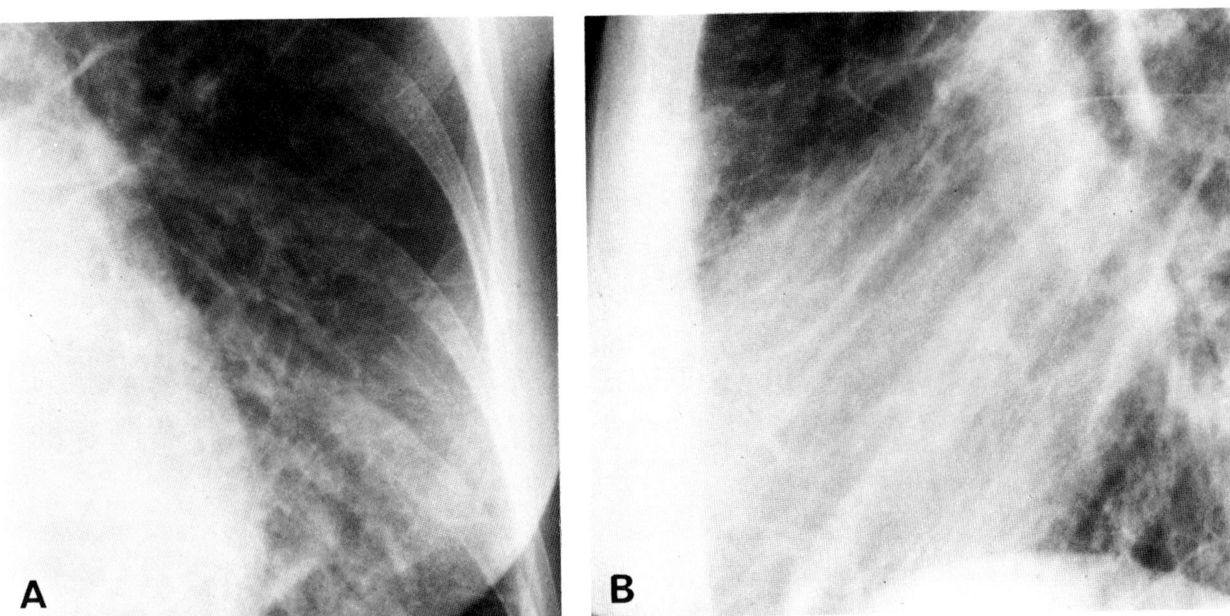

Fig. 22.6 Pulmonary interstitial oedema. (**A**) localized frontal view of the left base. (**B**) localized lateral view of the front of the chest. The horizontal basal peripheral line shadows are the 'B' lines probably due to oedema of the interlobular septa. The lines running in apparently random directions are the 'A' lines. In the lateral view the 'B' lines can be seen running horizontally at the back of the sternum together with 'A' lines. There is also thickening of the fissures indicating fluid within them.

hilum and thought to be due to oedema of the intercommunicating lymphatics. They are less frequently seen but have the same import as the B lines. They may also be seen behind the sternum rising up the chest on the lateral view.

Interstitial oedema is mainly seen in association with a rise in left atrial pressure from any cause; *mitral valve disease* either stenosis or incompetence, or obstruction at the mitral valve from a left atrial myxoma, all lead to a rise in left atrial pressure which is transmitted back to the pulmonary veins. *Left ventricular failure*, either from aortic disease, hypertension or disease of heart muscle, may be associated with the rise in left ventricular and hence left atrial pressure and pulmonary oedema. The non-failing left ventricle of *hypertrophic cardiomyopathy* may become so stiff that the high pressure required to distend it in diastole is transmitted back to the left atrium and leads to pulmonary venous hypertension. Rarely the obstruction may lie in the pulmonary veins in unusual forms of *constrictive pericarditis* or in *pulmonary veno-occlusive disease*. In this last condition the plain film illustrates the characteristic appearances of interstitial and alveolar oedema but there is no overt upper lobe blood diversion or evidence of left heart disease. Unless a lung biopsy is taken the diagnosis becomes one of exclusion. Interstitial lines are also a feature of a number of primarily lung diseases (see Part 2).

Once the left atrial pressure rises beyond the level at which the distended lymphatics can clear oedema fluid from the lungs, overt **alveolar pulmonary oedema** develops (Figs 22.7A and B). The classical appearance of this is of a confluent alveolar shadowing developing in both lungs and having a perihilar or 'bat's wing' appearance. The densest shadow appears around the hilar regions spreading off to an ill-defined periphery and sparing the bases of the lungs. Less commonly it may be localized to one lung, or part of the lung when its typical situation is in the right upper lobe. It may develop in the lung bases, or it may appear as a rather granular shadowing throughout the lungs without any overt perihilar concentration, or even as a peripherally distributed abnormal shadowing. Its association with a large heart, its rapid onset, rapid change with diuretic therapy, and often its extent, together with lack of fever, usually serve to differentiate it from infection.

Other features which may be seen in pulmonary oedema are blurring of the outline of the slightly distended hilum and blurring of the outlines of the central pulmonary vessels, due to perivascular oedema. Similar blurring may be seen around bronchi taken end on in the frontal chest X-ray, the so-called 'endobronchial cuffing'. These features go to support the diagnosis of pulmonary oedema.

The development of **pleural effusion** is common in the evolution of pulmonary oedema and may go to support the diagnosis. Pleural effusions may be of considerable size, and have their characteristic appearances in the costophrenic angles; however when very small they may appear as the lamellar shadow of a small parietal effusion lying against the outer wall of the thorax, deep in the costophrenic angles. Fluid in the fissures of the lung may be recognised as thickenings of the fissures in both the

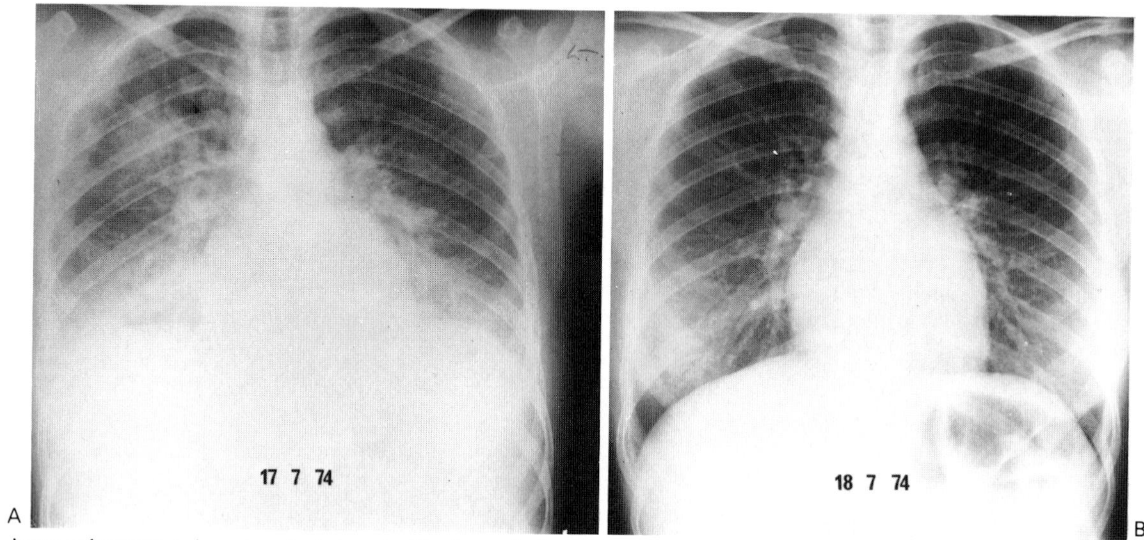

Fig. 22.7 Acute pulmonary oedema in mitral stenosis. The heart shadow is not large but shows the features of selective left atrial enlargement compatible with mitral valve disease. (**A**) On 17.7.74 there is extensive bilateral pulmonary shadowing, primarily perihilar, and associated with los of definition of the outline of the hila and vessels. (**B**) Within one day (18.7.74) this shadowing has cleared. The extensive nature of the shadowing, its perihilar rather than segmental distribution, and its rapidity of change of appearance, are the features which point to the diagnosis of pulmonary oedema.

frontal and lateral view and may go to support the diagnosis. Although pleural fluid may take any distribution it is relatively common for quite large effusions to collect in the fissures in the pulmonary oedema of cardiac failure where they may appear to resemble tumour masses on the frontal film. The nature of these 'disappearing tumours' is quite clear when a lateral view is taken.

Once diuretic therapy has begun, the relationship between rise in pulmonary venous pressure and radiological demonstration of pulmonary oedema is lost.

A sustained rise in left atrial pressure leads not only to distension of the upper lobe veins but also to constriction of the lower lobe veins and then the arteries, so that flow through the lungs is virtually confined to the upper lobes. These appearances are most commonly seen in long-standing mitral valve disease, the 'stag's antlers' appearance (Fig. 22.5).

Initially pulmonary venous hypertension is associated with a rise in pulmonary artery pressure equivalent to the rise in the pressure in the pulmonary veins, so that the pressure gradient across the lungs is normal, so-called *passive pulmonary hypertension*.

Ultimately obliterative changes in the pulmonary arterioles develop, leading to superimposed active pulmonary arterial hypertension which is thought to be some form of protective reaction to the lungs. This can be seen on the plain film (Fig. 22.5) when enlargement of the main pulmonary artery and the central pulmonary arteries develop, the changes being particularly marked in the upper lobe. When such changes are present, they indicate pulmonary arterial hypertension but their absence does not exclude it.

Long-standing pulmonary venous hypertension may be associated with the development of **haemosiderosis** (Fig. 22.8) which appears on the plain film as a series of fine punctate calcifications scattered throughout the lungs.

Very longstanding severe pulmonary venous hypertension may also be associated with the development of **pulmonary ossific nodules** (Fig. 22.5). These are small areas of bone formation in the lungs, never larger than 1 cm in diameter, the diameter of the secondary lobule. They often appear to have a trabecular structure.

PULMONARY ARTERIAL HYPERTENSION

This is considered to be present when the pulmonary artery pressure is over 30 mmHg systolic (and the pulmonary venous pressure is normal). In the absence of a shunt the pulmonary artery pressure can rise above the systemic levels.

When the pressure in the pulmonary artery approaches systemic levels a number of consequences develop. The right ventricle is unable to increase its output against this high pressure so that any fall in peripheral vascular resistance, such as that produced by exercise, leads to a fall in systemic blood pressure and may lead to syncope. This is the mechanism of hypotension and death associated with angiocardiography which produces a profound peripheral systemic vasodilatation. Low, fixed, cardiac output may lead to an anginal type of chest pain. Shortness of breath may be a feature. The high pulmonary artery pressure leads ultimately to right ventricular failure with dilatation and peripheral oedema. This clinical picture will of course

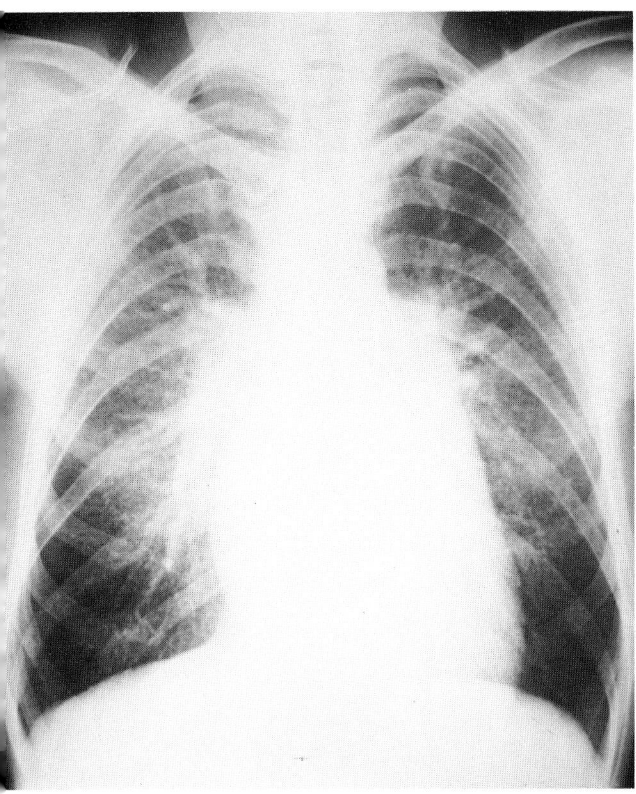

Fig. 22.8 Pulmonary haemosiderosis secondary to long-standing mitral valve disease. The fine granular background pattern to the lungs is typical of haemosiderosis. In addition there are changes suggestive of mitral valve disease with straightening of the left heart border and some upper lobe blood diversion.

be modified according to the nature of the underlying causative lung disorder.

Radiographic appearances. The plain film (Figs 22.9A–C) characteristically shows a large and often triangular heart. The main pulmonary artery and central pulmonary arteries are usually large and may be very large but taper rapidly to the periphery. Rarely the pulmonary vessels or heart may appear normal but it is rare for the main pulmonary artery to be inconspicuous.

Lung scanning usually shows normal perfusion and ventilation though rarely small peripheral perfusion defects may be seen.

PULMONARY EMBOLISM

This may lead to a variety of clinical pictures according to the size and number of the emboli and the underlying state of the circulation.

Acute massive pulmonary embolism

This occurs when one or more large pulmonary emboli, usually consisting of detached thrombus from the larger veins of the lower limb, impact in the central pulmonary arteries. It leads to the rapid onset of severe pulmonary obstruction, but this is usually associated with only a modest rise in pulmonary artery pressure as right ventricular dilatation and failure quickly ensues. The clinical onset is usually with some shortness of breath, hypotension and tachycardia and perhaps chest pain. A history suggestive of deep vein thrombosis of the legs may be present. The physical signs of a loud P2 and the ECG evidence of right ventricular strain may suggest the diagnosis, but the clinical picture could fit with myocardiac infarction, concealed haemorrhage or other cause of shock.

Radiographic appearances. The plain film may be helpful in this situation if it is of good quality and if the patient is otherwise fit (Fig. 22.10A). There may be a moderate increase in the heart size. The characteristic feature is the demonstration of *localized areas of under-perfusion* of the lung. These may be brought into relief by an apparent increase in perfusion of other segments. Large areas of one or both lungs may be affected. Increased density of the main pulmonary artery associated with peripheral cut-off vessels, though well recognized is exceptionally rare. Comparison with previous radiographs may be helpful in recognizing changes in the pulmonary vascular supply to the lungs. The characteristic changes are usually not recognized in poor quality films such as most portable X-rays; or when there is underlying heart disease, which is extremely frequent in association with pulmonary embolism; or if the embolization is so extensive it produces an overall diminution in pulmonary perfusion rather than localized hypoperfusion with compensatory hyperperfusion elsewhere. When the characteristic features are present they are helpful in diagnosis, but this is rather an infrequent finding.

The investigation of acute massive pulmonary embolism is according to the facilities available, the time of day at which the clinical picture developed and the clinical certainty of the clinician. The situation clinically may be so precarious and the diagnosis so certain that little more than an ECG and a plain X-ray may be taken before beginning treatment with anti-coagulants. The fatal pulmonary embolus is often not the one which brought the patient to medical attention, but one which follows soon after; if this can be prevented the patient should recover completely (Figs 22.11A and B). If the diagnosis is in doubt, it is usually quicker in most departments to organize emergency pulmonary angiography than pulmonary scanning and this should be the investigation of choice (Fig. 22.10B).

Sub-acute pulmonary embolism

When the emboli are smaller and fewer so that acute cor pulmonale does not develop immediately, changes have time to develop in the lungs. As the lungs have a second, bronchial, circulation, pulmonary infarction rarely develops. This is usually when a large vessel is occluded and there is impairment of the bronchial circulation, a feature

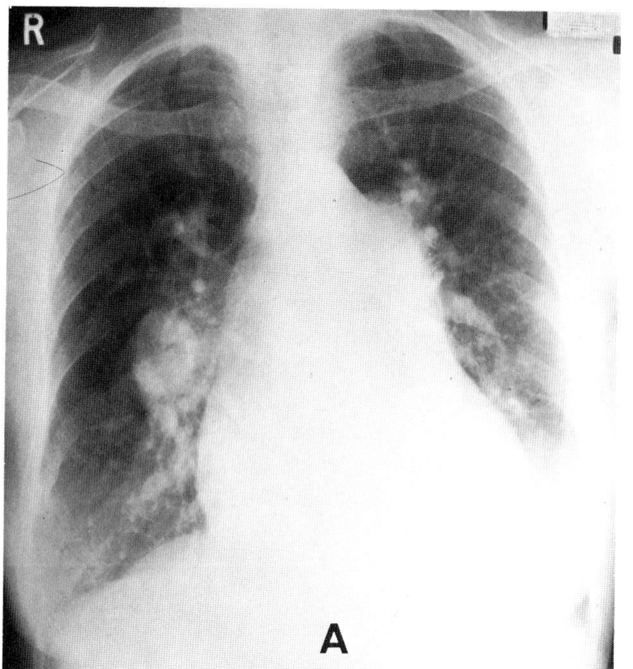

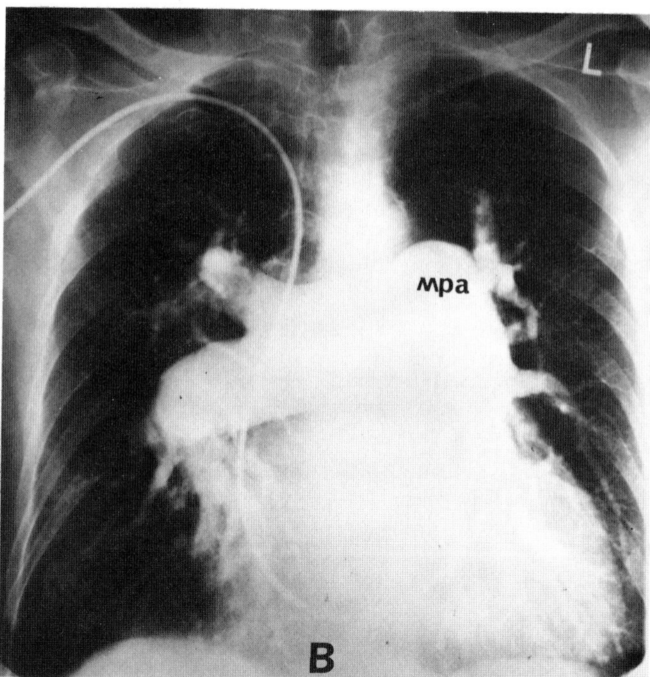

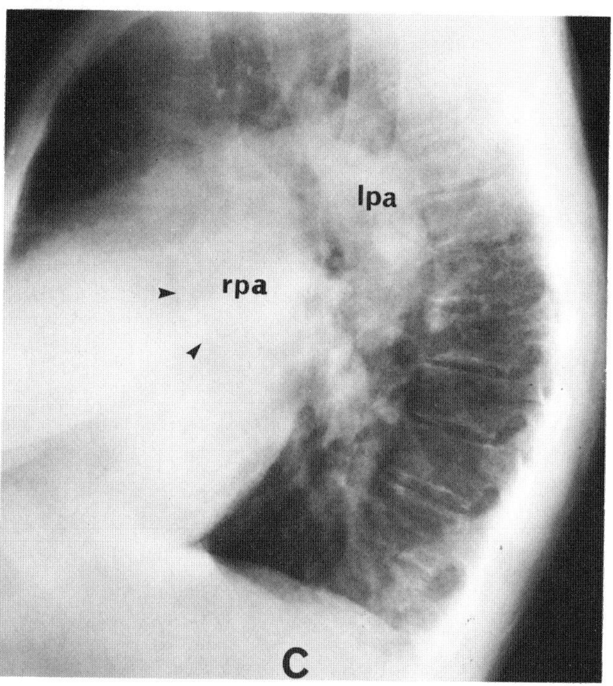

Fig. 22.9 Primary pulmonary hypertension. (**A**) Frontal chest film. The heart is enlarged with the triangular outline suggestive of right heart enlargement. The main pulmonary artery and central vessels are large but taper rapidly to the periphery. The enlarged right hilum is made up of an enlarged descending branch of the right pulmonary artery. (**B**) Frontal pulmonary arteriogram, same patient. This enables the main pulmonary artery to be identified, confirms the make-up of the right hilum, and illustrates the dramatic peripheral pruning of the pulmonary arteries. (**C**) Lateral chest film, same patient. This shows the enlarged right pulmonary artery (rpa) (arrows) and left pulmonary artery (lpa) and the right heart enlargement against the sternum.

which commonly occurs in association with heart failure. The usual sequence of events following occlusion of a pulmonary artery (Fig. 22.12), is that the unperfused lung ceases to aerate properly and this is associated with some reduction in volume. This is commonly seen on the plain film as an *elevation of the diaphragm* on the affected side. Over the next few days this hypoventilation may lead to areas of *collapse* which usually re-expand if the patient survives. Infarction itself may develop to some degree in the affected vascular segment of which the obstructed artery forms the apex and the pleural aspect the base. The infarction may be barely visible but may lead to a haemorrhagic *pleural effusion*, and this may be seen as a small fluid collection in the costophrenic angle. The infarction very rarely appears as the characteristic triangular shadow described in older textbooks. More commonly it appears as an area of rather nondescript *consolidation* whose chief characteristic is that it is associated with a pleural surface. This may only be apparent on the lateral view, and includes the surfaces of the fissures as well as the periphery of the lungs. These infarctions are usually partial and reversible in the course of time. They may disappear entirely or may heal to a linear scar. However if the infarction is large and there is impairment of bronchial perfusion, it may be irreversible and heal ultimately by scarring and *fibrosis* in the lungs.

The plain film appearances of pulmonary embolism with infarction, are largely confined to the lung bases, the right side being more commonly involved than the left.

Pulmonary embolism with infarction is associated with a sudden onset of chest pain, with haemoptysis and with

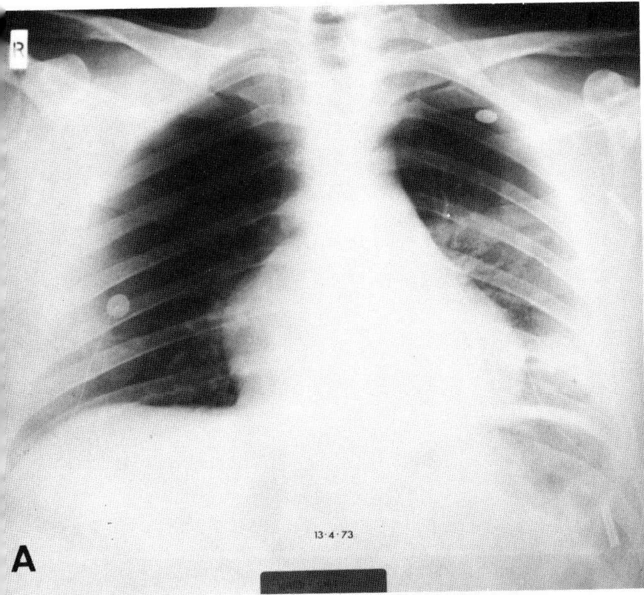

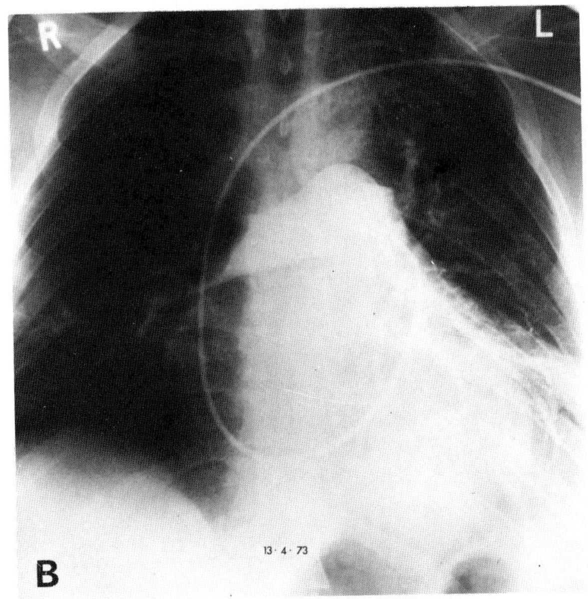

Fig. 22.10 Acute massive pulmonary embolism 13.4.73. (**A**) Frontal chest film (portable). The right lung and the left upper zone are hypertransradiant due to oligaemia, and there is overperfusion of the left mid and lower zones. (**B**) Pulmonary arteriogram, same patient. The leading edge of an embolus is seen impacted in the right pulmonary artery producing virtually complete obstruction. Another embolus is seen in the supply to the left upper lobe which is also impaired. Only the left lower lobe fills adequately with contrast.

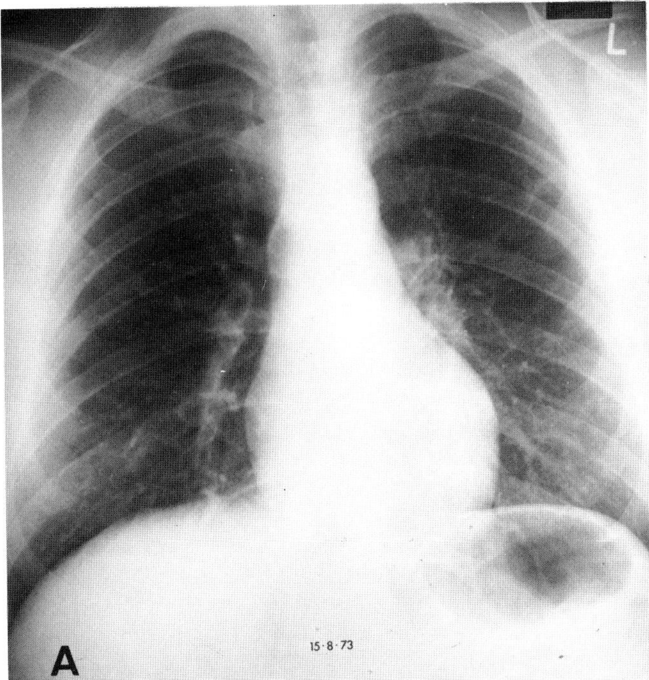

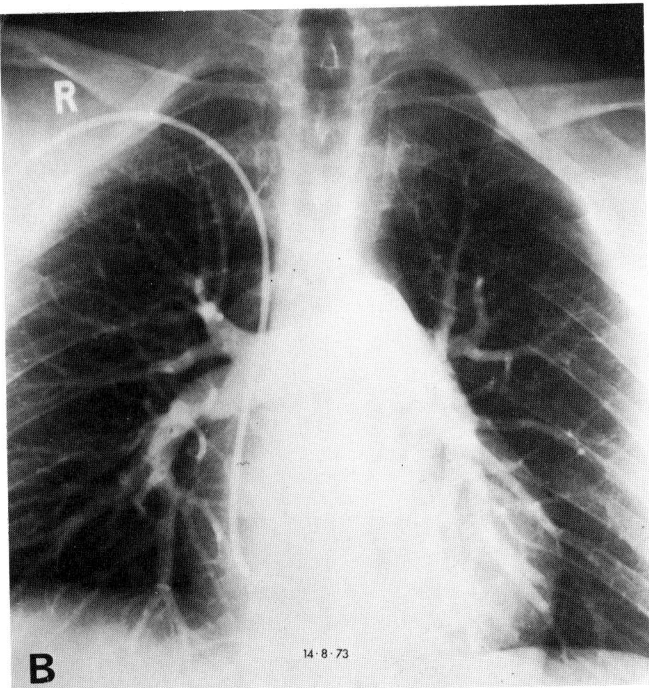

Fig. 22.11 Pulmonary embolism after effective treatment, 15.8.73. Same patient as Figure 22.10. (**A**) Frontal film. This is now entirely normal. (**B**) Pulmonary arteriogram. The pulmonary emboli have entirely resolved.

progressive increase in shortness of breath, as emboli arrive progressively and occlude the lung bed. A normal chest X-ray, even if of good quality, does not exclude the diagnosis which may be clinically difficult. It should be suspected in any case of what appears to be a chest infection which does not respond to antibiotics, or in which the shortness of breath seems excessive. It should be considered with any patient with chest pain and clinical indications of possible deep vein thrombosis. It may also be suspected in any patient, particularly in patients with heart failure, in whom the possibility of complicating pulmonary embolism arises, and in whom shortness of breath appears to be out of proportion to the underlying condition. It is in the

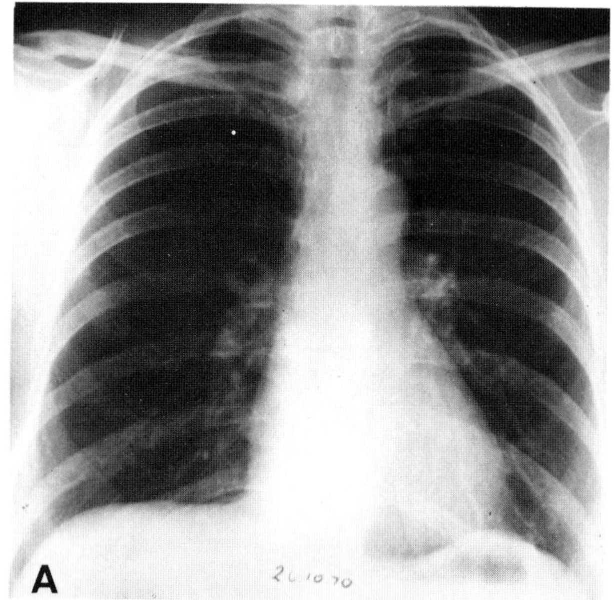

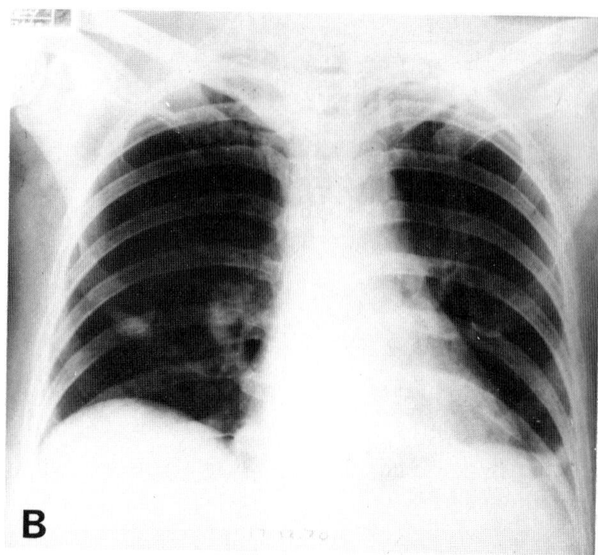

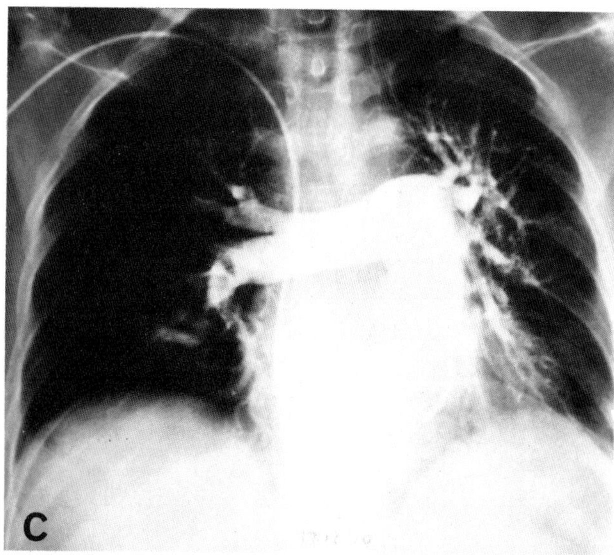

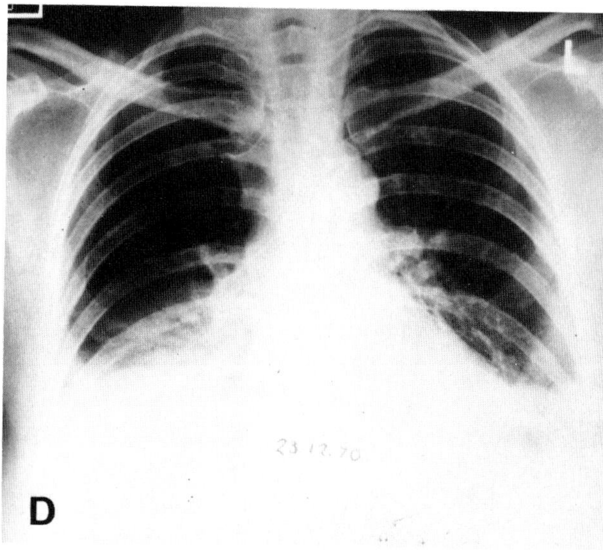

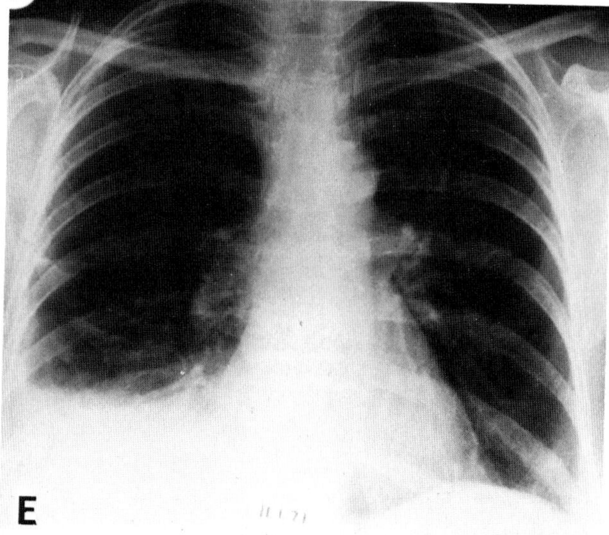

Fig. 22.12 Pulmonary embolism with infarction. (**A**) Frontal film 26.10.70. Preoperative when the chest X-ray was normal. (**B**) Frontal film 17.12.70. Following acute onset of chest pain and shortness of breath in the postoperative period. The right lung is obviously hypertransradiant and oligaemic and there is some filling in of the left costophrenic angle. (**C**) Pulmonary arteriogram performed at the same time. Emboli are sitting in the pulmonary arteries to the right lung which is oligaemic. There are probably emboli in arteries to the left lower zone. (**D**) Frontal film 23.12.70. Patchy basal consolidation and pleural fluid have appeared indicating the development of infarction. (**E**) Frontal film 11.1.71 following effective treatment. The infarction at the left base, which was reversible, has cleared. On the right more extensive infarction is still visible and line shadows of pulmonary scarring are developing.

ubacute pulmonary embolism that isotope lung scanning lays its major part.

sotope lung scanning

Modern methods of isotope imaging of the lung using a arge crystal gamma camera have enormously improved iagnostic accuracy in pulmonary embolism. Technetium-abelled albumin macroaggregates or microspheres injected ntravenously will impact in the lung in the absence of any ight to left shunt either cardiac or extracardiac. The listribution of these microspheres may be recorded by the amma camera. A normal perfusion isotope lung scan xcludes the diagnosis of pulmonary embolism from enous thrombus. If the perfusion lung scan shows the haracteristic wedged shape localized perfusion deficits hen pulmonary embolism becomes a possibility. Perfusion leficits can be caused by localized lung pathology such as nfections or areas of emphysema or they can be part of a attern of diffuse obstructive airways disease of the chronic ronchitis type. Multiple perfusion deficits involving parts of the lung which appear normal on the chest X-ray ncrease the suspicion of pulmonary embolism. At this tage it is desirable to perform a ventilation scan; much the nost effective is the inhalation of krypton 81m until equilibrium is reached and then recording the ventilation pattern with a gamma camera (Fig. 22.13). When the localized deficiencies of perfusion can be matched with deficiencies of ventilation the likely underlying cause is some form of lung disease, and if a chest film appears normal, then obstructive airways disease is most likely (Fig. 22.14). Where the ventilation remains normal yet a localized perfusion deficit is present pulmonary embolism is highly likely; if the mismatch is definite and the perfusion deficits typical (Fig. 22.15), then the diagnosis may be taken as proven and treatment instituted.

Pulmonary angiography

If the ventilation/perfusion findings are not typical or a full study cannot be performed, then it is desirable to proceed to angiography. Pulmonary angiography is usually performed by passing a catheter from a vein in the elbow through the heart to the main pulmonary artery. The pulmonary artery pressure can be recorded and then a pulmonary angiogram performed. A bolus of 50 ml at 25 ml/sec is usually satisfactory and a large film format rapid film changer with rapid early and slow delayed films gives whole lung cover and adequate definition.

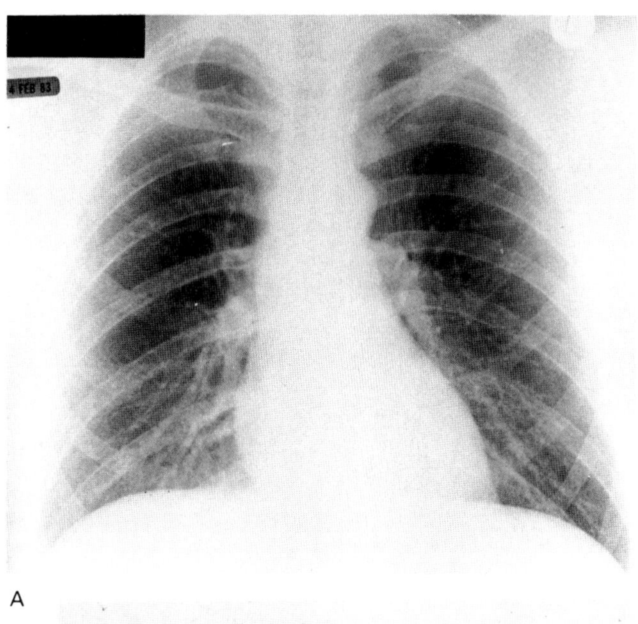

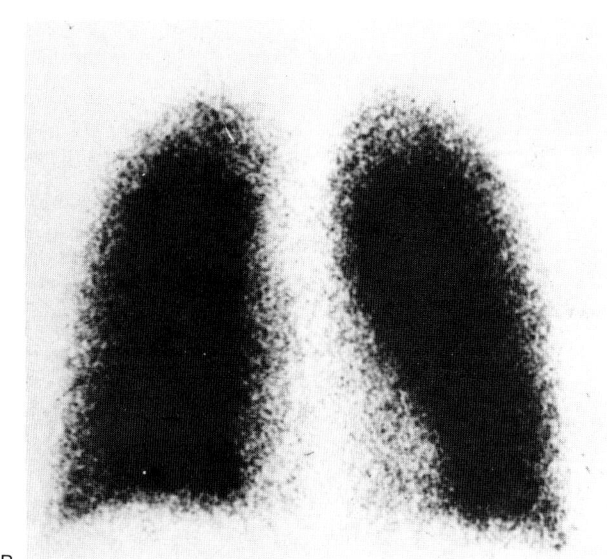

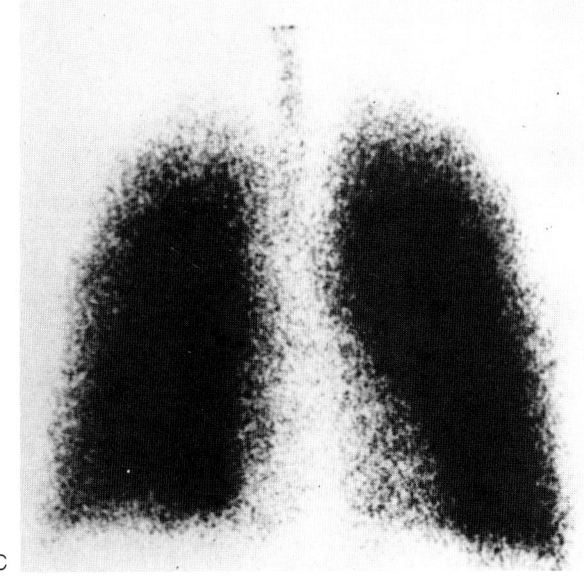

Fig. 22.13 Normal lung scan in a patient with acute chest pain. (**A**) Frontal film. This is normal. (**B**) Frontal perfusion scan. This shows even perfusion over the whole of both lungs. (**C**) Krypton-81m ventilation scan. This shows even ventilation over both lungs. Note the activity in the trachea which can be recognized in this type of ventilation scan. The even and matched distribution of isotope with perfusion and ventilation excludes the diagnosis of pulmonary embolism.

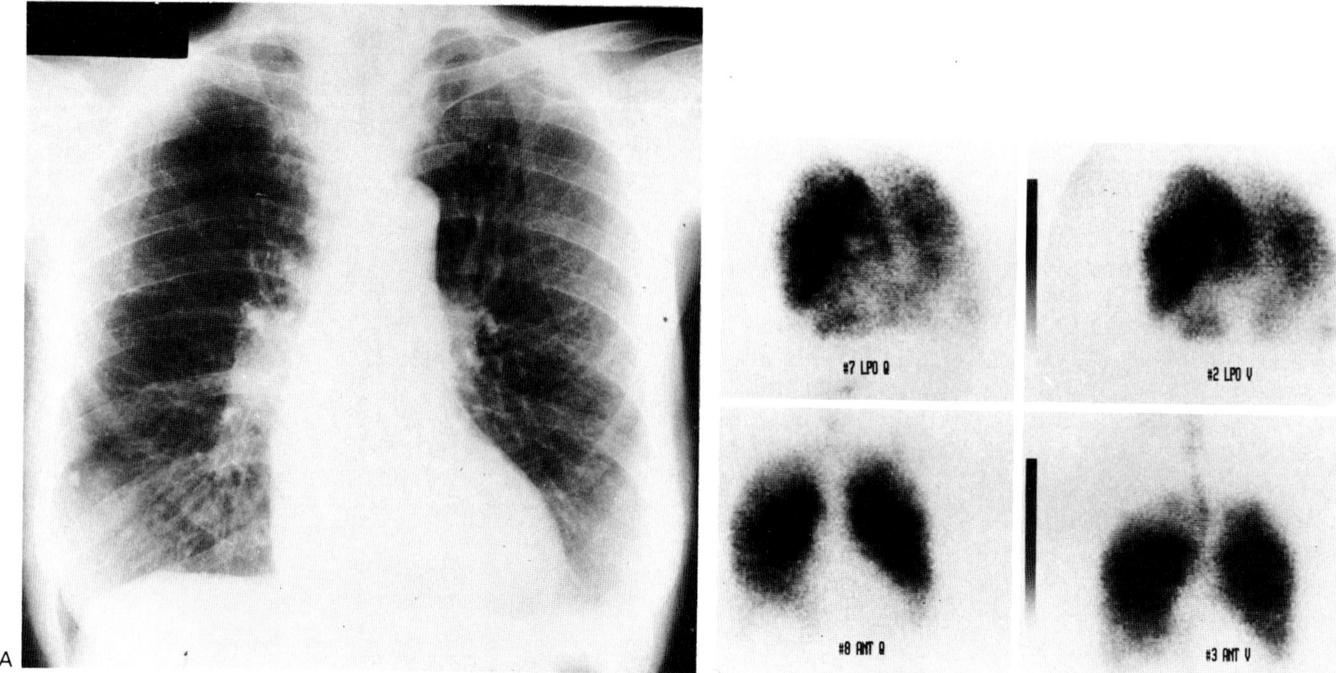

Fig. 22.14 Chronic obstructive airways disease. (**A**) Frontal film. Apart from a slight 'streakiness' of the lung markings which always raises the possibility of obstructive airways disease, the appearances are normal. (**B**) Computer reconstructions of perfusion and ventilation scans. Perfusion is on the left and ventilation on the right. Note that in the left posterior oblique (LPO) view there is a very large but matched defect of perfusion at the left base. The matching suggests that this is due to obstructive airways disease and not to pulmonary embolism.

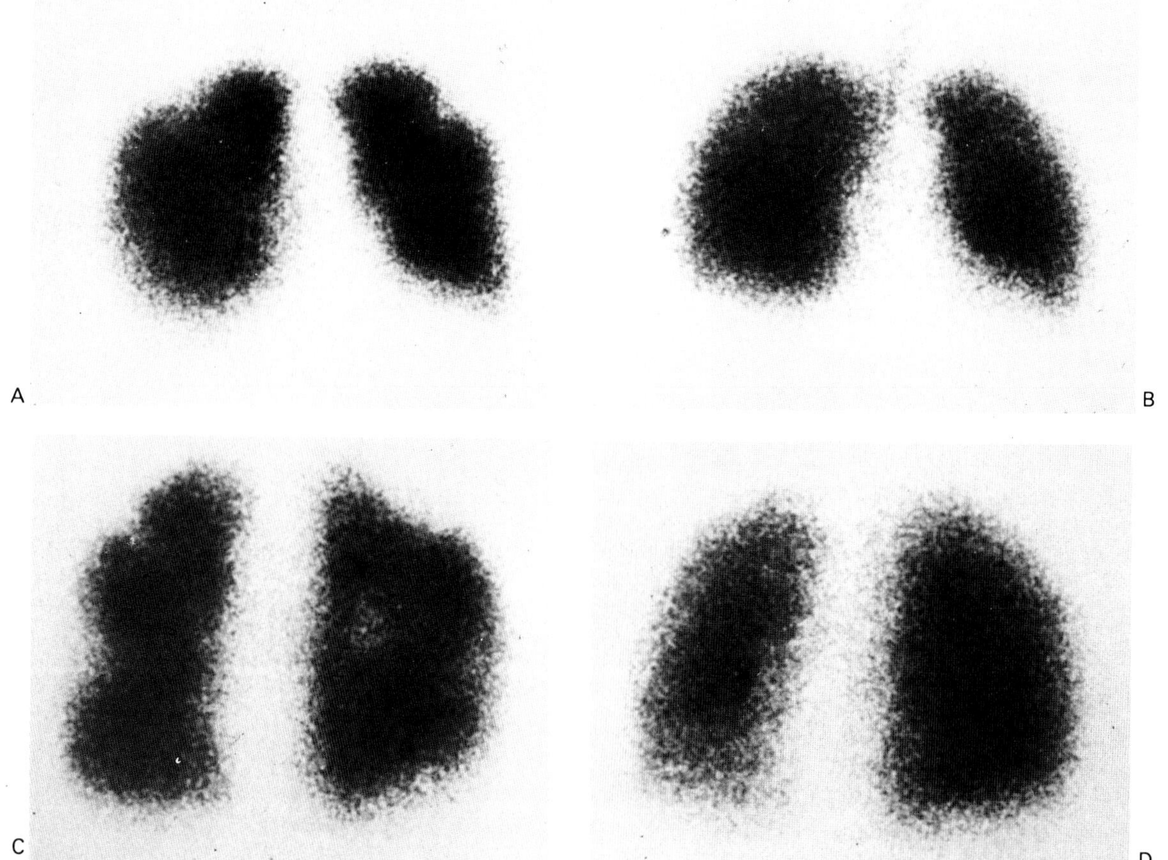

Fig. 22.15 Acute pulmonary embolism. (**A** and **B**) Frontal perfusion and ventilation scans. (**C** and **D**) Posterior perfusion and ventilation scans. Note the multiple wedge shaped deficits on both the frontal and posterior perfusion scans but the entirely normal distribution of the isotope in the frontal and posterior ventilation scans. These appearances are typical of acute pulmonary embolism. The plain film was normal.

Venous angiocardiography using a catheter in a peripheral vein and a larger bolus may give adequate visualization of the pulmonary arteries and this technique has now been upgraded by the use of *digital subtraction angiography* so that a fine catheter placed in the superior vena cava using a mechanical injector to give a large bolus of contrast gives adequate opacification of each lung in turn.

The right lung is usually well seen in the frontal view; the direct posterior inclination of the left pulmonary artery means that it, and its proximal branches, may be too foreshortened and a right posterior oblique which is usually obtained by raising the left shoulder towards the overhead tube, will unfold them. With sophisticated apparatus the AP film may be taken with cranial angulation of the X-ray tube to reduce the foreshortening of the central pulmonary vessels within the mediastinum.

Pulmonary emboli can usually be directly demonstrated as sharply demarcated intraluminal filling defects in the contrast-filled pulmonary arteries (Figs. 22.10B, 22.12C). When these are seen the diagnosis is certain. The presence of emboli reduces blood flow in the affected vessel so that parts of the lung may appear under-perfused, but similar appearances may be produced by abnormal lung and are only suggestive rather than specific. Reabsorbed pulmonary emboli from previous episodes may appear as irregular narrowings of vessels without the demonstration of the intraluminal filling defects. Normal pulmonary arteries down to the usual limits of the pulmonary arteriogram vessels of about 2–3 mm excludes recent pulmonary embolus.

Pulmonary emboli may be lysed rapidly by the local infusion of Streptokinase which may be necessary if the patient is in extremis as in massive pulmonary embolism. More usually the simple prevention of further pulmonary emboli by anticoagulant therapy is enough to save the patient's life and to promote the complete reabsorption of emboli. This takes place over a period of several weeks, and the subsequent pulmonary arteriogram may appear entirely normal (Figs 22.10B, 22.11B).

CHRONIC PULMONARY THROMBO-EMBOLISM

Established and irreversible pulmonary hypertension may develop as the result of continuing release of small emboli to the circulation. The patient presents with the clinical features of pulmonary hypertension and right heart failure though in the history there may be episodes of recurrent chest pain and haemoptysis and a history of deep vein thrombosis in the legs. This form of pulmonary embolism is characterized, commonly, by the presence of widespread small vessel disease in the lung and with associated localized obstructions of larger vessels.

The *plain film* will show the large main pulmonary artery which is usually seen in pulmonary hypertension and also enlargement of central vessels and peripheral pruning. This is of a patchy nature with some vessels remaining obviously enlarged and others small or absent and associated with hypertranslucent areas of the lungs (Fig. 22.16A).

The *isotope lung scan* will show widespread perfusion deficits with normal ventilation. *Cardiac catheterization* will reveal a pulmonary artery pressure which is markedly raised and may reach systemic levels, and *pulmonary angiography* shows several large vessels blocked proximally and with no distal perfusion of that segment of the lung, whereas other vessels are obviously enlarged and perfusing the remaining part of the lung. The disease may be so

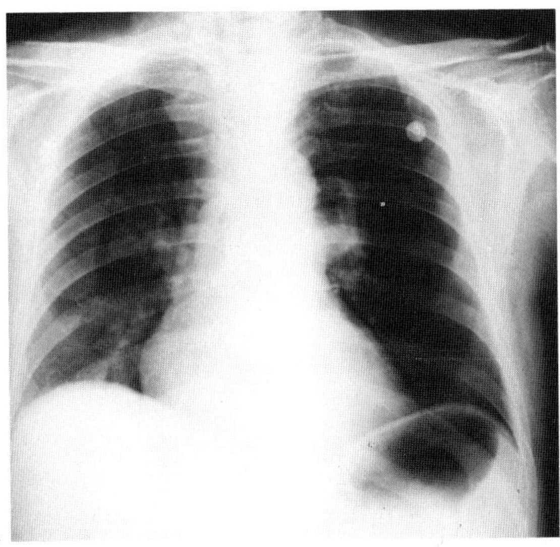

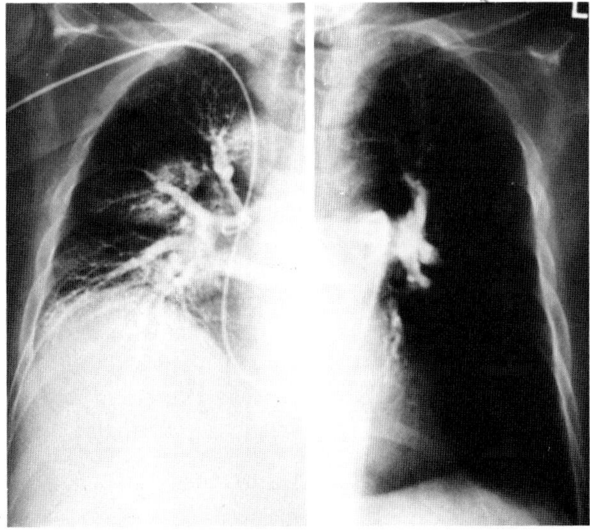

Fig. 22.16 Chronic pulmonary thrombo-embolism of the large vessel variety. (**A**) The frontal film shows a hypertransradiant left lung with areas of hypertransradiancy mixed with areas of increased perfusion in the right lung. (**B**) The pulmonary arteriogram of this patient shows obstructions of many of the large branches of the left pulmonary artery with irregularity, and rapid tapering of the arteries of the right lung, leading to patchy perfusion.

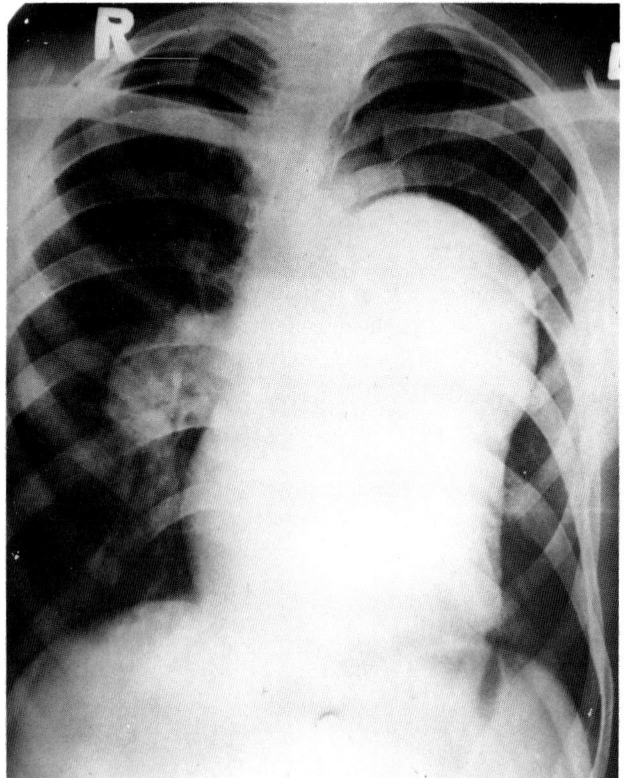

Fig. 22.17 Bilharzial pulmonary hypertension. Note the enormous enlargement of the main pulmonary artery. Some of the largest main pulmonary arteries are seen in this condition.

advanced that only one lobe of a lung appears to be adequately perfused (Fig. 22.16B).

Chronic pulmonary thrombo-embolism may also occur as a complication of *Bilharzia*. The plain film changes are often exceptionally gross with very extreme dilatation of the main and central pulmonary arteries and with marked pruning peripherally (Fig. 22.17).

Pulmonary hypertension may also result from *tumour emboli*, and the usual source is chorioncarcinoma.

FAT EMBOLISM

Fat embolism following major bone trauma may be associated with respiratory systems and a miliary or perihilar shadowing in the lungs. Fat globules may be seen in the sputum. However, the respiratory symptoms are more usually due to cerebral embolization occurring at the same time.

OTHER CAUSES OF PULMONARY ARTERIAL HYPERTENSION

Chronic bronchitis

Chronic bronchitis is defined as excessive sputum production associated with hypertrophy of the mucus glands of the bronchi. Acute infective exacerbations are extremely common. Superadded bronchospasm is also extremely frequent. In addition, infection of the abnormal bronchial mucosa leads to airways obstruction and in long-standing severe cases to hypercapnia and hypoxia with cyanosis, which in turn lead to a rise in pulmonary artery pressure and also to right heart failure with peripheral oedema, the so called 'blue bloater' type of patient.

Between acute attacks the plain film may look relatively normal, though the lungs are often overinflated. The heart appears small but the main and central pulmonary arteries often appear rather large. There may be evidence of emphysema with bullae and diaphragmatic adhesions and there may be scars of previous infections within the lung. In the acute phase the diaphragms rise and the lungs are no longer overdistended. The heart shadow increases in size and the main and central pulmonary arteries also enlarge. The increase in vessel size may occur out to the periphery of the lungs so that the appearances almost resemble those seen in a shunt. There may be fresh pulmonary consolidation. If the patient recovers these changes reverse and the appearances revert to those before the infection (Figs 22.18A and B).

Special investigations to make the diagnosis of chronic bronchitis are rarely indicated though its presence may complicate the interpretation of lung scans, if these have been performed to exclude pulmonary embolism. Perfusion deficits are common but they are usually associated with ventilation defects, and in experienced hands the exclusion of pulmonary embolism is not difficult.

Emphysema

Emphysema, the destruction of the terminal air spaces of the lung, often complicates chronic bronchitis but may occur alone. The usual pattern is of a dyspnoeic but not cyanosed patient, the so called 'pink puffer'. Rarely emphysema, especially when gross, may lead to hypercapnia and pulmonary hypertension and cor pulmonale.

Cystic fibrosis

With modern treatment many patients are surviving the inevitable severe respiratory infections to reach adolesence or beyond. In some of these patients characteristic cor pulmonale and pulmonary hypertension may develop with a large main and central pulmonary vessels against a background of overinflated lungs with the characteristic features of cystic fibrosis.

Other conditions

Pulmonary hypertension and right heart failure may be associated with *severe kyphoscoliosis* of the thoracic spine, particularly when it occurs in the high thoracic region. Hypercapnia and hypoxia may occur. The problem is primarily one of hypoventilation due to a combination of respiratory muscle difficulty and underdevelopment of

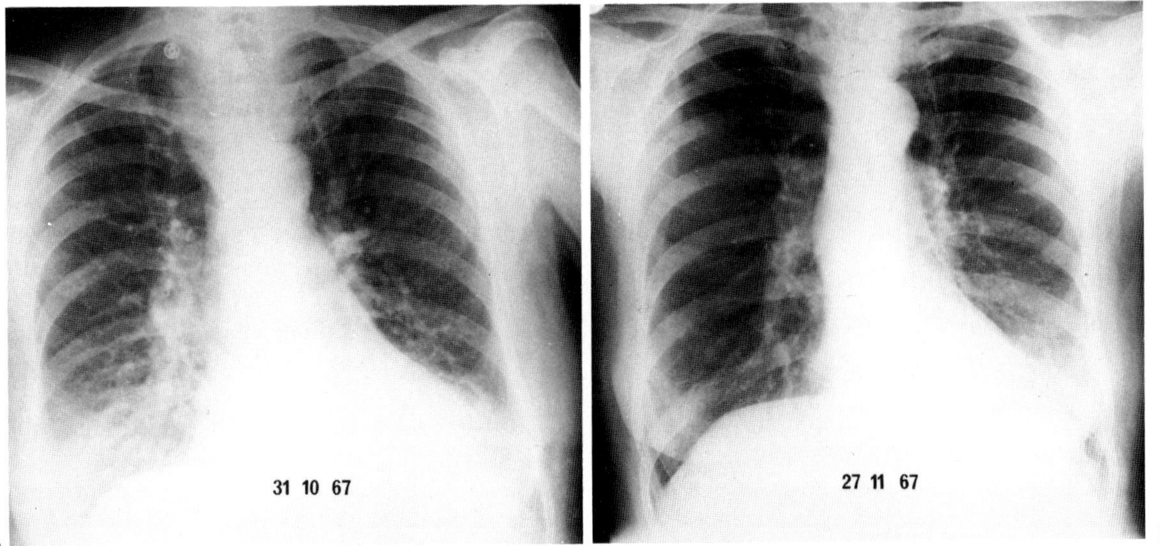

Fig. 22.18 Chronic obstructive airways disease with an acute exacerbation. (**A**) 13.10.67 — the heart is large and the pulmonary vessels increased in size and apparently in number, almost to resemble a shunt. (**B**) 27.11.67 — after resolution of the acute episode both the heart and the pulmonary vessels have reduced in size. Note however that the central vessels still remain quite large.

lung. In severe kyphoscoliosis the chest deformity is often so gross that no effective conclusions about the state of the lungs can be drawn from the usual plain films.

The *Pickwickian syndrome* consists of somnolence in an extremely obese patient. Polycythaemia is present and there may be right ventricular hypertrophy with right ventricular failure and associated pulmonary hypertension.

Ondine's curse is *idiopathic hypoventilation*. It occurs in young adult males and presents with lack of energy, somnolence, headache, shortness of breath on exertion and polycythaemia. The sufferers often stop breathing intermittently when they are asleep and this produces cyanosis. There may be pulmonary hypertension. The lungs are normal. A rather similar syndrome may occur in children with hypertrophy of the adenoids.

Pulmonary hypertension may also develop in patients who live at *high altitudes*.

CALCIFICATION OF PULMONARY ARTERIES

Calcification in pulmonary arteries can occur as a result of *atheroma* of the arterial wall, or in *thrombus* within arteries. Atheroma is almost always due to long sustained severe pulmonary hypertension and thus calcification may occur in the pulmonary arteries in those conditions in which this situation occurs. In addition the majority of cases of pulmonary artery thrombosis occur in conditions where pulmonary hypertension is a major manifestation and hence on many occasions pulmonary artery atheroma and thrombosis occur together. The characteristic appearance of pulmonary artery calcification is that of curvilinear calcifications, demonstrable by films of appropriate penetration, in the position of what are obviously enlarged central pulmonary arteries, and in addition there is peripheral pruning. Differentiation of pulmonary artery calcification, from the so-called 'egg shell calcification' of hilar glands is usually not in doubt.

PULMONARY ARTERY THROMBOSIS

Thrombosis of the main pulmonary artery or its branches is an uncommon complication of a variety of lung, heart and blood diseases. It may occur in association with parenchymal lung disease, with rheumatic or congenital heart disease, in association with sickle cell anaemia, polycythaemia, or even trauma to the lung. It may be found at post-mortem or demonstrated unsuspectedly by pulmonary angiography. There are no specific symptoms or signs, the occurrence being just part of the natural history of the underlying disease process. The **radiological appearances** depend on the extent of the thrombosis. Where a lobar or segmental artery alone is involved the plain chest X-ray will probably not reflect any change. Where a main pulmonary artery is entirely thrombosed the hilar shadow is thought to be dense and rather sharply defined, and slightly large. There will be marked reduction of the peripheral lung markings. It may be difficult to recognize these changes if the appearances of the lung are disorganized by the underlying precipitating disease.

The appearances at pulmonary angiography will vary according to the extent of the obstruction. Occlusion of a lobar or segmental vessel will be manifest by non-filling of this vessel, but without the classical leading edge of an embolus sign. Thrombosis of the main pulmonary artery will be revealed by a failure of any peripheral filling, and often by the demonstration of a filling defect within the main pulmonary artery, the thrombus itself. Again contrast medium will probably not trickle pass the intraluminal mass, pointing to this as an intrinsic thrombosis rather than an ill-fitting embolus.

ANEURYSMS OF THE PULMONARY ARTERIES

Dilatations of the pulmonary arteries are common in situations of altered pulmonary haemodynamics. They may occur in association with increased flow, as in atrial septal defect; with increased pulmonary artery pressure, as in long standing mitral valve disease; or when these factors are combined, particularly in patent ductus arteriosus. These dilatations may be visualized radiographically, but rarely exert a specific influence over the course of the underlying disease. *Aneurysms* of the pulmonary arteries, dilatations associated with abnormalities of the wall of the pulmonary artery, are rare. They may be due to syphilis, atheroma, mycotic embolization or other local disease of the arterial wall, or to trauma. These aneurysms may be asymptomatic, or may lead to recurrent chest pain and haemoptysis, presumably by peripheral embolization of the aneurysmal contents. It is this latter group of aneurysms which presents problems in differential diagnosis, because they are unilateral, and also have therapeutic implications.

Radiological appearances. In virtually all cases in which radiological examination of the chest has been performed, the aneurysm has been recognized as a rounded shadow in the hilum. It may grow to a large size, and be visible in the lateral view extending anterosuperiorly from the hilum. Curvilinear calcification may be demonstrated in its wall. Secondary lung abnormalities may be seen. In the cases where aneurysmal dilatation is associated with alterations of pulmonary haemodynamics due to heart disease, the pulmonary artery dilatations are commonly bilateral, and evidence of underlying cardiopulmonary abnormalities will usually be obvious. The chief differential diagnosis on plain film radiography is from a localized aortic aneurysm, which usually affects an older age group, and has a male sex preponderance. Bronchogenic carcinoma, or more rarely other lung or mediastinal masses, may also be considered in the differential diagnosis.

The diagnosis is confirmed by contrast examination. Any apparent increase in wall thickness is likely to be due to clot lining the aneurysm. Obstructions of peripheral arteries in relation to the aneurysms may be evidence of embolization. In the investigation of hilar mass by angiography it is important that filming should be carried on into the levophase so that if a mass fails to fill from the pulmonary artery it may be possible to determine its relationship to the opacified aorta.

SCIMITAR SYNDROME

The degree of haemodynamic abnormality associated with anomalous insertion of the pulmonary veins depends on the number of pulmonary veins which are abnormally draining, and the site into which they insert. Total anomalous pulmonary venous drainage usually presents as a cardiac emergency. The majority of forms of partial

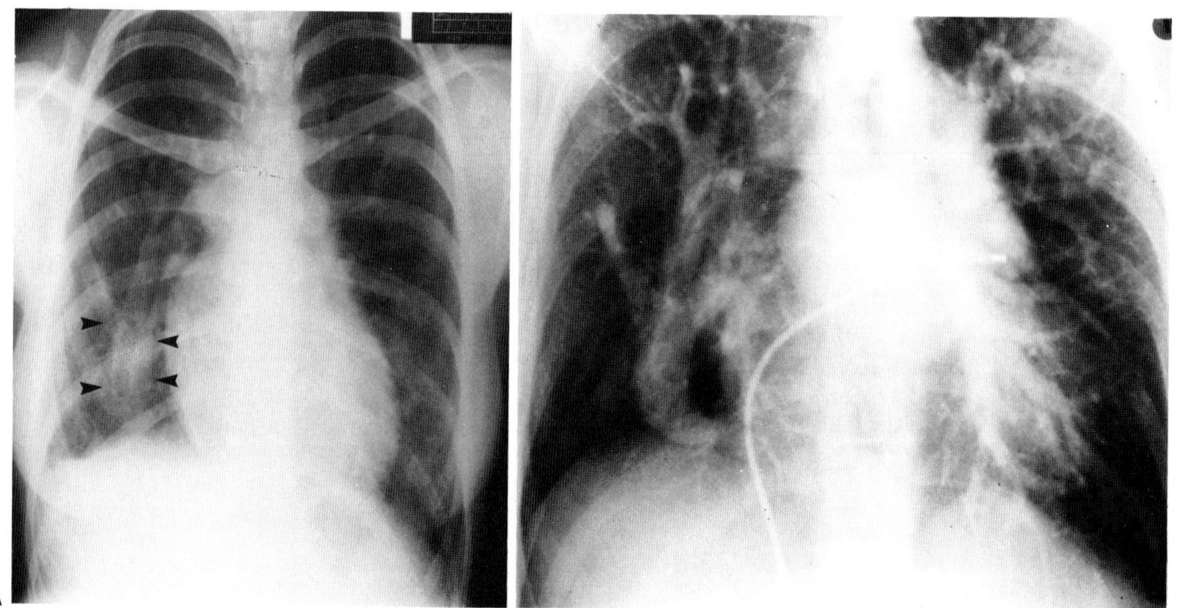

Fig. 22.19 Scimitar syndrome, the heart normally situated. (**A**) In the frontal film the scimitar is indicated by arrows. (**B**) It can be clearly identified in the levophase of the pulmonary angiogram. Almost the entire right lung drains anomalously to this vessel which is passing below the diaphragm.

anomalous venous drainage are associated with atrial septal defect and are considered in that section. The occurrence of an abnormal pulmonary vein draining the right lower lobe and inserting below the diaphragm, usually into the inferior vena cava, may occur in the absence of significant heart disease and may be considered separately. The condition may present with recurrent respiratory infection involving the right lower lobe of the lung and physical findings may reveal some crowding of the ribs of the right hemithorax and the presence of adventitial sounds in the right lung. The murmur of any associated *atrial septal defect* may also be heard as the condition commonly occurs in association with atrial septal defect.

Radiological appearances. The characteristic findings are those which give the syndrome the name; the abnormal pulmonary vein is visible as an inverted scimitar-shaped shadow of soft tissue density in the right lower zone terminating at or below the diaphragm. The shape is so characteristic that when seen the diagnosis of the nature of the abnormal shadow is rarely in doubt (Fig. 22.19). Where the right lower lobe is hypoplastic, as it may be when drained by an anomalous vein, and particularly when supplied by a systemic artery, the diagnosis may be complicated by displacement of the heart and mediastinal structures to the right, *dextroposition* of the heart. This may be so marked as to obscure the characteristic scimitar shadow unless good quality over-penetrated films are taken (Figs. 22.20, 22.21). The condition is not of course a true dextrocardia as the apex of the heart still remains pointing to the left. Scimitar syndrome is one of the several causes of dextroposition of the heart.

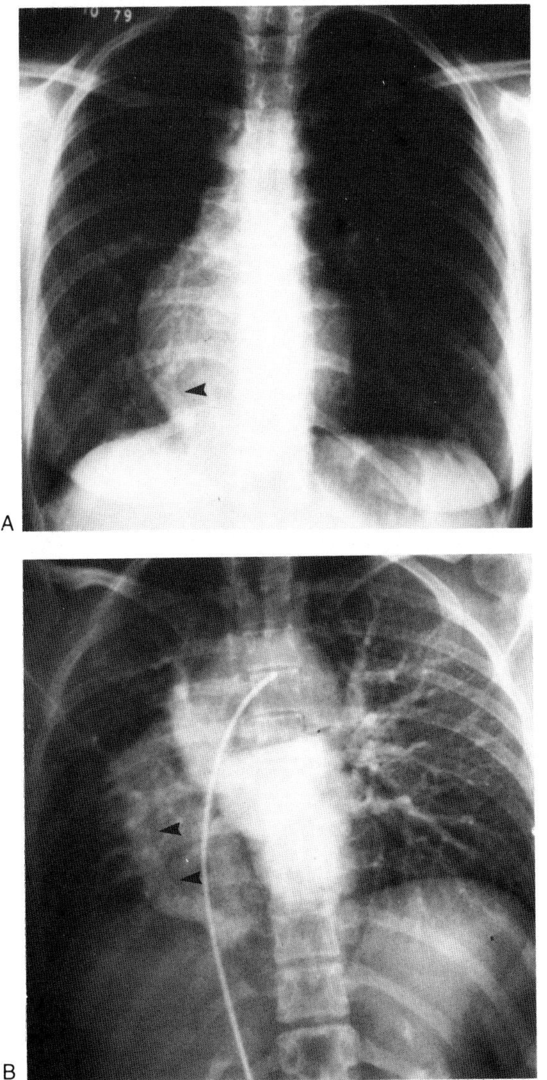

Fig. 22.20 Scimitar syndrome associated with dextroposition of the heart. (**A**) In the plain film the scimitar shadow (single arrow) is overlapped and largely concealed by the misplaced heart. (**B**) In the venous phase of the pulmonary angiogram, it can be clearly identified (paired arrows) passing below the diaphragm.

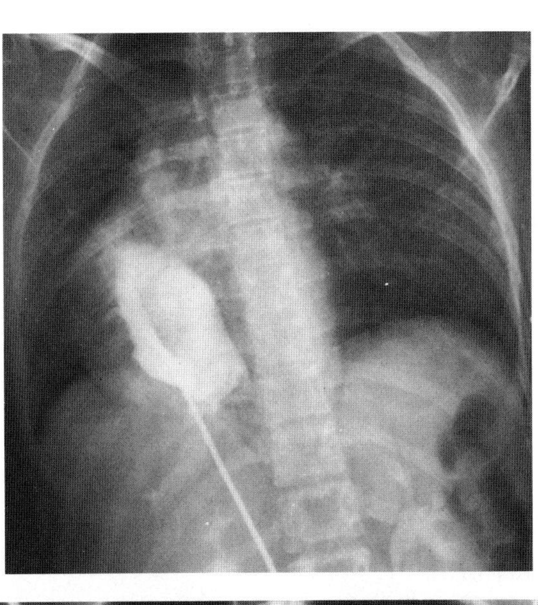

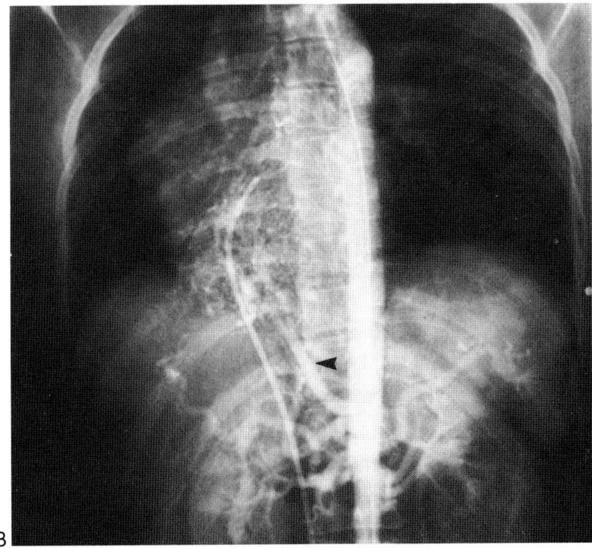

Fig. 22.21 Scimitar syndrome. (**A**) A venous catheter has been passed from the inferior vena cava into the abnormal vein. (**B**) Aortogram shows a systemic blood supply (arrow) ascending from the lumbar aorta through the diaphragm to supply part of the right lower lobe.

The appearances of the scimitar are pathognomonic. Investigation is only indicated to elucidate the presence of any associated intracardiac malformation or prior to surgery to determine which parts of the lung are drained by the abnormal vein, and how the arterial supply of the abnormal part of the lung is derived. For this reason the pre-operative assessment consists not only of selective pulmonary angiography filmed into the levophase to demonstrate the scimitar and its drainage, but also descending aortography to determine any element of systemic supply to the abnormal lung (Fig. 22.21B).

When the condition presents in the neonatal period it may lead to very severe symptoms and be difficult to treat.

RIGHT PULMONARY ARTERY — LEFT ATRIAL COMMUNICATION

This congenital malformation usually occurs as an isolated abnormality unassociated with other cardiac abnormalities. The communication is usually a saccular aneurysm of the descending branch of the right pulmonary artery which opens into the left atrium, though pulmonary venous abnormalities may also occur. Patients may present at any time from infancy to middle age. Symptoms are usually those of cyanosis and exertional dyspnoea. Emboli occur only rarely. About half of patients have rather non specific murmurs.

Over 75% of patients (Figs. 22.22, 22.23) have an abnormal density, visible at chest radiography and fluoroscopy, at the right heart border, below and behind

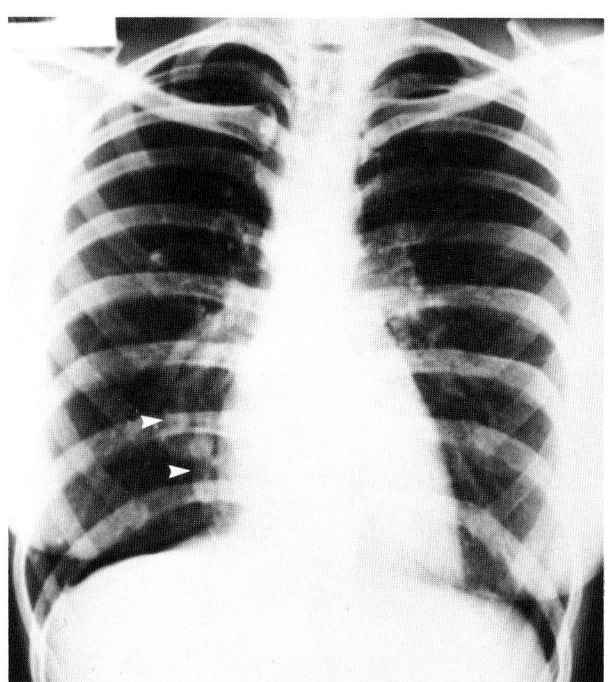

Fig. 22.22 Right pulmonary artery to left atrial communication. The white arrows indicate the abnormal density at the right heart border.

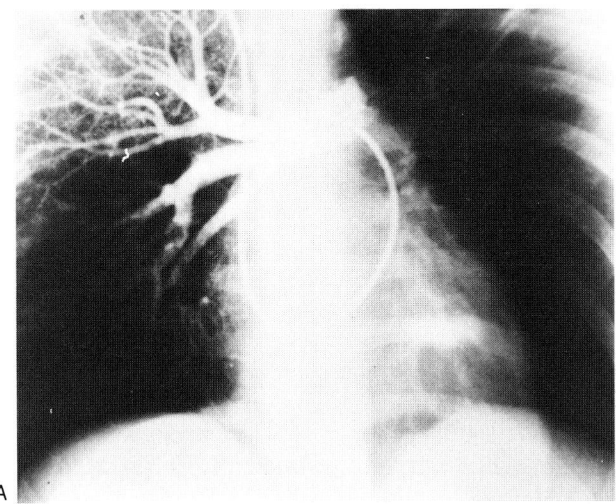

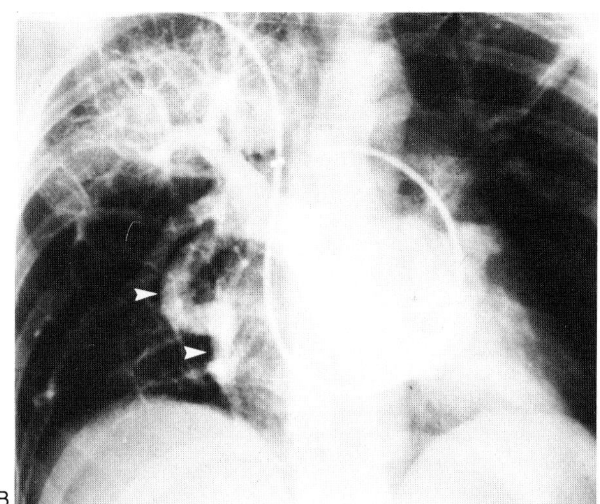

Fig. 22.23 (**A** and **B**) Right pulmonary artery to left atrial communication, pulmonary angiogram. In the venous phase the dilated right pulmonary artery (white arrows) has been opacified and is seen to be draining into the left atrium.

the right hilum, and this is the aneurysmal dilatation of the pulmonary artery. A cardiac catheter may be passed through the fistula to the left atrium. Pulmonary angiography will opacify the aneurysm and demonstrate its communication with the left atrium.

PULMONARY ARTERIO-VENOUS MALFORMATIONS

These are direct communications between the smaller pulmonary arteries and veins. The right to left shunt produced leads to dilatation of the terminations of these vessels. The lesions may be multiple, in one third of cases, and may show progressive enlargement. Also in one third of cases they are associated with telangiectasis elsewhere — Osler–Weber–Rendu disease.

The pulmonary lesions may be asymptomatic, or lead to dyspnoea or haemoptysis. The right to left shunt may be

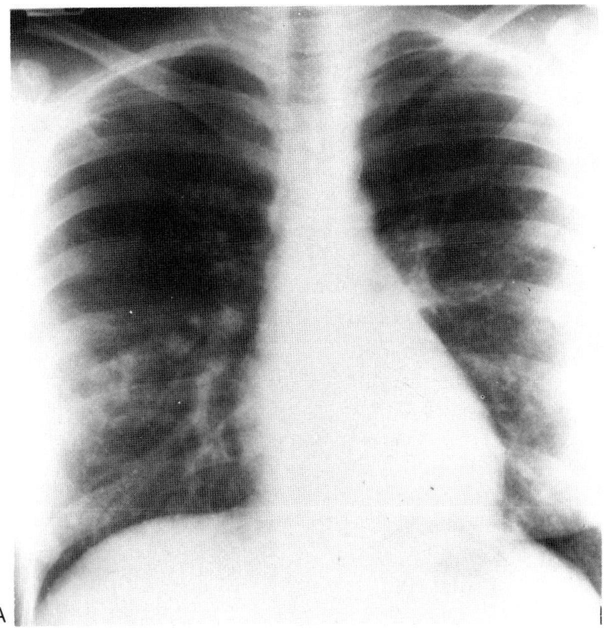

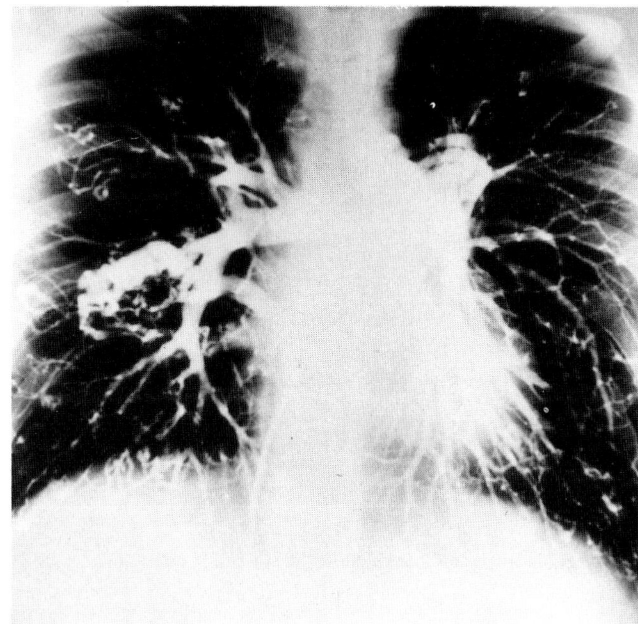

Fig. 22.24 Pulmonary arteriovenous malformations. (**A**) Frontal chest film. Abnormal pulmonary shadows, typically elongated, can be identified in the right mid zone. (**B**) Pulmonary arteriogram. The pulmonary arteriovenous malformations in the right mid zone, associated with premature venous filling, can be identified. Additional abnormal pulmonary vessels are clearly visible in the right upper zone and throughout the left lung.

complicated by polycythaemia, cyanosis and cerebral abscess. These may worsen as the lesions increase in size.

Radiological appearances. If the lesions are large and have led to dilatation of the peripheral pulmonary artery and vein a soft tissue density will be seen (Fig. 22.24A) which may change size if studied fluoroscopically during extremes of respiration. *Tomography* should be done to confirm the vascular nature of the lesion by demonstrating the supplying vessels, and reveal other small lesions not suspected on the standard chest X-ray.

The definitive investigation is *pulmonary angiography*, which is claimed to be both easy and helpful in this condition, as the high flow through the lesions aids in the opacification. It demonstrates enlargement of feeding arteries and draining veins and the direct connection between the two (Fig. 22.24B). There is no enlargement of the main pulmonary artery in uncomplicated arteriovenous malformations. Investigation should be performed if the condition is suspected prior to surgery, as if its nature is known, only a limited resection is required; also unsuspected lesions may be demonstrated.

PULMONARY VARIX

Localized dilatations of the pulmonary veins may occur with acquired or congenital heart disease, or may occur in asymptomatic patients, unassociated with cardiac abnormality. They are usually recognized as rounded or lobulated shadows often near the hila, on the chest X-ray,

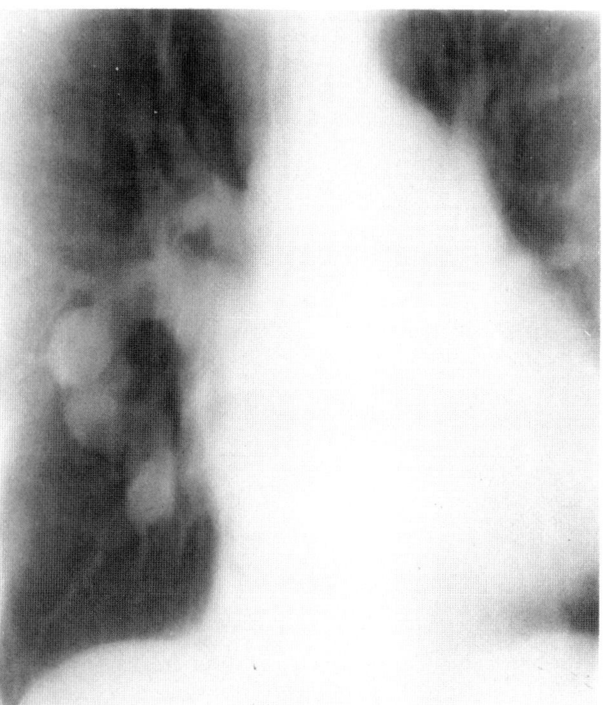

Fig. 22.25 Pulmonary varix. The AP tomogram shows the multiple rounded densities associated with the pulmonary veins which are typical of pulmonary varices. The venous nature of these was confirmed by angiography.

and which may be taken for some unrelated cause. Some may be seen to change size with respiration on *fluoroscopy*. *Tomography* may demonstrate the draining vein (Fig. 22.25), thus suggesting the diagnosis. Confirmation of the nature of the abnormal shadow is obtained by selective *pulmonary angiography*. The shadows show delayed filling with contrast after pulmonary artery injection and impaired drainage of the isolated vein. The appearances differ angiographically from those of arteriovenous malformation which shows early shunting and enlarged drainage veins. The difference is due to the by-passing of the capillary bed in arteriovenous malformations.

REFERENCES AND SUGGESTIONS FOR FURTHER READING

Fazio, F., Lavender, P. & Steiner, R. E. (1978) Krypton 81m ventilation and $^{99}Tc^{m}$ perfusion scans in chest disease. *American Journal of Radiology*, **130**, 421–428.

Grossman, Z. D., et al (1984) Digital subtraction angiography of the pulmonary arteries for the diagnosis of pulmonary embolism. *Radiology*, **150**, 843–844.

Harris, P. & Heath, D. (1978) *The Human Pulmonary Circulation*. Edinburgh and London: Churchill Livingstone.

Jefferson, K. & Rees, S. (1980) *Clinical Cardiac Radiology*, 2nd edn. London: Butterworths.

Raphael, M. J. (1970) Pulmonary angiography. *British Journal of Hospital Medicine*, 377–390.

Rees, S. (1981) Arterial connection of the lung. *Clinical Radiology*.

CHAPTER 23

ACQUIRED HEART DISEASE

VALVULAR HEART DISEASE

RHEUMATIC FEVER

This condition, now decreasing in incidence in the West, but still a major problem in developing countries, results from an abnormal response to group A streptococcal infection. The major clinical feature, flitting pains in the large joints, comes on about two to three weeks after a sore throat. There is no radiological evidence of joint destruction. Clinical evidence of carditis may be present and there may be radiological cardiomegaly, due either to carditis or to pericardial effusion. The acute phase usually regresses to an asymptomatic or quiescent phase lasting for many years, as chronic valve damage develops. The mitral is the commonest valve to be affected, followed by the aortic and then tricuspid valves. A history of rheumatic fever can be elicited in about half the patients with rheumatic valve disease. A similar valve disease may be seen after chorea.

MITRAL VALVE DISEASE

Mitral stenosis

Much the commonest cause of obstruction at the mitral valve is rheumatic fever. Stenosis develops by fusion of the leaflet commissures, thickening of the valve leaflets and shortening and thickening and adherence of the chordae tendineae, all of which restrict valve opening. Until the orifice is critically narrowed symptoms are few, then shortness of breath on exertion develops. Overt cardiac failure may not appear until the onset of atrial fibrillation. The clinical diagnosis is usually obvious, once the characteristic apical diastolic murmur is heard; however, a similar murmur may be heard in torrential aortic incompetence (the Austin–Flint murmur), in atrial septal defect (the patient, if elderly, may be in atrial fibrillation) and in other forms of mitral obstruction (left atrial myxoma, and congenital obstructions). The murmur may be inaudible in low output states or with tachycardia.

Radiographic appearances. The plain film signs are those of *selective left atrial enlargement*, which may vary from trivial to gross (Figs 23.1 and 23.2). Enlargement of the left atrial appendage is almost universally present as part of the left atrial enlargement and always suggests rheumatic mitral disease (as opposed to non-rheumatic). This enlargement may vary from a simple straightening of the left heart border to a very gross local protrusion (Fig. 23.3).

Mitral valve calcification indicates long-standing and usually severe mitral valve disease (Fig. 23.4). It is not commonly seen on the plain film. It is best seen in the lateral view between the left atrium and the left ventricle and is more rarely seen in the frontal view on an adequately penetrated film, in the position of the mitral valve. Image amplification fluroscopy is much the best way

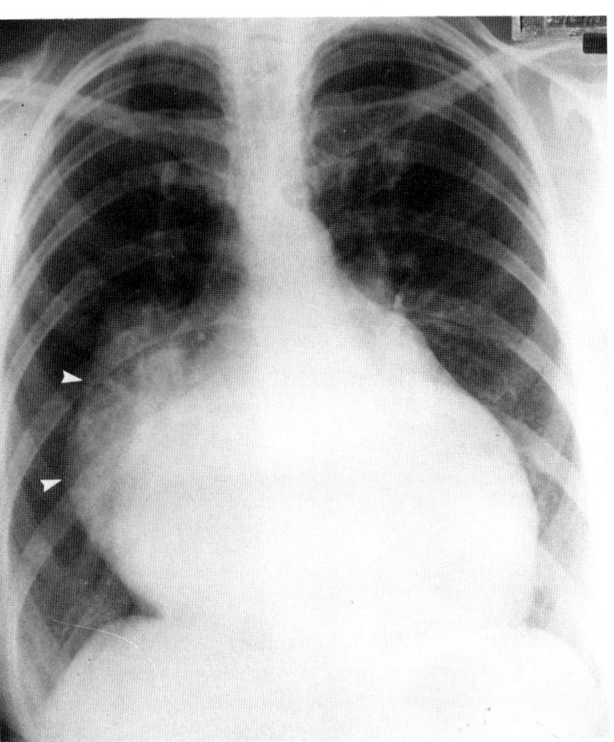

Fig. 23.1 Left atrial dilatation in mitral stenosis. The enlarged left atrium (arrows) extends beyond the right heart border. Note that the border of the right atrium can be identified where it is joined by the inferior vena cava coming up through the diaphragm.

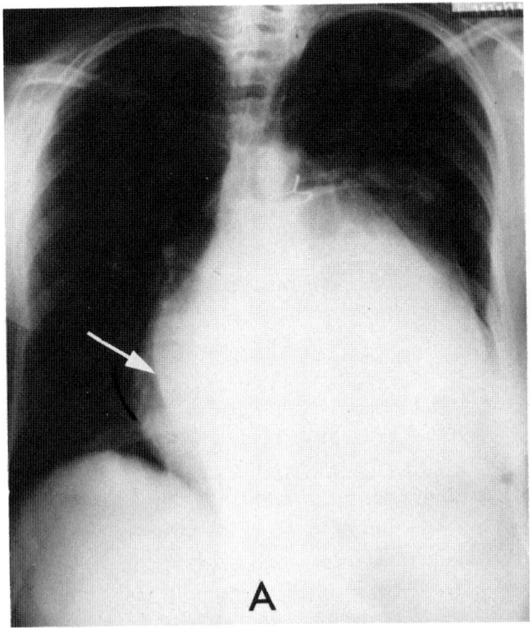

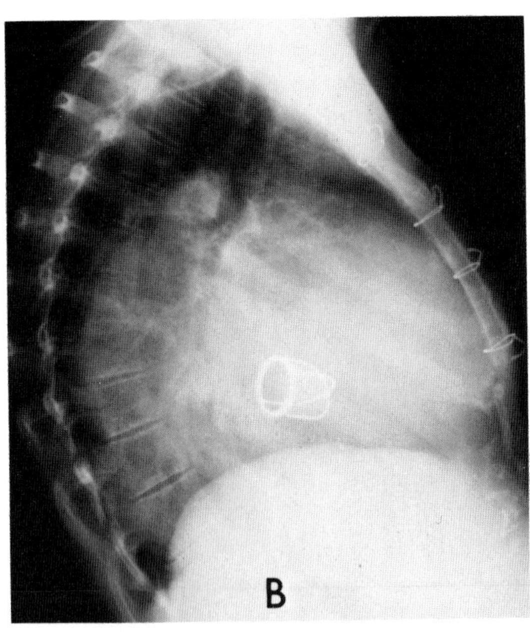

Fig. 23.2 Gross left atrial enlargement in association with a prosthetic mitral valve. (**A**) Frontal view. The double shadow of the left atrium, seen to the right of the spine, is indicated by an arrow. Note that the left atrium has so lifted up the left bronchus that it now goes upwards. (**B**) Lateral view. The prosthetic valve is more clearly seen. Again the left bronchus goes upwards. The right bronchus can also be seen in its normal position.

of detecting such calcification, locating it to the mitral valve, and identifying its movement towards the apex of the heart in diastole. It must be distinguished from the characteristically 'C' or 'J' shaped calcification which may occur in the mitral valve ring in the elderly. This may also be associated with a murmur but is of little haemodynamic importance (Fig. 23.5).

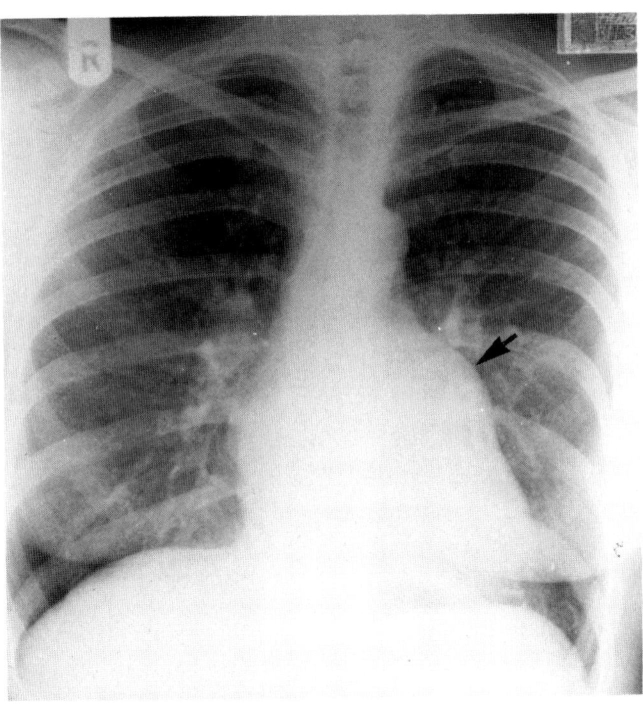

Fig. 23.3 Rheumatic mitral stenosis. This frontal film shows marked enlargement of the left atrial appendage (arrow).

Calcification may occur in the left atrium in longstanding mitral valve disease with atrial fibrillation (Fig. 23.6).

Marked *changes in the pulmonary circulation* resulting from the chronically raised left atrial pressure may be present (Ch. 22). Upper lobe blood diversion is seen in its most florid form, and is brought into prominence by lower lobe vascular constriction. Enlarged main and central pulmonary arteries and peripheral pruning indicate pulmonary arterial hypertension. Long-standing interstitial oedema with acute alveolar pulmonary oedema may be seen. *Haemosiderosis* and *ossific nodules* are mainly seen in rheumatic valve disease.

A very large or aneurysmal left atrium (one which reaches to within an inch of the chest wall) may be associated with segmental or lobar collapse from bronchial compression usually on the right (Fig. 23.7). The consolidation of pulmonary infarction may occur. Tracheobronchial calcification is also common in rheumatic mitral valve disease.

M mode echocardiography is reliable in documenting the presence of rheumatic mitral valve stenosis. The characteristic M mode echogram feature of rheumatic mitral stenosis (Fig. 23.8) is the reduced diastolic closure rate of the anterior mitral leaflet, which is held forward throughout diastole by the pressure gradient between left atrium and left ventricle. The abnormal movement of the posterior mitral cusp, which appears to move forward in parallel with the anterior one, is caused by the commissural fibrosis which retards the leaflet separation. Multiple intense

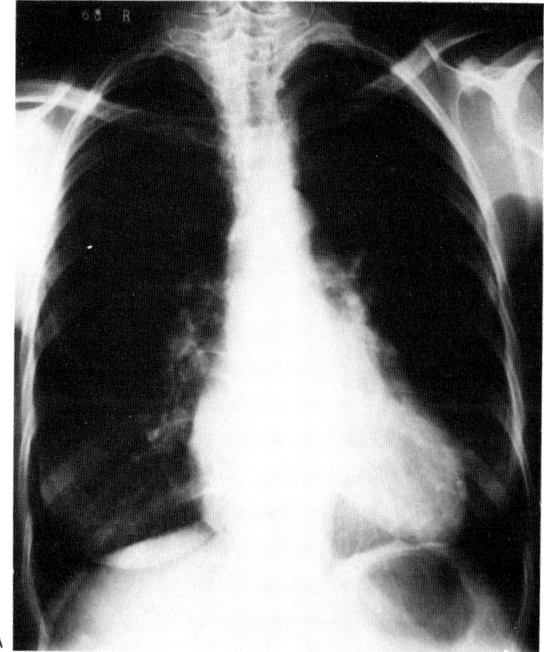

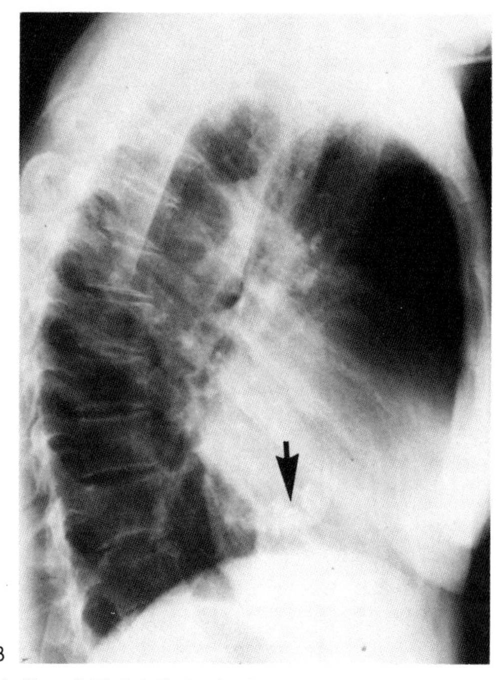

Fig. 23.4 (**A** and **B**) Calcified mitral valve in rheumatic mitral stenosis. The calcification is best seen in the lateral view (arrow).

echoes from the leaflet indicate fibrosis and/or calcification.

The distinctive motion of the *2DE* image of the leaflets is due to tethering of the leaflets by chordal and commissural fusion (Fig. 23.9). The presence of left atrial thrombus (Fig. 23.10) can also be documented.

Rheumatic mitral incompetence

Rheumatic mitral incompetence results from destruction of cusp tissue, mainly at the free edges, so that these do

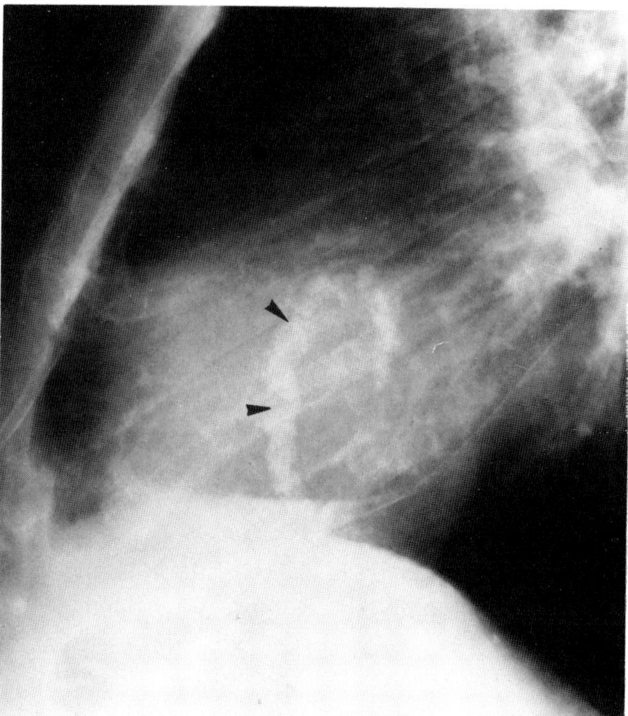

Fig. 23.5 Calcification in the mitral ring. In this lateral view the calcified mitral valve ring (arrows) appears as a characteristic C shape. It may take a J shape.

not meet and seal off the orifice, and also shortening of the chordae which holds the valve in the open position. The clinical presentation is with shortness of breath and the hallmark of the condition is the apical pan-systolic murmur radiating to the axilla. Symptoms may be precipitated by the development of atrial fibrillation. The murmur may be confused with that of non-rheumatic mitral incompetence or ventricular septal defect. When there is a murmur of associated mitral stenosis, or additional aortic valve disease, and a history of rheumatic fever, the diagnosis is obvious. Many patients have been diagnosed as having rheumatic fever when a murmur is first heard in childhood following an atypical febrile illness, and may turn out to have congenital heart disease.

The commonest result of rheumatic mitral valve disease is a valve which is both stenosed and incompetent, failing to open properly in diastole, and failing to adequately seal the mitral orifice in systole. The valve cannot be both severely stenosed and severely incompetent as stenosis limits the degree of incompetence that can develop.

Radiographic appearances. The plain film findings resemble those of mitral stenosis though the heart and particularly the left atrium is in general larger, and the left atrium may be very large or aneurysmal in mitral incompetence. It is not usually possible to identify specifically associated left ventricular enlargement due to mitral incompetence. If present, left ventricular enlargement is usually

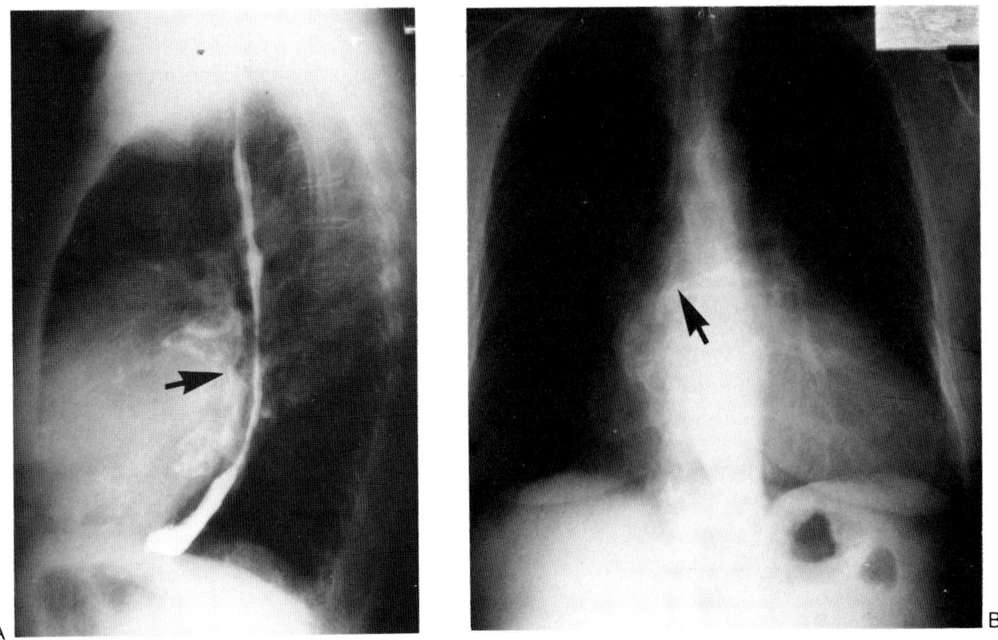

Fig. 23.6 (**A** and **B**) Calcified left atrium in chronic rheumatic mitral valve disease. In both lateral and frontal views curvilinear calcification (arrow) is identified in the position of the wall of the left atrium.

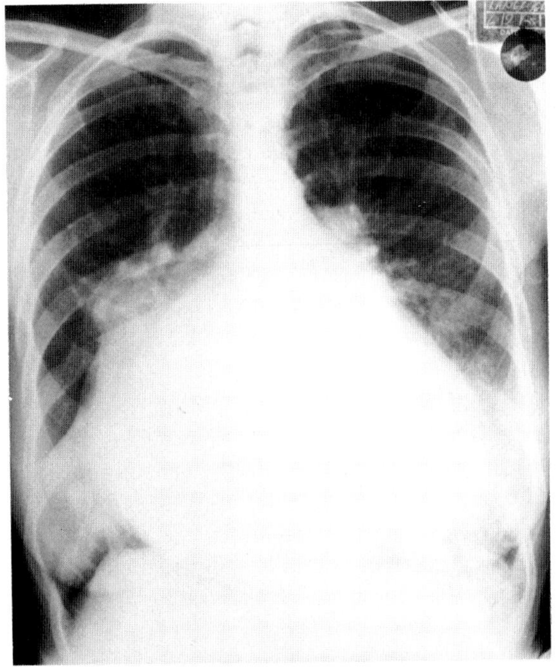

Fig. 23.7 Lobar collapse in association with left atrial enlargement. In this patient with a very large left atrium there is segmental collapse of the middle and part of the lower lobe on the right, due to bronchial compression.

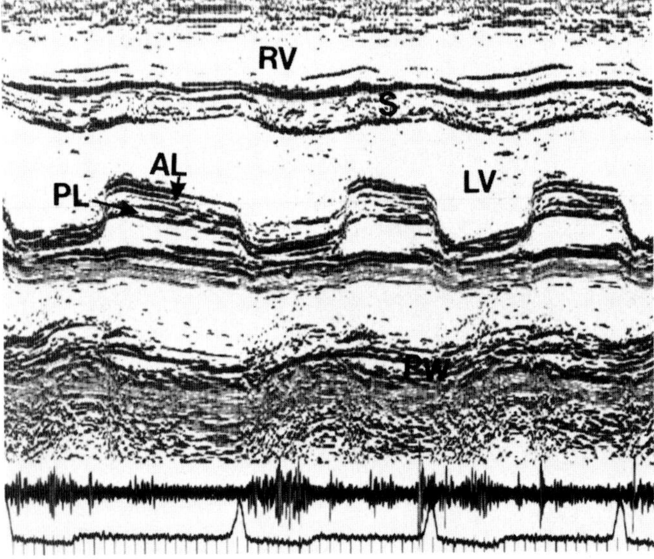

Fig. 23.8 Rheumatic mitral stenosis. The M-mode echocardiogram shows the characteristic features of this condition: the diastolic closure rate of the anterior mitral valve leaflet (AL) is reduced and the posterior leaflet (PL) moves forward in parallel with the anterior leaflet, due to commissural fibrosis which impedes leaflet separation. RV = right ventricle; LV = left ventricle; PW = posterior wall of the left ventricle.

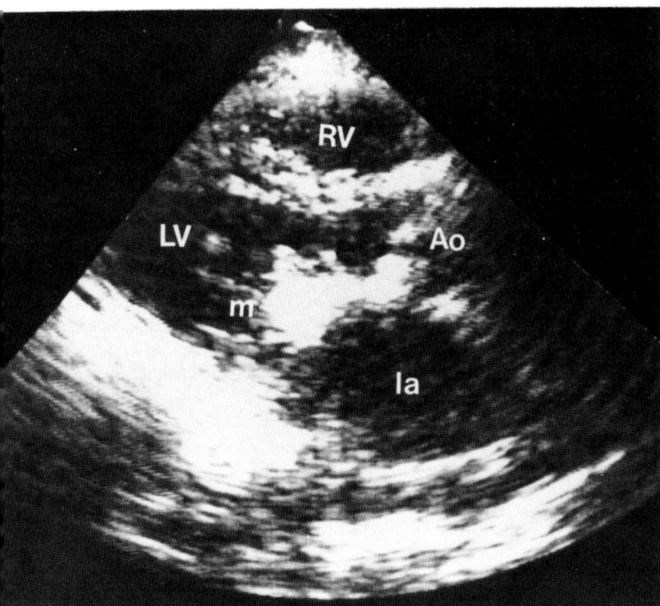

Fig. 23.9 Rheumatic mitral stenosis. The 2DE shows marked fibrosis and tethering of the mitral (m) leaflets due to chordal and commissural fusion. Ao = aorta; la = left atrium. Other lettering as in Figure 20.1.

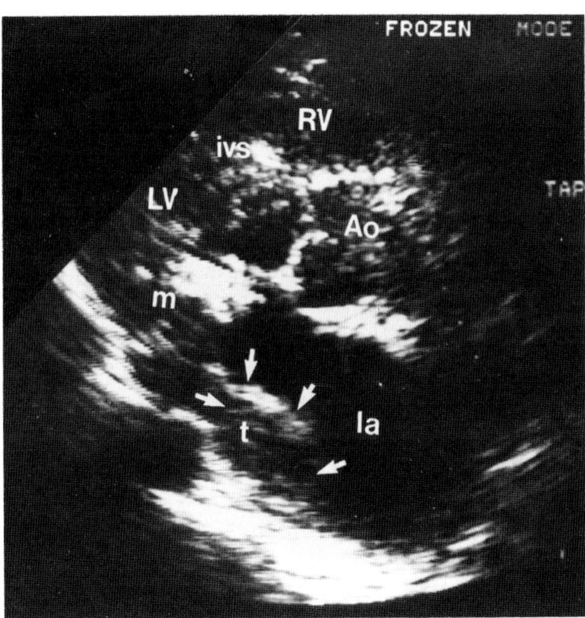

Fig. 23.10 Mitral stenosis. The 2DE demonstrates a large left atrial (la) cavity and the presence of atrial thrombosis (arrows). There is fibrosis and calcification of the mitral leaflets. ivs = interventricular septum. Other lettering as in Figure 20.1.

due to aortic valve disease. It is not possible to diagnose mitral incompetence by fluoroscopic demonstration of systolic expansion of the left atrium.

The *echocardiographic* assessment of mitral incompetence consists mainly in determining its aetiology. The severity of the regurgitation cannot be assessed by the appearances of the valve itself. Other features such as the extent of left atrial enlargement or exaggerated movement of the left ventricular walls may provide pointers to the severity of the valvular leak. Mitral regurgitation caused by chronic rheumatic carditis is usually associated with thickened, deformed and often calcified cusps (Fig. 23.9).

Non-rheumatic mitral incompetence

Two patterns of abnormality are commonly seen. In the commoner variety, *mucoid degeneration of the valve leaflets* allows redundant valve tissue to balloon into the left atrium in systole, and the same process may lead to elongation of the chordae. The ballooning of the valve produces an audible systolic click, and if chordal elongation is severe enough to impair apposition of the leaflets, mitral incompetence results.

Chordal rupture may also precipitate mitral incompetence by producing a flail leaflet (or part of a leaflet) so that apposition fails. This condition often progresses jerkily with groups of chordae rupturing and producing mitral incompetence, followed by compensatory left ventricular dilatation and then another episode of rupture.

Both types of mitral involvement may lead to cardiac failure which may be steadily or intermittently progressive, and may lead to death. There is a characteristic mid or late onset systolic murmur which may be initiated by a click. Atrial fibrillation is rarer than in rheumatic carditis. The differential diagnosis includes other causes of a late systolic murmur combined with left ventricular hypertrophy on the ECG, i.e. aortic stenosis and hypertrophic cardiomyopathy. Mitral incompetence in the course of ischaemic heart disease is considered below.

Radiographic appearances. The plain film appearances are very different from those in rheumatic mitral incompetence. In the acute phase the heart may be virtually normal in size and shape even in the presence of pulmonary oedema or other evidence of a high left atrial pressure (Fig. 23.11). If the patient survives to enter the chronic phase the heart enlarges with a left ventricular configuration. Left atrial enlargement is slight and the left atrial appendage is very rarely enlarged. Calcification does not occur. In the prolapsed mitral valve associated with the Marfan syndrome aortic root dilatation may be present.

Rarer causes of non-rheumatic mitral incompetence are those associated with a left atrial myxoma damaging the mitral valve, with bacterial endocarditis involving the mitral valve, with cardiac trauma damaging the mitral valve, with ischaemic heart disease involving the papillary muscles and with cardiomyopathy leading to mitral incompetence. Congenital causes are dealt with in Chapter 26.

Ultrasound is very useful in the diagnosis. The M mode echogram may show prolapse of the posterior mitral valve leaflet, or may recognize aortic stenosis or hypertrophic

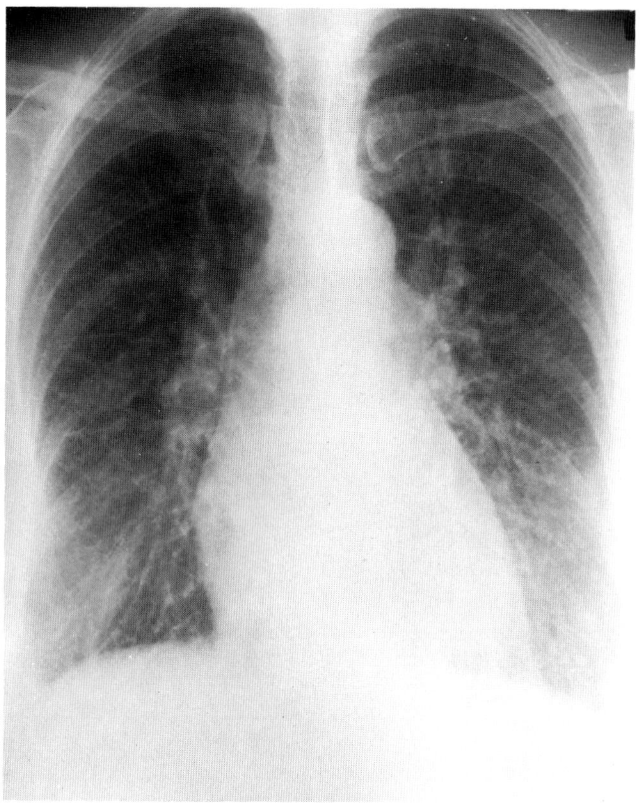

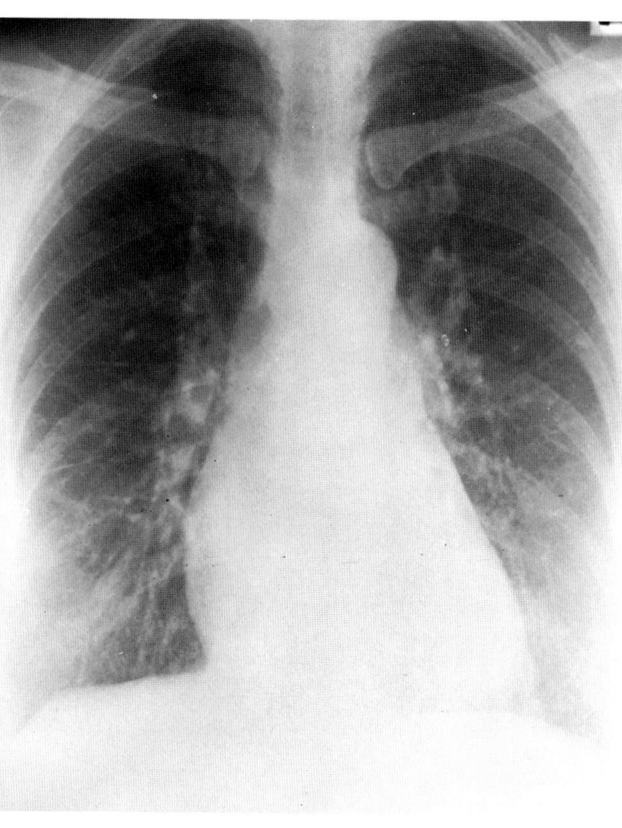

Fig. 23.11 Acute non-rheumatic mitral regurgitation. (**A**) Frontal view in the acute phase. The heart size is virtually normal, even in the presence of high left atrial pressure as evidenced by the preferential dilatation of the upper lobe vessels and interstitial oedema. (**B**) Frontal film 2 weeks later. This shows clearing of the oedema though upper lobe blood diversion can still be seen.

cardiomyopathy. It will also show the function of the left ventricle. 2DE is much more accurate in diagnosis, showing virtually all cases of prolapse of the mitral valve leaflet and also a flail mitral leaflet associated with chordal rupture. The essential feature is that the anterior and posterior leaflets do not appose properly in systole, usually because one or other has prolapsed back into the left atrium. These features are best observed by 2DE, which permits documentation of the striking bowing of the leaflets into the atrium (Fig. 23.12).

Cardiac catheterization and angiocardiography. Investigation is indicated for the diagnosis in those rare cases where it is in doubt, even after echocardiography.

Severity. Catheterization and angiocardiography are better able to assess the severity of the valve lesion than echocardiography. When severity is in doubt, or with associated lung disease as a possible cause of dyspnoea, and specially when more than one valve is abnormal, haemodynamic and angiographic investigation may be indicated. Additionally, they may help when it is not clear whether valve disease or impaired left ventricular function is the cause of the patient's symptoms, particularly after valve replacement.

Associated coronary artery disease. Coronary arteriography is routinely performed before surgery in patients with chest pain, ischaemic changes on the ECG, or when they are aged over 55. The severity of mitral valve obstruction is assessed by measuring the gradient across the mitral valve

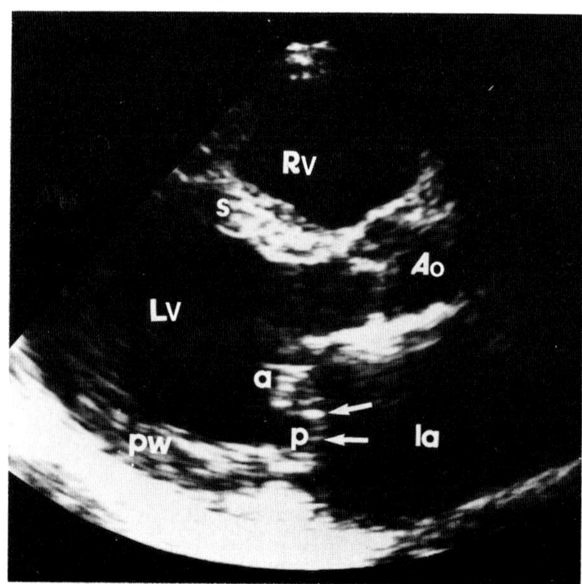

Fig. 23.12 Mitral valve prolapse. The 2DE shows striking bowing of the posterior (p) mitral leaflet into the left atrium (la) (arrows). Lettering as in Figure 20.1.

between simultaneously recorded indirect left atrial (wedged) pressure (or direct left atrial pressure recorded by transeptal catheter) and the left ventricular pressure obtained by retrograde catheterisation of the left ventricle across the aortic valve. The flow across the valve must also be measured by determining the cardiac output. If the gradient is low at rest, in patients clinically suspected of having significant mitral obstruction, it is usual to increase the cardiac output by exercise and check the gradient again.

Mitral incompetence is assessed by **cine left ventriculography** in the right anterior oblique projection. This projection brings the mitral valve into profile, and separates the left ventricle from left atrium. The severity of mitral regurgitation is estimated by the rapidity with which contrast passes across the mitral valve from left ventricle to left atrium to opacify the left atrium. Rapid passage of large quantities of contrast indicate that regurgitation is severe. In non-rheumatic mitral incompetence this feature can be misleading as the atrium is commonly small and opacifies rapidly with only slight regurgitation. In this situation pulmonary artery and left atrial pressures, if normal, suggest that regurgitation is not severe. The angiographic appearances of the mitral valve are of interest but rarely of significance. The normal mitral valve is flung widely open in diastole allowing an ill-defined broad front of non-opaque blood to enter the opacified left ventricle. If the valve is stenosed it is outlined by opaque blood on its ventricular aspect and non-opaque blood on its atrial aspect producing a domed valve if examined in profile (Fig. 23.13) or appearing as a filling defect under the aortic valve if seen *en face*.

The regurgitation of rheumatic mitral disease usually appears as one or more discrete jets of contrast passing through the mitral valve directly back into the left atrium (Fig. 23.14). Non-rheumatic mitral regurgitation appears

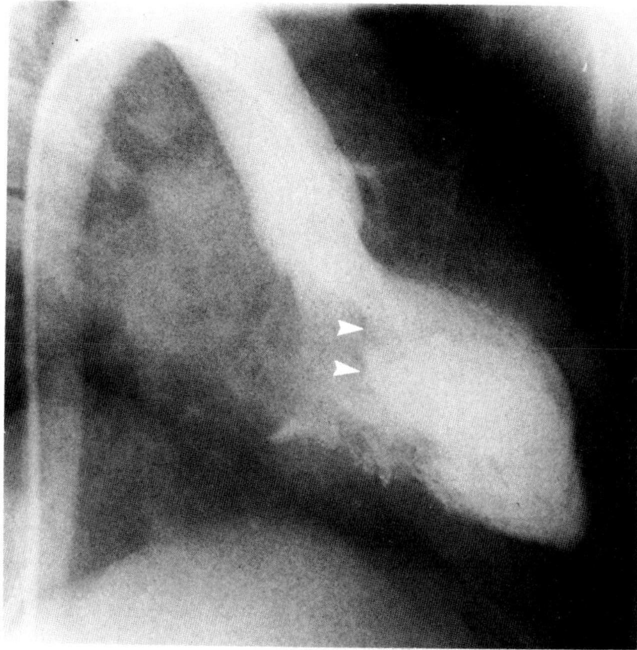

A

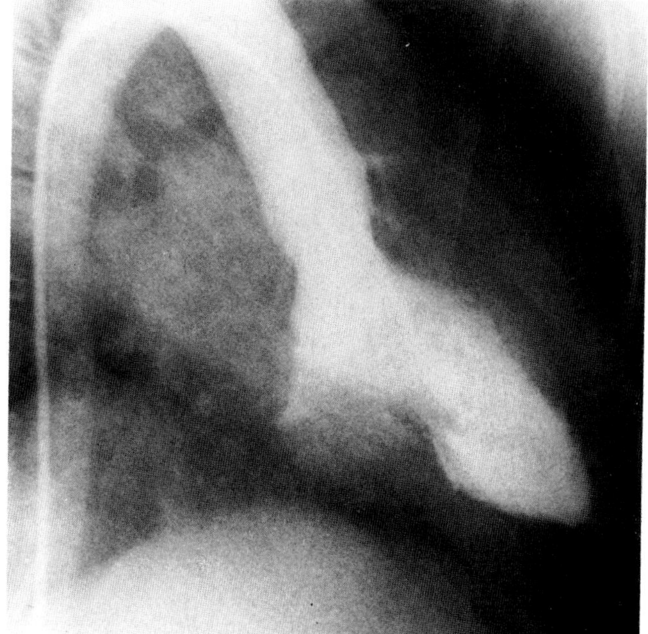

B

Fig. 23.13 Left ventriculography in mitral stenosis. (**A**) Right anterior oblique diastole. (**B**) Right anterior oblique systole. The mitral valve has closed normally in B. In A the stenosed valve is outlined by non-opaque blood on its atrial side so that it domes (arrows) into the ventricle in diastole.

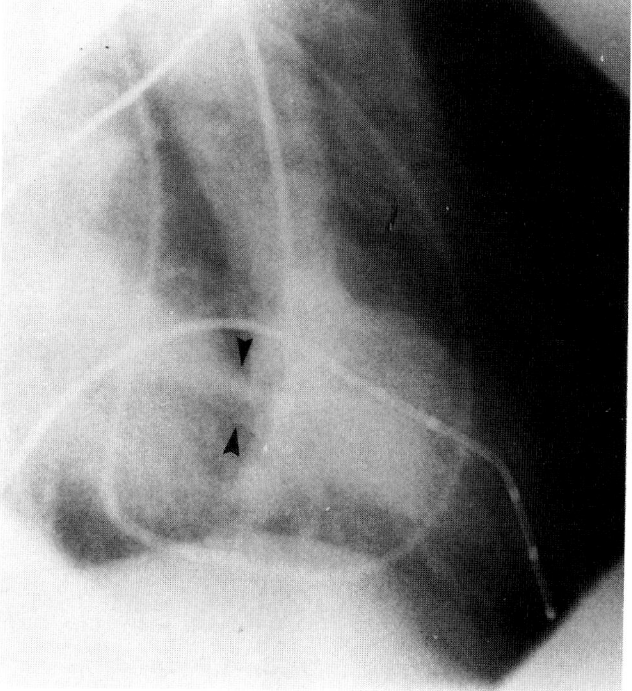

Fig. 23.14 Rheumatic mitral regurgitation. Left ventriculography in the RAO projection, systole. A discrete jet of mitral regurgitation (arrowed) passes through the closed mitral valve into the left atrium.

as a jet of contrast escaping under the flail edge of the mitral valve passing in a circular fashion around the wall of the left atrium.

A prolapsing mitral valve can be seen to balloon backwards into the left atrium during ventricular systole but it must be distinguished from the various crevices which appear in the left ventricle in the mitral valve area, by the fact that it must disappear entirely in ventricular diastole. When regurgitation occurs with a prolapsing valve, the prolapse may be demonstrated as developing in ventricular systole by angiography and the regurgitation may be seen to start only when prolapse has fully developed (Fig. 23.15). Thus angiography demonstrates that the prolapse itself is responsible for the click and the late onset of mitral incompetence. This explains the mid or late systolic onset of the systolic murmur which characterizes the condition.

Left ventricular function may be assessed from the cine left ventriculogram by the size of the ventricle and the degree of emptying that occurs with each beat, although in the presence of atrial fibrillation assessment may be difficult.

Coronary arteriography (see p. 597) will exclude or demonstrate associated atheromatous coronary artery disease. It may also demonstrate blood vessel formation in left atrial thrombus which is a not uncommon finding when it is performed for the investigation of long-standing rheumatic heart disease.

TRICUSPID VALVE DISEASE

This most commonly occurs late in the course of *rheumatic heart disease*. Tricuspid stenosis or tricuspid incompetence may be due to involvement of the valve by the rheumatic process, or triscuspid incompetence may be *functional*. Tricuspid disease may be suspected clinically when the jugular venous pressure is raised and its form abnormal, and

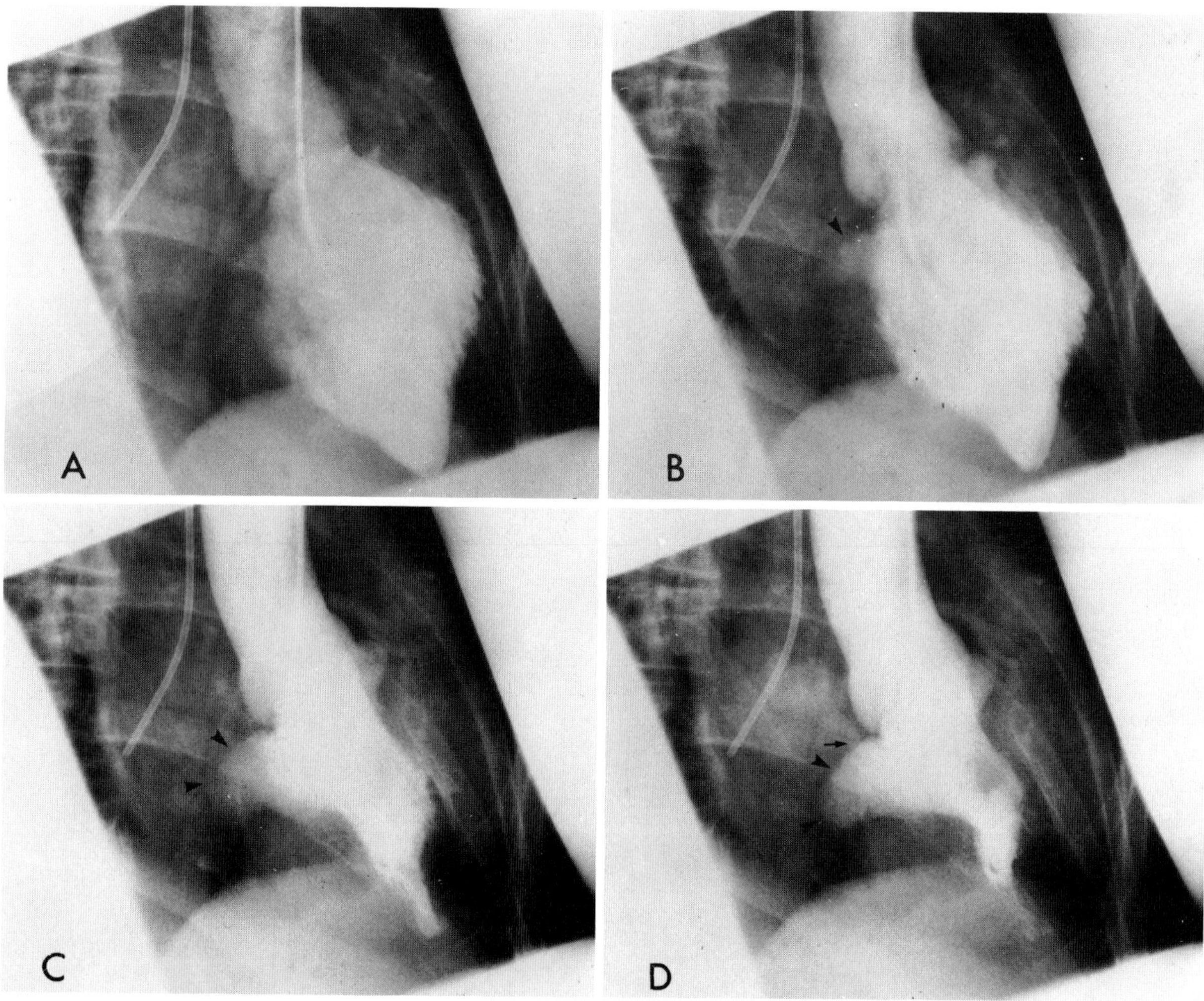

Fig. 23.15 Non-rheumatic mitral regurgitation due to prolapse of the mitral valve. Cine left ventriculography in the RAO protection. Frames (**A**), (**B**), (**C**) and (**D**) show progressive contraction from diastole in (**A**), to systole in (**D**). In (**A**) there is no evidence of prolapse of the mitral valve. As systole progresses prolapse of the posterior leaflet develops (arrowheads) and in (**D**) a small jet (arrow) of mitral regurgitation develops.

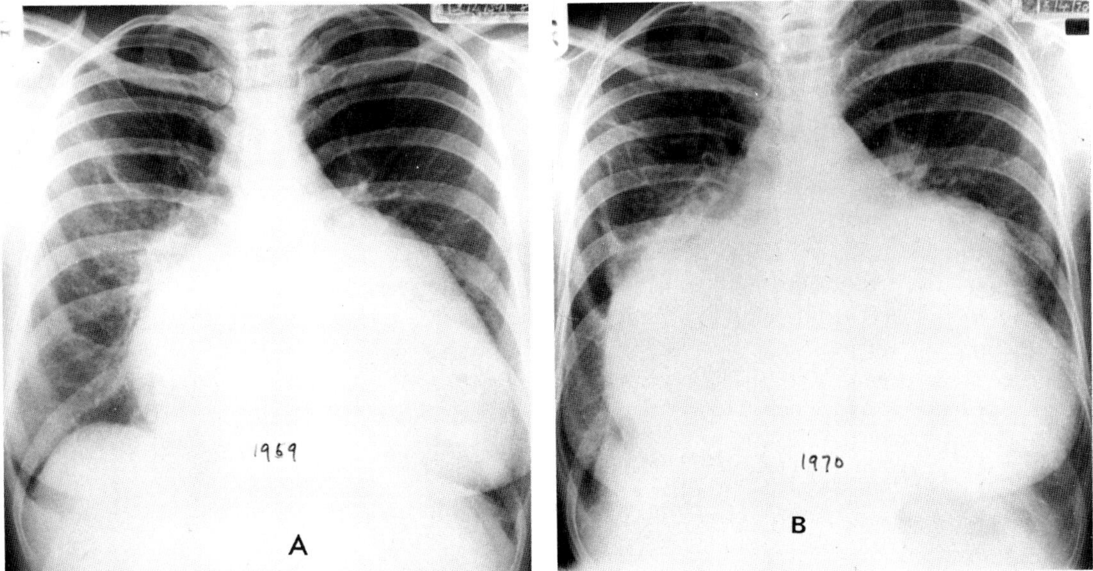

Fig. 23.16 Tricuspid valve disease. (**A**) 1959. The heart shadow is enlarged overall and there is a bulge in the position of the left atrial appendage and also a moderate bulge of the right heart border. (**B**) 1970. The left atrial appendage and left atrium have increased in size, but in addition there has been an enormous increase in the size of the right atrium, bulging to the right, as organic tricuspid stenosis has developed.

the liver is enlarged and pulsatile, while the murmurs closely resemble those of mitral valve disease.

The plain film shows enlargement of the right atrium bulging the heart shadow to the right (Fig. 23.16). Right atrial enlargement can usually be distinguished from left atrial enlargement due to mitral disease, by the entry of the inferior vena cava which limits its extent below.

The development of the characteristic murmur in a patient with a known *carcinoid syndrome* indicates the well-recognized development of tricuspid stenosis in this condition. It may be associated with a large right atrium on the plain film.

Bacterial endocarditis on the tricuspid valve is a common complication of intravenous *drug abuse*. The majority of the infections are staphylococcal, the main clinical and radiological manifestations appear in the lungs with extensive areas of consolidation often progressing rapidly to cavitation. In those patients who survive and develop significant tricuspid incompetence, right atrial enlargement may be detected on serial chest films.

M mode echocardiography is of no value in tricuspid disease as it rarely visualizes the tricuspid valve at all, and almost never completely, making interpretation of the findings virtually impossible. *2DE* visualizes the valve in the majority of cases and is able to show thickening of the valve when stenosed. It may also confirm the enlargement of the right atrium. Tricuspid incompetence may be detected by *contrast echocardiography* using the rapid intravenous injection of saline solution, which because of its contained microbubbles, acts as an ultrasound contrast agent. The presence of vegetations in the tricuspid valve and the diagnosis of tricuspid valve prolapse can also be ascertained by 2DE.

Cardiac catheterization and *angiocardiography* may be difficult to perform and interpret in tricuspid valve disease. Tricuspid stenosis is measured by simultaneous recording of right ventricular and right atrial pressures. As the pressures in diastole are low and the pressure gradients, even when significant, are small, pressures must be measured very carefully.

Right atrial angiography may reveal the large right atrium and thickened, domed, tricuspid valve leaflets, confirming that the tricuspid valve is abnormal. Right ventriculography will show tricuspid incompetence but the significance of the findings must be assessed carefully as some regurgitation may occur through the tricuspid valve during right ventriculography simply because the catheter, passed through the tricuspid valve, holds it open.

AORTIC VALVE DISEASE

The aortic valve may be stenotic or incompetent or both.

Aortic stenosis

This may occur as a congenitally stenotic valve or may develop in adult life either on the basis of a congenital bicuspid valve or from inflammatory commisural fusion which develops in the course of rheumatic heart disease.

Calcific aortic stenosis. This usually develops on the basis of a congenitally bicuspid valve, which may be detected in its mobile, pre-stenotic phase by its ejection click, there being no murmur. With deposition of calcium on the abnormal valve, beginning in the fourth decade, mobility (and the click) are lost, and stenosis develops. Valve calcification is invariable as it is the stenosing process (not as in mitral stenosis a result of the stenosis). This makes the cusps rigid and impedes the flow of blood.

Presentation is with shortness of breath, angina or syncope. The diagnosis is made on the basis of the slow rising plateau pulse, the ejection systolic murmur and thrill and the presence of left ventricular hypertrophy in the ECG.

Plain films may show rounding of the left ventricular apex indicative of left ventricular hypertrophy, post-stenotic dilatation of the ascending aorta, and, on the lateral film, calcification in the position of the aortic valve (Fig. 23.17).

In older patients, when the aorta has become unfolded and slightly dilated, localized post-stenotic dilatation may be difficult to detect. Significant aortic stenosis may be present with a virtually normal heart shadow though it is rare not to detect some evidence of ventricular enlargement in either frontal or lateral views.

M mode echocardiography (Fig. 23.18) shows a thickened, immobile aortic valve, but unless the characteristic box-shaped root echoes are identified, similar appearances may be obtained by a wrongly angled transducer. *Cross-sectional echocardiography* shows a thickened immobile valve with dense echoes indicative of calcium deposition (Fig. 23.18).

The haemodynamic severity of the aortic stenosis cannot be assessed by ultrasound, but it may show thickened ventricular walls, and permits the detection of various forms of subvalvar or supravalvar stenosis.

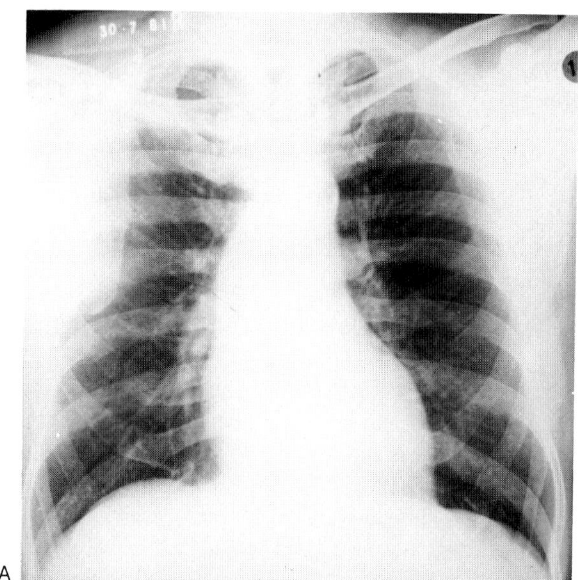

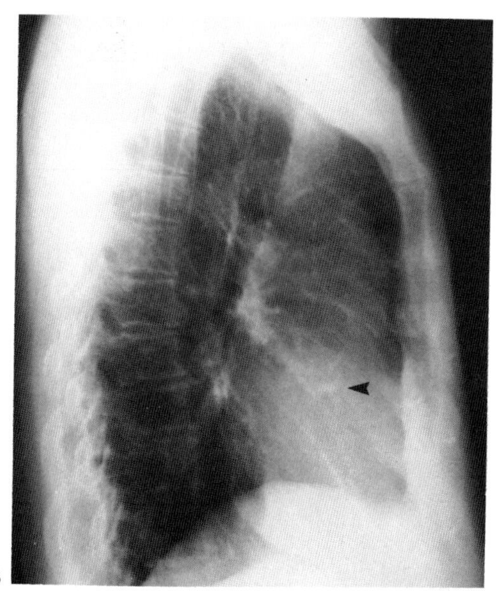

Fig. 23.17 Aortic stenosis. (**A**) Frontal film. This shows rounding of the left ventricular apex indicative of left ventricular hypertrophy, and also post-stenotic dilatation of the ascending aorta. (**B**) Lateral film. Calcification (arrowhead) is visible in the position of the aortic valve.

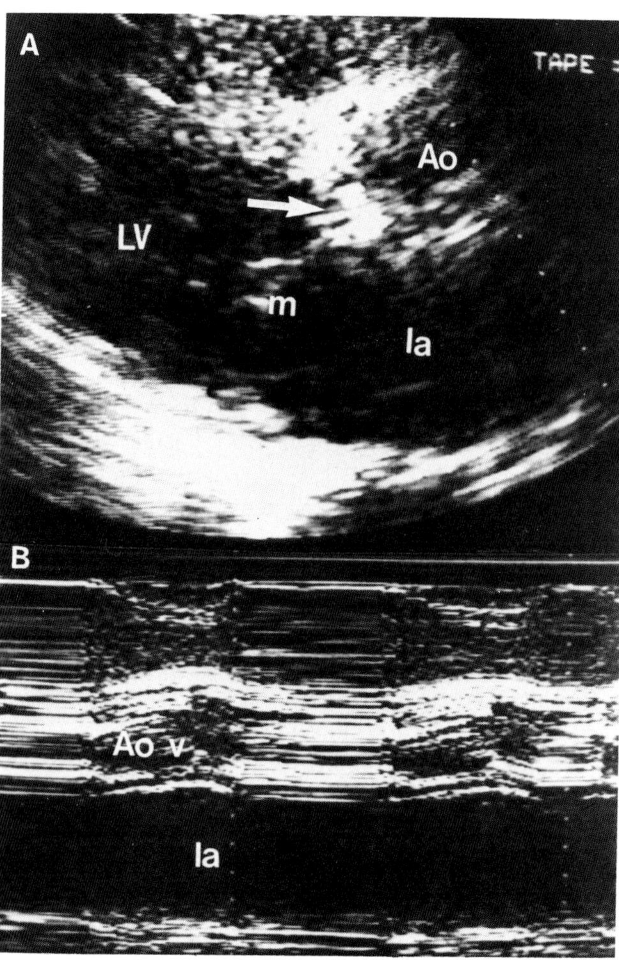

Fig. 23.18 Aortic stenosis. (**A**) Two dimensional echocardiographic study visualizing a thickened, immobile valve with dense echoes indicative of calcium deposition (arrow). (**B**) The M-mode echocardiogram also visualizes a thickened immobile aortic valve (AoV).

The clinical diagnosis is usually obvious when the characteristic murmur is heard, though rarely hypertrophic cardiomyopathy and non-rheumatic mitral regurgitation may have similar murmurs and also show left ventricular hypertrophy on the ECG.

In serious doubt, *fluoroscopy* will show valve calcification or exclude it. Note that the amount of calcium correlates only very roughly with the severity of the aortic stenosis.

Difficulty may be encountered when congestive cardiac failure has developed and cardiac output is so low that the characteristic murmur is not audible; the clinical picture may then resemble congestive cardiomyopathy; the presence of valve calcification on the lateral plain film may be the first indication of the diagnosis.

Rheumatic aortic stenosis. This is due to commisural fusion immobilizing the cusps. Calcification is frequently visible at image amplification fluoroscopy but is rarely more than a few flecks and is almost never seen on the plain film. Left ventricular hypertrophy may be seen on the plain film but post stenotic dilatation is rare. A history of rheumatic fever and evidence of mitral valve involvement either clinically or on echocardiography point to the diagnosis.

Aortic incompetence

This is most commonly due to damage to the aortic cusps by *rheumatic fever* or *endocarditis*, and it may occur *in association with aortic stenosis*. More rarely it may be due to primary disease of the aortic wall when this is involved by *aortitis* of any aetiology (syphilis being the best known) or due to an *aortic root aneurysm* occurring either alone or as part of Marfan's syndrome. *Dissecting aneurysm* reaching to the ascending aorta and valve ring may also precipitate aortic incompetence. The diagnosis is made clinically on the basis of the collapsing pulse and the detection of an early diastolic murmur.

Radiographic appearances. The appearances will vary depending on whether the aortic incompetence is chronic or of acute onset. In the *chronic* form the plain film shows a large heart with left ventricular configuration, and the heart size is commensurate with the severity of the aortic incompetence (Fig. 23.19). The aorta is often large in both ascending part and arch. Calcification of the aortic valve is not a feature of pure aortic incompetence but may be seen if aortic incompetence is combined with stenosis on a calcified, congenitally abnormal, valve. Aortic root abnormalities may show a localized aortic deformity, or what may appear to be simply a large ascending aorta bulging to the right of the mediastinum, or less often to the left. Sometimes the frontal film appears normal but an abnormal forward bulge of the root of the aorta may be seen on the lateral view (Fig. 23.20). Rarely no aortic abnormality may be detectable.

In *acute* aortic incompetence, usually due to bacterial endocarditis or aortic dissection, there may be congestive cardiac failure with a virtually normal sized heart, when this has not had time to dilate.

The diagnosis of aortic incompetence is usually obvious once the early diastolic murmur has been heard. Only in acute aortic incompetence may this be inaudible.

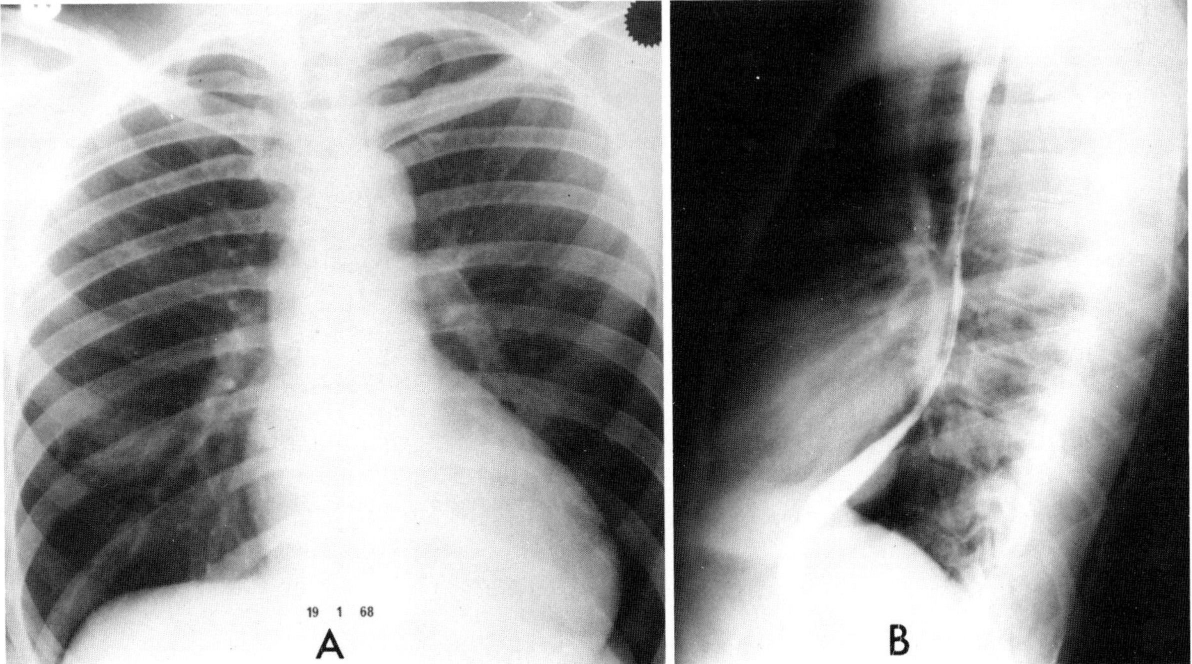

Fig. 23.19 Chronic aortic incompetence. (**A**) Frontal film. The heart shows gross left ventricular dilatation with elongation of the axis to the left. The aorta appears normal. (**B**) Lateral film. The enlarged left ventricle is visible behind the line of the barium-filled oesophagus.

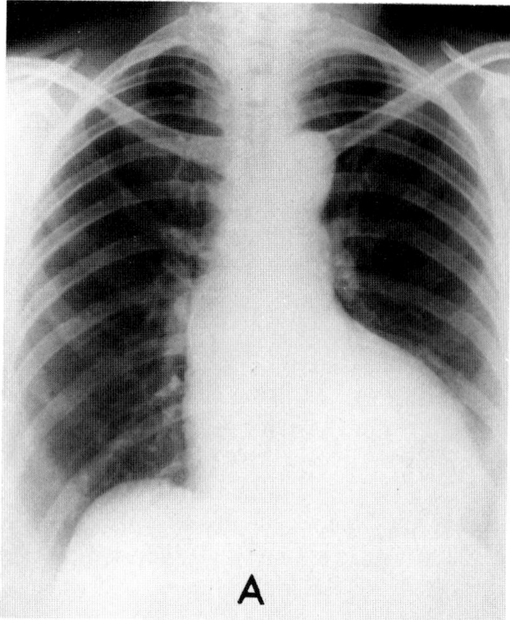

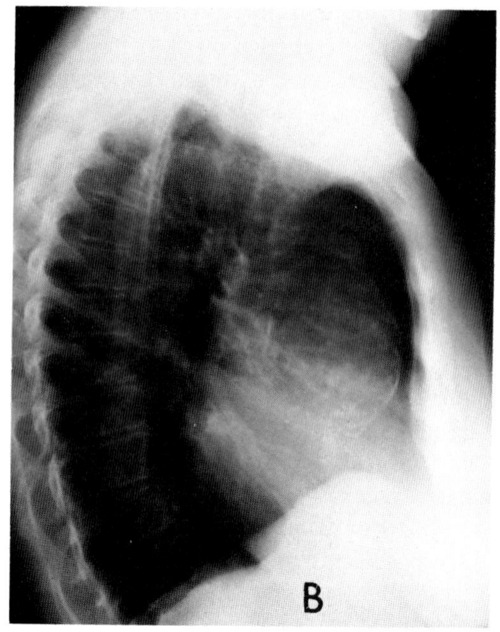

Fig. 23.20 Aortic incompetence due to syphilitic aortic root aneurysm. (**A**) Frontal view. This shows left ventricular dilatation extending to the left and only a slight prominence in the position of the ascending aorta with a barely visible rim of calcium. (**B**) Lateral view. This show a large saccular aortic root aneurysm clearly outlined by calcification.

M mode echocardiography shows the enlarged active left ventricle and may show premature closure of the mitral valve and flutter of its anterior leaflet. *2DE* may show an abnormal aortic valve and a large hyperdynamic left ventricle. The degree of aortic regurgitation cannot be quantified by ultrasound. Abnormalities of the aortic root may also be picked up on the 2DE which may recognize aortic root abscesses and vegetations in endocarditis.

Cardiac catheterization and angiocardiography

The severity of aortic stenosis is assessed by measuring the gradient across the aortic valve, and knowing the cardiac output. The left ventricular pressure may be obtained if the valve can be crossed retrogradely, or measured by a trans-septal approach. The aortic pressure is obtained by retrograde catheterization.

The angiographic visualization of the aortic valve is by retrograde root aortography using cine radiography in the left anterior oblique projection.

The normal aortic valve has three sinuses of Valsalva with three valve cusps which close in diastole so that no contrast leaks pass them into the left ventricle; in systole they fly open against the side of the aorta where they usually cannot be seen. The lowermost sinus of Valsalva seen on the aortogram is always the non-coronary.

Aortic stenosis. In lone calcific aortic stenosis calcification can almost invariably be seen and may be extremely gross. Even in rheumatic aortic stenosis small flecks of calcification are commonly seen in good quality cine-angiograms. The stenosed valve (Fig. 23.21) may be domed or simply show restricted opening. It is usually thickened so that the cusps can be well seen. The densely calcified valves are almost immobile during the cardiac cycle. The aortic root is often pinched in in rheumatic aortic valve disease.

The severity of aortic stenosis can only be estimated angiographically when a discrete negative jet of non opacified blood is seen. In the absence of a recognizable negative jet at root aortography (or a positive jet at left ventriculography) no conclusions can be drawn as the density of calcification bears only a very rough correlation with the severity of stenosis. A small negative jet indicates severe stenosis and a large negative jet insignificant stenosis.

Aortic incompetence. Aortic incompetence is categorized from the left anterior oblique cine-aortic root angiogram in 4 grades:

1. A small puff of contrast enters the left ventricle in diastole and is cleared immediately in systole.
2. The left ventricle is outlined with contrast in diastole but it is still cleared away in systole.
3. Progessively increasing opacification of the left ventricle occurs with each beat.
4. Massive immediate opacification of the left ventricle occurs.

Unfortunately there is no close correlation between this radiological assessment and the degree of aortic incompetence quantitated by measurement of the regurgitant flow by ventricular volume studies.

In diseases of the aortic cusps the appearances of the

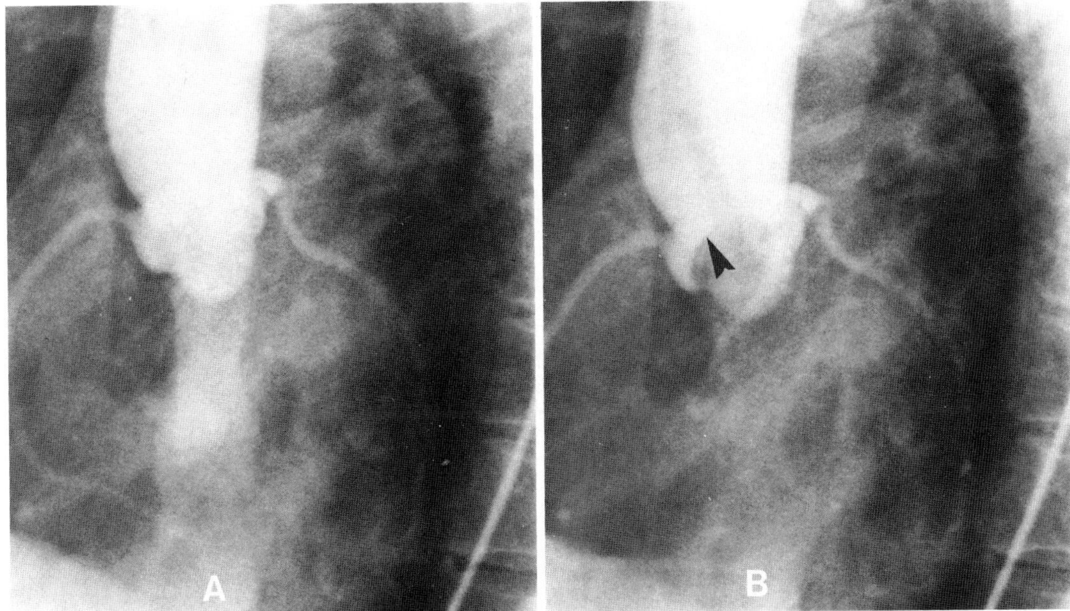

Fig. 23.21 Aortography in aortic stenosis, LAO projection. (**A**) Diastole. (**B**) Systole. In (**A**) the aortic valve appears largely normal and there is slight aortic regurgitation. In (**B**) the domed aortic valve (arrow) is clearly seen and passing through its centre is a negative jet of non-opaque blood, indicating the size of the orifice.

aortic regurgitation are largely non-specific except when there is a pin-hole jet of regurgitation through a valve cusp. This always raises the possibility of cusp perforation. Patients with rheumatic aortic incompetence may show evidence of 'doming' of the valve with commisural fusion. In acute bacterial endocarditis the nature of the pathological process may be suspected by recognizing paravalvar abscesses tracking into the septum (it is these that produce heart block, and indication for immediate surgery) or between the left ventricle and the left atrium.

When aortic wall disease is suspected investigation is always indicated. Dissections may be diagnosed by the tracking of contrast between the aortic wall and the elevated flap of intima (see Ch. 26). An aortic root aneurysm will be seen as a rather symmetrical fusiform dilatation of the aortic root involving the valve ring and often the cusps of the aortic valve (the so-called triple sinus aneurysm) but the dilatation usually stops short of the origin of the innominate artery. In Marfan's syndrome small intimal dissection may not be seen at aortography and attacks of acute chest pain probably represent small dissections even in the presence of a non-diagnostic arteriogram.

ISCHAEMIC HEART DISEASE

CORONARY ARTERIOGRAPHY

This is the radiological visualization of the coronary arteries (and left ventricle) by direct selective injection of contrast medium. It is the most sensitive and accurate method of studying disease in the coronary arteries and the effects of this disease on the heart, and a description of the technique and findings must be considered first.

TECHNIQUE

Two approaches are available to cannulate the coronary arteries. The most popular is the percutaneous femoral Seldinger technique using pre-shaped catheters, different for each coronary artery and for the left ventricle. Different configurations have been described by Judkins, Amplatz and Bourassa.

The earlier technique, that of Sones, required an arteriotomy of the right brachial artery and used a single soft tipped catheter which was buckled against the aortic valve and introduced into each coronary artery in turn, and into the left ventricle.

FILMING

High quality high resolution *cine filming* at 25 to 50 frames per second is now the standard method of recording the image. *Digital subtraction angiography* can however visualize a left ventricle either by central intravenous injection or by direct injection of low doses of contrast into the ventricle in the course of coronary arteriography. It is not yet clear whether the coronary arteries will be adequately visualized using subtraction techniques and aortic root injections, thus obviating the need for selective cannulation of the coronary arteries.

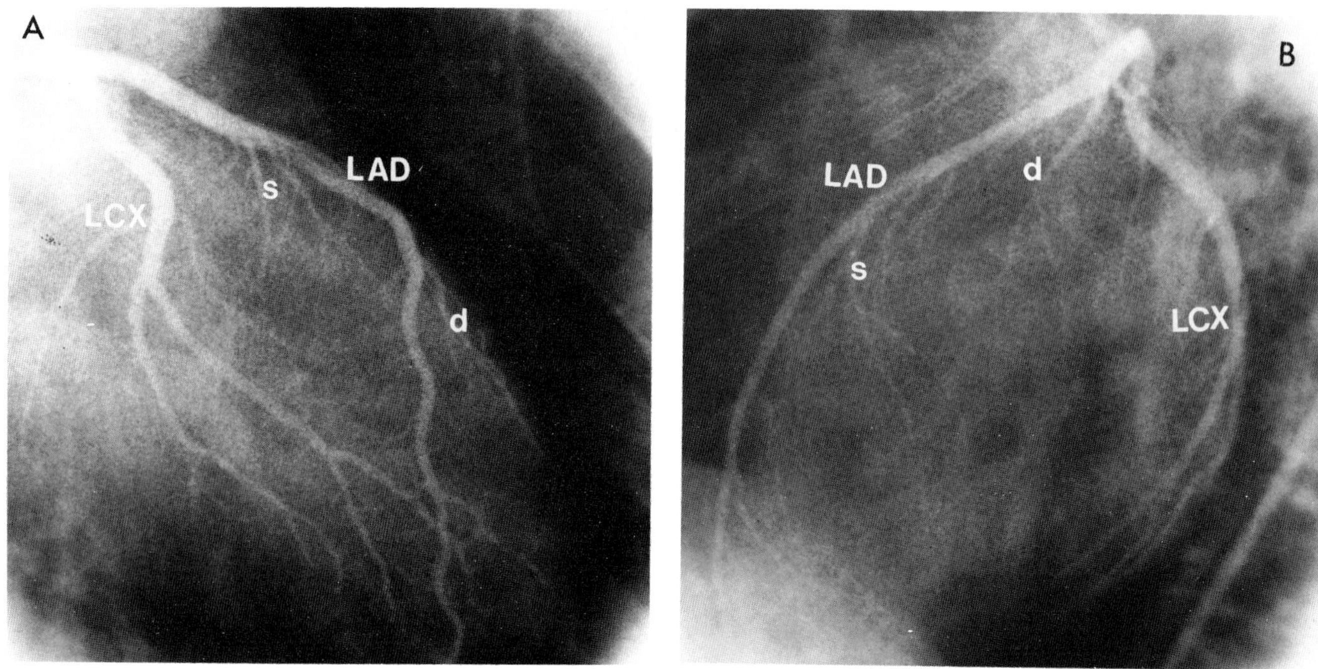

Fig. 23.22 Left coronary artery. (**A**) RAO view. (**B**) LAO view. The main stem, of variable length, passes to the left and divides into the anterior descending (LAD) and circumflex (LCX) branches. s = septal branch; d = diagonal branch.

Normal coronary anatomy

The *left coronary artery* (Fig. 23.22) comes off its sinus of Valsalva which is on the left and slightly posterior. The main stem, of variable length, passes to the left and divides into two.

The *anterior descending* coronary artery passes forward over the surface of the heart in the anterior interventricular groove (which marks the interventricular septum) and reaches to, and beyond, the apex of the heart to reach the inferior interventricular groove on the undersurface. Parallel *septal* branches descend from the anterior descending into the septum and *diagonal* branches to the free wall (as opposed to the septum) of the left ventricle pass to the left. The *circumflex* passes to the left in the left atrioventricular groove (which marks the atrioventricular valvar plane, separating atrial from ventricular part of the

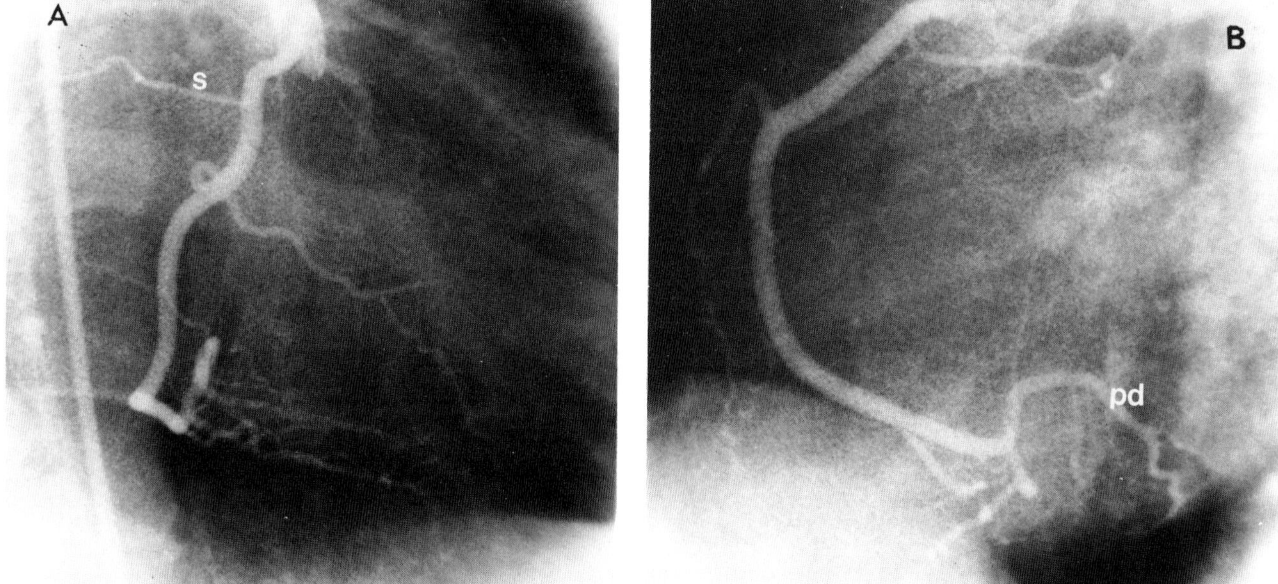

Fig. 23.23 Right coronary artery. (**A**) RAO view. (**B**) LAO view. The usual dominant right coronary artery gives off the posterior descending (pd) branch immediately before the crux of the heart. s = sinus node artery.

heart). It gives off forward running *obtuse marginal* branches to the left ventricular free wall, and normally terminates above the crux.

The *right coronary artery* (Fig. 23.23) comes off its sinus of Valsalva, in front and only slightly on the right, and passes forward and to the right to reach the right atrioventricular groove in which it encircles the right side of the heart. Its first branch, the *conus* branch is to the conus of the right ventricle; its second, which runs posteriorly, is the *sinus node artery* to the sinus node in the inter-atrial septum. Then come right ventricular branches. The usual *dominant* right coronary artery reaches the crux (the junction of the atrioventricular plane and the interventricular plane on the undersurface of the heart). Immediately before the crux it gives off the *posterior descending* coronary artery which runs forward in the inferior interventricular groove to supply the posterior septum. At the crux the right coronary artery loops into the myocardium, giving off the *atrioventricular node artery* at the apex of the loop before emerging back onto the surface of the heart. The right coronary artery then continues in the left atrioventricular groove supplying *posterolateral left ventricular branches* to the left ventricular free wall.

Normal variants. Variation of balance of the coronary arteries can make interpretation of the angiogram difficult. The common variation is *left dominance*. The circumflex branch of the left coronary artery is very large and extends around the back of the heart in the left atrioventricular groove until it reaches the crux where it supplies the posterior descending and atrioventricular nodal branches. The right coronary artery is consequentially small and supplies only the right ventricle, and may appear abnormal.

The circumflex rarely may be so large as to entirely replace the right coronary artery, or the right coronary artery may be so large that there is virtually no circumflex. Both may be large and the anterior descending very small.

Congenital anomalies. These abound in the coronary circulation. The circumflex may arise from the right coronary artery or from the right sinus of Valsalva; rarely the anterior descending may do this. Circumflex and anterior descending may have separate origins from the left coronary sinus of Valsalva. These anomalies lead to difficulties in catheterization but do not in themselves produce symptoms. Origin of the left coronary artery from the right sinus of Valsalva or of the right coronary artery from the left sinus of Valsalva may lead to symptoms if the artery is compressed.

Coronary disease

The normal coronary artery is a smoothly outlined, gently tapering structure at angiography. *Atheroma* appears as an irregularity of outline (Fig. 23.24A). When atheromatous plaques spread around the artery to form a stricture this can be identified and its severity evaluated (Fig. 23.24B). Angiography understates the extent of atheroma and the severity of stricture. Complete occlusions may be detected and the patency of the vessel beyond the complete occlusion identified as it opacifies by collateral flow (Fig. 23.25).

Spasm may also be seen during coronary arteriography. Catheter-induced spasm usually occurs as a smoothly tapered narrowing, usually in the right coronary artery, at the catheter tip. It is not usually associated with symptoms and may be relieved by Trinitrin. Spontaneous or drug-(Ergot preparations) induced spasm often begins at a rather minor atheromatous plaque and may progress to occlusion

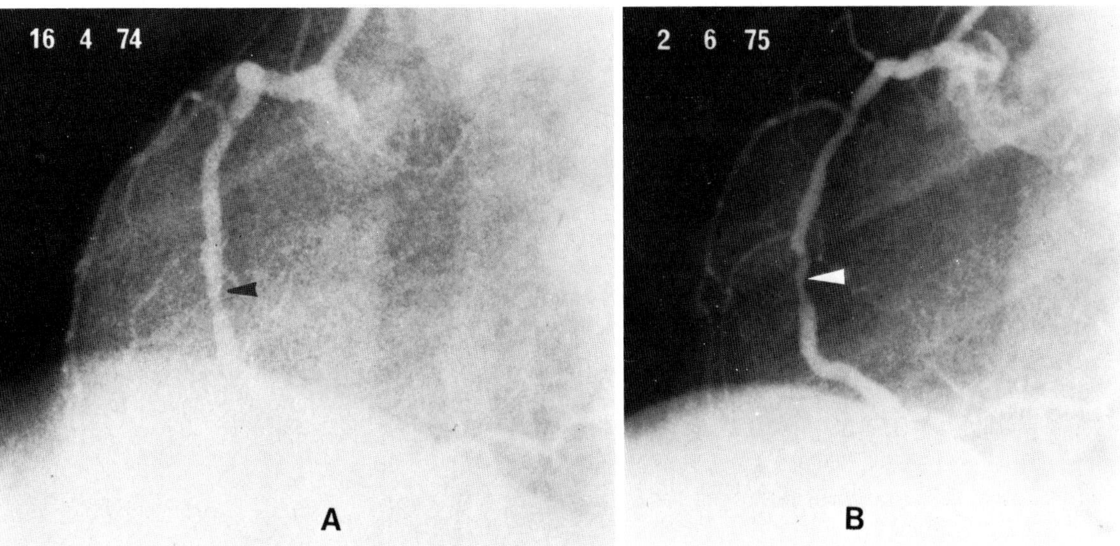

Fig. 23.24 Coronary artery disease. Right coronary artery, LAO view. (**A**) Atheromatous lesion in mid third of the right coronary, appearing as an irregularity of outline (arrow). (**B**) Restudy 14 months later, visualizing a severe stricture (arrow).

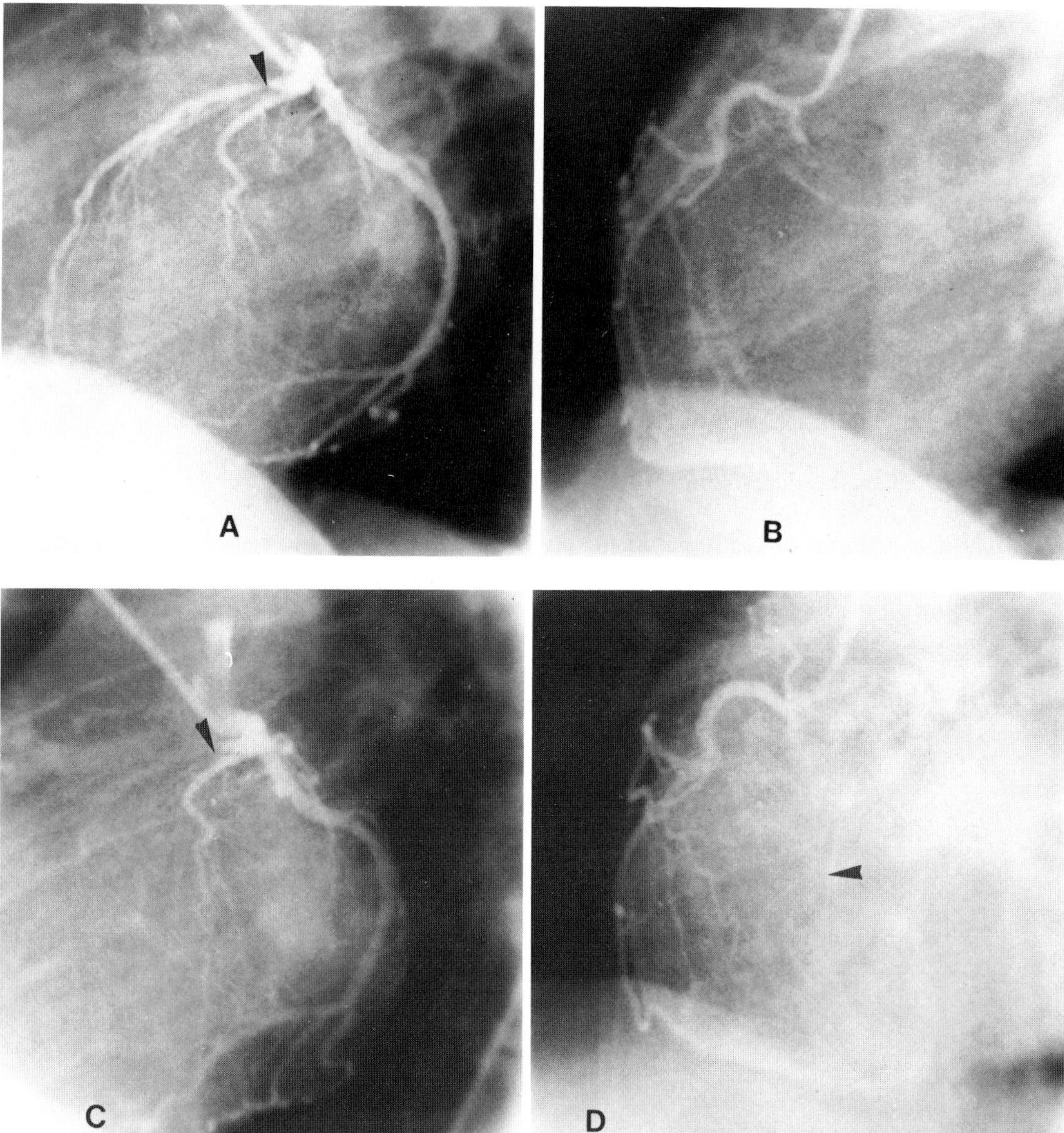

Fig. 23.25 Progression of coronary disease. Left anterior oblique views. (**A**) Left coronary artery. There is a critical narrowing at the origin of the anterior descending branch (arrow). (**B**) Right coronary artery. (**C** and **D**) correspond to a restudy performed 7 months later following an anterior infarction (see Fig. 23.27). The left coronary artery has become completely occluded (**C**, arrow) and fills via collaterals from the right coronary artery (**D**, arrow).

of the whole artery, often with the development of the patient's symptoms and ECG changes. It is usually relieved by Trinitrin.

Left ventriculography

The normal left ventricle is a carrot shaped structure with the aortic and mitral valves at its base (Fig. 23.26). It contracts concentrically with its anterior wall apex and inferior wall all moving equally inwards. Ischaemic heart disease produces localized abnormalities of wall movement (Figs 23.26 and 23.27), hypokinesia — reduced movement, akinesia — no movement and dyskinesia — paradoxical movement. Wall movement abnormalities are associated with overall impairment of function which can be seen on the angiogram as ventricular dilatation and poor emptying. Emptying is measured as the *ejection fraction* (stroke volume/diastolic volume) the proportion of the ventricle which empties with each beat, and in the normal is two thirds. Significantly impaired function would be represented by an ejection fraction of under 50%, proceeding to the very severest impairment, 10 to 20 %.

ANGINA PECTORIS

This is an episodic pain occuring almost anywhere above the diaphragm and thought to be due to transient myocar-

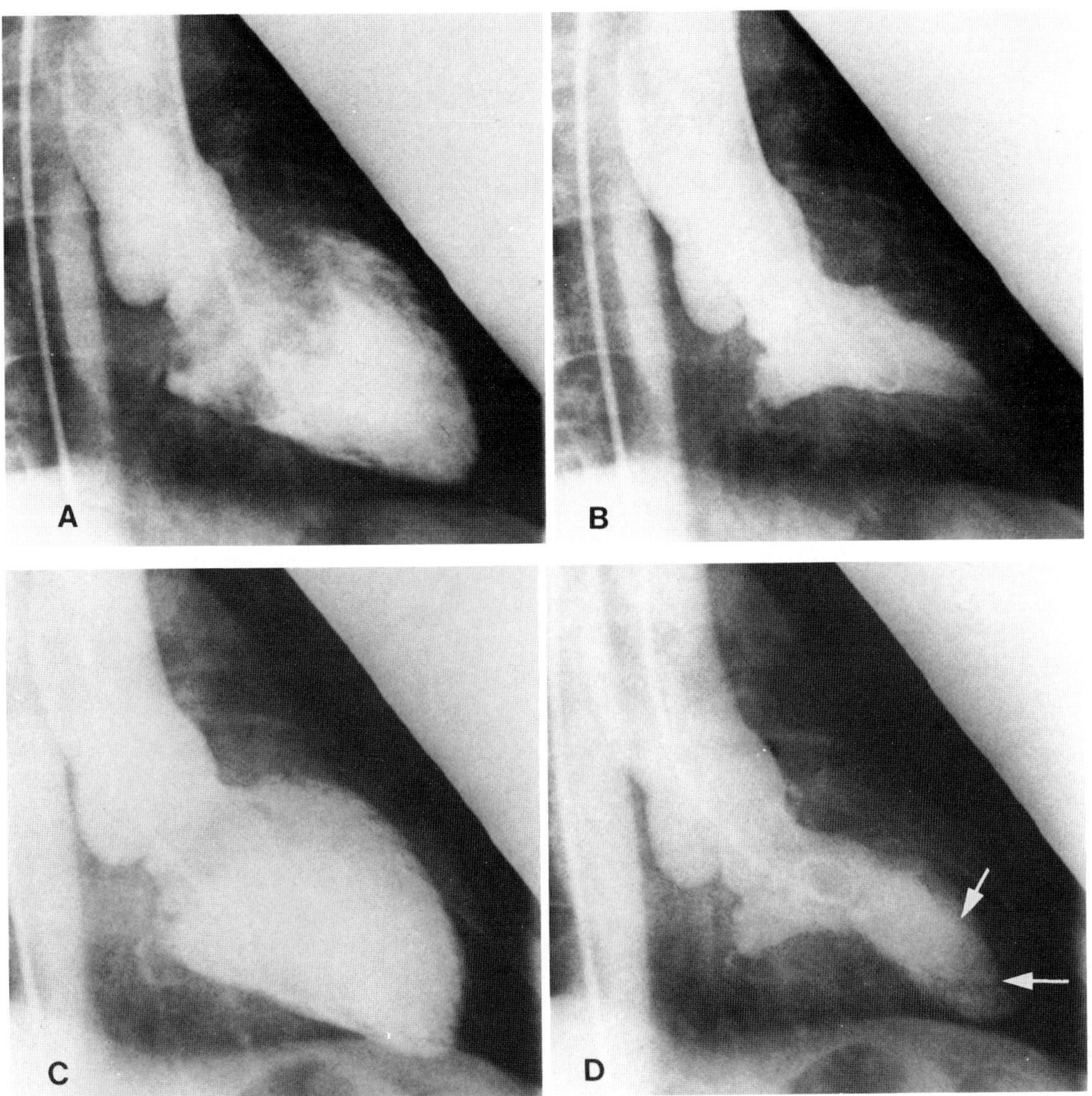

Fig. 23.26 Progression of coronary disease. Left ventriculogram (RAO views) (same patient as Fig. 23.25). (**A** and **B**) Initial study visualizes normal left ventricle which is a carrot-shaped structure (with the aortic and mitral valves in its base) and contracts concentrically. (**C** and **D**) Restudy 7 months later, following anterior infarction and occlusion of the left anterior descending coronary (see Figs 23.25C and 23.27). The left ventriculogram shows localised abnormality of wall movement in the antero-apical wall of the heart (arrows).

dial ischaemia. Classical angina is a crushing chest pain, often radiating to the left arm, brought on by exercise, and relieved by rest or Trinitrin. The ECG becomes abnormal during pain with ST segment depression. This condition is almost invariably associated with obstructed coronary arteries.

Prinzmetal's variant angina is an anginal pain, often coming on spontaneously, and associated with ST segment elevation on the ECG. The coronary arteries develop spasm during the pain but appear largely normal when the patient is symptom free.

Diagnosis of angina pectoris may be difficult when the pain develops in a bizarre site, such as the jaw, or when its relationship to exercise and relief by rest is unclear, as may occur in the many mixed patterns of angina which may be encountered.

Thallium scanning, performed during the ischaemic episode, may show a perfusion deficit which fills in at rest, supporting the idea that a localized area of myocardium becomes ischaemic, and that this is the cause of symptoms. Unfortunately thallium scanning is neither sensitive nor specific enough to be a particularly useful test in excluding the diagnosis of coronary artery disease though if its results are very positive it does support the diagnosis.

The *plain film* is normal in patients with uncomplicated angina pectoris unless there has been a previous myocardial infarction.

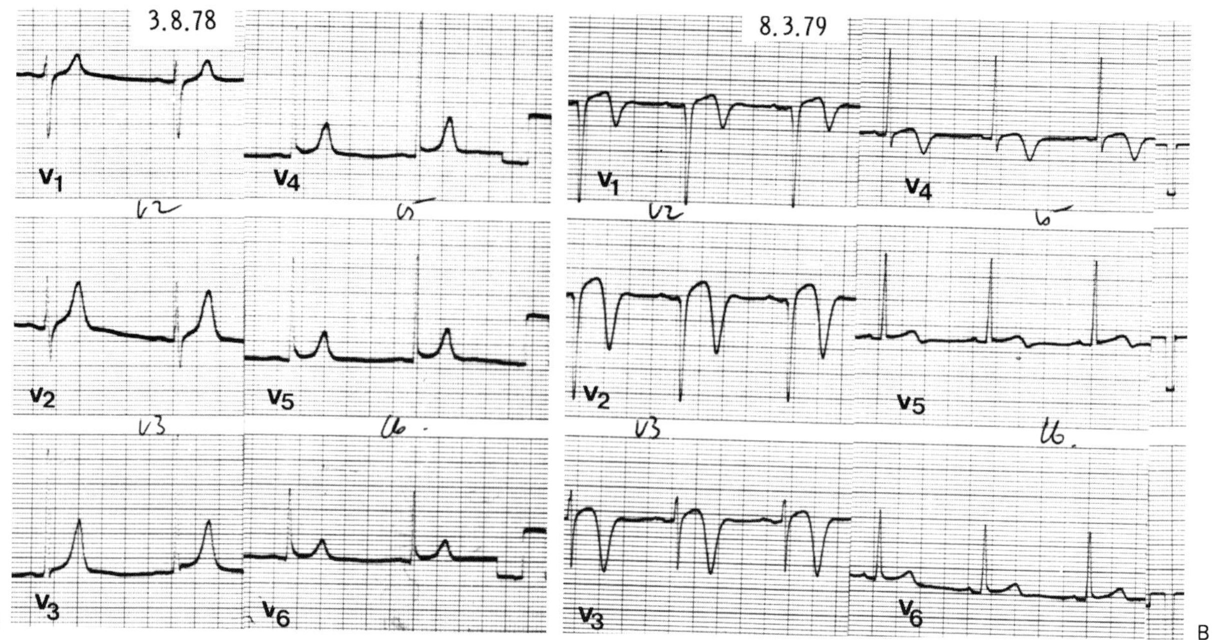

Fig. 23.27 Electrocardiographic tracings corresponding to the study in Figures 23.25 and 23.26. (**A**) Normal ECG obtained at the time of the initial angiographic assessment (precordial leads V1–V6). (**B**) The ECG shows an evolving anterior infarction following occlusion of the left anterior descending vessel (see Fig. 23.25C).

MYOCARDIAL INFARCTION

When ischaemia is severe enough to lead to death of muscle the syndrome of myocardial infarction results. The clinical features depend on the size of the infarction, the presence of arrythmias and the development of the mechanical complications of myocardial infarction.

Radiographic appearances. The *plain films* are initially ward unit portable films done anteroposterior, at short distance and often with low power apparatus.

They are thus usually of poor quality and with distorted geometry and heart size difficult to assess. The size of the heart will depend on the size of the current infarct and the

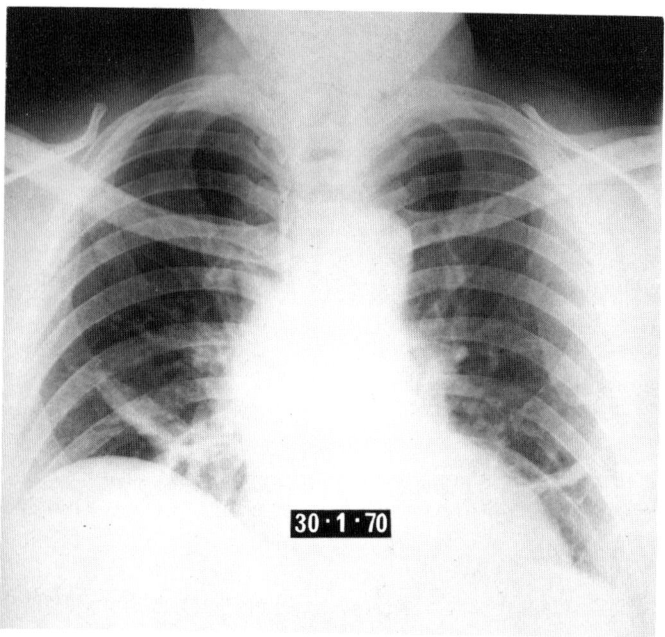

Fig. 23.28 Myocardial infarction. The chest X-ray demonstrates broad basal line shadows, probably areas of collapse due to diaphragmatic splinting from pain.

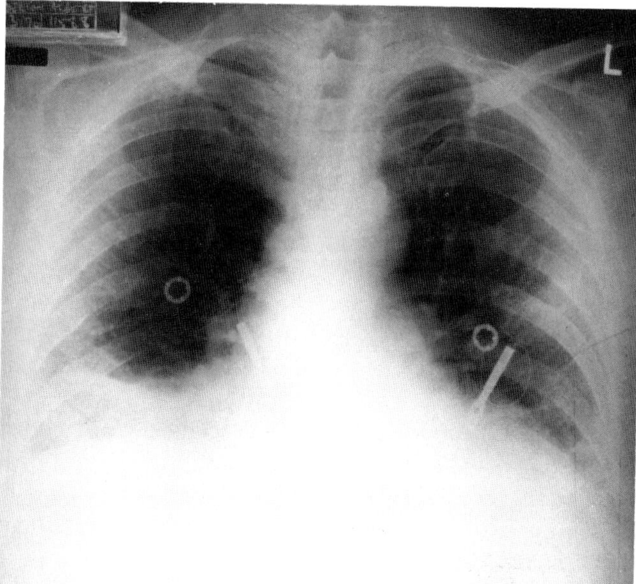

Fig. 23.29 Post-myocardial infarction (Dressler's) syndrome. Small effusions are seen in both costophrenic angles, together with ill-defined basal shadows resembling pulmonary infarcts.

effects of any previous infarctions. It may be small if the present infarct is the only one and is small, and large if the present infarct is large or there have been previous infarcts. The pulmonary vessels will reflect the haemodynamic disturbance with upper lobe blood diversion, interstitial and alveolar oedema, reflecting progressively more severe disturbance with higher left atrial pressure. Persisting pulmonary oedema or a large heart are both bad prognostic features.

In the convalescent phase a number of features may be seen. Ill-defined basal shadows beginning within a day or two of infarction and developing into broad basal line shadows are probably areas of collapse due to diaphragmatic splinting from pain (Fig. 23.28). *Dressler's syndrome* of pleuritis, pneumonitis and pericarditis comes on after 10 days with chest pain and fever (Fig. 23.29). Small effusions may be seen in the costophrenic angle, with ill-defined basal shadows resembling pulmonary infarcts, but the prompt response to aspirin or steroids usually makes the diagnosis obvious. Rarely a pericardial effusion may be so large as to cause tamponade. Dressler's syndrome may remit and relapse.

With recovery, departmental films may be taken. Coronary *calcification* may be identified by its parallel line appearance, usually best seen in the lateral view, in the position of the anterior descending or right coronary artery. It is much better seen at image amplification television fluoroscopy. Calcification may also be seen in old infarcts as a curvilinear density in the position of the wall of the left ventricle. Multiple infarctions produce congestive failure, 'ischaemic cardiomyopathy'. The heart is large with a left ventricular configuration, though all chambers are involved to some extent. Pulmonary oedema may be seen in untreated cases.

Ventricular aneurysm may develop about two months after a large infarction. Patients may present with congestive cardiac failure, angina, arrythmias, or may be asymptomatic. A variety of appearances may be seen, varying from an apparently normal heart shadow (rarely) through left ventricular enlargement, to a localized bulge of the apex of the heart (Fig. 23.30). The lungs will reflect the effects of treatment on the haemodynamic disturbance. In some cases curvilinear mural calcification may be seen, which always suggests an aneurysm and one of long-standing (Fig. 23.31). The diagnosis may be confirmed by *isotope ventriculography* either first pass or multiple gated studies,

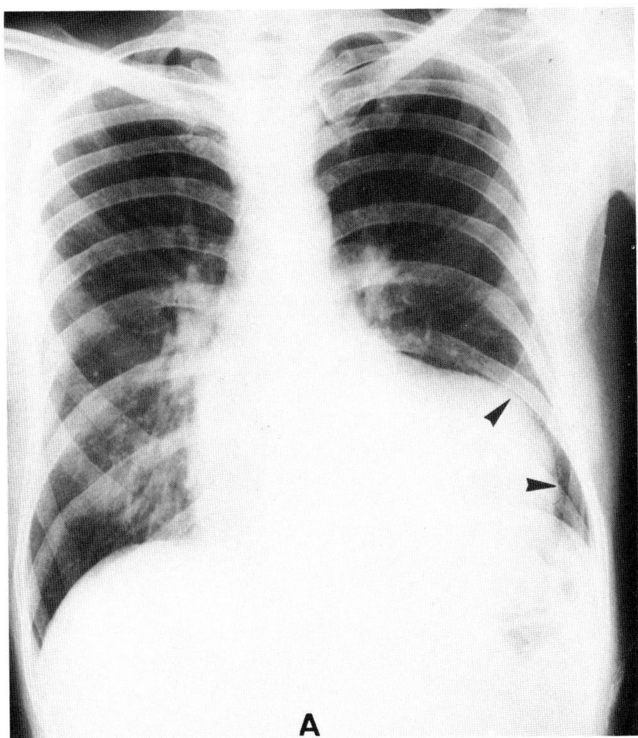

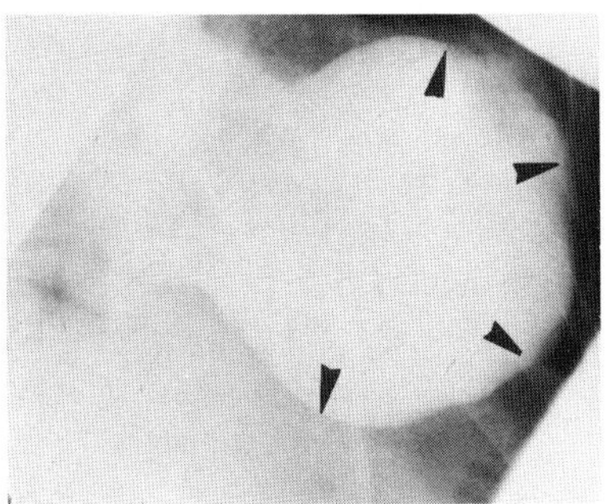

Fig. 23.30 Ventricular aneurysm. (**A**) The chest radiograph shows an enlarged heart with a localized bulge. (**B**) The aneurysm is clearly defined in the left ventriculogram which visualizes a large antero-apical dyskinetic area (arrows).

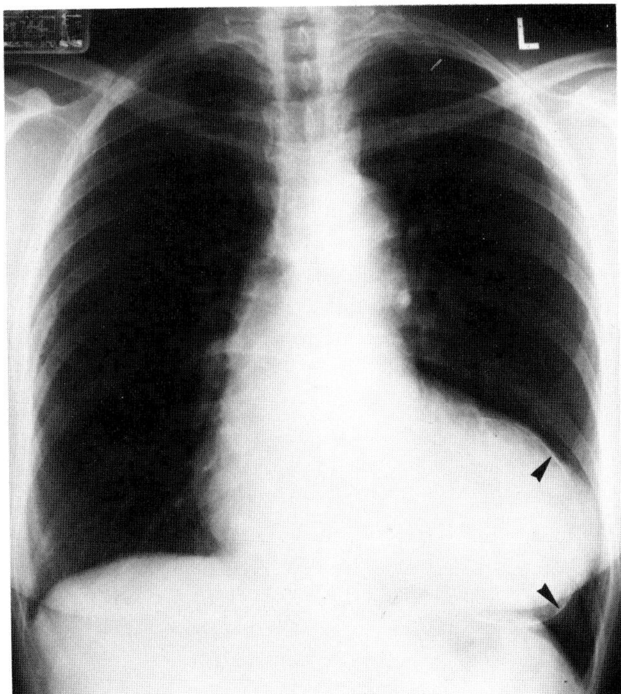

Fig. 23.31 Ventricular aneurysm. Cardiac enlargement and apical calcification (arrows) in a patient with a long-standing left ventricular aneurysm.

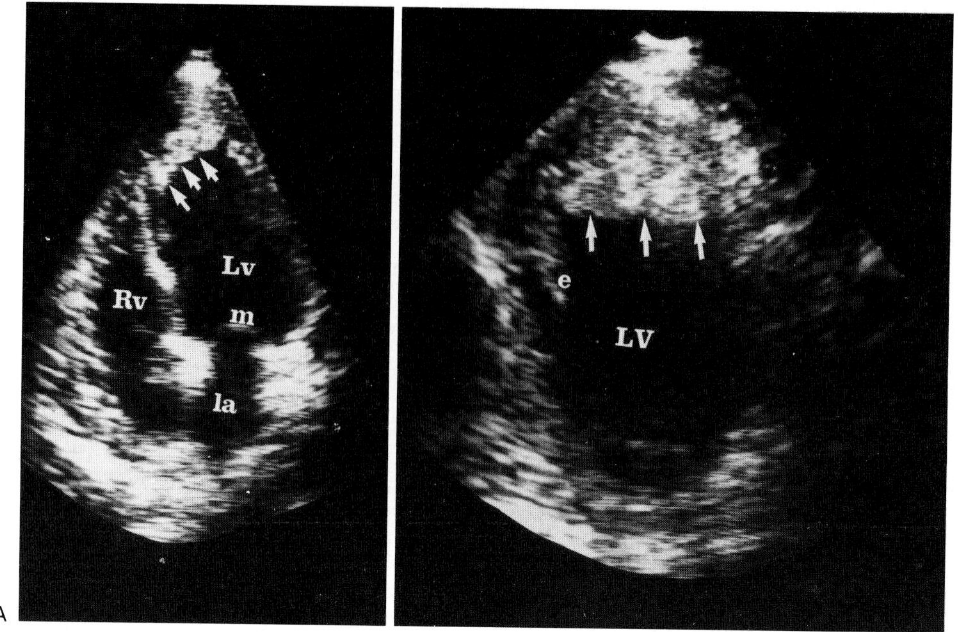

Fig. 23.32 (**A** and **B**) Ventricular aneurysm. The 2DE study (apical and short axis views) visualizes an antero-apical thinned out aneurysmal area with mural thrombus (arrows). e = endocardium. Lettering as in Figure 20.1.

cross-sectional echocardiography, which also shows clot (Fig. 23.32), or *CT scanning* which demonstrates the aneurysm and may also show intraventricular clot. Left ventriculography and coronary arteriography are usually performed pre-operatively.

Perforation of the ventricular septum following anterior myocardial infarction is marked by clinical deterioration and the development of a systolic murmur. The heart is usually large and the lungs show gross pulmonary oedema. *Echocardiography* shows not only the large and dyskinetic left ventricle but usually reveals the site of the perforation (see Fig. 23.33).

Left ventriculography and coronary arteriography are usually attempted pre-operatively if the patient's clinical condition permits. Pulmonary plethora may be seen in those few patients who survive long enough to develop it.

Post infarction mitral incompetence may be trivial if there is slight ischaemia of the papillary muscle, or catastrophic if the papillary muscle necroses and ruptures. This event is marked by sudden clinical deterioration and the development of a systolic murmur. The heart may be moderately enlarged but left atrial enlargement is not seen. There is usually gross pulmonary oedema. Cross-sectional echocardiography may demonstrate the size and function of the left ventricle in the presence of a flail mitral leaflet. Coronary angiography is usually performed pre-operatively.

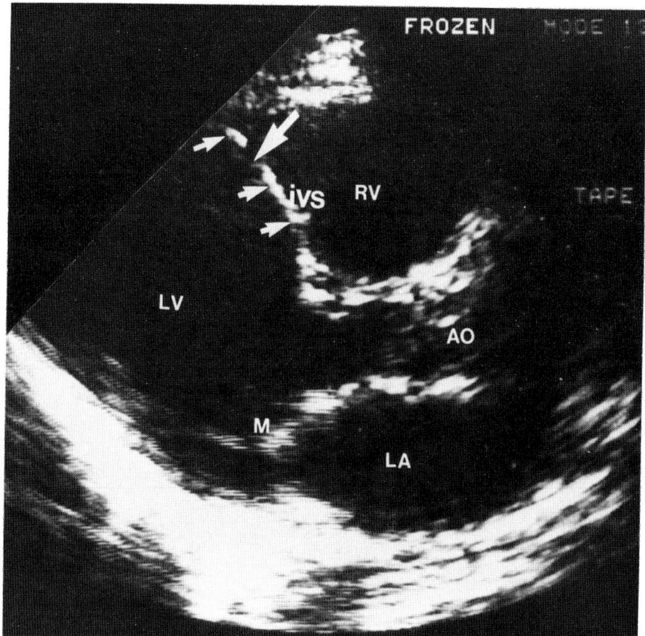

Fig. 23.33 Perforation of the interventricular septum in association with anterior myocardial infarction. The 2DE study reveals an antero-septal (ivs) thinned-out segment corresponding to the infarction (small arrows) and reveals the site of the perforation (long arrow). Lettering as in Figure 20.1.

CORONARY ARTERY SURGERY

The standard surgical procedure for the treatment of ischaemic heart disease is saphenous vein aorto-coronary bypass graft. The vein is attached end to side to the ascending aorta above and end to side to the coronary artery below, beyond the obstruction. Distal variations are used with Y grafts or jump grafts.

The indication for surgery, and hence the indications for pre-operative coronary arteriography are:

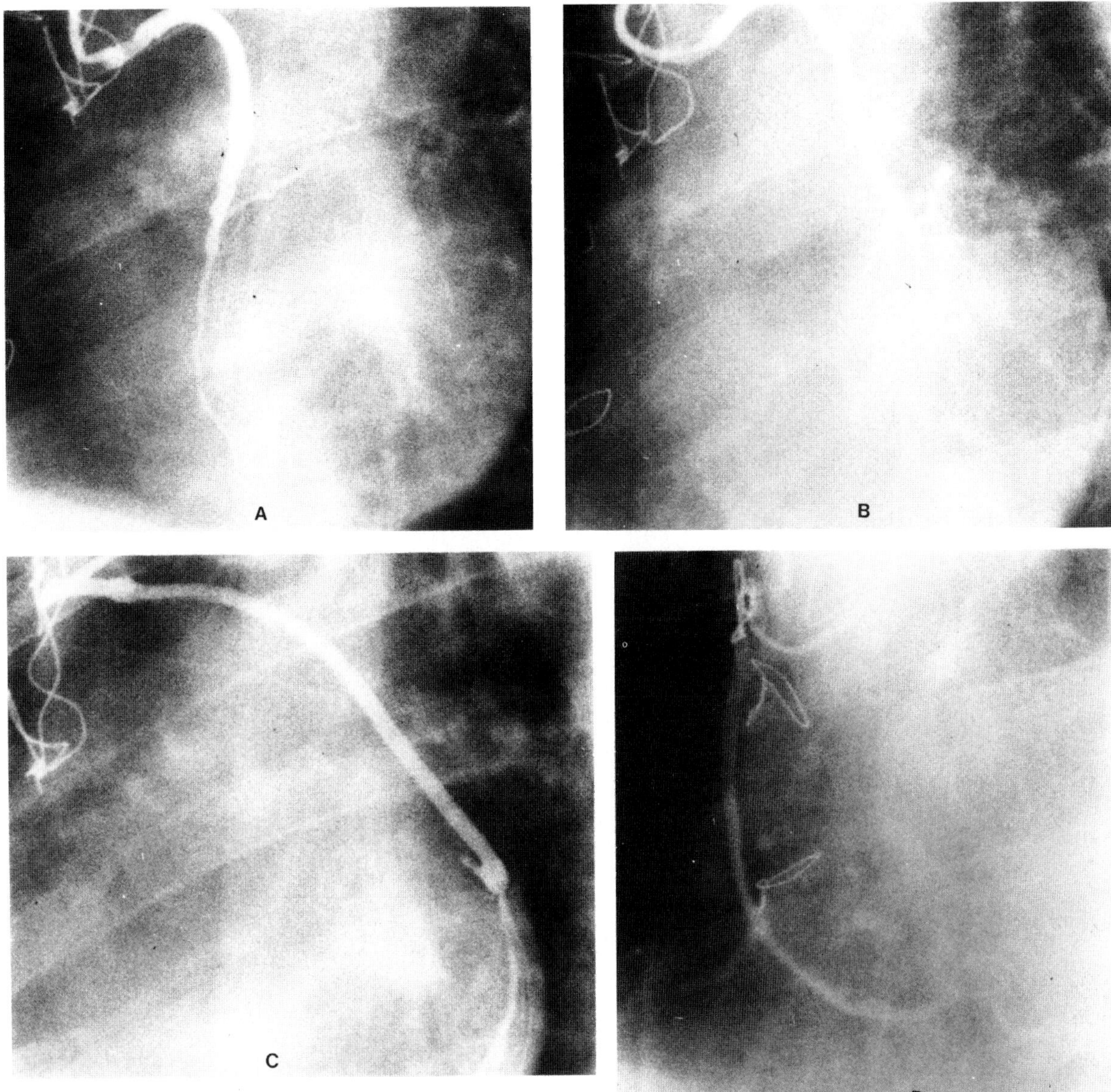

Fig. 23.34 Coronary artery surgery. Post-operative angiographic study (LAO projections) demonstrating patency of the vein grafts to the (**A**) left anterior descending, (**B**) diagonal, (**C**) circumflex, (**D**) right coronary arteries.

1. Angina unresponsive to medical treatment.
2. Post infarction ischaemia, either anginal or on exercise testing.
3. Mechanical complications.
4. Before valve surgery in patients with chest pain or aged over 50.

Coronary arteriography is also used post-operatively to study the state of the grafts and the state of the native coronary circulation, in cases where angina recurs (Fig. 23.34). Blocked grafts, strictured grafts and progress in the disease of the native circulation are all causes of unsuccessful relief of ischaemia.

Non-surgical interventions

Transluminal balloon dilatation coronary angioplasty (Gruntzig) is a significant advance in the management of coronary artery disease. The technique consists of using a large diameter guide catheter to introduce the small balloon catheter into the coronary artery and through the stricture. The indications for the procedure are as for bypass surgery. Severe single vessel non-occlusive strictures respond well with a high success rate (90%) (Fig. 23.35) initially and a low complication rate (3% emergency surgery). About 25% of strictures recur and can be redilated.

Streptokinase infusion either intravenous or intracoronary may be used to lyse thrombus in acute myocardiac infarction. It must be used within 2 hours and under

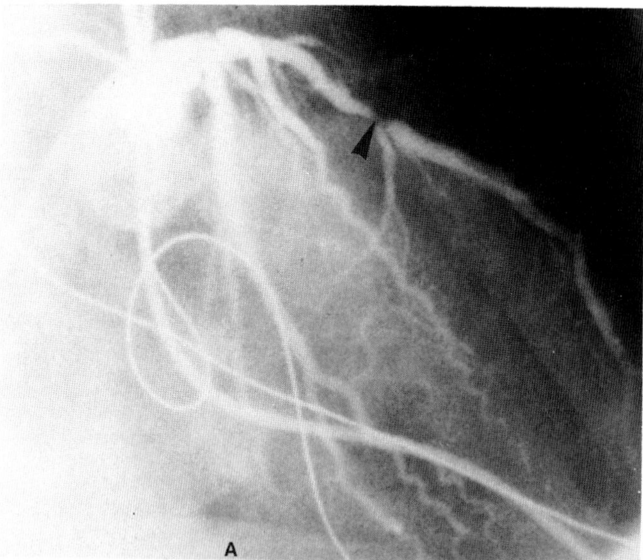

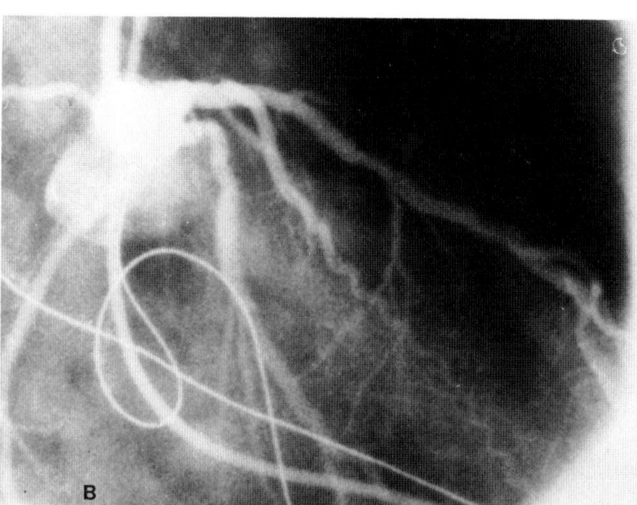

Fig. 23.35 Transluminal balloon dilatation coronary angioplasty. (**A**) Left coronary injection (RAO projection) visualises a localized, severe stenosis in the left anterior descending vessel (arrow). (**B**) The post-dilatation angiogram shows only a minor irregularity at the site of the stricture.

angiographic control. In these circumstances an occluded artery supplying infarcting myocardium can be re-opened and infarction limited or prevented.

HEART MUSCLE DISEASE

When heart failure occurs without recognizable mechanical cause the fault is presumed to be in the heart muscle itself. Heart muscle disease occuring in recognized association is so described, e.g. alcoholic heart disease. When there is no recognizable cause the condition is termed cardiomyopathy. Three varieties are recognized, *congestive* (*dilated*), *hypertrophic*, and *restrictive*.

CONGESTIVE (DILATED) CARDIOMYOPATHY

The hallmark of this condition is dilatation of the lef ventricle with impairment of emptying, i.e. a reduction ir the ejection fraction. Asymptomatic dilatation may b present for years, symptoms only developing when conges tive cardiac failure supervenes.

Presentation may be with congestive cardiac failure often manifesting as an attack of bronchitis, as a arrythmia or rarely with chest pain or even embolism fron clot in the left ventricle. The clinical findings of a thir sound gallop and an abnormal ECG indicate left ventricula disease.

The usual differential diagnosis is from other forms o congestive cardiac failure particularly ischaemic hear

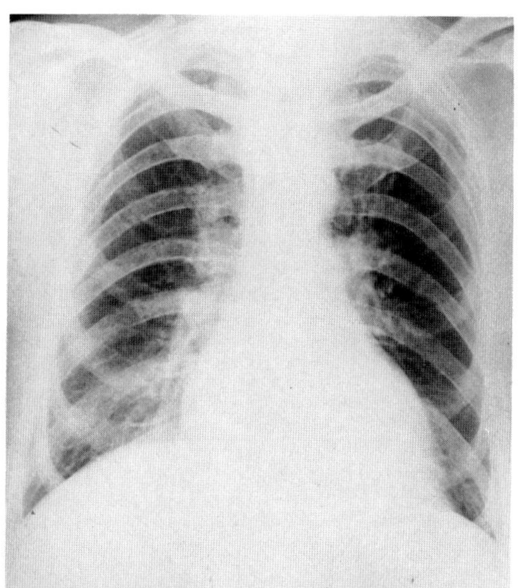

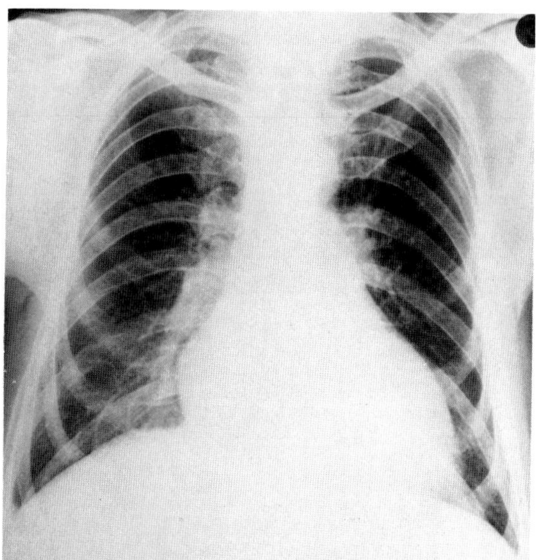

Fig. 23.36 Congestive cardiomyopathy. (**A**) The heart is only slightly large on 17.10.79. (**B**) Significant dilatation involving mainly the left ventricle has developed by 10.2.81.

disease, left ventricular aneurysm, silent aortic stenosis or even silent mitral stenosis. Ventricular dilatation may be associated with slight mitral regurgitation and a systolic murmur and occasionally it may be difficult to distinguish between congestive cardiomyopathy with some mitral regurgitation and mitral regurgitation leading to severe cardiac failure.

Radiographic appearances. The plain film almost always shows cardiac enlargement, which may be purely left ventricular (Fig. 23.36), or the heart may be globular in shape if all chambers are involved. Very rarely left ventricular enlargement may only be seen in the lateral view. The lungs will show evidence of raised left atrial pressure in the untreated patient. Patients usually respond to treatment with considerable clinical improvement, a reduction in heart size (rarely to normal) and the clearing of the lungs. Relapse however is usual and response to treatment less satisfactory with each relapse.

Isotope ventriculography usually demonstrates the dilated and poorly but concentrically contracting left ventricle. It will also exclude the surgically treatable possibility of left ventricular aneurysm.

M mode echocardiography usually demonstrates the large left ventricular cavity with poor wall movement, at least in the part that can be studied (Fig. 23.37). It should exclude silent aortic stenosis or silent mitral stenosis but not left ventricular aneurysm. *Cross-sectional echocardiography* should exclude all other possibilities and make a positive diagnosis of congestive cardiomyopathy (Fig. 23.37). It may also recognize intracavitary thrombus (Fig. 23.32).

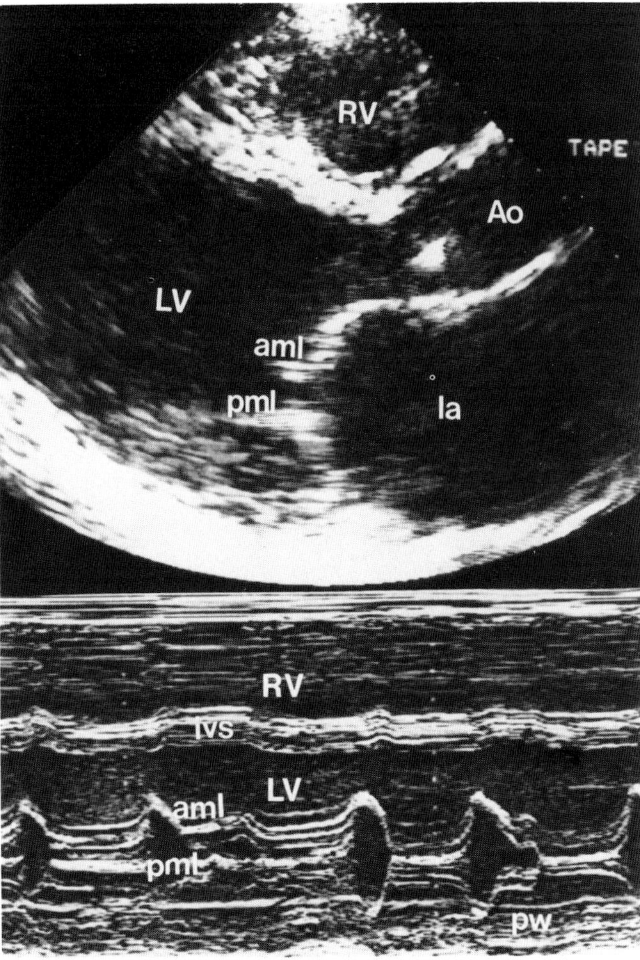

Fig. 23.37 Congestive cardiomyopathy. (**A**) The 2DE demonstrates a large left ventricular cavity with poor wall movement, together with limited opening of the mitral valve leaflets (aml, pml) due to the low cardiac output. (**B**) The M-mode echocardiogram visualises similar findings with abnormal septal (ivs) and posterior wall (pw) motion. Lettering as in Figure 20.1.

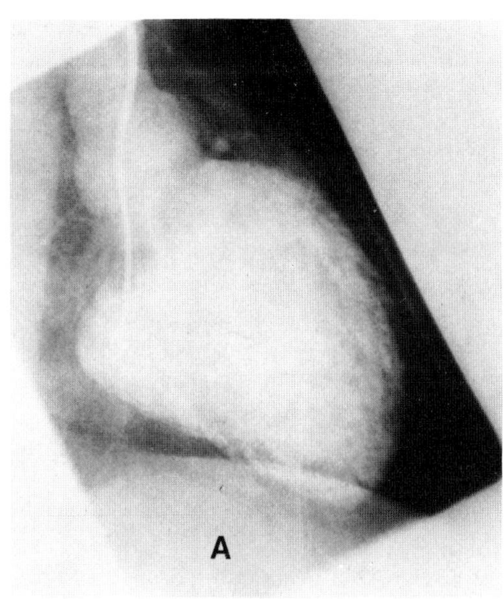

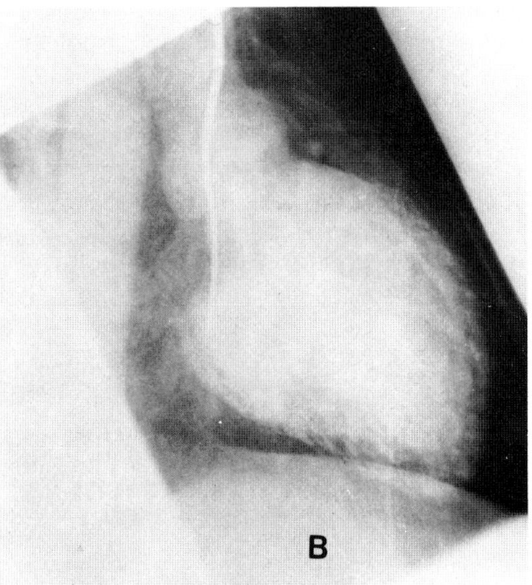

Fig. 23.38 Congestive cardiomyopathy. Left ventricular cine-angiogram (RAO view) corresponding to Figure 23.36B. (**A**) Diastolic and (**B**) Systolic frames demonstrate a large ventricular cavity with generalised reduction in wall motion.

Cardiac catheterization and *angiocardiography* are only indicated when the diagnosis is still in doubt. The dilated, poorly but concentrically contracting cavity of the left ventricle is usually obvious (Fig. 23.38); mitral and aortic stenosis and left ventricular aneurysm (Fig. 23.30) can all be excluded. In those cases complicated by mitral regurgitation the severity of this may be assessed and taken together with the degree of impairment of left ventricular contraction it is usually possible to distinguish between congestive cardiomyopathy and mitral regurgitation. The coronary arteries may also be studied at the same time.

HYPERTROPHIC CARDIOMYOPATHY

In this condition there is inappropriate hypertrophy of the myocardium occuring in the absence of any recognized stimulus. The hypertrophy is usually asymmetrical, and often concentrated in the upper septum, though all types of distribution of hypertrophy may be seen. The excessive muscle apparently contracts well.

The condition may present as sudden death; with shortness of breath due to difficulty in filling the hypertrophied stiff left ventricle; with angina; or with arrythmias. The pulse is characteristically jerky and the apex beat left ventricular with an atrial beat. Auscultation reveals a late systolic murmur and a fourth heart sound. The ECG usually shows gross left ventricular hypertrophy.

The *plain film* findings range from an apparently normal heart through a heart showing obvious left ventricular hypertrophy, often with a rather chunky outline to it (Fig. 23.39), to a globular heart with all chambers being involved. Evidence of raised left atrial pressure may be seen in the lungs.

The differential diagnosis usually lies between ischaemic heart disease, fixed aortic stenosis, non-rheumatic mitral regurgitation and hypertrophic cardiomyopathy.

On *M mode echocardiography*, the hypertrophy of the left ventricle usually involving the septum asymmetrically, can be identified together with the systolic anterior movement of the mitral valve, and this, with the demonstration of normal mitral and aortic valves, is enough to make the diagnosis (Fig. 23.40). A much better display of the anatomy is seen on the *cross-sectional echocardiogram* (Fig. 23.41).

Cardiac catheterization may reveal a high filling pressure and a variable intracavitary gradient which may be provoked by post-ectopic beats. *Angiocardiography* reveals a range of abnormalities from a left ventricle indistinguishable from normal to one which is of normal size but empties excessively, and with prominent papillary muscles and septum (Fig. 23.42), through to the grossly distorted ventricle almost resembling a myocardial tumour.

RESTRICTIVE CARDIOMYOPATHY

Mild forms of this may be encountered in patients being investigated for non-specific chest pain and found to have

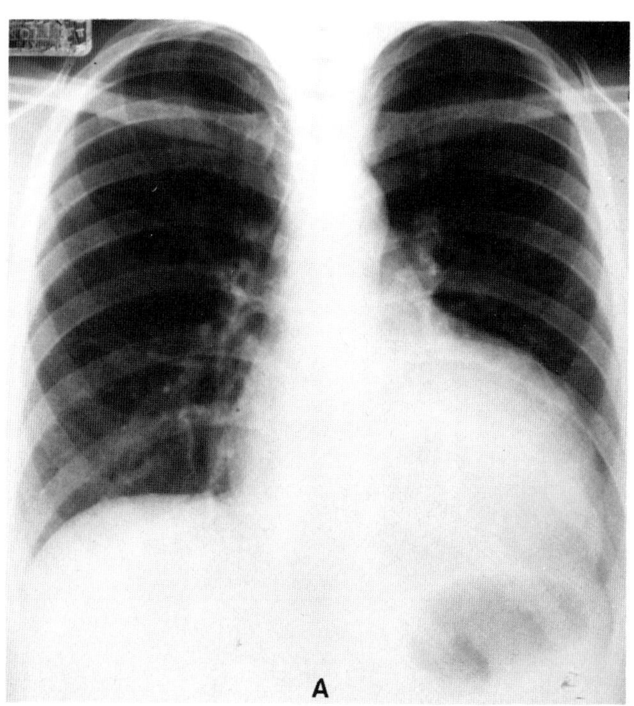

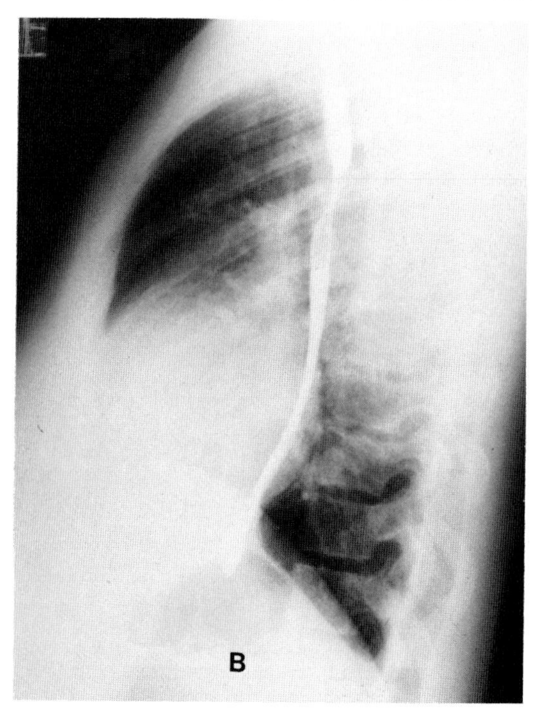

Fig. 23.39 Hypertrophic cardiomyopathy. (**A**) Frontal film. The heart shadow is markedly enlarged with an elongation of its axis to the left and rounding of the apex but with a rather bulky and irregular outline. (**B**) Lateral film. The enlarged left ventricle bulges back beyond the line of the barium-filled oesophagus.

In this patient the cavity of the ventricle (see Fig. 23.42) is normal in size and the bulk of the heart shadow is due to an enormous increase in thickness of the wall of the heart.

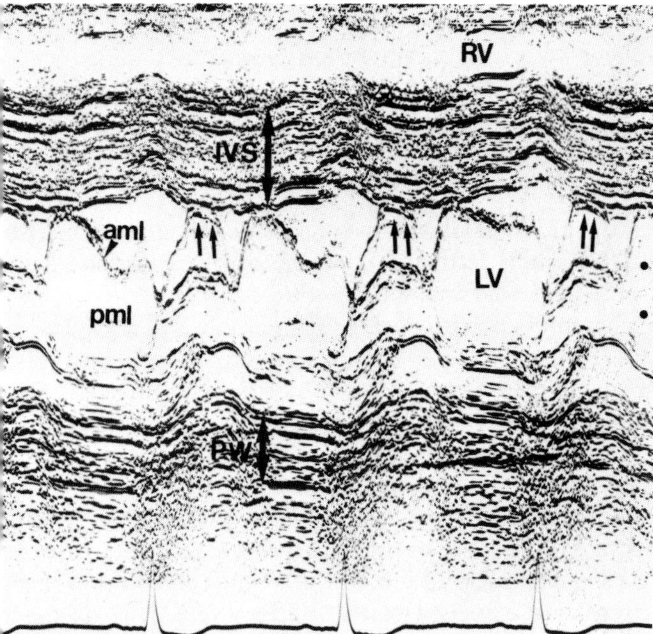

Fig. 23.40 Hypertrophic cardiomyopathy. The M-mode echocardiogram demonstrates hypertrophy of the left ventricle (LV) involving the septum (IVS) asymmetrically, together with systolic anterior movement of the anterior mitral leaflet (aml) (arrows). PW = posterior wall of the ventricle; pml = posterior mitral leaflet; RV = right ventricle.

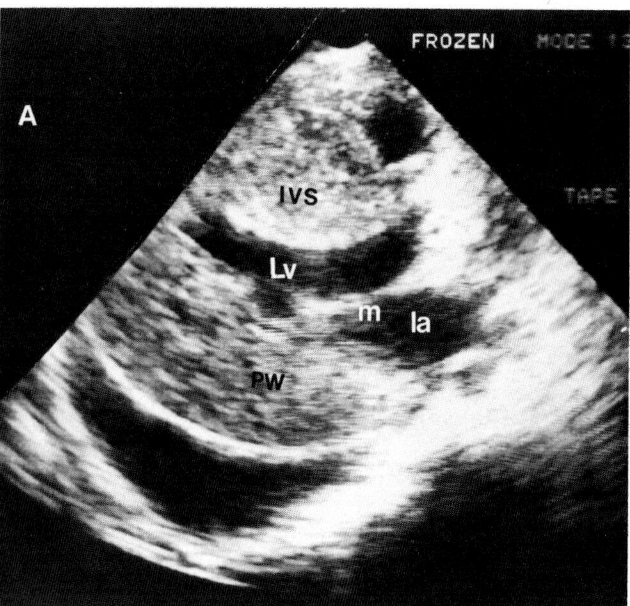

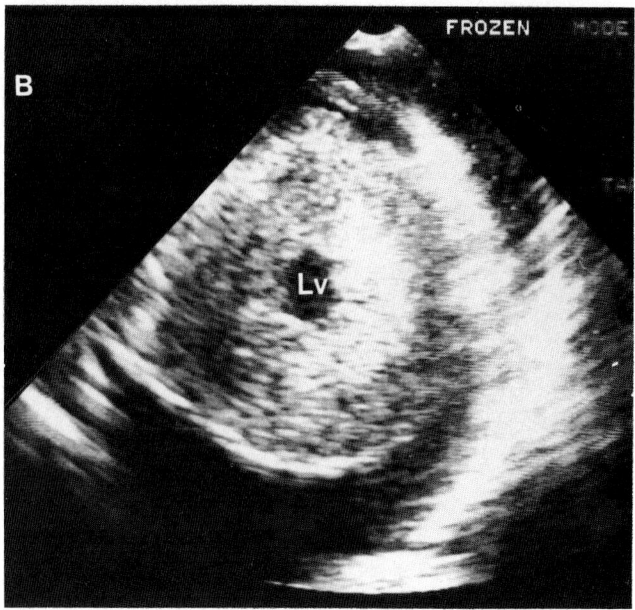

Fig. 23.41 Hypertrophic cardiomyopathy. The two dimensional echocardiogram visualizes the massive septal and posterior wall hypertrophy, almost obliterating the ventricular cavity. (**A**) Long axis view. (**B**) Short axis view.

a high end-diastolic filling pressure in the left ventricle with no other abnormality.

The most florid example is seen in the condition of *endomyocardial fibrosis*, which is usually identified in Africans, but is seen sporadically in Europeans under the name of *Leoffler's endocarditis*. The pathological process is the laying down of fibrous tissue on the inner aspects of the ventricles beginning at the apices and spreading to involve the inlet valves.

On the left side this leads to difficulty in filling the ventricle (but not of contraction or emptying) and mitral incompetence. On the right side there is a high filling pressure in the right ventricle and tricuspid incompetence and there may be a pericardial effusion. In left sided involvement the heart tends to be normal in size unless mitral regurgitation is severe. With right sided involvement the heart shadow is large and globular.

Findings of *angiocardiography* are characteristic with amputation and smoothing off of the apices of the ventricles and atrioventricular valvar regurgitation.

SPECIFIC HEART MUSCLE DISEASE

Abnormalities of heart muscle leading to a clinical syndrome similar to that of congestive cardiomyopathy may occur in a large variety of conditions.

Infections and collagen disorders

Viral myocarditis. This may be suggested when congestive cardiac failure occurs in relation to an obvious viral pyrexia (usually Coxsackie) particularly when there is a high, rising, antibody titre. However, cardiomyopathy may apparently begin with an influenza-like illness, or myocarditis may have no antecedent pyrexia. Endocardial biopsy, showing inflammatory cells eroding myocardial fibres is the most satisfactory diagnostic tool, and may indicate appropriate treatment.

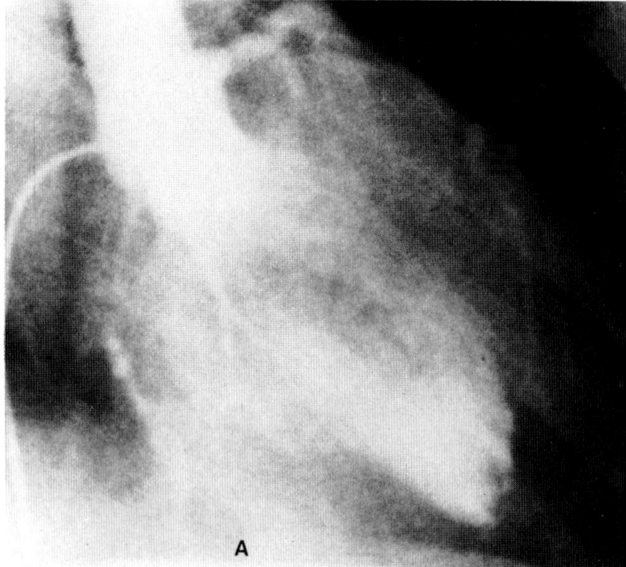

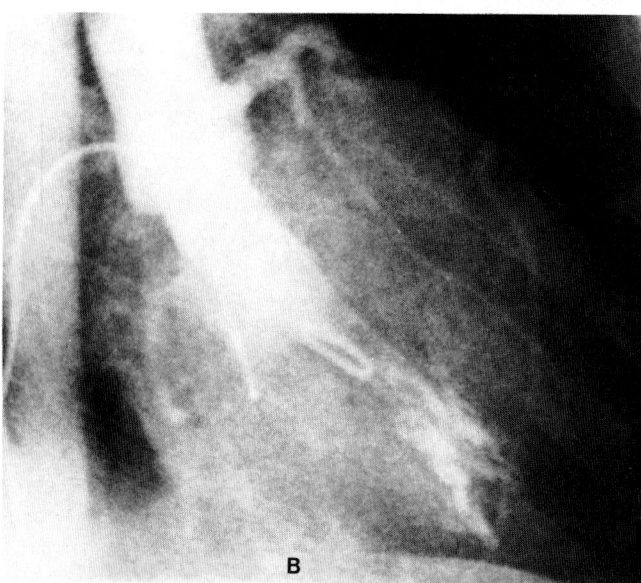

Fig. 23.42 Hypertrophic cardiomyopathy. Left ventricular cine-angiogram (RAO views). (**A**) Diastolic frame. (**B**) Systolic frame. *Note* the systolic obliteration of the ventricular cavity which results from the massive muscle hypertrophy.

Bacterial myocarditis. A toxic myocarditis may occur with severe bacterial infections and is a well-known complication of the exotoxin of diphtheria. Myocarditis may also occur in the course of bacterial endocarditis.

Parasites. Chagas's disease due to infection by *T. cruzi*, leads to a patchy fibrotic destruction of the myocardium causing left ventricular failure after a long latent period. The oesophagus may be involved producing appearances similar to those of achalasia. The disease is confined to Latin America.

Collagen diseases. Collagen diseases including rheumatic fever may involve the heart in their acute phase, leading to arrythmias or congestive cardiac failure. Systemic lupus erythematosus usually produces a pericardial (and pleural) effusion. It may also produce sterile vegetations (Libman-Sacks) on the mitral and aortic valves.

Myocardial infiltrations

Haemochromatosis. The deposition of iron in heart in this condition leads to congestive cardiac failure and is the cause of death of about one third of patients.

Sarcoidosis. Involvement of the heart by sarcoidosis is rare, but may precede the appearance of sarcoidosis elsewhere in the body by several years. The usual manifestation is an arrythmia but congestive cardiac failure may occur and rarely there may be mitral incompetence from papillary muscle involvement.

Amyloid heart disease. Amyloid may involve the heart alone or as part of a generalized disorder. There is severe cardiac failure, with low cardiac output and a low volume pulse. The patient is often murmur free. The diagnosis may be suspected when echocardiography demonstrates a left ventricle only slightly enlarged. It may be confirmed by endomyocardial biopsy.

Glycogen storage disease. This condition usually presents in the neonatal period with characteristic muscle weakness, but rarely the heart failure may appear first. The condition may be suspected by echocardiography or left ventriculography which shows a moderate cavity dilatation associated with gross wall thickening.

Metabolic disorders

Thyroid disease. Both forms of thyroid disease may lead to cardiac abnormalities. Myxoedema usually produces a pericardial effusion but there may be involvement of the heart muscle with cardiac dilatation. Thyrotoxicosis usually produces atrial fibrillation and should be suspected when this condition develops in the absence of mitral valve disease. Cardiac dilatation may also occur if thyrotoxicosis leads to high cardiac output failure.

Acromegaly. There is generally held to be a specific dilated cardiomyopathy in association with acromegaly but there is also a very high instance of hypertension and coronary artery disease.

Beri-beri This condition, due to a deficiency of thiamine leads to a high output, or much more rarely a low output cardiac failure. It usually responds to thiamine.

Drugs and poisons

Alcoholic heart disease. Alcoholic heart disease may be manifest by arrythmias or overt congestive cardiac failure A history of excessive intake of alcohol, and improvement when alcohol is forsaken, suggest the specific diagnosis.

Drugs. Beta blocking drugs in large doses may lead to cardiac dilatation or overt cardiac failure. It is not clear whether this only occurs in the presence of heart disease or could occur in a normal heart. The anthracycline antimitotic agents may lead to irreversable congestive cardiac failure. The effect is critically dose related.

Other conditions
Congestive cardiomyopathy may develop in a variety of heredo-familial *neuro-muscular disorders* and may be the cause of death. Congestive cardiomyopathy may also develop after pregnancy (*post-partum cardiomyopathy*). It usually responds to treatment but may relapse with subsequent pregnancies.

MISCELLANEOUS CONDITIONS

TUMOURS OF THE HEART

Secondary tumours, which commonly originate from breast or bronchus are much commoner than primary tumours. They are often silent and only recognized at necropsy. Involvement of the pericardium leading to pericardial effusion and tamponade is much commoner.

Primary tumours of the heart are rare and the majority are benign, consisting mainly of myxomas (50%) rhabdomyomas and fibromas. The clinical manifestations often depend on the site of origin. Intracavitary tumours are often pedunculated and cause obstruction whereas intramural tumours may infiltrate leading to arrythmias or cardiac failure.

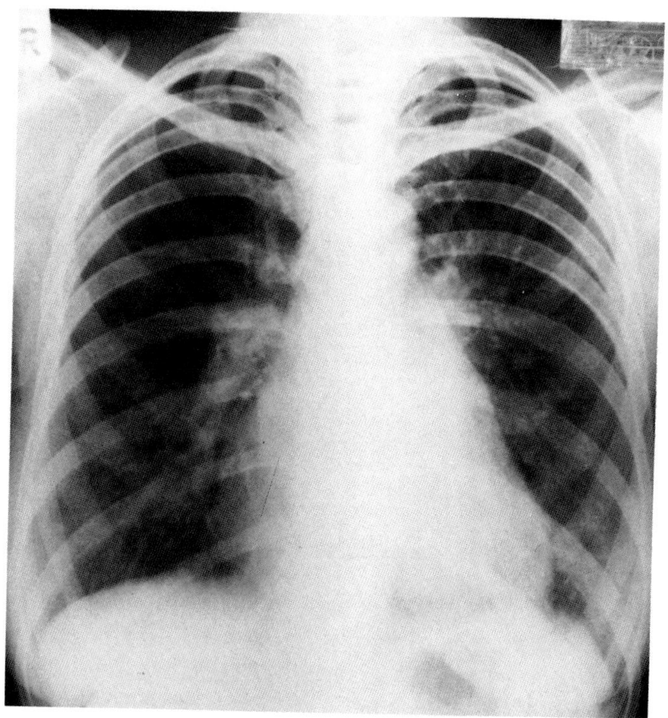

Fig. 23.43 Left atrial myxoma. The chest X-ray shows selective enlargement of the left atrium; the left atrial appendage is also enlarged.

MYXOMAS

The vast majority of these occur in the left atrium, originating from a pedicle attached to the left side of the interatrial septum. Three groups of symptoms may occur:

1. *Obstructive*. Presentation is with shortness of breath. Examination reveals the physical signs of mitral valve disease, though with normal rhythm. The physical signs may vary from day to day or with the position of the patient.

2. *Embolic*. Parts of the tumour may embolize producing stroke or limb ischaemia. On occasion the first diagnosis of myxoma has been histological examination of an embolectomy specimen.

3. *Systemic*. Fever, anaemia, a raised ESR, and sometimes finger clubbing may suggest the possibility of infective endocarditis, though blood cultures are sterile and splenomegaly does not occur.

Radiographic appearances. The plain film appearances may vary from a normal chest X-ray to an enlarged heart with selective left atrial enlargement, and the left atrial appendage may also be enlarged (Fig. 23.43). If obstruction is severe, upper lobe blood diversion or pulmonary oedema may be seen. Very rarely myxomas may be calcified and such calcification may be visible moving up and down in the atrium at fluoroscopy.

Though the diagnosis may be difficult to make clinically it should almost always be made at *echocardiography*. Correctly performed M mode echocardiography should show a virtually normal mitral valve in a patient suspected clinically of having mitral stenosis, and with a mass of echoes appearing in the mitral orifice in ventricular diastole (Fig. 23.44). The usual cause of error is an improperly performed examination rather than the rare sessile myxoma. Correctly performed 2DE should invariably identify the tumour in the left atrium (the commonest site), or anywhere else in the heart. The mobility of the pedunculated tumour, descending into the mitral valve in ventricular diastole is very typical.

Cardiac catheterisation and *angiocardiography* is no longer indicated if an echocardiogram has been correctly performed. In those occasions where the diagnosis is still in doubt, opacification of the left atrium by the levophase of a pulmonary artery angiogram will show the mobile filling defect (Fig. 23.45) and this may also be appreciated on left ventriculography.

Whenever the possibility of a myocardial tumour is in question, the first investigation is *cross-sectional echocardiography* (the M mode is really only useful for left atrial myxomas) and this will show any reactive pericardial effusion, any intracavitary mass (see Fig. 23.46) or any excessive wall thickening. Modern fourth generation *CT scanning* with short scanning times has also been used to demonstrate left atrial myxomas and would probably be

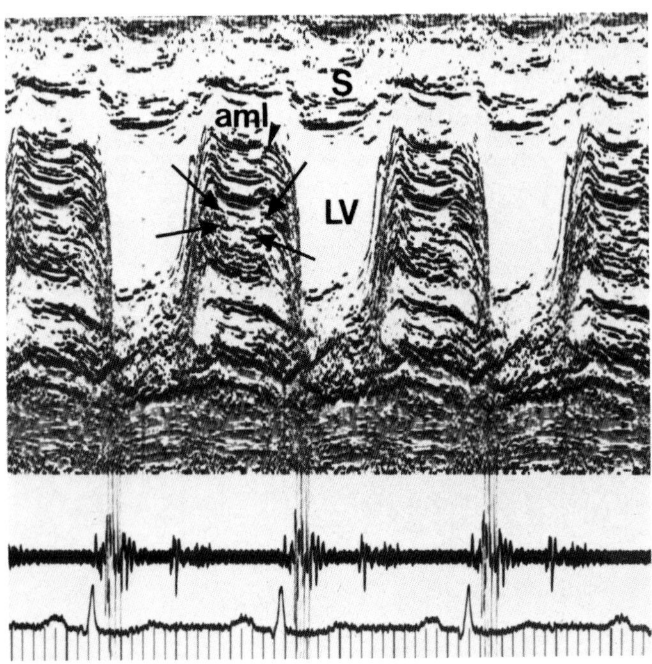

Fig. 23.44 Left atrial myxoma. The M-mode echocardiogram shows a normal anterior mitral valve leaflet (aml), with a mass of echoes appearing in the mitral orifice in diastole (arrows). S = septum; LV = left ventricle.

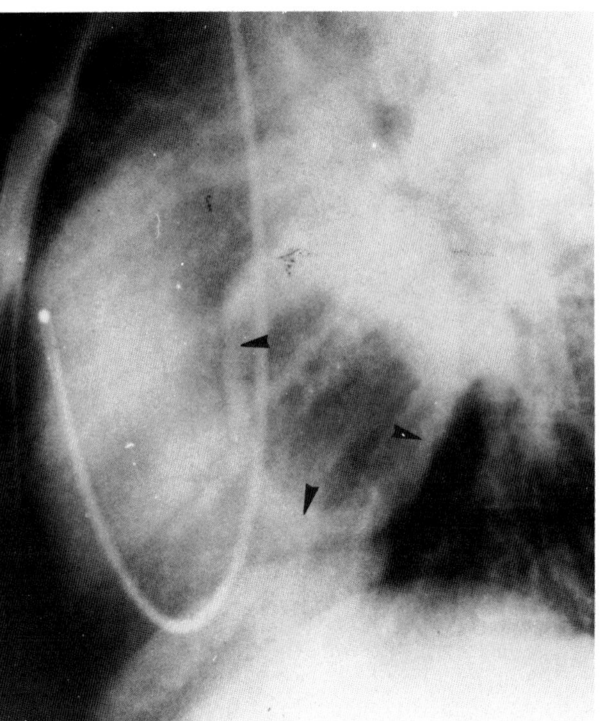

Fig. 23.45 Left atrial myxoma. The angiographic appearances of the left atrium following injection of contrast into the pulmonary artery, are characteristic: a mobile filling defect is clearly appreciated (arrows) (left lateral view).

useful in other forms of myocardial tumour. Angiocardiography and coronary arteriography may be helpful in defining the intracavitary extent of a tumour and also whether it has any pathological circulation from the coronary arteries. MRI is currently being evaluated.

TRAUMA TO THE HEART

Trauma to the heart may be either penetrating or blunt. **Penetrating injuries** usually lead to *haemopericardium* and tamponade, and require emergency drainage and possibly open surgery. Penetrating wounds may also damage the coronary arteries producing myocardial infarction, or disrupt the valves of the heart.

Blunt trauma may lead to myocardial contusion producing a similar clinical finding to myocardial infarction. The coronary arteries may be injured leading to the syndrome of myocardial infarction. The valves may be disrupted producing incompetence.

False aneurysms may result from trauma to the heart. They are characterized by an unusual origin from the left ventricle and a narrow neck. They require surgery as they may rupture.

ENDOCARDITIS

Bacterial (or rickettsial) infections may settle on abnormal valves on either side of the heart, or in congenital heart

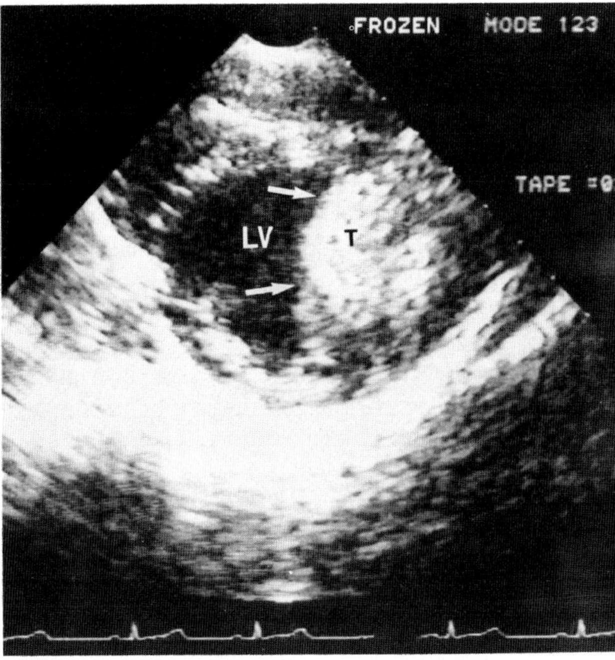

Fig. 23.46 Myocardial tumour. The two-dimensional echocardiogram (short axis view) demonstrates the presence of an intracavitary echo-dense mass (T) (arrows). LV = left ventricle.

sions such as the right ventricle opposite a ventricular septal defect; or on a patent ductus arteriosus. Resultant infection produces a protracted and, unless treated, fatal febrile illness.

M mode echocardiography has a low sensitivity in detecting vegetations in patients with proved bacterial endocarditis. Vegetations are best assessed by *2DE*, where they appear as rapidly oscillating masses that are either attached to or replace normal valve tissue. These masses can be localized to the individual leaflet, and the size and mobility of the lesion readily assessed. A large vegetation attached to the mitral leaflet prolapsing into the atrial cavity is shown in the illustration (Fig. 23.47). The diagnosis of bacterial vegetation was also suspected in the M mode study (Fig. 23.47).

An extremely small vegetation may be missed by *2DE*; improper gain settings may result in a false positive diagnosis. Furthermore, severely fibrotic, calcified or redundant valves may be incorrectly diagnosed as bacterial vegetation, and many patients have normal echocardiograms in the presence of confirmed infective endocarditis. The presence of a visible mass in the clinical setting of infective endocarditis does not always require surgical intervention; approximately 50% of the patients with this situation have been successfully treated medically.

Excavating abscesses may be identified by angiography or by echocardiography.

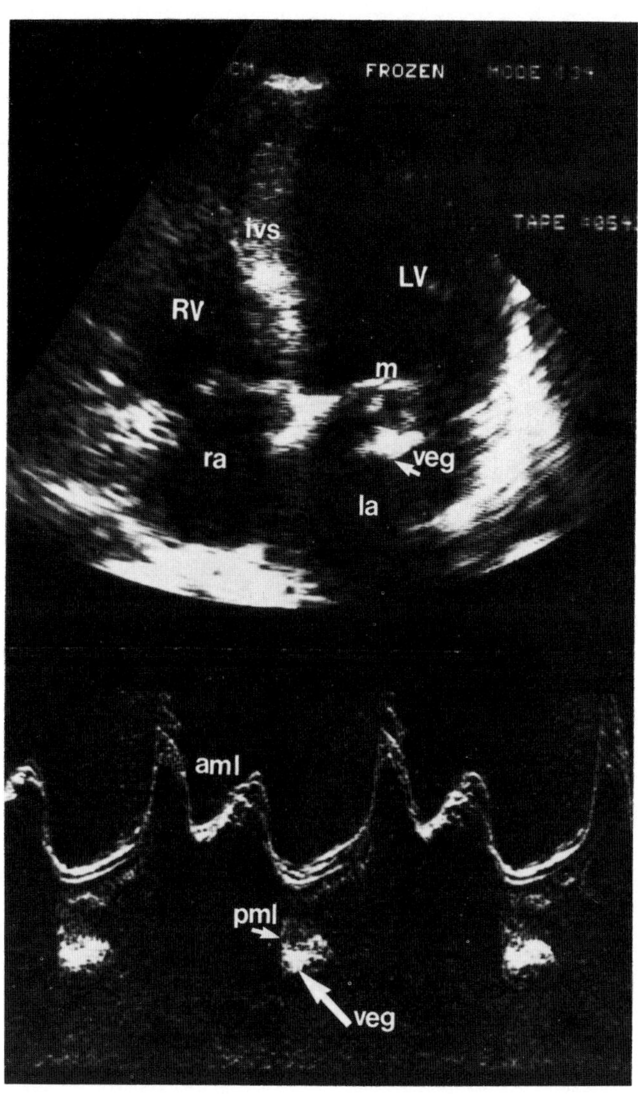

Fig. 23.47 Infective endocarditis. (**A**) The two-dimensional echocardiogram shows a large vegetation (veg) attached to the mitral (m) leaflet. (**B**) M-mode also documented the presence of a vegetation. RV = right ventricle; ivs =intra-ventricular septum; ra = right atrium, LV = left ventricle.

REFERENCES AND SUGGESTIONS FOR FURTHER READING

Braunwald, E: (ed.) (1984) *Heart Disease*. Philadelphia: W. B. Saunders.

Donaldson, R. M., Raphael, M. J. (1982) Missing coronary artery. *British Heart Journal*, **42**, 62–70.

Gensini, G. G. (1975) *Coronary Arteriography*. Mount Kisco, New York: Futura Publishing Co.

Hurst, J. J. (1982) *The Heart*, 5th edn. New York: McGraw Hill.

Jefferson, K., Rees, S. (1980) *Clinical Cardiac Radiology*, 2nd edn. London: Butterworths.

Raphael, M. J., Hawkin, D. R., Allwork, S. P. (1980) The angiographic anatomy of the coronary arteries. *British Journal of Surgery*, **67**, 181–187.

CHAPTER 24

CONGENITAL HEART DISEASE: GENERAL CONSIDERATIONS

Introduction

Many methods of classifying congenital heart disease have been proposed but in the main they have failed as too much emphasis has been placed on embryology. Recognizing that the heart consists of three segments, namely the atria, the ventricles and the great arteries, a descriptive scheme has been devised which not only includes all known possibilities but also has the potential to describe any as yet unrecorded. This method is known as **sequential chamber localization**.

The embryological development of the heart and its detailed anatomy will not be described in depth. Nevertheless morphological anatomy is an integral part of the correct recognition of heart chambers and great arteries enabling connections to be established. Hence sufficient detail will be included in this chapter to ensure that correct identification can be made. Where relevant, these features will also be included in the consideration of individual conditions (see Ch. 25). Thus, in order to diagnose congenital heart disease accurately, and in particular the more complex lesions, it is necessary to have a working understanding of sequential chamber localization. It is proposed in the present chapter to discuss general considerations and the principles of diagnosis. The subsequent chapter will describe in some detail specific conditions. The available diagnostic methods will be discussed and an attempt will be made to evaluate their relative merits in each condition.

THE NOMENCLATURE OF CONGENITAL HEART DISEASE

SEQUENTIAL CHAMBER LOCALIZATION

The terminology applied to simple lesions, such as pulmonary stenosis, secundum atrial septal defect and coarctation of the aorta, is well accepted and offers no problems. However, describing hearts with abnormal connections which are found in 30% of symptomatic infants presenting to a specialized unit, the ideal terminology should allow an easy, accurate and unambiguous description of any abnormality. A nomenclature based on chamber identification and connections (Shinebourne et a 1976) is used widely in the United Kingdom and Europe and many of the major centres in North America. When the sequential approach to diagnosis is applied, the first priority is to determine atrial situs. The connection between the atria and the ventricles and between the ventricles and the great arteries are then described. Next the relative positions of the two atria, the two ventricular chambers and the great arteries are identified. Finally additional anomalies are listed and any abnormal morphology stated. The various possibilities are shown in Table 24.1.

1. Atrial situs

In the normal heart the most distinctive features of the morphological right and left chambers are the attachments of the great veins. As, however, anomalous pulmonary and systemic venous drainage is relatively frequent in complex congenital heart disease, only the atrial appendages allow the unequivocal differentiation between morphological right and left atrial chambers. The right atrial appendage has the shape of a blunt triangle with a broad base. The left atrial appendage is much narrower having a restricted junction with the smooth-walled atrium. These morphological features are readily differentiated by angiocardiography in both the frontal and lateral projections. Whilst selective angiography of the left- and right-sided atria will allow the determination of atrial situs, this can result in the use of a volume of contrast media large enough to compromise the infant's circulation. For this reason, indirect methods of determining atrial situs are often preferred.

DETERMINATION OF ATRIAL SITUS

Situs solitus

The right atrium (systemic venous atrium) lies to the right of the left atrium. The right main bronchus is situated on the right side of the thorax. Normally the left main bronchus is twice the length of the right main bronchus

able 24.1 Sequential chamber localization

trial situs	1. Normal atrial arrangement (solitus) 2. Mirror image arrangement (inversus) 3. Dextro-isomerism 4. Levo-isomerism
trioventricular junction Type of atrioventricular connection:	
Biventricular atrioventricular connection	1. Concordant 2. Discordant 3. Ambiguus (atrial isomerism)
Univentricular atrioventricular connection Double inlet ventricle with	1. Left morphology 2. Right morphology 3. Indeterminate morphology
absent connection	1. Left 2. Right
Mode of atrioventricular connection	1. Two normal valves 2. Common valve 3. Overriding valve 4. Straddling valve 5. Stenotic valve 6. Imperforate valve
entricular relationships Position of RV chamber relative to LV chamber	1. Right/left orientation 2. Anterior/posterior orientation 3. Superior/inferior orientation
entriculoarterial junction Connection	1. Concordant 2. Discordant 3. Double outlet 4. Single outlet ventricle
Relations Position of aorta relative to pulmonary trunk	1. Right/left relations 2. Anterior/posterior relations
nfundibular morphology	1. Sub-aortic infundibulum 2. Sub-pulmonary infundibulum 3. Bilateral infundibulum 4. Bilaterally deficient infundibulum
ssociated malformations	1. Abnormalities of systemic or pulmonary venous return 2. Atrial abnormalities e.g. septal defects, diaphragm 3. Ventricular abnormalities, e.g. septal defects, diaphragm, muscle bar, cardiomyopathy 4. Great artery abnormalities: a. Valves — stenosis, prolapse, atresia b. Arterial trunk — stenosis including coarctation, hypoplasia, interruption c. Interarterial communication, e.g. ductus, aorta pulmonary window d. Coronary artery — anomalous origins e. Fistulous communication, e.g. rupture of sinus of Valsalva

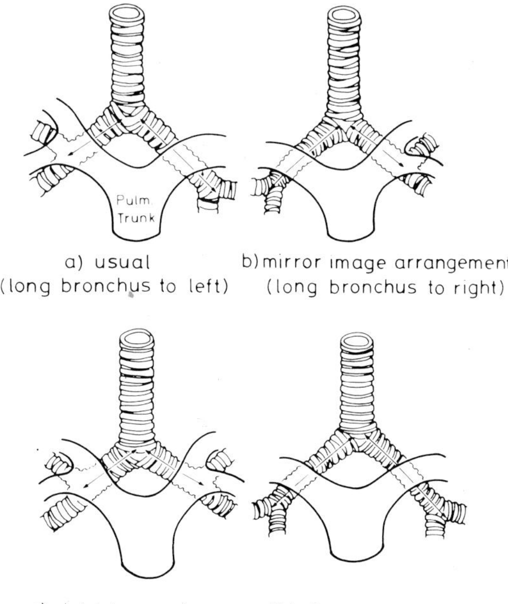

Fig. 24.1 Diagram of normal inversus and ambiguus bronchi

Fig. 24.1). In the abdomen, the liver is on the right and he spleen is on the left. Thus it may be possible to deter-nine atrial situs from plain films or tomograms Fig. 24.2A), though the use of a Cincinnati filter (tin 0.4 nm: copper 0.5 mm) yields higher diagnostic accuracy Fig. 24.2B). Atrial situs almost invariably follows the situs of the main bronchi (Partridge et al 1975). Less reliably, it is indicated by the situs of the abdominal viscera.

Situs inversus. If the situs of all the thoracic and abdominal viscera are inverted, then a mirror image of situs solitus is present. If the thoracic viscera are in the situs solitus position and the abdominal viscera inverted, this is known as *isolated situs solitus*. Conversely, if the thoracic viscera are inverted in the presence of solitus abdominal viscera, *isolated situs inversus* is present.

Levo-isomerism and dextro-isomerism. If atrial situs is indeterminate with either two right atria or two left atria present, this may be indicated by symmetrical bronchi. Two morphological right bronchi are accompanied by two morphological right atria (dextro-isomerism) and this is associated with asplenia. Similarly with two left bronchi, there are two left atria (levo-isomerism) and polysplenia is present (Macartney et al 1980). Partridge and colleagues (1975) have established the average length of the right and left main bronchi in relation to age allowing bronchi to be differentiated morphologically (Fig. 24.2C).

Echocardiography. Using cross-sectional echocardiography, horizontal sections through the abdomen at the level of the 12th dorsal vertebra will determine the position of the great arteries and from this situs can also be inferred (Fig. 24.3). In situs solitus, there is symmetrical arrangement of the two great vessels with the aorta recognized by its pulsation lying to the left of the spine and the inferior vena cava to the right. The mirror image arrangement

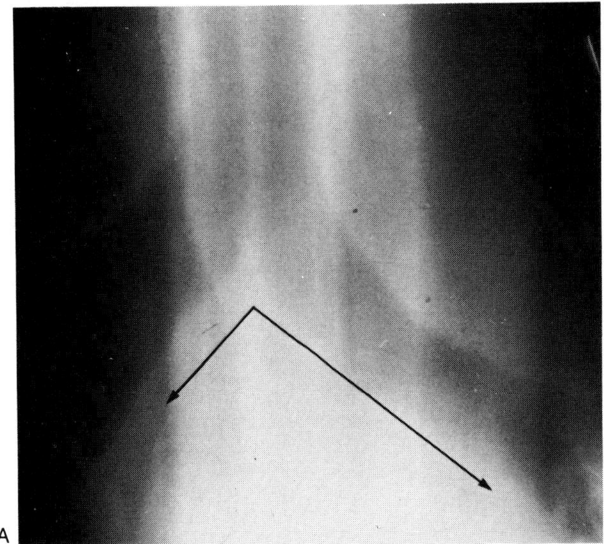

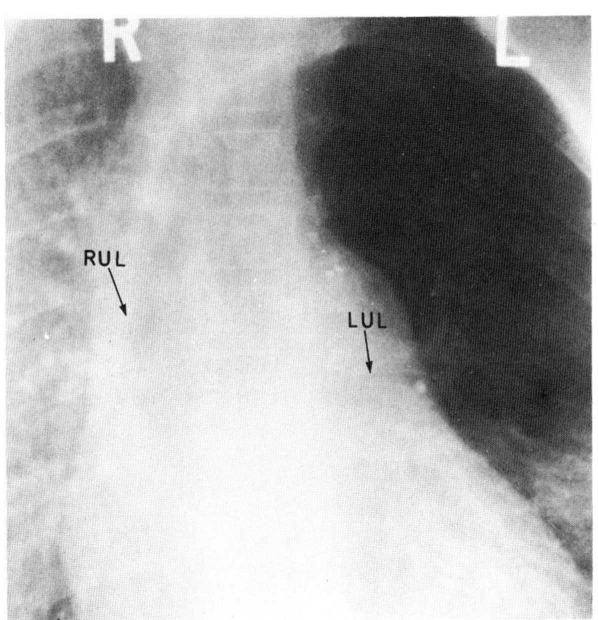

Fig. 24.2 A. Tomograph illustrating left main bronchus is twice length of right main bronchus as shown by arrows. Atrial situs almost invariably follows bronchial situs. **B.** Use of Cincinnati film outlining the right and left main bronchi. Note obstructive hyperinflation of L. upper lobe. **C.** Diagram relating bronchial lengths with age.

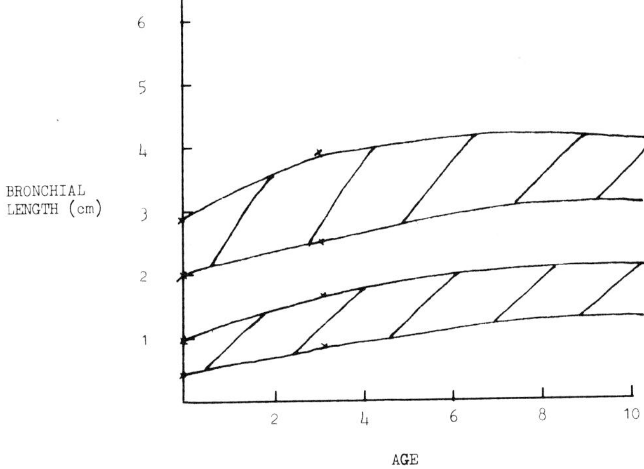

occurs in situs inversus. In the presence of right isomerism, the aorta and the inferior vena cava will both be on the same (usually left) side of the spine. In left isomerism, there is a central aorta and the azygos vein can be seen posterior to the aorta (Fig. 24.4). In addition all hepatic veins drain directly to the atria. The inferior vena cava is absent as there is no morphological right atrial component present. Experience has shown that the frequency of isomerism may be as high as 10% in symptomatic infants referred to a major paediatric cardiology centre. It is of interest that neonates with asplenia have a high incidence of pneumococcal sepsis.

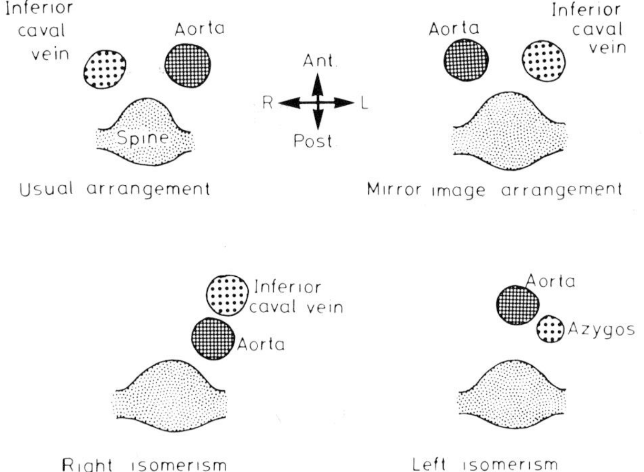

Fig. 24.3 Diagram of relative positions of abdominal great vessels to the spine in the four types of abdominal situs.

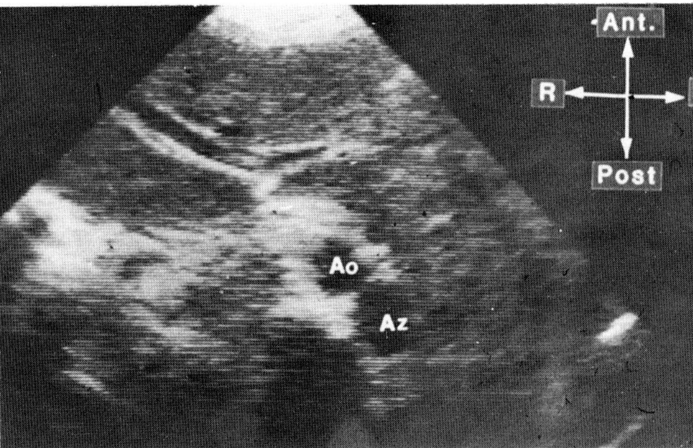

Fig. 24.4 Cross-sectional echocardiogram at level T12 in a patient with left isomerism.

2. Analysis of the atrioventricular junction

Having determined the arrangement of the atrial chambers, the atrioventricular connections are analysed which demands the determination of ventricular morphology.

3. Ventricular morphology

The morphological right ventricle is coarsely trabeculated (Fig. 24.40). The morphological left ventricle in contrast has a fine trabecular pattern and a smooth septal surface (Fig. 24.41). It is these different trabecular patterns which allow the right and left ventricles to be distinguished by angiography. In rare instances, a single chamber is found in the ventricular mass which has neither right nor left ventricular characteristics and this is then called a ventricular chamber of indeterminate morphology.

4. Atrioventricular connections

Having established atrial situs and ventricular morphology, it will be evident that in the majority of cases each atrium connects with a ventricle, i.e. the atrioventricular connection is biventricular. Atrioventricular concordance describes the connection of the morphological right atrium to the morphological right ventricle and the left atrium to the left ventricle. Conversely, atrioventricular discordance is present when atria connect to an inappropriate ventricle. The term 'ambiguus' atrioventricular connection is reserved for those hearts with isomeric atrial chambers when the terms concordant or discordant are not applicable. In some hearts the atria connect only to one chamber in the ventricular mass, a so-called univentricular atrioventricular connection (Fig. 24.5). This may occur in two circumstances: a) with double inlet connection and b) with an absent atrioventricular connection. In double inlet connection, both atria connect to the same ventricular chamber which may be left, right or of indeterminate morphology. With double inlet left ventricle, there will be an antero-superior rudimentary right ventricle. In hearts with double inlet right ventricle, there is a postero-inferior rudimentary left ventricle. Similarly, when there is absence of the left or right atrioventricular connection, the atria will still connect to a right, left or indeterminate ventricle.

The type of atrioventricular connection is readily determined by cross-sectional echocardiography using four chamber sections (see section on Echocardiography, p. 634). For biventricular hearts, the mitral and tricuspid valves can usually be distinguished as the septal leaflet of the latter is attached nearer to the apex of the heart (Fig. 24.6). Hence the left and right ventricles can be distinguished because embryologically the mitral valve develops as part of the left ventricle and the tricuspid valve as part of the right ventricle. In addition the left ventricle has two papillary muscles to which the mitral valve is attached by chordae. In contrast the tricuspid valve does not have discrete papillary muscles and chordae can be seen inserting directly into the right ventricular side of the interventricular septum (Fig. 24.7). In hearts with univentricular atrioventricular connection, the type of connection is easily identified as double inlet or absent connection (Rigby et al 1981).

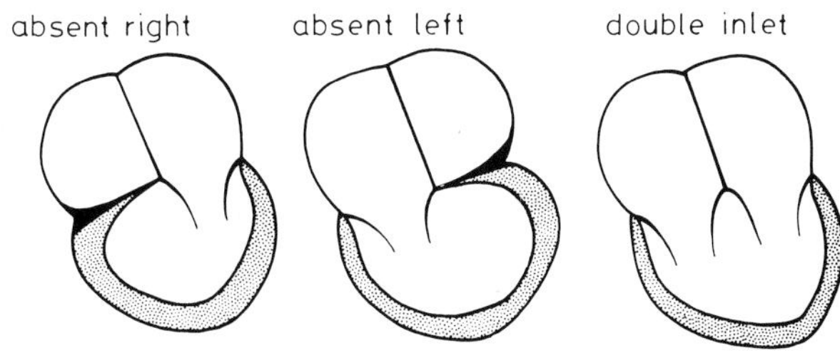

Fig. 24.5 Illustration of the three basic types of univentricular atrioventricular connection.

5. Mode of atrioventricular connection

The atrioventricular junction is that part of the heart where the atria connect to the ventricles. In the normal (concordant) heart it consists of two fibrous annulae which also support the leaflets of the mitral and tricuspid valves. This is known as the 'type' of connection. The morphology of the valves which guard the atrioventricular junction is referred to as the 'mode' of atrioventricular connection (Fig. 24.8). If the connection is biventricular, it may be via two valves one of which may be imperforate, override or straddle the ventricular septum or alternatively via a

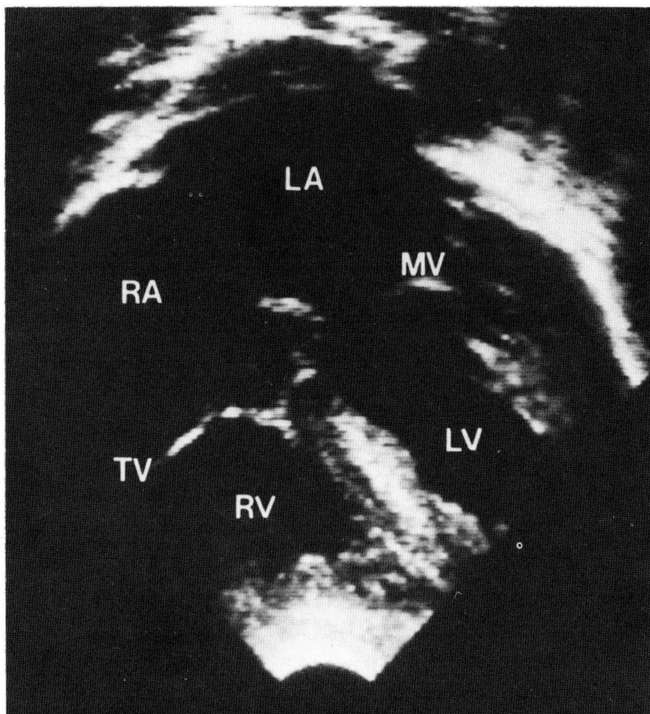

Fig. 24.6 Normal apical four-chamber cross-sectional echocardiogram demonstrating septal leaflet of tricuspid valve closer to the apex than the septal leaflet of the mitral valve.

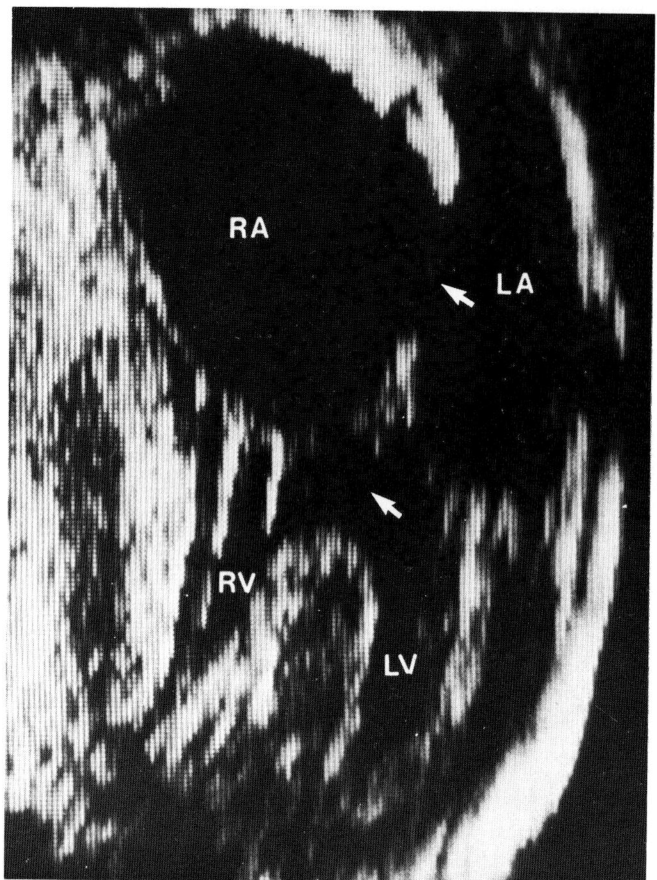

Fig. 24.7 Four-chamber cross-sectional echocardiogram showing a perimembranous inlet ventricular septal defect (lower arrow) and a secundum atrial septal defect (upper arrow). Chordal attachments of the tricuspid valve are seen inserting into the right ventricular side of the septum.

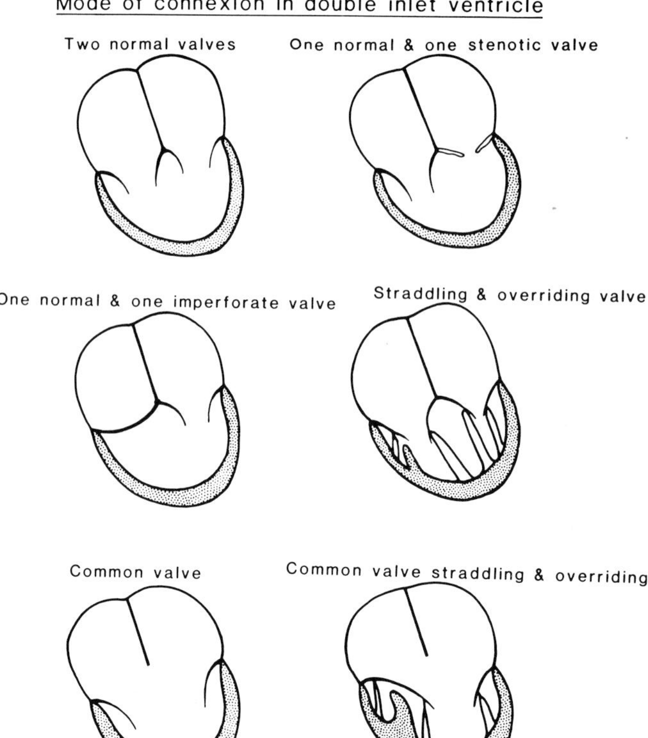

Fig. 24.8 Illustration of the various modes of atrioventricular connection in hearts with univentricular atrioventricular connection.

common valve which must both override and straddle the trabecular septum. Overriding valves are assigned to the ventricle to which they are most committed. Thus hearts with straddling and overriding valves can be categorized as having either a biventricular or a univentricular atrioventricular connection, depending upon the commitment of the overriding valve. Cross-sectional echocardiography is much superior to angiography in determining the mode of atrioventricular connection. The exact anatomical relations of the valves to the septum have considerable surgical implications.

6. The ventriculo-arterial junction

There are four possible types of ventriculo-arterial connection (Fig. 24.9). *Ventriculo-arterial concordance* describes the normal situation of the aorta arising from the morphological left ventricle and the pulmonary artery from the right ventricle. *Ventriculo-arterial discordance* describes the converse connection when the great arteries arise from inappropriate ventricles. *Double outlet ventricle* is present

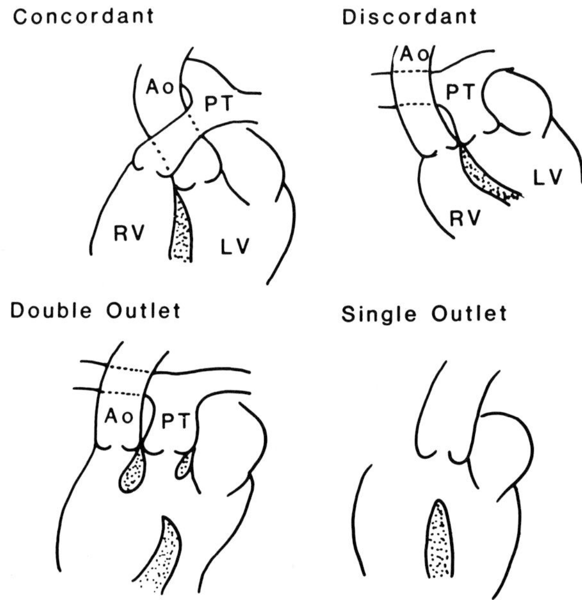

Fig. 24.9 Illustrations of the various types of ventriculo-arterial connection.

when both great arteries arise from the same chamber. Most commonly this would be from the right ventricle but hearts with double outlet left ventricle also exist and occasionally the great arteries arise from a single indeterminate ventricular chamber. For the purpose of categorization, great arteries are assigned to the chamber attached to more than 50% of their diameter. For example in tetralogy of Fallot, the aorta may override the septum by more than 50% so that it arises predominantly from the right ventricle. In this circumstance, the ventriculo-arterial connection will be double outlet right ventricle despite the tetralogy morphology. Finally, *single outlet* heart describes a solitary great artery, truncus arteriosus, aorta or pulmonary artery, arising from the left ventricle, right ventricle, or most commonly overriding the septum so that it is shared between the ventricular chambers. When describing the relationship of the great arteries, the position of the aortic valve relative to the pulmonary valve is described as either to the right or the left and lying either anteriorly or posteriorly. The third aspect of the ventriculo-arterial junction to be described is the presence or absence of a subpulmonary or subaortic infundibulum.

Although angiography gives the clearest definition of the great arteries, cross-sectional echocardiography will usually provide excellent visualization of the whole of the ascending aorta, its arch and proximal descending aorta together with the proximal pulmonary arteries. Both techniques readily allow the description of all aspects of the ventriculo-arterial junction.

EPIDEMIOLOGY AND CLINICAL PRESENTATION

EPIDEMIOLOGY

The incidence of congenital heart disease in Great Britain is 8 per 1000 live births. With improved diagnosis and treatment, the mortality in the first year of life may be as low as 0.6 to 0.8 per 1000 live births in some centres.

It appears that little is known about the specific aetiology of congenital heart disease but some 90 to 95% of cases can be explained by multifactorial inheritance. It is, however, well recognized that genetic defects are associated with congenital heart disease in 5% of cases. For example, Down's syndrome has a high incidence of septal and endocardial cushion defects. The XO-genetic form of Turner's syndrome (ovarian dysgenesis) is commonly associated with coarctation while the mosaic form (XX–XO) is associated with pulmonary stenosis. It is also well known that some maternal illnesses in the first three months of pregnancy, during the critical phase of cardiac development, are likely to give rise to congenital heart lesions. Rubella is probably the best known, the most common defects being peripheral pulmonary artery stenosis and patent ductus arteriosus.

Clinical presentation

Children with congenital heart disease are usually of normal height and weight unless they are cyanosed or in chronic heart failure. Impairment of growth reflects the extent of the underlying condition. The severity of symptoms correlates with the degree of functional disturbance. Thus the majority of patients who have a simple lesion such as a small ventricular septal defect have a normal growth rate. Even if the underlying lesion is complex but the pulmonary flow is normal, the patients are usually asymptomatic. Clinical presentation may occur at any age but if it is in the neonatal period, symptoms are likely to be severe. These may include heart failure, cyanosis and cardiogenic shock. Whilst children presenting at a later age may do so with severe symptoms, heart disease may also be recognized because of a murmur being heard on routine clinical examination or the presence of relatively minor symptoms. A large heart on a chest radiograph may also be observed following a radiological examination of the chest for some unconnected reason. Where there is disability, clinical, pathophysiological or imaging abnormalities may result from the following:

1. Increased or decreased pulmonary flow.
2. Volume or pressure overload of a ventricle.

Before discussing these in detail, brief definitions of commonly encountered terms will be given.

Oxygen saturation. This represents the percentage of oxyhaemoglobin present in the sample.

Partial pressure of oxygen. Oxygen represents 21% of the atmospheric pressure (760 mmHg). Thus, allowing for a reduction across the alveolar-arterial blood barrier, the partial pressure of oxygen is approximately 100 mmHg while breathing room air.

Oxygen content. This is the absolute amount of oxyhaemoglobin present together with the oxygen dissolved in the plasma. If the saturation is less than 91%, there is arterial desaturation which may lead to cyanosis. This will only be clinically detectable if at least 5 g of reduced haemoglobin are present.

Cyanosis. This may be either central or peripheral.

Central cyanosis. This occurs in the presence of a right to left shunt which bypasses the pulmonary capillary bed. These shunts may be due to either a cardiac abnormality or lung disease. Clinically, it may be difficult to distinguish between significant cyanotic heart disease or lung problems such as the respiratory distress syndrome in a neonate. This distinction can be achieved by allowing the baby to breathe 100% oxygen until an equilibrium state is reached. In the presence of cyanotic heart disease, the arterial $P\text{O}_2$ does not usually rise above 150 mmHg and never above 200 mmHg. If cyanosis occurs in the presence of primary lung disease, it is often possible to achieve an arterial $P\text{O}_2$ over 150 mmHg. However, there is a small group of patients with an intrapulmonary shunt in whom it is not possible to record values over 100 mm Hg.

Peripheral cyanosis. This is found where there is a low cardiac output, e.g. severe aortic stenosis. It is due to excess reduced haemoglobin as a result of capillary stasis.

Clubbing. The cause is uncertain but it may be related to connective soft tissue overgrowth secondary to oxygen desaturation. Clubbing does not occur under the age of 1 year. Hypertrophic pulmonary osteoarthropathy, in the presence of clubbing, is rare in cyanotic congenital heart disease. Correction of the underlying abnormality nearly always leads to resolution of the clubbing.

Polycythaemia. Persistent arterial desaturation stimulates the bone marrow leading to haemoglobin values greater than 15 g per 100 ml. Whilst initially increasing the oxygen carrying capacity of the blood when the packed cell volume exceeds 80%, this benefit is offset by the high viscosity which may result in venous thrombosis. This is particularly likely to occur with haemoglobin values higher than 21 g per 100 ml. Associated coagulation defects also give rise to increased bleeding risks at the time of surgery.

PULMONARY FLOW

Increased flow

In the normal person at rest only approximately one-third of the pulmonary capillary bed is open. On exercise more of the capillary bed opens up to accommodate the increased flow demand. The maximum flow rate that can be accommodated without an increase in pulmonary artery pressure is approximately 15 litres per minute. If the flow rate is above this, the pulmonary artery pressure must rise in order to overcome the resistance of the pulmonary vascular bed. This situation can occur in association with such conditions as hyperthyroidism. However, it is unusual for the pulmonary flow to increase to such an extent that pulmonary vascular resistance has to rise except in the presence of a very large left to right shunt. In the fetus, 90% of the right ventricular output passes through the ductus arteriosus into the systemic circulation and only about 10% of the right ventricular output perfuses the lungs. The reason is that the resistance to flow in the pulmonary circuit is greater than that in the systemic circuit. At birth when the lungs expand, the pulmonary vascular resistance falls to its normal level over about 10 days, reversing the ratio. During this time, there is mechanical expansion of the pulmonary capillary bed. There is a consequent rise in arterial Po_2 and alveolar Po_2. As a result, the pulmonary arterial pressure gradually falls to normal.

The factors which determine this course of events are not known with any certainty. In a very small number of cases, it is just possible that without any intrinsic cardiac abnormality, normal involution does not take place. These patients may have pulmonary artery pressures at or near systemic levels from birth (primary pulmonary hypertension). Where, however, there is an abnormal communication between the systemic and pulmonary circuits, the influence on the pulmonary resistance appears to be related to the size and situation of the defect.

Decreased pulmonary flow

In the presence of an intact atrial and ventricular septum right ventricular outflow tract obstruction will lead to an elevation of right ventricular pressure in order to overcome the obstruction. Prior to the onset of right ventricular failure, the right ventricular output is usually within normal limits and the lung fields show little or no deviation from normal. However, in the presence of a septal defect particulary in the ventricular septum, a right to left shunt is present secondary to the right ventricular outflow tract obstruction. Thus the pulmonary flow is diminished and oligaemia is visible on the plain film.

VOLUME OR PRESSURE OVERLOAD OF A VENTRICLE

Pressure overload

In the presence of increased obstruction to forward flow, concentric hypertrophy is found prior to the onset of frank ventricular failure except in neonates with critical obstruction when failure rapidly supervenes. In the presence of increased obstruction to forward flow, ventricular enlarge-

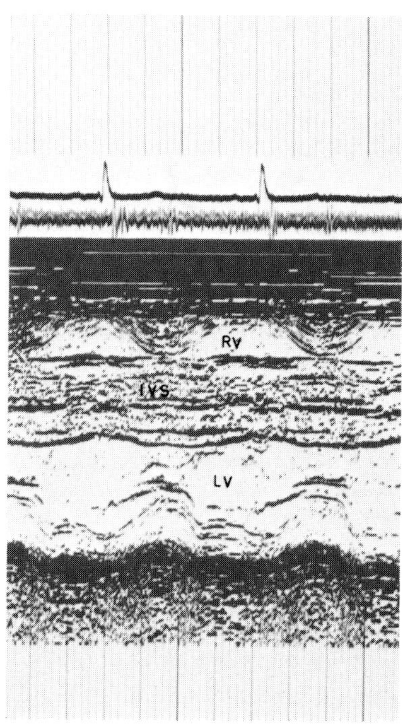

Fig. 24.10 M-mode Echocardiogram showing thickened left ventricular wall and i.v. septum.

ment is minimal and the chest radiograph often shows no significant abnormality. Echocardiography is much more sensitive in detecting hypertrophy and ventricular wall thickening can be clearly demonstrated (Fig. 24.10). The ability of the left ventricle to deal with obstruction is great and massive left ventricular hypertrophy may occur without symptoms being present. This can be regarded as a disadvantage because the absence of symptoms gives no warning of the presence of significant disease. It is in these cases that sudden death may occur due to ventricular fibrillation or asystole in a previously asymptomatic patient. If the obstruction occurs in the right ventricular outflow tract, symptoms such as dyspnoea and fatigue tend to appear early.

Volume overload

This occurs secondary either to incompetence of an atrioventricular or semilunar valve or in the presence of significant left to right shunting. The ventricle both dilates to accommodate the extra blood and hypertrophies in order to expel it. An increased volume of blood enters the ventricle in diastole either due to increased atrial volume secondary to an incompetent atrioventricular valve or through an incompetent semilunar valve (almost always the aortic valve). As a result, the heart is seen to be enlarged on the chest radiograph. If the abnormality is on the left side of the heart, the left ventricle may be both dilated and hypertrophied. This is by no means always so and both ventricles may be affected in the presence of a primary left-sided lesion due to strain on the right ventricle from associated pulmonary hypertension. As with pure hypertrophy of the ventricle, the echocardiogram is very sensitive in demonstrating a dilated ventricle (Fig. 24.11). Eventually, unless sudden death occurs, both obstruction to ventricular outflow and volume overloading terminate in fluid retention. Symptoms of left heart failure include dyspnoea on effort, orthopnoea and paroxysmal nocturnal dyspnoea with the usual signs of left heart failure on the radiograph. These are cardiac enlargement and pulmonary venous hypertension leading to pulmonary oedema (Fig. 24.12 A & B). Right heart failure results in excessive fatigue, sometimes dizziness, sometimes blurring of vision, vomiting and the triad of elevated peripheral venous pressure, an enlarged tender liver and peripheral oedema. Peripheral oedema, however, is rare in infants and young children and blurring of vision difficult, if not impossible, to detect in the younger age group. In the presence of right heart failure, the chest radiograph shows an enlarged heart but the lung fields are usually clear. As indicated above, right and left heart failure frequently coexist.

PULMONARY HYPERTENSION

The upper limits of the normal pulmonary arterial pressure are 25 to 30 mmHg in systole and 15 mmHg in diastole. At birth, the pulmonary systolic value is approximately at systemic value (60 mmHg) but usually falls to the normal value of 25 mmHg by the age of 10 days following a dramatic fall in the pulmonary vascular resistance. In the presence of a large ventricular septal defect, the pulmonary vascular resistance falls more slowly. Thus the onset of heart failure is usually delayed until the second month of life. By definition, pulmonary hypertension is present if the pulmonary artery pressure is above the normal value.

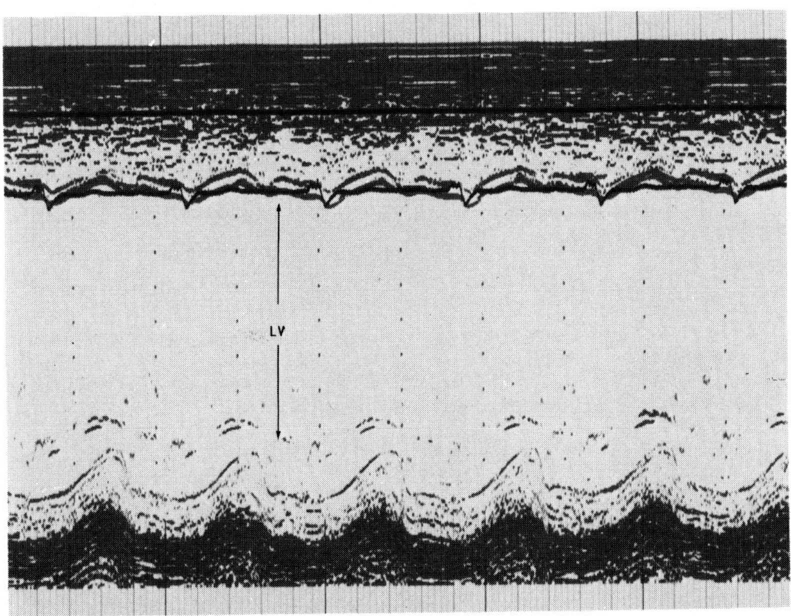

Fig. 24.11 M-mode Echocardiogram showing dilated left ventricular cavity (arrows).

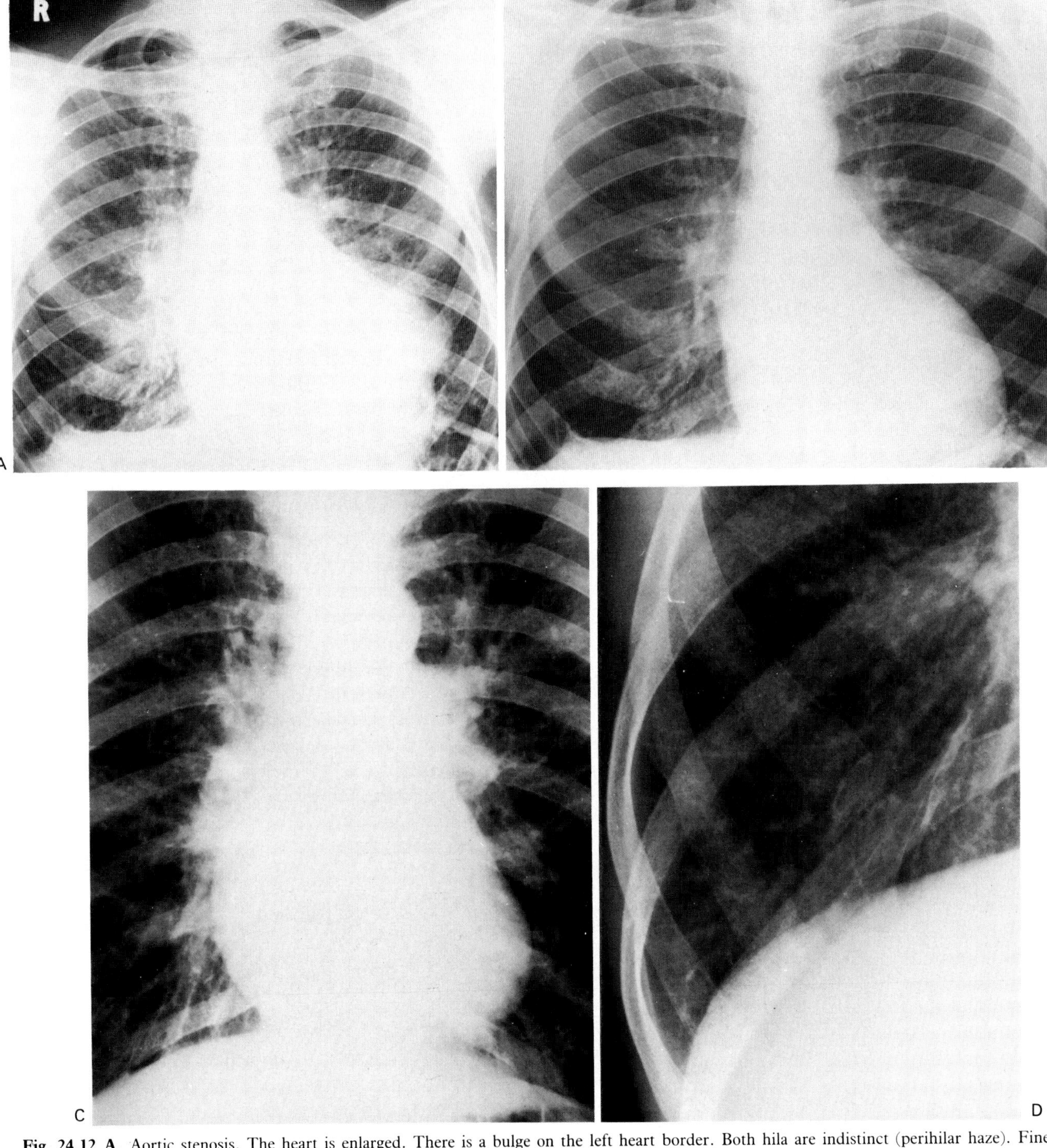

Fig. 24.12 A. Aortic stenosis. The heart is enlarged. There is a bulge on the left heart border. Both hila are indistinct (perihilar haze). Fine nodular shadowing is present in both mid-zones. The appearances are those of acute pulmonary oedema. **B.** Cardiac outline is smaller and the bulge has disappeared indicating a localised pericardial effusion. The perihilar haze has also resolved. This resolution is seen following diuretic therapy. **C.** Pulmonary venous hypertension indicated by upper lobe blood diversion. **D.** Septal lines extending out to the pleural surface and not continuous with pulmonary veins.

In practice, severe pulmonary arterial hypertension is seen in the following groups.

1. Infants with large left to right shunts.
2. Patients with left ventricular inflow tract obstruction, e.g. mitral stenosis or cor triatrium. These patients are symptomatic and if it can be established that irreversible changes in the pulmonary vascular bed are not present, then early surgical correction should be undertaken.

3. Established pulmonary vascular disease (Eisenmenger situation). These patients will initially be asymptomatic but will gradually develop effort intolerance, haemoptysis and syncope. Due to irreversible changes in the pulmonary vascular bed, they are not amenable to surgery.

Elevation of pulmonary vascular resistance

Elevated pulmonary vascular resistance may be regarded as reversible or irreversible. Hypoventilation, lung disease and hypoxia may lead to a reversible rise in pulmonary vascular resistance. If the underlying condition is successfully treated, the pulmonary vascular resistance will fall. The likelihood of success can be assessed by the response to breathing 100% oxygen. If a reversible condition is present, pulmonary vascular resistance will fall. If it does not fall, this indicates irreversible changes are present in the pulmonary vascular bed.

Increased pulmonary venous pressure

A rise in pulmonary venous pressure occurs secondary to any obstructive lesion on the left side of the heart, for example, aortic stenosis. Obstruction to left ventricular outflow results in a rise in left ventricular end-diastolic pressure and the left atrial pressure has to rise above this to ensure adequate left ventricular filling in diastole. The pulmonary venous pressure rises with the left atrial pressure and if it equals or exceeds the osmotic pressure of the plasma (above about 27 mmHg), exudation of fluid tends to occur into the lung parenchyma. Nevertheless, certain patients will tolerate chronic pressures of up to 30–35 mmHg without evidence of oedema. If the venous pressure rises very rapidly, acute pulmonary oedema occurs (Fig. 24.12A and B). In response to the rise in pulmonary venous pressures, reflex pulmonary venous constriction occurs. There is secondary rise in pressure in the pulmonary capillary bed and also in the pulmonary arteries. Further exudation of fluid is prevented when the extravascular osmotic pressure equals the pressure in the pulmonary veins. As older patients spend the majority of their time in the erect or semi-erect position, the added effect of gravity means that a critical pressure level is first reached in the capillary bed of the lower lobes. Reflex vasoconstriction, therefore, occurs first in this region and pulmonary blood flow is diverted to the upper zones. Thus the radiological phenomenon of upper lobe blood diversion is the first radiographic change indicating a rise in pulmonary venous pressure (Fig. 24.12C). It is probably detectable radiologically when the pulmonary venous pressure reaches 17–18 mmHg. This is followed by the development of septal lines (Fig. 24.12D). If the underlying condition persists, a functional constriction of the pulmonary arterioles is followed by organic occlusions leading to an elevated pulmonary vascular resistance and a consequent rise in pulmonary artery pressure which may reach systemic levels. The radiological changes in this situation are most commonly seen in association with acquired valve disease and ischaemic heart disease. They are described in Chapter 23. They are relatively uncommon in congenital heart disease but do occur following obstructive lesions on the left side of the heart.

AN APPROACH TO IMAGING TECHNIQUES IN THE INVESTIGATION OF CONGENITAL HEART DISEASE

In the management of congenital heart disease, much more information is required than can be obtained from a chest radiograph. Nevertheless, useful information may be present which may have an important bearing on the planning of subsequent investigations. Although it is only occasionally that it may be possible to make a definitive diagnosis such as coarctation of the aorta, the interpretation of the frontal radiograph does allow comment on heart size and chamber enlargement, bronchial and visceral situs and the vascular pattern of the lungs. The position of the aortic arch can be determined together with abnormalities in the position of the ascending aorta.

CLINICAL FEATURES

It is not essential before giving a radiological opinion on the plain film to have a complete clinical diagnosis. In fact this may not even be desirable; firstly, because it may influence the assessment unduly and secondly because it is not unknown for a preliminary clinical diagnosis to be incorrect. Nevertheless, it is important to know whether or not certain clinical signs are present.

1. Heart failure

Providing the patient is not in heart failure, it can be accepted that cardiac configuration and size as seen on the radiograph reflect the nature of the underlying abnormality. If, however, the patient is in failure, cardiac dilatation occurs and the heart size no longer accurately reflects the underlying lesion. Although the presence of failure largely nullifies the radiological assessment of heart size, the knowledge is in itself of value because certain conditions are more liable to result in heart failure at certain ages than others.

2. Pulmonary hypertension resulting from raised pulmonary vascular resistance

As has been described, pulmonary hypertension secondary to raised pulmonary vascular resistance can occur in infants and young children without any of the classical signs being present in the pulmonary vasculature. If this can be recognized clinically, which is not always easy, it is important this information should be available so that associated right ventricular hypertrophy and peripheral pulmonary oligaemia can be attributed to the correct cause. Further, different congenital heart conditions tend to develop pulmonary hypertension to different degrees and at different ages. This, in itself, is important in the radiological differential diagnosis.

3. Cyanosis

The presence of central cyanosis indicates that insufficient oxygenated blood is reaching the systemic circulation. This may be due to:

1. A right to left shunt related to either right ventricular outflow tract obstruction, e.g. Fallot's tetralogy or significantly raised pulmonary vascular resistance e.g. Eisenmenger situation.
2. Complete mixing of oxygenated and deoxygenated blood, e.g. single ventricle or total anomalous pulmonary venous return.
3. Failure of the pulmonary and systemic circuits to communicate as in transposition with intact ventricular septum.

4. Clinical course

Individual congenital abnormalities which have very similar radiological appearances often run very different courses and the knowledge of what is to be expected in each abnormality is of the greatest value in radiological interpretation. For example, right atrial and ventricular enlargement with pulmonary pleonaemia occurs in a number of congenital heart conditions including secundum atrial septal defect. If, however, these appearances are seen in early childhood in a patient who is not thriving because of a cardiac abnormality, it is unlikely that they are due to a secundum defect alone. It would be unusual for a patient with such an uncomplicated defect to present with severe symptoms at this age.

THE SIZE OF THE HEART AS SEEN ON THE FRONTAL RADIOGRAPH

As most patients with congenital heart disease are radiographed on a number of occasions, the cardiothoracic ratio provides a useful basis for the comparison of heart size over a period of time. Nevertheless, it must be appreciated that heart size is affected by respiration and in infants and young children, particularly if tachypnoeic, it may be difficult to obtain a full inspiration film. However, the heart may be anatomically grossly abnormal and yet not enlarged. Conversely in the first year of life, the normal heart may have a cardiothoracic ratio of up to 60%.

Cardiac configuration and on occasions, the identification of chamber enlargement, are more important than the transverse diameter of the heart. However, this measurement is not valueless. For example, in a patient who is cyanosed, a heart which is small is more likely to be due to Fallot's tetralogy than to transposition of the great arteries.

In the subsequent text, an indication will be given of the size of the heart to be expected in certain conditions. This should only be considered a very general guide as there are many exceptions.

ENLARGEMENT OF INDIVIDUAL CARDIAC CHAMBERS

In the preliminary assessment of cardiac abnormalities, the identification of which chamber or chambers are involved is of great importance. If this identification can be made with certainty and correlated with information obtained from the lungs and great arteries, then a sound basis for the correct diagnosis has been provided. The three important non-invasive techniques available for the preliminary assessment are:

1. The plain radiograph
2. The electrocardiogram
3. Echocardiography

If chamber enlargement is recognized radiologically, this is most frequently due to dilatation. Less commonly a combination of hypertrophy and dilatation may give rise to enlargement but it is unusual for this to be due to hypertrophy alone. Minor changes in chamber size may be difficult, if not impossible, to assess radiologically. However, electrocardiography and echocardiography are particularly sensitive techniques for demonstrating these small changes in size and such findings should be accepted in preference to a radiographic interpretation. The generally accepted criteria for an increase in specific chamber size as shown radiologically are indicated below and their value is critically discussed.

Left atrial enlargement

The left atrium is unique amongst the cardiac chambers in that increase in size, be it hypertrophy or dilatation, can be specifically recognized. This is due to the anatomical position of the left atrium on the posterior aspect of the heart. Increase in size, particularly if it is of any degree, occurs backwards, upwards and both to the left and to the right. An enlarged left atrium projects away from the main cardiac shadow and is surrounded by lung. This contrasting air–soft tissue density renders the left atrium visible on the radiograph as a double density lying behind the right heart border (Fig. 24.13). Even an early degree of atrial hypertrophy can be demonstrated. Increase in atrial size is less well seen behind the left heart border due to the merging of the left atrium with the left ventricle at the level of the mitral valve. However, the dilated left atrial appendage will present either as a straightening or

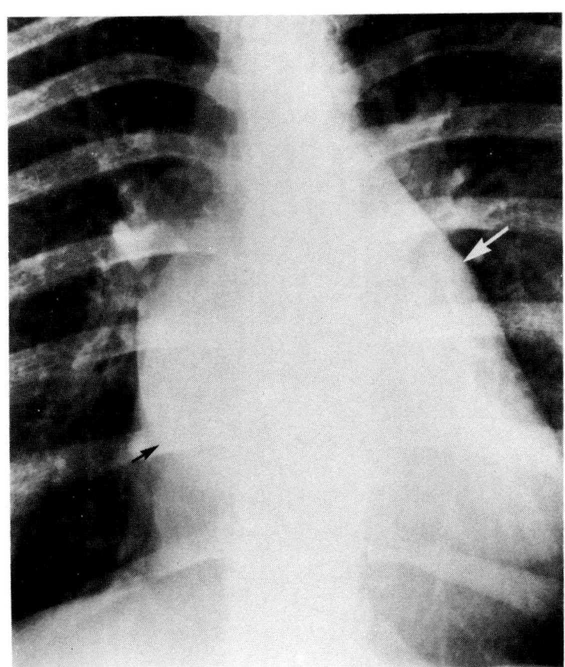

Fig. 24.13 Mitral stenosis. The double density behind the right heart order is due to an enlarged left atrium (black arrow) and the convexity on the left heart border represents a dilated left atrial appendage (white arrow).

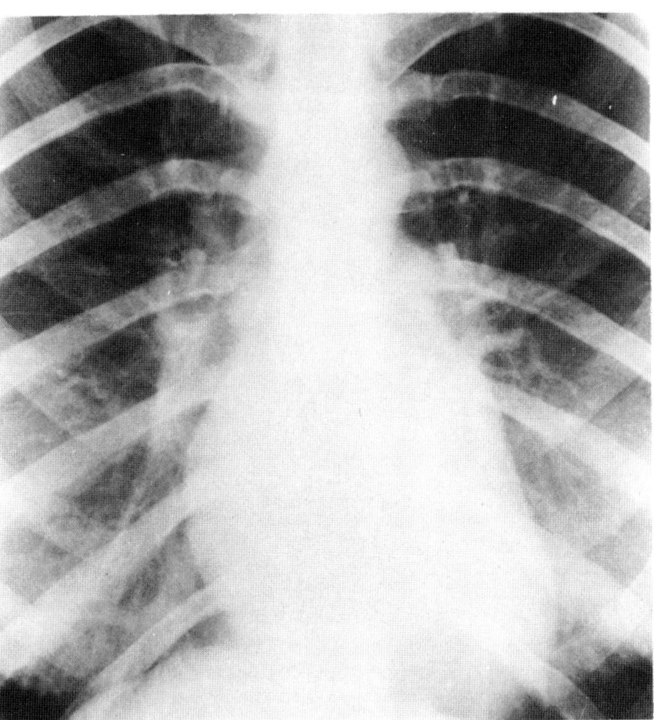

Fig. 24.14 Mitral stenosis. The bulge on the left heart border immediately below the pulmonary artery is due to dilated left atrial appendage.

definite convexity on the left heart border below the pulmonary artery (Fig. 24.14). Upward enlargement of the left atrium may elevate the left main bronchus (Fig. 24.15). A lateral radiograph will show a backward bulge below the left main bronchus which may also be displaced backwards (Fig. 24.16). It is important to note hat the double density behind the right heart border must not be confused with the shadow cast by a dilated aortic root lying anterior to the cardiac chambers. In the latter case, the density can be traced upwards into the right paratracheal region.

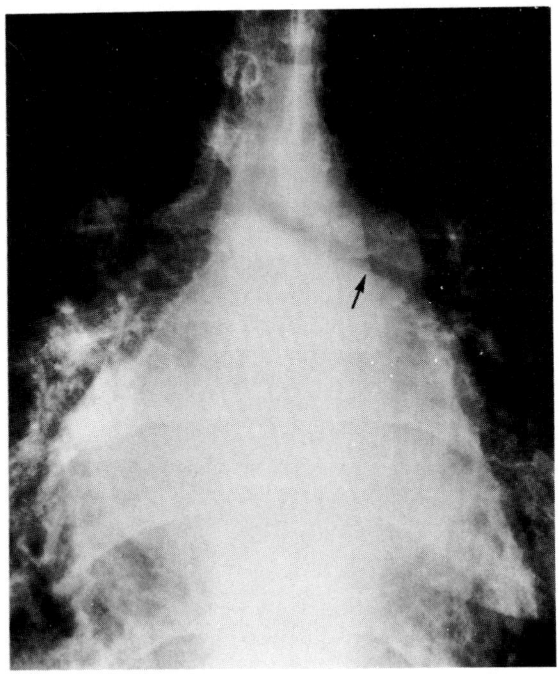

Fig. 24.15 Mitral stenosis and incompetence. The elevated left main bronchus (arrow) indicates an enlarged left atrium.

Right atrial enlargement

Increase in right atrial size is said to be recognized when the cardiac silhouette projects further to the right of the spine than usual (Fig. 24.17). Further right atrial enlargement may alter the silhouette so that the upper right atrial border projects almost horizontally. However, this appearance can also be due to right ventricular enlargement. Isolated right atrial dilatation is unusual and there is nearly always associated involvement of the right ventricle. Thus radiological assessment of right atrial size can be difficult.

Right ventricular enlargement

When the right ventricle hypertrophies or becomes enlarged, it causes the heart to rotate around its vertical axis so that in the postero-anterior view, the cardiac apex may rise above the diaphragm (Fig. 24.18). This appear-

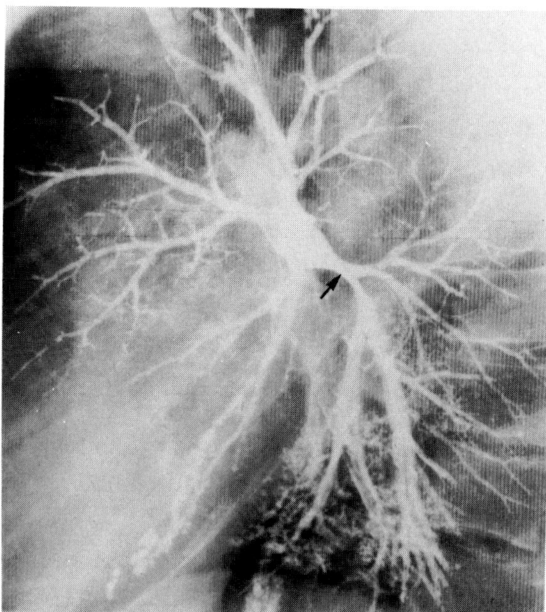

Fig. 24.16 Bronchogram in patient with mitral stenosis. The convex impression on the opacified left main bronchus (arrow) is due to the enlarged left atrium. This impression can also be seen on the plain films.

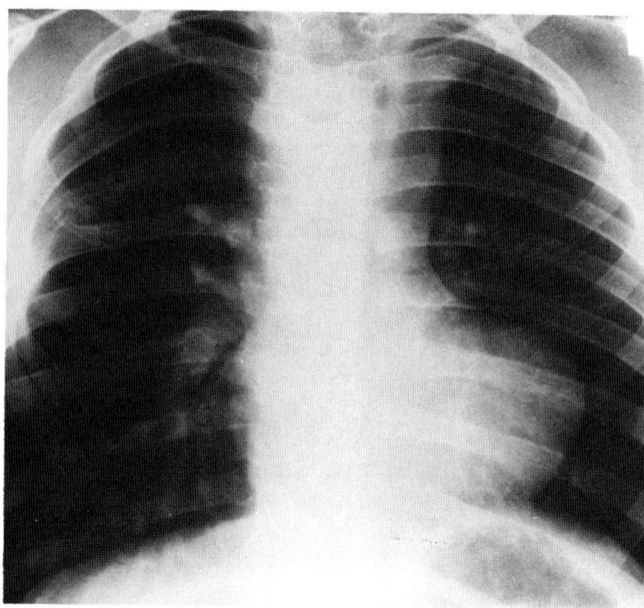

Fig. 24.18 Fallot's tetralogy. Note the elevated apex of the heart lying well above the diaphragm. The lung fields are oligaemic. There is a right aortic arch (occurs in 25% of Fallot's tetralogy). There is evidence of a right thoracotomy consistent with a previous systemic-pulmonary anastomosis.

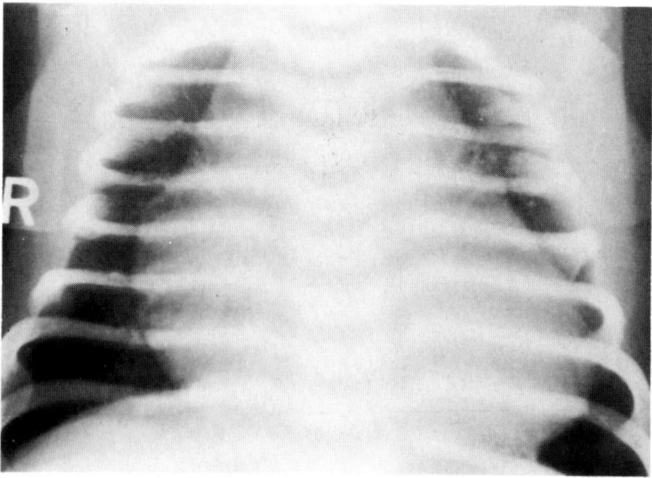

Fig. 24.17 Pulmonary stenosis with tricuspid incompetence. The right heart border projects to the right of the spine and the upper portion is horizontal.

ance of the elevated apex of the heart is seen only when the left ventricle is relatively underdeveloped as in Fallot's tetralogy. If right ventricular hypertrophy occurs in later life, e.g. secondary to primary lung disease, this appearance is not seen as the left ventricle has developed normally and prevents the right ventricle enlarging in an upward direction. In congenital heart disease, enlargement of the right ventricular outflow tract may result in the anterior border of the heart having an increased contact with the sternum though this may be simulated by enlargement of the right atrial appendage which in the lateral view overlies the outflow tract of the right ventricle.

Left ventricular enlargement

The heart rotates on its vertical axis in the opposite direction to the rotation of right ventricular enlargement. As a result, the apex is displaced downwards and outwards sometimes below the dome of the left hemidiaphragm (Fig. 24.19).

Whilst gross ventricular enlargement can usually be recognized radiologically minor degrees are difficult if not impossible to identify. They can, however, be accurately determined either by the electrocardiogram or by electrocardiography. Biventricular enlargement poses a particular problem as far as plain film radiography is concerned. If one ventricle is significantly more enlarged than the other, the findings are of enlargement of that ventricle and the changes in the second ventricle may be overlooked. In the presence of balanced biventricular enlargement, the transverse diameter of the heart is usually increased. The left ventricular element causes the cardiac apex to be displaced downwards and outwards whilst the right ventricular enlargement results in prominence in the region of the right ventricular outflow tract with a resulting convexity on the left cardiac border below the aortic knuckle. However, in minor degrees of balanced biventricular hypertrophy, difficulty may be experienced in deciding whether or not the heart is abnormal in exactly the same

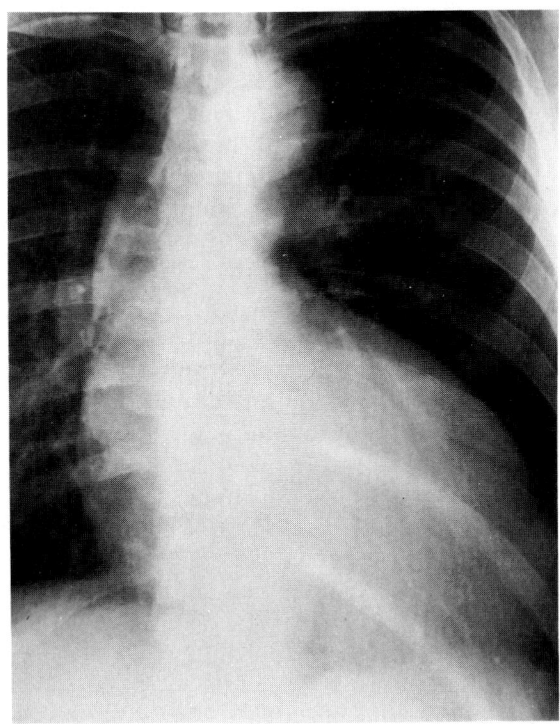

ig 24.19 Aortic incompetence. Left ventricular enlargement is shown y displacement of the apex downwards and outwards.

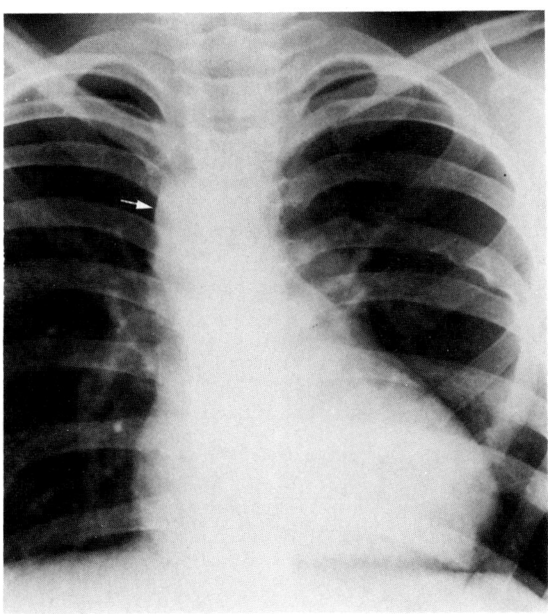

Fig. 24.20 Right ventral aorta uniting with right dorsal aorta. Note soft tissue density in right paratracheal region and absence of soft tissue shadow in left paratracheal region.

vay as difficulty may arise in interpreting an electrocardio- ram of such a case. However, the sensitivity of echo- ardiography often enables a diagnosis of biventricular nlargement to be made. Thus it will be seen that plain lm radiography plays a secondary role to the electrocar- liogram and to echocardiograhy in the accurate assessment f chamber enlargement. It is worth noting that, in the resence of a hypoplastic ventricle, such as in the hypo- lastic left heart syndrome, the configuration of the normal entricle is not particularly unusual. This is contrasted by he abnormal appearance of an enlarged or hypertrophied entricle as in Fallot's tetralogy or pulmonary atresia.

THE AORTA

n assessing the aorta, the following two points are of mportance:

1. Is the aortic arch left or right sided?
2. Is the aorta enlarged or small and where is the aortic root situated?

1. RIGHT AORTIC ARCH

The right ventral (ascending) most commonly unites with the right dorsal (descending) aorta (fig. 24.20). In the presence of congenital heart disease, this combination almost always indicates that a ventricular septal defect is present. Much less frequently, the right ventral aorta gives rise to a right aortic arch which immediately unites with the left dorsal aorta and this is rarely associated with congenital heart disease.

A penetrated or high kilovoltage film will almost always demonstrate the trachea and aortic arch enabling laterality to be established. Even if the arch cannot be clearly seen, its position can be inferred from the width of soft tissues on one or other side of the trachea. If doubt still exisits, a barium swallow will show an impression on the barium column on the side on which the arch lies.

2. THE SIZE OF THE AORTA AND POSITION OF THE AORTIC ROOT

a. Aortic size

Whilst dilatation of the ascending aorta can be assessed on the plain frontal film, a more accurate indication of size is obtained by echocardiography. Indeed, two-dimensional echocardiography (Tajik et al 1978) enables not only a measurement of size but also allows differentiation between the aorta and pulmonary artery. Thus the relative positions of the two great arteries can be established and also an estimation can be made of flow within them. Nevertheless, it must be pointed out that the aortic isthmus may be difficult to identify by echocardiography and it is for this reason that aortography may be necessary in some patients.

NORMAL NEONATAL AORTA

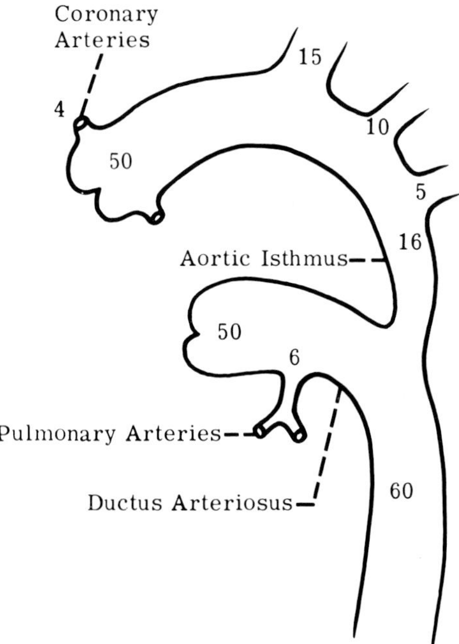

Fig. 24.21 Diagram to show the proportion of the combined fetal ventricular output that passes to aorta and pulmonary artery in the normal neonate at birth before closure of the ductus. The numerals indicate percentage flow traversing the vessels and the latter are drawn to indicate their approximate dimensions. (Courtesy of the *British Heart Journal* and E. A. Shinebourne and A. M. Elseed.)

Fetal flow patterns in the aorta

Shinebourne and Elseed (1974) have postulated a direc relationship between the fetal flow pattern and the size c the aortic isthmus. It has been shown that the dimensior of the great arteries reflect the flow through the (Heymann & Rudolph 1972). Figure 24.21 illustrates th normal fetal flow patterns. This indicates that only abo 16% of the cardiac output passes through the aorti isthmus which is narrow compared with the ascending an descending aorta. The junction between the isthmus an the descending aorta is characterized in the neonate by posterior indentation. It is the exaggeration of this inder tation that results in isolated juxta-ductal coarctation whic may well become haemodynamically significant when th duct closes (Fig. 24.22). Shinebourne and Elseed furthe noticed that in conditions with right ventricular outflo tract obstruction and a ventricular septal defect (Fallot tetralogy, pulmonary atresia and tricuspid atresia) coar tation did not occur. They suggested that the right to le shunt increased flow in the aorta and hence the isthmu (Fig. 24.23). As a result, the isthmal-aortic junction wa wider than in the normal and obstruction was unlikely. I contrast, mixing situations, such as transposition of th great arteries, with interatrial or interventricular commun cation are associated with a small aortic isthmus. Prior t birth, in a transposition situation, oxygenated blood fro the placenta, reaching the right heart via the inferior cav will shunt via the eustachian valve to the left ventricle an thence to the pulmonary artery. The relatively high *P*c

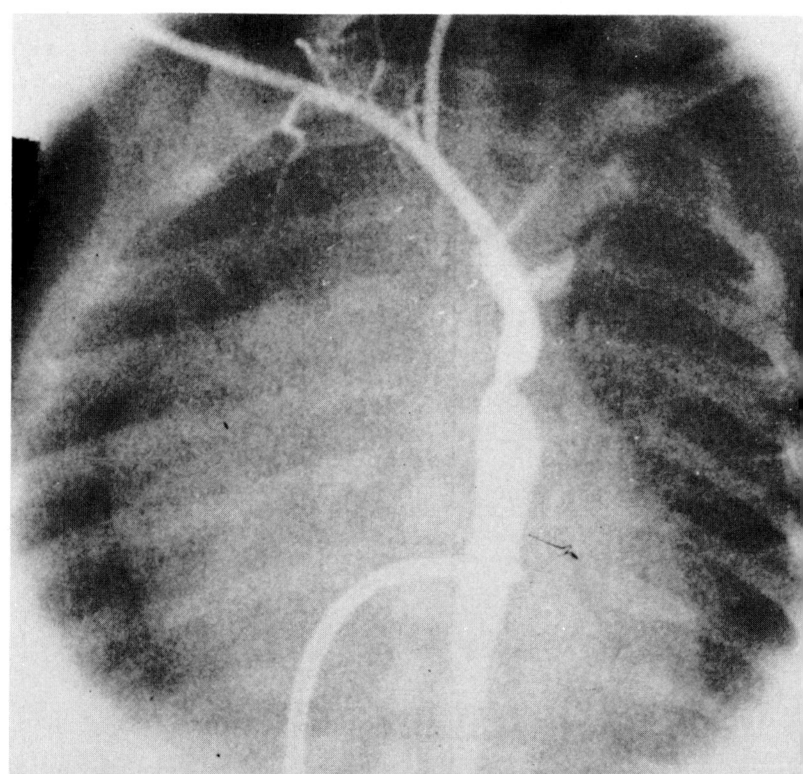

Fig. 24.22 Angiogram of isolated juxtaductal coarctation in oblique projection showing the posterior indentation which may cause significant obstruction when the duct closes.

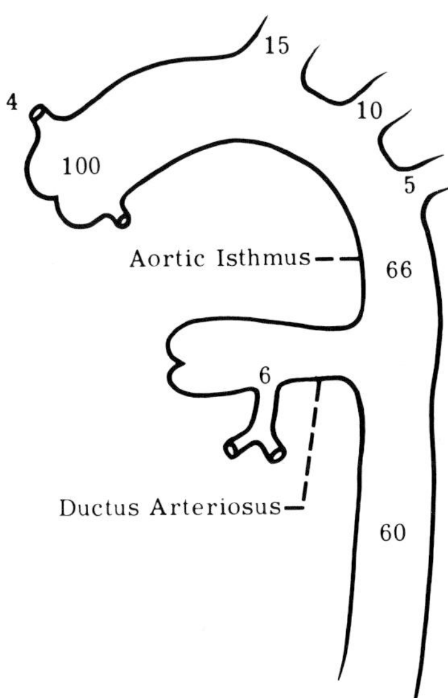

Fig. 24.23 Diagram to show the expected proportion of the combined fetal ventricular output that passes to aorta and pulmonary artery in a patient with pulmonary atresia. (Courtesy of the *British Heart Journal* and E. A. Shinebourne and A. M. Elseed.)

will lead to an increased pulmonary vasodilatation giving rise to increased pulmonary flow. There will be a corresponding decrease in aortic flow. As the head and neck arteries take their usual amount, isthmal flow is reduced with a consequent reduction in size (Fig. 24.24). This is demonstrated angiographically in Figure 24.25.

The size of the aorta or isthmus can be considered in relation to the pulmonary vessels:

i) With pulmonary oligaemia

A dilated ascending aorta and isthmus together with right ventricular hypertrophy and pulmonary oligaemia are diagnostic of right ventricular outflow tract obstruction with a ventricular septal defect.

ii) With pulmonary plethora

Plethoric lung fields indicate a left to right shunt. It has been suggested that a large aorta indicates an extracardiac shunt usually through a duct, whereas a normal or apparently small aorta represents an intracardiac communication. In fact, aortic size is not a reliable guide to the anatomical site of the shunt until late in childhood by which time the position of the defect has nearly always been identified. Nevertheless, the ratio of aortic diameter to that of the left atrium as seen on echocardiography has been used as an indicator of the magnitude of the shunt through a ductus. The greater the left atrial measurement in relation to the aorta (upper normal limit of ratio — aorta : left atrium — 1 : 1.3), the higher the flow (Baylan et al 1975, Silverman et al 1974).

It should be recognized that in truncus arteriosus and aortopulmonary window, there is frequently disparity in the size of the dilated ascending aorta compared with the small arch.

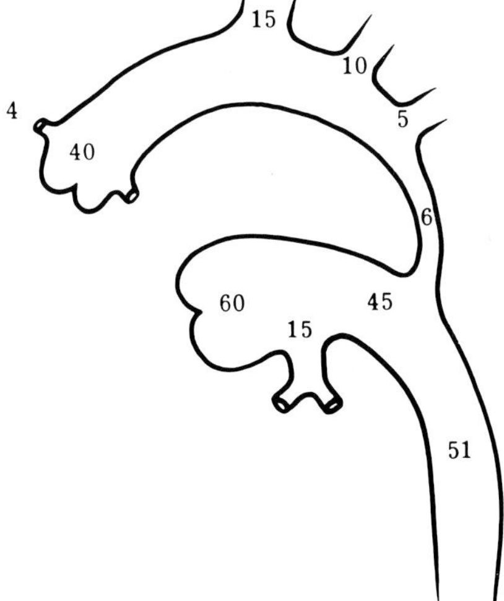

Fig. 24.24 Diagram to show the expected proportion of the combined fetal ventricular output that passes to aorta and pulmonary artery in a patient with ventriculo-arterial discordance (transposition of the great arteries) and a ventricular septal defect. (Courtesy of the *British Heart Journal* and E. A. Shinebourne and A. M. Elseed.)

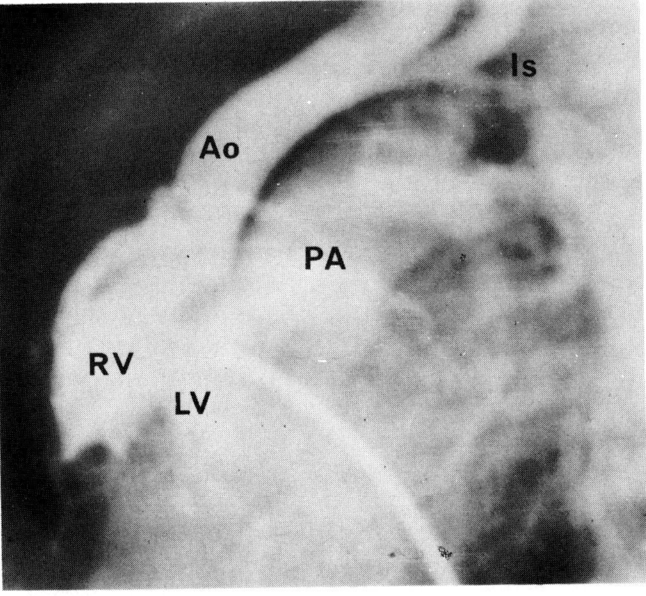

Fig. 24.25 Angiogram demonstrating right ventricle (RV), left ventricle (LV), aorta (Ao) and pulmonary artery (PA) in a patient with ventriculo-arterial discordance (transposition of the great arteries) and a ventricular septal defect. The PA is larger than the anterior aorta which has extreme narrowing at the isthmus (Is).

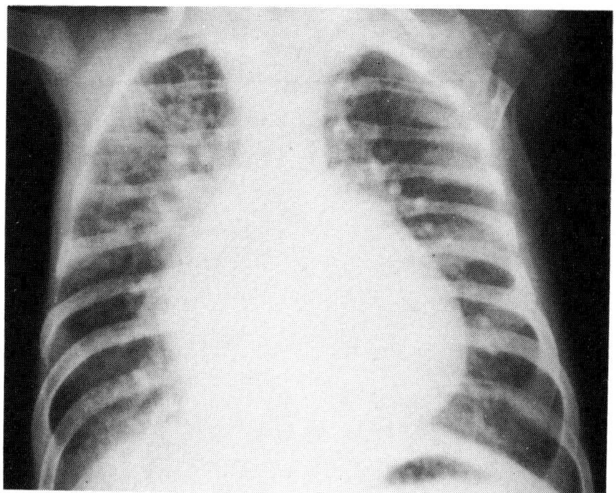

Fig. 24.26 The narrow pedicle of the heart seen in ventriculo-arterial discordance (transposition) due to the aorta lying almost directly in front of the pulmonary artery.

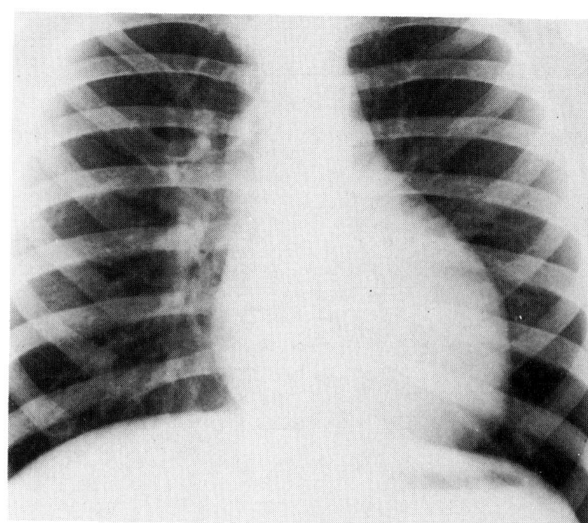

Fig. 24.27 Atrioventricular discordance and ventriculo-arterial discordance (corrected transposition). Plain film showing prominent straight left heart border due to l-malposition of ascending aorta.

iii) With normal pulmonary vessels

Dilatation of the aortic root with normal pulmonary vessels and left ventricular hypertrophy indicates the presence of aortic valve stenosis. Supravalve stenosis does not produce dilatation whereas subaortic stenosis does so but only rarely.

b. Position of aortic root

In complete transposition of the great arteries, the mediastinum may be narrow in the frontal view. When present, this outline is said to be characteristic (Fig. 24.26). It is, however, only seen in some 20% of cases (Counahan & Joseph 1973). The appearance is probably due to the aorta lying directly in front of the pulmonary artery although it has also been suggested that it may be due to a small thymic shadow in the sick child (Nogrady & Dunbar 1969). In congenitally corrected transposition, the ascending aorta is usually left sided. In this situation, the frontal radiograph will often show the upper left heart border to be straight. The aortic valve is in the position usually occupied by the pulmonary valve and the ascending aorta describes a smooth curve upwards with a slight outer concavity (Fig. 24.27). If the inferior vena cava is absent, a dilated azygos vein may simulate a right aortic arch (Fig. 24.29 A & B). In this situation, it should be possible to identify a normally positioned left arch as indicated earlier in this section.

PULMONARY VASCULATURE

In congenital heart disease, the pulmonary arteries and veins may present on the plain film with one of six specific patterns. The importance of recognizing these cannot be over emphasized and they are summarized below.

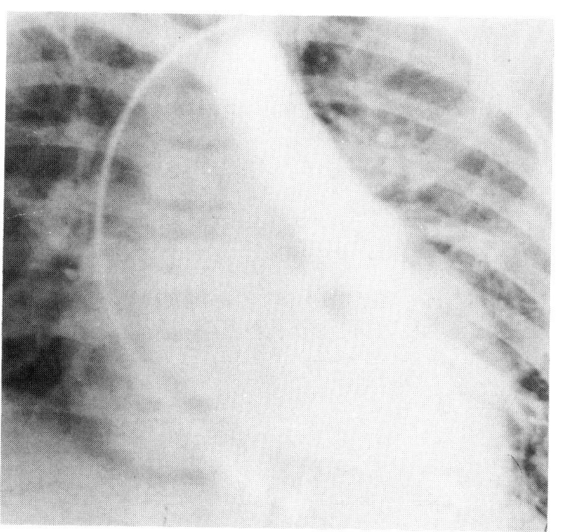

Fig. 24.28 Angiogram of patient with corrected transposition outlining ascending aorta in l-malposition forming left heart border. Aorta fills via LA and morphological RV.

1. The pulmonary vasculature may be **normal**.
2. **Pulmonary oligaemia** (Fig. 24.30). This indicates a reduced pulmonary flow and may occur in the following conditions:

   a. Right ventricular outflow tract obstruction with an interatrial or interventricular communication.
   b. Pulmonary hypertension.

All the classical radiological appearances of pulmonary hypertension may be seen and are described in Chapter 21. Nevertheless, it must be understood that these radiological changes rarely appear before the age of 5 years. Thus, although pulmonary artery pressure may be at systemic level, there may be little or no radiological evidence to suggest this except minimal peripheral oligaemia.

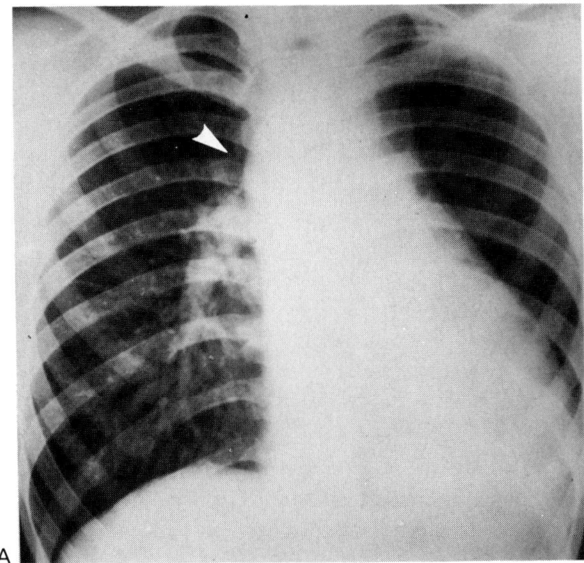

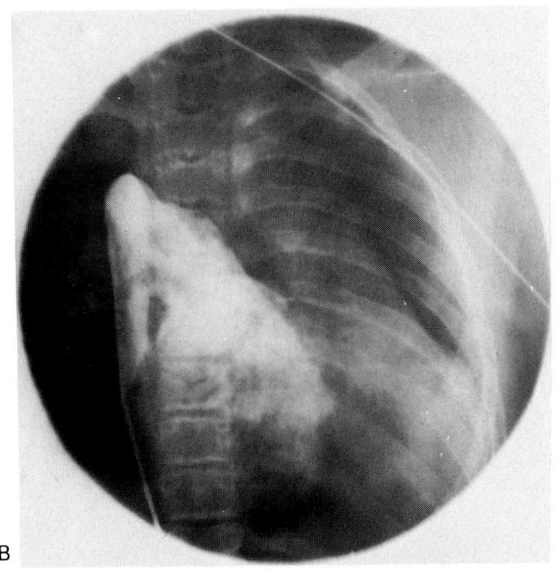

Fig. 24.29 A. Dilated azygos vein (arrowhead) simulating a right-sided aorta. **B.** Contrast injection confirming dilated azygos vein.

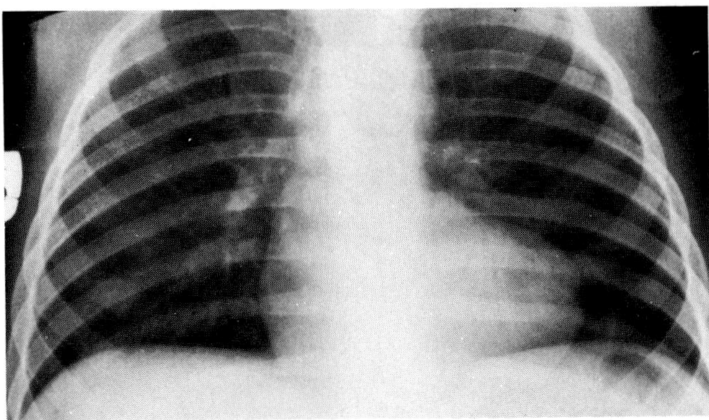

Fig. 24.30 Oligaemia due to reduced pulmonary flow in Fallot's tetralogy. The small main and peripheral pulmonary arteries should be noted.

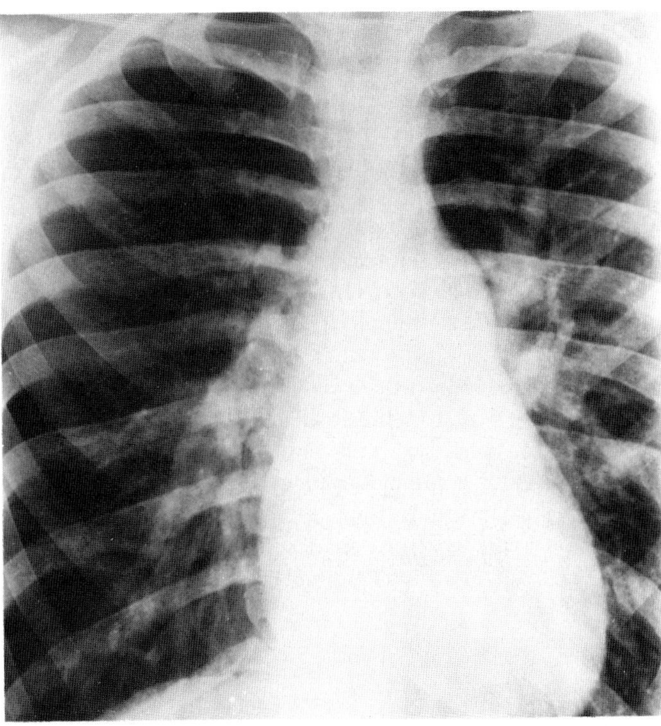

Fig. 24.31 ASD. Note displacement of heart to the left. The arteries and veins are dilated throughout the lung fields. The arteries dominate.

3. **Pulmonary plethora** (Fig. 24.31). This indicates an increase in pulmonary blood flow. The main pulmonary arteries are larger than normal with end on vessels close to the hilum being particularly well seen. Distal vessels are more visible than usual with branches extending out to the periphery of the lung. Although the pulmonary veins can easily be identified, they do not dominate as do the arteries. Despite the apparently well-defined radiological appearances, it may be extremely difficult to distinguish between plethora and pulmonary oedema in the neonatal age group; indeed they may both be present.

4. **Pulmonary venous congestion** (Fig. 24.12). This will occur in the presence of obstructive lesions on the left side of the heart and also secondary to congenital mitral incompetence and obstructed anomalous pulmonary venous return. In these situations, it is the pulmonary veins which dominate rather than the arteries. Upper lobe blood diversion is present and septal lines may be seen.

5. **Inequality in the pulmonary vasculature**, one lung being either more oligaemic or more plethoric than the other. Marked inequality of perfusion is usually due to an

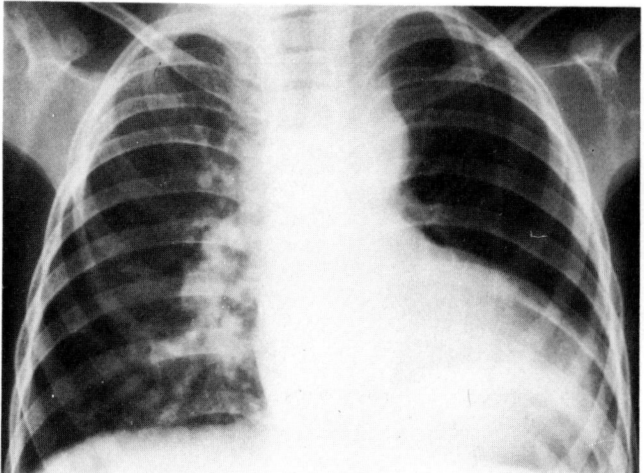

Fig. 24.32 Localized oligaemia in the left lung associated with peripheral pulmonary artery stenosis.

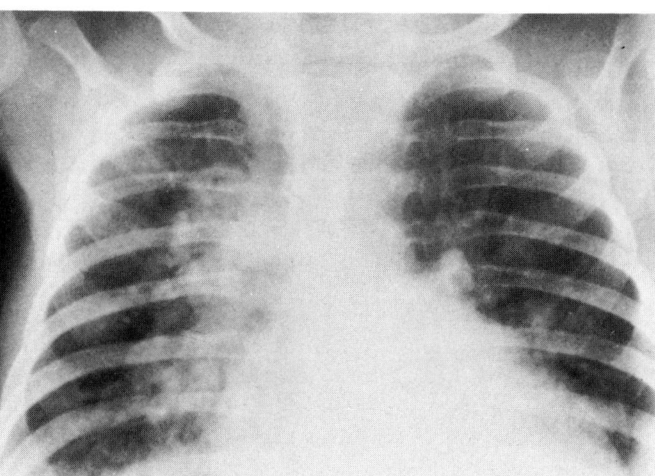

Fig. 24.33 Localized area of pleonaemia in the right middle and upper zone indicating presence of a VSD.

abnormality of the pulmonary arteries such as branch stenosis or congenital absence (Fig. 24.32). Bronchiolitis obliterans (Macleod's syndrome, Macleod 1954) with secondary hypoplasia of the pulmonary arteries may also give rise to unilateral pulmonary oligaemia or hypertransradiancy. Occasionally when both lungs are plethoric, pleonaemia may be particularly marked in the right middle and upper zones (Fig. 24.33). The reason for this is unknown but it almost always indicates a ventricular septal defect. Iatrogenic causes would include unilateral systemic-pulmonary artery shunt operations such as a Blalock operation.

6. **Abnormal pulmonary venous drainage**. The patterns of extracardiac and infradiaphragmatic total anomalous pulmonary venous return are described in Chapter 25 as is that of partial anomalous pulmonary venous return (Scimitar syndrome).

IDENTIFICATION OF PLETHORA AND OLIGAEMIA ON THE PLAIN FILM

Minor degrees of plethora or oligaemia may be very difficult to judge. Whilst it is not much help to say that accurate assessment is a matter of experience, there are two ways in which correct decisions can be reached.

Firstly, the medial two-thirds of each lung should be obscured and the lateral third carefully examined. The normal lung will have a few vessels in the periphery, whilst with oligaemia there will be no vessels visible and, with plethora, the vessels will be numerous. The second method is to identify the ring shadow of the anterior segmental bronchus of the upper lobe which is visible end on just lateral to the hilum. If the accompanying artery is the same diameter, the flow is normal; if the artery is smaller, there is oligaemia and if it is larger, then plethora is present (Fig. 24.34). If uncertainty still exists, direct comparison with a radiograph that is known to be normal will usually resolve the situation.

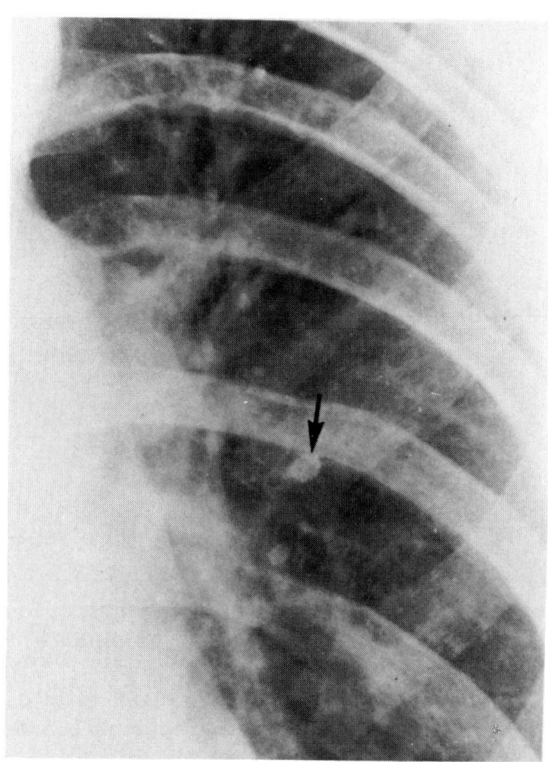

Fig. 24.34 Pulmonary artery seen *en face* (↓) is larger than the ring shadow of the adjacent bronchus medial to it in an otherwise unremarkable lung field. The patient had an ASD with a 3.5:1 shunt.

THE SKELETON

Rib notching

Certain skeletal abnormalities have well recognized associations with congenital heart disease and may be noted on the plain film. These are well described in *Clinical Cardiac Radiology* by Jefferson and Rees (1980), to which the reader is referred. The largest group of these abnormalities is *rib notching* (Fig. 24.35). The main causes are summarized in Table 24.2.

Table 24.2 Causes of rib notching

A Congenital heart disease
1. Coarctation of the aorta including the anomalous origin of Rt. subclavian artery
2. Right ventricular outflow tract obstruction with ventricular septal defect.
   a. Congenital, e.g. pulmonary atresia
   b. Acquired, e.g. systemic artery to pulmonary artery shunt operations

B Others
3. Superior vena caval obstruction
4. Neurofibromatosis

Notching is usually due to an attempt to bypass a *coarctation* by opening up a collateral circulation from the subclavian arteries to the distal aorta via the intercostal arteries. If the rib notching is absent on the left side, this indicates that the left subclavian artery is involved or originates below the coarctation. Absent notching on the right side indicates an anomalous origin of the right subclavian artery below the level of the coarctation.

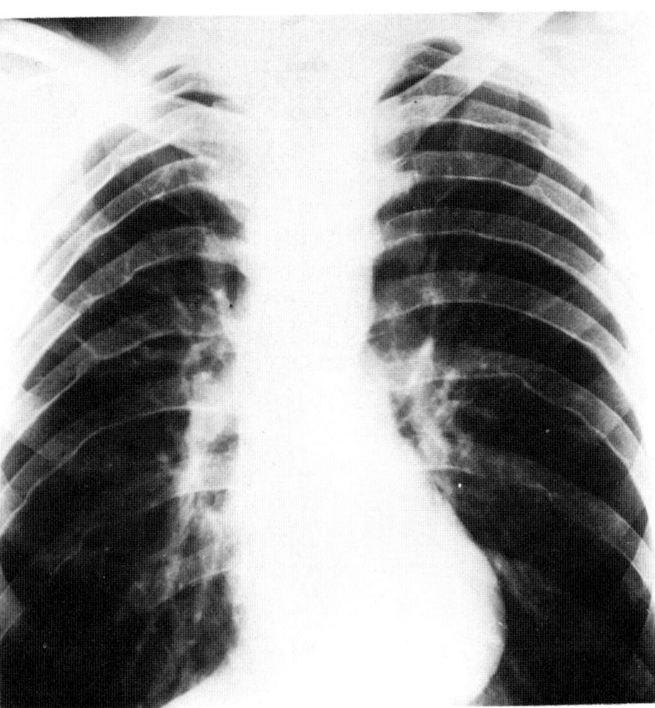

Fig. 24.35 Coarctation of the aorta. Note posterior rib notching extending from the fourth to the ninth ribs bilaterally.

The notching usually extends from the fourth to ninth ribs and is often asymmetrical. The notches are well defined, but with sclerosis being present, and vary in appearance from shallow to deep. They are situated on the posterior aspect of the ribs.

Rarely *right ventricular outflow tract obstruction* such as pulmonary atresia may lead to a systemic pulmonary artery anastomosis via the intercostal arteries with resulting rib notching. Notching is seen much more frequently following a subclavian–pulmonary artery anastomotic operation performed to improve pulmonary flow in the presence of right ventricular outflow tract obstruction (*Blalock operation*). These changes involve the first two or three ribs. They are unilateral and reflect an attempt to improve flow to the arm following division of the subclavian artery. The apparent absence of a subclavian steal syndrome is probably due to the young age of the patient and early development of anastomotic channels.

Whilst *venous obstruction* would not be expected to result in rib notching, this does occur occasionally with superior vena caval obstruction usually secondary to mediastinal fibrosis. Radiologically, it is indistinguishable from arterial notching. Pressure erosions from *neurofibromatosis* give a similar appearance though soft tissue opacities are usually visible.

Sternal depression and straight-back syndrome

Sternal depression (pectus excavatum) and the straight-back syndrome, where there is loss of the normal dorsal kyphosis, may cause compression of the heart between the sternum and the dorsal spine. Consequently, the heart may appear both enlarged and displaced to the left. The absence of any heart silhouette to the right of the spine, together with horizontal posterior ribs and relatively vertical anterior ribs, should suggest the possibility of bony compression. Atrial septal defects have a well-recognized association with a depressed sternum.

Premature sternal fusion and bowing of the sternum

Although premature fusion may be an isolated finding, 25% of patients have a ventricular septal defect. Anterior bowing of the sternum is seen secondary to a high pulmonary flow which is most often due to a large ventricular septal defect.

Scoliosis

A scoliosis is seen in congenital heart disease in a higher percentage of patients than would normally be expected. 15% of children with acyanotic shunts and 25% of those with cyanotic heart disease have an associated scoliosis.

Spine

Patients with Marfan's disease show posterior vertebral body scalloping and the vertebral bodies are often higher than they are wide. As the developmental abnormality in Marfan's is primarily that of a defect of connective tissue, aortic and mitral regurgitation may also occur and a dilated aorta often leading to dissection is frequently seen. Vertebral body abnormalities are also seen in the mucopolysaccharide diseases such as Morquio's disease.

THE ECHOCARDIOGRAPHIC APPROACH TO CONGENITAL HEART DISEASE

Until recently, cardiac catheterization and angiocardiography were considered to be the final arbiters in the diagnosis of congenital heart disease. Currently this is less appropriate because of the emergence of cross-sectional echocardiography as a generally available technique for diagnosis. This has meant that radical or palliative surgery can be undertaken on some patients without prior cardiac catheterization.

Echocardiography should be considered a routine investigation for all symptomatic infants and children with heart disease and for all patients undergoing cardiac catheterization and surgery. M-mode echocardiography was the first method to be employed and it is not yet outdated. Its importance lies in the resolution of depth and time, allowing accurate measurement of the diameters of the left ventricle, left atrium and aortic root, the thickness of the ventricular septum and the posterior left ventricular wall together with the systolic and diastolic function of the left ventricle (Table 24.3). *Cross-sectional* echocardiography is in essence the representation of cardiac morphology in life and often provides important additional information to that which may be obtained by angiocardiography. Particularly, the morphology of the atrioventricular junction in complex congenital heart disease is well demonstrated. In many instances, knowledge of the echocardiographic findings improves the information gained from cardiac catheterization and angiography by allowing the investigation to be planned in detail beforehand. If an echocardiogram is recorded during a peripheral or central injection of saline, blood or glucose, a contrast effect is produced as micro bubbles enter the heart. This technique of contrast echocardiography can be applied to both M mode and cross-sectional studies and may be used as a complement to angiocardiography at the time of cardiac catheterization (Valdez Cruz et al 1976). A right to left shunt will show bubbles crossing the septum (Fig. 24.36) whilst with a left to right shunt a negative jet is seen in the bubble stream. Whilst M mode echocardiography allows assessment of ventricular size and function, sequential segmental analysis is best achieved by means of cross-sectional (two-dimensional) echocardiography (Tajik et al 1978).

Table 24.3 Normal echocardiographic dimensions for infants and children. The weight is in kilograms and all other measurements are in centimetres. The numbers in parentheses are ±2 s. d. RVD = right ventricular dimension measured in diastole from the epicardial to right septal surface; LVD = left ventricular end-diastolic internal dimension from left septal surface to LV endocardium; AO = aortic root and LAD = left atrial dimension both measured in end-systole; Septum = septal thickness and LVW = LV wall thickness measured in end-diastole; PA = pulmonic root; RVOT = right ventricular outflow tract measured in end-systole.

	WEIGHT	HEIGHT	RVD	LVD	AO	LAD	SEPTUM	LVW	PA	RVOT
1 week–3 months	4.80 (1.55)	57.2 (4.8)	1.00 (0.19)	1.86 (0.31)	1.01 (0.15)	1.30 (0.27)	0.36 (0.06)	0.34 (0.08)	1.20 (0.20)	1.04 (0.24)
4–12 months	7.77 (1.80)	69.98 (3.98)	1.12 (0.18)	2.28 (0.36)	1.21 (0.14)	1.59 (0.33)	0.38 (0.08)	0.38 (0.08)	1.25 (0.09)	1.09 (0.32)
1–2 years	10.86 (2.15)	81.9 (6.6)	1.12 (0.22)	2.82 (0.26)	1.38 (0.15)	1.82 (0.30)	0.47 (0.09)	0.45 (0.09)	1.41 (0.33)	1.21 (0.22)
3–5 years	17.24 (2.28)	107.63 (4.8)	1.26 (0.26)	3.28 (0.31)	1.66 (0.20)	1.72 (0.38)	0.49 (0.08)	0.49 (0.12)	1.73 (0.21)	1.57 (0.31)
6–10 years	27.03 (6.4)	130.2 (11.8)	1.45 (0.30)	3.62 (0.35)	1.87 (0.19)	2.06 (0.28)	0.58 (0.12)	0.61 (0.12)	1.96 (0.40)	1.55 (0.30)
11–15 years	47.4 (12.3)	158.3 (10.9)	1.71 (0.32)	4.22 (0.41)	2.1 (0.31)	2.38 (0.44)	0.71 (0.17)	0.73 (0.15)	2.18 (0.14)	1.78 (0.37)
>15 years	64.03 (19.5)	167.3 (12.2)	1.78 (0.49)	4.39 (0.38)	2.46 (0.36)	2.78 (0.53)	0.79 (0.20)	0.79 (0.18)	2.25 (0.55)	1.91 (0.37)

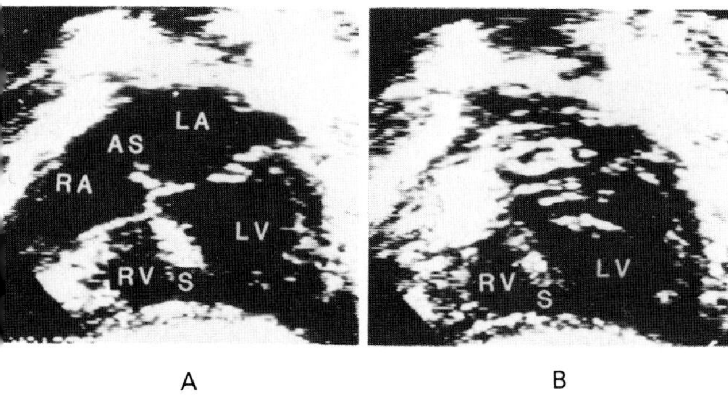

Fig. 24.36 Right atrial contrast echocardiogram showing right to left atrial shunt **A.** before and **B.** during injection.

Cross-sectional echocardiography is the most important method of diagnosing congenital heart disease by the ultrasound technique. The standard examinations are performed using the following entry ports:

1. The left parasternal region.
2. The apex.
3. The subcostal region.
4. The superstemal notch.

The transducer is placed so that the echo beam is either parallel or perpendicular to the major axis of the left ventricle and great arteries, these planes being described as either the long axis or the short axis (Tajik et al 1978). In the parasternal, apical or subcostal regions, a four chamber, a long axis, a short axis or an intermediate section can be recorded. With the transducer in the supra sternal notch, the aorta, pulmonary arteries and pulmonary veins can usually be visualized (Fig. 24.37).

ANGIOCARDIOGRAPHY

It is probably true to say that contrast angiographic studies remain the gold standard whereby definitive diagnoses are reached. Nevertheless, echocardiography is rapidly gaining

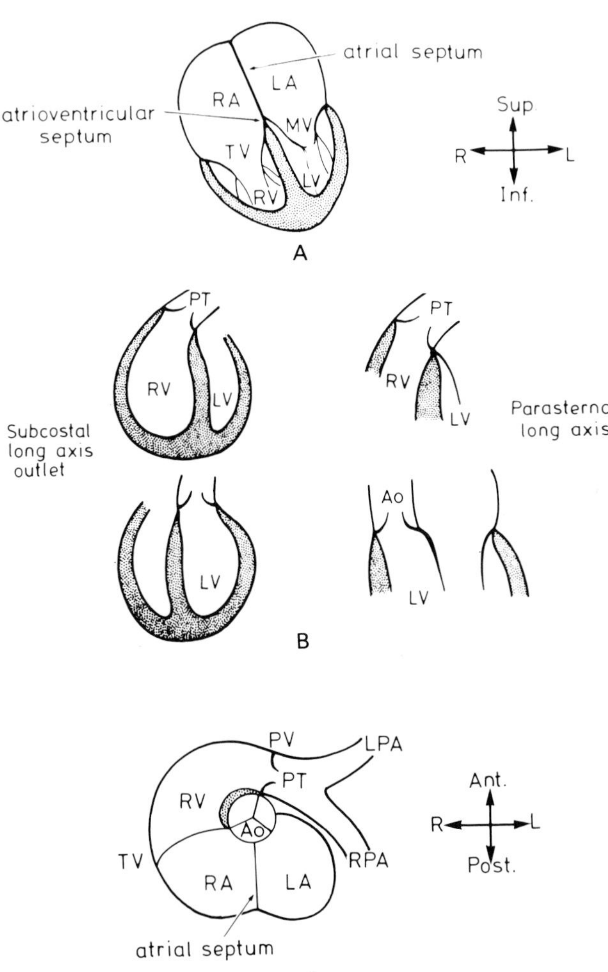

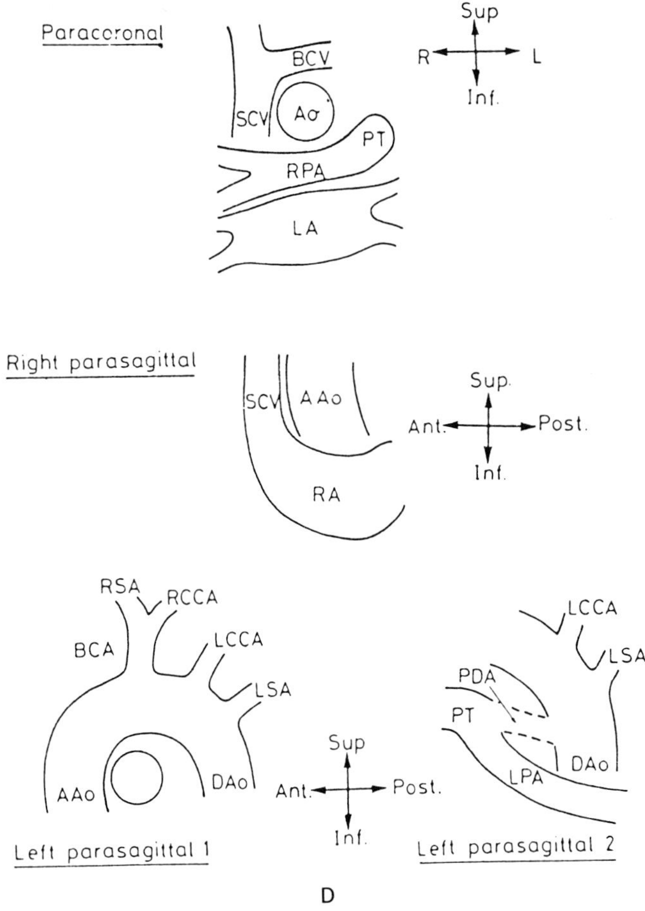

Fig. 24.37 Illustration of various echographic projections to illustrate **A.** four-chamber, **B.** long axis, **C.** short axis, and **D.** suprasternal views.

ground. It will be clear from the subsequent description of many conditions that echocardiography often yields sufficient information to form a firm diagnosis. Hence, it is essential to be clear what information angiocardiography may provide; the circumstances in which angiocardiography alone would give this information; and, finally, technically how best this information can be obtained.

The value of angiocardiography

It has been stated earlier that accurate and logical diagnosis in complex congenital heart disease is obtained by means of sequential chamber localization. Thus it is necessary to identify chamber morphology. Whilst this may be inferred from echocardiography, at present, it is only the angiographic demonstration of trabecular patterns that enables an accurate morphological identification of the ventricular chambers to be made. In addition, echocardiography does have the limitation that technically some patients may be extremely difficult to examine although this occurs much less frequently in children. Certainly, it should be possible to identify the atrioventricular valve, the semilunar valves and great arteries accurately by both methods. Nevertheless, the aortic arch and pulmonary veins can only be accurately identified on occasions by angiography. If structures are hypoplastic or even absent, it may be much more difficult to be certain as to their anatomical diagnosis using echocardiography. By the same token, small or multiple defects in the ventricular and atrial septa may not be accurately identified.

Angiographic appearances of the ventricles

Right ventricle. The right ventricle is quadrangular in shape (Fig. 24.38). Its base is on the diaphragm and the roof is formed by the crista supraventricularis lying between the tricuspid and pulmonary valves. The right ventricular outflow tract lies anteriorly and leads to the pulmonary valve which is positioned anterosuperiorly. The anterior wall of the outflow tract lies against the sternocostal surface of the chest wall and the posterior wall forms the right side of the ventricular septum.

The right ventricle consists of three portions. A short inflow portion, originating from the primitive ventricle, extends from the tricuspid valve to the trabecular zone (Fig. 24.39). The trabecular zone or body of the ventricle is excavated from the bulbus cordis. It is this section which has the coarse trabecular pattern, seen angiographically (Fig. 24.40), which is so characteristic of the morphological right ventricle. The right ventricular trabecular pattern is much more marked than the left ventricle so that a morphological distinction can be made.

The body of the right ventricle unites with the smooth-walled outflow tract which extends to the pulmonary valve and is known as the infundibulum.

The tricuspid valve, by definition, has three cusps, anterior, septal and mural. However, frequently only the two former can be identified at post-mortem and accurate angiographic recognition of individual cusps is impossible. In an ostium primum defect the so-called 'cleft' is a commisure which allows regurgitation from left ventricle

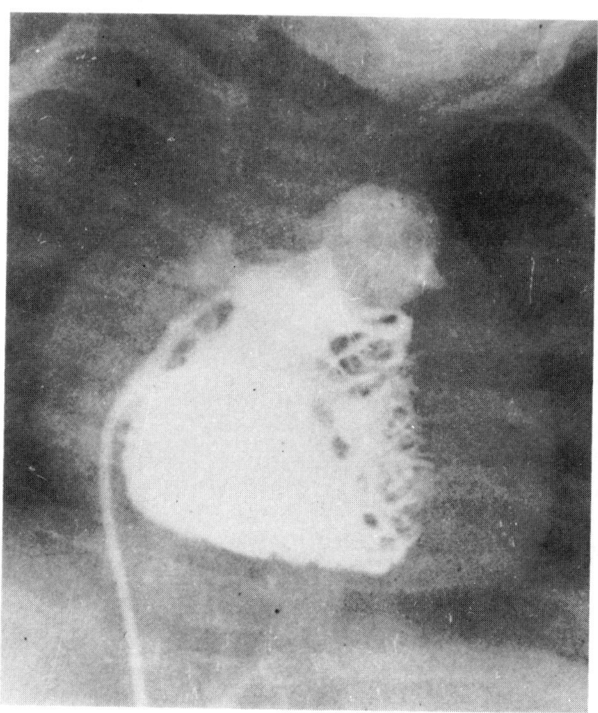

A

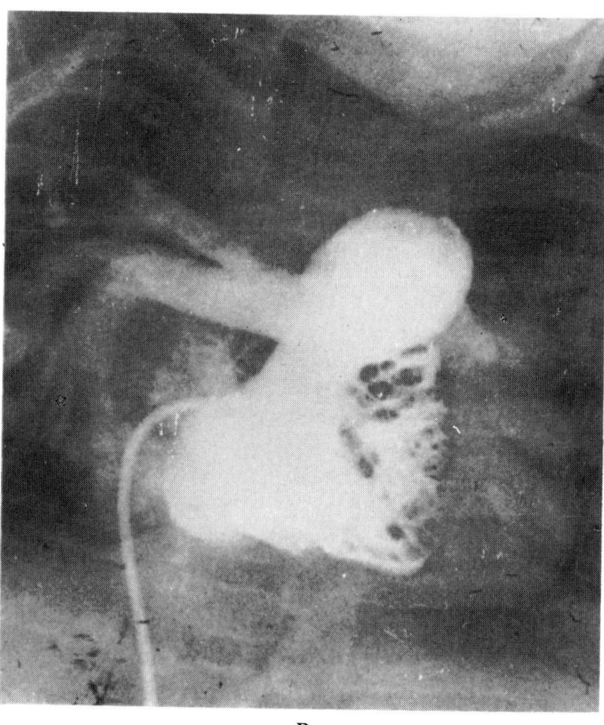

B

Fig. 24.38 Right ventricular angiocardiogram to show the normal anatomy. **A.** Diastole. **B.** Systole. The main pulmonary arteries are filling.

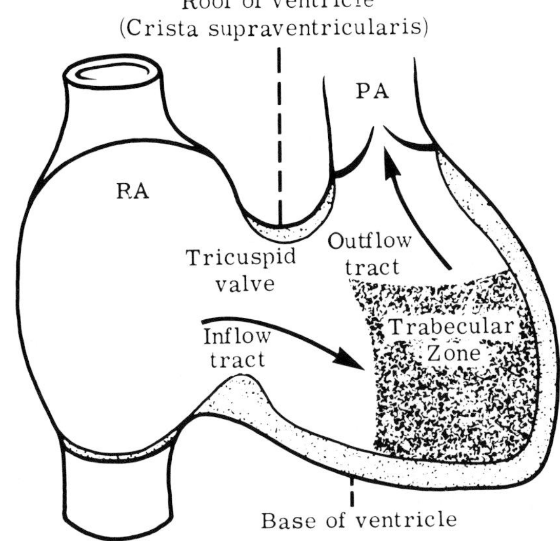

Fig. 24.39 Diagram to show the inflow and outflow tracts and trabecular zone of i.v. septum of the right ventricle (AP). (After *Quain's Anatomy*.)

to right atrium. A true cleft in the right atrioventricular valve, associated with a ventricular septal defect, may also allow regurgitation, from left ventricle to right atrium as in a Gerbode defect. The pulmonary valve has three cusps which can be seen angiographically. Two cusps lie anteriorly and one posteriorly. The pulmonary artery immediately above the cusps bulges to form the pulmonary sinuses of Valsalva.

Left ventricle. The left ventricle is conical with its point at the apex of the heart. The aortic and mitral valves lie at the base of the ventricle. As with the right ventricle, there is a short inflow portion merging with the trabecular zone. As already mentioned, the trabecular zone has a very much smoother pattern than that of the right ventricle (Fig. 24.41). It is the thick covering of numerous fine trabeculae which differs so markedly from the coarse pattern in the right ventricle that permit a clear distinction to be made. The left ventricle has a free lateral wall and a medial wall which forms the ventricular septum. The left ventricular wall is two to three times thicker than that of the right ventricle, a feature which is well seen echocardiographically (Fig. 24.37).

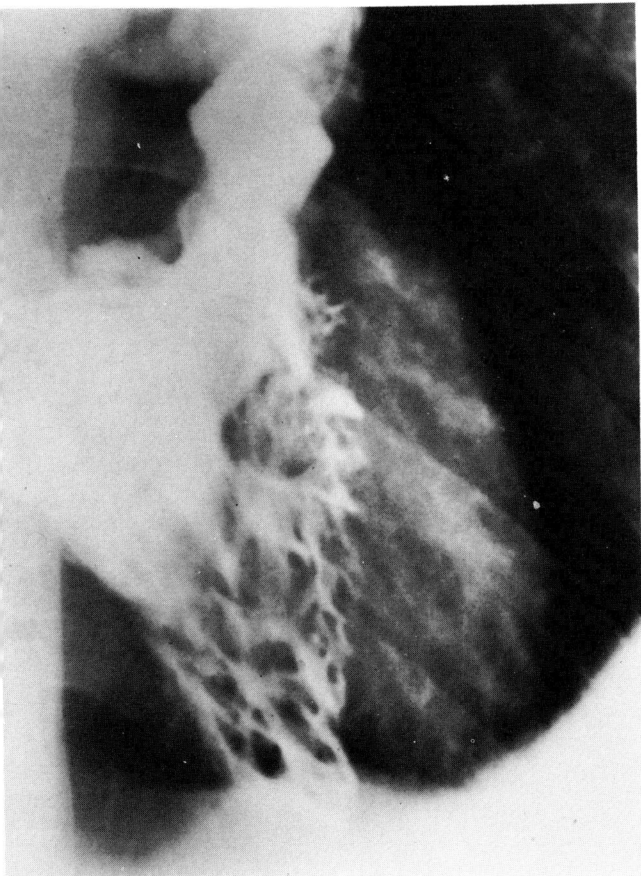

Fig. 24.40 Right ventricular angiocardiogram to demonstrate morphology showing smooth inflow and outflow tracts and central trabeculated zone.

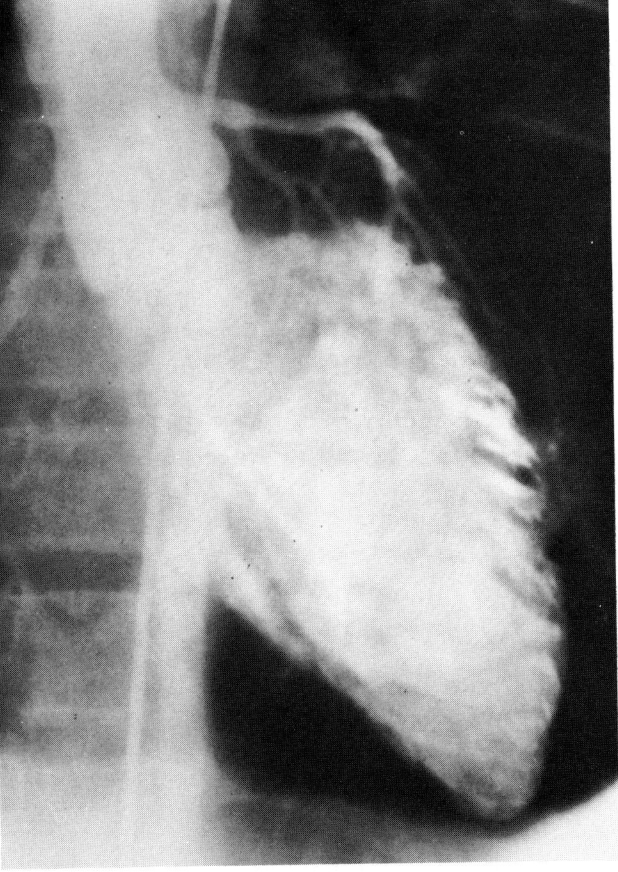

Fig. 24.41
Left ventricular angiocardiogram to show normal morphology (compare with Fig. 24.40). Note fine trabeculation.

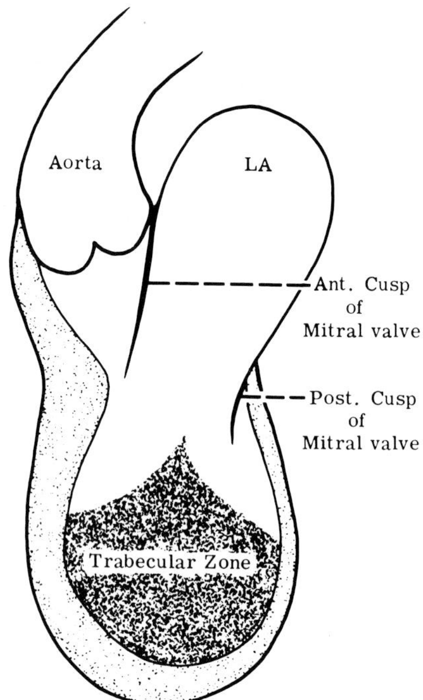

Fig. 24.42 A diagram showing the position of the anterior cusp of the mitral valve during atrial systole (lateral) (after *Quain's Anatomy*).

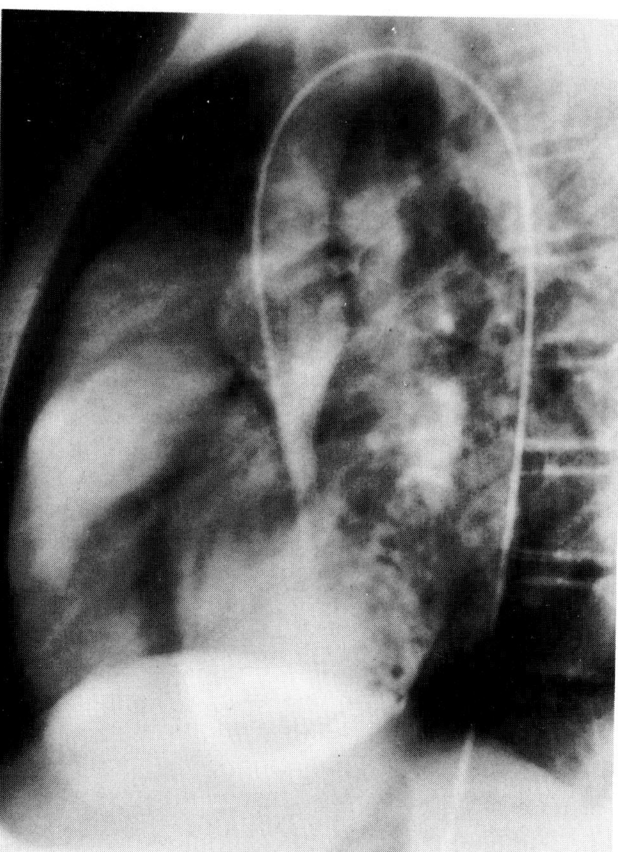

Fig. 24.43 Angiocardiogram demonstrating the anterior cusp of the mitral valve encroaching upon the left ventricular outflow tract during atrial systole. Aortomitral valve continuity is also seen.

The mitral valve. The mitral valve has an anterior cusp and a posterior cusp (Fig. 24.42), the latter frequently consisting of three small scallops. The anterior cusp is longer than the posterior and projects down to the left ventricle between the mitral and aortic orifices. In atrial systole (Fig. 24.43) the position of the anterior cusp can be seen clearly as it approximates towards the ventricular septum forming the characteristic cone shape seen on lateral angiocardiography. This view also demonstrates the continuity of the aortic and mitral valves already described (Fig. 24.42). This continuity is seen even more clearly on echocardiography (Fig. 24.37). Whilst the posterior cusp of the mitral valve cannot normally be identified angiographically, there is a tendency for one or more scallops to be redundant. In this situation, prolapse of the 'cusp' can easily be identified with the valve in profile in the right anterior oblique projection (Fig. 24.44). This can also be demonstrated echocardiographically (Fig. 24.45). Mitral incompetence may or may not be present.

The aortic valve. The aortic valve lies at the root of the aorta and has three cusps, one anterior and two posterior (Fig. 24.46). As with the pulmonary artery, the wall of the aorta bulges out adjacent to each cusp forming a sinus of Valsalva. The cusps are described in relation to the coronary arteries thus being termed the right coronary cusp (i.e. anterior), the left coronary cusp (i.e. left posterior) and the non-coronary cusp (i.e. right posterior).

The relationship of the aortic and pulmonary cusps is shown in Figure 24.47.

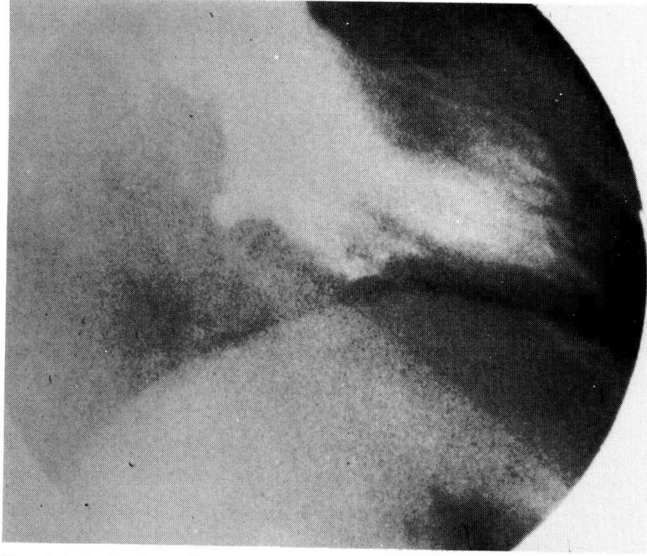

Fig. 24.44 Angiocardiogram showing prolapse of posterior cusp of mitral valve.

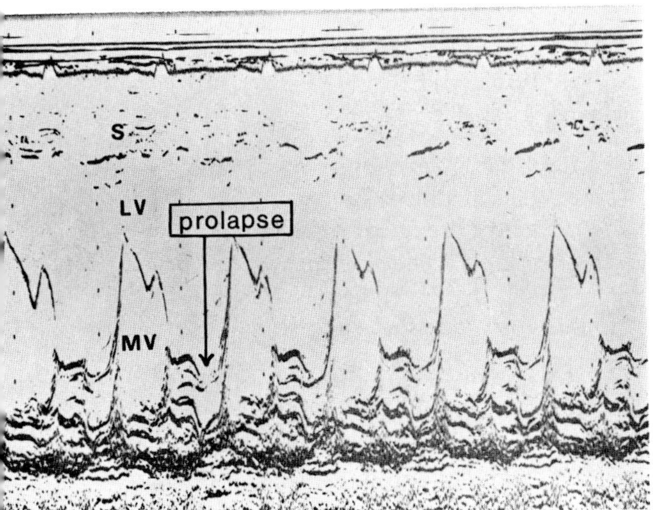

Fig. 24.45 Echocardiogram of mitral valve prolapse.

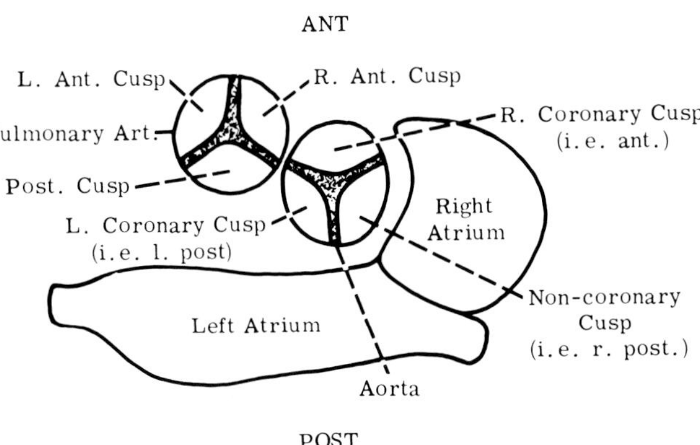

Fig. 24.46 Diagram showing relationships of the pulmonary artery and aorta to the atria. The cusps of the great arteries are also identified.

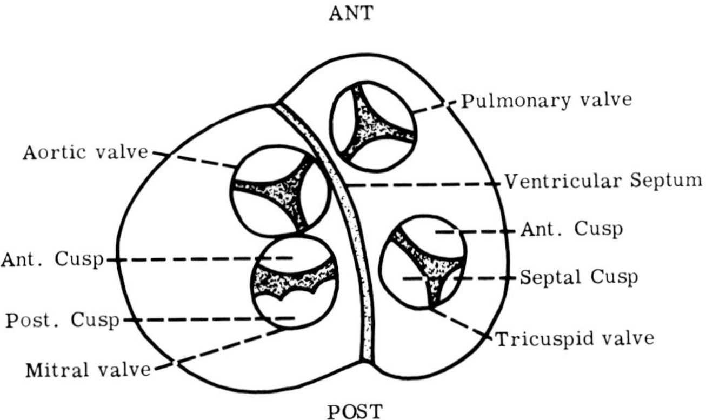

Fig. 24.47 A view of the base of the ventricle after removal of the atria to show the obliquity of the ventricular septum and the relationship of the mitral and tricuspid valve and also aortomitral continuity. (After *Quain's Anatomy*.)

The aortic cusps and the sinuses of Valsalva can be identified clearly both on left ventricular angiocardiography and in aortograms. They can easily be identified by noting that the lowest cusp is the non-coronary cusp and the right and left coronary cusps are seen on the right and left sides respectively.

ANGIOGRAPHY OF THE VENTRICULAR SEPTUM AND THE ATRIOVENTRICULAR VALVES

The ventricular septum is triangular in shape, its apex being at the apex of the heart with its base being fused posteriorly and superiorly with the atrial septum. Thus it slopes backwards and to the patient's right with the septum bulging into the cavity of the right ventricle. The septum is formed from two parts — the membranous and the muscular portions. The latter is divided into the inflow, the trabecular and the infundibular zones. These arise from the endocardial cushion, the primitive ventricle and the bulbus cordis respectively. The membranous portion of the septum varies considerably in size and shape but is nearly always present. It is well defined below, where it is sharply demarcated from the muscular portion of the septum, but above merges imperceptibly into the tissues of the aortic root. The membranous portion of the septum lies high in the septal wall and occupies the angle between the right coronary and non-coronary cusps of the aortic valve extending as far posteriorly as the origins of the anterior cusp and the mitral valve. From the right side, the membranous portion of the septum lies high between the tricuspid valve and the crista. It is crossed by the origin of the septal cusp of the tricuspid valve dividing it into an atrioventricular and interventricular component.

Defects in the ventricular septum

These can be classified as follows:

1. Perimembranous — adjacent to the central fibrous body and membranous septum.

   a. Inlet.
   b. Trabecular.
   c. Infundibular.
   d. Confluent.

2. Muscular defects (surrounded entirely by muscle).

   a. Inlet.
   b. Trabecular.
   c. Infundibular — may be associated with aortic regurgitation.
   d. Confluent.

Any of the defects described in 1 and 2 above may be isolated or occur in any combination.

3. Total absence of infundibular septum — the so-called doubly committed subarterial defect. This may also be associated with aortic regurgitation.
4. Malaligned defects.
   a. Malalignment of the atrial septum with the inlet ventricular septum giving rise to a double inlet ventricle or stradding atrioventricular valve.
   b. Malalignment of the trabecular septum with the infundibular septum giving rise to Fallot's tetralogy or double outlet ventricle.
5. Atrioventricular (Gerbode) defect. This communication between the left ventricle and the right atrium usually lies beneath the tricuspid valve and the communication is through a cleft within the valve.

The radiological investigation of the ventricular septum

The ventricular septum can be regarded topographically as consisting of two parts: 1. postero-inferior, 2. antero-superior.

The former is the more extensive and forms a wide angle with the latter. Clearly it is impossible to view both portions of the septum in one angiographic projection and from their orientation it will be apparent that they will not be clearly visualized on the standard projections (antero-posterior, lateral and oblique). Bargeron et al (1977) and Elliott et al (1977) have established the following views of the ventricles and septum which enable a more accurate spacial diagnosis of defects to be made.

1. **Long axial projection**. With the patient lying supine the C arm is rotated 65° into the left oblique position wit 25° of craniocaudal tilt (Fig. 24.48). This projectio demonstrates:

a. The infundibular septum
b. The trabecular septum.

It is useful for demonstrating:

a. Ventriculo-arterial connections
b. Infundibular ventricular septal defects
c. Trabecular ventricular septal defects.

2. **The right oblique projection**. The C arm is rotate 30° into the right oblique position with or without cranio caudal tilt (20°) (Fig. 24.48). An injection into the righ ventricle will demonstrate:

a. Infundibular morphology
b. The morphological anatomy of tetralogy of Fallot o double outlet right ventricle, the tricuspid valve and th right pulmonary artery.

Injection into the left ventricle will demonstrate the mitral valve and the long axis of the left ventricle.

3. **The four chamber projection**. The C arm is rotatec 40° in the left oblique position with 40° of craniocauda tilt (Fig. 24.48). This will demonstrate;

a. The atrial septum
b. Atrioventricular connections
c. The atrioventricular septum

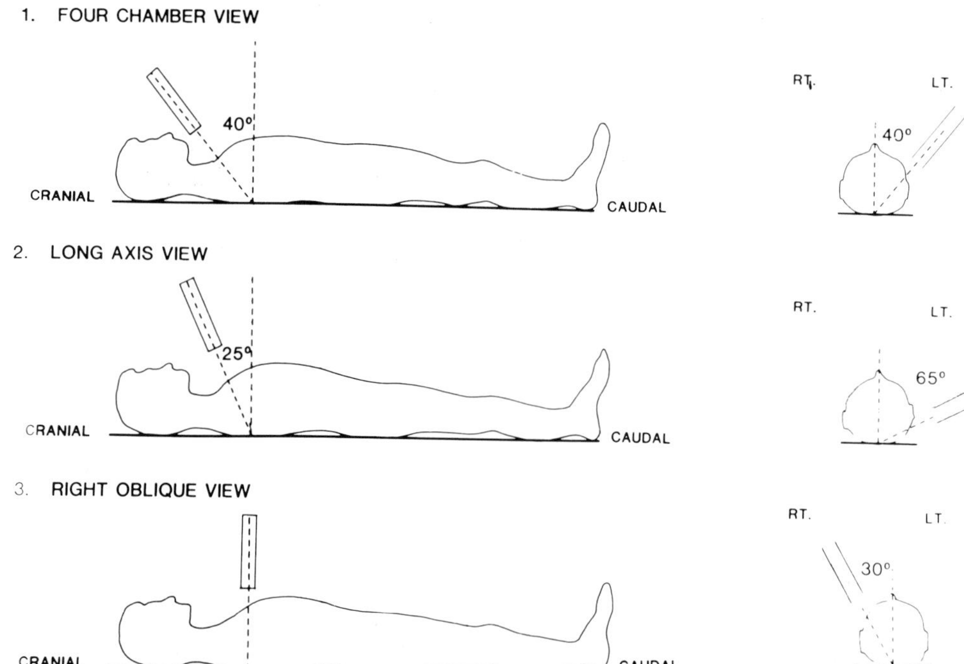

Fig. 24.48 Diagrams of four-chamber, long axial and right oblique projections.

4. The inlet ventricular septum
5. Trabecular septum.

It is useful for demonstrating perimembranous ventricular septal defects and also defects in the muscular and trabecular septa. It will also show atrioventricular septal defects and the bifurcation of the main pulmonary artery.

The identification of the site of the defect together with the ventricular morphology are taken into account in the establishment of a final diagnosis. The various ventricular septal defects are considered separately in association with ventricular morphology.

Volume of contrast agent to be used

Until recently, the only contrast agent available was an ionic compound containing a significant quantity of sodium. In small infants, particularly those with left ventricular failure, a sodium load was particularly undesirable. It was for this reason that the amount of contrast agent was limited, it being generally agreed that the total volume of contrast injected including test doses should not exceed 4 ml per kg body weight. Thus, for single injections, the following guidelines were used:

1. Shunt situations with a high flow rate: total volume to be injected — 2 ml per kg body weight.
2. Shunt situations with moderate flow or valve incompetence: total volume to be injected — 1.5 ml per kg body weight.
3. Ventricular or great artery injections without obstruction, incompetence or shunt: total volume to be injected — 1 ml per kg body weight.
4. Severe obstruction to outflow without a shunt situation: total volume to be injected — 0.5 ml per kg body weight.

Nevertheless even with these limitations, it was not unknown for an investigation to have to be terminated because the maximum safe limit of contrast had been reached before a diagnosis had been obtained. A repeat investigation then had to be performed with all its added risks. However, the introduction of the *non-ionic* contrast agents has revolutionized this situation as they enable a greater volume to be utilized. Indeed, it is probably safe to use twice the volume of the non-ionic agent compared with an ionic agent. Many centres now use the non-ionic agent routinely in infants and neonates undergoing angiocardiography.

Digital Subtraction Angiography

This computer-assisted technique undoubtedly leads to better detail in angiographic studies. It does not forgo the need for injections on the systemic side of the circulation but it does result in diagnostic images being obtained using a smaller volume of contrast. Thus a combination of the digital subtraction technique and non-ionic contrast agents now makes angiographic investigation of the neonate and small infant a much safer procedure than it was in the past.

RADIONUCLIDE IMAGING IN CONGENITAL HEART DISEASE

Although radionuclide investigations are relatively non-invasive, they have two drawbacks. They involve the use of ionizing radiation and the resolution of the technique is such that detailed anatomical analysis is not possible. As the majority of patients with clinical heart disease are young, echocardiography is usually technically possible though sedation may be necessary. However, some useful information can be obtained from radionuclide studies when it has not been possible to obtain a satisfactory echocardiogram.

The indications for radionuclide studies are:

1. Detection and quantification of shunts both from left to right and vice versa.
2. Assessment of the direction of flow within the heart and great vessels.
3. Assessment of ventricular size, morphology and function.
4. Assessment of myocardial perfusion.

Isotopes

The following are commonly employed:

1. Technetium-99m ($^{99}Tc^{m}$)-labelled red blood cells.
2. Carbon dioxide labelled with oxygen-15 ($^{15}O_2$) which is a positron emitter.
3. Thallium-201 (^{201}Tl).
4. Technetium-99m-labelled macroaggregates.

Left to right shunt

In the normal patient, the clearance of $^{99}Tc^{m}$ from the lung can be demonstrated by collecting counts from a given area of the lung. The activity is seen to fall off in a mono-exponential fashion. If a left to right shunt is present, the increased activity is seen as a late peak on a time activity curve. If the areas under the curves are calculated, pulmonary to systemic flow ratio can be derived (Treves 1980). The accuracy of the calculation depends, among other factors, on a good injection bolus and this fact is liable to result in error. In addition, it is not possible to detect shunts less than 1 to 1.2.

An alternative method is for the patient to breathe carbon dioxide labelled with oxygen-15, a positron emitter. $^{15}O_2$ is converted by carbonic anhydrase to $^{15}O_2$-labelled water which enters the pulmonary venous system. In the normal situation, there is an exponential decay in the activity in the lungs and washout occurs. In the presence of a left to right shunt, a second peak occurs due to recirculation. The size of the peak is proportional to the shunt which can then be calculated (Boucher et al 1977).

In practice shunts are usually calculated at cardiac catheterization but the isotope method is useful to check if there is any residual left to right communication following surgical closure of the defect.

Right to left shunting

Macroaggregated albumin (MAA) is labelled with $^{99}Tc^m$ and injected intravenously. Normally 97% of MAA is extracted by the pulmonary capillary bed on the first pass. In the presence of a right to left shunt, the number of counts recorded in systemic organs such as the kidneys, which receive 20% of the systemic output, is compared with the known injected activity and counts recorded from the lungs. Thus the magnitude of the right to left shunt can be calculated. The risk of significant embolisation must be borne in mind and the injected dose calculated accordingly.

The anatomy of pathophysiological communications

Using the first pass technique and accumulating data dynamically utilizing short time interval frames, the anatomy of the heart can be visualized. Thus it is possible to demonstrate early filling of the left ventricle simultaneous with right ventricular filling. Such a finding would indicate a right to left shunt as seen in Fallot's tetralogy. Unfortunately, due to the relatively long half-life of $^{99}Tc^m$ (6 hours), this technique is limited to three first-pass studies at any one time. However, it is possible that Iridium–191 with a half-life of 5 seconds may prove to be a much more satisfactory alternative (Treves et al 1980).

Coronary artery anomalies

Thallium-201 is valuable in assessing the degree of ischaemia that may occur in the presence of an anomalous origin of a coronary artery. The ischaemia may be related to a 'steal syndrome' if the anomalous origin arises from the low pressure pulmonary circulation. Global and regional wall abnormalities can also be recorded using $^{99}Tc^m$ gated blood pool studies.

MRI

MRI is currently being evaluated and already shows great promise as a new non-invasive technique for elucidating congenital heart lesions (Didier et al 1986).

REFERENCES AND SUGGESTIONS FOR FURTHER READING

Bargeron L. M., Elliott L. P., Soto B. et al (1977) Axial cineangiography in congenital heart disease: section I. Concept, technical and anatomic considerations. *Circulation*, **56**, 1075–1083.

Baylan B. G., Meyer, R. A. & Kaplan, S. (1975) The critically ill premature infant with persistent ductus arteriosus and pulmonary disease, an echocardiographic assessment. *Journal of Paediatrics*, **86**, 423–432.

Boucher C. A., Ahluwalia B. & Block P. C. (1977) Inhalation imaging with $15o_2$-labelled carbon dioxide for detection and quantitation of left to right shunts. *Circulation*, **56**, 632–640.

Counahan R. & Joseph M. (1973) The plain chest radiograph in d-transposition of the great arteries in the first month of life. *Journal of Paediatric Radiology*, **1**, 217–223.

Didier D., et al. (1986) Congenital heart disease: gated MR imaging in 72 patients. *Radiology*, **158(1)**, 227–235.

Elliott L. P., Bargeron L. M., Bream P. R. et al (1977) Axial cineangiography in congenital heart disease: section II. Specific lesions. *Circulation*, **56**, 1084–1093.

Heymann M. A. & Rudolph A. M. (1972) Effects of congenital heart disease on foetal and neonatal circulation. *Progress in Cardiovascular Diseases*, **15**, 115–143.

Jefferson K. E. & Rees R. S. O. (1980) The skeleton: The bony thorax in heart disease. In *Clinical Cardiac Radiology*, part III, ch. 13, pp. 125–133. London: Butterworths.

Macartney F. J., Zuberbuhler J. R., Anderson R. H. (1980) Morphological considerations pertaining to recognition of atrial isomerism. Consequences for sequential chamber localisation. *British Heart Journal*, **44**, 657–667.

Macleod W. M. (1954) Abnormal transradiancy of one lung. *Thorax*, **9**, 147.

Nogrady M. B., Dunbar J. S. (1969) Complete transposition of the great vessels, re-evaluation of the so-called typical configuration on plain films of the chest. *Journal de l'Association Canadienne des Radiologistis*, **20**, 124–131.

Partridge J. B., Scott O., Deverall P. B., Macartney F. J. (1975) Visualisation and measurements of the main bronchi by tomography as an objective indicator of thoracic situs in congenital heart disease. *Circulation*, **51**, 188–196.

Rigby M. L., Anderson R. H., Gibson D. et al (1981) Two dimensional echocardiographic categorisation of the univentricular heart. Ventricular morphology, type and mode of atrioventricular connection. *British Heart Journal*, **46**, 603–612.

Shinebourne E. A., Elseed A. M. (1974) Relationship between foetal flow patterns, coarctation of the aorta and pulmonary blood flow. *British Heart Journal*, **36**, 492–498.

Shinebourne E. A., Macartney F. J., Anderson R. H. (1976) Sequential chamber localisation — logical approach to diagnosis in congenital heart disease. *British Heart Journal*, **38**, 327–340.

Silverman, N. H., Lewis A. B., Heymann M. A. & Rudolph A. M. (1974) Echocardiographic assessment of ductus arteriosus shunt in premature infants. *Circulation*, **50**, 821–825.

Tajik A. J., Seward J. B., Hayler D. J. et al (1978) Two dimensional real-time ultrasonic imaging of the heart and great vessels. Technique, image orientation, structure identification and validation. *Mayo Clinic Proceedings*, **53**, 271–303.

Treves S. (1980) Detection and quantitation of cardiovascular shunts with commonly available radio nuclides. *Seminars in Nuclear Medicine*, **10**, 16–26.

Treves S., Cheng C., Samuel A. et al (1980) Iridium- 191 angiocardiography for the detection and quantification of left to right shunts. *Journal of Nuclear Medicine*, **21**, 1151–1157.

Valdez Cruz L. M. Pieroni D. R., Rowland J. M. et al (1976) Echocardiographic detection of intracardiac right to left shunts following peripheral vein injection. *Circulation*, **54**, 558–562.

CHAPTER 25

CONGENITAL HEART DISEASE — SPECIFIC CONDITIONS

SYSTEMIC VENOUS DRAINAGE

Anomalies of systemic venous return are not uncommon but they rarely cause any significant functional deficit. In utero, venous drainage into the sinus venosus takes place via the right and left cardinal, vitelline and umbilical veins. Development occurs (Fig. 25.1) so that:

1. The right and left cardinal veins join to form the superior vena cava.
2. The right vitelline vein forms the inferior vena cava.
3. The left horn of the sinus venosus forms the coronary sinus.
4. The left umbilical vein joins the right vitelline vein via the ductus venosus in utero and regresses after birth.

The sinus venosus is guarded by right and left venous valves. The right valve, the Eustachian valve, is important in fetal life, directing oxygenated blood from the inferior vena cava through the foramen ovale and thus bypassing the lungs.

ANOMALIES OF SYSTEMIC VENOUS RETURN

In the presence of an atrial septal defect, the occasional persistence of the Eustachian valve after birth will give rise to left atrial desaturation. If the left cardinal vein persists as a left superior vena cava, it will usually drain into the coronary sinus but will occasionally drain into the roof of the left atrium. A right superior vena cava may or may not be present. If so, it does not necessarily communicate with the left superior vena cava. If the right vitelline vein obliterates instead of the left vitelline vein, the inferior vena cava will drain to the coronary sinus.

If both vitelline veins fail to persist, venous drainage from the lower half of the body is via the right posterior cardinal vein — the azygos vein. This developmental anomaly is associated with left isomerism (see p. 615) and has clinical implications if cardiac catheterization is being considered from the groin. Very rarely both the superior and the inferior vena cavae may enter the left atrium resulting in *total anomalous systemic venous return*. This condition is also likely to be associated with left isomerism.

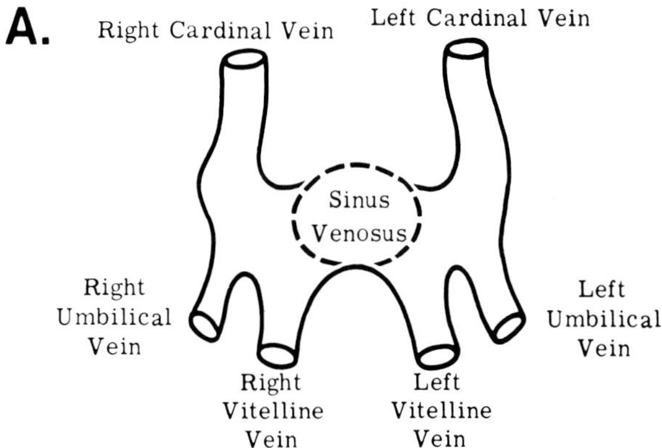

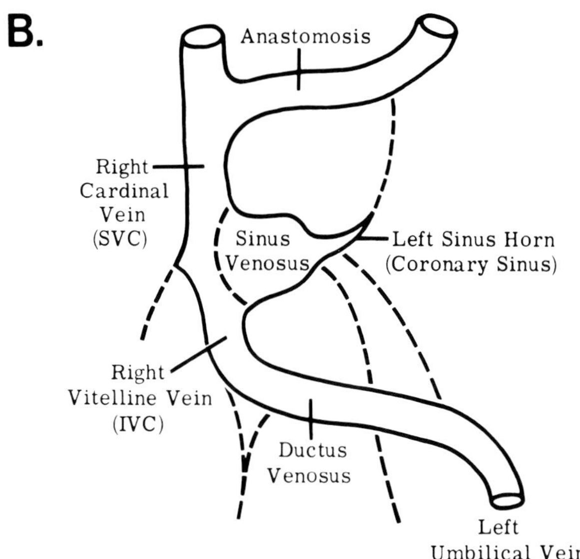

Fig. 25.1 Diagrammatic representation of sinus venosus and venous development (see text). (Courtesy of R H Anderson and *Price's Textbook of Medicine*.)

Clinical features. The majority of the anomalies described above do not have any significant clinical implications. It is only in those situations where a right to left shunt is present that cyanosis and desaturation may occur.

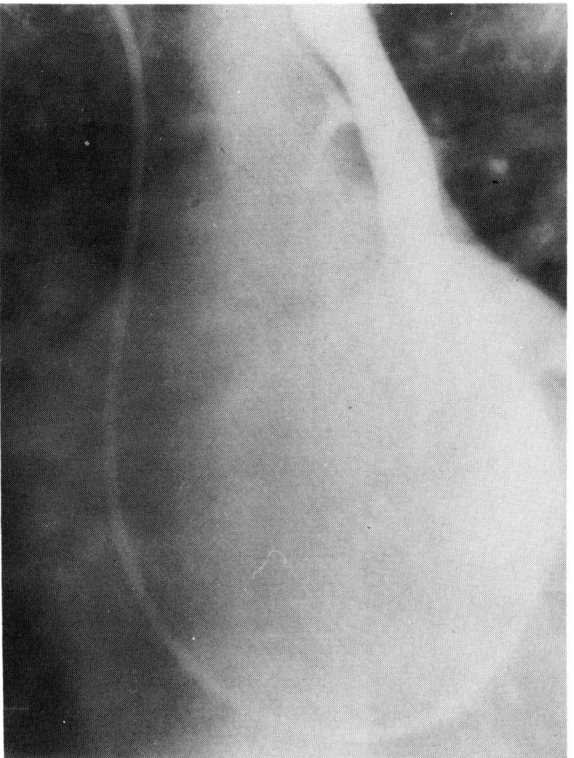

Fig. 25.2 Angiogram showing a fullness on the left side of the superior mediastinum due to a prominent left SVC.

These will include a *persistent Eustachian valve* and *total anomalous systemic venous return*.

The plain radiograph. This is often normal. A persistent left superior vena cava may give rise to fullness of the left side of the superior mediastinum (Fig. 25.2). If there is a significant right to left shunt, the lung fields may appear oligaemic.

Echocardiogram. Abnormal systemic venous return can be outlined by paracoronal suprasternal sections which will demonstrate a left superior vena cava or an azygos vein draining into the left superior vena cava (Figs 25.3, 25.4). The diagnosis of left isomerism with absent inferior vena

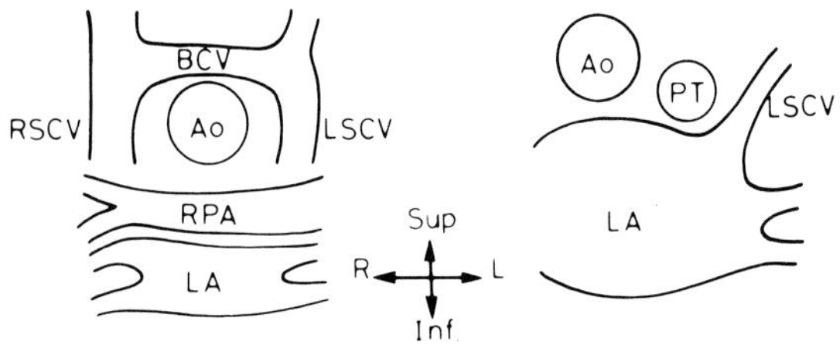

Fig. 25.3 Illustration of anomalous venous drainage.

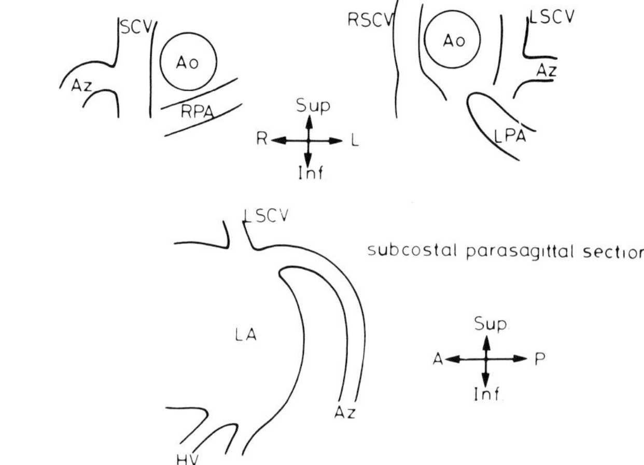

Fig. 25.4 Azygos vein in left atrial isomerism.

cava and venous drainage from the lower body via the azygos vein has been described in the section on sequential analysis (see p. 616).

Angiocardiography. The diagnosis of anomalous systemic venous return is usually made angiographically. As indicated above, it rarely has any significant effect in its own right but such anomalies are frequently associated with complex congenital heart abnormalities. Angiography in combination with echocardiography are the methods of choice for definitive diagnosis.

PULMONARY VENOUS ANOMALIES

Embryology and anatomy. The primary pulmonary vein arises from the posterior aspect of the left atrium uniting with the intrapulmonary veins which originate from the splanchnic plexus, thus allowing oxygenated pulmonary venous blood to reach the left atrium. Anomalies of pulmonary venous return occur when this union, either partially or completely, fails to happen. If the primary pulmonary vein is not fully incorporated into the posterior portion of the left atrium, it forms a separate chamber giving rise to the condition known as *cor triatriatum* (Fig. 25.5). There is almost always a pressure gradient between the primary pulmonary vein and the left atrium in this situation.

Union of the intrapulmonary veins with the caudal portion of the left cardinal vein gives rise to anomalous drainage to the coronary sinus via a persistent left superior vena cava. On the other hand, union with the cephalic portion of the left cardinal vein results in anomalous drainage, usually total, to the superior vena cava via the innominate (brachiocephalic) vein. Should the intrapulmonary veins remain united to the splanchnic veins, then drainage will occur anomalously into the portal system beneath the diaphragm.

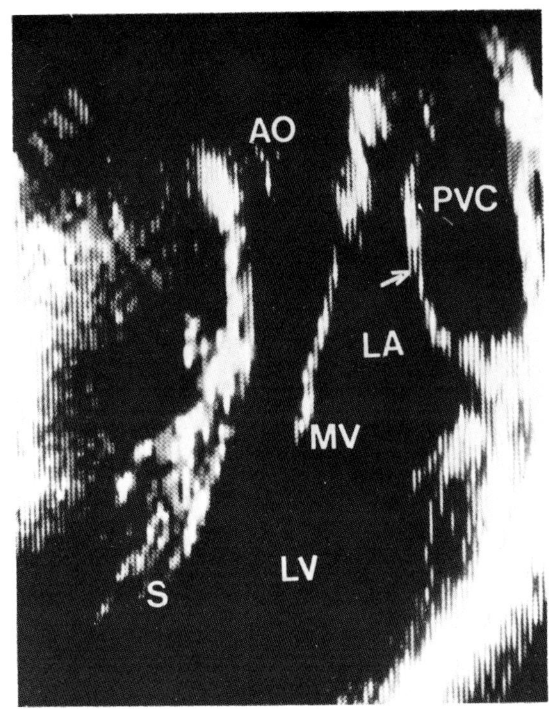

Fig. 25.5 Cross-sectional echocardiogram of a heart showing cor triatriatum. PVC — pulmonary venous confluence; arrow points to intra-atrial diaphragm.

TOTAL ANOMALOUS PULMONARY VENOUS DRAINAGE (TAPVR)

This is a relatively rare condition, accounting for less than 2% of all cardiac malformations (Keith et al 1967), in which the venous return from the lung drains, usually by a single trunk, into almost any part of the sinus venosus system. An associated septal defect is always present. The types of anomalous pulmonary venous return have been classified as follows:

Type 1 — Supracardiac return draining either into: a. the vertical vein which communicates with the brachiocephalic vein and the superior vena cava, or b. the azygos vein leading to the right superior vena cava. (Incidence: 55% of all TAPVR.)

Type 2 — Anomalous return at cardiac level, either into the coronary sinus or directly into the right atrium. (Incidence: 30% of all TAPVR.)

Type 3 — Infradiaphragmatic return draining into the portal system, a persistent ductus venosus or the inferior vena cava. (Incidence: 12% of all TAPVR.)

Type 4 — Draining at multiple levels. (Incidence: 3% of all TAPVR.)

Anatomy and physiology

Group A. In the presence of total anomalous return, a mixing situation occurs in the right atrium. Thus pulmonary venous blood is desaturated by the systemic venous return in the right atrium. For blood to enter the systemic circulation, an atrial septal defect must be present. As the right ventricular end-diastolic pressure is below that of the left ventricle, there is preferential flow through the right side of the heart. Hence high flow, pulmonary plethora and cyanosis are present. The increased pulmonary flow will eventually result in an elevated pulmonary vascular return if untreated.

Group B. Obstruction to pulmonary venous return may be seen in TAPVR types 1 and 3, particularly the latter. In type 1, if the vertical vein is kinked at its entry into the brachiocephalic vein or compressed by the left main bronchus, it may be obstructed. On the other hand, in type 3, infradiaphragmatic TAPVR, flow is frequently compromised as the descending vertical vein enters the portal system.

Clinical course. Obstructed TAPVR presents in the neonatal period with pulmonary oedema. If obstruction is absent, presentation with breathlessness and right ventricular failure occurs later but usually before the age of 6 months.

Imaging appearances

Plain radiograph. The appearances differ in the two groups.

Group A. Normal pulmonary vascular resistance and unobstructed pulmonary venous return

The cardiac configuration is that of an enlarged heart with right atrioventricular predominance. The increased flow through the lungs results in plethora. This appearance is identical with a large left to right shunt from any cause. The following features, which are peculiar to TAPVR, may be seen on the chest radiograph.

Type 1. (a) The figure of eight (Snowman) appearance (Fig. 25.6) is seen when the vertical vein unites with the brachiocephalic vein. Due to an increased flow, the brachiocephalic vein and the superior vena cava are dilated giving rise to the prominent superior contour of the mediastinum. This appearance is rarely seen in early infancy.

(b) If drainage is via the azygos vein, this vein may be enlarged.

Type 2. An abnormal contour may be seen on the right side of the heart similar in appearance to that formed by an enlarged left atrium. This is said to be due to an enlarged coronary sinus.

Differential diagnosis of group A. Patients with a high pulmonary blood flow and cyanosis secondary to TAPVR have to be distinguished from those with concordant atrioventricular and discordant ventriculo-arterial connections (complete transposition) and truncus arteriosus. If pulmonary arterial hypertension is present in any of this differential group, then pulmonary plethora will be replaced by dilated proximal pulmonary arteries and peripheral pruning.

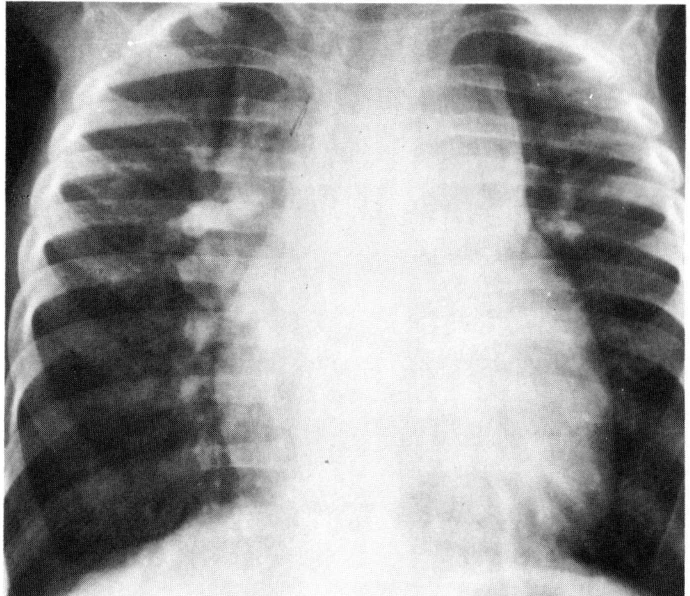

Fig. 25.6 Total anomalous pulmonary venous drainage. PA chest radiograph showing widening of the superior mediastinum forming a 'Snowman, figure-of-8 or cottage loaf' appearance. This is due to a dilated left innominate vein from increased flow. (See Fig. 25.9).

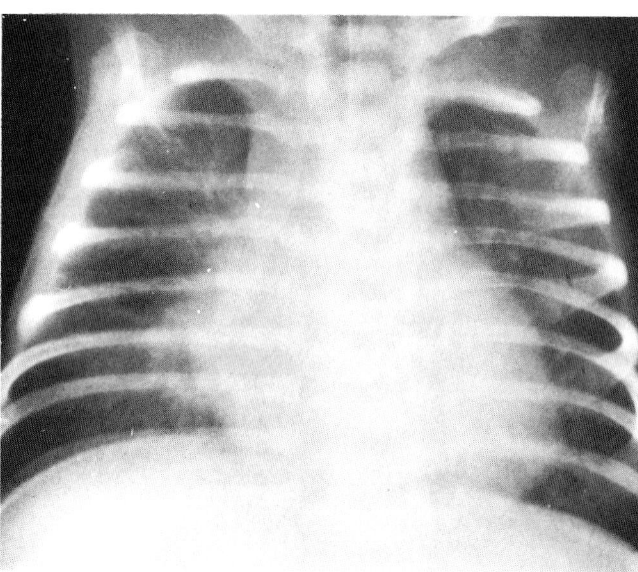

Fig. 25.7 Obstructed infra-diaphragmatic total anomalous pulmonary venous return. The heart is enlarged and there is a diffuse haze throughout both lungs indicating interstitial pulmonary oedema, secondary to obstruction of the descending common pulmonary vein as it enters the portal system.

Group B. Obstructed pulmonary venous return

In the presence of obstruction, the heart size is usually normal and gross pulmonary oedema is the dominating radiological feature of the patients who present in early infancy. The radiological appearance is that of coarse mottling obscuring details of pulmonary vessels (Fig. 25.7). Consequently, it may not be possible to recognize pulmonary venous hypertension. Thus, there may be considerable difficulty in differentiating between obstructed TAPVR (usually infradiaphragmatic), hyaline membrane disease, widespread respiratory infections including miliary tuberculosis and the hypoplastic left heart syndrome. Although the heart size is initially small, sooner rather than later, heart failure leading to cardiac dilatation occurs. Even if drainage is supracardiac, it is seldom that any of the radiological characteristics of types 1 and 2 can be identified.

Echocardiography. The characteristic echocardiographic features of TAPVR are demonstrated on a four-chamber section. The pulmonary veins are seen to join in a venous confluence superior to the left atrium (Fig. 25.8A). In supracardiac drainage, suprasternal para-coronal sections will show the venous confluence draining to the superior vena cava via dilated vertical and brachiocephalic veins. If the drainage is to the coronary sinus, a posterior four-chamber section will show the coronary sinus to be extremely dilated. In infradiaphragmatic drainage, a descending vein originating from the pulmonary vein confluence passes through the diaphragm parallel and in close proximity to the descending aorta to enter the inferior vena cava or hepatic portal vein. This

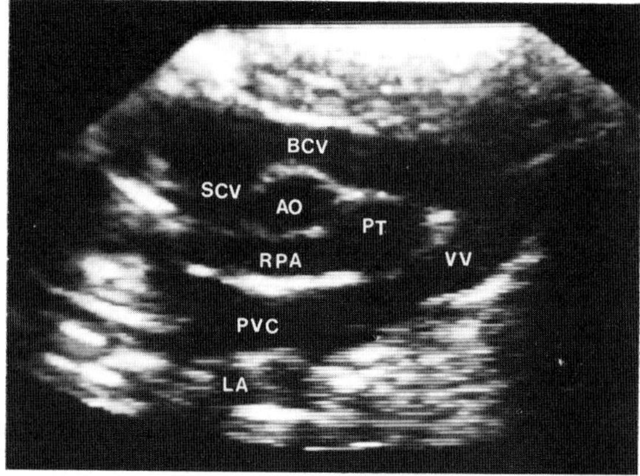

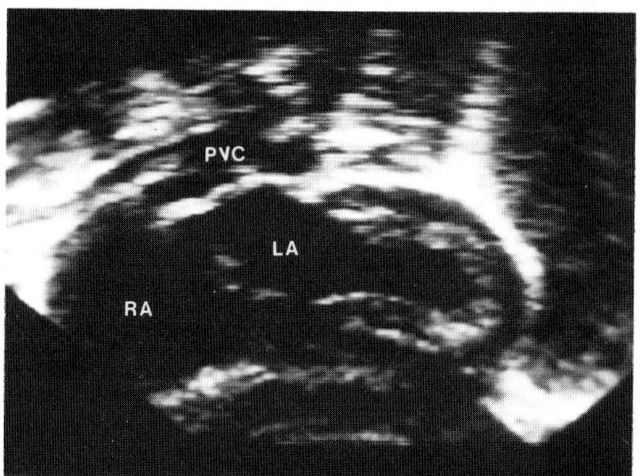

Fig. 25.8 A. and **B.** Suprasternal cross-sectional echocardiograms from a patient with supracardiac total anomalous pulmonary venous drainage. BCV Brachiocephalic vein; VV Vertical vein; PVC Pulmonary venous confluence.

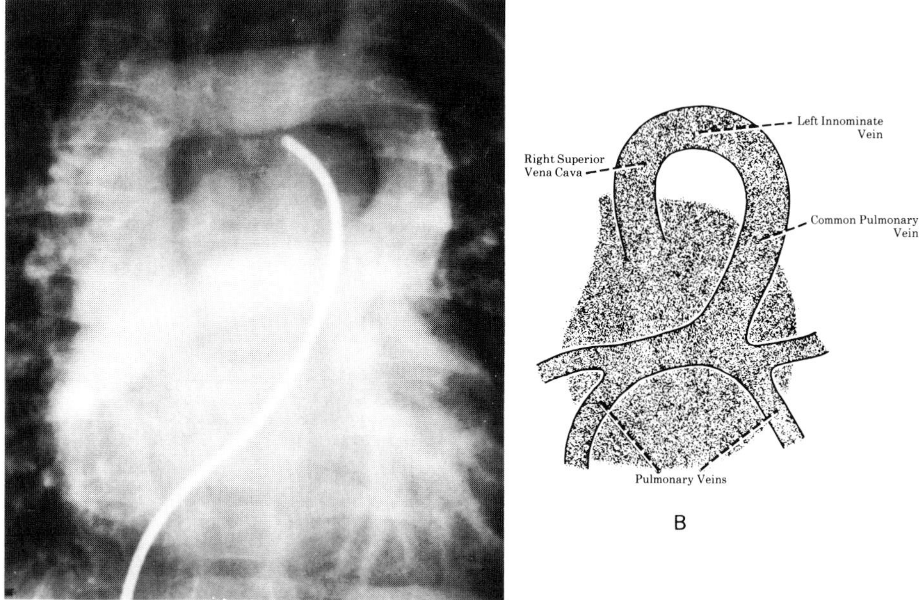

Fig. 25.9 A. and **B.** AP angiocardiogram demonstrating common pulmonary vein draining into left innominate vein which is dilated due to high flow.

descending vein is demonstrated by subcostal parasaggital section (Fig. 25.8B).

Angiocardiography. The anomalous venous return is demonstrated by injecting contrast into the main pulmonary artery and observing the drainage site of the pulmonary venous return (Fig. 25.9). It is essential to demonstrate good left ventricular function prior to total correction. This can be done either angiographically or by an echocardiogram.

Imaging technique of choice

As it is essential to identify accurately the anatomy and site of the anomalous venous return, it is almost always advisable to perform an angiogram. This is particularly important in cases of obstructed venous return especially if the venous return is of the infradiaphragmatic variety.

Management

Patients who have obstructed venous return, either supra- or infradiaphragmatic, require early surgical intervention. If there is no obstruction, operation can be delayed until the patient is older, but clearly it should be before there is irreversible change in the pulmonary vascular bed. Surgical correction of the anomalous drainage is by reimplanting the common venous channel into the left atrium and closing the associated septal defect.

ATRIAL SEPTAL DEFECT

Anatomy and embryology. Isolated atrial septal defects account for about 10% of all congenital heart disease. The defect occurs if the septum secundum fails to grow in order to obliterate the ostium secundum. The size varies from the smallest opening to almost complete absence of the septum, the average defect being 2–3 cm in diameter. The sinus venosus defect occurs if the right upper pulmonary vein over-rides the atrial septum and drains anomalously to the right atrium. This variety represents 5–10% of all atrial septal defects.

Physiology. Since the compliance of the left ventricle is greater than that of the right ventricle, systolic pressure in the left atrium is higher than that in the right atrium and a left to right shunt occurs. Thus blood returning from the lungs to the left atrium passes simultaneously to the left ventricle and the right atrium. Hence, in the right atrium, there is mixing of systemic and pulmonary venous return with a consequent increase in the volume passing through the right ventricle to the lungs.

The volume of the shunt depends both on the size of the defect and on the right atrial pressure which in turn relates to the right ventricular pressure and pulmonary vascular resistance.

Clinical. The majority of patients with this condition go through infancy and childhood with few if any symptoms and often the defect is only suspected when a murmur is heard at a routine examination. In later life, the clinical course depends largely on the size of the defect, small defects being well tolerated into middle and even old age. Occasionally these lesions are discovered as a result of atrial dysrythmias in the fifth or sixth decade. Patients with larger shunts may go into right heart failure aged 20–30, due either to a diastolic overload or to the development of an elevated pulmonary vascular resistance and pulmonary hypertension.

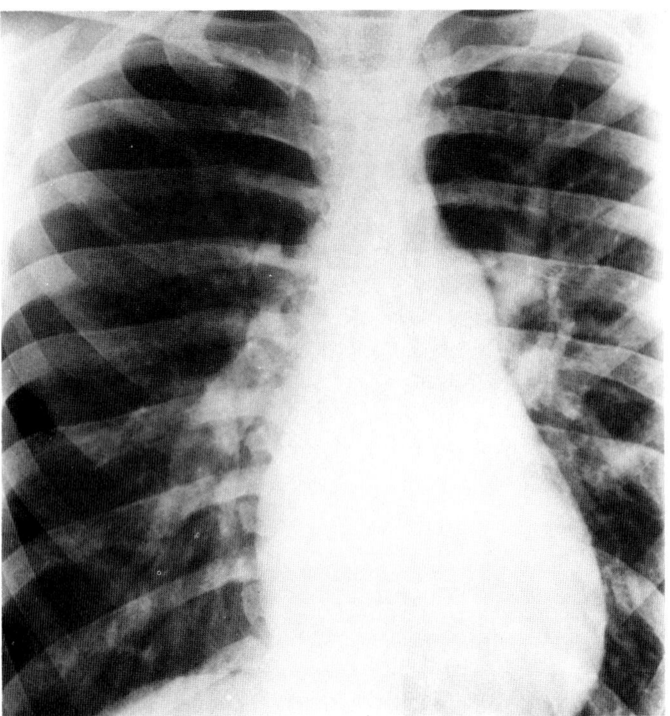

Fig. 25.10 PA film showing right atrioventricular enlargement with displacement of the heart to the left and apparently small aortic knuckle. Pulmonary plethora is also present.

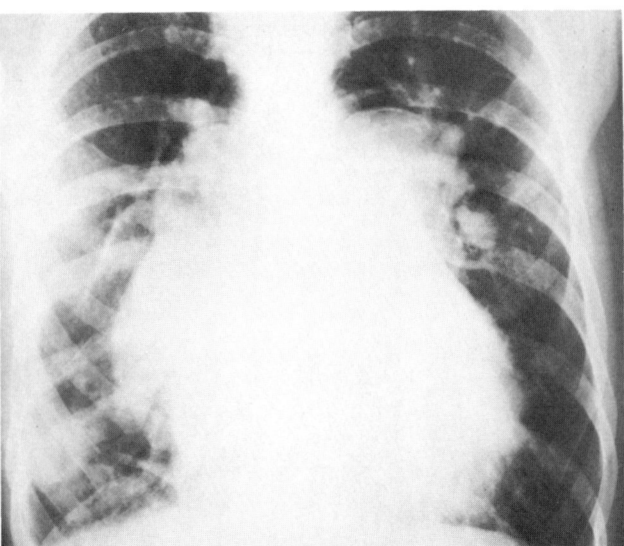

Fig. 25.12 Secundum ASD in later life (35 years) with the radiological changes of classical pulmonary hypertension. Note (a) the large proximal pulmonary arteries and marked peripheral pruning and (b) calcification in the main branches of the pulmonary artery, best seen at upper margin of l. hilum.

Imaging

Plain film. The increased volume load on the right side of the heart results in the right atrium and right ventricle being under strain. The characteristic cardiac configuration on the radiograph is that of right atrioventricular enlargement (Fig. 25.10). The right ventricle hypertrophies and dilates, leading to an anticlockwise rotation of the heart. Thus, in the frontal view, the right ventricle may form the left heart border. In addition, the arch of the aorta comes to lie more in the antero-posterior plane and as a result the aortic knuckle appears to be smaller than in the normal person. Angiography, however, confirms that the aorta is of normal size but lies within the mediastinum (Fig. 25.11).

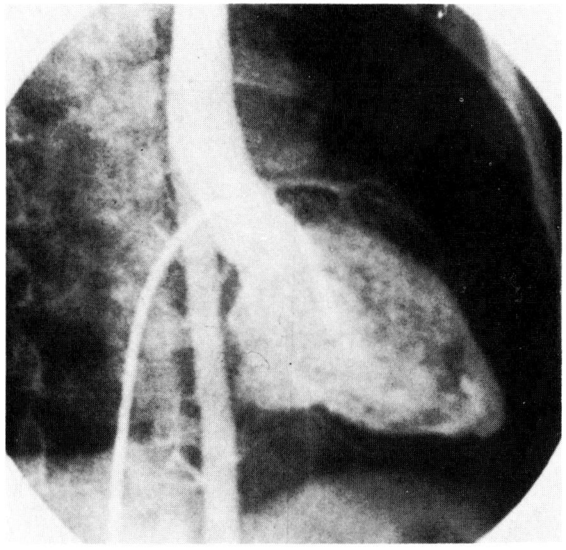

Fig. 25.11 Left ventricular angiocardiogram in patient with secundum ASD. Note (a) normal aortic dimensions, (b) catheter passing from right atrium through ASD to LA and LV.

Uncomplicated secundum defects usually show marked pleonaemia. Even large defects with a high pulmonary flow do not usually develop pulmonary hypertension until the second or third decade. It is later still before the more rarely seen Eisenmenger situation develops. Pulmonary hypertensive changes are due to gradual obliteration of the pulmonary vascular bed. This follows thrombotic episodes secondary to hypertrophy of the muscular component of

Fig. 25.13 **A.** Cross-sectional echocardiogram from a patient with an atrioventricular septal defect with two valves. There is right isomerism and complete absence of the atrial septum. **B.** Angiogram of LV injection in an osteum primum ASD. Note distance from inferior aspect of mitral valve to apex of ventricle is shorter than that from the superior aspect to the apex. Note also mitral regurgitation. **C.** 'Goose neck' deformity due to the anterior cusp of the atrioventricular valve floating up into the left ventricular outflow tract forming the lower border of the goose neck. The upper border of the goose neck is formed by the origin of the aorta and the superior margin of the left ventricular outflow tract. Film in diastole. **D.** Cross-sectional echocardiogram showing an atrioventricular septal defect with a common valve. **E.** LV angiogram in the four-chamber projection. VSD is seen to lie in the posterior portion of the inflow septum. The deficient ventricular septum is indicated by lack of visualization of the ventricular septal crest (see Fig. 25.17) and there is no communication between LV and RV underneath the aortic valve. The common A-V valve is seen as a non-opaque ring. Later frames would show contrast entering the atria through the valve ring (horizontal arrow with arrow head at either end). (Reproduced by courtesy of B. Soto.)

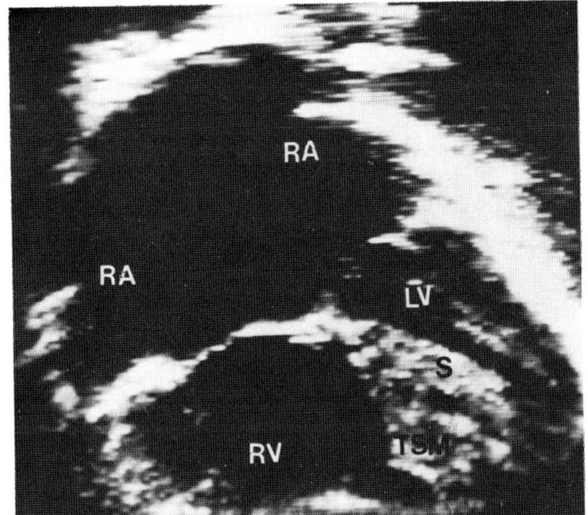

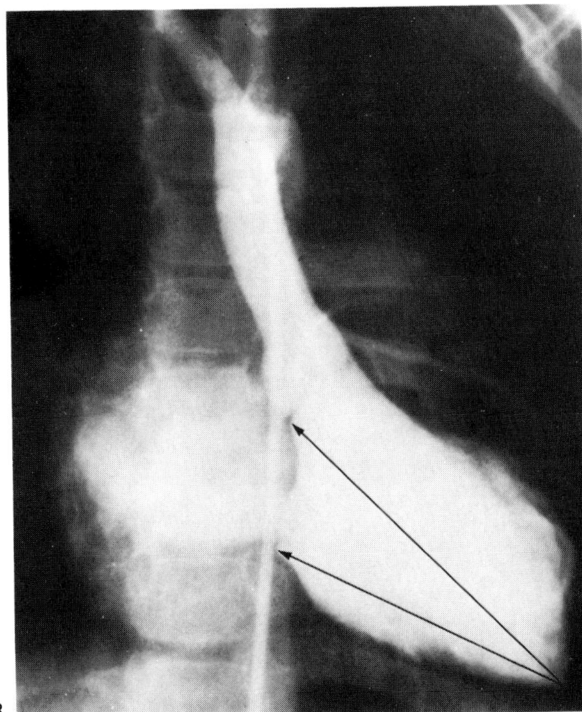

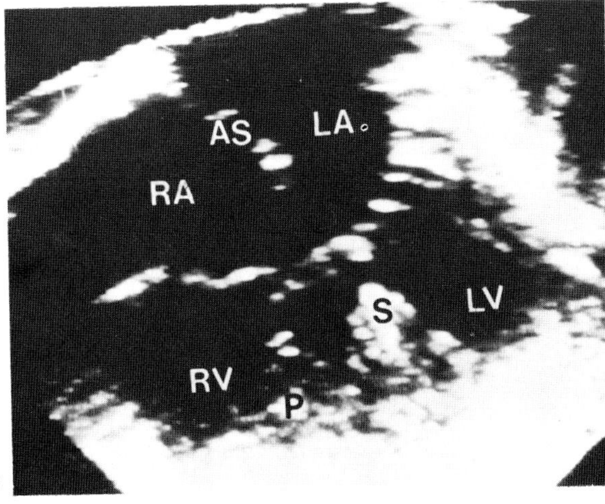

the walls of small vessels. Hypertrophy is consequent upon the long-standing, high-flow situation. This late and relatively slow development of severe pulmonary hypertension may very occasionally result in degenerative calcification in the main and proximal arteries (Fig. 25.12).

Echocardiography. All defects in the atrial septum can be demonstrated by subcostal four-chamber sections (Fig. 25.13).

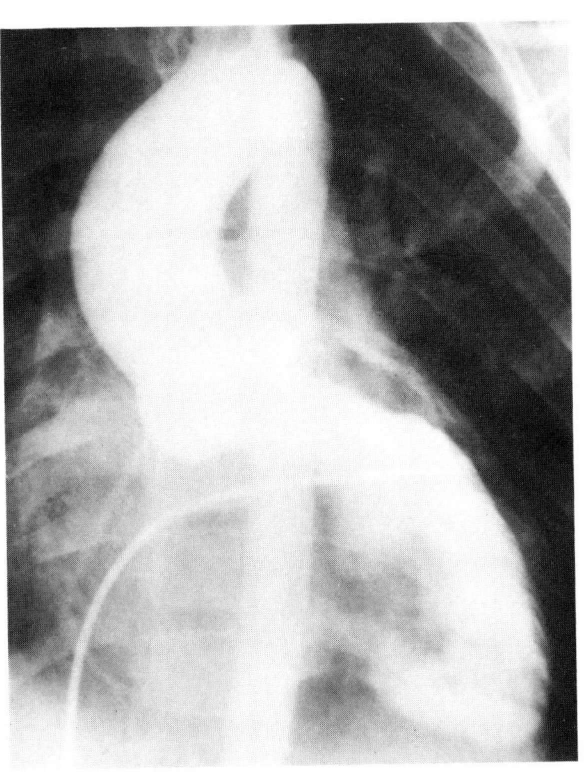

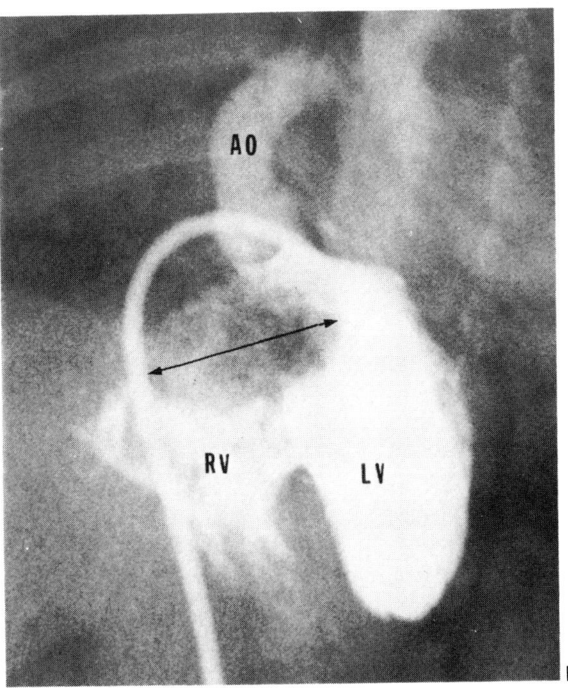

Cardiac catheterization. The diagnosis can be confirmed by demonstrating a rise in oxygen saturation in the right atrium and an increase in the ratio of the pulmonary to systemic flow rate. Angiographically, a pulmonary artery injection and flow-through to the left side of the heart will show the right atrium filling following left atrial opacification. Alternatively, a pulmonary vein can be selectively injected via a catheter passed through the defect. Using the four-chamber view (see p. 640), contrast will be seen passing from left to right across the superior portion of the atrial septum. Betriu et al (1975) have described an association between secundum atrial septal defects and partial prolapse of the posterior mitral valve leaflets. This combination may occur in up to 15% of patients with a secundum defect. Although the valves are usually competent, plication may occasionally be necessary, and it has become customary in some centres to perform a left ventricular angiogram as part of the investigation in order to assess mitral valve competence. This is performed by passing the catheter across the atrial septum and then through the mitral valve into the left ventricle.

Optimum imaging technique

Plain film findings will reveal a left to right shunt. The radiographic signs are sufficiently characteristic in the older patients to enable a fairly confident diagnosis of secundum atrial defect to be made. Nevertheless, this should be confirmed prior to surgery by echocardiography. If there is any clinical doubt as to the level of the pulmonary vascular resistance, cardiac catheterization can be used to determine this accurately.

Management. Closure of an atrial septal defect is usually recommended either aged 4–5, if it is diagnosed in infancy, or at the time of diagnosis, if found later in life. Surgery is aimed to prevent the development of irreversible changes in the pulmonary capillary bed, the onset of atrial fibrillation in the fifth or sixth decade and the more theoretical risk of subacute bacterial endocarditis at the site of the defect. However, it must be recognized that the diagnosis is sometimes made after the pulmonary vascular resistance has risen to a level which precludes surgery. Surgical mortality is very low, being less than 1%.

ATRIOVENTRICULAR SEPTAL DEFECTS

This group of anomalies is known by a variety of names, such as *endocardial cushion defect*, *atrioventricular canal malformations* and *atrioventricular defects*. The basic malformation is a deficiency of the atrioventricular part of the septum and on the basis of these observations the collective group of anomalies is probably better termed *atrioventricular septal defects*. The basic subdivision of atrioventricular septal defects is made on the basis of the valve leaflets which guard the malformed atrioventricular junction.

When the junction is guarded by separate right and left atrioventricular orifices, it is known as a *partial atrioventricular defect*. The most typical example is an ostium primum defect. If there is a common atrioventricular valve, a *complete defect* is present. Associated lesions are important. The most common of these is obstruction of the left ventricular outflow tract by atrioventricular tissue tags or alternatively discrete subaortic stenosis, tetralogy of Fallot, double outlet right ventricle, right atrial isomerism, complete transposition or congenitally corrected transposition together with hypoplasia of either the right or left ventricle.

PARTIAL ATRIOVENTRICULAR SEPTAL DEFECTS

Incidence, anatomy and physiology. This condition is widely known as the ostium primum type and accounts for approximately 20% of all atrial septal defects or 3% of all congenital heart disease. The anomaly is characterized by separate right and left atrioventricular orifices with a large defect between the lower edge of the atrial septum and the septal annulus of the separated valves.

Almost always there is a so-called 'cleft' between the anterior and posterior leaflets of the left atrioventricular valve which gives rise to varying degrees of mitral regurgitation. This 'cleft' is functionally a commissure. Both atrioventricular valves are attached to the crest of the inlet septum at the same level. In a few cases, small deficiencies occur at the site of the attachment of the leaflets, particularly the anterior leaflet, which permit interventricular communication.

Very occasionally hearts with well-formed primum atrial septum defects may have no cleft in the mitral valve or, alternatively, an isolated mitral cleft is the only stigma of an atrioventricular defect. The consequences of a partial atrioventricular septal defect are left to right atrial shunting and a varying degree of mitral regurgitation. Because of the cleft in the mitral valve, shunting from left ventricle to right atrium may also occur.

Clinical course. This depends on the degree of valve incompetence and whether or not congenital heart block is present. In the absence of heart block and incompetence, the clinical course is that of the secundum atrial defect. When mitral incompetence is present the clinical course is always more severe. The age of presentation depends on the severity. In contrast to patients with a secundum atrial defect who frequently do not have symptoms until the second or third decade, patients with a primum atrial septal defect often present between the ages of about 10 and 14.

The strain on the right ventricle, due to the left to right shunt at atrial level, is aggravated by tricuspid incompetence if present, and mitral incompetence places a load on the left ventricle. About 20% of patients have a significantly increased pulmonary vascular resistance.

A primum defect with valve incompetence is therefore a much more serious condition than a secundum defect. It also poses a more difficult technical problem for correction and, as a result, surgical mortality is higher.

Imaging

The plain film. When there is no significant valve incompetence, the appearances on the plain film resemble those of the secundum atrial septal defect showing right atrioventricular enlargement. If incompetence is present, the appearances depend on its degree. Mitral incompetence causes enlargement of the left ventricle but the left atrium does not increase in size as the regurgitant jet passes through the defect and strain is taken by the right atrium. Cardiac configuration is therefore that of biventricular and right atrial enlargement. The cardiothoracic ratio nearly always exceeds 1:2 and, as with the secundum defect, the aorta appears small. The lung fields are moderately pleoanaemic but by the second decade, radiological evidence of pulmonary hypertension and left ventricular failure may be seen.

Echocardiography. Subcostal or apical four-chamber sections demonstrate the morphology of the atrioventricular junction. There are separate right and left atrioventricular orifices, which are each at the same level, the valves being attached to the crest of the ventricular septum. In the majority of cases, there is a large defect between the lower edge of the atrial septum and the valve annulus so that part of this interatrial communication is within the ventricular mass (Fig. 25.13A). The left ventricular outflow tract is narrowed and subaortic stenosis is occasionally present. There may be a small interventricular communication at the site of the attachment of the left anterior leaflet and, rarely, the atrial septum is virtually intact. If there is a common atrium, right atrial isomerism is likely.

Angiography. The position of the interatrial defect can be accurately defined by the use of the four-chamber view (see p. 640) following a selective injection into the right upper pulmonary vein. The valve ring can be demonstrated in profile in the anterior projection when the degree of valve incompetence can be estimated (Fig. 25.13B).

COMPLETE ATRIOVENTRICULAR SEPTAL DEFECTS

Incidence, anatomy and physiology. Hearts with a common orifice account for approximately 60% of all cases of atrioventricular septal defects. There is lack of fusion of the anterior and posterior leaflets on the crest of the septum so that a ventricular septal defect is automatically present between the facing bridging leaflets. There is a common atrioventricular valve together with a defect between the lower edge of the atrial septum and the valve anulus. An inlet ventricular septal defect of variable size, depending upon the attachments of the bridging leaflets to the crest of the septum, and a narrow left ventricular outflow tract are also present. Complete atrioventricular septal defects allow left to right shunting at atrial and ventricular level. In addition there is a varying degree of mitral and/or tricuspid regurgitation frequently shunting from left ventricle to right atrium. The effect is to almost always produce severe congestive heart failure unless there is an associated tetralogy of Fallot when cyanosis predominates.

Clinical course. Complete atrioventricular septal defects usually present in early infancy with severe heart failure and surgery is almost always required. When there is a delay in the fall of the pulmonary vascular resistance, heart failure may not be the major feature and these infants may be relatively asymptomatic. Nevertheless, there is a tendency in this group for the early development of pulmonary hypertension.

Imaging

The plain film. The appearance on the plain film varies enormously depending on the degree of valve incompetence, the volume of the shunt and the presence or absence of heart failure.

Echocardiography. Subcostal and apical four-chamber sections readily demonstrate the morphology of the condition. The posterior bridging leaflet is frequently attached by a midline raphe to the crest of the ventricular septum though in some cases it may be free-floating. In the majority of patients, the anterior bridging leaflet is attached to a normally positioned medial papillary muscle on the right ventricular side of the septum (Fig. 25.13D). It is attached by multiple chordae to the crest of the septum. With increasing amounts of bridging of the anterior leaflet, the medial papillary muscle is displaced to the apex of the right ventricle and the bridging leaflet is less well attached to the crest. Hypoplasia of the left or right ventricle together with the appropriate component of the common orifice is an important variant which should be excluded.

Angiography. The following points can be demonstrated:

1. The anatomy of the atrioventricular valve. The characteristic findings in the atrioventricular canal defect were described by Baron et al (1964). These are a combination of the abnormal position of the aortic valve and the displaced and abnormally attached anterior leaflet of the common atrioventricular valve.
2. The presence or absence of a ventricular septal defect.
3. The direction of the atrioventricular and interventricular shunts.

Points 1 and 2 are best demonstrated in the anterior and long-axial projections. The four-chamber view will demonstrate the direction of the shunt.

The characteristic appearance described by Baron is the so-called 'goose neck' deformity seen in diastole (Fig. 25.13C). The anterior cusp of the atrioventricular valve floats up into the left ventricular outflow tract forming the lower border of the goose neck. As the origin of the aorta appears to be displaced superiorly taking a more vertical course than normal, its upper border together with the superior margin of the left ventricular outflow tract form the upper part of the goose neck. In systole, the anterior leaflet may be smooth but sometimes appears irregular due to abnormal chordae tendinae attachment. Often there is a definite cleft in the mid portion through which the regurgitant jet may pass. If so, it enters the right atrium directly due to the absence of the atrioventricular component of the septum. The abnormally placed mitral valve results in a reduction in the distance from the inferior aspects of the valve ring to the apex of the left ventricle. A further left ventricular injection in the long-axial position with the ventricular septum in profile will show the two components of the atrioventricular valve and confirm or exclude a ventricular septal defect. The four-chamber view shows the interventricular and atrioventricular communications (Fig. 25.13E) and the single atrioventricular valve ring.

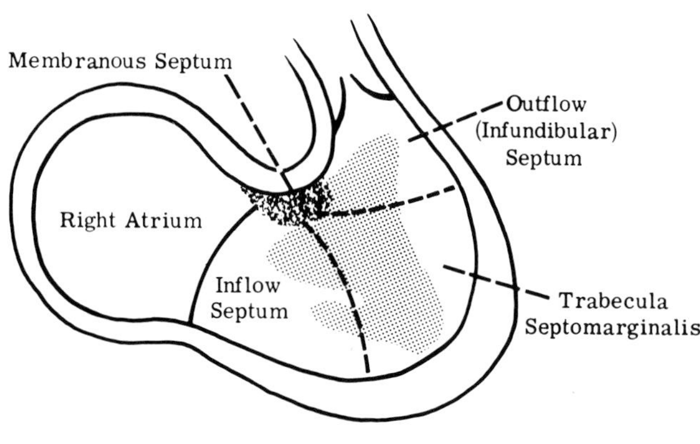

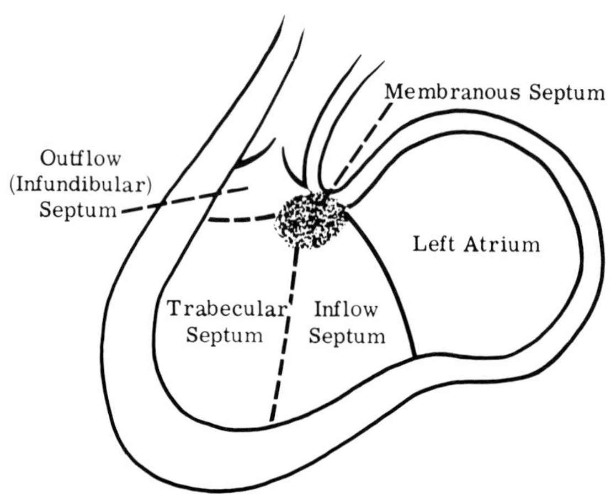

Fig. 25.14 Diagram to show inflow, outflow and trabecular zones of the muscular portion of the inter-ventricular septum from the ventricular aspects. (After Quain's Anatomy).

VENTRICULAR SEPTAL DEFECTS

Defects of the ventricular septum are the commonest type of congenital cardiac malformation. This section is confined to the so-called isolated ventricular septal defect, although there may be associated lesions such as atrial septal defect, pulmonary valve stenosis and coarctation of the aorta. This group accounts for 12% of all congenital heart disease.

A similar incidence of ventricular septal defect is found as part of complex congenital heart lesions such as tetralogy of Fallot, double inlet ventricle, absence of an atrioventricular connexion and double outlet ventricle. They are also frequently found in complete transposition, pulmonary atresia and atrioventricular discordance. Ventricular septal defects in these lesions have specific features which will be described in the appropriate sections.

Anatomy

The classification of isolated ventricular septal defects is a contentious topic. The terms 'infracristal' and 'supracristal' defects are in common use.

The so-called supracristal defect is placed in the outflow tract above the trabecular septomarginalis which in this instance qualifies as the crista. An infracristal defect is near to the central fibrous body above the trabecular septomarginalis but beneath the infundibular septum. The infracristal defect is thus named because, in this case, the infundibular septum is chosen as the crista. This nomenclature therefore seems illogical and an alternative classification which is now in common use has been adopted.

In this classification, the ventricular septum can be divided into membranous and muscular portions, the former being extremely small. The *muscular* septum can be considered as having three parts: an inlet component separating the ventricular inlet portions; a trabecular part separating the apical zones and a third outlet component separating the outflow tracts of the right and left ventricles (Figs 24.39 and 25.14). In congenitally malformed hearts, defects are found in all parts of the ventricular septum, but they can be grouped into three basic types (Table 25.1).

Perimembranous defects are found around the central fibrous body which is the area of the heart where the tricuspid, mitral and aortic valves are in fibrous continuity. In the past these have been termed membranous defects because it was argued that they resulted from absence of the interventricular component of the membranous septum. In practice, these defects are considerably larger

Table 25.1 Classification of ventricular septal defects

Trabecular		Perimembranous
		Muscular Mid-trabecular Apical Multiple
*Outlet (subarterial)	Beneath one artery (subaortic/subpulmonary)	Perimembranous
		Muscular
	Doubly committed	Perimembranous
		Muscular rim
*Inlet		Perimembranous
		Muscular
*Confluent		Perimembranous
		Muscular

* may be associated with malalignment

than this structure. When the embryonic muscular interventricular septum closes, there is no membranous component. We prefer, therefore, to avoid 'membranous defect'. Without a doubt, however, these defects are partly bordered by the membranous septum and thus the term 'perimembranous' is preferred.

The defects are always beneath the aortic valve and they may involve mainly the inlet septum, or the trabecular septum or may divide the trabecular and outlet septa with the latter deviated into the right ventricle. Alternatively, it can be a combination of any or all of these in which case the term confluent perimembranous defect is used.

The inlet perimembranous defect lies beneath the septal leaflets of the tricuspid and mitral valves. The long axis of the perimembranous trabecular defect is directed towards the ventricular apex. Not infrequently, the septal leaflet of the tricuspid valve is a cleft in the area of the defect or there may be an anomalous attachment of tricuspid valve tissue so that direct shunting from the left ventricle to the right atrium may occur. Such defects are sometimes known as *Gerbode defects* which in the past have been thought to be a deficiency in the atrioventricular septum but this is probably very rarely the case.

Infundibular perimembranous defects result either from malalignment between the infundibular septum and the trabecular septum or hypoplasia of the former. Characteristically the aortic valve overrides the trabecular septum.

Muscular ventricular septal defects have completely muscular borders but, like perimembranous defects, they can be subclassified depending on their position within the muscular septum. Multiple small apical trabecular defects produce the condition known as 'Swiss cheese septum'. Infundibular muscular defects are less common but may allow prolapse of the right coronary cusp of the aortic valve giving rise to aortic regurgitation.

Doubly committed subarterial defects are found directly beneath the aortic and pulmonary valves which are in continuity with each other in the roof of the defect. As in the case of muscular infundibular defects, there is a capacity for prolapse of the right coronary cusp of the aortic valve and aortic regurgitation is a common complication.

Clinical features

For the most part, the clinical presentation of an isolated ventricular septal defect depends upon its size and it is the large defects, occurring in less than 10% of patients, that require surgery. At birth, pulmonary vascular resistance is high. In the presence of a large defect it falls gradually so that the clinical features of fluid retention or heart failure classically do not develop until the second or third month of life. Failure to gain weight with adequate medical treatment is an absolute indication for surgery.

Characteristically, in these patients, there is a large left to right shunt with a high pulmonary blood flow and a mean pulmonary artery pressure at least two-thirds that in the aorta. Many centres now adopt a conservative approach to management and in practice many relatively large ventricular septal defects will undergo spontaneous closure. Overall, approximately 70% of defects will close spontaneously.

In perimembranous defects, this is often by the apposition of tricuspid valve tissue and in muscular trabecular defects either by fibrosis around the margins of the defect or by ingrowth of myocardium. It appears that the muscular infundibular defect and doubly committed subarterial defects do not close spontaneously. In these cases, the development of aortic regurgitation is an absolute indication for surgical closure but it may be that prophylactic surgery may help to prevent this complication.

One of the major reasons for early surgical closure of large ventricular septal defects is to prevent the development of the *Eisenmenger syndrome*, which is, in practice, a rare complication of isolated ventricular septal defects. Rarely, patients with the Eisenmenger syndrome and a ventricular septal defect do not develop symptoms during infancy and as a consequence present later in childhood. It is likely that in these cases the pulmonary vascular resistance has never fallen.

Imaging

Plain film. Small ventricular septal defects which present as a chance finding on clinical examination have a normal chest radiograph. It is not until the pulmonary to systemic flow rate ratio is of the order of 2.5 : 1 that changes are visible on the radiograph (Fig. 25.15). As the flow ratio increases the heart becomes enlarged and the lung fields increasingly plethoric. Both the aorta and the pulmonary artery tend to increase in size although the latter is more

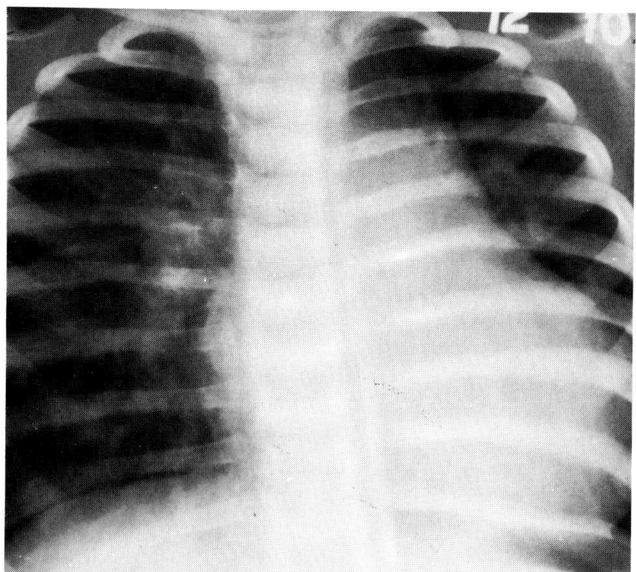

Fig. 25.15 VSD. Large heart and marked plethora due to low pulmonary vascular resistance and large defect. Pulmonary: systemic flow 4:1.

noticeable. Nevertheless, it is usually difficult to identify increase is size of the great arteries before the age of 4 or 5. Prior to this age, the heart and mediastinum are non-specifically enlarged.

Echocardiography. Four-chamber echocardiographic sections from subcostal and apical positions will identify the central fibrous body (often considered the 'crux' by echocardiographers) and distinguish between a perimembraneous inlet defect (Fig. 25.16A) and a muscular inlet defect (Fig. 25.16B). By scanning anteriorly from the subcostal four-chamber section, perimembranous trabecular defects can be identified, together with the doubly committed subarterial defects illustrating absence of the infundibular septum with aortic and pulmonary valves in fibrous continuity. From the apical and four-chamber sections, clockwise rotation of the transducer to a long axis projection will identify the infundibular or outlet septum revealing the presence of defects in this area. In addition, perimembranous defects extending into the outlet septum, together with those ventricular septal defects associated with malalignment of the outlet septum, can be seen using the same approach. Doubly committed subarterial defects can be recognized and distinguished from muscular outlet defects as muscle can be identified between the aortic and the pulmonary valves. Intermediate sections between the apical and parasternal four-chamber and long axis sections will identify perimembranous trabecular defects. Apical muscular trabecular defects are usually best identified from an apical four-chamber section but cross-sectional echocardiography may sometimes fail to demonstrate the so-called 'Swiss cheese variety' and angiocardiography has an important place in diagnosing this defect.

Angiocardiography. With the use of axial angiocardiography (see Ch. 24, p. 640), the basic types of ventricular septal defects can be recognized. Long axial projections of left ventriculograms illustrate the subaortic position of perimembranous ventricular septal defects (Fig. 25.17A). When it can be shown that the defect does not extend to the aortic valve and central fibrous body, it should be presumed that the defect is not perimembranous. This is particularly obvious in cases of muscular defects in the trabecular septum where an extensive area of septum

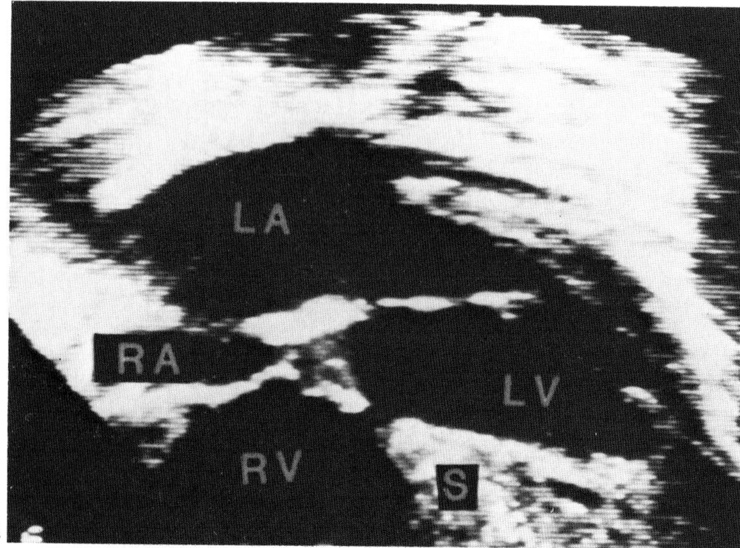

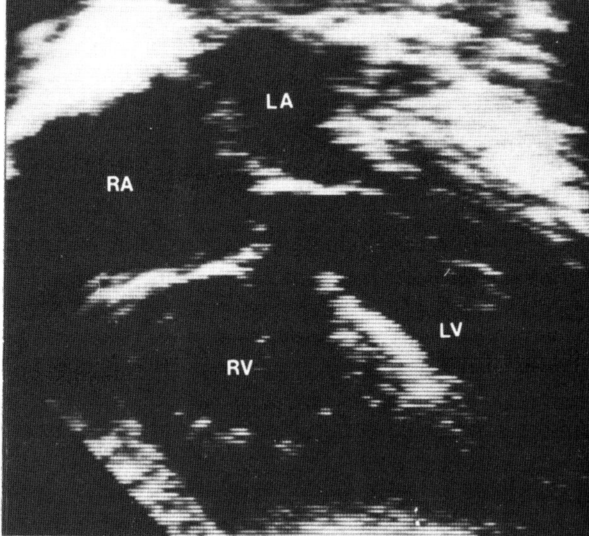

Fig. 25.16 A Cross-sectional echocardiogram showing a muscular inlet ventricular septal defect. **B** Cross-sectional echocardiogram showing a perimembranous inlet ventricular septal defect.

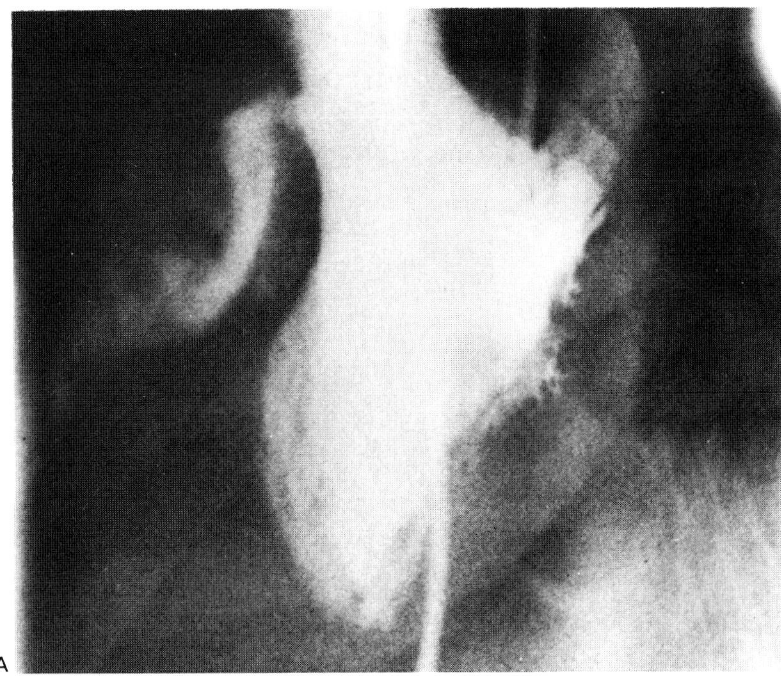

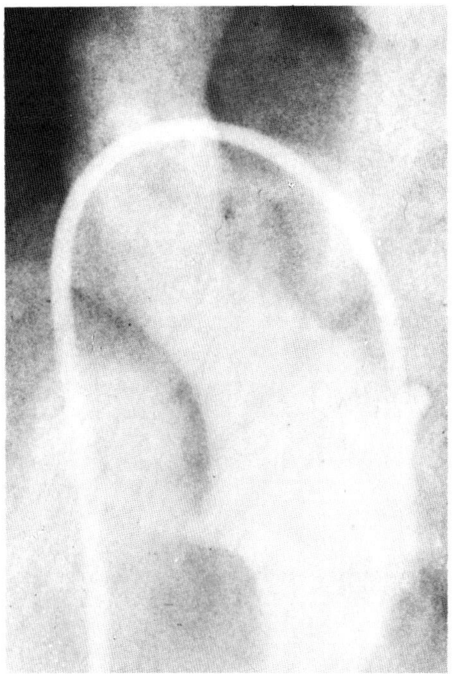

Fig. 25.17 A. Left ventriculogram from a patient with a small perimembranous ventricular septal defect. **B.** Left ventricular angiogram from a patient with a muscular trabecular ventricular septal defect.

separates the defect from the aortic valve (Fig. 25.17B). When there is a perimembranous inlet defect, not only will it be subaortic, but contrast will be seen to be trapped beneath the septal leaflet of the tricuspid valve as it passes through the defect. For other types of perimembranous defect, the majority of the contrast will be seen superior to the septal leaflet of the tricuspid valve. For doubly committed subarterial ventricular septal defects, the absence of the infundibular septum is best recognized employing the right anterior oblique projection.

Optimum imaging technique

Echocardiography is the optimal imaging technique for demonstrating the anatomy of the single ventricular septal defect. However, it is well recognized that it may fail to demonstrate smaller additional defects in the trabecular septum. Thus left ventricular angiography is mandatory in patients being considered for surgery.

TETRALOGY OF FALLOT

Tetralogy of Fallot describes a combination of anatomical features which together produce a characteristic morphological entity. It is the most common type of cyanotic heart disease and accounts for approximately 10% of all infants and children undergoing cardiac surgery.

Anatomy. The characteristic morphological abnormality in tetralogy of Fallot is anterior deviation of the infundibular septum. At one stroke this anterior deviation produces the ventricular septal defect, infundibular pulmonary stenosis and overriding of the aorta (Fig. 25.18). The right ventricular hypertrophy is a natural consequence of these features. Hearts with a ventricular septal defect and pulmonary valve stenosis or infundibular stenosis but without aortic override are not necessarily examples of tetralogy of Fallot. The degree of aortic over-ride shows marked variation in hearts exhibiting the morphological features of teralogy. In some cases the degree of override is such that both the aorta and pulmonary artery arise predominantly from the right ventricle. Hence for the purposes of categorization of the ventriculo-arterial connection, tetralogy of Fallot can exist with either ventriculo-arterial concordance or with double outlet right ventricle. Usually the ventricular septal defect is a perimembranous confluent defect extending to the infundibular septum (see above). In some examples of tetralogy with a muscular ventricular septal defect, the infundibular septum itself may be absent so that the defect becomes subarterial or what has been called supracristal. Varying degrees of hypoplasia of the pulmonary artery are almost always present. Associated anomalies are frequent in tetralogy, the most important being an atrioventricular septal defect with common orifice, absence of the pulmonary valve or absence of one pulmonary artery. A secundum atrial septal defect is a less significant association and it is sometimes called 'pentalogy of Fallot'.

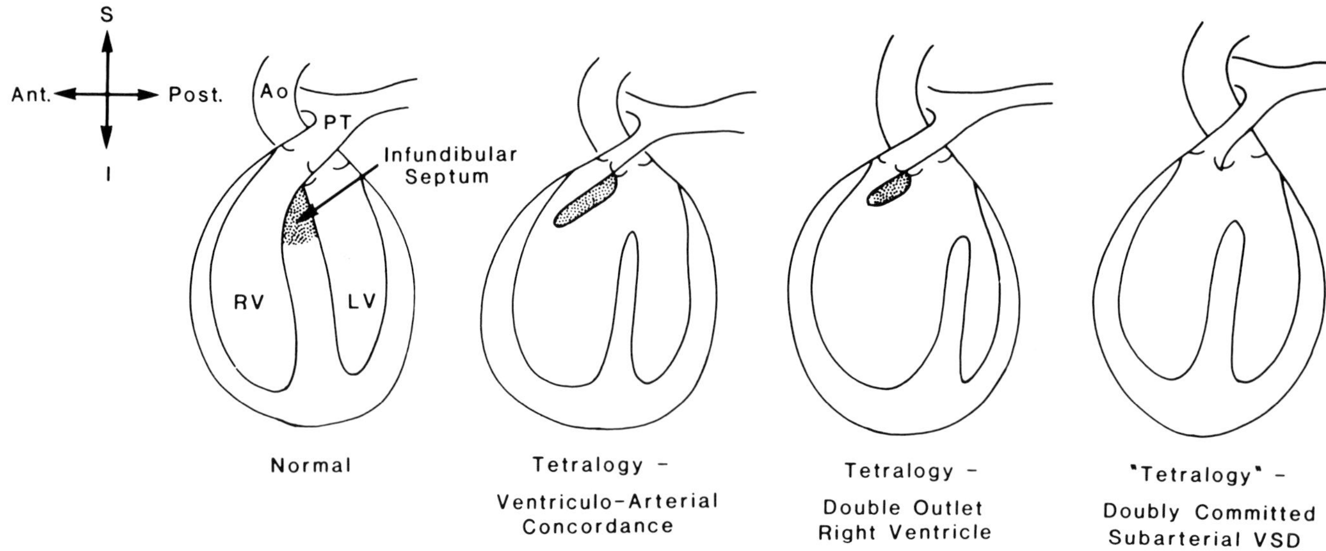

Fig. 25.18 Illustration of a normal heart and various types of tetralogy of Fallot.

Physiology. In tetralogy of Fallot, the ventricular septal defect is large and offers little resistance to flow so that the systolic pressures in the ventricles are equal. The direction and magnitude of blood flow through the defect depends upon the systemic resistance and the resistance imposed by the pulmonary stenosis. Thus very severe infundibular pulmonary stenosis gives rise to a large right to left shunt and to severe cyanosis. On the other hand mild or moderate infundibular obstruction will be accompanied by a predominantly left to right shunt and the initial presentation in infancy may be more like a simple isolated ventricular septal defect.

Clinical features. The mode and age of presentation are both dependent on the severity of the infundibular obstruction. When there is severe infundibular stenosis at birth, the neonate presents as an emergency with profound cyanosis. At the other extreme, with negligible infundibular stenosis, a large left to right shunt may present during the second or third month of life which may even cause heart failure. Most commonly a systolic murmur is heard in an otherwise asymptomatic child, but cyanosis tends to develop during the first year with increasing infundibular obstruction. Hypercyanotic spells related to muscular spasm of a severely stenotic infundibulum are a common complication and an absolute indication for further investigation and surgery.

Imaging

Plain films. The heart size is usually within normal limits providing right ventricular failure is not present. The outline can be characteristic and has been described as the 'boot-shaped heart'. This is due to the presence of right ventricular hypertrophy and a relatively hypoplastic left ventricle. The dominant hypertrophied right ventricle presents radiographically with the apex elevated above the diaphragm giving the 'boot-shaped' appearance. A marked pulmonary bay is present due to the hypoplastic main pulmonary artery (Fig. 25.19). The pulmonary vessels show oligaemia. If the right ventricular outflow tract obstruction is relatively mild leading to a left to right shunt the features described above will not be present. The cardiac outline often appears normal and in the presence of a left to right shunt there will be pulmonary plethora.

Approximately 25% of patients with Fallot's tetralogy have a right aortic arch which is seen as a prominence on the right side of the mediastinum.

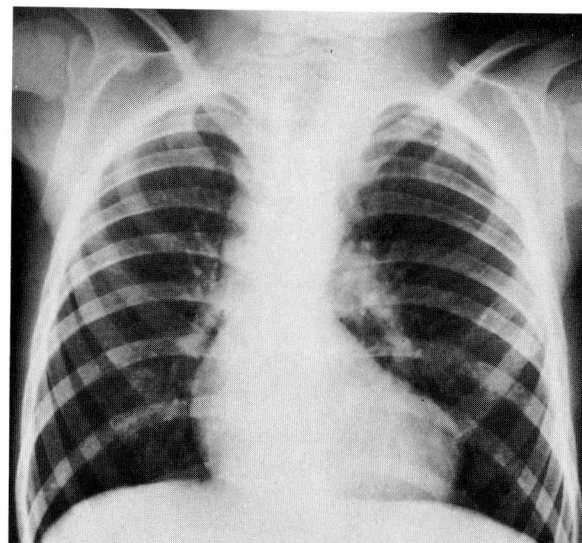

Fig. 25.19 Fallot's tetralogy. Note marked pulmonary bay and oligaemic lung fields.

If these patients have presented in infancy with severe right ventricular outflow tract obstruction and have required palliative surgery in the form of a Blalock (systemic to pulmonary artery shunt) operation, notching on the first four ribs may be seen due to the formation of a collateral circulation following division of the subclavian artery, the proximal portion of which is anastomosed to the pulmonary artery (Fig. 25.20).

Echocardiography. Parasternal and apical four-chamber sections demonstrate the posterior extension of a perimembranous ventricular septal defect into the inlet septum. Parasternal long axis views will show the aorta over-riding the ventricular septum and, with a clockwise rotation of the transducer to demonstrate the right ventricular outflow tract, the infundibular stenosis will be evident (Fig. 25.21A & B). Suprasternal short axis and long axis sections can be used to demonstrate the left and right pulmonary arteries so that their size can be compared with the descending aorta at the level of the diaphragm.

Angiocardiography. All the features of a typical outflow tract anatomy in tetralogy of Fallot are readily seen in the elongated right anterior oblique projection (Fig. 25.22A). A long axis projection of the left or right ventricular injection will demonstrate the ventricular septal defect, the aortic override and the size and distribution of the pulmonary arteries (Fig. 25.22B). As well as the usual perimembranous ventricular septal defect, one or more apical muscular trabecular defects are occasionally seen. These are best demonstrated by a left ventricular injection. In some severe cases of tetralogy, a well-developed bronchopulmonary circulation may be present (see p. 658 — pulmonary atresia).

Optimum imaging technique

In the sick neonate, an acceptable anatomical diagnosis can be made by echocardiography. This will usually enable a palliative systemic to pulmonary artery shunt operation to be performed. However, if total correction is being planned, most centres will carry out angiography to

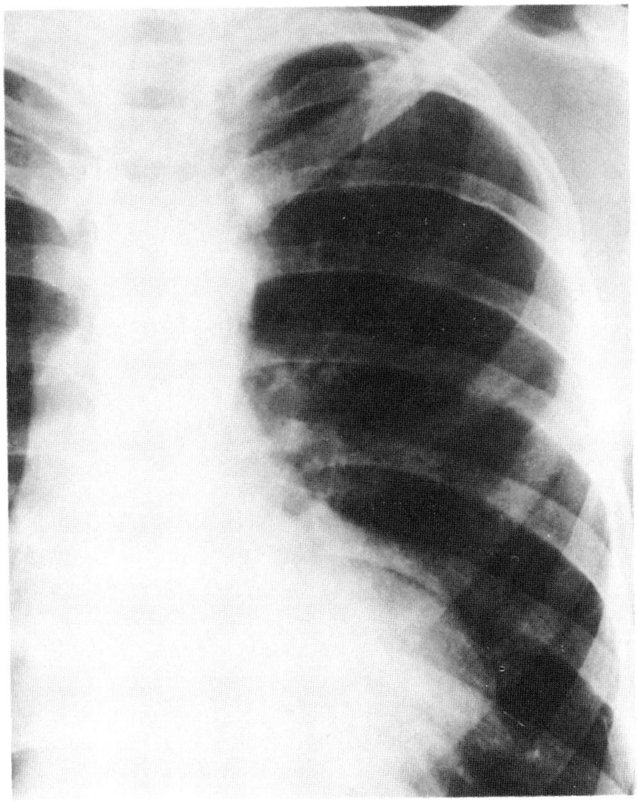

Fig. 25.20 Unilateral rib notching on upper four left ribs following a Blalock anastomosis palliating Fallot's tetralogy. Note pulmonary bay and elevated apex of heart.

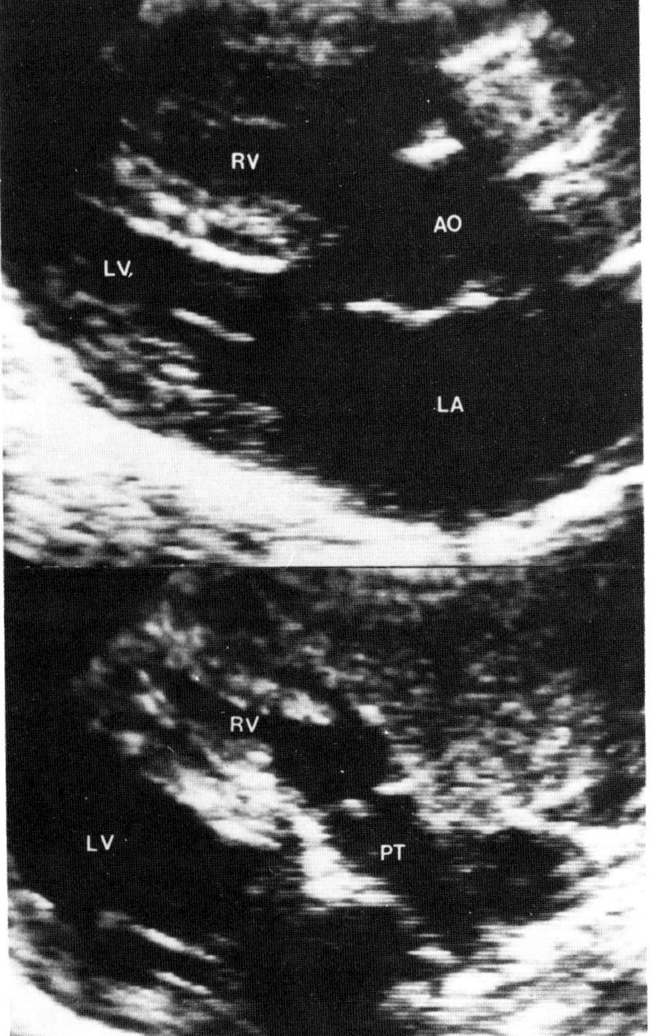

Fig. 25.21 Parasternal long axis cross-sectional echocardiogram from a patient with tetralogy of Fallot illustrating (**A**) over-riding aorta and (**B**) infundibular pulmonary stenosis. PT = pulmonary trunk.

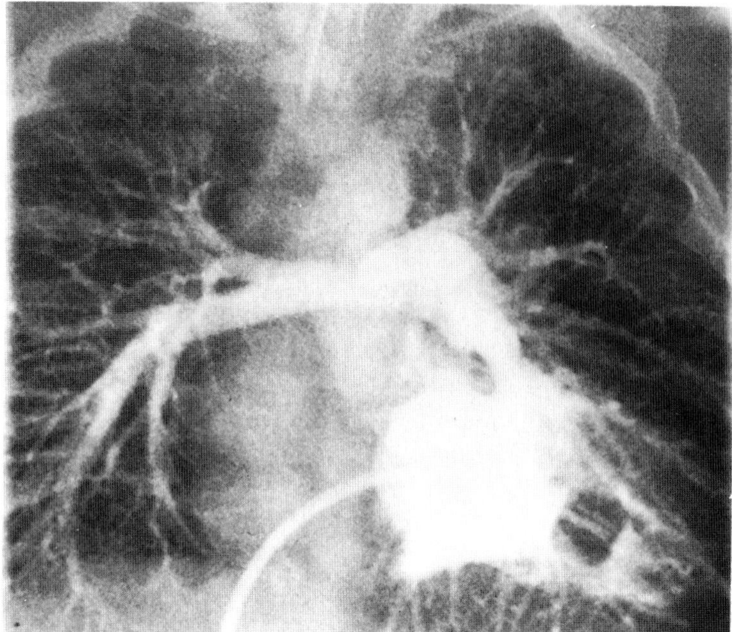

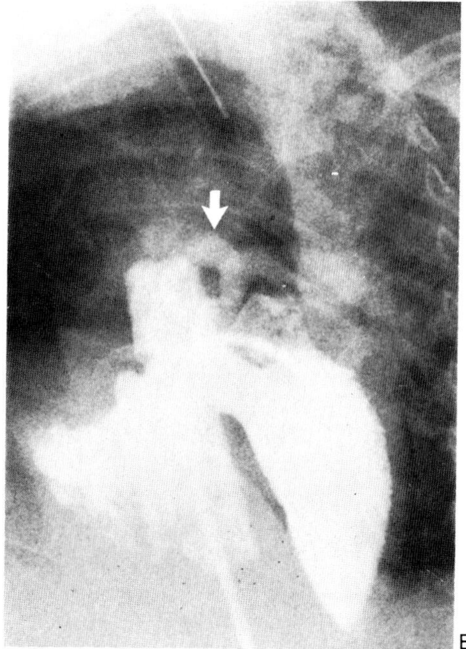

Fig. 25.22 A. Right ventriculogram in right oblique projection illustrating infundibular stenosis of patient with tetralogy of Fallot. **B.** Left ventriculogram in four chamber projection demonstrating a perimembranous ventricular septal defect in a patient with tetralogy of Fallot. Small pulmonary arteries are also seen (arrow).

demonstrate the right ventricular outflow tract and pulmonary arteries. A further left ventriculogram is employed to demonstrate accurately the number of ventricular septal defects, which may be multiple in up to 5% of patients. It is worth noting that *digital angiography* may well replace conventional angiograms for the detailed demonstration of the pulmonary arteries.

PULMONARY ATRESIA WITH VENTRICULAR SEPTAL DEFECT

Pulmonary atresia may exist with either an intact ventricular septum or a ventricular septal defect. Those cases with an intact septum are described in the section on hypoplastic right ventricle and will not be considered further at this point. Pulmonary atresia with a ventricular septal defect is in essence an extreme tetralogy of Fallot with anterior deviation of the infundibular septum giving rise to a ventricular septal defect and aortic override. It is important to remember that pulmonary atresia may exist also in hearts with abnormal connections. For example, it is commonly associated with classical tricuspid atresia. It may also occur in hearts with double inlet ventricle and is seen quite commonly when the aorta arises from the right ventricle.

Anatomy. The greatest variability in the morphology of pulmonary atresia with ventricular septal defect is the arrangement of the pulmonary arteries and the source of the pulmonary blood supply. The various possibilities are represented in Figure 25.23. Pulmonary blood supply may occur as follows:

1. Through one or both pulmonary arteries via a unilateral or bilateral ductus arteriosus.
2. Via major aortopulmonary collateral arteries.
3. By multiple small bronchial artery anastomoses with the distal pulmonary arteries (rare).

Even when the proximal (intrapericardial) pulmonary arteries are absent, there are always intrapulmonary arteries present which may receive the blood from any of the above sources. In order to plan surgical correction, it is important to demonstrate the pulmonary blood flow in detail distinguishing between multifocal and unifocal supplies.

Physiology. The ventricular septal defect is large and offers little resistance to flow so that the systolic pressures in the ventricles are equal. All of the output of the right ventricle enters the aorta and as a consequence, pulmonary blood flow must be maintained either through a ductus, via aortopulmonary collaterals or by bronchial collaterals in the manner already described.

Clinical features. Pulmonary atresia with a ventricular septal defect presents during the first few days of life with severe hypoxia if pulmonary blood flow is maintained only via the ductus arteriosus. However, in those cases in which pulmonary blood supply depends on aortopulmonary collateral vessels, the clinical presentation is extremely variable. When the pulmonary blood flow is low, extreme

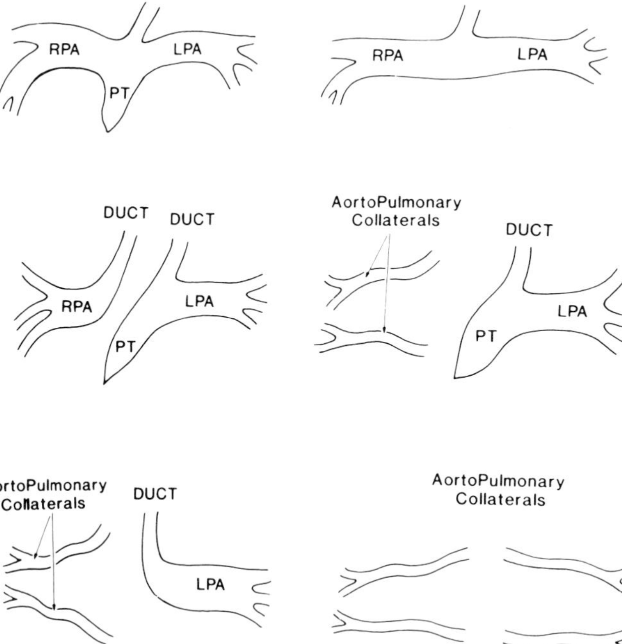

Fig. 25.23 Diagram of the various types of pulmonary atresia.

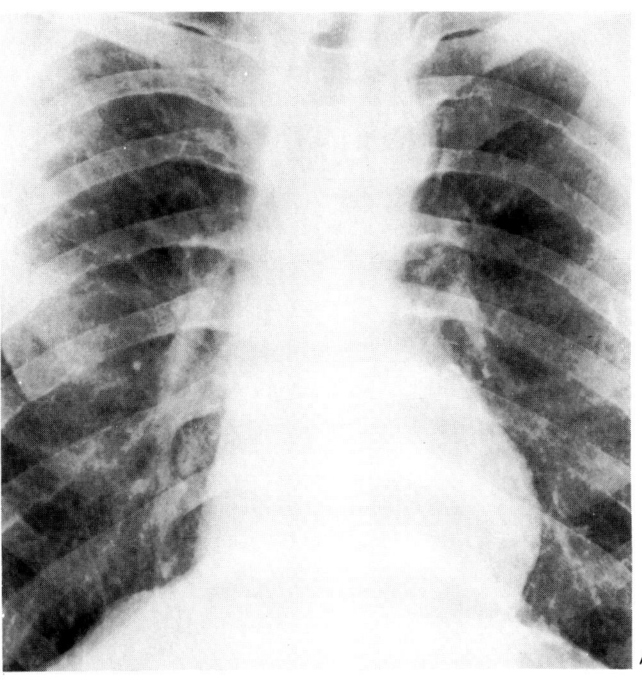

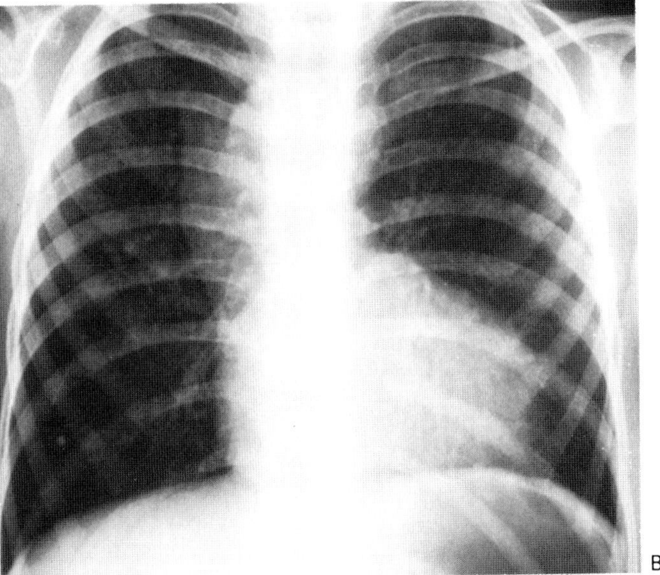

Fig. 25.24 A. Pulmonary atresia. Plain film of patient aged 40 with no previous surgery showing pulmonary bay, large aortic knuckle and marked rib notching. **B.** Pulmonary atresia with broncho-pulmonary collaterals. Right aortic arch and pulmonary bay indicating right ventricular outflow tract obstruction. Nodular shadowing in the right lung due to broncho-pulmonary collaterals. Collaterals absent in the L. lung which appears relatively oligaemic.

hypoxia may be the presenting feature in the neonatal period. Relatively high pulmonary blood flow causes less marked cyanosis resulting in a later presentation. Occasionally pulmonary blood flow is so high that heart failure develops in early infancy.

Imaging

Plain film. The plain film provides useful information for diagnosis. The most important constant findings are the normal or near normal heart size and reduction of lung markings. There is a right aortic arch in approximately 30% of cases. The classical heart contour shows slight elevation of the apex, a pulmonary artery bay and prominent aortic knuckle (Fig. 24.24A). Although the lung markings are usually reduced, a rather granular appearance is often evident in the presence of aortopulmonary collaterals (Fig. 25.24B). If the collaterals are large, there may be excessive pulmonary flow.

Echocardiography. Cross-sectional echocardiography will demonstrate the large ventricular septal defect with aortic override and proximal pulmonary arteries if they are present. However, it is of limited value in the precise diagnosis of the peripheral pulmonary blood supply.

Angiography. All the features of the typical outflow tract anatomy in pulmonary atresia with ventricular septal defect are seen when a right ventriculogram is performed in the elongated right anterior oblique projection (Fig. 25.25A). A left or right ventriculogram in the long axial projection identifies the ventricular septal defect, excludes additional muscular septal defects, demonstrates the aortic override and may allow visualization of the pulmonary trunk and the proximal right and left pulmonary arteries when present (Fig. 25.25B). In order

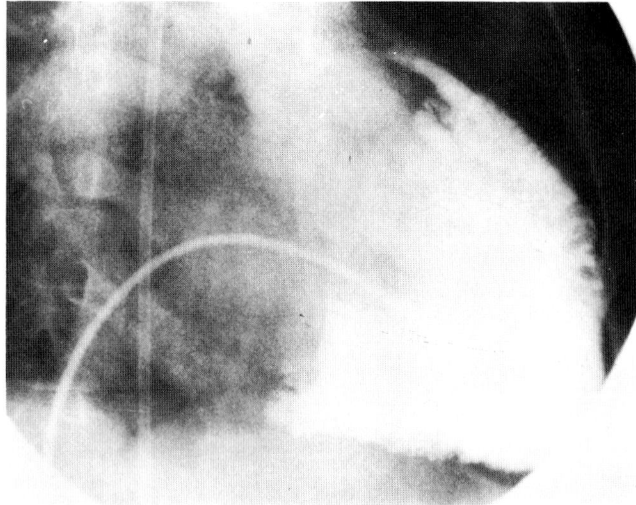

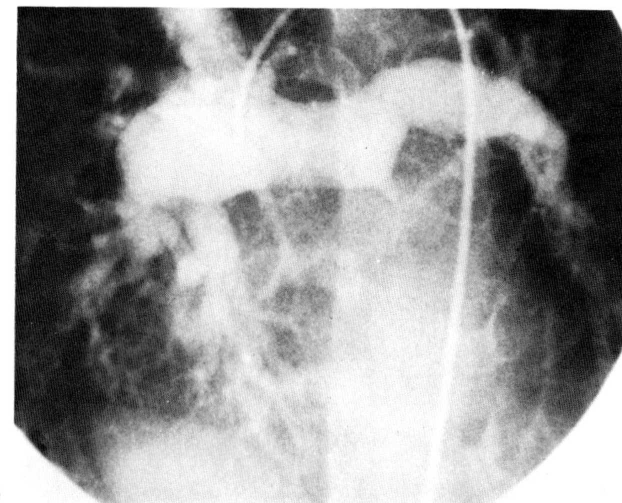

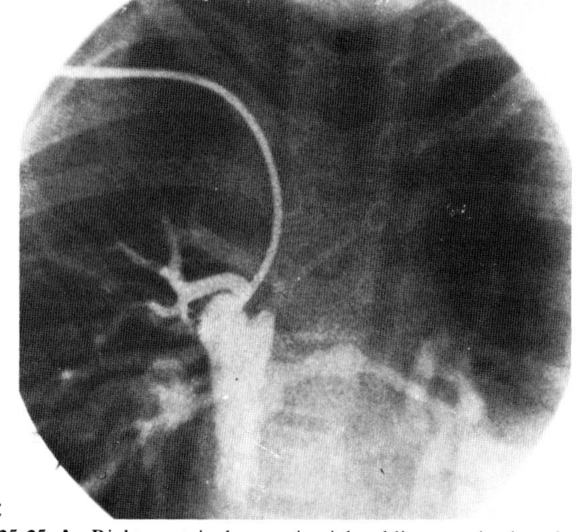

Fig. 25.25 A. Right ventriculogram in right oblique projection showing blind ending right ventricular outflow tract in a patient with pulmonary atresia and ventricular septal defect. **B.** Angiogram through a right Blalock anastomosis demonstrating the right and left pulmonary arteries and absence of the pulmonary trunk in the same patient with pulmonary atresia. **C.** Aortogram in a patient with pulmonary atresia and a ventricular septal defect demonstrating systemic pulmonary collateral arteries.

to demonstrate the pulmonary blood supply, an aortogram is the minimum requirement. When there are aortopulmonary collaterals, selective injections into each of these are desirable to demonstrate the exact blood supply to each lung (Fig. 25.25C). In a few instances, when the proximal pulmonary arteries are present but are not well demonstrated by aortography, pulmonary venous wedge angiography can be performed. By this method the proximal pulmonary arteries can be demonstrated by retrograde flow.

Optimum imaging technique

The demonstration of the proximal pulmonary arteries and the pulmonary blood supply is essential in all patients with pulmonary atresia. An aortogram and selective injections into the aortopulmonary collaterals when appropriate are also essential. Digital subtraction techniques may be of considerable help in making the precise diagnosis.

ATRIOVENTRICULAR DISCORDANCE AND CONGENITALLY CORRECTED TRANSPOSITION

The term atrioventricular discordance describes an atrioventricular connection in which the morphological right atrium is connected to the morphological left ventricle via the mitral valve and the morphological left atrium is connected to the morphological right ventricle via the tricuspid valve. Such hearts are sometimes described as having 'ventricular inversion' although this is a misnomer because atrioventricular discordance can exist with normally positioned ventricles, either with situs inversus of the atria or with the 'criss-cross' heart. Conversely, the presence of 'ventricular inversion' does not always mean that atrioventricular discordance is present. Atrioventricular discordance can exist either with situs solitus or situs inversus but not with atrial isomerism. These conditions may coexist with any ventriculo-arterial connection.

Congenitally corrected transposition is characterized by the combination of both atrioventricular and ventriculo-arterial discordance. Thus it can exist as either situs solitus or inversus. This condition is also known as L-transposition, a term which most authorities prefer not to use.

Anatomy. It has already been stated that congenitally corrected transposition describes an abnormality of both the atrioventricular and ventriculo-arterial connections. Additional lesions occur in the majority of cases. The most common is a *ventricular septal defect* which may be positioned anywhere in the septum but is usually a perimembranous defect overridden by the pulmonary trunk. *Pulmonary stenosis* is present in just under half of these cases and may be valvar or subvalvar. The most frequent atrioventricular valve malformation is an Ebstein-like anomaly of the morphological tricuspid valve. Usually the valve is dysplastic and allows regurgitation. Less commonly there may be straddling of the septum by either trioventricular valve. Malposition of the heart within the horax is frequent.

While atrioventricular discordance is most commonly ound in association with congenitally corrected transposition, it can also exist with pulmonary atresia, double outlet right ventricle, ventriculo-arterial concordance, double outlet left ventricle or truncus arteriosus.

Physiology and clinical findings. The clinical presentation of congenitally corrected transposition depends upon the associated anomalies. When only a ventricular septal defect is present the clinical features will be as for an isolated ventricular septal defect and will depend upon the size of that defect. Pulmonary stenosis associated with a ventricular septal defect may result in cyanosis when the clinical features may mimic tetralogy of Fallot. Occasionally the clinical presentation may be as isolated heart block. Rarely, incompetence of the tricuspid valve functioning as the systemic atrioventricular valve may be the only abnormality and the clinical presentation will be very much like that of mitral incompetence in a heart with normal connection.

Imaging

Plain film. In the presence of the usual atrial arrangement (solitus), the cardiac position and orientation of the apex are variable. A prominent left upper cardiac border, due to a left-sided ascending aorta, may be visible (Fig. 25.26). In the presence of ventricular septal defect, the heart size may be enlarged and there may be evidence of increased pulmonary blood flow. If there is pulmonary stenosis, pulmonary oligaemia may be evident.

Echocardiogram. Cross-sectional echocardiography readily allows the diagnosis of congenitally corrected transposition to be made. In the presence of situs solitus, an apical four-chamber section shows the mirror image of the usual offsetting of the atrioventricular valves (Fig. 25.27A). Thus the septal leaflet of the left (tricuspid) valve is attached nearer to the apex of the heart than the septal leaflet of the right (mitral) valve. In the presence of a perimembranous septal defect, the atrioventricular valves are in continuity with the central fibrous body and therefore lose their usual relationship (Fig. 25.27B) though the tricuspid valve can be recognized by its chordal attachments to the ventricular septum. Parasternal long axis and short axis sections establish the presence of ventriculo-arterial discordance demonstrating the relative positions of the aorta and the pulmonary artery.

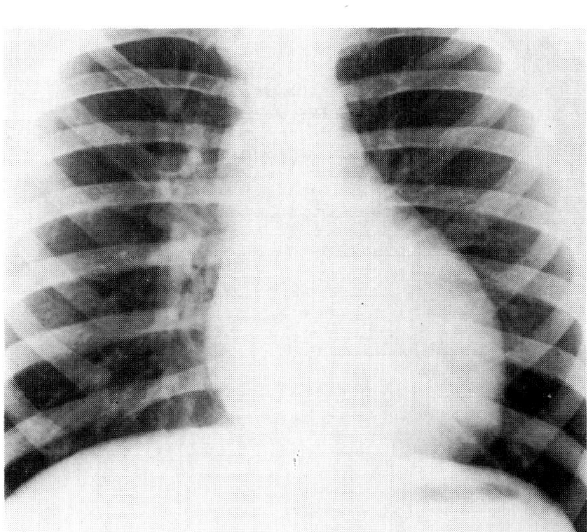

Fig. 25.26 Atrioventricular discordance with ventrio-arterial discordance (corrected transposition). Plain film showing prominent straight left heart border due to L-malposition of the ascending aorta. Some cardiac enlargement and mild pulmonary plethora is present.

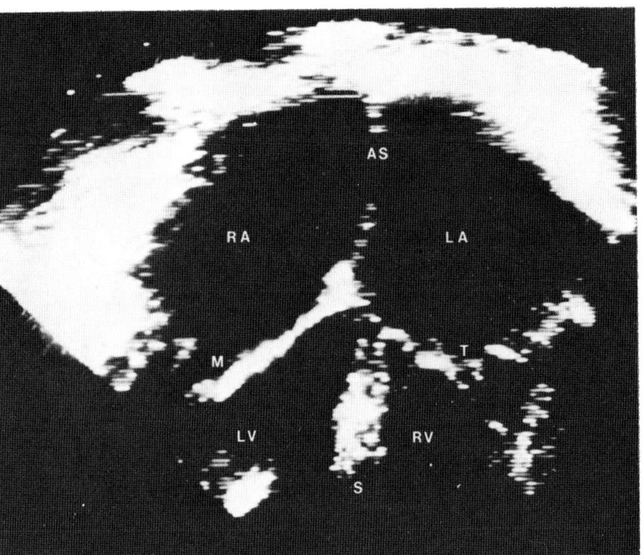

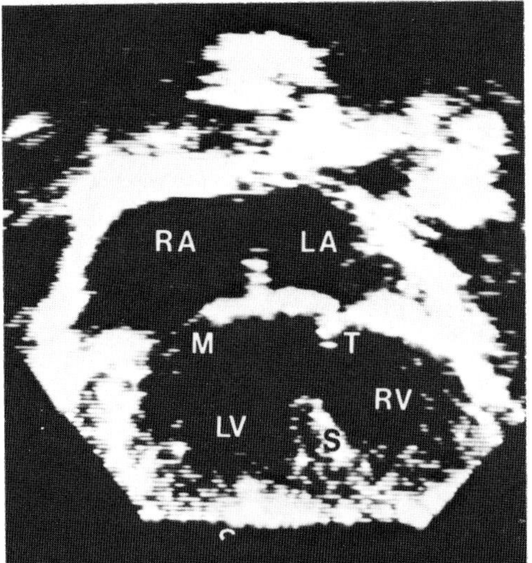

Fig. 25.27 A. Cross-sectional echocardiogram illustrating atrioventricular discordance with usual atrial arrangement. **B.** Cross-sectional echocardiogram illustrating atrioventricular discordance with usual atrial arrangement and a large perimembranous ventricular septal defect.

Angiography. In hearts with the usual atrial arrangement (solitus) and typical congenitally corrected transposition, ventriculography in the antero-posterior projection reveals a left-sided morphological right ventricle, a right-sided morphological left ventricle and ventriculo-arterial discordance characteristically with a left-sided anterior aorta (Fig. 25.28). In this projection, the ventricular septum and the left ventricular outflow tract are clearly demonstrated allowing the recognition of a ventricular septal defect and subpulmonary stenosis if present.

Optimum imaging technique

It is invariably possible to establish the diagnosis by cross-sectional echocardiography, but for those patients requiring surgery it is the usual practice to perform cardiac catheterization and angiography.

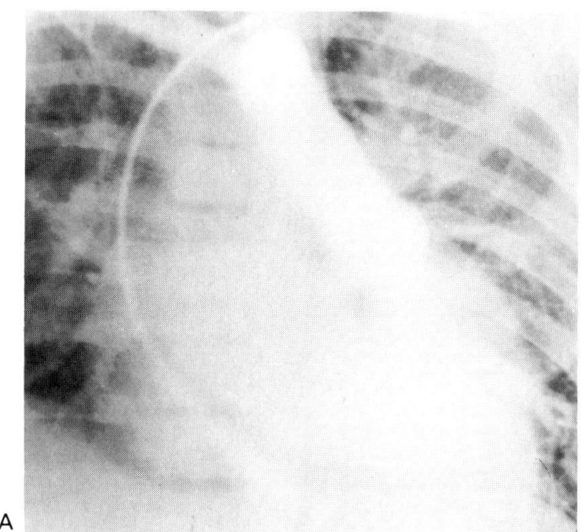

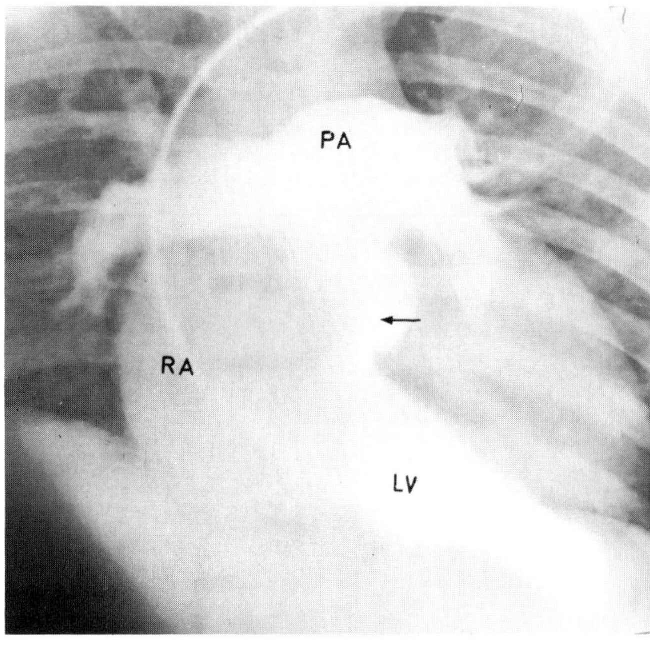

Fig. 25.28 A. Contrast in the morphological right ventricle demonstrates an anterior ascending aorta arising from it. **B.** Injection into the posterior morphological left ventricle demonstrates the posterior pulmonary artery arising from that ventricle. Note associated pulmonary valve stenosis (←).

COMPLETE TRANSPOSITION

There has been considerable controversy surrounding the definition of transposition, but it is now generally accepted that the term complete transposition describes a combination of atrioventricular concordance and ventriculo-arterial discordance. The major advantage of this approach is that it excludes from consideration cases in which ventriculo-arterial discordance is associated with other atrioventricular connections such as atrioventricular discordance, double inlet ventricle, ambiguus atrioventricular connection or absent connection. Certainly ventriculo-arterial discordance with any of these atrioventricular connections can justifiably be termed transposition but the clinical problems posed are quite different from those produced by complete transposition.

COMPLETE TRANSPOSITION WITH INTACT VENTRICULAR SEPTUM

Incidence, anatomy and physiology. Complete transposition accounts for approximately 5% of all symptomatic infants presenting with congenital heart disease. The systemic venous return enters the right atrium and from there blood passes to the right ventricle and aorta. The pulmonary venous return enters the left atrium, passes through the mitral valve to the morphological left ventricle and then enters the pulmonary trunk to be distributed to the lungs.

Without a mixing site for systemic venous and pulmonary venous blood, the prognosis is grave but the introduction of the technique of balloon atrial septostomy performed at cardiac catheterization to create an atrial septal defect, has ensured survival in infancy for the majority of patients and has revolutionized treatment of complete transposition. This approach enables early palliative management and permits definitive surgery to be performed at a later date.

There may be considerable variation in the anatomy of hearts with complete transposition. Usually, the aortic valve is anterior and to the right of the pulmonary valve but cases are frequently encountered in which the aortic valve is directly anterior to the pulmonary valve or even to the left of it. When the ventricular septum is intact, the aortic valve has a complete muscular infundibulum.

The emergence of an anatomical correction (the switch operation) for complete transposition has highlighted the need for a thorough understanding of the anatomy of the coronary arteries and a detailed description is readily availɔle elsewhere (Vlodaver et al 1975, Grittenberger et al ɔ83). The most important associated lesions are more kely to occur in the presence of a ventricular septal efect, but if the septum is intact, then aortic coarctation or ulmonary stenosis (valvar, subvalvar or supravalvar) may e encountered.

Clinical features. Complete transposition presents in the arly neonatal period with severe cyanosis and over 50% f cases present on the first day of life. The typical clinical eatures are severe cyanosis associated with a progressive etabolic acidosis and tachypnoea. The definitive treatment is balloon atrial septostomy performed at cardiac atheterization.

maging techniques

Plain film. The typical features are cardiomegaly with ıcreased pulmonary vascular markings and an egg-shaped ardiac silhouette with a narrow superior mediastinum Fig. 25.29). These, however, are not always present and

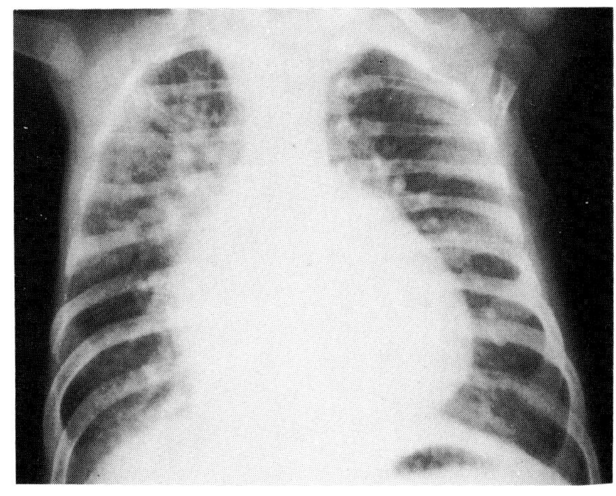

ig. 25.29 The narrow pedicle of the heart seen in ventriculo-arterial iscordance (complete transposition) due to the aorta lying almost irectly in front of the pulmonary artery.

certainly during the first two days of life, cardiomegaly and increased pulmonary vascular markings may be absent.

Echocardiography. Subcostal long axis views demonstrating the ventricular outflow tracts and great arteries readily show that the pulmonary artery arises from the morphological left ventricle and the aorta from the right ventricle (Fig. 25.30). Short axis sections through the great arteries demonstrate the relationship of the aorta to the pulmonary artery.

Angiography. The major role of cardiac catheterization is to allow *balloon atrial septostomy* to be performed in a patient already diagnosed as having complete transposition by echocardiography. It is also particularly important to measure the left ventricular pressure in patients being considered for the *switch operation* and this investigation also allows the quantitation of the severity of associated pulmonary stenosis. Angiography will demonstrate both the ventriculo-arterial discordant connection (Fig. 25.31), together with any associated lesions such as right ventricular dysfunction, coronary artery anomalies and coarctation of the aorta.

Optimum imaging technique

Echocardiography readily allows the diagnosis of complete transposition and will almost always demonstrate coarctation of the aorta when present and a ductus arteriosus. Some cardiologists now prefer to perform atrial septostomy at the time of cardiac catheterization and to avoid angiography, particularly in sick infants.

COMPLETE TRANSPOSITION WITH VENTRICULAR SEPTAL DEFECT

When complete transposition is associated with a ventricular septal defect, the clinical presentation is with cyanosis from birth but typically these infants develop heart failure during the second month of life. The most common type

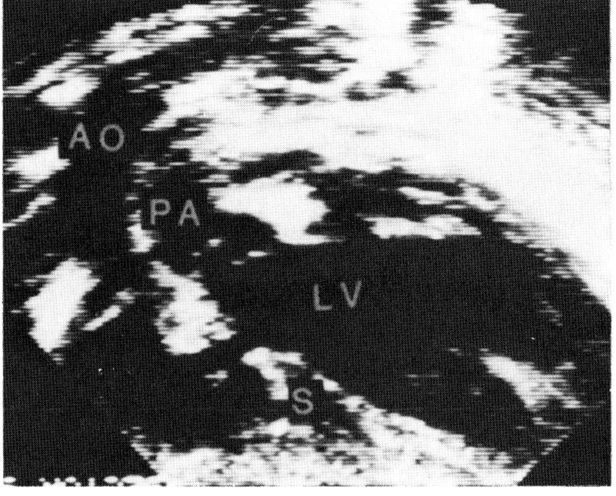

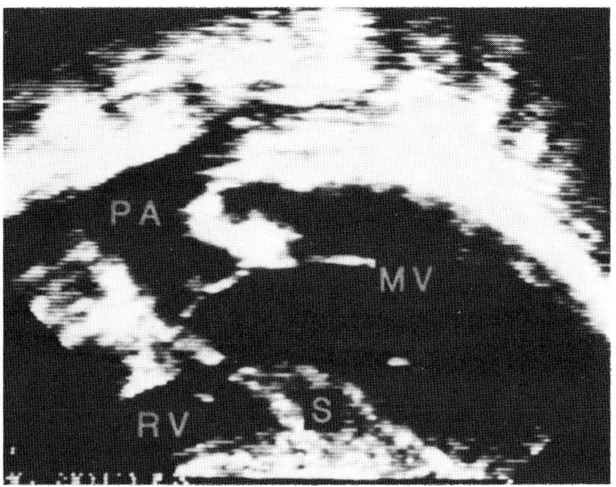

ig. 25.30 **A.** and **B.** Cross-sectional echocardiogram from a patient with complete transposition and a small muscular ventricular septal defect, howing pulmonary artery arising from left ventricle.

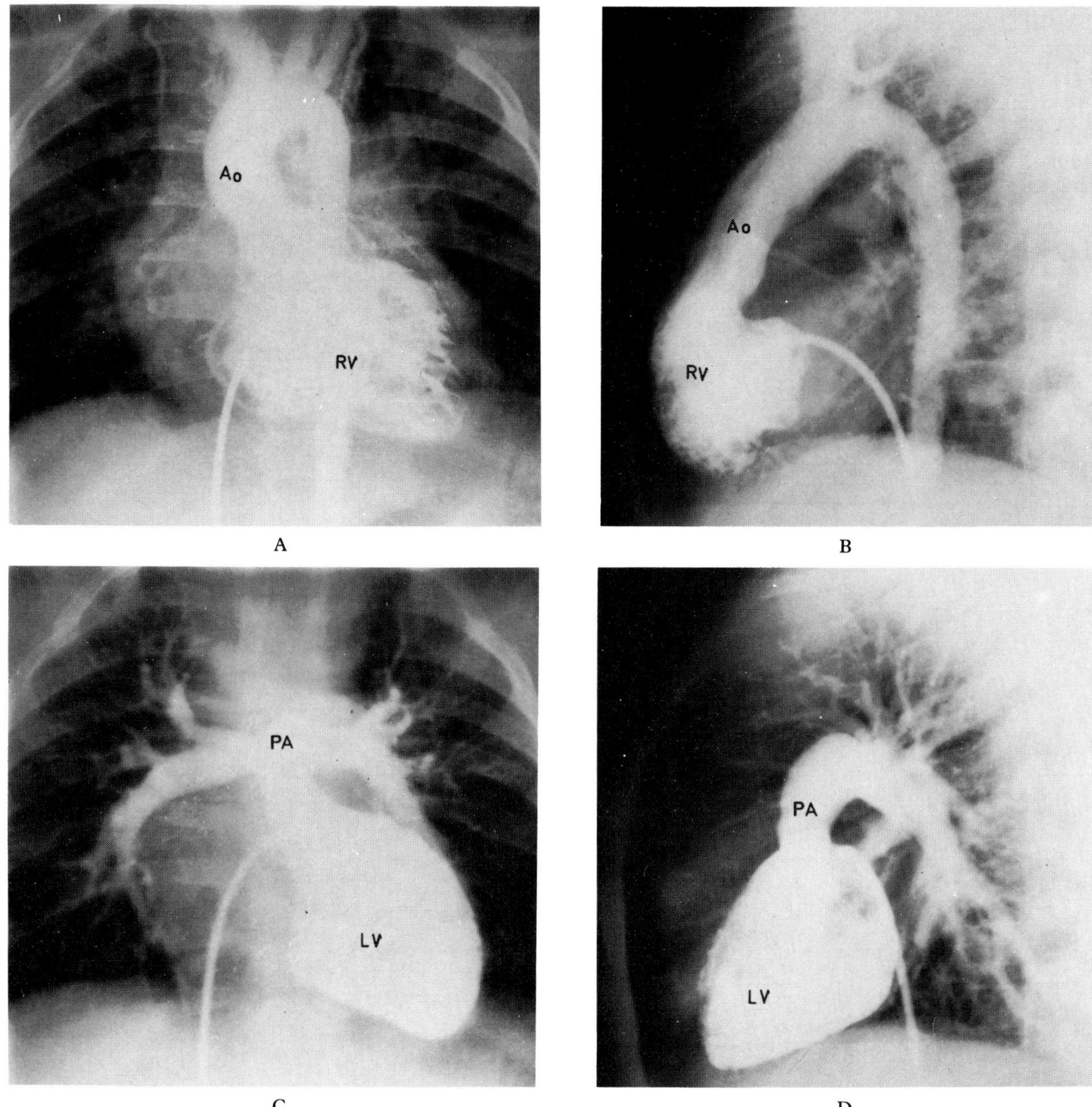

Fig. 25.31 Atrioventricular concordance with ventriculo-arterial discordance (complete transposition) with D-relations of the great arteries. **A.** and **B.** The morphological right atrium connects with the morphological right ventricle which supports the aorta. **C** & **D** The morphological left atrium connects with the morphological left ventricle which supports the pulmonary artery. The aorta lies to the right of the pulmonary artery and is thus D-related.

of ventricular septal defect is an infundibular malalignment defect associated with anterior deviation of the infundibular septum. The anatomy of such a defect is readily demonstrated both by echocardiography and ventriculography. Coarctation is much more likely to occur in the presence of a ventricular septal defect. When there is a posterior deviation of the infundibular septum, left ventricular outflow tract obstruction is likely to occur.

DOUBLE OUTLET VENTRICLE

Any heart in which more than half of both arterial valve are connected to the same ventricle can be considered t have a double outlet from that ventricle. Double outlet lef ventricle is exceedingly rare but double outlet righ ventricle is more common (3% of patients presenting wit symptomatic congenital heart disease) and will b considered here in some detail. It is important to realiz that double outlet ventricle is a ventriculo-arterial connec tion that can exist with any atrioventricular connection Thus, it may occur in the setting of not only atrioven tricular concordance but also atrioventricular discordance ambiguus atrioventricular connection and in hearts wit univentricular atrioventricular connections. In this section only double outlet right ventricle with atrioventricular concordance will be considered. Any description of double outlet right ventricle must also include the relative positions of the great arteries and the presence or absence of a subarterial infundibulum.

Anatomy. The basic division of hearts with double outlet right ventricle depends upon the position of the ventricular septal defect. This may be subaortic, subpulmonary, doubly committed or non-committed. Figure 25.32 illustrates the possibilities that may occur. In hearts with a subaortic defect, the aorta is usually posterior and to the right of the pulmonary artery or side by side and to the right. Typically such hearts are described with a bilateral infundibulum and a ventricular septal defect is usually surrounded entirely by muscle although occasionally it may be perimembranous. When such a perimembranous defect is associated with anterior deviation of the infundibular septum, then the diagnosis is tetralogy of Fallot but with double outlet right ventricle. Occasionally a subaortic ventricular septal defect may become restrictive or even close completely. Pulmonary valve stenosis is also frequent.

In hearts with a subpulmonary defect, the aorta is usually anterior and to the right and in this situation it is the pulmonary valve which is likely to override the septum. This situation is also known as the *Taussig-Bing malformation*. Subaortic stenosis and coarctation of the aorta occur quite frequently with subpulmonary ventricular septal defect.

A doubly committed ventricular septal defect occurs beneath both great arteries because the infundibular septum is deficient. A 'non-committed' ventricular septal defect in double outlet right ventricle may be a muscular defect remote from the great arteries or a perimembranous defect with tricuspid valve tissue inserting into the infundibular septum between the left ventricle and the great arteries. The latter defect is particularly difficult to repair surgically.

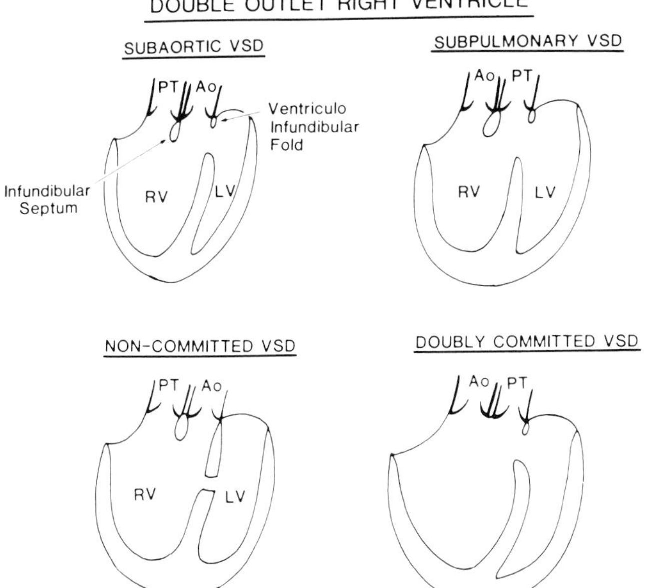

Fig. 25.32 Illustration of the various types of double outlet right ventricle.

Physiology and clinical features. Double outlet right ventricle represents 3% of symptomatic congenital heart disease presenting in the first year of life. The majority of hearts with this condition have a large unrestrictive ventricular septal defect so that the pressures in the right and left ventricles are equal. A small or restrictive ventricular septal defect allows limited egress of blood from the left ventricle so that there is considerable elevation of left atrial and pulmonary venous pressure. In the presence of the usual large ventricular septal defect, a subaortic defect gives rise to the clinical features of an isolated ventricular septal defect and a subpulmonary defect mimics the clinical features of transposition with a ventricular septal defect and marked desaturation. A subaortic defect with infundibular stenosis may produce the typical features of tetralogy of Fallot whilst the subpulmonary defect may be associated with subaortic stenosis and coarctation of the aorta.

Imaging

Plain film. There are no pathognomonic features of double outlet right ventricle on the plain chest radiograph. The appearances merely reflect the amount of pulmonary blood flow so that in the absence of pulmonary stenosis, pulmonary vascular markings are increased and the heart size is enlarged. On the other hand pulmonary stenosis is likely to be associated with oligaemic lung fields and a normal heart size.

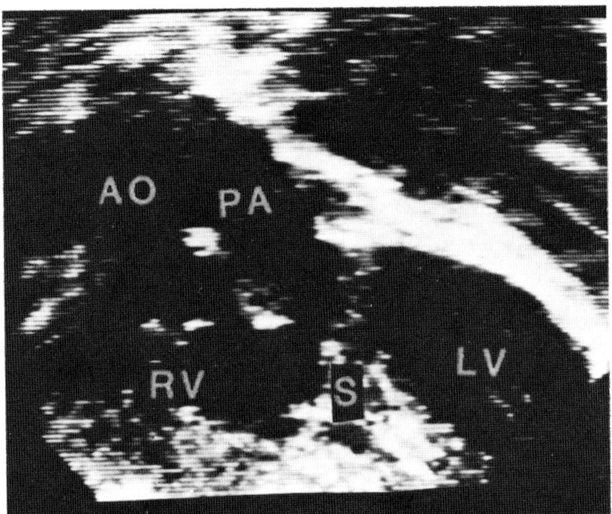

Fig. 25.33 Cross-sectional echocardiogram illustrating double outlet right ventricle.

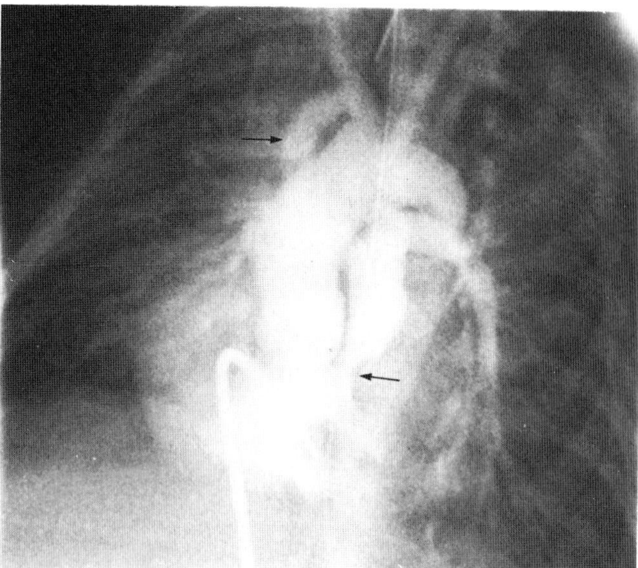

Fig. 25.34 Angiogram of double outlet right ventricle. Long axial projection showing anterior aorta and posterior pulmonary artery arising from morphological right ventricle. Note narrowed infundibulum below pulmonary valve (←) causing obstruction to pulmonary flow and consequent right Blalock shunt (→).

Echocardiography. Subcostal and parasternal long axis projections will demonstrate the site of the ventricular septal defect but the ventriculo-arterial connection itself is best demonstrated from the parasternal position (Fig. 25.33).

Angiography. A left or right ventriculogram in the long axial projection identifies the ventricular septal defect, excludes additional muscular septal defects and demonstrates both great arteries arising primarily from the right ventricle (Fig. 25.34).

Optimum imaging technique

The diagnosis can almost always be readily established by cross-sectional echocardiography but, in the presence of severe subpulmonary or subaortic stenosis, angiography will demonstrate more clearly the pulmonary arteries and the aortic arch.

HYPOPLASIA OF THE RIGHT VENTRICLE

For the purpose of classification of congenital heart disease used in this section, the term 'hypoplasia of a ventricle' refers to one which is normally constituted, that has an inlet, trabecular and outlet portion but in which the whole ventricular structure is underdeveloped. Thus, the right ventricle in tricuspid atresia, or in association with double inlet left ventricle, is excluded because in these circumstances it is rudimentary rather than hypoplastic, as the inlet portion is absent. Whilst a hypoplastic right ventricle is nearly always associated with pulmonary atresia in the presence of an intact ventricular septum, it may also be associated with a small tricuspid valve, normal outflow tract and gross hypoplasia of the trabecular component of the ventricle.

Anatomy. Pulmonary atresia with intact septum is associated with varying degrees of right ventricular hypoplasia. The tricuspid valve and annulus are small and anomalies of the tricuspid valve itself are frequent, the most common being gross dysplasia or *Ebstein's anomaly*. The pulmonary atresia is of two types: the infundibulum may be patent to the level of an imperforate pulmonary valve membrane, or the infundibulum itself may be atretic so that the pulmonary trunk arises from the ventricular mass, widening as it ascends to end blindly.

Incidence, physiology and clinical features. Pulmonary atresia with intact septum accounts for 1.9% of all symptomatic infants with congenital heart disease and 4.7% of those neonates presenting during the first week of life. Because of the obstruction in the right ventricular outflow tract, blood exits by one or both of two possible routes. The first is through intramyocardial sinusoids to the coronary arterial system with retrograde flow into the aorta. This can be demonstrated angiographically. Secondly, there may be varying degrees of tricuspid regurgitation. Regardless of the detailed anatomy of the right ventricle, the basic pathway of the circulation is similar and depends upon a right to left shunt at atrial level through the foramen ovale maintaining pulmonary blood flow via the ductus arteriosus. The predominant clinical feature is progressive neonatal cyanosis due to a closing ductus. This almost always is evident within the first 24 hours of life. The imminent closure of the ductus arteriosus causes severe hypoxia with metabolic acidosis and treatment with intravenous E-type prostaglandins, in order to keep the duct open, is life saving.

Imaging

Plain film. The typical appearances are mild cardiomegaly, because of the right atrial and left ventricular enlargement, and diminished pulmonary vascular markings. The cardiac contour typically shows a prominent right cardiac border, a concave pulmonary artery bay and a prominent convexity of the cardiac apex.

Echocardiogram. The apical or subcostal four-chamber section has the appearance of a hypoplastic right ventricle and a small tricuspid valve. The parasternal section through the aortic root demonstrates the presence or absence of the right ventricular infundibulum, the pulmonary valve membrane and the main pulmonary artery with its bifurcation.

Angiography. A right ventriculogram should be performed using only a small amount of contrast medium. Typically, the right ventricle is small and there may be some degree of tricuspid regurgitation. There may be a right ventricular infundibulum and contrast may be seen lling the coronary arteries and ascending aorta via sinusids. The pulmonary arteries opacify via the ductus and re usually of a good size.

Optimum imaging technique

The diagnosis can be readily established in the neonate by ross-sectional echocardiography and in the majority of ases palliative surgery can be undertaken without the need for cardiac catheterization. When radical surgery is ontemplated later in life, angiography is essential in order o assess the pulmonary arteries.

DOUBLE INLET VENTRICLE

The classification of hearts with double inlet ventricles or absence of an atrioventricular connection is a contentious opic and numerous classifications have been applied in the past (Anderson et al 1983). For the purpose of this chapter, hearts with double inlet ventricle are defined as those in which both atria are in direct or potential communication with the same ventricle. Whatever the classification or nomenclature employed, most of these hearts have two chambers in their ventricular mass. If the rudimentary chamber is given ventricular status, then, in the majority of hearts with double inlet connection, it is not the heart which is univentricular but the atrioventricular connection. The '*univentricular atrioventricular connection*' is therefore a generic term given to a group of anomalies whose unifying feature is the atria connecting to only one ventricle. Included in this group are not only hearts with double inlet ventricle but also those with absent right or left atrioventricular connection. The latter will be discussed subsequently.

When considering the ventricular mass in hearts with double inlet ventricle, it is necessary to consider the trabecular pattern of the main and rudimentary ventricular chambers and their relationships. When the univentricular connection is to a morphological left ventricle, the rudimentary right ventricle is found in an antero-superior position and can be left sided, right sided or occasionally directly anterior. In double inlet right ventricle, the rudimentary left ventricle is positioned postero-inferiorly usually to the left but sometimes directly posterior. When it is impossible to identify a second chamber within the ventricular mass, then it is most likely that the univentricular connection is to a ventricle of indeterminate morphology. Thus it is evident that the corner stone of the diagnosis of ventricular morphology of hearts with double inlet ventricle is the identification of the trabecular pattern of the main chamber and the position of the rudimentary ventricle. It is important, nevertheless, to realize that the diagnosis of double inlet ventricle is incomplete unless the atrial situs and the ventriculo-arterial connection has been described and the mode of atrioventricular connection determined. The mode of connection in these hearts may be via two atrioventricular valves or a common valve and has been described fully on page 617.

Incidence, physiology and clinical features. Double inlet ventricles occur in 4.3% of symptomatic infants presenting with congenital heart disease in the first year of life. The clinical features and presentation depend upon pulmonary blood flow. When there is associated pulmonary stenosis, cyanosis is often severe and the presentation occurs during the first month of life. In the absence of pulmonary stenosis there is mild cyanosis with heart failure, and tachypnoea is the prominent clinical feature. These infants present typically during the second and third months of life.

Imaging

Plain film. There is no typical chest radiographic appearance associated with the diagnosis of double inlet ventricle. When there is associated pulmonary stenosis, the heart size may be normal and pulmonary oligaemia may be present. Without pulmonary stenosis, cardiomegaly is the usual finding together with increased lung vascularity.

Echocardiography. Four-chamber sections readily demonstrate the type and mode of atrioventricular connection and the position of the rudimentary ventricle lying either to the right or left (Fig. 25.35). Parasternal long axis sections will demonstrate an anterior rudimentary right ventricle in hearts with double inlet left ventricle and a posterior rudimentary left ventricle in hearts with double inlet right ventricle.

Angiography. Angiograms of the main ventricular chamber should be performed to profile the septum so that ventricular morphology, ventricular relationships and the size of any interventricular communication can be seen. In

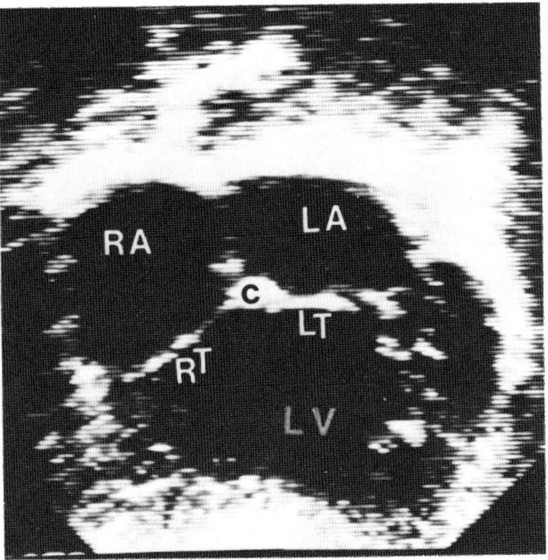

Fig. 25.35 Four-chamber cross-sectional echocardiogram illustrating double inlet left ventricle in which the mode of connection is through two atrioventricular valves.

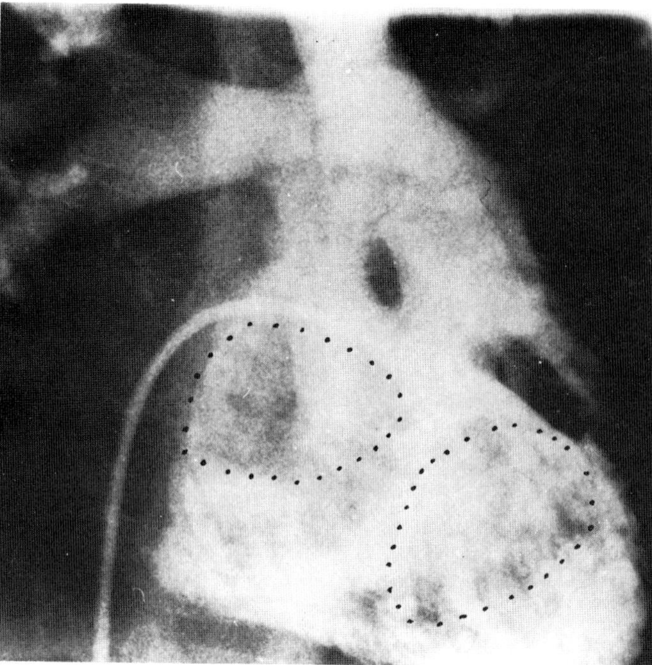

Fig. 25.36 Injection into a morphological left ventricle. Both atrioventricular valves are outlined by non-opacified blood and are seen to enter the ventricle.

order to demonstrate these features and the ventricular arterial connections, it may be necessary to perform two separate injections so that antero-posterior, lateral and left anterior oblique projections can be recorded (Fig. 25.36). Compared with cross-sectional echocardiography, angiography enables a better demonstration of the trabecular pattern of the ventricles to be obtained. Nevertheless, the same principles of diagnosis remain because in double inlet left ventricle, a rudimentary right ventricle is found in the antero-superior position while in double inlet right ventricle, the rudimentary left ventricle is posterior and inferior. In cases where the morphology of the main chamber is uncertain, this can be inferred from the position of the rudimentary ventricle. The trabecular pattern of a solitary rudimentary indeterminate left ventricle is also characteristic and lies between the morphological appearances of either a right or left ventricle. Nevertheless, difficulties may be encountered in distinguishing this relatively rare type from a right ventricular chamber with a tiny rudimentary left ventricle.

Optimum imaging technique

In infancy it is usually possible to establish the diagnosis by cross-sectional echocardiography alone so that, if necessary, palliative surgery can be undertaken. If associated abnormalities of the great arteries are suspected, angiography may be required. When radical surgery, such as ventricular septation or an anastomosis of the right atrium to a pulmonary artery, is contemplated, cardiac catheterization and angiography are mandatory.

TRICUSPID ATRESIA

The term classical tricuspid atresia is reserved for those hearts in which there is complete absence of the right atrioventricular connection. In this circumstance, the left atrium connects to the left ventricle and there is a rudimentary right ventricle. These hearts can therefore be included among those with univentricular connection.

Incidence, anatomy and physiology. Tricuspid atresia accounts for approximately 4% of all symptomatic infants with congenital heart disease. The great majority of examples have absence of the right atrioventricular connection but in some cases there is an imperforate tricuspid valve membrane so that the right atrium is in potential communication with either the right ventricle in cases of atrioventricular concordance or the left ventricle in cases of double inlet left ventricle. Most commonly the ventriculo-arterial connection is either concordant or discordant but occasionally both great arteries may arise from the left ventricle or rudimentary right ventricle and tricuspid atresia may also be associated with pulmonary atresia. With ventriculo-arterial concordance, there is commonly subpulmonary stenosis. When the ventriculo-arterial connection is discordant, subpulmonary stenosis is unusual, but subaortic stenosis may occur and coarctation of the aorta is a relatively frequent association. In the presence of tricuspid atresia, there is an obligatory right to left atrial shunt with admixture of systemic and pulmonary venous blood in the left atrium. As a consequence,

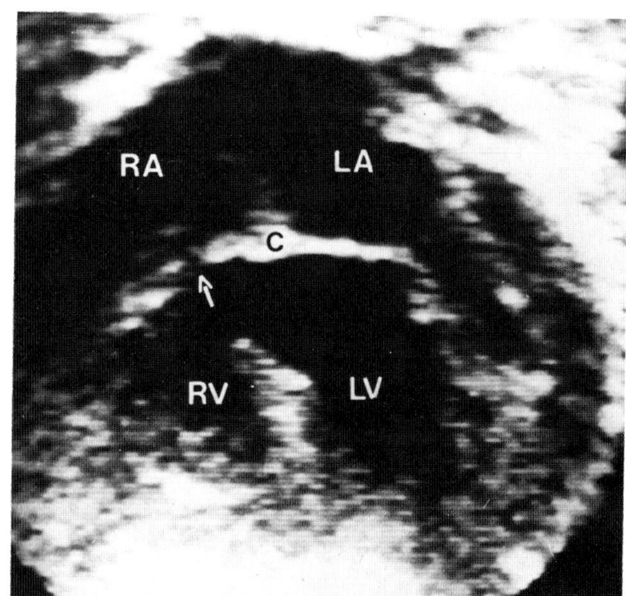

Fig. 25.37 Four-chamber cross-sectional echocardiogram illustrating tricuspid atresia. There is complete absence of the right atrioventricular connection (arrow).

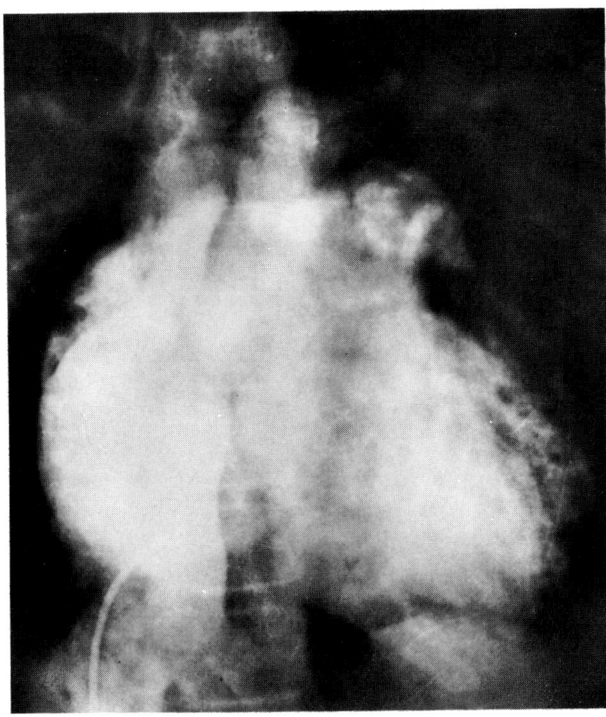

A

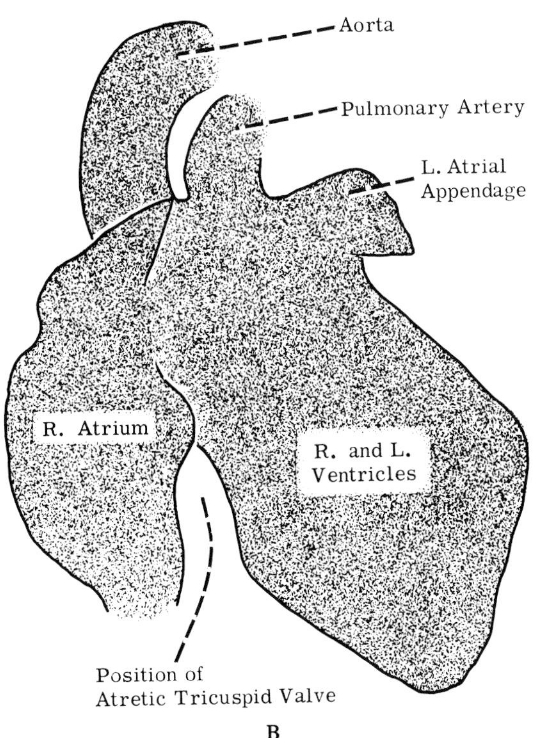

B

Fig. 25.38 A. and **B.** Tricuspid atresia. Injection into the right atrium shows contrast passing across the atrial septum to outline the LA and LV. There is an absent right atrioventricular valve. **C.** Injection into the left ventricle demonstrates the ventricular septal defect and the size of the outflow portion of the right ventricle.

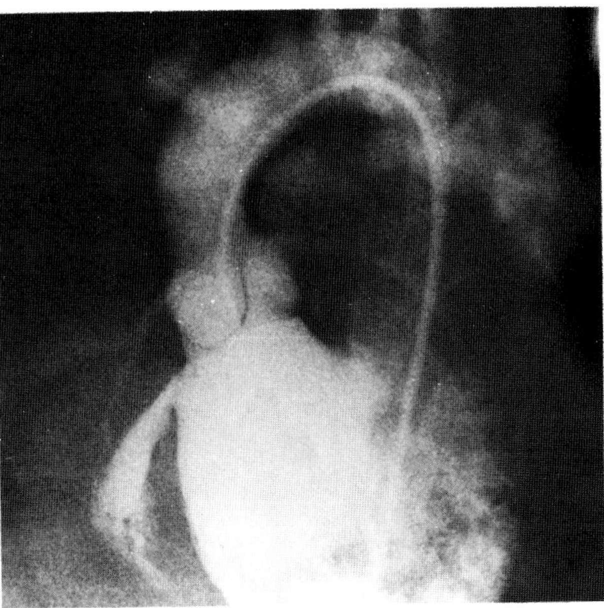

C

cyanosis is always present but is more severe in the presence of subpulmonary stenosis. The clinical features are dependent upon the presence or absence of pulmonary stenosis and its severity. Thus, with severe pulmonary stenosis, there is marked cyanosis from birth but without pulmonary stenosis the presenting feature is heart failure usually during the second month of life. Most commonly this is associated with ventriculo-arterial discordance, but in a few cases it may be the presenting feature of hearts with vetriculo-arterial concordance.

Imaging

Plain film. There are no characteristic findings on the chest radiograph. However, in the presence of severe cyanosis, there is likely to be a normal heart size and oligaemic lung fields. On the other hand, heart failure will be associated with cardiomegaly and increased pulmonary vascular markings.

Echocardiography. The anatomy of the atrioventricular junction is readily demonstrated by four-chamber sections. These demonstrate complete absence of the right atrioventricular connection with sulcus tissue interposing between the floor of the right atrium and the ventricular mass (Fig. 25.37). There is therefore no potential communication between the right atrium and the ventricle. In most cases subcostal and parasternal long axis sections readily demonstrate ventriculo-arterial connection.

Angiography. For the angiographic demonstration of tricuspid atresia, the minimum requirements are a right atrial injection in the antero-posterior and lateral projections, a left ventriculogram in the four-chamber projection and an aortogram to exclude coarctation of the aorta and demonstrate any ductus arteriosus (Fig. 25.38).

Optimum imaging technique

In most cases of tricuspid atresia, it is possible to perform palliative surgery without the necessity for cardiac catheterization and angiography. When there is severe cyanosis, a Blalock Taussig anastomosis is required and in the presence of heart failure, pulmonary artery banding is the treatment of choice. Prior to definitive surgery by the Fontan operation, cardiac catheterization is mandatory in order to measure the pulmonary artery pressure and to demonstrate any gradient across the interventricular communication.

PULMONARY STENOSES

SUPRAVALVAR STENOSIS

In this rare condition, there is a membrane with an aperture of varying size situated in the main pulmonary trunk. It usually lies about 1 cm above the pulmonary valve. The valve and the right ventricular outflow tract are usually normal. However, minor degrees of supravalvar muscular narrowing are frequently observed in tetralogy of Fallot.

VALVAR AND INFUNDIBULAR STENOSIS

Incidence, anatomy and physiology. These are common conditions accounting for 10–15% of all patients with congenital heart disease. Valvar stenosis, with or without functional infundibular obstruction, is 5–10 times as common as organic infundibular stenosis. However, approximately equal numbers of the two groups actually require surgery. In valvar stenosis, the cusps of the pulmonary valve are thickened and fused into a membrane with a variable sized aperture. Whilst the aperture is usually central, it may also be eccentric. In addition, the valve ring may be small. Poststenotic dilatation of the main pulmonary artery may also occur.

In organic infundibular stenosis, there is a muscular ring in the infundibular portion of the right ventricular outflow tract. There is often an associated degree of hypoplasia of the outflow tract. Functional infundibular obstruction may occur secondary to valve stenosis. As the right ventricular muscle hypertrophies in order to overcome the obstruction at valve level, the infundibular walls may become so thickened that in ventricular systole, they approximate towards each other, thus causing obstruction. In extreme cases, this functional stenosis may cause total obstruction of the flow into the pulmonary artery long before the end of ventricular systole.

Valvar and organic infundibular stenosis may occur separately or coexist. With increasing obstruction to outflow, systolic pressure in the right ventricle rises. The level reached depends on the degree of obstruction and the age of the patient but pressures of up to 200 mmHg have been recorded. The onset of right ventricular failure is heralded by a rise in right ventricular end diastolic pressure and this is reflected by an elevation of right atrial systolic pressure. In the presence of a patent foramen ovale or atrial septal defect, a right to left shunt may occur. This usually happens secondary to pulmonary valve stenosis and is rare in the presence of organic infundibular obstruction.

Clinical course. Clinical presentation is intimately related to the severity of the stenosis. Neonates with only a pinhole orifice or critical stenosis, will develop right heart failure in the first few days of life. However, if the pressure gradient across the valve is less than 40 mmHg, the patient may have few, if any, symptoms throughout childhood and adolescence. Nevertheless, the majority of symptomatic patients lie between these two groups often presenting in early childhood. If there is an intra-atrial communication even if only potential such as with a patent foramen ovale central cyanosis may occur as a right to left shunt across the atrial septum develops.

Imaging

Plain film. The radiographic appearances depend not only on the anatomical site but also on the degree of obstruction. Thus, if obstruction is at valve level, there is poststenotic dilatation of the main pulmonary artery extending to the left pulmonary artery and this may be quite marked (Fig. 25.39). As with aortic valve obstruction, the degree of dilatation bears no relation to the extent of obstruction. On the other hand, organic infundibular stenosis may be associated with a hypoplastic outflow tract which is seen as a deep concave bay on the left heart border between the aortic knuckle and the hypertrophied right ventricle (Fig. 25.40). The presence of a poststenotic dilatation and cyanosis is usually associated with a right to left shunt at atrial level. However, a pulmonary bay and

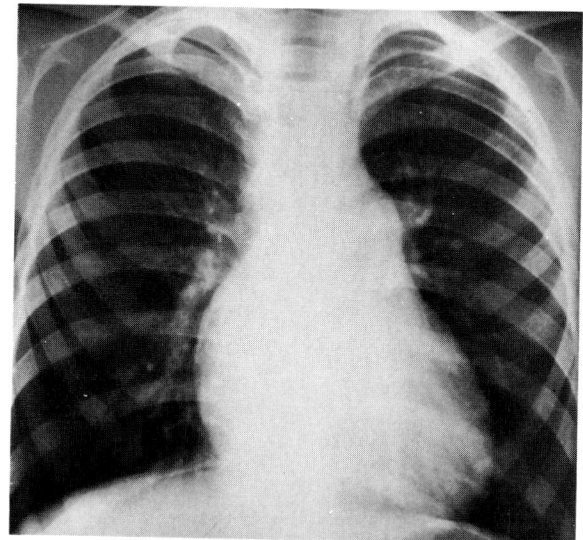

Fig. 25.39 Pulmonary valve stenosis with intact ventricular septum. Note poststenotic dilation of the pulmonary artery. The oligaemic lung fields were due to a shunt at atrial level.

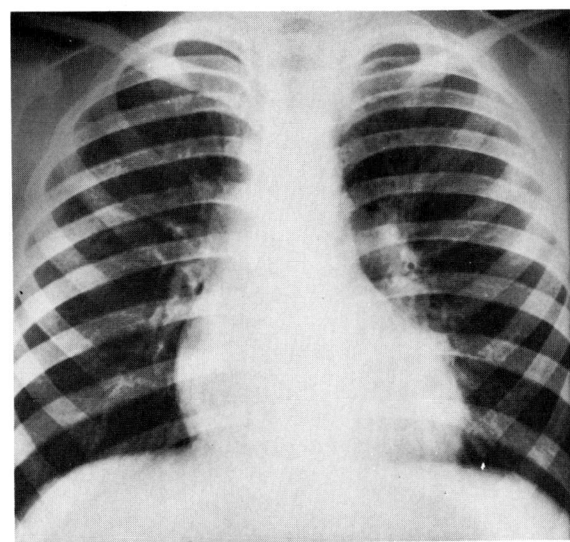

Fig. 25.40 Infundibular pulmonary stenosis with intact ventricular septum. Note concave pulmonary bay due to a hypoplastic right ventricular outflow tract.

cyanosis almost invariably indicates an intraventricular communication, e.g. Fallot's tetralogy. In addition to poststenotic dilatation and a pulmonary bay, the following radiological appearances may be seen and these are related to the degree of obstruction.

1. Right ventricular hypertrophy and dilatation. If the stenosis is mild (the pressure gradient across the valve is 30 mmHg or less), the cardiac configuration is normal. As the gradient increases, right ventricular hypertrophy occurs. Eventually, this may be so marked that the left heart border is formed by the right ventricle. A significant overall increase in heart size is not seen prior to right heart failure. However, right ventricular hypertrophy does lead to rotation of the heart with the left ventricle and aortic arch rotating into the mediastinum. Consequently, the aortic arch may appear small on the postero-anterior view. If frank right-sided failure occurs, the heart dilates and appears enlarged on the chest radiograph.

2. Right atrial enlargement. With moderate to severe stenosis, the right atrial pressure is elevated so that it exceeds right ventricular end-diastolic pressure thus enabling right ventricular filling to take place in diastole. As a result, some right atrial enlargement may be seen but if functional tricuspid incompetence is present then the right atrial enlargement is often marked.

3. Pulmonary oligaemia. Prior to the onset of heart failure, the cardiac output will be normal in the presence of an intact ventricular septum. Hence the pulmonary vascular pattern will be normal. It is only with the onset of right ventricular failure that the lungs become oligaemic. On the other hand, if there is a ventricular septal defect with a right to left shunt, the lungs will be oligaemic. This situation occurs in Fallot's tetralogy.

4. Heart size. This is within normal limits unless right heart failure develops when dilatation occurs.

Echocardiogram. The pulmonary valve may be difficult to visualize by echocardiography, but, if identified, its size can be estimated together with any cusp thickening and immobility. The right ventricular cavity size, wall thickness and outflow tract can also be measured. The presence or absence of the defect in either the atrial or ventricular septum will be apparent.

Angiography. If the echocardiogram is equivocal, a right ventricular injection will demonstrate the anatomy as outlined above (Fig. 25.41A). If the stenosis is critical, there is the theoretical danger of pulmonary vascular vasodilatation with acute low output failure occurring following a contrast injection. This can be avoided by the use of as small a volume of non-ionic contrast medium as possible. In this way the added complication of a sodium overload is avoided.

If the right ventricular pressure is equal to or above systemic pressure, this indicates severe or even critical obstruction. The infundibular region is likely to be particularly irritable with a high risk of catheter-induced dysrhythmias. Thus a hand contrast injection under the pulmonary valve is probably advisable in the most severe cases.

Optimum imaging technique

Although echocardiography often yields diagnostic information in neonates, if corrective surgery is being contemplated, it is necessary to perform both a right and left ventriculogram in order to assess the right ventricular outflow tract, the ventricular septum and left ventricular size and function.

Management

A small group of patients with critical pulmonary valve stenosis present as neonates and the condition can almost always be diagnosed by echocardiography. In older children, the severity is more accurately assessed at cardiac catheterization when the right ventricular pressure can be measured. If this is at or near systemic level, significant obstruction can be inferred even if it is not possible to cross the valve. If a gradient of more than 40 mmHg is measured across the valve, pulmonary valvotomy is performed. A closed balloon valvotomy may be performed after the age of 1 year and this technique is currently being evaluated (Fig. 25.41B and C). An open valvotomy also enables relief of infundibular stenosis if this is indicated.

PULMONARY VALVE STENOSIS AND VENTRICULAR SEPTAL DEFECTS

The combination is uncommon. Its presence may be suggested on the plain film and it can be confirmed angio-

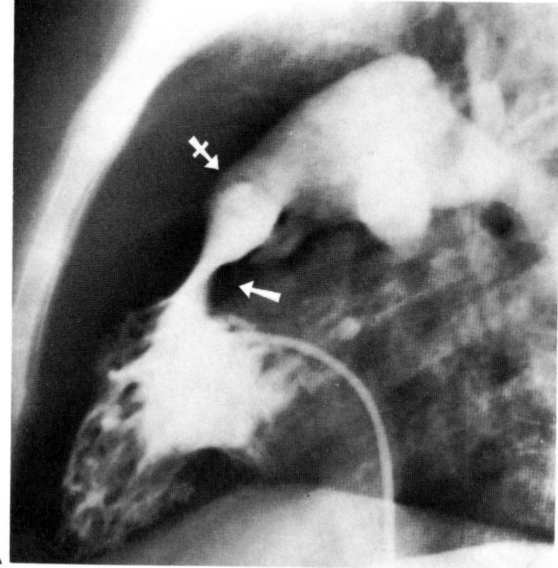

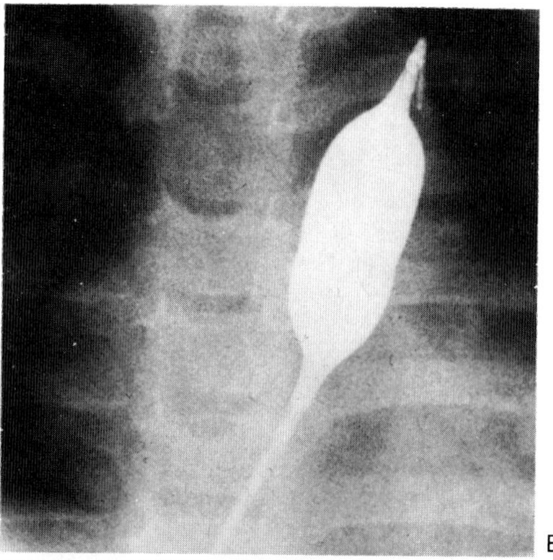

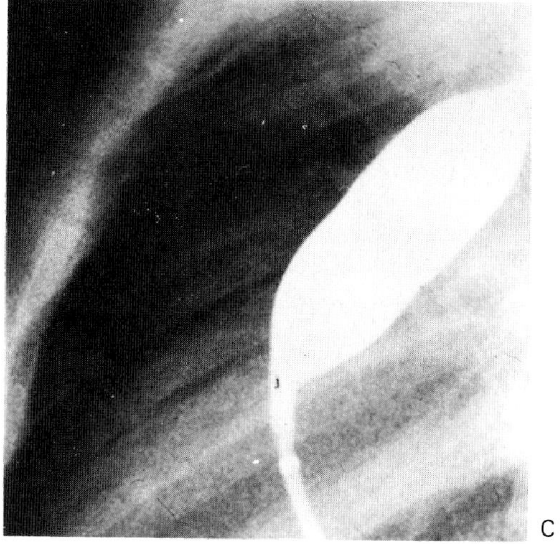

Fig. 25.41 A. Pulmonary valve stenosis with secondary infundibular narrowing showing poststenotic dilatation of the main and left pulmonary arteries. **B.** and **C.** Antero-posterior and lateral cine frames from a patient undergoing balloon pulmonary valvotomy.

graphically where it should be distinguished from Fallot's tetralogy. As the right ventricular infundibulum is not hypoplastic, the infundibular septum is normally positioned and the aortic root lies posterior to the ventricular septal defect which is perimembranous. Prolapse of the septal cusp of the tricuspid valve through the perimembranous defect may be present as an associated lesion. Thus, although right ventricular pressure may be higher than that in the left ventricle, a right to left shunt only occurs in very early systole. Similarly, if the defect, be it either single or multiple, lies in the muscular septum, a shunt will only occur briefly in early systole before the defect is occluded. Thus with either of these two conditions, the clinical presentation and course is essentially that of pulmonary valve stenosis with an intact ventricular septum.

PULMONARY INCOMPETENCE

Rarely, incompetence may be associated with an absent pulmonary valve syndrome, a condition in which the basic morphology is that of tetralogy of Fallot with gross dilatation of the central pulmonary arteries. However, it is seen more frequently following pulmonary valvotomy and also as a functional event secondary to peripheral pulmonary vascular disease. Occasionally it may be seen as an isolated phenomenon. The true incidence of congenital pulmonary incompetence is unknown but it may account for some cases of 'idiopathic' dilatation of the main pulmonary artery. Most often, no specific therapy is required though in cases of congenital absence of the pulmonary valve, a homograft or Xenograft valve replacement has been advocated.

THE AORTIC STENOSES

SUPRAVALVE STENOSIS

Anatomy and physiology. In this rare condition, the aortic lumen is narrowed 1–2 cm above the valve. The narrowing may involve the entire thickness of the aortic wall, resulting in a hypoplastic ascending aorta. Alternatively, there may be a membrane or diaphragm partially occluding the aortic lumen, in which case the external appearance of the aorta is normal. Occasionally, both defects may be present. As with aortic valve stenosis, the left ventricle hypertrophies to overcome the obstruction.

Clinical course. In the neonatal period, if the obstruction is critical, the presentation is very similar to the hypoplastic left heart syndrome. However, most cases present in childhood with clinical evidence of left ventricular outflow tract obstruction. The condition may be

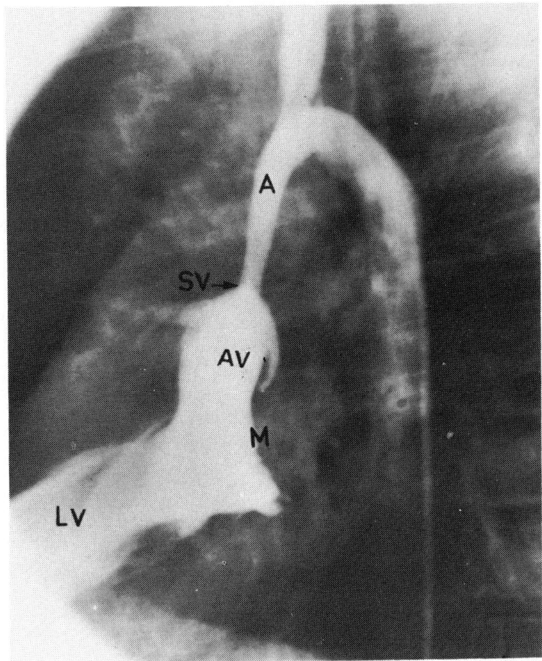

Fig. 25.42 Supravalve aortic stenosis. A = aorta: AV = aortic valve: SV = site of supravalve stenosis: M = mitral valve orifice: LV = left ventricle.

familial and associated with hypocalcaemia. If so, other vascular anomalies may be seen in up to 60% of cases. These include pulmonary and renal artery stenosis together with coarctation and the child may have a characteristic elfin facies with impaired intellect.

Imaging

The heart size is normal prior to the onset of left ventricular failure. A hypoplastic aorta will be evident on the plain film. Post stenotic dilatation is not seen with a hypoplastic aorta but may be present in association with a supravalve diaphragm. Radiological evidence of idiopathic hypocalcaemia may be evident in the skeleton. Both echocardiography and angiography will demonstrate the supravalve obstruction but angiography is mandatory to fully assess the aortic arch and the pulmonary, the coronary and renal arteries (Fig. 25.42).

Management

Surgical resection of the diaphragm is possible and this has a better prognosis than attempts to relieve obstruction due to a hypoplastic segment.

VALVE STENOSIS

Incidence, anatomy and physiology. In recent years, a vast majority of cases of aortic valve disease presenting in the United Kingdom have been of *congenital* origin. *Acquired* aortic valve disease has become increasingly rare. As a group, aortic stenosis accounts for some 3–5% of all congenital heart disease. Two-thirds are at valve level and one-third are subvalvar. As indicated above, supravalve lesions are rare. Aortic valve lesions are five times as common in men as in women.

In congenital aortic stenosis, the valve may be truly bicuspid or tricuspid with fusion of one or more commissures. With advancing age, the endocardium along the edges of the cusps and sinuses of Valsalva becomes thickened, irregular and calcified in 80% to 85% of abnormal valves.

The calcification may extend downwards, migrating along fibrous connections towards the mitral valve. It may also enter the region of the bundle of His leading to conduction defects. Calcification almost always indicates significant obstruction of the left ventricular outflow tract. As the aortic valve orifice has to be reduced to about a quarter of its natural size before any haemodynamic effect occurs, calcification must represent narrowing to this degree. The pressure gradient may range from a few millimetres up to 150 mm of mercury. As the stenotic valve cusps are relatively immobile, some associated aortic regurgitation is common. Left ventricular hypertrophy develops in response to the obstruction at aortic valve level and ejection of blood through a stenotic valve ring gives rise to turbulence and poststenotic dilatation of the ascending aorta.

Myocardial ischaemia is probably secondary to reduced diastolic coronary artery flow and to a degree of coronary artery compression during diastole. The natural history of aortic valve stenosis is that the severity of the condition progresses with age. Thus, in practice, echocardiography and angiography may need to be repeated.

There are two significant groups of patients: those presenting as neonates or in childhood and those first seen in the fifth and sixth decades. It is difficult to estimate the relative frequencies of these two groups but the latter may represent the majority.

Left ventricular hypertrophy and significant stenosis may be established before the symptoms of breathlessness, syncope or angina appear. The onset of these symptoms is thought to coincide with the valve cusps becoming rigid. Once symptoms are present, deterioration is rapid and, without treatment, most patients die within two years due to either dysrhythmias or heart failure. In addition, the abnormal structure of the valve renders it liable to infection and bacterial endocarditis and this complication may occur at any age.

Imaging

Plain film. *a. Heart size.* Systolic overload leads to left ventricular hypertrophy without an increase in heart size in compensated aortic valve disease. However, the left heart border may be prominent (Fig. 25.43). Once failure supervenes, cardiac dilatation and enlargement occurs. With imminent left ventricular failure, the left ventricular

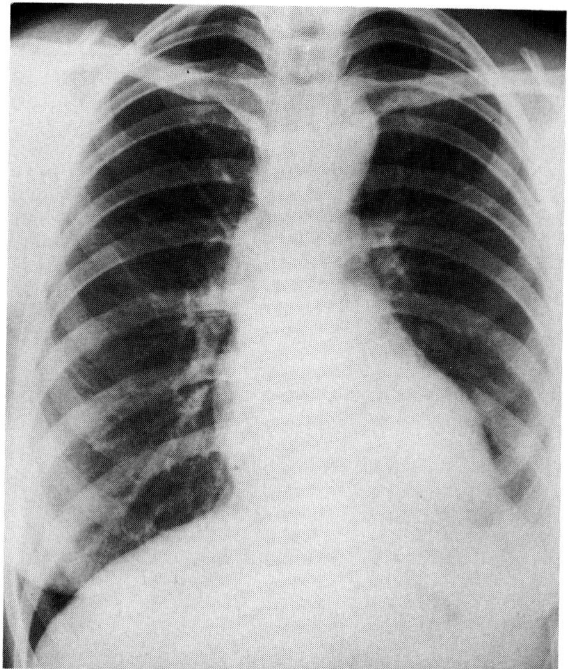

Fig. 25.43 Aortic valve stenosis. Note (a) Normal size of heart with configurations suggesting left ventricular hypertrophy, (b) Poststenotic dilatation of ascending aorta.

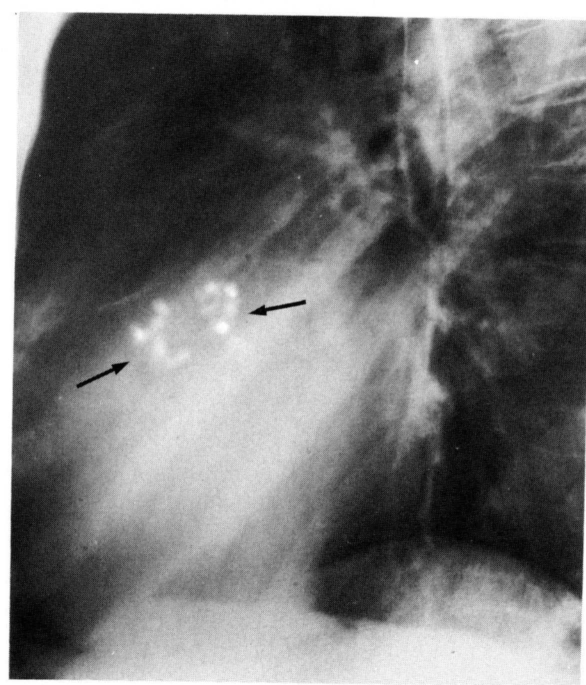

Fig. 25.44 Calcified aortic valve seen on the lateral view.

end-diastolic pressure rises and consequently left atrial pressure must increase to maintain left ventricular filling. Thus there may be some left atrial enlargement secondary to hypertrophy and if visible, this may herald left ventricular decompensation.

b. Poststenotic dilatation. The aortic root dilates just above the valve in response to turbulence but there is no direct relationship to the pressure gradient. Indeed, with a large gradient, there may be relatively little turbulence. Dilatation is related to the turbulence, ejection jet and the ageing degeneration of the elastic fibres in the aorta which occurs over the age of 40. Thus, in latter years, true poststenotic dilatation may be difficult to identify (Jefferson & Rees 1980).

c. Calcification. Calcification of a stenotic aortic valve usually occurs over the age of 40. Indeed, if absent, the diagnosis should be reviewed. Aortic valve calcification may be difficult to identify on the PA view as it overlies the spine. This is particularly true if a high kV technique is used. The lateral film is the projection of choice (Fig. 25.44). The distinction between aortic and mitral valve calcification can be made on the plain film if a line is drawn from the junction of the sternum and the diaphragm to the carina. There is a tendency for calcium to migrate within the tissues and, therefore, if the majority of the calcium lies above and superior to the line, it is situated predominantly in the aortic valve. If it lies inferior and posterior, then it is the mitral valve which is involved. If doubt exists, the presence and site of calcification can be confirmed by fluoroscopy (including at cardiac catheterization). Dynamically aortic valve calcification has a characteristic up and down movement in the long axis of the body whilst the mitral valve calcification has a dancing side to side movement. It should be pointed out that if calcium is identified radiographically, it is always much more extensive at operation.

Echocardiography. The domed aortic valve can be identified together with any calcium that may be present. Left ventricular hypertrophy will also be visible. The presence of cavity obliteration in systole indicates severe obstruction (Fig. 25.45).

Angiography. If the aortic valve can be crossed, the gradient should be measured. A left ventricular angiogram will demonstrate wall motion and when combined with an aortogram will identify the cusps which may be seen to dome in systole and be thickened with restricted movements (Fig. 25.46). Any associated regurgitation can also be assessed. As many of these patients are in an age group where ischaemic heart disease is common, the symptoms may be difficult if not impossible to distinguish. Thus concomitant coronary arteriography is frequently performed.

Optimum imaging technique

Angiography is not usually performed in patients under the age of 40, as echocardiography will demonstrate both the left ventricular wall motion, an abnormal valve and the subvalvar region. In the older age group, as coronary

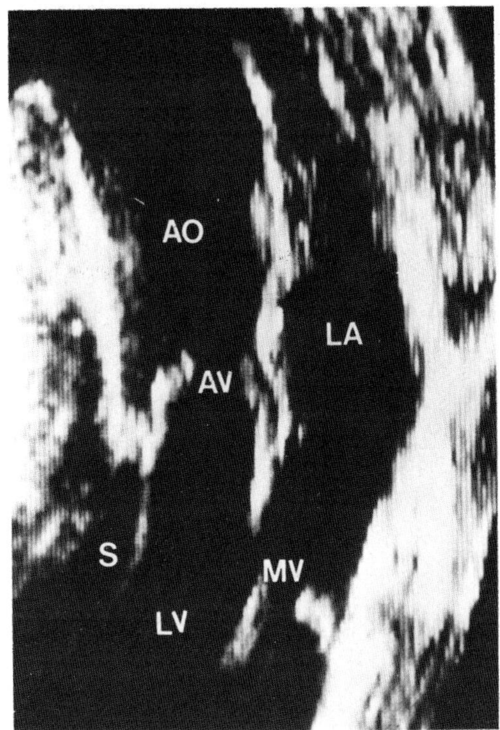

Fig. 25.45 Cross-sectional echocardiogram illustrating doming of the aortic valve in aortic valve stenosis.

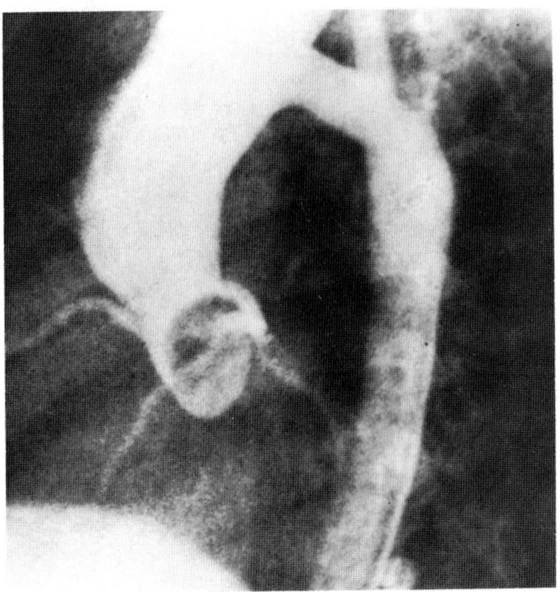

Fig. 25.46 Aortogram showing thickening and doming of aortic valve cusps in systole.

arteriography is often required, the aortic valve may be assessed angiographically at the same time.

Management

Calcified valves require valve replacement with associated coronary artery bypass grafting and pacing where indicated. In children and adolescents with isolated valve stenosis, valvotomy or valve reconstruction may be attempted as a holding procedure whilst the patient is still growing.

ATYPICAL AORTIC VALVE STENOSIS

Somerville and Ross (1977) have described a group of young patients between the ages of 4 and 16 (18% of their total series of aortic valve stenosis) in whom not only was the aortic valve abnormal but the septal hypertrophy and subvalve obstruction were present. The aortic root was small and had an abnormal histology. Even at this early age, they advocated excision of the valve and aortic root and replacement with a homograft. The plain film appearances are similar to those of aortic valve stenosis.

DIAPHRAGMATIC SUBVALVE STENOSIS

Anatomy and physiology. This condition, which is related to incomplete involution of the bulbus cordis, consists of a diaphragm which extends across the outflow tract of the left ventricle, usually within 2 cm of the aortic valve. The degree of obstruction depends on the size of the aperture in the diaphragm. If the diaphragm is immediately below the aortic valve, the jet through the aperture may damage the aortic cusps and cause superadded valvar stenosis or incompetence, the latter being the more common. The diaphragm may also interfere directly with aortic valve closure.

Clinical course. Many of these patients remain well throughout early childhood but they tend to show evidence of left heart obstruction at about the age of 10–12, or earlier if valve damage has occurred. They are particularly prone to bacterial endocarditis. If the diagnosis is made before irreversible changes have occurred in the left ventricle or aortic valve or before the condition has been complicated by the occurrence of bacterial endocarditis, then the diaphragm can simply be excised at operation.

Imaging

There is left ventricular hypertrophy at plain X-ray with a normal cardiothoracic ratio until failure occurs. The aortic arch is normal, there being no poststenotic dilatation of the aortic root unless the aortic valve has been damaged by turbulent blood passing through the small aperture in the diaphragm. The diagnosis may be confirmed by either echocardiography or left ventricular angiography demonstrating the subvalve diaphragm (Fig. 25.47).

FIBROMUSCULAR SUBVALVE STENOSIS

In this condition, which is relatively rare, there is a thickened elevated fibrous ring at the junction of the outflow and muscular paths of the left ventricle. The origin of this condition is not clear and it is often difficult to distinguish

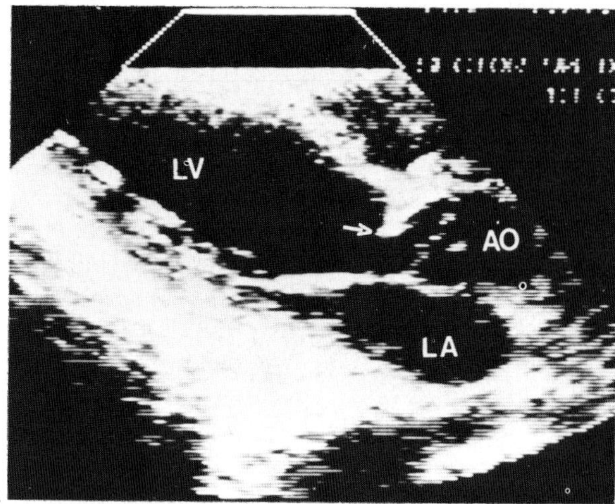

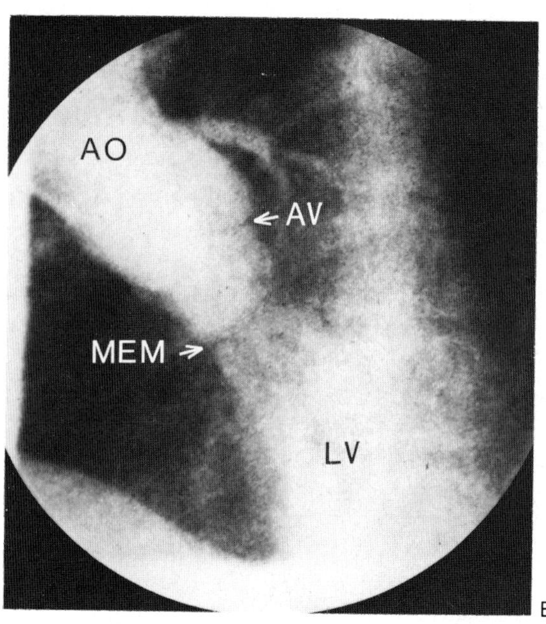

Fig. 25.47 A. Long axis parasternal cross-sectional echocardiogram showing discrete subaortic stenosis (arrow). **B.** LV angiogram of diaphragmatic subaortic stenosis due to failure of complete excavation at the junction of the primitive ventricle and the bulbus cordis.

from the fibrous ridge which develops in the same situation in hypertrophic obstructive cardiomyopathy.

The clinical course and radiological findings on the plain film are similar to those of diaphragmatic obstruction, except that the valve damage does not develop and the patients tend to present in an older age group. The level of the gradient can be identified by a withdrawal trace at cardiac catheterization. If ventricular hypertrophy has occurred, the radiological appearances on the left ventricular angiogram are indistinguishable from those seen in the left ventricle in hypertrophic obstructive cardiomyopathy.

HYPERTROPHIC OBSTRUCTIVE CARDIOMYOPATHY (HOCM) (Idiopathic hypertrophic subaortic stenosis: IHSS)

Most writers regard this as a congenital abnormality. However, it has already been described in the section on acquired heart disease (Ch. 23, p. 608).

AORTIC INCOMPETENCE

Aortic incompetence may be associated with ventricular septal defect, with bicuspid valve and with aneurysm or rupture of the sinus of Valsalva.

Fenestration of the aortic cusps is a very rare condition in which congenital defects exist in the cusps so that incompetence occurs. In *Marfan's syndrome* regurgitation occurs due to the dilatation of the aortic ring. In both conditions, left ventricular hypertrophy and enlargement due to diastolic overload are present. In Marfan's disease, there is usually also marked dilatation of the ascending thoracic aorta, and dissection may occur (see Ch. 26).

TRUNCUS ARTERIOSUS

Truncus arteriosus may be defined as a single arterial trunk leaving the base of the heart via a single arterial valve to supply the systemic, pulmonary and coronary circulations. If the ascending aorta gives rise to one pulmonary artery and the other pulmonary artery arises directly from the right ventricle via a second arterial valve, then such a heart is best described as having anomalous origin of one pulmonary artery rather than 'hemitruncus'.

Anatomy. Although truncus arteriosus can exist with any atrioventricular connection, most frequently it will be found with atrioventricular concordance. Almost always there is a ventricular septal defect as a consequence of the absence of the infundibular septum. The truncal valve usually overrides the ventricular septum so that it arises from both the right and left ventricles although it can be predominantly committed to one or the other. A major variation in truncus is found in the pattern of origin of the pulmonary and aortic tributaries from the ascending trunk. Three basic types are illustrated in Figure 25.48A. Truncus type 4 is described with the pulmonary blood flow originating from the descending aorta but it is preferable to call this condition pulmonary atresia with ventricular septal defect and a systemic pulmonary collateral supply to the lungs. Anomalies of the aorta are common in truncus and include interruption of the aortic arch and a right aortic arcb.

Incidence, physiology and clinical features. Truncus arteriosus is found in approximately 1% of symptomatic infants with congenital heart disease. There is a large unrestrictive ventricular septal defect so that pressures in the right and left ventricles are equal and similarly the free

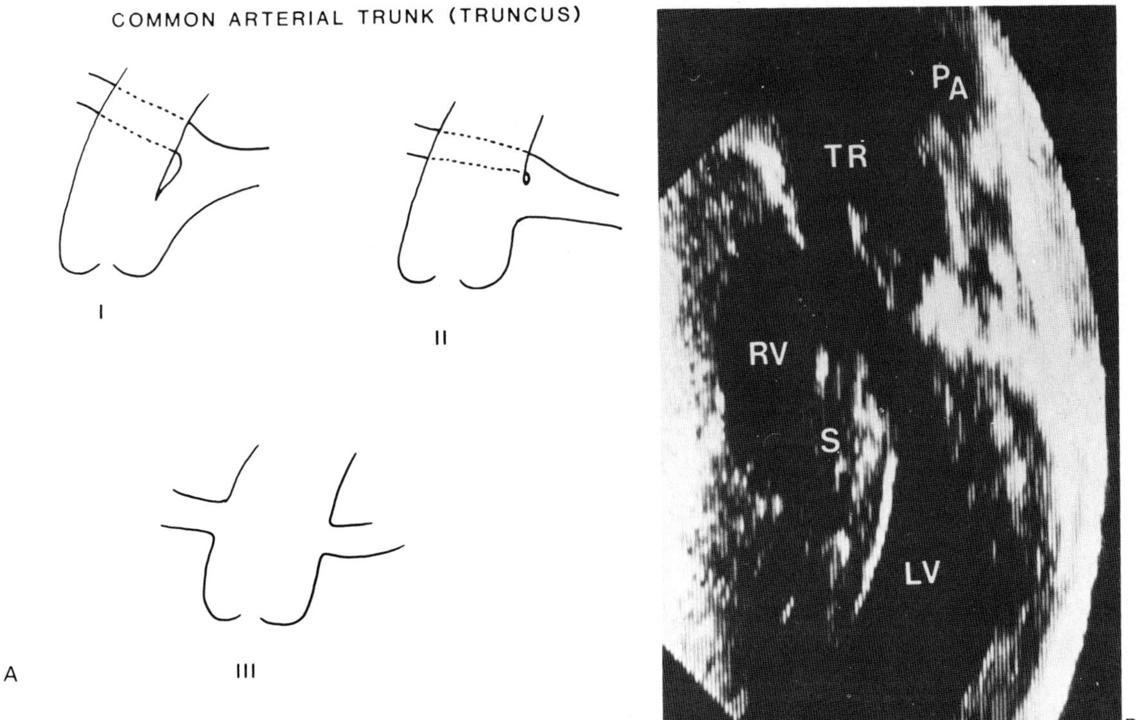

Fig. 25.48 A. Illustration of the various types of common arterial trunk. **B.** Subcostal long axis cross-sectional echocardiogram showing a common arterial trunk which over-rides the ventricular septum. There is a doubly committed ventricular septal defect and the pulmonary trunk arises posteriorly from the common arterial trunk.

communication between the aorta and pulmonary artery is also associated with equal pressures in these vessels. Typically the symptoms of congestive cardiac failure develop as the pulmonary vascular resistance falls so that from the age of about 2 months, tachypnoea, chest infections, poor feeding and failure to thrive are common.

Imaging

Plain film. Typically the chest radiograph shows cardiac enlargement with increased pulmonary vascular markings and enlargement of the left atrium. A right aortic arch is present in approximately 30% of patients.

Echocardiogram. Cross-sectional echocardiography readily allows the demonstration of a single arterial trunk arising from the ventricular mass and overriding the septum. A suprasternal long axis section will show the aorta and pulmonary artery arising from the common trunk but it may be difficult to demonstrate the exact pulmonary artery anatomy (Fig. 25.48B).

Angiography. It is now a common practice for radical corrective surgery to be performed in early infancy and this can be undertaken without prior cardiac catheterization. A major advantage of angiocardiography is that a selective injection into the trunk may demonstrate the exact anatomy of the pulmonary arteries, exclude branch stenosis of these vessels and allow the demonstration of any truncal valve incompetence (Fig. 25.49). It is the high flow and large cardiac output that makes accurate angiographic detail difficult to achieve.

Optimum imaging technique

For the most part cross-sectional echocardiography alone will allow the diagnosis of truncus arteriosus to be made. Thus taking into consideration clinical data, angiography will not usually be necessary.

THE HYPOPLASTIC LEFT HEART SYNDROME

Hypoplasia of the left ventricle associated with a *hypoplastic mitral valve* is found most frequently with *aortic atresia*. This group of anomalies is collectively called the hypoplastic left heart syndrome. The clinical presentation is in the first week of life with severe heart failure and a metabolic acidosis. The condition is rarely compatible with life beyond the age of 10 days.

Imaging. Cross-sectional echocardiography allows a precise diagnosis to be made and typically subcostal and apical four-chamber sections demonstrate the very small left ventricle and hypoplastic mitral valve (Fig. 25.50). In the majority of cases the left atrium is of normal size but has a thick wall and the flap valve of the atrial septum is usually herniated into the right atrium through an associ-

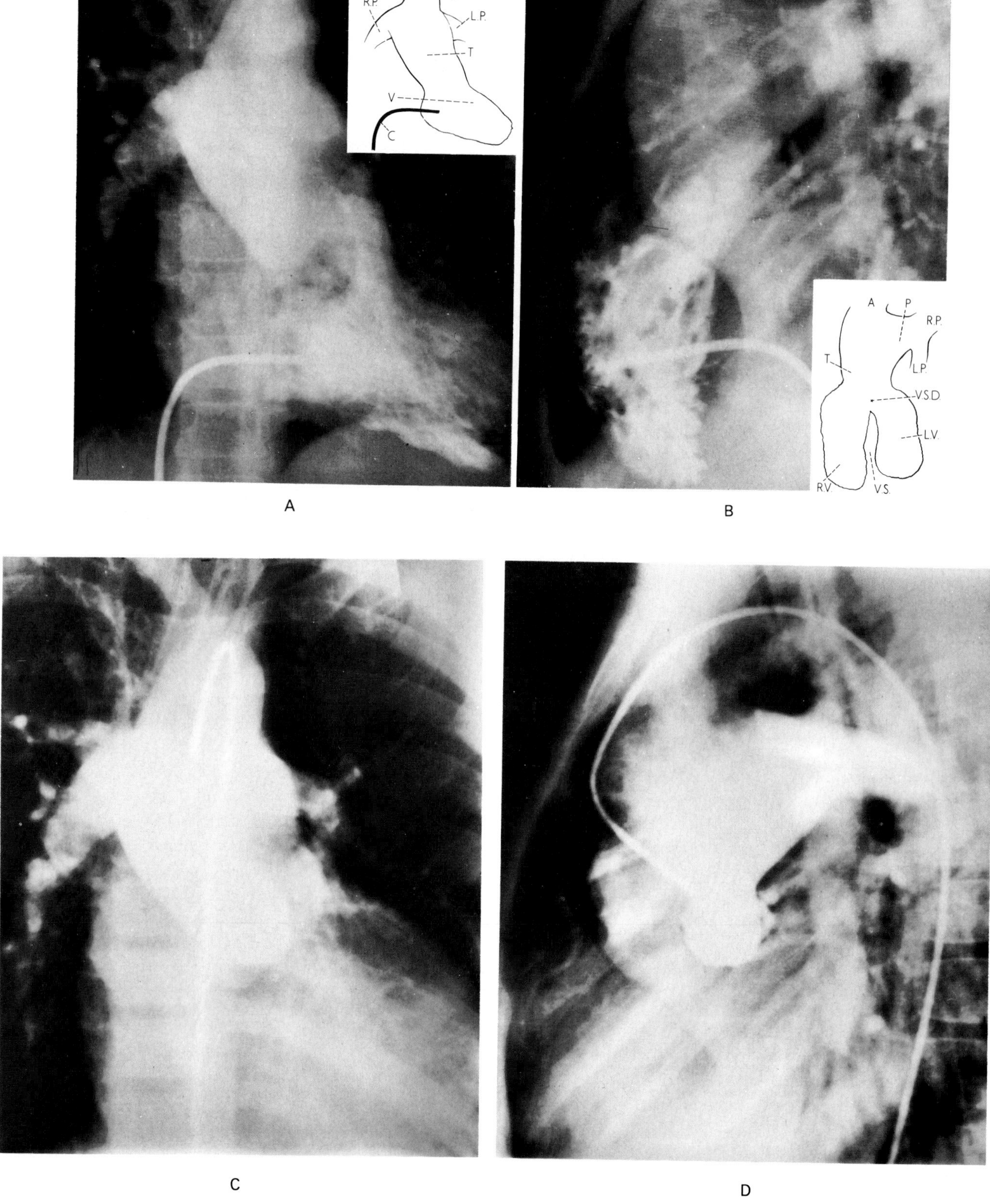

Fig. 25.49 A. Truncus arteriosus. Right ventricular angiogram showing single trunk over-riding VSD and confirming two ventricles. **B.** Lateral view showing posterior origin of pulmonary artery from the trunk. **C.** and **D.** Retrograde aortogram showing truncus and confirming posterior origins of pulmonary arteries from trunk. (**C.** = AP view, **D.** = lateral view.) *Diagrams*: A = aorta; P = pulmonary artery; RP & LP = right and left pulmonary arteries; T = truncus arteriosus; RV = right ventricle; LV = left ventricle; VSD = ventricular septal defect; VS = ventricular septum; C = catheter.

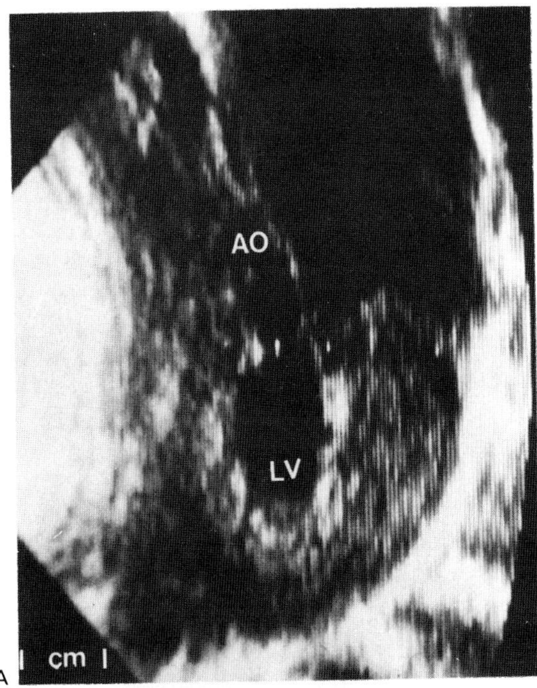

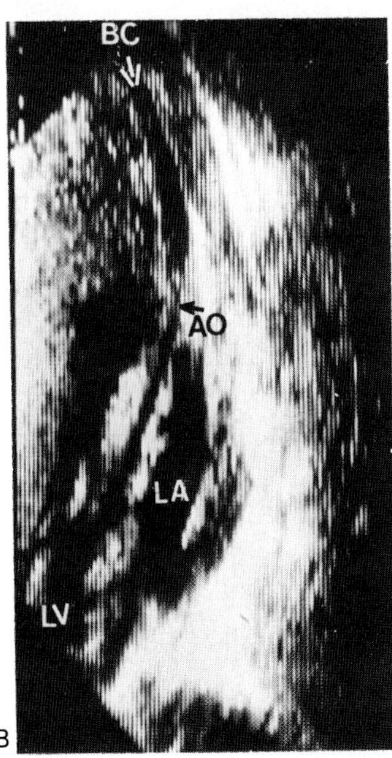

Fig. 25.50 A. and **B.** Two cross-sectional echocardiograms from an infant with the hypoplastic left heart syndrome showing severe aortic hypoplasia and severe hypoplasia of the left ventricle.

ated atrial septal defect. Parasternal long axis sections demonstrate the hypoplastic aorta, and the atretic aortic valve. In most institutions, cardiac catheterization and angiography are not undertaken when the diagnosis has been made by cross-sectional echocardiography. Nevertheless a selective aortogram will demonstrate severe hypoplasia of the ascending aorta as shown in Figure 25.51.

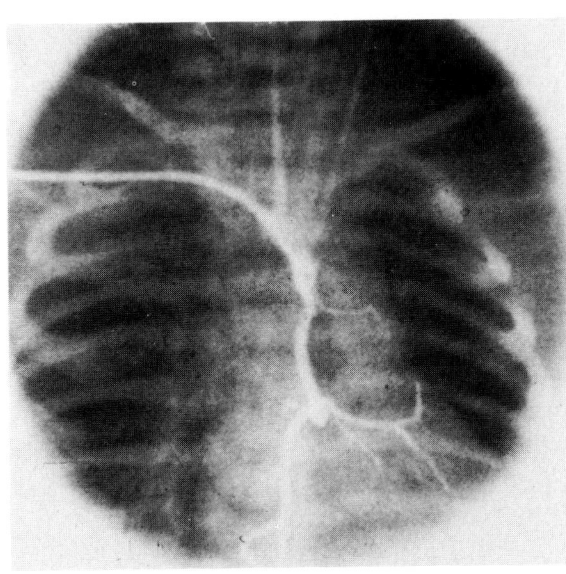

Fig. 25.51 Hypoplastic left heart syndrome — aortic atresia. Aortic arch injection outlining markedly hypoplastic ascending aorta with coronary arteries filling retrogradely.

ANOMALIES OF THE GREAT ARTERIES AND ASSOCIATED ABNORMALITIES

AORTOPULMONARY COMMUNICATIONS

It must be remembered that, although there are a number of aortopulmonary communications, ductus arteriosus accounts for 98%. Whilst the exact diagnosis is important in each individual case, the real significance lies in the possible differential diagnosis.

DUCTUS ARTERIOSUS

Incidence, anatomy and physiology. This is a common condition being the second most frequent in Wood's series of 900 cases of congenital heart disease (1960). The function of the ductus and the related fetal flow patterns have already been described (see p. 628). The ductus originates at the bifurcation of the main pulmonary artery extending upwards to the inferior aspect of the aortic arch opposite the origin of the subclavian artery. It should be appreciated that if the aortic arch is right sided, then the ductus may communicate directly with the left subclavian artery (Fig. 25.52) rather than the aortic arch (see radiological appearances). The flow through the ductus is in direct proportion to the cross-sectional area and inversely related to the pulmonary vascular resistance. Thus, if the pulmonary and systemic vascular resistances are balanced, the shunt may be small. In this situation, an elevated pulmonary artery saturation may not be detected and the communication is only demonstrated by angiography.

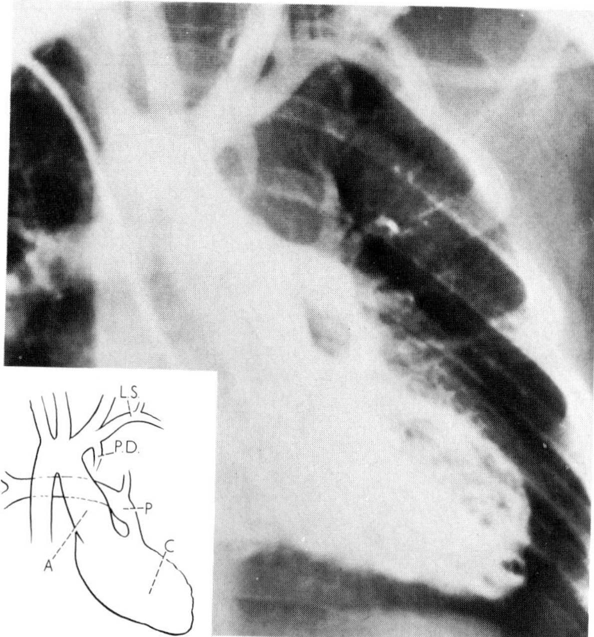

Fig. 25.52 Angiogram showing ductus arising from left subclavian artery in association with right aortic arch. *Diagram*: A = aorta; P = pulmonary artery; C = primitive ventricle; LS = left subclavian artery; PD = ductus.

Systemic vascular resistance is higher than that in the pulmonary bed in the majority of patients. Hence pulmonary artery pressure is normal or only slightly elevated and flow occurs through the ductus in both systole and diastole giving rise to a continuous (machinery) murmur. The pulmonary to systemic flow ratio is usually more than 1.5 to 1 and may be as high as 4 or 5 to 1. In approximately 10% of all ductus cases, pulmonary artery pressures are elevated as a result of high flow and raised pulmonary vascular resistance. This may occur at an early age. Depending upon the exact level of pulmonary artery pressure, flow may only occur in systole and a continuous murmur is no longer present. If the pulmonary vascular resistance rises above systemic vascular resistance, reversal of flow occurs (the Eisenmenger situation). The resulting right to left shunt leads to relative cyanosis of the lower half of the body (differential cyanosis).

Clinical course. Most patients with an uncomplicated persistent ductus remain relatively asymptomatic throughout childhood. If the duct diameter is large with a considerable flow, then dyspnoea, fatigue and failure to thrive may become increasingly noticeable. The dangers of heart failure, pulmonary vascular disease and bacterial endocarditis are always present. Without treatment, many patients will become increasingly disabled. This may become apparent during early childhood and certainly so by the late teens or early twenties. Occasionally, however, if pulmonary and systemic vascular resistances are almost balanced, patients will survive to adult life with a very small left to right shunt and virtually no symptoms. In this clinical situation, the duct may calcify.

Imaging features

Plain film. Changes on the chest radiograph depend on the size of the shunt and volume of flow. If these are small, the heart and lung fields will be normal. With increasing flow, the strain falls on the left atrium and left ventricle with subsequent enlargement of these chambers. This may be difficult to detect in that the cardiothoracic ratio rarely exceeds 50%. Although a prominent aortic arch is visible in older patients, this is not usually noted under the age of 10. If the pulmonary to systemic flow ratio is more than 2 to 1, plethora will be visible in the lung fields. If the flow ratio is higher, the likelihood of irreversible changes in the pulmonary vascular bed increases. The changes become more apparent with increasing age and electrocardiographic evidence of right ventricular hypertrophy will also be present. Irreversible changes in the pulmonary vascular bed will occur in about 10% of untreated patients and may lead to the Eisenmenger situation. The radiographic appearances of these haemodynamic states have been described on page 567.

If the ductus has calcified, this will be visible as a 'comma'-shaped density lying inside the line of the aortic arch in the frontal view (Fig. 25.53).

Echocardiography. In the neonate, it is frequently possible to visualize the ductus by a suprasternal parasaggital section as shown in Figure 25.54. However, if the pulmonary artery is large or the ductus small, its identification may prove difficult.

Angiography. Whilst the ductus can be demonstrated by passing a catheter via the pulmonary artery through the

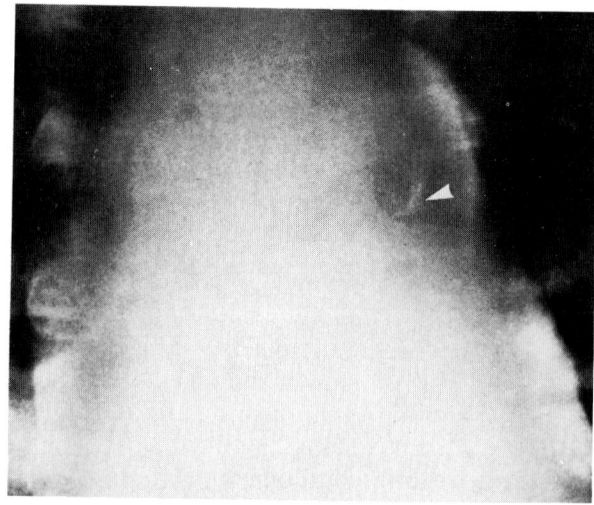

Fig. 25.53 Calcium in ductus. Note shape of calcium, which is lying well within lateral wall of aorta (arrow).

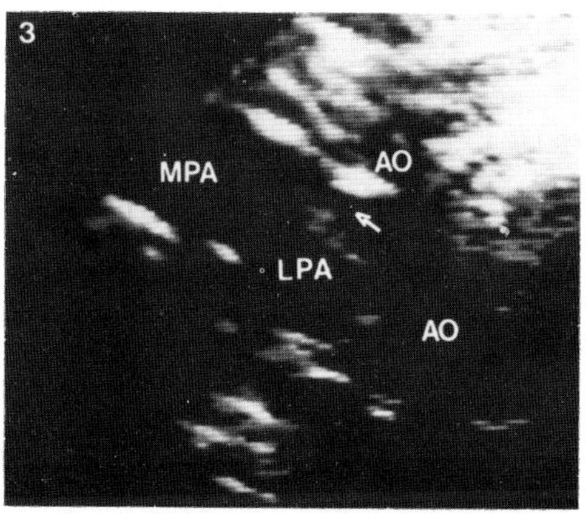

Fig. 25.54 Suprasternal parasagittal cross-sectional echocardiogram showing an arterial ductus (arrow).

ductus and on down the descending aorta, it is usual to confirm its presence angiographically for the following reasons:

1. To confirm or exclude the ductus in the presence of a ventricular septal defect. If the pulmonary vascular resistance is sufficiently high to abolish the diastolic component of the machinery murmur, it may not be possible to distinguish between the two conditions clinically.
2. In early infancy, when a continuous murmur may be absent due to persisting elevation of pulmonary vascular resistance.
3. To distinguish between the ductus and other aortopulmonary communications.

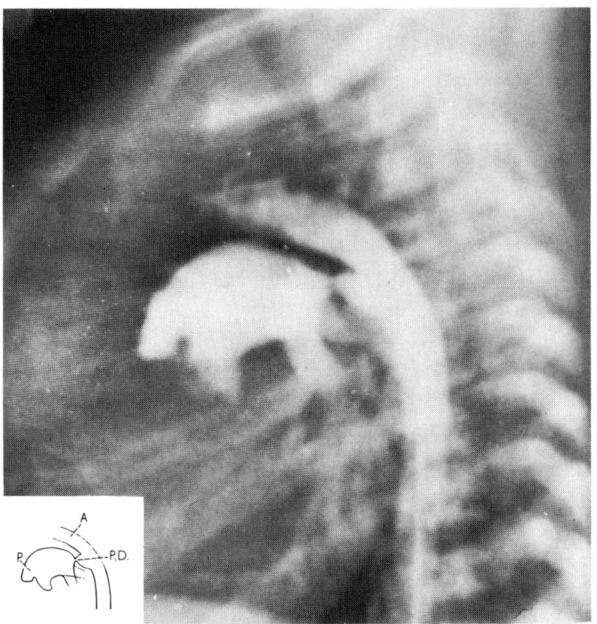

Fig. 25.55 Retrograde aortogram showing ductus. *Diagram*: A = aorta; P = pulmonary artery; PD = ductus.

As the aim of aortography is to demonstrate the site of the aortopulmonary communication, all the proximal aorta must be outlined from the level of the aortic valve to the left subclavian artery. The arch should be visualized in the left anterior oblique projection. If the duct is small it may be necessary to repeat the injection with a catheter tip lying in the aortic isthmus just proximal to the origin of the ductus (Fig. 24.55). Even if the systemic and pulmonary circulations are balanced, a pressure injection will temporarily create a left to right shunt. If systemic desaturation is present indicating a right to left shunt, then the duct can be demonstrated by an injection into the main pulmonary artery with subsequent outlining of the descending aorta.

Optimum imaging technique
As it may be difficult to identify the ductus by echocardiography especially if it is small or the pulmonary artery is large, cine-aortography in the left anterior oblique projection is frequently the investigation of choice. In doubtful cases, it may be necessary to inject with a catheter tip lying just proximal to the ductal origin.

Management
As there is always a risk of irreversible pulmonary vascular disease, a ductus should be closed. Of course, this presupposes that irreversible pulmonary vascular disease is not already present. The small but well-recognized risk of subacute bacterial endocarditis endorses this management policy. In infants, children and young adults, the ductus is ligated via a left thoracotomy. However, if the ductus is calcified, there is a risk of the ligatures cutting through the ductus with consequent torrential haemorrhage. It is for this reason that patching the ductus from within the aorta has been advocated.

AORTOPULMONARY WINDOW

Incidence, anatomy, embryology and physiology. This rare anomaly occurs if there is only partial division of the truncus arteriosus into an anterior pulmonary artery and a posterior aorta. If present, this communication lies immediately above the aortic valve. Both the aortic and pulmonary valves are normal and usually there is no associated ventricular septal defect. If a shunt is present, the direction and volume will depend on the size of the defect and the pulmonary vascular resistance.

Clinical course. Large defects giving rise to a big left to right shunt present in infancy with heart failure. Patients who present later are usually considerably disabled and, without treatment, death tends to occur in the second decade from heart failure due to elevated pulmonary vascular resistance. However, occasionally if the shunt is very small, patients may remain symptom free and the condition is often not detected until quite late in adult life.

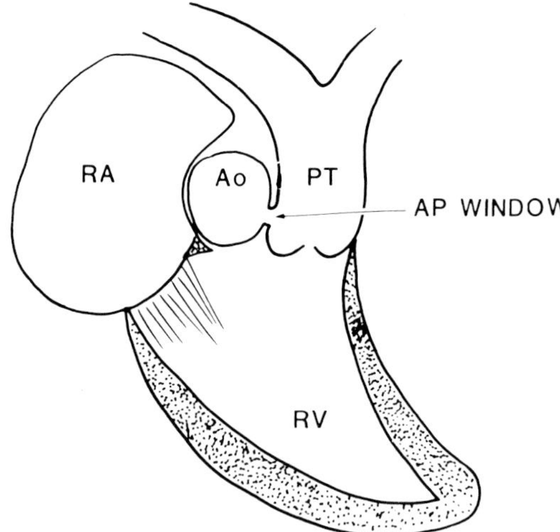

Fig. 25.56 Diagram of subcostal long axis cross-sectional echocardiogram showing aortopulmonary window.

Imaging

Plain film. The heart is frequently enlarged. If it is possible to distinguish a large aortic root with a relatively small aortic arch in the presence of a left to right shunt, this is a strong pointer towards an aortopulmonary window. The lung vascular pattern is that of plethora often with evidence of pulmonary hypertension.

Echocardiography. Whilst it is sometimes possible to demonstrate this anomaly by echocardiography (Fig. 25.56), the main value of echocardiography is to exclude ventricular septal defect and to demonstrate normal semilunar valves.

Angiography. An aortogram is mandatory to demonstrate that the site of the defect is above the semilunar valves, thus distinguishing it from truncus arteriosus.

Optimum imaging technique

Echocardiography will normally demonstrate the ventricular septum and semilunar valves. However, angiographic detail of the aortopulmonary communication is almost always necessary.

Management

Irreversible pulmonary vascular disease may develop at a young age and it is to prevent this complication that early diagnosis and surgical correction are essential. As the condition is seen infrequently, accurate figures are not easily available for operative mortality.

RUPTURED SINUS OF VALSALVA

Incidence, anatomy and physiology. A fistulous communication between an aortic sinus of Valsalva and the pulmonary circulation is seen in less than 1% of patients with symptomatic congenital heart disease. The communication may be present from birth or may occur later in life often in early adolescence, rupturing through a region of congenital weakness. Communications may occur as follows:

1. Right sinus → right ventricular outflow tract.
2. Non-coronary sinus → right atrium.
3. Left sinus i) anterior → main pulmonary artery.
   ii) posterior → left atrium.

Rupture occurs most frequently through the right sinus of Valsalva.

Clinical course. If a communication is present at birth the condition presents as a left to right shunt and differentiation from a ductus may be extremely difficult. If rupture occurs as the later event, the presenting symptoms are precordial pain, dyspnoea and a continuous murmur. Ventricular failure and even death may follow rapidly.

Imaging features

Plain film. If the condition is present from birth, the lung fields will show evidence of a left to right shunt, the exact findings depending on the vascular resistance (see p. 567). If the sinus ruptures later in life, pulmonary oedema is likely to be the presenting feature on the plain film. If the sinus is aneurysmal, this may present as an enlarged aortic root. In the very rare event of the communication being from the aortic root into the left atrium, the radiograph may be normal.

Echocardiography and angiography. Whilst echocardiography may demonstrate the defect, an aortogram is usually required for confirmation (Fig. 25.57).

Management

This is by surgical closure of the communication.

ANOMALOUS ORIGIN OF THE CORONARY ARTERY OR CORONARY ARTERY FISTULA

This condition consists either of the right coronary artery arising from the right atrium or right ventricle or alternatively the left coronary artery arising from the pulmonary artery. Due to the low pressure of the right side of the heart flow in the coronary is reversed, resulting in a left to right shunt. Systemic blood from the other coronary artery is supplied via collateral communications. In addition to the shunt, myocardial ischaemia frequently occurs secondary to the run off into the low pressure pulmonary circulation.

Clinical course. Whilst many of these patients remain asymptomatic, if the shunt is sufficiently large, myocardial ischaemia, confirmed electrocardiographically, may progress to cardiac enlargement and heart failure.

Imaging. The heart may enlarge with evidence of left ventricular failure. Coronary arteriography defines the

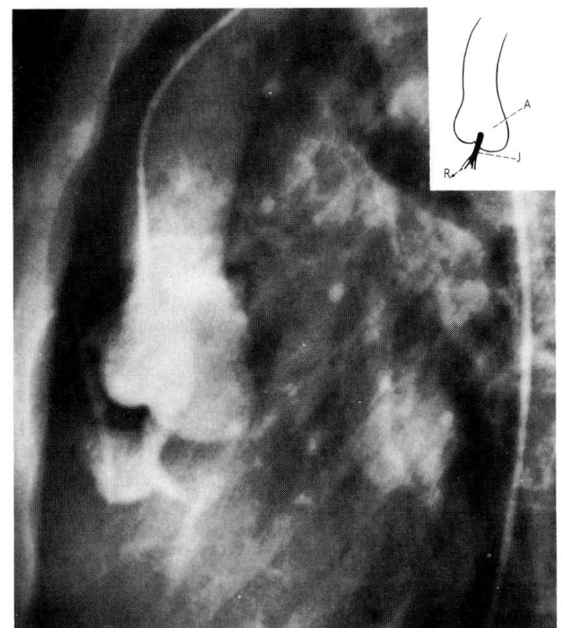

Fig. 25.57 Rupture of sinus of Valsalva. Aortogram showing rupture of right coronary sinus into RV. *Diagram*: A = aortic root; J = jet passing through ruptured sinus; R = right ventricle.

lesion and is the definitive investigation (Fig. 25.58) except in infants where an aortogram may yield sufficient information.

Management. For symptomatic infants with incipient infarction, implantation of the anomalous artery into the aorta is the operation of choice. In older patients where the problem is predominantly a left to right shunt, ligation of the artery can be performed.

COARCTATION OF THE AORTA

Incidence, anatomy and physiology. Isolated coarctation and coarctation with a ventricular septal defect are seen in more than 10% of symptomatic infants referred to specialist paediatric centres. Older children and adults with this condition may also present with hypertension. As has been indicated by Shinebourne and Elseed (1974), 'classical' coarctation occurs in the juxtaductal position. There is a 'thickening' of the postero-lateral wall of the aorta, opposite the origin of the ductus, resulting in a decrease of the lumen of the aorta. Whilst the duct remains open, significant obstruction does not occur. However, following duct closure, the aorta may be constricted at this level. The degree of constriction depends to some extent on the size of the aortic isthmus — the portion of the aorta between the head and neck arteries and the origin of the ductus. The size of the isthmus, like all other vessels, is flow dependant. Hence, it may be small in the presence of left ventricular outflow tract obstruction, e.g. aortic stenosis. If the flow in the aortic arch is increased, for instance in the presence of right ventricular outflow tract obstruction, e.g. Fallot's tetralogy or pulmonary atresia, the isthmus will be large and an associated coarctation extremely rare.

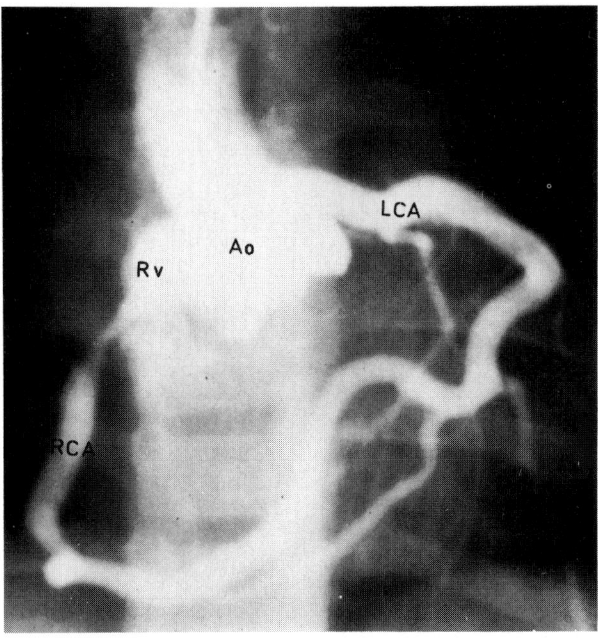

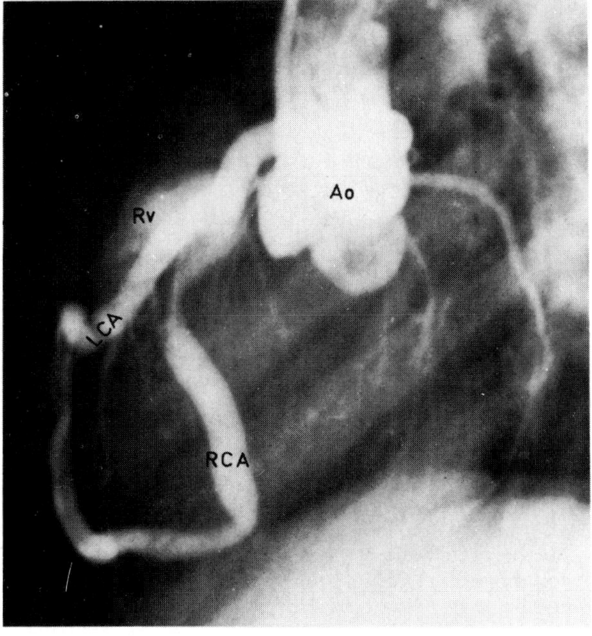

Fig. 25.58 **A** & **B** Aortic root injection showing left coronary artery arising normally. The artery is dilated and fills the right coronary artery retrogradely. The latter arises anomalously from the right ventricular outflow tract. (Reproduced by courtesy of Dr B Strickland.)

Associated aortic valve lesions are not uncommon occurring in approximately 10% of cases. Failure of the ductus to close may occur in up to 15% of cases. The left subclavian artery also may be involved in a coarctation. If the isthmal narrowing is marked, the coarctation may appear to extend proximally but it should be appreciated that this appearance is the combination of two separate defects. Rarely, narrowed areas may be present in the descending thoracic or abdominal portions of the aorta. These are due to a different pathogenesis. The thoracic lesions present in a similar way to classical coarctation but the abdominal variety usually give rise to abdominal or peripheral claudication. A ventricular septal defect is found in 40% of patients with coarctation and the condition has also been described in conjunction with Turner's syndrome (Nora et al 1970).

Clinical course. Many patients present in early infancy though some are asymptomatic until at least their late teens or early twenties, when coarctation may be detected at a routine medical examination. In this situation, there may be asymptomatic hypertension, delayed or absent femoral pulses or a bruit, usually around the scapulae, arising from a well-developed collateral circulation. Left ventricular hypertrophy will be apparent on the electrocardiogram. Hypertension in the young person should always raise the possibility of coarctation. There is usually little or no delay in physical development.

Patients who present with pulmonary oedema in the neonatal age group have to be distinguished from those with a large left to right shunt, aortic valve disease, the hypoplastic left heart syndrome and obstructed total anomalous pulmonary venous return.

Imaging appearances

Plain film. Symptomatic infants may show cardiomegaly and pulmonary venous hypertension. However, provided left heart failure has not supervened, the plain film will usually show the cardiac outline to be within normal limits but with prominence of the left heart border suggesting left ventricular hypertrophy. The classical abnormality is that of rib notching (see Fig. 24.35). Rib notching is not pathognomonic for coarctation as it also occurs in a number of other conditions — see Table 25.2.

Table 25.2 Causes of rib notching

1. Coarctation (this may be unilateral — see text)
2. Superior vena cava obstruction
3. Severe right ventricular outflow tract obstruction, e.g. Fallot's tetralogy or pulmonary atresia
4. Systemic-pulmonary artery shunt operations (notching is unilateral)
5. Neurofibromatosis

It should be appreciated that coarctation is by far the most common cause of rib notching. Collateral circulation, bypassing the obstruction, is through the costocervical trunk and internal mammary arteries arising from the subclavian artery. The costocervical trunk supplies the first two intercostal arteries which, together with the internal mammary artery, anastomose with the remaining intercostal arteries and the flow through these latter vessels is retrograde supplying the distal aorta. It is the intercostal arteries, having become tortuous and hypertrophied which cause the rib notching. The notching, which is nearly always bilateral, usually occurs on the fourth to eighth ribs posteriorly. Occasionally the third and ninth ribs are also involved. Notching may be unilateral on the right side if the left subclavian artery is involved in the coarctation. The notching will be unilateral on the left side if there is an aberrant origin of the right subclavian artery arising from the descending aorta below the coarctation. Rib notching is rarely present before the age of 10 to 12 years though it has been recognized in a patient as young as 3.

As the volume of blood carried by the head and neck arteries is greater than normal, these increase in size. This may be apparent on the radiograph if the left paravertebral shadow is widened due to the hypertrophied left subclavian artery. Occasionally, the descending aorta is clearly seen below the coarctation when a poststenotic dilatation may be apparent. This dilatation is aneurysmal in about 4% of cases.

Echocardiography. Echocardiography is an unreliable method for demonstrating coarctation. However, it will identify an associated ventricular septal defect and exclude aortic interruption.

Angiography. The anatomy can be outlined prior to surgical correction by means of an aortogram in the left oblique position in adults. Biplane studies may be carried out in children. A catheter should be positioned to outline the aortic valve as well as the arch in order to confirm or exclude aortic valve disease and arch interruptions. A left ventricular injection may also be included to assess the ventricular septum. The approach to the aorta is usually via the right arm, although it is possible to cross a mild obstruction from below. Not only is it important to make the diagnosis of coarctation, it is also essential to identify the relationship of the coarctation to the left subclavian artery. Occasionally the left subclavian artery is involved in the coarctation and if this is so, the surgical technique has to be planned accordingly (Fig. 25.59).

Optimum imaging technique

Whilst it may be possible to obtain adequate information from an echocardiogram, angiography should be undertaken if doubt persists.

Management

Once the anatomy of the coarctation and associated arteries have been satisfactorily identified, relief of the obstruction is always indicated. In the neonatal period, it may be

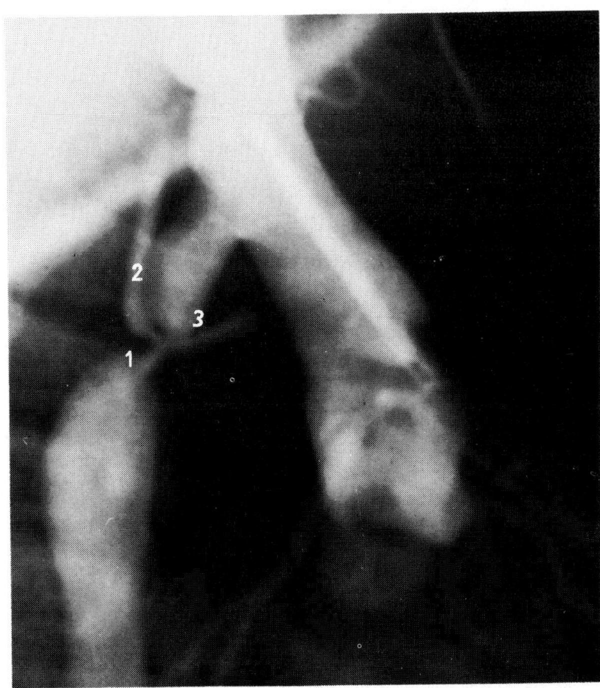

Fig. 25.59 Coarctation of the aorta. An aortic root injection outlines the coarctation at the juxtaductal site. Note (1) posterior indentation of the aorta: (2) left subclavian artery involved in the coarctation: and (3) small ductus still patent.

necessary to operate as an emergency procedure. In the adult, repair of the coarctation will relieve left heart strain and reduce the risk of bacterial endocarditis.

Pseudocoarctation
This occurs most commonly in elderly patients when it is due to kinking of the aorta secondary to atherosclerosis. It is also occasionally seen in children. There is no pressure gradient or rib notching and this condition should not be confused with true coarctation.

PERIPHERAL PULMONARY ARTERY STENOSES

A *single stenosis* of either of the main branches of the pulmonary artery or of the peripheral branches is not uncommon and may occur either as an isolated defect or, more commonly, in association with a congenital cardiac abnormality. This may either be a malformation of the outflow tract to the right ventricle or supravalvar aortic stenosis associated with hypercalcaemia and mental retardation.

Multiple stenoses in the branches of the pulmonary artery giving rise to proximal pulmonary artery hypertension is a much rarer condition. It is often associated with arteriovenous malformations in the lungs. Clinical symptoms are those of right heart obstruction, sometimes associated with haemoptysis from the arteriovenous malformations. The radiological appearances are those of right atrioventricular enlargement with normal hilar vessels and occasionally with prominent peripheral pulmonary arteries, due to post-stenotic dilatation distal to the multiple strictures. Occasionally peripheral pulmonary artery stenosis may complicate other types of congenital heart disease, particularly Fallot's tetralogy. There is also an association with conditions such as congenital rubella and infantile hypercalcaemia (William's syndrome) (Fig. 25.60).

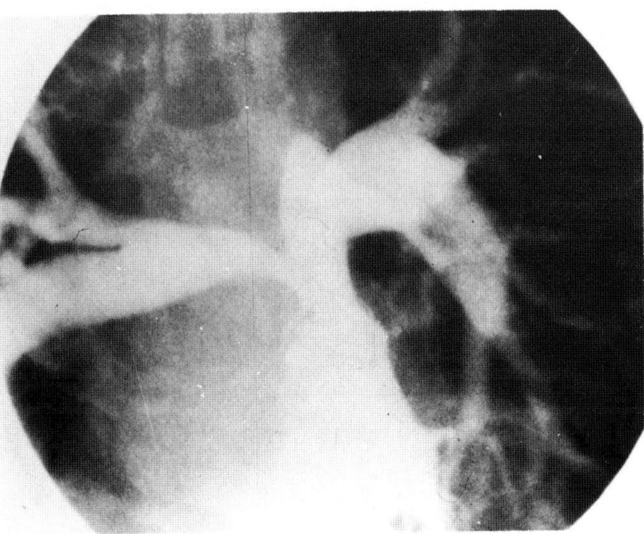

Fig. 25.60 Pulmonary arteriogram in four-chamber projection from a patient with peripheral pulmonary artery stenoses.

VASCULAR RINGS

Anatomy and physiology. Vascular rings are rare, being seen in less than 1% of symptomatic children. The rings may be formed in a number of ways and these are illustrated by the diagrams in Appendix C. They can be classified into two groups, being those with either a left or a right descending aorta. The group with the left descending aorta includes the aberrant right subclavian artery arising from the descending aorta, and also the aberrant left pulmonary artery which arises directly from the right pulmonary artery.

Clinical. If the ring is causing tracheal compression, the patient will present with stridor in the neonatal period.

Imaging features

Plain film. The presence of a right aortic arch should alert the clinician to the possibility of a vascular ring. The right arch, which is particularly well seen in a high kV film, is recognized by increased density in the right paratracheal region. There is insufficient opacification in the left paratracheal region to account for an aortic arch and descending aorta on that side. Although the level of 'cross over' of the descending aorta from the right side of the spine to the left side is variable, it is usually in the lower thorax relatively close to the left-sided aortic hiatus (in patients with situs solitus — see p. 614). Thus the right paraspinal line will be prominent whereas that on the left side may be difficult to identify.

Barium swallow. With improved film technique and development of echocardiography, the barium swallow is now only of importance in the assessment of vascular rings. The position of the aortic arch can be confirmed and an aberrant right subclavian artery or aberrant left pulmonary artery identified (see diagrams in Appendix C).

Echocardiography. Whilst the right aortic arch can be identified by echocardiography, it may be extremely difficult to demonstrate smaller arteries completing the rings. This will depend both on the size of the vessels and their patency. Thus where a 'ductus' is represented only by a ligamentum arteriosum, echocardiography will be of no help.

Angiography. If the plain film and barium swallow suggest a vascular ring, angiography may demonstrate abnormality of the aortic arch. Indeed, many centres consider an aortogram essential prior to surgery (see diagrams in Appendix C).

Optimum imaging technique

The plain film and barium swallow are accepted screening procedures. If these do not indicate, or at least suggest, a ring, no further action is necessary. If a ring appears to be present, this should be confirmed angiographically.

Management. If the ring is causing stridor, the obstruction should be relieved surgically.

REFERENCES AND SUGGESTIONS FOR FURTHER READING

Anderson, R. H., MacCartney, F. J., Tynam M. et al (1983) Univentricular atrioventricular connection: single ventricle trap unsprung. *Paediatric Cardiology*, **4**, 273–280

Baron, M. G., Wolfe, B. S., Steinfield, L., Van Mierop, L. H. S. (1964) Endocardial cushion defects, specific diagnosis by angiocardiography. *American Journal of Cardiology*, **13**, 162–175

Betriu, A., Wigle, E. D., Felderhof, C. H., McLoughlin, M. J. (1975) Prolapse of the posterior leaflet of the mitral valve associated with secundum atrial septal defects. *American Journal of Cardiology*, **35**, 363–369

Dickinson, D. F., Arnold, R., Wilkinson, J. L. (1981) Ventricular septal defects in children born in Liverpool 1960–1969. Valuation of natural cause and surgical implication in an unselected population. *British Heart Journal*, **46**, 47–54

Grittenberger de Groot, A. C., Sauer, U., Oppenheimer-Decker, A., Quaegerbeur, J. (1983) Coronary arterial anatomy in transposition of the great arteries: a morphological study. *Paediatric Cardiology*, **4**, Supplement I, 15–21

Jefferson, K. E., Rees, R. S. O. (1980) *Clinical Cardiac Radiology*. London: Butterworth

Keith, J. D., Rowe, R. D, Vlad, P. (1967) *Heart Disease in Infancy and Childhood*. New York: MacMillan

Nora, J., Torres, F., Sinha, A., McNamara, D. (1970) Characteristic cardiovascular anomalies of XO Turner's syndrome, XX and XY phenotype and XO, XX Turner mosaic. *American Journal of Radiology*, **25**, 639

Scott, D. J., Rigby, M. L., Miller, G. A. H., Shinebourne, E. A. (1984) The presentation of symptomatic heart disease in infancy based on 10 years experience (1973–82). Implication for the provision of services. *British Heart Journal*, **52**, 248–257

Shinebourne, E. A., Elseed, A. M. (1974) Relations between foetal blood flow patterns, coarctation of the aorta and pulmonary blood flow. *British Heart Journal*, **36**, 492–498

Somerville, J., Ross, D. N. (1977) Atypical aortic valve stenosis — a diffused and congenital cardiovascular disease — recognition and surgical management. *British Heart Journal* **39**, 390

Vlovader, Z., Neufield, H. N., Edwards, J. E. (1975) *Coronary Variations in the Normal Heart and in Congenital Heart Disease*. New York: Academic Press

Wood, P. (1960) *Diseases of the Heart and Circulation*, p. 360. London: Eyre & Spottiswoode

CHAPTER 26

ARTERIOGRAPHY AND THERAPEUTIC ANGIOGRAPHY

Historical

It is a remarkable fact that arteriography of the human body was achieved within one month of Roentgen announcing his discovery of X-rays in December 1895. Haschek and Lindenthal published the first angiogram of an amputated hand in January 1896. Such post-mortem injections were copied elsewhere, but a quarter of a century passed by before the next major advances. Orfin published *An X-ray Atlas of the Systemic Arteries of the Body* based on post-mortem injections in 1920, which may have stimulated workers in several different countries to attempt in vivo angiography. This was finally achieved in the 1920s.

In 1923 Sicard and Forrestier in France, after animal experiments, injected a small amount of Lipiodol into a human femoral vein and watched its transit to the heart and lungs. There were no ill effects to the patient apart from transient coughing. In the same year Berberich and Hirsch in Germany produced the first true arteriograms and venograms in living humans by injecting strontium bromide into the upper limb. In 1924 Brooks in the USA produced the first femoral arteriogram by injecting sodium iodide. Soon after Moniz carried out his classic work on human cerebral angiography which was published in 1928, and in 1929 Dos Santos described lumbar aortography. In the early 1930s organic iodides were developed and began to be used for angiography.

The first cardiac catheterization was carried out by Forssman in Germany in 1929 and in 1936 Amiaille first opacified the heart chambers in man using a catheter. In 1937 Castellanos, Pereiras and Garcia described the use of right heart angiography in the diagnosis of congenital heart defects, whilst in 1941 Farinas first described retrograde catheter angiography.

Although all the basic work had now been done it was not until the 1950s that arteriography became widely used in medicine. Much of the credit goes to Scandinavian workers who developed percutaneous techniques of injection in the 1940s. Seldinger's ingenious method of percutaneous catheterization was first described in 1953, and the stage was now set for more widespread adoption of angiography.

TECHNIQUES OF IMAGING ARTERIES

These now include:

1. Direct arteriography by needle puncture or arterial catheterization.
2. Imaging of arteries by ultrasound.
3. Imaging of arteries by isotopes.
4. Imaging of arteries by CT and by MR.
5. Venous arteriography, i.e. visualization of arteries following injection of contrast into the venous system.
6. Digital subtraction angiography (DSA).

The vast majority of arterial investigations have been, and continue to be, carried out by direct arteriography.

Ultrasound has been mostly used to demonstrate abdominal aneurysms. It is also used to confirm and show the size of peripheral aneurysms. The method can also demonstrate internal carotid occlusions or stenosis. With the latter conditions however few surgeons would proceed to surgery purely on ultrasound findings and where surgery is to be performed direct arteriography or DSA is usually required.

Isotope angiography will also show abdominal aneurysms or major arterial occlusions. It has also been used to show the patency of arterial grafts. Resolution, however, is relatively poor and intraluminal clot cannot be shown. The method is especially useful in patients with a known iodine sensitivity which precludes the use of conventional contrast media.

Computed tomography is a non-invasive method of demonstrating major vascular lesions, such as thoracic or abdominal aneurysms. It is usual, however, to inject an i.v. bolus of contrast prior to the examination to improve definition and show intraluminal clot or other abnormalities. With this technique aneurysms and dissecting aneurysms can be shown, and the anatomy of coarctation is well demonstrated. The patency of coronary or other arterial grafts can also be shown by CT.

Magnetic resonance has already proved very effective for the demonstration of major vascular lesions and is still being evaluated (see Ch. 68).

Venous arteriography was used in the past as a method of showing major vessels such as the aorta without the hazards of direct arteriography. Using a large i.v. bolus of contrast and subtraction films of the appropriate area adequate visualization of the aorta and great vessels could often be obtained. The method was a forerunner of the more sophisticated digital subtraction angiography.

Digital subtraction angiography (DSA) is similar to the technique just described but uses computers to obtain rapid digital information of the contrast bolus as it passes through the arteries. The information is obtained from an intensifier screened image. The computer is able to subtract the bones and other structures leaving only the opacified vessels on the analogue images obtained (Fig. 26.45).

Using intravenous injection the method can be performed on an outpatient basis and it is now widely used as a screening procedure for such lesions as renal artery stenosis or carotid artery stenosis and thrombosis. DSA is also valuable as a less invasive method for left ventriculography, and for postoperative angiography of all kinds. Thus it has been used to check the patency of grafts, in the follow up of angioplasty, and in the follow up of aneurysms treated operatively. The technique is also being increasingly applied to direct arteriography where its main function is to reduce the dose and volume of contrast medium used.

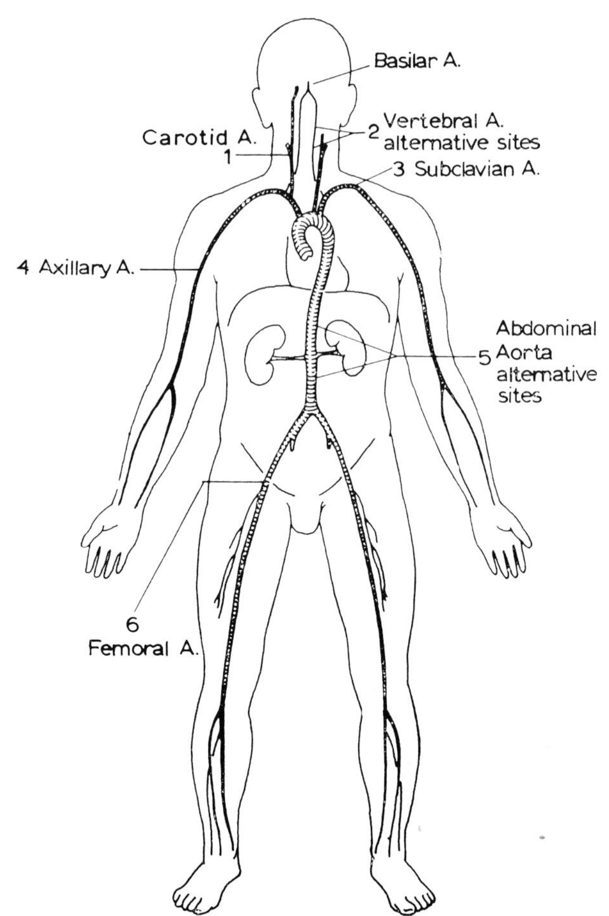

Fig. 26.1 Sites of arterial puncture. 1. Carotid artery. 2. Vertebral artery showing alternative sites. 3. Subclavian artery. 4. Axillary artery. 5. Abdominal aorta showing alternative sites. 6. Common femoral artery. Sites of percutaneous catheterization. 6. Common femoral artery. 4. Axillary artery. 1. Carotid artery (rarely used).

DIRECT ARTERIOGRAPHY

There are two basic techniques in widespread use for direct arteriography:

1. Percutaneous needle puncture.
2. Percutaneous arterial catheterization.

The sites of arterial puncture are illustrated in Figure 26.1.

PERCUTANEOUS NEEDLE PUNCTURE

The method has been applied to most areas of the body, and the investigations practised for the different areas include, or have included:

1. Head and neck:
   a. Common carotid arteriography
   b. Vertebral arteriography.
2. The upper limb:
   a. Subclavian arteriography
   b. Axillary arteriography
   c. Brachial arteriography.
3. The lower limb:
   Femoral arteriography.
4. The abdomen:
   Lumbar aortography.

Needle puncture of the thoracic aorta has been practised in the past, but it was soon discarded as dangerous and replaced by percutaneous catheter techniques. Puncture of the subclavian or axillary artery was generally preferred to brachial artery puncture but is now rarely used, having also been replaced by transfemoral catheter techniques. Cerebral angiography also, which was widely practised by direct needle puncture techniques for many years, is now mainly performed by transfemoral catheter techniques.

Arteriogram needles are usually of 18 British standard wire gauge (s.w.g.) (external diameter 1.2 mm) for routine work involving the carotid, vertebral, femoral, subclavian, and axillary arteries, although occasionally, and with children, the smaller 19 British s.w.g. (external diameter 1.0 mm) needle is used. For lumbar aortography a larger needle of 16 British s.w.g. (external diameter 1.6 mm) is used. All needles are about 12 cm long, with the exception of the aortogram needle, which is about 20 cm in length.

It is important that the syringes should not be directly attached to the needle but joined to it by flexible plastic tubing. Such connecting systems are usually 20–30 cm in length. Plastic disposable syringes are usually used for hand injections and vary in capacity from 10 to 30 ml.

Direct needle puncture is now used mainly for lumbar aortography and femoral arteriography. Its use in the other areas mentioned above is now merely as a back up alternative technique when catheter methods fail or are impractical for technical reasons.

PERCUTANEOUS ARTERIAL CATHETERIZATION

Simple catheterization. Percutaneous arterial catheterization is based upon the original work of Seldinger (1953) in Stockholm. The use of a Seldinger-type needle and guide wire permits the introduction of catheters percutaneously into arteries. The original Seldinger needle consists of a cannula with a central needle and stillette. Immediately after its introduction we modified this to a simpler needle of the same calibre as the cannula and with a shield mount (Seldinger-Sutton needle). The basic technique is illustrated in Figure 26.2. The most useful sites for the insertion of catheters into the arterial tree are:

1. The femoral artery in the groin.
2. The axillary artery in the axilla.

Percutaneous catheters have also been inserted into the arterial system from the brachial artery just above the elbow, and from the common carotid artery in the neck. In practice the femoral or axillary arteries permit investigation of most areas. Thus a catheter passed from the femoral artery can be sited:

1. In the ipsilateral iliac artery.
2. High or low in the abdominal aorta.
3. High or low in the thoracic aorta.

Under image intensifier control a transfemoral catheter can also be passed up into the left subclavian artery in younger patients and on into the left vertebral artery if required. It can also be passed around the aortic arch into the ascending aorta. A transaxillary catheter can be passed into a subclavian artery and on the right side into the innominate artery, or into the aortic arch. It can sometimes be passed straight into a vertebral artery, particularly on the right side.

Selective arterial catheterization is a refinement of the technique just described. Radiopaque catheters are preshaped for catheterization of individual branches of the aorta or great vessels. The method has been very widely used for renal angiography. It has also been extensively used for investigation of the coeliac axis, superior mesenteric and inferior mesenteric arteries. Other vessels which are frequently catheterized are the major branches of the aortic arch (innominate, left common carotid and left subclavian arteries). Selective catheterization of the right subclavian and right common carotid arteries is also possible, as is catheterization of the internal carotid, external carotid and vertebral arteries. Preshaped torque control catheters (Judkins or 'head hunter' catheters) have been widely used for this purpose, as have the similar Cook catheters. The Simmonds sidewinder catheter is also a useful catheter for selective work involving the splanchnic vessels. For selective carotid and vertebral angiography the small Mani-type catheters are now widely used. Cerebral angiography is discussed in detail in Chapter 59.

Many of the newer catheters are of the small French 5 gauge and are safer and less traumatic than the older 7 or 8 French gauge catheters.

Percutaneous selective coronary arteriography using Judkins catheters has now largely replaced the alternative cut down technique of Mason Somes. Among smaller vessels which can be selectively catheterized are the internal mammary and thyroid axis arteries. Spinal angiography is also feasible by injection of the costocervical and intercostal arteries as well as the vertebral and lumbar arteries. Even tiny arteries like the bronchial or the adrenal arteries can be selectively injected.

Superselective arterial catheterization is the term used for catheterization of branches of the coeliac axis such as the splenic, hepatic or gastroduodenal artery. This is achieved by advancing the catheter from the coeliac axis into its main branches. Superselective catheterization can also be carried out in branches of any of the major vessels including the external carotid artery and is being increasingly practised for embolization.

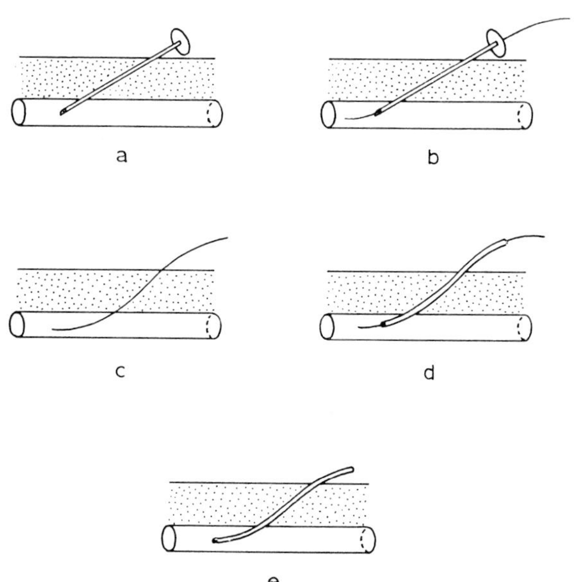

Fig. 26.2 Diagram to illustrate technique of percutaneous catheter insertion using the Seldinger-Sutton needle. (a) Needle inserted into artery. (b) Guide passed through needle into artery. (c) Needle withdrawn leaving guide in artery. (d) Catheter passed over guide into artery. (e) Guide withdrawn leaving catheter in artery.

Arterial cannulation is similar to arterial catheterization, but the Seldinger cannula is advanced along the guide-wire so that its distal 2 or 3 cm lie along the lumen of the artery. Injections are then made directly through the cannula. The method has been mainly used for cerebral angiography (Ch. 59) but can also be applied to other vessels. For this technique Sheldon replaced the central Seldinger needle by a pointed trocar with the aid of which the arterial wall is first penetrated by the cannula. He also uses a very short guide-wire preset to a desired length by a movable restraining chuck at its hind end. The cannula is advanced along the arterial lumen, and once inserted it has the advantage that it is unlikely to become displaced as needles occasionally are. There is also less possibility of periarterial injection or subintimal injection.

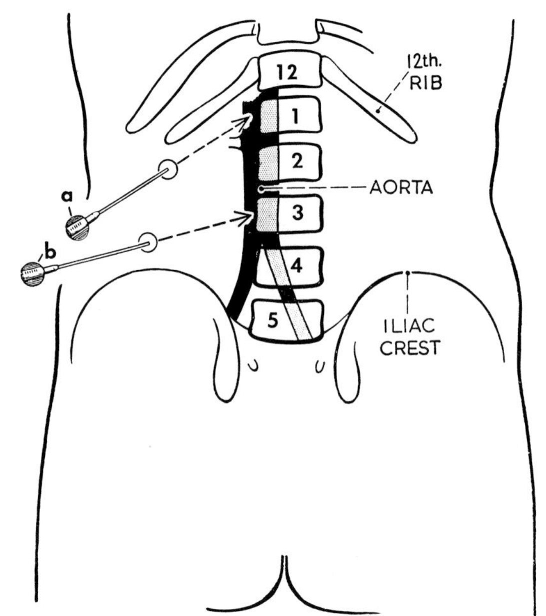

Fig. 26.3 Lumbar aortography: site of puncture. (a) High puncture. (b) Low puncture.

TECHNIQUE OF ARTERIAL PUNCTURE

The technique used for arterial needle puncture or catheterization is similar for most of the arteries injected.

The *common femoral artery* is usually punctured in the groin. The *axillary artery* is punctured in the axilla, with the patient's arm abducted. The *common carotid artery* is generally punctured below the carotid bifurcation.

In all the above cases the artery is fixed by the index and middle fingers of the palpating hand. Some workers prefer to fix the vessel by holding the fingers across the artery and others by placing the fingers along the course of the vessel. This is largely a matter of personal preference and experience. Several of the arteries listed above are not accessible to palpation and different methods must therefore be used to localize and puncture them.

The *abdominal aorta* is approached from the left lumbar region with the patient lying prone. It is customary to take a preliminary X-ray film with markers placed over the lumbar spines so as to localize the levels of the vertebrae. Depending on the purpose of the injection, the operator punctures at different levels (Fig. 26.3). For renal angiography the puncture is made at above L.1. or opposite the L.1/2 disc space, i.e. about or just above the origin of the renal arteries. A similar point or one a little higher (D.12–L.1) is chosen when aortography is being performed to demonstrate an abdominal aneurysm or an aortic thrombosis. In cases of low aortic or iliac disease the puncture is usually made below the renal arteries (at about the upper border of L.3).

Once the point of puncture has been chosen, the needle is inserted from the flank at about a hand's breadth from the midline. For the higher puncture the needle is inserted obliquely upwards at an angle of about 45° but this angle is reduced for the lower punctures. In the latter case the skin puncture may also be made an inch or so farther out than with the higher punctures.

The *subclavian artery* may be punctured as it passes over the first rib. A skin puncture is made just behind the centre of the clavicle and the needle passed obliquely downwards to strike the anterior end of the first rib. By using this as a guide the needle may be cautiously brought backwards along the rib and the subclavian artery entered. In this way it should be possible to avoid the brachial plexus or the apex of the lung. Alternatively the subclavian artery may be approached from below the clavicle. However direct subclavian puncture is now rarely required, since most workers prefer to inject the subclavian artery by transfemoral catheterization.

The *vertebral artery* can be punctured in the neck and several different approaches have been used (Ch. 59). It is now general practice to inject the vertebral artery by percutaneous catheterization, direct puncture being reserved for occasional cases where catheterization fails.

With all the above arteries the procedure, once the artery has been punctured, is similar. Successful puncture is marked by a rapid pulsation of arterial blood through the needle into the plastic tubing. The force with which this takes place will vary according to the size of the artery, but even with such small arteries as the vertebral the blood is under a definite arterial pressure which will readily and spontaneously press backwards the piston of the attached syringe.

As soon as this backflow of arterial blood is perceived, an assistant injects saline through the plastic system and needle into the artery. He continues to do this intermittently during the whole course of the investigation except for the actual contrast injections. The aim is to ensure that the needle remains correctly positioned in the artery and that it is kept clear of blood which may clot in the needle or plastic tubing. Injection of contrast medium, in doses as described below, can then be made at the appropriate moment and after preparing the radiological apparatus for serial X-rays.

TECHNIQUE OF PERCUTANEOUS CATHETERIZATION

The modified Seldinger's method as used by the writer is as follows, and can be divided into three stages (Fig. 26.2).

1. The artery (usually the femoral, less commonly the axillary) is punctured by a thin-walled Sutton needle. This has plastic tubing and a syringe attached, exactly as in the technique for simple needle arterial puncture. Once the needle is in the arterial lumen, saline is injected until all is ready for stage 2.
2. The plastic tubing and syringe are detached from the needle, which is held steady with its tip in the arterial lumen. There will be an immediate spurting of blood from the exposed end of the needle. The guide wire which has a flexible tip in front is at once inserted through the needle and passed for a few centimetres along the artery till the stiff part is in the lumen. Holding the guide-wire firmly in this position the needle is then drawn backwards along it and off the guide-wire. Firm manual pressure is meanwhile applied through gauze swabs around the site of puncture in order to prevent haematoma formation. At this stage the guide-wire has been introduced percutaneously into the artery and all is ready for the final stage.
3. The catheter, which has been specially prepared and has a syringe attachment fixed at its hind end, is now passed along the guide-wire into the arterial lumen. The catheter is shorter in length than the guide-wire and as its front end reaches the tip of the guide-wire the latter protrudes backwards from the back end of the catheter. When the catheter is definitely in the arterial lumen the guide-wire can easily be extracted. Once the guide-wire is extracted there is a rush of arterial blood backwards through the catheter. A saline-loaded syringe, or a saline drip system, is immediately attached to the catheter and the latter is cleared of blood. Flow can be established or turned off by means of a tap at the catheter syringe attachment. The catheter can now be passed along the artery so that its tip lies at any desired level. In tortuous or atheromatous vessels it may be necessary to use special guides with flexible 'J' tips in order to advance the catheter through a difficult area and reach the desired level. Saline perfusion of the catheter is maintained either by slow hand injection, or by an automatic drip system. Heparinized saline is routinely used in order to counteract the tendency to clot formation around the catheter tip.

TECHNIQUE OF SELECTIVE ARTERIAL CATHETERIZATION

The catheter is introduced into the aorta by the Seldinger percutaneous technique just described. The catheters used are radiopaque and can be observed on the fluorescent screen. Their consistency is such that they can be preshaped to any desired form, for introduction into specific branches of the aorta. They are preshaped by dipping in sterile hot water and then setting them in sterile cold water after moulding. Alternatively, commercially made preshaped catheters can be used. Once the catheter is in the aortic lumen the radiologist observes its tip by screening with an image intensifier. By manipulating the free end, the tip is guided into the orifice of the artery chosen for injection. The use of an image intensifier is essential for this part of the procedure. Final manipulation of the catheter tip may also require special 'J' tip guide wires. These are made with varying curves of 3, 7 or 15 mm in diameter. Guide-wires with special long floppy tips may also help in certain circumstances.

This technique enables excellent angiograms to be obtained free of any overlying vascular shadows, and utilizing only small quantities of low concentration contrast medium. Thus an excellent renal arteriogram can be obtained with only 8 ml of low concentration contrast.

RADIOGRAPHIC APPARATUS

Arteriography usually requires rapid serial films of the area being investigated. In some areas, e.g. the lower limb, four serial films taken within about 5 to 8 seconds are usually adequate. In other areas, e.g. the aortic arch, films taken at three or four per second for 3 or 4 seconds may be necessary. In certain situations and with such lesions as arteriovenous fistula multiple rapid serial films may also be necessary.

Many types of serial changer are on the market for peripheral and cerebral studies. For studies requiring rapid serial work either the Schonander cut film changer or the Elema roll-film rapid serial unit are usually used. The former allows speeds of up to six films per second, the latter even faster speeds (up to 12 films per second). The smaller Puck changer permits speeds of three films per second which is adequate for most cases. Fine focus, high power tubes are vital in angiography to permit magnification techniques. Subtraction techniques are also widely used.

Arteriography is now being widely practised using DSA equipment. This has the advantage of reducing both the volume and the concentration of contrast medium used. Resolution is less than can be obtained with the best conventional techniques but is adequate in most cases.

Injection apparatus

Hand injection is perfectly satisfactory for many forms of

arteriography, but pressure injection with special apparatus is essential for thoracic aortography, for catheter flush abdominal aortography and angiocardiography. It is also necessary for DSA using intravenous injections. Sophisticated and versatile apparatus commercially available for this purpose include the Swedish Cisal and the American Cordis and Medrad injectors.

ANAESTHESIA

Most angiographic procedures can be carried out under local anaesthesia, but with the more complex investigations basal sedation may be necessary. The drugs used vary in different centres. Some drugs, such as Pethidine, are more liable than others to produce a hypotensive reaction in the patient and should therefore be used with caution, particularly if arterial stenosis is suspected.

General anaesthesia is usually necessary with children and may be required with difficult or nervous patients. General anaesthesia undoubtedly adds to the hazards of the procedure, since the patient is unable to react to misplaced injections or test doses. Further, subintimal stripping or damage to the arterial wall may not be recognized until after the films are inspected or the patient comes round from the anaesthetic. With a conscious patient symptoms and untoward reactions are at once apparent, and the procedure can be stopped immediately.

CONTRAST MEDIA

As noted above the first contrast media used for in vivo angiography were Lipiodol and strontium bromide in 1923 followed by sodium iodide in 1924. Thorotrast (a 25% solution of thorium dioxide) was widely used in the 1930s for angiography after Moniz employed it successfully for cerebral angiography in 1932. This substance, though an excellent contrast medium, is unfortunately radioactive. It was taken up by the reticuloendothelial system and stored in the body for an indefinite period. Much of the Thorotrast was taken up by the spleen and plain X-ray of the abdomen showed a characteristic picture. An X-ray of the abdomen taken many years after the injection still showed this appearance, which can be regarded as diagnostic. It consisted of multiple fine stippled opacities throughout the whole spleen, resembling miliary calcification (Fig. 26.4).

In experimental animals malignant changes have supervened following Thorotrast injections and isolated cases have also been reported in humans. As a result the substance is no longer used.

The major breakthrough in contrast media came with the development of organic iodide preparations. Swick (1929) demonstrated that Uroselectan (Iopax), which contained 1 atom of iodine per molecule, was a reliable agent for intravenous urography. Soon after Abrodil

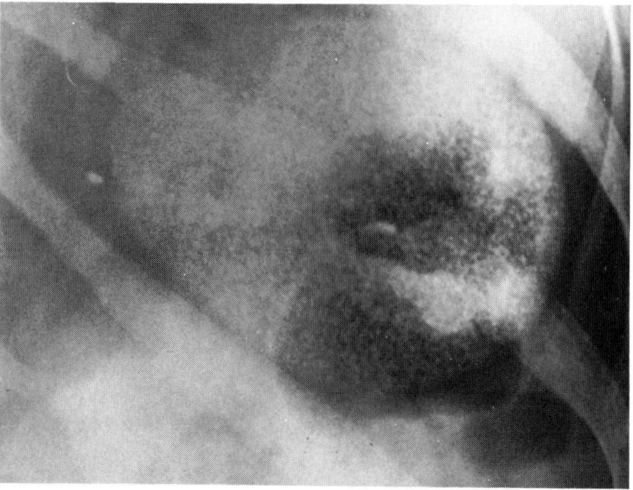

Fig. 26.4 Thorotrast spleen.

(Skiodan) and later Per Abrodil (Diodrast; Diodone) were synthesized and were employed for angiography. They were widely used in the late 1930s and through the 1940s. In the mid-1950s they were replaced by Renografin (Urografin) and Hypaque which were less toxic but more viscous, and later by Conray and Triosil. These four contrast media, all of which are tri-iodinated, have been widely used for angiography over the last 20 years. Their chemical formulae and other characteristics are listed in Table 26.1.

Although generally satisfactory, these contrast media do not represent the ideal water-soluble contrast medium. The ideal contrast medium should be completely non-toxic and completely painless to the patient. It should also be of low viscosity and easy to inject. Further steps along the road to such an ideal contrast agent have been made in recent years with the introduction of so-called 'non-ionic' contrast media. This owes much to the work of the Swedish radiologist Almen who developed the non-ionic metrizamide (Amipaque). This revolutionized the practice of myelography by replacing Myodil. The substance was not widely used for angiography owing to its high cost and problems of preparation before use. However, the new generation of low osmolality products (Table 26.2) do not suffer from these defects, and are now being generally used for angiography since they are available in sterile solution in ampoules and are much cheaper. They include iopamidol and iohexol which are non-ionic monomeric agents and ioxaglate which is a monomeric salt of a monoacid dimer. All these new media are relatively painless and produce little patient discomfort, reducing the need for general anaesthesia. They also produce fewer toxic side effects, and are now the contrast media of choice for most angiography procedures.

The reduced discomfort and toxicity are related to their low osmolality which is much closer to that of plasma than were the older contrast media. At an iodine concentration

Table 26.1 Intravascular contrast media

Product	Formula	I_2 Content g/ml	Viscosity at 37°C
Hypaque 45	(a) Sodium Diatrizoate 45% w/v	0.27	2.1
Hypaque 65	(b) Sodium diatrizoate 25% w/v and N-methylglucamine salt of diatrizoic acid 50% w/v		8.4
Hypaque 85	As above but (a) 28.33% w/v (b) 56.67% w/v	0.44	12.2
Urografin 290	Mixture of the sodium and the methylglucamine salts of diatrizoic acid in the proportion 10 to 66	0.44	8.4
Urografin 370	Mixture of the sodium and the methylglucamine salts of diatrizoic acid in the proportion 10 to 66	0.37	8.5
Urografin 310 (Angiografin)	Meglumine amidotrizoate 65%	0.306	5.1
Conray 280	Iothalamate 60% w/v	0.28	4.0
Conray 325	Sodium Iothalamate 54% w/v	0.325	2.7
Conray 420	Sodium Iothalamate 70% w/v	0.42	5.4
Cardio-Conray	Meglumine Iothalamate 52%. Na Iothalomate 26% w/v	0.40	8.6
Triosil 280	Meglumine Metrizoate 59% w/v (with Ca)	0.28	4.0
Triosil 370	Meglumine Metriozoate (with Na and Ca)	0.37	8.5
Triosil 350	Sodium Metrizoate 52% w/v (with Meglumine, Ca, or Mag.)	0.35	3.4
Triosil 440	Sodium Metriozoate 66% w/v (with Meglumine, Ca or Mag.)	0.44	6.6

Table 26.2 Low osmolality contrast media

Product	General formula	Ratio I atoms to particles in solution	I content mg/ml	Viscosity at 37 °C
Iopamidol [Niopam] Non-ionic	R_3; I, I; R_1, R_2; I	3:1	200 300 370	2.0 4.7 8.6
Iohexol [Omnipaque] Non-ionic	Similar to above but with different radicles R_1, R_2 or R_3	3:1	240 280 300 350	3.3 4.8 6.1 10.6
Ioxaglate [Hexabrix] Ionic	R_3; COO^- {Na^+ or $Meglumine^+$}; I, I, I, I; R_1, R_2; I, I	6:2 [= 3:1]	320	7.5

of 280 mg per ml all these products have less than one-third the osmolality of Conray. They measure only 470–490 mmol/kg H_2O compared with 1500 for Conray, and 300 for plasma.

Osmolality is proportional to the ratio — iodine atoms: number of particles in solution. The older conventional hyperosmolar contrast media have an iodine atom: particle ratio of 3:2. The new non-ionic contrast media (iohexol and iopamidol) have a ratio of 3:1 and do not ionize in solution. Ioxaglate as a mono-acid dimer does ionize in solution but also has a similar high iodine atom: particle ratio of 6 : 2 (= 3 : 1). This is why all three new products have similar low osmolality.

DOSAGE

The last generation of organic iodide contrast media (Table 26.1) were solutions of salts of iodinated organic acids. The recommended maximum doses of Conray or other proprietary preparations (Urografin, Trosil, Hypaque) depended on the individual vessel being injected and its size and blood flow as well as on the target organ.

Peripheral and smaller arteries

The smaller the vessel and the lower its flow rate the

Table 26.3 Recommended doses of Conray 280 or equivalent (smaller arteries)

Femoral artery	20 ml
Subclavian (or axillary) artery	20 ml
Carotid artery	10 ml
Vertebral artery	8 ml
Renal artery	10 ml
Inferior mesenteric artery	15 ml
Intercostal artery	3 ml
Bronchial artery	5 ml

smaller is the volume and concentration of contrast and the slower the speed of injection. The recommended doses are listed in Table 26.3. In most vessels the same injection can be safely repeated after a short interval.

For cerebral angiography we regarded Urografin 310 as the preferable contrast medium and for coronary angiography Triosil 370, since there is experimental evidence that these media were least toxic in these sites. The coronary arteriography injection doses varied from 4 to 8 ml per injection depending on the state of the patient and individual vessel flow.

The new low osmolality products iopamidol (Niopam), iohexol (Omnipaque) and ioxaglate (Hexabrix) have undergone widespread clinical trials in the last few years and, as noted above, offer significant advantages over the older contrast media.

The only apparent drawback to their use is cost, which is still considerably greater than that of the older media. Hopefully, this will be overcome with increased usage. The doses used for peripheral and smaller vessels are identical to those used for the older media.

Larger vessels

1. The *abdominal aorta* (either by lumbar aortography or by catheter aortography). 30 ml of 65% Hypaque or Conray 420 (or equivalent of other proprietary preparations) is safe, delivered in 1.5 or 2 seconds for a high injection (above the renal arteries), provided both kidneys are functioning normally. If there is severe renal impairment or only one functioning kidney, caution should be observed and the maximum dose should not exceed 20 ml of Hypaque 65.

Similar precautions should be observed if an aortic thrombosis is present and most of the injected contrast medium will enter the renal arteries. For a low aortic injection (used either for pelvic angiography or for serial angiography of the lower limbs) 25 ml of 65% Hypaque or equivalent preparation is usually adequate delivered in 1.5 seconds.

The normal *coeliac axis* and *superior mesenteric* arteries both have high flow rates and can tolerate injections of 30 ml of 65% Hypaque (or equivalents) at one injection. Some workers recommend doses as high as 50 ml for the demonstration of the venous side of the visceral circulation. Speed of injection is about 8 ml per second.

2. *Arch aortography*. For injections into the aortic arch the highest concentrations of contrast media are used. The usual dose is about 40 ml of contrast (Hypaque 65 or 85, Triosil 370 or 440, or Conray 420) delivered at 20 ml per second.

In the last two or three years the doses recommended above have also been used with the new low osmolality contrast media, using them in their higher available concentrations which are iopamidol 370, iohexol 350 and Hexabrix 320. These new products appear to offer significant advantages in patient tolerance and lower toxicity and are now the contrast media of choice.

The above recommended doses are within normal tolerance limits. They have been used for some 20 000 angiograms performed in the author's departments and we have seen no complications attributable to the toxicity of the contrast medium.

PHARMACOANGIOGRAPHY

Pharmacoangiography aims to improve the diagnostic value of angiograms by modifying blood flow to target organs with vasoactive drugs.

Vasodilators are used to reverse vasospasm, to increase the size of arterioles and collaterals and to improve the visualization of the venous return. They will also enhance the outline of non-vascular lesions such as cysts. They have been most frequently used in arterioportography for better visualization of the portal circulation following splenic or coeliac arteriography. They have also been used to improve the filling of distal vessels in arteriography of the limbs.

The vasodilators used include Priscoline (Tolazoline) for the splanchnic, femoral and brachial arteries, prostaglandin E_1 in the femoral artery and bradykinin in the renal and superior mesenteric arteries.

In healthy patients Priscoline is normally given as a 25 mg bolus into the splanchnic vessels and as a 12 mg bolus into limb vessels. Priscoline can produce hypotension and cardiac arrythmias and must be used with caution in cardiac patients.

Vasoconstrictors help to differentiate normal from tumour vessels since only the former will react to them. The most widely used is Epinephrine (adrenaline) which is administered for both renal and splanchnic arteriography. Vasopressin and Angiotensin have also been used as vasoconstrictors. Epinephrine is administered as a 3–6 μg bolus into the renal artery, and as a 5–8 μg bolus into splanchnic vessels.

Epinephrine increases blood pressure and peripheral resistance and must therefore be used with caution in patients with cardiac disease, when it may be contraindicated. It is the responsibility of the radiologist to ensure that any of the above drugs are used in safe doses and that the patient's cardiac status does not contraindicate their use.

In cerebral angiography a similar effect can be obtained by *hyperventilation*. Normal cerebral vessels respond readily to hyperoxaemia and hypocapnoea by constricting, while tumour vessels show no response. Hyperventilation is usually performed by the anaesthetist when cerebral arteriograms are being done under general anaesthesia.

COMPLICATIONS

Many complications have been described as a result of

arteriography, particularly in its early days. However, many of the investigations previously regarded as potentially dangerous are now undertaken as routine procedures and their morbidity has become negligible. On the other hand, new dangers have arisen with the investigation of new areas and the introduction of newer and more complex techniques for opacifying internal vessels, and with the development of interventional angiography. The complications are summarized in Table 26.4.

Table 26.4 Complications of arteriography

General
1. Acute anaphylaxis
2. Minor allergic reactions (urticaria, coughing, sneezing)
3. Severe hypotension (leading to thrombosis of stenosed arteries)
4. Septicaemia
5. Air embolus
6. Catheter clot embolus
7. Cotton fibre emboli
8. Vagal inhibition

Local
1. Haemorrhage at the puncture site — haematoma
2. Pseudoaneurysm formation at the puncture site
3. AV fistula formation at the puncture site
4. Perivascular contrast injection
5. Local thrombosis due to:
   a. subintimal injection and local dissection
   b. severe trauma to arterial wall with local clot
   c. 'stripping' of catheter tip clots
6. Local infection
7. Damage to nerves or nerve roots
8. Damage to organs, usually from excess of contrast medium
   a. brain
   b. spinal cord
   c. kidneys
   d. bowel
   e. testis
   f. pancreas
   g. cisterna chyli (from lumbar aortogram needle, leading to chylothorax)
   h. lung or pleura (haemothorax)
   i. heart
   j. skin
9. Fracture and loss of guide-wire tips.
10. Knot formation in catheters
11. Embolization accidents
12. Angioplasty accidents

This formidable list of complications emphasizes that arteriography is best undertaken at centres where large numbers are performed and the investigations are best conducted by radiologists with considerable training and experience in this field. In this way accidents and complications will be kept down to a minimum.

A full discussion of the complications of arteriography will be found in specialist monographs, but attention is directed below to a few of the more important complications.

Damage to arterial walls. This usually results from a traumatic needle or catheter puncture. The intima may be stripped from the media, particularly if saline or contrast is injected into the arterial wall (Figs 26.5, 26.7). In small vessels this can result in actual occlusion and thrombosis. Many of the cases of hemiplegia reported as complications of carotid angiography were undoubtedly due to this cause as were many reported occlusions of the femoral artery. The use of short bevelled needles together with skill and experience are the major means of preventing these accidents.

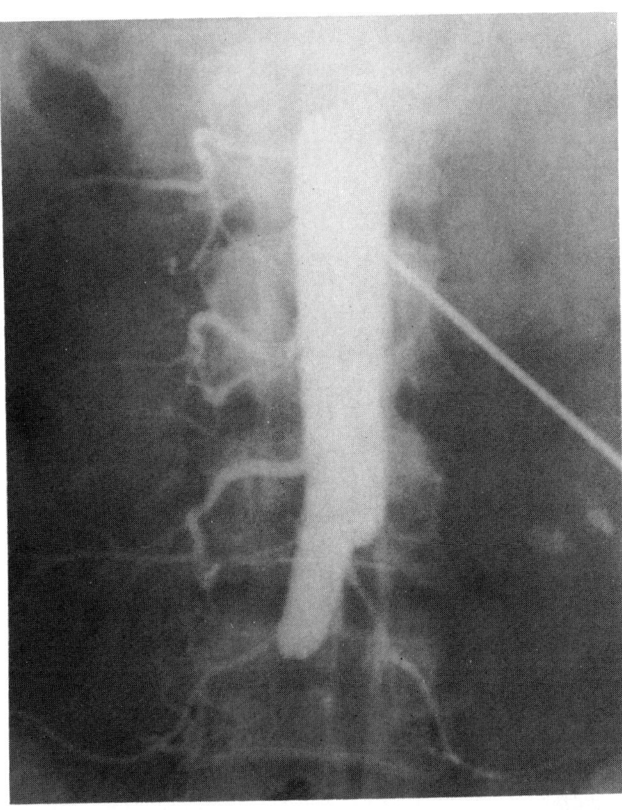

Fig. 26.5 Subintimal contrast injection at lumbar aortography. Most of the contrast lies in the wall of the aorta and right common iliac artery. A small amount is intraluminal and outlines lumbar arteries. Contrast in the aortic wall persists on serial films.

There is little doubt that general anaesthesia adds to this risk, since extravasation or subintimal injection may not be suspected until the X-ray films are developed and inspected. If the patient is being examined under local anaesthesia the patient's reaction and subjective symptoms may provide immediate warning of such mishaps, and prevent repetition of misplaced injections. *Perivascular injection* (Fig. 26.6) is relatively harmless, though it may prove quite painful to the patient being examined under local anaesthesia.

Severe hypotensive reactions. Such reactions may occur with any arteriographic examination, but particularly with the more complex catheter investigations and with lumbar aortography. They should be carefully watched for, since patients with severe arterial disease may have lesions in many vessels. If there is a severe stenosis, the hypotension may lead to thrombosis of the diseased artery.

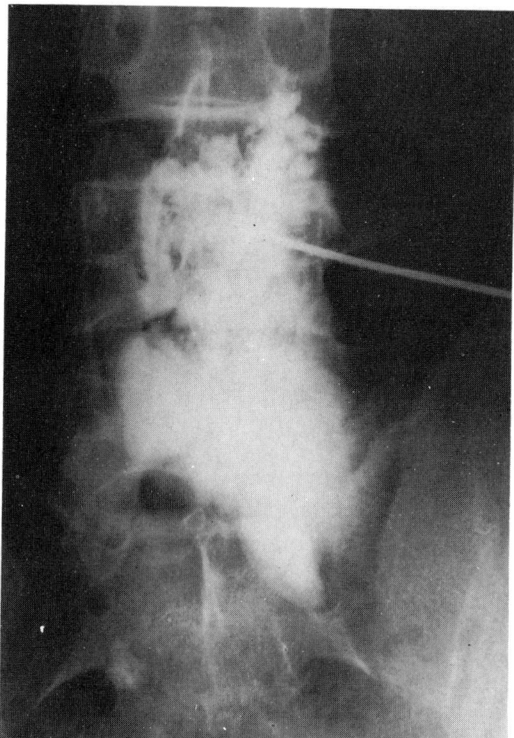

Fig. 26.6 Perivascular contrast injection at lumbar aortography.

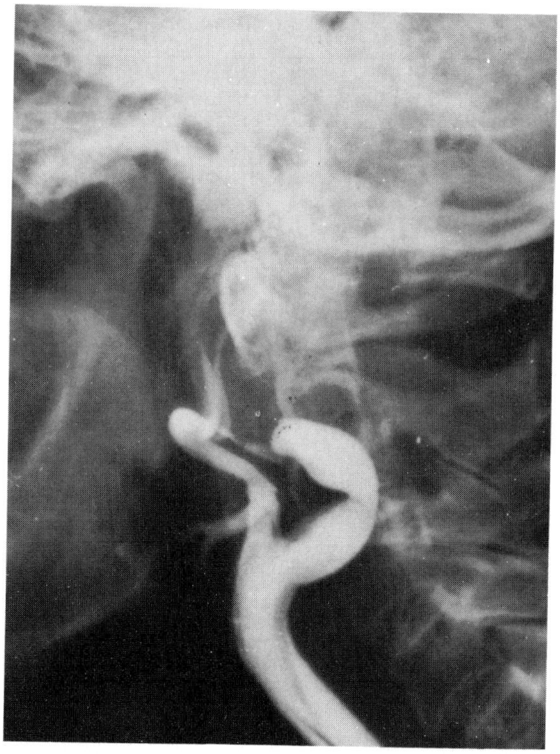

Fig. 26.7 Subintimal contrast injection at needle common carotid arteriogram. Contrast persists in the arterial wall on serial films. Note linear translucencies caused by displaced intima.

Coronary infarction, or hemiplegia from thrombosis of a diseased internal carotid, may result.

Hypotension may also occur several hours after the arteriogram, and the patient must be kept under observation in the ward for the postoperative period. We consider it unwise to perform major vascular investigations on outpatients, and always keep the patient in hospital overnight following such a procedure.

Thrombosis of arteries. As noted above, this can result from severe trauma to the arterial wall at the arterial puncture. It may also result from subintimal injection of the contrast medium with the formation of a local dissecting aneurysm (Fig. 26.7). Another possible mechanism for arterial thrombosis is the formation of clot at the end of a catheter. This is then stripped from the catheter tip as the catheter is extracted from the artery and forms a focus for local thrombosis.

Whichever of the three mechanisms described above is responsible there is little doubt that thrombosis of arteries at the site of arterial puncture bears a direct relationship to the skill and experience of the operator and to the adequacy of the patient's cardiovascular system. Patients with severe atheromatous disease and poor cardiac output are at greater risk.

In this sort of patient the angiogram must only be performed either by or under the careful supervision of an experienced angiographer.

It should be noted that local arterial thrombosis can occur as readily with operative cut-down techniques as with the percutaneous Seldinger technique. Thus brachial thrombosis was a not infrequent complication of the operative use of the brachial artery by cardiologists for left ventriculography or for the Mason Somes technique of selective coronary arteriography.

Systemic heparinization is recommended to counter thrombosis and catheter clot formation. As soon as the catheter is in the aorta 3000 units of heparin are injected. The procedure is useful in prolonged catheterizations and rarely causes a bleeding problem. If it does this can be countered by administering 10 mg protamine sulphate per 1000 units of heparin used.

Allergy. The minor allergic reactions rarely give rise to any serious concern but any radiologist performing angiography should be prepared for the prompt treatment of a major hypersensitivity reaction. This will mean the administration of a corticoid, e.g. Dexamethasone 10–20 mg intravenously, and, if necessary, artificial respiration with positive pressure and oxygen. For oedema of the glottis 0–5 mg of adrenalin subcutaneously or intramuscularly is recommended, together with the slow intravenous injection of an antihistamine. Arrangements should also be ready beforehand for the emergency treatment of such catastrophies as cardiac arrest, ventricular fibrillation or collapse with circulatory insufficiency.

Air embolus has undoubtedly been an unrecognized cause of fatalities in the past. Air can easily enter a large steel or other opaque syringe without being recognized and can easily be injected, particularly if the syringe is positioned with its nozzle horizontal or upward. Great care must be taken in the loading of syringes with contrast medium and the injection should be made with the syringe in the nozzle-down position.

Catheter clot embolus. Clot embolus to the brain has been recorded in catheter techniques where the catheter tip lies in or proximal to the great vessels. These include left ventriculography, coronary arteriography and 'head hunter' catheterization of the cerebral and subclavian arteries. Speedy and skilful catheterization and the use of small catheters are important factors in preventing this complication. Systemic heparinization is also a useful prophylactic measure.

Vagal inhibition may occur after a major contrast injection and has been encountered at intravenous urography and intravenous cholangiography. It is characterized by collapse of the patient with *bradycardia*. This helps to distinguish it from circulatory collapse in acute allergy, which is usually associated with tachycardia. The distinction is of vital importance since the latter is often treated with adrenalin, which is contraindicated in vagal inhibition where atropine is the drug of choice and may be life-saving.

Haematoma should be relatively uncommon if small needles are routinely used and catheter tips are tapered. They are more likely to occur in hypertensive patients. After arterial puncture firm pressure at the operative site is required until all oozing has stopped. The puncture site should also be inspected some hours after the angiogram and on the following morning. The patient should also be told to report back if further swelling or oozing occurs. False aneurysms or pulsating haematomas can occur in such circumstances and will require surgical treatment. It is important to ensure that patients have been taken off any anticoagulant drugs in advance so that the prothrombin time falls to normal before percutaneous catheterization is performed.

Damage to nerves. The axillary artery is closely related to branches of the brachial plexus and many cases of damage to the brachial plexus following transaxillary catheterization have been recorded resulting in severe disability. Most have been due to plexus compression by haematomas or false aneurysms, though trauma during arterial puncture may be responsible in some cases. Transaxillary catheterization should only be undertaken by senior and experienced arteriographers and postoperative observation for signs of haematoma or nerve damage should be maintained for at least 24 hours. If symptoms of paresis appear and progress they are usually due to a haematoma or false aneurysm and urgent decompression of the neurovascular sheath is required as the only way to prevent permanent paralysis.

Damage to organs. Angiographic *deaths* have occurred from damage to the brain and from damage to the kidneys and bowel. In most cases the cause has been either arterial thrombosis from the causes mentioned above, or local organ damage from an excess of contrast medium. Knowledge of the correct dosage is therefore mandatory, as is the acquisition of adequate skills in the techniques of arteriography.

Unilateral brain damage has resulted in *hemiplegia*, both transient and permanent. *Cortical blindness*, occasionally permanent but fortunately in most cases transient, has followed vertebral angiography, especially with catheter techniques.

Spinal cord damage is a rare and tragic complication of arteriography where an excessive dose of contrast has entered a main artery of supply to the spinal cord. Thus *paraplegia* has been recorded after abdominal or lumbar aortography, presumably from injection of the artery of Adamkewicz, which supplies the cord from the region of D.8 downwards. This may arise from one of the lower intercostals or from one of the upper lumbar arteries. *Tetraplegia* has resulted from thyroid axis angiography to demonstrate parathyroid adenoma. In such cases contrast has been incidentally injected into the deep cervical artery supplying the cord. Tetraplegia has also resulted from vertebral angiography. It has been suggested that such cases should be treated by immediate replacement of cerebrospinal fluid by isotonic saline, and by systemic steroids, though the value of such procedures is doubted by some.

Coronary arteriography carries the special complications of vagal inhibition, ventricular fibrillation, cardiac asystole or myocardial infarction. All of these are potentially fatal unless immediate treatment is at hand.

Embolization and **angioplasty** also carry special risks which are discussed below.

THERAPEUTIC ANGIOGRAPHY

The use of angiographic techniques for therapy as well as for purely diagnostic purposes has increased in recent years. Therapeutic angiography includes the following techniques:

1. Transluminal angioplasty
2. Embolization
3. Balloon occlusion
4. Intra-arterial drug therapy.

TRANSLUMINAL ANGIOPLASTY

A method for dilating arterial stenoses or recanalizing occluded arterial segments was first introduced by Dotter and Judkins in 1964. A guide wire was passed through the lesion and coaxial catheters were then passed along it to produce dilatation of the narrowed lumen.

A major advance in this field was the introduction of the dilatable double-lumen balloon catheter by Gruntzig in 1976. These dilatable balloon catheters were first used in femoral and iliac lesions, but their use was later extended to several other areas, particularly the renal and coronary arteries. They have also been used in the abdominal aorta and splanchnic arteries and in the great vessels. They are not, however, recommended for the carotid arteries owing to the special dangers of peripheral embolus or occlusion of flow in the internal carotid.

The type of case most suitable for dilatation by a Gruntzig balloon catheter is one with a localized stenosis. However, multiple stenoses and localized occlusions can also be treated by the method. Occlusions longer than 8–10 cm are not regarded as suitable.

The balloons are cylindrical with a smooth outer surface and allow considerable radial force to be exerted on the arterial lesion with only minimal increase in balloon diameter as the inflation pressure is increased (Fig. 26.8).

Originally it was thought that balloon angioplasty compressed and redistributed the atheromatous material along the vessel wall. However, experimental work on animals and cadavers has shown that the increase in size of the arterial lumen is due to splitting of the intima followed by retraction of the plaque on either side over the next few weeks. There is also slight stretching of the media resulting in permanent slight local increase in arterial diameter (Fig. 26.9).

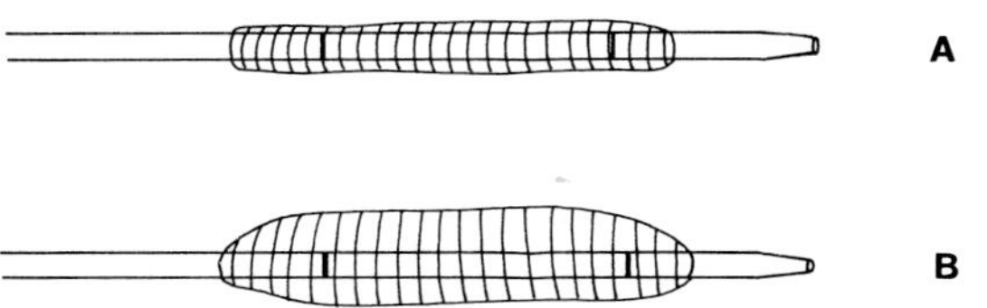

Fig. 26.8 Diagram of Gruntzig type balloon catheter. **A.** with balloon deflated. **B.** After balloon dilatation.

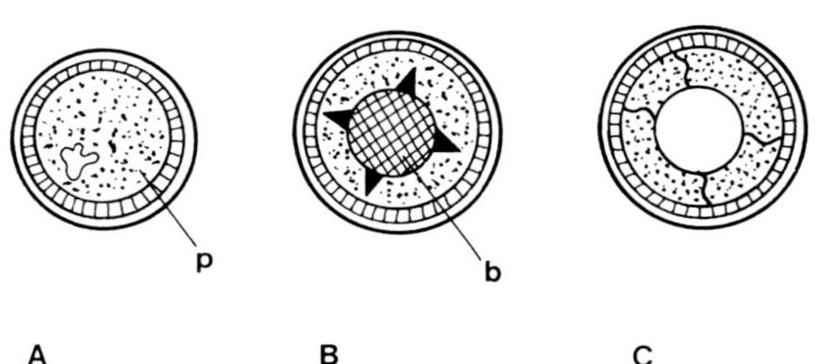

Fig. 26.9 Mechanism of angioplasty. **A.** before angioplasty, — p = atheromatous plaque. **B.** Dilated balloon (b) dilates lumen and artery allowing fissuring of plaque and redistribution around dilated lumen. Volume of plaque is unchanged. **C.** Late result.

Gruntzig balloon catheters have a double lumen, one communicating with the circumferential balloon for inflation and deflation, and one communicating with the catheter end hole. The balloon is inflated with a mixture of equal amounts of contrast and saline to give both low viscosity and radiographic visibility. The latest balloons will withstand pressures of up to 10 or 12 atmospheres, which is the maximum pressure advised. A pressure gauge is helpful to ensure that maximum pressures are not exceeded. Balloon lengths and diameters are carefully chosen to match the arteries and lesions being treated.

Femoral and popliteal angioplasty. A high antegrade femoral puncture is used. There is a tendency for the guide-wire to enter the profunda instead of the superficial femoral artery. This can be countered by abduction and external rotation of the limb and by the use of a 6 mm J guide-wire to select the superficial femoral artery. Gruntzig balloons of 4 or 5 mm diameter are usually used on a size 7F catheter.

Iliac angioplasty (Fig. 26.10). A standard retrograde femoral puncture is used and this is usually possible even with a damped or absent pulse. Balloons of 6, 7 or 8 mm diameter may be required and the latter usually require 9F catheters.

Renal artery angioplasty. A 7F catheter with a 4 or 5 mm balloon is used. Standard catheters may not readily enter the renal artery even over an exchange guide-wire, and coaxial catheters have therefore been used. However, the procedure has been simplified by the introduction in 1983 of 7F Simmons type 'sidewinder' balloon catheters (Figs 26.11, 26.12). These are turned in the aortic arch and brought down to the abdominal aorta where they will readily enter the renal or splanchnic arteries. Stenosis at the anastomosis of a renal artery transplant or even in a segmental branch can also be corrected by percutaneous angioplasty.

Coronary angioplasty. This requires the use of coaxial guiding catheters through which the balloon catheters are introduced. The balloons are 2, 3 and 3.7 mm in diameter. Coronary angioplasty is discussed in Chapter 23.

Aortic angioplasty has been performed on patients with severe aortic stenosis by using two 8 mm balloons side by side.

Intra-arterial pressure recording

This is a most important aspect of the Gruntzig procedure. Pressure should be recorded proximal to the lesion (or in

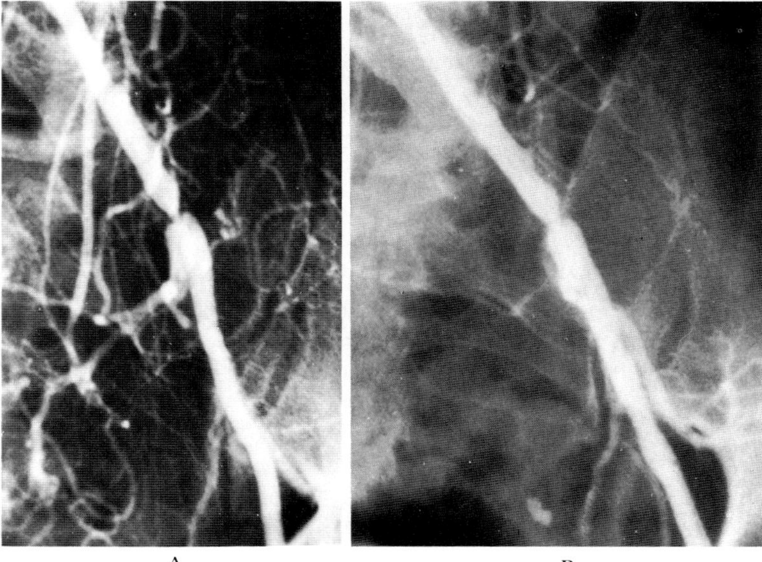

Fig. 26.10 Gruntzig catheter dilatation of arterial stenosis. **A.** Before. **B.** After. Slight narrowing persists but the pressure gradient was abolished.

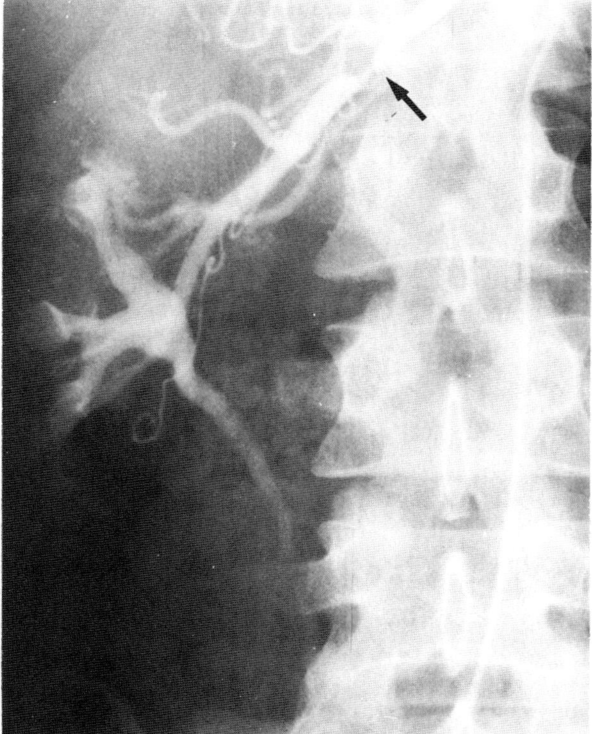

Fig. 26.11 Renal angioplasty. Before dilatation there is a severe localized stenosis about 4 cm from the origin of the right renal artery (arrow).

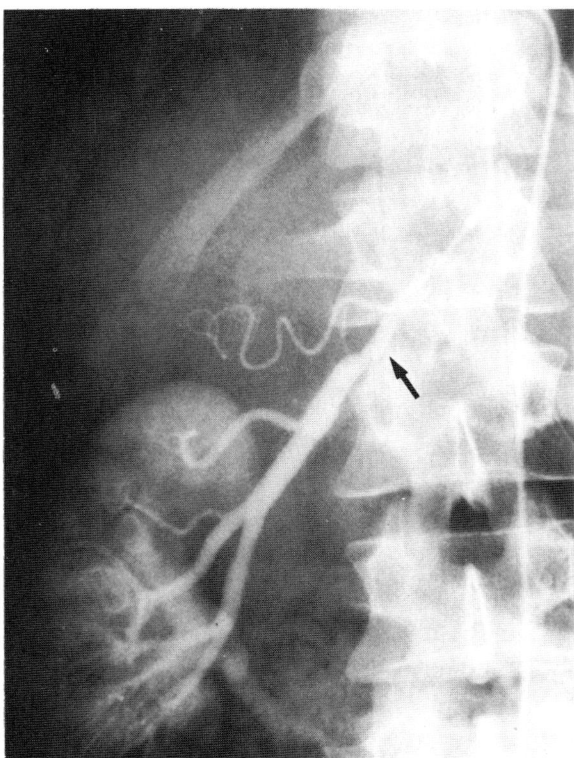

Fig. 26.12 After dilatation only slight narrowing remains. Note the sidewinder balloon catheter withdrawn proximal to the stenosis. The deflated balloon lies between the two metal markers. The pressure gradient was abolished and b.p. fell to normal.

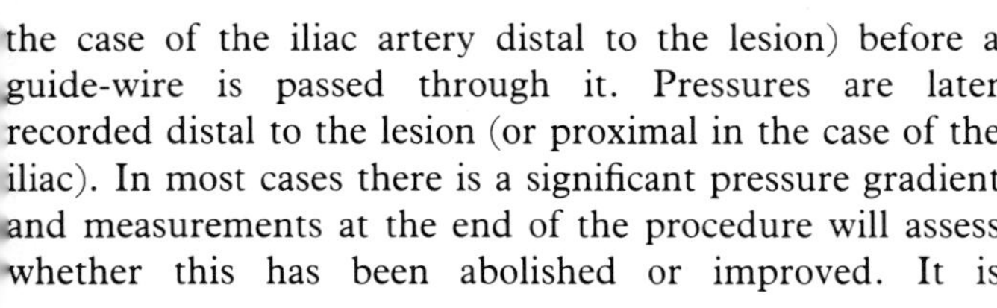

the case of the iliac artery distal to the lesion) before a guide-wire is passed through it. Pressures are later recorded distal to the lesion (or proximal in the case of the iliac). In most cases there is a significant pressure gradient and measurements at the end of the procedure will assess whether this has been abolished or improved. It is important that the lesion is only traversed once by the guide wire. If a catheter has to be withdrawn through it for exchange or other purposes this must only be done with the guide-wire replaced before the catheter is withdrawn. In this way the possibility of complications such as local dissection is much reduced.

Angiograms performed immediately following angioplasty may appear disappointing because of intimal fissures suggesting dissection, but the pressure recordings are the best guide to successful results, and later angiography will show a more normal appearance.

Anticoagulants

Heparinization. In order to reduce the possibility of thrombosis or embolus 5000 units of heparin are injected through the catheter once the lesion has been passed. For coronary angioplasty heparin 10 000 units i.v. is used. *Aspirin* therapy is usually recommended for 24 hours before and for 6 months after angioplasty. Some workers also recommend long-term anticoagulation with Warfarin from the second postoperative day.

It is desirable that non-ionic contrast media should be used for control preoperative and postoperative angiography since they are less likely to irritate the traumatized intima as well as being more comfortable for the patient.

Complications

Local dissection. The guide-wire or catheter may pass subintimally and produce a local dissection, which may go on to a local thrombosis.

Embolization may occur especially during the recanalization of occluded vessels.

Arterial perforation by the guide-wire has been recorded particularly with small vessels or in the renal artery.

Balloon rupture is occasionally seen. If the rupture is longitudinal the balloon can usually be removed without problems, but if it is horizontal and peels back around the catheter the help of a surgeon may be required.

Local arterial trauma with haematoma, false aneurysm or thrombosis may all occur at the puncture site as with any form of arterial catheterization, particularly with large catheters or coaxial sheaths.

Spasm is not uncommon in femoropopliteal angioplasty particularly if the guide-wire is passed below the knee. It can be guarded against by giving 50 mg of Lignocaine intra-arterially before the catheter traverses the lesion. If spasm is encountered Tolazoline (10–20 mg) can also be administered.

These complications emphasize that the procedure should not be lightly undertaken, and that surgical help must always be available to treat complications should they arise. In the case of renal or coronary angioplasty immediate emergency surgery may be required.

Results of angioplasty

There has now been extensive experience of angioplasty by the Gruntzig balloon technique at many centres in Europe and North America. As regards the *femoral and popliteal* arteries the primary success rate is about 90% with a 3-year patency rate of just over 70%. In the iliacs the primary success rate is just over 90%, and 3-year patency is over 80%. In both cases the results are similar to those achieved by surgery. Angioplasty, however, has no reported mortality whilst that of surgery is 1–4% in different series. Complications requiring further surgery are similar in both angioplasty and surgery (about 3%).

Renal angioplasty has been less widely practised. The main indication is renal artery stenosis with secondary hypertension which cannot be adequately controlled by drugs. The success rate with angioplasty seems so far to be very similar to that of direct surgery. As with surgery better results are obtained with fibromuscular hyperplasia than with atheromatous stenosis (75% cure or improvement rate against 40%).

EMBOLIZATION

Deliberate transcatheter arterial occlusion has been increasingly practised in the last decade and has become an important branch of interventional radiology.

A wide variety of particulate materials has been used for this purpose. They include *biological* (muscle slips, fibrous tissue, fat, lyodura and autologous clot); *gelatin and fibre* (Gelfoam, Oxycel, Avilene—Ivalon); *metallic* (stainless steel balls, silastic coated metal balls, carbon microspheres, metal filings and barium particles) and *plastic* (polyvinyl alcohol, silastic spheres, polystyrene spheres, acrylic spheres, Sephadex particles). In addition tiny *steel coils* with attached fibre strands have been successfully used for arterial occlusions, as has *Bucrylate*, an organic adhesive or 'superglue', which can be delivered intra-arterially by a catheter technique. Vascular occlusion and tissue infarction and ablation have also been obtained by injecting high doses of *hyperosmolic contrast media, absolute alcohol* or other sclerosing agents. Finally *detachable balloons* have been used to occlude vessels.

Of all the particulate substances mentioned above those which have proved most acceptable and have been most widely used include autologous clot, Gelfoam, Avilene and polyvinyl alcohol. Some of the other substances mentioned (steel coils, Bucrylate, absolute alcohol) also have enthusiastic advocates. The method used in a particular situation depends largely on local skills and preferences. There are many dangers and possible complications attached to the procedure and it is clear that embolization should only be practised by experienced angiographers.

The permanence of the vascular occlusion varies with the different substances used. Autologous clot is rapidly reabsorbed and its effect lasted only hours or days. It was also of little use in patients with poor blood clotting. Though it was once widely used for gastrointestinal haemorrhage it was largely replaced by longer lasting agents. Gelfoam and Avilene produce occlusions lasting many days or weeks, but in most cases are resorbed in three months or so. Polyvinyl alcohol, steel coils, Bucrylate and absolute alcohol produce more permanent effects.

Clinical indications. These include:

1. Haemorrhage
2. Occlusion of arteriovenous malformation
3. Occlusion of arteriovenous fistula and aneurysm
4. Neoplasm — infarction or reduction of blood flow
5. Organ ablation e.g. medical nephrectomy or splenectomy
6. Treatment of varicocele.

Haemorrhage

Upper gastrointestinal haemorrhage can be treated by vasopressin infusions as described below (p. 703). However, when vasopressin fails to control gastroduodenal haemorrhage, embolic therapy should be considered. Many now consider embolic therapy as the primary treatment of choice for bleeding from chronic duodenal ulcer. A rich collateral blood supply will normally protect from the danger of infarction, but great caution is necessary in the postoperative situation where major vessels have been ligated, or where surgery and vascular ligation are about to follow. The site of bleeding is first demonstrated by superselective angiography and depending on the site, embolization of the left gastric, gastroduodenal or pancreaticoduodenal arteries will be performed.

Embolization has also been performed in bleeding from lesions in the territory of both the superior and inferior mesenteric arteries but is more dangerous because of the difficulty of superselective catheterization. Normally such lesions are best treated by vasopressin infusions.

Pelvic haemorrhage may be difficult to control in carcinoma of the bladder or of the cervix, or in a postradiation or post-traumatic situation. Such haemorrhage can be controlled by embolization of one or both internal iliacs, or their branches.

Renal haemorrhage, either from trauma or neoplasm, has also been controlled by superselective embolization (Fig. 26.13), as has *hepatic haemorrhage* (Fig. 35.24).

There are many other sites and situations where embolization has been practised or considered, e.g. external carotid artery branches in *epistaxis* or in bleeding from *head and neck tumours*, and the bronchial arteries in severe *haemoptysis*. In all cases care must be taken that the procedure is as superselective as possible and the dangers of infarction or backflow guarded against. In some situations temporary balloon catheter vascular occlusions of a major vessel may offer a simpler alternative.

Arteriovenous malformations

Embolization may be the only method of treating many of these lesions or can provide an alternative to major radical surgery. Small lesions respond well provided a good superselective approach to the main feeding vessels can be obtained. Larger lesions are more difficult to treat owing to the multiple nature of the feeding vessels and the rapid arteriovenous shunting. Such lesions may require more than one session and even these may result in only partial success.

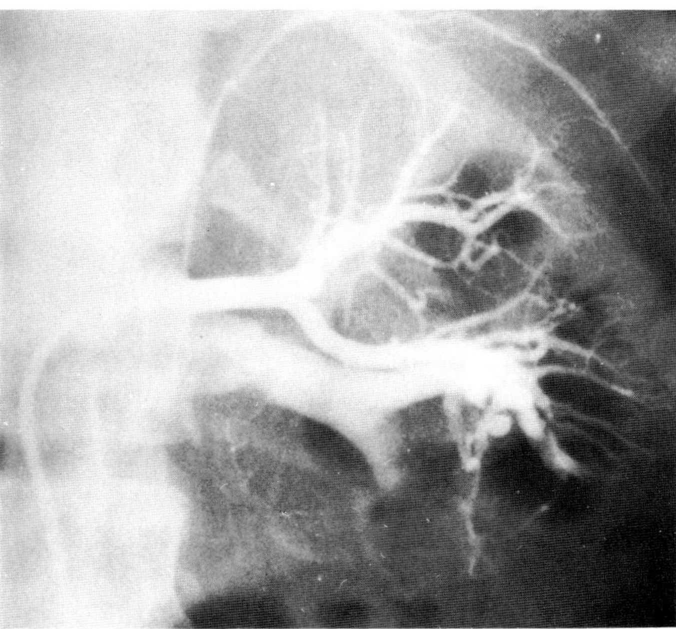
A

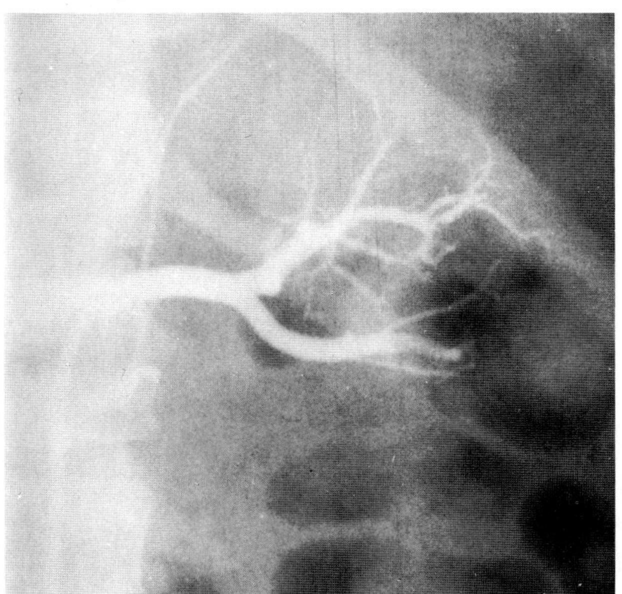
B

Fig. 26.13 Patient with severe haematuria following renal biopsy. **A.** Angiogram shows traumatic AV fistula. **B.** Fistula closed following embolization.

Arteriovenous fistula (Figs 26.13, 26.14)

Small arteriovenous fistulas can be closed with emboli provided the feeding vessels can be superselectively catheterized. With larger fistulae there is a danger of pulmonary emboli. Detachable balloons have also been

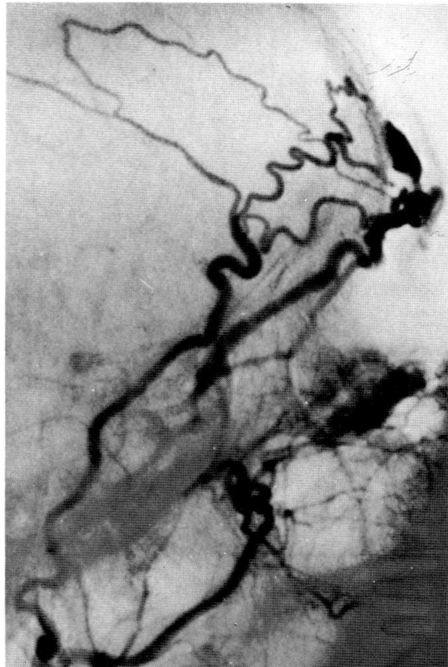

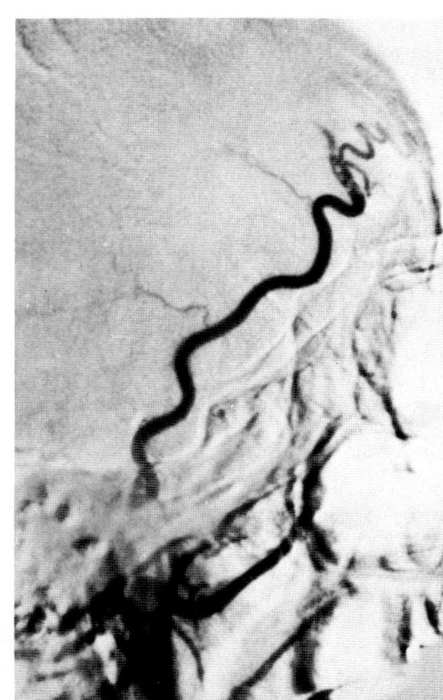

Fig. 26.14 AV fistula of scalp with drainage to superior ophthalmic vein **A.** Before. **B.** After embolization.

used for closure of arteriovenous fistula, particularly with caroticocavernous fistula (see Ch. 61).

Aneurysms

Aneurysms and false aneurysms of non-vital arteries can be occluded by embolization of the aneurysm or its feeding artery and the technique has been successfully used in patients with aneurysm of a hepatic (Fig. 35.24) or renal artery branch. In such cases there is little danger even if the segmental feeding artery is occluded, but there are considerable dangers with more vital arteries. Nevertheless the technique has been used in neuroradiology (see Ch. 61) and even with aneurysms of the abdominal aorta.

Neoplasms

Embolization has also been used in the treatment of tumours, either for infarction of the tumour, or as a preoperative measure to reduce the blood supply of vascular tumours (Fig. 26.15). The most widespread use has been in *renal carcinomas*. It is suggested that, even in inoperable cases, embolization of renal tumours may stimulate an immune response. It also reduces tumour bulk and may stop haematuria. Embolization of renal tumours is usually followed by flank pain lasting some 48 hours and requiring relief by narcotics. There may also be mild fever for several days, accompanied by nausea or vomiting, and transient hypertension may be seen. Other complications are discussed below.

Liver tumours. Both primary and secondary liver tumours have been treated by embolization (Ch. 35, p. 998). The liver is extremely vascular and, apart from the hepatic and portal blood supplies, has multiple collateral pathways. Normal liver receives some 75% of its blood supply from the portal system and only 25% from the hepatic artery. In liver neoplasms the situation is reversed and 96% of the tumour blood supply comes from the hepatic artery. Selective hepatic artery embolization is a relatively safe procedure in inoperable primary carcinoma or as a preoperative measure in operable cases. It is also useful in the treatment of deposits not responding to chemotherapy.

Embolization has also been used but less commonly with a variety of other neoplasms including *bone* tumours. Small *adrenal* tumours have been infarcted by retrograde venous injection of an excess of contrast and *parathyroid* adenomas have also been destroyed by superselective arterial contrast injections.

Organ ablation

Embolization of both the kidney and the spleen have been used as alternatives to surgical nephrectomy and splenectomy. The latter procedure, however, has been complicated by a high incidence of splenic abscess.

Varicocele

Testicular varicocele has been treated by selective left testicular vein catheterization. A percutaneous catheter is passed from the groin to the left renal vein and thence into the left testicular vein. The latter is then occluded by a detachable balloon or a sclerosant. The technique has been particularly used in the treatment of infertility in men with varicoceles.

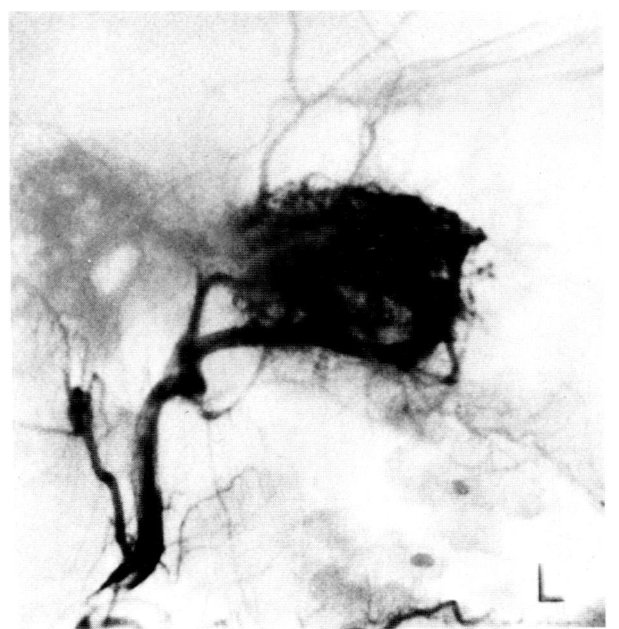

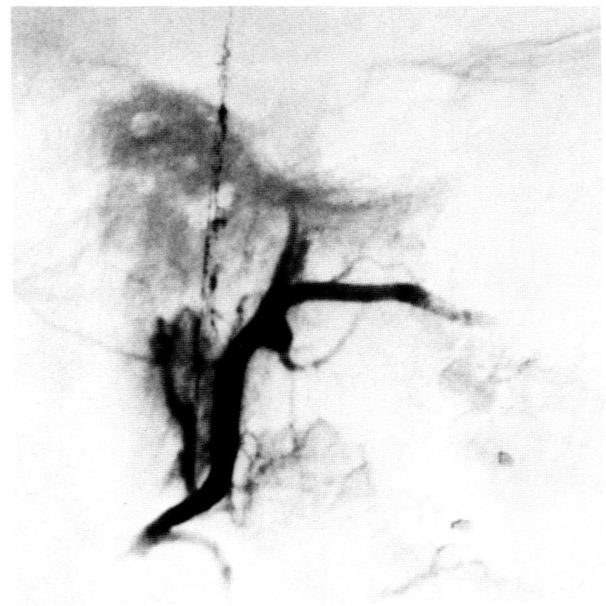

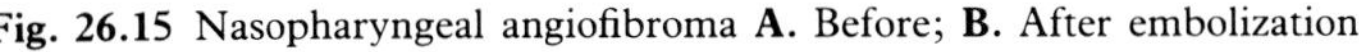

Fig. 26.15 Nasopharyngeal angiofibroma **A.** Before; **B.** After embolization.

Complications

Apart from the complications which may occur with all varieties of percutaneous angiography, embolization has special hazards associated with the procedure. The main danger is undesired *ischaemia* and even *tissue necrosis* in the target area, or elsewhere in the body. The latter can occur from backflow of particles or misplacement of the catheter tip. It should be guarded against by careful monitoring of the particulate injections on the screen using contrast with the injections and using multiple small doses rather than one or more large doses. The danger of reflux is greatest near the end of the procedure as the capillary bed becomes progressively blocked. A further safeguard is the use of a balloon catheter to block the afferent vessels whilst delivering the particles.

The complications recorded have included lower limb ischaemia and gangrene; gut necrosis; splenic infarction and abscess; hepatic infarction and abscess; pulmonary infarction; renal infarction, abscess and anuria; and spinal cord infarction.

There are special dangers associated with the use of steel coils (*arterial perforations, loss of coils* to the aorta or other vessels) and of bucrylate (internal catheter gluing). Neuroradiological procedures also carry special hazards (see Ch. 61).

BALLOON CATHETER ARTERIAL OCCLUSION

Double-lumen balloon catheters with an inflatable balloon near their tips are available for percutaneous introduction as with simple catheters. These catheters can be used for temporary occlusion of blood vessels. The method can be used in the control of internal haemorrhage and even large arteries can be occluded by this means. We have used this technique as an alternative to embolization prior to surgery in cases of highly vascular hypernephromas. The catheter is introduced directly before the patient is sent to the operating theatre and enables the surgeon to operate in an almost bloodless field (Fig. 26.16). The balloon is deflated and the catheter removed immediately following surgery.

Detachable balloon catheters (Debrun 1979) are becoming more widely used (Fig. 26.17). The main indication is the closure of arteriovenous fistula, and particularly carotico-cavernous fistula (see Ch. 61). They have also been used in the treatment of intracranial aneurysms.

INTRA-ARTERIAL DRUG THERAPY

Intra-arterial chemotherapy. Maximal therapeutic doses of cytotoxic drugs may be delivered directly to tumours by selective arterial catheterization. The technique has been used for inoperable tumours, particularly liver metastases (Figs 26.18 and 35.25) and for presurgical treatment of large tumours.

Intra-arterial therapy by vasoconstrictors. This method has been mainly used for the control of acute gastrointestinal haemorrhage by slow infusion of vasoconstrictors (Baum et al 1973). Vasopressin has been mainly used after angiographic demonstration of contrast extravasation at the bleeding point. Selective infusion into the left gastric artery usually controls bleeding from Mallory-Weiss tears or from gastritis and stress ulcers in the upper

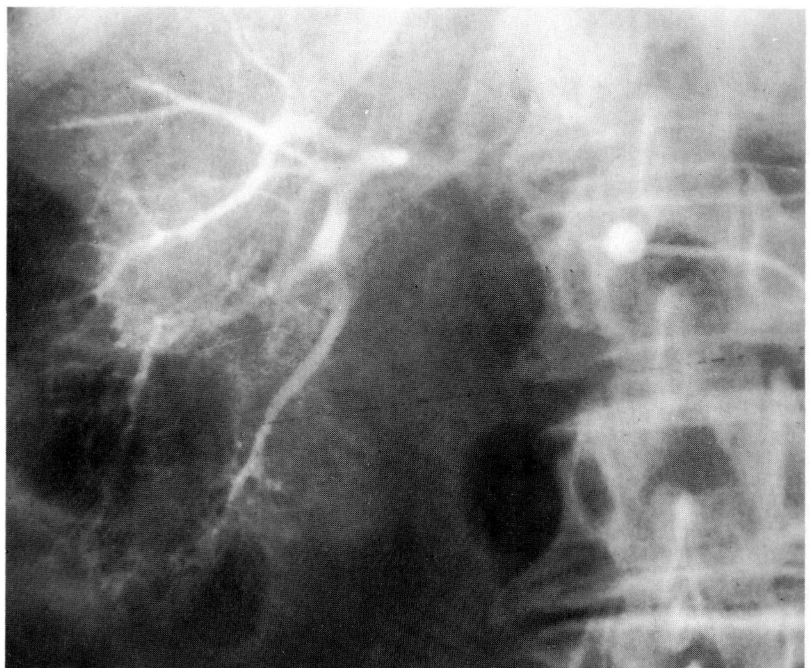

Fig. 26.16 Balloon catheter occluding right renal artery prior to surgery. A small dose of contrast is lingering in the arteries 10 seconds after injection, confirming occlusion of lumen.

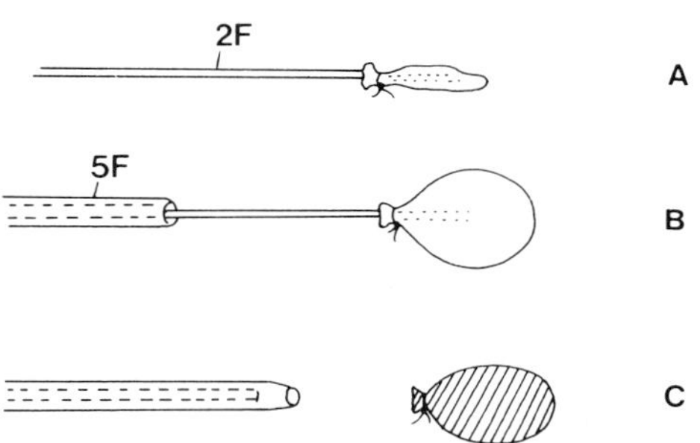

Fig. 26.17 Principle of Debrun detachable balloon. A. A latex balloon is attached to the end of a 2F Teflon catheter by a latex ligature. B. The balloon can be inflated with contrast after introduction through a 5F catheter. C. Before detachment balloon is filled with liquid silicone. Once the silicone has hardened, the balloon is detached by advancing the 5F catheter to push it off the smaller 2F catheter.

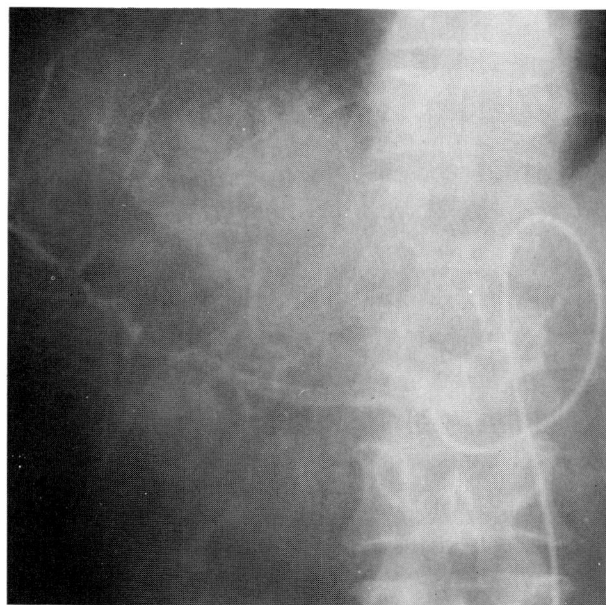

Fig. 26.18 Small catheter selectively inserted into right hepatic artery arising from superior mesenteric artery. The catheter was left in site for several days for infusion of cytotoxic drugs. Multiple liver secondaries. The site was confirmed by small contrast injection.

part of the stomach. Infusion into the common hepatic artery is used in antral lesions and into the gastroduodenal artery in duodenal bleeding. The superior mesenteric and inferior mesenteric can also be used for the control of lesions in their respective territories. Dosage for vasopressin is 0.2 units per minute and for epinephrine 8–30 μg per minute. Initial duration is 20–40 minutes but may have to be prolonged, particularly in older arteriosclerotic patients.

The method is very successful in controlling small vessel and capillary haemorrhage as in mucosal tears, stress ulcers and colonic diverticula, but less so when large arteries are involved as in chronic peptic ulcers, or where haemocoagulation defects exist. Superior mesenteric artery infusion can also be used for the control of venous bleeding from oesophageal or gastric varices in portal hypertension. The aim in these cases is to reduce portal venous pressure by reducing portal flow and thus to stop the bleeding and avoid emergency surgery. The technique frequently succeeds in the presence of normal haemocoagulation, but not in patients with severe cirrhosis and major clotting defects. In these cases the alternative technique of percutaneous transhepatic portal venography with direct embolization of the left coronary vein is preferable.

Complications of vasopressin therapy include water retention (ADH effect), which may require management by diuretics and electrolyte replacement. Abdominal cramp and diarrhoea may also occur as may cardiotoxic effects (hypertension, bradycardia or arrhythmia). The drug must therefore be used with caution in patients with cardiac disease.

INDICATIONS

The indications for arteriography of the central nervous system are discussed in later chapters and those for coronary arteriography have already been dealt with. Elsewhere in the body the indications vary with different organs and anatomical regions, but can be described under the major headings of **a**. vascular lesions and **b**. tumours and suspected tumours.

Vascular lesions. These will be discussed under the following subheadings:

1. Congenital
2. Aneurysms
3. Stenoses and thromboses
4. Embolus
5. Angiomatous malformations
6. Arteriovenous fistula
7. Haemorrhage.

Tumours and suspected tumours. These will be discussed under the particular organ or area involved. Angiography of tumours is also discussed in more or less detail in some of the chapters devoted to individual organs. In particular, cerebral tumours are described fully in Chapter 60, adrenal tumours in Chapter 36, and hepatic and pancreatic tumours in Chapter 35.

VASCULAR LESIONS

CONGENITAL

Congenital anomalies of the vascular system are common. Anomalies of the aortic arch itself have already been discussed (Ch. 25). Its great branches can also show variations. Some are particularly common and these are illustrated in Chapter 59. The common anatomical variations of the peripheral arterial system are well described in most textbooks of anatomy. However, attention is drawn to a few which have practical significance.

The *brachial* artery occasionally divides into its radial and ulnar branches at a high level and this was of some practical importance when brachial arteriography was more widely practised. In the lower limb the *popliteal* artery not infrequently divides into its posterior tibial and anterior tibial branches above the knee joint. Very occasionally the main blood supply to the lower limb instead of passing through the normal femoral artery passes through a *persistent primitive sciatic* artery.

This vessel persists from fetal life and, when present in an adult, is seen as a large vessel arising from a dilated hypogastric artery and passing through the greater sciatic notch. It then passes down behind the femoral neck and femur to join the popliteal artery. The true femoral artery is hypoplastic and may terminate in the thigh, as the profunda femoris.

Congenital anomalies of the *renal* arterial supply are not infrequent. Some 25% of kidneys examined by arteriography are found to have an accessory artery supplying the kidney. This of course makes such kidneys useless as renal grafts. Occasionally three arteries to one kidney are shown at angiography, but the demonstration of four arteries is very rare. Horseshoe and ectopic kidneys usually have an anomalous blood supply including arteries arising from the common iliac artery.

Anomalies of the arterial supply to the *liver* are also very frequent. The classical anatomical model of the common hepatic artery arising from the coeliac axis and dividing into right and left hepatic branches to supply the whole liver is found in only some half of patients examined.

Some 20% of patients have a right hepatic or accessory right hepatic artery arising from the superior mesenteric and a similar proportion have a left hepatic or accessory left hepatic artery arising from the left gastric artery. About 2% of patients have a common hepatic artery arising from the superior mesenteric artery.

Other major branches of the coeliac axis, i.e. the *splenic* and *left gastric* arteries may occasionally arise from the aorta as separate branches.

The *bronchial* arteries which arise on the anterior surface of the aorta just below the carina are double on the left in 60% of cases and on the right in 30% of patients.

Anomalies of the arterial supply to the brain are

discussed elsewhere (Ch. 59), but it should be noted that there are great variations in the size and adequacy of the components of the circle of Willis,

Coarctation of the aorta. In this anomaly there is a congenital stenosis just distal to the origin of the ligamentum arteriosum. The condition is discussed in detail in Chapter 25.

Poststenotic aneurysms occur as complications in about 4% of cases. Atypical forms of coarctation are relatively rare and include patients with infantile arches proximal to the stenosis, involving a fairly long segment of aorta, and patients with stenosis in atypical sites. These include the descending aorta or the abdominal aorta. So-called 'abdominal coarctation' may involve the origins of splanchnic vessels or the renal arteries (Fig. 26.19).

Pseudocoarctation or lateral **buckling** of the aorta is an unusual condition which can be mistaken for a rounded mass in the region of the aortic knuckle. The lesion appears to be associated with a sharp kink at the junction of arch and descending aorta in the region of the ligamentum arteriosum. Buckling of the aorta may also occur in the mid arch. This is best recognized in the lateral view.

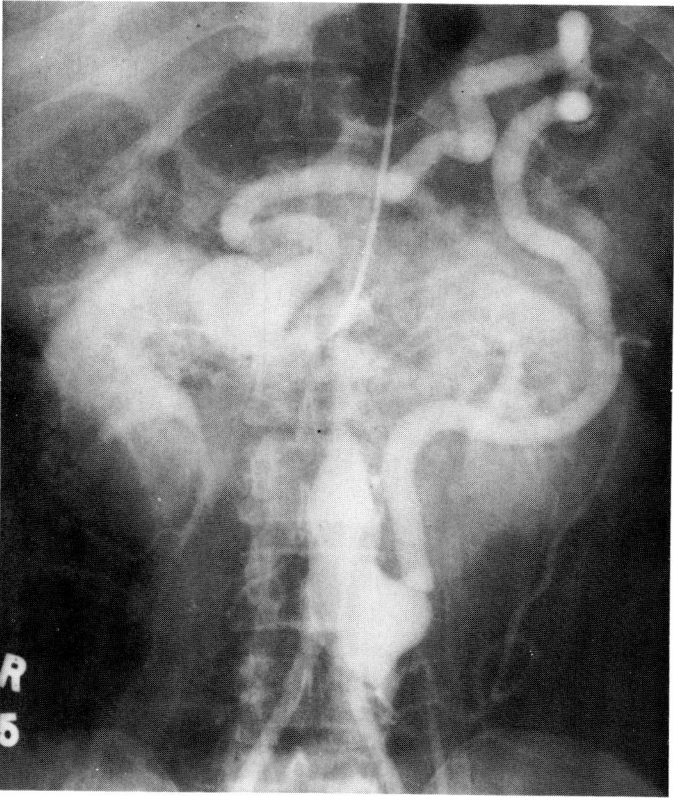

Fig. 26.19 Abdominal coarctation with involvement of the superior mesenteric origin. There is a collateral circulation through the artery of Drummond from the left colic branch of the inferior mesenteric to the middle colic branch of the superior mesenteric. Owing to the increased flow, aneurysms have developed at both ends of the collateral. (Courtesy of Dr. R. Eban).

Vascular rings around the oesophagus can be of many different types and the commonest lesions are illustrated diagrammatically in Appendix C. Study of the barium-filled oesophagus is often very helpful in elucidating these cases.

Hypoplasia of the aorta is sometimes found as a chance finding. It may be associated with Marfan's syndrome where there is a mesodermal defect and medial degeneration of the aorta. However, in Marfan's syndrome the aorta will eventually dilate because of the medial defect and dissecting aneurysms may also occur, especially in the ascending aorta.

ANEURYSMS

Aneurysms can be classified into the following main groups:

1. Congenital
2. Infective (mycotic or syphilitic)
3. Degenerative
4. Traumatic
5. Poststenotic
6. Dissecting
7. Miscellaneous (necrotizing vasculitis).

Congenital aneurysms are most commonly seen in the intracranial circulation. Whilst it is probable that these aneurysms are basically due to a defect in the muscular coat at points of arterial bifurcations, it is clear from clinical experience that other factors such as age, atheroma and hypertension are also of great significance in their pathogenesis. They are further discussed in Chapter 60. So-called congenital aneurysms have also been described in most areas of the body, but they are relatively rare in comparison with other forms of aneurysm.

Infective aneurysms may be classified as mycotic or syphilitic.

Mycotic aneurysms are nearly always due to bacterial endocarditis. They may involve any artery in the body, and the author has seen examples at the junction of the aorta and inferior mesenteric artery, in the common femoral artery, in the popliteal and the posterior tibial artery, in the middle cerebral artery and in the hand (Figs 26.20, 26.21, 26.22).

Mycotic aneurysms can grow very rapidly in size and, in one example seen by us, a common femoral aneurysm reached a diameter of 5 cm in 3 weeks. Surgical intervention is necessary in these cases to prevent rupture.

Syphilitic aneurysms were once extremely common in clinical and surgical practice. With the advent of antibiotics and the early treatment of syphilis they have become relatively rare in this country. However, they may still be encountered and can involve arteries in any part of the body. The commonest artery to be involved is the thoracic aorta and aneurysms here may reach a very large

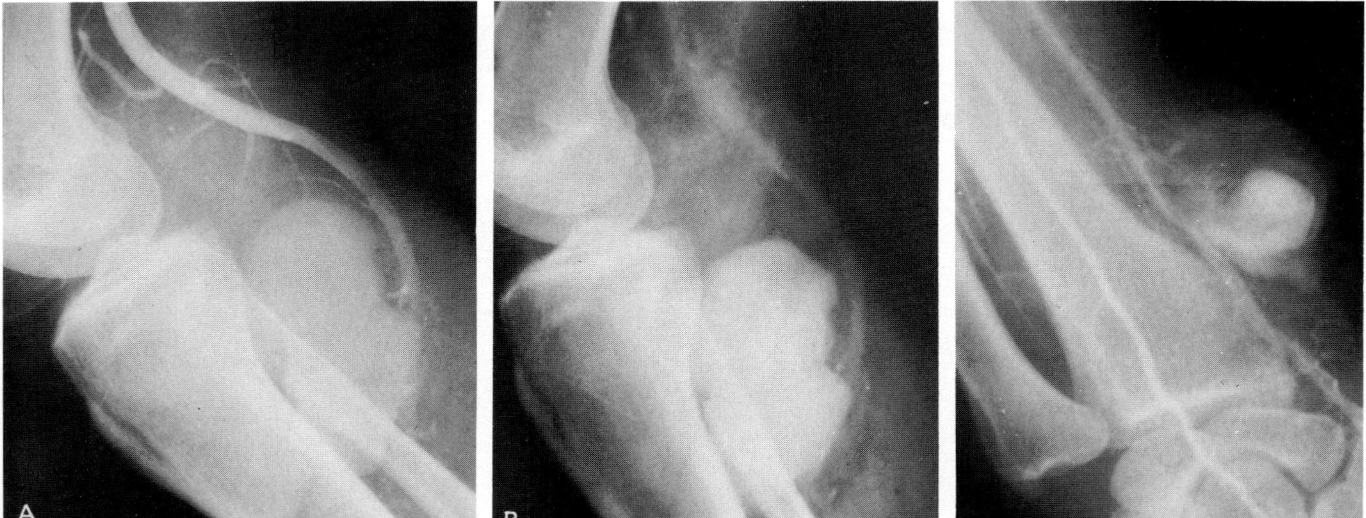

Fig. 26.20 A. and **B.** Mycotic aneurysm in the lower popliteal artery.

Fig. 26.21 Mycotic aneurysm of the lower end of the ulnar artery.

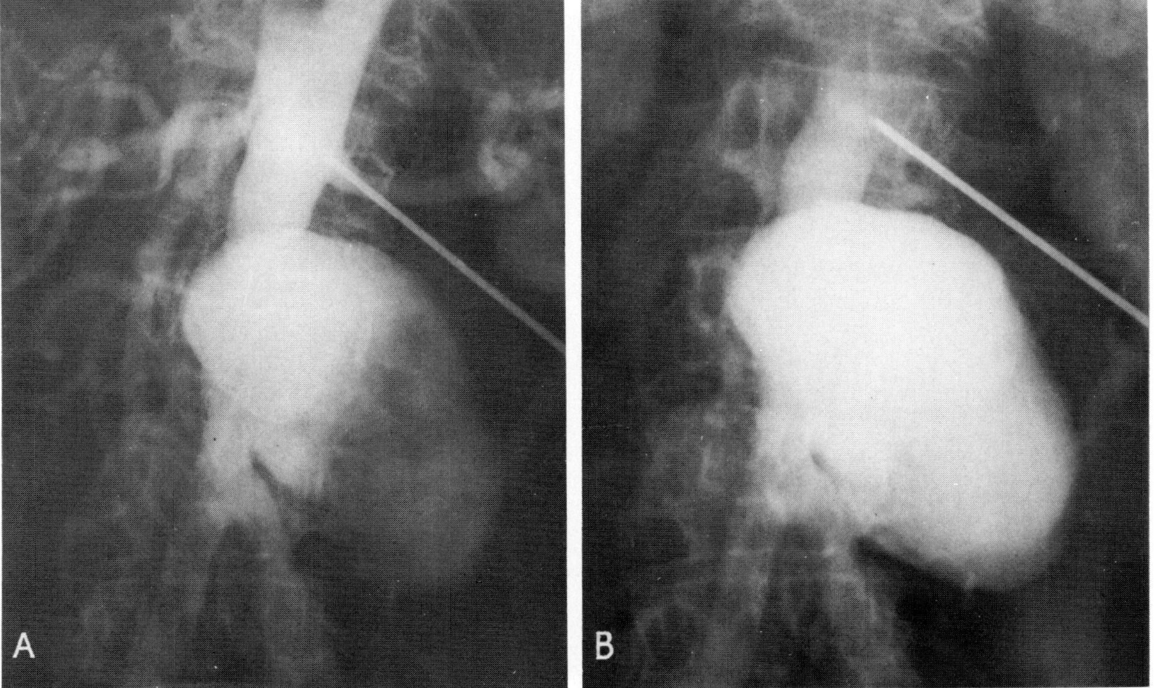

Fig. 26.22 A. and **B.** Mycotic aneurysm at the origin of the inferior mesenteric artery.

size (Fig. 26.23). Syphilitic aneurysms are of course still common in undeveloped countries.

Advances in vascular surgery in recent years have rendered many aneurysms of the thoracic aorta, which were previously considered inoperable, suitable for surgical treatment and cure.

It is sometimes difficult to differentiate by simple X-ray between a thoracic aortic aneurysm and a mediastinal tumour or cyst. In these cases angiography enables a firm diagnosis to be made and is a necessary prerequisite to corrective surgery.

Apart from arteriography confirmation of the diagnosis is of course possible by DSA or by less invasive imaging techniques. Thus CT will show thoracic aneurysms well,

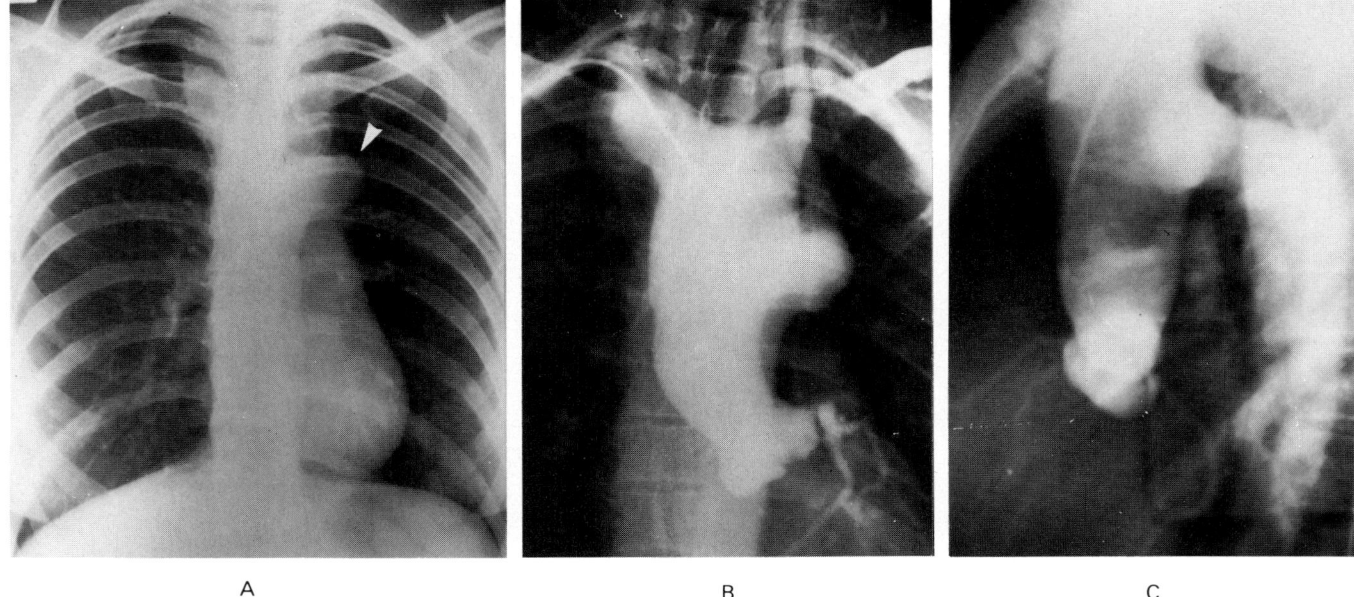

Fig. 26.23 **A.** chest film showing aortic knuckle (arrow) apparently displaced downwards by suptra-aortic mass. **B.** and **C.** Angiogram shows that this is due to an aneurysm of the arch and innominate artery.

as will NMR. Nuclear angiography will also show thoracic aneurysms, though it will not demonstrate the wall of clot such aneurysms may contain. Ultrasound, though very useful in the case of abdominal and peripheral aneurysms, is little used for thoracic aneurysms because of the overlying rib cage.

Degenerative aneurysms result from atheroma. They are commoner in men than women, reflecting the increased sex incidence of atheroma in males. The commonest site is the abdominal aorta (Figs 26.24, 26.26). Other common sites are the iliac arteries and the popliteal arteries (Fig. 26.25) though such atheromatous aneurysms

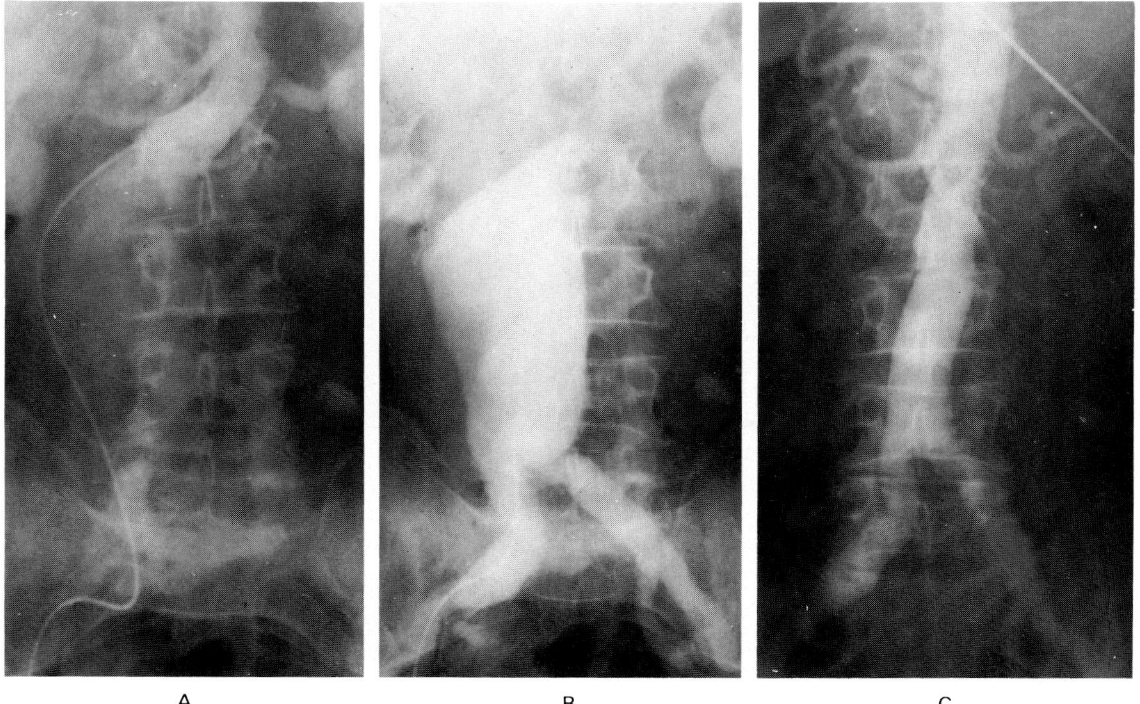

Fig. 26.24 Degenerative aneurysm of the abdominal aorta. **A.** and **B.** Before operation. **C.** After operation.

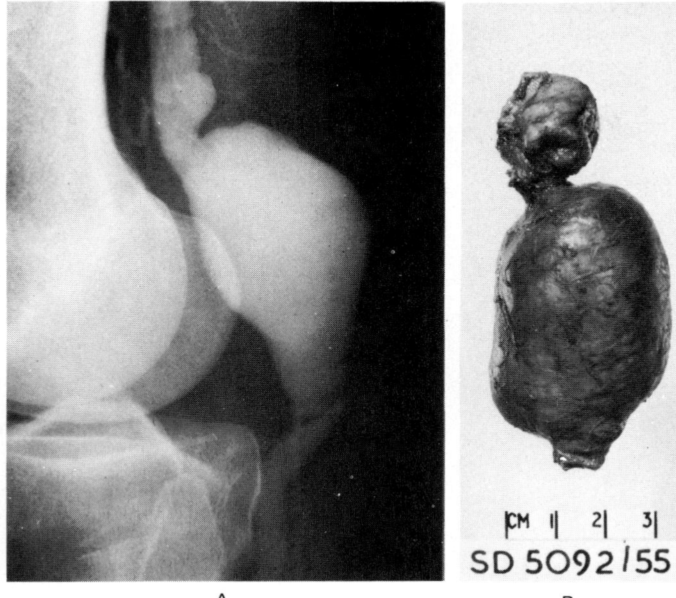

Fig. 26.25 A. Popliteal aneurysm shown by angiography. **B.** excised specimen.

may be seen anywhere in the body including the femoral and basilar arteries. They are also becoming commoner in the thoracic aorta and, together with traumatic and dissecting aneurysms, have replaced syphilis as the main cause of thoracic aneurysm in Western countries. Degenerative thoracic aneurysms involve the descending aorta or distal arch and rarely affect the ascending aorta.

Degenerative aneurysms are often fusiform resulting in a generalized dilatation or ectasia of the vessels, but may become saccular particularly in the sites mentioned above. Such saccular aneurysms are liable to rupture with serious results. The aneurysms may also form a nidus for intraluminal clot, and this may become detached leading to embolic occlusion of more peripheral vessels.

Atheroma is probably a factor in the production of many of the so-called 'congenital' berry aneurysms which are found in the cerebral circulation. It may also be a factor in the production of the rare renal artery aneurysm. The latter may be associated with hypertension, and hypertension itself may be another causative factor in the development of degenerative aneurysms.

Ultrasound is the simplest method of confirming a diagnosis of abdominal aortic aneurysms (Fig. 26.26) and it is widely used for preliminary assessment and follow-up. Nuclear angiography will also show the lumen well (Fig. 26.27) but not the wall of the clot.

CT has the advantage of showing both the lumen and the wall of clot; it also shows the relationship to the renal arteries, which is important to the surgeon and evidence of leakage. Further direct measurement of the size of the aneurysm in all planes and of its lumen, is possible by CT (Fig. 26.28); MRI, if available, can provide similar information.

The methods used now vary in different centres and depend to some extent on local availability of equipment and expertise. Where DSA is available, it is being increasingly used as an alternative to direct angiography.

Traumatic aneurysms can occur wherever an arterial wall is subject to injury. Such aneurysms are commonest in the limbs (Fig. 26.29) although they are also encountered in the thorax, abdomen and head and neck.

Traumatic aneurysm of the thoracic aorta is being increasingly encountered following crush injuries of the chest. If the condition is suspected clinically a simple X-ray will often show broadening of the mediastinum from

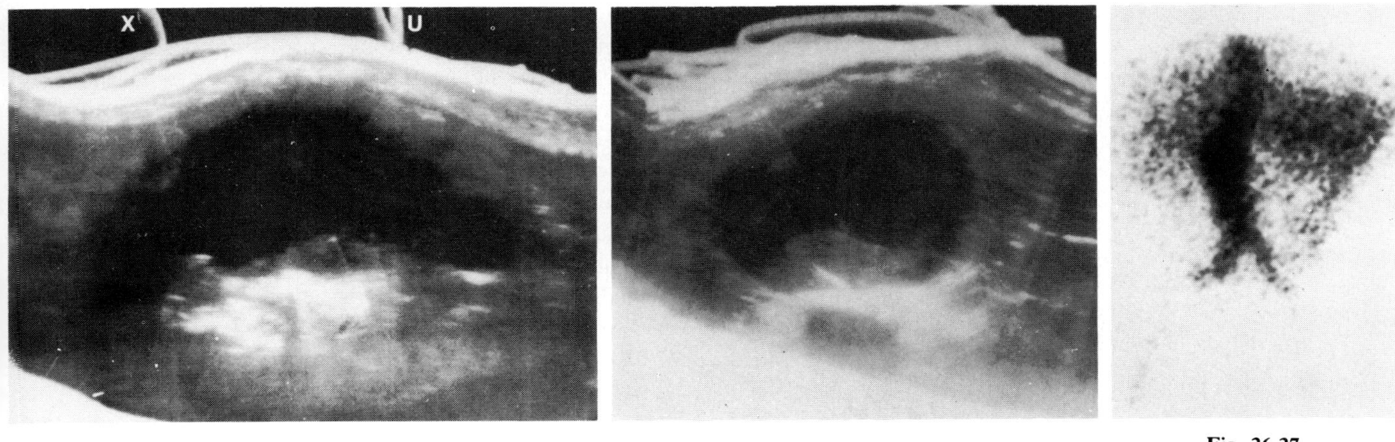

Fig. 26.27

Fig. 26.26 Aortic aneurysm shown by ultrasound. It is not usually possible to assess the relationship to the renal arteries by this method, or clearly to define the relationship to the bifuration of the iliacs. **A.** Longitudinal scan. **B.** Transverse scan.

Fig. 26.27 Nuclear angiogram showing aneurysm of the abdominal aorta. This method gives a good idea of the lumen but not of the wall of clot.

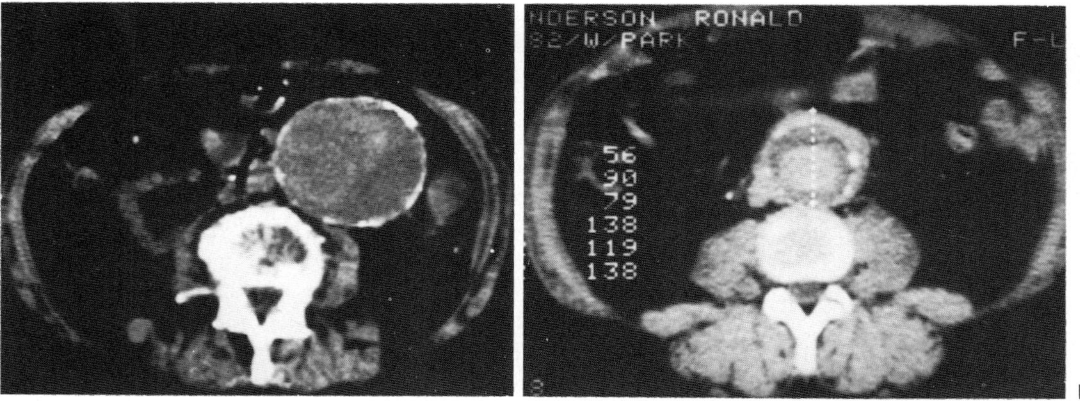

Fig. 26.28 **A.** CT scan of lower abdomen shows a huge abdominal aneurysm with a diameter of 8.5 cm and a calcified wall. **B.** CT scan of lower abdomen in another patient after i.v. contrast shows the lumen of a medium-sized aneurysm with a wall of clot. The diameter as measured by the electronic cursor is 5.6 cm. The wall is thickened and irregular and enhances with contrast, features of so-called 'inflammatory' aneurysm or perianeurysmal fibrosis.

haematoma, and emergency angiography or DSA is justified to confirm the diagnosis prior to surgery.

Automobile accidents have led to a great increase in the incidence of these traumatic thoracic aortic aneurysms. The shearing effect of the deceleration injury usually involves the isthmus of the aorta near the ligamentum arteriosum. Although such injuries are usually fatal, about 20% of cases survive temporarily by the formation of a periaortic haematoma and false aneurysm (Fig. 26.30). This is due to temporary containment by the periadventitial mediastinal tissues or because the adventitia has not yet ruptured.

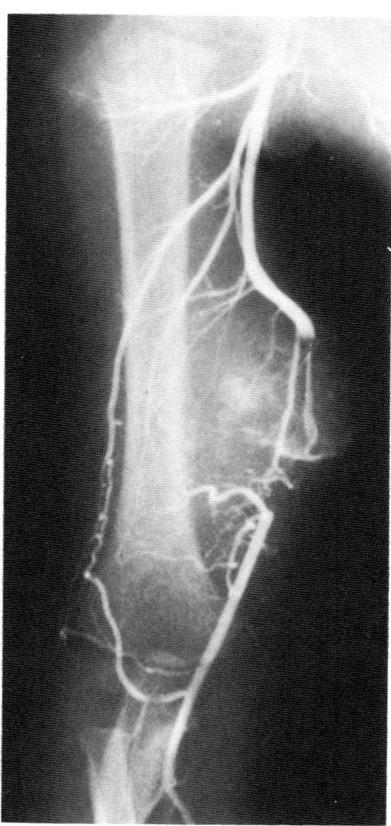

Fig. 26.29 Traumatic false aneurysm with rupture of the brachial artery in a child, following fall while carrying a glass milk bottle.

It is vital to recognize such cases before secondary rupture because 30% will die in 24 hours and another 30% within a week. The chance of proceeding to chronic aneurysm formation in untreated cases was put at only 2% in a review of 262 cases at the American Armed Forces Institute of Pathology.

Most of these cases are suffering from multiple injuries but salvage is possible by early diagnosis and treatment. As noted above, simple X-ray of the chest may show broadening of the mediastinum but this may be difficult to assess in portable or emergency X-rays. Arteriography will show a false aneurysm, usually near the isthmus, but the signs may be more subtle, consisting merely of mural irregularity or an intimal flap at the site of the tear (Fig. 26.30B). A small ductus diverticulum should be readily differentiated by its smooth wall.

Dissecting aneurysms are mainly encountered in the aorta and hypertension is the main predisposing cause. The incidence in the USA has been estimated at 5–10 cases per million of population annually. Males are mainly affected and they are usually aged between 50 and 70 years. In one series only 5% of cases were below the age of 40. These younger patients were often associated with Marfan's syndrome, or, in females, with pregnancy. Apart from hypertension, atheroma, Marfan's syndrome and pregnancy there are also associations with aortic stenosis, bicuspid aortic valves and coarctation.

The dissection usually commences in the aortic arch or ascending aorta and extends peripherally. DeBakey has classified dissection into three groups (Fig. 26.31).

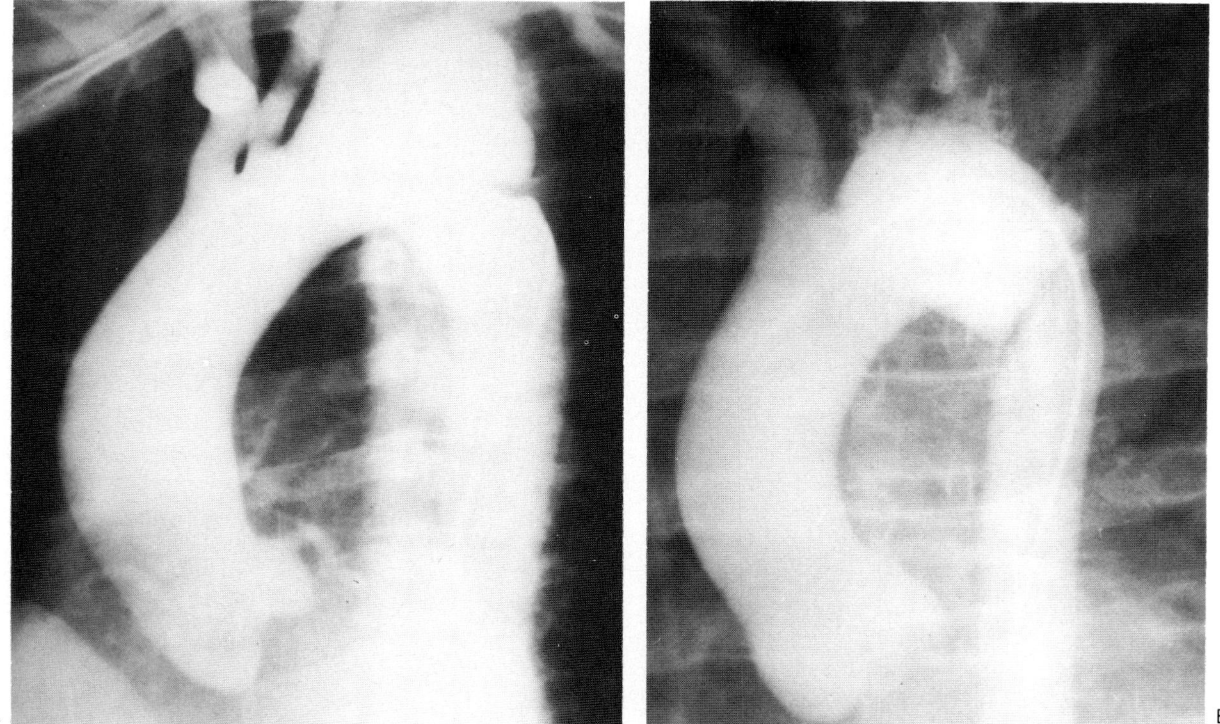

Fig. 26.30 A. and **B.** Traumatic false aneurysms of the aortic arch. Two different cases. Note intimal flaps.

Type 1 commences in the ascending aorta and extends through the arch and descending aorta to the iliacs (Fig. 26.32). Type II also commences in the ascending aorta but does not extend beyond it. Type III commences in the distal arch and extends down to the iliacs (Fig. 26.33).

DeBakey's type II is the least common and is usually associated with Marfan's syndrome. It forms about 10% of the cases seen, the other 90% being fairly evenly shared by the other two types.

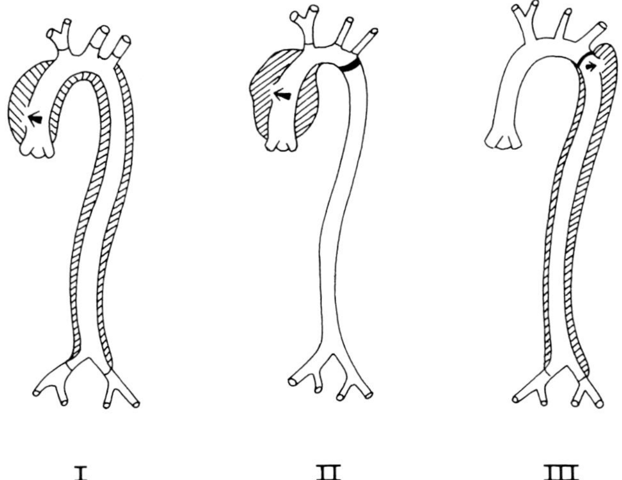

Fig. 26.31 Diagram showing types of dissecting aneurysms (see text).

From the surgical viewpoint a better classification is into type A, which includes all cases involving the ascending aorta, and type B, which includes all other cases (see below).

The clinical features in classical cases are well known and include sudden agonizing pain in the chest. As the dissection tracks along the aorta it may involve and obstruct major branches. Hemiplegia and vertebral symptoms may result from involvement of cerebral vessels and paraplegia from involvement of intercostal or lumbar arteries supplying the cord. Ischaemia of one or both legs can follow iliac involvement. Proximal dissection may rupture into the pericardium with cardiac tamponade, or may involve the coronaries causing ischaemia. Involvement of coeliac axis or superior mesenteric may give rise to abdominal pain, pancreatitis or mesenteric ischaemia; renal artery involvement may precipitate acute hypertension or anuria.

It is important to realize that many cases may be atypical and the diagnosis may easily be missed. The majority of cases are fatal within a few days, but occasionally the dissection appears to cure itself by spontaneous re-entry into the aorta at a lower level giving rise to the so-called 'double barrel' aorta. We have encountered several cases where the presence of a chronic dissection of this type came as a surprise to the referring physician.

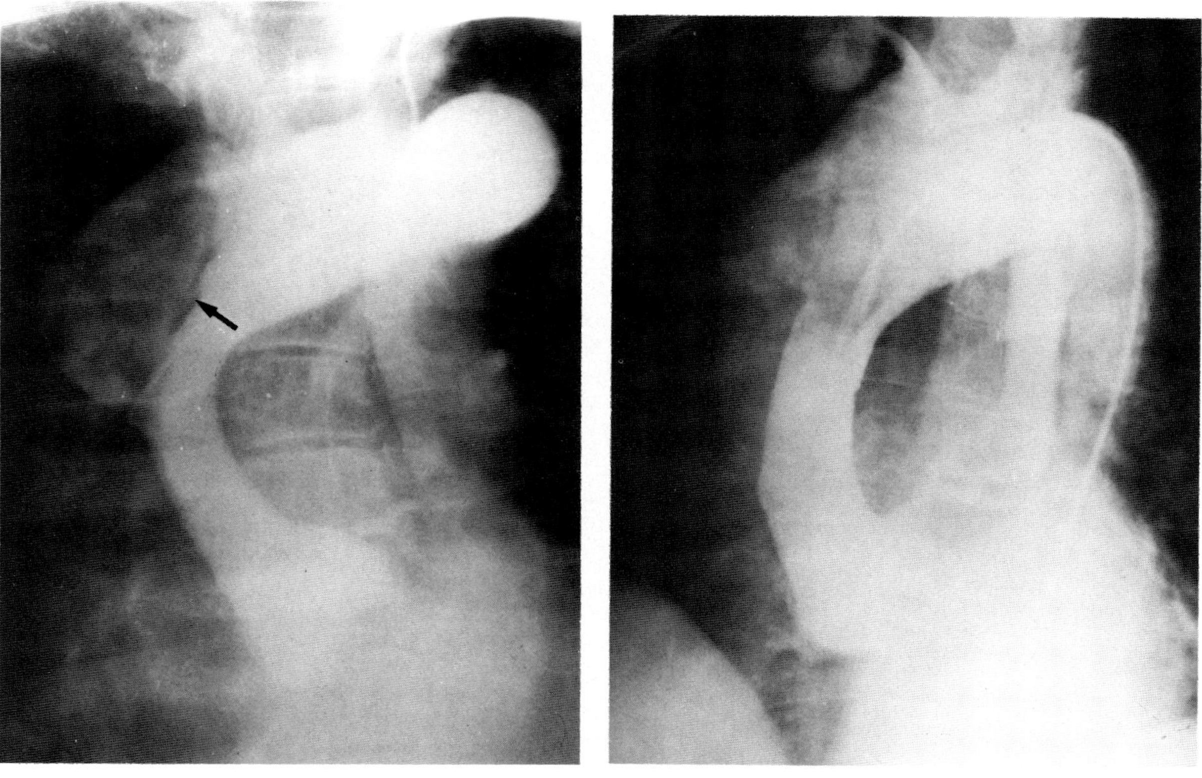

Fig. 26.32 Type I dissections. Two cases. **A.** The dissection is compressing the true lumen of both the ascending and descending aorta. A small amount of contrast is seen entering the dissection through the tear in the intima of the ascending aorta (arrow). **B.** Contrast is entering the false lumen separated by intimal flap in descending aorta.

It is our experience that the clinical diagnosis of dissecting aneurysm is made more frequently than such lesions are actually present. On the other hand, the diagnosis is occasionally missed when the history is atypical. Radiology can therefore be of great help in establishing the diagnosis.

Dissecting aneurysms of the thoracic aorta carry a grave prognosis with some 30% of patients dying within 24 hours, and a further 50% in the next few days or weeks. Only 20% of patients survive beyond 6 weeks and half of these will die from subsequent rupture of the aneurysm. The best prognosis rests with type III dissections not involving the ascending aorta.

Present opinion favours medical treatment in these cases, but surgery is indicated in cases involving the ascending aorta. The survival rate in one series of ascending aorta dissections treated by surgery was 64% as against a medical treatment survival rate of 22%. There is thus some urgency in establishing the diagnosis and in localization of the dissection in all suspected cases.

Imaging findings. Simple X-ray of the chest may show widening of the mediastinum, though this may be difficult to assess in portable supine films. More characteristic is localized dilatation of the thoracic aorta involving the aortic knuckle and upper descending aorta. This may give rise to a prominent 'hump' sign due to the outward projection of the aortic knuckle. Lateral and anterior displacement of the trachea may also be seen on the plain film. The descending aorta often bulges to the left and can appear lobulated. If a recent previous chest X-ray is available for direct comparison the change in outline is virtually diagnostic.

Medial displacement of the calcified intima at the aortic knuckle may be recognized in a small proportion of patients, and a pleural effusion due to haemothorax is present in about 20% of cases. In patients with Marfan's syndrome, which is associated with DeBakey's type II dissection, localized bulging of the ascending aorta to the right may be obvious on the simple chest film.

In recent years *CT* has been increasingly used as a non-invasive method of confirming the diagnosis of dissecting aneurysm. Intravenous contrast medium should be administered provided the patient's renal and cardiovascular state permits. In typical cases the dilated aorta with true and false lumen separated by an intimal flap can be readily identified, as can thrombi and intimal calcification (Figs 26.34 A and B).

Ultrasound has also been used to successfully demonstrate the intimal flap in dissecting aneurysms, and can help to confirm the diagnosis.

MRI can also show dissections and may eventually supplant other methods.

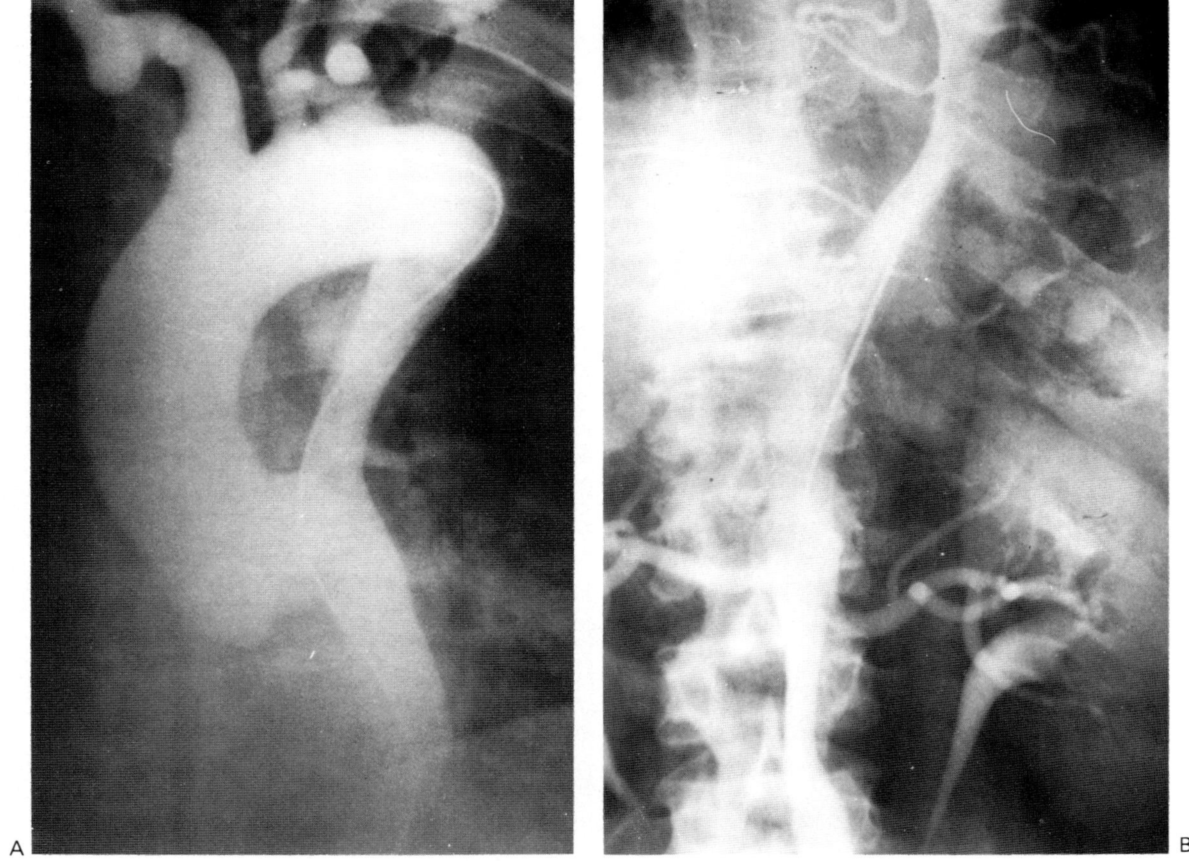

Fig. 26.33 Type III dissection. **A.** The dissection commences in the distal arch and compresses the descending aorta. **B.** Irregular compression of the lower thoracic and abdominal aorta. Both renal arteries fill well but the coeliac and superior mesenteric arteries are not identified and appear compressed. They are probably perfused by the dissection, which shows faint opacification.

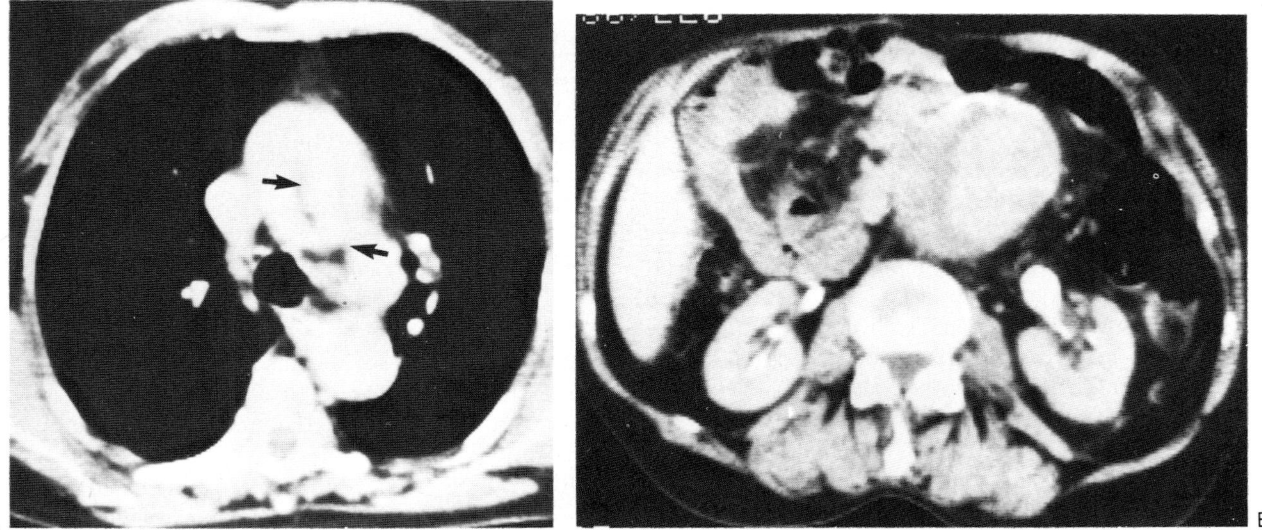

Fig. 26.34 **A.** Dissecting aneurysm shown by CT postcontrast; both true and false lumen are opacified but are separated by displaced intimal flaps (arrows) in the dilated ascending aorta (W 512 L 60). **B.** Dissection involving abdominal aorta, which shows fusiform aneurysmal dilatation. Contrast in both true and false lumens separated by intimal flap (W512 L38).

Arteriography has been most widely used to confirm the diagnosis and will provide very accurate anatomical information. The author has investigated a series of over 100 suspected cases of dissecting aneurysm by direct arteriography. An interesting feature was the significant proportion of negative angiograms (10%), confirming that the clinical diagnosis is not always justified, and that differential diagnosis from cardiac or other lesions can sometimes be difficult.

Arteriography was performed by the transfemoral route, or by the right transaxillary route where this was not possible. The catheter should be passed to the aortic root so that the whole of the thoracic aorta can be visualized. This enables aortic insufficiency with regurgitation into the left ventricle to be recognized. Patients who show no filling of the false lumen with the catheter tip proximal to the site of the intimal tear (Fig. 26.33) have a much better prognosis and showed a 90% survival rate in one series.

Usually, both the true and the false lumen of the aorta will be outlined by contrast. The displaced intima appears as a linear band separating the two channels, and the intimal tear as the point where the two channels communicate and contrast enters the false from the true lumen (Fig. 26.32 A and B). Less commonly, only the true channel is outlined and is deformed by the presence of the false channel, which contains solid blood clot or stagnant blood with no re-entry into the true lumen at a lower level (Fig. 26.33).

The catheter is then withdrawn to the dorsilumbar junction and an abdominal series obtained to define the lower limit of the dissection and assess involvement of splanchnic, renal and iliac vessels (Figs 26.33B and 26.35). Injections made here, or in the thoracic aorta below the level of the tear, will outline only the true lumen. The latter may show the 'twisted tape' sign due to the true lumen being constricted in different planes at different levels as the dissection spirals around the aorta. It should be appreciated that, in these circumstances, vessels which appear to be occluded may be patent and perfused by the dissection.

The thoracic aorta is the main site of dissecting aneurysm, but the lesion is occasionally encountered as an isolated finding in peripheral vessels. In our material we have seen examples in the renal and iliac arteries and localized to the abdominal aorta. Localized dissection in the common carotid artery is also well documented.

Localized iatrogenic arterial dissection as a complication of arteriography has been mentioned above. These can be relatively benign and will usually resolve spontaneously, particularly when the dissection is minor in degree or produced by retrograde instrumentation so that bloodflow tends to flatten rather than fill the intimal flap.

Necrotizing vasculitis. The mysterious disease *polyarteritis nodosa* is associated with necrotizing vasculitis. As the process advances the vascular walls weaken and aneurysm formation occurs in small vessels. These nodose lesions have a predilection for the bifurcations of small vessels but may occur anywhere along their lengths. Any artery in the body can be involved, including the vasa nervorum, and this accounts for the protean clinical manifestation.

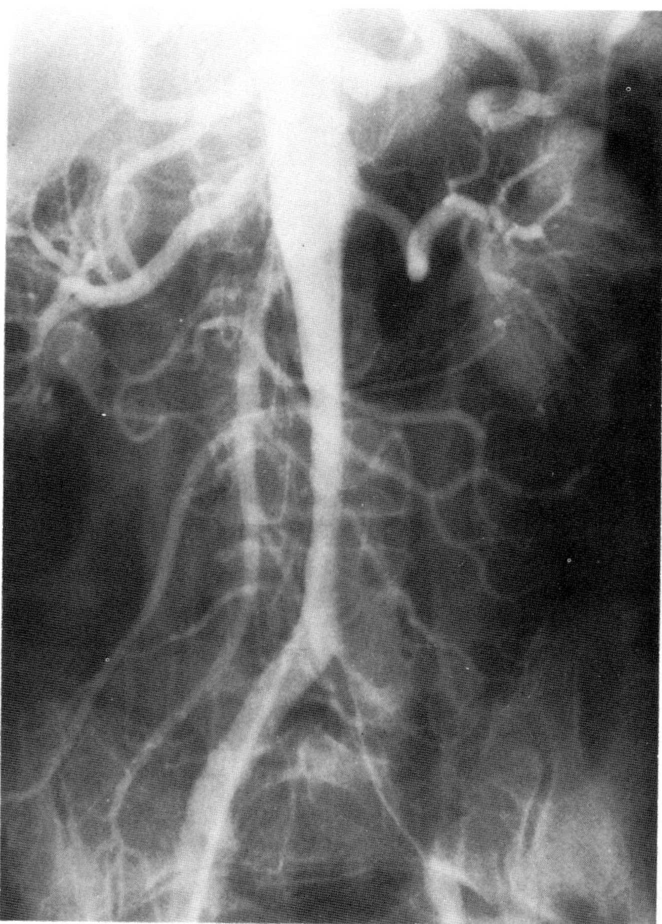

Fig. 26.35 Dissecting aneurysm. Abdominal series shows good filling of splanchnic and renal vessels but the lower abdominal aorta and left common iliac artery are obstructed. The latter forms the lower limit of the dissection.

The kidneys are very frequently involved and hypertension is seen in over 70% of cases. Multiple small aneurysms at renal angiography are characteristic (Fig. 43.5A) but are not invariably found. The small aneurysms may rupture giving rise to perinephric haematomas. Small aneurysms of other splanchnic vessels can also rupture. In our experience visceral and renal angiography has proved a valuable diagnostic technique since the demonstration of small multiple aneurysms is almost diagnostic.

Other rarer causes of similar small aneurysms are *Wegener's granulomatosis*, *systemic lupus erythematosus* and *atrial myxoma emboli*. Necrotizing arteritis has also been reported following *drug abuse*, particularly metamphetamine.

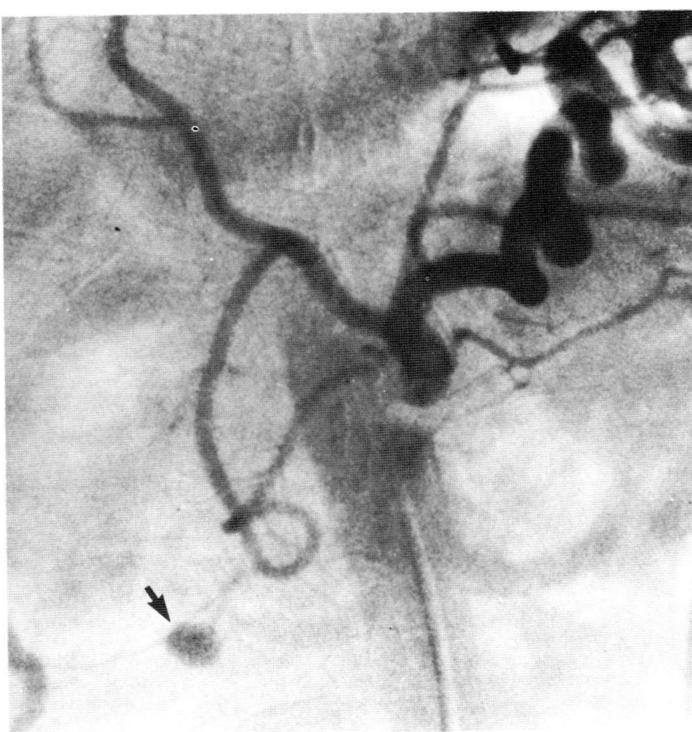

Fig. 26.36 Aneurysm of the pancreatico-duodenal arcade (arrow) secondary to acute pancreatitis (subtraction film).

Small aneurysms may also be seen as a complication of *pancreatitis* when they may involve small vessels supplying, or adjacent to, the pancreas (Fig. 26.36). Again, these aneurysms may rupture with serious consequences.

STENOSES AND THROMBOSES

Stenoses in arteries are most commonly the result of atheroma. Congenital stenosis of arteries also occurs. This is well known as the cause of *coarctation of the thoracic aorta* and less well known as the cause of the rare *abdominal coarctation of the aorta*. In the latter condition the origins of renal or major splanchnic vessels may be involved. Congenital stenoses have also been described in other vessels including the pulmonary arteries.

Atheroma is the commonest cause of stenotic vascular disease in clinical practice. There is a predominantly male sex incidence though females are by no means exempt, particularly in the older age groups. The atheromatous plaque may encroach upon the lumen of an artery. Further narrowing of the vessel may be produced by subintimal haemorrhage beneath the plaque, and eventual thrombosis may result. The clinical effects depend upon the vessel affected. There are certain sites of election for such atheromatous arterial stenosis and different clinical syndromes arise according to the vessel affected. Lesions of greater clinical importance involve:

1. The internal carotid origin and the vertebral origin. Lesions of these vessels give rise to cerebrovascular insufficiency and are discussed in greater detail in Chapter 60.
2. The coronary arteries, giving rise to cardiac ischaemia (Ch. 23).
3. The renal arteries, where hypertension may result.
4. The femoral and popliteal arteries.
5. The iliac arteries.
6. The abdominal aorta.

With lesions involving the abdominal aorta, iliac or lower limb arteries, intermittent claudication is the cardinal presenting symptom. Atheromatous stenosis also occurs in the upper limb but is of lesser clinical significance.

Atheromatous thrombosis of the abdominal aorta (Leriche syndrome) is not uncommon and we have personally encountered over 150 cases. Once a thrombosis of the abdominal aorta occurs it will slowly extend upwards, but in most cases it will stop short at the renal arteries (Fig. 26.37). Occasionally the origin of a renal artery may be involved and secondary hypertension result. Atheromatous thrombosis of the femoral or iliac arteries is extremely common (Fig. 26.38).

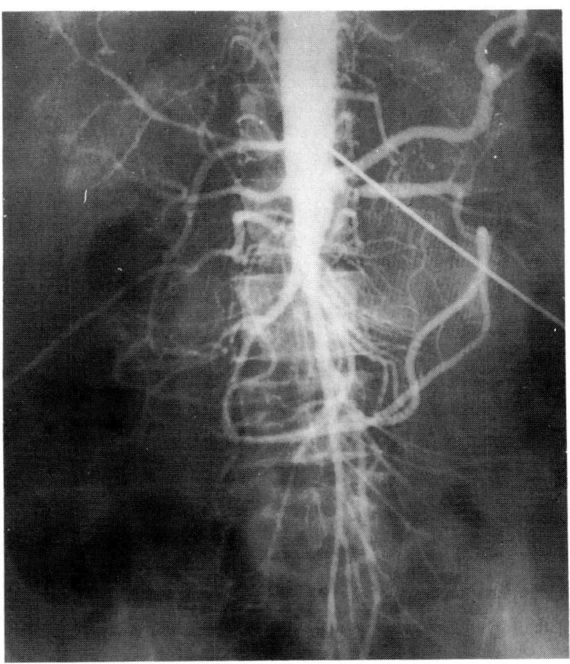

Fig. 26.37 Aortic thrombosis. There is also atheromatous stenosis of the left renal artery and filling of the inferior mesenteric from the artery of Drummond.

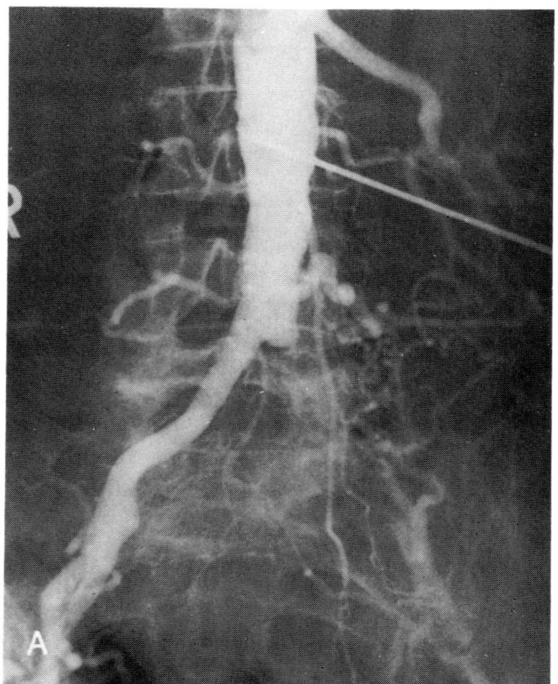

Fig. 26.38 Iliac thrombosis due to atheroma.

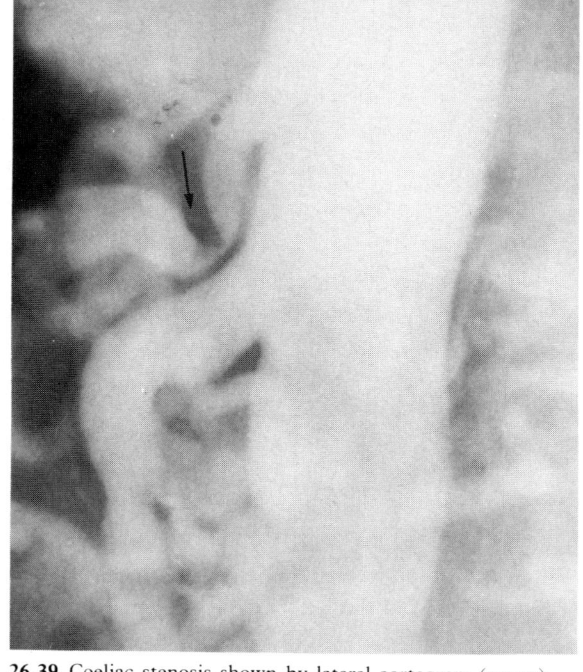

Fig. 26.39 Coeliac stenosis shown by lateral aortogram (arrow).

So-called *primary popliteal thrombosis* in young males may be due to atheroma, but can be caused by the rare popliteal cyst or by popliteal entrapment by an anomalous tendon.

Popliteal cysts usually occur in young males, the average age of onset of symptoms being 36 years. They present with calf claudication due to popliteal stenosis, which may later go on to thrombosis. The angiogram shows healthy arteries with a smooth narrowing suggesting external compression. The cyst is mucin-secreting and lies in the wall of the artery. It is thought to be due to developmental inclusion of mucin-secreting synovial cells derived from capsular synovial cells of the knee joint. Similar lesions have been seen in other arteries including the common iliac, radial and ulnar arteries.

Popliteal entrapment also occurs mainly in young males and is due to trapping of the popliteal artery by an anomalous tendon of the medial head of gastrocnemius. As noted patients usually present with acute thrombosis.

Atheromatous stenosis of the origins of the coeliac axis and mesenteric arteries has been cited as a possible cause of gastrointestinal dysfunction. Fibromuscular hyperplasia has also been described in these vessels. The coeliac axis may also be narrowed at its origin by external compression either by the median arcuate ligament of the diaphragm, or by coeliac plexus fibrosis giving rise to the so-called '*coeliac compression syndrome*' (Fig. 26.39). It should be realized however, that the inferior mesenteric artery can be completely occluded without referable symptoms as frequently happens in the Leriche syndrome. This is because there is an excellent collateral circulation from the superior mesenteric and other vessels. Stenosis and occlusion of the other splanchnic vessels can also occur without symptoms. We have even encountered patients with both coeliac axis and superior mesenteric artery occluded in whom the inferior mesenteric supplied an adequate collateral circulation (Figs 26.19, 26.40).

Coronary stenosis and **thrombosis** is extremely common. Coronary arteriography is now widely practised in this investigation and is discussed in detail in Chapter 23, as is the use of coronary angioplasty by the Gruntzig technique.

Renal artery stenosis. Ischaemia of the kidney is an important and sometimes remediable cause of hypertension. The commonest cause is atheroma of the origin of the renal artery (Fig. 26.41 A and B). It may also occur with other lesions and of these *fibromuscular hyperplasia* is the one most frequently encountered. This is a rare disease of unknown aetiology, further discussed below. The artery shows irregular muscular hypertrophy and luminal narrowing (Fig. 26.42 A and B).

Rare causes of renal artery stenosis are *extrinsic pressure* by fibrous bands or tumours, *neurofibromatosis* and so-called *congenital hypoplasia*. As noted above, *aortic thrombosis* may be complicated by stenosis of a renal origin. Takayashu syndrome, a *non-specific aortitis*, may also be complicated by renal artery stenosis, as may the rare *abdominal coarctation*.

Whatever the cause of the renal ischaemia, secondary

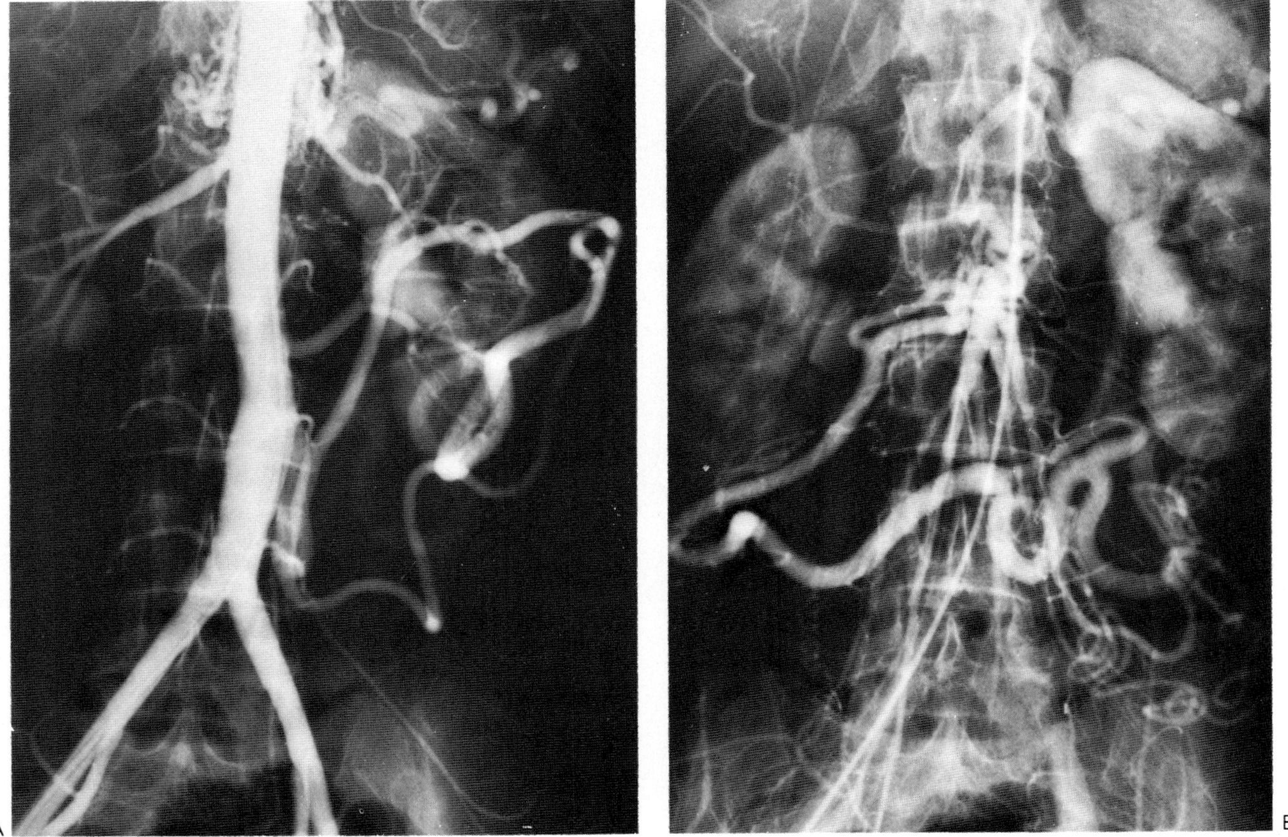

Fig. 26.40 A. Occlusion of coeliac and superior mesenteric arteries. Separate origin of splenic artery and low origin of right renal artery. Hypertrophied artery of Drummond arising from inferior mesenteric. **B.** Artery of Drummond supplies superior mesenteric origin and then hepatic artery through pancreatic arcades.

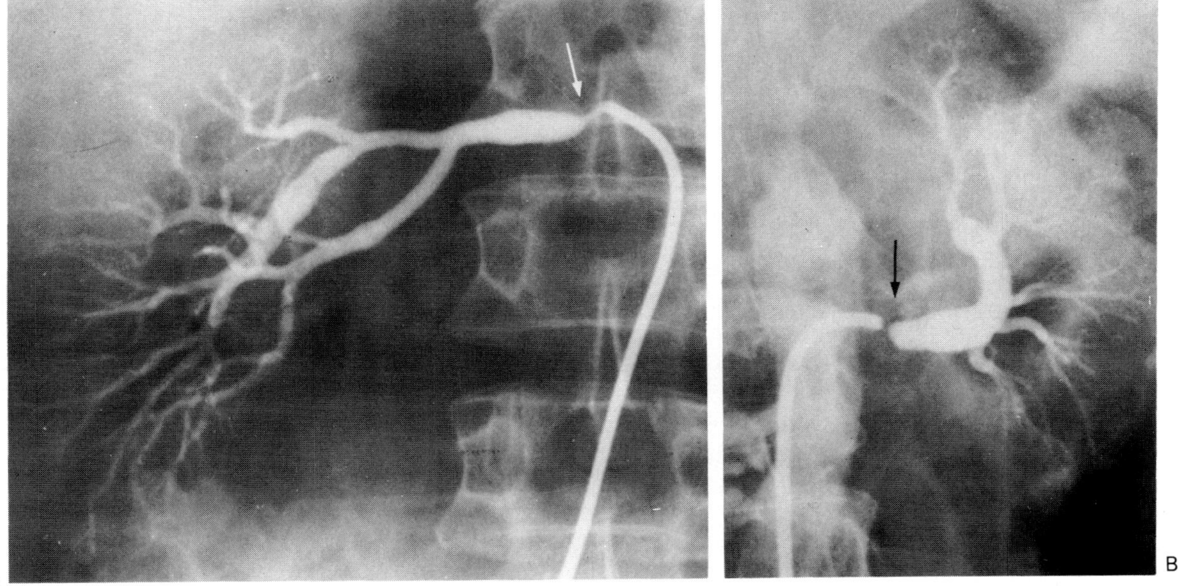

Fig. 26.41 A. Renal artery stenosis due to atheroma. **B.** Renal artery stenosis. Note poststenotic dilation of the renal artery.

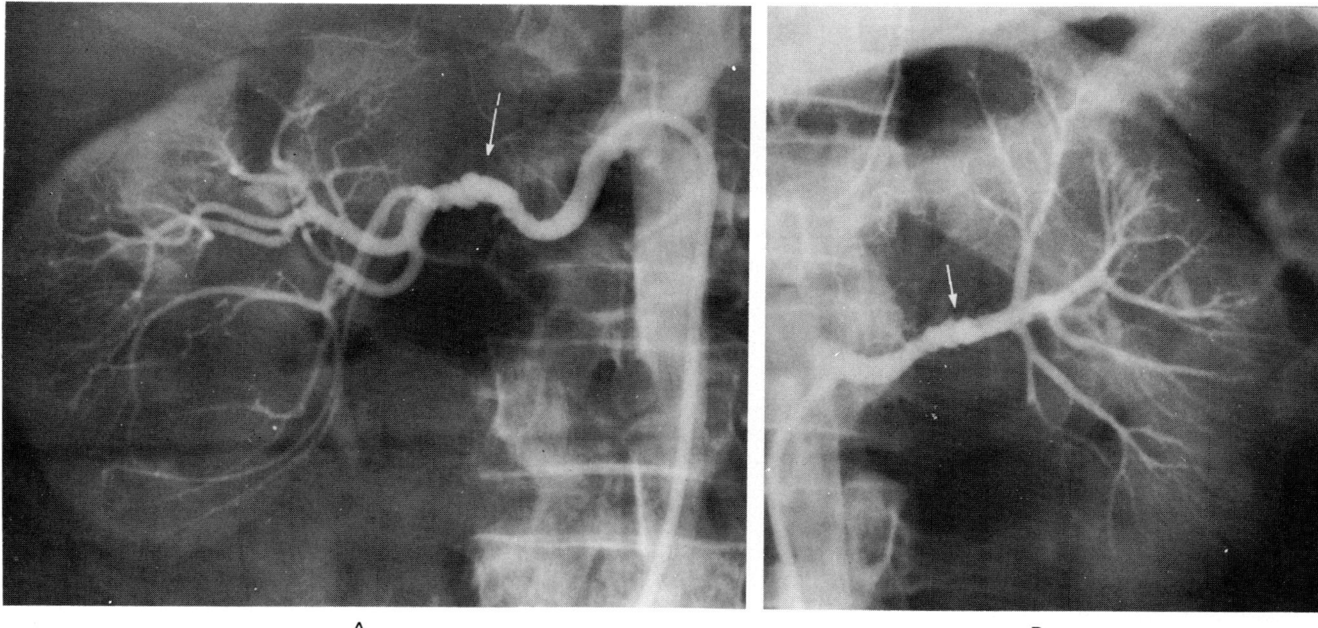

Fig. 26.42 A. and **B.** Renal artery fibromuscular hyperplasia (arrows).

changes usually develop in the kidney and these may be recognized at plain X-ray and at intravenous pyelography. The affected kidney is usually smaller than its normal fellow but remains smooth in contour. A high proportion of these cases also show increased concentration of the contrast medium on the affected side with rather small spindly calyces. This is because the ischaemic kidney will reabsorb water well although the volume of glomerular filtrate is smaller. There is often also a slight initial delay in excretion of contrast on the affected side because of the reduced blood flow. This is best demonstrated on early films taken 1, 2 and 3 minutes after injection of the contrast medium. The differences in concentration of the contrast medium on the two sides can also be exaggerated by so-called 'water load IVP'. In this examination about 500 ml of water is drunk just before the contrast injection. This promotes a diuresis which may accentuate the difference in concentration of contrast medium in the calyces and pelves on the two sides.

It has already been noted that renal artery stenosis can now be treated by the radiologist using the Gruntzig technique of percutaneous catheterization and balloon dilatation of the stenosis. Figure 26.11 illustrates a case of hypertension in a young man where simple dilatation produced an immediate and dramatic improvement. The blood pressure remained at normal levels on follow-up two years later. The method has the advantage that it can be repeated should stenosis recur.

In recent years there has been increasing use of DSA as a screening technique for demonstrating or excluding a diagnosis of renal artery stenosis.

Subclavian stenosis. Compression of the subclavian artery at the root of the neck is seen in the *thoracic inlet syndrome* and may be associated with various anomalies. These include cervical rib and anomalous first rib which will be obvious at simple X-ray. In many cases however there is no obvious cause on plain X-ray and the compression is due to a fibrous band or the scalenus anticus muscle.

Clinically these patients may present with ischaemic hands, with Reynaud's phenomenon or with peripheral emboli, usually involving the digits. The latter arise from clot which usually forms in poststenotic aneurysms. These are quite common in our experience and are usually fusiform though they can be saccular (Fig. 26.43 A and B). Thrombosis of the subclavian artery can also occur (Fig. 26.44).

Radiological investigation is usually by subclavian arteriography following transfemoral catheterization. Important features of the examination are arteriography with the limb first in neutral position, and then with the artery stretched by Adson's manoeuvre. The latter consists of fully abducting the arm with the head turned to the opposite side. In cases with minimal or doubtful changes at standard arteriography Adson's manoeuvre will often show clear evidence of compression (Fig. 26.45 A and B).

DSA now offers a less invasive method of showing these lesions (Fig. 26.45).

Reynaud's phenomenon. This may occur in healthy individuals as an abnormal response to cold (spastic type). The lesion may also be secondary to organic disease of the arteries both major and minor. Table 26.5 lists the

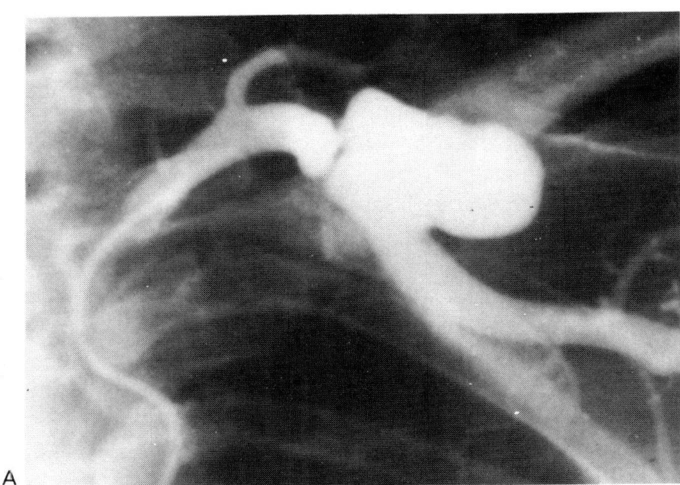

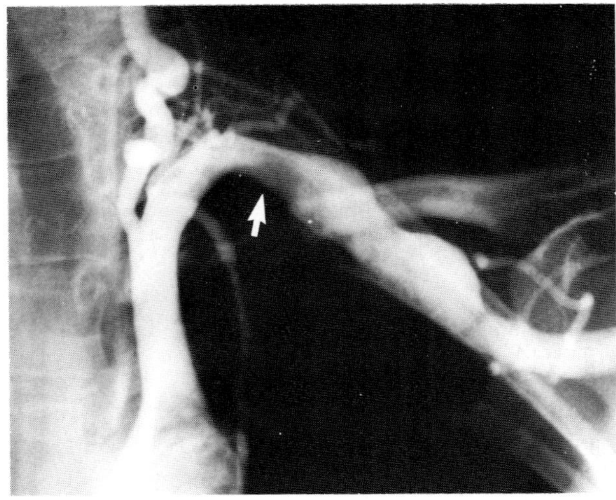

Fig. 26.43 Subclavian stenosis with poststenotic aneurysm formation. **A.** Saccular. **B.** Fusiform aneurysm.

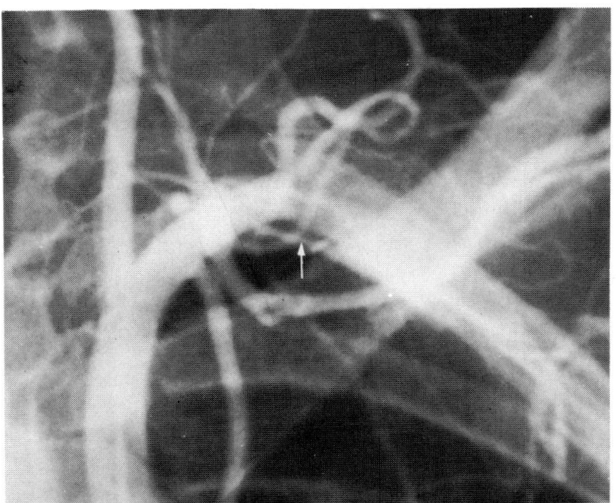

Fig. 26.44 Subclavian thrombosis (arrow).

numerous diseases which have been associated with Reynaud's phenomenon and organic digital ischaemia.

Atheromatous lesions in the upper limb are usually less marked and less disabling than in the lower limbs since the collateral circulation around the shoulder and elbows is so good. Nevertheless, atheroma is found quite frequently in the proximal and peripheral arteries of the upper limb. The commonest proximal segment to be occluded is the first part of the left subclavian artery. We have often

Fig. 26.45 Right subclavian artery shown by DSA. **A.** In neutral position there is slight fusiform aneurysmal dilatation, but no obvious stenosis. **B.** With Adson's manoeuvre there is marked obstruction.

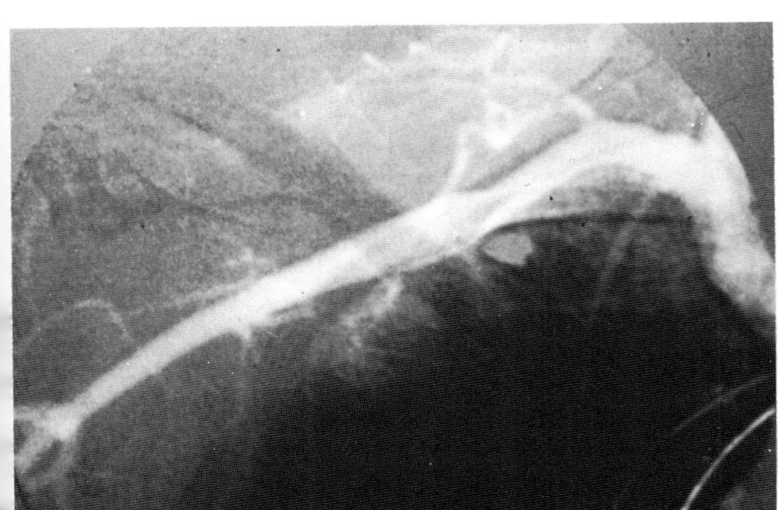

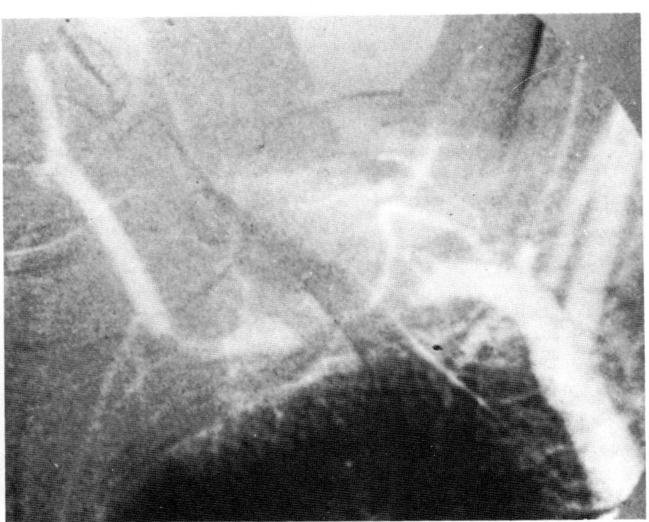

Table 26.5 Digital ischaemia and Reynaud's phenomenon

1. Lesions of major vessels (often with small vessel emboli)
Atheroma
Takayashu disease
Non-specific arteritis
African idiopathic aortitis
Thoracic inlet syndrome
Buerger's disease
Fibromuscular hyperplasia
2. Collagen disorder
Scleroderma
DLE
Rheumatoid arthritis
Polyarteritis nodosa
3. Blood disorders
Polycythaemia
Sickle cell disease
Cryoagglutination
The contraceptive pill
PVC poisoning
4. Specific conditions
Reynaud's phenomenon (spastic type)
Vibrating tools
Ergotism

discovered occlusions here as symptomless chance findings in patients being investigated for cerebrovascular lesions. When the first part of the left subclavian is occluded there is, in most cases, an excellent collateral flow to the arm by reverse flow down the left vertebral. This arrangement has been christened 'subclavian steal' by American workers on the basis that blood is being stolen from the brain to supply the upper limb.

We reviewed our first 30 cases of this syndrome and found very little correlation between the subclavian steal and cerebral symptoms. The left brachial pulse was often surprisingly good though blood pressure in the affected limb was usually slightly less than in the normal limb. The same phenomenon may occur on the right side but is less frequent as the proximal segment of the right subclavian is shorter than the left. Occlusion of the innominate artery can also occur leading to both right subclavian and right carotid steal.

Atheromatous occlusions are also met with in the distal upper limb vessels. In the digital vessels they can give rise to severe symptoms of localized ischaemia which may require amputation. Most cases of localized ischaemia of a digit in elderly men are due to this aetiology though there are other potential causes of the syndrome.

Generalized ischaemia of the fingers is more likely to be due to generalized disease such as scleroderma.

Buerger's disease has always been a controversial subject since the original description in 1908. The diagnosis of Buerger's disease, or 'thromboangiitis obliterans', became increasingly popular in the 1920s and 1940s and was made on clinical grounds in most cases of peripheral gangrene and ischaemia. It was also made in cases of thrombosis of the internal carotid artery. Thus, Moniz (1931) in his original monograph described the first cases of internal carotid thrombosis to be shown by angiography and made the erroneous assumption that these were due to 'thromboangiitis obliterans'!

As a healthy reaction to overdiagnosis of Buerger's disease, Wessler et al (1960) pointed out that in most of the cases examined by them the pathological lesions were indistinguishable from those due to atheroma with peripheral thrombosis. This gave rise to the view held by some that Buerger's disease was a myth and most so-called cases were due to atheroma.

Angiographic studies, however, have shown that whatever the nature of the specific lesions in Buerger's disease there is little doubt that it is a separate entity. It occurs in a much younger age group than does atheroma and many of our patients have been in their 20s and 30s. Although atheroma has a predominantly male sex incidence it is also found in females and the incidence is increasing with the more widespread habit of cigarette addiction in women. On the other hand, Buerger's disease is virtually confined to males, and female cases are very rare. There is also however, a direct connection with heavy cigarette smoking. Angiographically the appearances are characteristic and quite unlike those of atheroma. The lesions affect the distal vessels which become totally occluded and the occlusions then spread upwards in the limbs. Above the level of the blocks the major vessels seem smooth-walled and healthy with no evidence of disease and no suggestion of atheroma (Fig. 26.46). Often one or more long tortuous collaterals are seen following the course of a main calf artery, and it has been suggested that these are due to hypertrophy of the vasa vasorum.

Spasm. An unusual form of peripheral vascular disease occasionally diagnosed is diffuse peripheral spasm due to *Ergot poisoning*. The patients are suffering from migraine, have been overdosed and then present with peripheral ischaemia usually in the lower limbs, though the arms can be affected. In two patients seen by us, the diagnosis was not suspected until angiography had been performed. The appearances at arteriography are quite characteristic, and show the large vessels in the lower limb below the common femoral arteries contracting down to narrow, thread-like structures. Recovery to normal is rapid once the patient is taken off Ergotamine. Similar changes may occur in the upper limbs, but are less common, and spasm has also been recorded in splanchnic vessels.

Localized spasm of peripheral arteries is sometimes seen at arteriography, usually in smaller vessels with a prominent muscular coat, and is thought to be caused by irritation from the catheter tip or a local high concentration of contrast medium. It is characteristically found just distal to the tip of the catheter and should not be mistaken for a true stenosis. Its spastic nature is usually revealed by repeating the injection with the catheter withdrawn to a more proximal position.

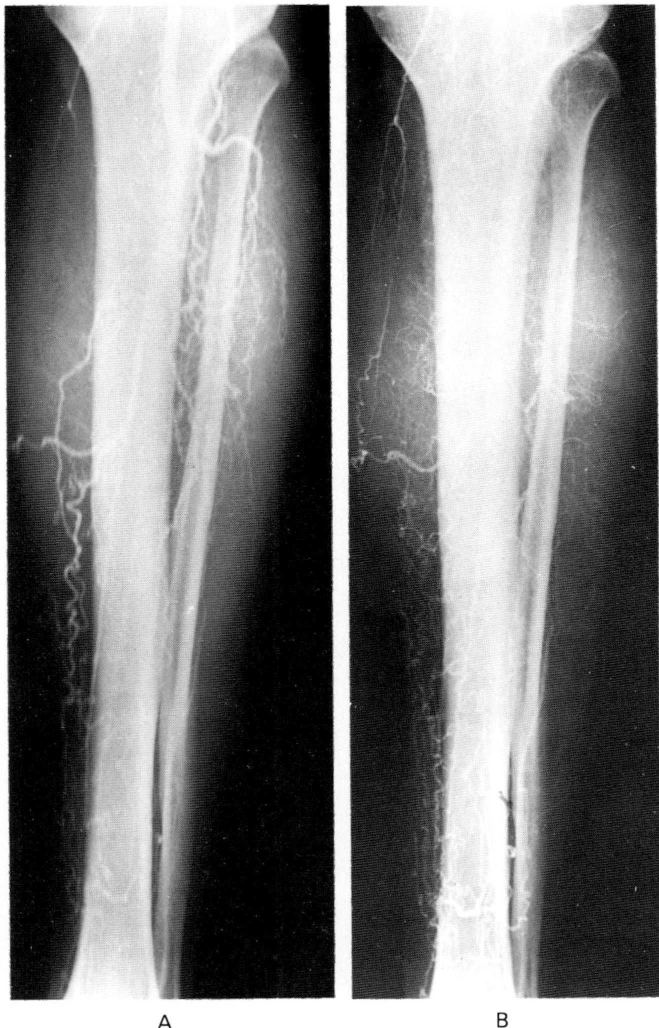

Fig. 26.46 A. and **B.** Buerger's disease. Femoral arteriography showed normal smooth-walled femoral and popliteal arteries, but occlusion of the calf vessels with collaterals.

Beaded spasm is a descriptive term applied to an unusual appearance seen most frequently in the femoral and popliteal arteries, but also encountered in other vessels including the iliac and splanchnic arteries. The condition has also been called 'standing' or 'stationary arterial waves' or arterial beading. It does not appear to represent true pathology and may be a physical phenomenon due to arterial pressure waves, though this is debated. In our experience it has been most frequently seen in the femoral arteries of patients with Buerger's disease and obliterated calf vessels. The regular and perfectly symmetrical nature of the beading, which has been likened to a 'chain of pearls' helps to distinguish it from the less regular and asymmetrical appearance of fibromuscular hyperplasia.

Fibromuscular hyperplasia is an unusual arterial disease first described in the renal arteries. Here the lesion is most frequently seen in young adult females and is a significant

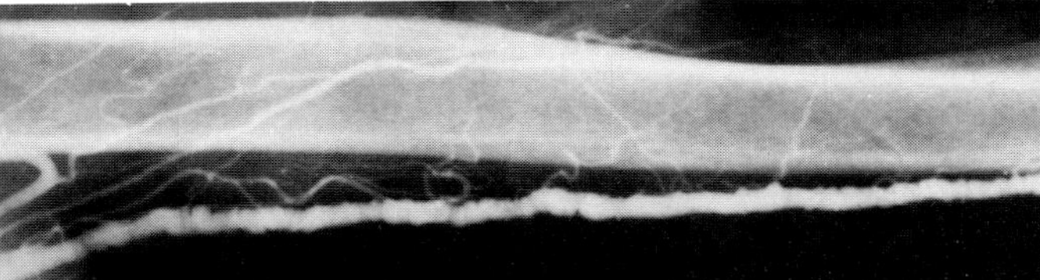

Fig. 26.47 Fibromuscular hyperlasia of the brachial artery. Female aged 50 presenting with digital ischaemia.

cause of renal artery stenosis and hypertension. The disease is characterized angiographically by an irregular beaded appearance of the artery with stenoses and sacculations. The latter are sometimes aneurysmal. The stenoses may be severe enough to cause renal ischaemia and hypertension.

While the lesions are presumably of congenital origin their exact cause remains a mystery (Fig. 26.42). They have also been demonstrated in other vessels, including the splanchnic arteries, and we have encountered examples in the superior mesenteric, coeliac and external iliac arteries. Cases have also been described in the literature in the internal carotid artery but the lesion appears to be rare in the vessels of the limbs. However, we have personally encountered a very striking case in the brachial arteries of a middle-aged female, presenting with digital ischaemia (Fig. 26.47).

EMBOLUS

Embolus of the systemic system is most commonly seen with atrial fibrillation and intra-atrial clot. The commonest cause of this complication is mitral valve disease. Embolus

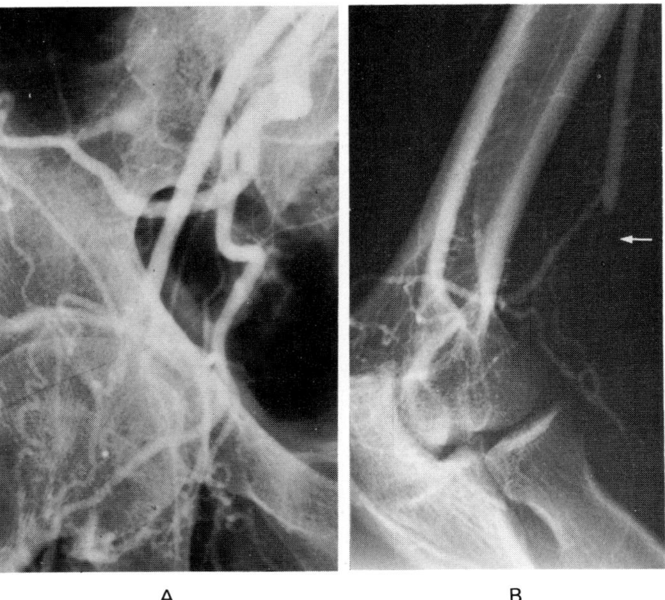

Fig. 26.48 A. Embolic occlusion of the iliac artery. **B.** Embolic occlusion of the brachial artery.

may also result from clot formation in the left ventricle following cardiac infarction. Emboli may also be detached from mural thrombus forming on atheromatous plaques or in aneurysms. The rare paradoxical embolus results from a clot arising in a peripheral vein passing through a septal defect to reach the left side of the heart. The intracardiac defect across which an embolus reaches the left side of the heart is almost always a patent foramen ovale, which is present in nearly one-third of the population. Normally right to left shunting is prevented by a valve at the foramen, and the fact that pressure in the left atrium is higher than that in the right. Thus, the only way in which paradoxical embolus can occur is when right atrial pressure exceeds left atrial pressure. This can occur from massive pulmonary embolus or from chronic lung disease.

Clinically it may be difficult to distinguish an acute embolus from an acute thrombosis, but with most cases of embolus there is clinical evidence of the predisposing cause. Peripheral emboli in the limbs usually have quite a good prognosis even with conservative treatment. Surgery may be required with the larger and more proximal emboli, such as aortic bifurcation or iliac bifurcation embolus. Angiography will localize the lesions with complete accuracy (Fig. 26.48). Cerebral emboli are discussed in Chapter 60.

ANGIOMATOUS MALFORMATIONS

(synonyms: angioma; congenital arteriovenous fistula)

In this condition there are direct communications between arterioles and venules without the interposition of a capillary bed. The lesion is congenital and in our experience is most common in the cerebral circulation though it can occur anywhere in the body. The cerebral lesions are

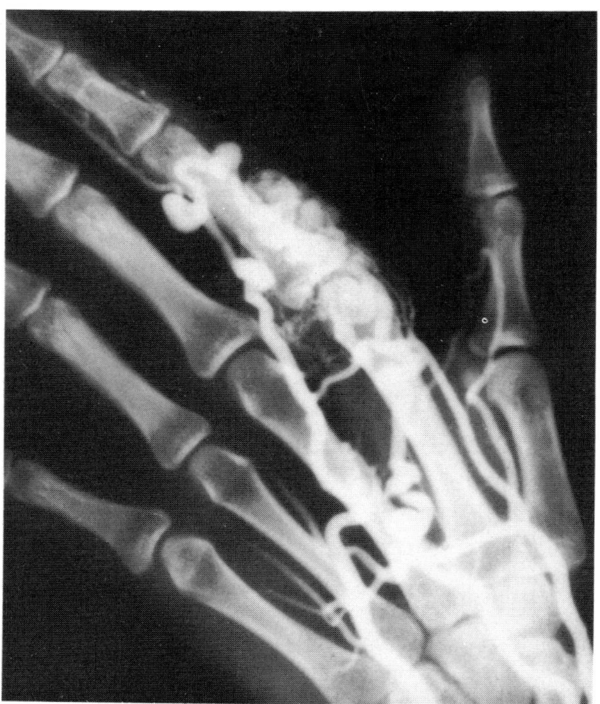

Fig. 26.49 Angioma of the hand.

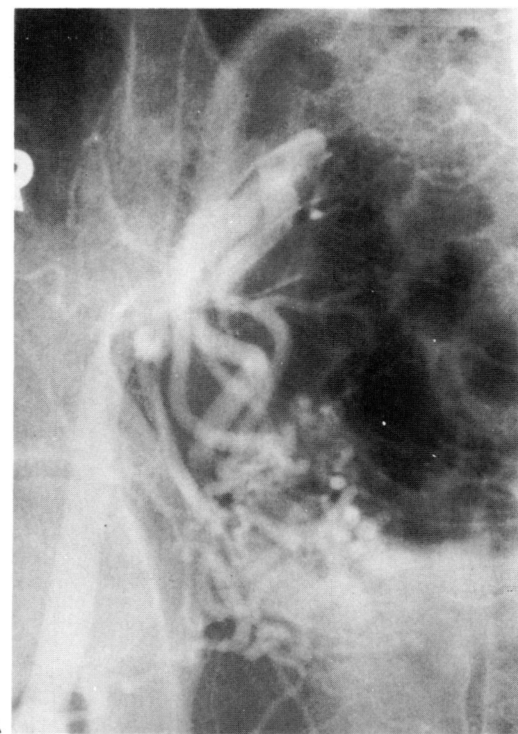

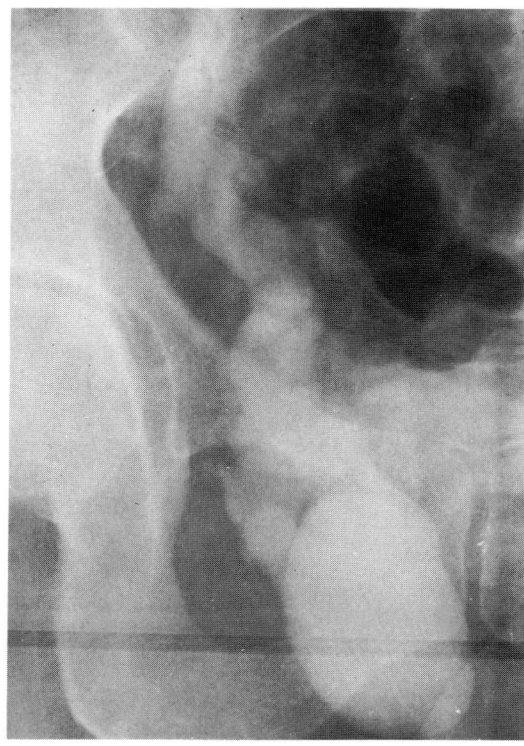

Fig. 26.50 A. and **B.** Angioma of the pelvis, presenting as vulval swelling. Aneurysmal dilatation of draining vein.

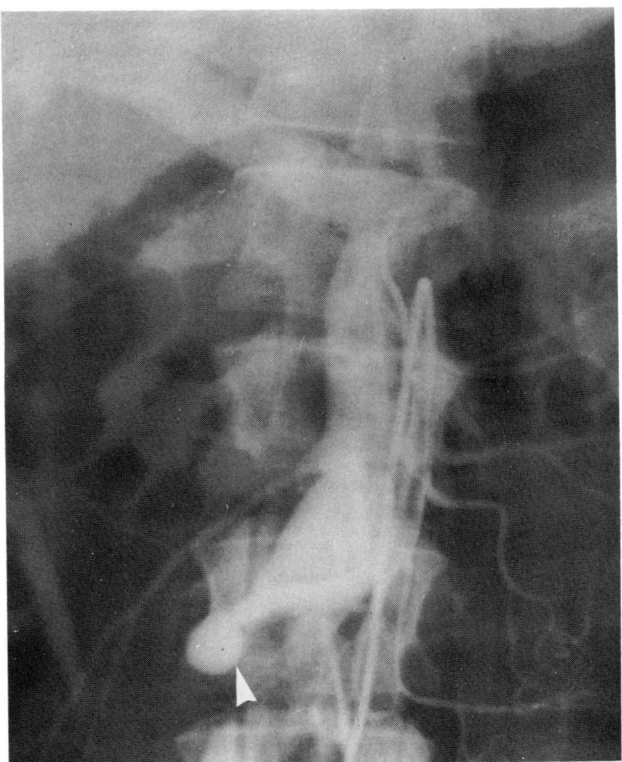

Fig. 26.51 Mesenteric-portal fistula (arrowed) shown by selective superior mesenteric injection. There is rapid filling of dilated superior mesenteric and portal veins. The lesion followed a crush injury to the abdomen.

discussed in detail in Chapter 60. These lesions must be distinguished from acquired communications between arteries and veins or arteriovenous fistula which is discussed below.

Figures 26.49, 26.50 and 26.54 show angiomatous malformations presenting in the hand, pelvis and bowel, respectively. The angiographic features are the presence of hypertrophied arteries leading to the lesion and filling early. Dilated veins are also shown filling early and draining the lesion. They may often be seen in the arterial phase and long before normal veins would fill. Larger angiomas can provide a considerable arteriovenous shunt and this may produce a high output cardiac failure. This complication is, however, rare and is only seen with very large angiomas.

Smaller angiomas at fine vessel level may be more difficult to demonstrate by angiography, particularly those with low flow or at precapillary level. Superselective angiography and magnification techniques may be necessary in such cases.

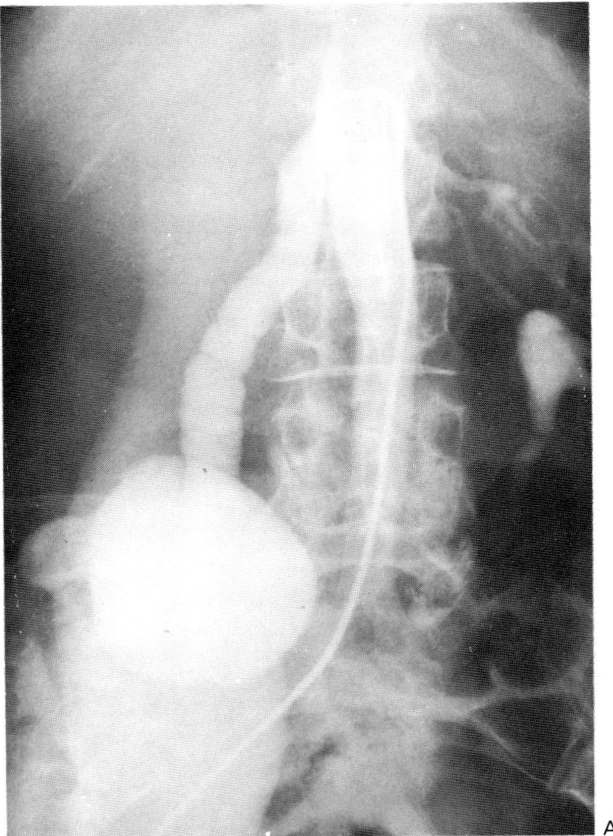

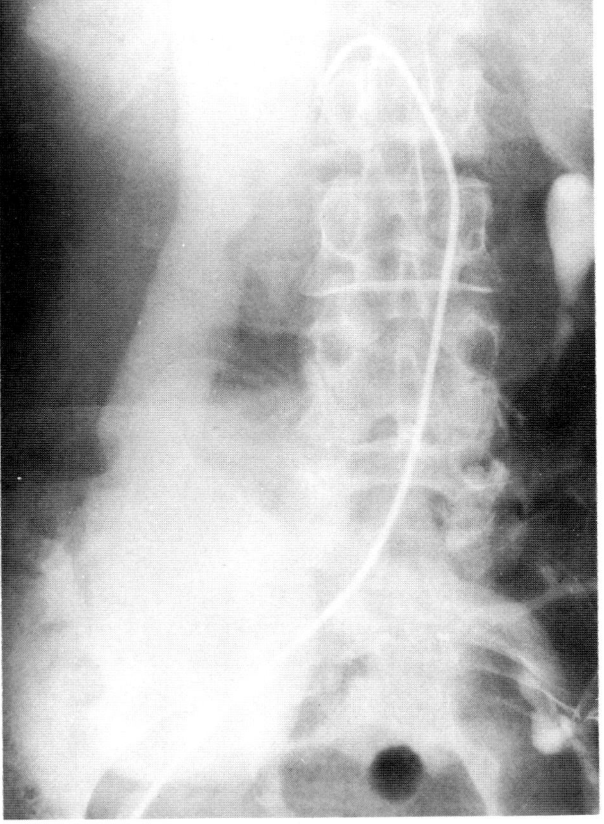

Fig. 26.52 Giant renal AV fistula. Possibly due to rupture of an aneurysm associated with fibromuscular hyperplasia. The patient presented with heart failure and a pulsating mass clinically thought to be pelvic. **A.** Arterial phase. **B.** Venous phase showing dilated IVC.

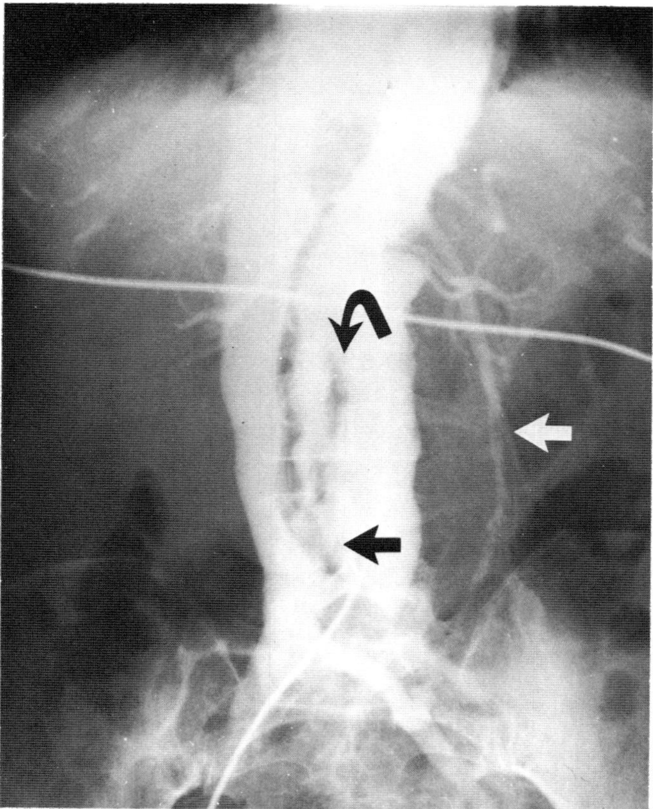

Fig. 26.53 Aortocaval fistula following spontaneous rupture of an abdominal aortic aneurysm. The superior mesenteric is displaced by the aneurysm containing mural thrombus (white arrow). The fistula into the IVC is marked by the black arrow. The curved arrow suggests an intimal flap in the aneurysm. (From Gregson et al 1983. Spontaneous aortocaval fistulae. *Clinical Radiology* **34**: 683–687, Fig. 1. Reproduced with permission of the Editor of *Clinical Radiology*.)

ARTERIOVENOUS FISTULA

Arteriovenous fistula is most commonly of *traumatic* origin. Gunshot wounds or other penetrating injuries are the most frequent cause but the lesion can follow non-penetrating trauma (Fig. 26.51). Such fistulae can occur anywhere in the body and we have encountered them in all anatomical sites from the foot to the scalp.

Spontaneous arteriovenous fistula can also occur from rupture of a diseased artery into an adjacent vein though this is much less frequent (Fig. 26.52). A common site for spontaneous arteriovenous fistula is the cavernous sinus where it gives rise to pulsating exophthalmos. This is presumably due to rupture of a carotid aneurysm in the cavernous sinus and is discussed in Chapter 60. Spontaneous arteriovenous fistula can also occur from rupture of an abdominal aneurysm leading to aortocaval fistula (Fig. 26.53). These can provide difficult diagnostic problems and the diagnosis can be easily missed.

So-called *congenital* arteriovenous fistula is sometimes seen in infants and children, but it is difficult in these cases to exclude previous trauma. We have seen such fistulae involving the thoracic aorta and azygos system in a small girl, and involving the vertebral artery in a small boy.

Iatrogenic arteriovenous fistula, apart from those deliberately induced for dialysis, has followed a number of surgical procedures including orthopaedic operations on the hip, ankle and spine. Thus aortocaval and ilio-iliac fistula have been seen following lumbar disc surgery, and renal arteriovenous fistula may be seen as a complication of renal biopsy (Fig. 26.13). Arteriography has given rise to arteriovenous fistula at the site of arterial puncture and has been recorded in the brachial and vertebral arteries, and rarely in the femoral artery.

A traumatic arteriovenous fistula develops hypertrophied veins draining it. It may be extremely difficult to localize at operation, and arteriography is therefore invaluable in the preoperative assessment. As with angiomas, the dilated arteries fill early and the dilated veins will usually fill in the arterial phase. Rapid serial films and the injection of large quantities of contrast may be necessary to show these lesions fully.

A large traumatic arteriovenous fistula can lead to a high cardiac output state and this may result in cardiac failure unless successfully treated.

In recent years, small arteriovenous fistulas have been increasingly treated by embolization as described above (Fig. 26.13).

HAEMORRHAGE

Angiography has proved extremely helpful in the control of patients with acute gastrointestinal haemorrhage.

Upper gastrointestinal haemorrhage. Treatment will depend on the state of the patient and the degree of haemorrhage. In patients with massive haemorrhage and severe collapse, whose lives are in obvious danger despite attempted resuscitation, laparotomy will be indicated. Patients in a less serious and more stable condition with acute upper gastrointestinal tract bleeding will be examined by endoscopy in the first place. Angiography will be reserved for cases requiring embolization or pharmacological therapy.

Patients of an intermediate group considered too ill or uncooperative for endoscopy, and who are bleeding briskly, may be investigated by angiography. It should be pointed out that the rate of blood loss must be about 5–6 ml a minute to show at arteriography, though a superselective injection could show bleeds as slow as 1 ml a minute. The characteristic angiographic appearance is a smear of contrast extravasation persisting at the site of the bleed, whether from a peptic ulcer, Mallory-Weiss tear or gastritis. Treatment of these cases by embolization or pharmacological therapy has been discussed above.

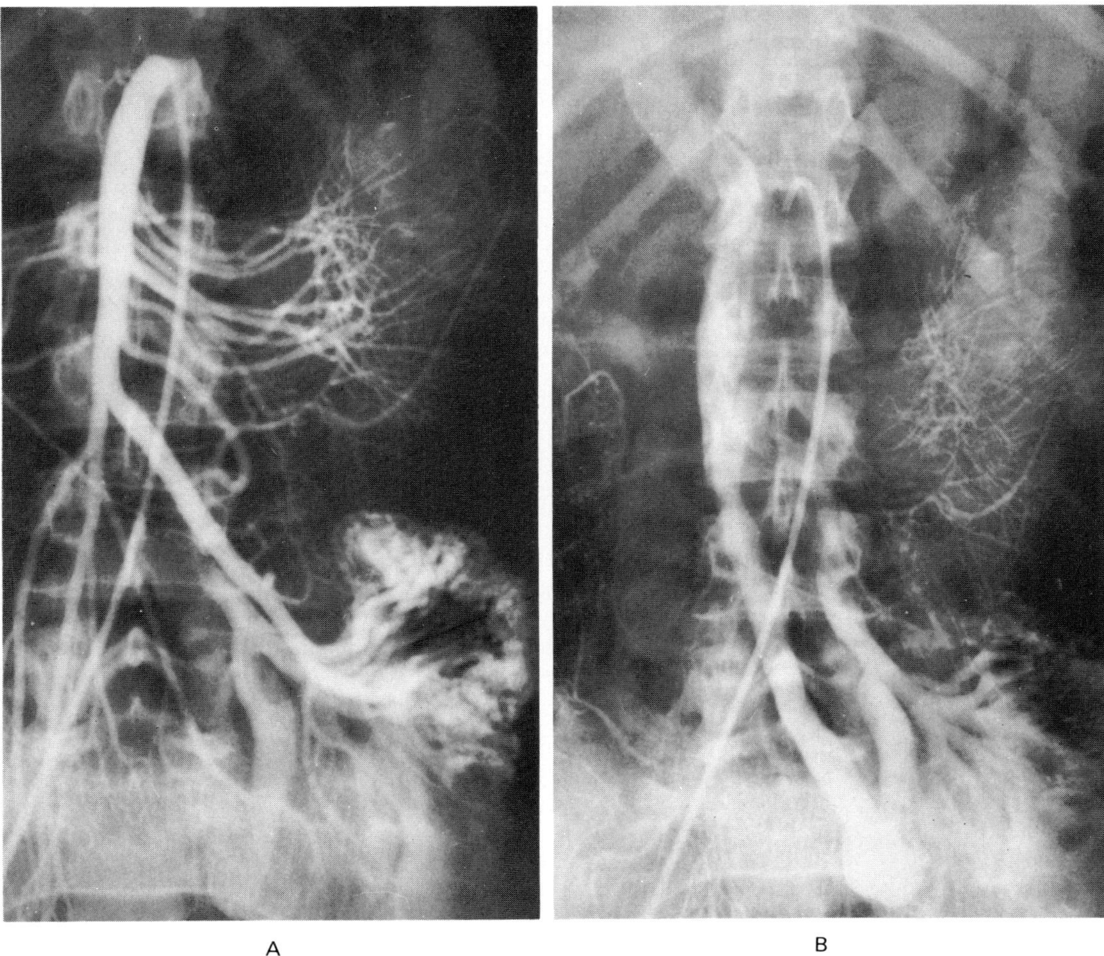

Fig. 26.54 A. and **B.** Angioma of the small bowel with high volume shunting into the portal system. Female of 24 with repeated attacks of melaena. In the previous 10 years she had had four barium enemas and five barium follow-throughs with negative findings. Large angiomas like this are unusual, small areas of dysplasia being more common.

Another indication for angiography is the individual with persistent bouts of haemorrhage either from the small or large bowel where all conventional methods of examination have failed to demonstrate a causative lesion (Fig. 26.54).

Lower gastrointestinal tract haemorrhage. Persistent haemorrhage from the distal bowel is usually investigated first by proctosigmoidoscopy to rule out lesions in the rectum and distal sigmoid. However, it should be noted that colonic carcinoma and polyps rarely present with severe bleeding.

Many patients with acute severe rectal bleeding and no other symptoms are suffering from colonic diverticula. When such diverticula bleed they are usually on the right side, though diverticula are in fact more numerous in the sigmoid. Bleeding from colonic diverticula has been controlled by intra-arterial vasopressin. Another cause of bleeding in elderly patients is a small area of vascular ectasia in the right colon. Such lesions are often small and require good quality angiograms for their demonstration. Arteriovenous shunting with rapid vein filling should always raise suspicion of such a lesion.

Radioisotope scanning is a useful method of demonstrating the site of lower gastrointestinal bleeding in a simple and non-invasive way and can be performed as a preliminary to angiography if time permits. It is claimed that bleeding at rates as low as 0.1 ml per minute can be detected by the use of such agents as $^{99}Tc^{m}$ sulphur colloid or of $^{99}Tc^{m}$-labelled red cells.

NEOPLASMS AND MASS LESIONS

Angiography has proved of great value in the diagnosis of neoplasms and other mass lesions. The value of the method has varied in different organs, but has proved greatest in organs like the brain or kidney which are deep seated or not readily accessible to clinical examination.

The value of angiography in the diagnosis of tumours arises from three facts. *First*, tumours have circulations which may differ from that of the organ in which they arise. This results in abnormal or 'pathological' vessels being outlined by contrast during arteriography, thus localizing and identifying the neoplasm. Arteriovenous shunting with early filling of tumour drainage veins is a frequent feature of the more malignant and vascular tumours. *Second*, the growth of the tumour may displace and deform the normal vessels at its periphery. The stretched or distorted vessel enables the lesions to be localized. *Third*, tumours may involve arteries of supply, producing 'cuffing' and irregular narrowing of the affected artery.

The so-called 'pathological vessels' are in some cases specific to a particular tumour and this may result in pathological diagnosis being possible from the angiogram, e.g. the meningioma 'smear' seen in cerebral angiography.

Angiography is of course an invasive diagnostic technique with potential hazards. The newer imaging techniques of isotope scanning, ultrasound, CT and MRI are preferable as primary investigations in most mass lesions. In many cases they can supply a clear-cut answer to the diagnostic problems. However, they have by no means replaced angiography, which is still widely used to complement the non-invasive investigations or provide further information. The scope of angiography has at the same time been extended by the new therapeutic techniques described above.

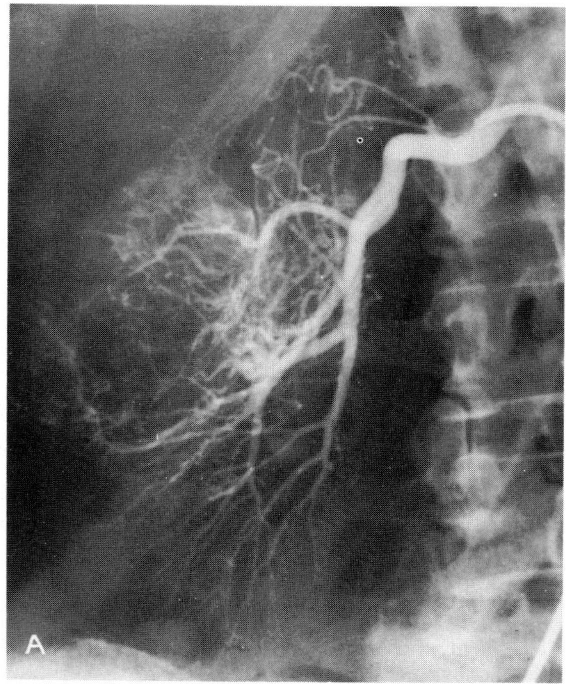

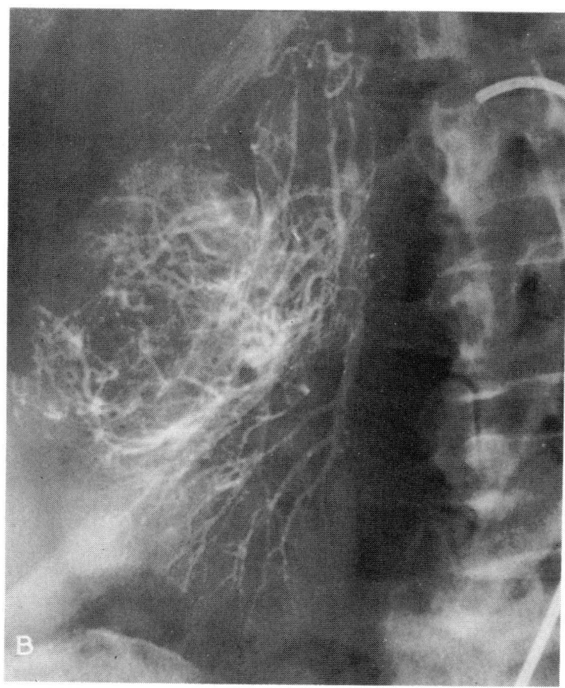

Fig. 26.55 Renal carcinoma showing pathological vessels.

RENAL MASSES

For many years arteriography was the method of choice for elucidating the nature of mass lesions in the kidney. Ultrasound or CT now offer non-invasive methods of demonstrating renal masses and differentiating between cysts and neoplasms, and either method will now provide a definitive diagnosis.

Ultrasound has the advantage of being cheaper and, if a cyst is demonstrated, can be followed immediately by cyst puncture and aspiration under ultrasound control. CT will provide more information about a neoplasm, including local infiltration and glandular involvement.

Renal angiography nevertheless is still quite widely used in cases of renal carcinoma. This is to assess the vascularity of the tumour and its suitability for preoperative embolization, and also for embolization in the treatment of non-operable cases.

Renal carcinoma is often a highly vascular tumour and the demonstration of typical pathological vessels in a renal expanding lesion is diagnostic (Fig. 26.55). Occasionally these tumours may be so vascular as to closely resemble angiomatous malformations (Fig. 26.56).

It should be remembered, however, that renal carcinoma may occasionally be non-vascular, in which case it may prove difficult to differentiate it angiographically from a cyst (Fig. 26.57). However, in these cases one can sometimes recognize tortuous or irregular vessels entering the periphery of the avascular cyst-like mass.

Epinephrine has been used at some centres to help elucidate cases where angiography is equivocal. Doses as high as 10–25 mg have been used, but these are unnecess-

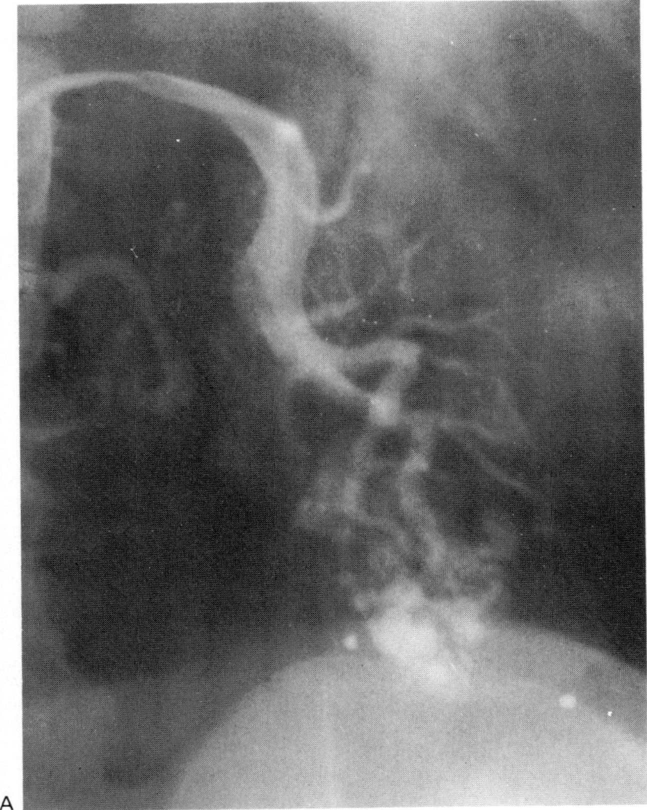

A

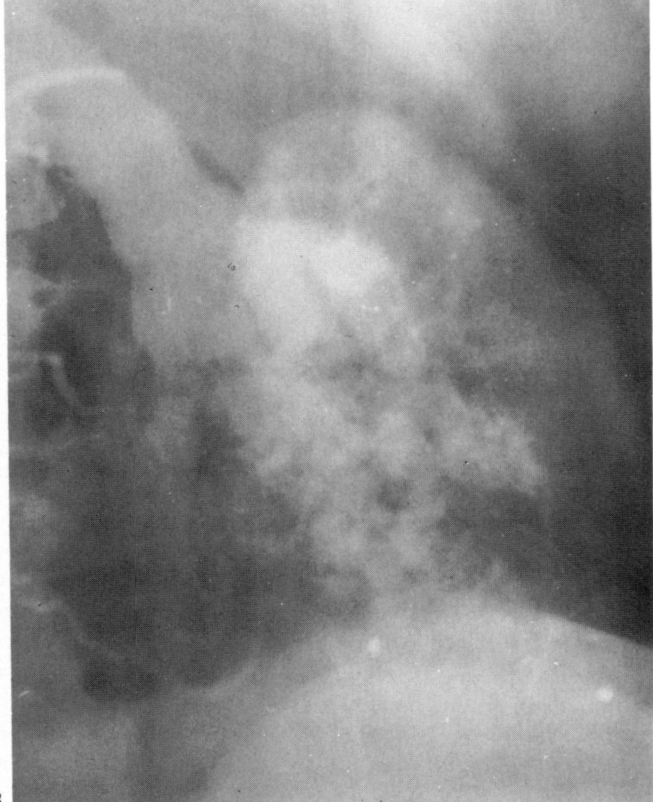

B

Fig. 26.56 Highly vascular renal carcinoma resembling angioma. Note huge drainage vein in nephrogram phase.

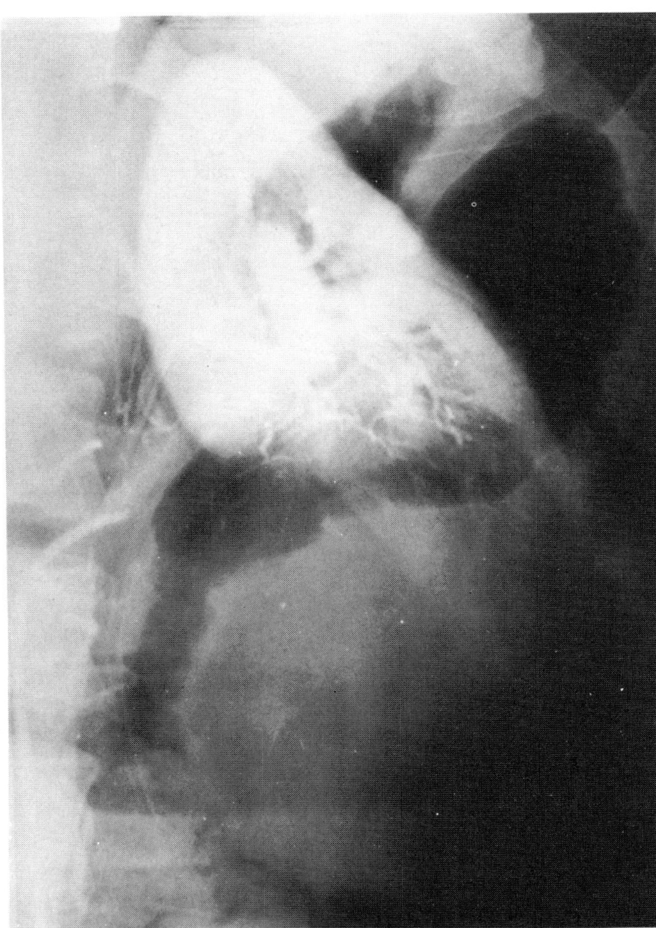

Fig. 26.57 Avascular carcinoma simulating cyst. Note: there is no evidence of pathological vessels in the tumour but the vessels at its upper margin are tortuous and not stretched as one would expect with a cyst.

ary, and satisfactory results are obtained with doses as low as 2–5 mg (Ekelund et al 1978). There is also a danger that the larger doses can shut down the normal arterial trunks supplying small peripheral tumours, leading to false negative diagnoses. The small dose is administered via the catheter in 10 ml of saline and followed 10–30 seconds later by the usual 8–10 ml of contrast medium. The adrenalin will close down the normal peripheral vessels, but not the abnormal neoplastic vessels which now stand out sharply in a relatively bloodless field. Since blood flow is reduced there is also less dilution of the contrast medium.

In contrast to renal carcinoma *renal cysts* generally appear as rounded avascular lesions best identified in the nephrogram phase. The cortex at the margin of the cyst may be displaced laterally and compressed, producing a beak-like projection of opacified cortex (Fig. 26.58). Further, the normal arteries will be stretched around the margin of the cyst in the arterial phase.

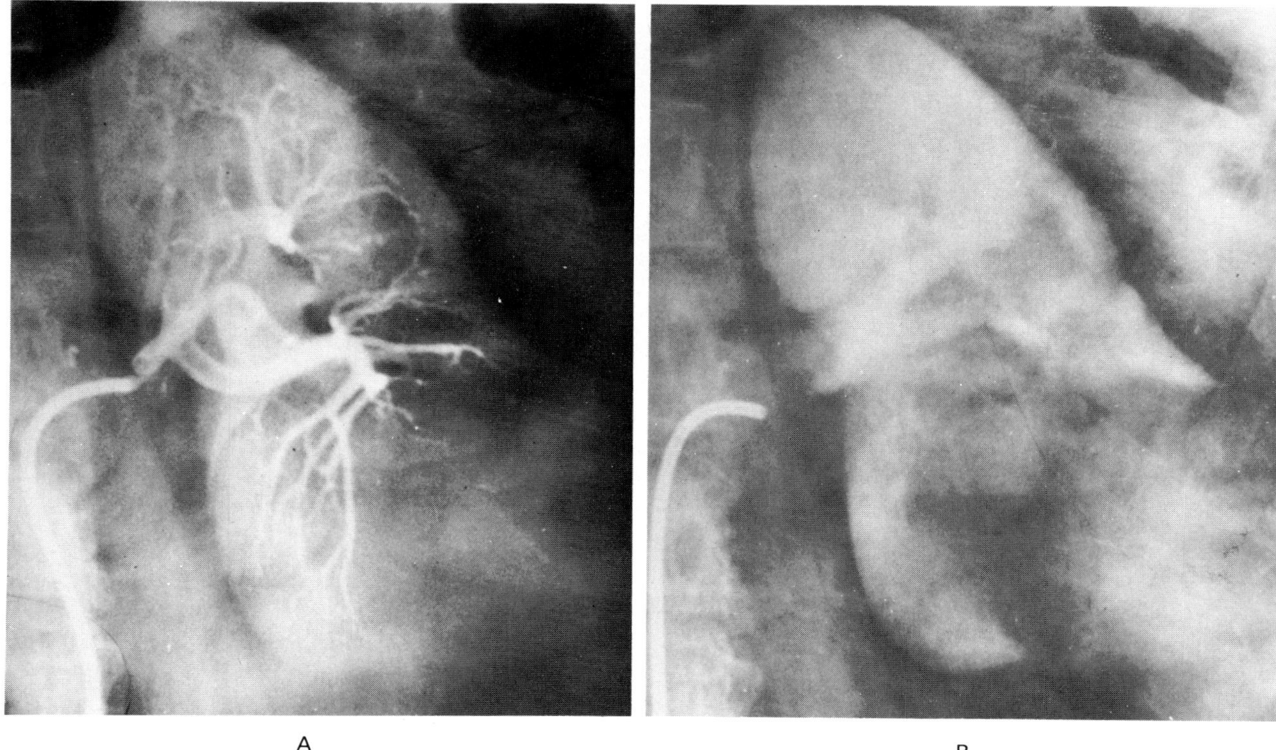

A B

Fig. 26.58 Renal cyst. Note displaced arteries in arterial phase and displaced cortex in nephrogram phase (beak sign).

Carcinoma of the renal pelvis is relatively avascular but has been identified with good quality selective arteriograms, as has the rare carcinoma of the ureter. In these cases one or more abnormal small tortuous vessels leading to the tumour are the diagnostic feature.

Wilms tumour (nephroblastoma) occurs in infants up to about 5 years of age, though it has occasionally been described in adults. Some 10% of cases are bilateral. The tumour is composed of both sarcomatous and carcinomatous elements and can reach a very large size. Differential diagnosis is usually from neuroblastoma. Although investigation is now by ultrasound or CT, angiography will also differentiate the two by showing a pathological circulation either in a distorted kidney or above a normal kidney. While a pathological circulation may be demonstrated, it should be appreciated that both these tumours can be nonvascular. However, diagnosis is still possible from the appearance of the nephrogram.

Renal angiography has also been of great value in the past in the assessment of various benign conditions which can simulate tumours and is still occasionally used for this purpose when ultrasound or CT are equivocal or nondiagnostic. These conditions include the so-called '*dromedary hump*', a bulge from the lateral surface of the kidney usually on the left side. Angiography will show that this merely represents normal renal tissue. *Pseudotumour* (cortical unfolding, or focal hypertrophy) is an unusual congenital lesion causing displacement of the calyces on the pyelogram and displacement of arteries on the angiogram. The infolded cortical tissue, however, shows a normal dense blush in the nephrogram phase.

True benign tumours of the kidney are rare but important in differential diagnosis. *Adenomas* are usually small and subcapsular in situation. There is a rare form of *giant benign renal adenoma* which at angiography is sharply circumscribed and separate from adjacent normal renal tissue. Angiography shows the lesion well but there is no arteriovenous shunting or puddling as with a hypernephroma.

Angiomyolipoma (*hamartoma*) is also a tumour which is histologically benign, though the angiogram usually shows a very vascular lesion which can be mistaken for a carcinoma. Hamartomas of this type occur in tuberous sclerosis (epiloia) when they may be multiple. *Xanthogranulomatous pyelonephritis* is a chronic inflammatory condition of the kidney, which also produces a vascular angiogram resembling neoplasm.

Renal oncocytoma have been described as rare benign tumours resembling hypernephroma, but well encapsulated and sometimes showing a 'spoke-wheel' pattern. The existence of this entity remains controversial and they are considered by some to be low grade hypernephromas.

Even rarer is the renin-secreting *juxtraglomerular cell tumour*, occasionally found in hypertensive patients. At angiography the tumour appears as a cortical defect resembling a small cyst in the nephrogram phase. A few fine vessels to the tumour may be identified as may the bulge in the surface of the kidney. Renin assay of the renal vein helps to confirm the diagnosis by showing consistently higher concentrations on the affected side.

Renal angiography has also proved valuable in the investigation and diagnosis of **vascular lesions.** Renal artery *stenosis* and *thrombosis*, and renal *arteriovenous fistula* have been discussed above. Renal artery *aneurysms* may also be encountered, most commonly in association with hypertension, or with *fibromuscular hyperplasia*. *Embolus* and *angiomatous malformation* have also been demonstrated by renal angiography.

Characteristic angiographic appearances can also be demonstrated in various other renal lesions, and this was particularly valuable in the investigation of the unilateral non-functioning kidney. *Hydronephrosis* showed a small renal artery with its branches stretched and splayed around the dilated pelvis and calyces. The nephrogram phase showed only a small rim of functioning renal tissue. *Polycystic renal disease* also showed splayed arterial branches, but the cysts are usually evident as multiple small rounded defects in the nephrogram phase. Ultrasound and CT are now the primary investigations of choice in these conditions.

Renal graft arteriography. The treatment of renal failure by cadaver kidney graft is now widespread and live donor grafts are also occasionally used. Where a live donor is used it is wise to do a preliminary flush aortogram to ensure that the kidney to be used has only one artery of supply since multiple arteries occur in 25% of kidneys. The grafted kidney is usually placed in the right iliac fossa and its artery is anastomosed to the patient's internal iliac artery.

The commonest cause of failure of a transplant kidney is renal rejection which can be immediate or delayed. Sometimes it is clinically difficult to differentiate between rejection of the graft and other complications affecting renal function.

A graft arteriogram will show whether the transplanted kidney is perfusing normally and demonstrate such complications as renal artery stenosis at the junction of the patient's internal iliac artery and the grafted renal artery (Fig. 26.59). Generalized small vessel occlusions, which are usually due to rejection, will be demonstrated, as will impaired perfusion, or thrombosis of the main artery.

Kidney transplant arteriography can be performed by injection of a large bolus of contrast medium (20 ml of 65% Hypaque or equivalent) into the common iliac artery. Selective angiography with an end hole catheter will give better visualization. This is achieved by using a catheter with a small preshaped curve at its tip that can be manipulated into the origin of the internal iliac artery. More

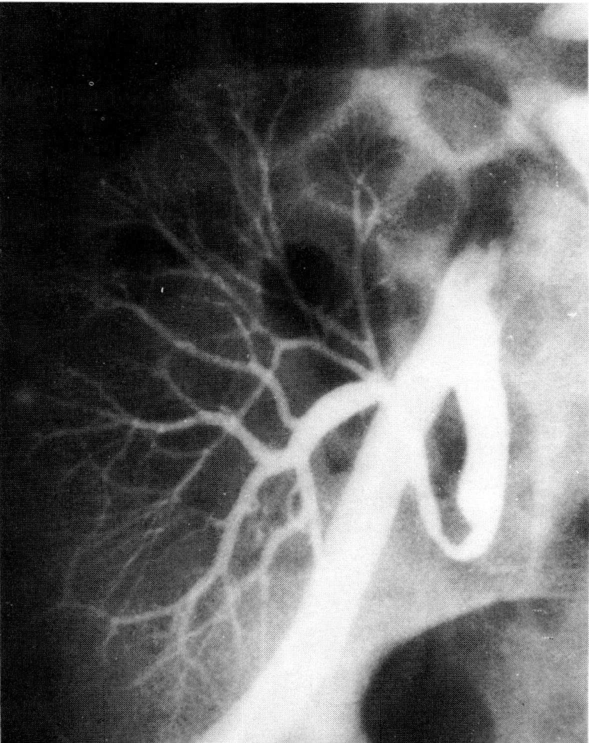

Fig. 26.59 Renal graft arteriogram. The patient developed secondary hypertension and a bruit. The arteriogram shows an unusual stenosis of the proximal segment of the graft artery.

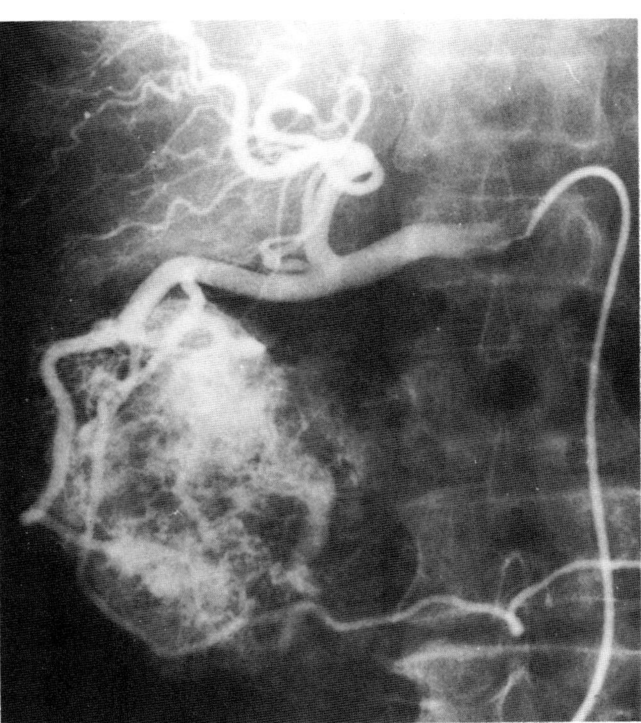

Fig. 26.60 Pancreatic cystadenoma showing florid pathological circulation in the haed of the pancreas.

recently DSA has permitted graft arteriography using minimal doses of contrast.

ADRENAL TUMOURS

CT is now the method of choice for demonstrating adrenal tumours (see Ch. 36). Angiography was widely used for many years in the diagnosis of these lesions but now has only a limited place for the assessment of the occasional problem case. Arteriography was most used in the assessment of *phaeochromocytoma*, but was also useful in *carcinoma* and *neuroblastomas*. Small *adenomas* of the type seen in Conn's syndrome or Cushing's syndrome were usually diagnosed by adrenal phlebography, but again CT has become the investigation of choice and the procedure is now little used.

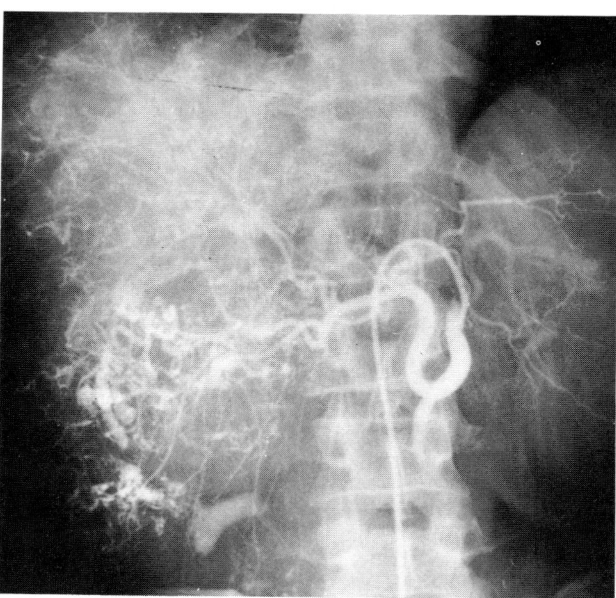

Fig. 26.61 Selective hepatic arteriogram. A large vascular tumour is shown in the lower part of the right lobe of the liver. Histology primary hepatoma.

PANCREATIC TUMOURS

Pancreatic tumours can be identified at arteriography using the technique of superselective coeliac axis and/or superior mesenteric arteriography. Highly vascular tumours such as

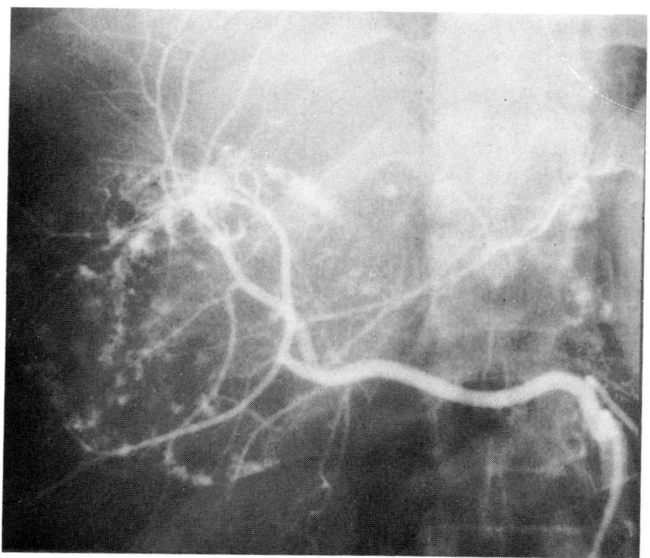

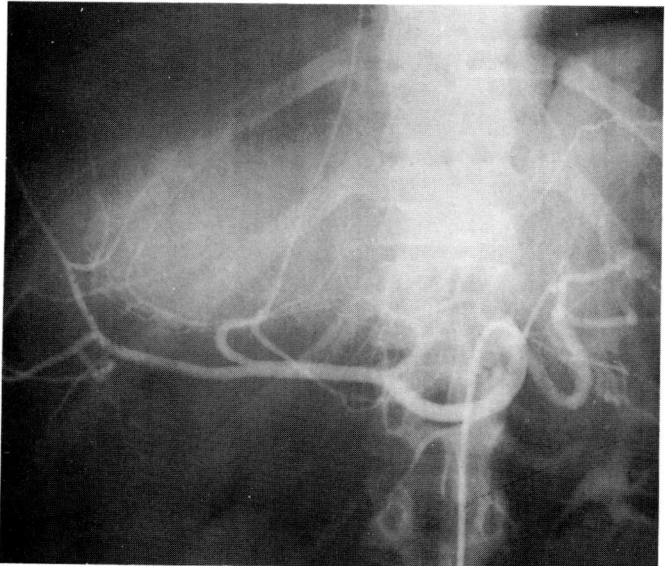

Fig. 26.62 Non-vascular mass in liver. This proved to be an amoebic abscess. Examination performed before ultrasound available.

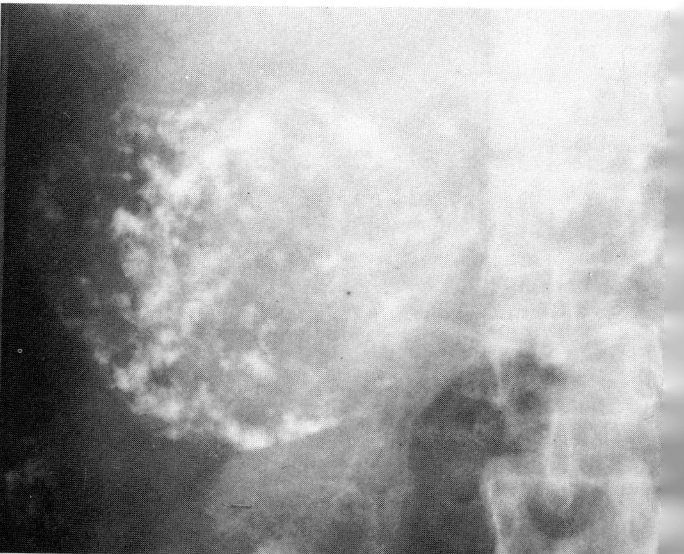

Fig. 26.63A. and **B**. Vascular lesion simulating tumour in the liver. Haemangioma. Note absence of drainage veins or AV shunting and persistence of contrast in late phase.

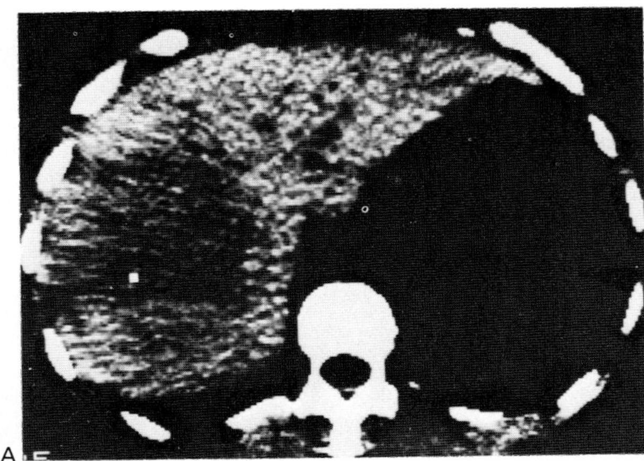

Fig. 26.64 Hepatic adenomas **A.** CT shows large low-density mass in right lobe of liver (W134 L67). **B.** and **C.** Angiogram shows vascular mass with smaller mass in lower part of right lobe.

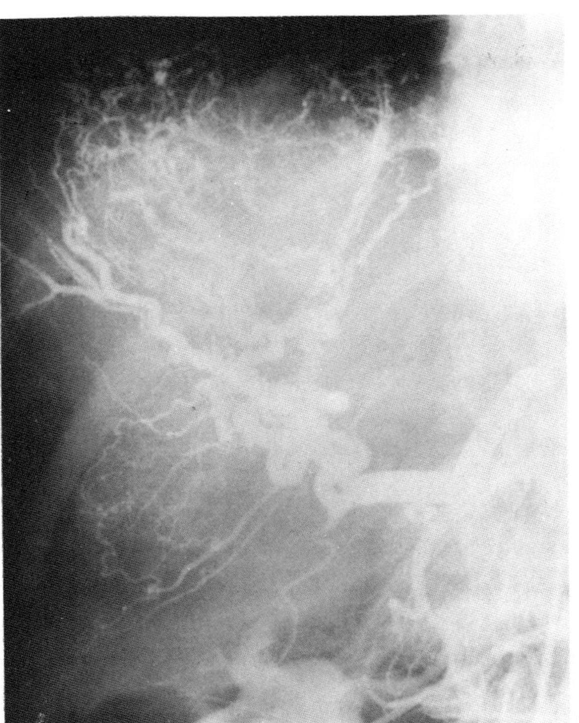

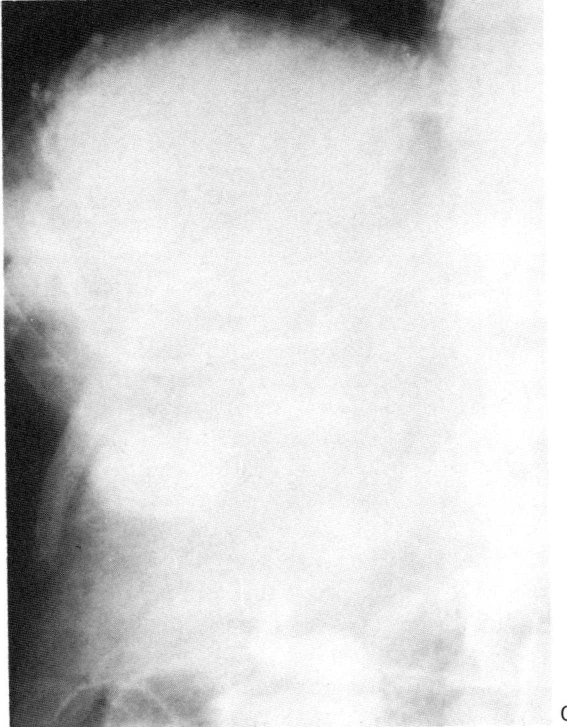

cystadenoma may be diagnosed by the demonstration of pathological vessels (Fig. 26.60). In *carcinoma*, which is relatively avascular, displacement of vessels supplying the pancreas or involvement of their walls by tumour can be demonstrated.

Islet cell adenomas in the pancreas have also been shown by angiography. Despite their usually small size they may stand out clearly as a rounded blush of contrast in the late arterial or capillary phase. It has been claimed that only the more vascular tumours will be demonstrated. However, superselective angiography of pancreatic arteries of supply will often show even the less vascular tumours (Clouse et al 1977). Large islet cell adenomas are occasionally seen and can be very vascular.

Pancreatic hormone-producing tumours can also be identified by venous blood sampling and assay from the pancreatic drainage veins. The samples are obtained by transphepatic portal catheterization as described below (Ch. 35).

Ultrasound, CT and ERP have now largely replaced angiography in the diagnosis of all but the small pancreatic mass lesions. The subject is discussed in detail in Chapter 35.

HEPATIC TUMOURS

The primary investigation of liver masses is now by ultrasound, CT or isotope scanning and all three of these imaging methods can provide valuable information. They are discussed in detail in Chapters 35, 65, 66 and 67.

There is still, however, a place for angiography in the control of these cases, either for treatment by embolization or chemotherapy, or for elucidation of the occasional problem case.

Selective hepatic angiography can demonstrate both primary and secondary carcinoma of the liver. Malignant tumours usually show a well-marked pathological circu-

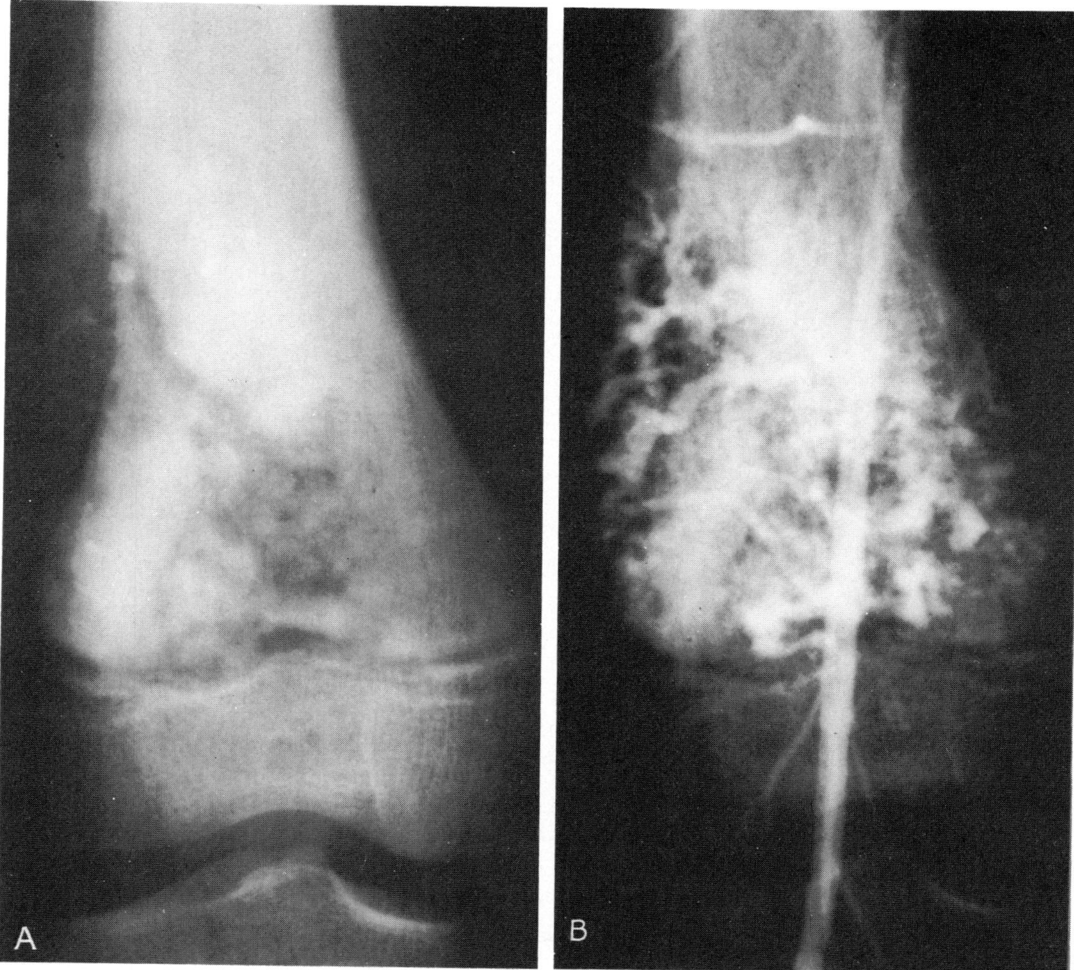

Fig. 26.65 A. and **B.** Osteogenic sarcoma showing pathological vessels with arteriovenous shunting.

lation (Fig. 26.61). However, such tumours are occasionally non-vascular and are then difficult to differentiate from benign expanding lesions. The latter tend merely to stretch and displace branches of the hepatic artery (Fig. 26.62).

Haemangioma is the most common benign tumour of the liver and also shows an abnormal circulation. Since these lesions may be multiple they can be mistaken for malignant tumours at echosound and isotope scanning and at angiography. Differentiation, however, is possible on the angiogram since the feeding vessels are normal in size and there is slow flow in the tumour with large vascular spaces and no early arteriovenous shunting (Fig. 26.63).

Hepatic adenomas may also occur and have been described following hormonal treatment with the contraceptive pill or androgens. Their vascular pattern is more regular than that of a malignant tumour and they usually stand out as encapsulated tumours in the hepatogram phase (Fig. 26.64).

TUMOURS OF BONE AND SOFT TISSUES

Arteriography has proved valuable in the diagnosis and differential diagnosis of bone tumours, of retroperitoneal masses and of soft-tissue masses in all parts of the body.

The newer techniques of imaging have reduced the need for arteriography, but have not completely superseded it, particularly if embolization is being considered.

Malignant tumours

Malignant bone tumours are often highly vascular (Fig. 26.65) and the angiographic appearances may be pathognomonic.

Ateriography will often give a much better impression of the total extent of a malignant bone tumour than will plain X-rays (Fig. 26.66).

Secondary deposits in bone vary in their vascularity. Some are relatively non-vascular, others are highly vascular.

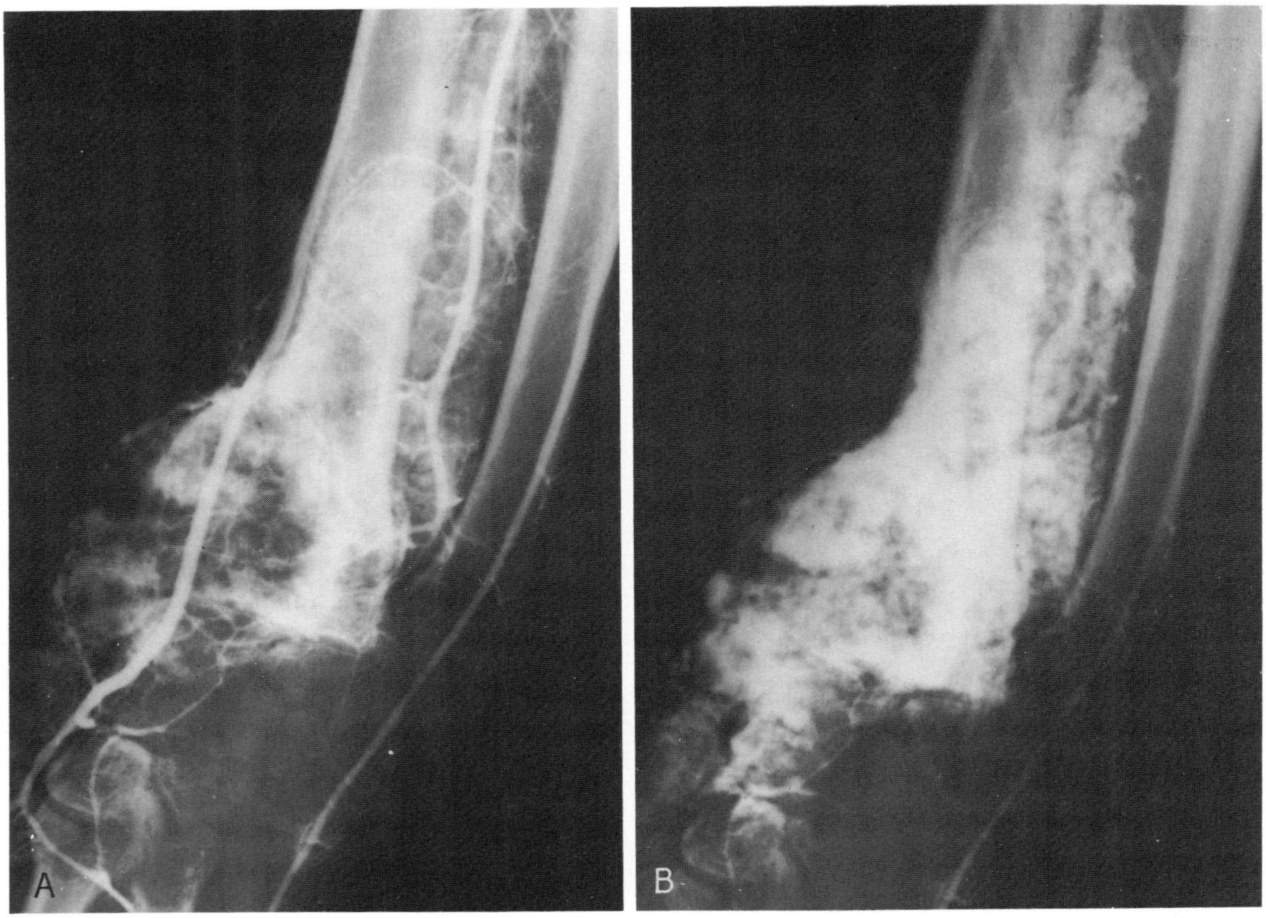

Fig. 26.66 A. and **B.** Malignant osteoclastoma. Note spread outside bone.

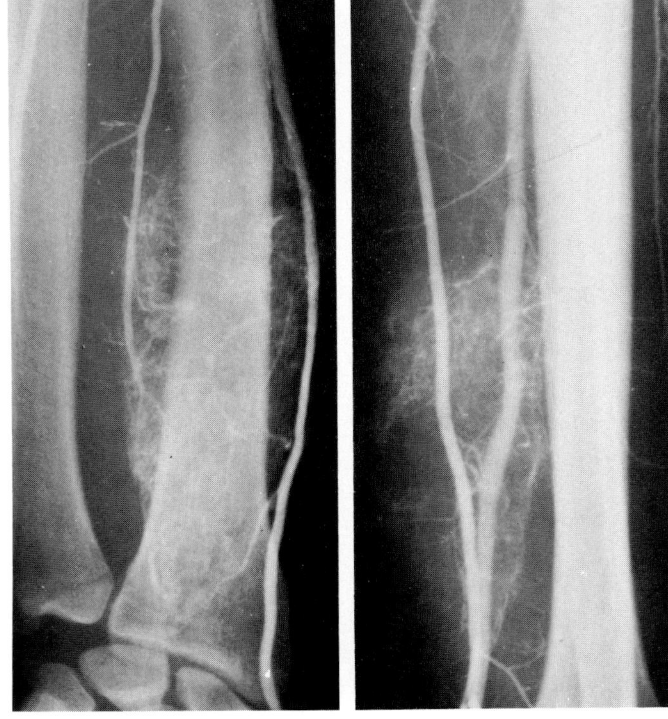

Fig. 26.67 Malignant tumour of the forearm (rhabdomyosarcoma). **A.** AP view. **B.** Lateral view.

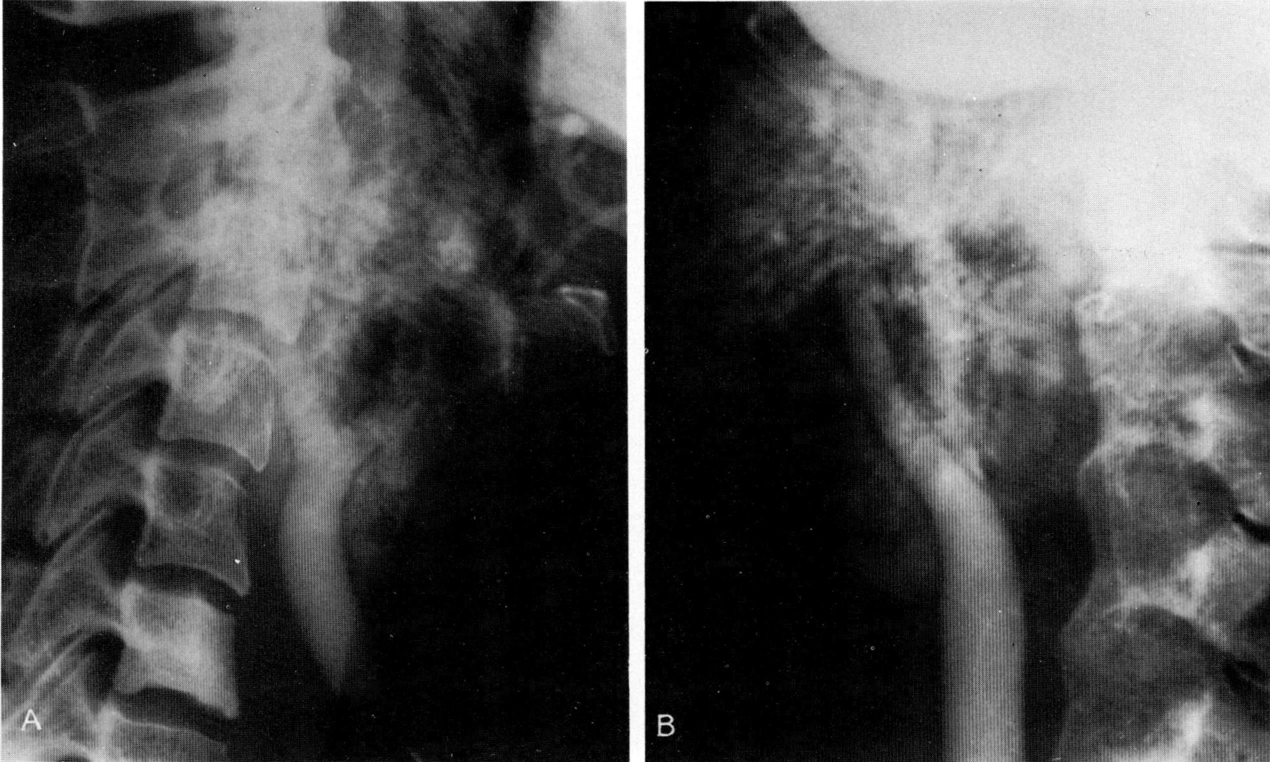

Fig. 26.68 A. and **B.** Carotid body tumour.

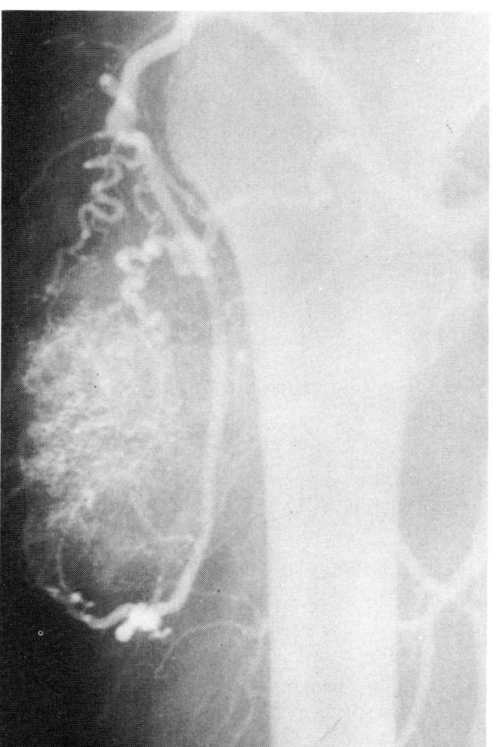

Fig. 26.69 Haemangiopericytoma. Patient presented with a lump in the thigh. This vascular tumour was highly malignant and metastasized rapidly.

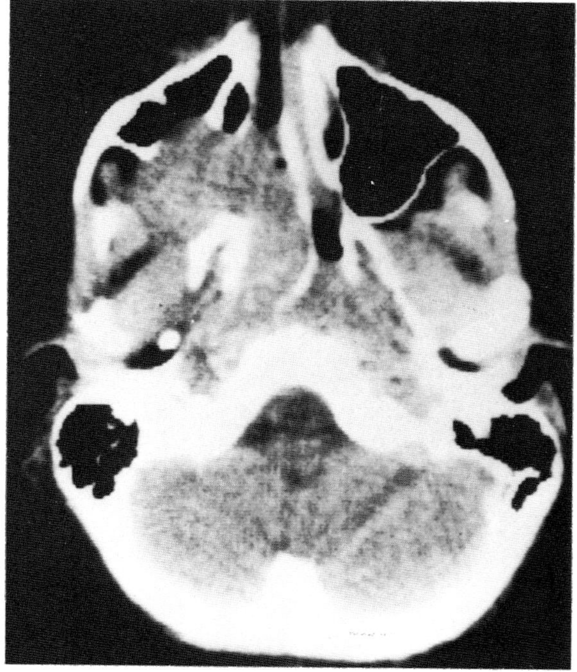

Fig. 26.70 Nasopharyngeal angiofibroma. CT shows large mass deforming right antrum and nares (W256 L36). Same case as Figure 26.15.

Secondary hypernephroma and secondary thyroid carcinoma have been amongst the most vascular lesions we have encountered. Isolated cases of secondary hypernephroma have even been encountered which presented as superficial pulsating masses and clinically resembled aneurysms or arteriovenous malformations.

Soft tissue *sarcomas* are usually well demonstrated by angiography when highly malignant (Fig. 26.67). However, with fibrosarcoma and tumours of low grade malignancy it is unusual to demonstrate pathological vessels, though local stretched vessels may be recognized.

Chromaffinoma. These rare tumours are usually seen at the carotid bifurcation, when they are known as *carotid body tumours*. They are extremely vascular and show a characteristic appearance at angiography (Fig. 26.68). Clinically they are sometimes mistaken for local aneurysms. Conversely, the rare aneurysms which occur in this situation are sometimes mistaken for carotid body tumours.

Another site for these chromaffinomas is at the base of the skull where they arise from the glomus jugulare and are known as *glomus jugulare tumours*. Clinically these tumours are usually associated with the presence of a cherry-red polyp protruding into the drum. They are also highly vascular and show angiographic appearances similar to those of the carotid body tumour. Careful superselective angiography of the external carotid artery with subtraction films may be necessary to show their full extent. Embolization may be required in extensive inoperable cases, and prior to surgery in others (see Ch. 61).

Rarely these tumours have been described in other situations but again they show angiographic appearances characteristic of the carotid body tumours. Cases have been demonstrated by angiography high in the neck (*glomus vagale tumour*) over the aortic arch (*aortic body tumour*) and in the pelvis.

Haemangiopericytoma is a rare tumour of small blood vessels which may occur anywhere in the body where there are capillaries, but is seen mainly in the soft tissues. The tumour may be benign, but is sometimes malignant. The appearances at angiography vary from the poorly vascularized to the excessively vascular, and the vascularity may be related to the degree of malignancy (Fig. 26.69).

Juvenile angiofibromas (nasopharyngeal angiofibromas) are highly vascular tumours presenting in the nasopharyngeal area of adolescent males. They may invade the antrum and produce swelling in the cheek. They are best shown by CT, which is now the primary investigation of choice (Fig. 26.70), but they are also well shown by superselective angiography of the external carotid artery. Surgery which may otherwise be hazardous, can be aided by prior embolization of the main feeding vessels (Fig. 26.15). They are further discussed in Chapter 48.

REFERENCES AND SUGGESTIONS FOR FURTHER READING

See end of Chapter 27.

CHAPTER 27

PHLEBOGRAPHY

The types of contrast phlebography used in clinical practice include:

1. Phlebography of the lower limb
2. Pelvic phlebography and inferior vena cavography
3. Hepatic, renal and adrenal phlebography
4. Phlebography of the upper limb and superior vena cava
5. Intraosseous phlebography
6. Portal phlebography
7. Spinal phlebography.

The investigations listed use direct contrast phlebography. Indirect phlebography can be achieved by serial fliming following arteriography. The latter method is the one routinely used for the demonstration of the cerebral veins following cerebral angiography and commonly for the demonstration of the renal veins following selective renal arteriography. It is also used for portal phlebography following selective coeliac or splenic arteriography — so-called *arterioportography*. Other imaging techniques have been used in the investigation of the venous system but have only limited application.

Radio-isotope phlebography can be performed as a prelude to a perfusion lung scan in suspected pulmonary embolus. Half the dose of $^{99}Tc^{m}$ is injected into each foot simultaneously and the passage of the isotope up the legs and through the abdomen recorded. The resulting images may show evidence of venous obstruction or a normal deep venous system. Delayed scans are also obtained of the calf and thigh to demonstrate local hold up suggesting venous obstruction. Radio-isotope phlebography offers an alternative technique in patients with iodine sensitivity or other contraindications to formal phlebography. ^{125}I-fibrinogen has also been widely used to diagnose deep vein thrombosis. In this case, however, the isotope is injected into an arm vein and is later taken up by the developing thrombosis. Recordings are made over the calf, popliteal and femoral veins and will demonstrate local increase of uptake. False positives may be obtained over wounds, haematomas and cellulitis, but the test has a high degree of accuracy with large recent thrombi and is relatively easy to perform.

Doppler ultrasound has attractions as a non-invasive technique for diagnosing venous thrombosis. Doppler flow signals can be recognised over the femoral, popliteal and posterior tibial veins. Deep vein thrombosis is suggested when signals are absent or when muscle compression of the thigh does not produce the expected increase in femoral vein blood flow. In expert hands a high degree of accuracy is claimed though smaller lesions in the calf are difficult to identify by this method.

Real time or B scan ultrasound will demonstrate well such deep-seated structures as the inferior vena cava or portal vein but, generally speaking, has little place in the investigation of most of the lesions discussed in this chapter.

CT will demonstrate the major veins well, but usually requires contrast injections for the confirmation of such lesions as caval thrombosis, and in view of its cost can hardly be justified for routine use.

MRI also shows major vessels well and does not require contrast injections. However, it is also costly and not yet freely available (see Ch. 68).

DSA is limited in the area that can be examined at one time but will reduce contrast dosage in areas where it can be used.

Capnocavography. The introduction of 60–100 cc of pure carbon dioxide gas into the left femoral vein with the patient in the left lateral decubitus position has been used in the past for studying the inferior vena cava in patients with sensitivity to iodine. The development of isotopes and ultrasound rendered the technique obsolete.

THE LOWER LIMB

Indications. Phlebography of the lower limb is practised at most medical centres for the following purposes:

1. To demonstrate deep vein thrombosis in the calf, thigh, pelvis or inferior vena cava.
2. To show suspected venous obstruction by tumour or extrinsic pressure.
3. To investigate secondary or recurrent varicose veins thought to be associated with an abnormality of the deep

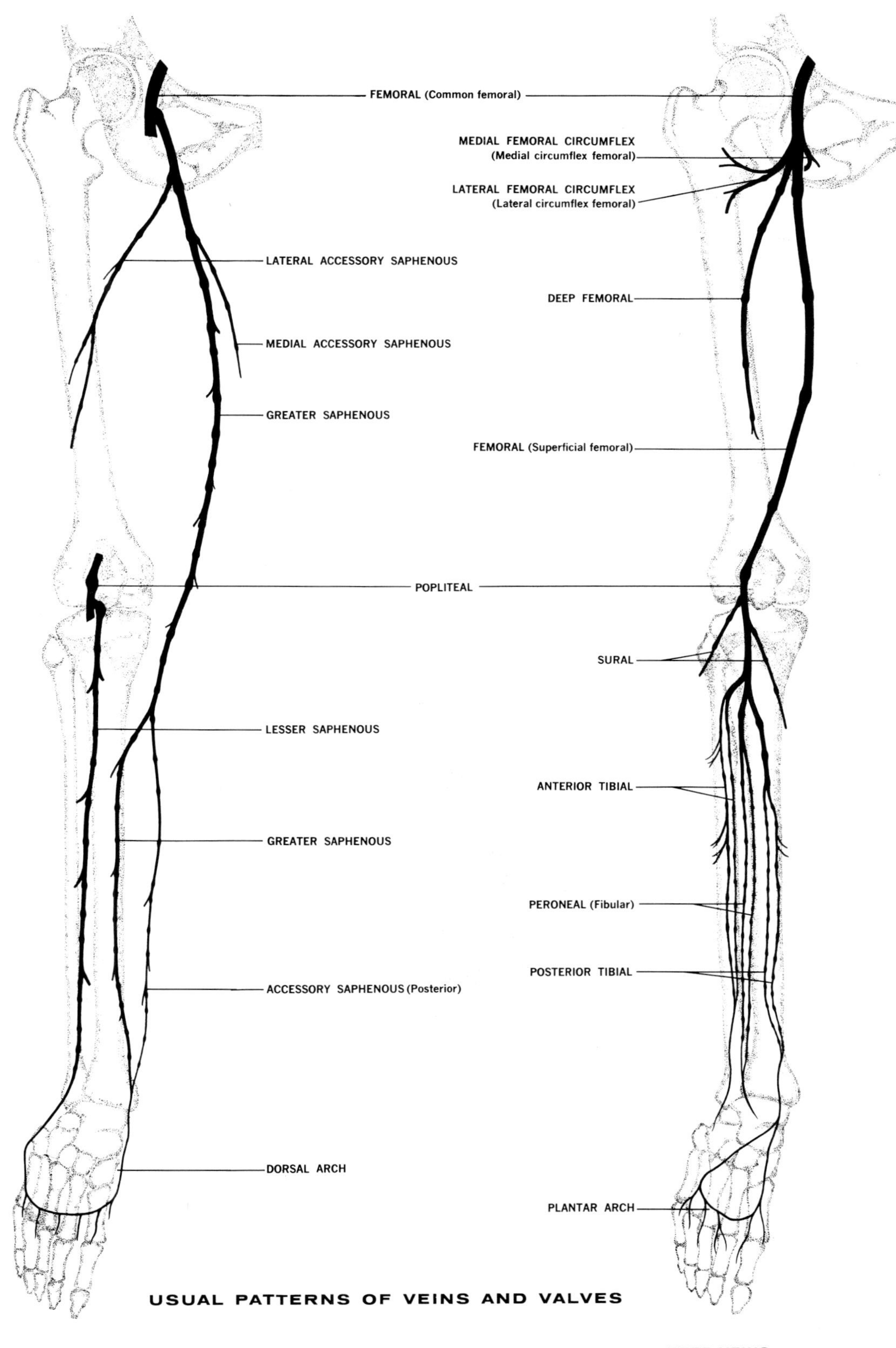

Fig. 27.1 Diagram of the deep and superficial veins of the lower limb. (Copyright Eastman Kodak Co. Reprinted courtesy of Health Sciences Division, Eastman Kodak Co.)

venous system such as post-thrombotic destruction of valves and associated incompetent perforators, or with inadequate surgery.

4. To investigate swollen legs where the differential diagnosis between lymphoedema, cellulitis, and venous incompetence or obstruction, is not clear.

5. To investigate varicose ulcers in the post-thrombotic syndrome.

6. To outline venous malformations.

Suspected deep vein thrombosis is probably the commonest cause for patient referral and in most cases there is strong clinical evidence for the lesion. In some cases, however, e.g. in patients with repeated pulmonary emboli but no obvious source, the investigation may be undertaken to exclude the lower limb as a source of emboli.

Normal anatomy. The venous drainage of the lower limb can be divided into two separate systems, the deep veins and the superficial veins. These are connected by the communicating veins (Figs 27.1, 27.2).

The *deep* veins in the calf follow the same distribution as the main arteries but are usually double, forming the anterior tibial, posterior tibial, and peroneal veins. The calf veins, or sural veins, arise in calf muscles and emerge from them to join the peroneal, posterior tibial or popliteal veins.

The communicating veins are usually small and paired and connect the superficial and deep veins. Normally they are extremely narrow, but they can become quite large when hypertrophied. They are valved so that blood only flows from the superficial to the deep veins. Under pathological conditions they can become incompetent permitting reverse flow from the deep to the superficial veins (Fig. 27.3).

The popliteal vein is a smooth large vessel lying behind the knee and passing up into the femoral vein which follows the course of the femoral artery. The femoral vein is sometimes double, or the profunda vein, which usually lies in the upper two-thirds of the thigh, may connect in its lower part with the femoral or popliteal vein. Perforating or communicating veins in the thigh are normally small, but if incompetent may be demonstrated connecting the superficial and deep veins in the lower third of the thigh (Fig. 27.4).

The *superficial* leg veins drain into the saphenous veins. The short saphenous vein passes up the lateral side of the leg to the knee, where it passes deeply to join the popliteal

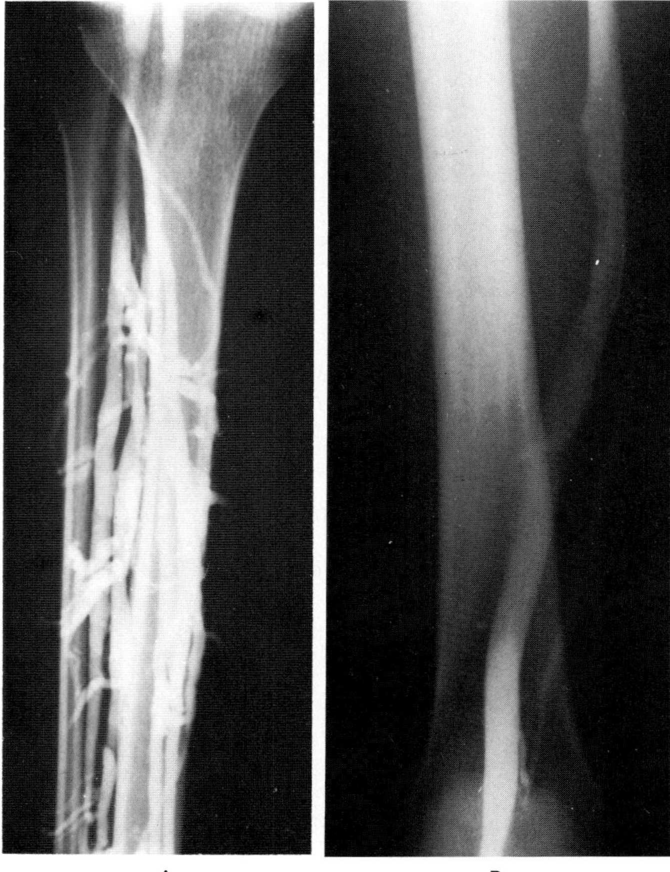

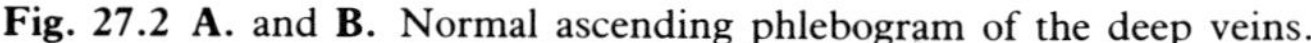

Fig. 27.2 A. and **B.** Normal ascending phlebogram of the deep veins.

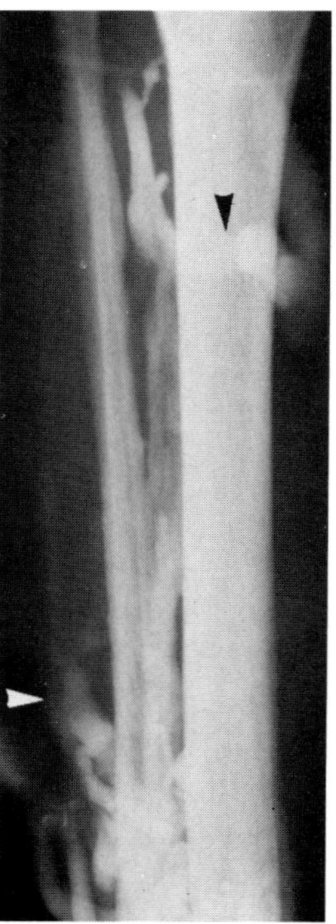

Fig. 27.3 Incompetent perforating veins in the calf (arrows).

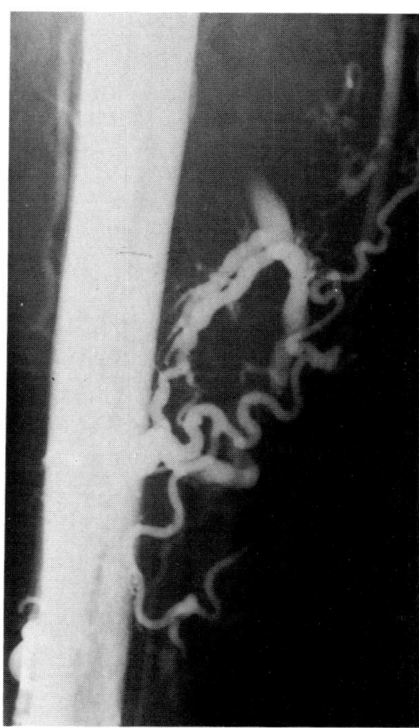

Fig. 27.4 Incompetent perforating veins in the thigh.

vein. The long saphenous passes up the medial side of the calf and thigh and then joins the femoral vein below the groin.

The venous system can be regarded as a blood reservoir and normally contains some two-thirds of the body blood, largely in the lower limbs. Flow to the heart depends on the pressure gradient between the veins and right atrium, and is assisted by the muscle contractions, particularly in the calf, acting as a pump. The veins themselves can also actively contract and help onward flow of blood. The valves are also of great importance in preventing retrograde flow, and their destruction or damage by thrombosis has serious haemodynamic consequences leading to venous incompetence.

Technique

1. **Ascending phlebography**. A large number of different techniques have been described in the literature. No standard technique has been generally accepted. The technique used by us has been modified over the years and is as follows. A small needle is inserted percutaneously into a vein on the dorsum of the foot. Occasionally this may prove impossible and the needle may have to be inserted by cut down. If the foot is swollen or oedematous, prior bed rest with the foot elevated is desirable to reduce the swelling. Once the needle is in position, compression is applied just above the ankle and also just above the knee by tourniquets or by inflatable cuffs. The pressure used is just sufficient to occlude the superficial veins completely without affecting the patency of the deep veins.

Contrast medium (40–50 ml) is then injected by hand pressure. In some cases more contrast may be required to obtain adequate filling of the femoral and iliac veins, but it should rarely be necessary to use more than 80–100 ml. In the past, 65% Hypaque or equivalent other media have been used. However, the newer contrast media with low osmolality are now being increasingly used (see Ch. 26) and these are better tolerated by the patient and less likely to produce complications.

Since the foot veins are usually punctured with small butterfly needles (21 British standard wire gauge) the injection can take 20–30 seconds. Flow is monitored by observation with an image intensifier and films obtained at appropriate moments as the veins are sequentially filled. Whilst some workers conduct the examination with the patient supine others insist that the patient should be tilted on the table into a 30° to 60° feet-down position. This is mainly to prevent layering of contrast posteriorly giving rise to artefactual filling defects and to ensure mixing of blood and contrast. The foot and leg should be medially rotated to separate the tibia and fibula and the deep veins of the calf. The weight should not be borne by the foot being injected, so that the calf muscles remain relaxed and their veins can be filled with contrast.

2. **Descending phlebography**. This is less frequently practised but is occasionally used with the patient supine on a tilting table and his feet against the footrest. The femoral vein is punctured at the groin and, with the needle in situ, the patient is then tilted to the erect or near erect position and contrast injected. If the patient performs the Valsalva manoeuvre, contrast will reflux down an incompetent femoral vein into the popliteal vein. It has been claimed, however, that contrast will sometimes flow past competent valves, though it is usually possible to assess the degree of true incompetence and show the valves clearly, particularly when they are competent (Fig. 27.5).

Complications. A few patients tolerated the procedure badly with the older contrast media and complained of pain and discomfort in the calf with ascending phlebography. Nausea, vomiting and minor allergic reactions were also occasionally seen as with all contrast media. The new low osmolality contrast media are better tolerated and give rise to little discomfort.

Care should be taken to ensure there is no contrast extravasation at the site of puncture as this can be quite painful, and with large volume extravasation the consequences, particularly in an ischaemic or oedematous foot, can be serious. Skin necrosis has been recorded from this accident.

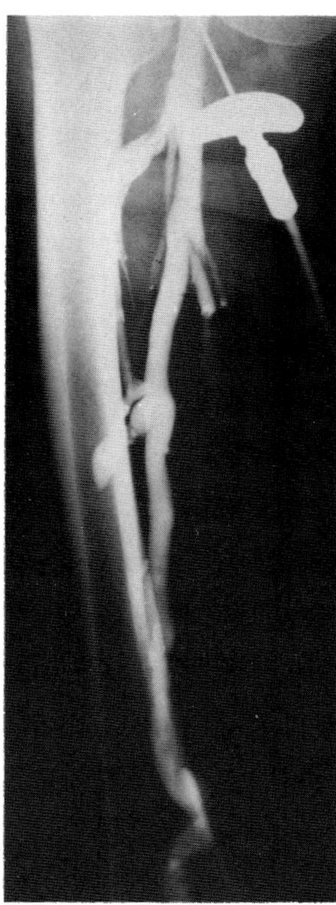

Fig. 27.5 Descending phlebogram showing incompetent valves and reflux down to the popliteal vein.

Phlebitis and postphlebography venous thrombosis can occur where large volumes of high concentration contrast are used. This should be guarded against by flushing out residual contrast with saline at the end of the procedure, and by using the new low osmolality contrast media.

Radiological findings. In the normal patient the deep veins of the calf are outlined by contrast at ascending phlebography with cuffs inflated; three paired veins accompanying the peroneal, posterior and anterior tibial arteries can be recognized, the last being smaller than the others. There is no filling of the superficial or communicating veins (Fig. 27.2), but with progressive injections of contrast there will be varying degrees of filling of the soleal muscle veins which are typically large and valveless and drain into the peroneal and posterior tibial veins. There may also be filling of the gastrocnemius veins, which are valved and usually multiple, running a downward course from their points of entry into the upper popliteal vein.

The popliteal vein is single and commences near the knee joint passing upwards to become the femoral vein. Views of the calf are usually obtained in both AP and lateral projections. Valves are usually obvious in the distended veins but can be accentuated by the patient performing the Valsalva manoeuvre.

A good quality ascending phlebogram will also demonstrate the iliac veins and inferior vena cava, but these are best shown by releasing the tourniquet and manually compressing the calf to improve the upward flow of contrast at the same time as the pelvic exposure is made. This ensures a good bolus of contrast entering the iliac veins. If the suspected lesion affects only the pelvic veins or inferior vena cava direct pelvic phlebography is to be preferred (see below).

Deep vein thrombosis

Venous thrombosis appears to be multifactorial in origin and is associated with slowing of the blood flow and an increased liability to blood coagulation. Conditions known to predispose include malignant disease, age, obesity, trauma and surgery, as well as prolonged immobilization, myocardial infarction and congestive heart failure.

The risk of deep vein thrombosis is particularly high after abdominal and pelvic surgery, and even higher after operations on the hip, knee or femur. It becomes even greater if there is associated myocardial infarction or congestive heart failure. The thrombosis may be bilateral in some 30% of patients.

Clinically, symptoms are present only if there is significant obstruction or inflammation produced by the thrombosis and it is claimed that 50% or more of cases are silent and symptomless.

The main danger is pulmonary embolus, and the incidence in the USA of this complication is over 500 000 cases per annum. The mortality in different series ranges from 10 to 30%.

The vast majority of these emboli arise from the leg veins. As already noted, half the cases show no prodromal leg symptoms before the embolus occurs.

Acute thrombosis of the deep veins appears as filling defects within the veins, the defect often being outlined by a marginal layer of contrast. Views in more than one plane may show that the clot is adherent to the vein at some point in one or other plane. Upward extension of the clot may be seen lying more freely in the lumen, and such a floating tail is likely to embolize. Adherent clot is regarded as relatively less dangerous. Clot may be identified in calf veins only, or involving the popliteal and femoral veins or in the iliac veins and inferior vena cava (Figs 27.6–27.9).

True clot defects should be distinguished from

1. artefacts due to layering,
2. streaming from the entry of large non-opacified tributary veins, and
3. turbulence around valves.

Films in more than one plane, the Valsalva manoeuvre and multiple films all help in this respect as do large doses of contrast and the semi-erect position.

Acute thrombosis is later followed by clot retraction, thrombolysis and recanalization, but the venous valves are damaged and destroyed so that the vein becomes irregular

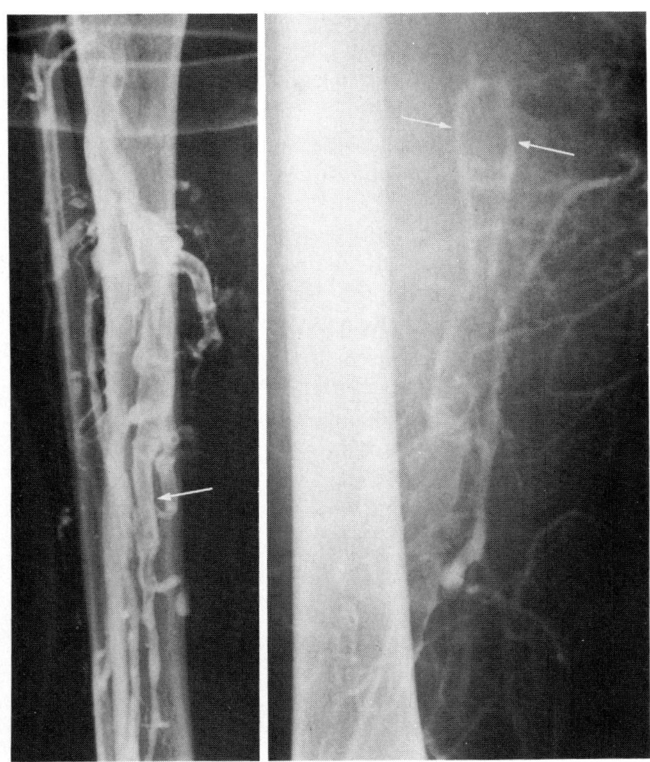

Fig. 27.6 Fig. 27.7

Figs 27.6 and **27.7** Phlebogram showing venous thrombosis (**Fig. 27.6**) in deep veins of the calf, and (**Fig. 27.7**) in the femoral vein. The clot shows as central filling defects with marginal contrast (arrows).

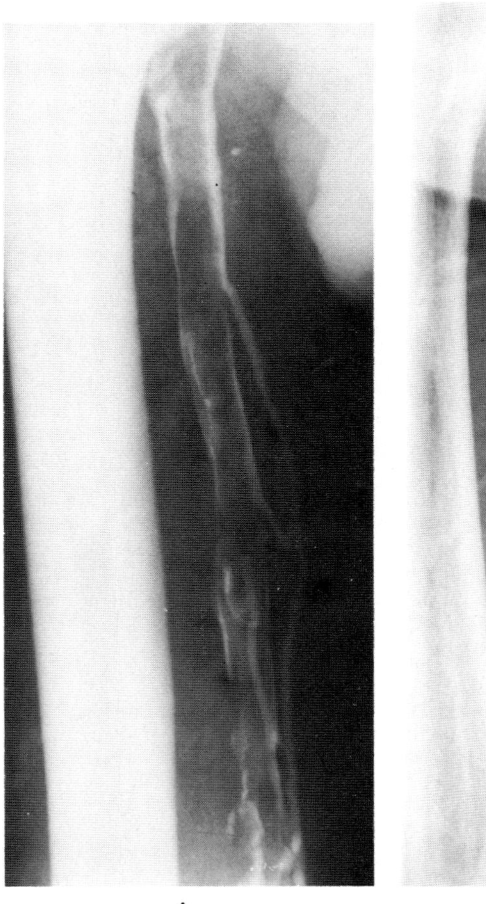

A B

Fig. 27.9 Extensive clot in the femoral vein.

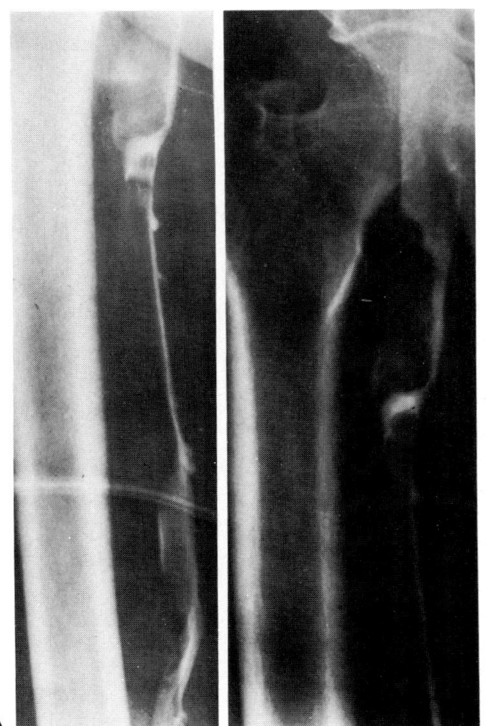

A B

Fig. 27.8 A. and **B.** Extensive clot in the femoral vein adherent in part.

and incompetent. Some veins are severely stenosed or occluded and in these cases venous return is largely by dilated collaterals. In either case a *post-thrombotic syndrome* may develop characterized by swelling and pain in the affected leg. Eventually this may lead to induration and ulceration. This is usually on the medial aspect of the ankle, but is occasionally lateral in position. This is related to the fact that the medial aspect of the lower third of the leg just above the ankle is the site for a group of communicating veins usually three in number. As these are at the most dependent part of the limb the increased pressure from incompetence and partial obstruction is greatest here and is accentuated by the pressure from calf muscle contractions.

Phlebography in patients with post-thrombotic states will show involved veins to be irregular and incompetent. In severe cases the major veins may be occluded in whole or in part and replaced by numerous collateral veins.

Recurrent varicose veins. The recurrence of varicose veins after surgery is a frequent clinical problem and may occur several years later. In these patients a useful

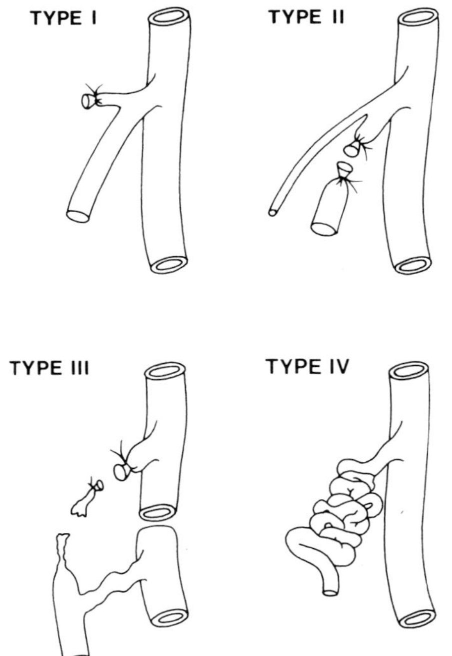

Fig. 27.10 The four types of recurrence in the thigh are shown diagrammatically. More than one type may apply in a given patient. (Reproduced with permission from Starnes et al. (1984) *Clinical Radiology*, **35**, 96.)

procedure is direct injection of one or more of the superficial thigh varicose veins to demonstrate their distribution and the pattern of recurrences at the groin following the previous high ligation of the long saphenous vein. A recent study has shown that there are several mechanisms but the most usual a tortuous leash of recanalized vein and not a missed tributary of the long saphenous or a missed perforating vein (Fig. 27.10). The procedure may have the additional bonus of sclerosing the recanalized trunk and producing a clinical cure.

CONGENITAL ANOMALIES

Duplication of the popliteal or femoral vein or of both is not infrequent, as is duplication of the long saphenous vein. Congenital *absence* of the posterior tibial veins is another anomaly that is not infrequent. In this case veins are usually seen passing laterally above the ankle to drain into the peroneal veins.

Congenital absence of the venous valves is described in the major veins giving rise to venous stasis (primary deep venous insufficiency) and should be considered when children or teenagers present with varicosities or chronic leg swelling. However, such a diagnosis should be made with caution as previously unrecognized deep vein thrombosis with recanalization cannot always be excluded. It is claimed that such recanalization can sometimes result in apparently normal-looking veins without the usual irregularities seen in the post-thrombotic syndrome.

Kippell-Trenaunay syndrome. This is characterized by a naevus with hypertrophy of bones and soft tissues of affected limbs, usually legs, though arms may also be affected. There is venous dysplasia and the normal venous return is replaced by persistence of a more primitive system, usually a large lateral venous channel in the leg, or a single large medial venous channel in the arm (Fig. 27.27). These can be associated with superficial varicosities. The large drainage vein is often valveless and shows sluggish flow.

Other anomalies. A large *varix* or venous aneurysm can occur anywhere in the venous system. Such lesions are not uncommon at the termination of the long or short saphenous veins. Superficial or deep venous varices or '*venous angioma*' are sometimes seen, such lesions having no obvious connection with an arterial lesion. Their anatomy is well shown by simple phlebography.

THE PELVIS AND ABDOMEN

As noted above, the iliac veins and inferior vena cava are quite well shown by good quality ascending phlebograms from the foot, and their demonstration should be part of all such investigations. However, they can be more constantly and clearly demonstrated by direct femoral phlebography, which is the technique of choice where the lesion is known to be intra-abdominal. The method is also used in the occasional cases where ascending phlebography from the foot has failed to clearly exclude or confirm clot in the iliacs or inferior vena cava because of poor contrast for technical or other reasons.

The lesions shown by pelvic and inferior caval phlebography include:

1. Acute thrombosis with recent clot, or post-thrombotic sequelae with partial obstruction and collateral circulation.
2. Obstruction by neoplastic or glandular masses, usually by extrinsic pressure, but also by tumour invasion as in hypernephromas.
3. Extrinsic pressure from large benign tumours or other lesions, e.g. lymphocele, aneurysms, retroperitoneal fibrosis, haematoma.
4. Obstruction of the left common iliac vein by pressure from the right common iliac artery (so-called 'lymphoedema praecox').
5. Post-traumatic or radiotherapy venous damage.
6. Pelvic varicosities.
7. Congenital anomalies.

Technique. The iliac veins and inferior vena cava are well shown by direct injection into the femoral veins of 30–40 ml of contrast on each side. Both veins are injected at the same time unless only one iliac vein is obstructed and it is desired to show collateral and bypass drainage pathways clearly (Fig. 27.16). A unilateral injection will also suffice if only the inferior vena cava is under examination. The injection is made through a large needle inserted into the femoral vein at the groin, or after percutaneous insertion of a catheter which is passed 2–3 inches up the vein.

To obtain good filling, contrast is injected rapidly as a bolus, taking 2–4 seconds for the 40 ml on each side. Serial films of the abdomen are obtained at the rate of 1 a second for 5 seconds as normal flow is rapid. Better and more prolonged filling can be obtained if the patient performs the Valsalva manoeuvre.

Radiographic appearances. The normal external and common iliac veins and inferior vena cava are valveless and appear as large contrast-filled tubes. There may be a slight extrinsic pressure defect at the termination of the left common iliac where it is crossed by the overlying right common iliac artery. Occasionally the artery can partially obstruct venous flow (see below). The internal iliac veins do contain valves and are not normally demonstrated. The Valsalva manoeuvre will fill their terminations and sometimes provides better filling, but this is unusual. Streamlining by non-opacified blood may be seen where large veins such as the renal veins enter the inferior vena cava. Figure 27.11 illustrates the normal superior vena cava and its connections.

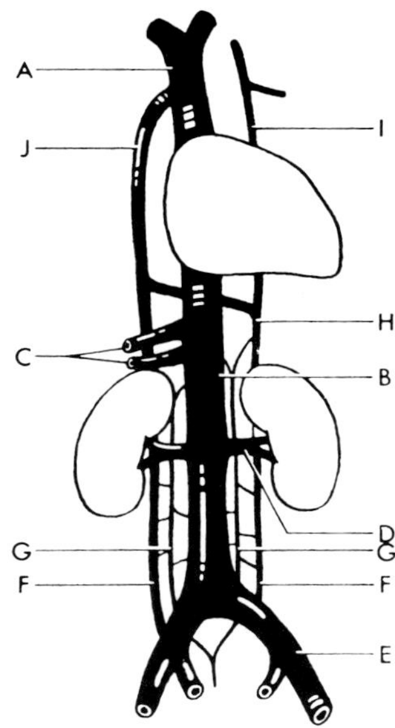

Fig. 27.11 Diagram showing venous drainage and connections of the inferior vena cava. A = superior vena cava. B = inferior vena cava. C = hepatic veins. D = renal veins. E = iliac veins. F = ascending lumbar veins. G = vertebral venous plexus. H = hemiazygos vein. I = ascending hemiazygos vein. J = azygos vein.

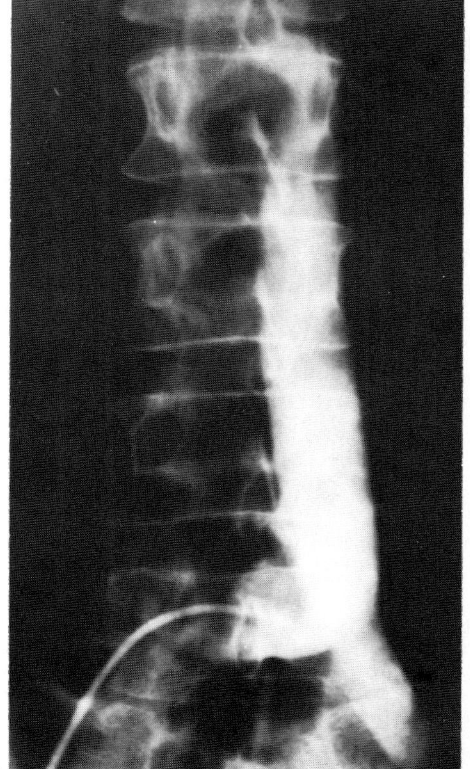

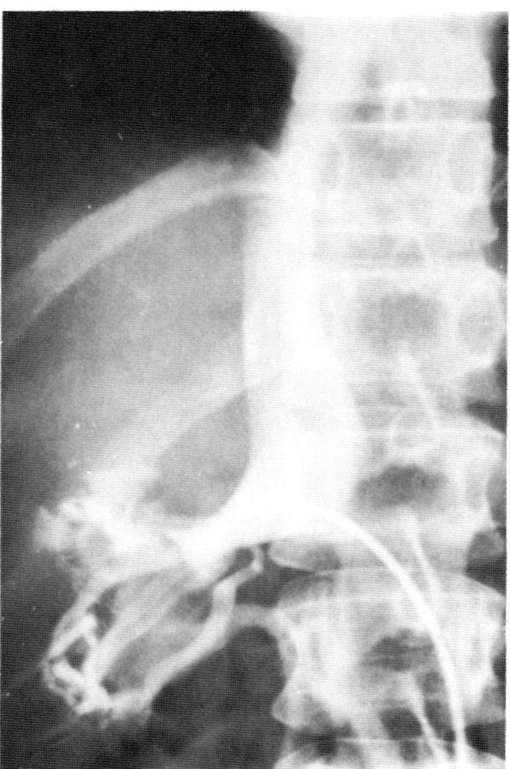

Fig. 27.12 A. Left-sided inferior vena cava as a chance finding in a patient undergoing renal vein catheterization. **B.** The catheter has passed over to the right renal vein through the left IVC draining into the left renal vein; the upper part of the IVC is normally sited.

Congenital anomalies of the inferior vena cava occur in less than 1% of patients, but the incidence is higher in patients with congenital heart disease.

Left-sided inferior vena cava is the commonest of these anomalies. In these cases the left-sided vena cava terminates in the left renal vein, which then usually drains into a normally sited terminal segment of the inferior vena cava (Fig. 27.12). Less frequent is a *double inferior vena cava* with the right larger than the left, or both equal in size. The left cava again terminates in the left renal vein (Fig. 27.13). Occasionally a left inferior vena cava may drain into the lumbar and hemiazygos systems, the coronary sinus or the left atrium. The supra renal segment of a normal or abnormal infrarenal IVC occasionally drains into the azygos vein or the hemiazygos vein instead of passing through the liver. This anomaly has been recognized at CT, when it is shown behind the diaphragmatic crura adjacent to the aorta as it enters the thorax.

Both *agenesis* and *hypoplasia* of the inferior vena cava have been described. In these cases blood from the pelvis and lower limbs drains mainly into the lumbar, hemiazygos and azygos veins, which act as collaterals.

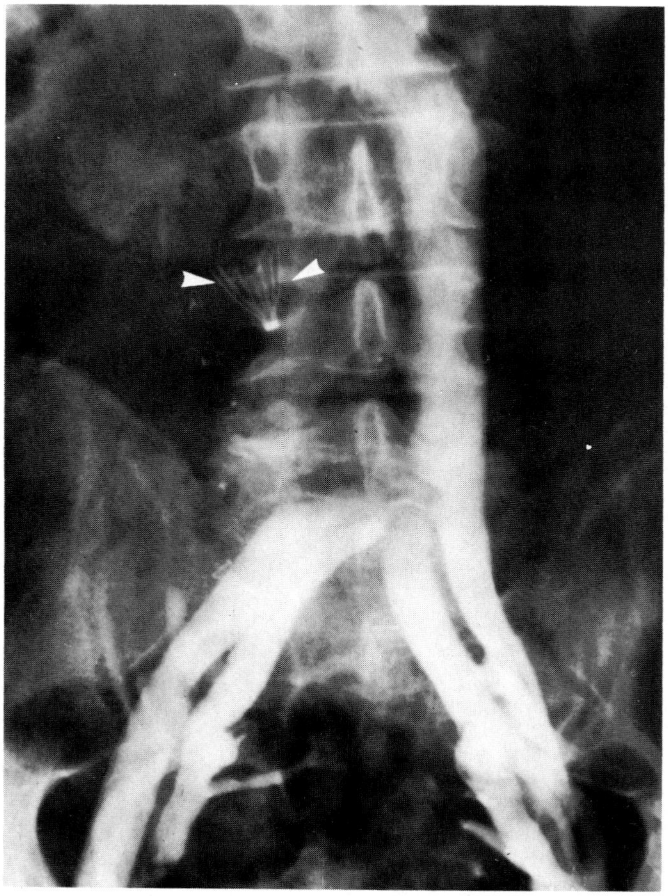

Thrombosis of the iliacs or inferior vena cava in the acute phase shows similar appearances to those described above in lower limb thrombosis, i.e. clot defect occupying most of the lumen with attachment to the vein wall (Fig. 27.14A), or, more dangerously, with a tail of clot extending into the lumen. In the latter case surgery may be indicated to prevent emboli passing to the lung. In the past this consisted of plication of the inferior vena cava, an operation superseded by the transvenous insertion of filters (see below). Collateral bridging vessels will be seen dependent on the site and extent of obstruction.

Complete thrombosis of the inferior vena cava is occasionally seen and there is then a collateral circulation utilizing a wide variety of collaterals including the lumbar and azygos veins, the vertebral plexus, the anterior abdominal wall veins, the retroperitoneal or even mesenteric veins (Fig. 27.15). Such complete thrombosis usually extends to the level of the renal veins which remain patent. The upper limit can be demonstrated by retrograde phlebography from above a catheter being passed from the arm through the right auricle to the upper inferior vena cava.

Recanalization of the iliacs and inferior vena cava may occur after complete thrombosis when the vessels will appear smaller and more irregular with evidence of collateral vessels (Fig. 27.16).

Glandular and neoplastic masses can produce considerable distortion of the iliacs and inferior vena cava. Large benign masses can produce marked displacement with little obstruction when only the inferior vena cava is affected (Fig. 36.25), but the iliacs are more easily obstructed by extrinsic pressure (Fig. 27.17). In the past, inferior vena cavography was widely used to assess para-aortic glandular involvement in reticulosis in conjunction with lymphangiography, but with the development of CT and ultrasound this is no longer indicated.

Renal vein invasion by hypernephroma is quite common and tumour may then spread into the inferior vena cava. Such tumour spread is well shown by inferior vena cavography (Fig. 27.18) or by CT.

Fig. 27.14 A. Recent clot obstructing left common iliac and partially obstructing lower inferior vena cava. **B.** Thrombosis of IVC and common iliacs with collateral circulation. Some irregular recanalization of common iliacs.

Fig. 27.15 A. & **B.** Thrombosis of IVC and common iliacs. Collateral drainage from the right leg via internal iliacs and haemorrhoidal plexus → inferior mesenteric vein → portal vein. **C.** Same patient. Collateral drainage from the left leg mainly via ascending lumbar veins and vertebral venous plexus.

Fig. 27.13 Double inferior vena cava. A Mobin-Uddin umbrella (arrowed) has been inserted in the normal right-sided IVC. Postoperative phlebogram shows an unsuspected double inferior vena cava with the right side now occluded.

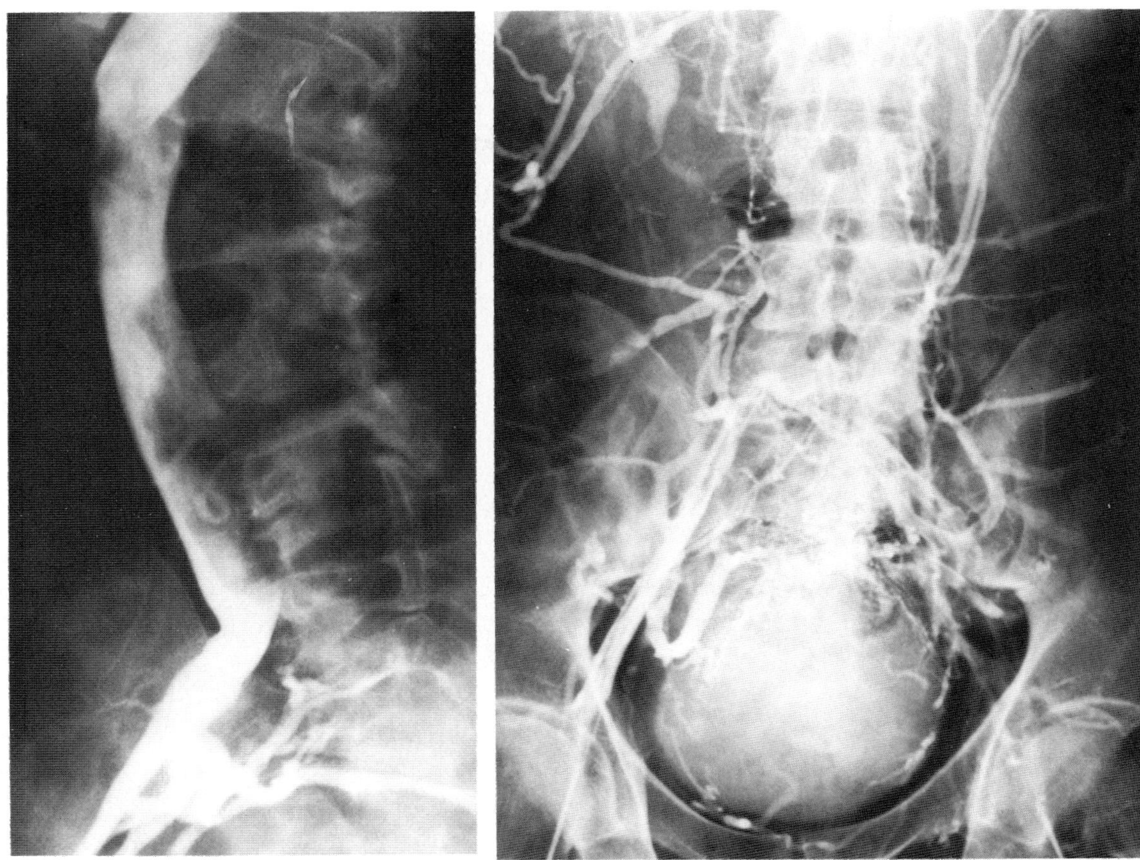

Fig. 27.14A

Fig. 27.14B

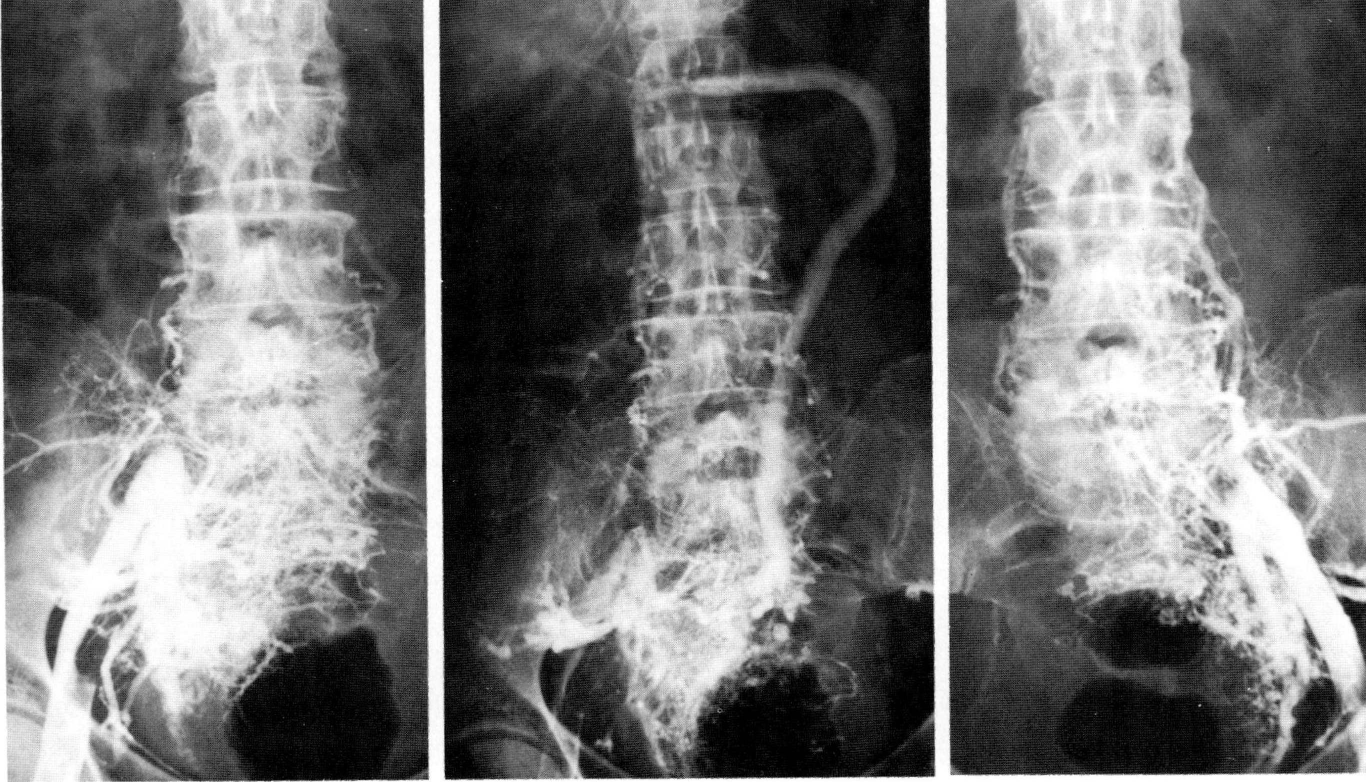

Fig. 27.15A

Fig. 27.15B

Fig. 27.15C

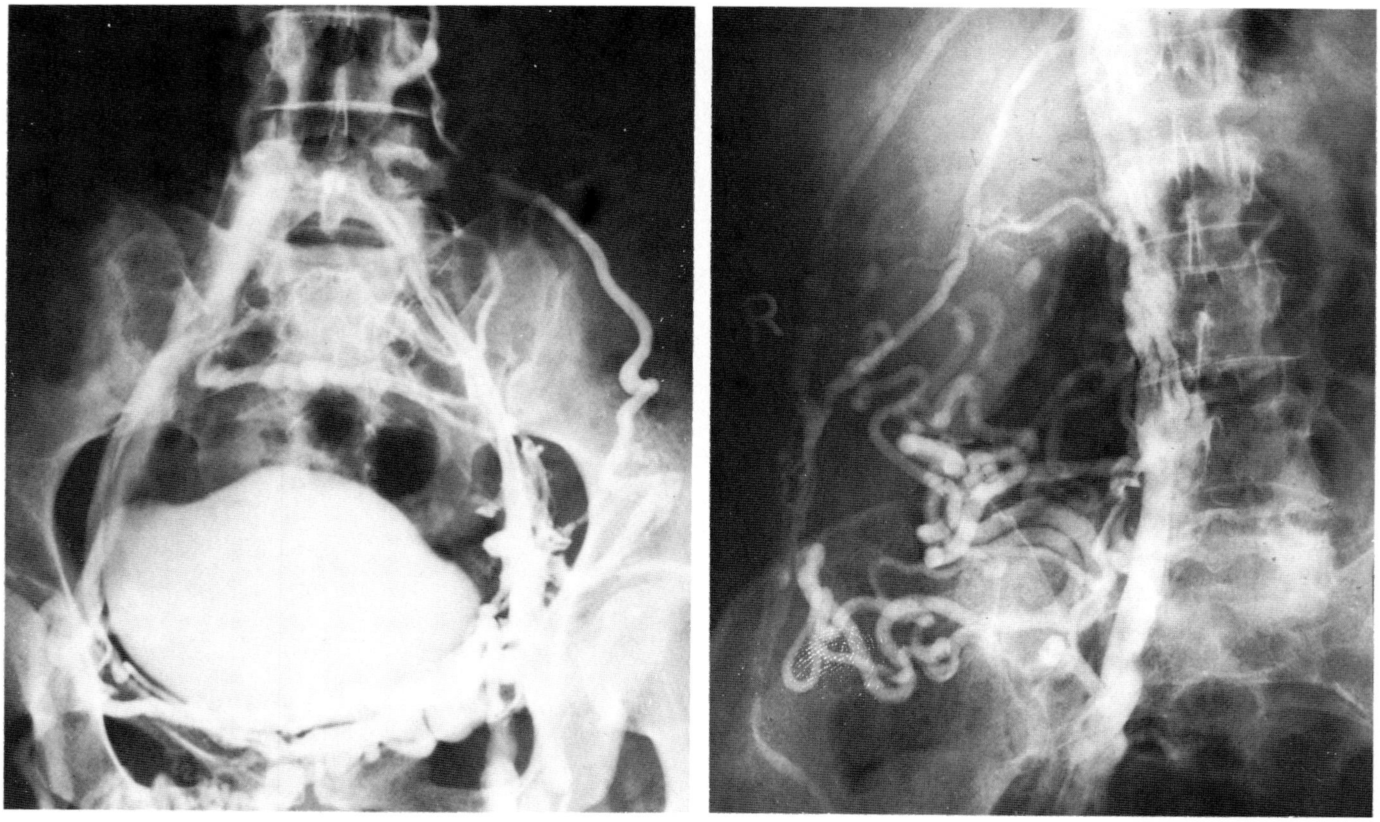

Fig. 27.16 A. Thrombosis of left iliac veins with partial recanalization and drainage of the left leg mainly by collaterals to the right iliacs via pubic veins. **B.** Thrombosis of IVC with recanalization and collateral circulation.

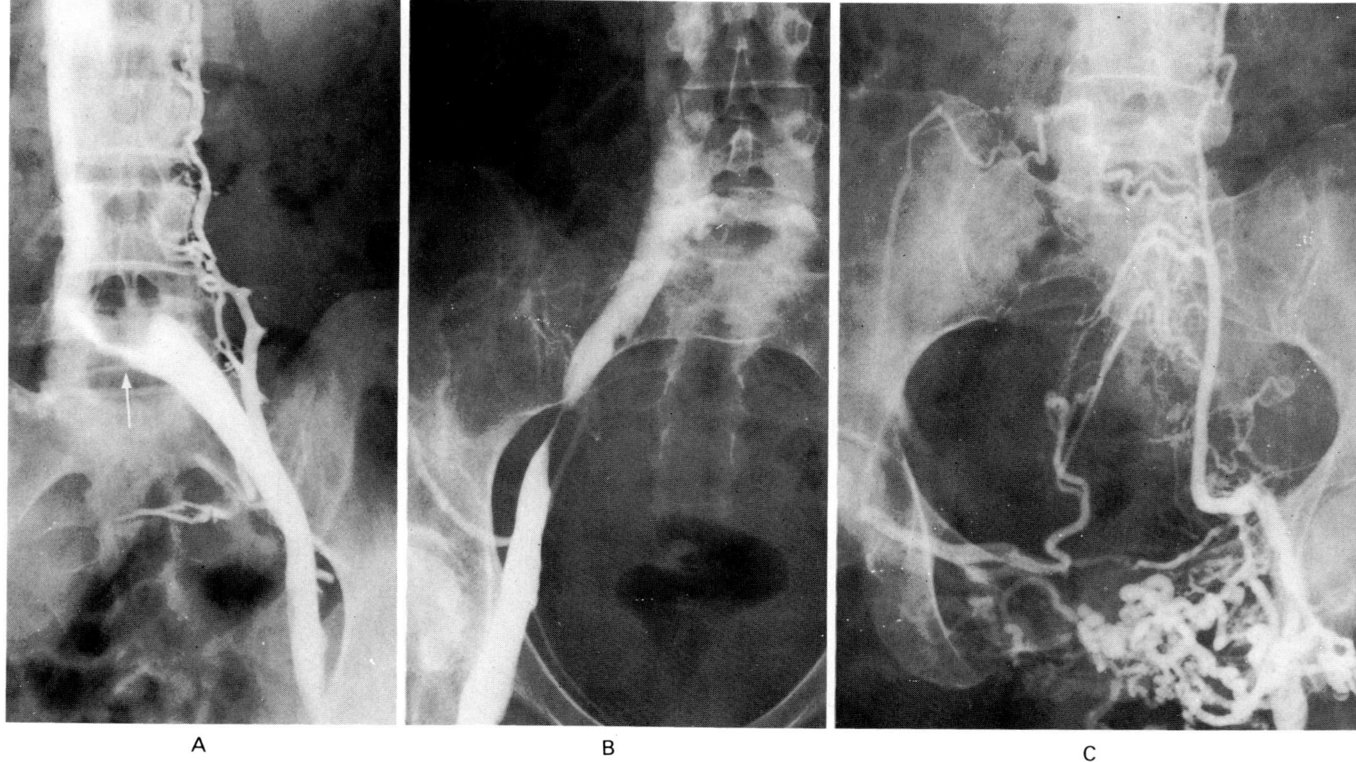

Fig. 27.17 A. Obstruction of the left common iliac vein by pressure from the right common iliac artery (arrow). Note collateral circulation via ascending lumbar vein. **B.** Iliac vein obstruction by glandular mass. **C.** Obstruction of left iliac veins in a patient with carcinoma of the cervix treated by radiotherapy.

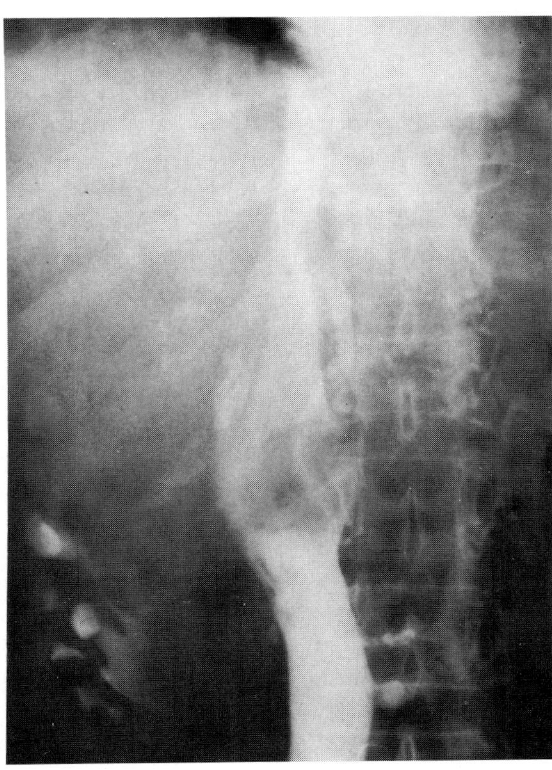

Fig. 27.18 Invasion of IVC by hypernephroma spreading up right renal vein.

THERAPEUTIC INTERRUPTION OF THE INFERIOR VENA CAVA

Pulmonary embolus is a major cause of death. It is estimated that there are 630 000 cases per annum in the USA with some 200 000 deaths. In untreated cases the recurrence rate is said to be 60% with a significant further mortality rate (22%). Most cases are treated by anticoagulation, with thrombolysis by strepo-kinase, or pulmonary embolectomy indicated in cases of massive pulmonary embolus. If anticoagulation is contraindicated, or fails to prevent recurrence then caval interruption should be considered, since over 90% of emboli arise from the leg veins.

Therapeutic interruption of the inferior vena cava to prevent further pulmonary emboli was first practised in 1945 by operative occlusion. Later operative partial interruption was practised by suture partition, bead compression and external fenestrated clipping. Because of the risks involved to seriously ill patients from general anaesthesia and laparotomy, these operations were gradually replaced by a simpler technique. This involved transvenous insertion of devices from the right internal jugular vein after operative cut down under local anaesthesia. The devices used include:

1. The Mobin-Uddin umbrella filter (1967) (see Fig. 27.13)
2. The Kimray-Greenfield filter (1973)
3. The Hunter detachable balloon (1975)

The procedure is best carried out by a radiologist and surgeon in cooperation. A preliminary inferior vena cavogram is necessary to confirm patency, to demonstrate possible anomalies and to show the level of the lowest renal vein. The device is passed down below the renal veins before being detached and stabilized. In some cases filters have been introduced from a femoral vein approach.

More recently, attempts have been made to develop filters which can be introduced percutaneously. The most promising of these is the 'bird nest filter' (Cook Inc) devised by Roehm et al. This can be introduced through a sheath and an 8F catheter. It consists of four stainless steel wires 0.18 mm wide by 25 cm long. The filter has two fine wire hooks at each end which can be fixed to the caval wall. The whole procedure can be rapidly performed by a radiologist and, if preliminary reports are confirmed, will undoubtedly become the procedure of choice.

MISCELLANEOUS ABDOMINAL CONDITIONS

Vulval varices are seen in pregnancy in 1 or 2% of patients and persist in a small proportion of cases, some of whom complain of discomfort requiring surgery. In some cases phlebography by direct injection of the varix will be required to show the anatomy and drainage. This is mainly into the internal pudendal and obturator veins and thence to the internal iliac, but there may be partial drainage to the external pudendal and femoral veins.

Lymphoedema Praecox was the term used for swelling of the left leg, usually occurring in young females and associated with partial obstruction of the left common iliac vein by the right common iliac artery passing over it (Fig. 27.17A).

Pelvic varicosities in the utero-vaginal plexus and in the broad ligament are said to be fairly common and have been cited as a cause of the 'pelvic congestion syndrome'. They can also be associated with vulval varices. High-dose bilateral femoral phlebography with simultaneous compression of the inferior vena cava has been recommended to demonstrate these pelvic varicosities well, but is not always successful.

Gonadal veins (ovarian and testicular veins). The right gonadal vein crosses in front of the ureter at the level of L.4 as it passes up and medially to enter the inferior vena cava below the right renal vein. When hypertrophied the ovarian vein can cause obstruction to the ureter giving rise to the so-called '*ovarian vein syndrome*'. This remains a controversial subject and the existence of this entity is not generally accepted.

The left gonadal vein usually drains into the left renal vein. Both gonadal veins can be demonstrated by passing a catheter into their upper ends from a transfemoral vein approach and injecting contrast. Varicoceles, which occur mainly on the left side, have been treated by percutaneous embolization of their drainage veins. Considerable success has been claimed for this procedure in the treatment of varicocele associated with male infertility.

Hepatic vein obstruction (Budd-Chiari syndrome). Following the passage of a catheter into the upper part of the inferior vena cava, the hepatic veins can often be demonstrated by a forced contrast injection, particularly if the patient performs the Valsalva manoeuvre during injection. Failure to fill the hepatic veins provides some evidence of thrombosis as occurs in the Budd-Chiari syndrome. In this condition the hepatic venous drainage is obstructed by tumour or thrombosis and a collateral circulation develops through the periumbilical veins. At inferior vena cavography, the upper inferior vena cava may be seen to be compressed or obstructed (Fig. 27.19) when a tumour is responsible.

Direct *hepatic phlebography* is performed by passing a catheter from the arm through the right auricle and into a hepatic vein. In the Budd-Chiari syndrome the normal wedged hepatic vein pattern is replaced by fine collateral vessels ('spider's web network'), or actual occlusions may be shown (see Ch. 35).

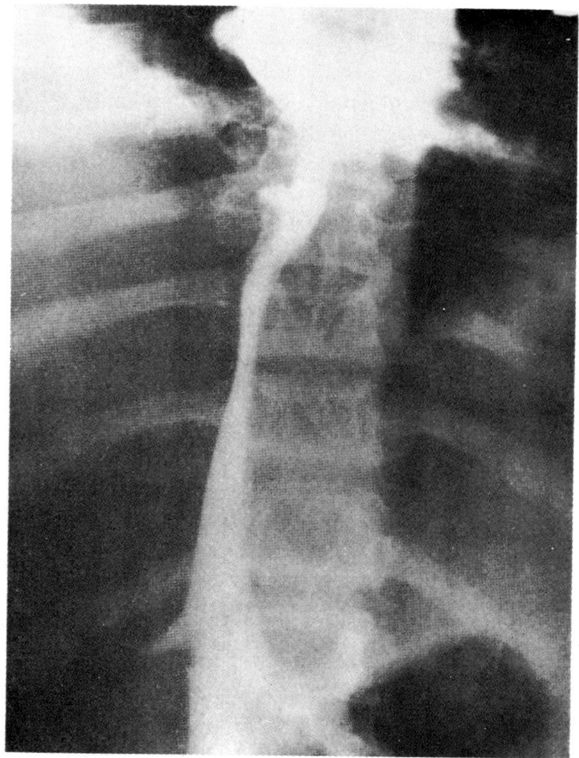

Fig. 27.19 Obstruction of hepatic veins with compression and distortion of upper IVC by liver neoplasm resulting in Budd-Chiari syndrome. The patient was performing the Valsalva manoeuvre. Note reflux filling of renal veins.

Renal phlebography. The renal veins can be selectively catheterized using the Seldinger percutaneous technique. A forced injection of 10 ml of contrast will show the venous drainage of most of the kidney and will thus confirm or exclude a renal vein thrombosis (Fig. 27.12B). The method has also been used to demonstrate mass lesions in the kidney, but these are better shown by other techniques.

The renal veins can also be shown by serial films taken after selective renal arteriography. The normal renal veins usually show well by this method. If they do not and a collateral venous drainage is also shown, this is good presumptive evidence of main renal vein occlusion.

It is important to realize that there may be more than one renal vein on either side, and attempts should always be made to identify and catheterize accessory veins. On the left side 7% of individuals have a lower accessory vein which is smaller than the normal upper vein and is retroaortic in position. The two veins form a circumaortic ring with the lower one usually entering the inferior vena cava at L.3–4 (Fig. 27.20).

Renal vein thrombosis has also been investigated by inferior vena cavography. In the normal inferior vena cavogram 'streamlining' effects are usually visible when the large renal veins enter the inferior vena cava. Absence of this normal streamlining effect is thought to be very suggestive of renal vein thrombosis, particularly when unilateral. Direct renal phlebography will prove the diagnosis conclusively.

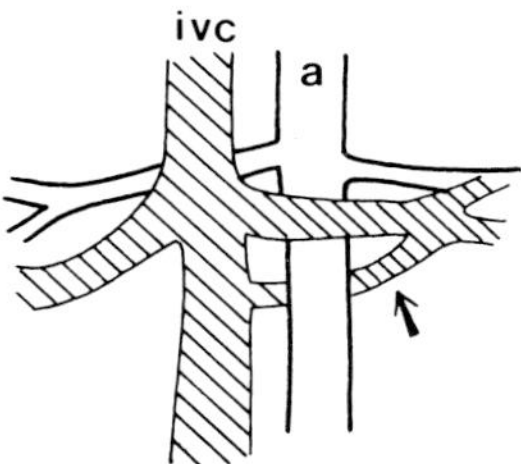

Fig. 27.20 Circumaortic ring formed by renal veins. a = aorta, IVC = inferior vena cava.

Renal vein thrombosis is common in dehydrated infants with diarrhoea. It also occurs in adults in association with inferior vena caval thrombosis, or thrombotic disease elsewhere. Occasionally it is seen with pyelonephritis or other renal disease. The affected kidney is usually enlarged from venous engorgement and the nephrotic syndrome may result. The vein itself is narrowed and irregular and the small peripheral veins may be occluded.

As noted above, hypernephroma frequently involves the renal vein and tumour may extend into the inferior vena cava (Fig. 27.18). The renal vein may also be occluded or compressed by extrinsic tumour masses or aneurysm, or by retroperitoneal fibrosis.

Renal vein renin. In cases of renal artery stenosis or suspected renal ischaemia it is helpful to assay the renin in the renal venous blood from the suspected kidney. This is obtained by percutaneous catheterization of the renal veins using the Seldinger technique. Samples are obtained from an arm vein at the same time so that comparisons can be made with peripheral venous blood.

Adrenal vein phlebography. The adrenal veins can be selectively catheterized using special catheters. Small tumours have been demonstrated by this means, when other methods have failed. In our experience the method has proved of most value in the diagnosis of small Conn's tumours in primary hyperaldosteronism. The method is discussed in greater detail in Chapter 36, but has now been superseded by CT.

UPPER LIMB AND SUPERIOR VENA CAVA

The usual indications for investigation of the venous drainage of the arm and superior vena cava are:

1. Oedema of the upper limb thought to be associated with venous thrombosis or obstruction, in order to demonstrate the site of obstruction, in either the axillary, subclavian or innominate veins.
2. Superior vena caval obstruction.
3. Demonstration of the full anatomy of venous angiomas or varices.
4. Demonstration of congenital venous anomalies as in the Klippel-Trenaunay syndrome.

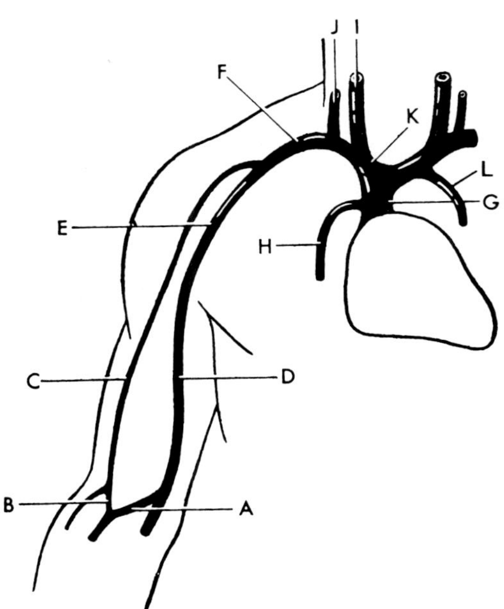

Fig. 27.21 Diagram showing venous drainage of the arm. A = median basilar vein. B = median cephalic vein. C = cephalic vein. D = basilic vein. E = axillary vein. F = subclavian vein. G = superior vena cava. H = azygos vein. I = internal jugular vein. J = external jugular vein. K = innominate vein. L = hemiazygos vein.

Technique. A vein at the elbow is catheterized and a catheter advanced several inches up the arm. This can be done percutaneously in most cases though occasionally a cut down exposure may be necessary. It is best to use the median basilic vein, since this will make it possible to opacify the axillary vein. Use of the median cephalic vein will of course bypass the basilic and axillary veins, since the cephalic vein does not join the subclavian vein until it has pierced the clavipectoral fascia (Fig. 27.21).

Some 30 ml of contrast medium are injected within 2 seconds, using a pressure injector if necessary. A rapid rate of injection is essential, since otherwise the contrast will fail to show the superior vena cava well. It is rapidly diluted in the thorax by the large blood flow from the head and neck and contralateral upper limb.

Serial films are taken at speeds of 1 or 2 films per second.

Another technique which can be used where percutaneous puncture of an elbow vein proves difficult is similar to that used for ascending phlebography of the lower limb. A vein on the dorsum of the hand is percutaneously punctured with a fine needle of the type routinely used by anaesthetists (B.S.W. gauge 21 or 23).

A tourniquet is applied just above the elbow and some 30 ml of contrast medium injected. The tourniquet is then released and the forearm massaged to ensure that a good bolus of contrast is delivered to the large veins in 2 seconds.

Radiographic appearances. The normal findings are illustrated in Figure 27.22.

Left-sided superior vena cava is an important congenital anomaly in which the superior vena cava lies on the left and drains into the coronary sinus. It may occur alone or in association with congenital heart disease. Occasionally there is a *double superior vena cava*, the right draining normally to the right auricle, and the left into the coronary sinus (Fig. 27.23).

Where a localized thrombosis is present in a major drainage vein, such as the axillary or subclavian vein, the blockage is usually well shown together with the collateral circulation which develops to bypass the lesion (Fig. 27.24).

Superior vena caval obstruction. This is characterized by venous engorgement of the head, neck and arms. The involvement of the superior vena cava by malignant glands can be recognized well before clinical evidence of superior vena caval obstruction ensues. In these cases extrinsic pressure defects on the vein will be seen. In the past, superior vena cavography has been used to assess suitability of cases of bronchial carcinoma for surgery, and to exclude clinically silent mediastinal glandular involvement. However, CT now provides a less invasive method of assessing mediastinal glandular involvement. DSA will also enable the superior vena cava to be checked using only a small amount of low concentration contrast medium. Isotope scanning can also confirm caval obstruction.

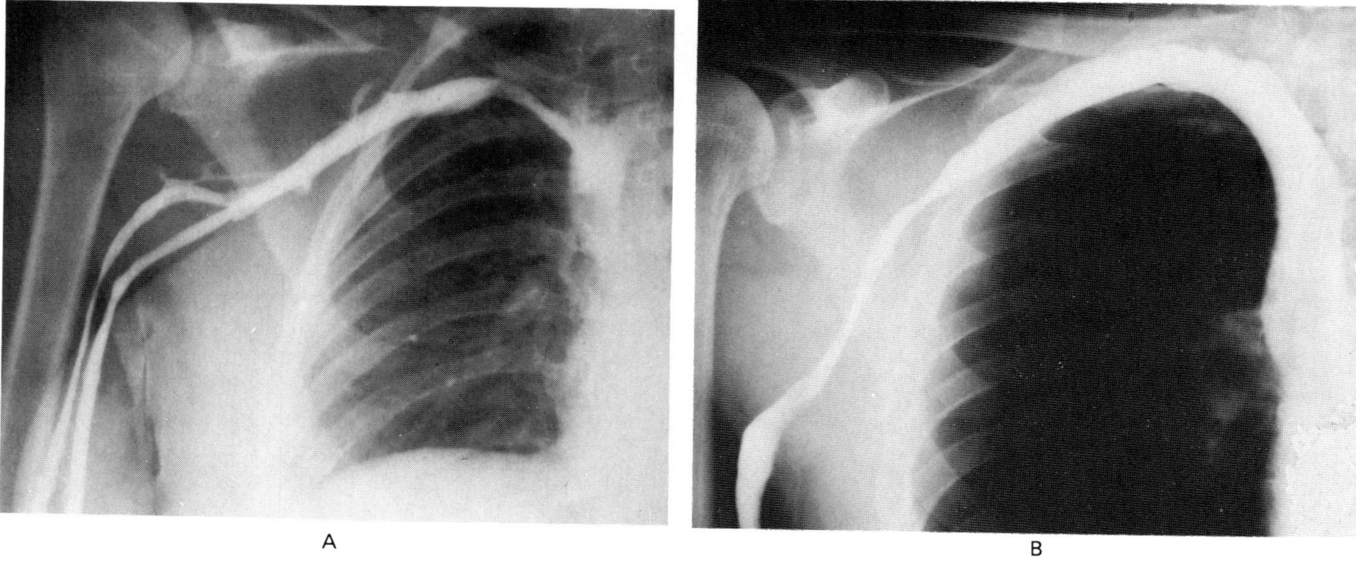

Fig. 27.22 A. Arm phlebogram showing normal appearances. **B.** Normal arm phlebogram — different case.

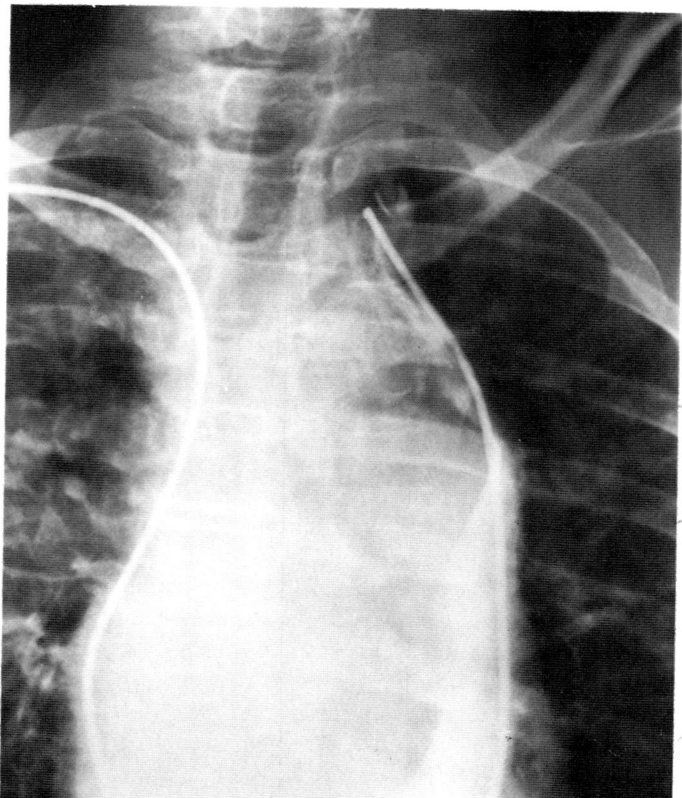

Fig. 27.23 Double superior vena cava. A catheter has been passed from the right arm for pulmonary angiography. Instead of entering the ventricle it has passed through the dilated coronary sinus and into the left superior vena cava draining into it, as evident on contrast injection. Note the widened mediastinum.

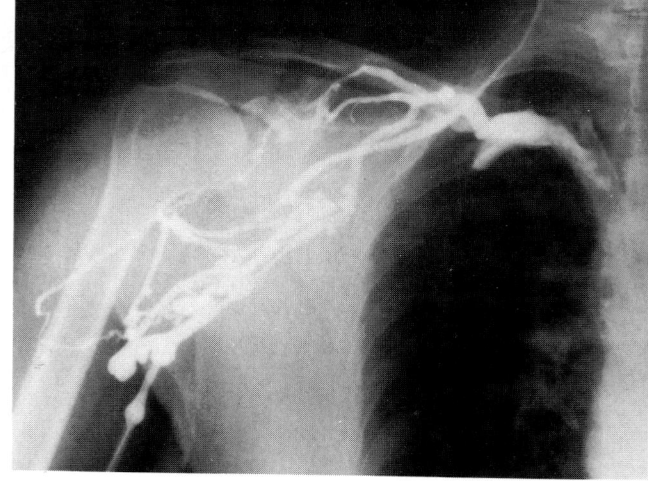

Fig. 27.24 Arm phlebogram showing obstruction in the axillary and subclavian veins.

The majority of patients (over 95%) with superior vena caval obstruction are suffering from *malignant neoplasm* (Fig. 27.25). Of these, about 80% have carcinoma of the lung and about 20% are suffering from lymphomas.

The small group of patients with *benign* superior vena caval obstruction are usually suffering from *fibrosing mediastinitis* (Fig. 27.26). These patients present with a relatively slow onset permitting the development of multiple collaterals. The aetiology is either unknown (idiopathic) or it is granulomatous. In this country the latter cases are usually *tuberculous*, but in North America

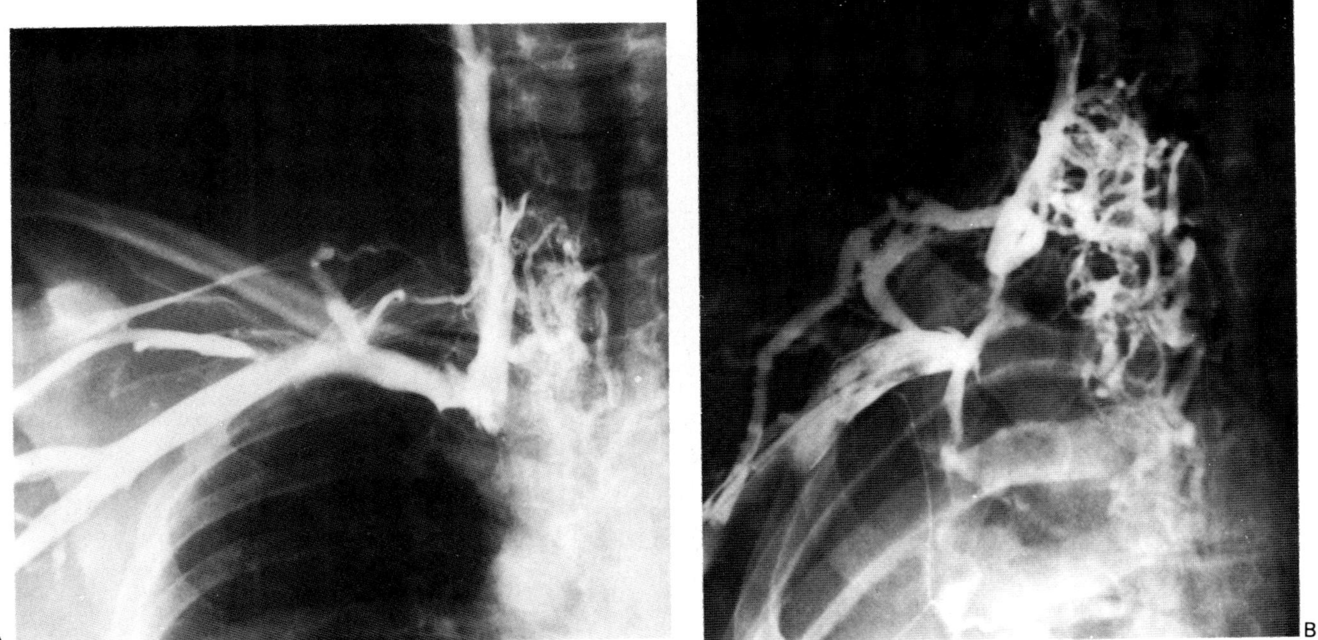

Fig. 27.25 A. Right arm phlebogram confirms malignant occlusion of innominate and SVC with reflux up right internal jugular, and vertebral collaterals. **B.** Occlusion of SVC innominate and termination of right subclavian vein. Collaterals to the vertebral vein and vertebral plexus.

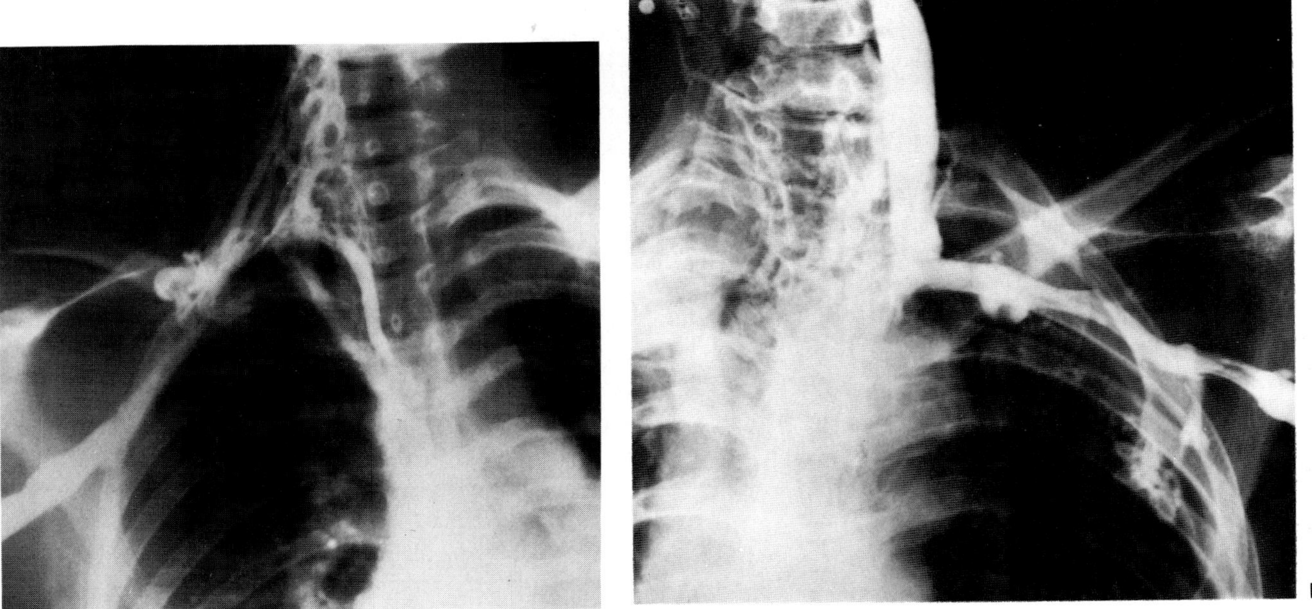

Fig. 27.26 A. Right arm phlebogram in fibrosing mediastinitis with involvement of SVC and right innominate vein. **B.** Left arm phlebogram in patient with fibrosing mediastinitis (tuberculous). Note kinked trachea. SVC and left innominate occluded. Collateral circulation via left internal jugular and vertebral plexus.

histoplasmosis is also a cause of the syndrome. Very rarely thrombosis of the superior vena cava is seen as a complication of ventriculo-atrial shunts. Compression of the superior vena cava may also be occasionally seen with aneurysm and other non-malignant mediastinal masses.

The *Klippel-Trenaunay syndrome* has been noted above (p. 742). The appearances in the affected upper limb of a patient with this condition are illustrated in Figure 27.27. Multiple phleboliths were present in addition to the venous dysplasia.

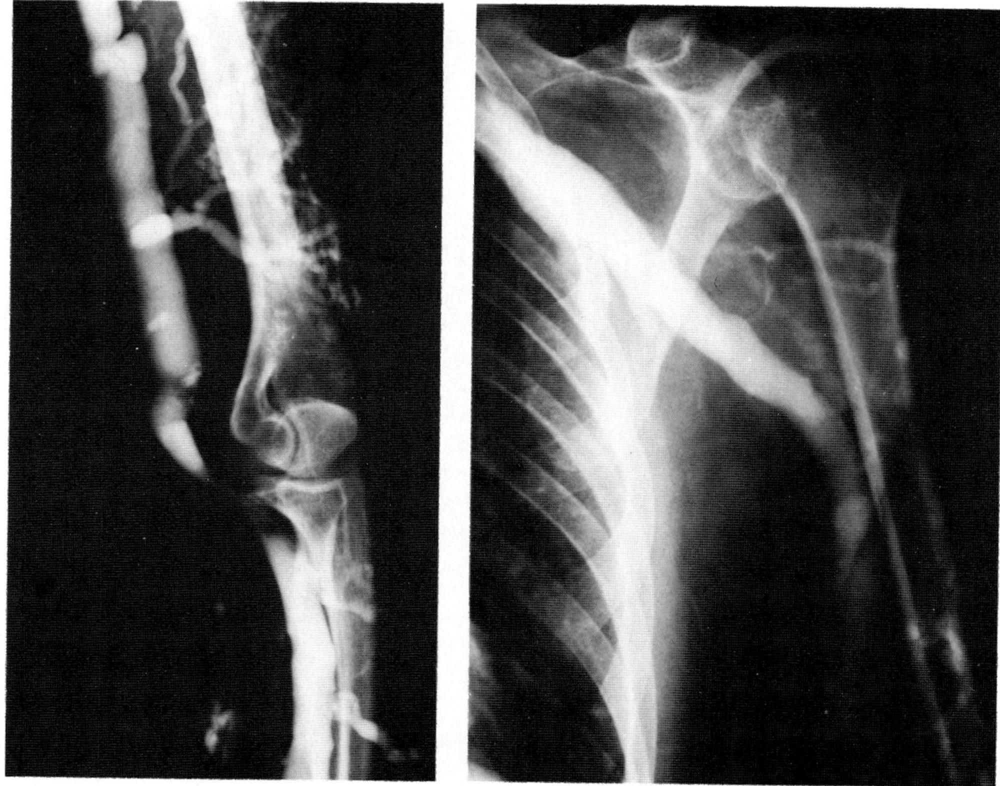

Fig. 27.27 A. & B. Klipped-Trenaunay syndrome involving left arm. Drainage is via a single medial vein which appears valveless with very sluggish flow.

INTRAOSSEOUS PHLEBOGRAPHY

Contrast can be readily injected into bone marrow and passes thence to the venous drainage. This fact has been made use of in the technique of intraosseous phlebography. A strong needle is passed through the bone cortex. A bone marrow type of needle is generally adequate for superficial bones, but a longer needle is necessary for bones situated deeply. The needle may be inserted by hard pressure or by sharp blows. Some workers prefer to perform this investigation under general anaesthesia, though others do it under local anaesthesia.

Once the needle is in situ, blood is aspirated from the bone marrow and up to 20 ml of 45% Hypaque or its equivalent are injected as rapidly as possible by hand. Most of the contrast usually passes into the venous sinusoids and drains into small veins. It then passes into larger trunks which emerge from the bone and enter the adjacent deep veins.

Complications. Faulty insertion of the needle has resulted in perforation of adjacent structures and, according to the bone being injected, these have included bladder, spinal cord and aorta. These complications have occurred during attempts to inject the superior pubic rami or the spinal vertebrae. The introduction of infection with resulting osteomyelitis is another possible complication.

Indications. Osseous phlebography has been mainly used for demonstrating the veins of the leg by injecting either the medial or lateral surfaces of the calcaneum, the medial malleolus or the lateral malleolus. For the thigh, injections have been made into the tibial tubercle or a femoral condyle. For pelvic phlebography and the demonstration of the inferior vena cava, injections have been made into the greater trochanter. The superficial ramus of the pubis had been used to demonstrate the pudendal, vesical, prostatic and presacral venous plexuses. The anterior superior iliac spine has also been used.

In the upper limb injections have been made into the olecranon process and the lower end of the radius. The acromion process has also been used for the cephalic and axillary veins. Contrast material has also been injected into the spinous process of the vertebrae to show the external and internal spinal venous plexuses.

Azygography can be performed by injection of contrast into one of the lower ribs, whence it passes to an intercostal vein.

The method has had some enthusiastic advocates but has not found general acceptance, and most workers prefer the safer techniques of phlebography described above.

PORTAL PHLEBOGRAPHY

The portal circulation, which is illustrated diagrammatically in Figure 27.28, can be outlined by four different methods:

1. Percutaneous splenic puncture
2. Operative mesenteric phlebography
3. Arterioportography
4. Transhepatic portal phlebography

1. **Percutaneous splenic puncture**. This technique has been widely used in the investigation of portal hypertension or suspected portal hypertension. It is also used in some cases of splenic enlargement where thrombosis in the splenic vein or portal system is thought to be a factor.

Technique. The usual landmark for percutaneous puncture of the spleen is in the 10th or 11th interspace in the mid-axillary line. The needle is passed inwards and upwards, and where the spleen is enlarged puncture is fairly easy. Usually the needle point can be felt puncturing the splenic capsule, and once it is in the splenic pulp a backflow of blood into the connecting tubing takes place. If portal pressure is very high the reflux of blood may be at considerable pressure. It is possible to measure the intrasplenic pressure by attaching the connecting tubing to a manometer and many workers practice this routinely.

For the contrast injection 20 to 50 ml of water-soluble iodide contrast medium is used. Better contrast is obtained by using high concentrations such as 85% Hypaque, or 440 Triosil, though lower concentrations can also be used.

Serial films are taken commencing about half-way through the injection of the contrast medium. Rates of 1 to 2 films per second for up to 10 seconds are generally adequate.

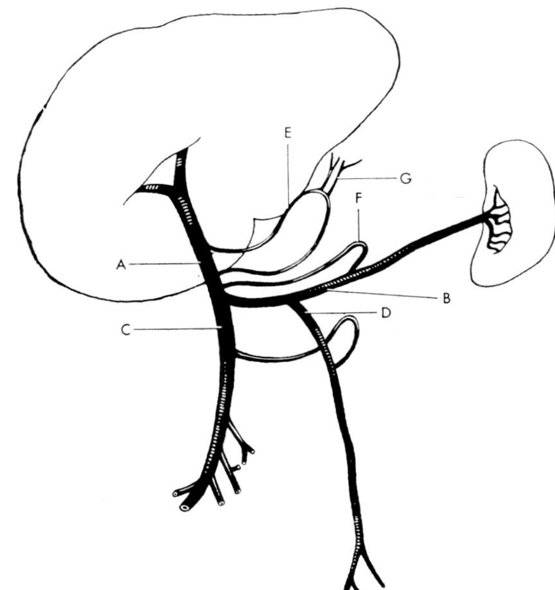

Fig. 27.28 Diagram of the portal circulation A = portal vein. B = splenic vein. C = superior mesenteric vein. D = inferior mesenteric vein. E = left gastric vein. F = gastroepiploic vein. G = oesophageal vein.

Where needle puncture is practised the needle is kept in the spleen for the minimum period necessary to complete the investigation. This is normally not more than 2 or 3 minutes. The procedure can be aided by the use of an image intensifier. This enables a small test dose to be given before the main injection and so permits more accurate siting of the needle tip. It also prevents the occasional accident of subcapsular extravasation of the contrast medium. Whilst the needle is in situ the patient is warned not to breathe too deeply and use only shallow respiration.

Some workers prefer to introduce a catheter into the spleen, either of polythene or of Teflon. This is done in the same way as for percutaneous needle puncture. The catheter is fitted tightly over the puncture needle, and the latter is withdrawn once its tip is in the correct position. If a catheter is inserted percutaneously it can of course remain in the spleen for a longer period than a needle.

Complications. Rupture of the spleen requiring splenectomy has been reported following the procedure. Therefore, unless laparotomy is to be proceeded with immediately after the splenic phlebogram, the patient should be carefully observed for a few days after the investigation for any sign of splenic rupture.

Occasionally the needle tip is badly positioned and a major injection of contrast medium has been made into the subcapsular region of the spleen. Less commonly, injections have been made into the peritoneum, and even into the colon. Apart from localized pain, these accidents appear to have had no serious consequences.

Indications. The main value of splenic phlebography is in the investigation of portal hypertension. Most cases are due to cirrhosis of the liver, but it is sometimes impossible to differentiate clinically between intrahepatic and extrahepatic portal obstruction. Where this problem arises, portal phlebography will often provide a clear-cut and unequivocal answer by showing a patent portal vein (Fig. 27.29).

If surgery is contemplated it will also provide the surgeon with valuable information by demonstrating the size of the portal vein and whether or not it is possible to anastomose it to the inferior vena cava. It will also show the size and shape of the splenic vein if the alternative operation of a splenorenal anastomosis is being considered.

Postoperative splenic phlebograms are occasionally performed to demonstrate the patency of a surgical anastomosis (Fig. 27.30).

Extrahepatic portal obstruction can result from tumours primary or secondary at the liver hilum. It can also result from portal vein thrombosis and this can occur in cases of cirrhosis, as can splenic vein thrombosis. A thrombosed or partially thrombosed portal vein can result in the development of collateral veins (Fig. 27.31), a condition once thought to be congenital and termed 'cavernoma' of the portal vein. It is thus clear that non-visualization of the

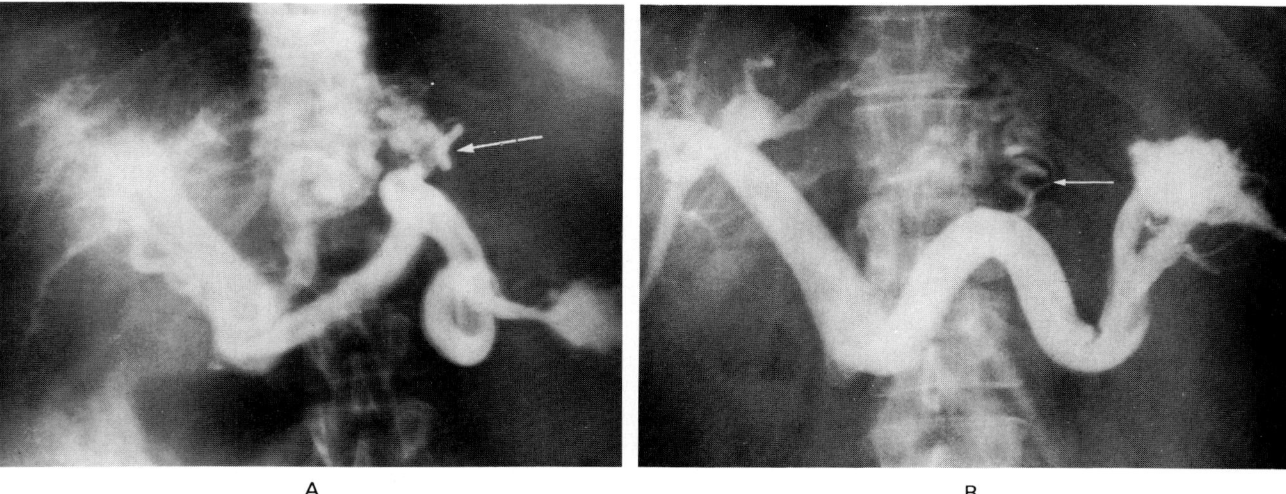

Fig. 27.29 A. and **B.** Splenic phlebograms showing gastric varices (arrow). The portal vein is patent in both cases.

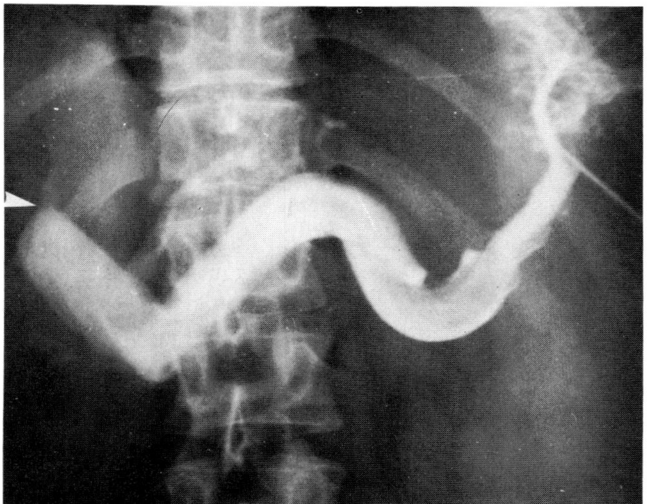

Fig. 27.30 Postoperative splenic phlebogram showing shunt of contrast from portal vein into inferior vena cava (arrow).

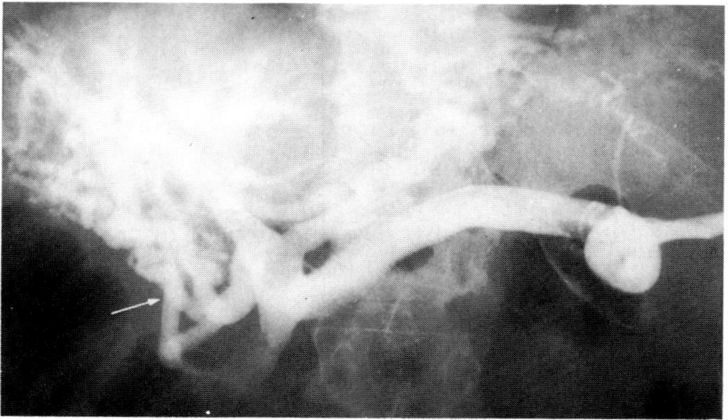

Fig. 27.31 Splenic phlebogram showing gastric varices. The portal vein is thrombosed and replaced by collaterals (arrow).

portal vein at splenic phlebography can be due to several causes and does not exclude a diagnosis of cirrhosis.

It is also important to realize that the portal vein may occasionally fail to outline, even when patent, if there is a major collateral circulation into which the splenic blood is being diverted. In these cases most of the portal blood is derived from the mesenteric circulation. Thus, where the portal vein has failed to show at a splenic phlebogram, or where the splenic vein itself appears obstructed, it may be necessary to perform arterial portography or even an operative mesenteric phlebogram to decide whether or not the portal vein is patent (Fig. 27.32)

Umbilical sepsis in infants is another cause of portal vein thrombosis. Recanalization may follow with a collateral circulation resulting in so-called cavernoma of the portal vein as described above.

Splenic phlebography has also been used in the past for demonstrating the morphology of the liver, in particular its vascular pattern in suspected neoplasms both primary or secondary and in cases of cirrhosis.

Radiological appearances. In cases of portal hypertension due to cirrhosis of the liver or to posthepatic portal obstruction the splenic and portal veins are normally well demonstrated, the latter being large in calibre. The collateral circulation is usually well shown also, and where gastric or oesophageal varices are present these can be clearly outlined (Fig. 27.29). In most cases, portal venography gives a better and more accurate demonstration of oesophageal varices than does the simpler examination of barium swallow. Sometimes, however, cases occur with excellent demonstration of oesopheageal varices by barium swallow where these failed to show well at portal venography.

Distortion of the intrahepatic vascular pattern may be seen in cases of cirrhosis, but this can be difficult to interpret.

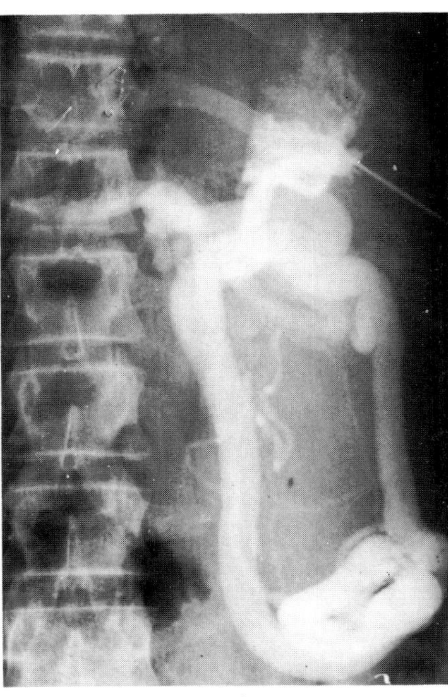
A

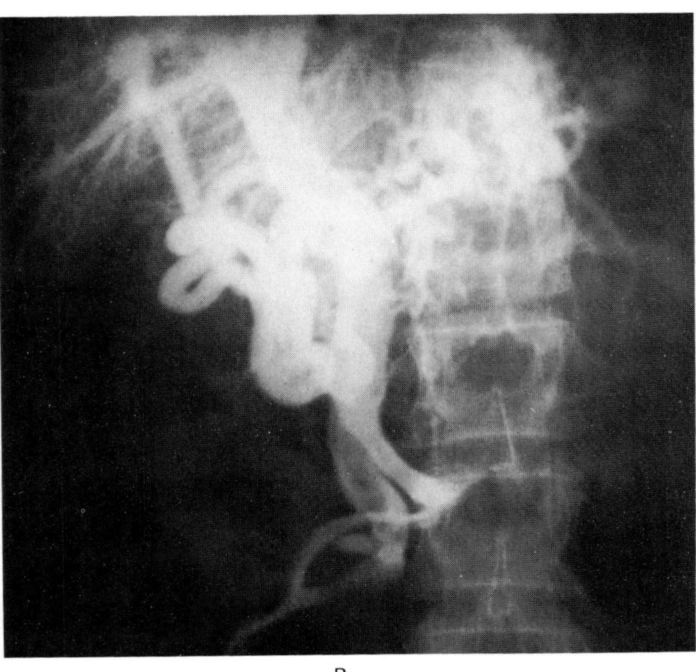
B

Fig. 27.32 A. Splenic phlebogram showing collateral circulation through huge inferior mesenteric vein. The splenic vein was occluded distally. **B.** Operative superior mesenteric phlebogram showing patent portal vein in the same case.

The widespread use of splenic venography has demonstrated the existence of numerous other collateral venous channels beside the well-recognized ones.

2. **Operative mesenteric phlebography.** In this method the portal system is demonstrated by injecting a mesenteric vein at laparotomy. As noted above the technique may be required to prove patency of the portal vein where the findings at percutaneous splenic phlebography has been inconclusive (Fig. 27.32).

Some early workers used the operative technique as a routine, but most preferred the percutaneous technique as the primary procedure.

3. **Arterioportography.** Advocates of this method prefer it because it obviates the dangers of direct splenic puncture and because the information obtained comprises both arterial and venous phases and can show the whole portal system. It can also contribute to the planning of shunt surgery. The normal technique is to catheterize the coeliac axis and then inject from a superselective position of the catheter tip in the splenic artery. 30–60 ml of contrast are injected at a rate of 10 ml per second and serial films obtained in the arterial and venous phase. If the patient's condition permits, the common hepatic artery can also be injected to show the state of the liver and pancreas with late films to demonstrate any possible hepaticofugal flow in the portal veins. If required, the left gastric artery can be injected to show varices and the superior mesenteric artery can also be injected to demonstrate the superior mesenteric vein. It may be essential to show this if mesocaval shunting is being considered.

There is no doubt that thorough arterioportography provides more information than simple splenic phlebography but it can be a prolonged and technically difficult procedure compared with simple direct splenic phlebography. It also requires good quality subtraction films to show the portal circulation well. Even with these, definition is never as clear as with the direct splenic method.

DSA can now be used to improve the definition of arterioportography. It also permits adequate visualization with much smaller doses of contrast medium.

4. **Transhepatic portal phlebography.** The main collateral venous supply of gastro-oesophageal varices may be visualized by percutaneous transhepatic catheterization of the portal vein (Fig. 27.33). Apart from being demonstrated by injection through the percutaneous catheter the varices can be selectively catheterized and obliterated by embolization (Lunderquist & Vang 1974, Viamonte et al 1977). The major indication is severe cirrhosis in patients in whom surgery is contraindicated. After successful obliteration of varices, surgery may be performed electively or deferred. The long-term effectiveness of this method has not yet been established.

The method of transhepatic portal phlebography has also been used for the purpose of obtaining venous samples for assay from the pancreatic drainage veins into the splenic and superior mesenteric veins. These assays are helpful in the localization of pancreatic hormone producing tumours. The method is discussed in greater detail in Chapter 35.

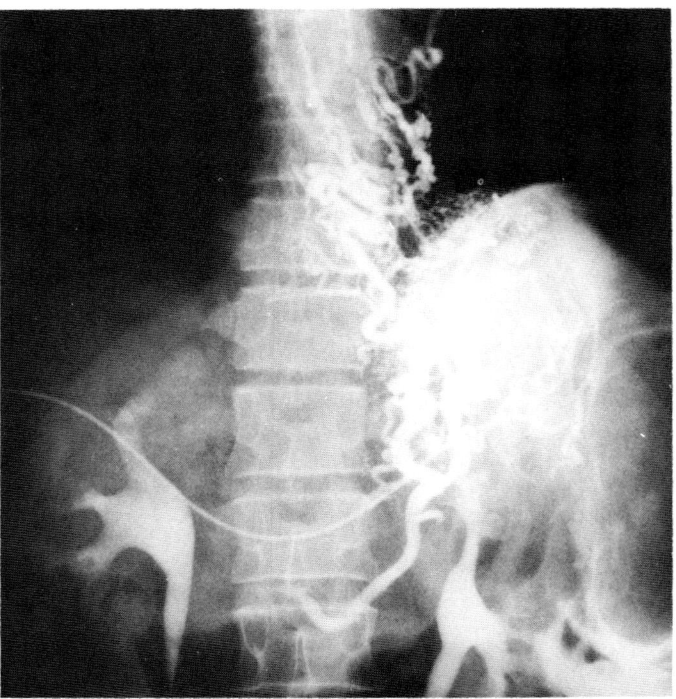

Fig. 27.33 Varices demonstrated by transhepatic portal vein catheterization.

SPINAL PHLEBOGRAPHY

The epidural veins in the spinal canal can be demonstrated by spinal phlebography. The main use of this method has been for the lumbar region where it has proved a useful addition to conventional methods of investigating disc protrusions.

Myelography and even radiculography will occasionally prove negative in cases of disc protrusion, usually where the disc lies laterally or there is a large epidural space. In these cases the spinal phlebogram can sometimes confirm strong clinical suspicion that a lesion is present despite the negative radiculogram. With the increasing use of CT and MRI for spinal disc problems, the method may soon become obsolete (see Chs 58 and 68).

Technique. A short 5F catheter is introduced via the femoral vein by Seldinger technique and passed into a lateral sacral vein on the opposite side. A similar catheter is passed into an ascending lumbar vein on the same side since simultaneous injection of contrast material into an ascending lumbar vein on one side and a lateral sacral vein on the other side often gives the best results. The contrast injection is made with abdominal compression of the inferior vena cava so as to force the contrast into the lumbar sacral and epidural veins. Disc herniation is diagnosed from complete interruption of an epidural vein or partial interruption or displacement. Deformity or interruption of the veins in the intravertebral foramina are also significant (veins of the lateral foramina). These veins connect the ascending lumbar and ascending epidural veins at each disc level (Fig. 27.34).

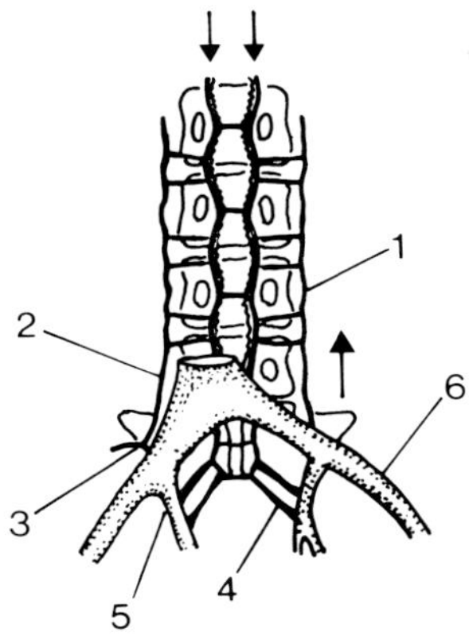

Fig. 27.34 Diagram of lumbar spinal veins (after Theron et al 1976).

REFERENCES AND SUGGESTIONS FOR FURTHER READING

Major text-books

Abrams H. L. (ed.) 1983 *Angiography*, 3rd ed. Boston: Little Brown

Athanasioulis C. A. et al. (eds) (1982) *Interventional Radiology*. Philadelphia: Saunders

Reuter R. S., Redman R. H. (1977) *Gastro-intestinal Angiography*, 2nd edn. Philadelphia: Saunders

References of historical interest

Berberich J., Hirsch S. (1923) Die Rontgenographische Darstellung der Arterien und Venen am lebenden Menschen. *Klinische Wochenschrift*, 2226–2228

Brooks B. (1924) Intra-arterial injection of sodium iodide. *Journal of the American Medical Association*, **82**, 1016–1019

Doby T. (1976) *Development of Angiography*. Littleton, Mass.: Publishing Sciences Group Inc.

Dos Santos R., Lamas A. C., Caldas J. P. (1931) *Arteriographie des membres et de le aorte abdominale*. Paris: Masson

Farinas P. L. (1941) A new technique for the arteriographic examination of the abdominal aorta and its branches. *American Journal of Roentgenology*, **46**, 641–645

Forssman W. (1929) Die Sondierung der Rechten Hertzens. *Klinishce Wochenschrift*, **8**, 2087–2089

Haschek E., Lindenthal T. O. (1896) Ein Beitrag zur praktischen Verwerthung der Photographie nach Rontgen. Wiener *Klinishe Wochenschrift* **9**, 63–4, Jan. 23, 1896

Moniz E. (1931) *Diagnostic des tumeurs cerebrals et epreuve de l'encephalographie arterielle*. Paris: Masson

Orrin H. C. (1920) *X-ray Atlas of the Systemic Arteries of the Human Body*. London: Bailliere Tindall & Cox

Seldinger S. (1953) Catheter replacement of the needle in percutaneous *arteriography*. *Acta Radiologica*, **39**, 368–376

Serbinenko F. A. (1974) Balloon catheterization and occlusion of major cerebral vessels. *Journal of Neurosurgery*, **41**:1, 125–145

Sicard J. A., Forestier J. (1932) *The Use of Lipiodol in Diagnosis and Treatment*. London: Oxford University Press
Sutton D. (1962) *Arteriography*. Edinburgh: Livingstone

References

Ansell G. (1976) *Complications in Diagnostic Radiology*. Oxford: Blackwell
Chuang V. P., Wallace S. (1981) Hepatic artery embolization in the treatment of hepatic neoplasms. *Radiology*, **140**, 51–58
Dawson P., Grainger R. G., Pitfield J. (1983) The new low osmolar contrast media. *Clinical Radiology*, **34**, 221–226
Debrun G., Legre J., Kasbarian M., et al. (1979) Endovascular occlusion of vertebral fistulae by detachable balloons with conservation of vertebral blood flow. *Radiology*, **130**, 141–147
Ekelund L., Gerlock J., Ogoncharenko V. (1978) The epinephrine effect in renal angiography revisited. *Clinical Radiology*, **29**, 387–392
Goodwin J. D., Hertfkens R. L., et al. (1980) Evaluation of dissections and aneurysms of the thoracic aorta by conventional and dynamic CT scanning. *Radiology*, **136**, 125
Gregson R. H. S., Sutton D., Brennan J., et al (1983) Spontaneous aorto-caval fistula. *Clinical Radiology*, **34**, 683–687
Gruntzig A. (1978)Transluminal dilatation of coronary artery stenosis. *Lancet*, **1**, 263
Gruntzig A., et al. (1978) Treatment of renovascular hypertension with percutaneous transluminal dilatation of a renal artery stenosis. *Lancet*, **i**, 801
Herlinger H. (1978) Arterioportography. *Clinical Radiology*, **29**, 255–275
Hobbs J. T. (ed.) (1977) *The Treatment of Venous Disorders*. Philadelphia: Lippincott
Lang E. K. (1981) Transcatheter embolization of pelvic vessels for control of intractable haemorrhage. *Clinical Radiology*, **35**, 85–93
Lea Thomas M. (1982) *Phlebography of the Lower Limb*. Edinburgh: Churchill Livingstone
Lunderquist A., Vang J. (1974) Transhepatic catheterization and obliteration of the coronary vein in patients with portal hypertension and oesophageal varices. *New England Journal of Medicine*, **291**: 646–649
Mandell V. S. et al. (1985) Persistent sciatic artery. *American Journal of Roentgenology*, **144**, 245–249
Miller D. C., Stinson E. B., Oyer P. E., et al. (1979) Operative treatment of aortic dissections: experience with 125 patients. *Journal of Thoracic and Cardiovascular Surgery*, **78**, 365
O'Halpin D., Legge D., MacErlain D. P. (1984) Therapeutic arterial embolization: Report of five years experience. *Clinical Radiology*, **35**, 85–93
Royal S. A., Callen P. W. (1979) CT evaluation of anomalies of the I.V.C. and left renal vein. *American Journal of Roentgenology*, **132**, 759–763
Sutton D., North E. (1977) Unusual AV Communications presenting as Cardiac Murmurs in Infancy *British Journal of Radiology*, **50**, 871
Starnes H. F., Vallance R., Hamilton D. N. H. (1984) Recurrent varicose veins: a radiological approach to investigation. *Clinical Radiology*, **35**, 95–99
Theron J., Houteville J. P., Ammerich H., et al, (1976) Lumbar phlebography by catheterization of the lateral sacral and ascending lumbar veins with abdominal compression. *Neuroradiology*, **11**, 175–182
Viamonte M., et al. (1977) Transhepatic obliteration of gastro-oesophageal varices. *American Journal of Roentgenology*, **129**, 237–241
Wallace S. et al. (1981) Embolization of renal carcinomas: experience with 100 patients. *Radiology*, **138**, 563
Wells I. P., Hammonds J. C., Franklin K. (1983) Embolization of hypernephromas: a simple technique using ethanol. *Clinical Radiology*, **34**, 689–692
Wilbur A C et al. (1985) Adventitial cystic disease of the Popliteal Artery Radiology 155: 63–4
Zeitler E., Gruntzig W., Schoop W. (1978) *Percutaneous Vascular Recanalization*. Berlin: Springer

CHAPTER 28

THE LYMPHATIC SYSTEM

Developments in imaging techniques in recent years have challenged the traditional role of lymphangiography in the assessment of lymphatic disease. CT scanning, in particular, is being more frequently used in the initial assessment of patients with suspected nodal disease. Lymphangiography, however, remains the only method capable of visualizing the internal architecture of the lymphatic vessels and nodes and still plays a very important role especially in the evaluation of the lymphoedemas. The anatomy of the lymphatic system and the technique of lymphangiography will be briefly described followed by discussion of the disorders of the lymphatic system and the role of the various imaging modalities.

LYMPHANGIOGRAPHY

The first description of a method for the in vivo demonstration of lymphatic vessels was by Kinmonth in 1952 using water-soluble contrast. This was extended by Wallace et al. in 1962 to a full examination of the lymphatic channels and glands by injecting oily contrast medium. This made it possible to investigate nodal disease as well as the lymphoedemas.

Indications for lymphangiography

1. The investigation of primary and secondary lymphoedema.
2. The detection of metastases in cases of malignant disease, e.g. melanoma, seminoma of the testicles, carcinoma of the female genital tract and bladder tumours.
3. To check efficient gland clearance at operation (portable films can be taken in theatre).
4. The diagnosis and staging of the reticuloses and checking progress during therapy by taking follow-up films. The contrast remains in the glands for 6 months to 2 years in pathological cases.
5. Miscellaneous conditions such as chylothorax, thoracic duct injuries, filariasis, chyluria and lymphocele formation may be investigated.
6. The intralymphatic route may be used for chemotherapy in cases of melanoma.

Contraindications

Iodine sensitivity and a definite history of allergy are absolute contraindications. In severe pulmonary disease with reduced respiratory reserve, oily lymphangiography should be avoided.

Severe skin sepsis, and especially epidermophytosis, should be treated beforehand. Lymphoedematous legs are very prone to sepsis.

If the leg or arm is very oedematous, successful cannulation is less likely and every effort should be made to reduce the oedema by preliminary bed rest and limb elevation.

TECHNIQUE

The procedure is performed in the radiology department with television monitoring. If the leg or arm is oedematous it is necessary to have it elevated for approximately 48 hours before attempting to cannulate a lymphatic. In the presence of oedema there may be no lymphatic uptake of the patent blue violet dye used to delineate the lymphatics and no lymphatics may be found on exploration.

The patient should have an empty bladder before the examination is begun as he will be immobilized for some time. The patient and the ward sister should be warned that the patent blue dye will cause an overall greyish-green skin discolouration which will fade within 24 to 48 hours. The urine is also discoloured blue.

Before commencing the examination a decision is made as to whether a water-soluble or oily contrast medium is to be used. This will depend on the presenting problem. However, in either technique the initial stages of the examination are identical and consist of demonstrating a lymphatic vessel, dissecting it and cannulating it.

The foot is thoroughly cleansed and 0.5 ml of patent blue violet 2.5% are injected subcutaneously into two toe or finger webs. The foot or hand is actively or passively exercised for 5 minutes. The dye is taken up by the lymphatic vessels draining the area injected which are clearly seen through the skin on the dorsum of the foot or hand. In some cases of lymphoedema, instead of lymphatic vessel delineation the dye may diffuse through the foot in the subcutaneous tissues. When this occurs it is not possible in many of the cases to isolate a lymphatic vessel and the procedure may have to be abandoned. This is seen most often in lymphatic hypoplasia and aplasia. However, even in the presence of diffuse skin staining it is worthwhile making an exploratory incision beyond the edge of the dye as occasionally a single lymphatic may be found.

Having outlined the lymphatics with the patent blue dye, a suitable one is chosen for cannulation and local anaesthetic is injected subcutaneously over it. An incision is made on the dorsum of the foot in a transverse direction through the anaesthetized skin. The transverse incision is chosen as it has the advantage that it can easily be enlarged in either direction to isolate a companion lymphatic if failure to cannulate the first vessel occurs. The selected lymphatic is dissected free from its surrounding structures by using blunt dissection with small mosquito forceps in the line of the lymphatic. When the lymphatic vessel has been isolated the tip of a pair of mosquito forceps is slipped beneath it. This is used to steady the lymphatic during manipulation and to apply countertraction when inserting the needle. In addition, some very fine catgut is passed beneath the lymphatic and left in situ, ready to tie the needle in place after insertion. The cannula used is the St Thomas' type, 27G, prepacked, sterilized and disposable. Before use the tube is filled with saline. The needle is introduced along the lymphatic and saline is gently injected. Any leakage from the lymphatic will be obvious and implies an imperfect puncture. The injection should immediately cease and another attempt at a clean puncture should be made. It is remarkable how well the lymphatic vessel will tolerate a number of unsuccessful punctures. When the needle has been satisfactorily placed in the lymphatic and no leakage occurs on injection, the catgut is tied around the needle, securing it in place. The tubing can be held in position by loose adhesive strapping in the form of a bridge.

Before injecting oily contrast it is wise to check that there is satisfactory lymphatic filling. A few millilitres of a water-soluble contrast are injected and observed on the television screen. This is especially important for the less experienced operator to avoid the inadvertent cannulation of a small venule.

Ultra fluid Lipiodol is the oily medium used and no more than 6–10 ml should be injected into each limb (3–4 ml are sufficient for the upper limb). The rate of injection should be 7 ml per hour. A pump system is required to introduce the oil. Various types of pump are available, from a simple gravity feed system to a variable speed electrically driven pump. During the injection the progress of contrast can be checked on the television screen and particular note is taken of any possible lymphatico-venous communication. When the injection has been completed the needle is removed, the incision is sutured and a sterile dressing is applied. In the investigation of pelvic and abdominal glands, both lower limbs are cannulated and infused at the same time.

When necessary, the procedure can be performed on the wards and check films taken with a portable X-ray machine. The radiographs that are taken in the X-ray department with the overcouch tube are the following:

1. Antero-posterior view of groin and pelvis.
2. Lateral pelvis.
3. Antero-posterior abdomen.
4. Oblique pelvis and abdomen.
5. Lateral abdomen.
6. Chest.

On occasion it may be helpful to have an AP with 45° caudal angulation view. The oblique views are particularly helpful in cases where overlapping of glands creates a difficulty in diagnosis.

Where doubt exists about normality of a gland or a possible translucency, then tomography may be performed.

These first films are taken immediately after the oily infusion has been completed to show the lymphatic phase. Further films are taken at 24 hours, when the lymphatic vessels will have emptied and glandular filling will be more complete.

An intravenous injection of contrast may be given to delineate the kidneys and ureters. This information may be useful to the radiotherapist.

The same principle is applied in lymphangiography of the upper limbs.

Testicular lymphangiography may be indicated in cases of testicular tumours. A laterally placed gland opposite L1 or L2 may only fill by injecting spermatic cord vessels. Metastases to this region can occur in testicular tumours.

In cases of primary lymphoedema when only water-soluble contrast is used, the injection is made by hand and a mechanical pump is not needed. The flow is observed on the television screen and films are taken during the injection. Conray 280 is a suitable contrast medium.

COMPLICATIONS

1. Allergic reactions. Reaction to iodine occurs in 0.1% of cases and varies from a mild urticarial rash to severe oedema, bronchospasm and circulatory collapse. Reactions may occur to the local anaesthetic or the patent blue dye.

2. Wound infection.

3. Lymphangitis. This may be chemical or bacterial and occurs more commonly in lymphoedema.

4. Fever. This is normally mild and follows oily injections.

5. Nausea and vomiting.

6. Lymphatic rupture. This may occur if the contrast injection is too forceful or rapid (Fig. 28.1).

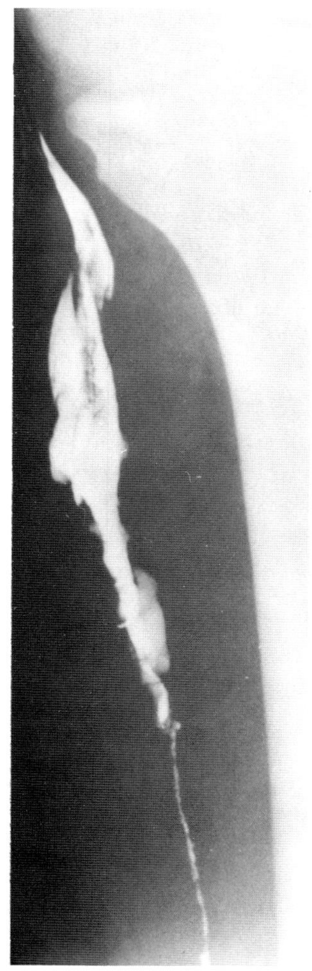

Fig. 28.1 Perilymphatic contrast medial to the tibia following rupture of the lymphatic due to high injection pressure.

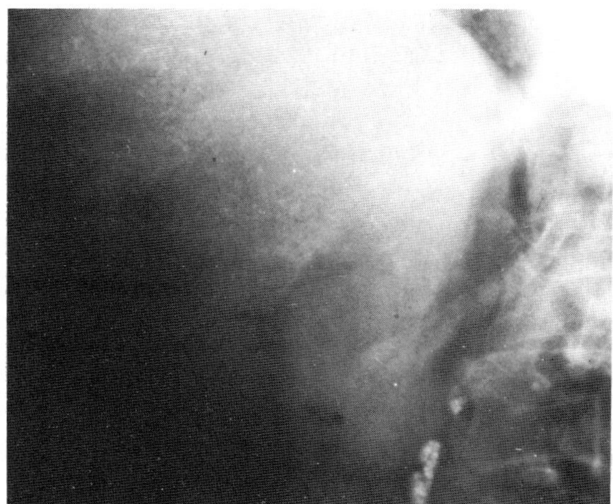

Fig. 28.2 Oily contrast in the liver from lymphaticoportal communications following pelvic clearance for gynaecological malignancy.

7. Accidental venous injection of oil. Television screening during the early stages should detect oil in the veins and the procedure should be stopped.

8. Pulmonary oil embolism. Fine embolization into the lungs occurs in all cases as the thoracic duct opens into the venous system and miliary or reticular oil deposits are seen in the lungs after 24 hours in about 10% of patients. Small oil emboli reduce the capillary bed available for diffusion of gases and cause an alveolar-capillary block. The maximum decrease occurs between 3 and 72 hours. This is of no clinical consequence in the vast majority of patients. In some however, more severe oil embolization may occur leading to cough, pain, fever, oedema and sometimes collapse. These severe complications occur more frequently when excessive quantities of the oily contrast are used and in the presence of lymphatic obstruction with lymphaticovenous communications. In these cases smaller doses of contrast should be used and careful monitoring is advisable.

9. Hepatic oil embolism. This is rarely a cause of symptoms. It occurs in lymphatic obstruction with lymphaticoportal anastomoses. The incidence is approximately 0.2% and stippled densities may be seen in the liver (Fig. 28.2).

10. Cerebral oil embolism. This is rare and more likely to occur in patients receiving radiotherapy at the time of the procedure. Lymphangiography should not be performed during radiotherapy or on patients who have had radiotherapy to the lungs recently.

NORMAL ANATOMY

Lower limbs and abdomen. The lymphatic vessels from the subcutaneous tissues of the foot form three major groups at the ankle. The *antero-medial* group accompanies the long saphenous vein on the medial aspect; the *antero-lateral* group accompanies the peroneal vessels and crosses over to the medial aspect to join the first group and drain into the superficial inguinal nodes. The *posterior* group runs close to the short saphenous and drains into the popliteal nodes and the deep inguinal nodes. The vessels remain approximately the same size but branch and rebranch as they pass upwards.

Both the deep and superficial inguinal glands continue into the external iliac glands. Occasionally a lymphatic channel may bypass the inguinal nodes to enter the pelvic nodes. This variant has some importance in assessing the spread of cancer.

In the pelvis the lymphatics form three channels around the external iliac artery and enter the external iliac glands. The efferent vessels form three chains around the common iliac vessels and enter the common iliac glands. The efferent vessels from both common iliac glands join at the sacrum and enter the para-aortic group which are in four situations: right para-aortic, left para-aortic, retroaortic, and preaortic.

The efferent vessels from the abdominal viscera join the vessels from the para-aortic region to enter the cisterna chyli at the level of L2–T12 and then continue into the thorax as the thoracic duct. The duct traverses the thoracic spine to the left at T5 level and, in the vast majority of people, enters the venous system at the junction of the left internal jugular and the left subclavian veins. There are many variations in the anatomy of this termination.

In the chest the thoracic duct receives tributaries from the posterior mediastinum and the posterior intercostal lymphatics. It is joined by the left jugular trunk from the neck and the left subclavian trunk. An accessory duct may be found on the left which opens independently. The thoracic duct may open as one, two or multiple channels. It may enter the subclavian vein directly or the innominate vein or even join the venous system on the right.

Upper limb. The channels formed by the superficial vessels in the dorsal and palmar aspects of the hand pass vertically upwards in two major groups. The *medial ulnar* group which accompanies the basilic vein to the antecubital fossa and then pierces the deep fascia to end in the axillary glands. The *lateral radial* group closely accompanies the cephalic vein and ends in the axillary and infra-clavicular nodes.

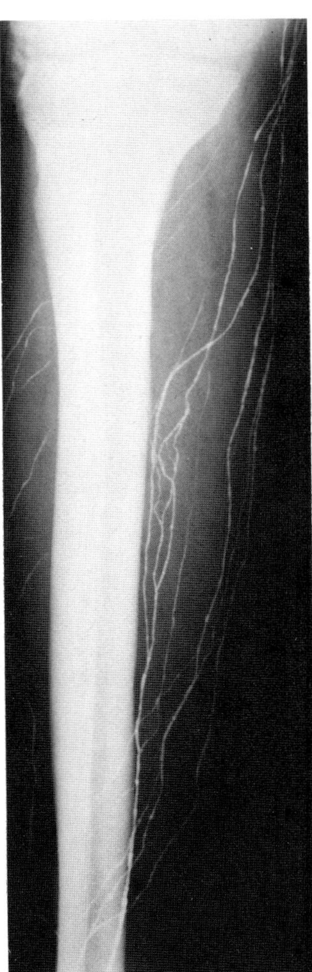

Fig. 28.3 Normal lymphatic channels in the calf. The beaded appearance of the lymphatics is due to small valves.

Normal radiographic appearances

The examination demonstrates a lymphatic phase seen on the early films, and a nodal phase seen on the 24-hour films when the lymphatic vessels have emptied.

The lymphatic vessels of the limb form fine channels which contain tiny valves ensuring the centripetal flow of the lymph. These valves are so numerous that they give the lymphatics a sacculated appearance. The lymphatic vessels in the calf vary from 5 to 15 in number (Fig. 28.3). The efferent vessels from one group of glands may bypass the next set of glands to a higher group. An example of this is shown in Figure 28.4. Ectopic glands are sometimes present in the thigh as seen in Figure 28.5.

Figure 28.6 shows the lymphatic phase in the groin and pelvis. Figures 28.7 and 28.8 show the nodal phase of the abdomen and pelvis in the antero-posterior and oblique projections. The lateral film of the abdomen (Fig. 28.9) demonstrates the relationship of the lymphatic pathways to the spine. Cross-flow channels exist between the two sides and these become more prominent in the presence of obstruction.

There is no constant pattern of node anatomy in the pelvis or abdomen. The nodes are frequently different in distribution on both sides in the same patient. There is

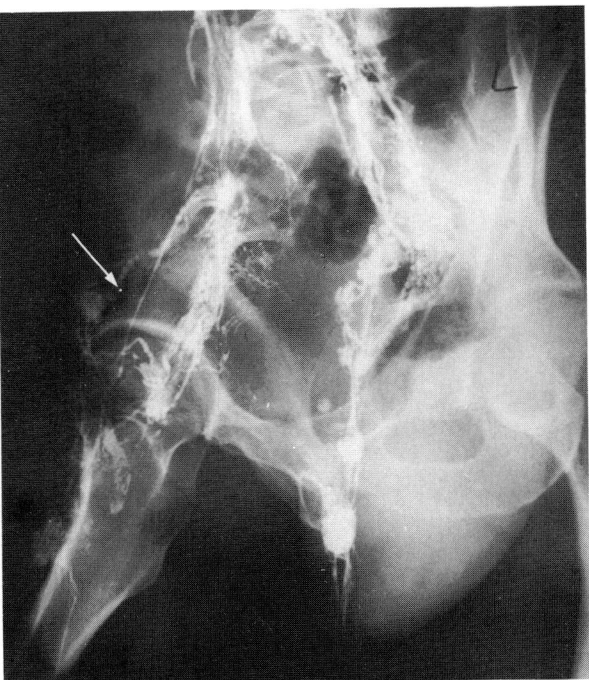

Fig. 28.4 Oblique view of the pelvis showing lymph vessel on the right bypassing the inguinal nodes (arrow).

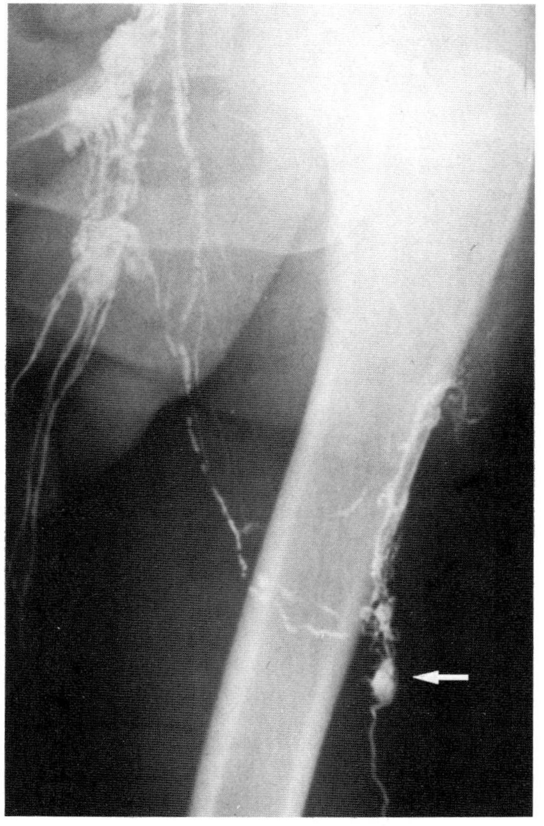

Fig. 28.5

Fig. 28.6

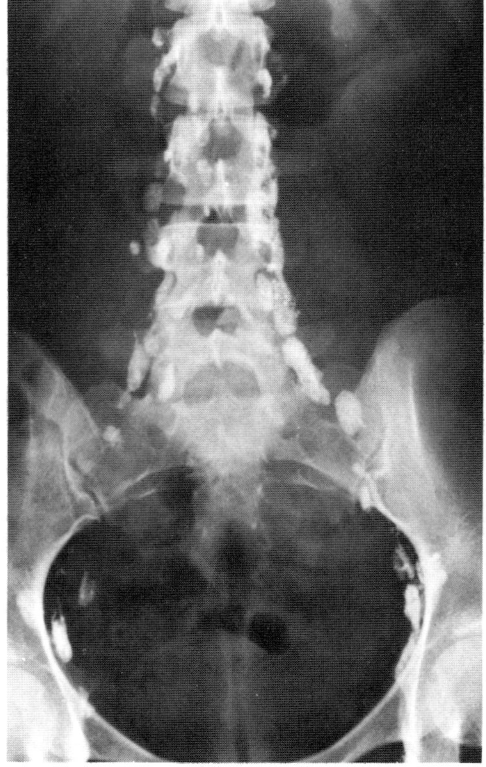

Fig. 28.7

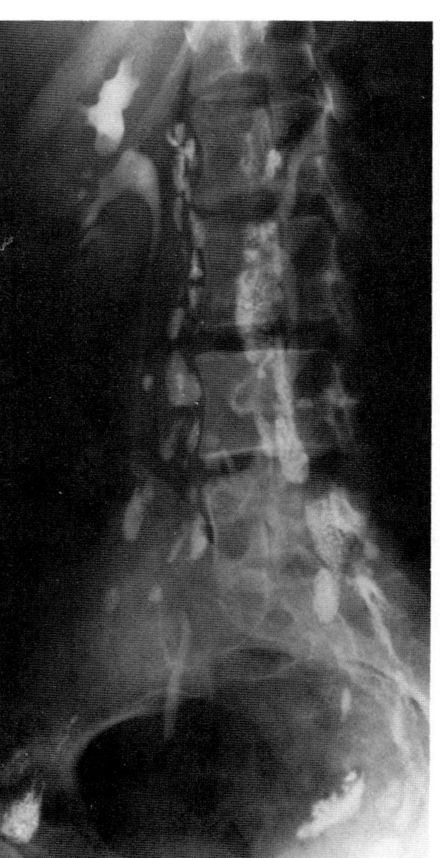

Fig. 28.8

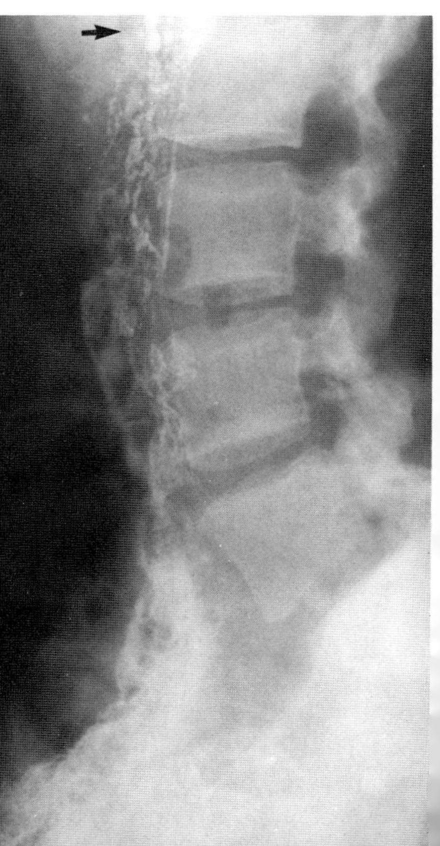

Fig. 28.9

Fig. 28.5 Filling of an unusual ectopic gland in the lateral aspect of the thigh. (See also Fig. 28.25.)

Fig. 28.6 Normal appearance of the lymphatic channels in the pelvis during the lymphatic phase.

Fig. 28.7 Normal abdominal and pelvic nodes in the nodal phase.

Fig. 28.8 Normal nodes. The oblique view shows the glands without overlap. A simultaneous IVU shows the position of the ureters in relation to the glands.

Fig. 28.9 The lateral projection shows the position of the lymphatic channels in relation to the spine. The lower part of the cisterna chyli is also seen (→).

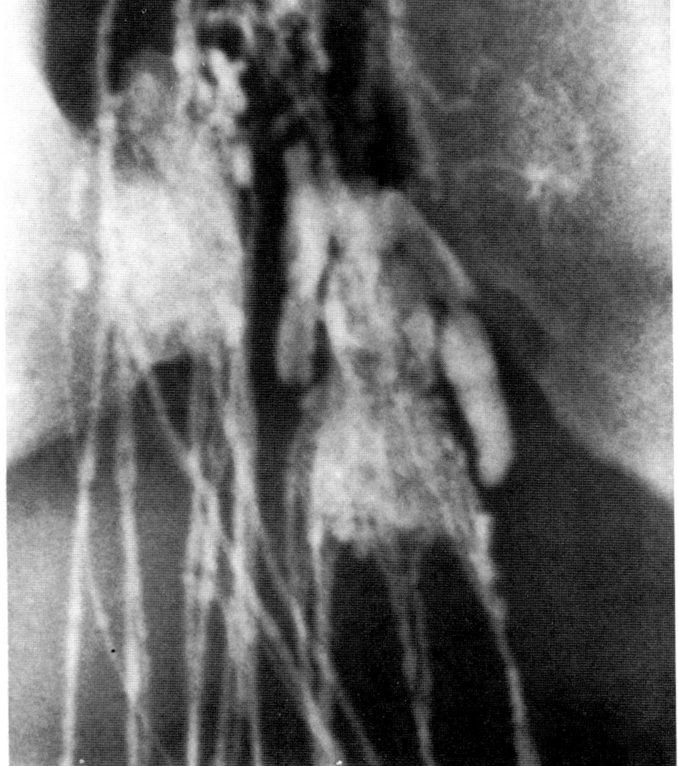

Fig. 28.10 Normal inguinal glands — lymphatic phase.

frequently better filling of the left para-aortic glands up to L1 level while the right para-aortic glands frequently stop at L3.

The normal lymph node can be round, oval or bean-shaped and has a regular outline and a mottled granular appearance in the nodal phase with afferent and efferent vessels in the lymphatic phase (Figs 28.10 and 28.11).

The normal gland measures 1–3 cm in length but assessment of size can be difficult when glands are closely approximated. The para-aortic glands do not normally extend laterally beyond the transverse processes of the lumbar vertebrae.

Fibrolipomatosis of the glands is a benign degenerative process commonly seen in older patients and affects the inguinal and axillary glands in particular. This may result in filling defects seen in the glands in the nodal phase simulating metastatic deposits. However, comparison with a film obtained in the lymphatic phase will show that the defect is due to afferent and efferent vessels, (Figs 28.12–28.15). Follow-up films will confirm the static nature of the defect.

The *cisterna chyli* forms at L2–T12 level from the aortic and intestinal lymphatics (Fig. 28.16). It varies in length from 5 to 7 cm and continues into the thoracic duct which passes through the aortic opening into the thorax and crosses to the left at the level of T5 to open into the venous angle (Figs 28.17 and 28.18). Some filling of the cervical and mediastinal glands may occur.

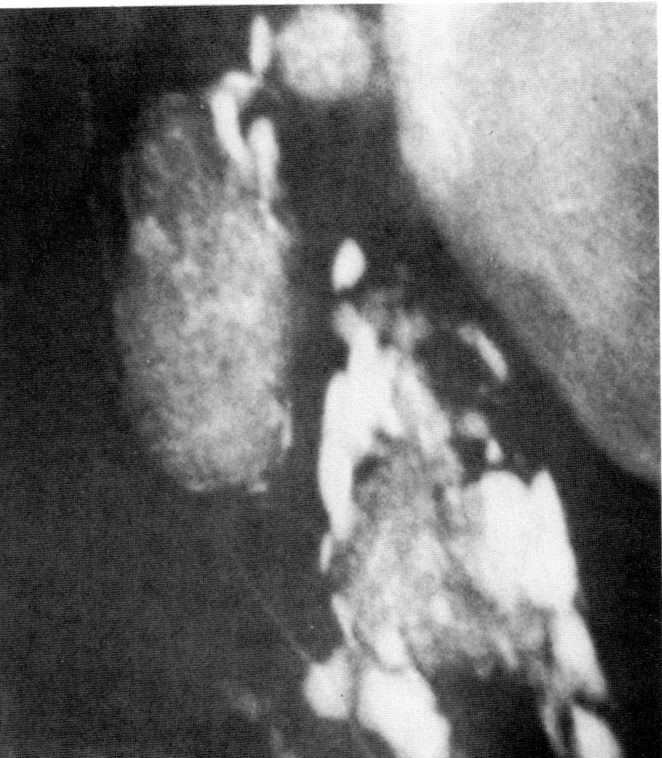

Fig. 28.11 Normal inguinal glands — nodal phase.

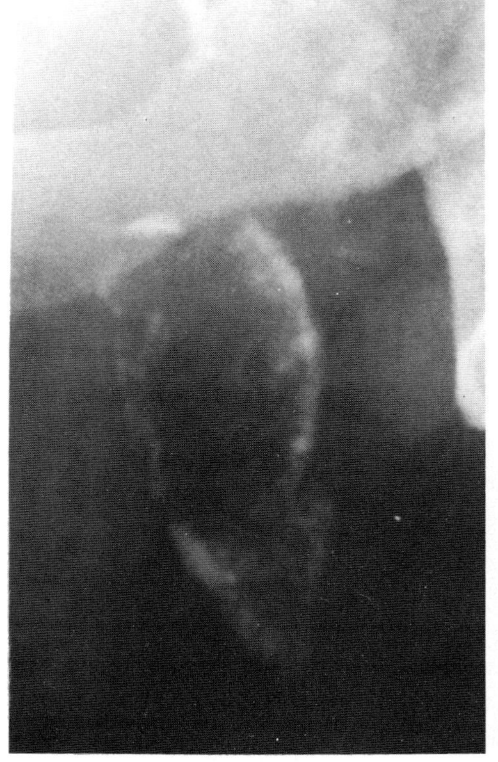

Fig. 28.12

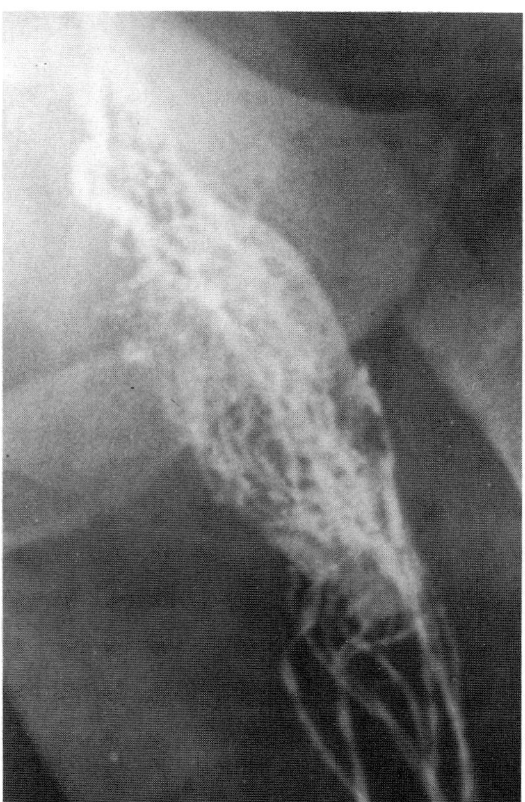

Fig. 28.13

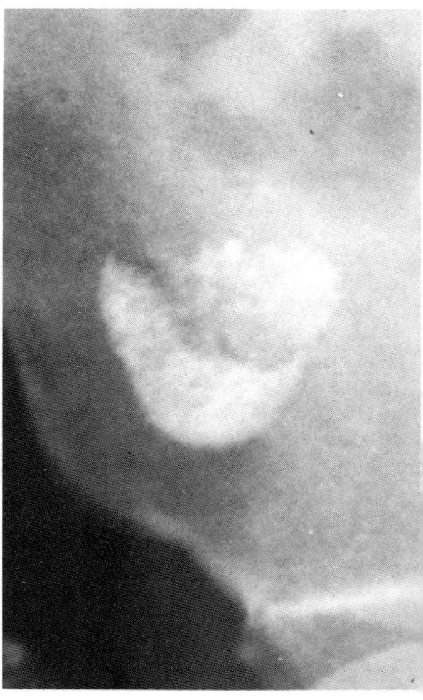

Fig. 28.14

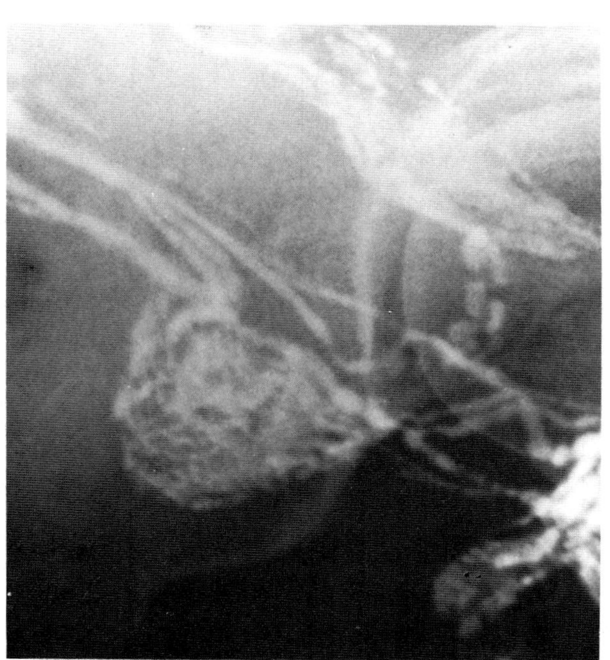

Fig. 28.15

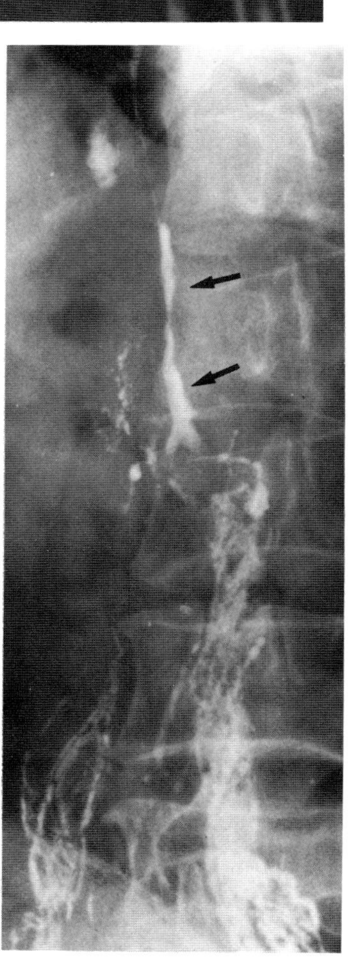

Fig. 28.16

Fig. 28.17

Fig. 28.12 Large central filling defect in an inguinal gland simulating a deposit.

Fig. 28.13 The same gland in the lymphatic phase. The defect is due to afferent and efferent channels. Fibrolipomatosis.

Fig. 28.14 Large eccentric defect in an external iliac node due to fibrolipomatosis.

Fig. 28.15 The lymphatic phase shows efferent lymphatics in the defect.

Fig. 28.16 The normal cisterna chyli (arrows). The lower part of the thoracic duct can be seen.

Fig. 28.17 Normal thoracic duct. There is filling of the posterior intercostal nodes (▲) (occurs in 10–20% of cases) and left hilar glands (◆) (uncommon).

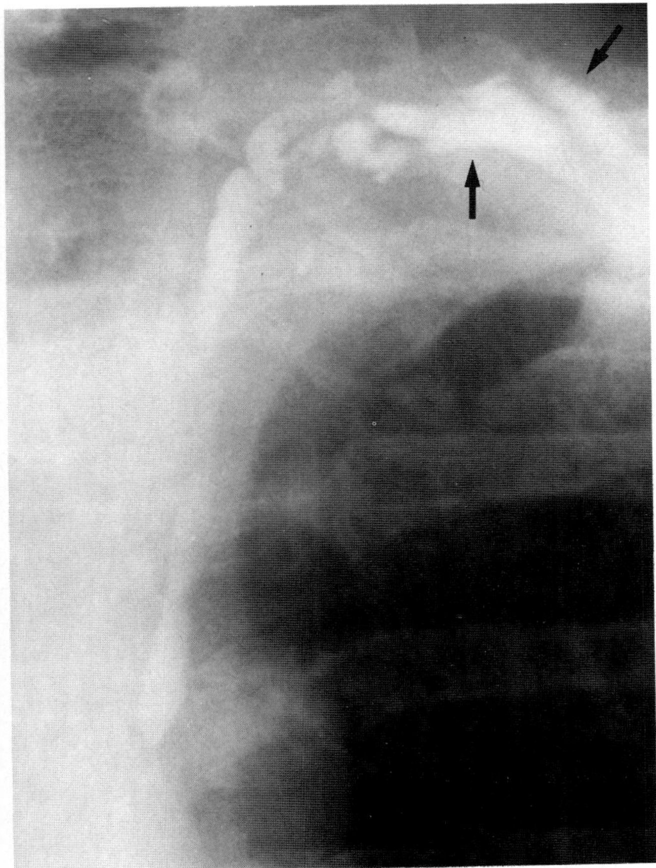

Fig. 28.18 The upper end of the thoracic duct. The beaded appearance is due to valves. Some of the supraclavicular glands are visualized (arrows).

DISEASES OF THE LYMPHATIC CHANNELS

Primary lymphoedema: Lymphoedema can be classified according to the age of onset into: congenita, praecox and tarda.

1. *Lymphoedema congenita*. This may be present at birth and includes the hereditary *Milroy's disease*. It can be associated with other congenital anomalies of the vascular system and gonadal dysgenesis.

2. *Lymphoedema praecox*. This is the commonest form of lymphoedema and is much more common in females. The oedema may occur spontaneously or may be precipitated by trauma, surgery, infection or pregnancy. These stress factors render the abnormal lymphatic system, which had been coping, insufficient.

3. *Lymphoedema tarda*. The symptoms appear after the age of 35 years.

Kinmonth classifies the radiological appearances into two main groups:

1. *Hypoplasia*. The vessels are few or small (Figs 28.19 and 28.20). This is seen in 90% of cases and includes *aplasia*, a severe form in which no lymphatic can be found.

2. *Hyperplasia*. The vessels are enlarged and tortuous (Fig. 28.21). These changes are seen in 10% of patients.

Dermal backflow may be seen in both hypoplasia and hyperplasia (Fig. 28.22).

Two other groups are worthy of mention:

1. *Lymphangiopathia obliterans* is a disorder of unknown aetiology described by Kaindl et al (1960). There is degeneration of the intima of the lymphatics leading to narrowing of the lumen and ultimately complete occlusion (Fig. 28.23). This disorder is commoner in young females.

2. *Lymphatica porosa*. In this condition contrast is seen to diffuse out of the lymphatic channels, causing blurring of their outlines (Fig. 28.24). This is probably another factor contributing to the inadequacy of the lymphatic system in some cases of primary lymphoedema.

The findings in a series of 100 patients seen at St Mary's Hospital, London, were classified as follows:

Lymphatic hypoplasia	56%	72%
Lymphatic aplasia	16%	
Lymphangiectasis	5%	
Lymphatica porosa	7%	
Lymphangiopathia obliterans	5%	
Trauma	5%	
Normal	6%	

Attention has recently been directed to the role of lymph node pathology in patients with primary lymphoedema as abnormal lymph nodes may be seen on the nodal phase films obtained in these patients. A study by Kinmonth and Wolfe (1980) showed the presence of significant fibrosis in the nodes in most cases of primary lymphoedema and

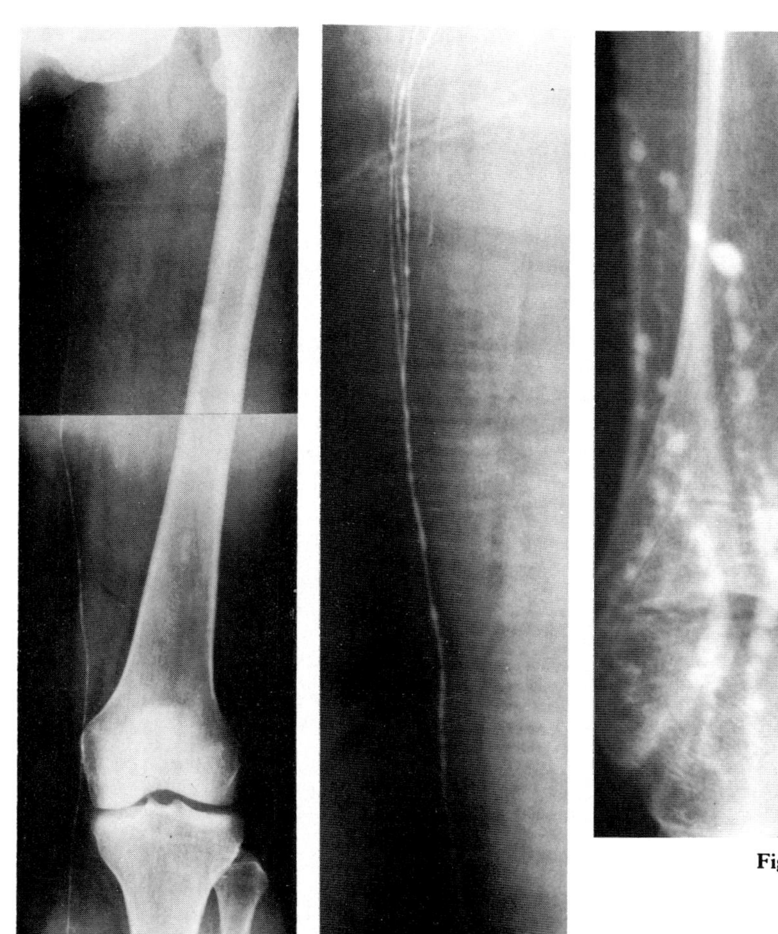

Fig. 28.19

Fig. 28.20

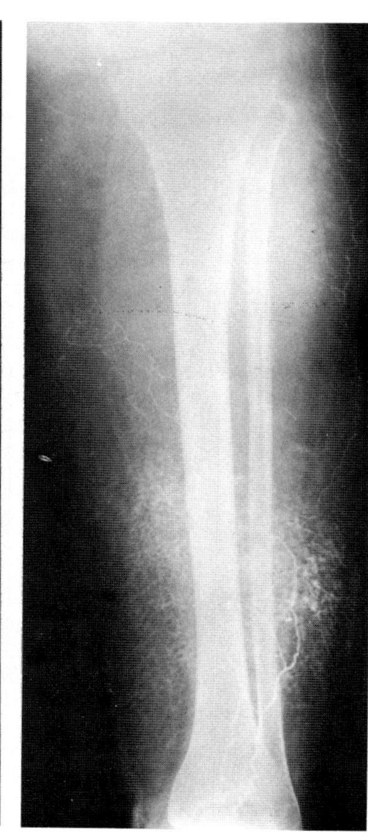

Fig. 28.21

Fig. 28.22

Fig. 28.19 Hypoplasia; single lymphatic.

Fig. 28.20 Hypoplasia; single lymphatic in the lower thigh. Only four lymphatics are visible in the groin.

Fig. 28.21 Lymphangiectasia with large varicose tortuous lymphatics.

Fig. 28.22 Marked dermal backflow in a case of hypoplasia.

Fig. 28.23 Lymphangiopathia obliterans. The abnormal lymphatics terminate abruptly in the upper arm.

suggested that nodal fibrosis may be the most important single pathological factor in primary hypoplastic lymphoedema.

Secondary lymphoedema. Stagnation of contrast and filling of side channels and lymphaticovenous communications indicate obstruction to lymphatic flow.

Surgical excision of lymph nodes, as in radical mastectomy and extensive traumatic skin loss, can produce

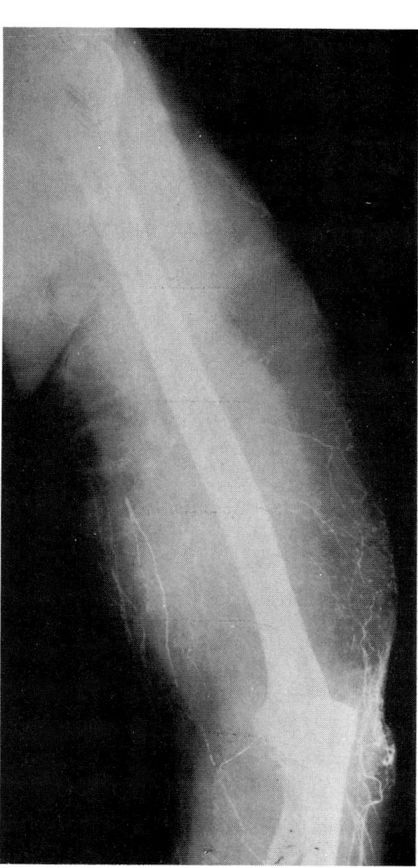

Fig. 28.23

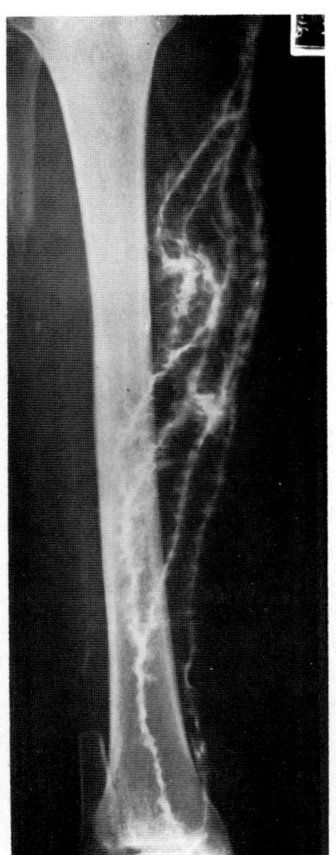

Fig. 28.24

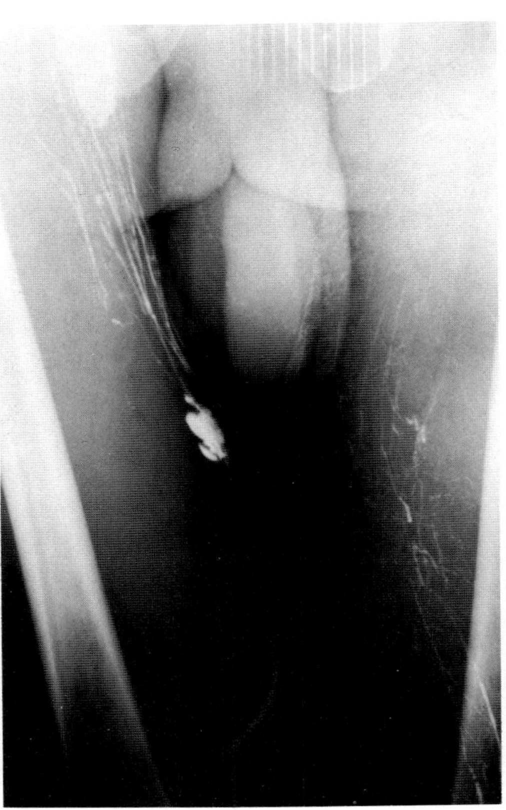

Fig. 28.25

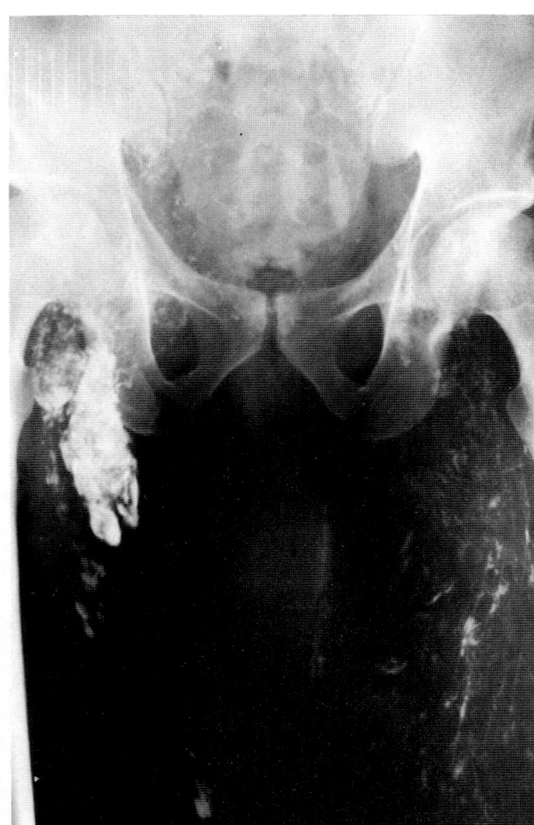

Fig. 28.26

Fig. 28.24 Leaking lymphatics (lymphatica porosa). Note the blurred outline of the lymphatics.

Fig. 28.25 Damaged lymphatics in the left thigh following surgery and deep radiotherapy in a patient with lymphoma. There is a mid-thigh ectopic gland on the right.

Fig. 28.26 Film in the nodal phase showing the abnormal lymphatics on the left. Abnormal glands are seen in the pelvis.

oedema. Radiation alone does not cause much damage. However, high doses coupled with surgical intervention could result in disruption of the lymphatic channels and destruction of the tumour-invaded lymph nodes, resulting in stagnation (Figs 28.25 and 28.26).

Malignancy in itself may block the lymphatic channels (Fig. 28.27).

Isotope scanning in the lymphoedemas. Labelled colloidal compounds, such as $^{99}Tc^{m}$-antimony sulphide colloid, when injected in the subcutaneous tissue of the foot, are taken up by the lymphatic channels and lymph nodes.

Interruption of the flow of isotope may be seen in cases of lymphoedema and in postsurgery follow up. The rate of

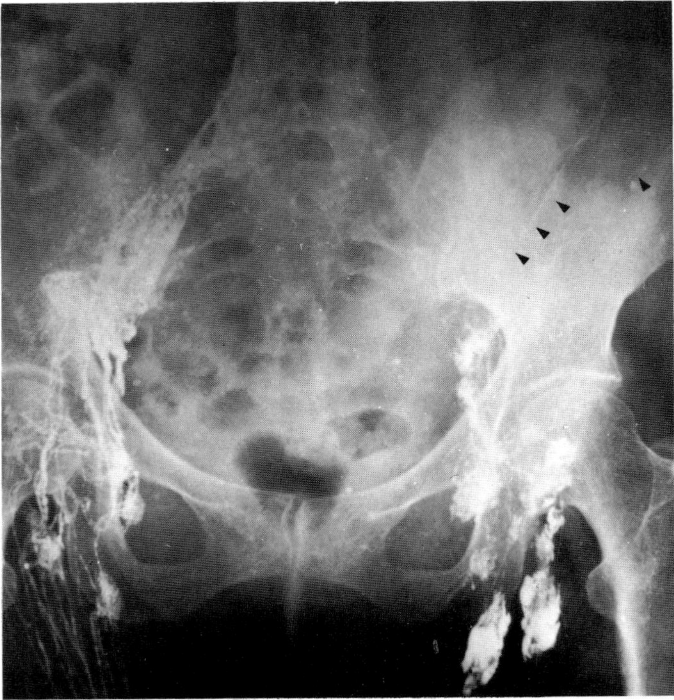

Fig. 28.27 Carcinoma of the cervix involving the left common iliac glands. The lymphatic drainage is through side channels (▲).

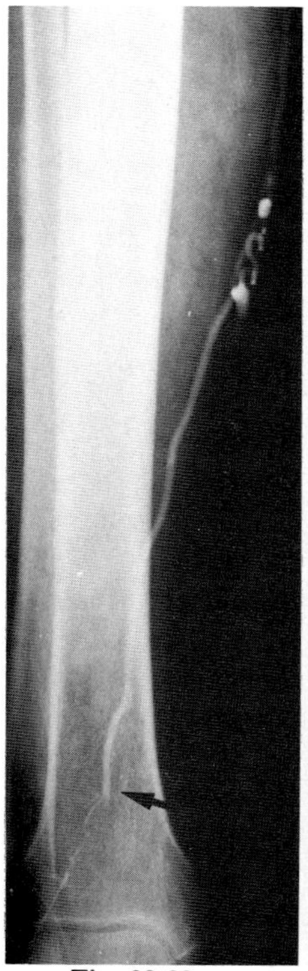

Fig. 28.28 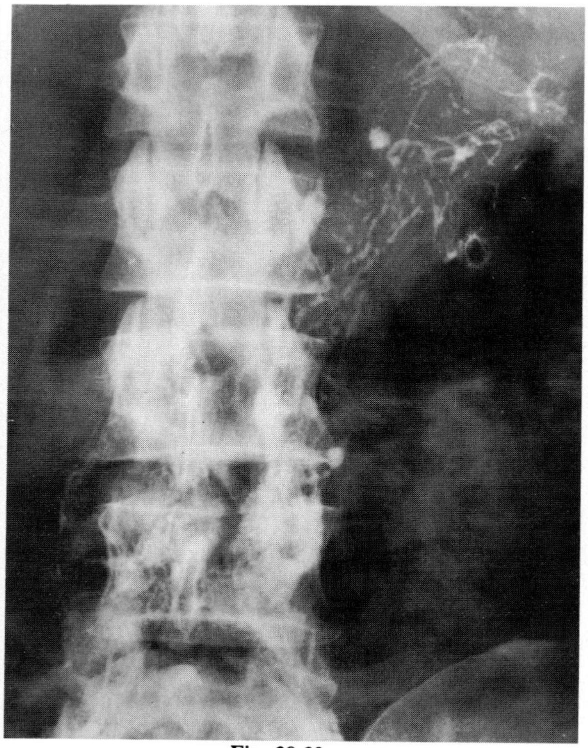 **Fig. 28.29** 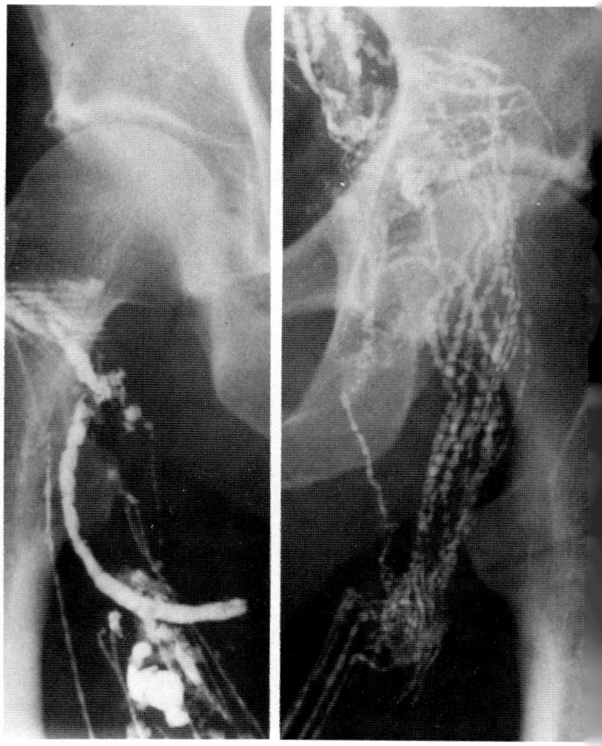 R L **Fig. 28.30**

Fig. 28.28 Lymphaticovenous fistula (←) in the lower leg in a case of severe hypoplasia.

Fig. 28.29 Left lymphatic-renal shunt in a case of chyluria due to filariasis.

Fig. 28.30 Right lymphaticocutaneous fistula following surgery. The dense contrast in the right inguinal glands indicates stasis.

drainage can be quantified to permit accurate assessment of progress.

The experimental results have so far been encouraging but lymphangiography remains the procedure of choice in the investigation of the lymphoedemas.

Lymphatic fistulae. Surgery, tumour invasion, trauma and infestation may block the lymphatic drainage through the thoracic duct. *Lymphaticovenous communications* may then open up (Fig. 28.28). Ascites due to *chyloperitoneal communications* and *chylothorax* may also occur.

Chyluria is most frequently due to filariasis and although non-filarial chyluria can occur, it is rare. Figure 28.29 shows a lymphatic–renal shunt in a case of chyluria due to filariasis.

Lymphaticocutaneous fistulae are usually secondary to surgical interference with the lymphatic channels (Fig. 28.30). The purpose of lymphangiography in these cases is to:

1. Establish the diagnosis and demonstrate the site of fistula.
2. Assess the extent of the lymphatic disease. This may influence the prognosis and determine the treatment.
3. Try and demonstrate the site of the lymphatic block.

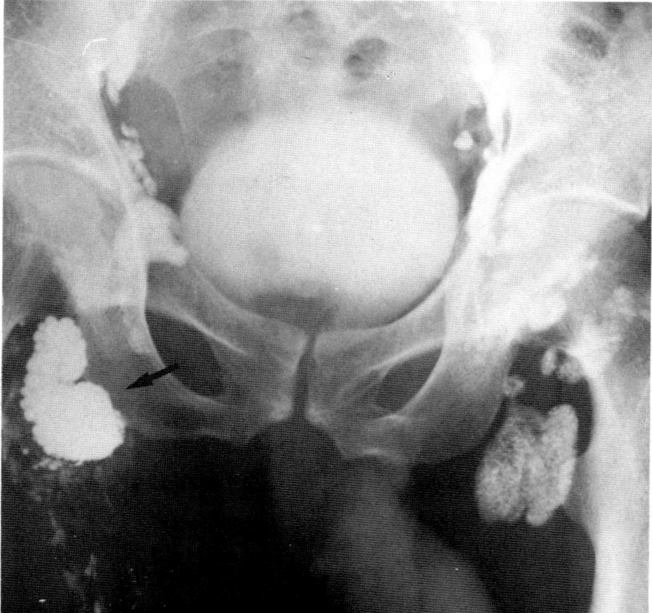

Fig. 28.31 Right inguinal lymphocele (←) following surgery. The oily contrast forms globules in the lymph (caviar sign). There is reactive hyperplasia of the left inguinal glands.

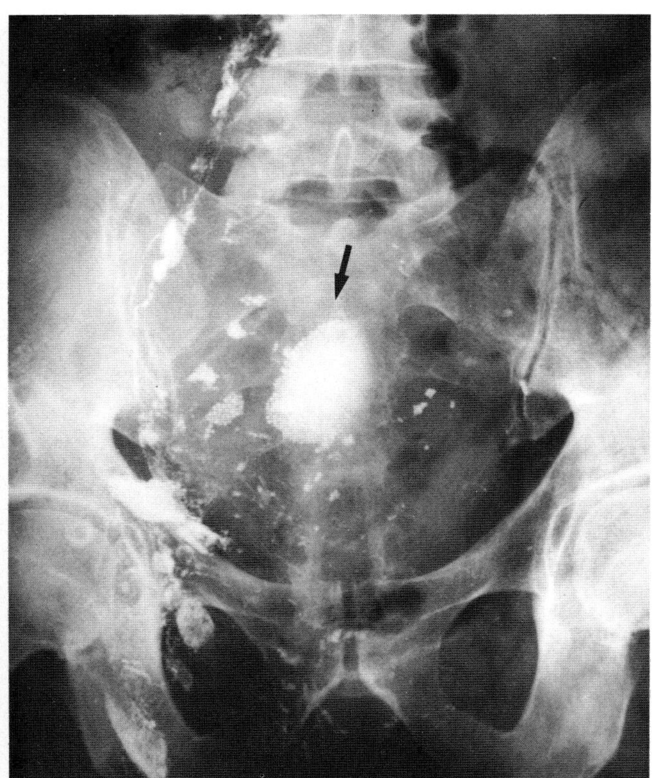

Fig. 28.32 Pelvic lymphocele (↓) in a renal graft recipient. Note the caviar sign in the lymphocele and the abnormal lymphatic channels in the pelvis.

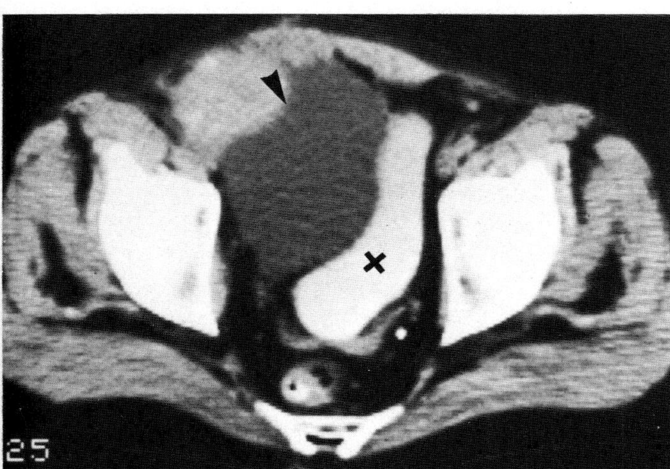

Fig. 28.33 Large pelvic lymphocele (▼) compressing the opacified bladder (×) in a renal graft recipient (W:256, L:35).

Lymphoceles. These may occur secondary to glandular removal particularly in the pelvis in gynaecological operations and renal transplantation. The leakage of lymph may result in a loculated collection causing symptoms by pressing on the adjacent pelvic organs. These lymphoceles can be visualized by lymphography (Figs 28.31 and 28.32), but this should be reserved for cases in which ultrasound and CT scanning are unhelpful, since the latter can readily show these lesions. Figure 28.33 shows a large pelvic lymphocele in a renal graft recipient compressing the bladder and causing ureteric obstruction.

DISEASES OF THE LYMPH NODES

Benign disease.

1. *Fibrolipomatosis.* This condition has been described above (p. 763).

2. *Inflammatory disease.* The changes are non-specific and may take the form of generalized enlargement associated with coarsening of the granular pattern due to multiple small filling defects. These changes may be seen in viral illnesses, collagen diseases, syphilis and lymphogranuloma venereum (Fig. 28.34).

Filling defects simulating malignant deposits may be seen in caseating nodal tuberculosis. Sarcoidosis, on the other hand, can cause generalized enlargement of the glands with a reticular pattern similar to that seen in lymphoma.

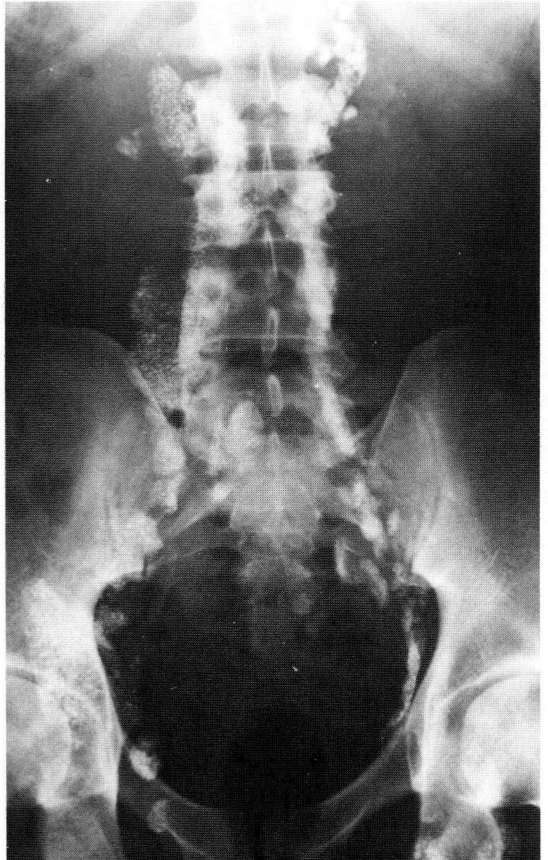

Fig. 28.34 Enlarged pelvic and para-aortic glands with a reticular pattern in a case of lymphogranuloma venereum.

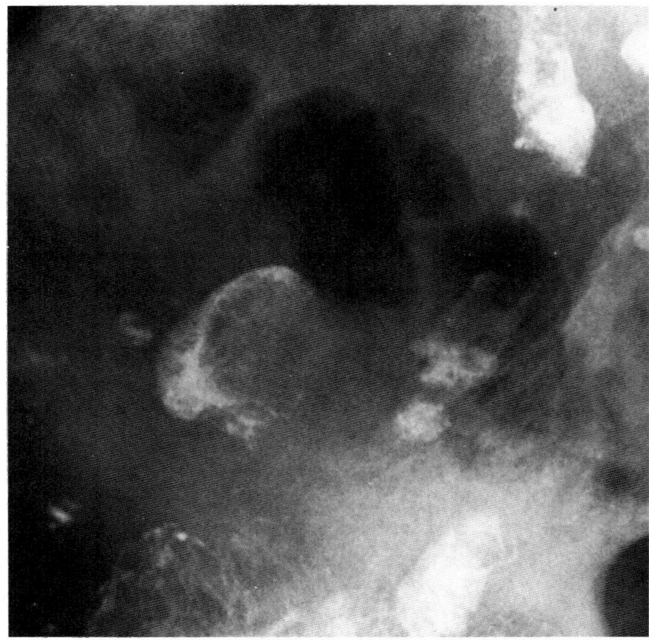

Fig. 28.35 Large melanoma deposit in the nodal phase in an external iliac gland.

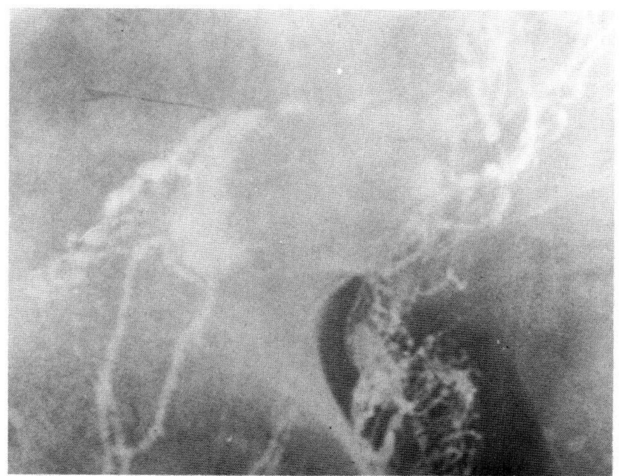

Fig. 28.36 The same node in the lymphatic phase. (Compare with Figs 28.14 and 28.15.)

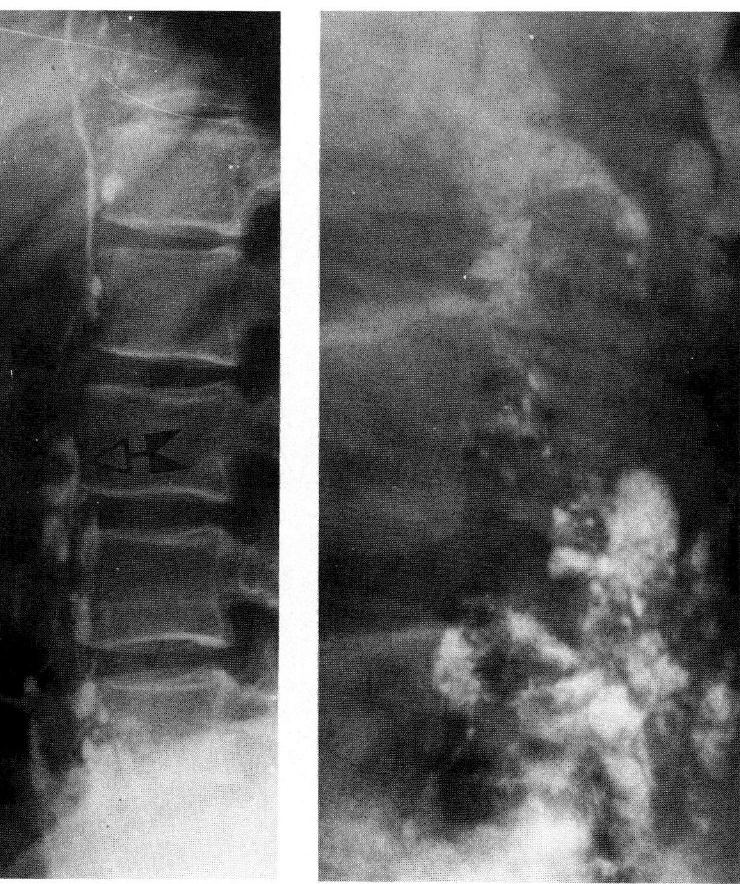

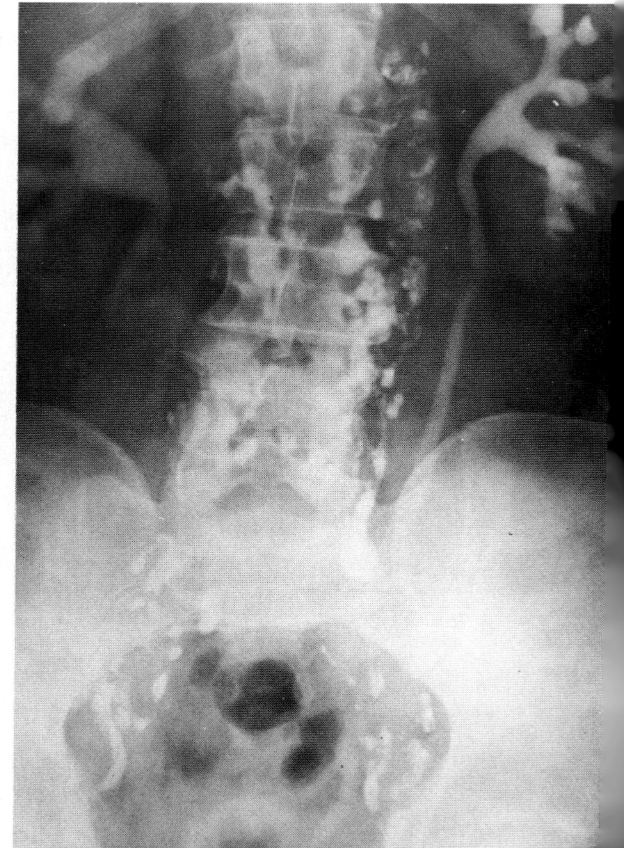

Fig. 28.37

Fig. 28.38

Fig. 28.39

Malignant metastases:

The typical changes of malignancy on lymphangiography include enlargement of the involved gland, filling defects within the gland, obstruction of the lymphatic drainage and displacement of the nodes and channels. The presence of a globular filling defect is the most specific feature of malignancy on lymphangiography.

Knowledge of the drainage routes of a particular tumour is essential in the assessment of the lymphangiogram. The primary drainage routes of some of the commonly investigated tumours are summarized in Table 28.1.

Table 28.1 Primary drainage routes of some common tumours

Site of tumour	Primary lymph drainage
Testis	Para-aortic. External iliac in advanced disease
Prostate	Internal, external & common iliac
Bladder	Internal, external & common iliac
Body of uterus	External iliac, para-aortic
Uterine cervix	External iliac, internal iliac

Figures 28.35 and 28.36 show a large secondary deposit from a malignant melanoma in the foot. Figure 28.37 shows a deposit from a testicular tumour seen well only on the lateral film. Figure 28.38 is a close-up of para-aortic glands involved by uterine carcinoma. Figure 28.39 shows the relationship of the ureters to enlarged para-aortic nodes in carcinoma of the bladder, while Figure 28.40 shows the changes of testicular teratoma in the para-aortic glands. Figure 28.41 is of a deposit visualized by tomography during lymphangiography.

The lymph node metastases of different types of tumour may appear identical. Testicular seminoma may mimic the lymphomas. It should of course be realized that a negative lymphangiogram does not exclude metastatic disease.

The reticuloses

Lymphangiography has an important role in the diagnosis and staging of the reticuloses. The technique will not distinguish between the different varieties of reticuloses. Hodgkin's disease, non-Hodgkin's lymphomas and reticulum cell sarcoma may all produce similar defects.

The most characteristic appearance is the soap bubble or foamy pattern seen in cases of Hodgkin's disease (Fig. 28.42). Figures 28.43 and 28.44 show a coarse reticular pattern in both the lymphatic and nodal phases in a case of non-Hodgkin's lymphoma. Less commonly, filling

Fig. 28.37 A single deposit from testicular tumour in the para-aortic nodes (arrow). This was visible only in the lateral projection.

Fig. 28.38 Multiple deposits in the para-aortic nodes from carcinoma of the body of the uterus.

Fig. 28.39 Pelvic and para-aortic deposits from carcinoma of the bladder. A simultaneous IVU demonstrates the irregular bladder and the position of the ureters.

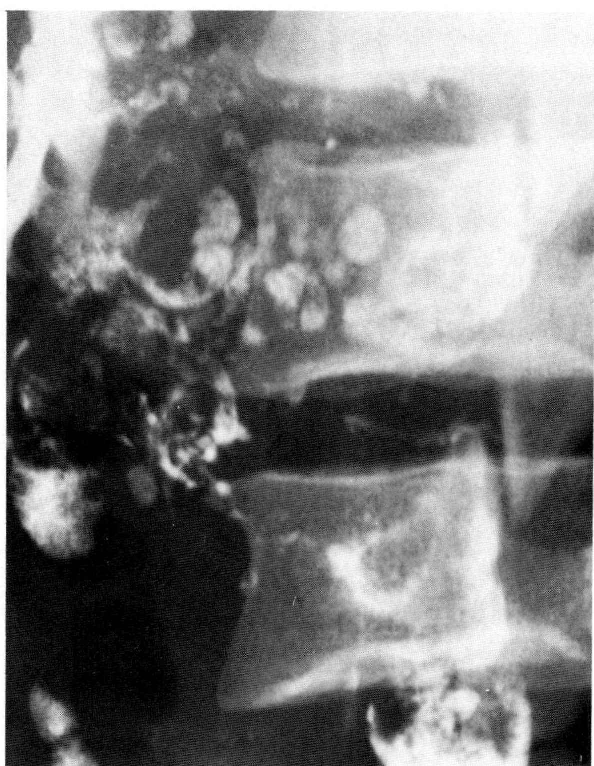

Fig. 28.40 Deposits from testicular teratoma.

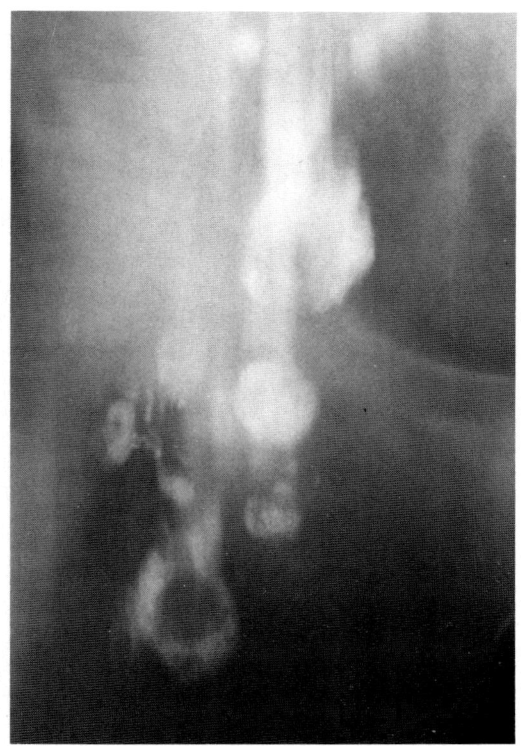

Fig. 28.41 Tomogram of melanoma deposits in the right groin.

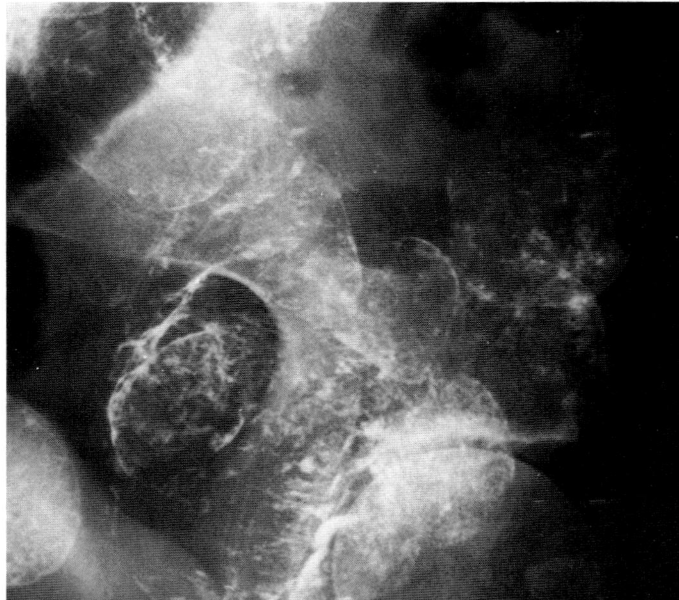

Fig. 28.42 Pelvic nodes showing the soap-bubble appearance in a case of Hodgkin's disease.

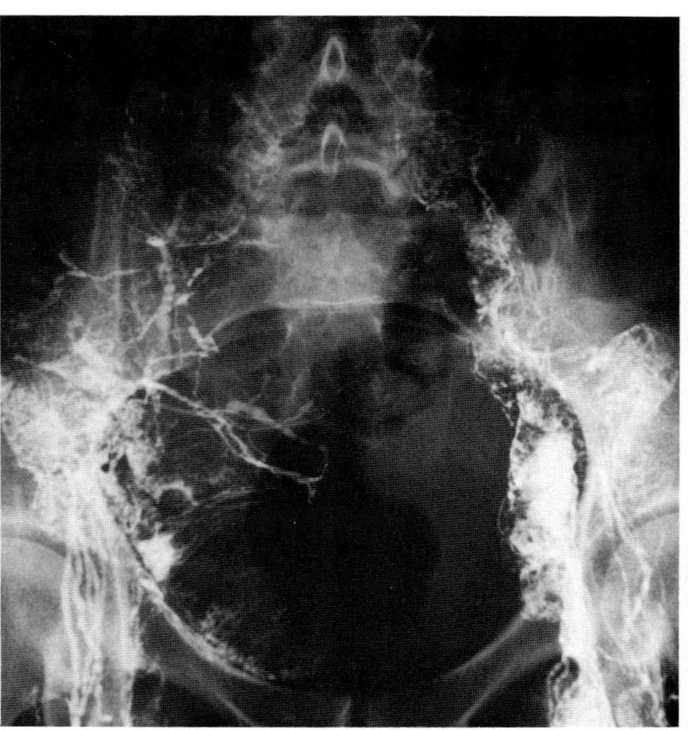

Fig. 28.43 Non-Hodgkin's lymphoma — the lymphatic phase.

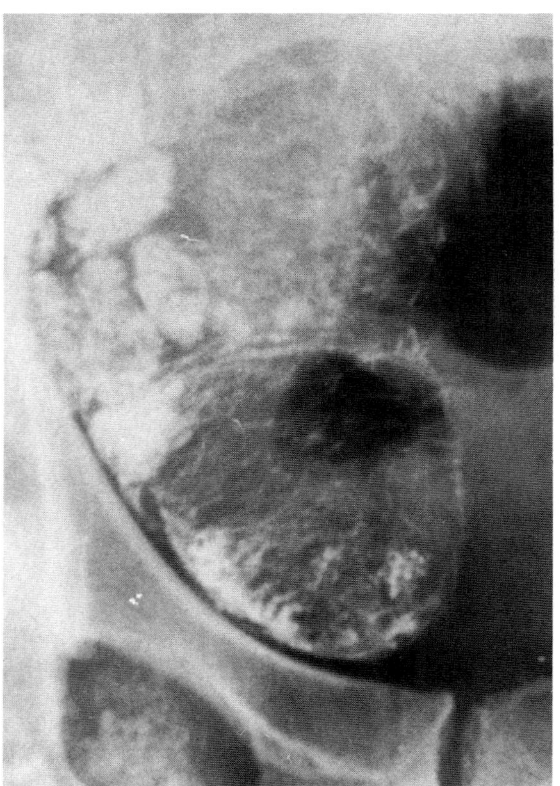

Fig. 28.44 Non-Hodgkin's lymphoma — same case. The nodal phase shows the reticular pattern in the glands.

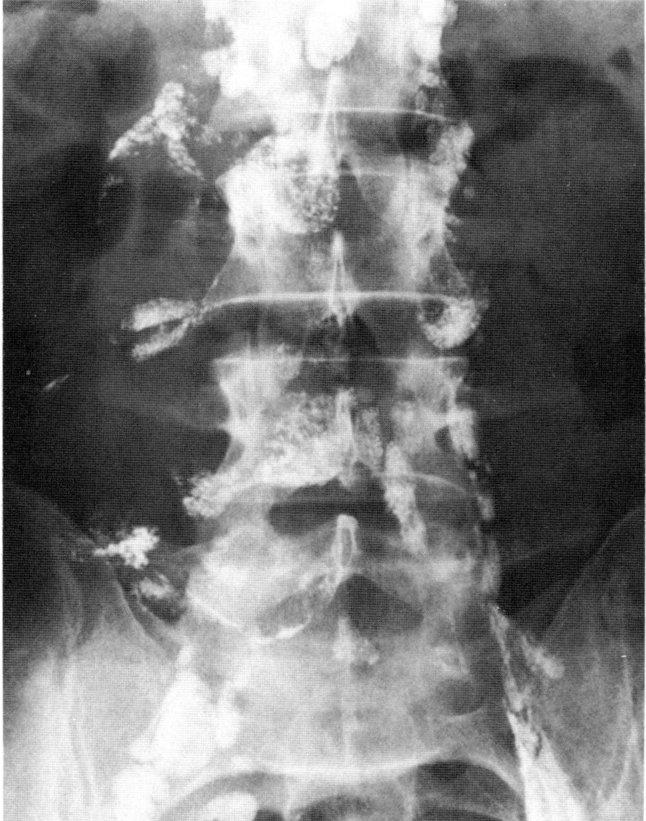

Fig. 28.45 Large filling defects in para-aortic nodes in a case of Hodgkin's disease.

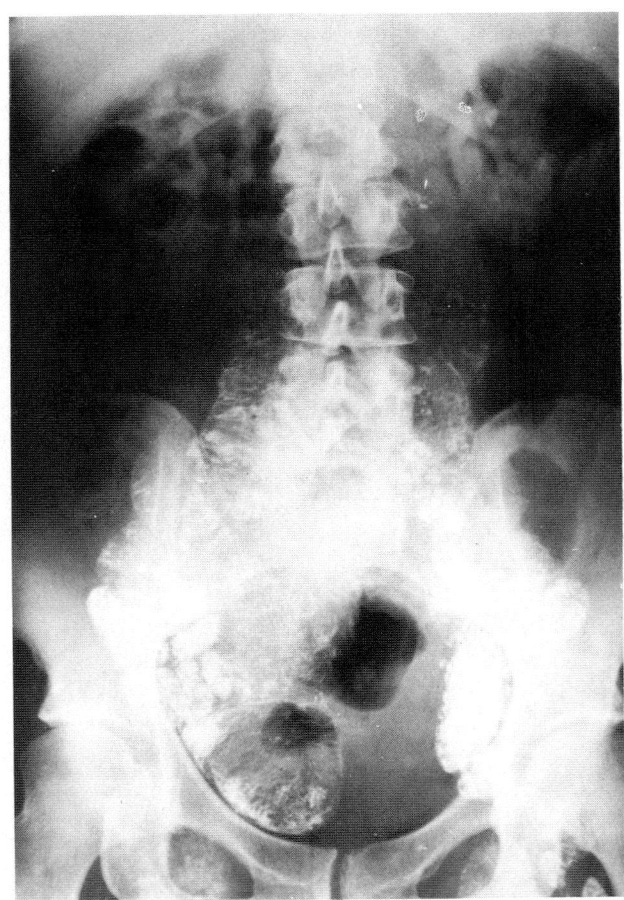

Fig. 28.46 Non-Hodgkin's lymphoma. The involved pelvic and lower para-aortic glands are well filled. There is no filling of the high para-aortic nodes, which have been completely destroyed by the tumour.

defects simulating carcinoma can be seen in the involved glands, making the diagnosis more difficult (Fig. 28.45). Non-filling of a chain of glands may occur due to replacement by lymphoma causing obstruction to the flow (Fig. 28.46). Progress under treatment may be assessed by follow up films (Figs 28.47 and 28.48). Lymphatic leukaemia can produce glandular enlargement and irregularities similar to those seen in the reticuloses.

The accuracy of lymphangiography in nodal disease

It is important to remember, before accuracy is discussed, that a negative lymphangiogram does not exclude nodal disease. The accuracy of lymphangiography in the various tumours has been the subject of many investigations and is generally believed to be around 90%. False-negative lymphangiograms are encountered in two situations:

1. The deposits are too small to be visualized (deposits as small as 4 mm can be detected on lymphangiography).

2. Non-filling of the involved node chains. For example, the internal iliac glands are the first group to be involved in prostatic carcinoma and cervical cancer. These glands do not routinely fill on pedal lymphangiography and pelvic

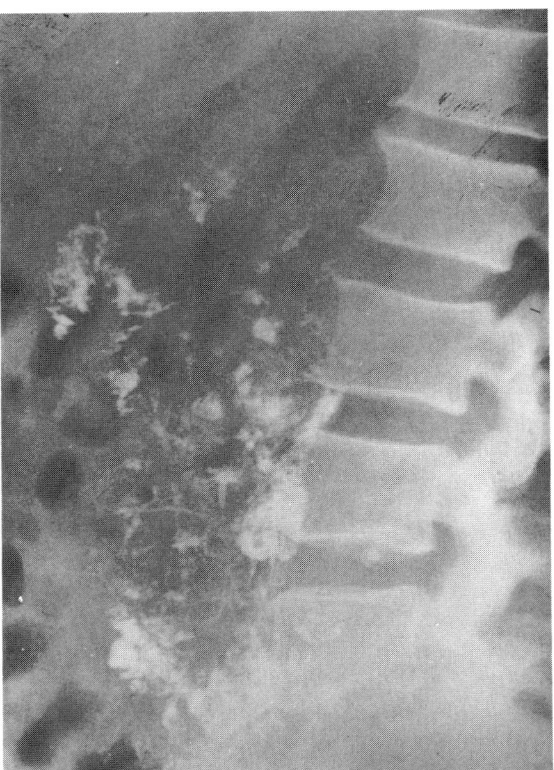

Fig. 28.47 Lateral view — nodal phase — reticulosis before therapy.

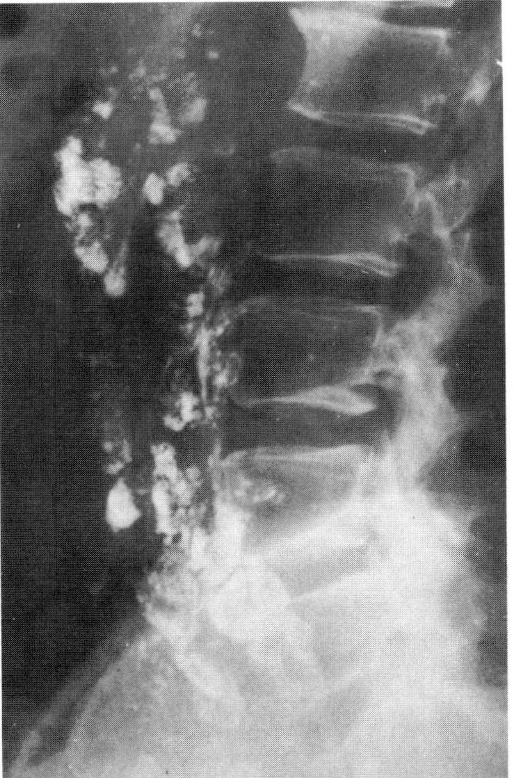

Fig. 28.48 Lateral view during irradiation therapy. Glandular mass smaller and glands smaller resulting in increased density of individual glands.

disease is therefore difficult to detect. The same principle applies to the high para-aortic glands in testicular tumours.

In the reticuloses, it has been found that the lymphangiogram demonstrated the presence of unsuspected nodal disease below the diaphragm in about 20% of patients with Hodgkin's disease leading to a change in staging and treatment. Progressive disease can also be detected on serial follow-up films after lymphangiography.

CT SCANNING IN LYMPH NODE DISEASE

CT has several advantages over lymphangiography:

1. It is non-invasive.
2. It demonstrates extranodal as well as nodal disease and allows visualization of other affected organs such as the liver, adrenal glands and lungs.
3. It demonstrates involvement of certain glandular groups that do not normally opacify on lymphangiography such as the internal iliac glands in the pelvis; the retrocrural, high para-aortic, portal and mesenteric glands in the abdomen; and the mediastinal glands in the thorax.
4. The true bulk of the nodal disease can be assessed. This may be important as in testicular teratoma staging.

CT scanning is, on the other hand, expensive and the changes in nodal disease are non-specific, the only diagnostic criterion for abnormality being glandular enlargement.

Tumour-invaded glands that are not enlarged will not be identified on CT. This explains the lower accuracy rate of CT scanning compared to lymphangiography in abdominal malignancies.

CT will, nevertheless, give more useful information about the patient in a single examination than any other imaging modality and it should, if available, be used as the first investigation in nodal disease (Figs 28.49–28.55). Negative or equivocal scans can be supplemented by lymphangiography if clinically indicated.

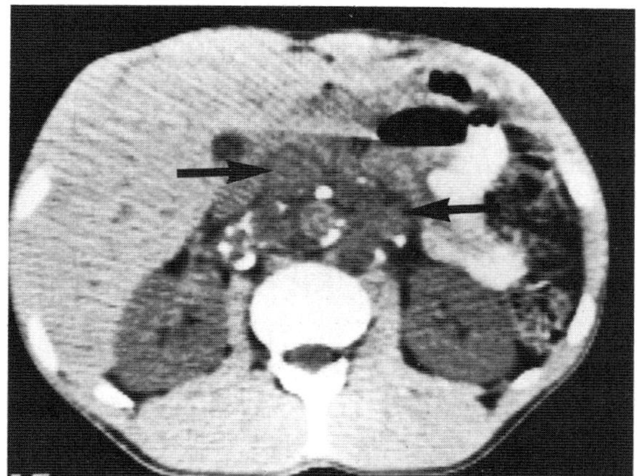

Fig. 28.49 CT scan at the level of the renal hila following lymphangiography in a patient with testicular seminoma. Enlarged para-aortic nodes (→ ←) some containing contrast (W:256, L:45).

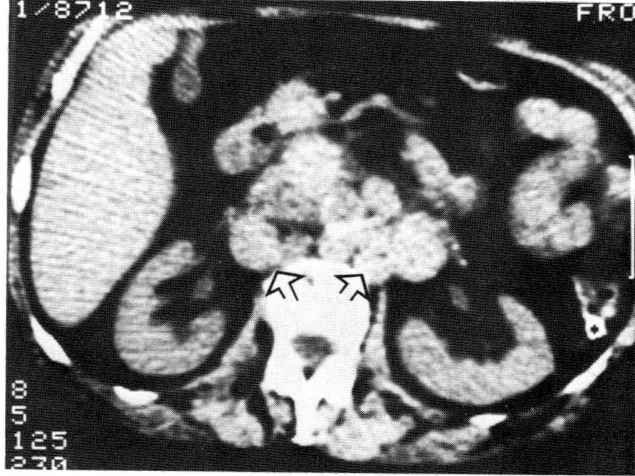

Fig. 28.51 Large para-aortic nodes (arrows) displacing the calcified aorta anteriorly in a case of Hodgkin's disease (W:256, L:45).

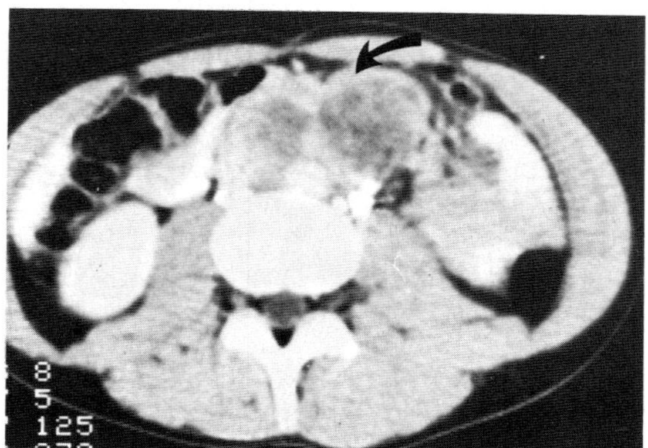

Fig. 28.50 CT at the level of L3/4 following lymphangiography in a patient with testicular teratoma. A large mass of para-aortic glands (arrow). These were not visible on lymphangiography. The relatively necrotic centre of the mass is visible after intravenous contrast (W:256, L:65).

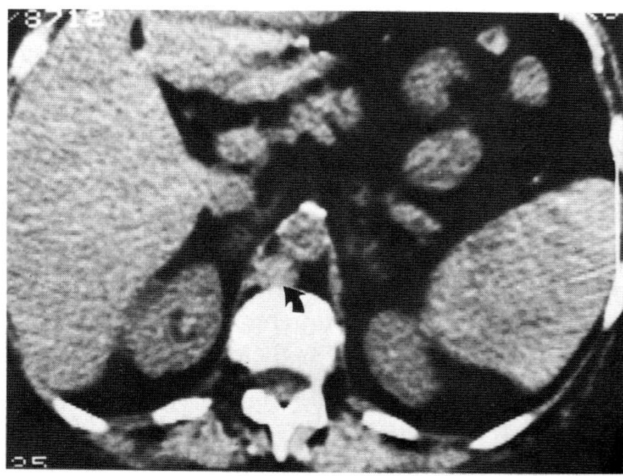

Fig. 28.52 A large retrocrural node (arrow) in a case of Hodgkin's disease. The spleen is also enlarged (W:256, L:45).

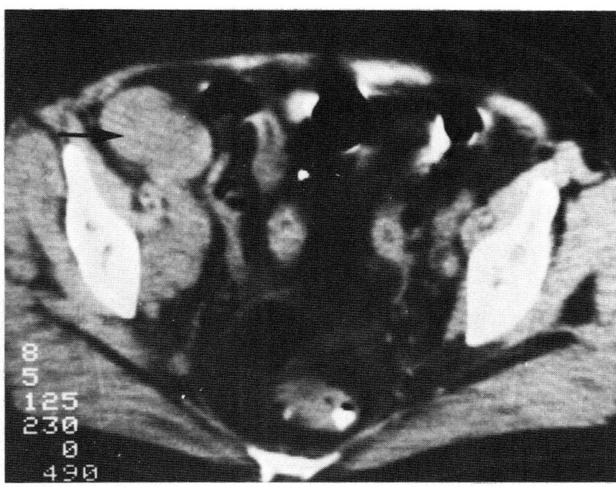

Fig. 28.53 Enlarged right iliac nodes (→). Hodgkin's disease (W:512, L:45).

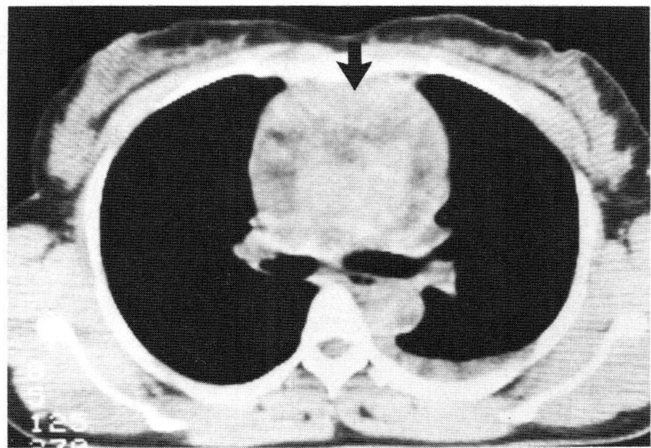

Fig. 28.54 Enlarged anterior mediastinal glands (↓) at the level of the carina (W:512, L:45).

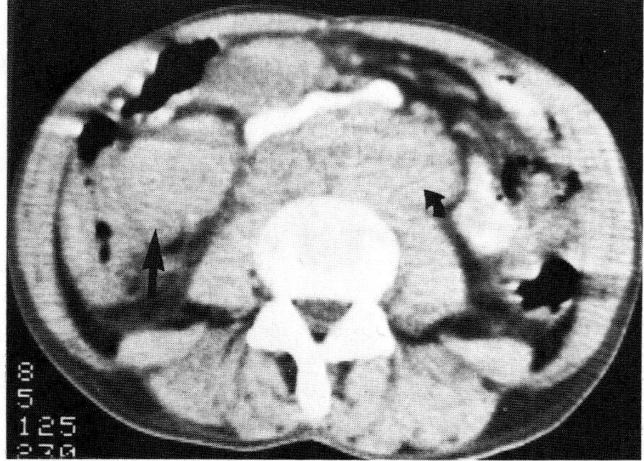

Fig. 28.55 Enlarged para-aortic (curved arrow) and mesenteric (↑) nodes in a case of non-Hodgkin's lymphoma. The bowel is sandwiched between the enlarged nodes (W:512, L:35).

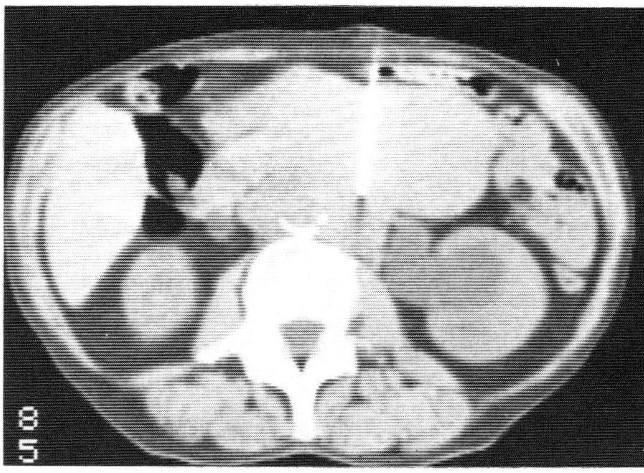

Fig. 28.56 CT scan to show the position of the biopsy needle in a large para-aortic mass causing hydronephrosis on the left. Hodgkin's disease (W:512, L:36).

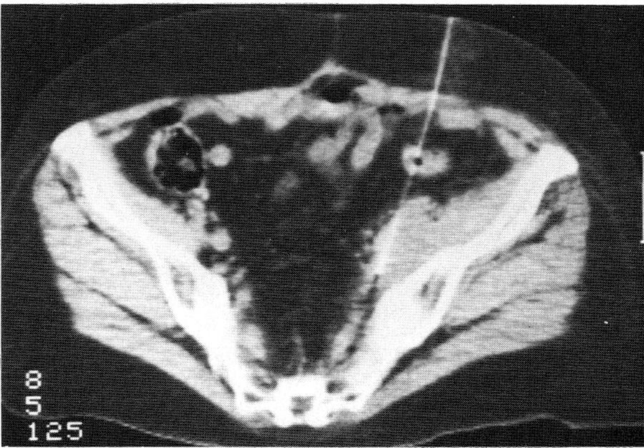

Fig. 28.57 Biopsy of left pelvic nodal mass in a case of recurrent uterine carcinoma (W:512, L:50).

Percutaneous biopsy can be performed under CT control to help establish the diagnosis, stage the tumour or establish the presence of viable tissue after radiotherapy. A cytological or histological specimen can be obtained depending on the type of needle used. A 95% diagnostic yield may be expected in metastatic nodal disease. Making a definite tissue diagnosis in lymphomas is more difficult and this is reflected in the lower diagnostic yield of around 50%. CT control of percutaneous biopsy is illustrated in Figure 28.56, which shows a biopsy procedure on a large para-aortic mass. Figure 28.57 shows a biopsy of a pelvic glandular mass.

ULTRASOUND IN NODAL DISEASE

Para-aortic and pelvic nodes can be assessed by ultrasound, although interference from bowel gas may cause some difficulty. Portal nodes are usually visualized through the liver window. It is also possible to scan the liver and other

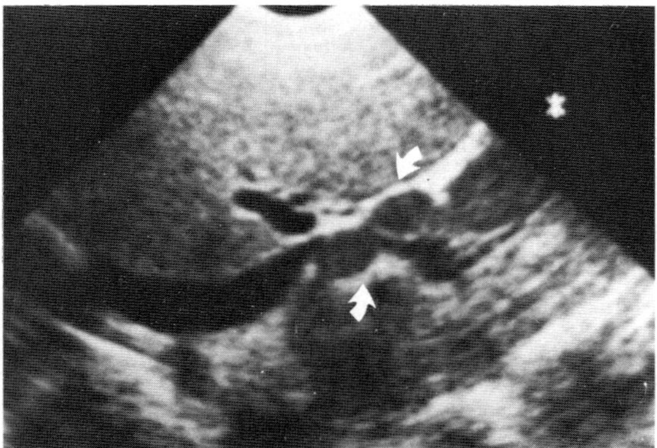

Fig. 28.58 Longitudinal ultrasound scan showing enlarged glands (arrows) compressing the IVC in a patient with metastatic bronchial carcinoma.

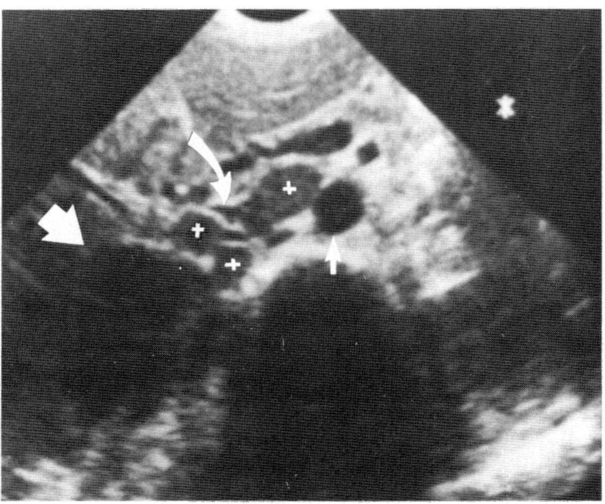

Fig. 28.59 Transverse section on the same patient at the level of the splenic vein. The enlarged glands (+) are seen to the right of the aorta (straight arrow). The IVC (curved arrow) is compressed. A large right adrenal deposit (thick arrow) is also visible.

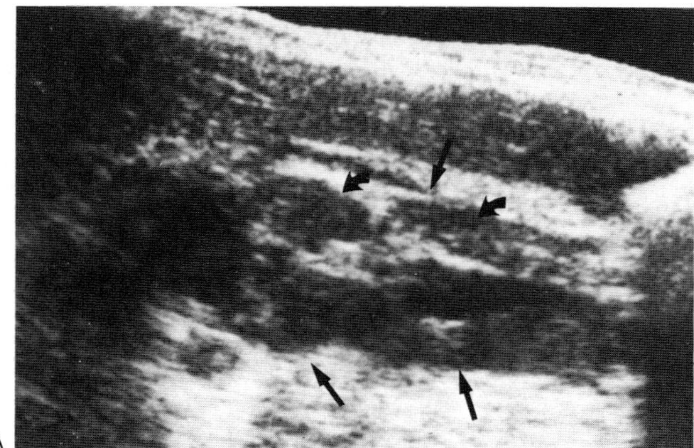

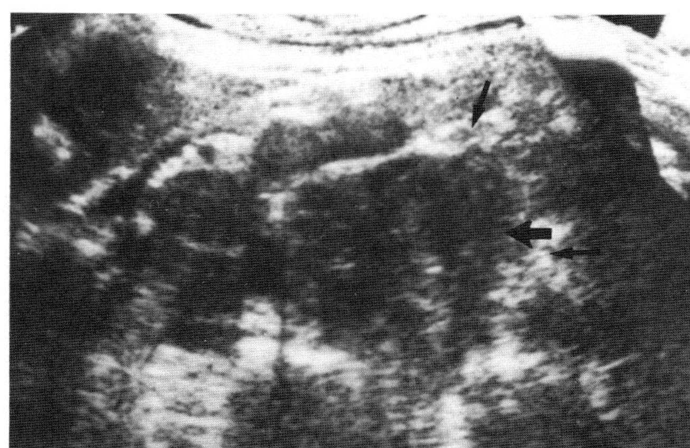

Fig. 28.60 A. Longitudinal ultrasound scan showing enlarged para-aortic glands (arrows) in a case of Hodgkin's disease. **B.** Transverse section on the upper abdomen in the same patient showing the enlarged glands (arrows).

abdominal organs at the same time. Ultrasound is more readily available than CT and less costly, but it is operator-dependent. Abnormal glands have to be enlarged to be visualized and usually have no specific ultrasonic features (Figs 28.58–28.60).

Quantification studies (tissue characterization) in ultrasound are still in the research stage. Advances in this field may make it possible to assess the response of nodal and organ deposits to therapy by measuring the change in the speed of sound waves through the tissues.

Ultrasound, in expert hands, is a useful screening method, particularly if CT is not available, and can be used to guide needle biopsies.

ISOTOPE SCANNING IN NODAL DISEASE

The availability of new colloidal compounds such as $^{99}Tc^{m}$ antimony sulphide has made it possible to obtain diagnostic isotope images of the lymphatic system. The main advantage of this method is its ability to delineate the regional drainage of certain areas by injecting the labelled compound subcutaneously. This is particularly useful in the preoperative assessment of the regional drainage in malignant melanomas and internal mammary disease in breast cancer. The use of this method has been extended to abdominal malignancies and some of the workers claim a high accuracy rate in the prediction of pelvic disease in gynaecological malignancies. Difficulties in the interpretation of the images have restricted the use of this method. The recent development of labelled specific monoclonal antibodies to some tumours is likely to improve tumour diagnosis and treatment in the future.

MAGNETIC RESONANCE IMAGING IN NODAL DISEASE

The role of MRI in the lymphatic system is not yet clear.

However, this new modality offers two theoretical advantages:

1. The use of non-ionizing radiation.
2. Histological diagnosis based on tissue characteristics may be possible since different tumours appear to have different relaxation times.

Clinically, enlarged nodes can be clearly visualized in the mediastinum, abdomen and pelvis. The use of different pulse sequences allows differentiation between blood vessels and lymph nodes. This can be useful in assessing difficult areas such as the mediastinum and pulmonary hila (see Ch. 68).

REFERENCES AND SUGGESTIONS FOR FURTHER READING

Brascho, D. J., Durant, J. R., & Green, L. E. (1977) The accuracy of retroperitoneal ultrasonography in Hodgkin's disease and non-Hodgkin's lymphoma. *Radiology*, **125**: 485–487

Cohen, A. M., Creviston, S., LiPuma, J. P., Bryan, P. J., & Alfidi, R. J. (1983) NMR evaluation of hilar and mediastinal lymphadenopathy. *Radiology*, **148**: 739–742

Craig, O. (1969) Primary lymphoedema and lymphatica porosa. *Radiology*, **92**: 1216–1222

Craig, O. (1970) Radiology of lymphatic disorders. *British Journal of Hospital Medicine*, **2**: 276–282

Dooms, G. C., Hricak, H., Crooks, L. E., & Higgins, C. B. (1984) Magnetic resonance imaging of the lymph nodes. Comparison with CT. Radiology, **153**: 719–728

Dooms, G. C., Hricak, H., Moseley, M. E., Fisher, M., Higgins, C. B. (1985) Characterization of lymphadenopathy by magnetic resonance relaxation time: Preliminary results. Radiology, **155**: 691–697

Ennis, M. G., & MacErlean, D. P. (1980) Percutaneous aspiration biopsy of abdomen and retroperitoneum. *Clinical Radiology*, **31**: 611–616

Freeman, L. M., Blaufox, M. D., & Ege, G. N. (eds) (1983) Interstitial lymphoscintigraphy. *Seminars in Nuclear Medicine*, **13**: 1

Gothlin, J. H., Rupp, N., Rothenberger, K. H., & MacIntosh, P. K. (1981) Percutaneous biopsy of retroperitoneal lymph nodes. A multicentric study. *European Journal of Radiology*, **1**: 46–50

Jing, B. S., Wallace, S., & Zornoza, J. (1982) Metastases to the retroperitoneal and pelvic lymph nodes: computed tomography and lymphangiography. *Radiologic Clinics of North America*, **20**: 3: 511–530

Kaindl, F., Mannheimer, E., Pfleger-Schwarz, L., & Thurnhee, B. L. (1960) *Lymphangiographie und lymphadenographie der extremitaten*. Stuttgart: Thieme

Kinmonth, J. B. (1952) Lymphangiography in man. A method of outlining lymphatic trunks at operation. *Clinical Science*, **11**: 13

Kinmonth, J. B., & Wolfe, J. H. (1980) Fibrosis in the lymph nodes in primary lymphoedema. *Annals of The Royal College of Surgeons of England*, **62**: 344–354

Kinmonth, J. B. (1982) *The Lymphatics: Surgery, Lymphography and Disorders of the Chyle and Lymph Systems*. London: Edward Arnold

Lee, J. K. T., Heiken, J. P., Ling, D. L., Glazer, H. S., Balfe, D. M., Levitt, R. G., Thomas Dixon, W., & Murphy, W. A. Jr. (1984) Magnetic resonance imaging of abdominal and pelvic lymphadenopathy. Radiology, **153**: 181–188

Lerski, R. A. (1982) Ultrasonic tissue characterization. *Diagnostic Imaging*, **51**: 238–248

Parker, B. R., Blank, N., & Castellino, R. A. (1974) Lymphangiographic appearance of benign conditions simulating lymphoma. *Radiology*, **111**: 267–274

Porter, L. L., & Hande, K. R. (1983) Potential uses of NMR in clinical oncology. In: Partin, C. L., James, A. E., Rollo, F. D., & Price, R. R. (eds) *Nuclear Magnetic Resonance Imaging*, pp. 349–353. W. B. Saunders Company

Schellinger, D., Miller, W. E., Harrison, E. G. Jr, & Kiely, J. M. (1974) Lymphographic patterns of the subtypes of malignant lymphoma including Hodgkin's disease. *Radiology*, **111**: 257–266

Wallace, S., Jackson, L., & Dodd, C. D. (1965) Lymphangiogram interpretation. *Radiologic Clinics of North America*, **3**: 467–485

PART 4

THE GASTROINTESTINAL TRACT AND ABDOMEN

CHAPTER 29

THE SALIVARY GLANDS, PHARYNX AND OESOPHAGUS

THE SALIVARY GLANDS

Technique of examination

The paired parotid and submandibular glands are best investigated by conventional radiographic means.

The parotid gland is located behind the angle of the mandible, with a large single duct (Stenson's) opening on a papilla on the buccal mucosa opposite the second upper molar tooth. Anteroposterior (normal and soft tissue exposure), tangential, lateral and lateral oblique plain radiographs are useful for showing calculi and soft tissue swelling.

The submandibular gland lies below the mandible and can be seen best in a lateral oblique view. This is supplemented by a lateral view obtained with the patient's finger in the mouth depressing the tongue; the purpose of this manoeuvre being to push the submandibular gland into sight beneath the mandible. The single submandibular duct (Wharton's) opens on a papilla at the side of the frenulum beneath the tongue, and is best demonstrated free of superimposed mandible by placing an occlusal film in the mouth and using a submentovertical type of projection. This is frequently the only view to show a calculus situated in the anterior part of the submandibular duct (Fig. 29.1).

Sialography. A series of plain films is necessary before proceeding to sialography. The examination is usually performed with the patient lying on a conventional skull table with the operator seated by the head. Good lighting and suitable instruments are required. The appropriate duct orifice is located and, if necessary, dilated with a metal probe. When the orifice is difficult to identify, a drop of lemon juice on the tongue will stimulate salivation and reveal its location. Intubation of a duct can be achieved by several methods. Most operators use either a blunt-tipped slightly angulated metal cannula, or a fine thin-walled

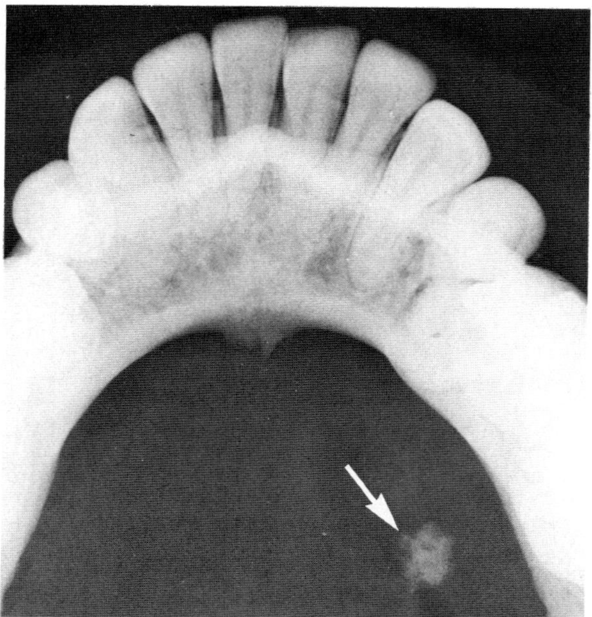

Fig. 29.1 Stone in submandibular duct shown on intraoral view. (Courtesy of Miss Ruth Donaldson.)

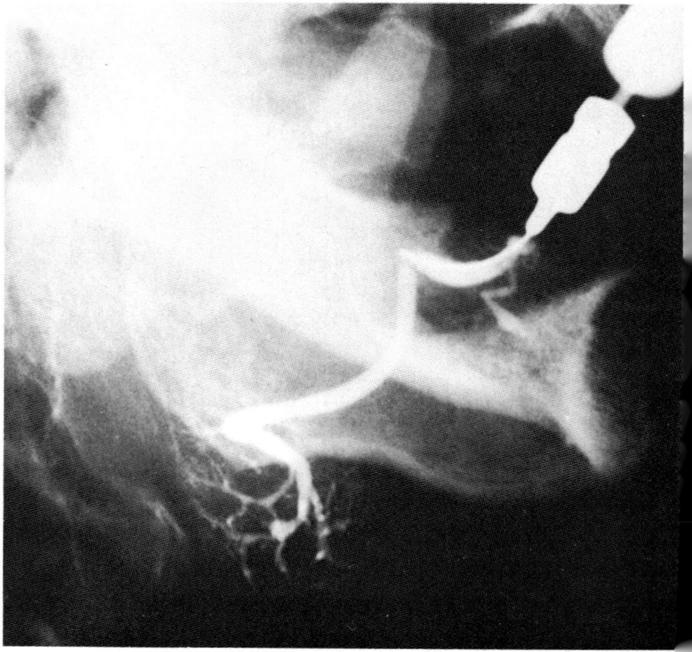

Fig. 29.2 Normal submandibular sialogram. Lateral oblique view.

polythene catheter with a tapered end connected to a 2 cc glass syringe. Generally a parotid duct is easier to enter than a submandibular duct. Approximately 0.5–1.5 cc of the chosen contrast medium is slowly injected by hand until the patient indicates, by a previously arranged signal, that distension of the gland is being felt. Most radiologists use either iodized oil fluid injection (Lipiodol ultrafluid) or a water-soluble medium. A series of radiographs matching the controls is then obtained (Fig. 29.2). During the exposures it is customary, when using a catheter, to leave it held in place between the patient's closed lips, but a metal cannula is usually removed immediately following the contrast injection. Some operators conduct the examination under fluoroscopic control, taking spot films in suitable projections as required. When satisfactory radiographs have been obtained, the patient is given a few drops of lemon juice to stimulate salivation and an 'after lemon' film is taken 5 minutes later. Normally on this film very little contrast medium is seen remaining in the ducts.

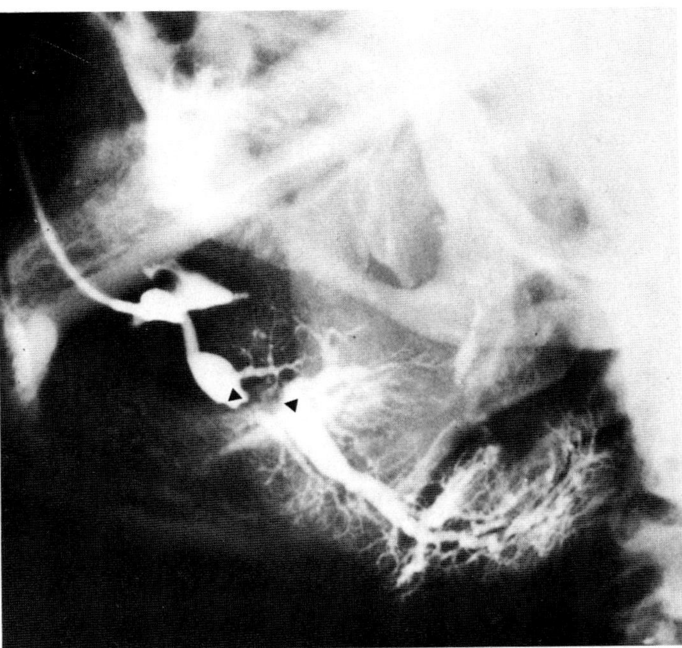

Fig. 29.3 Obstructive sialectasis. Parotid sialogram demonstrating a non-opaque calculus in the main duct (between the arrow heads). The stone is producing obstruction and the main duct is dilated. The peripheral duct system is normal. (Courtesy of Dr G J S Parkin.)

SALIVARY DISEASE: STONES, INFLAMMATION, NEOPLASM

Salivary disorders may be classified according to their sialographic appearance into *inflammatory diseases* and *mass lesions*. Sialography is contraindicated in acute parotitis. Chronic non-neoplastic enlargement of the salivary glands may be divided into chronic obstructive sialectasis (sialodochiectasis) and chronic non-obstructive sialectasis.

Chronic obstructive sialectasis results from two main causes: calculi and strictures.

Stones may be solitary or multiple. The majority are opaque and may be seen on plain radiographs. The incidence of stones is much higher in the submandibular glands, but multiple calculi are more frequent in the parotid glands. Sialography can identify and locate opaque and non-opaque calculi and associated strictures in the duct system. When a stone is large enough to produce obstruction (generally when it exceeds 3 mm in a main duct), dilatation of the proximal ducts occurs (Fig. 29.3). Secondary infection may lead to irregular collections of contrast medium within small cavities in the gland.

Strictures involving the main duct may be single or multiple; a stricture of the orifice of Stenson's duct is not uncommon. Tooth extractions and ill-fitting dentures are frequently the cause. Strictures may also be a sequel to surgery, inflammatory disease or trauma. When a stricture is present the main duct and its tributaries are dilated proximal to the point of obstruction and contrast medium is seen to be retained on 'after lemon' films. When there are multiple strictures the main duct when filled with contrast medium has the appearance of a string of sausages.

Chronic non-obstructive sialectasis occurs in a heterogenous group of chronic inflammatory diseases that produce enlargement of the major salivary glands clinically resembling a neoplasm, from which they may be distinguished by sialography. The group includes *recurrent sialadenitis* in children, recurrent *pyogenic parotitis* in adults, *Sjögren's syndrome* and *Mikulicz's disease*. The clinical features of each of these diseases are distinctive, but radiographic appearances are similar.

Preliminary radiographs usually show soft tissue swelling, and fine, nodular, calcific densities may be present in affected glands. The degree of sialectasis has been classified into grades according to severity:

1. In the *normal* sialogram the ducts are evenly distributed and gently tapered.
2. The earliest finding in sialectasis is a '*pruned tree*' appearance, with stretched and tapered intraglandular ducts, and non-filling of the acini (Fig. 29.4).
3. *Punctate* sialectasis consists of punctate dilatations (less than 1 mm in size) of the peripheral ducts (Fig. 29.5).
4. In *globular* sialectasis the peripheral ducts exhibit globular dilatations (1–2 mm in size), and the intraglandular ducts are irregular, deformed and sparse (Fig. 29.6).
5. *Cavitating* sialectasis results from coalescence of the globules into cavities (Fig. 29.7).
6. The final stage of the disease is *destructive* sialectasis. A bizarre pattern of filling with pooling of contrast medium results from complete destruction of the gland (Fig. 29.7). The pattern simulates a malignant neoplasm and stones may be present.

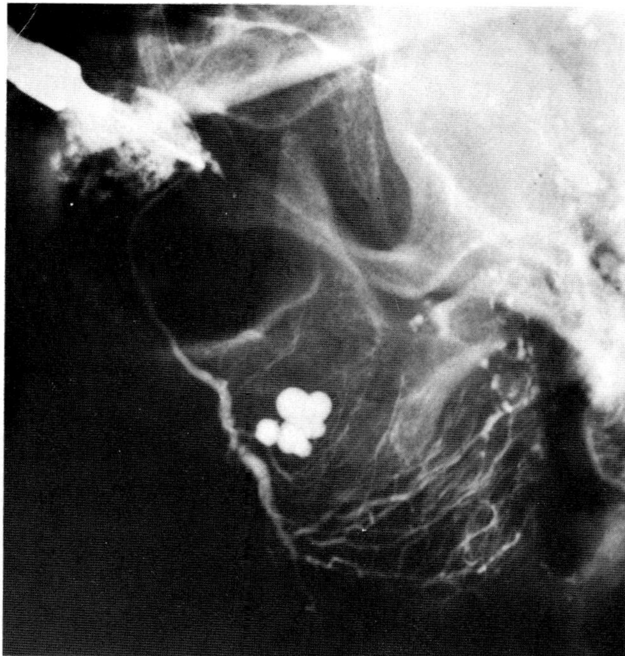

Fig. 29.4 Grade 2 sialectasis. Parotid sialogram showing irregular, sparse intraglandular ducts. Localised globular sialectasis results from obstruction of a small peripheral branch. (Courtesy of Dr G J S Parkin.)

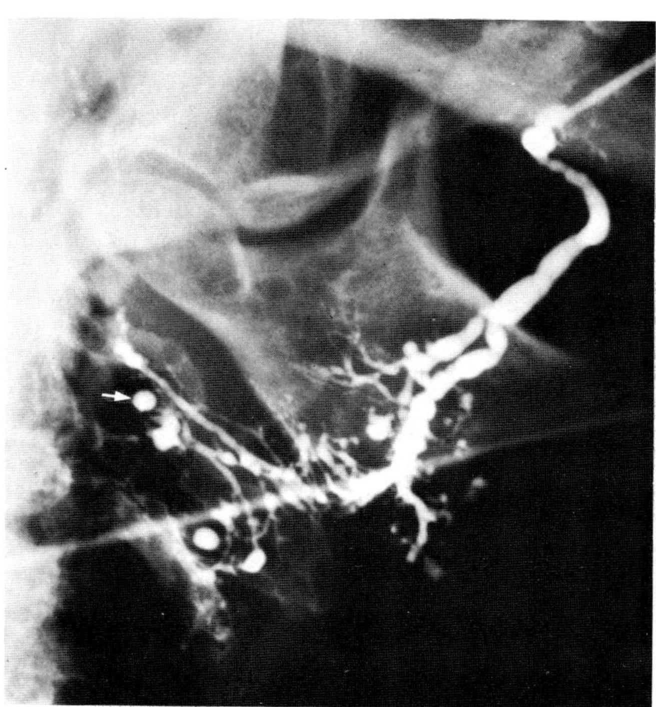

Fig. 29.6 Grade 4 sialectasis. Parotid sialogram showing globular sialectasis. Collections of contrast medium 1–2 mm in size, are evenly distributed throughout the gland (one of them has been identified with an arrow). The intraglandular ducts are stunted, irregular and sparse.

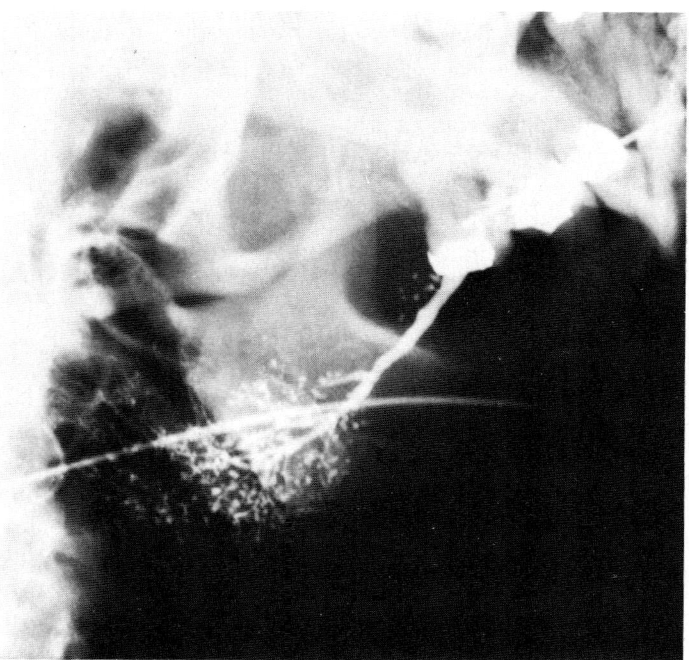

Fig. 29.5 Grade 3 sialectasis. Parotid sialogram showing punctate sialectasis. The peripheral branches of the intraglandular ducts have not filled, and there are numerous small collections of contrast medium evenly distributed throughout the gland. (Courtesy of Dr G J S Parkin.)

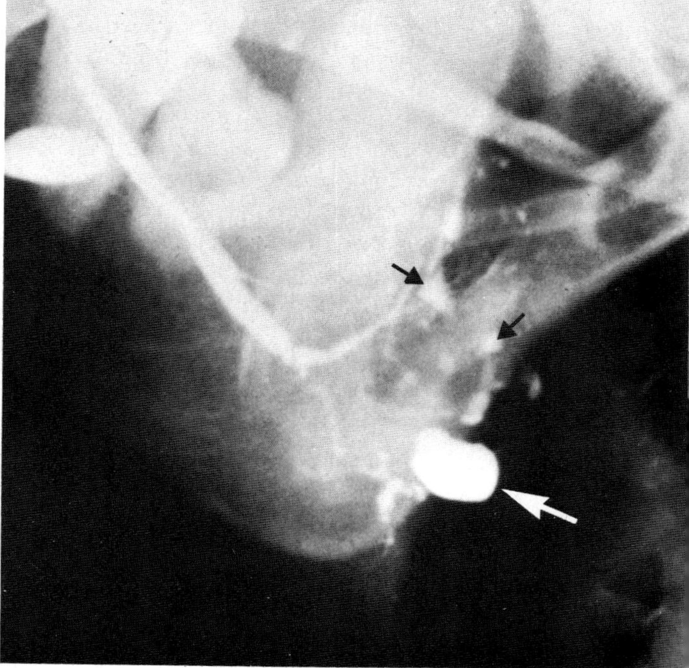

Fig. 29.7 Grade 5 and 6 sialectasis. Parotid sialogram showing cavitating and destructive sialectasis. There is a large cavity indicated by a white arrow. There are also numerous small irregular collections of contrast medium (e.g. black arrows) thoughout the gland, almost entirely replacing the normal intraglandular duct system. (Courtesy of Dr G J S Parkin.)

Sialography is a useful means of differentiating intrinsic from extrinsic salivary masses. A normal sialogram indicates that a mass is extraglandular.

Salivary gland tumours are relatively uncommon, 80% occurring in the parotid glands. The most common salivary gland tumour is the *mixed salivary tumour*, the majority of which are benign. *Carcinoma* and *adenoma* are rare. The distinction on sialography between benign and malignant tumours is unreliable. In general, benign neoplasms are encapsulated with displacement of the stretched ducts around a circumscribed filling defect in the parenchyma of the gland (Fig. 29.8). Most malignant tumours are infiltrative, producing an irregular filling defect with duct distortion and pooling of contrast medium. However, some malignant tumours may be encapsulated and indistinguishable from a benign tumour.

Ultrasound (US), computed tomography (CT) and scintigraphy have been used to investigate salivary gland disorders, but their value is secondary to that of plain radiography and sialography, and is mainly directed towards showing the extent of spread of invasive tumours.

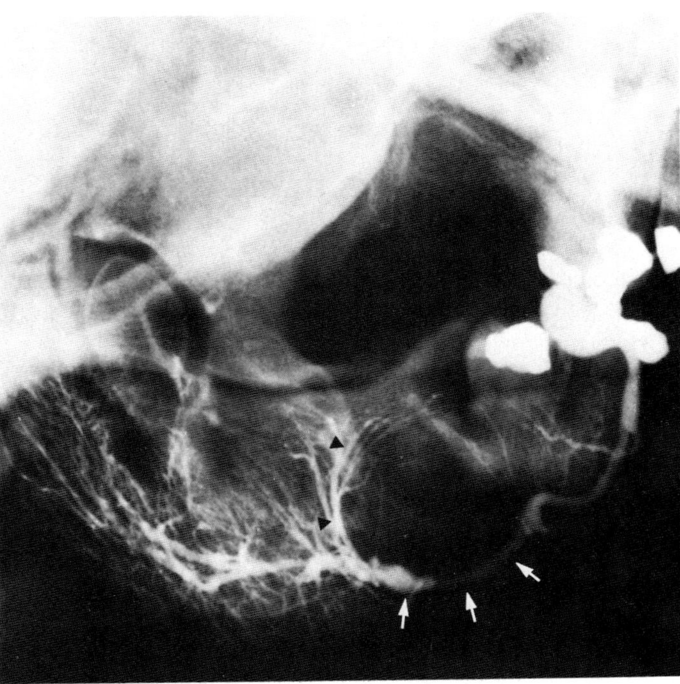

Fig. 29.8 Parotid sialogram showing a 2.5 cm diameter benign salivary tumour in the anterior part of the gland, which is displacing the main duct (white arrows) downwards, and the intraglandular ducts (black arrow heads) backwards. The site of the tumour is devoid of ducts and acinar filling. The remainder of the gland is normal.

PHARYNX AND OESOPHAGUS

THE UPPER OESOPHAGUS

Technique of examination

From a radiological viewpoint the oesophagus can be divided into three anatomical parts: the *upper oesophagus* (consisting of the hypopharynx and the cervical oesophagus), the *thoracic oesophagus*, and the region around the *oesophagogastric junction*. The hypopharynx extends from the epiglottis to the level of the cricoid cartilage opposite the 6th cervical vertebra where it becomes the cervical oesophagus, which continues into the thoracic inlet where it becomes the thoracic oesophagus.

Some lesions occur at any level, whilst others have a predisposition, or are specific to, certain sites. A familiarity with the normal radiographic appearances at all levels is necessary for accurate interpretation. Under some circumstances plain radiography has an important role, but the mainstay of diagnosis is the barium swallow (syn: contrast oesophagography). The technique of examination varies according to the anatomical region under investigation, and is also dependent upon the nature of the suspected abnormality.

It is convenient to examine the hypopharynx and cervical oesophagus together. Lateral soft tissue radiographs of the neck are useful in detecting radiopaque foreign bodies, soft tissue swelling and associated disease in the cervical spine. A barium swallow is the usual method for studying disorders of swallowing, anatomical abnormalities and disease. A rapid sequence technique is necessary in order to ensure that the region is seen fully distended. Cine radiography employed in the frontal and lateral projections at frame speeds of 50–100 per second, and videotape recording, are the best techniques for investigating disorders of swallowing. Photofluorography at 4–6 frames per second is suitable when a structural abnormality is suspected. Conventional spot film radiography with precise timing of the exposures can successfully demonstrate structural abnormalities in patients who are able to swallow barium to order.

With the fluoroscopic table upright, the patient takes a large mouthful of barium and retains it in the mouth. The patient's head is then positioned facing straight forwards with the chin slightly raised, and the fluoroscopic explorator is correctly sited over the mouth and neck. The motion recording device is started, the patient swallows, and progress of the bolus through the upper oesophagus is recorded. Immediately afterwards, with the patient breathing quietly a spot film is taken in the same position to show **the hypopharynx** distended with air and coated with barium. The sequence is then repeated with the patient in the lateral position or slightly oblique in order to clear the overlying shoulders. The anatomy of the hypopharynx is best appreciated on the frontal view (Fig. 29.9). Superiorly the epiglottis is seen as a barium-coated smooth mound superimposed over the paired dependent pouches of the valleculae. The lateral boundaries of the hypopharynx are the outer margins of the two pyriform sinuses, each having a pointed inferior

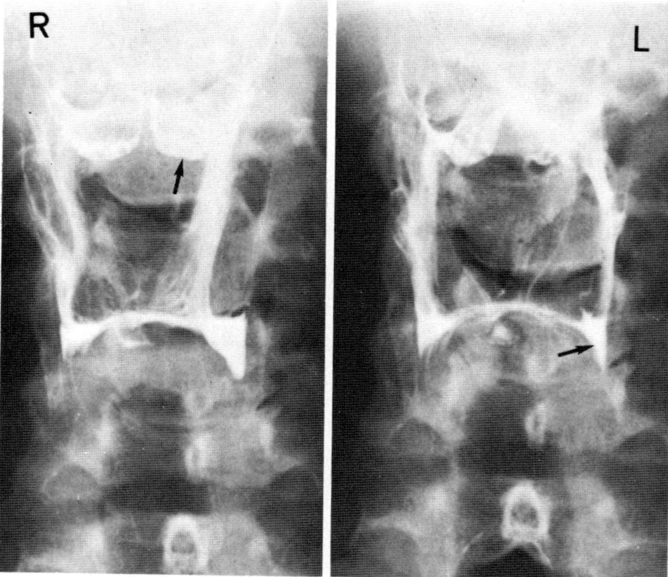

Fig. 29.9 Frontal view of the normal hypopharynx demonstrated after a mouthful of barium has passed down the oesophagus. The upper arrow indicates the valleculum, and the lower arrow points to the inferior recess of the pyriform sinus.

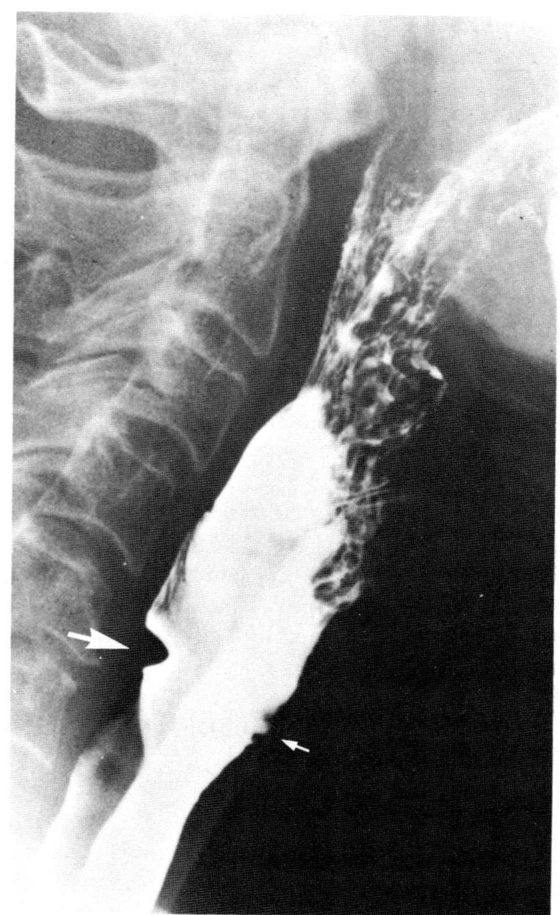

Fig. 29.10 Barium swallow showing the cervical oesophagus. Lateral view. The small irregular anterior indentation (small arrow) is a normal venous plexus. The well-defined posterior impression (large arrow) is produced by thickening of the transverse portion of the cricopharyngeus muscle. (Courtesy of Dr J L Isaacs.)

recess, with an arched inter-connecting line forming the inferior boundary. The lateral view of the hypopharynx is more complex due to superimposition of structures. The epiglottis is seen antero-superiorly with the superimposed aryepiglottic folds passing downwards and backwards from the epiglottis to the arytenoid cartilages. The pyriform sinuses are also superimposed. When distended with barium the posterior wall of the hypopharynx is well seen in profile parallel to the cervical spine, making this projection particularly useful for showing retropharyngeal masses. Inferiorly the transverse portion of the cricophrayngeus muscle causes a smooth posterior indentation at the pharyngo-oesophageal junction.

The cervical oesophagus is a featureless tube which transmits a barium bolus with great rapidity. Its only notable feature is the presence on its anterior wall of a venous plexus that forms an irregular nodular indentation in the post-cricoid region (Fig. 29.10). This normal structure should not be mistaken for a web or a neoplasm.

THE UPPER OESOPHAGUS:

Functional abnormalities in the act of swallowing mainly comprise cricopharyngeal dysfunction, misdirected swallowing and epiglottic dysfunction. In *cricopharyngeal dysfunction* (syn: *cricopharyngeal achalasia*) there is incomplete or improperly timed upper oesophageal sphincter relaxation. Thickening of the transverse band of the cricopharyngeus muscle produces a prominent, rounded, extrinsic impression in the posterior wall of the barium-filled oesophagus, which may result in obstruction and dysphagia (Fig. 29.10). It is possible that hypertrophy of this segment of muscle initiates the formation of a pharyngeal pouch. Patients with laryngeal speech following laryngectomy sometimes develop dysphagia due to gross hypertrophy of the cricopharyngeus muscle.

Another cause of dysphagia which occurs secondary to poliomyelitis and other neurological diseases is *pharyngeal constrictor paresis*, in which there is an interruption of normal propulsive pharyngeal peristalsis.

Structural abnormalities. The great majority of structural abnormalities occurring in the hypopharynx and cervical oesophagus fall under one of four headings: (1) webs, (2) neoplasm, (3) retropharyngeal abscess, and (4) diverticula.

Webs

Three varieties of oesophageal web may be recognized:

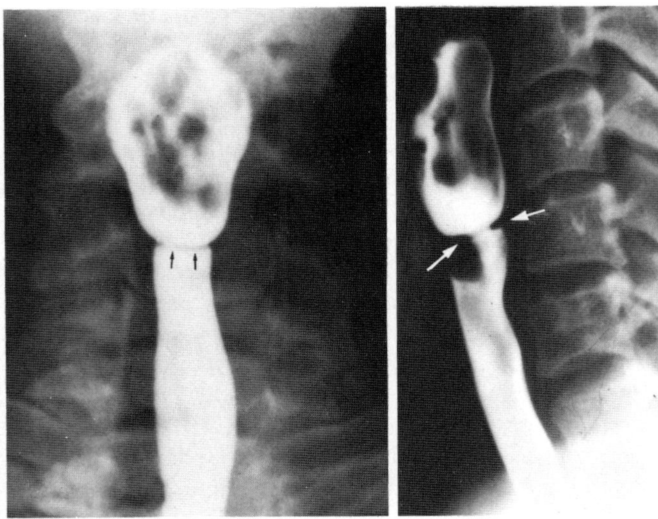

Fig. 29.11 A concentric upper oesophageal web seen in both the frontal and lateral projections (arrows). The way in which the web narrows the lumen is well seen in the lateral view.

1. an incidental finding (sometimes called 'non-specific'),
2. a component of the Plummer-Vinson syndrome,
3. associated with some miscellaneous specific conditions.

Webs are semicircular membranes of variable size, 1–2 mm thick, consisting of plications of normal squamous mucosa without inflammation. They commonly arise from the anterior wall of the cervical oesophagus just below the cricopharyngeus (Fig. 29.11). Multiple webs are fairly common. Webs also occur infrequently in the mid or lower oesophagus. Most are best seen with the patient swallowing a large bolus of barium in the lateral position; many are also visible in other projections. Cine radiography is the most sensitive method of detection.

Webs in the upper oesophagus are a common incidental finding, especially in females over 50 years of age. They are common amongst patients with dysphagia due to concomitant functional abnormalities in the act of swallowing, and may themselves be a cause of dysphagia when large enough to produce obstruction (Fig. 29.12). Postcricoid webs are associated with the Plummer-Vinson syndrome (syn: Paterson-Brown-Kelly syndrome), although frequently the full blown syndrome is absent. In the majority of cases there is an iron deficiency anaemia or a low serum iron with a low iron binding capacity. The relationship of postcricoid webs to carcinoma is controversial, and the evidence that such webs are premalignant is not as strong as previously thought. Webs may occur together with a carcinoma of the larynx, oesophagus or stomach. They have also been recorded in pernicious anaemia, and they may occur as a complication of certain skin diseases such as epidermolysis bullosa and benign pemphigoid.

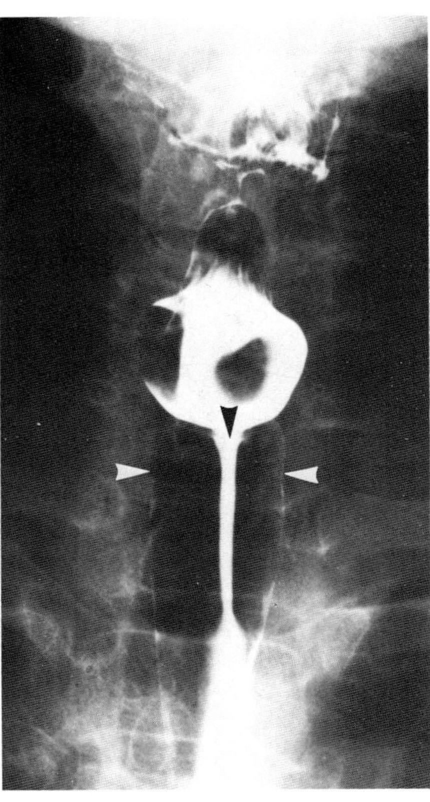

Fig. 29.12 Postcricoid web. Frontal view showing obstruction with 'jet' effect of the narrow barium stream passing through the small orifice in the web (black arrowhead). The white arrowheads indicate the full width of the oesophagus below the web. (Courtesy of Dr A Chapman.)

Neoplasm

Most tumours arising in the upper oesophagus are *squamous-cell carcinomas*. *Sarcomas* also occur. Diagnosis is usually by direct visual or endoscopic means. Radiological investigation is directed towards determining the site and extent of disease. On barium swallow a carcinoma produces an irregular intraluminal mass, or deformity with loss of normal distensibility and narrowing caused by tumour infiltration (Fig. 29.13). In selected cases CT may provide useful information on staging and response to radiotherapy.

Retropharyngeal abscess

A retropharyngeal abscess is an inflammatory mass located between the pharynx or cervical oesophagus and the cervical spine, usually resulting from tonsillitis, traumatic pharyngitis or infection of the cervical spine. Perforation may be caused by trauma from a swallowed foreign body or instrumentation. Vertebral infection is usually tuberculous or staphylococcal, with disc space narrowing and bone destruction. A retropharyngeal abscess is seen in the lateral projection as a soft tissue mass sometimes containing bubbles of gas. According to the size and level of the mass, there is an impression in the posterior wall of the hypo-

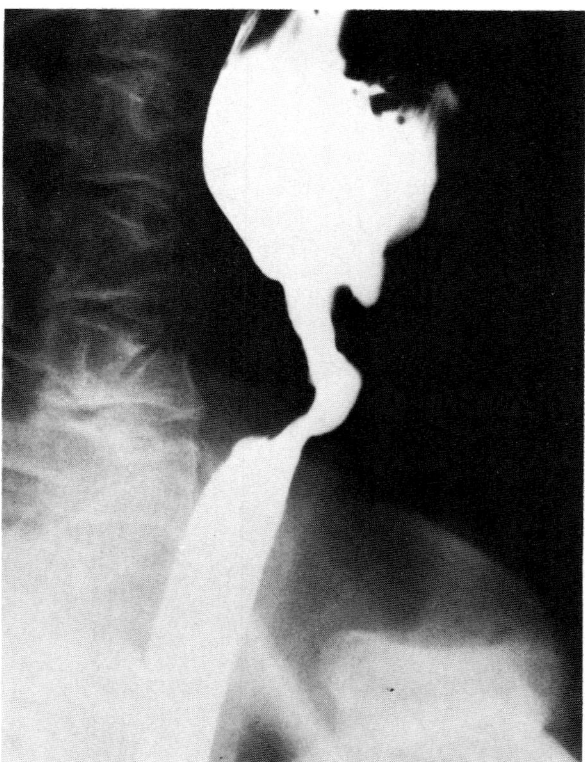

Fig. 29.13 Postcricoid carcinoma. Lateral view showing irregular narrowing.

pharynx or cervical oesophagus, and forward displacement of the pharynx, oesophagus and trachea may occur.

DIVERTICULA

The great majority of oesophageal diverticula are acquired, seldom developing before the age of 40 years. Small diverticula are usually symptomless, but dysphagia may be present with larger ones. Oesophageal diverticula are generally false, being formed by the projection of a pouch of mucosa through the muscularis. They may be classified according to their anatomical site into *posterior* and *lateral pharyngeal*, *thoracic* and *epiphrenic*.

Posterior pharyngeal diverticula (syn: Zenker's diverticulum, pharyngeal pouch) are relatively common and originate just proximal to the upper oesophageal sphincter through the dehiscence between the oblique and transverse fibres of the inferior constrictor muscle of the pharynx. These pouches are either asymptomatic or manifest in the elderly with dysphagia and regurgitation of undigested food. There is considerable variation in size with some pouches becoming very large. Aspiration results in pneumonic changes at the lung bases (the so-called 'spill-over' syndrome). Erect plain radiographs of the neck often show a gas-fluid level in the pouch. A barium swallow confirms the posterior position of the pouch, usually to the left, displacing the oesophagus forward (Fig. 29.14). As a result

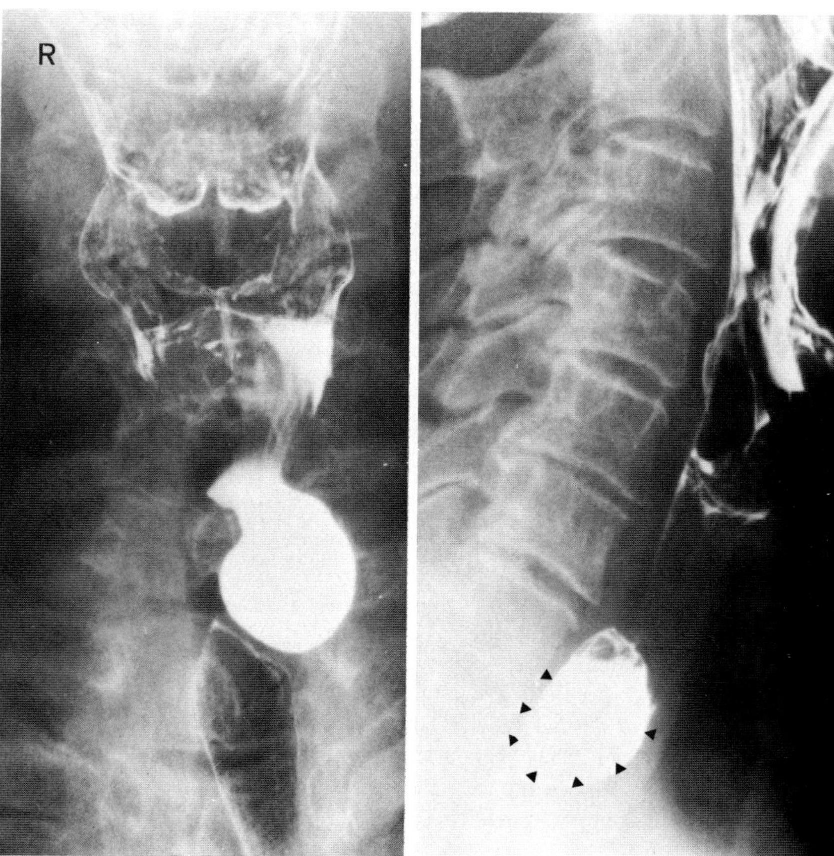

Fig. 29.14 Posterior pharyngeal diverticulum seen on the frontal view to be extending towards the patient's left. The diverticulum remains filled with barium after the rest of the swallowed bolus has passed.

of the oesophageal displacement the pouch comes to lie in the line of the swallowed foodstuff. Consequently an endoscope is liable to enter the pouch in preference to passing down the normal channel, with the danger of perforation.

Lateral pharyngeal diverticula are uncommon, and there is some confusion over terminology. Most are bulges (syn: pouches, pharyngoceles, ears) occurring through the thyrohyoid membrane; these are small, bilaterally symmetrical and of no clinical importance. Lateral bulges may also occur in the tonsillar fossa in glassblowers and trumpet players. The rare congenital lateral pharyngeal diverticula are true branchial cleft cysts and sinuses that arise in the pharynx and end blindly in the neck.

Diverticula in the **thoracic oesophagus** are pulsion or traction in origin. Pulsion diverticula arise as a consequence of the ageing process or result from an underlying motility disorder. Rarely pulsion diverticula may be congenital. Traction diverticula, associated with mediastinal tuberculous glands, are uncommon. Diverticula are usually wide necked and project in any direction except posteriorly where the spine is located (Fig. 29.15). They are usually demonstrated best by barium swallow in the prone position.

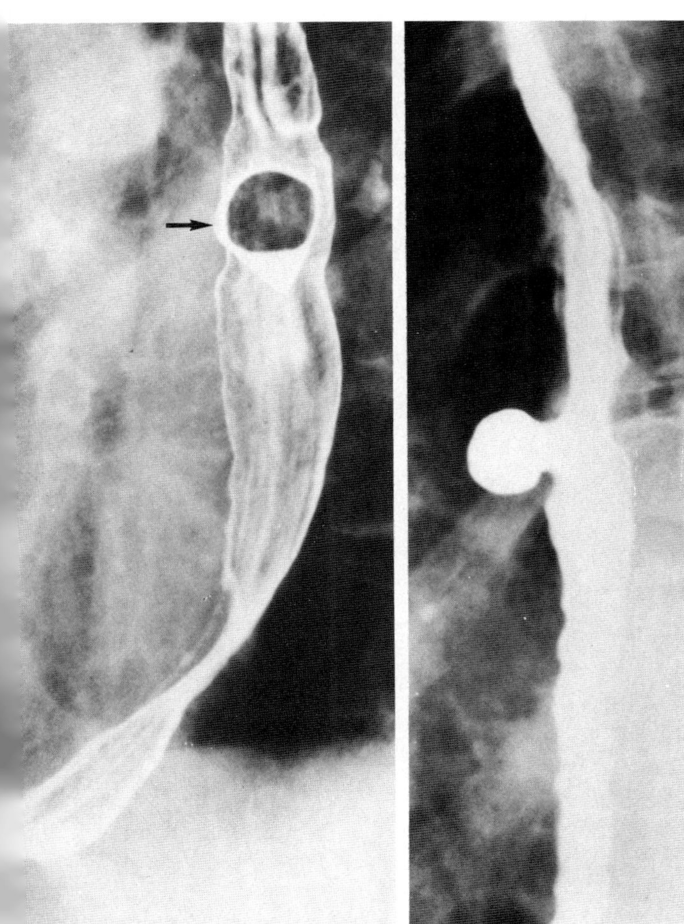

Fig. 29.15 Mid-oesophageal diverticulum seen *en face* on the left, and in profile on the right.

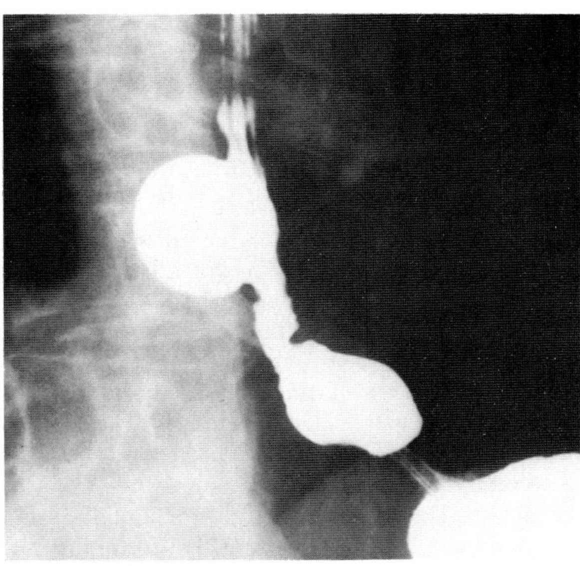

Fig. 29.16 Large lower oesophageal diverticulum associated with disordered motility of the oesophagus.

Diverticula at the lower end of the oesophagus (**epiphrenic**) generally project to the right, are often best seen in the supine position, and are frequently associated with severe tertiary oesophageal contractions (Fig. 29.16).

MOTOR DISORDERS OF THE OESOPHAGUS

Fluoroscopy of patients swallowing barium whilst in the standing and recumbent positions is a useful procedure in the assessment of motor disorders of the oesophagus. Unless specifically indicated for diagnostic purposes a hypotonic drug, e.g. Buscopan (hyoscine-n-butylbromide) should not be given. Peristaltic contractions in the body of the oesophagus and sphincteric mechanisms at both ends comprise normal oesophageal motility. The upper oesophageal sphincter (cricopharyngeus) acts as an important barrier preventing reflux of oesophageal contents into the pharynx, and aspiration of air into the oesophagus during respiration. The lower oesophageal sphincter forms the major barrier to gastro-oesophageal reflux. In the oesophagus the primary peristaltic wave begins with the act of swallowing and proceeds along the oesophagus to the cardia. The main secondary propulsive waves start at the level of the aortic knuckle and proceed rhythmically to the cardia and are followed by a wave of relaxation.

The normal oesophageal motility pattern may be disordered in several ways. Peristalsis may be lost, weakened or replaced by non-progressive *tertiary contractions*. Sphincteric action may be accentuated by an impairment of relaxation; conversely, over-relaxation of the lower oesophageal sphincter allows excessive gastro-oesophageal reflux. In most cases of disordered motility several combinations of these abnormalities occur. There is evidence that primary oesophageal motility disorders constitute a spectrum of conditions consisting of *achalasia*, *diffuse oesophageal spasm* and *intermediate types*. The latter are characterized by varying degrees of peristaltic abnormality and sphincter relaxation deficiency. Evolution of one disorder to another has been reported. However, some authorities believe that achalasia and diffuse oesophageal spasm are completely separate entities and do not subscribe to the idea of intermediate types and evolution.

Tertiary contractions are non-propulsive, uncoordinated contractions of the circular muscle that cause the outline of the barium-filled oesophagus to be indented by a series of rings (Fig. 29.17). The contractions may last for a few seconds before relaxation occurs, to be followed by another series. This symptomless disorder is quite common in the elderly and is generally of no clinical importance. In its severest form smooth pouches or pseudodiverticula appear between the contracted areas. The asymmetrical series of barium-filled pouches and contractions has given rise to the descriptive term 'corkscrew oesophagus'. Some authors incorporate tertiary contractions and corkscrew oesophagus within the term 'curling phenomenon'.

Symptomatic diffuse oesophageal spasm is characterized by intermittent chest pain and dysphagia in the absence of a demonstrable organic lesion, and by abnormal non-peristaltic contractions. It is important for the patient that this condition should be differentiated from angina pectoris. Diagnosis is based on a combination of clinical symptoms and manometric abnormalities together with the immediate relief of pain and spasm by Buscopan (20 mg i.v.). The appearances on barium swallow are characterized by severe contractions that obliterate the lumen and force barium back up the oesophagus (Fig. 29.18). This retrograde propulsion is accentuated by a failure of relaxation of the cardia. The disorder usually affects the lower two thirds of the oesophagus. Swallowing barium sometimes initiates spasm, and the radiologist is able to relate the patient's pain to the simultaneous fluoroscopic appearances.

Symptomatic oesophageal peristalsis is a syndrome characterized by angina-like chest pain due to accentuated

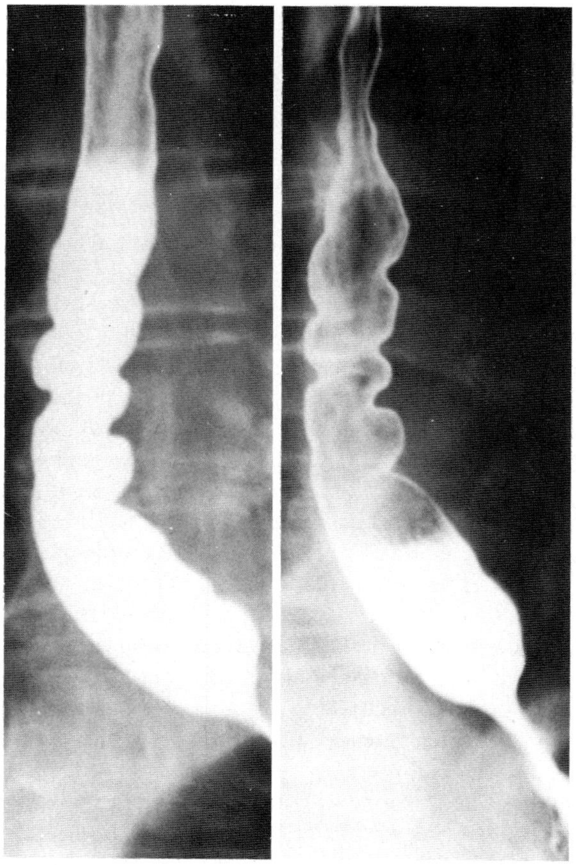

Fig. 29.17 Tertiary contractions of the oesophagus seen as a series of asymmetrical indentations resembling the shape of a corkscrew. Smooth tapering of the lower end of the oesophagus suggests a diagnosis of vigorous achalasia.

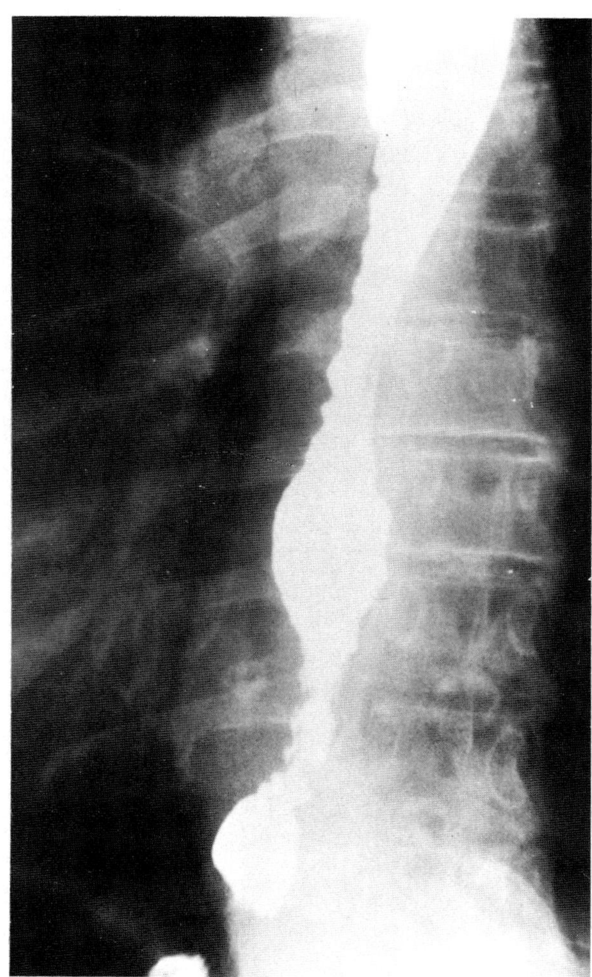

Fig. 29.18 Symptomatic diffuse oesophageal spasm. Severe contractions have forced the barium back up the oesophagus whilst the cardia has failed to relax.

peristaltic contractions. Manometric criteria have been proposed for diagnosis.

Achalasia. The motor disorder of the oesophagus most familiar to radiologists is achalasia. Loss of propulsive peristaltic contractions together with defective sphincter relaxation results in stasis of food and a progressively dilating and tortuous oesophagus. The condition usually presents in adults ranging in age between 30 and 50 years. Dysphagia for both fluids and solids is the most prominent symptom. Diagnosis is by means of clinical, radiographic and manometric data. Provocation tests may be useful in early cases; the oesophagus of most patients with achalasia is hypersensitive to cholinergic drugs such as intravenous Carbachol (or Mecholyl in some countries) which produce oesophageal spasm and pain.

The radiological appearances vary according to the severity of the condition. In the early stages the oesophagus is only slightly dilated throughout its length, with weakened peristalsis and delay in emptying of barium into the stomach. When standing, barium collects in the lower oesophagus and passes into the stomach intermittently in small spurts. The lower end of the oesophagus is smoothly tapered in a form that has been likened to a rat's tail. Later these features are accentuated (Fig. 29.19). In advanced cases dilatation is gross with an oesophageal diameter in excess of 10 cm. This is accompanied by elongation of the oesophagus resulting in a winding tortuous course. Chest radiography at this stage shows the wall of the dilated oesophagus outlined by air as a characteristic linear opacity, indented by the azygos vein, to the right of the superior mediastinum, and as a 'double shadow' behind the heart. An air-fluid level produced by air above liquid oesophageal contents or a mottled appearance of translucencies and densities due to a mixture of air and food, may be visible in the mediastinum. Signs of pneumonia and fibrosis are often seen at the lung bases due to the aspiration of oesophageal contents. Lung abscess and empyema may also result. There is little or no air in the stomach due to the lower oesophageal waterseal.

Narrowing of the lower end of the oesophagus is not specific to achalasia, although the presence of defective peristalsis and dilatation make this diagnosis likely (Fig. 29.20A). An achalasia pattern is often found in *Chaga's disease*, due to destruction of the myenteric plexus by the protozoan *Trypanosoma cruzi*. *Carcinoma* of the oesophagus or stomach can produce an identical narrowing, either by direct involvement or by destruction of the myenteric plexus (Fig. 29.20B and C). Achalasia has also been reported in association with carcinomas of the pancreas, bronchus and stomach; the mechanism of this type of achalasia is not firmly established *Extrinsic involvement* of the lower end of the oesophagus simulating achalasia also occurs in carcinoma of the tail of the pancreas (Fig. 29.20D), metastatic carcinoma (usually from an intra-abdominal primary) and lymphoma. Carcinoma of the

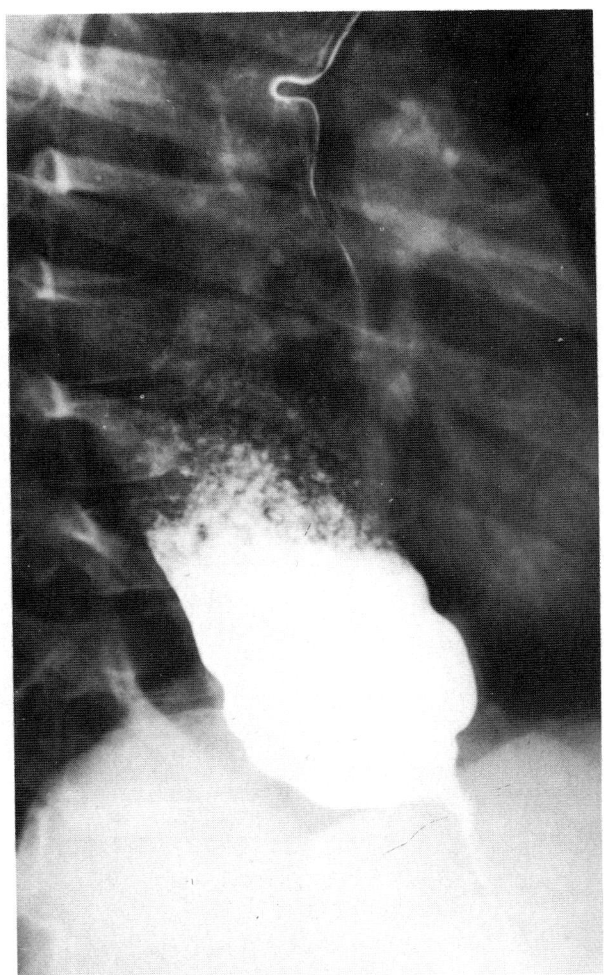

Fig. 29.19 Achalasia with typical tapered narrowing of the lower end of the oesophagus producing obstruction. Lateral view. Barium has accumulated in the dilated oesophagus; the mottled appearance at the top of the dense barium pool is due to floating retained fluid and food. No air is seen in the gastric fundus.

oesophagus is also a complication of long-standing achalasia (Fig. 29.21). Food residues often make this diagnosis extremely difficult, and aspiration of the oesophagus may be necessary in order to obtain a satisfactory barium examination. Therefore all cases of newly diagnosed achalasia should be subjected to oesophagoscopy and biopsy to exclude malignancy, and reviewed at regular intervals.

The normal methods of treatment of achalasia; dilatation by mercury bougie, transluminal balloon dilatation, endoscopic myotomy and Heller's myotomy all have a success rate of about 75%. Perforation and gastro-oesophageal reflux are the two major complications of these procedures.

Vigorous achalasia is believed by some authorities to occupy the part of the spectrum of oesophageal motility disorders between diffuse oesophageal spasm and achalasia; others consider it to be an early stage of achalasia. It tends to occur in a younger age group than 'full blown' achalasia and is characterized by high amplitude contractions which may alternate with tertiary contractions in an oesophagus of normal calibre. Smooth tapering of the lower oesophagus is seen as in achalasia.

Presbyoesophagus is the name given to a fairly common disorder of oesophageal motility associated with ageing. Peristalsis is diminished or absent, the lower oesophageal

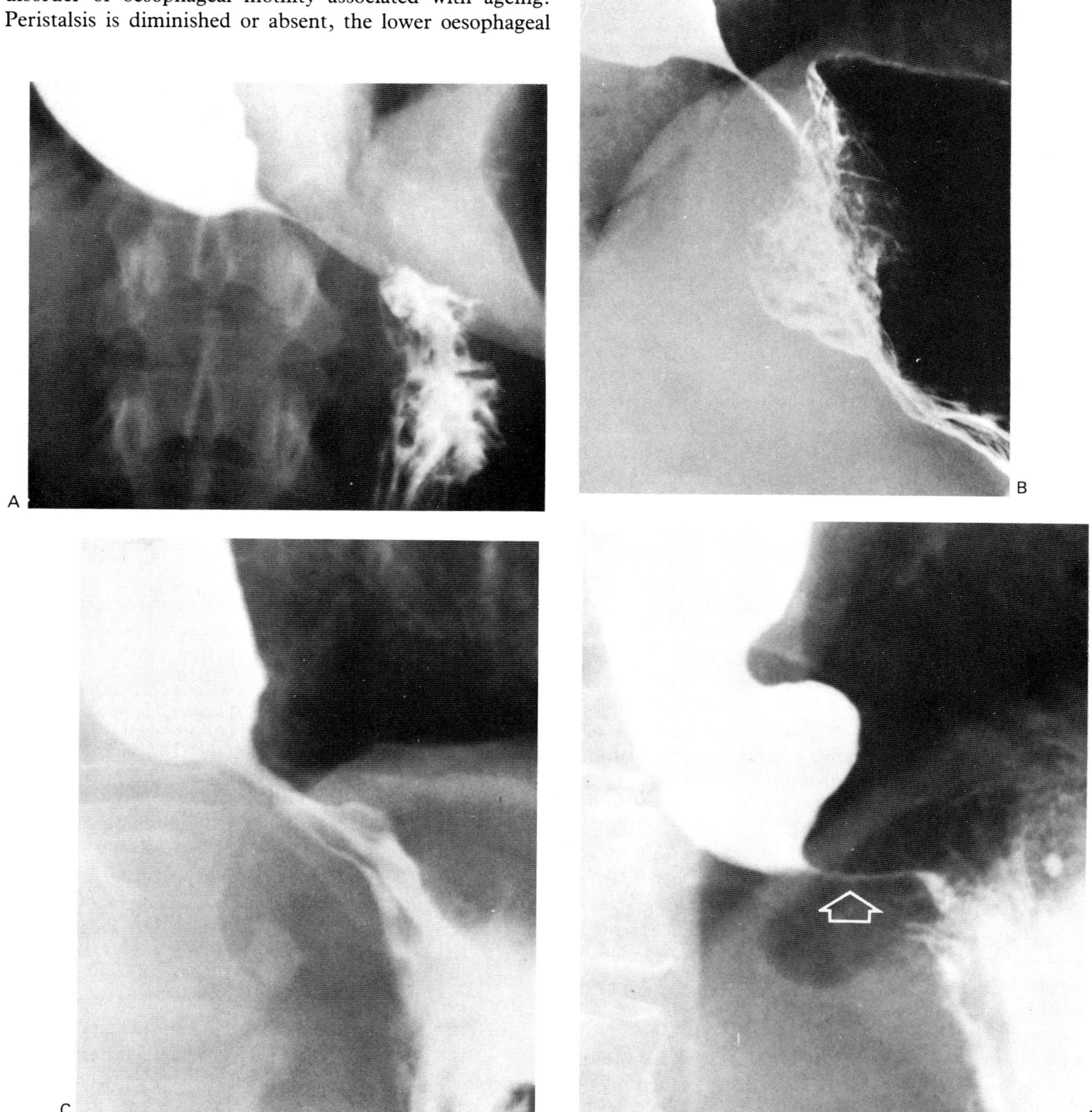

Fig. 29.20 A series of cases to show the resemblance of achalasia to malignant involvement of the cardia. **A.** Achalasia. **B.** Narrowing of the cardia with an associated filling defect in the gastric fundus due to carcinoma of the stomach extending to involve the lower end of the oesophagus. **C.** Narrowing of the cardia due to infiltrating squamous carcinoma of the lower end of the oesophagus. **D.** Narrowing of the cardia due to a large carcinoma of the tail of the pancreas extending to the oesophageal hiatus. Note that the dilated oesophagus is at a right angle to the tapered narrowing at its lower end. This right-angled configuration is absent in achalasia. (Courtesy of Dr N Joffe and the Editor of *Clinical Radiology*.)

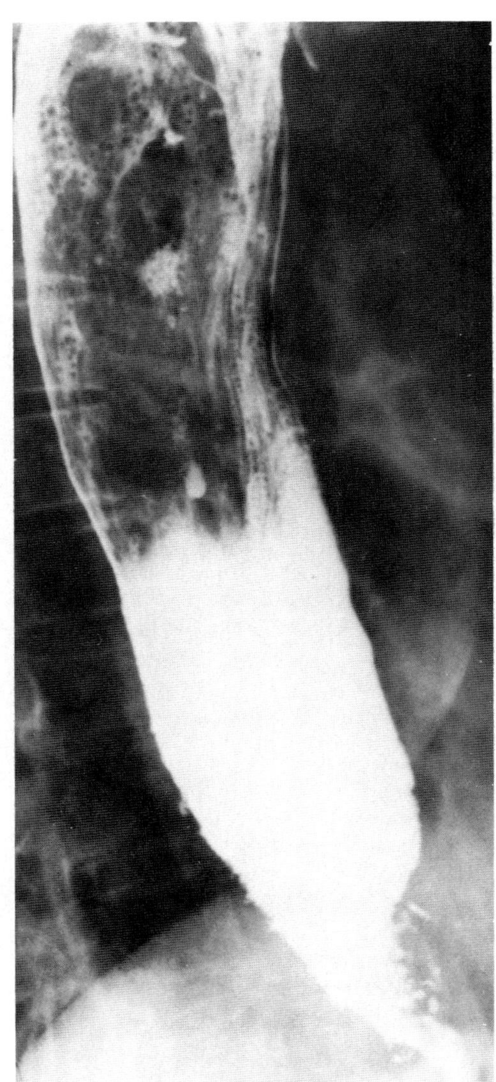

Fig. 29.21 Achalasia with irregular ragged lower end of the oesophagus due to carcinomatous change.

sphincter segment may fail to relax, and the oesophagus is usually slightly dilated. Tertiary contractions may occur. The condition is often symptomless, although the occasional patient may complain of dysphagia. Distinction from achalasia is made on grounds of age and severity, presbyoesophagus being a mild condition of the elderly.

Secondary disorders of oesophageal motility are associated with many conditions. *Postoperative* dysphagia is a recognized sequel to bilateral *truncal vagotomy*. Mild symptoms may occur in as many as 10% of patients, and the dysphagia is severe in about 1%. Dysphagia for solids is first noticed about 10 days after vagotomy, usually disappearing within 2 months. Barium swallow shows mild oesophageal dilatation and persistent tapered narrowing of the lower end. The syndrome has been attributed to post-operative oedema and haematoma. *Metabolic* disorders such as *diabetes* and *chronic alcoholism*, particularly when associated with peripheral neuropathy, may cause abnormal oesophageal motor function. Barium swallow shows diminished peristalsis, non-propulsive contractions and delayed oesophageal emptying. Clinical symptoms are usually absent. Dysphagia may occur in a large number of *neuromuscular disorders*. There is no specific pattern but diminished peristalsis, non-propulsive contractions and delayed oesophageal emptying are frequently observed. Pronounced pharyngeal abnormalities may also be present.

Oesophageal involvement is quite common in patients with *scleroderma*. Diminished or absent peristalsis with associated slight dilatation of the lower half of the oesophagus is commonly present. Hiatus hernia, gastro-oesophageal reflux and peptic stricture may also be found. To appreciate the motility defect it is necessary to examine the patient by barium swallow in the Trendelenburg (head down) position, because in scleroderma when the oesophagus is affected the patient is unable to swallow uphill. Following examination of the oesophagus it is worthwhile following the barium into the duodenum and small bowel in order to detect more extensive involvement. A barium enema is the best way of showing the characteristic pseudo-diverticula of scleroderma in the large bowel. Chest radiography may show pulmonary fibrosis, and there may be characteristic bone and soft tissue changes in the hands.

THE NORMAL LOWER END OF THE OESOPHAGUS: THE OESOPHAGOGASTRIC JUNCTION

Our understanding of the radiological anatomy and function of the lower end of the oesophagus and the oesophagogastric junction has been confused by the inconsistent application of names to a variety of appearances. Agreement is still lacking in some areas but a simplified version of what now seems to be the general view (Fig. 29.22) is as follows:

1. The *diaphragmatic hiatus* (hiatus) is the normal opening in the diaphragm which transmits the oesophagus and stomach. It does not mark the oesophagogastric junction. The *phrenico-oesophageal membrane* normally tethers the distal oesophagus to the diaphragm at the hiatus. The precise identification of the hiatus is not always easy as it may lie above the apparent radiographic intersection of the barium-filled oesophagus and diaphragm. Its location may be demonstrated best on deep inspiration, which causes 'pinching' of the oesophagus by the diaphragm (see 6).

2. The *oesophagogastric junction* (syn: *cardia*) may be identified on a barium swallow by a thin transverse mucosal fold known as *ring B* (syn: *mucosal ring, gastro-oesophageal ring*) (Fig. 29.22). In normal adults the oesophagogastric junction can be within 2 cm above or below the hiatus.

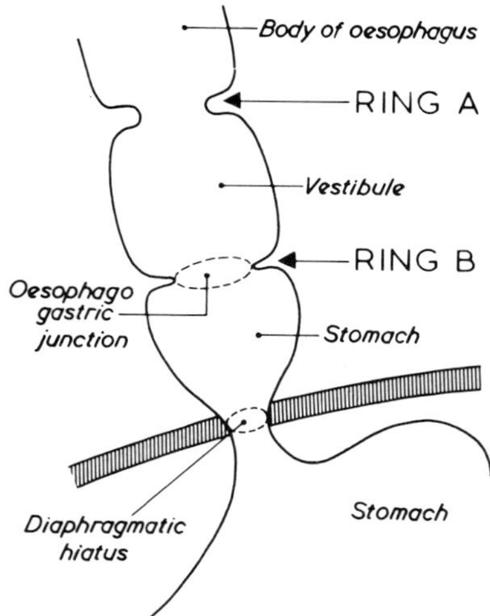

Fig. 29.22 Diagrammatic representation of the lower end of the oesophagus. Ring B may normally be within 2 cm above (as depicted here) or below the hiatus. Thus the oesophageal vestibule may normally be entirely above, or straddle, the diaphragmatic hiatus.

3. The oesophagogastric junction is located at the top of the *sling fibres of the stomach*. These are the innermost muscle fibres of the stomach which constitute the lesser curvature and loop up around the notch between the lower oesophagus and the gastric fundus (the left oesophagogastric angle) thus forming the *cardiac incisura* which may be seen when there is a sliding hiatus hernia (Fig. 29.23).

4. The change from squamous (oesophageal) to columnar (gastric) epithelium in the distal oesophagus is marked by an irregular line known as the *transition fold line* (syn: *the Z line*), at which gastric rugae (or areae gastricae) abruptly give way to straight oesophageal folds. This line does not always coincide with the oesophagogastric junction.

5. Proximal to ring B (usually by about 2–4 cm) is a thicker ring produced by active muscle contraction and known as *ring A* (syn: the *inferior oesophageal sphincter*, the *tubulo-vestibular junction*) (Fig. 29.22).

6. The more distensible lower end of the oesophagus between ring A and ring B is called the *vestibule*, which also constitutes the *lower oesophageal sphincter segment* or *high pressure zone*. The vestibule thus comprises the distal 2–4 cm of the oesophagus immediately above the oesophagogastric junction. The vestibule is not fixed in position and may normally be located above or straddle the hiatus. In inspiration the vestibule may be stretched, with the margins of the diaphragmatic hiatus squeezing (or 'pinching') its lower end to produce *the submerged or empty segment*, which is therefore located within the hiatus. The body of the oesophagus above the vestibule is known as the *tubular oesophagus*.

It is important to appreciate that in many normal subjects rings A and B may not be seen. Consequently the site of the oesophagogastric junction and vestibule cannot always be precisely determined and may have to be assumed.

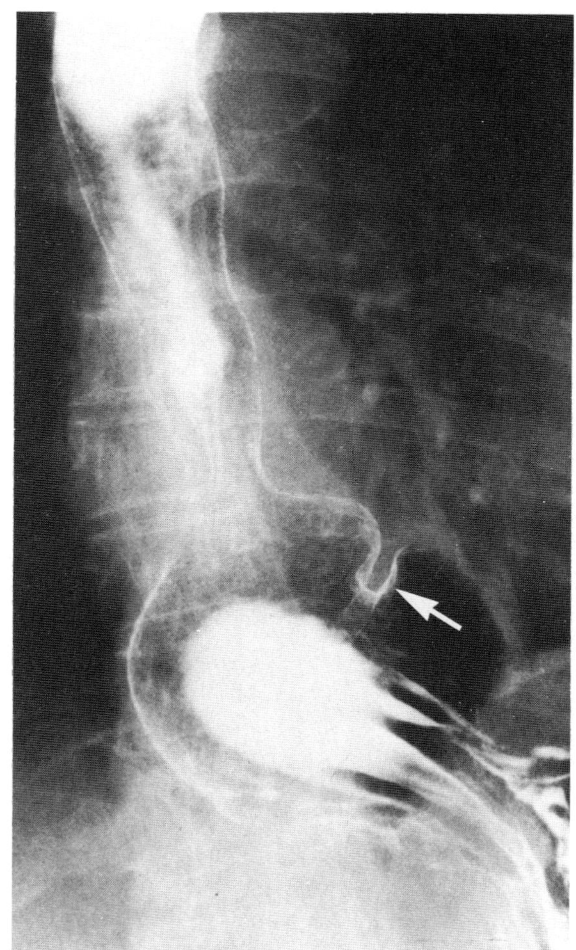

Fig. 29.23 Sliding hiatus hernia with cardiac incisura (arrowed) produced by the sling fibres of the stomach.

7. Additional names which have been given to the vestibular region include the *cardiac oesophagus* (= the lower 3 cm of the oesophagus above the cardia), and the *phrenic ampulla* (syn: ampulla). The latter term is best avoided because authors have variously described it as being synonymous with the vestibule or part of the vestibule, or also including part of the body of the oesophagus (above ring A) plus herniated stomach.

Other authors have further complicated matters by defining the oesophagogastric junction as a segment about 5 cm long between the body of the oesophagus and the stomach, corresponding to what most authors call the vestibule. They call the upper part of this tract the phrenic ampulla, which extends down to the diaphragmatic hiatus. The lower part between the ampulla and the body of the stomach is intra-abdominal in location and designated as the 'submerged segment' or 'abdominal gullet'. To avoid confusion most radiologists may prefer not to use the terms or interpretations applied in this paragraph.

8. Descriptions of *Schatzki's ring* in the literature are conflicting. In practice, experienced radiologists often find it difficult to differentiate between a Schatzki's ring, a prominent A or B ring and an annular peptic stricture at the oesophagogastric junction. Hence the frequent usage of the imprecise term 'lower oesophageal ring' which includes them all (Fig. 29.24). On fluoroscopy Schatzki's ring is seen as an annular narrowing at, or near, the oesophagogastric junction, variously described in different accounts as either transient or fixed, and either with or without significant inflammation and fibrosis. Whatever the truth of the matter, for practical purposes it is sufficient to think of Schatzki's ring as a rare condition consisting of a ring at the oesophago-gastric junction which is always associated with a small sliding hiatus hernia, and is most consistently demonstrated when the oesophagus is distended. It may be symptomless or liable to produce obstruction and dysphagia when its lumen is less than 20 mm in diameter.

9. The muscular ring in Barrett's syndrome (columnar-lined oesophagus) resembles a high A ring. The oesophagus below the ring is lined with columnar epithelium.

The preceding account of the anatomical landmarks at the lower end of the oesophagus has been given in an attempt to assist in the understanding of a complicated region. However, radiologists will find that in practice it is unnecessary to define all the landmarks described. A familiarity with the normal appearances, which comes with experience, is sufficient.

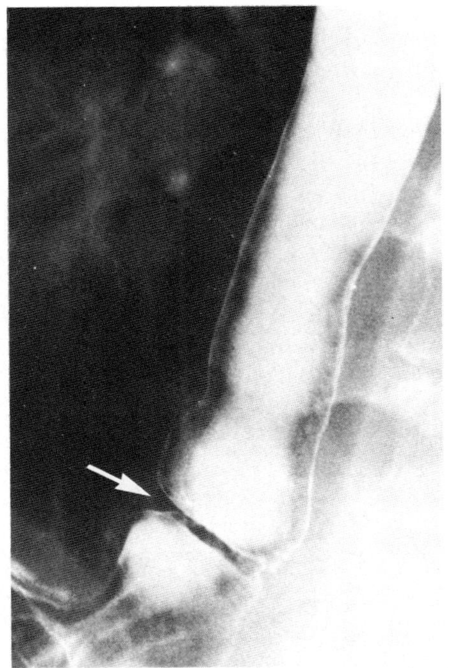

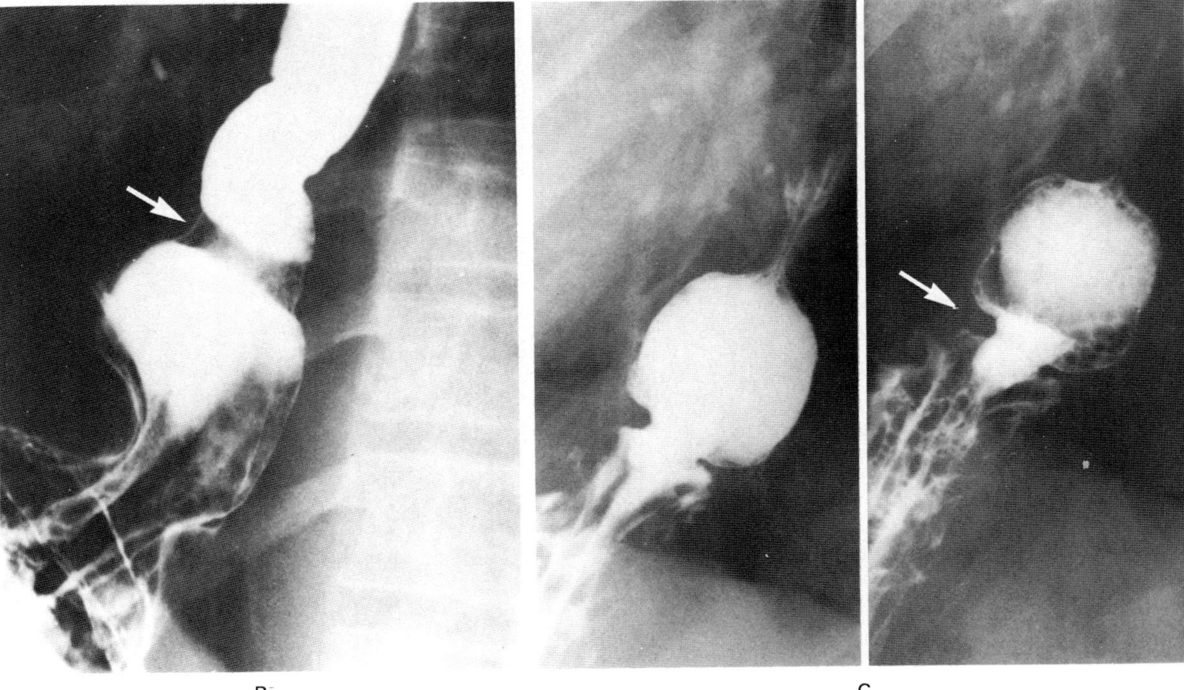

Fig. 29.24 Lower oesophageal rings: illustrating difficulties in nomenclature (see text). **A.** Small sliding hiatus hernia with accentuated but normal ring B. **B.** Small sliding hiatus hernia with a prominent abnormally thickened, but non-obstructing, ring B. **C.** Small sliding hiatus hernia with a Schatzki's ring, showing a bolus of bread soaked in barium sticking at the ring. The ring is located at the site of ring B at the oesophagogastric junction, with the barium-filled vestibule seen above it. (Courtesy of Dr A Chapman.)

HIATUS HERNIA, GASTRO-OESOPHAGEAL REFLUX, OESOPHAGITIS: DIFFERENTIAL DIAGNOSIS

Herniation of part of the stomach through the diaphragmatic hiatus is common. Four types of hernia have been distinguished; sliding (axial), short oesophagus, para-oesophageal and thoracic stomach.

Sliding hiatus hernia

By far the most frequent type is the sliding hiatus hernia, defined as being present when any stomach at all protrudes through the hiatus into the chest in a child, or when more than 2 cm of stomach protrudes into the chest of an adult. Thus, in the normal adult, the gastro-oesophageal junction may be situated within 2 cm of the hiatus, and the presence of a small gastric protrusion is not considered sufficient to constitute a hernia. The oesophagus is attached to the diaphragm by the phrenico-oesophageal membrane. The firmness of this attachment diminishes with advancing age, and in adults with a sliding hiatus hernia the normal elasticity is lost as the membrane is replaced by fibrous tissue, so that when the stomach 'rides up' it is not retracted.

The radiological diagnosis of a sliding hiatus hernia in an adult depends upon the demonstration on a barium swallow of at least one of the following features:

1. A pouch of stomach above the hiatus of more than 2 cm (Fig. 29.25). Large and medium-sized hernias are easily identified, whereas the detection of small hernias is often difficult.
2. Three or more gastric folds seen passing from the stomach across the hiatus (Fig. 29.26).
3. The Z-line is located above the hiatus, i.e. areae gastricae are seen above the hiatus (Fig. 29.27A).
4. A wide hiatus, measuring more than 3 cm in diameter (Fig. 29.26).
5. A sign consisting of a gastric fundal fold crossing the cardia and ending in a polypoid protuberance in the distal oesophagus (Fig. 29.27B). This appearance, known as the polyp and fold complex, is seen specifically in patients with gastro-oesophageal reflux, but the mechanism of its production is uncertain.

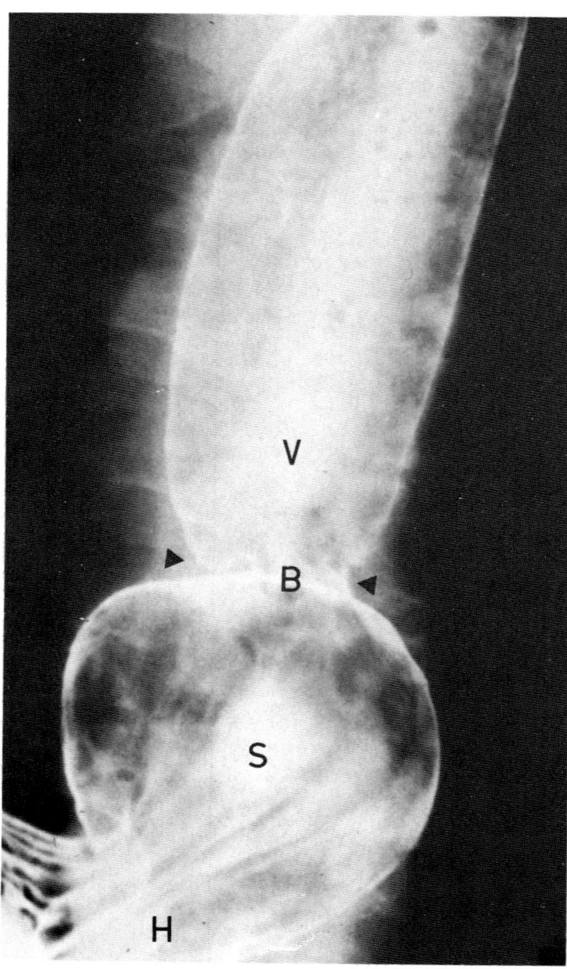

Fig. 29.25 The radiographic features of a sliding hiatus hernia. H = hiatus, more than 3 cm wide with at least three gastric folds seen extending across the hiatus. S = stomach forming the hernia. B = ring B, the oesophagogastric junction. V = vestibule. Ring A is not visible.

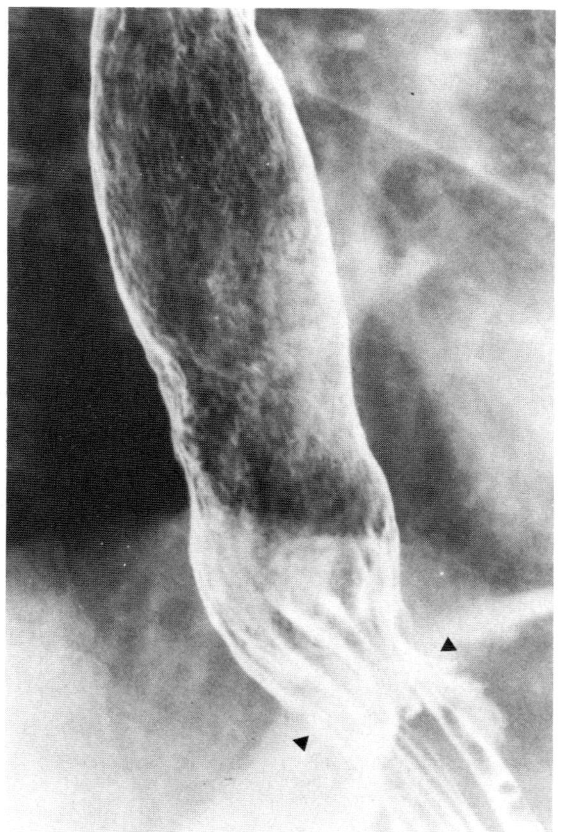

Fig. 29.26 Sliding hiatus hernia with peptic oesophagitis. The hiatus (between the arrowheads) is wide (>3 cm) and at least three gastric folds are seen extending across it. The oesophageal mucosa is coarsely granular indicating oesophagitis.

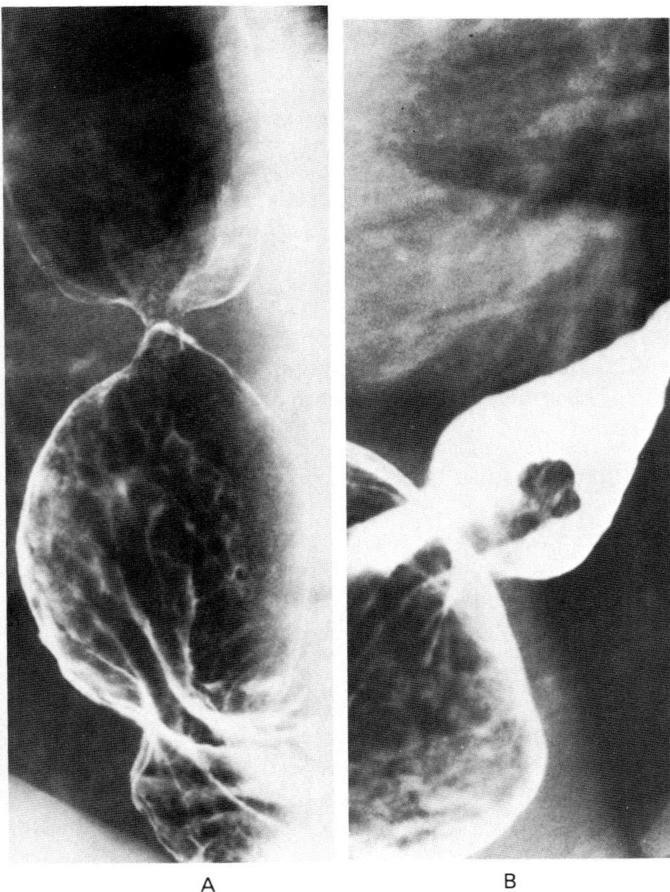

Fig. 29.27 A. Sliding hiatus hernia containing areae gastricae. Short tight peptic stricture at oesophagogastric junction. (Courtesy of Dr A Chapman.) **B.** Polyp and fold complex occurring in association with gastro-oesophageal reflux (Courtesy of Dr A. Grundy.)

Sliding hiatus hernias range in size from small pouches to very large hernias comprising all of the stomach and most of the duodenum. Small hernias usually reduce in the standing or sitting posture, and appear in the recumbent position. Movement of the stomach up and down within the hiatus may lead to the development of an ulcer on the lesser curvature. Large sliding hiatus hernias often become 'fixed' with the stomach remaining permanently in the thorax. Such hernias can be seen behind the heart on a sufficiently penetrated plain chest radiograph.

It is important for the radiologist to appreciate that small sliding hiatus hernias are often without clinical significance especially in the elderly, and that vigorous efforts to demonstrate small hernias should not be undertaken. If there is any doubt in the radiologist's mind as to whether a small hernia is present or not, he should report in the negative. In the barium examination of the lower oesophagus in patients with symptoms of reflux the detection of peptic oesophagitis is the primary concern, and more important than the demonstration of gastro-oesophageal reflux (which may occur without producing oesophagitis), or the detection of a hiatus hernia. The barium swallow should therefore be conducted with these priorities in mind.

The patient first swallows a gas-producing agent, immediately followed by a number of large mouthfuls of barium whilst standing in the frontal and right anterior oblique (RAO) positions. Exposures are made of the lower oesophagus just after each bolus of barium has passed into the stomach at a time when the oesophagus is coated with barium and distended with air. The examination is then continued with the patient in a horizontal position. Most examiners use a pillow or some comfortable compression device beneath the abdomen of the prone patient. Barium is then fed through a drinking straw and the lower end of the oesophagus is observed in both respiratory phases as the patient is rotated into various positions. There are many individual variations on this routine, but the Valsalva manoeuvre and the Trendelenburg (head down) position are no longer generally employed, nor is forcible manual compression of the upper abdomen with a gloved hand. Radiographic exposures are made at opportune moments. Whether to give a hypotonic agent, e.g. Buscopan 20 mg i.v., and at what stage in the procedure, are decisions that depend upon the preferences of the individual radiologist and the particular clinical features. Where the prime concern is the detection of oesophagitis the use of Buscopan is likely to be advantageous.

Any *hiatus hernia* of clinical importance will be shown by gentle passive means as a rounded dilatation above the hiatus which retains barium for longer than would be expected of the normal lower oesophagus. There is sometimes a prominent notch (the cardiac incisura) at the left oesophagogastric angle due to the pull of the sling fibres of the stomach, and the resulting para-oesophageal pouch mimics a para-oesophageal hernia or diverticulum (Fig. 29.23). This may incorrectly give rise to the term 'mixed' hiatus hernia because of the resemblance to a combined sliding and para-oesophageal hernia.

The supine left *anterior* oblique (LAO) position seems to be the best for demonstrating a sliding hiatus hernia and *gastro-oesophageal reflux*. Reflux is the involuntary, unconscious passage of gastric content into the oesophagus and fluoroscopic observation of this event by the radiologist is necessary for diagnosis. The flow of barium may be initiated by the patient changing position, swallowing saliva or by the 'siphonage' manoeuvre whereby the patient swallows one or two mouthfuls of water given through a straw. However, it should be remembered that taking water will compromise the subsequent performance of a double contrast examination of the stomach and duodenum. The presence of barium in the oesophagus is not sufficient to indicate reflux, because it may not have come from the stomach. The mechanism of oesophageal closure and the prevention of gastro-oesophageal reflux is complex. The acuteness of the gastro-oesophageal angle, the pressure of the right crus of the diaphragm and the tone of the lower oesophageal sphincter have all been credited with a role. The presence of a hiatus hernia undoubtedly disturbs this mechanism and reflux of gastric contents usually occurs. Reflux can also result from the presence of an indwelling oesophagogastric tube.

A comprehensive clinical history should always be the cornerstone of the diagnosis of gastro-oesophageal reflux. A barium swallow is the test most commonly used to detect reflux, but is unreliable. In a recent study radiographic reflux was demonstrated in only 58% of the most severely symptomatic patients. In another study the occurrence of radiographic reflux was noted in approximately 25% of patients who had no symptoms of reflux. Radiology alone is therefore not of great value in the diagnosis of reflux. For this reason other tests have been developed including the acid perfusion test, oesophageal manometry, the standard acid reflux test, the acid-clearance test, 24-hour pH monitoring and radioisotope studies. However, none of these tests as presently performed is entirely satisfactory and, for practical reasons, a clinical history, barium swallow and endoscopy will continue to be the basic tools of the clinician.

Oesophagitis

The significance of gastro-oesophageal reflux is the liability of the acid gastric contents to produce oesophagitis. **Reflux oesophagitis** (syn: *peptic oesophagitis*) is characterized by three abnormalities:

1. Incontinence of the cardia.
2. Frequent reflux of gastric contents into the oesophagus.
3. Inflammatory damage to the oesophageal mucosa.

A sliding hiatus hernia is often associated.

The normal mucosa of the fully distended oesophagus, as demonstrated in double contrast, looks smooth en face and in profile (Fig. 29.28A). Occasionally fine, close transverse lines are seen representing contraction of the muscularis mucosae, and an association has been reported between this appearance and reflux. In the undistended state, smooth, crisply outlined longitudinal folds are seen.

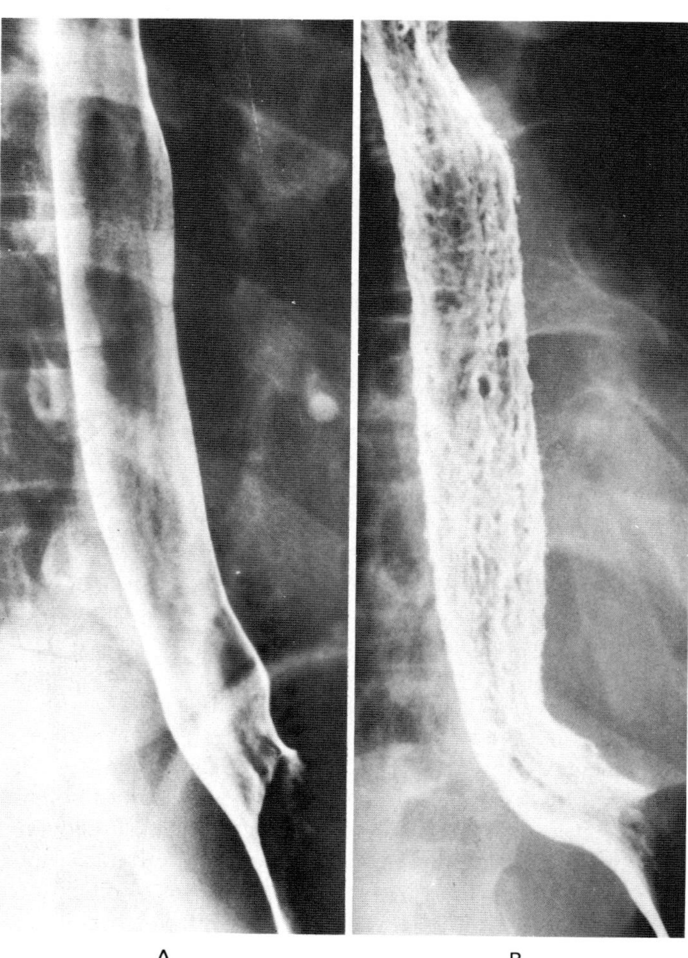

Fig. 29.28 Peptic oesophagitis. Comparison of normal mucosa (**A**) with severe ulcerative peptic oesophagitis (**B**). (Courtesy of Dr R A Lowe.)

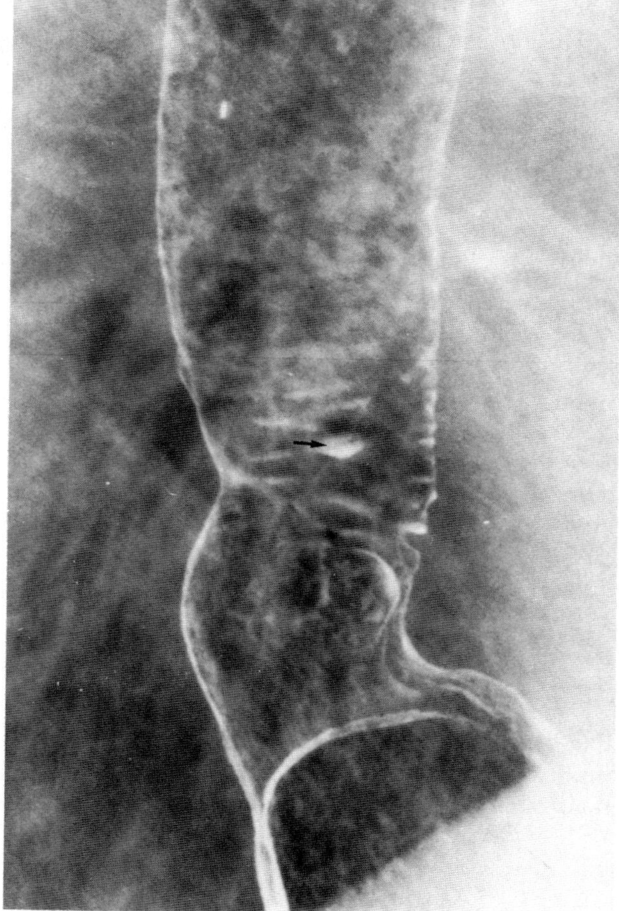

Fig. 29.29 Peptic oesophagitis associated with sliding hiatus hernia. A rounded ulcer (arrow) and linear ulcers and scars are present.

In very mild oesophagitis the only mucosal change is hyperaemia, which can be detected by endoscopy but not by radiology. However, in most cases of symptomatic oesophagitis, inflammatory changes consisting of *granular mucosa*, *ulceration* and *nodules* can be consistently demonstrated by double contrast barium examination with intravenous Buscopan (Fig. 29.28B). The normal homogenous, smooth barium coating is replaced in oesophagitis by a granular, 'smudged' or patchy appearance. Erosions are seen as multiple tiny specks of barium. Ulcers are larger and may be rounded, spicular, linear, band shaped or 'collar stud' in form. Transverse linear scars are common (Fig. 29.29). In severe disease ulceration may be accompanied by a nodular or 'cobblestone' appearance. In the uncommon proliferative form of reflux oesophagitis inflammatory polyps produce irregular intraluminal filling defects simulating carcinoma. On single contrast examination the mucosal folds are thickened and distorted by oedema, and in profile the margins of the distended oesophagus are serrated. In severe cases the folds are obliterated.

Untreated, chronic oesophagitis leads to *fibrosis* and *stricture* formation (Fig. 29.30). The differentiation of a peptic stricture from a stricture due to carcinoma of the oesophagus is an important consideration. A *peptic stricture* is normally associated with a sliding hiatus hernia and gastro-oesophageal reflux is likely to be present, but carcinoma may also be accompanied by hernia and reflux. Peptic strictures are almost always located in the oesophagus immediately above the cardia and their length is variable. The upper end is tapering and the mucosal changes of oesophagitis are usually present either in the stricture itself or

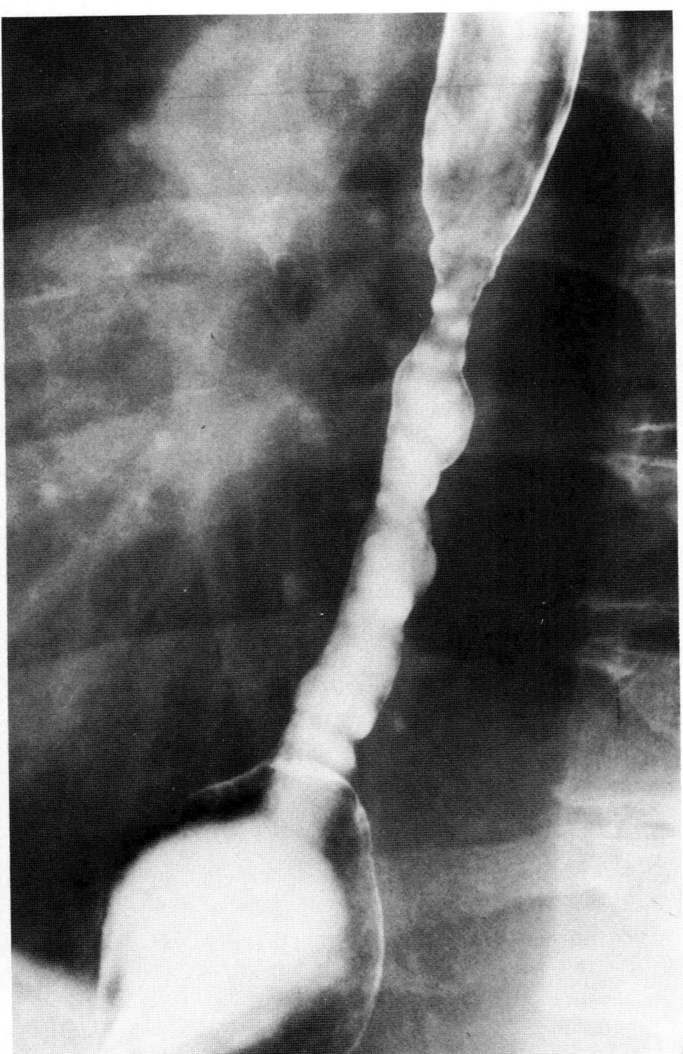

Fig. 29.30 Chronic peptic stricture. There is a sliding hiatus hernia with a long stricture of the oesophagus immediately proximal to it. The margins of the stricture have a slightly saccular appearance. The mucosa looks normal with no sign of active oesophagitis.

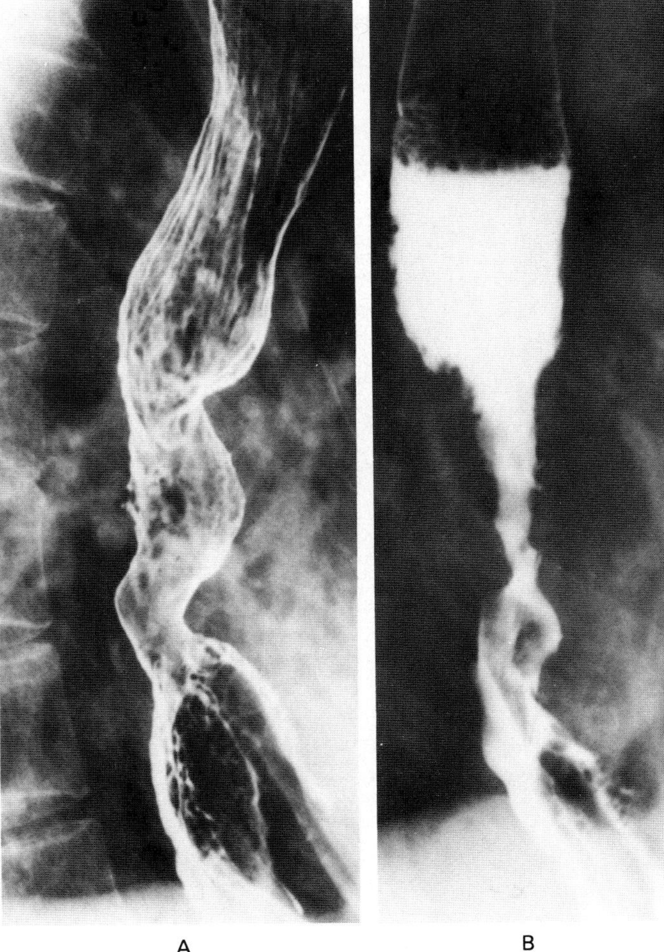

Fig. 29.31 Comparison of peptic stricture (**A**), with oesophageal carcinoma (**B**). In both cases a stricture is situated immediately above a sliding hiatus hernia. In **A** there are signs of oesophagitis in the stricture and proximal to it. The mucosa is not destroyed and the stricture merges imperceptibly with oesophagus and hernia at its ends. In **B** there are no signs of oesophagitis. The margins of the stricture and one wall of the oesophagus above the stricture are ragged, and the mucosa is destroyed.

in the oesophagus above it (Fig. 29.31A). A *carcinoma* can usually be differentiated by its shouldered ends, mucosal destruction and irregular channel with intraluminal filling defects (Fig. 29.31B). However, the distinction by radiology is sometimes extremely difficult, and in view of this many clinicians choose to perform fibre-optic endoscopy with biopsy on all oesophageal strictures, however benign they may look radiographically. Nevertheless a double contrast barium swallow with Buscopan should be performed before endoscopy in order to:

1. Confirm the presence, anatomical position and length of a stricture. Barium will pass through a tight stricture that cannot be penetrated by an endoscope, and will therefore show the whole length of the stricture and beyond.
2. Provide a reasonably accurate provisional diagnosis.
3. Indicate the degree of obstruction.
4. Show the anatomy of the stomach (useful before surgery), and the presence of other lesions such as hiatus hernia and oesophageal diverticulum (which could make endoscopy hazardous).

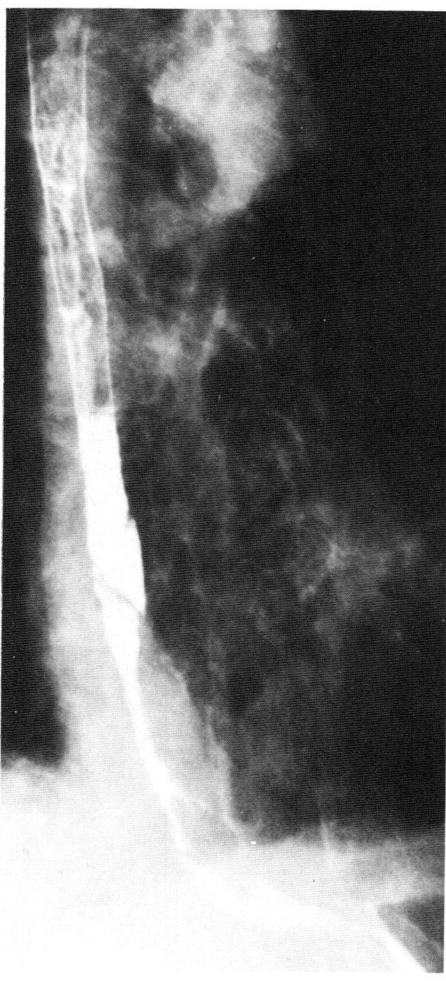

Fig. 29.32 Peptic oesophagitis with a long ragged stricture and mucosal sloughing resulting from the presence of a nasogastric tube. (Courtesy of Dr A Chapman.)

Prolonged **nasogastric intubation** produces severe peptic oesophagitis with stricture formation (Fig. 29.32). The presence of the tube renders the lower oesophageal sphincter incompetent and interferes with normal peristalsis, thus facilitating reflux. The consequent oesophagitis is especially severe when gastric surgery results in reflux of bile into the stomach and thence into the oesophagus.

Barrett's syndrome (syn: *Barrett oesophagus, columnar-lined oesophagus*) is an acquired condition characterized by progressive columnar metaplasia of the distal oesophagus due to chronic reflux oesophagitis. There is often an associated hiatus hernia. Ulceration progressing to stricture formation is common. Strictures may be long or short, and located at any level in the oesophagus, but always at the junction of squamous and columnar epithelium (Fig. 29.33A). Levine et al. (1983) have described a delicate reticular pattern in the oesophagus, which they believe to be specific to this condition (Fig. 29.33B). There is strong evidence that Barrett's syndrome is a premalignant condition associated with an increased incidence of adenocarcinoma. Barrett's syndrome is most commonly seen in middle-aged or elderly individuals, and patients may present with reflux-related symptoms or dysphagia if there is a stricture. The condition is probably more common than generally appreciated, and in one large series 10% of those with reflux oesophagitis had pathological evidence of columnar metaplasia.

Intramural pseudodiverticulosis is an uncommon condition characterized by the presence of multiple small outpouchings due to dilated mucous glands. The radiographic features are variable. In some cases, a series of flask-like pouches resembling small diverticula are seen, ranging in size up to about 0.5 cm (Fig. 29.34A). In other cases the projections are much smaller and more numerous, simulating extensive deep ulceration (Fig. 29.34B). A variable length of oesophagus is affected. Sliding hiatus hernia, stricture, secondary infection with *Candida albicans* and diabetes are common accompaniments. Most authors consider the condition to be a sequel to any type of severe oesophagitis. However, at the time of diagnosis the patient may be symptomless. The features on a barium swallow are usually permanent.

Infectious oesophagitis. Whilst peptic oesophagitis is the most frequent form, oesophagitis may also be caused by many infectious agents. The list includes moniliasis, tuberculosis, herpes simplex and other viral and bacterial organisms. Most patients who develop infectious oesophagitis are *debilitated* by malignant disease, diabetes, alcohol, renal failure or immunosuppressant, cytotoxic or steroid therapy. The most common organism infecting the oesophagus is *Candida albicans*, a yeast that causes *moniliasis*. Dysphagia is a frequent symptom, and about half the

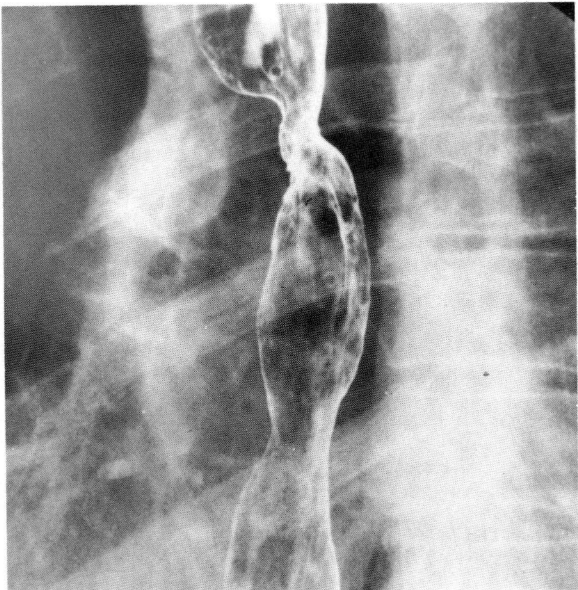

Fig. 29.33A

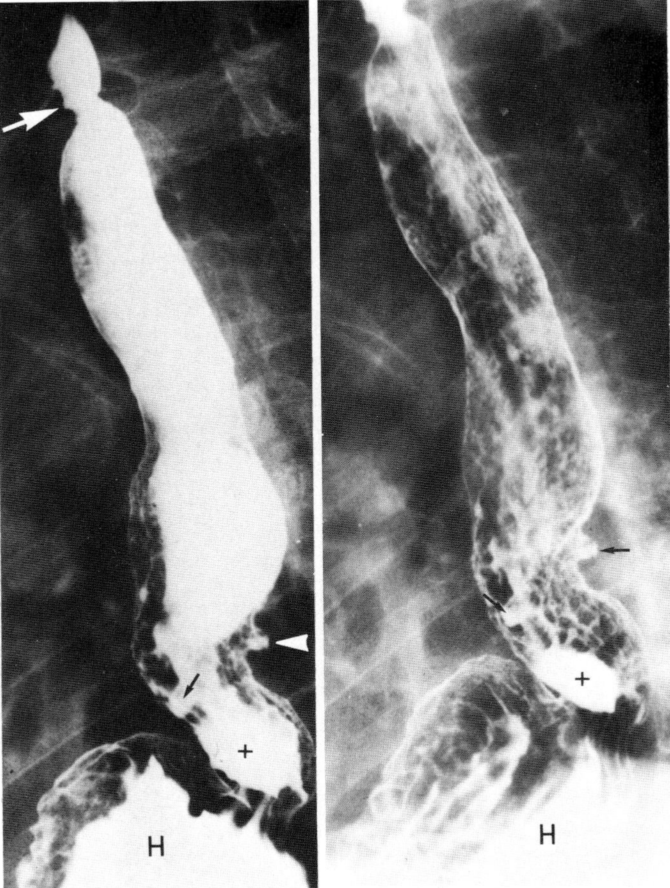

Fig. 29.33B

Fig. 29.33 Barrett's oesophagus. **A.** Barrett's oesophagus stricture situated in the proximal thoracic oesophagus. There are slight mucosal changes at the site of the stricture but elsewhere in the oesophagus the mucosa looks normal. A sliding hiatus hernia was present. **B.** The features illustrated are typical. Sliding hiatus hernia (H). Severe peptic oesophagitis with several ulcers (two are arrowed) at the lower end of the oesophagus. The collection of barium marked (+) is the result of pooling in the deformed lower oesophagus, and is not an ulcer. A large area of the mucosa has a coarse reticular appearance which is reported to be characteristic of this condition (see text). High in the oesophagus, at the junction of columnar and squamous epithelium is a short ulcerated stricture (top arrow). (Courtesy of Dr D J Lintott.)

patients have oral thrush. Barium examination usually shows extensive disease consisting of mucosal irregularity with thickened folds, nodules, 'cobblestones', plaques and ulcers which together produce a 'shaggy' appearance in profile (Fig. 29.35). Prompt clinical relief follows treatment with the fungicidal drug nystatin. Identical appearances are produced by infection with *Herpes simplex*, a self-limiting disease diagnosed by cytology. *Tuberculous* oesophagitis is uncommon and has highly variable radiographic findings. Ulceration, narrowing, skip lesions, sinuses, fistulae and mediastinal lymphadenopathy are all found. The diagnosis is made by culturing the organism.

A large number of **drugs** have been implicated in the causation of oesophagitis. The list includes slow-release potassium chloride, tetracycline and emepronium bromide. The characteristic clinical presentation is sudden dysphagia and retrosternal pain within 8 hours of ingesting the drug. Double contrast radiography shows a collection of erosions or ulcers (Fig. 29.36A) often in the region of the aortic arch. A repeat examination one week after withdrawal of the medication generally shows complete resolution.

Ingestion of *caustic agents* is another important cause of severe oesophagitis. Strong alkalis like caustic soda can produce deep coagulation necrosis within minutes, whereas necrosis from acids tends to be more superficial. The severity of damage obviously varies according to the identity, quantity and concentration of the ingested substance. Generally, long segments of the oesophagus are involved with a predisposition for sites of normal narrowing. In the acute stages a water-soluble contrast agent should be used for investigation because of the possibility of perforation. Later, if necessary, barium can be given. The oesophagus is hypotonic from the beginning, with ulceration and strictures (Fig. 29.36B) developing later. Contemporary involvement of the gastric antrum may also be present.

Oesophagitis is liable to follow *mediastinal irradiation*. Patients receiving Adriamycin (doxorubicin) or Actinomycin D are particularly susceptible to this complication of radiotherapy. Typically mild heartburn or dysphagia occur several weeks after the onset of treatment, and a barium swallow shows abnormal motility with or without mucosal oedema. Strictures are uncommon, and develop 4–8 months following completion of radiotherapy. Ulceration, pseudodiverticula and fistulae may also occur.

Other conditions may be occasionally associated with oesophagitis such as **bullous dermatosis** (e.g. *pemphigus*

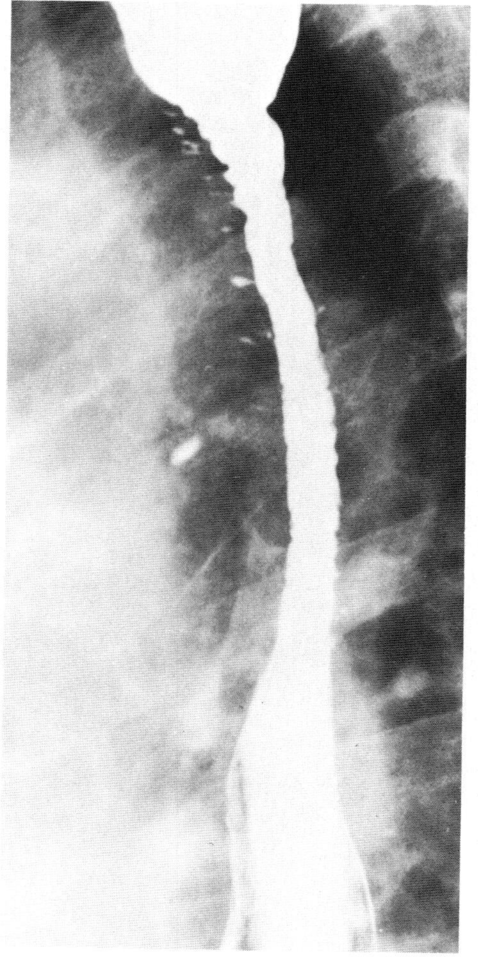

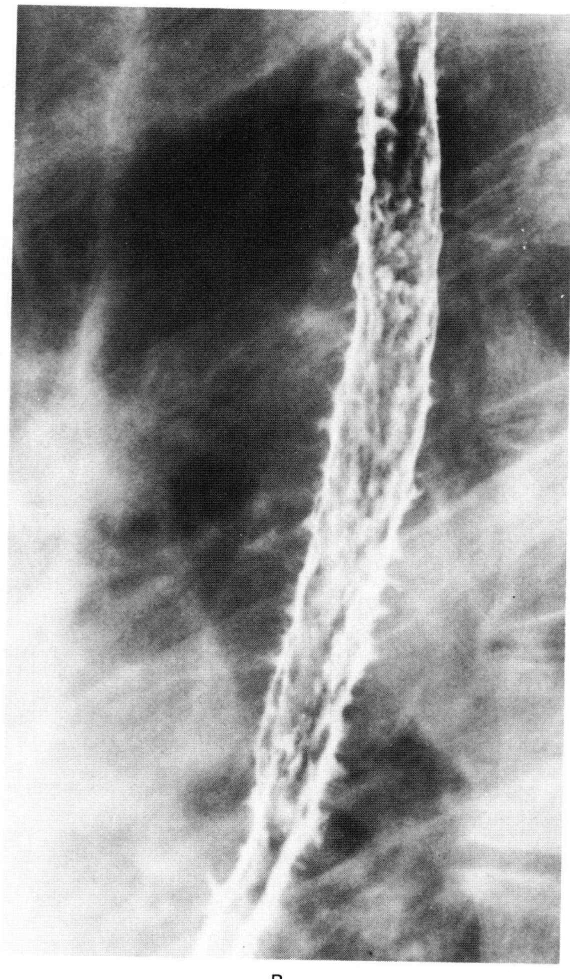

Fig. 29.34 Intramural pseudodiverticulosis. **A.** Mid oesophageal peptic stricture with small flask shaped projections **B.** Extensive involvement with pseudodiverticulosis resembling deep ulceration. An incidental finding in a patient without oesophageal symptoms. (Courtesy of Dr A Chapman.)

and *epidermolysis bullosa dystrophia*), **Behçet's disease** and **Crohn's disease**. The oesophageal lesions of the bullous dermatoses consist of vesicles, bullae and ulcers. During the acute stage bullae may produce multiple oesophageal filling defects on barium examination. Later ulceration may lead to stricture formation. In Behçet's disease ulceration and perforation have been recorded. The morphology of Crohn's oesophagitis is the same as the disease elsewhere in the intestinal tract.

Short oesophagus

The short oesophagus type of hiatus hernia (also axial) resembles the sliding variety except that the oesophagus is shortened and the cardia is situated on the summit of the herniated fundus. Some cases are congenital, but in the majority shortening is believed to be the result of reflux oesophagitis associated with a sliding hiatus hernia. Differentiation from the regular variety of sliding hiatus hernia may, therefore, be extremely difficult, and the only importance of recognizing that the oesophagus is short is the influence that this will have on surgical treatment.

Para-oesophageal hernia

The para-oesophageal (syn: rolling) hiatus hernia is much less frequent than the sliding variety. As its name implies the cardia remains beneath the diaphragm whilst the fundus herniates through the hiatus to lie alongside the lower oesophagus (Fig. 29.37). There is therefore only a slight predisposition to reflux, and the most frequent complication is anaemia from chronic bleeding. Most para-oesophageal hernias are not reducible.

Thoracic stomach

In another uncommon variety of hiatus hernia the entire stomach, or the major portion of it, lies above the diaphragm. The significance of a thoracic stomach is its liability to volvulus and respiratory embarrassment.

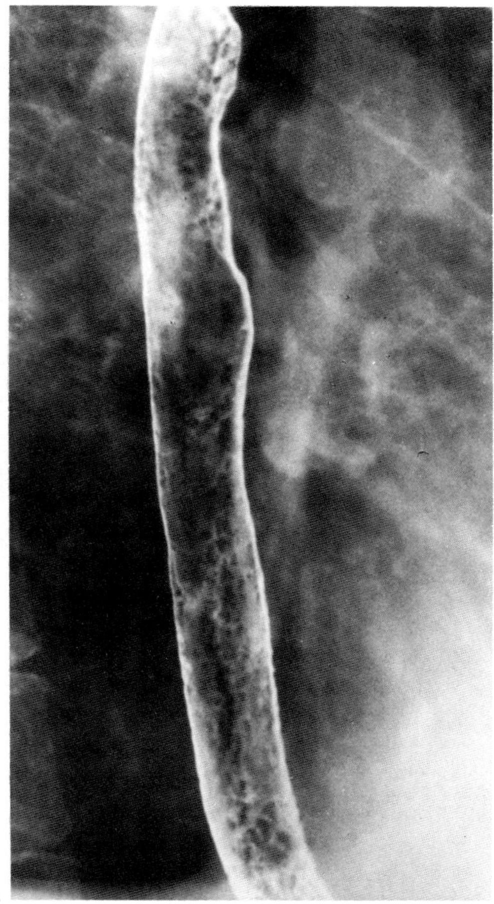

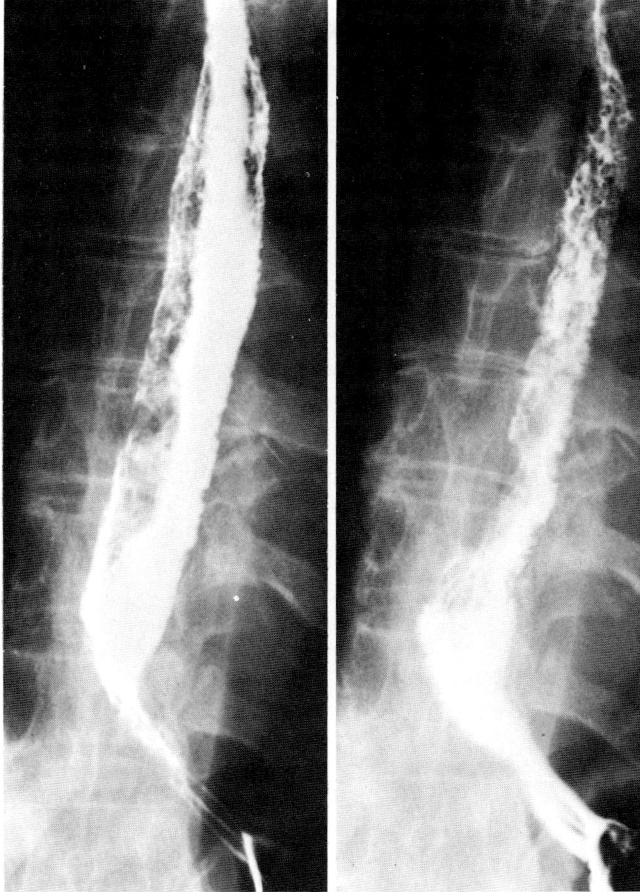

Fig. 29.35 Monilia oesophagitis. **A.** Mild infection with small plaques and patchy mucosal granularity involving the whole length of the oesophagus. (Courtesy of Drs G M Fraser and P M Earnshaw, and the Editor of *Clinical Radiology*.) **B.** Plaque-like filling defects and ulceration. These severe changes of monilia oesophagitis are in an elderly debilitated patient on antibiotics. (Courtesy of Dr S F Millward.)

Postoperative appearances

The radiologist should be familiar with the appearances following hiatus hernia repair. In the *Belsey* operation, which is designed to repair a sliding hernia and prevent reflux, the gastric fundus is fixed around the lower oesophagus for approximately two thirds of its circumference. In the *Nissen* fundoplication the gastric fundus is wrapped around both sides of the lower oesophagus and sutured together anteriorly. A barium swallow after fundoplication shows angulation and narrowing of the lower oesophagus, and a pseudotumour involving the cardia (Fig. 29.38). Knowledge of the nature of prior surgery and the typical radiographic appearance is necessary to avoid confusing the surgically fashioned soft tissue mass with a carcinoma of the cardia.

CONGENITAL DIAPHRAGMATIC HERNIA

Herniation of abdominal viscera into the thoracic cavity may occur through:

1. A normal anatomical orifice in the diaphragm (hiatus hernia, which is considered in the preceding account).
2. A congenital defect (Bochdalek and Morgagni hernia). Failure of complete closure of the diaphragm during development produces a defect through which the thoracic and abdominal cavities are in direct communication.
3. A diaphragmatic tear.

A hernia through the foramen of **Bochdalek** is a common diaphragmatic hernia in infants and may present as a respiratory emergency immediately after birth. In other instances the herniation may not be noticed until adult life. The radiographic findings depend upon the size of the defect and the contents of the hernia. The defect lies posterolaterally, and is due to incomplete closure of the pleuroperitoneal membrane. Plain radiographs of the chest (PA, penetrated PA and left lateral) show herniated gut usually on the left side, and this can be confirmed by barium studies. On the left the hernia may contain the spleen or kidney, and in the absence of herniated bowel the resulting solid opacity in the chest may be a diagnostic problem.

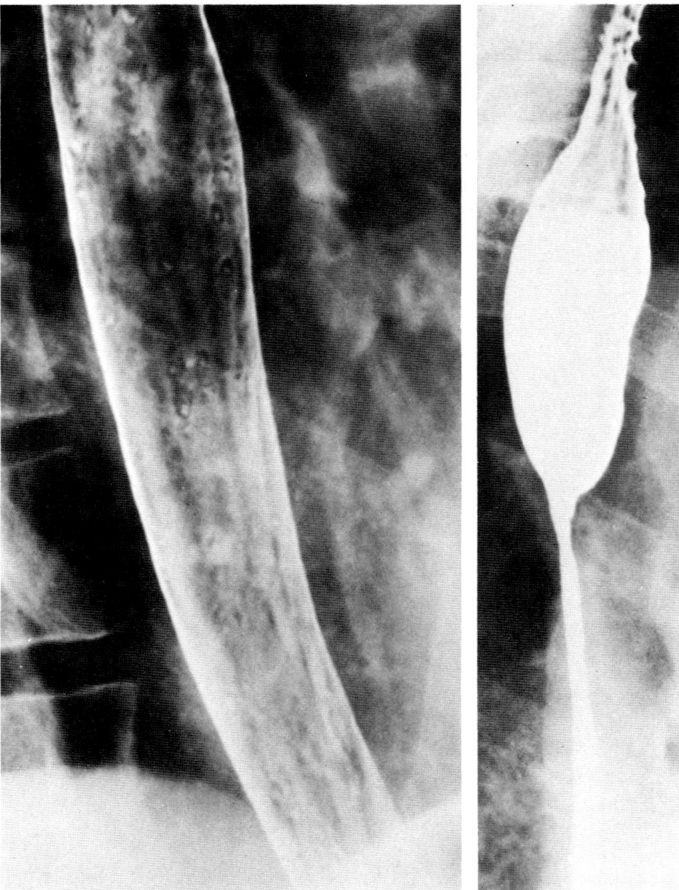

Fig. 29.36 A. Drug-induced oesophagitis. There are multiple discrete erosions resembling aphthoid ulcers. The patient was taking oral naproxen for rheumatoid arthritis. (Courtesy of Drs G M Fraser and P M Earnshaw, and the Editor of *Clinical Radiology*.) **B.** Mid oesophageal corrosive stricture resulting from swallowing lye as a child (Courtesy of Dr A. Chapman.)

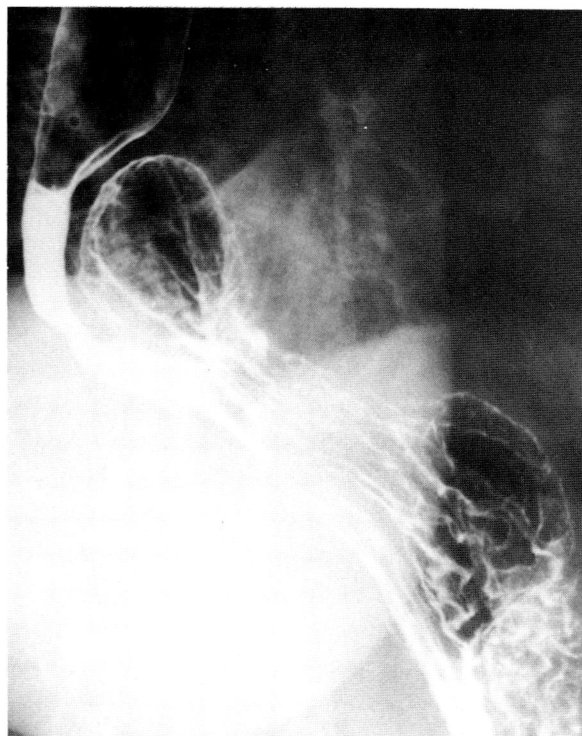

Fig. 29.37 A para-oesophageal (rolling) hiatus hernia. The cardia is in a normal position and the fundus of the stomach lies alongside the lower oesophagus above the diaphragm.

A hernia through the foramen of **Morgagni** resulting from incomplete attachment of the diaphragm to the sternum is the least common diaphragmatic hernia. Most Morgagni hernias are situated anteriorly to the left of the mid-line and are asymptomatic. The contents of the hernia may include extraperitoneal fat, omentum and transverse colon. Plain radiographs are usually sufficient for diagnosis.

CARCINOMA OF THE OESOPHAGUS

Carcinoma is the most common tumour of the oesophagus. There are wide geographical variations in its incidence. The two most important causes in Great Britain are alcohol and tobacco, which may account for as many as 90% of cases. Most patients present over the age of 60 years with dysphagia and weight loss. The vast majority of tumours are *squamous carcinomas*, which are most frequent in the lower two thirds of the oesophagus. The remainder are

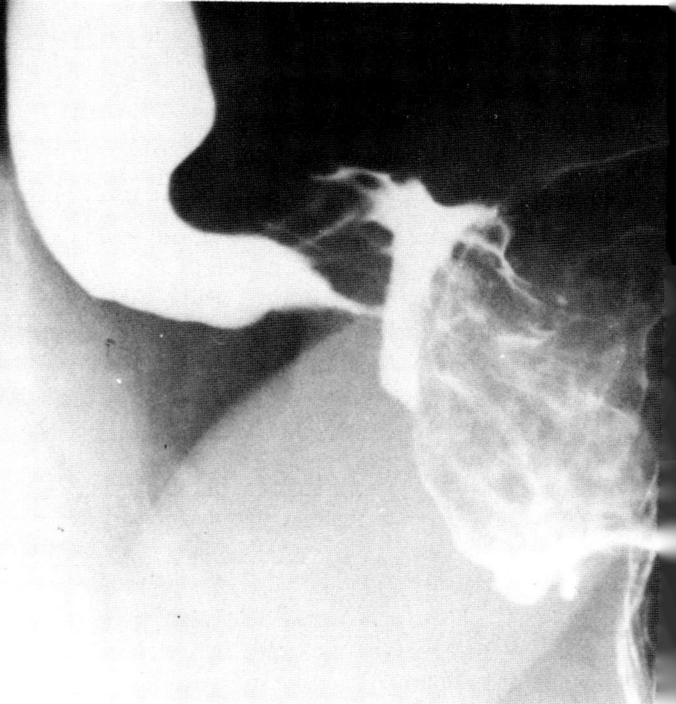

Fig. 29.38 Post-fundoplication pseudotumour. There is narrowing and deformity of the cardia with a filling defect in the fundus of the stomach. Unlike a carcinoma the mass appears to be composed of mucosal folds.

adenocarcinomas arising at the lower end of the oesophagus from gastric epithelium. Prognosis is generally poor.

Oesophageal carcinoma presents a wide variety of morphological appearances on barium swallow (Figs 29.39, 29.40 and 29.41). Evaluation of large carcinomas is accomplished as readily by single contrast examination as double contrast. Most small tumours are shown better on double contrast. Early lesions are detected as an area of mucosal irregularity, or a small plaque, nodule, polyp or ulcer (Fig. 29.39). These may be an incidental finding in patients with symptoms arising from some other gastrointestinal condition. Pathologists are now able to recognize precancerous lesions in the oesophageal mucosa comparable to the dysplasia and carcinoma *in situ* that are found in the cervix uteri. Whether it will be possible for these changes to be detected radiographically has yet to be determined, but it seems unlikely. Most advanced lesions are strictures with abrupt shouldered ends, mucosal destruction and intraluminal filling defects (Fig. 29.40A). Ulceration and necrosis often produce an irregular, ragged channel (Fig. 29.40B). Obstruction is common. Other advanced lesions are predominantly polypoid and proliferative, with a large irregular intraluminal mass (Fig. 29.41). Occasionally varicoid tumours simulate varices (Fig. 29.46). Infrequently a carcinoma of the oesophagus presents as a smooth fusiform stricture with tapered ends resembling a peptic or caustic stricture.

Carcinoma at different sites in the oesophagus often shows special features. For example a tumour at the distal end of the oesophagus can produce an appearance simulating achalasia (Fig. 29.20C). Therefore if a person over the age of 50 years presents with apparent achalasia, carcinoma should be suspected even if oesophagoscopy and biopsy are negative. Postcricoid carcinoma occurs predominantly in females, and is sometimes associated with the Plummer-Vinson syndrome (Fig. 29.13). A soft tissue mass may be visible in the neck on a lateral radiograph. Aspiration of ingested material into the lungs is liable to occur. With tumours of the middle third of the oesophagus sinuses often develop in the late stages, and there may be fistulation to the tracheobronchial tree. A chest radiograph may show a mediastinal mass, aspiration pneumonia or pulmonary and bone metastases.

Radiology has an important role in the selection of patients for palliative intubation, surgical resection or radiotherapy. The great majority of malignant tumours of

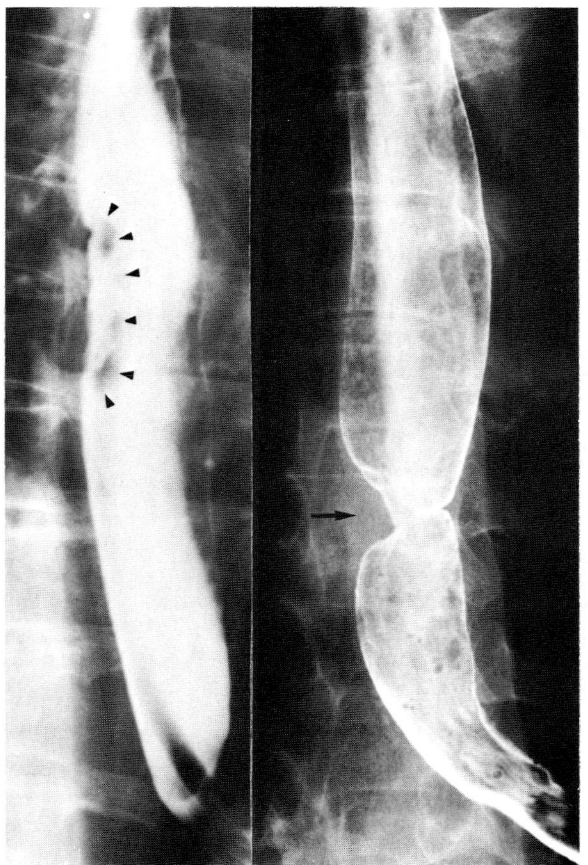

Fig. 29.39 Squamous carcinoma of the oesophagus. **A.** Shallow ulcer with tumour rim. **B.** Small filling defect resembling an intramural lesion. (Courtesy of Dr D A Ward.)

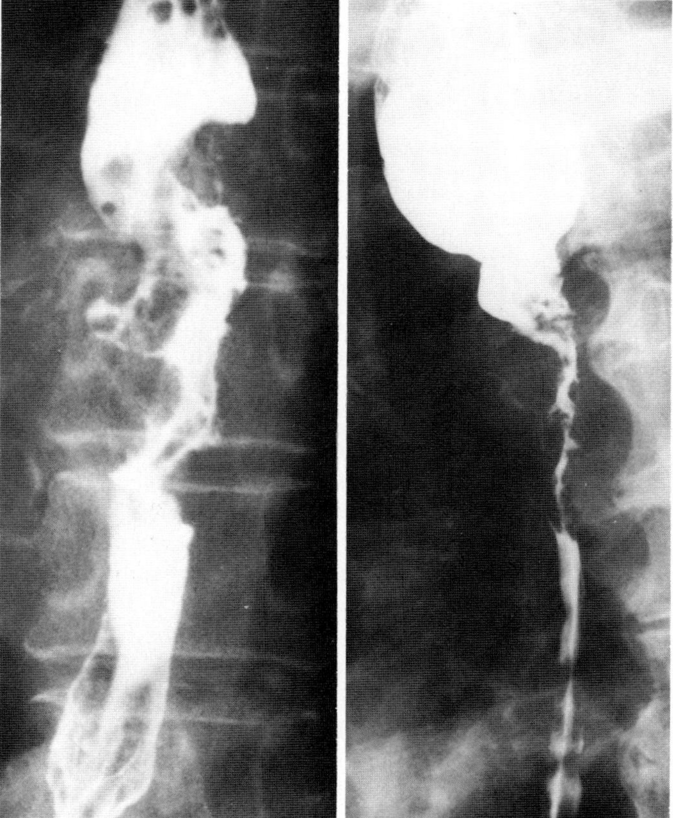

Fig. 29.40 Squamous carcinoma of the oesophagus. Advanced lesions. **A.** Stricture with mucosal destruction, irregular intraluminal filling defects, and 'shouldering'. **B.** Tight irregular stricture which is producing considerable obstruction.

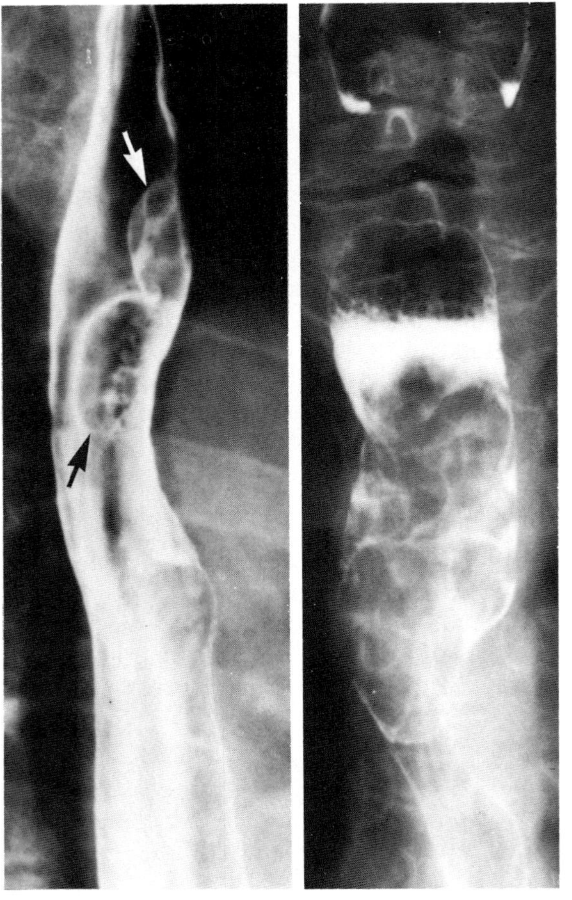

Fig. 29.41 Squamous carcinoma of the mid-oesophagus. **A.** Two tumour nodules with surface ulceration. (Courtesy of Dr R Edwards.) **B.** An irregular polypoidal intraluminal filling defect which is producing obstruction.

the oesophagus are squamous-cell carcinomas. Their anatomical position has an important influence on treatment and prognosis. The more distal the tumour the better the prognosis, because distal tumours are less often inoperable and are easier to resect. From a practical viewpoint *tumour size* is the most important prognostic indicator and determinant of operability. 50% of oesophageal carcinomas less than 5 cm in length already have lymph node metastases, while 90% of those longer than 5 cm have metastases. Therefore 5 cm is the upper limit with a realistic prospect of cure. Consequently the role of the barium swallow is to identify, locate and define the tumour.

To produce maximum information it is necessary to demonstrate the whole length of the tumour. The double contrast technique using a hypotonic agent such as Buscopan intravenously is often particularly helpful in producing distension of the normal oesophagus (or gastric fundus) on either side of the lesion, thus defining the full macroscopic extent of the abnormality. Prognosis is also dependent upon *histology*, and in general adenocarcinomas have a worse prognosis than squamous-cell tumours. A tumour found to be involving the stomach around the cardia as well as the lower oesophagus is almost certainly an adenocarcinoma arising either in the stomach, or in the oesophagus from an area of gastric metaplasia (Fig. 29.42).

The usual sequence of investigation of patients with suspected oesophageal carcinoma is barium swallow, chest

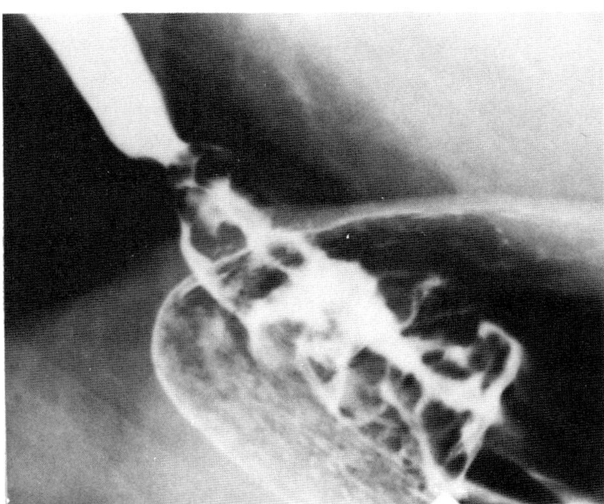

Fig. 29.42 Adenocarcinoma of the fundus of the stomach extending proximally to involve the lower oesophagus. Irregular, nodular, intraluminal filling defects are present.

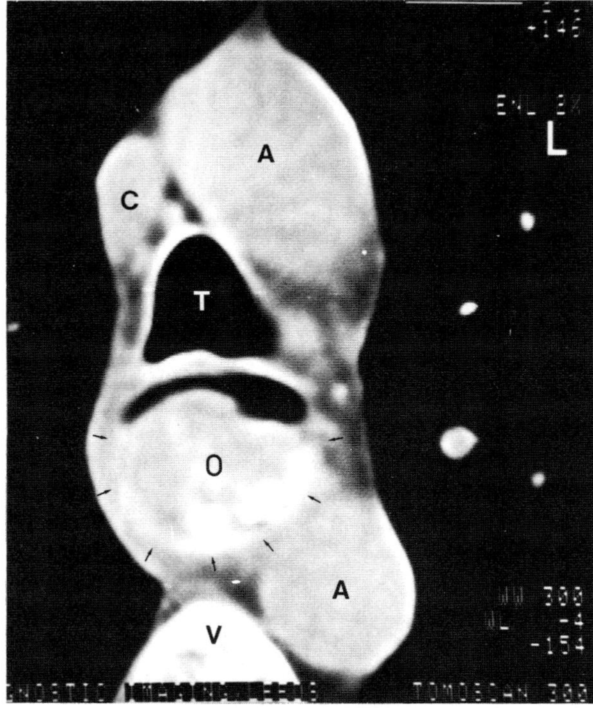

Fig. 29.43 Carcinoma of the oesophagus investigated by CT. The tumour (arrows) has been demonstrated within the oesophageal lumen. There is no evidence of any extension into the mediastinum. This information is useful when considering possible treatment.
V = vertebra, A = aorta, T = trachea, C = superior vena cava,
O = oesophageal tumour. (Courtesy of Dr P J Robinson.)

radiography, oesophagoscopy with biopsy, and CT. *Computed tomography* is a useful method for staging carcinoma of the oesophagus and cardia and the extent of extraoesophageal tumour infiltration can be accurately defined (Fig. 29.43). This information determines whether surgical or conservative treatment is the most appropriate, and allows better planning for surgical or radiation therapy. *Endoluminal ultrasonic scanning* can be used to evaluate the degree of tumour infiltration in the muscular wall and surrounding tissues. With further technical developments this could become a valuable additional diagnostic tool in the evaluation of oesophageal tumours.

For the minority who are considered suitable for resection many methods have been employed to bridge the gap after oesophagectomy, with jejunum, stomach and colon most frequently used. Radiological examination with a water-soluble contrast agent is useful for the investigation of suspected leaks or obstruction at an anastomosis during the early postoperative period. The majority of patients are unsuitable for curative surgery and temporary palliation may be provided by radiotherapy, or intubation when dysphagia becomes a problem. Oesophageal tubes of the Celestin, Atkinson or Livingstone type are often used to re-establish a clear passage from the proximal oesophagus to the stomach in malignant stricture. The placement of an oesophageal tube can be conveniently accomplished under fluoroscopic control. Complications are common and related either to operative technique or to the physical presence of the tube within the stricture. Water-soluble contrast examination shows the tube's position and its patency, and will demonstrate a perforation.

MISCELLANEOUS OESOPHAGEAL TUMOURS: CYSTS: VARICES

Leiomyoma is the most common benign tumour of the oesophagus, generally occurring as a solitary mass lesion in the lower third of the oesophagus. Barium swallow examination demonstrates a smooth, broad-based filling defect bulging into the oesophageal lumen, with intact mucosa over its surface (Fig. 29.44). A large extrinsic soft tissue mass component, sometimes containing calcification, is often present. Rare morphological varieties include a lobulated or pedunculated intraluminal lesion, an annular form and multiple tumours. Malignant potential is negligible. Other benign submucosal neoplasms such as *neurofibroma*, *fibroma* and *lipoma* are extremely rare.

Many different non-neoplastic mass lesions have been found in the oesophagus.

Fibrovascular polyps are of mixed histology and are therefore classified by some pathologists as hamartomas. They generally develop in the upper third of the oesophagus, are often quite large and pedunculated, and frequently produce dysphagia and bleeding.

Inflammatory oesophageal polyps (composed of granulation and fibrous tissue) are a component of the proliferative form of reflux peptic oesophagitis. Oesophagoscopy with biopsy is usually necessary to distinguish inflammatory polyps from carcinoma.

Several varieties of cystic lesion occur in the oesophagus.

Retention cysts or mucoceles are acquired and caused by ductal obstruction of an oesophageal mucous gland. They are commonly solitary but may be multiple, with a tendency to occur in the lower oesophagus. Radiographically a retention cyst resembles a small leiomyoma.

Oesophageal duplication is a rare congenital anomaly. About two thirds present in childhood, and the remainder are usually an incidental finding in adults. Most duplications are segmental and located in the lower posterior mediastinum. Two types occur, *intramural cysts* arising from persistent vacuoles, and *neuroenteric cysts* derived from the notochord. The latter are commonly associated with cervical and thoracic spinal abnormalities. Plain radiographs of the chest often show an oesophageal duplication as a posterior mediastinal mass. On barium swallow the features are those of an extrinsic or intramural mass and resemble leiomyoma. Rarely, when the whole oesophagus is involved, the duplication may communicate to produce a 'double-barrel' oesophagus.

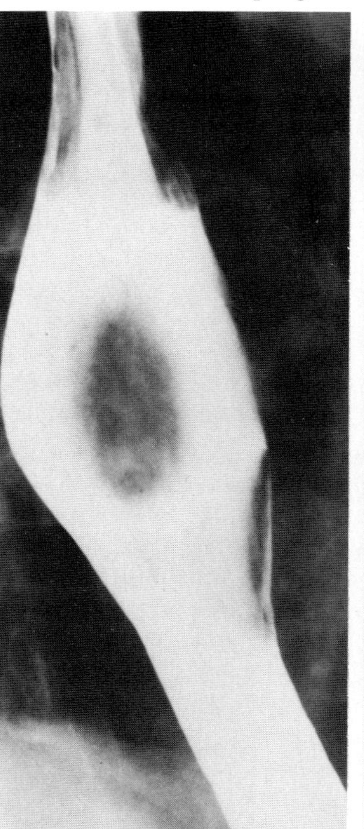

A

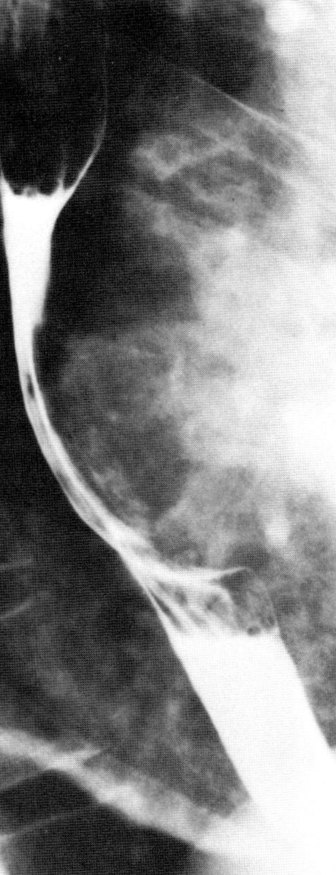

B

Fig. 29.44 A. and **B.** Leiomyoma of the oesophagus. Two views showing features typical of an intramural or extrinsic lesion. There is a broad-based filling defect bulging into the lumen and displacing the oesophagus. (Courtesy of Dr A Chapman.)

Oesophageal varices comprising dilated submucosal veins in the lower oesophagus occur chiefly as a consequence of portal hypertension in cirrhosis of the liver. Such varices result from increased collateral blood flow, via the azygos vein, between the intra-abdominal portal venous system and the intrathoracic superior vena cava.

The demonstration of varices by barium swallow is highly dependent upon technique. The following factors are important:

1. The detection rate is increased by the administration of an anticholinergic agent such as Buscopan 20 mg i.v. immediately beforehand.
2. Fairly thick or high density barium should be used. The administration of a gas-producing agent is optional.
3. Multiple spot films of the oesophagus should be taken:
   a. in various projections
   b. with the patient in various positions, e.g. supine, prone, erect, 45° semirecumbent
   c. in different phases of respiration and with the Valsalva or Mueller manoeuvre.

   No single position or manoeuvre gives uniformly superior results, hence the use of a full permutation.
4. Exposures should be made with the oesophagus slightly underdistended as it collapses down following the passage of a barium bolus. Overfilling of the oesophagus with barium or gas produces distension which may obliterate the varices.

Using the technique described, a detection rate of approximately 90% can be expected. It is worth remembering that while varices can be diagnosed on a single film they cannot be excluded on any number of films.

The appearance of varices is characteristic. Beaded or serpiginous translucent filling defects are seen *en face* resembling earthworms lying in the lumen of the oesophagus (Fig. 29.45). In profile varices may appear as a line of nodular or scalloped filling defects. Oesophageal varices seldom cause any symptoms other than upper gastrointestinal bleeding which may be torrential. The demonstration of varices in a patient with haematemesis does not necessarily establish the origin of bleeding, because about a third of such patients bleed from another cause such as a peptic ulcer. Endoscopy or arteriography may determine the site of bleeding.

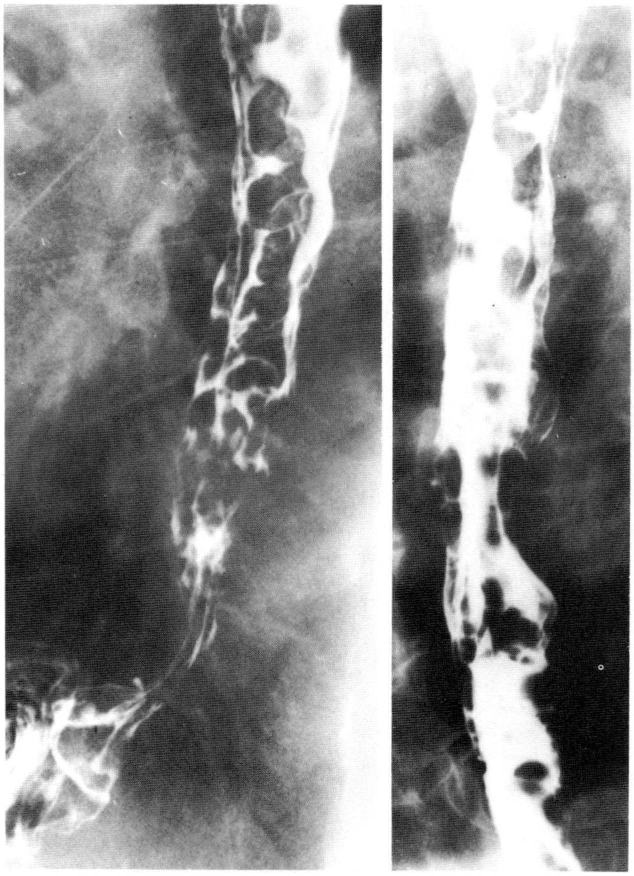

Fig. 29.45 Oesophageal varices. Typical worm-like filling defects. **A.** Non-distended oesophagus following passage of barium. **B.** Same case with barium.

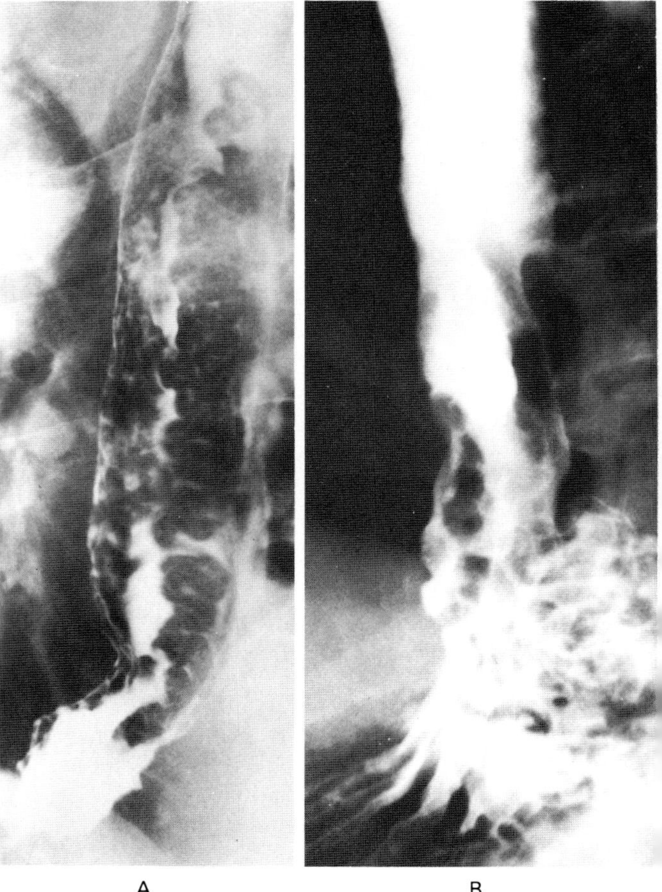

Fig. 29.46 Carcinoma resembling oesophageal varices. **A.** Varices seen as filling defects resembling thickened mucosal folds with erosions. **B.** Adenocarcinoma involving the lower end of the oesophagus with filling defects resembling varices. (Courtesy of Dr H Irving.)

Several other conditions, notably oesophagitis and carcinoma, can simulate the radiographic appearance of oesophageal varices. Clinical factors are usually helpful in diagnosis. Oesophagoscopy may be necessary in doubtful cases. In practice, the main problem is in deciding whether varices are present or not. In most cases, when filling defects are shown, the appearances are sufficiently characteristic to enable a confident diagnosis of varices to be made. In *oesophagitis* there is usually a mucosal abnormality in addition to thickened folds, and a sliding hiatus hernia with gastro-oesophageal reflux is invariably present. The varicoid form of oesophageal *carcinoma* is characterized by fixed thickened mucosal folds, with rigidity and loss of peristalsis of the affected area (Fig. 29.46). Rarely *lymphoma* presents as a submucosal tumour with thickened nodular folds. Other evidence of lymphoma is commonly present elsewhere in the body.

EXTRINSIC LESIONS AFFECTING THE OESOPHAGUS

The oesophagus traverses the posterior part of the middle mediastinum, and is therefore closely related in places to the aorta and its branches, the tracheobronchial tree, the heart, the lungs and lymph nodes. Benign neoplasms of adjacent organs, lymph nodes and vascular anomalies tend to displace or impress the oesophagus, whereas malignant tumours and inflammatory conditions such as mediastinal tuberculosis may also involve and invade it.

There are two normal impressions on the left anterolateral aspect of the thoracic oesophagus which are seen best in the RAO view due respectively to the *aortic arch* and the *left main bronchus*. A wide variety of vascular anomalies of the aorta and its major branches, and of the pulmonary vessels, can also cause extrinsic impressions on the barium-filled oesophagus.

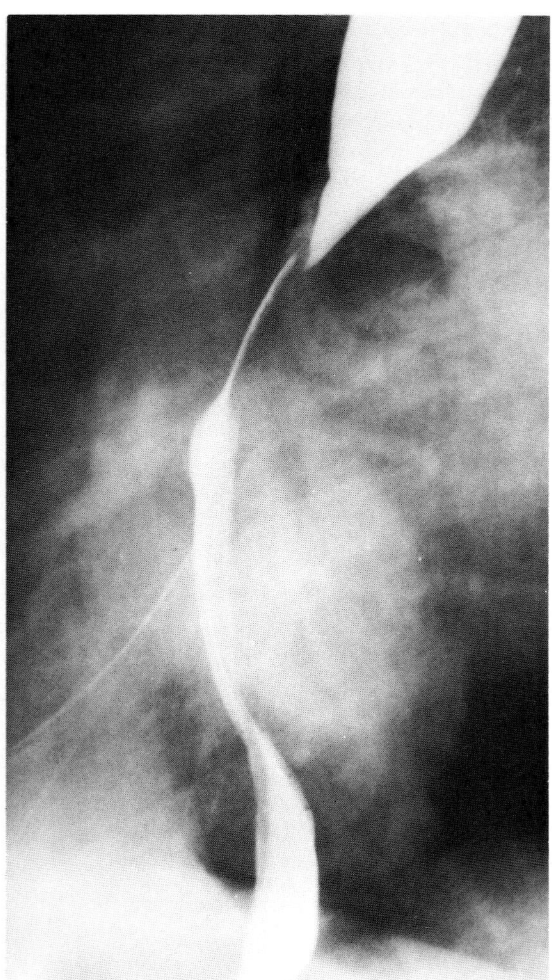

Fig. 29.47 Oesophageal displacement by an extrinsic mass: an atheromatous aneurysm of the aorta. Lateral view showing oesophagus narrowed and displaced anteriorly by the aneurysm.

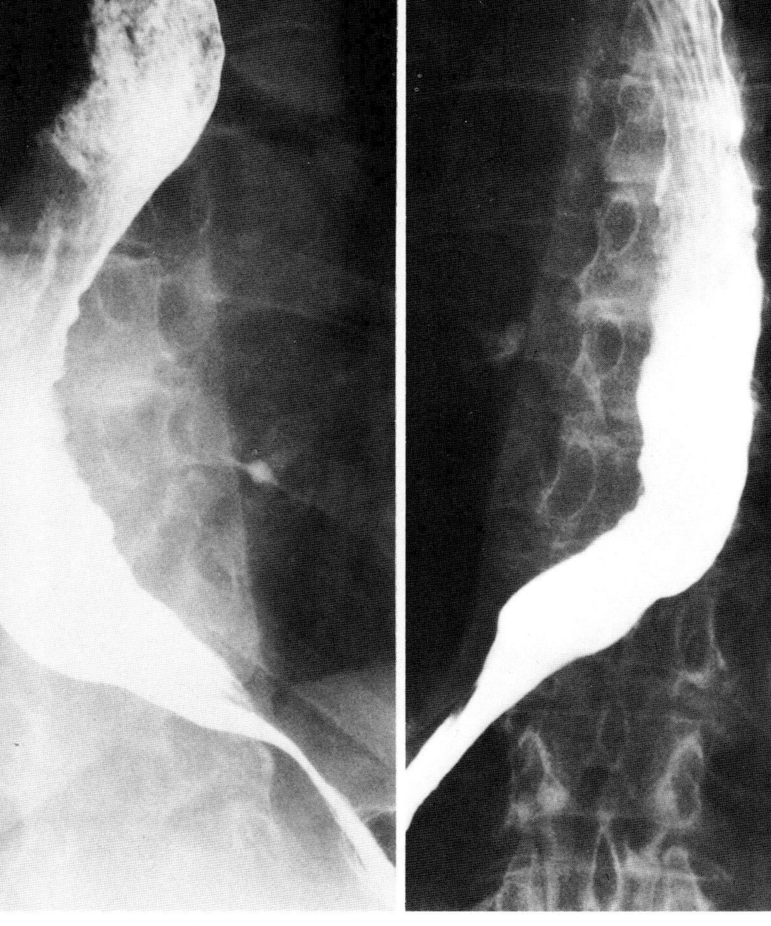

Fig. 29.48 Lower oesophageal obstruction produced by compression from an atheromatous aorta. **A.** Erect. Obstruction with tapered lower end of the oesophagus (simulating achalasia). **B.** Prone. Obstruction relieved. (Courtesy of Dr A Chapman.)

The most common aortic anomaly is a *right-sided aortic arch* and descending aorta. The oesophagus is indented on its right side by the aortic knuckle and the usual characteristic left aortic arch impression is absent. The left subclavian artery may impress the oesophagus posteriorly as it passes behind it. In *coarctation of the aorta* a reversed three impression may be produced on the left side of the oesophagus by the prestenotic and poststenotic dilatation.

Aneurysms of the aortic arch and descending aorta frequently give rise to dysphagia and cause considerable localized displacement of the oesophagus (Fig. 29.47). As the aorta becomes *atheromatous* it assumes a tortuous course and displaces the lower end of the oesophagus anteriorly and to the side. Transient intermittent obstruction may occur, sufficient on rare occasions to produce dysphagia. Fluoroscopy of the barium-filled oesophagus shows the characteristic transmitted pulsations, and obstruction in the erect and supine positions may be seen to be relieved by turning the patient prone (Fig. 29.48).

The most common non-aortic vascular impression on the oesophagus is an *aberrant right subclavian artery*. This is usually an incidental finding, but occasionally it produces dysphagia. The aberrant vessel arises from the aortic arch distal to the origin of the left subclavian artery, and passes upwards and to the right behind the oesophagus giving rise to a characteristic smooth, oblique indentation on the posterior wall of the barium-filled oesophagus (Fig. 29.49).

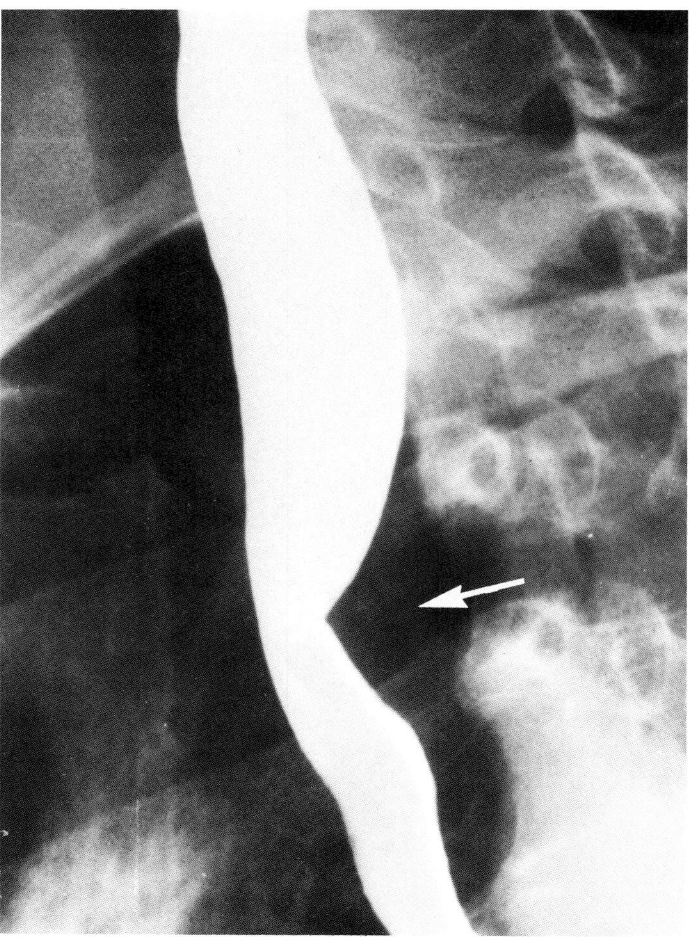

Fig. 29.49 Aberrant right subclavian artery producing characteristic extrinsic defect in the oesophagus just above the level of the aortic arch. Left anterior oblique view.

The *left atrium* is in direct contact with the anterior aspect of the oesophagus. Therefore enlargement of this chamber from whatever cause produces a characteristic anterior impression and posterior displacement of the barium-filled oesophagus below the carina. This is best seen with the patient in the lateral or RAO projections. There is also some displacement of the oesophagus to the right. Enlargement of the *left ventricle* produces a similar indentation but at a lower level. An enlarged left atrium can cause partial obstruction to a bolus of food or tablet, and cases have been recorded of tablets (usually containing potassium chloride) lodging in the oesophagus and giving rise to ulceration and stricture formation.

Displacement of the middle third of the oesophagus by a mediastinal mass is best recognized on frontal and lateral views of the barium-filled oesophagus taken with the patient recumbent. The most frequent cause is *mediastinal lymphadenopathy*, particularly enlarged subcarinal nodes, from lymphoma, metastases from carcinoma of the bronchus or infection (Fig. 29.50). Extension of malignancy or infection such as tuberculosis may involve the oesophagus to produce a stricture resembling a primary carcinoma. Other masses in the middle or posterior mediastinum that indent the oesophagus include primary tumours and cysts of the mediastinum, abscess and haematoma.

Enlargement of the *thyroid gland* frequently displaces the upper oesophagus and trachea to one side, and produces narrowing. A large *parathyroid tumour* also causes a lateral indentation in the barium-filled oesophagus.

Shift of the mediastinum from whatever cause displaces the oesophagus accordingly. Fibrosis of a lung apex resulting from tuberculosis will draw the oesophagus towards it.

A RADIOLOGICAL APPROACH TO THE DIFFERENTIAL DIAGNOSIS OF OESOPHAGEAL STRICTURES

For accurate diagnosis of oesophageal strictures the following procedure should be followed:

1. A full clinical history is taken. The length and nature of symptoms, such as dysphagia, heartburn and weight loss, are important. Some histories are diagnostic, e.g. swallowing a piece of bone, drinking a corrosive substance or recent radiotherapy. A physical examination is also necessary.

2. Plain radiographs of the chest (PA, penetrated PA and lateral) are taken to show evidence of achalasia mediastinal mass or secondary lung changes.

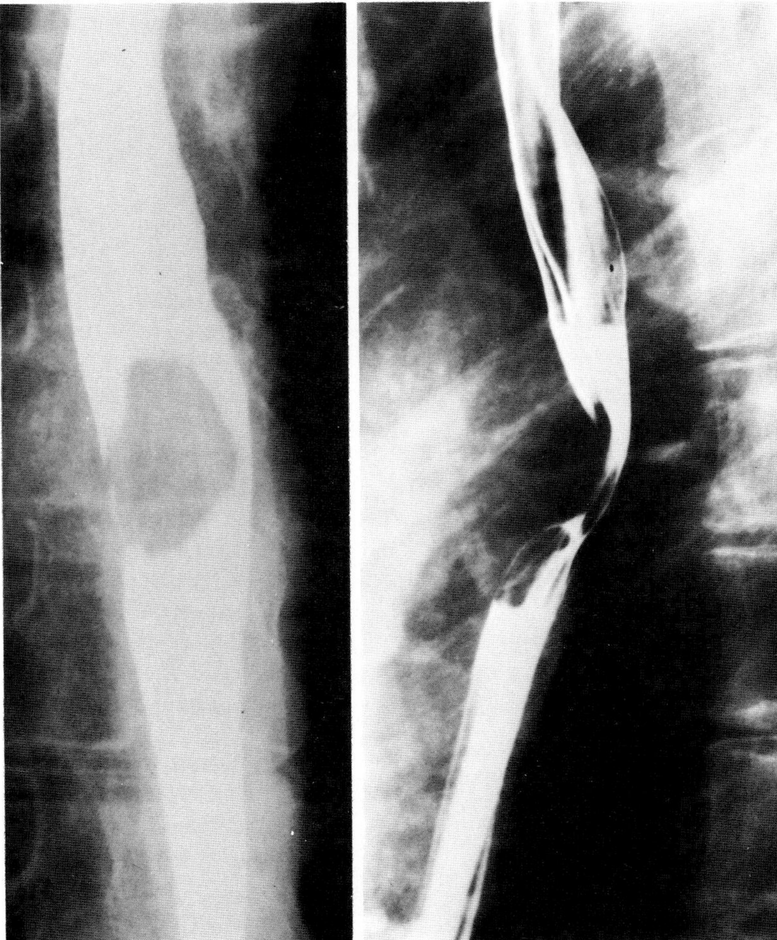

Fig. 29.50 Extrinsic mass involving the thoracic oesophagus. Frontal and lateral views demonstrate an anterior impression. The preoperative radiological diagnosis was leiomyoma (see Fig. 29.44). At surgery an enlarged tuberculous mediastinal lymph node was found to be adherent to the oesophagus.

3. A properly conducted barium examination of the whole length of the oesophagus and of the stomach is performed, and the following radiographic information about the stricture is obtained: its site, length, shape (is it intrinsic or extrinsic?), state of the mucosa in its body (is it present, thickened, ulcerated or destroyed?), presence or absence of intraluminal filling defects, shape of the ends (tapered or shouldered?) and the degree of obstruction. Any abnormality in the remainder of the oesophagus and stomach is detected and noted, and especially the presence or absence of a sliding hiatus hernia, gastro-oesophageal reflux or motility disorder.

4. Judging from the information obtained strictures are placed into one of the following five groups.

a. primary oesophageal carcinoma
b. peptic stricture
c. an extrinsic lesion
d. some other characteristic pathology
e. diagnosis still uncertain.

The majority of cases will have the characteristic features of an oesophageal carcinoma or peptic stricture. For these oesophagoscopy and biopsy is usually advisable to confirm the radiological diagnosis, and determine histology. If necessary, extrinsic lesions can be examined further by CT or angiography. When the clinical data and radiographic appearances are characteristic of a particular condition further investigation and management is dependent upon its nature. For those few cases where the diagnosis remains in doubt oesophagoscopy and biopsy will usually be conclusive, but a very small residue will defy diagnosis.

FOREIGN BODIES AND INJURY

Many sorts of foreign bodies are swallowed by young children, psychiatric patients and normal adults. Most pass through the alimentary tract without lodging, but sharp objects such as *open safety pins* may arrest in the oesophagus. Metallic or dense foreign bodies are obvious on plain radiography. Non-opaque foreign bodies can be demonstrated by swallowing a small quantity of barium.

The most common foreign body encountered in adults is an unchewed *meat bolus* arrested at a site of anatomical or pathological narrowing. Complete obstruction by an

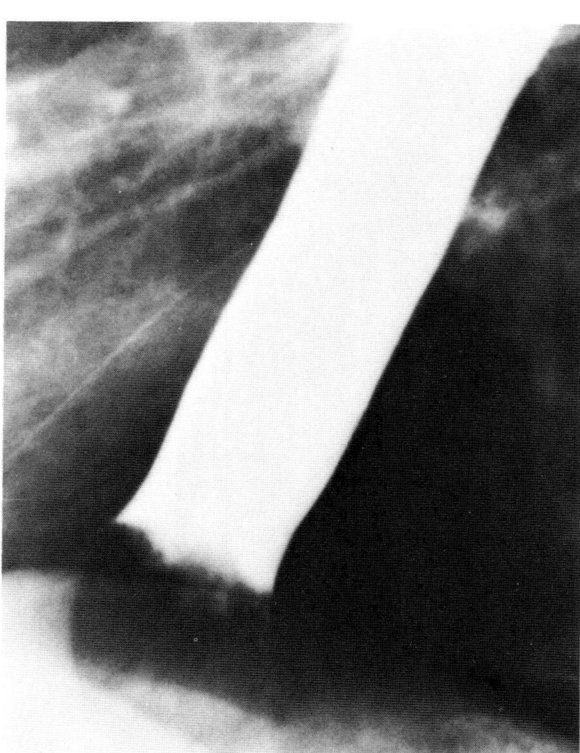

Fig. 29.51 Lower oesophageal obstruction produced by impaction of a foreign body just above the cardia. A large meat bolus was removed.

Fig. 29.52 Perforation of the oesophagus demonstrated with Gastrografin. **A**. Localized leak resulting from endoscopic trauma. (Courtesy of Dr G J S Parkin.) **B**. Penetrated chest radiograph taken with a horizontal beam, with the patient in the decubitus right side down position after swallowing Gastrografin. Endoscopic perforation resulting in a mediastinal abscess (large arrow), which communicates with a large pleural fluid collection (small arrows). Some Gastrografin is also seen in the fundus of the stomach. (Courtesy of Dr G J S Parkin.)

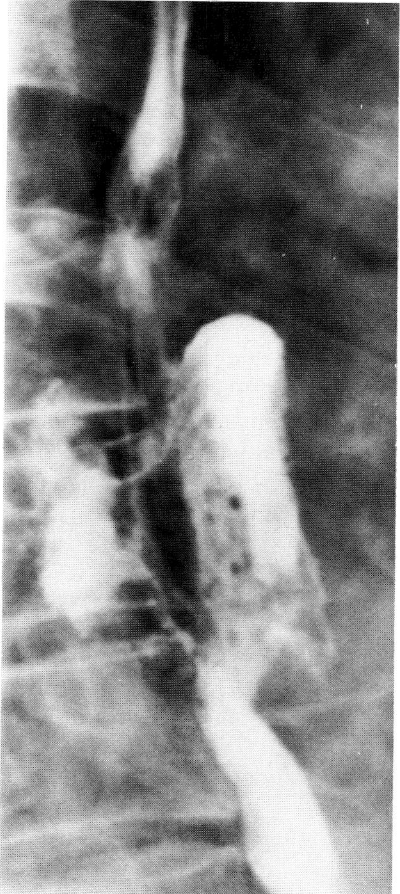

Fig. 29.52A

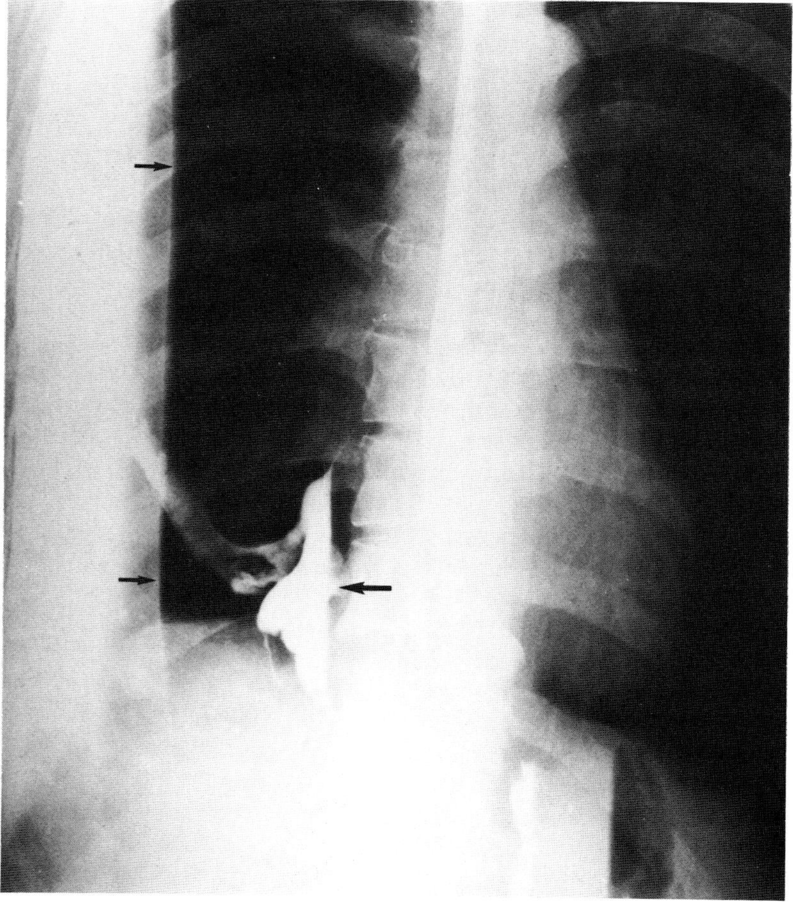

Fig. 29.52B

intraluminal filling defect, such as a lump of meat, may simulate neoplasm but the history is usually diagnostic (Fig. 29.51). Following removal of a foreign body by oesophagoscopy it is necessary to exclude a pathological narrowing as the cause of hold up.

Pieces of *impacted bone* are a particular problem. The favourite site of impaction is in the cervical oesophagus. Plain radiography may show bones of sufficient density, but care must be taken not to mistake normal laryngeal cartilage ossification for a foreign body. Meat and chicken bones are more likely to be detected on plain radiographs than fish bones, which are generally less opaque, although those from fish with bony skeletons (as opposed to cartilaginous skeletons) may be detectable. When plain radiography and barium swallow are unsuccessful in locating a possible impacted bone the patient should be asked to swallow a piece of barium-soaked bread or cotton wool. Delay in passage of this fibre bolus will indicate the site of the impacted object.

Oesophageal injury is not uncommon and may be iatrogenic, self-inflicted or the result of violence. The most frequent cause of perforation of the oesophagus in adults is *endoscopy*, either with or without biopsy. A diverticulum or a stricture predispose to this complication. Other common iatrogenic causes are *dilatation procedures* (e.g. in achalasia), attempted endotracheal or nasogastric *intubation* and *para-oesophageal surgery* (e.g. vagotomy). Traumatic perforation also results from *penetrating injuries* (e.g. stab wounds) or less frequently *blunt trauma*. Perforation due to a *swallowed foreign body* mainly occurs in infants and psychiatric patients. Oesophageal perforation is rarely caused by *peptic oesophagitis, caustic ingestion, malignant neoplasm* or following *radiotherapy*.

Initial chest radiographs taken within minutes of perforation are often normal, and soft tissue emphysema, mediastinal widening, pleural effusion, pneumothorax and abscess formation may not be detected until later. The site of oesophageal perforation (Fig. 29.52A) and any interconnecting mediastinal and pleural spaces are reliably demonstrated by a water-soluble contrast medium (e.g. Gastrografin) swallow. Fluoroscopy should be supplemented by radiographs taken with a *horizontal beam* with the patient in the prone, supine, right and left decubitus positions (Fig. 29.52B). If the procedure reveals no gross abnormality barium should be given for a better demonstration of mucosal detail.

Spontaneous oesophageal rupture results from trauma caused by stresses such as vomiting or straining (*Boerhaave's syndrome*) and occurs at the distal oesophagus on the left side.

When the tear is superficial and limited to the mucosa, the term *Mallory-Weiss syndrome* is applied. Mallory-Weiss tears frequently involve the gastric fundus as well as the lower end of the oesophagus (Fig. 29.53), and are often not demonstrated on a barium swallow. The condition usually causes bleeding which may be shown by selective coeliac arteriography, the localization of the bleeding site depending upon the detection of extravasated contrast medium.

A third syndrome resulting from forcible vomiting occurs when a mucosal tear produces an *intramural haematoma*. The radiographic appearances on a barium swallow depend upon the extent of the haematoma. When this is localized, a filling defect is produced resembling an intramural tumour such as a leiomyoma. An extensive haematoma tracks in all directions to encase and narrow the oesophageal lumen. Rarely, a haematoma ruptures into the oesophagus at a distance from the original tear in a manner resembling a dissection of the aorta. When this happens the mucosa is outlined on both sides by barium, creating a double lumen and the 'mucosal stripe sign'. As mucosal tears heal and haematomas resolve, the barium appearances return to normal over the course of a few weeks. Other causes of oesophageal haematoma include instrumentation, anticoagulant therapy and other defects in blood clotting.

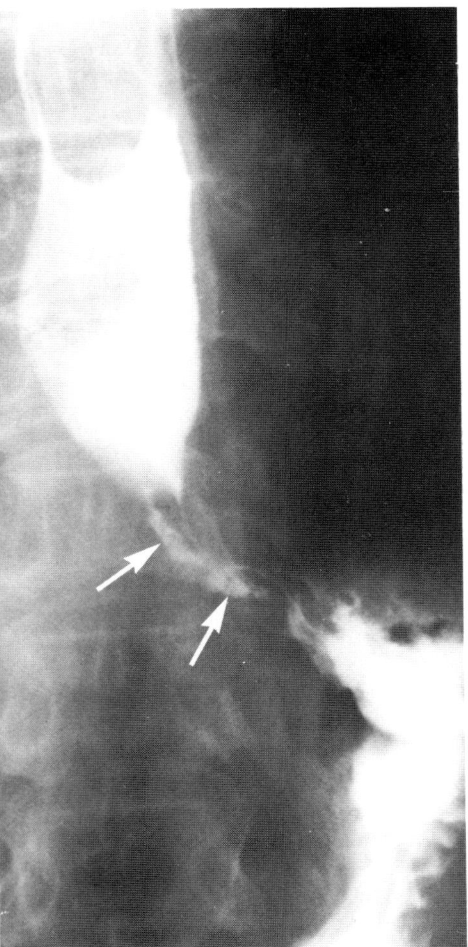

Fig. 29.53 The Mallory-Weiss syndrome. Tear in the oesophagus at its lower end caused by vomiting. Barium (arrowed) has tracked through the defect to lie beneath the mucosa. Translucencies filling the oesophageal lumen proximal to the tear are blood clots.

REFERENCES AND SUGGESTED FURTHER READING

Cho, S. -R., Sanders, M. M., Turner, M. A., Liu, C. -I., & Kipreos, B. E. (1981) Oesophageal intramural pseudodiverticulosis. *Gastrointestinal Radiology*, **6**, 9–14

Creteur, V., Laufer, I., Kressel, H. Y., Caroline, D. F., Goren, R. A., Evans, K. A., Glick, S. N., & Gatenby, R. A. (1983) Drug-induced oesophagitis detected by double contrast radiography. *Radiology*, **147**, 365–368

Donner, M. W., Saba, G. P., & Martinez, C. R. (1981) Diffuse diseases of the oesophagus: A practical approach. *Seminars in Roentgenology*, **16**, 198–213

Eisenberg, R. L. (1983) *Gastrointestinal Radiology*. J. B. Lippincott Company

Ekberg, O. (1981) Cervical oesophageal webs in patients with dysphagia. *Clinical Radiology*, **32**, 633–641

Gelfand, D. W., & Ott, D. J. (1981) Anatomy and technique in evaluating the oesophagus. *Seminars in Roentgenology, 16,1*, pp. 168–182. Grune and Stratton Inc, New York

Itai, Y., Kogure, T., Okuyama, Y., & Akiyama, H. (1977) Diffuse finely nodular lesions of the oesophagus. *American Journal of Roentgenology*, **128**, 563–568

Jewell, D. P., & Selby, W. S. (1982) Oesophageal carcinoma. Oesophageal motility. *Topics in Gastroenterology, 10*, pp. 3–76. Blackwell Scientific Publications. Oxford, London, Edinburgh, Boston, Melbourne

Kressel, H. Y., Glick, S. N., Laufer, I., & Banner, M. (1981) Radiologic features of oesophagitis. *Gastrointestinal Radiology*, **6** 103–109

Laufer, I. (1979) *Double Contrast Gastrointestinal Radiology*. W. B. Saunders Company, London, Philadelphia, Toronto

Laufer, I. (1982) Radiology of oesophagitis. *Radiologic Clinics of North America*, 20,4, pp. 687–699. W. B. Saunders Company, London, Philadelphia, Toronto

Lepke, R. A., & Libshitz, H. I. (1983) Radiation-induced injury of the oesophagus. *Radiology*, **148**, 375–378

Levine, M. S., Kressel, H. Y., Caroline, D. F., Laufer, I., Herlinger, H., & Thompson, J. J. (1983) Barrett oesophagus: Reticular pattern of the mucosa. *Radiology*, **147**, 663–667

Lewicki, A. M., & Moore, J. P. (1975) Oesophageal moniliasis. A review of common and less frequent characteristics. *American Journal of Radiology*, **125**, 218–225

Lipinski, J. K., Conway, S. S., Kottler, R. E., & Werner, D. I. (1982) The radiology of oesophageal tubes for malignant strictures. *Clinical Radiology*, **33**, 453–459

Margulis, A. R., & Burhenne, H. J. (1983) *Alimentary Tract Radiology*, 3rd edn. C. V. Mosby Company, St Louis, Toronto, London

Parkin, G. J. S. (1973) The radiology of perforated oesophagus. *Clinical Radiology*, **24**, 324–332

Tegtmeyer, C. J. & Keats, E. T. (1981) The salivary glands. In: Telplick, J. G., & Haskin, M. D. (eds) *Surgical Radiology*, *3*, pp. 2582–2596 W. B. Saunders Company, London, Philadelphia, Toronto

Trenkner, S. W., & Laüfer, I. (1984) Double contrast examination of the oesophagus, stomach and duodenum. *Clinics in Gastroenterology*, 13(1), 41–73

Vantrappen, G., & Hellemans, J. (1982) Oesophageal spasm and other muscular dysfunction. *Clinics in Gastroenterology, 11, 3*, pp. 453–477 W. B. Saunders Company, London, Philadelphia, Toronto

Zaino, C., & Beneventano, T. C. (1977) *Radiologic Examination of the Orohypopharynx and Oesophagus*. Springer-Verlag, New York

CHAPTER 30

THE STOMACH AND DUODENUM

BARIUM EXAMINATION

The dual cornerstones of diagnosis of disease in the upper gastrointestinal tract are the complementary techniques of barium examination and fibre-optic endoscopy. The achievement of high quality gastrointestinal contrast studies is dependent upon many factors. The essential basic requirements for optimum results are described below.

EQUIPMENT AND MATERIALS

Equipment. The generator, overhead X-ray tube, image intensifier and fluoroscopic viewing system ('TV' chain) should be carefully chosen, bearing in mind the need for fine detail, consistent results and durability. Standard fluoroscopic equipment with a simple three-phase generator and 1 mm focal spot are usually employed.

Special consideration should be given to the selection of the recording system. Most radiologists prefer a conventional spot film device, with a capacity for producing full frame radiographs of the stomach, split vertically for the oesophagus and duodenal loop, and quartered for the duodenal cap. In North America it is customary to combine a spot film examination with radiographs obtained from a conventional overhead tube and bucky system. An alternative system is photofluorography which employs a 'photospot camera' producing 100 mm cut film or 105 mm roll film format. The advantages of this system include the capacity for either single exposures or frame rates of up to 12 per second, the ability to choose different sizes of image, cassette-free ease of use, very short exposure times which eliminate movement blurr, and a reduction in patient irradiation. Problems with image quality, processing and reliability appear to have been largely overcome. Although cine cameras and videotape recorders are not often used in gastrointestinal work, they are particularly useful in the examination of the swallowing act and its disorders. The possible role of digital radiography in gastrointestinal radiology is currently being investigated.

The choice of fluoroscopic table depends upon the radiologist's preference for conventional or remote control fluoroscopy. The superior radiographic quality of the remote systems has to be balanced against the advantage with a conventional unit of having the radiologist close by the patient. The importance of properly matched components and regular maintenance should not be forgotten.

Radiographic technique. High kilovoltage (120–150 kV) is usual for the conventional barium meal. A lower kilovoltage (70–120 kV) is employed for double contrast.

Contrast media. One general-purpose barium sulphate product will not suffice for all examinations. Manufacturers have developed suitable preparations for the double contrast barium meal. There are many factors which affect the performance of a barium sulphate medium. These include the size of the particles, the charge on the particles, the type of water in which the barium is suspended, the nature and qualities of any additives, the purity of the barium, the settling and flocculation characteristics, viscosity, pH, palatability, date of manufacture and storage qualities, and the way the product is prepared and dispensed to the patient in the X-ray room. A high-density, concentrated barium suspension with low viscosity for better fluidity is chosen for double contrast examination. Most radiologists use a 200–250% weight/volume concentration for double contrast, and a much lower concentration for single contrast.

Gas-producing agents. Several such agents are available releasing carbon dioxide in the stomach quickly and consistently, and incorporating an antifoaming agent. Sodium bicarbonate is the basic ingredient plus citric or tartaric acid.

Pharmacological aids. 10–20 mg of *Buscopan* (hyoscine-N-butylbromide) or 0.1–0.2 mg of *glucagon* are given intravenously to induce hypotonia and improve distension.

METHODS

Patient preparation: X-ray room organization. The preliminaries to a barium meal are as important as the examination itself. The clinician's request for radiological consultation should include the relevant points in the patient's history and physical examination, the suspected diagnosis or the conditions that are to be excluded, details of previous X-ray examinations especially barium studies and their findings, and a note of any previous thoracic or abdominal surgery.

Patients who are to have a barium meal should be given instructions beforehand; outpatients can be given an information sheet when they book their examination. Fasting is necessary for at least 8 hours, and patients should also abstain from smoking. Some radiologists also like to give a laxative for two nights before the examination in order to clear the colon of faeces which might otherwise obscure or impress the part under examination. In order to avoid fetal irradiation women of childbearing age should be questioned about the possibility of pregnancy.

The organization of the X-ray room and the radiographic team is the responsibility of the radiologist. For the sake of efficiency departmental routines should be formulated and carried out, so that every member of the team knows precisely what to do. This is facilitated if radiologists agree to use the same agents and procedures, whilst retaining some individual freedom of action when necessary. A typical session may last about 1½ hours and comprise 6 booked patients at 10-minute intervals. This leaves sufficient time, if required, for additional acute cases. If possible, difficult or complicated cases should be last on the list. Ideally, in a large department, one room should be devoted exclusively to barium meals with four sessions a day, each conducted by a different radiologist. In small departments a more flexible arrangement is necessary. A system whereby one radiologist alternates fluoroscopy for barium meals and double contrast enemas between two rooms is successfully employed in some departments.

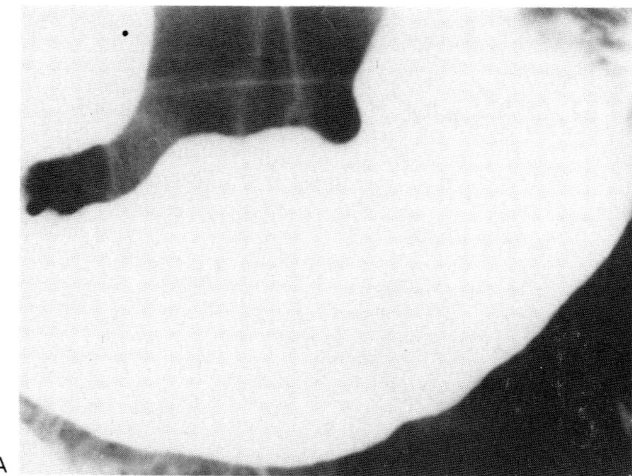

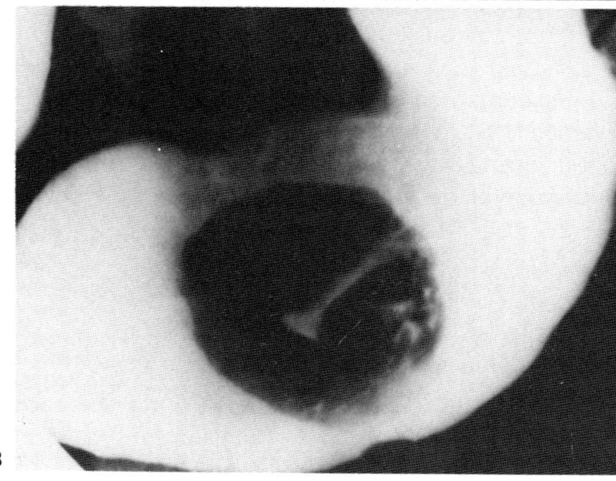

Fig. 30.1 Illustration of technique: The value of compression. A large plaque-like ulcerating carcinoma is present in the body of the stomach. **A**. Tumour obscured by barium pool. **B**. With compression the barium pool is thinned to reveal the tumour.

BARIUM MEAL TECHNIQUES

There are two basic types of barium meal, namely single contrast and double contrast. Individual radiologists adopt their own ways of conducting each of these methods. The **single contrast examination** is the traditional method. Mucosal views of the stomach are obtained with a small quantity of high-density barium. The remainder of the examination is performed with a large volume of dilute barium which produces the necessary distension. Fluoroscopy is an essential part of the procedure, combined with graded compression and exposure of spot films with the patient in appropriate positions. The method does not tolerate standardization, and its success is very dependent upon operator skills. Information is obtained from observation of peristalsis and other motor activity, from the barium profile, and from the *en face* surface under compression (Fig. 30.1). The effectiveness of palpation or compression with a device may be limited by the rib cage, obesity, abdominal wounds from recent surgery, and restricted access to the patient resulting from apparatus design. Fistulae and obstruction are especially well demonstrated.

Worldwide progress in fibre-optic endoscopy revealed the high error rate of the conventional single contrast examination, and stimulated the Japanese to develop the **double contrast barium meal**. Their success in detecting early gastric carcinoma by this technique inspired British, European and North American radiologists to follow their method. The double contrast technique has proved to be of particular value in the detection of mild peptic oesophagitis, early gastric cancer, small gastric and duodenal ulcers, linear ulcers, ulcer scars, erosive gastritis, duodenitis, pathology in the second part of the duodenum, and in the examination of the postoperative stomach.

The routine double contrast barium meal is a general purpose study of the upper gastrointestinal tract from the pharynx to the duodenojejunal flexure. For optimum results separate examinations would be required for:

1. the hypopharynx and cervical oesophagus
2. the mid and lower oesophagus and cardia
3. the stomach
4. the duodenum.

The reason for this is that the technique of examination, and the quantity and quality of the barium preparation, is different in the four regions. Obviously, to perform four separate examinations in every patient is impractical, and also unnecessary. A compromise is achieved by concentrating on the stomach first because this is the area where technique is most critical. When satisfactory radiographs of the stomach have been obtained the focus shifts to the duodenum, and then, if necessary, extra barium can be given for a more detailed examination of the pharynx and oesophagus. Also, whilst employing the general-purpose examination the radiologist concentrates on the site of likely abnormality. When there is uncertainty at the completion of the examination about the presence or nature of a possible abnormality, the alternatives are either endoscopy or a repeat barium study a few days later focusing on the suspect area.

A small quantity of high-density barium sulphate is used to demonstrate fine mucosal detail. Distension and double contrast are achieved with a gas-producing agent. A hyptonic drug may be administered to maintain distension and inhibit peristalsis. Maximum information is obtained from the radiographs, fluoroscopy being used mainly for positioning the patient and directing the movement of the barium pool across the mucosa. Fluoroscopy should be limited to the minimum necessary. In most patients the method is very amenable to standardization. Whilst operator skill is important, it is possible for relatively inexperienced radiologists to perform good quality double contrast examinations at an early stage of their training. This method is therefore better suited than the single contrast technique to departments that undertake training. Interpretation of the radiographs requires considerable skill, and an experienced radiologist is necessary to check the reporting of junior staff.

Even amongst experienced radiologists there is evidence in favour of double viewing of double contrast barium examinations because most errors are perceptive. There are often practical reasons why all examinations cannot be viewed by two radiologists, but double viewing by the same person is always possible. The first viewing takes place at the completion of the examination before the patient leaves the department. This gives the operator the opportunity of getting the patient back into the X-ray room for 'a second look' if there is any area that has not been adequately demonstrated, or if a possible abnormality needs closer scrutiny. The second viewing is during formal reporting.

The greatest attribute of the double contrast barium meal is in showing **mucosal detail**. The conduct of the examination is therefore directed towards this end. The quality of the mucosal coating depends to a large extent on the type of barium being used. Also, coating is impaired by fluid or mucus within the intestinal lumen. By repeatedly turning the patient in the recumbent position the barium pool can be used to wash mucus from the wall of the stomach and improve coating.

It is important to obtain radiographs with the patient in the *supine* and *prone* positions so that a lesion will be on the dependent surface on at least one of them. A shallow barium pool outlines a protruding lesion (e.g. polyp) on the dependent surface as a radiolucent filling defect, and a depressed lesion (e.g. ulcer) is shown as a barium collection. A deep barium pool will obscure both protrusions and depressions, hence the importance of shifting the barium pool from side to side to thin it out and uncover abnormalities. Displacement of the pool from over a lesion can also be achieved by graded compression; a manoeuvre which is especially useful in the gastric antrum. In general, lesions on the non-dependent surface are less obvious than on the dependent surface because the film of barium is much thinner, and there is no pool with which the radiologist can work. A protruding lesion on a non-dependent surface is slightly opaque and etched in white. An ulcer crater on the same surface is empty of barium and therefore seen as a thin white ring around a central translucency. An adequate number of projections should be obtained to show each portion of the stomach free of overlapping barium-filled loops of duodenum and proximal jejunum. Multiple projections are also necessary in order to see lesions in profile. Erect views are useful for showing lesions in the fundus of the stomach, polyps with stalks and barium in ulcer craters.

Distension is also an important factor in the detection of lesions in the gastrointestinal tract. Incomplete distension can easily obscure lesions; and barium trapped between adjacent folds, or a collapsed viscus, can simulate ulceration or neoplasm. Overdistension can also obscure lesions by effacement, but with good mucosal coating this is much less of a problem than underdistension. The optimum degree of distension is that which just effaces the normal gastric mucosal folds. In most patients this means ingesting an effervescent agent that produces 300 to 400 cc of gas. This quantity of gas on average distends the gastric fundus to 10 cm, the mid-body to 7 cm and the duodenal loop to 4 cm. Distension is improved by using a hypotonic drug.

Whilst conforming to the principles of good technique, there are many different ways of performing a double contrast barium meal. Radiologists in training will develop their own technique based upon that of their teachers and departmental protocols. The basic routine technique should be varied if necessary to take account of each particular clinical problem, and to clarify any abnormalities detected on fluoroscopy. The procedure outlined below is the approach employed by the author, but it should be appreciated that only rarely is precisely the same sequence of manoeuvres carried out on consecutive patients because the circumstances are seldom identical.

An effervescent agent is administered, and the shoeless patient immediately guided onto the footplate of the erect fluoroscopic table facing the standing radiologist. The radiologist can supplement the history on the request card by asking the patient questions as the examination proceeds.

A plastic cup containing about 60 cc of a high density barium mixture is given into the left hand. Rapid fluoroscopy of the chest, diaphragm and upper abdomen is performed in order to detect any gross abnormality. The patient then swallows the barium under fluoroscopic observation, and two or more exposures (frontal and right anterior oblique on a split 24 cm × 30 cm radiograph) are taken of the mid and lower oesophagus. To capture the **oesophagus** distended with air and coated with barium, it is necessary to make the exposure just after a large bolus of barium has passed.

The barium cup is retrieved and the table lowered to the horizontal position. A pillow is placed under the patient's head. Brief fluoroscopy indicates whether barium has entered the duodenum, and if not the patient is turned on to the right side. Ideally only a small quantity of barium is required in the duodenum at this stage, as the barium-filled duodenum and jejunal loops may obscure the stomach.

As soon as the cap fills the patient is turned on to the left side to empty the antrum of barium, and then in the supine position 20 mg of *Buscopan* are administered intravenously. If a suitable vein is not available the injection is made into the deltoid muscle. The hypotonic effect is almost immediate and lasts for approximately 10–15 minutes. *Prostatic enlargement* and suspected *glaucoma* are theoretical contraindications to Buscopan. In practice the danger of precipitating urinary retention by giving Buscopan in this dosage is remote and may be ignored. Previously diagnosed glaucoma will have been controlled by drugs or surgical treatment, and will not be adversely affected. If the patient has glaucoma unknowingly the radiologist will not have the necessary skill and specialized equipment for diagnosis, but fortunately only the uncommon closed-angle variety of glaucoma is liable to be exacerbated by Buscopan.

The patient is then turned to the left into the prone position, via the right side up in order to prevent too much barium entering the duodenum. A pillow is slipped under the abdomen, and a film of the **whole stomach and duodenum** is taken to show anterior wall lesions. In the same position the patient is then given another 50–60 ml of barium mixture to drink through a straw, and a further two exposures are made of the lower end of the oesophagus. When there is any question of hiatus hernia, gastro-oesophageal reflux or oesophagitis additional manoeuvres are carried out as described in the previous chapter. However, if for any reason a detailed examination of the oesophagus is required, this is best delayed until after films of the stomach and duodenum have been obtained, when large quantities of barium can be given without compromising the rest of the examination.

The patient is now turned from the prone position via the right side up to the supine right anterior oblique (RAO) position and a film is taken of the stomach and duodenum. Rotation of the patient from side to side, or through a complete turn, washes the mucosa and improves coating, sometimes at the expense of flooding the duodenum with barium. These manoeuvres are performed whenever fluoroscopy suggests that mucosal coating could be improved, or if it is necessary to wash barium over a suspected lesion. The fundus of the stomach is next emptied of barium by turning the patient on to the right side. A film is taken in the right lateral position followed by a left anterior oblique. A straight supine view completes the routine supine series of stomach films. The lateral and LAO films show best the fundus, the straight view the mid-part, and the RAO film the lesser curvature and antrum of the stomach and the duodenal cap and loop. Generally, this latter view is the most useful of the entire series. The frequent changes in the patient's position are best achieved with some assistance. By grasping the patient's hips the radiologist can control both the direction of movement and the final position. The presence of an assistant at the head end is also useful to rotate the shoulders and 'unwind' the arms.

The radiologist's attention now focuses on the **duodenal cap**. An average of four exposures are made (on a 'serial' film) with the patient in various positions including prone and RAO. The prone — right side up — RAO sequence is again usefully employed to produce maximum distension and coating of the cap and second part of the duodenum. Two views of the duodenal loop are then obtained (on a split film) in the RAO and prone positions. Fluoroscopy of the stomach and duodenum is repeated at this stage and additional exposures are made if necessary.

The table is elevated to 45°, and a film is taken with the patient turned into the LAO position. This view gives a good demonstration *en face* of the cardia and upper part of the lesser curvature of the stomach. The table is then brought back into the upright position, taking care to ensure that the patient's feet are firmly on the foot plate and his balance is steady. The radiologist's left hand can be used to steady the patient whilst the right hand operates the elevator switch. Two films of the gas-filled fundus are obtained in the frontal and RAO positions. This normally completes the examination.

The patient is assisted off the step and resumes his place in the waiting room whilst the films are developed. When the radiologist has checked that these are satisfactory the patient is allowed to leave the department. Outpatients with Buscopan-induced blurred vision (which rarely lasts more than ½ hour and does not affect distance vision) are warned of the possible dangers of driving a vehicle or operating machinery within 1 hour. A laxative is given to assist evacuation of the barium.

This routine procedure as described above is capable of infinite variation according to individual radiologist's preferences, and clinical circumstances. When a particular area is seen on fluoroscopy to be especially well demonstrated a film should be taken immediately, without strictly adhering to the routine sequence; an opportunity to obtain a good picture is sometimes not repeated. Whenever a problem arises the radiologist should not hesitate to obtain additional views, give more barium or gas, palpate, compress, or do anything that will further the diagnosis.

Young et al (1985) have suggested that a minimum number of views are unnecessary for a routine examination of the stomach and duodenum. In a series of 738 patients, three double contrast views of the stomach (supine, RAO and right lateral) diagnosed 96% of *reported* gastric abnormalities, while double contrast views of the duodenum diagnosed 93% of *reported* duodenal lesions.

Tubeless **hypotonic duodenography** performed as part of the routine double contrast barium meal or as a specific examination of the duodenum is almost always successful. Rarely, persistent pylorospasm, poor coating, poor distension, or an unusual position of the duodenal loop lead to failure. In these circumstances intubation of the duodenum is necessary. A hypotonic agent is administered and approximately 50–100 ml of barium suspension is injected down the tube with the patient lying on the right side, followed in the RAO position by as much air as is necessary for distension. The tube is then removed and radiographs are obtained in the usual manner.

The **biphasic barium meal examination** is a modification of the double contrast technique which aims to incorporate the possible advantages of the single contrast method. Double contrast films are taken first in the usual way. A large quantity of dilute barium is then given, and oesophageal motility is observed. Additional spot films of the stomach and duodenum with compression are obtained. Some radiologists conclude the procedure with several overhead radiographs.

Difficult patients. The handling of ill, frail, immobile or elderly persons presents problems that require patience and experience. The first essential is a sufficient number of assistants. It is also necessary for the radiologist to have a clear idea of what the clinician would like to have excluded; for instance, obstruction, carcinoma of the stomach or peptic ulceration. The examination should be conducted expeditiously with the likely pathology in mind, because a long and arduous examination may have a harmful effect on the patient. The experienced radiologist should 'cut corners' and not hesitate to omit any part of the procedure that is impractical, such as the effervescent mixture, hypotonic agent, drinking through a straw, turning on the table or particular projections. The purpose of this type of examination is to detect a major lesion and not to demonstrate trivial abnormalities. As soon as the cause of the patient's symptoms has been found, or the questions asked by the clinician have been answered, the examination should be concluded and the patient returned to the ward.

The double contrast barium meal and endoscopy

There is controversy over whether the patient with symptoms referable to the upper gastrointestinal tract should be investigated first by endoscopy or radiology. Mendelson (1985) has suggested that the choice of primary investigation should be tailored to the symptom complex of the individual patient. *Endoscopy* is preferred for those with acute haemorrhage, aged over 50 years at the onset of 'dyspepsia', constant or daily pain, weight loss, vomiting, symptoms of oesophagitis, suspected recurrent disease following surgery, suspected non-bleeding varices, and for unco-operative patients. A *double contrast barium meal* is recommended first for those aged under 50 years with 'simple' dyspepsia (no constant or daily pain, weight loss or vomiting), dysphagia, symptoms of reflux or hiatus hernia, and to delineate the gross anatomy after surgery. For most patients only one of the investigations is necessary, but in a substantial minority double contrast radiology and endoscopy provide complementary information, and both will be required.

THE NORMAL STOMACH AND DUODENUM

The stomach is a J-shaped hollow viscus (Fig. 30.2) consisting of a fundus, body and antrum, communicating with the oesophagus by the cardia and with the duodenal cap (syn: bulb) by the pyloric canal (syn: pylorus). In profile the stomach is outlined by a lesser and a greater curvature. The incisura angularis marks the intersection on the lesser curvature of the body and antrum. There are three normal features that should be regularly identified on a double contrast barium meal. With adequate coating of the mucosa the surface pattern of the *areae gastricae* is demonstrated (Fig. 30.3). This varies from a fine reticular appearance to coarse nodularity, usually best seen in the distal two thirds of the stomach. The mucosa lining the fundus and body of the stomach is normally thrown into numerous *longitudinal folds* or *rugae*, which are most prominent along the greater curvature and run predominantly in the direction of the long axis of the stomach (Fig. 30.2). Folds are more obvious when the stomach is underdistended and may be completely obliterated by distension with barium and gas, especially under the influence of a

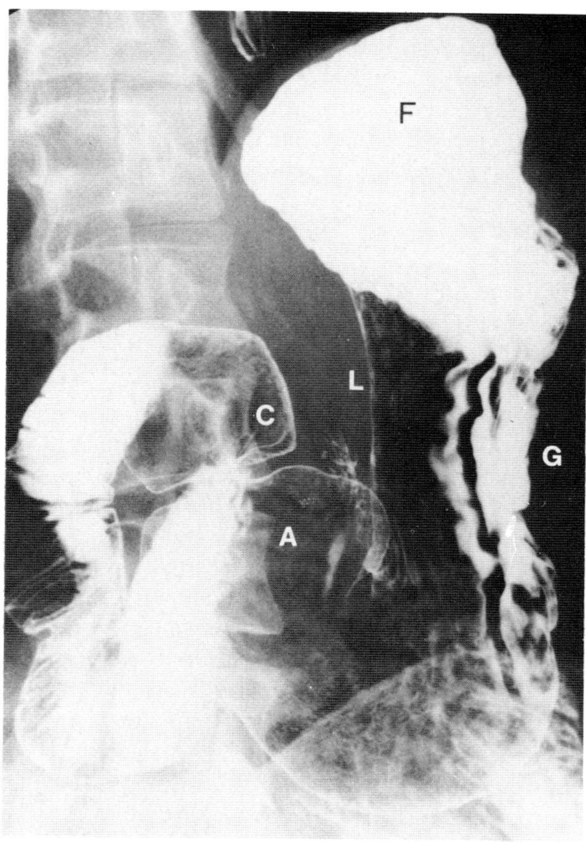

Fig. 30.2 Double contrast barium meal. Normal stomach and duodenum. Supine right anterior oblique position. In this position barium accumulates in the gastric fundus (F); the antrum (A) and duodenal cap (C) are shown in double contrast. L and G indicate the lesser and greater curvatures. Longitudinal mucosal folds (rugae) are present near the greater curvature.

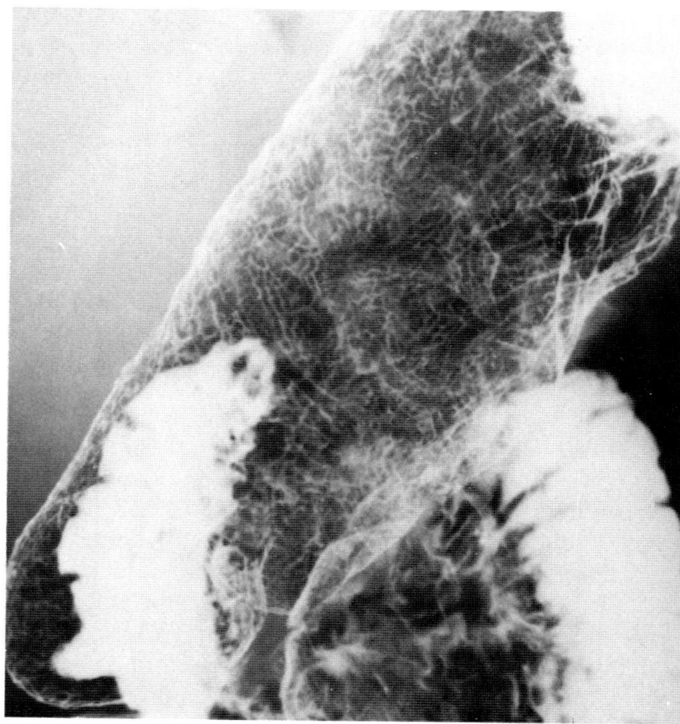

Fig. 30.3 Areae gastricae. Normal reticular pattern produced by areae gastricae. The appearance in this case is slightly coarser than usually seen. Supine left anterior oblique position.

hypotonic agent. The *gastric cardia* lies on the posteromedial aspect of the fundus about 5 cm below its summit. Viewed *en face* in the LAO position short folds are seen radiating to the oesophageal orifice in a form resembling a rosette, and frequently a curved mucosal fold forms a hood over the cardia. Rarely a small filling defect is present representing a protrusion of the distal oesophagus into the stomach.

The duodenum extends from the pylorus to the duodenojejunal flexure. The radiographic duodenum consists of a cap immediately beyond the pylorus, a second part (or descending duodenum) which lies in a C-shaped curve to the right of the spine, and a third part (or horizontal duodenum, consisting of the anatomical third and fourth parts) which crosses the spine from right to left to join the jejunum at the duodenojejunal flexure. It is customary to refer to the second part and the proximal portion of the third part, which encompass the head of the pancreas, as the *duodenal loop* or sweep.

The normal duodenal cap has a symmetrical triangular or acorn shape, with clearly defined borders in profile and an even coating of barium *en face* on double contrast views (Fig. 30.4A). A fine velvety reticular appearance is often seen due to the presence of villi (Fig. 30.4B). Villi are usually more obvious in the second and third part of the duodenum than in the cap. *Mucosal folds* are not seen in the normal distended cap, but when the cap is in a collapsed state the mucosal pattern becomes obvious.

Mucosal folds are a normal feature of the duodenum beyond the cap, and are visible with all degrees of distension. On the normal double contrast hypotonic duodenogram (Fig. 30.5) folds are seen as narrow 2 mm wide translucent bands extending across the whole width of the duodenum. They are straight, slightly wavy or branched in the shape of a Y on its side. At the bowel edge folds seen in cross-section produce small notches. *The papilla of Vater* (syn: major duodenal papilla), which normally measures up to 1.5 cm in diameter, projects into the lumen on the inner side of the second part of the duodenum (Fig. 30.5). Three further landmarks have been identified in the vicinity of the papilla, namely the promontory, the straight segment and the longitudinal fold. Both the promontory and the straight segment are visualized in profile. *The promontory*

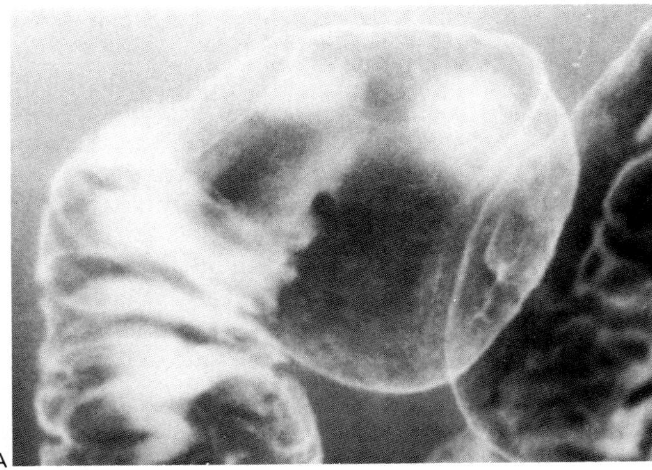

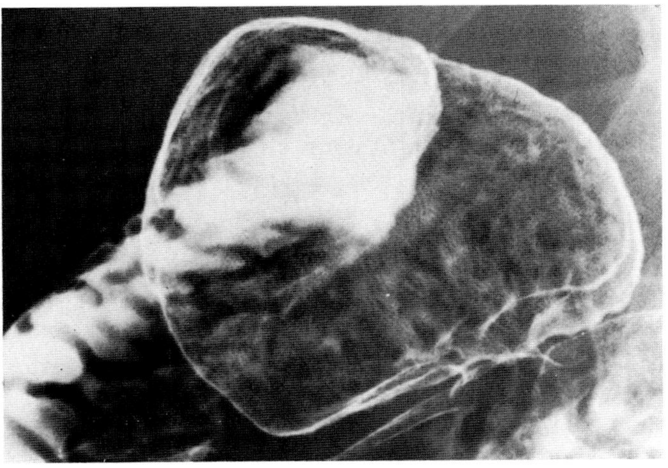

Fig. 30.4 The normal duodenal cap seen by double contrast. The mucosa has a velvety appearance due to the presence of villi. **A.** Surface coating, almost homogenous. **B.** A fine reticular pattern is present.

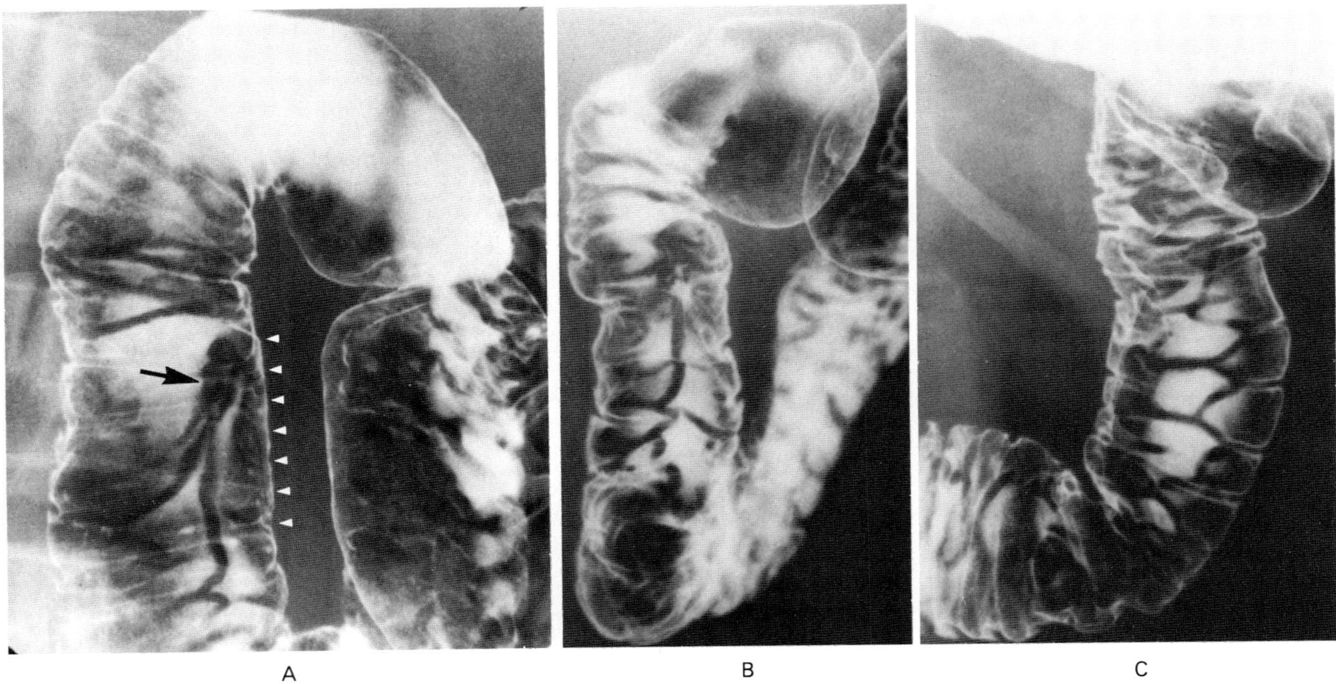

Fig. 30.5 The normal duodenal cap and loop. Hypotonic duodenogram obtained as part of the routine double contrast barium meal. **A** and **B** are supine right anterior oblique and **C** is prone. **A.** Seen *en face*, the papilla of Vater (black arrow) with longitudinal and oblique folds extending below it. The straight segment is indicated by white arrowheads. **B.** and **C.** The arrangement of the transverse mucosal folds is shown in **C.** The papilla and longitudinal fold are seen in **B.**

is a shoulder-like projection of the medial wall of the duodenum close to the papilla, and *the straight segment* is a smooth portion of wall several centimetres in length immediately distal to the promontory (Fig. 30.5). *The longitudinal fold* extends for several centimetres below the papilla of Vater in a direction parallel to the straight segment. The longitudinal fold and the papilla are visualized *en face* in a form resembling a tailed comet (Fig. 30.5). Usually one or two of these landmarks are recognized on hypotonic duodenography, but it is uncommon for all three to be seen together. Additional folds may be present near the papilla of Vater, and occasionally an accessory papilla (syn: minor duodenal papilla, papilla of Santorini) is seen 2 cm proximal to it.

GASTRIC DISPLACEMENT: EXTRINSIC MASSES:VOLVULUS

Enlargement of any one of the structures forming the gastric bed readily produces changes in the barium- or gas-filled stomach, and the manner in which the shape and position of the stomach is altered indicates which organ is enlarged.

Enlargement of the *spleen* usually causes a forward and medial displacement of the stomach, and a splenic impression on the fundus may simulate a submucosal gastric tumour. A left subphrenic abscess produces a similar appearance (Fig. 30.6). A large mass originating in the left *kidney* usually displaces the stomach forwards, but can also displace it to the left and produce an impression on the lesser curvature.

Lesions causing enlargement of the left lobe of the *liver* lie anterior to the stomach and cause backward displacement of the fundus and body. Enlargement of the right lobe of the liver may displace the stomach to the left and posteriorly, but more often produces an impression on the lesser curvature.

Large tumours or cysts of the body or tail of the *pancreas* produce forward displacement of the stomach. To detect such displacement it is essential that horizontal beam radiographs should be taken with the patient supine so that the barium-filled stomach can fall backwards on the enlarged pancreas. Pancreatic cysts arising in the gastric bed usually present through the lesser omentum displacing the stomach forwards and stretching the lesser curvature around the cyst. More rarely cystadenomas, especially when affecting the distal half of the body of the pancreas, present below the stomach causing an upward indentation of the greater curvature. Smaller and more solid pancreatic tumours may not present above or below the stomach but, merely by forward displacement, show an impression in the mid-part of the stomach simulating a submucosal gastric tumour. Lesions of the head of the pancreas may produce a smooth pressure defect on the greater curvature of the gastric antrum (the pad sign), displacing it upward and forward (Fig. 30.69B).

Any intra-abdominal mass if large enough may displace the stomach. Such masses include ovarian cysts, mesenteric cysts, retroperitoneal tumours, e.g. sarcomas, and aortic aneurysms. A suspicion of an extrinsic impression or displacement of the stomach on a barium meal should be

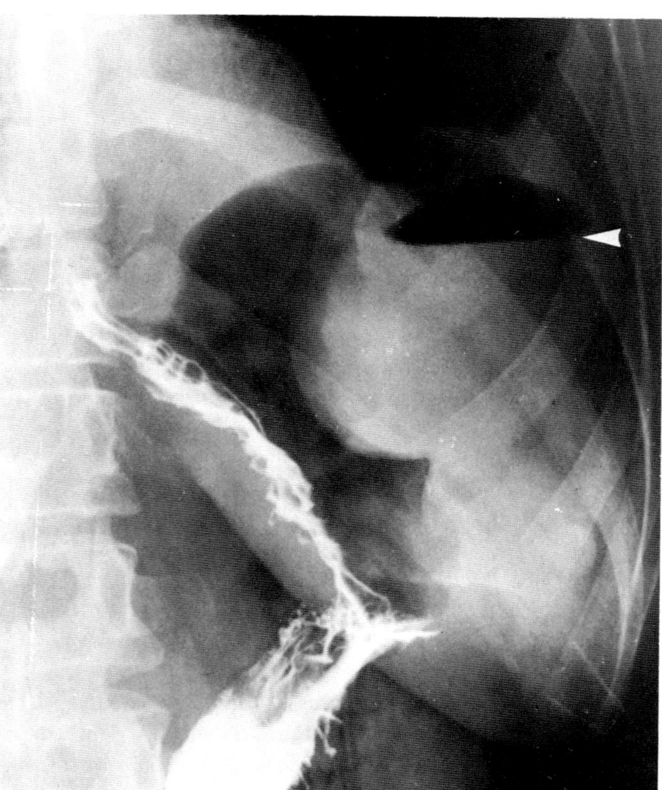

Fig. 30.6 Gastric extrinsic mass. Large subphrenic abscess (with fluid level) producing an extrinsic impression in the gas-filled gastric fundus. One mouthful of barium outlines the lesser curvature of the stomach. There is also a small left pleural effusion.

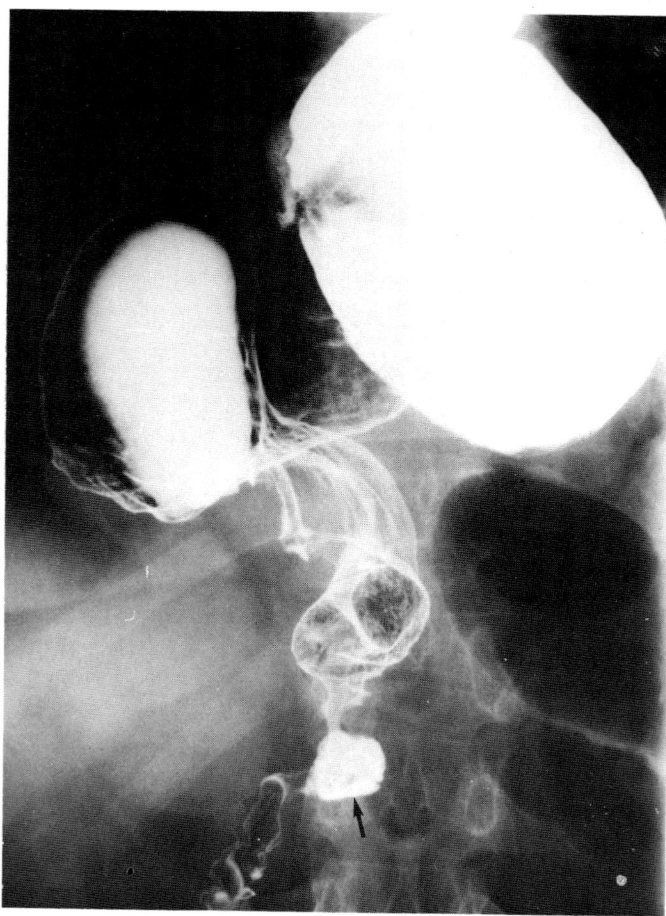

Fig. 30.7 Organo-axial volvulus of an intrathoracic stomach. The greater curvature is folded upwards and to the right. There is a giant duodenal ulcer (arrowed) which perforated 10 days later.

followed by examination with ultrasound (US) or computed tomography (CT) to determine the origin and extent of any mass.

Volvulus of the stomach is classified into two types according to the plane around which rotation occurs. *Organo-axial* volvulus occurs around an axis through the cardio-oesophageal junction and pyloric canal, and *axial* (*or mesentero-axial*) volvulus occurs around a vertical axis through the cardio-oesophageal junction. In the vast majority of cases rotation is along the organo-axial line with the greater curvature of the stomach twisting upwards and to the right (Fig. 30.7). As a result the antrum and duodenal cap are directed downwards and backwards. This type of volvulus is particularly liable to occur when the stomach is in a diaphragmatic hernia, and eventration of the left diaphragm is a common association. Organo-axial volvulus can simulate the normal variant of *'cup and spill'* (*cascade*) *stomach* (Fig. 30.8). This variant can be readily appreciated on erect lateral views when the dependent part of the fundus which forms the 'cup' component lies posteriorly. As it fills with barium the level in the fundus rises until spilling occurs into the body of the stomach, and barium 'cascades' down the lesser curvature and posterior wall. Organo-axial volvulus has also to be distinguished from deformity due to external adhesions and displacement of the stomach by an extrinsic mass.

Minor degrees of torsion of the stomach without obstruction are often asymptomatic. Volvulus may be chronic and intermittent, but the acute type is the most significant and represents an acute surgical emergency. Plain films in gastric volvulus show a gas- or fluid-distended viscus in the upper abdomen or chest, with one or more fluid levels in horizontal beam views. A barium swallow shows obstruction at the lower end of the oesophagus or in the body of the stomach depending upon the site of the twist.

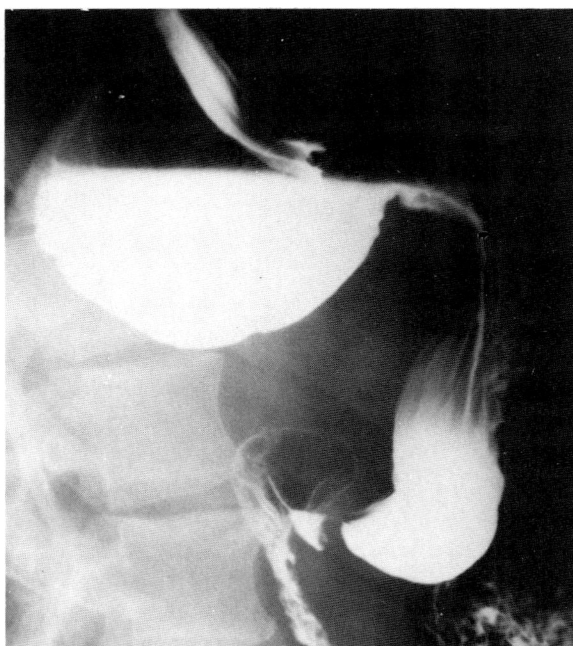

Fig. 30.8 'Cup and spill' or 'cascade' stomach. Erect lateral view showing barium pooling in the drooping fundus (cup) and spilling over into the body of the stomach (cascading down the lesser curvature).

DUODENAL DISPLACEMENT AND IMPRESSIONS

The position of the duodenal loop may vary from the norm for *congenital* reasons, or as a result of *displacement by a mass* in a nearby organ.

Duodenum inversum is an uncommon developmental anomaly of little clinical significance in which abnormal peritoneal fixation allows the third part of the duodenum to pass across the abdomen above the cap (Fig. 30.9A).

Variations in peritoneal fixation produce either right or left paraduodenal fossae. **Paraduodenal hernias** are the commonest form of internal hernia. In the more common left-sided variety loops of small bowel pass into the paraduodenal fossa above the duodenojejunal flexure where incarceration may occur. Plain films and small bowel barium studies are helpful in diagnosis.

The duodenal cap and loop are closely related to other organs in the upper abdomen. Enlargement or **mass lesions** of the gall bladder, liver, right kidney (Fig. 30.9B), right adrenal, pancreas or colon are liable to affect the duodenum.

A normal gall bladder can produce an impression on the right upper quadrant of the duodenal cap; a distended gall bladder or abscess around the gall bladder may impress and displace the second part of the duodenum to the left. The common bile duct, even when normal, can produce a band or rounded impression on the duodenal cap, and a dilated duct makes a larger impression.

Hepatic and renal enlargement produce similar effects. Also, direct invasion of the second part of the duodenum by a malignant renal tumour results in narrowing, mucosal destruction, ulceration and intraluminal filling defects. The effects of pancreatic enlargement on the duodenum are considered on page 860. The transverse colon crosses the second part of the duodenum so that a colonic carcinoma near the hepatic flexure may impress, displace or invade it, and a duodeno-colic fistula may develop.

Examination by US, CT or angiography is often helpful in determining the precise origin and nature of any mass which is displacing the duodenum.

The third part of the duodenum lies in a fixed position in a closed compartment bounded anteriorly by the root of the mesentery, which carries the superior mesenteric vessel sheath (artery, vein, nerve), and posteriorly by the aorta and lumbar spine. Any factor that obliterates this compartment can produce narrowing of the third part of the duodenum with consequent obstruction. This is known as the **superior mesenteric artery syndrome**. Even in normal

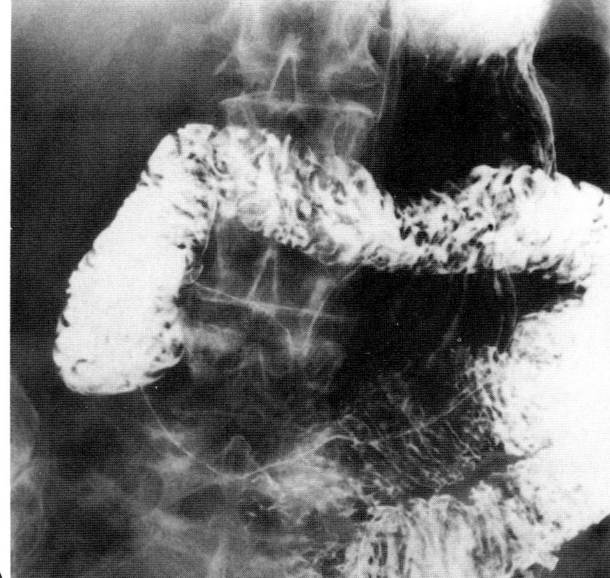

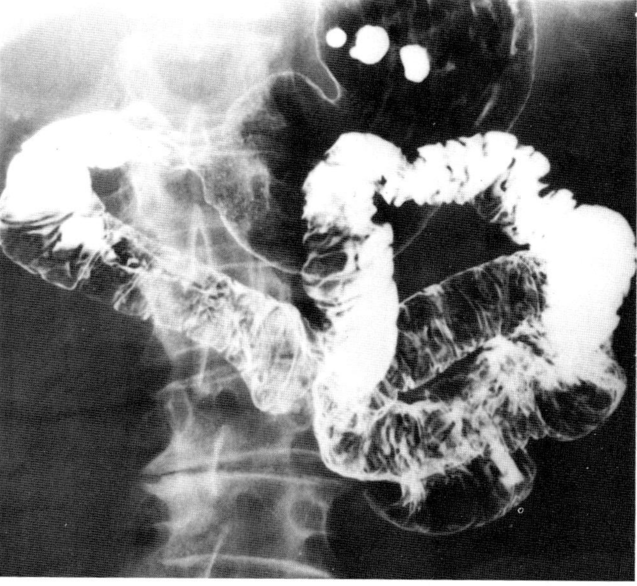

Fig. 30.9 Duodenal displacement. **A.** Congenital. Duodenum inversum. The second part passes upwards, and the third part passes across the spine in a higher position than usual, anterior to the body of the stomach. **B.** Acquired. The second part of the duodenum is displaced upwards and medially by a large right hydronephrosis. (Opacities overlying the stomach are due to barium from a previous examination in diverticula in the transverse colon.)

subjects there is often a transient delay in the passage of barium through the duodenum where it lies in front of the vertebral column in the angle between the superior mesenteric artery and aorta. Numerous cases of this syndrome have been reported, but the exact nature of the condition is not entirely understood. An association has been reported with peptic ulceration, prolonged bed rest (often in a body plaster cast), severe weight loss, diminished duodenal peristalsis (e.g. scleroderma), inflammation and fibrosis in the root of the mesentery (e.g. pancreatitis, Crohn's disease) and retroperitoneal tumours and masses (e.g. carcinoma of the pancreas, aortic aneurysm).

Regardless of the underlying pathology barium examination shows dilatation of the duodenum proximal to a broad vertical band-like pressure defect across the third part of the duodenum overlying the spine (Fig. 30.10). On fluoroscopy vigorous to-and-fro peristalsis is seen proximal to the obstruction (except in scleroderma). In some cases the obstruction is related to posture and by turning the patient prone or on to the left side the 'obstruction' is

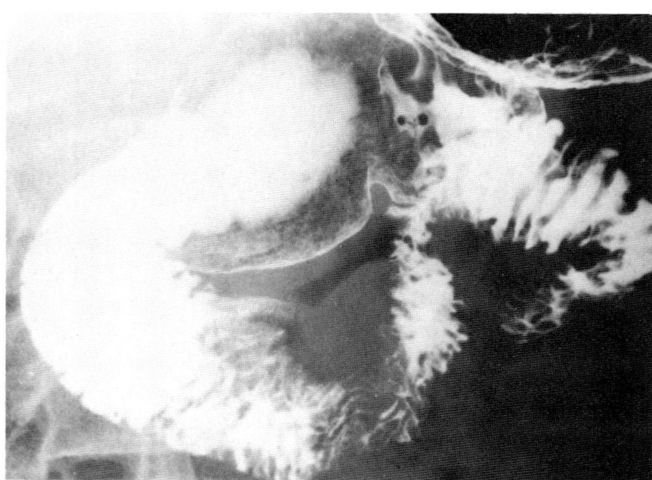

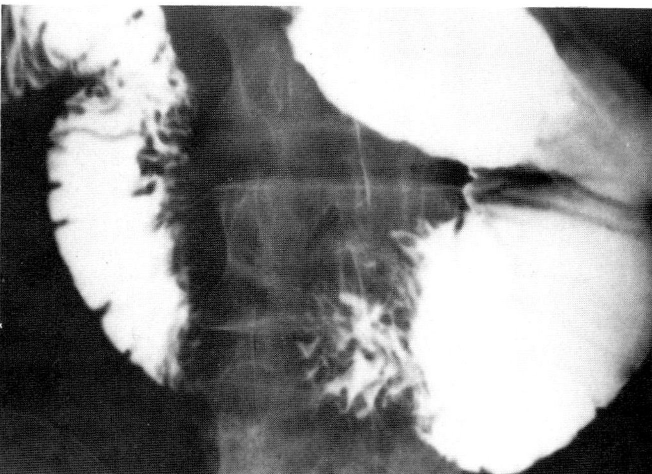

Fig. 30.10 Superior mesenteric artery syndrome caused by carcinoma of the pancreas invading the root of the mesentery. **A.** Supine position. Compression of the third part of the duodenum. **B.** Prone position. The compression persists and dilatation of the proximal duodenum is accentuated. (Courtesy of Drs J R Anderson, P M Earnshaw and G M Fraser, and the Editor of *Clinical Radiology*.)

released and barium will proceed. The attacks of abdominal pain and vomiting encountered in this condition are frequently intermittent, and the radiological features are best demonstrated during an attack. Recent controversy has centred around whether some cases of this condition are a localized form of chronic idiopathic intestinal pseudo-obstruction, a syndrome of diverse pathophysiology characterized by recurrent obstructive symptoms without evidence of mechanical obstruction.

MISCELLANEOUS STRUCTURAL ABNORMALITIES OF THE STOMACH AND DUODENUM

There are two forms of **hypertrophic pyloric stenosis**: the infantile (see Ch. 37) and the adult. The cause of the rare *adult* type is obscure, but a congenital deficiency in the longitudinal muscle of the pylorus with hypertrophy of the circular muscle has been postulated. Some cases are associated with antral gastritis or chronic gastric ulceration and result from long continued spasm. The features on barium examination are similar to those seen in the infantile form. The pyloric canal and distal antrum are narrowed and elongated with a niche between the two segments (Fig. 30.11A). An indentation in the base of the duodenal cap is often present due to the impression of the hypertrophied muscle. The proximal end of the stenosis is abrupt. Gastric outflow obstruction may result. The differentiation of this condition from an annular carcinoma of the antrum is assisted by detecting a slight change in calibre of the narrowed area on fluoroscopy, and longitudinal mucosal folds along the channel.

An **antral diaphragm** consists of a thin diaphragm with a small central opening extending across the whole width of the lumen of the gastric antrum (Fig. 30.11B). This rare condition may be an incidental finding or a cause of gastric outflow obstruction.

Diverticula of the stomach are invariably single and located on the posterior wall of the fundus close to the cardia (Fig. 30.12A). It is thought that they are probably acquired lesions due to a localized area of muscle weakness. Most diverticula are small but occasionally large ones are seen. Each consists of a smooth-walled pouch connected to the stomach by a narrower neck traversed by mucosal folds. Like other diverticula in the intestinal tract barium is liable to be retained in the pouch long after the remainder of the stomach has emptied. Gastric diverticula are symptomless and should not be mistaken for ulcers. A diverticulum is distinguished from an ulcer by its characteristic shape and location, and by the absence of secondary signs of ulceration such as an ulcer mound or radiating folds.

Rarely, diverticula occur in other sites, particularly on the greater curvature of the antrum in association with pancreatic rests (Fig. 30.12B).

Duodenal diverticula are demonstrated on barium meal examination in approximately 5% of cases and are usually an incidental finding without clinical significance. Diverticula occur most commonly along the inner border of the duodenal loop and are often multiple (Fig. 30.13). The average diameter is between 2 and 3 cm. They may contain food residues and often retain barium for several weeks. Complications such as biliary obstruction, perforation and bleeding are rare. With the advent of endoscopic papillotomy, para-ampullary diverticula have attained greater significance and may perforate or bleed following papillotomy if the endoscopist is not aware of their presence.

PEPTIC ULCERATION

Peptic ulcer disease is a major problem in the Western world with a prevalence in Great Britain of 10.4% for men and 4.9% for women. Significant factors in the incidence of peptic ulceration include a familial history, cigarette

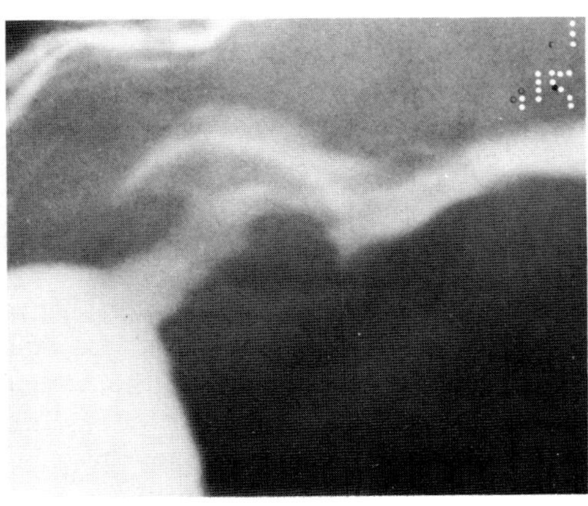

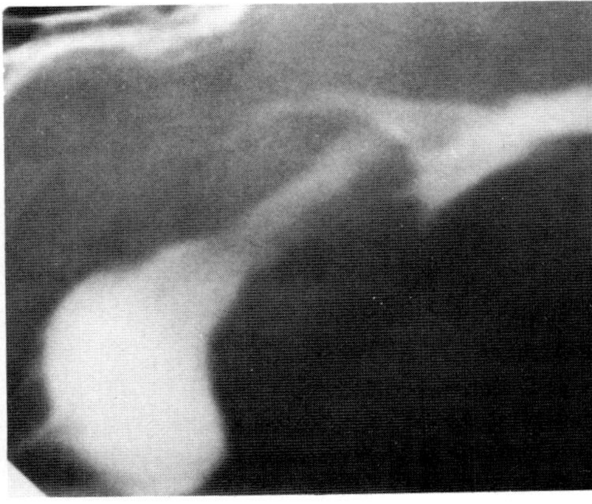

A

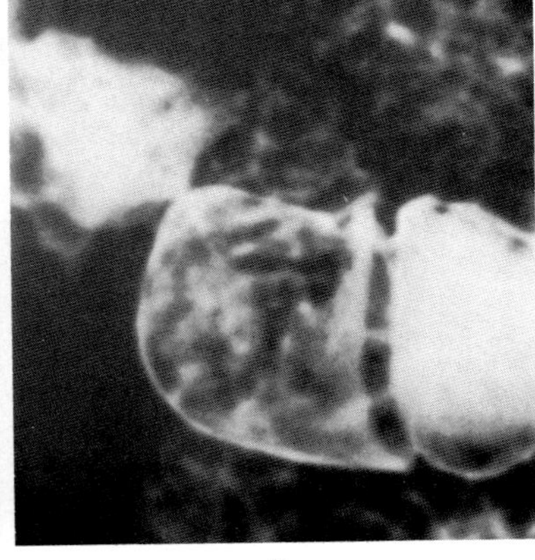

B

Fig. 30.11 Conditions which may obstruct gastric emptying. **A**. Adult hypertrophic pyloric stenosis. Two consecutive serial exposures show an elongated pyloric canal with an umbrella shaped defect at the base of the duodenal cap. (Prone views.) **B**. An antral diaphragm.

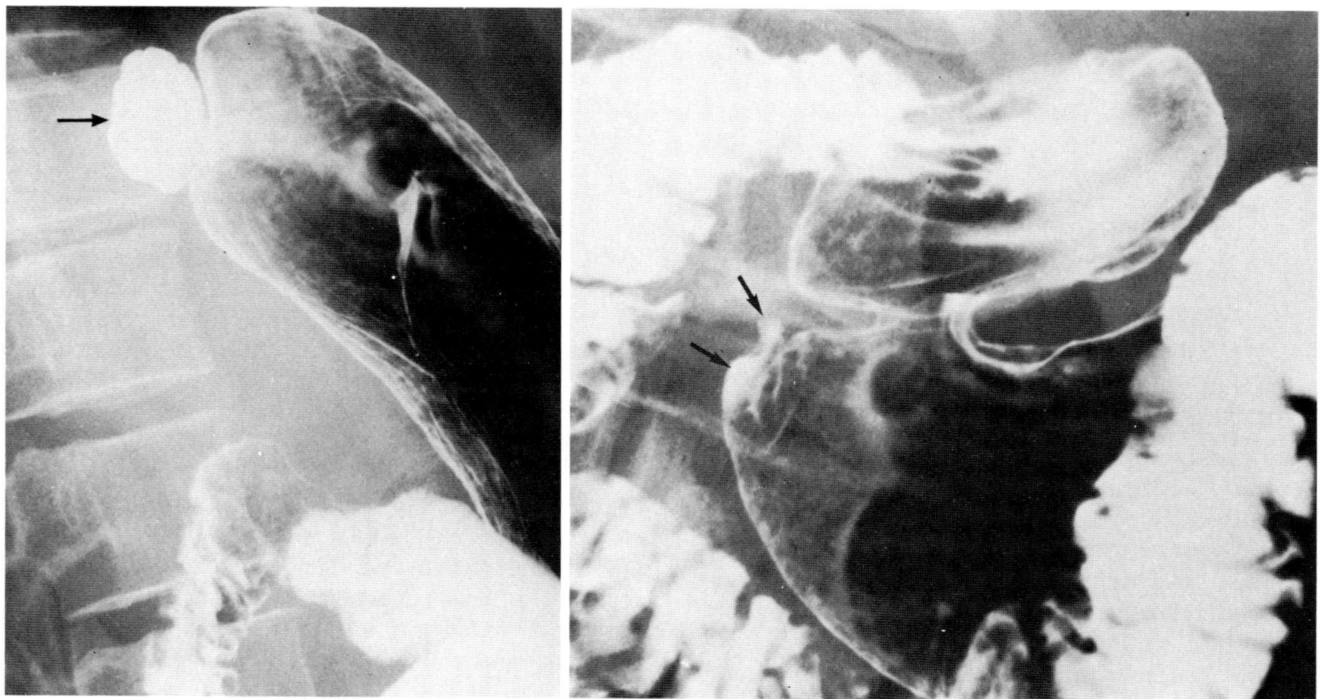

Fig. 30.12 Gastric diverticula. **A**. Erect lateral view showing a barium-filled diverticulum situated in the typical site. **B**. Diverticulum associated with pancreatic rest situated in typical location in the antrum (Courtesy of Dr D.J. Lintoff)

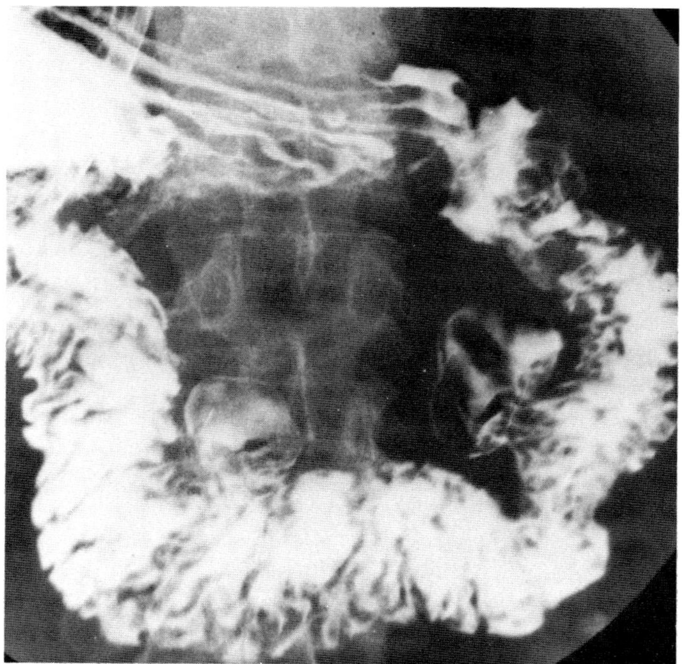

Fig. 30.13 Duodenal diverticula. Two diverticula are present in the second and third parts of the duodenum. Prone view.

smoking, alcohol consumption, certain drugs and some chronic diseases such as emphysema and renal failure. The pathogenesis of peptic ulcer remains elusive, but generally duodenal ulcers are associated with an increased acid production and gastric ulcers perhaps with decreased mucosal resistance.

In clinical practice duodenal ulcers are three or four times more common than gastric ulcers. In approximately 20% of cases of gastric ulceration the ulcers are multiple, and combined gastric and duodenal ulceration is common. The incidence of multiple duodenal ulcers is about 10%.

Symptoms are varied and non-specific, but most patients give a history of recurrent episodes of epigastric pain. However, some patients with active duodenal ulcers who present with acute bleeding have no previous history of digestive complaints. Gastric and duodenal ulceration, and gastritis and duodenitis without identifiable ulcers, may all produce similar symptoms.

Peptic disease also occurs in the lower oesophagus, usually as a result of gastro-oesophageal reflux associated with a sliding hiatus hernia. Therefore the radiologist should perform a detailed examination of the lower oesophagus, stomach and duodenum in all cases of suspected peptic ulceration.

Radiographic appearances

The hallmark of peptic ulceration is an ulcer crater, which

may be demonstrated on a barium meal examination in profile, obliquely or *en face*. With the **single contrast technique** ulcers are seen as collections of barium. As the majority of gastric ulcers occur on the posterior aspect of the lesser curvature of the stomach, they are usually best demonstrated in profile by a bolus of swallowed barium flowing down the wall of the stomach with the patient standing in the RAO position. The barium-filled ulcer crater is readily seen projecting from the line of the lesser curvature. Ulcers at other sites may be shown in profile with the patient in various positions.

An ulcer crater is demonstrated *en face* with the single contrast method by applying graded compression over the site of the ulcer with a compression device or lead gloved hand which displaces the surrounding pool of barium to reveal the barium-filled crater. Compression is especially useful in the distal half of the stomach and in the duodenum, whereas the rib cage prevents compression of the gastric fundus. The same principles apply to single contrast examination of the duodenal cap, where a series of compression 'spot' films are taken with the patient standing in positions ranging from frontal, through both obliques to lateral. Most operators using the single contrast method also seek to obtain double contrast views of the duodenal cap by utilizing the air that is normally swallowed with the barium. With the patient in the supine RAO position air rises from the stomach to distend the duodenal cap which is at a higher level. Prone compression views normally complete the cap series.

With the **double contrast technique**, as previously described, gastric and duodenal ulcers are radiographed containing varying amounts of barium according to the position of the patient, the location of the ulcer and the technique of the operator. For example, an ulcer on the posterior wall of the stomach normally fills with barium when the patient is supine, because in this position the posterior wall is dependent. The operator can fill and empty the crater by alternately raising each side of the patient with a rocking motion, and can skilfully move the barium pool across the ulcerated area in order to demonstrate the crater and coat the surrounding mucosa. An ulcer on the non-dependent surface (e.g. the anterior wall when the patient is supine) when seen *en face* appears as a round translucency within a narrow white ring produced by the outline of the barium-coated rim and side-wall of the crater. Duodenal ulcers occur most frequently in the cap, and like gastric ulcers they are seen *en face* as either collections of barium or rings according to their position (Fig. 30.14A & B). Ulcers are seen in profile either filled or coated with barium.

In general, information about ulcer craters can be obtained equally well by single or double contrast technique, but the latter gives a clearer demonstration *en face* of the ulcer brim and surrounding mucosa.

Most benign gastric and duodenal ulcers are *round* or *oval*, *en face*, but shallow or healing ulcers may assume a wide variety of shapes. Occasionally, if the mucosal edge is less undercut in parts of the ulcer crater, only a fragment of the ring appears giving rise to an *arc* sign. *Linear* ulcers of variable length are regularly seen on endoscopy, and with good technique and diligent searching they are being identified more frequently on double contrast barium

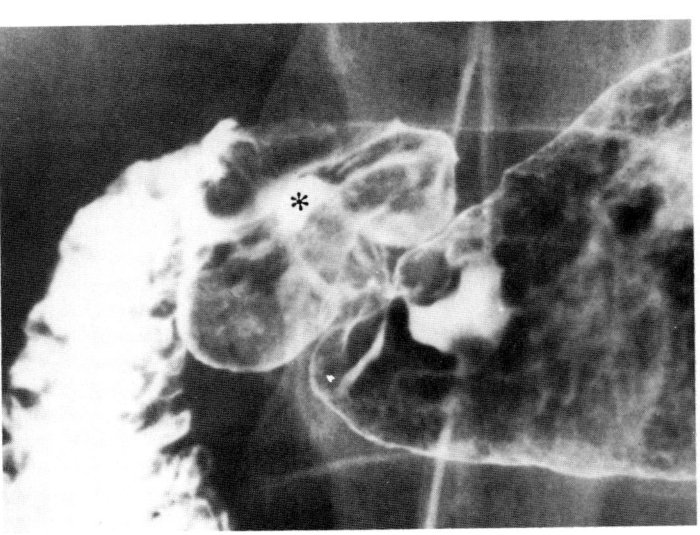

A

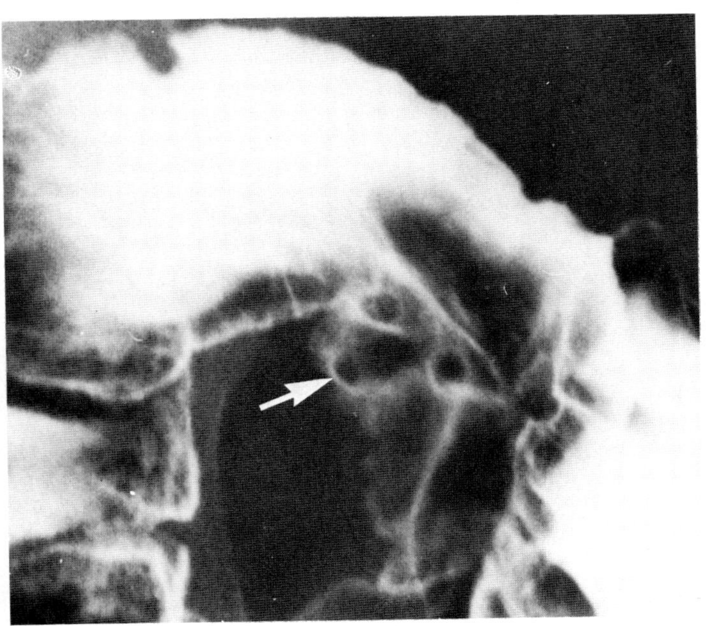

B

Fig. 30.14 Duodenal ulceration: Comparison of appearance of anterior and posterior wall craters. **A.** Supine view. Central barium-filled posterior wall ulcer crater (*) with radiating folds. The duodenal cap has distended well and is not deformed. The collection of barium in the gastric antrum is not an ulcer, and results from pooling of barium between slightly oedematous mucosal folds. **B.** Supine view. Three anterior wall ulcer craters are demonstrated as rings (one marked with arrow). Several radiating folds are present.

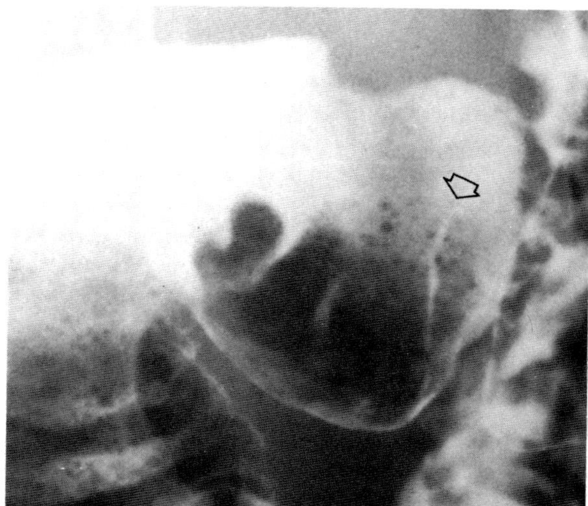

Fig. 30.15 Linear duodenal ulceration. A linear ulcer about 2 cm in length extends across the cap (beneath the arrow). Supine view.

meals, especially with compression. However, the differentiation of a linear ulcer from a mucosal fold or scar is sometimes impossible. Long linear ulcers often straddle the lesser curvature of the stomach, and may be associated with short perpendicular folds and with scarring. Short linear ulcers also occur in the stomach and in the duodenal cap. Linear ulcers comprise 6–7% of duodenal ulcers and are invariably transversely orientated in the cap (Fig. 30.15).

The brim of a gastric ulcer when seen in profile may show one of the following features:

1. *Hampton's line* is a thin (1 mm wide) lucent line across the neck of the ulcer, which represents the intact but undercut mucosa around the mouth of a benign ulcer crater.
2. An *ulcer collar* is similar to Hampton's line, but thicker, due to oedematous tissue surrounding the ulcer crater (Fig. 30.16A).
3. An *ulcer mound* is a prominent ulcer collar produced when the inflammatory reaction is severe.

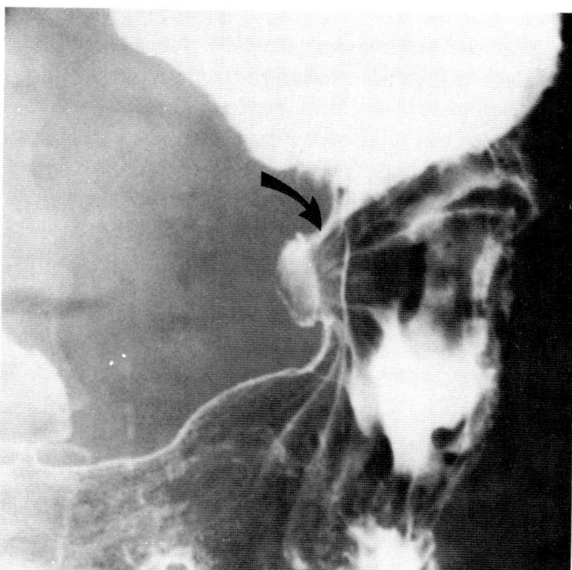

Fig. 30.16 A

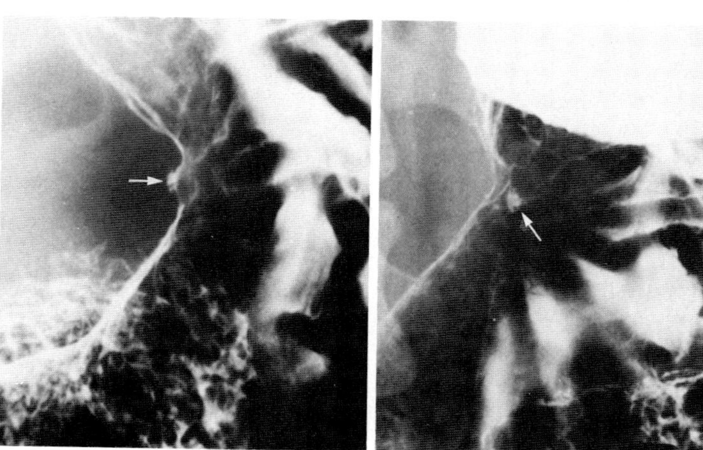

Fig. 30.16 B

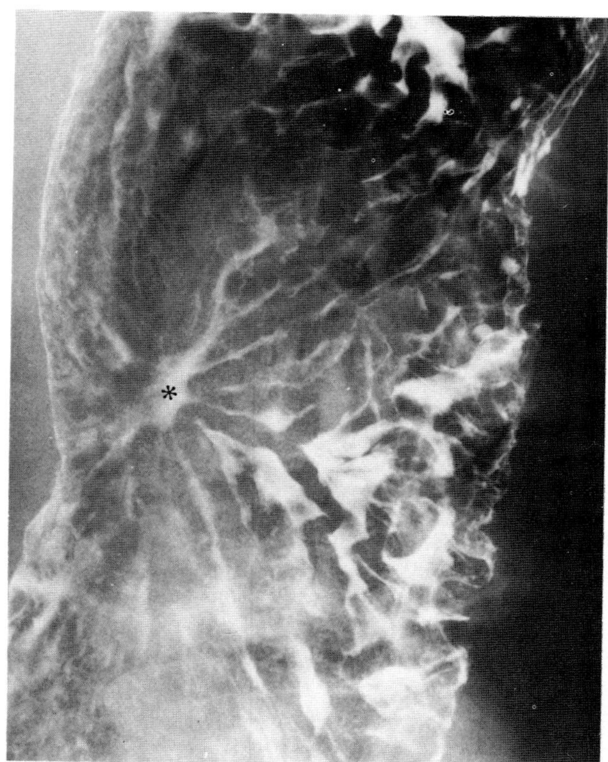

Fig. 30.16 C

Fig. 30.16 Benign gastric ulceration: Typical appearances.
A. Moderately large mid-lesser curvature ulcer demonstrated in profile. The ulcer crater is projecting outside the wall of the stomach, radiating mucosal folds extend to the edge of the crater, and there is a clearly defined ulcer collar (beneath the arrow). **B.** Small posterior lesser curvature ulcer (arrowed). In profile (left) the crater projects outside the wall of the stomach. *En face*, oedema around the ulcer (the ulcer mound) prevents radiating mucosal folds from reaching the edge of the crater. **C.** Small posterior wall ulcer (*) demonstrated *en face*. Radiating mucosal folds extend to the edge of the crater.

An ulcer collar or mound at the brim of a crater may also be seen *en face* as a translucent halo surrounding the ulcer crater (Fig. 30.16B). A mound of oedema is also quite frequently seen around a duodenal ulcer.

It is important to evaluate the mucosa in the area around a gastric ulcer crater and its brim. Two particular features may be identified; *normal areae gastricae* and *radiating mucosal folds* or scars. The latter are best seen *en face* by double contrast as thin white lines extending outwards from the edge of an ulcer crater (Fig. 30.16C), or outer margin of an ulcer mound if appreciable inflammatory oedema is present. In the stomach the sighting of lines may point to an ulcer crater or scar which might otherwise have been overlooked.

Radiographic analysis of gastric ulcers: benign v. malignant

It is estimated that only about 5% of all gastric ulcers are malignant, and therefore the chance of any individual ulcer being a carcinoma is small. Nevertheless the differentiation of benign from malignant ulcers is obviously important, and is the main purpose of careful observation of every gastric ulcer. Most malignant gastric ulcers are primary carcinomatous ulcers produced when a pre-existing carcinoma undergoes ulceration during its development. Rarely malignant change may occur in a previously benign chronic peptic ulcer to produce a secondarily malignant ulcer.

In the radiographic evaluation of a gastric ulcer an analysis is necessary of 1. the crater profile, 2. the ulcer brim and 3. the surrounding mucosa.

The crater profile. In a study of the radiographic diagnosis of benign and malignant gastric ulcers it has been found that most ulcers can be divided into two simplified types based on their profile appearances (Fig. 30.17), viz. projecting and non-projecting (intraluminal). Very small or shallow ulcers are not amenable to inclusion in this classification. To demonstrate projection of an ulcer it is usually necessary to turn the patient into an oblique or lateral position. By this means it can be seen whether the ulcer crater projects beyond the line of the stomach wall on either side of it; this line usually being formed by the lesser curvature.

Projecting ulcers are almost always benign (Fig. 30.16A), but the rare secondarily malignant ulcers (malignant change in a previously benign chronic peptic ulcer) are usually of this type, and occasionally a benign-looking projecting ulcer is a primary carcinomatous ulcer.

Non-projecting gastric ulcers (with the exception of those located on the greater curvature (Fig. 30.18)) are almost always malignant, because in order for an ulcer to be intraluminal (i.e. seen in all projections to lie within the normal outline of the stomach), it must be formed within an intraluminal mass or elevated tumour rim (Fig. 30.19). Also most malignant ulcers are non-projecting.

The combination of an intraluminal ulcer crater surrounded by an elevated rim of tumour produces a

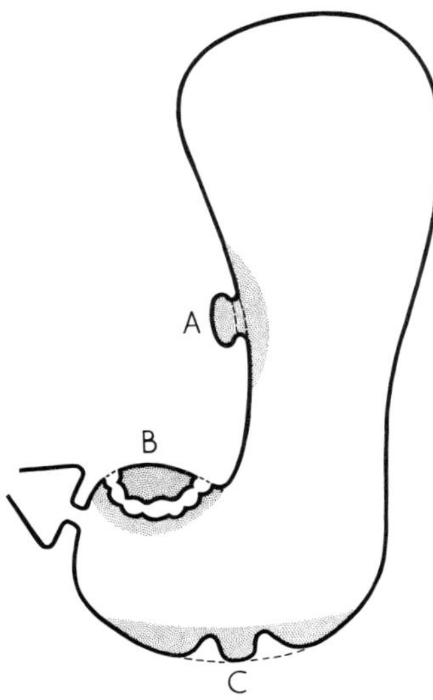

Fig. 30.17 Diagram illustrating three characteristic types of gastric ulcer. The shading represents barium. **A.** Benign, projecting, lesser curvature ulcer with collar (broken lines). **B.** Malignant, intraluminal ulcer with irregular, nodular tumour rim. **C.** Non-projecting benign greater curvature ulcer.

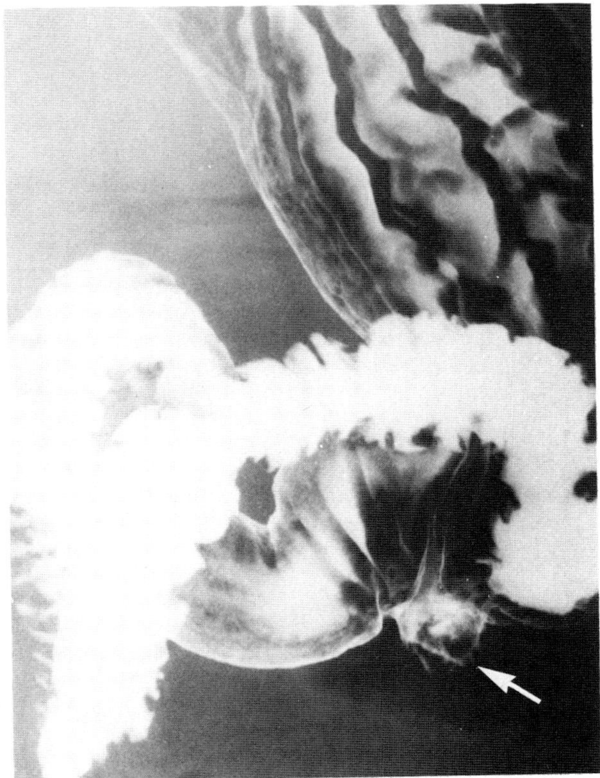

Fig. 30.18 Benign gastric ulcer on the greater curvature. The ulcer crater (arrow) projects only slightly from the line of the greater curvature. It has an irregular base and contains several filling defects. At least two radiating mucosal folds extend to the edge of the crater. It is typical of benign ulcers in this location to be non-projecting. (Courtesy of Dr R Lowe.)

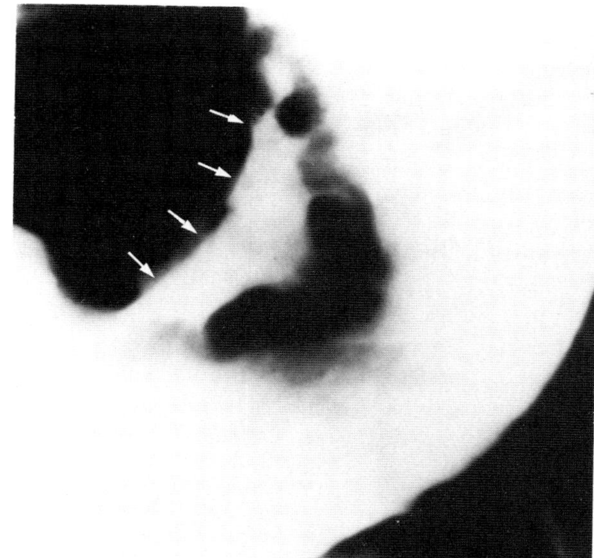

Fig. 30.19 Malignant gastric ulcer. Single contrast examination. The appearances are typical, and strongly diagnostic of malignancy. The ulcer is situated close to the lesser curvature and near the incisura angularis. The arrows indicate the base of the ulcer in line with the lesser curvature i.e. the crater is non-projecting. The translucent tumour mound around the crater is nodular and of variable width. There is no clearly defined 'meniscus', but the curve of the interface between ulcer and tumour mound is convex towards the lumen.

curved interface resembling a meniscus and called *Carman's meniscus sign*. By means of compression and positioning the patient under fluoroscopic control it is possible to 'fold' and superimpose the two halves of an ulcer as it 'saddles' the lesser curvature of the stomach. In profile the floor of the crater forms the straight external edge or 'fold' in line with the adjacent curvature. The meniscus component of this uncommon sign is the cause of considerable confusion. Whether the meniscus is concave or convex towards the lumen is mainly dependent upon the site of the ulcer relative to the incisura angularis. The reason for this is difficult to explain but is related to the way in which the examiner can alter the radiographic representation by positioning the patient and by palpation. Most carcinomatous ulcers exhibiting Carman's meniscus sign are distal to the incisura, with the meniscus convex towards the lumen. A malignant ulcer near the lesser curvature proximal to the incisura usually has a meniscus concave towards the lumen. This rare sign, if correctly interpreted, is a reliable indicator of malignancy.

The ulcer brim. The mound of oedema at the brim of a benign ulcer crater is smooth and clearly defined, whereas a malignant ulcer is characterized by an irregular nodular or ill-defined tumour mound.

The surrounding mucosa. When radiating folds reach the edge of an ulcer it is very likely to be benign (Fig. 30.16A & C). However, if a mound of oedema is present at the brim of a benign ulcer the folds usually terminate at the outer edge of the mound (Fig. 30.16B). The presence of clubbing, irregularity, thickening or amputation of folds is suggestive of malignancy. An assessment is also made of the areae gastricae of the mucosa around an ulcer, and if normal areae gastricae can be seen extending to the edge of an ulcer then malignancy is very unlikely.

In summary:

1. 95% of gastric ulcers are benign.
2. Projecting ulcers are common, and nearly always benign.
3. Non-projecting ulcers are uncommon, and nearly always malignant (but see 5).
4. Most malignant ulcers are non-projecting.
5. Greater curvature ulcers are infrequent, and most of them are benign, irrespective of whether they are projecting or non-projecting.
6. Carman's meniscus sign is rare, but when correctly interpreted is a reliable indicator of malignancy.
7. An ulcer with radiating folds which reach the edge of the crater is nearly always benign.

Management policy for ulcers

This has been revolutionized by the advent of the fibre-optic endoscope. Everybody agrees that all **gastric ulcers** must be followed up until healed. Most authorities advocate fibre-optic endoscopy with multiple biopsies of all gastric ulcers with repeat endoscopy at intervals until complete healing occurs. Others use the barium meal for follow-up purposes after an initial endoscopy has produced satisfactory biopsy specimens showing no sign of carcinoma. As the great majority of gastric ulcers are benign a third body of opinion favours restricting endoscopy to those few cases which do not conform on the initial or follow-up barium meal examination to the characteristic radiographic appearances of benignancy.

It is important to be aware of the limitations of endoscopy imposed by observer error, faulty technique and the inadequacy of forceps biopsy. In one recent series (Fraser & Earnshaw 1983) 13% of gastric ulcers were not identified at the initial endoscopy. Of these 7 ulcers, 3 were high on the lesser curvature just below the cardia and 2 were at the incisura. It is likely that further technical developments in endoscope design will improve accuracy. Histological reports on biopsy material can also be unreliable. Radiology and endoscopy are therefore complementary techniques that should be employed sensibly, whilst bearing in mind the clinical features of each particular case.

Surgery is indicated when biopsy for carcinoma is positive, for some very large benign ulcers, for ulcers of any size where healing is protracted, and when significant complications arise. Even at surgery it may not be possible to differentiate between a chronic benign gastric ulcer and a carcinomatous ulcer. The microscopical examination of frozen sections of an ulcer obtained on the operating table are a useful guide to the surgeon, but are not infallible.

For practical purposes all **duodenal ulcers** are benign. An initial barium meal or endoscopy is necessary for diagnosis, but unless there is a change in symptoms follow-up barium examinations are not required.

Ulcers at unusual sites

Pyloric canal ulcers are relatively uncommon and nearly always benign (Fig. 30.20). Most of them are small, but associated spasm frequently produces gastric outflow obstruction. The term *juxtapyloric* is used to include ulcers not only in the pyloric canal but also close to it, either at the base of the duodenal cap or in the distal gastric antrum. As a result of accompanying spasm and deformity it is often difficult to precisely localize these ulcers.

Postbulbar ulcers are uncommon, probably accounting for less than 5% of duodenal ulcers. They usually present with pain and haemorrhage. Typically a crater of about 1 cm diameter is present in the second part of the duodenum just beyond the cap, with associated intense annular spasm or fibrosis and abrupt 'shoulders' simulating a carcinoma of the duodenum or annular pancreas (Fig. 30.21). Healing by fibrosis produces a deep incisura or ring-like narrowing.

Ulcer healing

Most patients with peptic ulceration undergo treatment with an H_2 histamine receptor antagonist such as cimetidine which blocks the stimulation of acid secretion. The manifestations of healing **gastric ulcers** are related to the size, depth, site and chronicity of the ulcer. Initially the crater becomes smaller and any surrounding ulcer mound due to inflammatory oedema disappears. This allows radiating folds which may previously have stopped short at the outer edge of the ulcer mound to continue to the rim of the crater. Progressive healing often results in the formation of a small residual depression known as an ulcer scar with radiating folds (Fig. 30.22A).

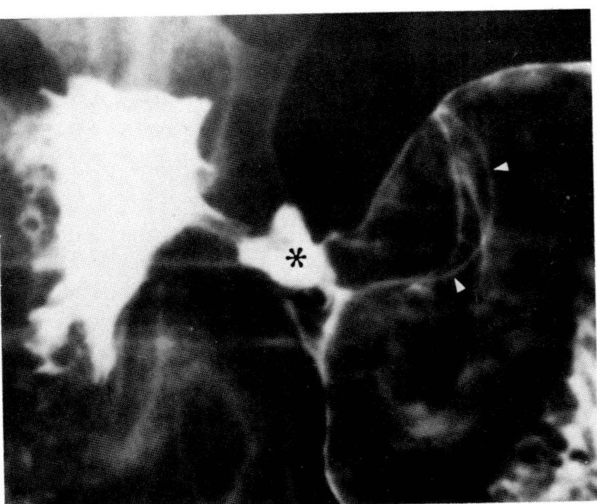

Fig. 30.20 Benign pyloric ulceration. An ulcer crater (*) is present in the posterior wall of the pyloric canal. An associated inflammatory mass is producing an impression (white arrowheads) on the gastric antrum.

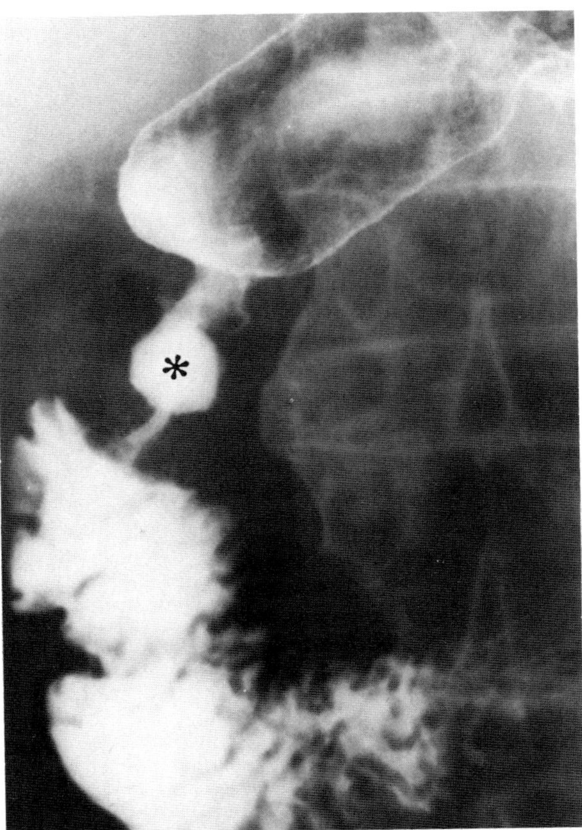

Fig. 30.21 Postbulbar duodenal ulcer. Characteristic appearance with ulcer crater (*) in the middle of a stricture produced by spasm and oedema.

Small ulcers often heal without any scarring, the appearances returning entirely to normal. Occasionally radiating folds persist in the absence of an ulcer scar. A collection of barium within a depressed ulcer scar can simulate an active ulcer crater, and endoscopy is necessary to confirm complete healing.

Ulcers on the lesser curvature are particularly liable to exhibit prominent scarring, which may take one of several forms. An *incisura* is seen as a band-like translucency extending towards the ulcer from the greater curvature opposite; quite small ulcers may be associated with prominent incisuras. When an ulcer heals a permanent *constriction* may remain dividing the stomach into two chambers and giving rise to the description *'hour-glass stomach'* (Fig. 30.22B). Longitudinal scarring and contraction of the lesser curvature also occurs leading to elevation of the antrum and duodenal cap which become apparently 'hitched up' to produce an appearance which has been likened to a tea pot or watering can. Other forms of bizarre

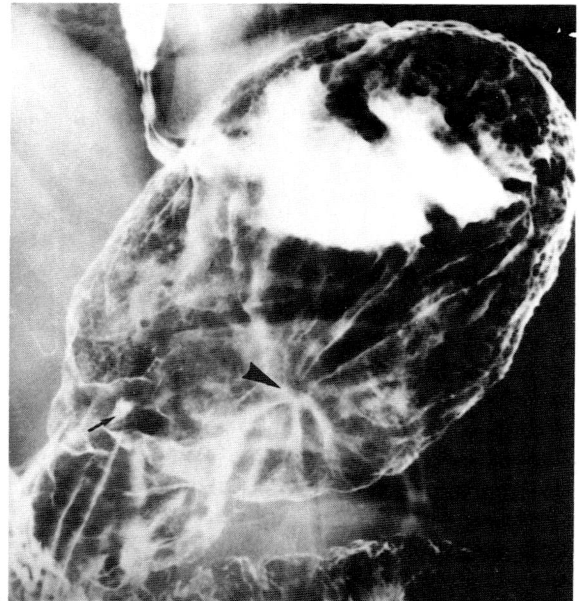

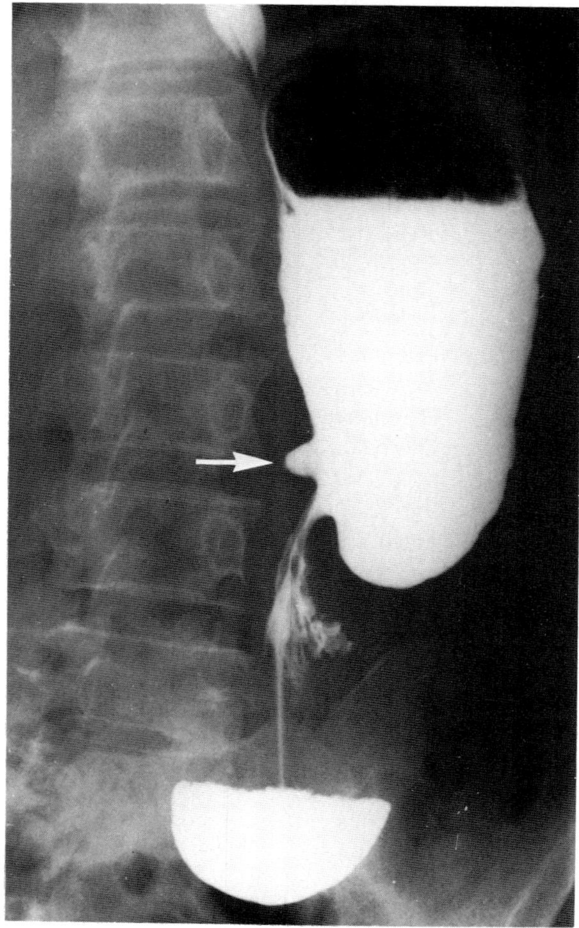

Fig. 30.22 Healing benign gastric ulcers. **A.** Ulcer scar (arrowhead). Mucosal folds radiate towards a scar at the site of a previous ulcer crater. A small crater (arrow) is also present. **B.** Incisura and 'hourglass' stomach. A typical benign ulcer on the mid-lesser curvature of the stomach is associated with a prominent incisura which divides the stomach into two, and is producing obstruction.

deformity may result from scarring following chronic penetration and perforation of large lesser curvature ulcers.

Small **duodenal ulcers** may heal without scarring, but commonly radiating folds persist. Contraction of scars towards the site of a healing (Fig. 30.23A) or healed ulcer produces characteristic pouches known as pseudodiverticula. Many patterns of scarring occur ranging from a grossly narrowed almost obliterated channel to a regular symmetrical arrangement of pseudodiverticula resembling the shape of a clover leaf (Fig. 30.23B). The detection of an ulcer crater in a severely deformed cap, and the differentiation of a pseudodiverticulum from a large ulcer is sometimes very difficult; the presence of radiating folds from an ulcer crater is usually the best discriminator.

COMPLICATIONS OF PEPTIC ULCERATION

Bleeding

In patients presenting with haematemesis and melaena the history may lead to a correct diagnosis of the underlying disorder, but more frequently the actual site of haemorrhage cannot be localized. The major sources of upper gastrointestinal (GI) bleeding are *oesophageal varices*, *oesophagitis*, the *Mallory-Weiss syndrome*, *peptic ulcers* (gastric and duodenal), *haemorrhagic* or *drug-induced erosive gastritis*, and *neoplasms*.

The site of active upper GI bleeding can usually be identified by **endoscopic examination** of the oesophagus stomach and duodenum. Success in identifying a bleeding site is dependent upon the timing of the examination. Definite evidence that a particular lesion was responsible for bleeding has been found in about 70% of those endoscoped within 12 hrs of admission but in only 40% of those studied after that time. Similar results have been achieved by double contrast barium examination. It is necessary to appreciate that the site of bleeding is not determined by the detection of a lesion but by the identification of active bleeding. For example, up to 50% of patients with massive bleeding and known cirrhosis bleed from a non-variceal cause.

The *radiological signs* indicating that a particular lesion is the site of recent or continued bleeding are:

1. Blood clot seen as an irregular translucent defect (the so-called Berg's nodule) in the base of a barium-filled ulcer crater, or forming over a bleeding point (Fig. 30.24A).
2. An artery in the base of an ulcer, seen as a small, round, translucent defect (Fig. 30.24B).
3. Active bleeding detected on fluoroscopy by the identification of non-opaque blood displacing the barium in a manner likened to 'larval flow' (Fig. 30.24C).

In most centres the primary procedure for investigating patients with upper GI bleeding is endoscopy. Barium examination is not used much in acute bleeding because it

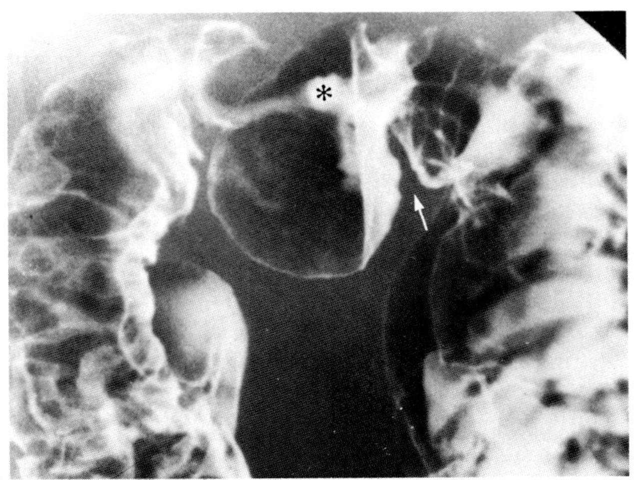

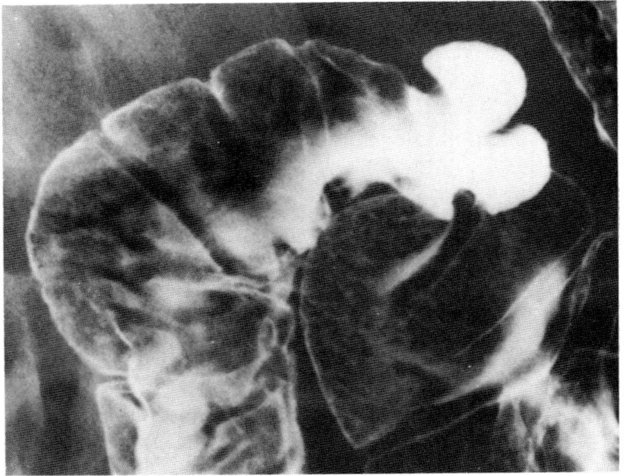

Fig. 30.23 Healing duodenal ulcers. **A.** Supine view. An ulcer crater (*) is associated with deformity of the cap. A deep incisura is present inferiorly (arrow). **B.** Scarring of the duodenal cap resulting from a chronic duodenal ulcer which has now healed. The pouches produced by the scarring resemble the shape of a clover leaf.

interferes with other investigations (e.g. angiography) for several days.

In selected cases *endoscopic haemostasis* may be attempted by means of electrocoagulation or continuous wave argon ion lasers. Continued development of laser technology is likely to make this technique more generally available than at present.

For patients not responding adequately to conservative management and with signs of active bleeding, *angiography* should be considered as a prelude to vasoconstrictor therapy or surgery. The lowest rate of haemorrhage detectable by angiography is generally accepted as 0.5 ml/min, but in clinical practice a higher rate is usually necessary. Nasogastric aspiration in the angiography suite will indicate if bleeding is active and will also allow estimation of the rate of blood loss. The Seldinger technique via the femoral artery is employed and a coeliac arteriogram and appropriate selective studies are performed. The detection of extravasated contrast material in the gut lumen precisely localizes the bleeding point. It is then possible to attempt to undertake *transcatheter haemostasis*. The two methods which have been successfully applied are vasoconstrictor and embolic therapy. *Vasopressin* (*Pitressin*) is administered selectively by direct intra-arterial injection into a bleeding vessel. A number of agents have been employed for *embolic therapy*, including autogenous clot, Gelfoam and steel coils.

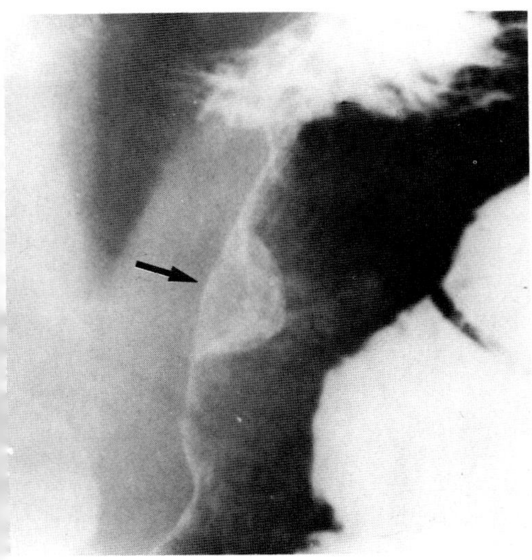

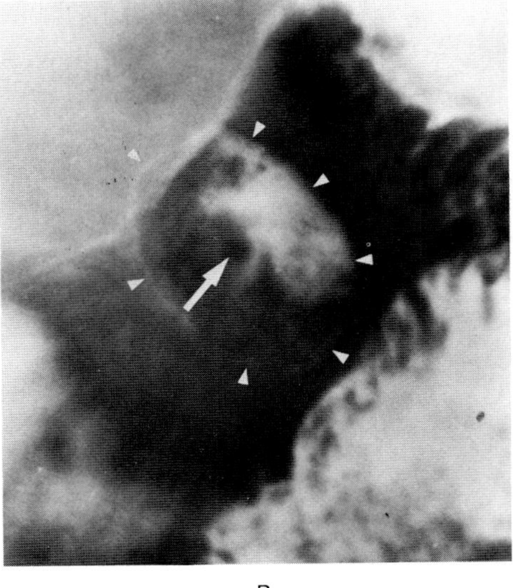

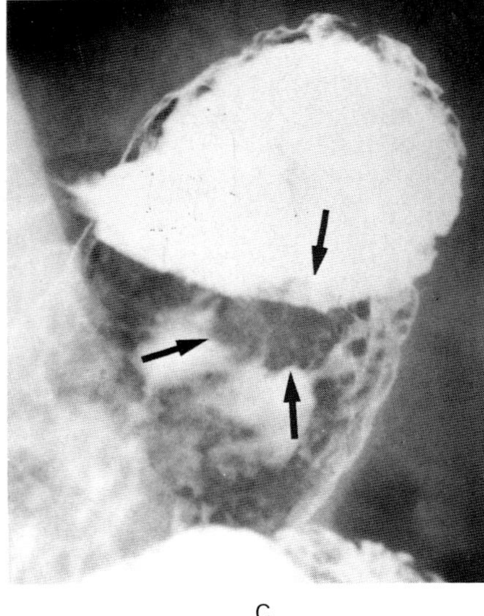

Fig. 30.24 Signs of acute gastrointestinal bleeding. **A.** An appearance simulating a polyp, but in fact due to a blood clot adherent over a bleeding site. **B.** Large lesser curvature gastric ulcer with a small round central lucency (large arrow) due to a bleeding artery in the base of the ulcer. **C.** Active bleeding seen as an area of gastric mucosa which fails to coat with barium (arrows). Barium is constantly washed away by the non-opaque blood. (Courtesy of Dr G M Fraser, and the Editor of *Clinical Radiology*.)

If transcatheter haemostasis is unsuccessful, surgery is necessary.

Another method of detecting upper GI bleeding is with *radioisotopes*. Several radionuclides have been tried including ^{131}I-labelled albumin, ^{51}Cr-labelled RBC and ^{99}Tc^{m} sulphur colloid, all with some success. Further developments are likely.

Within any medical institution the policy for investigation and treatment of acute upper GI bleeding is dependent upon clinical factors and the local availability of skilled personnel and facilities for undertaking endoscopic and angiographic examinations. A clinical history, physical examination and resuscitation of the patient always precede any other procedures. Patients with slow or arrested bleeding are usually subjected to endoscopy or double contrast barium meal preferably within 12 h of the bleed, or on the next available session. Those with active bleeding are endoscoped as soon as possible, immediately followed by angiography and angiographic haemostasis if a bleeding point has been localized. Surgery is undertaken if necessary.

Perforation

Perforation of an ulcer into the peritoneal cavity or into adjacent organs usually results in an 'acute abdomen'. Free intraperitoneal gas is reliably identified by supine and horizontal beam plain radiography. The erect PA chest film is the most valuable in demonstrating free gas which will be seen in approximately 70% of perforated ulcers. A decubitus view of the abdomen with the patient's right side uppermost is a useful alternative for those not fit enough to stand. The use of a water-soluble contrast agent has been advocated in suspected ulcer perforation by Fraser (1983, personal communication). Oral Gastrografin will increase the diagnostic accuracy to the region of 96%. Radiographs taken following Gastrografin will also differentiate between perforated ulcer and acute pancreatitis in the majority of cases. This can be very helpful (especially to junior surgical staff in the middle of the night) when there is clinical doubt and before the result of the serum amylase estimation is available.

Penetration

Chronic ulcers may extend to penetrate adjacent organs. Whilst the great majority of gastric ulcers are less than 2 cm in diameter, and duodenal ulcers less than 1 cm, giant ulcers occur in both locations.

Most *giant gastric ulcers* occur in elderly patients and arise high on the lesser curvature, excavating posteriorly into the bed of the pancreas (Fig. 30.25). The demon-

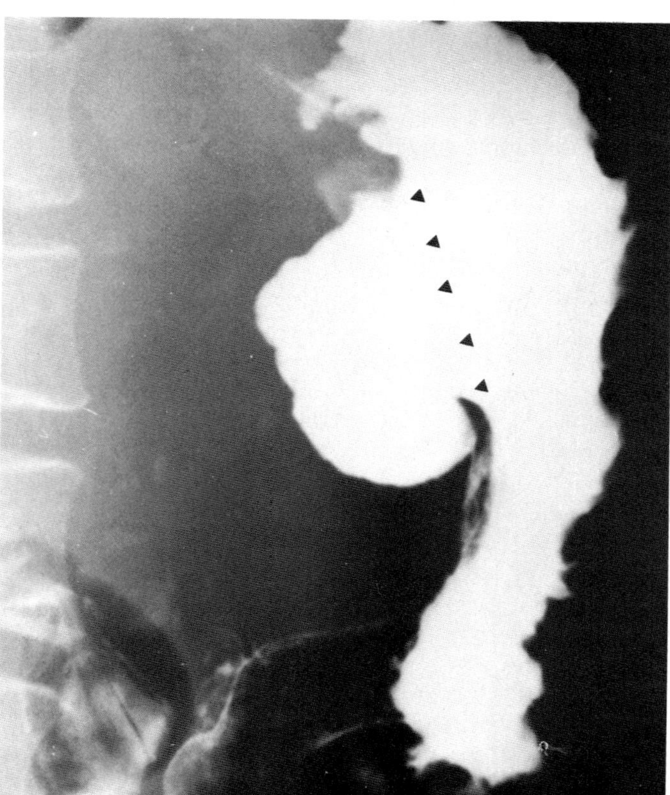

Fig. 30.25 Giant benign lesser curvature gastric ulcer projecting from the posterior wall of the stomach and penetrating into the pancreas.

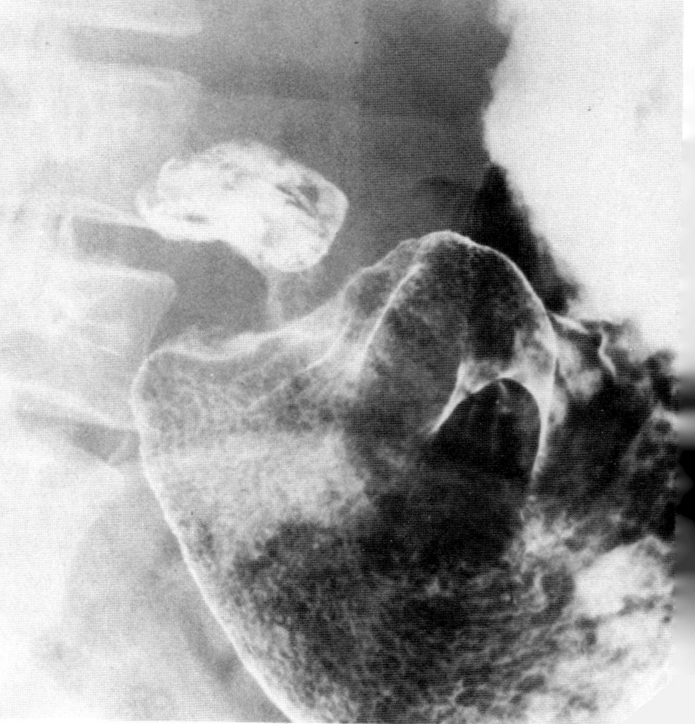

Fig. 30.26 Giant duodenal ulcer replacing the duodenal cap. Translucencies within the ulcer are due to food and other debris. An associated inflammatory mass surrounding the ulcer crater is responsible for the extrinsic impression in the distal gastric antrum. (Courtesy of Dr D J Lintott.)

stration on an erect film of a fluid level in a gastric ulcer almost invariably means that the ulcer has penetrated through the gastric wall.

Giant duodenal ulcers are by definition more than 2 cm in diameter. They are often difficult to diagnose because the crater may replace and thus simulate the barium-filled duodenal cap (Fig. 30.26). However, unlike a normal cap, a giant ulcer has a tendency to retain barium, and maintains a fairly constant size and shape throughout the course of the examination; it is usually rounded in shape, and often contains debris but not mucosa.

Duodenal ulcers, especially large ones, have a tendency to be surrounded by an inflammatory mass arising in response to penetration and chronic perforation. This mass may compress the lumen of the duodenal cap and produce a pressure defect in the adjacent gastric antrum simulating carcinoma of the stomach, but the presence of duodenal involvement makes the latter diagnosis unlikely.

Fistulae arise from penetration of a duodenal ulcer into the biliary tract (Fig. 30.27), or from a gastric ulcer eroding into the colon usually at the splenic flexure.

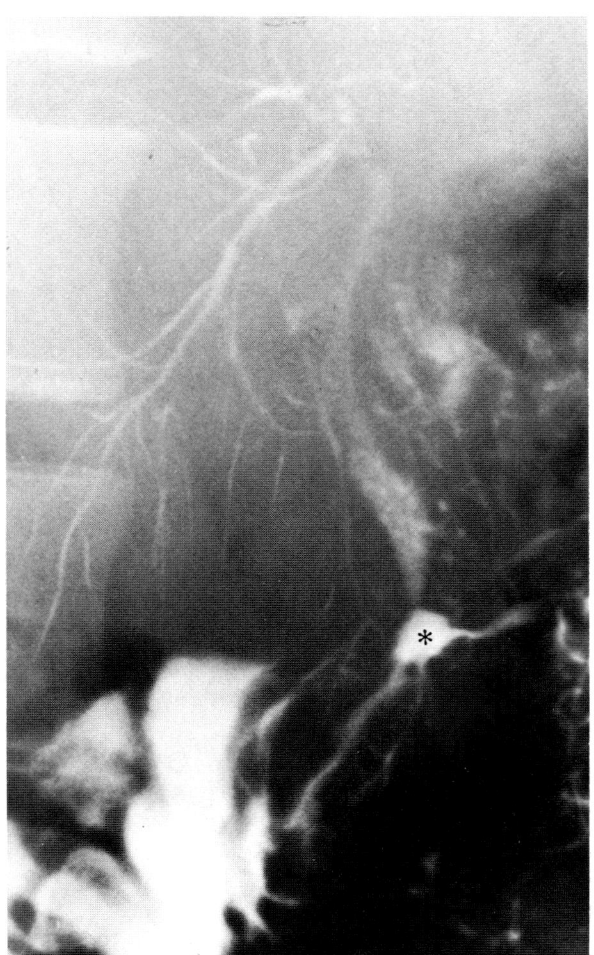

Fig. 30.27 Duodenal ulcer (*) eroding into the common bile duct. Barium is seen in the biliary tree.

Obstruction

Juxtapyloric ulcers with associated spasm or fibrosis produce gastric outflow obstruction (*pyloric stenosis*). As a result the stomach is distended with fluid and food, and this can be determined on plain radiography. If necessary a mouthful of barium can be given for confirmation, and on fluoroscopy the barium is seen dispersing into the pool of fluid lying within the distended atonic stomach (Fig. 30.28A). In these circumstances it is unlikely that the cause of obstruction will be accurately identified at this stage. It is advisable therefore to hospitalize the patient for gastric aspiration and lavage prior to a repeat barium examination a few days later when the stomach will be empty and have recovered some of its tone (Fig. 30.28B).

By positioning the patient in the prone oblique position with the right side down barium will almost always pass through the obstruction and allow its nature to be determined. The main causes of gastric outflow obstruction are scarring and stenosis due to *juxtapyloric* or *duodenal ulceration*, and *carcinoma* of the gastric antrum or pyloric canal. Differentiation between benign ulcer and carcinoma by barium meal can be difficult and endoscopy with biopsy may be necessary.

POSTOPERATIVE RADIOLOGY

The great majority of patients undergoing gastric surgery do so because of peptic ulcer disease or carcinoma of the stomach. Each surgeon's skill and training largely determines what particular operation is performed. Surgical procedures for peptic disease fall into three main groups: 1. gastrectomy, 2. vagotomy and 3. drainage procedures.

There are many varieties of **partial gastrectomy**. The more common surgical eponyms used in Great Britain and North America are as follows:

Billroth I — Partial gastrectomy (antrectomy) with gastroduodenostomy (Fig. 30.29A).

Billroth II — Partial gastrectomy (antrectomy) with gastrojejunostomy.

Polya — Partial gastrectomy (antrectomy) with gastrojejunostomy, using the entire cut end of the stomach for the anastomosis (Fig. 30.29B).

Hofmeister — A Polya with a restricted stoma, and partial closure of the cut end of the stomach.

Vagotomy may be truncal, selective (total gastric) or highly selective (proximal gastric). Truncal and selective vagotomy require an added drainage procedure either a pyloroplasty or gastroenterostomy, in order to assist gastric emptying. A drainage procedure is not necessary with a highly selective vagotomy because the vagal fibres to the gastric antrum are left intact so that the 'antral pump' is

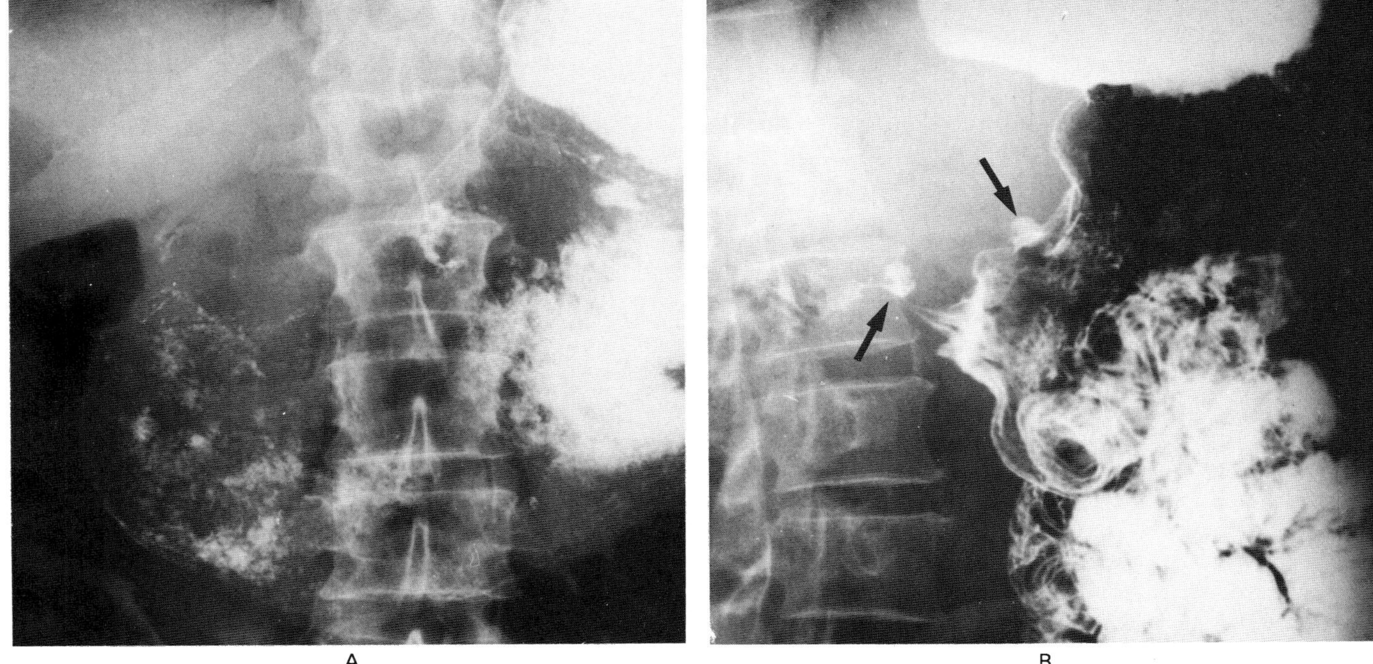

Fig. 30.28 Illustration of technique in gastric outflow obstruction. **A.** Distended stomach with outflow obstruction. Retained fluid gastric contents prevent adequate barium examination. **B.** One week later following repeated aspiration and lavage. The stomach is now smaller, having regained its normal tone and activity. Gastric emptying is rapid. Two ulcers are demonstrated (arrows), one on the lesser curvature of the stomach and the other at the base of the duodenal cap (juxtapyloric) associated with considerable scarring.

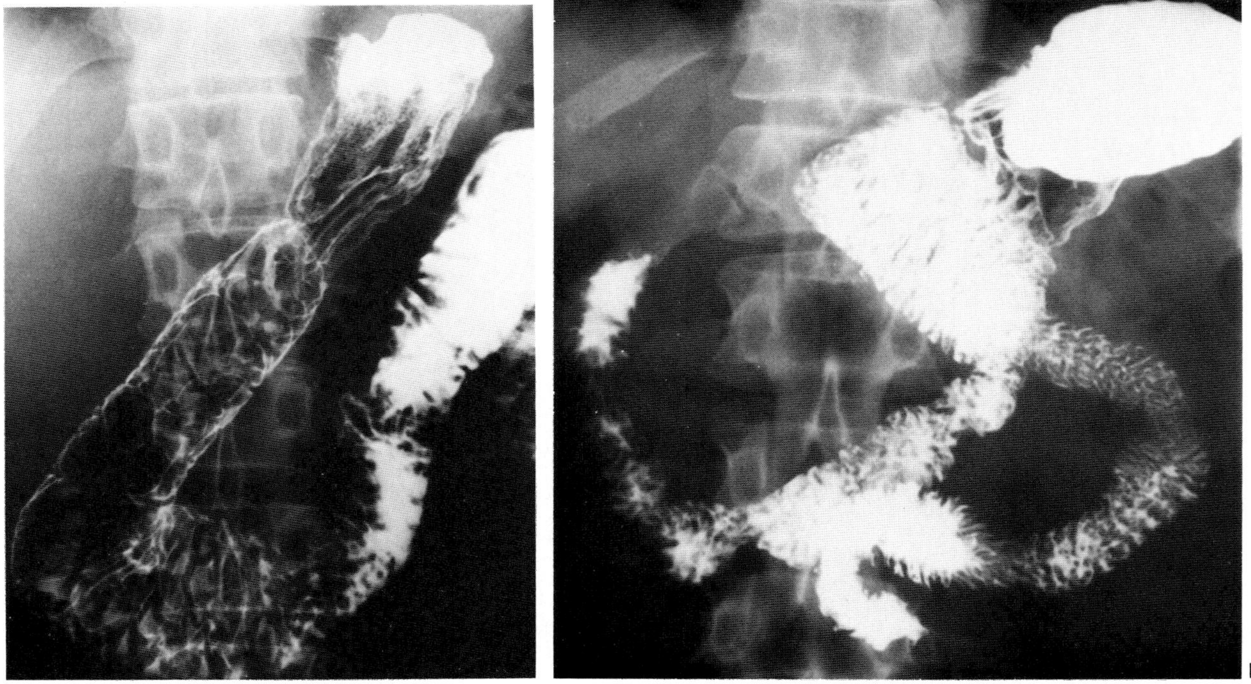

Fig. 30.29 Normal postoperative barium examinations following partial gastrectomy. **A.** Bilroth I. **B.** Polya. (Moynihan modification with left to right direction of anastomosis.)

still active in emptying the stomach. Many surgeons routinely combine vagotomy with partial gastrectomy.

The usual method of **pyloroplasty** consists of making a longitudinal incision in the line of the pyloric canal extending for a length of about 5 cm on either side of the pylorus, and then sewing the cut edges at right angles to the incision. This results in a widened channel with two large pouches or 'ears' (Fig. 30.30).

The most common variety of gastroenterostomy is, in fact, a **gastrojejunostomy**, whereby a loop of proximal jejunum is anastomosed posteriorly to the 'sump' of the stomach to produce a 'short circuit', whilst leaving the normal gastric outflow route intact (Fig. 30.31).

Another frequently performed operation is a **Roux-en-Y** procedure consisting of an end to side jejunojejunostomy (Fig. 30.32). This technique is usually employed following a total or subtotal gastrectomy, and provides a route back into the normal channel for bile and pancreatic secretions, whilst at the same time reducing the susceptibility to bile reflux into the gastric remnant or oesophagus. This is achieved by relocating the blind loop into which the common bile duct opens in a more distal position.

Many disorders follow surgery to the gastrointestinal tract. For accurate diagnosis the radiologist must have the relevant clinical and surgical details, and in particular an indication from the surgeon as to what he thinks may be wrong, or what he would like to exclude. The radiologist is then in a position to tailor his technique accordingly, and to focus his attention on the likely site of abnormality. Also the selection of the most appropriate technique depends upon the questions that need answering. The great majority of cases fall into two main groups:

1. *Early problems*: usually leakage from suture lines, obstruction or disordered function.
2. *Late problems*: usually mechanical, bleeding, ulceration, recurrence of tumour or disordered function.

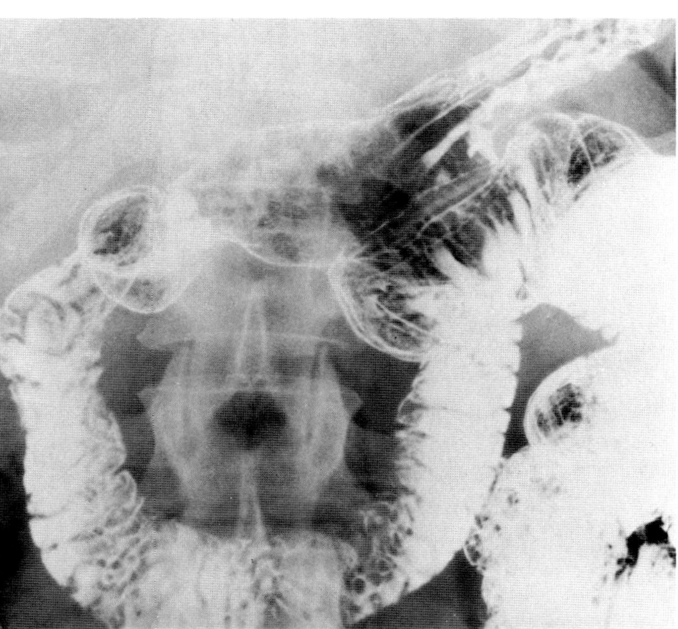

Fig. 30.31 Gastroenterostomy. A gastrojejunostomy with a wide stoma.

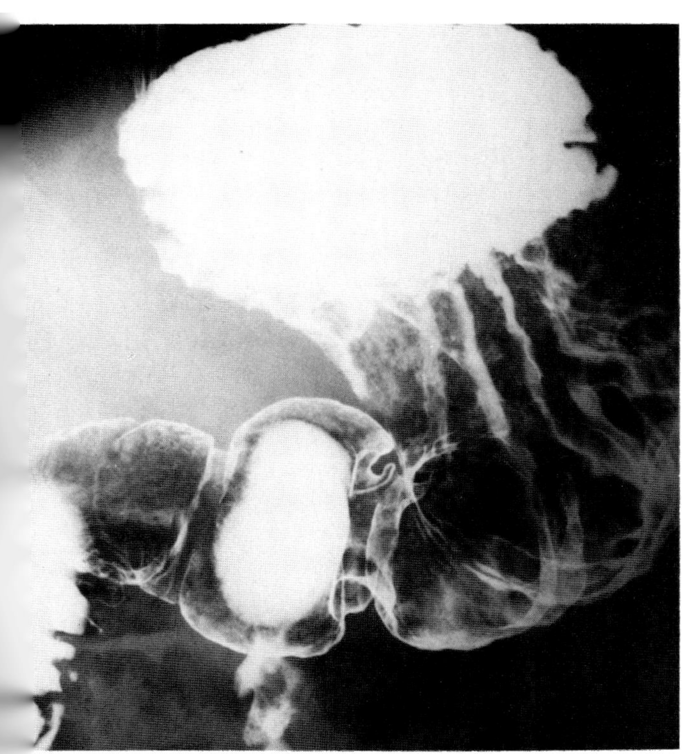

Fig. 30.30 Pyloroplasty. A wide gastroduodenal channel has been produced. (Courtesy of Dr A Chapman.)

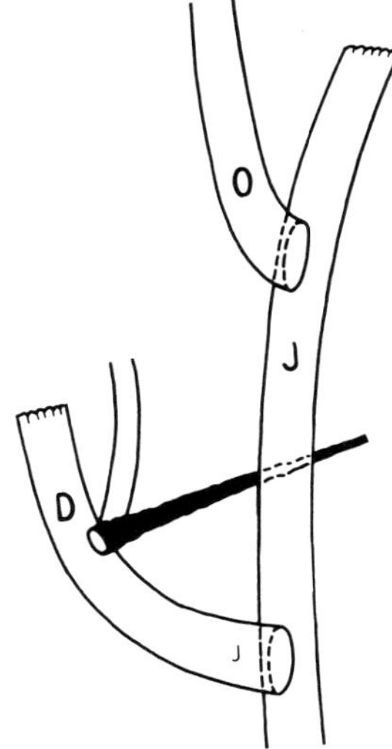

Fig. 30.32 Diagram illustrating the Roux-en-Y procedure (not to scale). A total gastrectomy has been performed with an end to side oesophagojejunostomy, and lower down is the roux-en-Y consisting of an end to side jejunojejunostomy. O = oesophagus, D = duodenum, J = jejunum.

There is controversy about the relative merits of endoscopy and contrast examination after gastric or duodenal surgery. Most authorities agree that contrast studies are to be preferred during the early postoperative period for showing the origin and extent of leakage, the site and degree of obstruction, and atony. Later, if there is haemorrhage or if stomal ulceration or tumour recurrence are suspected, endoscopy is the primary procedure of choice. However, in expert hands the double contrast barium meal still has a useful role.

Plain abdominal radiographs are useful before any postoperative contrast study in order to show:

1. air-fluid levels indicating obstruction or abscess
2. distended bowel
3. free intraperitoneal air
4. metallic surgical material such as sutures and clips which are a guide to previous operative procedures, suture lines and anastomoses
5. retained foreign bodies, e.g. surgical instruments and swabs (sponges) with opaque markers.

The immediate postoperative examination

A water-soluble contrast medium, such as Gastrografin, is suitable for most cases, but a low osmolar agent is preferable in neonates or when there is a risk of contrast entering the bronchial tree.

Most patients soon after a surgical operation on the abdomen are weak and uncomfortable, and those coming for radiological examination are likely to be suffering from low morale because they are aware that 'something has gone wrong' with the operation. Such patients therefore need especially careful handling. They should arrive in the radiology department suitably attired without need for undressing. The X-ray room should be ready to receive the patient immediately and all preparations for the examination should be carried out beforehand. The team of assistants should be ready; at least two helpers are necessary to handle the contrast, lift, manipulate, assist and support the patient, and look after the paraphernalia of stands, tubes, wires, bottles and bags. The examination should be conducted in a manner dependent upon the state of the patient, the operative procedure that has been performed and the clinical factors. It should be performed as rapidly as possible and terminated as soon as the necessary information has been obtained.

Bearing in mind that *suspected leakage* or *obstruction* are the most likely indications for contrast studies in the early postoperative period it is necessary to examine the patient supine, on both sides, and erect or semi erect. Contrast may be conveniently administered via a nasogastric tube which is likely to be in place, or else by mouth. Hypotonic agents such as Buscopan are contraindicated. Spot films are taken at opportune moments. The radiographs should be processed quickly whilst the patient remains lying on the table, and as soon as they are seen to be satisfactory the patient is returned to the ward after a few words of encouragement from the radiologist about the findings. To give an appreciation of the sequence of events it is helpful to number the radiographs in the order that they are taken.

Gastric outflow obstruction resulting from oedema and haematoma around the stoma may follow partial gastrectomy and gastroenterostomy, especially posterior gastrojejunostomy. Some degree of gastric stasis is normal for a few days after surgery on the stomach. Gastrografin examination is indicated if gastric retention persists for longer than four or five days, and this will readily distinguish between obstruction at the stoma and gastric atony with a patent anastomosis. As stomal oedema subsides patency is established and a further laparotomy is avoided.

The commonest early complication to be encountered following gastroenterostomy is **efferent loop obstruction** due to haematoma or oedema at the stoma. This leads to '*afferent loop circuit*' movement of Gastrografin through the pylorus, duodenum, afferent loop and back into the stomach via the unobstructed afferent loop side of the stoma.

Following partial gastrectomy, jejunal obstruction may result from a postgastrectomy internal hernia and contrast will not enter the affected loop.

In suspected **duodenal stump rupture** or **anastomotic leakage** radiographic examination with a water-soluble contrast agent is indicated, because early surgical intervention is necessary. Rupture of the duodenal stump is one of the gravest complications of gastric surgery and occurs without warning any time during the first three weeks after operation. Stump leakage may produce a sinus to a right subphrenic abscess. Anastomotic leakage following partial gastrectomy usually occurs on the lesser curvature angle and may result from an area of ischaemia. A sinus may lead to a left subphrenic abscess.

The late postoperative examination

This is performed using a standard barium sulphate preparation by either a single or double contrast technique according to the anticipated abnormality.

Single contrast examination is the method of choice when one is looking for a fistula or for the direction and rate of flow. Under fluoroscopic control the patient should first be given one mouthful of barium to swallow in the standing position. This will reveal the nature of the operative procedure and the presence or absence of obstruction. The examination should then be continued with the table in a horizontal position. Further barium administration combined with appropriate posturing of the patient and palpation will enable the gastric remnant, stoma and small bowel loops to be filled and examined.

Double contrast barium meal is the technique of choice in most circumstances. The postoperative examination is less amenable to standardization than the regular examination and is conducted at all stages according to the questions that need to be answered and the nature of the surgery that has been performed. For instance, following partial gastrectomy for peptic ulcer disease the most frequent questions are, 'Is there any stomal ulceration?' and, 'Is the stomach emptying properly?' An outline of the procedure usually adopted by the author is as follows:

An initial mouthful of high-density barium is given under fluoroscopic control with the patient standing as for the single contrast method. Several exposures are made to record the direction and rate of flow. Then a gas-producing mixture is administered and the table lowered to a horizontal position. Films of the stoma are obtained at this early stage before it becomes obscured by barium-filled loops of small bowel. Additional barium is next given through a straw with the patient either prone or lying on one side. The pharynx and oesophagus are examined in this position and then, depending upon the operative procedure, further attention is given to gastric emptying, stomal function and filling of afferent and efferent loops of small bowel. Further exposures are made at opportune moments as required. The timing of administration of Buscopan is dependent upon the particular circumstances of each individual examination.

In the presence of a *gastroenterostomy* it is necessary to examine both the normal channel and the stoma. Usually barium will preferentially leave the stomach via the new route. Then by turning the patient on to the right side whilst drinking barium through a straw, it is usually possible to fill the antrum, duodenal cap and loop via the normal route (Fig. 30.31). In the years following an effective gastroenterostomy the old route atrophies with the antrum becoming narrowed and tubular. Scarring of the duodenal cap by ulceration, for which the operative procedure was performed, is permanent.

LATE COMPLICATIONS

Following surgery for peptic disease, problems arising outside the immediate postoperative period for which a double contrast barium meal may be performed include obstruction (including bezoars and intussusception), haemorrhage, postoperative ulcer disease, retained gastric antrum, fistula, postgastrectomy syndromes (including dumping and malabsorption) and afferent loop obstruction.

Barium examination is useful in suspected **stomal obstruction**. The site and degree of obstruction are readily determined, and in most cases the cause. *Prolapse of gastric mucosa* through the stoma is usually symptomless, but can produce partial obstruction. A polypoid mucosal filling defect in the stoma is shown with barium. *Jejunogastric intussusception* may be acute or chronic. Barium examination characteristically shows obstruction and a filling defect in the stomach above the stoma which can be identified as jejunum by the striated 'coil-spring' appearance of the oedematous valvulae conniventes (Fig. 30.33A). There is a tendency for **gastric bezoars** to follow gastric surgery, particularly partial gastrectomy with vagotomy, and these can obstruct the stoma. Most are due to a mass of matted vegetable or fruit pith (*phytobezoar*). Barium outlines the mass and penetrates the interstices producing a characteristic appearance (Fig. 30.33B). Gastric bezoars can also occur in the intact stomach (Fig. 30.51) including matted hair (*trichobezoar*).

Peptic oesophagitis from gastro oesophageal reflux, and oesophageal stricture resulting from acid gastric contents tracking up alongside an indwelling nasogastric tube are liable to occur following gastric surgery. *Gastritis* due to reflux of bile salts into the stomach is common following some operations, but usually subsides within a few weeks. If there is gastro-oesophageal reflux a bile oesophagitis results.

There are many causes of post-gastrectomy **haemorrhage**. *Ulceration* and *haemorrhagic gastritis* account for the majority. Endoscopy is the initial procedure of choice. In acute cases the site of bleeding is often successfully demonstrated by arteriography. A double contrast barium meal may be worthwhile in selected less acute cases.

Ulceration after gastric surgery for peptic disease may be due to recurrence at the original site, or more frequently at a new site (and therefore not recurrent) in the jejunum just distal to the anastomosis. These are known as marginal, stomal, or anastomotic ulcers (Fig. 30.34). This complication occurs most frequently following surgery for duodenal ulceration. The Bilroth I type of partial gastrectomy is particularly prone to stomal ulceration unless vagotomy is also performed, and is therefore mainly used in the treatment of gastric ulcers.

Signs of stomal ulceration on barium examination include an ulcer crater, radiating folds, stomal narrowing, thickened jejunal mucosal folds, irritability and spasm. Endoscopy is the procedure of choice when a stomal ulcer is suspected, but in expert hands a double contrast barium meal with Buscopan is almost as successful, showing an ulcer crater in about 50% of cases and indirect signs of ulceration such as mucosal fold thickening and irritability in a further 30%.

The identification of an ulcer crater following surgery is difficult for several reasons. With a freely patent stoma adequate distension is often not possible, flooding of jejunal loops with barium obscures the stoma; surgical deformities and in particular mucosal pouches simulate ulcer craters and some ulcers are extremely small and easily hidden amongst mucosal folds.

When following gastric surgery of the Polya variety a portion of the gastric antrum is unintentionally left behind at the end of the afferent loop, a source of gastrin remains. Acid production therefore continues, and marginal ulceration results. The **retained gastric antrum** can be detected

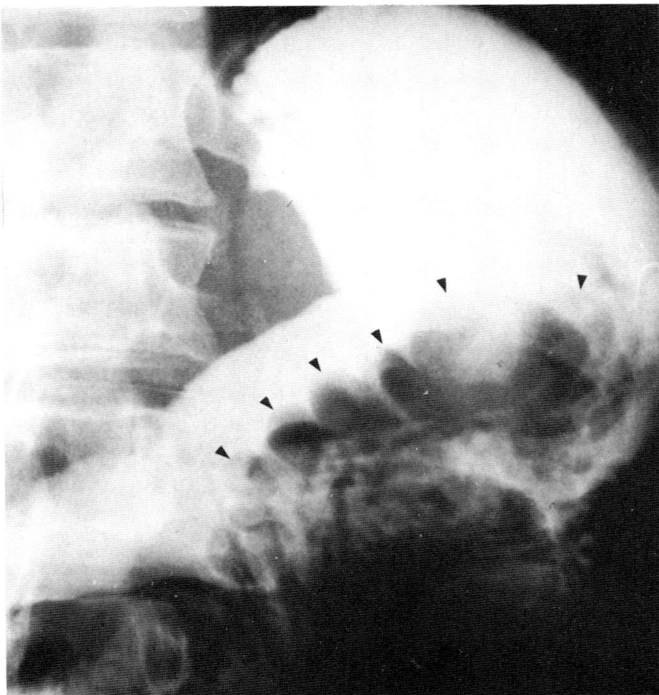

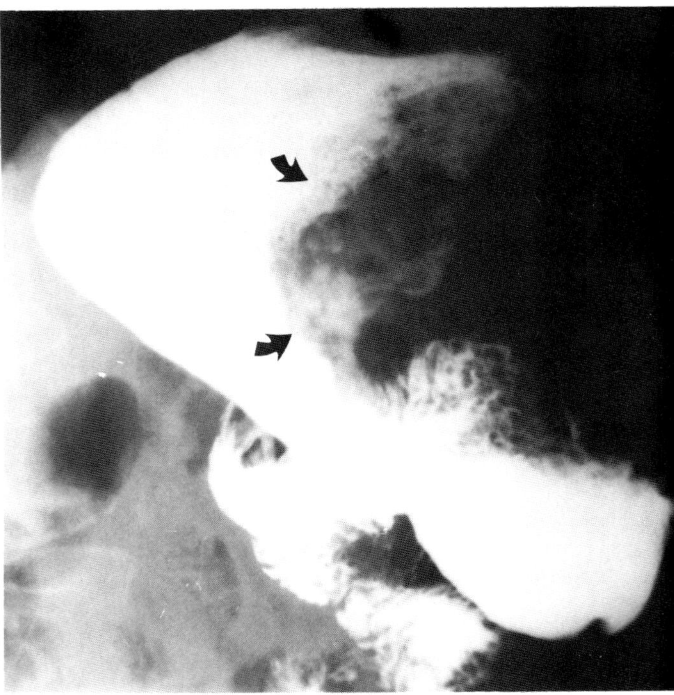

Fig. 30.33 Complications following gastric surgery. **A.** Retrograde jejunogastric intussusception following gastrojejunostomy. The loops of jejunum within the stomach (arrowed) have a characteristic 'coiled-spring' appearance. **B.** Bezoar formation following partial gastrectomy. There is a large filling defect (arrowed) in the gastric remnant due to a phytobezoar.

radiographically if there is sufficient filling of the afferent loop to allow barium to reflux from the duodenum via the pylorus into the antrum.

A chronic marginal ulcer is the commonest cause of a **gastrojejunocolic fistula**. A barium enema is more likely to show such a fistula than a meal. Less frequently a gastrocolic fistula is produced by extension and necrosis of a carcinoma either of the stomach or colon. A history of previous gastric surgery, particularly gastroenterostomy, is strong evidence that a chronic marginal ulcer is the cause of a fistula even when such an ulcer cannot be demonstrated.

Following resection or short-circuit operations on the stomach the patient may suffer from abdominal distension, nausea, sweating and faintness, which are symptoms of **the postgastrectomy syndrome**. The syndrome comprises mechanical dumping, the early postprandial dumping syndrome and late postprandial hypoglycaemia. Studies using a mixture of barium and food or glucose have been undertaken and the gastric emptying rate, small bowel transit time and contrast dilution have been recorded. However, the findings are inconsistent and therefore not generally regarded as useful.

After a Polya gastrectomy barium is seen to enter both the afferent and efferent loops, although most of it goes down the efferent loop. Appropriate posturing of the patient will usually enable the afferent loop to be filled. **The afferent loop syndrome** is characterized by postpran-

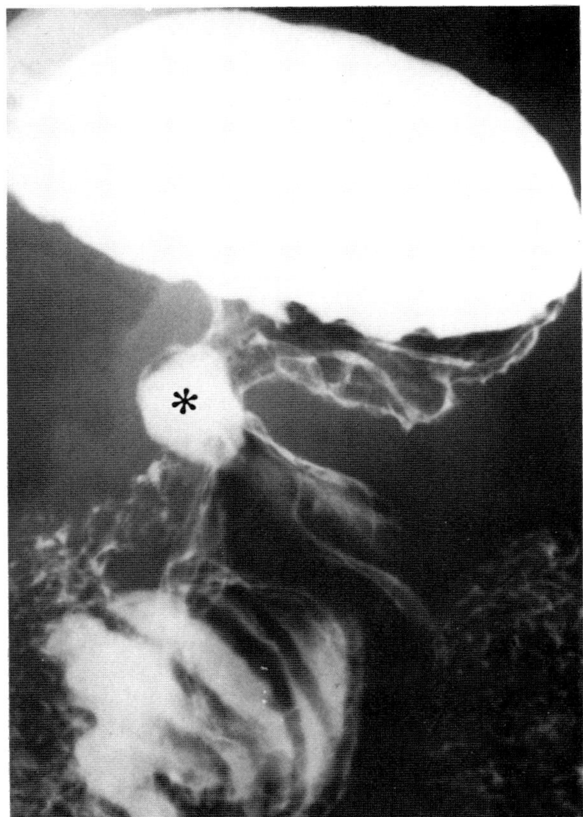

Fig. 30.34 Stomal (marginal) ulcer (*) with scarring following Polya partial gastrectomy.

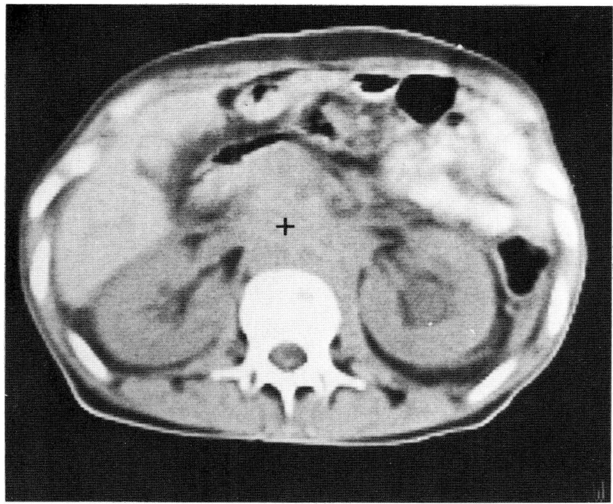

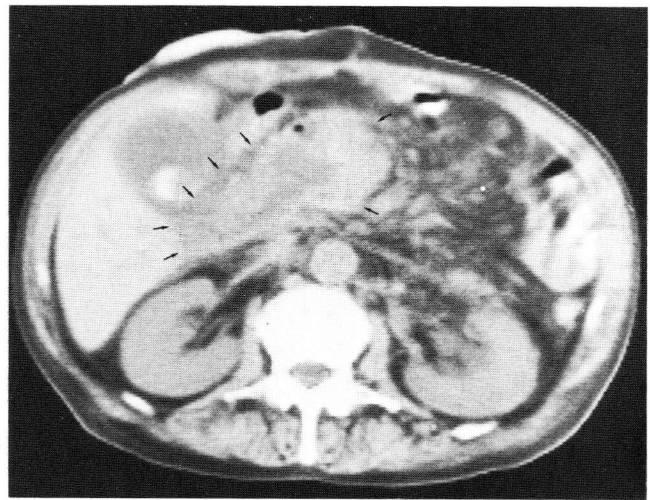

Fig. 30.35 Recurrent gastric carcinoma: CT examination. **A.** Previous total gastrectomy and Roux-en-Y for carcinoma. A mass of recurrent tumour (+) is shown around the aorta and inferior vena cava extending up into the porta hepatis. **B.** Total gastrectomy for carcinoma. A recurrent tumour mass is shown at the porta hepatis (arrowed). (Courtesy of Dr P J Robinson.)

dial epigastric fullness relieved by bilious vomiting. Stasis in the afferent loop is present, leading to bacterial overgrowth and anaemia. The usual cause is twisting or kinking near the origin of the loop. The distended afferent loop may be evident as a fluid-filled structure on plain radiography, US or CT. Barium examination may detect the point of obstruction, and sometimes in partial obstruction barium will enter and show the distended loop.

Post-tumour surgery

Surgery for malignant gastric tumours is often more radical than for peptic disease, and the choice of procedure is dictated by the extent of involvement. Total gastrectomy with oesophagojejunal anastomosis and fashioning of a Roux-en-Y loop may be necessary for extensive disease (Fig. 30.32), but with a distal carcinoma it is sometimes possible to retain the fundus of the stomach and perform a subtotal gastrectomy usually accompanied by a Roux-en-Y to prevent troublesome bile reflux. Gastroenterostomy is a common palliative procedure when a distal gastric carcinoma is producing outflow obstruction.

Diagnosis of **recurrent carcinoma** following surgery is difficult, with a reported success rate for barium examination of only about 50%. Mucosal destruction, ulceration, intraluminal filling defects, narrowing of an anastomosis, rigidity and stricture formation are all signs of malignancy which may not be obvious when the tumour recurrence is extrinsic. In such cases CT is valuable for defining the exogastric mass (Fig. 30.35).

Also difficult is the radiological diagnosis of **primary gastric carcinoma** developing after partial gastrectomy or gastroenterostomy. The risk of gastric malignancy following a gastroenterostomy for peptic ulceration is increased sixfold (Fig. 30.36). The interval between surgery and the development of a carcinoma may be prolonged, and statistically the risk appears to become greater after an interval of 15–20 years. There is also a slightly increased risk of carcinoma developing after a partial gastrectomy.

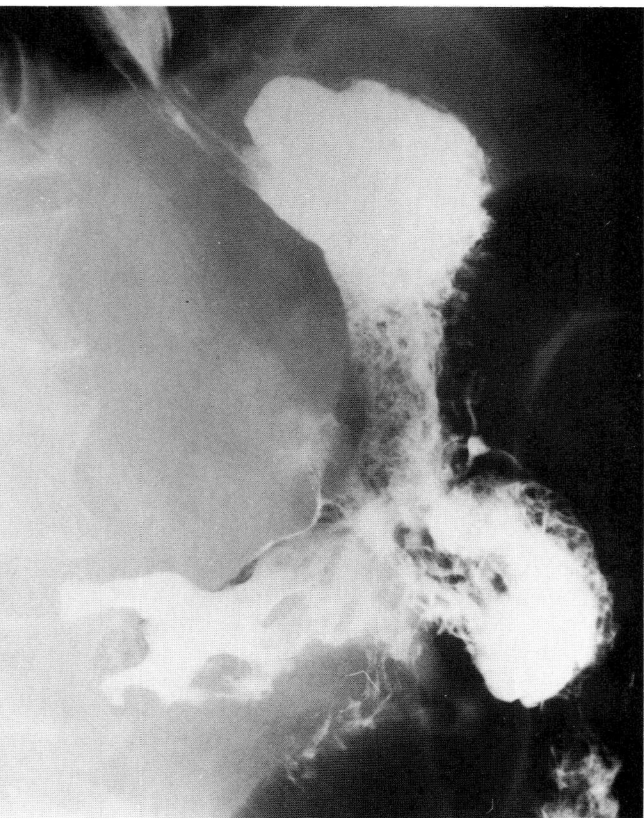

Fig. 30.36 Gastric carcinoma presenting 15 years after gastroenterostomy for duodenal ulcer. The tumour is seen to be involving the stomach distal to the anastomosis. (Courtesy of Dr S F Millward.)

In addition to ulcer and cancer surgery, there are a number of other surgical procedures that may produce complications amenable to radiological diagnosis. Some form of *gastric bypass* is now the operation of choice for the surgical management of obesity. Leaks from the anastomotic line are the most feared complication and lead to the greatest morbidity. Outflow obstruction, reflux oesophagitis and gallstones are the most common other complications.

AORTO-ENTERIC FISTULA

Aorto-enteric fistulae occur either following the spontaneous rupture of an aortic aneurysm into the duodenum or following aortic reconstructive surgery. 80% of aorto-enteric fistulae are seen in the duodenum, due to the susceptibility of the fixed third part of the duodenum to pressure necrosis from an adjacent pulsating aorta or aortic graft. The most important presenting symptom is bleeding. Endoscopy, selective arteriography and barium meal examination have all been successfully employed in diagnosis. Gregson and Craig (1983) recommend endoscopy as the initial investigation in order to detect ulceration and exclude other causes of bleeding, followed by barium examination of the stomach and small bowel to demonstrate the site of the fistula. Signs demonstrated on barium studies include ulceration, a filling defect in the third part of the duodenum, an extrinsic mass impressing the bowel and the presence of a Dacron graft outlined by barium in an irregular cavity.

GASTRITIS

ACUTE AND CHRONIC: DIFFERENTIAL DIAGNOSIS

The term 'gastritis' is used to describe a variety of conditions affecting the gastric mucosa, some of which are inflammatory in origin and some of which are not. The confusion that exists about gastritis, and especially chronic gastritis, arises mainly because of the poor correlation between symptoms and endoscopic, radiological and histological findings. The role of radiology in gastritis is secondary to that of endoscopy. Sometimes a confident radiological diagnosis of gastritis can be made on the basis of characteristic findings on barium meal examination in a patient with compatible clinical features, but usually endoscopy with multiple biopsies is necessary for confirmation and more importantly to exclude serious pathology which may simulate the radiographic appearances of gastritis. Gastritis may be acute or chronic.

Acute gastritis

Acute erosive (haemorrhagic) gastritis is characterized by mucosal oedema and erosions. An *erosion* is defined as an epithelial defect that does not penetrate beyond the muscularis mucosae (whereas an *ulcer* is a defect of the full thickness of the mucosa that may extend into deeper layers of the stomach). Erosive gastritis forms part of the spectrum of peptic disease, but is also caused by other factors including stress, trauma, analgesics, steroids, alcohol, Crohn's disease, candidiasis, viral infections and bile reflux. The clinical presentation of erosive gastritis is extremely variable ranging from an incidental finding in an asymptomatic patient, to acute bleeding, or severe incapacitating anorexia, abdominal pain and weight loss. Gastric erosions may be acute and transitory with a duration of a few days, or in the case of complete erosions they may become chronic. Erosive gastritis accounts for up to 20% of cases of acute upper gastrointestinal bleeding. Erosions are frequently found at endoscopy and in symptomatic patients an incidence of 11% has been reported. The reported incidence using the double contrast barium meal with compression is between 2% and 10%.

Gastric erosions are classified as complete (varioliform) or incomplete. A *complete erosion* is accompanied by a surrounding mound of mucosal oedema, and is therefore elevated. Radiographically complete erosions are seen *en face* in double contrast or on compression views as a small central spot of barium surrounded by a translucent halo producing a 'target' or 'bull's eye' lesion (Fig. 30.37A). In most cases erosions are multiple with mounds of similar size ranging up to about 1 cm in diameter. The lesions may be localized to the gastric antrum or scattered diffusely throughout the stomach, with a tendency to be aligned in rows along mucosal folds. In the healing phase the disappearance of erosions may precede the subsidence of the mucosal mound resulting in scalloping of the affected mucosal folds.

By custom small complete erosions are often referred to as *'aphthoid' ulcers* because of their resemblance to ulcers of this name occurring in the mouth; and some authors use the term 'aphthoid' (syn: aphthous) ulcer for any complete erosion irrespective of size. Whilst aphthoid ulcers are found in many different conditions they are particularly associated with Crohn's disease, and to avoid confusion it is suggested that within the alimentary tract the term 'aphthoid ulcer' should be confined to this disease.

An *incomplete erosion* has no surrounding mucosal mound or translucent halo and is therefore flat and much more difficult to detect radiologically (Fig. 30.37B).

There are several other less common forms of acute gastritis. Severe acute gastritis results from the swallowing of *corrosive substances* such as strong alkalis or acids. Mucosal oedema in the initial stages progresses to fibrosis and contraction. The most frequent site of involvement is the gastric antrum where the features resemble scirrhous carcinoma. Similar changes result from *radiation injury*. *Phlegmonous gastritis* is an acute, fulminating infection of the stomach with necrosis; in survivors healing occurs with fibrosis.

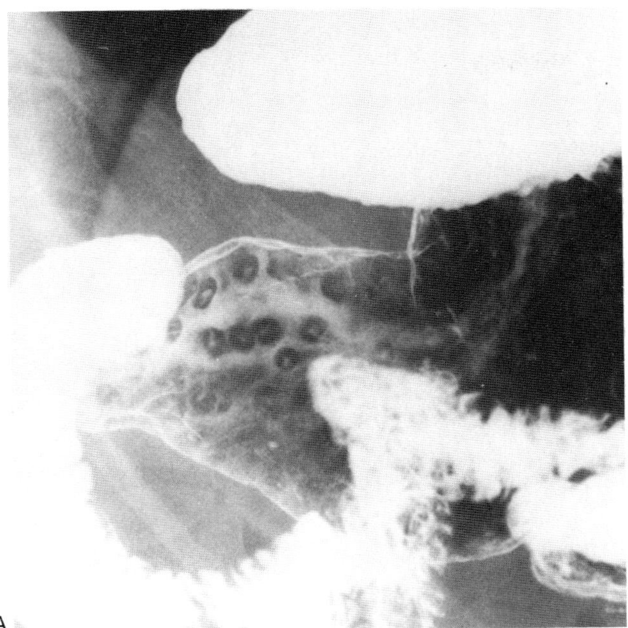
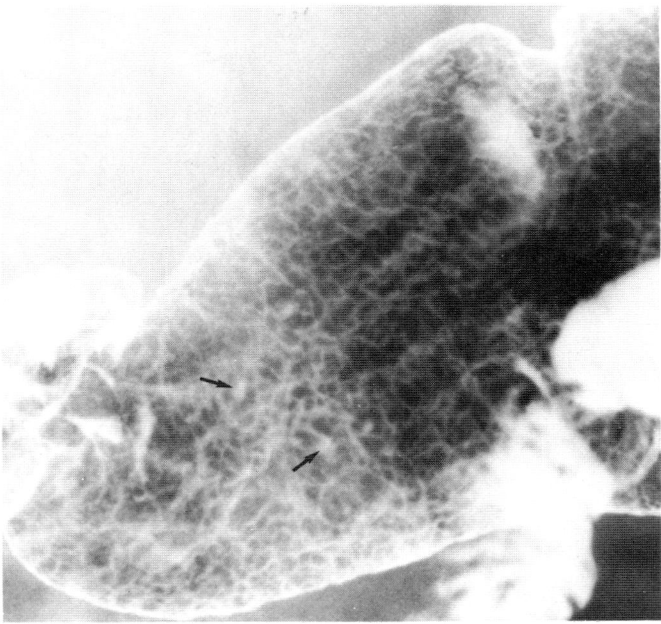

Fig. 30.37 Erosive gastritis. **A.** Numerous erosions are present in the stomach, best seen in two rows in the antrum. Each erosion consists of a small central collection of barium surrounded by a translucent ring (a small 'target' lesion). By definition these are 'complete' erosions (see text). **B.** Prominent areae gastricae with several small 'incomplete' erosions (two of the erosions are indicated with arrows).

Emphysematous gastritis with multiple gas bubbles or streaks within the wall of the stomach is a rare finding that may occur as a complication of corrosive and phlegmonous gastritis. Gas in the stomach wall is also found in the benign condition pneumatosis cystoides intestinalis, and following mucosal damage by ulceration or intubation especially in the presence of gastric outflow obstruction.

Damage to the mucosa by *freezing*, *ischaemia* and *parasitic infestation* are other causes of mucosal oedema and thickening. An unusual infestation of the stomach found in Japan is *acute anisakiasis*, a form of visceral larva migrans acquired by the ingestion of raw or poorly cooked fish containing larvae of the nematode anisakis. Thickened mucosal folds in the stomach and in the duodenum are also a manifestation of *acute pancreatitis*.

Chronic gastritis

Chronic gastritis may be either atrophic or hypertrophic *Chronic atrophic gastritis* encompasses a spectrum of pathological changes including chronic superficial gastritis, atrophic gastritis and gastric atrophy, all of which are associated with a high incidence of gastric carcinoma. The reported findings on double contrast barium meal examination include the presence of large irregular areae gastricae, areas of mucosa devoid of areae gastricae and the absence of the mucosal folds normally present on the greater curvature and fundus of the undistended stomach. The most sensitive method of diagnosis is endoscopy with multiple biopsies. Radiology plays a minor role. Discrepancies between clinical, radiological, endoscopic and pathological findings are frequent.

The diagnosis of *chronic hypertrophic gastritis* is subject to similar difficulties. The key finding is thickening and tortuosity of the mucosal folds (hyperrugosity) which may be localized or generalized. In gross cases the presence of thickened folds is indisputable, but there is a wide variation in normal size and normal folds can be substantial. As a general rule folds in the antrum with a width in excess of 0.5 cm and along the greater curvature and fundus more than 1.5 cm, are likely to be abnormal. Generalized rugal thickening is associated with high acid output, heavy beer consumption and excessive smoking.

Similar appearances are seen in the *Zollinger-Ellison syndrome* which is due to a non-beta islet cell tumour of the pancreas. The gastrointestinal changes in this syndrome result from the marked hypersecretion of hydrochloric acid by the stomach. In addition to the rugal changes, there is increased gastric fluid secretion, fulminating peptic ulceration (often multiple and in atypical locations, e.g. jejunum),thickened coarse duodenal folds and changes in the small intestine resembling malabsorption (Fig. 30.38). A variety of infiltrative processes can also result in the radiographic pattern of thickened gastric folds. These include lymphoma, eosinophilic gastritis, Crohn's disease, sarcoidosis, tuberculosis, syphilis and amyloid disease.

A particular form of localized hypertrophic gastritis known as *Ménétrièr's disease* is characterized by an excessive secretion of mucus by the stomach and a considerable loss

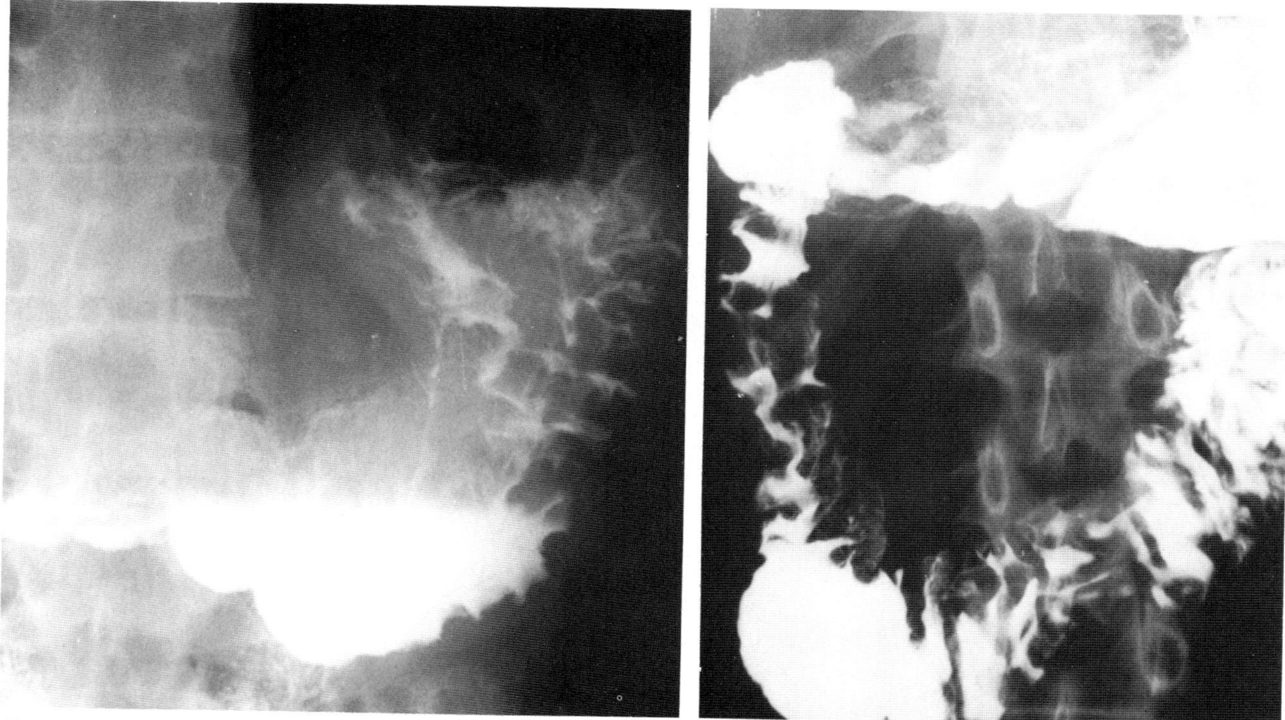

Fig. 30.38 The Zollinger-Ellison syndrome. **A.** Stomach. Large quantity of resting fluid and thickened gastric mucosal folds. **B.** Duodenum. Thickened mucosal folds.

of protein may occur. Histological changes are confined to the mucosa, and the lesser curvature and antrum are spared. The massive localized thickening of rugae in this condition (Fig. 30.39) simulates a mass of polyps, a polypoid carcinoma, lymphoma, gastric varices or the intragastric prolapse of a sliding hiatus hernia. The softness and mobility of thickened rugae and the absence of ulceration or an extraluminal mass helps in differentiation from lymphoma and carcinoma. A mass of polyps usually shows rounded or lobulated filling defects.

To be differentiated from localized hypertrophic gastritis are gastric varices and intragastric prolapse of a sliding hiatus hernia. In portal hypertension *varices* of the gastric fundus are nearly as frequent as varices of the oesophagus although more difficult to demonstrate. The presence of gastric varices without oesophageal varices indicates isolated splenic vein occlusion. Radiographically fundal varices are best demonstrated using a small quantity of barium and a double contrast technique with intravenous Buscopan. Overdistension of the stomach is liable to obliterate varices and should be avoided. Varices are seen as multiple smooth serpiginous filling defects similar in appearance to those occurring in the oesophagus (Fig. 30.40A). Their changing size and shape usually distinguishes varices from thickened folds.

Also to be considered is a fundal filling defect at the cardia consisting of a bunch of mucosal folds due to *intra-*

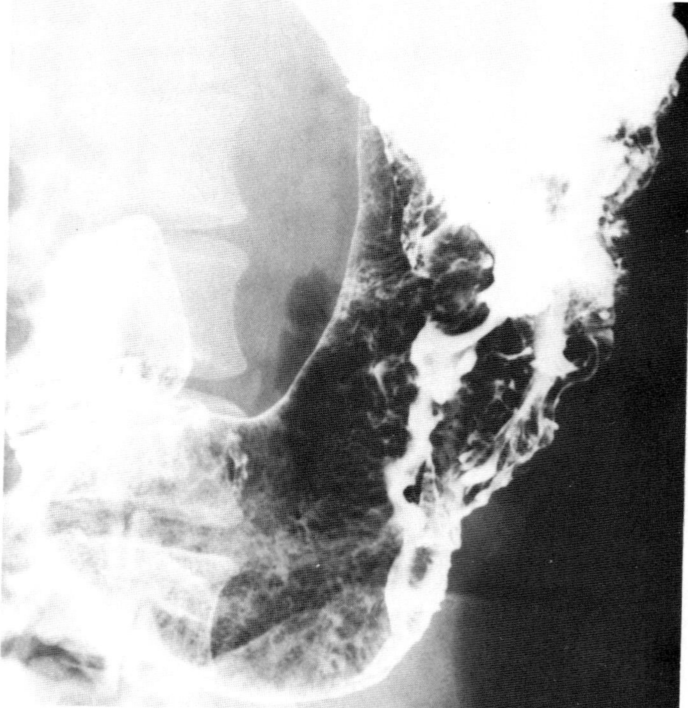

Fig. 30.39 Ménétrièr's disease. Thickened, distorted mucosal folds (rugae) are present along the greater curvature of the body of the stomach. The appearances are not specific to Ménétrier's disease but may be seen in any form of hypertrophic gastritis. Differentiation from lymphoma may be difficult. (Courtesy of Dr D J Lintott.)

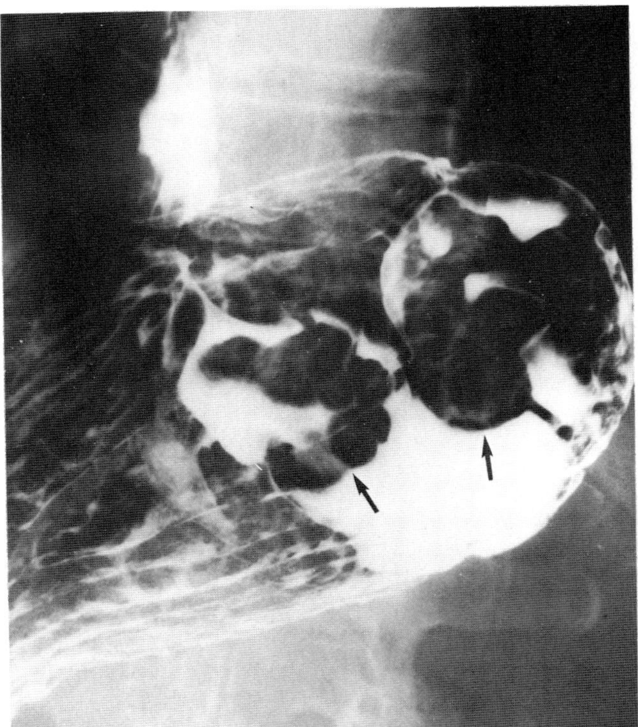

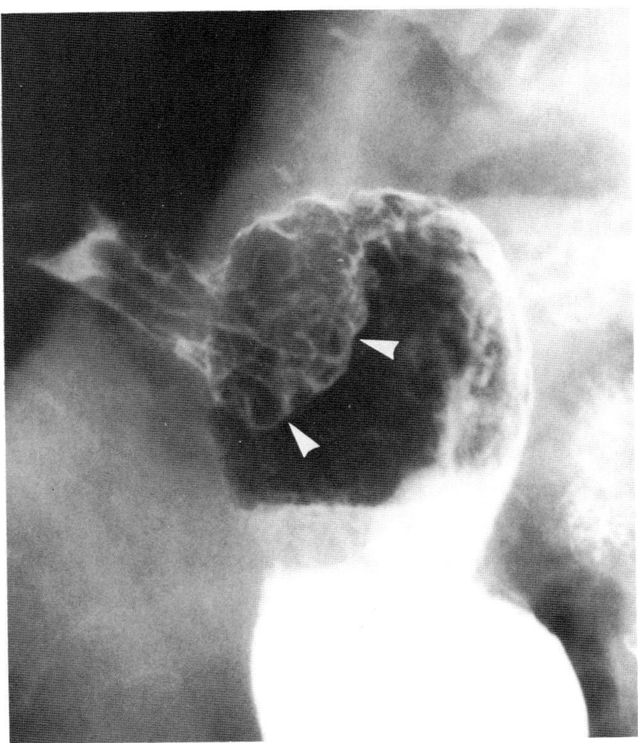

Fig. 30.40 Pseudotumours of the gastric fundus. **A.** Gastric fundal varices. Filling defects (arrowed) resembling a bunch of enlarged nodular mucosal folds. (Courtesy of Dr G M Fraser and the Editor of *Clinical Radiology*.) **B.** Intragastric prolapse of a sliding hiatus hernia. The mass (arrowed) appears to be composed of a mass of mucosal folds, and vanishes when the hernia is reduced above the diaphragm in the recumbent posture.

gastric prolapse of a sliding hiatus hernia (Fig. 30.40B). This characteristic defect is best seen on double contrast examination with the patient standing, and proof of its origin is obtained by examining the patient prone which will cause the fundal defect to vanish as the hernia is produced in its usual position above the diaphragm.

Antral gastritis is characterized by narrowing of the gastric antrum with obliteration of the normal prepyloric 'shoulders', thickened mucosa either in the form of nodular longitudinal folds or bunches, and erosions (Fig. 30.41). Sometimes narrowing and mucosal changes occur independently. Coexisting duodenal ulceration or duodenitis is often present. It has been reported that patients with antral gastritis usually have epigastric pain unrelated to eating and unaffected by antacids. Evidence suggests that antral gastritis is part of the spectrum of peptic ulcer disease and that in most cases there is a generalized histological gastritis, with more severe changes sufficient to produce mucosal fold enlargement in the antrum.

The differential diagnosis of antral gastritis includes carcinoma of the stomach and peptic ulceration (Fig. 30.41). In antral gastritis, unlike carcinoma, the mucosal folds are intact, there is no sharply defined proximal shouldering and the calibre of the narrowed antrum varies slightly during the course of the examination. The effects of gastric ulceration can mimic antral gastritis. The presence of narrowing of the antrum should initiate a search for a lesser curvature benign gastric ulcer which frequently produces antral spasm (Fig. 30.42). Narrowing may persist due to thickening of the wall of the antrum after the ulcer itself has healed. A gastric ulcer in the prepyloric region may produce in its neighbourhood thickened folds, spasm, scarring and deformity, and these appearances may be indistinguishable from antral gastritis. Other rare causes of antral narrowing such as lymphoma, Crohn's disease, tuberculosis, syphilis, eosinophilic gastritis and sarcoidosis should be considered. In all cases of apparent antral gastritis where there is any doubt about the diagnosis confirmation should be sought by endoscopy and biopsy.

DUODENITIS: COARSE DUODENAL MUCOSAL FOLDS: COBBLESTONE CAP: NODULAR CAP

The clinical importance of duodenal inflammation in the absence of chronic ulceration has been debated for many years, and remains controversial. A simplified version of what now seems to be generally agreed on the basis of the data at present available is as follows.

Duodenitis is a clinical entity which can give rise to dyspepsia and, on rare occasions, gastrointestinal haemorrhage. Duodenitis may also be present without clinical

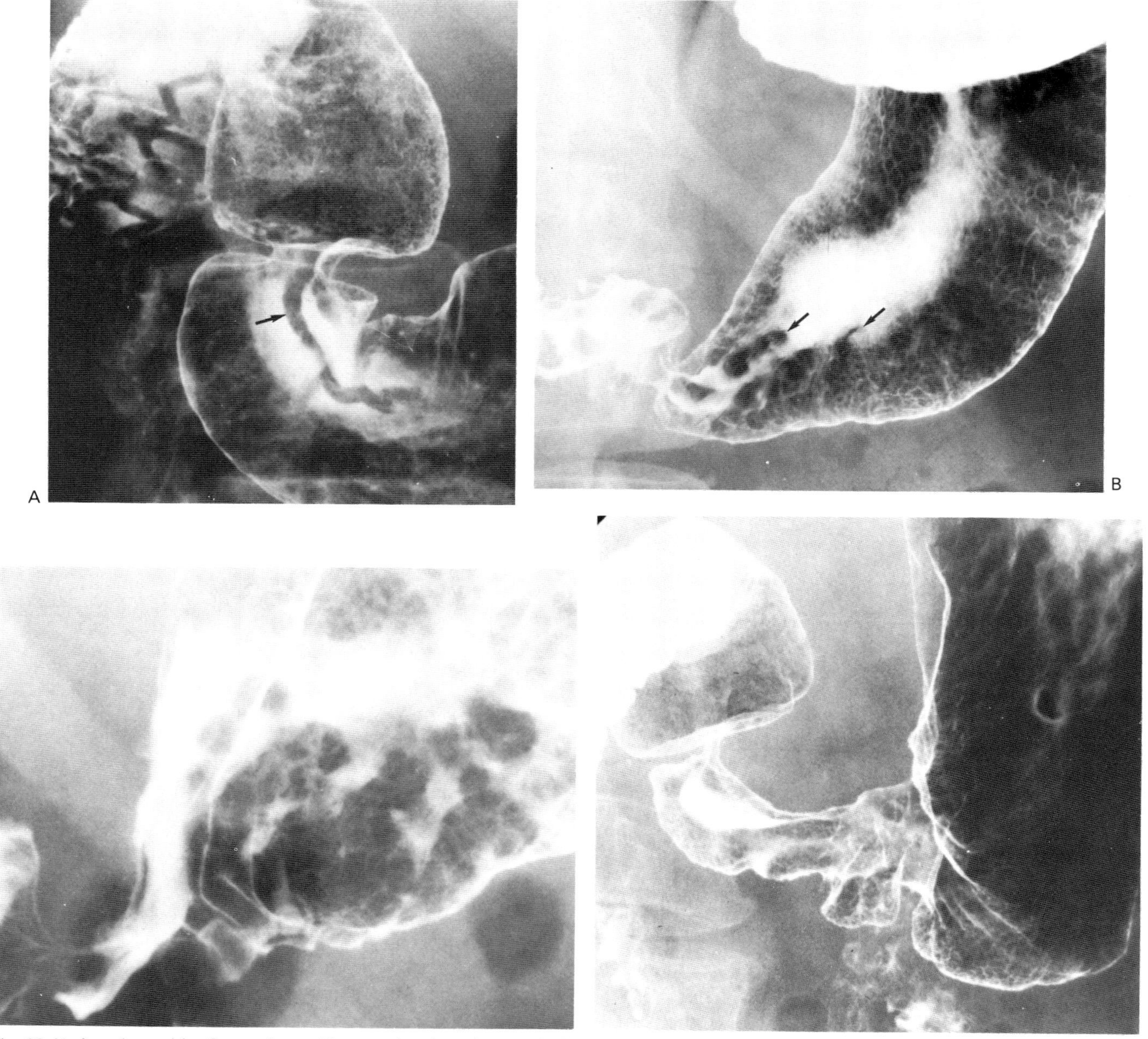

Fig. 30.41 Antral gastritis. Comparison with normal and carcinoma. **A.** The normal gastric antrum when distended is either devoid of mucosal folds or contains one or two small longitudinal folds (arrowed). The distal antrum has prominent 'shoulders' parallel to the base of the duodenal cap. **B.** Antral gastritis. Two thickened, nodular mucosal folds are present (arrowed), and the antrum is cone shaped. The mucosa in the duodenal cap is also thickened (duodenitis). **C.** Severe antral gastritis. The normal antral mucosa is replaced by a mass of thickened nodular mucosal folds. Cone-shaped narrowing of the antrum completely obliterates the normal distal 'shoulders'. **D.** Antral carcinoma. The mucosa is destroyed. Narrowing is concentric and not cone shaped, and the proximal end of the tumour is sharply defined. One shoulder is retained and the other is obliterated.

symptoms. It appears that duodenitis is part of the spectrum of duodenal ulcer disease occurring in some patients independent of duodenal ulceration, whilst in others it may precede ulceration or remain after ulceration has healed. The terms erosive duodenitis, peptic duodenitis and non-specific duodenitis have also been applied to this condition. Like duodenal ulceration the disease predominantly affects the duodenal cap.

Developments in cytological and histological techniques and interpretation have led to more accurate pathological diagnosis of duodenitis. Two problems which have been identified are the wide variation in histological findings that can occur in the duodenal mucosa of asymptomatic subjects, and the fact that duodenitis is a focal disease. It is therefore necessary for the endoscopist to see that biopsy specimens come from an abnormal-looking area. Taking

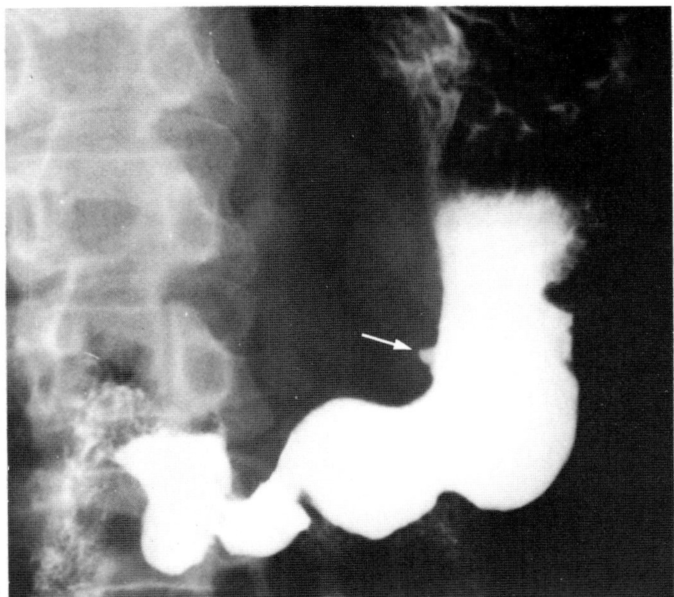

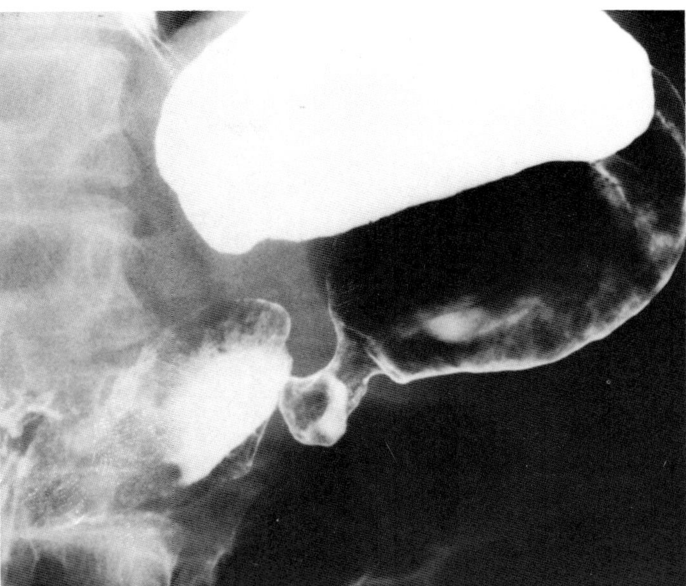

Fig. 30.42 Narrowing of the gastric antrum. Comparison of ulcer spasm and carcinoma. **A.** Spasm secondary to a lesser curvature benign gastric ulcer. **B.** Antral carcinoma.

these factors into account a good correlation has been reported between endoscopic duodenitis and a group of histological features, except in mild disease (Joffe et al. 1978). Notwithstanding these encouraging results, many gastroenterologists still find considerable discrepancies between symptoms, endoscopy, radiology and histology.

The contribution of radiology to the diagnosis of duodenitis is subservient to that of endoscopy. Mild grades cannot be reliably demonstrated by radiographic means. Double contrast examination is the most sensitive technique; the use of a hypotonic agent assists detection. Several radiological signs of duodenitis have been described. Those which correlate best with the endoscopic appearances are erosions and coarse mucosal folds.

Erosions are seen *en face* on double contrast as tiny specks of barium often without a surrounding translucent halo, and are by definition diagnostic of erosive duodenitis. Erosions may occur either on a background of normal duodenal mucosa or thickened folds (Fig. 30.43A & D).

Coarse mucosal folds in the cap occur in two forms. Firstly as *thickened folds* seen as slightly wavy band-shaped filling defects a few centimetres long by approximately 0.5–1 cm wide (Fig. 30.43B & C). Secondly as multiple round or oval translucent defects measuring between 0.5 and 1 cm in diameter; an appearance that has been given the descriptive name of '*cobblestone cap*' (Fig. 30.44A & B). Usually the 'cobblestones' are localized to the cap, but they may extend further into the duodenum. The coarse mucosal fold pattern is susceptible to obliteration by overdistension or compression. Without Buscopan the cap is usually irritable. Coarse mucosal folds are an indirect sign of duodenitis, and are due to spastic contraction of the muscularis induced by a high concentration of acid in the duodenum. In association with erosions and coarse folds there is often in duodenitis a defect in barium coating of the mucosa which becomes granular, patchy and nonhomogenous.

It is important to appreciate that there are other causes of erosions and coarse mucosal folds in the duodenum. For instance the diagnosis of Crohn's disease (Crohn's duodenitis) should be considered whenever erosions (aphthoid ulcers) are found. Also 'cobblestone cap' can be produced by *hyperplasia of Brunner's glands*; an uncommon condition associated with atypical upper abdominal symptoms. In this condition the 'cobblestones' are constant and the duodenal cap is not irritable. At surgery multiple small nodules are found confirming the radiographic appearance, and histological examination shows the characteristic hyperplasia of Brunner's glands (Fig. 30.44C).

Other causes of thickening of the mucosal folds in the duodenum, particularly beyond the cap, are the Zollinger-Ellison syndrome, pancreatitis, infestation by parasites such as *Strongyloides* and *Giardia*, Crohn's disease, chronic renal failure, mucoviscidosis, neoplastic infiltration such as lymphoma, varices, intramural haemorrhage, and diffuse infiltrative disorders such as Whipple's disease, amyloidosis and intestinal lymphangiectasia.

To be distinguished from 'cobblestone cap' are two other conditions characterized by multiple small nodules predominantly in the duodenal cap ('nodular cap').

Nodular lymphoid hyperplasia in the gastrointestinal tract is characterized by proliferation of lymphoid aggregates, and is a relatively common normal finding in the terminal ileum in young people. Some cases are associated with

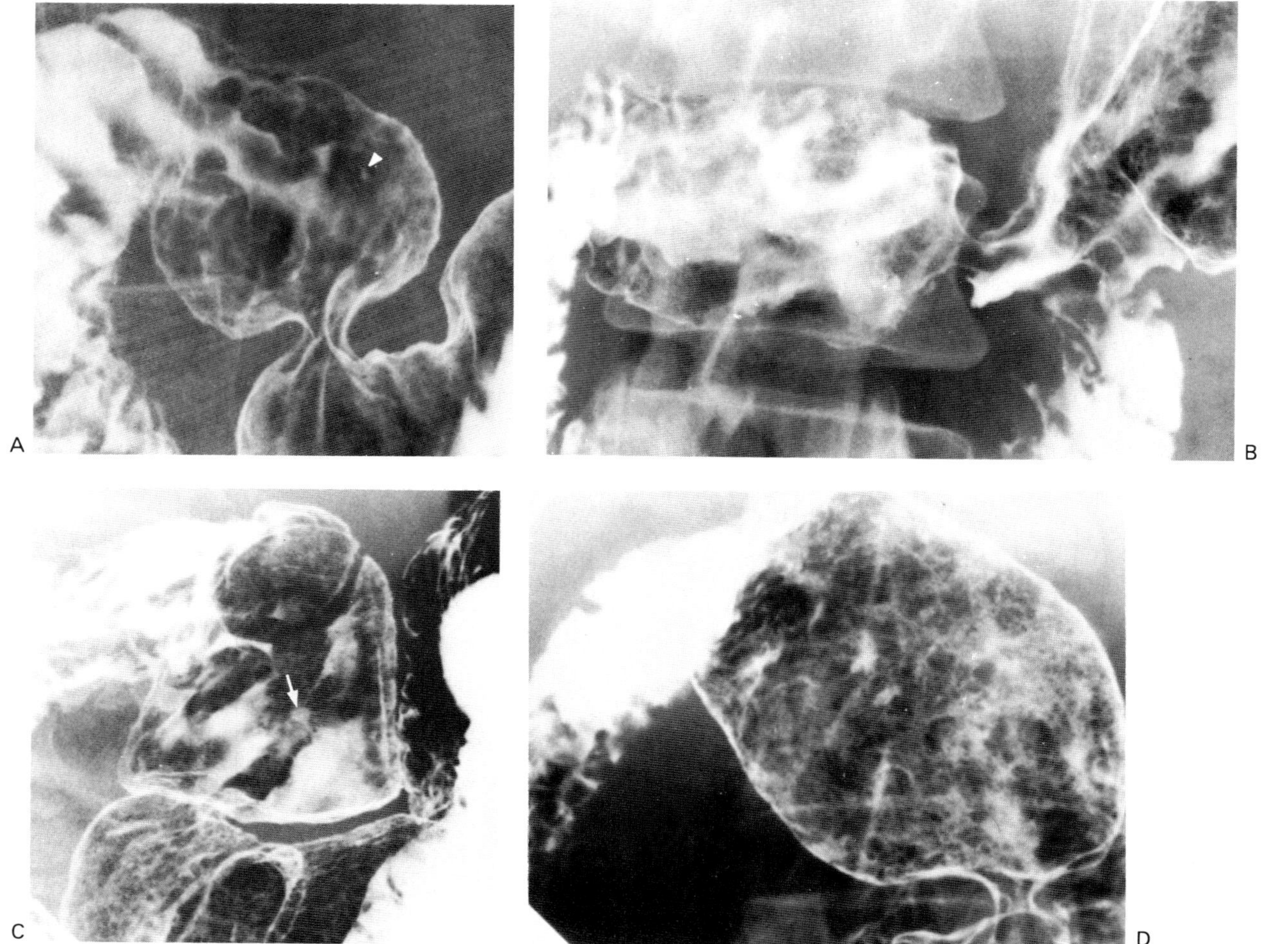

Fig. 30.43 Duodenitis. Typical appearances in cap. **A.** Slightly coarsened mucosa with patchy barium coating and several erosions (one indicated). (Courtesy of Dr D J Lintott.) **B.** Thickened ill-defined mucosal folds with poor mucosal coating with barium. Not a 'cobblestone' pattern. No erosions or ulcers seen. There are similar changes in the gastric antrum (antral gastritis). **C.** Coarsened mucosa with small ulcer (arrow). **D.** Background reticular pattern (villi) with several superimposed erosions and ulcers of various shapes. Patient has Crohn's disease of the ileum, but duodenal biopsy showed non-specific inflammatory changes only.

Giardia infection and hypogammaglobulinaemia. Double contrast barium examination shows multiple round nodules with a uniform size (about 2 mm) and shape, evenly distributed throughout the duodenum (Fig. 30.45). The nodules are usually seen most clearly on gas distended views of the cap.

Heterotopic gastric mucosa (syn: gastric metaplasia) is quite a common finding on histological examination of the duodenal cap, and is being demonstrated radiographically much more frequently since the advent of double contrast hypotonic duodenography. Multiple small nodules of various shapes and sizes ranging from 1 to 6 mm are present extending from the pylorus towards the apex of the cap (Fig. 30.46). The condition is unlikely to be of any clinical significance. The differential diagnosis includes air bubbles which are round, mobile and inconstant.

Another rare cause of small nodules in the duodenal cap is *Crohn's disease*.

CARCINOMA OF THE STOMACH

EARLY AND ADVANCED: DIFFERENTIAL DIAGNOSIS

Carcinoma of the stomach is the second most common malignant tumour of the gastrointestinal tract in Great Britain. Men are affected twice as often as women. The incidence of the disease varies greatly from race to race. Early symptoms are usually vague and indefinite comprising loss of appetite, epigastric discomfort and pain, weight loss and the symptoms of anaemia. There is, therefore, a delay before most patients seek medical advice and, all too frequently, a further delay in diagnosis while symptomatic treatment is prescribed. Generally prognosis is poor.

Stimulated by the high incidence and poor prognosis of gastric cancer in Japan, the modern technique of double contrast radiography of the stomach was devised by

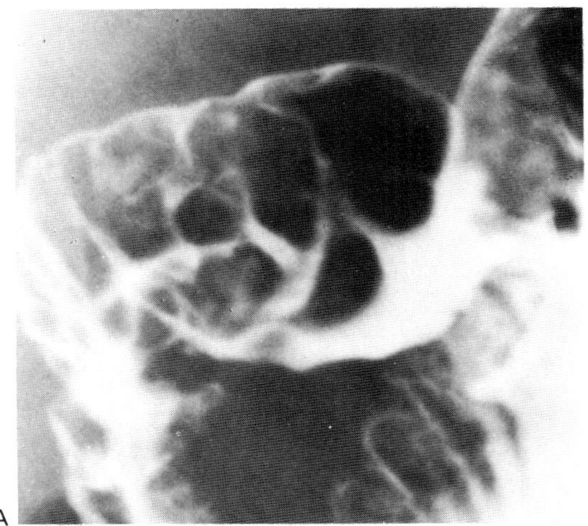

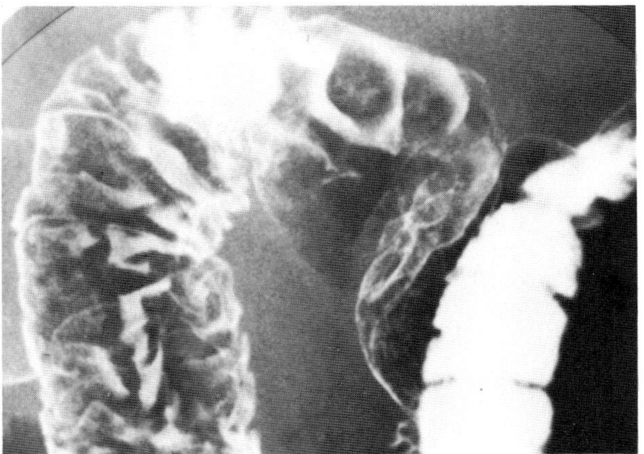

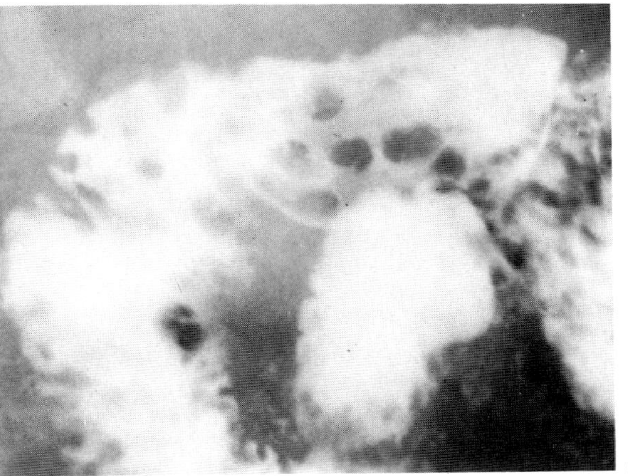

Fig. 30.44 'Cobblestone' cap due to duodenitis and hyperplasia of Brunner's glands. **A.** Duodenitis. The nodules are of different sizes, closely bunched and due to swollen mucosa. (Courtesy of Dr G M Fraser.) **B.** Duodenitis. Two large nodules are seen due to enlargement of a single mucosal fold. (Courtesy of Dr J Virjee.) **C.** Hyperplasia of Brunner's glands. The nodules are clearly defined, discrete and randomly distributed in the duodenal cap and postbulbar region. (Courtesy of Dr A Schulman.)

Shirakabe and his co-workers more than 20 years ago, with the aim of detecting cancer at an early curable stage.

Early gastric cancer

Early gastric cancer is defined as, 'carcinoma in which invasion is limited to the mucosa and submucosa without regard for the presence of lymph node and distant metastases'. A report from the Cancer Institute Hospital in Tokyo has shown that the 5-year survival rate of those with early gastric cancer ranges from 95% when the tumour is limited to the mucosa to 78% in polypoid cancers with submucosal involvement.

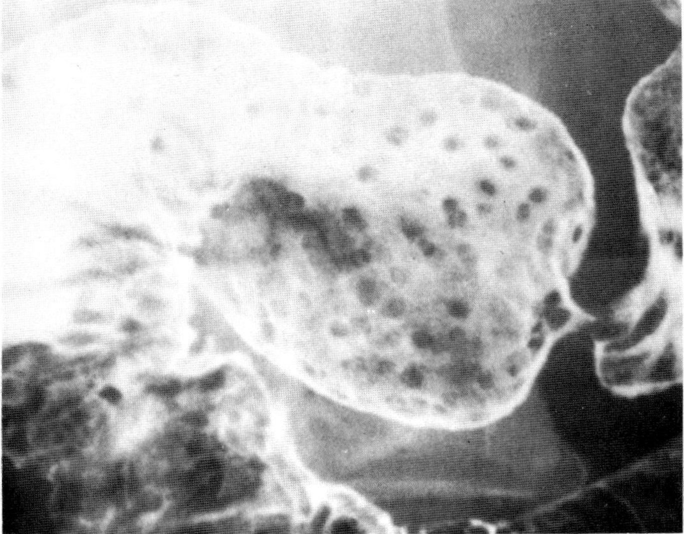

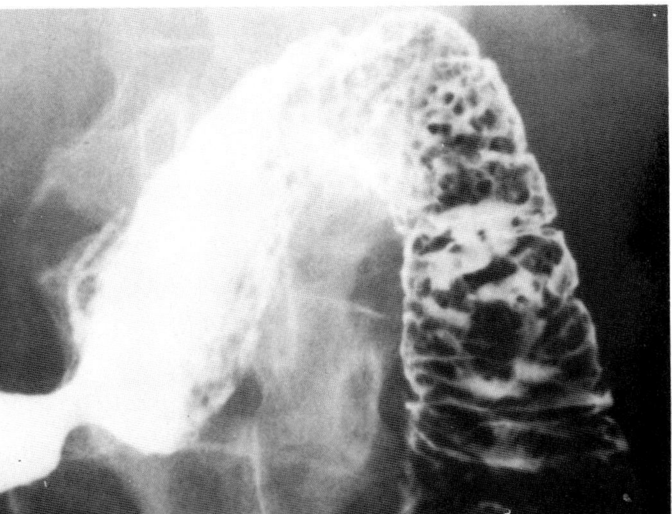

Fig. 30.45 Nodular lymphoid hyperplasia is characterized by numerous small nodules all of the same size and evenly distributed. **A.** Small round nodules evenly distributed throughout the duodenal cap. (Courtesy of Dr J Virjee.) **B.** Different case to **A.** Prone view. The nodules can be seen to extend into the second part of the duodenum.

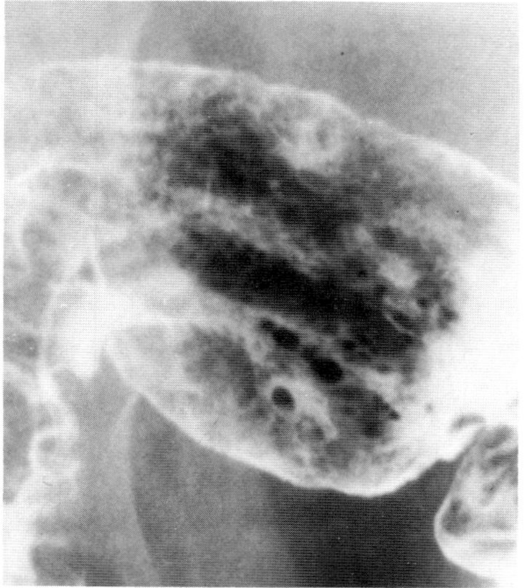

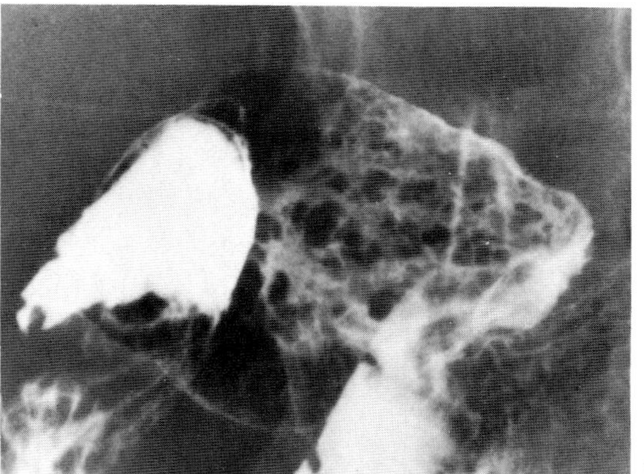

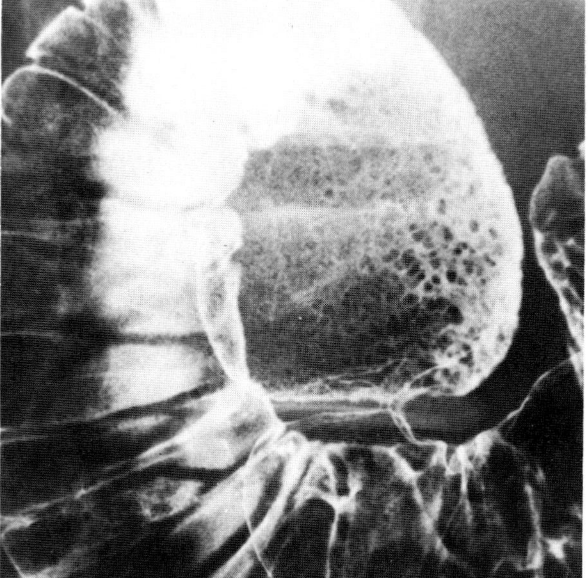

Fig. 30.46 Gastric metaplasia. The presence of gastric epithelium in the duodenal cap produces small nodules of various sizes and shapes extending from the pylorus towards the apex of the cap. **A.** Several nodules of different sizes almost entirely confined to the proximal half of the cap. (Courtesy of Dr G M Fraser.) **B.** A cluster of irregularly shaped nodules of different sizes occupy more than half of the cap, the remainder of the cap being normal. **C.** A cluster of very small nodules with the same characteristics as **A** and **B**, and mainly occupying the same area of the cap as in **B**. (Courtesy of Dr J Virjee.)

The macroscopic classification of early gastric cancer, based upon the appearance of exised specimens, endoscopy and barium examinations, comprises three basic types according to the amount of protrusion or depression of the tumour. Combinations of types are frequent (Fig. 30.47). A summarized version of the classification is as follows:

Type I Polypoid (>0.5 cm in height)

Type II Superficial
- a. elevated (<0.5 cm in height)
- b. flat
- c. depressed (shallow, superficial ulceration)

Type III Excavated (with prominent depression usually due to ulceration)

The diagnosis of *polypoid early cancer* is made from high-quality double contrast radiographs with graded compression over the lesion. Most lesions are between 1 cm and 4 cm in diameter, with a granular surface pattern and lobulated contour. A critical observation is that in early polypoid cancer where invasion is limited to the submucosa the surface pattern of the tumour is comparable to the surrounding mucosa and the areae gastricae are preserved. As tumour infiltration extends deeper than the submucosa the similarity of the surface pattern disappears and erosions and ulceration are seen.

A radiological diagnosis of *excavated early cancer* is based upon an analysis of the ulceration and the surrounding mucosal surface. Generally ulcers are irregular with ill-defined, serrated or spicular margins (Fig. 30.47A). The presence of converging folds assists diagnosis firstly by drawing the observer's attention to a small area of ulceration and secondly by showing characteristic abnormalities of the folds such as tapering, clubbing, amputation and fusion (Fig. 30.47B).

In Britain a diagnosis of early gastric cancer is rarely made. There are three main reasons for this.

1. The incidence of gastric carcinoma is considerably less than in Japan.

2. Barium meals or fibre-optic endoscopy are only performed on symptomatic patients in whom any disease is likely to be fairly advanced, thus the detection of an early gastric cancer is usually incidental in someone with symptoms from another cause.

3. The standard barium meal examination is a general purpose procedure whereby the gut is examined from the

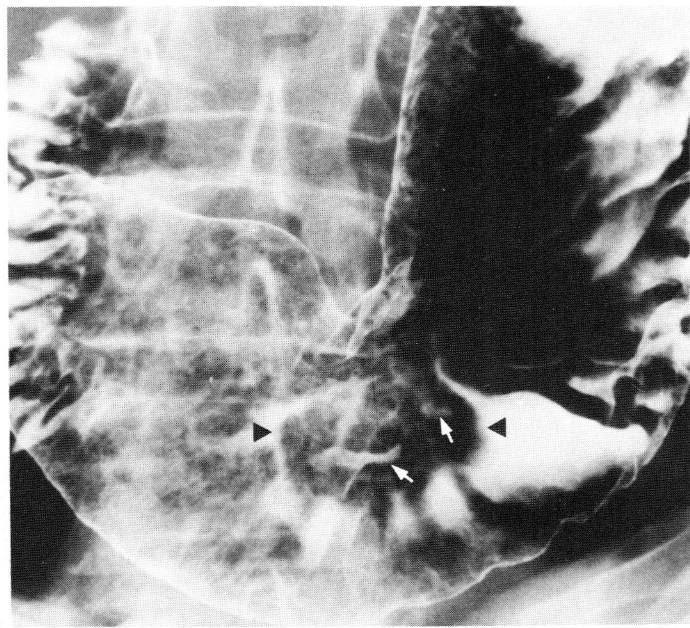

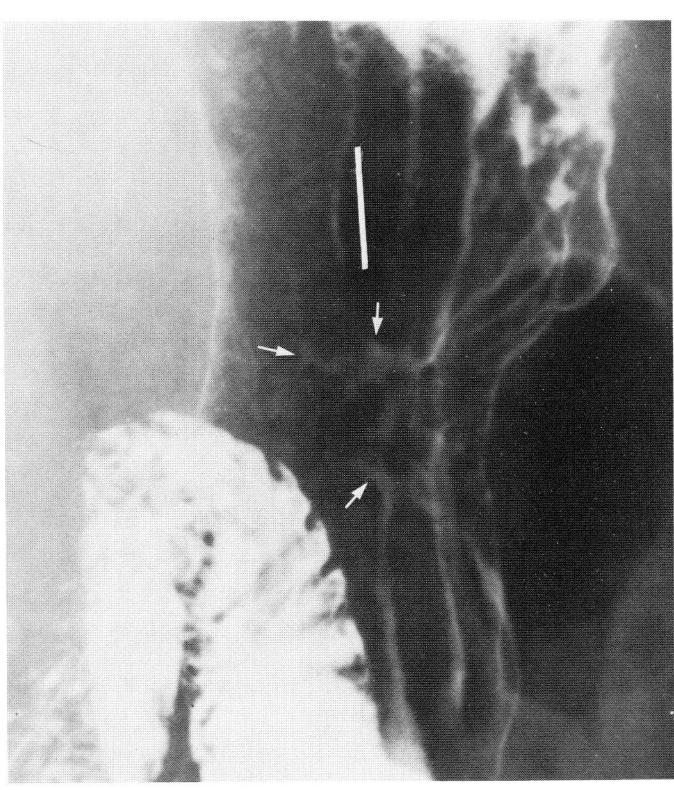

Fig. 30.47 Early gastric carcinoma: Mixed types (see text). **A.** An elevated tumour (between the black arrowheads) is outlined by barium. Two small irregular ulcers are present (white arrows). **B.** The tumour comprises a group of nodules and several small irregular areas of ulceration (arrowed). The mucosal folds (on either side of the vertical white line) are amputated at their lower ends.

pharynx to the duodenojejunal flexure. This is not the optimum examination for the detection of an early gastric carcinoma because the amount of barium and the sequence and nature of the manoeuvres employed to show for instance a suspected hiatus hernia or duodenal ulcer are not the same as would be chosen to exclusively examine the stomach. For these reasons the tumour is usually well advanced by the time the diagnosis is established.

Advanced gastric cancer

Advanced gastric carcinomas, based on their morphological characteristics, are *infiltrative*, *nodular*, *fungating*, *ulcerating* or a combination of each. The key radiological signs on barium examination are narrowing, loss of peristalsis, mucosal destruction, ulceration and intraluminal filling defects.

The **infiltrating** gastric carcinoma spreads in or beneath the mucosa. Many of these tumours evoke a pronounced fibrous tissue response and are therefore known as *scirrhous* carcinomas. The gastric wall becomes thickened and rigid at the site of the tumour and there is loss of peristalsis. The normal mucosal pattern is destroyed and replaced by an amorphous granular or nodular appearance. On a single contrast barium examination these features may be appreciated by careful observation and palpation under fluoroscopic control. Using double contrast the lack of distensibility of the involved part of the stomach and the altered surface pattern of the tumour will be demonstrated. Scirrhous carcinoma may be localized or generalized.

In the *localized form* a stricture develops usually with abrupt shouldered ends (Fig. 30.48A). When this involves the gastric antrum, as is frequently the case, outflow obstruction eventually results. Usually the diagnosis is obvious, but sometimes the stigmata of malignancy are less florid and the antrum is seen to be merely narrowed with loss of peristalsis. In these cases consideration should be given to other conditions, mostly of a chronic inflammatory nature, which can produce a similar appearance. These include lymphoma, Crohn's disease, tuberculosis, syphilis, amyloidosis, sarcoidosis, eosinophilic gastroenteritis, the ingestion of corrosives and the effect of irradiation. Other conditions which can produce narrowing of the gastric antrum are involvement by extension of malignancy or infection from surrounding organs for example carcinoma of the pancreas, or a duodenal ulcer with a surrounding inflammatory mass. The presence of an exogastric mass is usually obvious in such cases and points to the correct diagnosis. Computed tomography or US can be performed for confirmation. Also to be considered are antral gastritis, spasm or residual scarring from a benign gastric ulcer either in the antrum itself or higher up the lesser curvature, and atrophic antrum following gastroenterostomy. In these conditions there is no sign of an exogastric mass or of mucosal destruction.

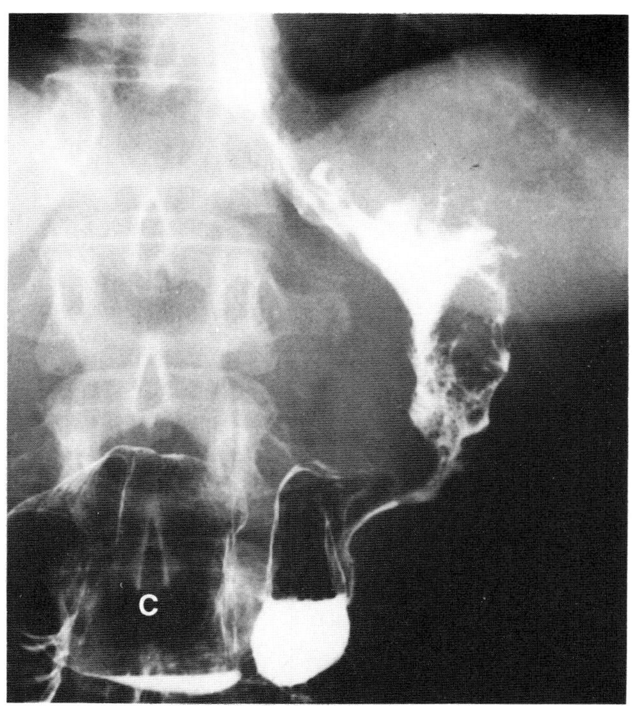

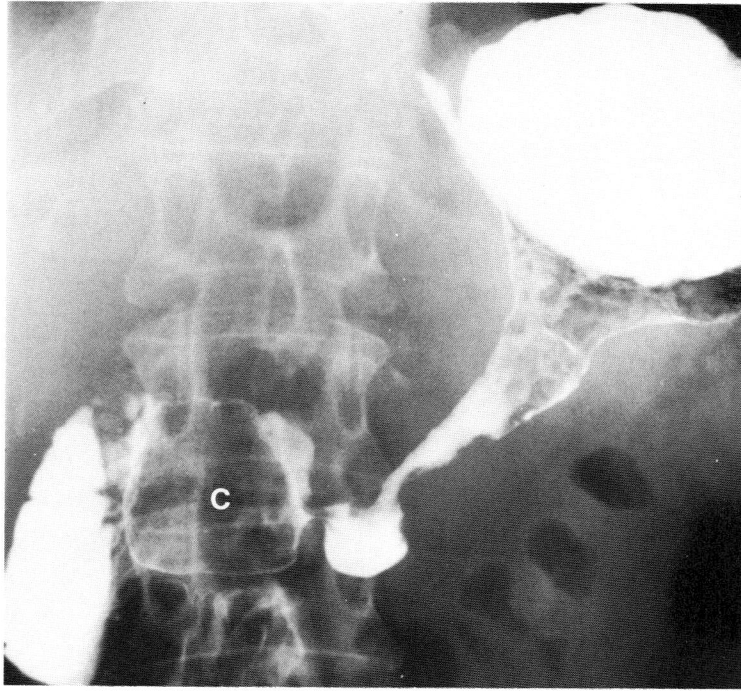

Fig. 30.48 Advanced gastric carcinoma. Typical appearances of scirrhous tumours. (C = duodenal cap.) **A.** Scirrhous tumour involving the distal two thirds of the stomach, with mucosal destruction and stricture formation. **B.** Linitis plastica. Almost all of the stomach is involved, with thickening of the wall and narrowing of the lumen.

In the *generalized form* of scirrhous carcinoma diagnosis may be difficult because the margins of the tumour are ill defined. Eventually the whole of the stomach is affected to an extent where the thickened wall encroaches on the lumen to produce a uniform narrowing known as *'leather bottle stomach'* or *'linitis plastica'* (Fig. 30.48B). The stomach is thus transformed into a tube through which fluid rapidly passes, and obstruction is not a feature.

Not all infiltrating carcinomas are scirrhous; in **superficial erosive spreading carcinoma** there is an absence of fibrosis (Fig. 30.49). The mucosal pattern is usually destroyed over the surface of the tumour, but occasionally the tumour may spread beneath the mucosa. In these rare cases the mucosal folds are retained and may be thickened simulating lymphomatous infiltration. There is also a tendency to ulceration and small polypoid filling defects may be present. In the early stages before the changes become florid diagnosis is difficult but worthwhile, because of the relatively good prognosis following surgery.

Nodular carcinomas consist of raised nodules of growth, sometimes discrete but often confluent, which frequently progress to an ulcerated form (Fig. 30.50A & B).

The **fungating** type of gastric carcinoma produces an irregular intraluminal mass which may become ulcerated and necrotic as it develops (Fig. 30.50C). The diagnosis is usually obvious but other less common advanced malignant conditions such as leiomyosarcoma (see page 854) and lymphoma (see page 855) can produce the same appearance.

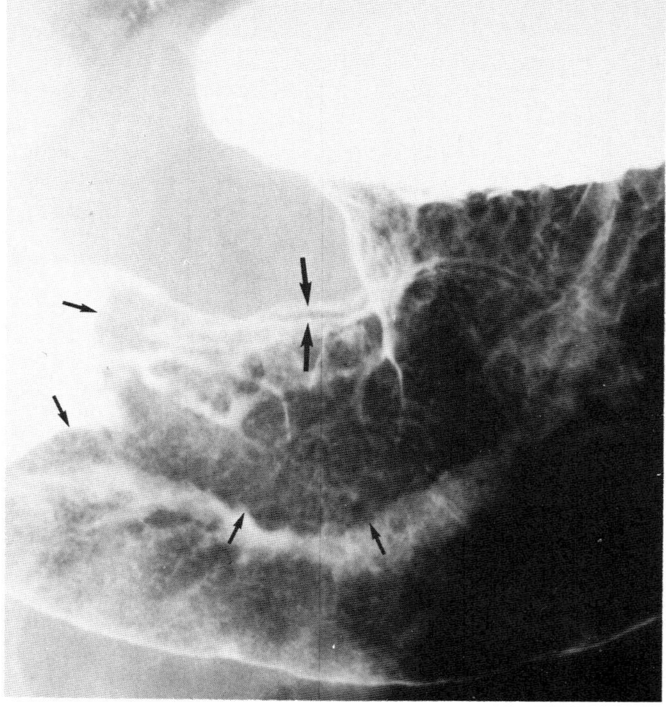

Fig. 30.49 Superficial spreading gastric carcinoma outlined by a film of barium (small arrows). On the horizontal lesser curvature there are double lines (large arrows). These two parallel white lines represent the profiles of the normally distended gastric wall and the adjacent wall restricted by malignant infiltration. In the area beneath the large arrows is a group of tumour nodules.

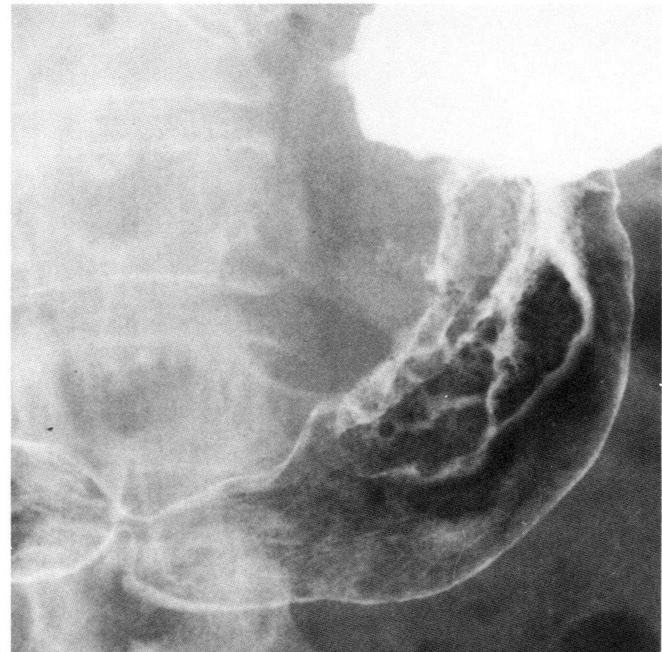

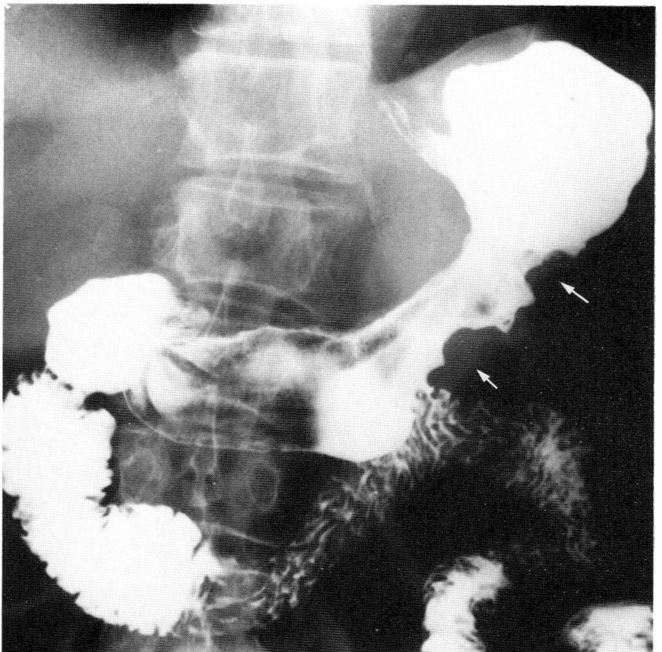

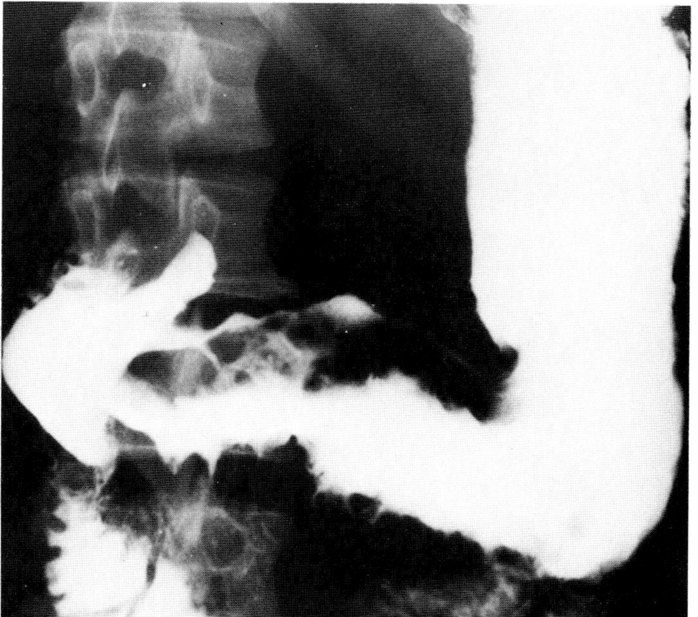

Fig. 30.50 Advanced gastric carcinoma. Typical variety of appearances. **A.** Plaque-like nodular tumour involving most of the middle third of the stomach. **B.** Large nodular filling defects along the middle third of the greater curvature of the stomach with mucosal destruction and lumenal narrowing. This pattern resembles lymphoma and hypertrophic gastritis. **C.** The distal half of the stomach is involved by a large irregular, ulcerated filling defect.

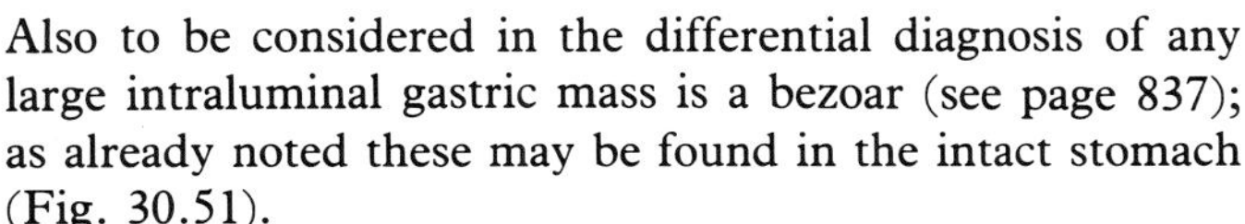

Also to be considered in the differential diagnosis of any large intraluminal gastric mass is a bezoar (see page 837); as already noted these may be found in the intact stomach (Fig. 30.51).

Ulcerating *carcinomas* (syn: primary carcinomatous ulcer) present as shallow ulcers with raised edges and infiltration of the surrounding tissues. It is clear from the preceding account that 'ulcerating carcinoma' is not the only type of gastric carcinoma in which ulceration occurs. Others include early gastric carcinoma types II (c) and III; malignant transformation of a chronic benign peptic ulcer; and ulceration occurring in a nodular or fungating tumour or in superficial erosive spreading carcinoma to such an extent that ulceration becomes the predominant feature.

Many gastric carcinomas, especially at an advanced stage, show features of more than one of the basic morphological types. Large, fungating, ulcerated tumours are found, producing both luminal narrowing and an extraluminal mass (Fig. 30.50C). Barium may enter irregular necrotic cavities within a tumour or associated inflammatory mass. Extension to adjacent organs may produce *fistulae*, especially to the transverse colon.

The role of the radiologist in suspected gastric cancer is to detect an abnormality, and, with the assistance of fluoroscopy, too produce a series of radiographs for analysis. As a policy, whenever there is a suspicion of an abnormality that could possibly be neoplastic, endoscopy with multiple biopsies should be the next procedure. For a full radiological assessment of a gastric carcinoma, and in order to determine suitability for surgical resection, it is necessary to decide:

1. Whether a tumour is producing obstruction

2. What are the tumour's basic morphological characteristics, viz. infiltrating, nodular, fungating, ulcerating or a combination of each
3. The extent of involvement of the stomach
4. If the oesophagus or duodenum are involved
5. The size of any extragastric tumour component, or abscess
6. The extent of spread of disease to adjacent organs and structures
7. Evidence of metastases, e.g. to lungs and liver.

The first four of these items of information are best obtained by double contrast barium meal, items 5 and 6, by CT and item 7 by a variety of means.

Computed tomography and ultrasound. The examination of malignant gastric tumours by CT provides useful preoperative information. Masses in the wall of the stomach and large ulcers are shown, but the main use of CT is to indicate the extent of extragastric spread of malignancy (Fig. 30.52A). Enlarged lymph nodes, abscesses and involvement of adjacent organs and structures are well demonstrated by CT. Also, metastases in the liver can be detected. Similar, but in general less accurate, information is also obtained by US. Carcinomas of the gut tube characteristically appear as a sonolucent periphery with a densely echogenic central zone (Fig. 30.52B). However, similar findings have been noted in cases of benign peptic ulceration, Crohn's disease, gastric lymphoma and metastatic disease to the stomach; and a multitude of colonic diseases including carcinoma. *Endoluminal ultrasonic scanning* can be used to evaluate the degree of tumour infiltration in the muscular wall and surrounding tissues. With further tech-

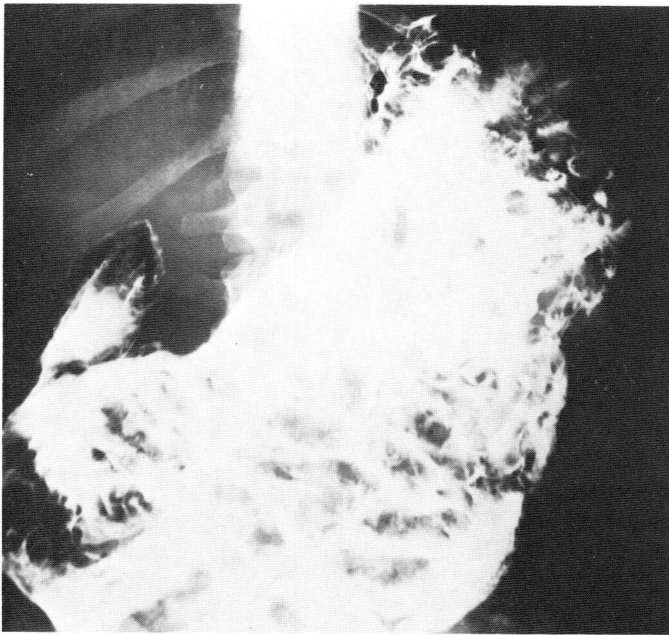

Fig. 30.51 A most unusual bezoar. A male aged 35 years presented with a history of vomiting for 4 days, getting worse. The barium meal shows multiple filling defects in a distended stomach. After this, further questioning revealed that in an attempt to smuggle marijuana through Customs, the patient had wrapped small amounts in cellophane and then dipped them in latex before swallowing them (1.5 kg!). Presumably the latex had not fully set and reacted with the gastric secretions to form a large mass in the stomach. The same evening, following the barium meal, he was admitted to hospital because of perforation. At operation a large coagulated mass of latex containing capsules of cellophane was removed. There were multiple ulcers in the stomach with perforation. Recovery was uneventful. (Courtesy of Dr Ben Green.)

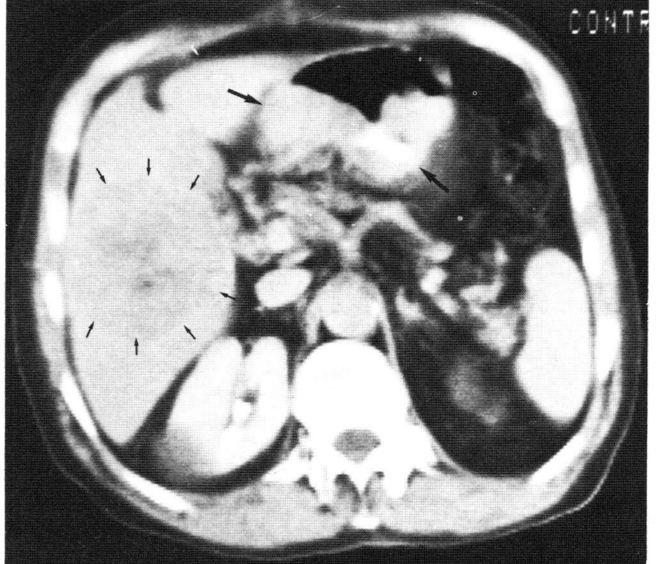

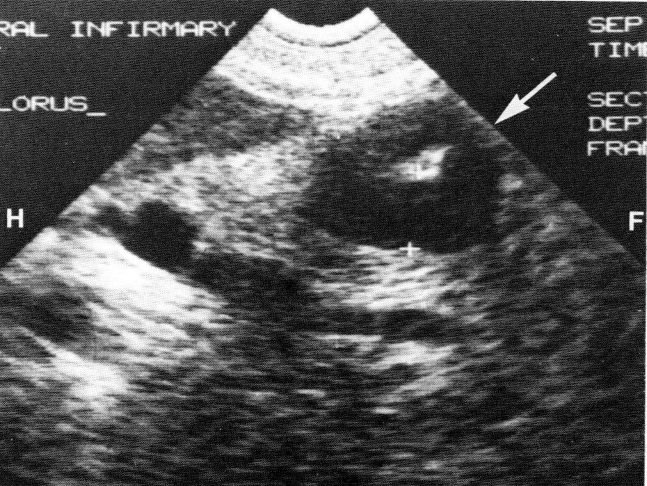

Fig. 30.52 **A**. Gastric carcinoma: CT examination. Gastric tumour (large arrows) with hepatic metastases (small arrows) in a patient presenting with right upper quadrant abdominal pain and fever. (Courtesy of Dr P J Robinson.) **B**. Gastric carcinoma demonstrated by US. Longitudinal scan (H = head, F = feet). The antral tumour (arrowed) has a target appearance; the thickened wall is seen as a sonolucent peripheral band with a densely echogenic core. (Courtesy of Dr J K Watters.)

nical developments this could become a valuable additional diagnostic tool in the evaluation of gastrointestinal tract tumours.

The value of CT and US in suspected malignant disease of the stomach is therefore as follows:

1. To confirm the diagnosis in some doubtful cases by showing thickening of the stomach wall.
2. To demonstrate the extent (if any) of extragastric disease, the involvement of adjacent organs, and ascites.
3. To detect metastases in the liver and lungs.
4. In the investigation of an abdominal mass of uncertain origin, to determine its origin and indicate which diagnostic procedure should be performed next.
5. As guidance for percutaneous needle biopsy to enable material to be obtained for histological or cytological examination.

MISCELLANEOUS GASTRIC TUMOURS AND INFILTRATIONS

Benign gastric polyps are uncommon, but with the increased use of double contrast technique they are being detected more frequently. Histologically they may be classified as 1. *regenerative* (*hyperplastic*), 2. *neoplastic* (*adenomatous*) or 3. *hamartomas*. The majority are hyperplastic, and these are usually small, multiple and evenly distributed throughout the stomach (Fig. 30.53A & B). Adenomas tend to be larger and are characteristically single lesions located in the gastric antrum (Fig. 30.53C). The most important difference between hyperplastic and adenomatous polyps is that whereas hyperplastic polyps have no significant cancer potential, adenomas have a definite liability to carcinomatous transformation. The incidence of malignancy in adenomas is related to size with a significant risk in those over 2 cm in diameter. Furthermore both hyperplastic and adenomatous polyps tend to develop in patients with chronic atrophic gastritis, a condition known to be associated with a high incidence of gastric carcinoma. Thus even if a gastric polyp is proved to be benign, the entire stomach must be carefully examined for the possibility of a coexisting carcinoma (Eisenberg 1983).

The polyposis syndromes which are characterized by polyps in the colon may be associated with gastric involvement. The polyps of *familial polyposis* (syn: adenomatosis

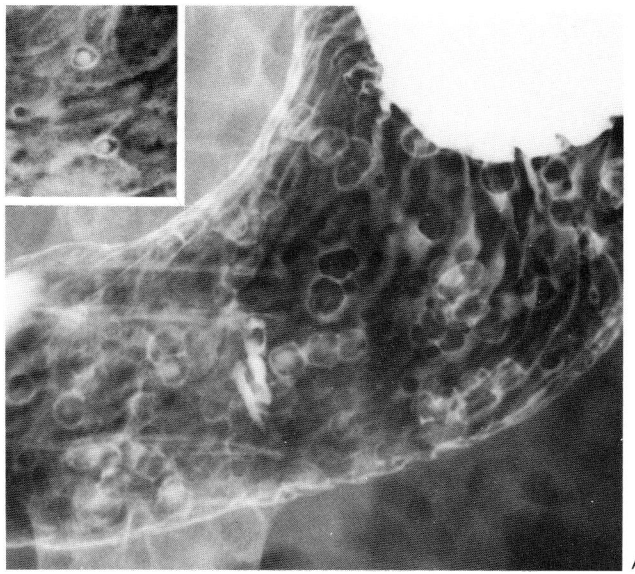

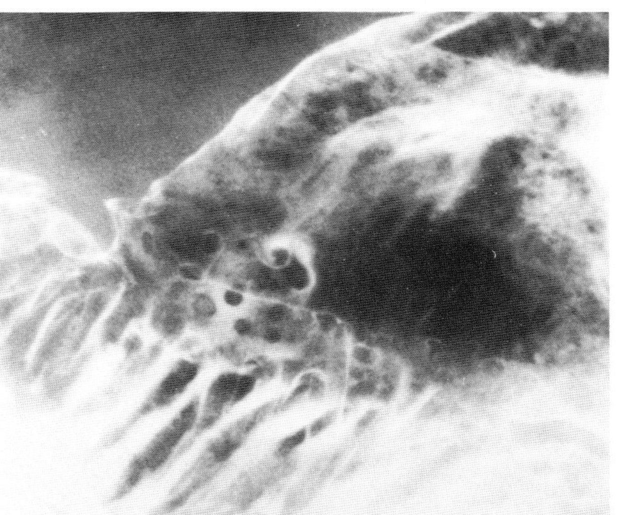

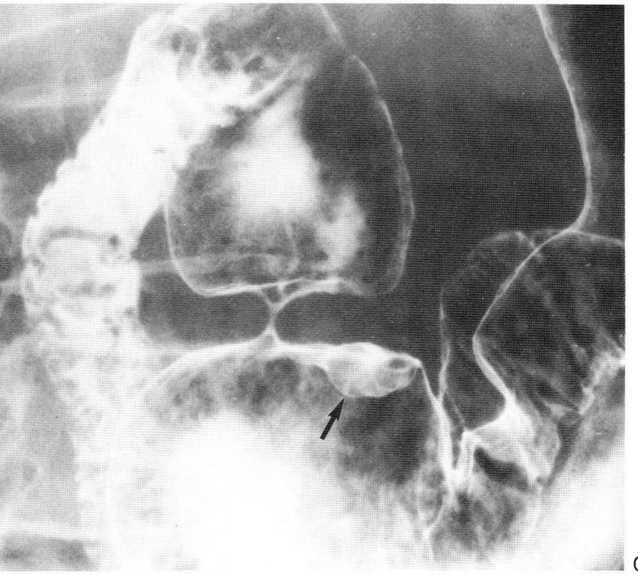

Fig. 30.53 Gastric polyps. **A**. Multiple benign hyperplastic polyps of various sizes evenly distributed throughout the stomach. Inset shows barium pooling on umbilicated polyps (a different case). Hamartomas may have an identical appearance. (Courtesy of Dr P M Chennells.) **B**. Small hyperplastic polyps, all of similar size in a group just proximal to a gastrojejunal stoma. (Courtesy of Dr S F Millward.) **C**. Solitary benign pedunculated adenomatous polyp in the gastric antrum. (Courtesy of Dr C E Williams.)

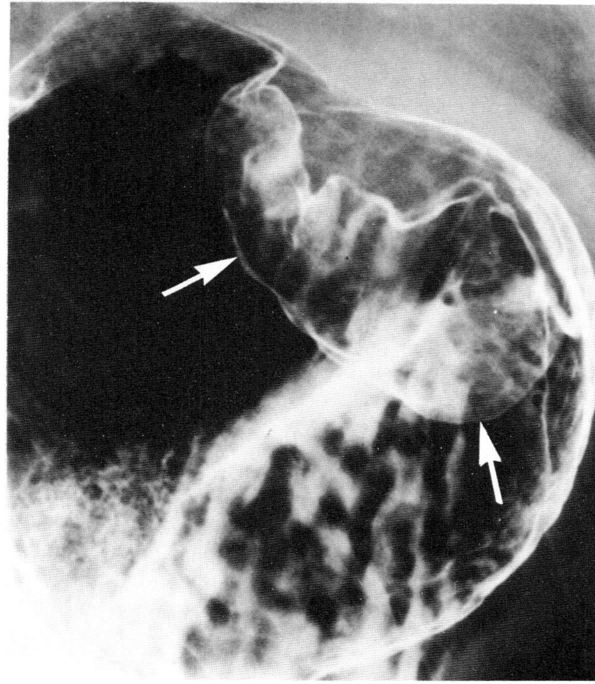

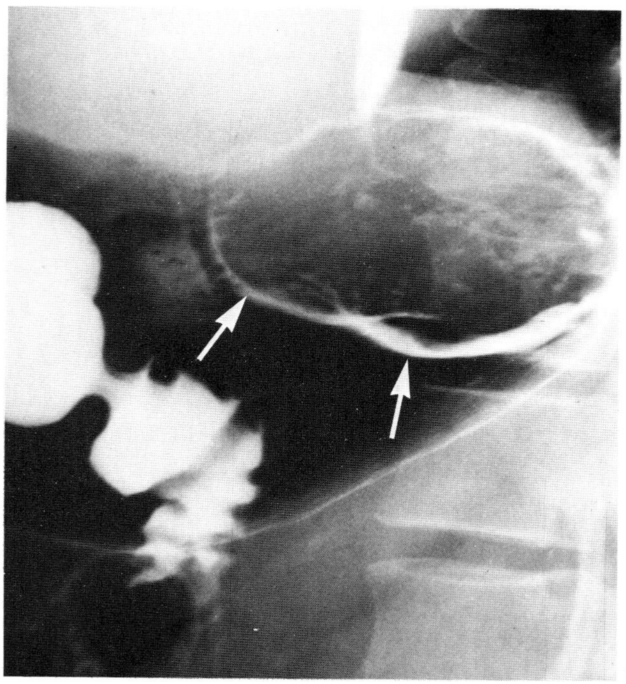

Fig. 30.54 Intramural tumours: Comparison of gastric leiomyoma with carcinoma. **A.** Benign leiomyoma producing a clearly defined filling defect in the gastric fundus typical of an intramural tumour. **B.** Gastric carcinoma in the form of a spherical mass in the gastric fundus resembling a leiomyoma.

coli) are adenomas and potentially malignant. In the *Cronkhite-Canada syndrome* (polyposis coli, nail and hair changes) polyps are benign and may regress. *Peutz-Jeghers* polyps are benign hamartomas.

Most gastric polyps are asymptomatic but bleeding sometimes occurs, and the pedunculated variety when situated near the pylorus are liable to prolapse through the pyloric canal into the duodenum producing intermittent obstruction. The radiographic features of gastric polyps are similar to those seen in the colon and described in detail in Chapter 32. A sessile polyp has a smooth, rounded dome and a base applied to the mucosal surface of the stomach, and the pedunculated variety has a head and a stalk by which it is attached (Fig. 30.53C). Some benign sessile polyps have a smooth shallow surface depression which may contain a small pool of barium when in the dependent position (Fig. 30.53B).

Intramural gastric tumours are uncommon and include *leiomyomas*, *neurofibromas* and *lipomas*, all of which may become sarcomatous. **Leiomyomas** are seen most frequently, usually as broad-based filling defects bulging into the gastric lumen (Fig. 30.54). Many leiomyomas are large with a substantial extraluminal component. Calcification and malignant transformation are usually features of the larger tumours, but the radiographic differentiation between benign and malignant tumours is unreliable. The mucosal surface of a leiomyoma is usually intact except in its centre where a depression or ulcer may occur. The central white barium collection with its surrounding translucent halo representing the tumour mass produces an appearance when viewed *en face* likened to a '*bull's eye*' or '*target*'.

This appearance is not specific to leiomyoma and results from ulceration or umbilication of any spherical or oval mass. A solitary large target lesion is most likely to be

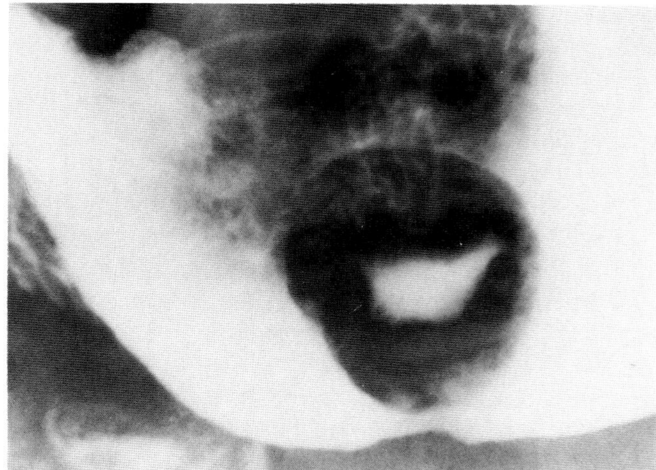

Fig. 30.55 Gastric 'target' lesion. An ulcerating spherical tumour in the body of the stomach. This pattern is typical of leiomyoma and of metastasis from melanoma, but the diagnosis in this case is primary gastric carcinoma.

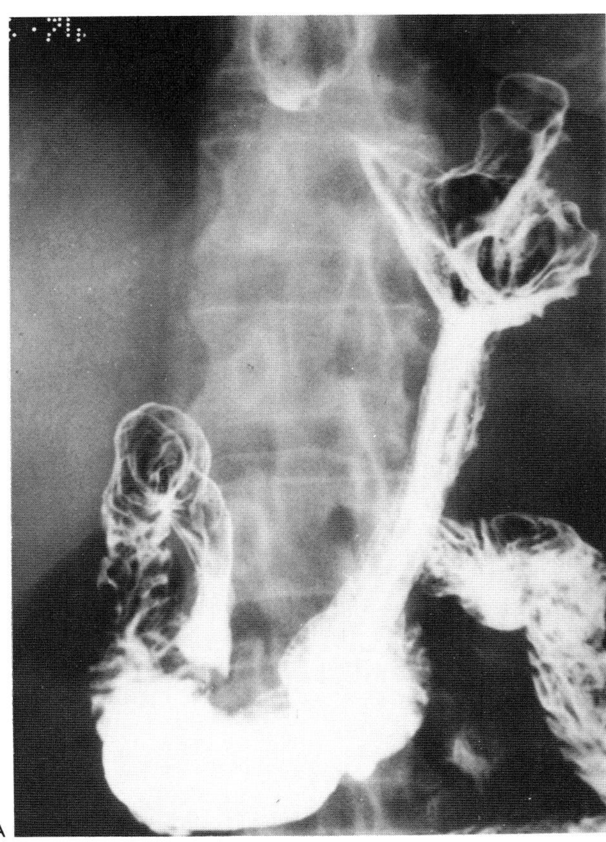

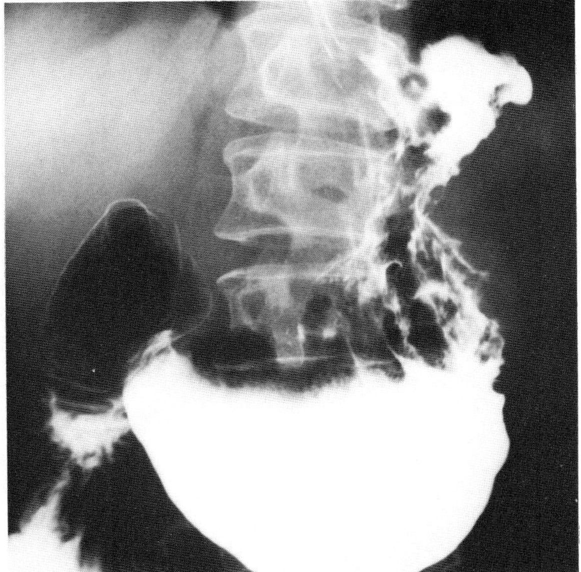

Fig. 30.56 Metastatic disease of the stomach. Two different cases, but both from primary carcinoma of the ovary. **A**. The fundus is encased by tumour, but not invaded. Endoscopy was twice negative. **B.** The fundus and body of the stomach is encased and invaded by metastatic carcinoma. Mucosal destruction and infiltration is present with ulceration. The appearances are indistinguishable from primary gastric carcinoma.

a primary gastric carcinoma (Fig. 30.55), metastasis or leiomyoma. Other rarer causes include lymphoma, carcinoid tumour, ectopic pancreas, and eosinophilic granuloma. Multiple target lesions in the gastrointestinal tract are highly suggestive of metastatic disease, especially melanoma. Multiple ulcerating metastases may also originate from carcinomas of the breast, bronchus, kidney and Kaposi's sarcoma. The most common cause of small target lesions in the stomach is erosive gastritis, but dimpled polyps should also be considered.

The main differential diagnosis of a non-ulcerating leiomyoma is from *primary gastric carcinoma*, *metastasis* and an *extrinsic mass*. Whatever its radiographic appearance the most likely diagnosis of any sizeable gastric tumour is primary carcinoma.

Metastatic disease manifests as mass lesions, but also occurs as an extrinsic encasement (Fig. 30.56A) and in an infiltrative form indistinguishable from a primary gastric carcinoma (Fig. 30.56B). The stomach can also be involved directly by malignant disease originating in neighbouring organs such as the pancreas and transverse colon. Initially an extrinsic mass may be demonstrated, but as spread occurs the stomach becomes fixed and ulceration may progress to fistula formation usually to the colon. Leiomyosarcoma can produce an identical appearance. An extrinsic impression on the stomach produced by enlargement of the liver, spleen, pancreas or kidney simulates a submucosal tumour with a large extrinsic component, and US, CT or angiography may be necessary for diagnosis.

Lymphoma involves the stomach in a number of ways and may be indistinguishable from gastric carcinoma. Differentiation is usually made by the detection of additional lymphomatous deposits either elsewhere in the intestinal tract or in other systems. Computed tomography has a useful role in this respect (Fig. 30.57). Also most

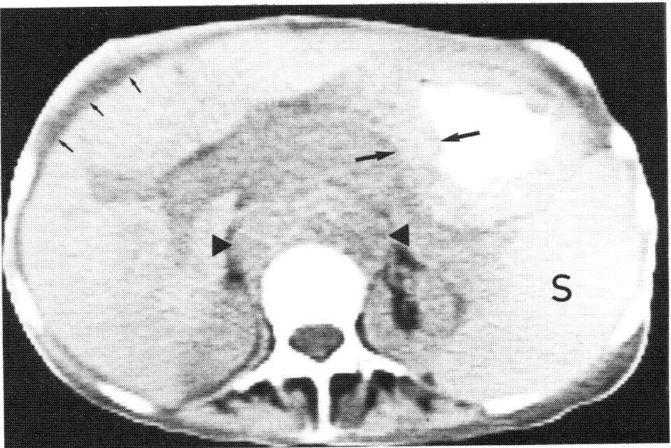

Fig. 30.57 Non-Hodgkins lymphoma. CT shows diffuse gastric wall thickening (arrows), ascites (small arrows), splenomegaly (S) and enlarged para-aortic lymph nodes (between two arrowheads) with a neoplastic mass extending anteriorly. (Courtesy of Dr P J Robinson.)

patients with lymphoma are younger than those with gastric carcinoma. Particular features on a barium meal that suggest the diagnosis of gastric lymphoma are thickened mucosal folds, ulceration, an associated extraluminal mass and extension of the disease into the duodenum (Fig. 30.58). A rare condition that can be mistaken for lymphoma both radiologically and histologically is *pseudolymphoma*, which is a benign proliferation of lymphoid tissue produced as a reaction to peptic ulceration.

Granulomatous diseases with gastric involvement are uncommon and include Crohn's disease, tuberculosis, sarcoidosis, histoplasmosis, syphilis and eosinophilic gastritis. The radiographic manifestations of all of these conditions are similar, consisting of narrowing of the lumen accompanied by mucosal changes. The main differential diagnosis is carcinoma.

In Great Britain the granulomatous disease most likely to affect the stomach is *Crohn's disease* in the indigenous population, and *tuberculosis* in those originating from the Indian subcontinent. The earliest changes of Crohn's disease discernible on the double contrast barium meal are small superficial erosions (aphthoid ulcers), seen *en face* as tiny specks of barium surrounded by translucent halos. Gastric erosions are not specific to Crohn's disease and are more commonly due to other conditions such as erosive gastritis and coeliac disease. In established Crohn's disease deep ulceration, thickened mucosal folds and a cobblestone surface pattern are seen (Fig. 30.59). Narrowing of the gastric antrum is a common feature, and frequently the adjacent duodenum is also involved to produce by obliteration of the normal configuration an appearance known as '*pseudo-Bilroth I*' because of the resemblance to this post-surgical state. Differentiation of tuberculosis from Crohn's and the other granulomatous diseases is made by identification of the tubercle bacillus and by response to anti-

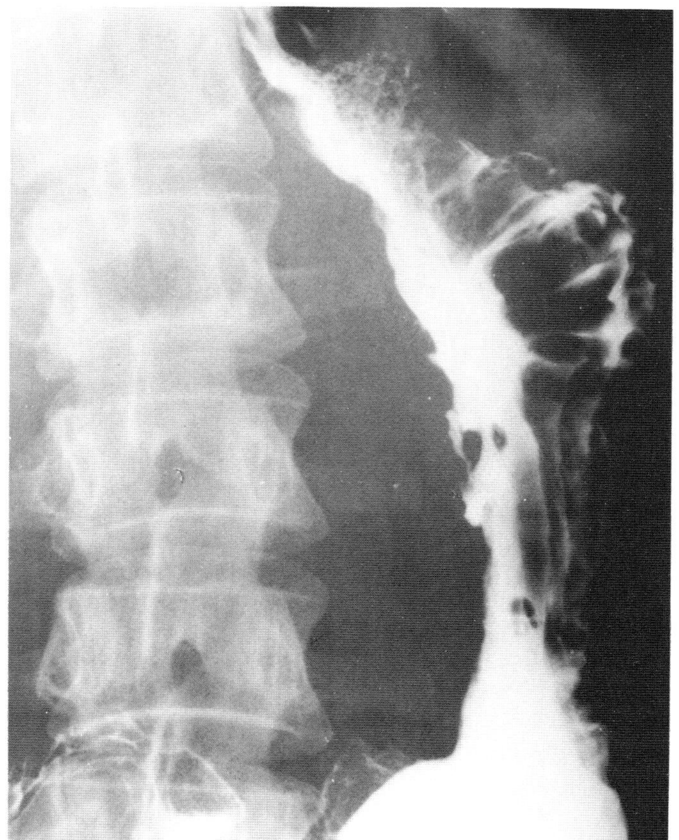

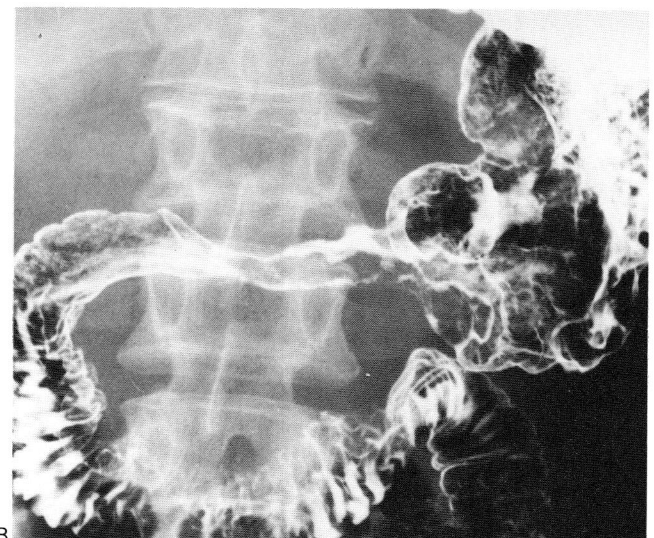

Fig. 30.58 Gastric lymphoma. **A.** The proximal lesser curvature of the stomach is irregular and ulcerated with thick mucosal folds in the fundus. **B.** An irregular stricture is present in the distal stomach, also involving the duodenal cap. A large associated soft tissue mass is producing an impression on the inside of the duodenal loop.

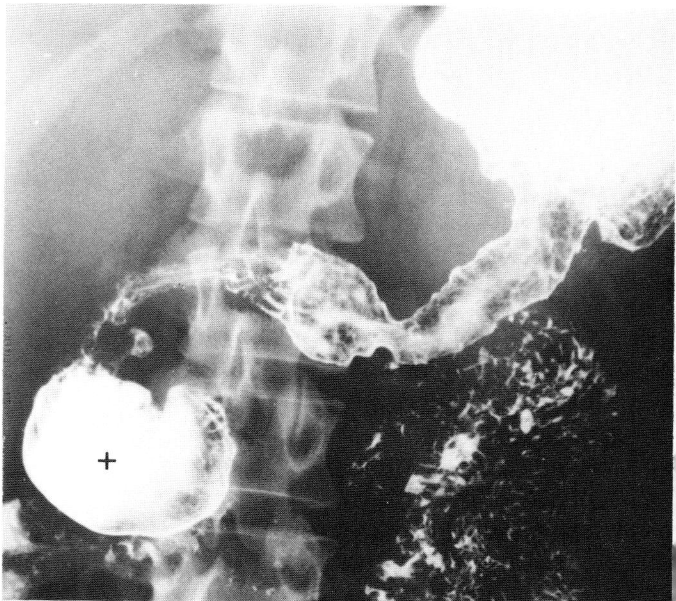

Fig. 30.59 Gastroduodenal Crohn's disease. Narrowing and irregularity of the distal two thirds of the stomach simulates gastric carcinoma. There are two strictures in the duodenum, separated by a short segment of dilated duodenum (+).

tuberculous therapy. In most cases of Crohn's disease and tuberculosis there is other evidence of the disease in the intestinal tract especially in the ileocaecal region. There may be coexistent gastric and pulmonary tuberculosis.

Eosinophilic gastritis is a rare granulomatous disease which also affects the small bowel, hence the term eosinophilic gastroenteritis. Eosinophilia is usually present and the condition is believed to be an allergy. Barium examination is non specific, showing narrowing of the antrum with thickened mucosal folds.

DUODENAL TUMOURS

The demonstration of ulcers, tumours and other lesions in the duodenal cap and loop is conveniently achieved by tubeless hypotonic duodenography performed as an integral part of the routine double contrast barium meal. The second part of the duodenum can be regularly demonstrated with the patient in the supine RAO and prone positions. Almost 90% of tumours in the duodenal cap are benign. In the duodenal loop the incidence of benign and malignant tumours is approximately equal, and in the remainder of the duodenum malignant tumours predominate.

Benign duodenal neoplasms are often asymptomatic, but ulceration with haemorrhage and abdominal pain may occur, and intraluminal tumours may undergo intussusception. The commonest benign tumour of the duodenum is the *adenoma*. Most adenomatous polyps are less than 1 cm in diameter, and are either sessile or pedunculated with the same morphological features as elsewhere in the bowel. Villous adenomas are rare with a high malignant potential, appearing radiographically as lobulated filling defects with a network of barium-coated fronds. Small *hamartomatous* polyps may be found in patients with the Peutz-Jeghers syndrome. *Leiomyomas* are intramural tumours bulging into the lumen of the duodenum with intact mucosa over their surface except when ulcerated (Fig. 30.60). *Lipomas* are translucent submucosal tumours which may be pedunculated, and liable to change shape under the influence of palpation, gravity and peristalsis. Benign or malignant *carcinoid tumours* are usually single, lobulated and located in the duodenal cap or postbulbar region (Fig. 30.61).

Primary malignancy of the duodenum is relatively uncommon compared with the stomach. Weight loss and anorexia are frequent presenting symptoms, and bleeding and obstruction also occur. Tumours involving the papilla of Vater produce obstructive jaundice. The most common primary malignant duodenal tumour is an adenocarcinoma, followed by leiomyosarcoma. *Adenocarcinomas* occur most frequently in the third (transverse) part of the duodenum, and around the ampulla of Vater. Stenosing, ulcerating and polypoid forms are seen with features resembling adenocarcinoma elsewhere in the gastrointestinal tract (Fig. 30.62).

Secondary cancer produces similar appearances either by metastasis, or extension from a contiguous cancer of an adjacent organ such as the pancreas (Fig. 30.63). It may not be possible to distinguish between a primary carcinoma of the duodenum and a carcinoma of the pancreas invading the duodenum. Metastases are frequently multiple, have a large extrinsic mass component and may be accompanied by widespread peritoneal metastatic disease with malignant ascites. Duodenal filling defects with central necrosis and ulceration ('target' or 'bull's eye' lesions) suggest leiomyoma or haematogenous metastases, particularly melanoma.

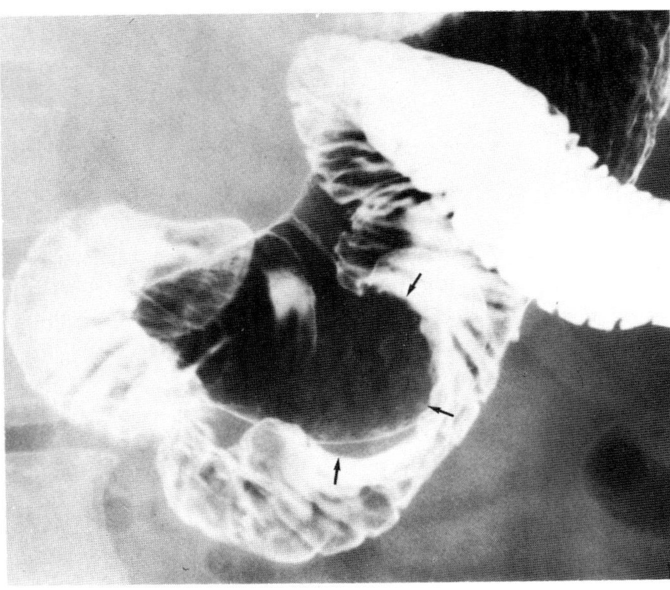

Fig. 30.60 Duodenal leiomyoma. Extrinsic filling defect in the inner aspect of the third part of the duodenum showing the typical form of an intramural tumour. (Courtesy of Dr B M Carey.)

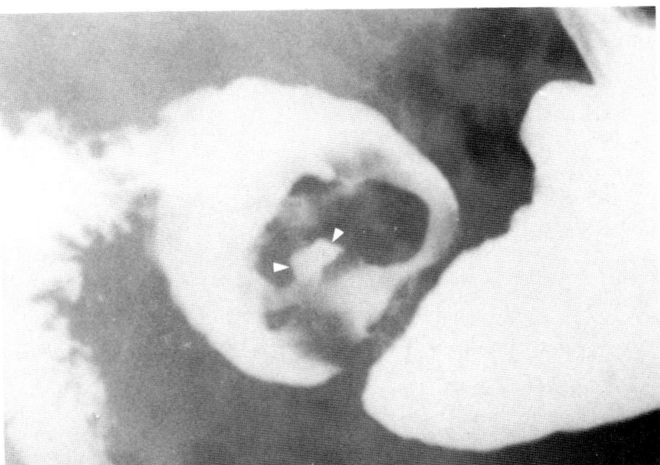

Fig. 30.61 Duodenal carcinoid tumour. An irregular, lobulated filling defect with central ulceration (arrows) is present in the duodenal cap. Leiomyoma, melanoma, metastasis and duodenal ulcer with oedema can produce this appearance.

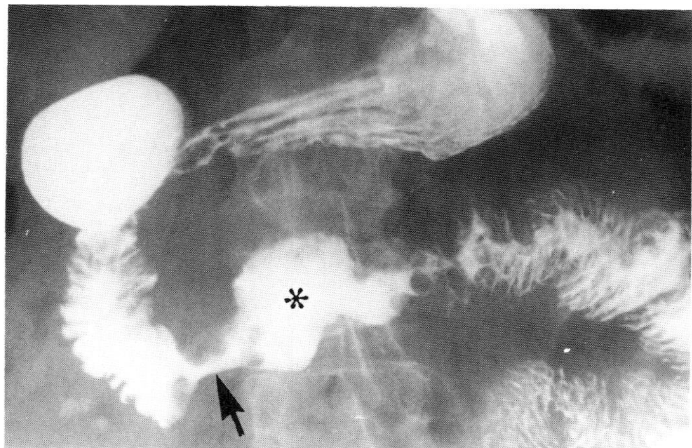

Fig. 30.62
Primary carcinoma of the third part of the duodenum. The tumour is large, comprising a stricture (arrowed), a necrotic cavity (*), and a soft tissue mass. The mass is compressing the small bowel at the duodenojejunal flexure and elevating the distal part of the greater curvature of the stomach.

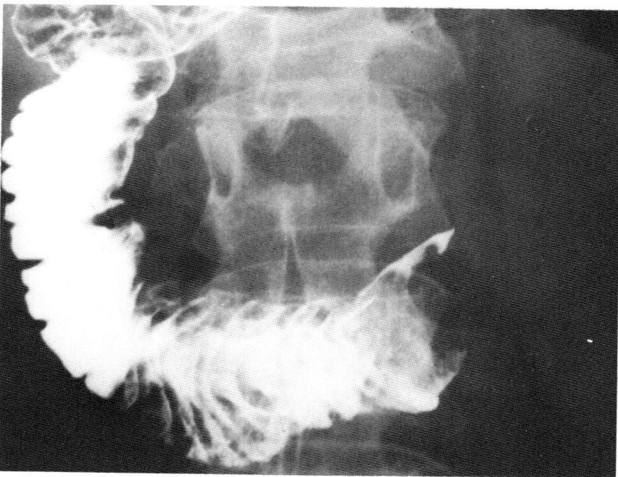

Fig. 30.63 Carcinoma of the pancreas producing complete obstruction of the third part of the duodenum. An associated soft tissue mass is compressing the duodenum proximal to the point of obstruction. A primary carcinoma of the duodenum or a metastasis can give an identical appearance.

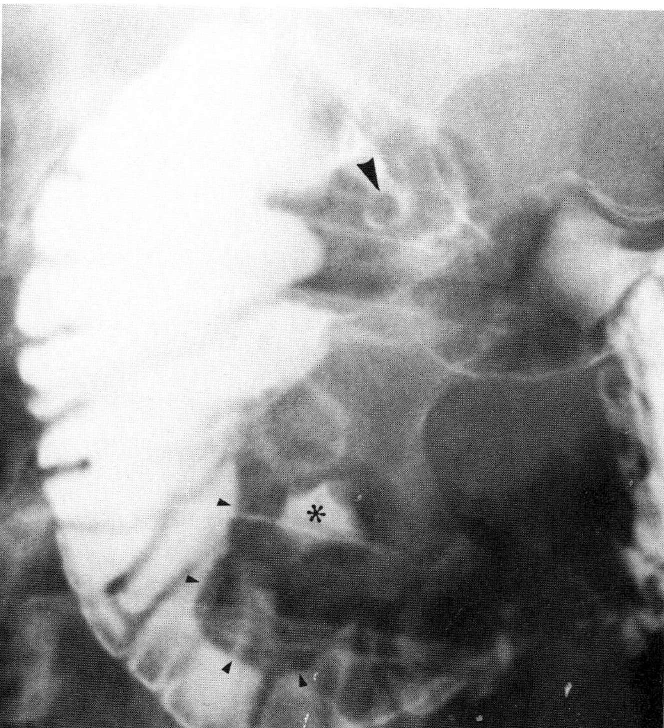

Fig. 30.64 Duodenal leiomyosarcoma. The patient presented with haematemesis. There is an ulcerating (*) tumour in the third part of the duodenum which was found at operation to be a leiomyosarcoma. The cause of the bleeding however was an anterior wall duodenal ulcer (large arrowhead).

Leiomyosarcomas cannot be reliably differentiated from their benign counterpart by radiographic means, and generally present as lobulated intramural filling defects, often with central ulceration (Fig. 30.64). *Primary lymphoma* of the duodenum is rare, presenting as a polypoid mass, thickened folds or multiple nodules.

MISCELLANEOUS DUODENAL FILLING DEFECTS AND INFILTRATIONS: DIFFERENTIAL DIAGNOSIS

Other conditions that simulate a duodenal neoplasm by appearing as filling defects on barium examination may be conveniently grouped as either located in the duodenal cap or beyond.

Defects in the duodenal cap

These include a prolapsed pedunculated antral polyp, gastric mucosal fold prolapse, adenomas and cysts of Brunner's glands, extrinsic impression by a distended gallbladder, flexure defect pseudotumour, oedema around an ulcer crater, blood clot and food residue.

The head of a *pedunculated polyp* with its base attached to the gastric antrum, may occasionally pass through the pylorus and come to lie in the duodenal cap (Fig. 30.65). Upper abdominal discomfort and intermittent obstruction may result. The characteristic morphology of such a polyp is usually obvious on fluoroscopy and on the radiographs. Similarly, *redundant mucosa* in the gastric antrum can prolapse through the pylorus under the influence of peristalsis resulting in a lobulated umbrella-shaped filling defect at the base of the duodenal cap. Mucosal folds can usually be traced from the antrum. The condition is not generally considered to be of any clinical significance. *Adenomas and cysts of Brunner's glands* are rare tumours which present radiologically as solitary filling defects in the duodenum. The *flexure defect pseudotumour* is a normal finding due to bunching of mucosal folds at the apex of the cap where the

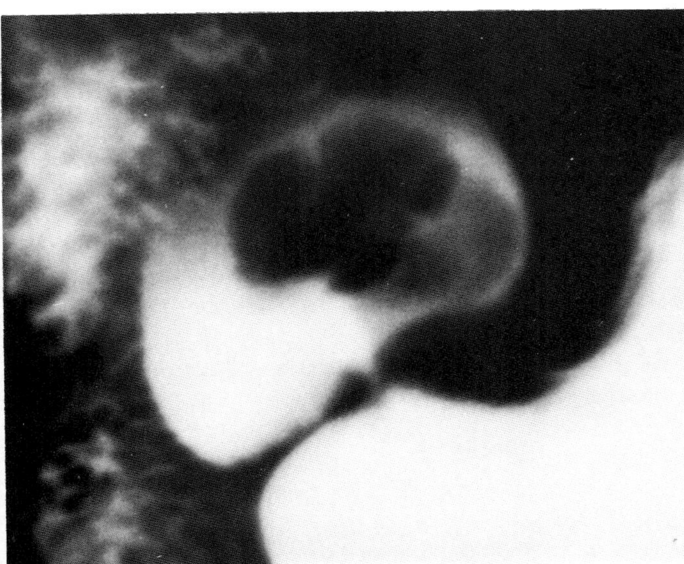

Fig. 30.65 Pedunculated gastric polyp. The head of the polyp has prolapsed through the pyloric canal to produce a translucent filling defect in the duodenal cap.

direction of the duodenum changes acutely (Fig. 30.66). Oedema around an ulcer crater (*the ulcer mound*) can be prominent and simulate an ulcerated tumour. Differentiation can usually be made because the ulcer mound is relatively shallow, and there are often secondary signs of ulceration such as radiating folds or scars. *Blood clots* or *food residue* in the cap are usually mobile and may change in shape throughout the course of a barium examination.

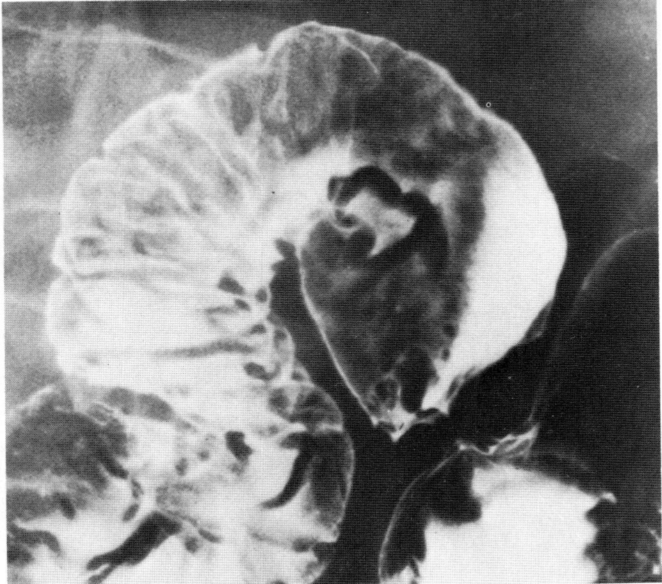

Fig. 30.66 Pseudotumour at the apex of the duodenal cap, and produced by bunching of folds as the duodenum changes directions.

A bleeding lesion may be identified to account for blood clot. Food residues in the duodenum are rare except when there is obstruction.

Lesions in the duodenum beyond the cap

These are usually single, and include aberrant pancreatic tissue (ectopic pancreas), annular pancreas, an enlarged papilla of Vater, perivaterian carcinoma, choledochocele and duplication cyst. Multiple filling defects may be produced by varices and haematomas. Lesions of the pancreas also affect the duodenal loop.

Ectopic pancreas (syn: pancreatic rest) is an embryological anomaly that can present as a filling defect resembling a sessile polyp. Pancreatic rests are usually single and occur most frequently in the gastric antrum. Those found in the duodenum are usually in the cap or second part. A characteristic radiographic sign of ectopic pancreas is a central barium collection resembling an ulcer crater, but in fact due to filling of miniature duct-like structures present in the nodules of pancreatic tissue. The condition is generally asymptomatic, although bleeding is a possibility.

Annular pancreas results from overdevelopment of the uncinate process of the head of the gland leading to the formation of a ring of pancreatic tissue surrounding the duodenum. The radiographic appearance of an annular pancreas in adults is a pronounced notch-like defect in the lateral wall of the second part of the duodenum causing an eccentric narrowing of the lumen without ulceration (Fig. 30.67). Obstruction may occur.

The papilla of Vater projects into the lumen on the inner side of the second part of the duodenum at or just below the promontory, and is best demonstrated by hypotonic duodenography (Fig. 30.5). Enlargement of the papilla is usually due to oedema produced by impaction of a gall stone in the distal common bile duct, or pancreatitis. An oedematous papilla has the shape of a half pea which may become more spherical when swelling is gross, in differentiation from a perivaterian carcinoma where the filling defect is usually irregular, nodular and ulcerated.

Perivaterian carcinoma is a collective term which includes a number of malignancies arising in the duodenum, distal common bile duct, ampulla or pancreas which can either extend to involve the papilla or produce a separate intraluminal tumour mass simulating the papilla.

A choledochocele is a rare cystic dilatation of the intraduodenal portion of the common bile duct producing a smooth extrinsic impression on the inner wall of the second part of the duodenum. A dilated obstructed *common bile duct* may also indent the duodenum.

Duodenal *duplication cysts* can appear as intramural filling defects, but usually present as abdominal masses in childhood.

Duodenal varices occurring in portal hypertension are almost always associated with oesophageal varices, and

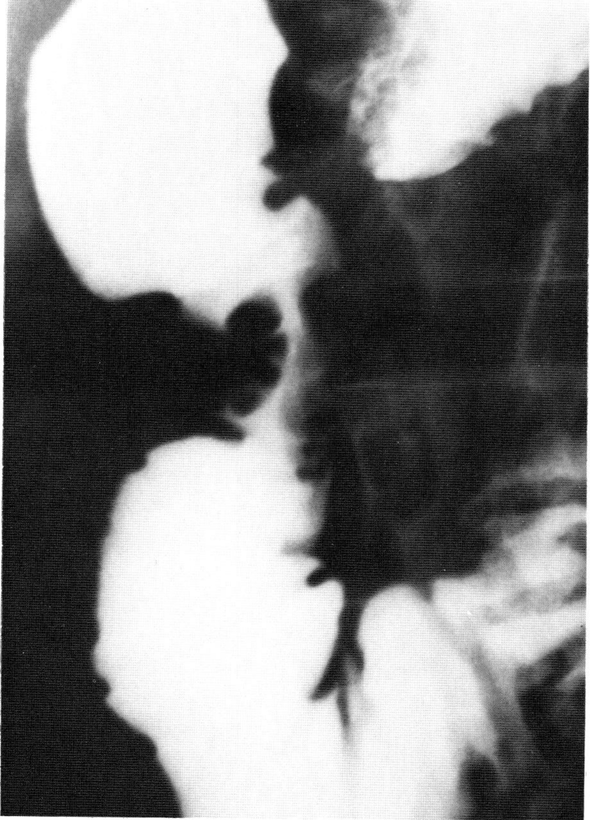

Fig. 30.67 Annular pancreas producing characteristic eccentric narrowing of the second part of the duodenum, with a prominent filling defect on its lateral aspect. (Courtesy of Dr D J Lintott.)

produce serpiginous thickening of mucosal folds. Intramural and submucosal duodenal **haematomas** can occur from trauma, or from bleeding in those receiving anticoagulants or with a bleeding diathesis. Frequently the jejunum is also involved. A series of semilunar filling defects resembling a row of 'thumb prints' is characteristic. A more generalized oedema may produce thickening of mucosal folds and an appearance likened in profile to a '*picket fence*'. The duodenum is susceptible to injury by blunt abdominal trauma because of its fixity and its position in front of the vertebral column. Bleeding into the duodenal wall produces an intramural mass that may be large enough to cause obstruction.

By the time **carcinoma of the pancreas** affects the duodenum the prospects of surgical cure are remote. Methods of examination capable of diagnosing tumours at a very early stage are necessary and these are described in Chapter 35. The most common manifestation of pancreatic cancer is painless jaundice resulting from obstruction of the lower end of the common bile duct. Approximately 70% of pancreatic carcinomas arise in the head of the gland and tend to affect the duodenal loop by compressing the mucosal folds along its inner border to produce a 'double-contour' effect, and by widening its sweep. The tethering influence of the ampulla of Vater is responsible for the expanded loop assuming a reversed 3 configuration known as *Frostberg's sign* (Fig. 30.68). Other signs of abnormality along the inner duodenal border comprise nodularity, spiculation and flattening with fold effacement. Further tumour growth may proceed to invasion of the duodenum with mucosal destruction and ulceration (Fig. 30.69A). Distortion of a duodenal diverticulum by compression from a pancreatic mass is an infrequent finding (Fig. 30.69B).

A mass in the head of the pancreas may also produce a pressure defect in the greater curvature of the antrum of the stomach known as the 'pad sign' (Fig. 30.69B). A carcinoma arising in the body or tail of the pancreas may involve the third part of the duodenum (Fig. 30.63), and displace the stomach forwards.

Acute inflammatory disease in the upper abdomen such as *pancreatitis and cholecystitis* frequently produces secondary changes on the duodenum, usually the second part. Spasm and mucosal oedema narrow the duodenal lumen. Enlargement of the head of the pancreas in acute pancreatitis enlarges the duodenal loop in a similar manner to carcinoma. A *pancreatic pseudocyst* may simulate a carcinoma by its mass effect on the stomach or duodenum according to its location. Barium studies have limited discriminatory value and examination by US or CT is more informative.

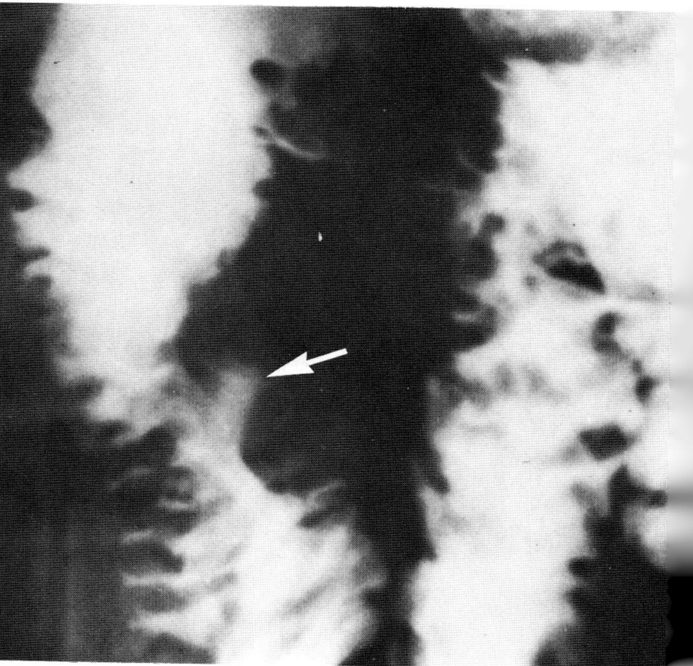

Fig. 30.68 The Frostberg reversed 3 sign characteristic of a tumour of the head of the pancreas. In this case the cause is a periampullary carcinoid tumour. The arrow indicates the site of the ampulla, (and the central limb of the reversed 3). (Courtesy of Dr A Schulman.)

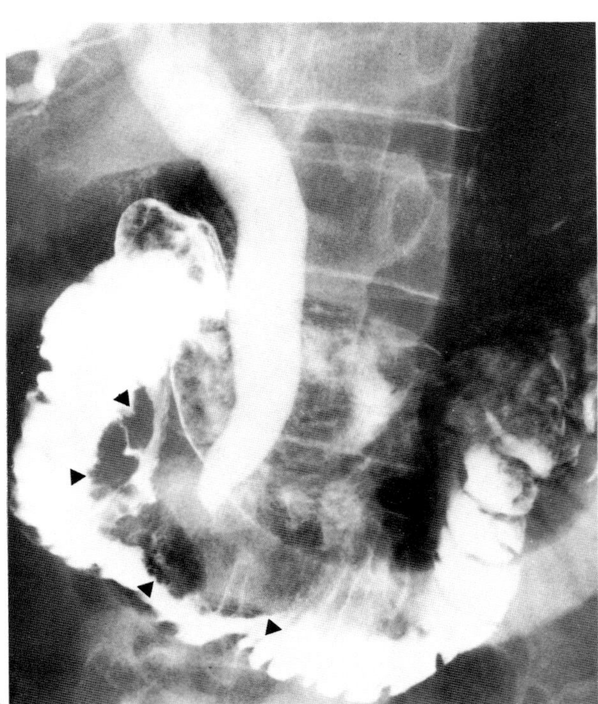

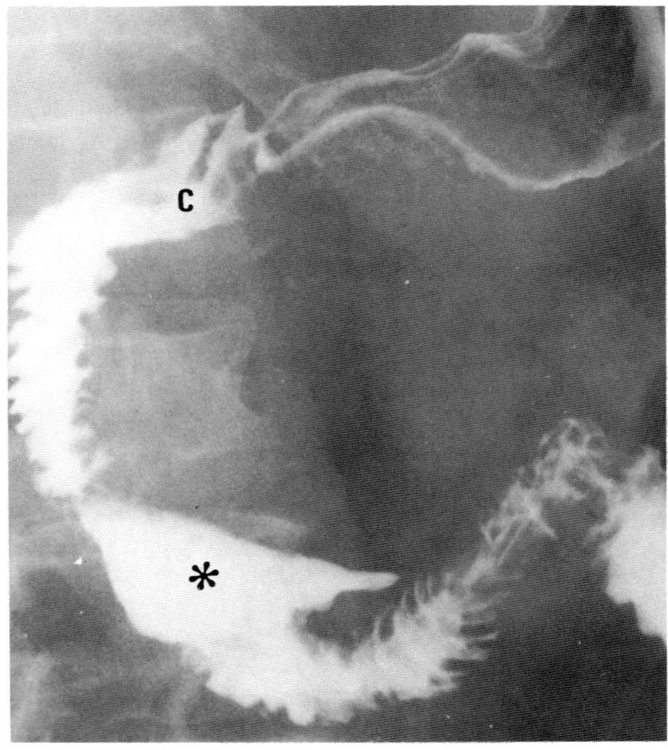

Fig. 30.69 Carcinoma of the pancreas. **A.** Carcinoma of the head of the pancreas invading the medial wall of the duodenal loop. A percutaneous transhepatic cholangiogram performed with the barium study shows the common bile duct obstructed at its lower end. (Courtesy of Dr A Chapman.) **B.** Pancreatic tumour producing an impression on a duodenal diverticulum (*), and also impressing and elevating the gastric antrum (the pad sign). C = duodenal cap.

REFERENCES AND SUGGESTED FURTHER READING

Alavi, A., Arger, P. H. (1980) Radioisotopic detection and localisation of gastrointestinal bleeding. In: *Multiple Imaging Procedures, 3. Abdomen*, pp. 121–142. New York: Grune and Stratton Inc.

Anderson, J. R., Earnshaw, P. M., & Fraser, G. M. (1982) Extrinsic compression of the third part of the duodenum. *Clinical Radiology*, **33**, 75–81

Beckley, D. E. (1974) Alimentary tract metastases from malignant melanoma. *Clinical Radiology*, **25**, 385–390

Beggs. I., & Freeman, A. H. (1982) Excavated tumours of the gut. *Clinical Radiology*, **33**, 523–528

Craig, O., & Gregson, R. (1981) Primary lymphoma of the gastrointestinal tract. *Clinical Radiology*, **32**, 63–71

de Roos, A., & Op den Orth, J. O. (1982) Linear niches in the duodenal bulb. *American Journal of Radiology*, **140**, 941–944

Eisenberg, R. L. (1983) *Gastrointestinal Radiology* J. B. Lippincott Company

Franken, E. A. (1973) Caustic damage of the gastrointestinal tract. *American Journal of Radiology*, **118**, 77–85

Fraser, G. M. (1978) The double contrast barium meal in patients with acute upper gastrointestinal bleeding. *Clinical Radiology*, **29**, 625–634

Fraser, G. M., & Earnshaw, P. M. (1983) The double contrast barium meal: A correlation with endoscopy. *Clinical Radiology*, **341**, 121–131

Gelfand, D. W. (1984) *Gastrointestinal Radiology*. Edinburgh: Churchill, Livingstone

Gordon, R., Laufer, I., & Kressel, H. Y. (1980) Gastric polyps found on routine double contrast examination of the stomach. *Radiology*, **134**, 27–30

Gregson, R., & Craig, O. (1983) Aorto-enteric fistulae: The role of radiology. *Clinical Radiology*, **34**, 65–72

Joffe, S. N., Lee, F. D., & Blumgart, L. H. (1978) Duodenitis. In: *Clinics in Gastroenterology*, *7,3*, pp. 635–650. London, Philadelpia, Toronto: W. B. Saunders Company.

Komaiko, M. S. (1979) Gastric neoplasm: Ultrasound and CT evaluation. *Gastrointestinal Radiology*, **4**, 131–137

Laufer, I. (1979) *Double Contrast Gastrointestinal Radiology*. London, Philadelphia, Toronto: W. B. Saunders Company

Laufer, I., Hamilton, J., & Mullens, J. E. (1975) Demonstration of superficial gastric erosions by double contrast radiography. *Gastroenterology*, **68**, 387–391

Margulis, A. R., &Burthenne, H. J. (1983) *Alimentary Tract Radiology*, 3rd edn. St Louis, Toronto, London: The C. V. Mosby Company.

Mendelson, R. M. (1985) Horses for courses in the upper GI Tract: an approach to diagnosis: *Radiology Now*, **7**, 13–16

Morson, B. C., & Dawson, I. M. P. (1979) *Gastrointestinal Pathology*. Oxford: Blackwell Scientific Publications.

Press, A. J. (1975) Practical significance of gastric rugal folds. *American Journal of Radiology*, **125**, 172–183

Salter, R. H., Girdwood, T. G., Scott-Harden, W. G., & Cole, T. P. (1978) Endoscopic and radiological assessment of recurrent ulceration after peptic ulcer surgery. *British Journal of Radiology*, **51**, 257–259

Stevenson, G. W. (1977) The distribution of gastric ulcers: Double contrast barium meal and endoscopy findings. *Clinical Radiology*, **28**, 617–622

Stevenson, G. W. (1978) Gastroduodenal lesions in Crohn's disease. *Gut*, **19**, 962–966

Wolfe, B. S. (1971) Observations on Roentgen features of benign and malignant gastric ulcers. *Seminars in Roentgenology*, **6**, 140–150

Young, J. W., Ginthner, T. P., & Keramati, B. (1985) The competitive barium meal. *Clinical Radiology*, **36**, 43–46

CHAPTER 31

THE SMALL BOWEL

Imaging of the small bowel is performed by conventional radiological techniques in the vast majority of cases. The newer imaging techniques have only a minor and auxiliary role in selected cases.

The radiological investigation of the small intestine is not easy since there are some 6.7 metres (22 feet) of rhythmically contracting coiled tube to be examined, of which only the extreme ends are fixed in position. By comparison, the stomach and colon are easy to examine by well established double contrast techniques and can also be examined by endoscopy. Nevertheless reliable and accurate examination of the small intestine is essential since it is the main organ of absorption into the body and it is the only part of the gut we cannot live without.

Since the radiological examination of the small bowel is time-consuming and involves the patient in considerable X-irradiation it should never become a routine addendum to a barium meal examination. Most patients with clinical evidence of small bowel disease do not need detailed examination of the stomach and the chances of finding small bowel pathology in a patient with symptoms referable to the stomach or duodenum are small. Moreover, examination of the stomach and small intestine are not easily combined, since double contrast examination of the stomach requires a relatively small volume of high-density barium whereas the examination of the small bowel requires a large volume of more dilute barium. A 'follow-through examination', consisting of a few overcouch films taken at predetermined intervals without fluoroscopy, is not an adequate examination of the small intestine. The exact indication for the examination, together with details of any previous abdominal surgery, should be known before the examination begins so that the most suitable technique to investigate the specific problem can be chosen.

There are many different ways of examining the small bowel, each having enthusiastic advocates. The method of choice often depends on the reason for the examination. As each method has a different appearance in the normal as well as in disease, it is essential that the radiologist should be thoroughly familiar with the methods he is using. Although the techniques vary in detail, the following principles are common to them all:

1. The small intestine should be demonstrated in continuity by a continuous column of barium sulphate mixture (Fig. 31.1).
2. When any abnormality is seen on a supine film, an erect horizontal ray film should be taken at the same time and the two films examined and diagnosed together.
3. Whenever possible, the small bowel should be examined when distended as well as when collapsed.
4. Overlapping coils should be separated by taking prone or oblique projections and by applying general or local abdominal compression.

Contrast medium

The exact composition of commercial barium sulphate preparations is a trade secret and may be changed by the manufacturers without reference to the radiologists who use them. Since the radiological appearance and the

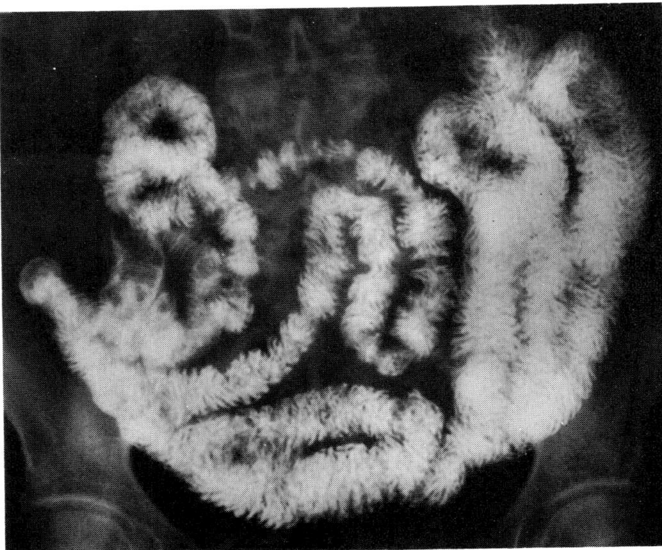

Fig. 31.1 Normal small bowel meal showing the continuous feathery pattern of the small intestine.

interpretation of the findings depend to some extent upon the composition of the preparation this is not a desirable situation. Most modern barium preparations are designed to resist flocculation when mixed with intestinal contents. This is, however, variable, and many preparations will flocculate in infants and children and to some extent in adults, particularly if the transit time is very long. Another variable is the osmolarity of the contrast medium when in the small bowel. Many barium sulphate preparations become concentrated when in the small intestine by the extraction of water, while others contain a hydroscopic agent such as carboxymethylcellulose which retains water within the lumen of the small intestine giving a more bulky appearance and tending to distend the small intestine.

Water-soluble contrast media such as Gastrografin have been advocated, particularly in suspected incomplete small bowel obstruction. However, its high osmolarity and consequent dilution in the small bowel make it quite unsuitable as a contrast medium. The resulting large volume of dilute contrast medium shows neither the site of the obstruction nor any detail of the mucosal pattern. A small volume (e.g. 10 ml) of Gastrografin may be added to barium sulphate preparation in order to increase the bulk of the contrast medium and to hasten transit into the colon. *Magnesium sulphate* 10–15 g will have a similar effect and will also prevent the barium becoming inspissated in the colon (Fig. 31.46). This can be helpful, particularly in bedridden or elderly patients who may have difficulty getting rid of the barium from the colon.

Most barium preparations are approximately isotonic and may give useful information in patients with subacute small bowel obstruction. They will never complete an incomplete obstruction of the small bowel, but should be used with caution if colonic obstruction is suspected.

TECHNIQUES OF EXAMINATION

The barium sulphate may be given by mouth, as in the *small bowel meal*, or following intubation of the duodenum or the first loop of jejunum, as in the *small bowel enema*, which can produce either a single or a double contrast examination. In many centres the small bowel is examined by the conventional method of the small bowel meal and the small bowel enema is reserved for patients with specific problems in whom the simple technique has not provided sufficient information.

The small bowel meal

The aim is to outline the small intestine throughout its length by a continuous column of barium in the shortest possible time with the least upset to the patient (Fig. 31.1). There is a wide variation in transit time in the normal small bowel, so that the actual time taken for barium to pass from the duodenum to the caecum is of little significance, especially if an accelerating agent has been used. Flocculation of barium may occur if the transit time is very long. Although there are many minor variations in technique the following principles are worth observing:

1. Enough barium sulphate preparation should be given for there to be some in the stomach throughout the examination. The presence of barium in the antrum acts as a stimulus to peristalsis, helping to propel the barium along the small intestine and shorten the examination time. If the stomach is found to be empty when most of the small bowel has been outlined, but the barium has not yet reached the caecum, a dry meal (e.g. a sandwich and a small cup of coffee) may be given instead of more barium sulphate in order to propel the barium on its way. On average, between 10 and 20 ounces (280–560 g) of barium sulphate, diluted to approximately 45% w/v, is required to outline the small bowel. If very dilute barium is used the excess added water will soon be removed in the jejunum and passed from the body as urine, unless a hydroscopic agent is present in, or added to, the barium preparation. A small volume, e.g. 10 ml of Gastrografin, may be added as an accelerator. This is insufficient to affect the osmolarity or stability of the mixture.

2. During the whole of the examination, except during fluoroscopy, the patient should lie in the right lateral decubitus position. This ensures that barium leaves the stomach in a continuous column since no air can leave until all the barium has left and care is taken to ensure that there is always barium in the stomach throughout the examination. It also reduces the time of the examination since barium in the antrum acts as a stimulus to peristalsis. In the upright or supine position, gas and barium leave a hypotonic stomach intermittently giving rise to an interrupted column of barium in the small bowel which makes interpretation difficult.

3. The rate of gastric emptying can be assessed during preliminary fluoroscopy and films taken at intervals determined by this and by the particular reason for the examination. Films taken with the patient supine with a fine focus undercouch tube and well coned to avoid scatter are sufficient if the appearances are normal but should be supplemented by horizontal ray films if any abnormality is seen on fluoroscopy. Localized views, using compression, are invaluable, particularly in showing the terminal ileum. The examination in most cases should be completed in $1-1\frac{1}{2}$ hours. Some normal patients fill their terminal ileum within 20 minutes, others take up to 4 hours. Slow transit is found in some patients on antidepressants and antispasmodic drugs.

4. The most reliable method of shortening the examination is by using *metoclopramide*, which acts by increasing peristaltic activity in the stomach and proximal small bowel, causing rapid gastric emptying and small bowel filling. Its action is most reliable when given intravenously

(10 mg), or intramuscularly. When given by mouth, it should be taken either before the meal is begun or with the first few mouthfuls of barium, since it is only effective after it has been absorbed from the small intestine. This oral route is less reliable than the intravenous route. Provided sufficient barium preparation is given to fill the whole of the small bowel and the patient lies on his right side, the examination should be completed within 75 minutes, barium often reaching the terminal ileum much sooner than this. The fact that metoclopramide has been given should be recorded in the report and preferably on the films, as its administration modifies the radiological appearances, causing an increase in tone of the small bowel which appears more contracted then normal. *Domperidone* 10 mg may be used as an accelerator instead of metoclopramide and is said to cause less drowsiness. If the caecum has not been reached after 60 minutes, a further dose of an accelerating agent may be given. Patients who are hypokalaemic, on certain drugs, or have had a vagotomy, may show no hastening effect from metoclopramide.

5. Full-length radiographs should be taken at intervals to demonstrate the whole length of the small intestine. In addition, all patients should be examined fluoroscopically with local spot films taken of areas of interest. The mobility and pliability of individual loops together with any localized tenderness can be assessed by palpation. Once the barium column has reached the caecum, the caecum and terminal ileum can sometimes be better demonstrated following insufflation of the colon by air per rectum — the peroral pneumocolon.

Small bowel enema

The small bowel enema is performed by the introduction of barium sulphate preparation directly into the small bowel through a nasogastric tube passed through the pylorus into the duodenum or first loop of jejunum. A Bilbao-Dotter duodenal tube is suitable since it has a guidewire of the correct rigidity. The tube may be introduced through the mouth or nostril into the stomach when the guidewire is passed down its lumen to within a few centimetres of the tip. Gentle but continuous pressure by the tip of the tube on the pylorus usually results in the pylorus relaxing and the tip passing into the duodenum. Firm manual pressure on the epigastrium may help at this stage. The guidewire is then removed and the tube, now more flexible, is manoeuvred into the third part of the duodenum. It may be difficult to get the tube beyond the descending limb of the duodenum because of the presence of a lax duodenum or duodenal diverticulum. The examination may still be carried out, but reflux into the stomach is more likely to occur and this tends to spoil the examination. A small bowel enema may be carried out in children, provided the technique is modified and adequate sedation is given before and during the examination (Ratcliffe 1983).

Single contrast enteroclysis

This technique has now been further simplified by Sellink (1983), who emphasizes the importance of emptying the colon by dieting and the use of laxatives before the examination, since a loaded caecum delays small bowel transit and makes it necessary to use a larger volume of barium.

A flocculation-resistant barium sulphate preparation without hyperosmolar additives is used. The barium concentration is varied according to the thickness of the patient's abdomen. For the obese patient, 42% w/v is recommended, reducing to 28% w/v in thin patients: these concentrations refer to specific gravity of 1.32 and 1.23. A constant flow-rate through the catheter of 70 ml per minute is considered ideal since an infusion at a rate faster than this tends to cause nausea and reflux of contrast into the stomach. A total volume of approximately 700 ml is required to outline the whole of the small bowel.

In addition to scout films of the intestine (Fig. 31.2), it is important to take local compression views of all parts of the small intestine and not only the terminal ileum (Miller & Sellink 1979). This single contrast method is simple but there may be difficulty in demonstrating the distal loops of ileum and the amount of distension is not so great as with the double contrast methods.

Water double-contrast small bowel enema

In order to overcome the lack of distension of the bowel in the single contrast method, Sellink has used 600 ml or more of water after the barium has reached the distal ileum. This will produce better distension of ileal loops but the excessive dilution with water leads to a disintegration

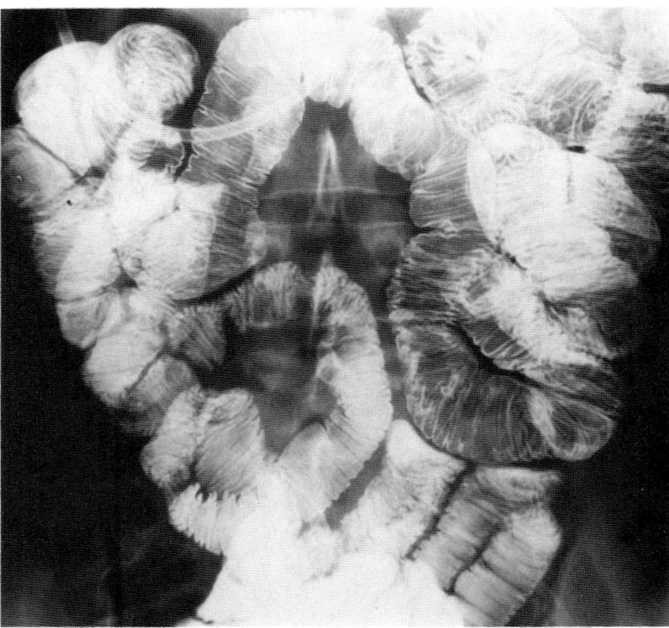

Fig. 31.2 Normal small bowel enema, using barium sulphate 35% w/v, showing the jejunum and proximal ileum moderately distended in continuity.

of the barium suspension particularly in the ileum. Moreover, the double contrast effect lasts only a very short time.

Air double contrast enema

In this method a small volume of more concentrated barium suspension is used than in the single contrast method. A 60% w/v suspension of barium, to which Simethicone antifoam has been added, is instilled at the rate of 60 ml per minute to a total volume of 400–500 ml. During the filling process, fluoroscopic spot films are taken as required. Air is then injected at the rate of 100 ml per minute to a total of 700–1000 ml. Double contrast films of the jejunum are taken first. An injection of glucagon is given once sufficient air has reached the caecum. Double contrast views of the more distal small bowel are then taken. This air contrast method can give exquisite detail of the jejunum, but is less reliable in the ileum. It does not have the advantage of a double contrast examination of the colon since most of the films have to be taken with a vertical ray and horizontal ray lateral decubitus films are impracticable since the loops tend to crowd together in this position.

Methylcellulose double contrast small bowel enema

A 0.5% solution of methylcellulose, injected after the introduction of barium sulphate suspension, is capable of propelling it towards the colon, leaving behind a thin barium coating on the intestinal mucosa (Herlinger 1978). Barium suspension 85% w/v is injected at the rate of 80–100 ml per minute to a total volume of 150–200 ml. More may be used if the patient is stout or if the diagnostic problem specifically relates to the distal ileum. Considerably more may have to be given, up to 400 ml if there is small bowel dilatation with excess fluid. A cooled solution of 0.5% methylcellulose is then introduced at about 100–150 ml per minute. This is continued until a sufficient degree of transradiancy has been achieved in the distal and terminal ileum. Normally 1 or 2 litres of methylcellulose solution are injected. Intermittent fluoroscopy is employed with the patient being rotated as necessary. Individual loops are palpated to assess mobility, adhesions and pliability. Spot films with compression are taken as necessary. By this method a double contrast is produced between the high density coating of barium on the mucosa and the low density of the fluid distending the lumen. The degree of distension is greater than is obtained by other methods and there is plenty of time to study the bowel in detail and to take all necessary radiographs (Fig. 31.3).

NORMAL ANATOMY

The normal jejunum and ileum are arranged compactly in the centre of the abdomen into a series of loops. Although at first sight the position of the individual loops appears to be haphazard, the general arrangement is fairly constant owing to the attachment of the small intestine to the posterior abdominal wall by the mesentery. The root of the mesentery, where it is attached to the posterior abdominal wall, is about 15 cm long and extends from the lower border of the pancreas at the level of the second lumbar vertebra to the right iliac fossa near the right sacral iliac joint (Fig. 33.25).

The mesentery is thickest at its base where it contains fat and fibrous tissue as well as major blood vessels supplying the small intestine, lymphatics, lymph nodes and nerves. The unattached edge of the mesentery, where it is attached to the small intestine, is about 6 metres long and is 40 times longer than its root. The length of the mesentery, measured from its root to the edge attached to the intestine, is about 25–30 cm and is greater in the centre of the small intestine than at either end. Thus, about 6.7 m of small intestine is suspended from a fan-shaped ligament about 25 cm long with a base about 15 cm long, extending from the left border of L2 down to the right sacro-iliac joint area.

Loops of jejunum normally occupy the left upper abdomen and those of the ileum the right lower abdomen but the mesentery is of such a length that the loops are able to move freely within the abdominal cavity. This means that the position occupied by any one portion of the small bowel, with the exception of the beginning of the jejunum and the end of the ileum, cannot be determined with certainty. This variation in position of the intestinal loops is difficult to recognize on routine barium examination

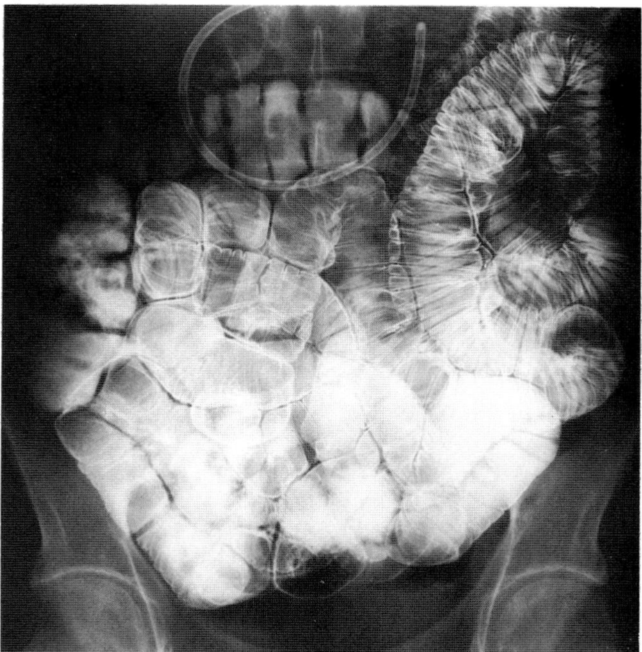

Fig. 31.3 Normal small bowel enema, using barium and methyl cellulose, showing distension of the distal jejunum and ileum with some barium in the colon.

because the loops tend to look alike and cannot always be traced in continuity.

The importance of recognizing the mesenteric and antimesenteric borders of the intestine has been emphasized by Meyers, who has pointed out that certain pathological conditions preferentially occur on one or other border. Consideration of the basic normal anatomy allows us to determine with a fair degree of certainty the mesenteric and antimesenteric borders on a radiograph of the barium-filled small bowel. If the small bowel were the same length as the root of the mesentery, it would extend in a straight line from the duodenojejunal junction to the ileocaecal valve, so that the mesenteric border would lie posteriorly and the antimesenteric border anteriorly. But the intestine is much longer than this so that most of it lies either superiorly and to the right, or inferiorly and to the left of our imaginary line, in which case the mesenteric border will be rotated to lie on the concave side of each loop facing towards the root of the mesentery. The further the loop from the root of the mesentery the more pronounced this effect will be. Thus, the concave margin of a loop of small bowel facing towards the root of the mesentery is the mesenteric border and the convex margin of a loop of small bowel facing away from the root of the mesentery is the antimesenteric border. Those loops of small bowel lying immediately in front of the root of the mesentery have the mesenteric border posteriorly and the antimesenteric border anteriorly.

The significance of recognizing the mesenteric and antimesenteric borders of the small intestine has been emphasized by Meyers, because some pathological conditions selectively favour one site rather than the other.

1. Diverticulosis of the small intestine

Diverticulosis, which is practically limited to the duodenum and jejunum, consists of pulsion diverticulae which extend into the mesentery at the site of the penetration of the bowel wall by the vasa recta which enter on the mesenteric border (Fig. 31.37).

2. Meckel's diverticulum

A Meckel's diverticulum represents the remnant of the vitelline duct (omphalomesenteric duct). It therefore occurs on the antimesenteric border of the ileum (Fig. 31.5).

3. Intestinal duplication

Duplication, enteric or enterogenous cysts may, but usually do not, communicate with the adjacent gut. These, whether they communicate or not, lie on the mesenteric border of the normal small intestine and may displace it or cause haemorrhage by interference with blood supply.

4. Metastases

Transperitoneal metastases spread throughout the abdomen following the pathways of the ascitic fluid. They tend to collect and then grow at the sites where peritoneal fluid tends to pool and collect. In the mid-abdomen, pooling occurs within the peritoneal recesses of the mesenteric ruffles; the most consistent pool forms at the termination of the small bowel mesentery at the ileocolic junction. Seeded metastases tend to lodge and grow on the mesenteric borders of the small bowel and tend to involve the distal ileal loops.

Haematogenous metastases, commonly those from melanoma, tend to occur on the antimesenteric border, presumably because the small tumour emboli lodge and subsequently grow within the smaller arterial branches on the antimesenteric border of the intestine.

5. Lymphoma

Lymphomatous masses tend to occur in the distal small bowel and extend into the mesentery, thus deforming and displacing the concave borders of the small bowel loops (Fig. 31.24).

6. Regional enteritis

As long ago as 1932, Crohn, Ginzburg and Oppenheimer found that the small linear ulcerations of regional enteritis tended to lie on the mesenteric side of the intestine and certainly the radiological findings of mucosal irregularies, ulcers, rigidity and sinuses tend to occur most on the concave mesenteric border. The antimesenteric border is commonly less involved and may remain more pliable thus giving rise to a skip lesion or a pseudosaccular pouch.

7. Bleeding

Intramural haemorrhage, whether localized giving rise to 'thumb prints', or diffuse causing a 'stacked coin appearance', tends to arise on the mesenteric border of the gut (Fig. 31.20). If, as a result of the haemorrhage, contraction of the mesentery occurs, pseudosacculation may occur on the antimesenteric borders.

CONGENITAL ABNORMALITIES

Malrotation of the small bowel may be complete or incomplete. In the *complete* form the colon lies on the left side of the abdominal cavity and the small bowel on the right. This may occur in association with a complete situs inversus. *Partial* malrotation results in the caecum and ascending colon, only being displaced to the left with the jejunum lying on the right upper abdomen below the liver (Fig. 31.4). Both these congenital variants can readily be recognized on small bowel meal examination.

Internal herniations into paraduodenal fossae and other peritoneal pockets are recognized by an immobility and relative fixity of a coil or several coils of small bowel. These internal herniations are usually seen on the right side in the region of the descending portion of the duodenum or near

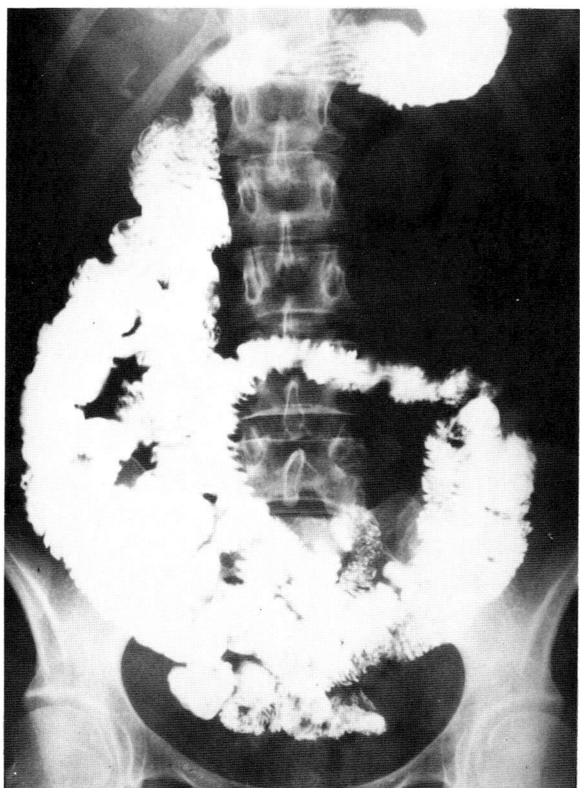

Fig. 31.4 Malrotation. The jejunum and proximal ileum lie to the right of the spine and the colon to the left.

the ligamentum of Treitz on the left. Occasionally almost the whole of the small bowel may lie within an internal hernia. The fixed position of the coils in serial films or in fluoroscopy enables the herniation to be identified. Unless mechanical obstruction develops in an internal hernia, they are usually completely asymptomatic.

Duplication of various parts of the small intestine may occur with or without communication with the main intestinal lumen. When there is no communication the duplication may take the form of a cyst filled with clear fluid lying alongside the mesenteric border of the gut and displacing it. When there is a connection between the duplication and the main lumen, barium may enter the duplication and be retained in it after the rest of the barium has passed along the intestine.

Meckel's diverticulum occurs in 1.5% of subjects, but is seldom recognized by radiological methods. Clinically, the diverticulum may present with melaena due to ulceration of ectopic gastric mucosa in its wall, as an acute intra-abdominal inflammatory condition like appendicitis, or as the initial cause of an intussusception in childhood. It may also become involved in a femoral hernia and become strangulated without giving rise to intestinal obstruction.

Bleeding from a Meckel's diverticulum may be recognized by an *isotopic* method following injection of $^{99}Tc^{m}$-sodium pertechnetate and, if brisk, by *selective angiography* of the superior mesenteric artery. A Meckel's diverticulum is seldom recognized on a small bowel meal because there is no significant hold-up and the barium residue remaining in the Meckel's diverticulum is very small since it has a wide neck and empties readily. It can more easily be demonstrated by a small bowel enema or reflux small bowel examination (Fig. 31.5). Extremely rarely, it may appear as a large gas-filled viscus with a fluid level on the horizontal ray film.

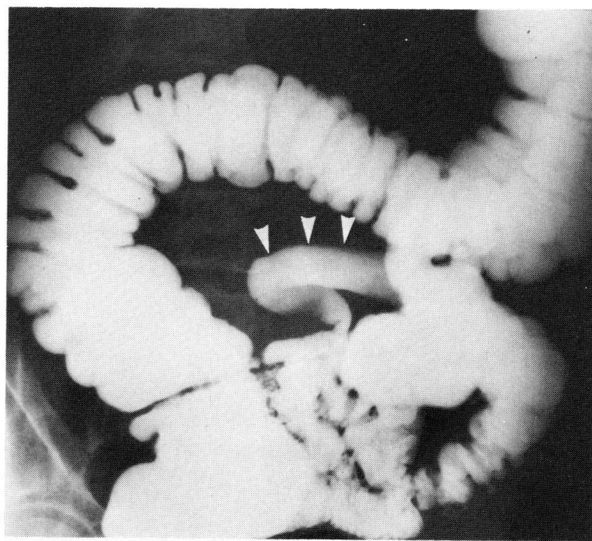

Fig. 31.5 Meckel's diverticulum (arrows) shown by barium enema with reflux of barium into the terminal ileum.

PARASITIC INFESTATION OF THE SMALL BOWEL

Parasitic infestation of the small bowel is usually due to infestation of the duodenum with a tape worm (*Taenia saginata, Taenia solium*) or of the duodenum and jejunum with *Giardia lamblia* or of the jejunum and ileum with the round worm (*Ascaris lumbricoides*). Hook worm infestation of the duodenum with *Ankylostoma duodenale* is also a common finding in some tropical areas.

Giardia lamblia, a flagellated protozoan, is a common parasite of the human proximal small bowel. In most instances it is not responsible for any symptoms, but severe infestation may cause acute diarrhoea and steatorrhoea, particularly in patients with some immune deficiency. The organisms inhabit the duodenum and proximal jejunum where they become attached to the mucosa. In patients with symptoms, there may be thickening of the mucosal folds in the proximal jejunum with rapid transit of barium which may make the affected area of gut difficult to demonstrate (Fig. 31.6). Both the clinical features and radiological appearances are reversible following appropriate treatment and the elimination of the parasites.

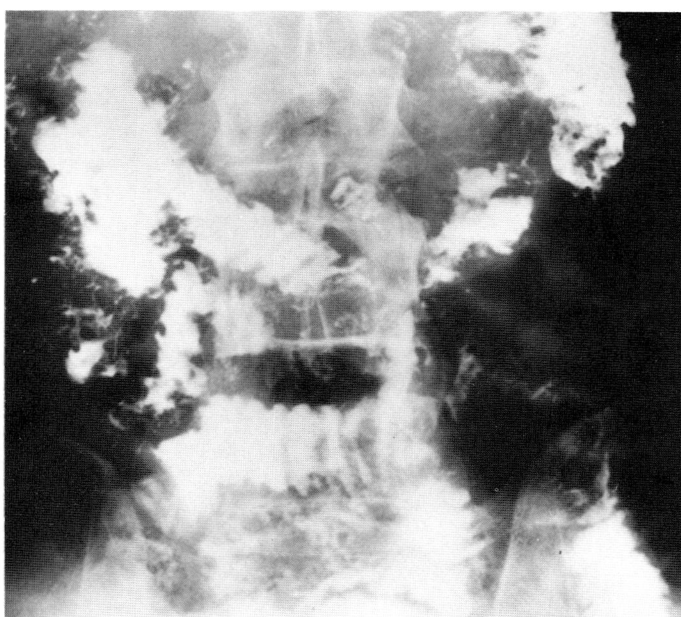

Fig. 31.6 Giardiasis. Young male with acute onset of steatorrhoea. Thickening of mucosal folds in the jejunum. Responded to Metronidazole.

Tape worms inhabit the proximal small bowel and, although the patient is usually asymptomatic, the worms may be responsible for abdominal pain and distension, flatulence and nausea. The head of the worm in the duodenum is seldom demonstrated but occasionally a particularly long worm may become folded upon itself, when it may give rise to longitudinal radiolucent stripes in the distal jejunum or ileum. Unlike the round worm, the tape worm has no alimentary canal and so cannot ingest the barium.

Hook worms tend to inhabit the proximal small bowel where they become attached to the mucosa, causing chronic inflammation and anaemia. In the acute stage there may be abdominal tenderness and discomfort, anorexia, nausea and vomiting. In chronic cases, diarrhoea, steatorrhoea and anaemia may occur. The radiological findings resemble those of giardiasis with thickening and distortion of the mucosal folds in the proximal small bowel.

Round worm infestation is common in tropical areas but may be seen in any part of the world. In children the worms may multiply to such an extent as to form conglomerate masses which may give rise to intestinal obstruction. Trapping of intestinal gas between these masses of worms may give rise to appearances suggesting coiled locks of hair, the so-called 'Medusa locks', which can sometimes be seen on plain films of the abdomen. In the adult the degree of worm infestation is seldom severe enough to produce any abnormal appearance on the plain films but the worms may be seen on small bowel barium examination. The adult worm casts a negative shadow in the barium-filled intestine (Fig. 31.7). Less frequently, a central thin thread of barium indicates that the worm has ingested some of the barium into its own alimentary canal.

Strongyloides stercoralis infestation of the small bowel may give rise to changes similar to those seen in hook worm infestation, but because the parasites are not just attached

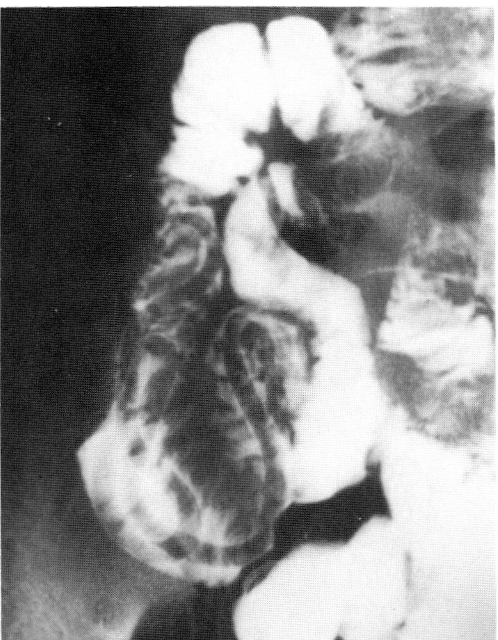

Fig. 31.7 Roundworm. The adult worm casts a negative shadow in the barium-filled intestine. (Courtesy Dr Louise Sheppard.)

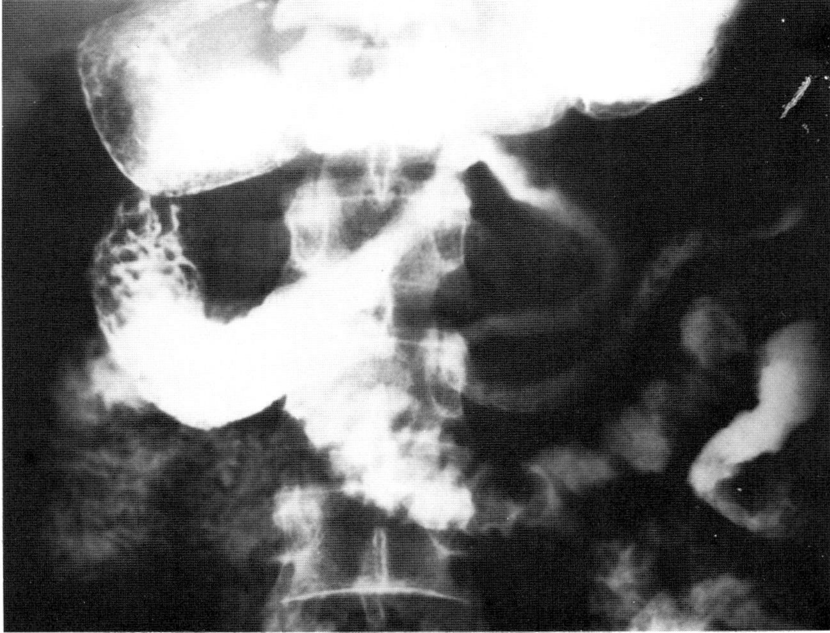

Fig. 31.8 Strongyloides infestation. There is marked thickening, narrowing and irregularity of the proximal jejunum.

to the mucosa but may penetrate into the wall of the gut and give rise to inflammation, fibrosis and granuloma formation the changes may be much more severe. Thickening and rigidity of localized segments of jejunum may be seen and these may give rise to stenosis and obstruction (Fig. 31.8). The ileum is commonly normal.

ULCERS OF THE SMALL BOWEL

Ulceration of the small bowel is usually part of a generalized *enteritis*, e.g. paratyphoid or typhoid fever, but a solitary ulcer may result as a sequel of the enteric-coated *potassium* tablets administered in the treatment of hypertension. It has been suggested that the liberation of potassium locally in the small bowel results in local venous thrombosis, which may give rise to necrosis and solitary ulceration. Such ulcers develop circumferentially around the bowel wall and can be demonstrated on barium films. They may perforate and present as an acute abdomen, or as a more slowly developing granulomatous lesion around the ulcer giving rise to small bowel obstruction. In other cases, healing of the ulcer may result in a fibrous stricture which may give rise to small bowel obstruction.

ACUTE INTESTINAL INFECTIONS

Acute inflammatory lesions of the small bowel, when due to specific infections, e.g. typhoid or paratyphoid infection, or non-specific infections, are only investigated radiologically when the diagnosis has not been suspected clinically. The radiological signs are those of intestinal hurry and increased motility of the small bowel. Erect films may reveal isolated small fluid levels dispersed in a disorderly pattern all over the abdomen, but there is no proportionate gas distension of the bowel such as seen in true mechanical obstruction.

REGIONAL ENTERITIS (CROHN'S DISEASE)

Pathology

Regional enteritis (Crohn's disease) is a chronic granulomatous condition which may affect any part of the gut from the stomach to the anus, but is most commonly seen in the terminal ileum and colon. It was first described in 1932 by Crohn, Ginzburg and Oppenheimer under the name regional ileitis. Before that date the condition was confused with intestinal tuberculosis with which it has clinical, pathological and radiological features in common. It may be difficult to distinguish the conditions even today.

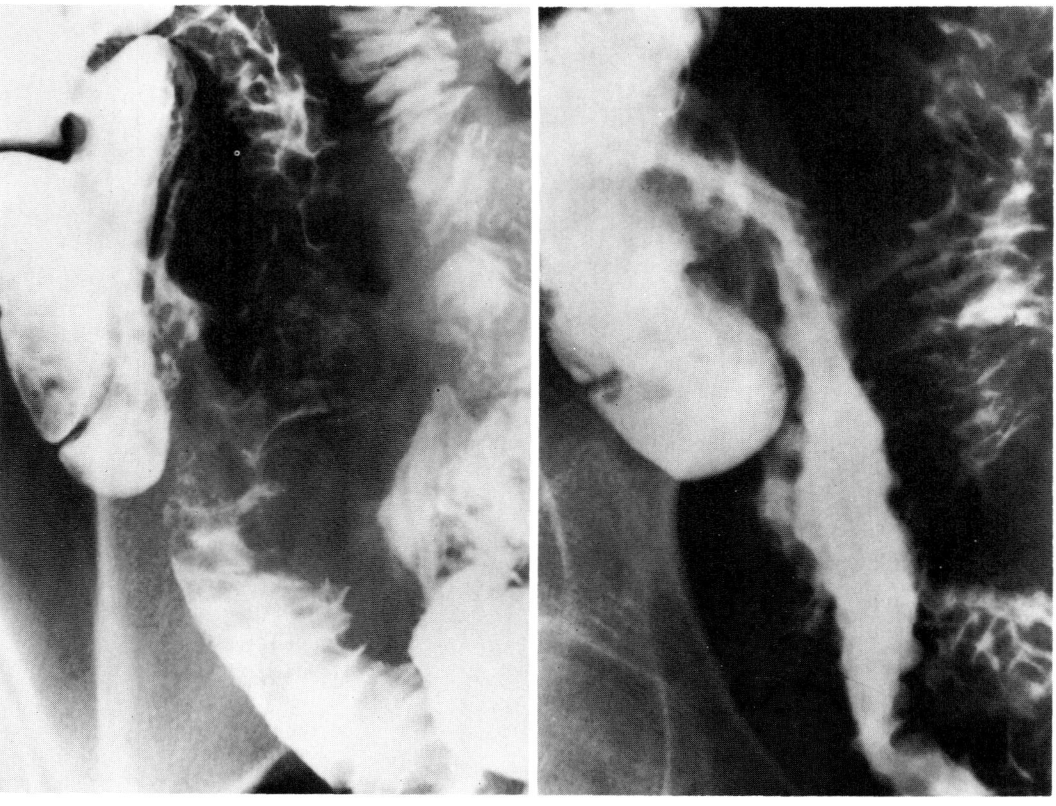

Fig. 31.9 A. Crohn's disease of terminal ileum showing oedematous mucosa and deep ulceration. **B.** Crohn's disease of terminal ileum showing ulceration. The affected loop is slightly dilated and has a thickened wall.

The affected bowel is sharply demarcated from the normal. Several separate areas of disease (*skip lesions*) may be present in the bowel separated by lengths of normal intestine. In some affected loops of intestine one side of the bowel may be ulcerated while the opposite side is normal or less affected. The bowel wall is thickened, congested and rigid, its lumen usually narrowed and ulcerated (Fig. 31.9A & B). The mucosa may have a cobblestone appearance due to the intersection of longitudinal and transverse ulcers. The attached mesentery is thickened and mesenteric lymph nodes enlarged. Affected loops become matted together so that perforation into the peritoneal cavity is rare but fistulae between loops and to adjacent viscera are common. Sinuses form in the skin of the abdominal wall. Abscesses often form between affected loops and may rupture into the bladder or vagina or into the retroperitoneal tissue, causing fibrosis and ureteric obstruction.

Histologically there is a chronic granulomatous inflammatory reaction with oedema and fibrosis affecting all coats of the intestinal wall. Deep fissured ulcers may extend into the submucosa and muscular layers. Non-caseating granulomas containing multinucleated giant cells, epitheloid and mononuclear cells may be seen in most resected specimens, but the ease with which they are found varies and they are not essential for diagnosis.

Clinical presentation

Regional enteritis may present at any age but is most commonly seen in the second and third decade. The onset may be acute, resembling acute appendicitis, or insidious leading to chronic ill health. Diarrhoea, colic, low grade fever, anaemia due to blood loss, anorexia and loss of weight are common in the less acute cases. A common finding on clinical examination is a tender abdominal mass in the right lower quadrant due to thickened bowel and mesentery and lymph nodes. Sometimes an intra-abdominal abscess is present. Perianal abscess or fistula are common and may precede evident involvement of the intestine. Subacute obstruction is very common, but complete obstruction requiring immediate surgery is rare. Malnutrition may be severe, especially in complicated cases following multiple resections or exclusion operations.

Patients with regional enteritis may have a variety of associated conditions, such as small superficial aphthous ulcers or fistula in ano. An arthropathy particularly affecting the sacro-iliac joints, sclerosing cholangitis and toxic dilatation of the colon may all occur but are less common than with ulcerative colitis. Other differential features are listed in Table 31.1.

Management and prognosis

Most patients follow a long chronic course with low-grade disability. Antibiotics do not appear to affect the course of the disease, but may be used if there is abscess formation. Steroids may relieve symptoms, particularly in the acute exacerbations, but do not alter the long-term natural history of the disease.

Surgery is reserved for the management of complications, including fistulas between the bowel and the viscera and abdominal abscesses. Recurrence of the disease following resection of affected intestine is not uncommon and usually occurs just proximal to the anastomosis (Fig. 31.13). Short circuit operations with side-to-side anastomoses, with the

Table 31.1 Comparison of Crohn's disease and ulcerative colitis

	Ulcerative colitis	Crohn's disease
Clinical features		
Rectal bleeding	Virtually always	50%
Abdominal pain	Uncommon	50%
Abdominal mass	Never	Common at some stage
Anal lesion	25%	75%
Colon involved	Distal colon always	Predominantly right-sided
Colonic features		
Distribution of lesions	Rectum in 95% in continuity	Rectum in 30% Discontinuous; normal patches in diseased areas, symmetrical
Ulceration	Shallow and granular	Deep, rose-thorn
Haustra	Lost early in disease	Incomplete loss
Small bowel	If involved, in continuity with caecum Ileo-caecal valve patulous Terminal ileum dilated	Often discontinuous Ileo-caecal valve narrow or normal Terminal ileum stenosed and thickened
Complications		
Fistula and sinuses	Never	Common
Toxic dilatation	Common	Rare
Perforation	Uncommon	Rare
Carcinoma of colon	High risk in total colitis	Rare
Associated conditions	Arthritis Sclerosing cholangitis	

formation of an antiperistaltic stagnant loop, is best avoided. An exclusion operation, with the formation of an isoperistaltic blind loop, may be necessary sometimes as an emergency procedure, or when the bowel is so matted together that resection is not possible.

Radiological features

The radiological appearances in regional enteritis reflect the various pathological lesions of this condition. In the early stages, or in bowel that is only slightly affected, *aphthous ulcers* may be demonstrated. These are seen as minute collections of barium surrounded by a small halo of raised oedematous mucosa. These are more easily demonstrated in the colon when it is fully distended than in the small intestine.

Oedema of the mucosa and submucosa results in thickening and blunting of the mucosal folds, with the smoothing out or effacement of the primary folds, the valvulae conniventes, as well as the secondary folds. Congestion and oedema of the muscular layers causes *rigidity* and *thickening* of the walls so that the lumen of affected loops appear separated from neighbouring loops, whether normal or abnormal. Thus the abnormal loops 'stand out' from the rest because of their abnormally thick wall (Fig. 31.9). This is best seen when all the intestinal loops are filled by a continuous column of barium (Fig. 31.10).

Ulceration, when seen *en face*, appears as longitudinal and transverse streaks of barium in deep fissured crevices giving a cobblestone appearance best seen in the jejunum. When seen in profile, these ulcers (Fig. 31.10) appear deep and fissured, so called *rose-thorn ulcers*. *Stenotic areas* are common and are often multiple and may vary in length from less than a centimetre to 15–20 cm in length (Fig. 31.12). Subacute obstruction with proximal *dilatation* is common, but complete obstruction is surprisingly uncommon considering the length and narrowness of the strictures sometimes demonstrated. As fibrosis continues, the ulceration may become less severe so that the intestine becomes a long, thick-walled rigid tube with a central lumen and devoid of peristalsis (Fig. 31.11). The partially obstructed proximal small bowel becomes dilated (Fig. 31.9).

Adjacent loops of bowel may become matted together and *fistulae* develop between them. Ileoileal fistulae are difficult to demonstrate but ileocolic fistulae may be easily shown by barium enema examination (Fig. 31.14). Intra-abdominal abscesses or enlarged lymph nodes in the mesentery may displace loops of bowel around a mass which is found to be tender on palpation. Fistulae may form between the gut and the bladder giving rise to serious urinary infection and pneumaturia. *Sinuses* may form from the intestine to the vagina or abdominal wall. Sinograms are usually better than small bowel examinations for showing the site of the leak from the small intestine. The retroperitoneal tissues may become involved giving rise to *retroperitoneal fibrosis* with obstruction of the right ureter or iliac veins.

Dilatation of loops of bowel may be a particularly prominent feature of ileal involvement. The duodenum is rarely involved unless there is widespread disease elsewhere in the bowel or unless a duodeno-colic fistula has formed (Fig. 31.14).

The acuteness of the clinical presentation influences the radiological appearance. These may be grouped into:

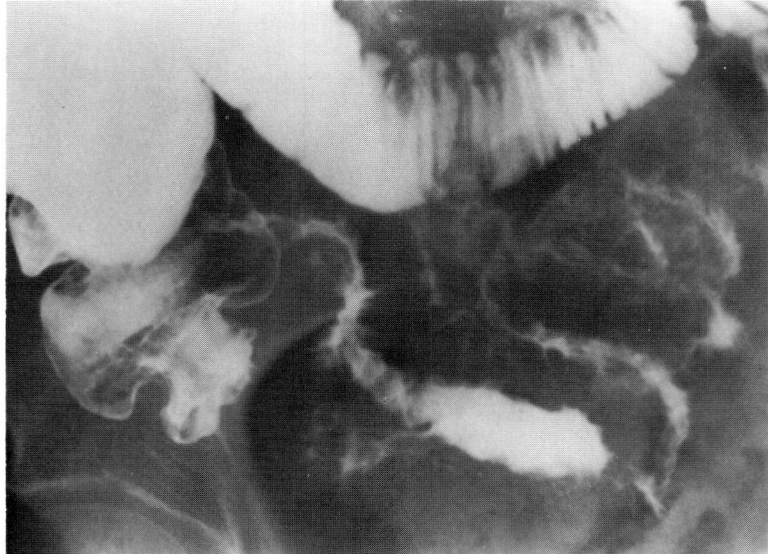

Fig. 31.10 Crohn's disease. There is extensive involvement of the distal ileum, the walls of which are grossly thickened. There is dilatation of proximal loops. The medial wall of the caecum is affected.

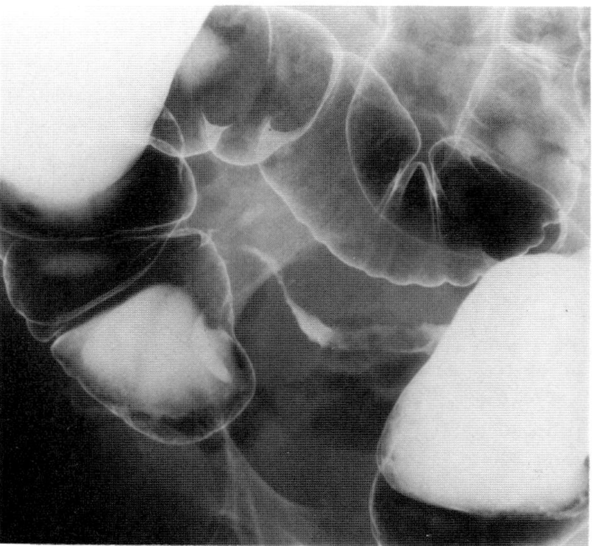

Fig. 31.11 Crohn's disease. Barium enema showing narrowing of the terminal ileum which has a grossly thickened wall separating it from the adjacent loops of bowel, giving rise to the 'string sign'.

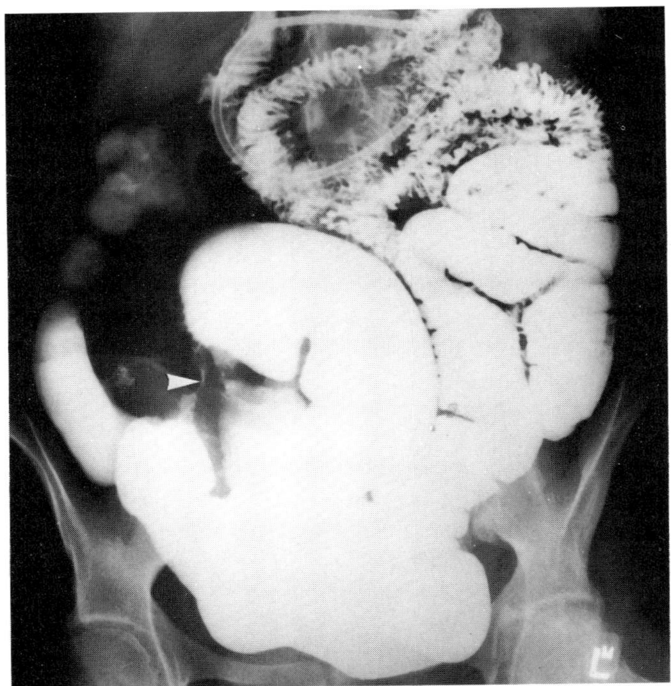

Fig. 31.12 Crohn's disease. Small bowel enema showing grossly dilated loops of ileum proximal to a number of short strictures.

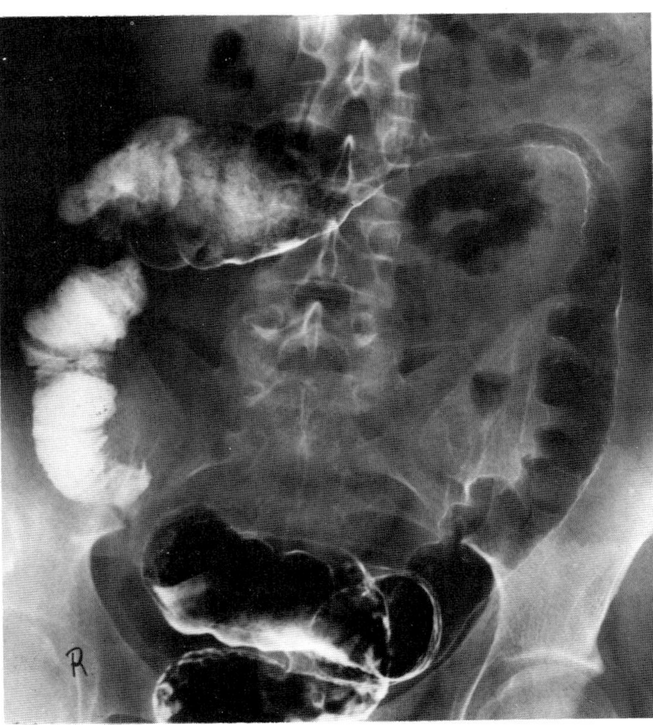

Fig. 31.13 Crohn's disease. The patient has had a partial ileocolostomy with end-to-end anastomosis. There is a stricture at the anastomosis due to a recurrence of the disease. The splenic flexure is narrowed and there is pseudodiverticular formation in the descending colon.

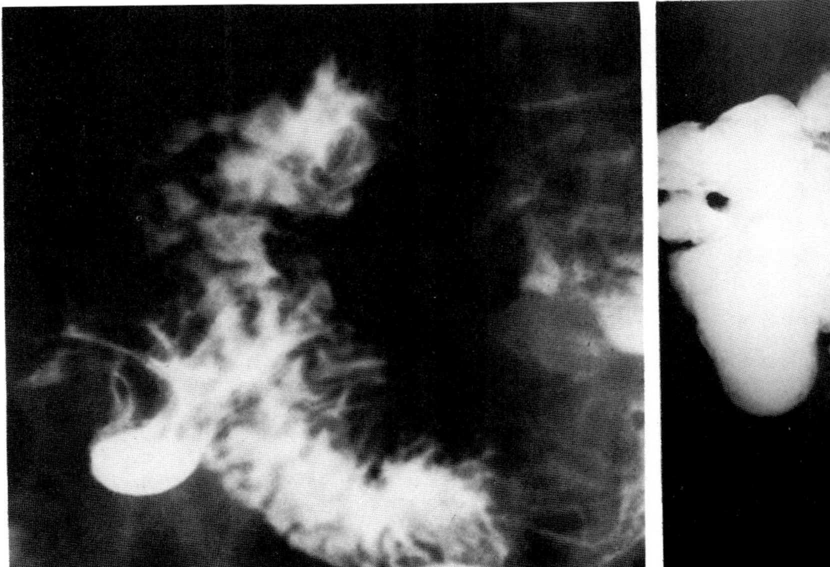

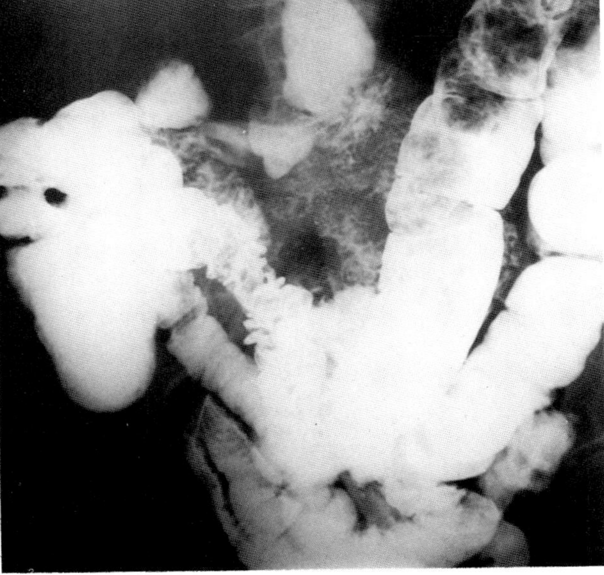

Fig. 31.14 Crohn's disease with duodenocolic fistula. **A.** Barium meal showing the second part of the duodenum with transient filling of a very small part of the colon. **B.** Barium enema examination showing filling of the stomach and small intestine from the colon through the fistula.

1. Acute. The symptoms and signs mimic those of an acute appendicitis and the radiological examination usually does not involve contrast studies but is confined to plain films of the acute abdomen. At this stage plain films show a single or a few small isolated fluid levels in the terminal ileum, sometimes with a suggestion of a soft tissue mass, indistinguishable from that seen in acute appendicitis or acute enteritis.

2. Subacute. The commoner clinical presentation is one of a tender mass in the right iliac fossa, sometimes associated with fever, general malaise and frequently with colicky abdominal pain and diarrhoea. At this stage the radiological appearances are due to subacute inflammatory changes in the terminal ileum which is swollen, thickened and ulcerated. It is tender on palpation and the mucosal pattern is destroyed, with a cobblestone appearance of the mucosa and rose-thorn ulceration seen *en face* and marginal rose-thorn ulcers. There may be some dilatation of the proximal ileum due to a degree of obstruction.

3. Chronic. In the later stages of the disease the patient has commonly had several subacute attacks with partial obstruction and pain and tenderness. By this stage there is commonly a fixed inflammatory mass often with external sinus formation or chronic internal fistulae, usually into adjoining loops of bowel. Classically at this stage the radiological features are of long narrow segments of rather featureless bowel without obvious ulceration. The bowel may be separated by small abscesses and there may be narrow fistulous tracks extending in various directions. Extension of the disease into the bladder may give rise to serious urinary infection and pneumaturia, or if the retroperitoneal tissues are involved there may be retroperitoneal fibrosis with obstruction of the right ureter or iliac veins.

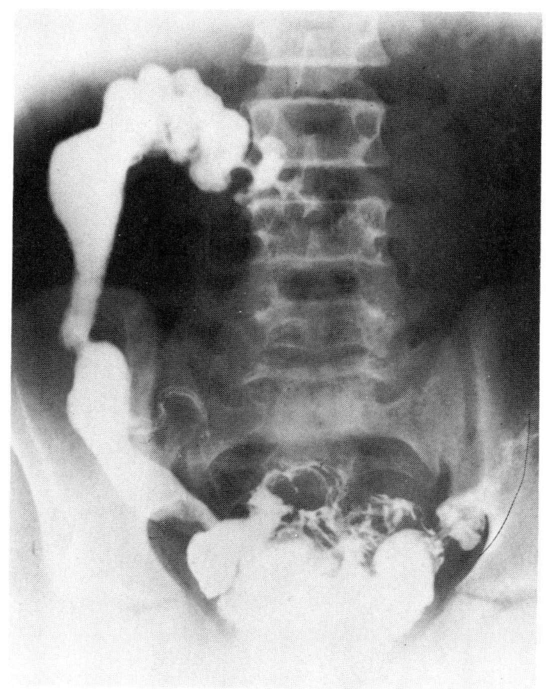

Fig. 31.15 Tuberculosis of the caecum in a boy aged 14 years. The caecum is very contracted and the terminal ileum moderately dilated.

Differential diagnosis

In many cases of regional enteritis the appearances are characteristic and the diagnosis not difficult. A number of conditions may display features seen in some cases of regional enteritis.

Lymphosarcoma may simulate the non-stenotic stage of regional ileitis with ulceration, thickening and blunting of folds (Fig. 31.25). There may be fistula formation. However, in lymphosarcoma the lumen tends to be eccentric, intralumenal nodules are common and stenotic areas are rare (Fig. 31.31). Hodgkin's disease can have a similar appearance to lymphosarcoma but, being more fibrotic, stenotic lesions are more common and fistulae rarely occur.

Tuberculosis of the small bowel may simulate regional enteritis completely. Stenotic lesions are common and may be multiple. The terminal ileum, caecum and ascending colon are often affected in continuity and both fistulae and sinuses may occur (Fig. 31.15). Generally, in tuberculosis the stenotic lesions are shorter and the caecum is more contracted than in regional ileitis (Fig. 31.16). Although there may be obvious pulmonary tuberculosis, this is not necessarily the case and the differentiation of the two conditions may be very different.

Segmental *infarction* of the small bowel may show rapid changes with severe oedema, ulceration and spasm proceeding to a fibrotic stricture. The progression is rapid and the history may be helpful. Similar changes, indistinguishable from regional ileitis, may be seen in *radiation* ileitis (Figs 31.57 and 31.58). Rarely, *carcinoid tumours* may

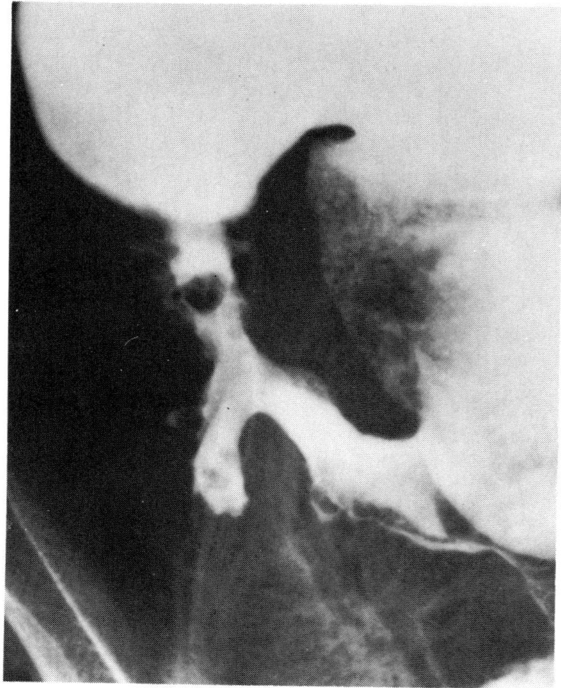

Fig. 31.16 Tuberculosis affecting the terminal ileum, caecum and ascending colon. The caecum and ascending colon are fibrosed and contracted and the ileocaecal valve is patulous.

be multiple and cause stenotic lesions in the ileum (Fig. 31.39).

The fine nodulation of *lymphonodular hyperplasia* may simulate Crohn's disease, but the changes tend to be more diffuse and obstruction does not occur (Fig. 31.17). There may be an associated immune deficiency (Fig. 31.18).

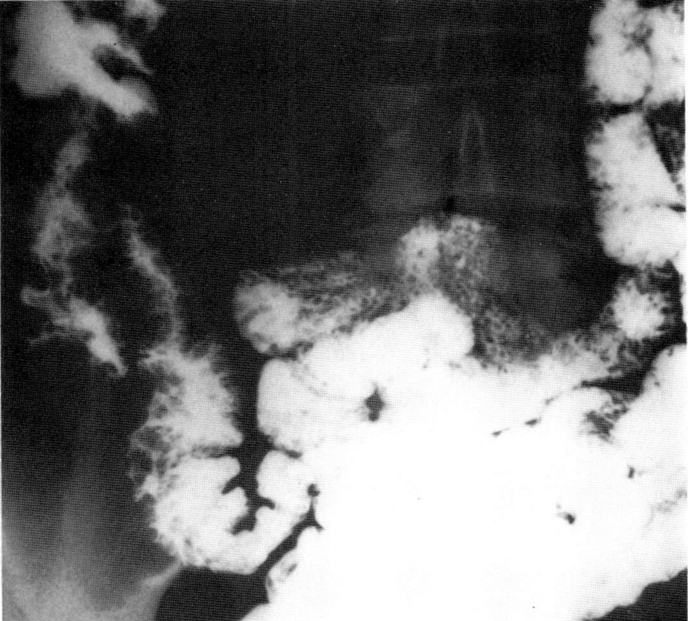

Fig. 31.17 Nodular lymphoid hyperplasia. There is extensive fine nodulation throughout the distal and terminal ileum and the ascending colon.

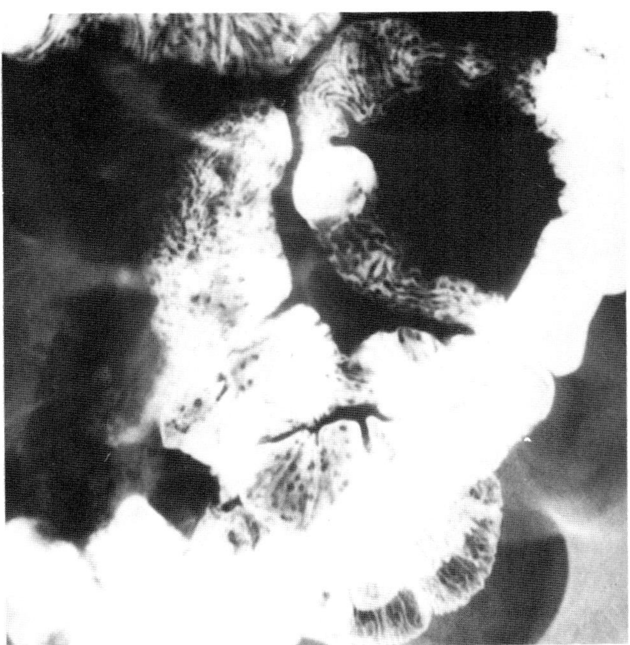

Fig. 31.18 Nodular lymphoid hyperplasia in a patient with hypogammaglobulinaemia. Fine nodulation was demonstrated throughout most of the small intestine.

VASCULAR LESIONS

Haemorrhage into the wall of the small bowel

Bleeding into the wall of the small bowel can cause a number of radiological appearances. If the blood spreads along the wall of the small bowel it may give rise to a uniform regular thickening of the folds of the small bowel with a sharply delineated margin. This parallel arrangement produces a spike-like appearance simulating a 'stack of coins' or 'picket fence' (Fig. 31.19A & B). These appearances are more obvious in the jejunum than in the ileum because of the greater prominence of the valvulae conniventes in the jejunum. If the blood clots and forms

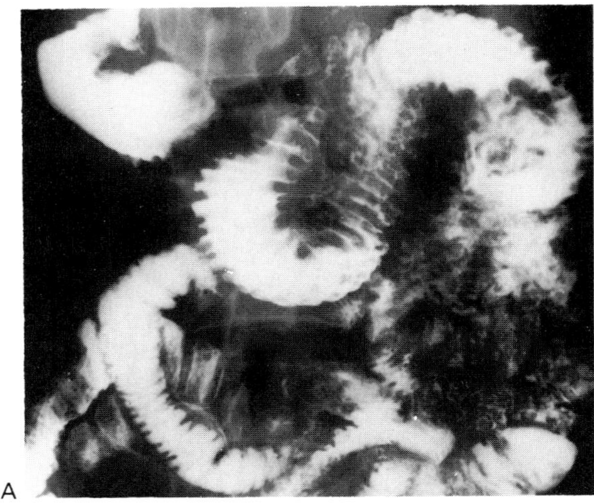

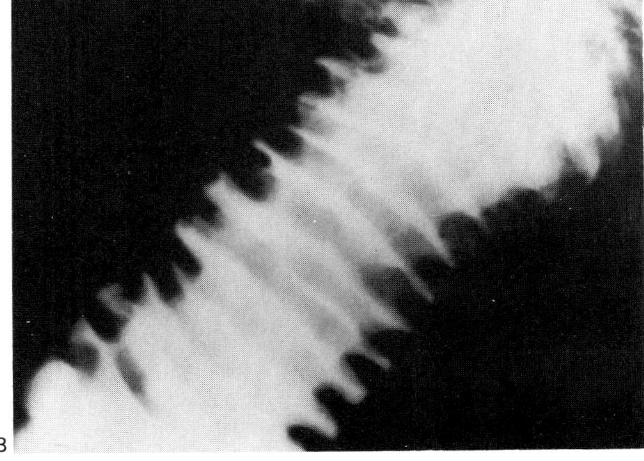

Fig. 31.19 A. Spontaneous intramural haematoma of the jejunum in a male of 45 years who was a known haemophiliac since childhood. Sudden onset of colicky pain followed by melaena. **B.** Dilated loop of proximal jejunal with broad, coarse transverse folds resembling a 'picket fence'.

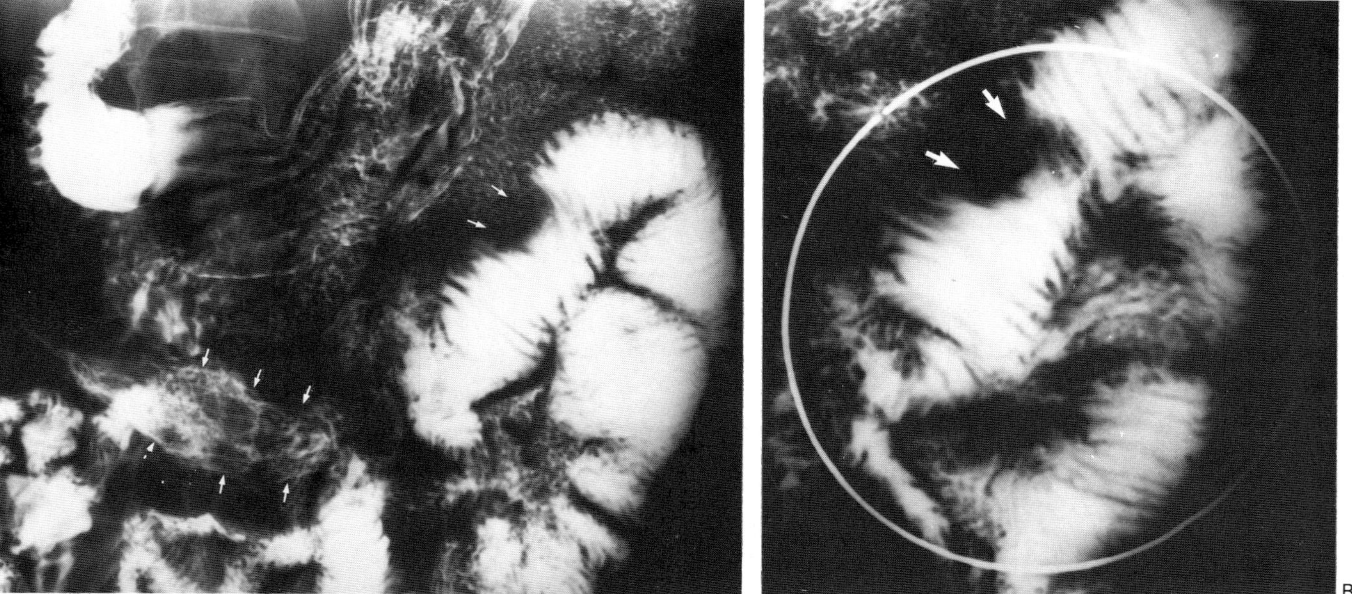

Fig. 31.20 Angioneurotic oedema. Young male presenting with recurrent attacks of colicky pain sometimes associated with melaena. **A.** Intramural haemorrhage into the jejunum. **B.** Local view of marginal 'thumb print' due to local haematoma.

a local haematoma, marginal thumbprinting may be seen (Fig. 31.20A & B). If bleeding into the mesentery has also occurred, an extrinsic mass effect may be seen with flattening of the folds on the mesenteric side of the bowel and separation of bowel loops around the mass. This appearance is most likely to occur in a bleeding diathesis such as haemophilia and in patients on anticoagulant therapy.

Bowel ischaemia

Primary vascular lesions affecting the small bowel may cause acute or chronic ischaemia. Acute ischaemia may result from arterial embolization or thrombosis of an atheromatous artery. It presents as a surgical emergency. Initially there may be a local ileus and oedema of the affected segment of gut. This may improve spontaneously or progress to gangrene, rupture of the gut wall and generalized peritonitis. The plain films will show dilated fluid-filled loops of small bowel, possibly with air in their wall. Later there may be free gas in the peritoneal cavity. If the gut becomes infected with gas-forming organisms, gas may be seen in the portal vein or in the intrahepatic branches, usually a sign of impending death (Fig. 31.21). Less severe, and sometimes transient, changes may be seen following venous thrombosis in women using a hormonal contraceptive pill.

In acute ischaemia barium examination is contraindicated. In a few cases emergency angiography has demonstrated the cause, usually an embolus in a major vessel, and allowed restorative vascular surgery. Most patients with acute ischaemia of gut are dealt with as a surgical emerg-

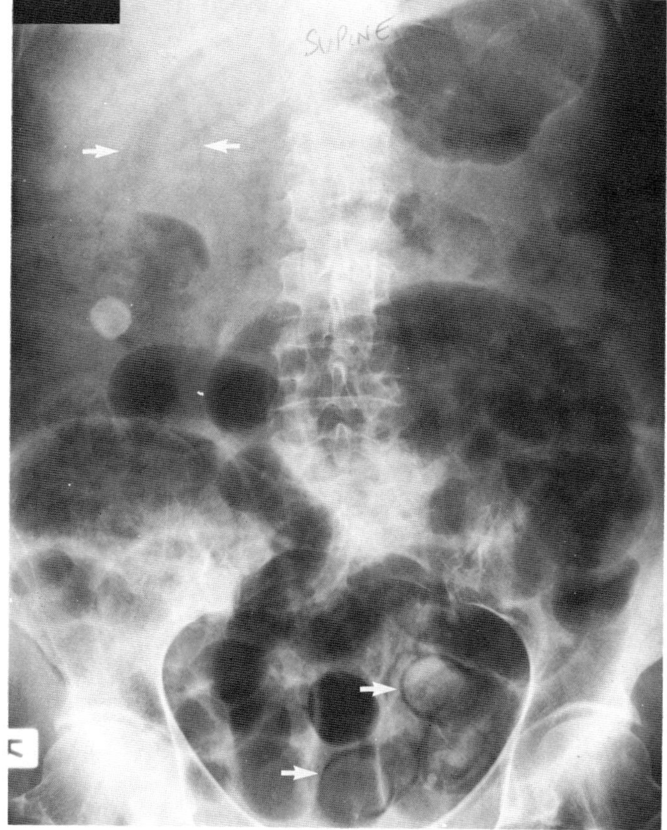

Fig. 31.21 Mesenteric infarction. Gas is seen in the wall of the small bowel within the pelvis and in the branches of the portal vein in the liver (arrows).

ency, the aim being to preserve as much viable gut as possible, and arteriography is not undertaken.

Chronic ischaemia may result from atheromatous narrowing of arterial ostia, an arteritis, fibromuscular hyperplasia or pressure on the coeliac axis artery by a band or the crus of the diaphragm. There is such a rich anastomosis between the coeliac axis and the superior and inferior mesenteric arteries that a gradual narrowing or occlusion of one main vessel may give rise to no symptoms and is often a chance finding at aortography. If two major vessels are affected, mid-gut ischaemia may result.

Unfortunately, the symptoms of chronic ischaemia, so-called intestinal angina, are rather non-specific so that it is difficult to select the right patients for full angiographic examination. Pain occurring regularly at a fixed time after meals, steatorrhoea and severe loss of weight may occur. An abdominal bruit may be heard. It is likely that many cases of ischaemia pass unrecognized.

Plain films may be normal or show dilatation of loops of small bowel. Barium examination may show thickened, rigid loops of intestine some being dilated with thickened oedematous folds. A featureless 'hose-pipe' small bowel appearance has also been described. The appearances may very closely mimic coeliac disease or even regional enteritis.

A main-stream aortogram, to show the overall circulation and anastomoses, is essential, but it is the lateral view of the aorta which gives the most information about the pathological anatomy and the exact site of the stenotic lesions. The gut is supplied by three main arteries with rich anastomotic connections, the coeliac axis, the superior and inferior mesenteric arteries. It is necessary for at least two of these arteries to be narrowed significantly for symptoms to occur. The lateral view shows the site and the extent of the stenosis and the anterior view the attempt at collateral circulation.

Reconstructive arterial surgery is hazardous and not uniformly successful. Percutaneous angioplasty by arterial dilatation of a localized arterial stenosis offers greater hope of success. Relief of symptoms may sometimes follow operation for pressure on the coeliac axis artery from a band or the crus of the diaphragm.

Infarction of bowel due to mesenteric venous thrombosis may be even more difficult to recognize unless there are venous thromboses elsewhere in the body. A barium small bowel examination may show distorted inactive segments of bowel with 'finger-print' deformities in the wall caused by mucosal and submucosal haemorrhages. Other manifestations of bowel ischaemia, including ulceration, sacculation and stricture formation, may occur.

Vasculitis

Vasculitis may compromise the blood supply to a segment or the whole of the small bowel and cause ischaemic or haemorrhagic changes in the bowel wall. In systemic connective tissue diseases (rheumatoid arthritis, polyarteritis nodosa, systemic lupus erythematosus and dermatomyositis), the arteries, arterioles or veins of the small bowel may be involved by a necrotizing vasculitis. This may give rise to massive multiple infarctions and perforation.

Henoch-Schonlein syndrome is an acute recurring arteritis in which purpura, abdominal pain, renal disease and joint pain occur. The disease tends to be self-limiting, but frequently recurs. Like other forms of vasculitis, there may be irregular thickening of the folds of the small bowel, evidence of oedema and haemorrhage with thumb-printing and dilution of contrast (Fig. 31.20).

Haemorrhage into the wall of the small bowel may occur in other conditions, such as idiopathic thrombocytopenic purpura and rarely in thromboangiitis obliterans.

TRAUMA

The increasing use of safety belts in cars has resulted in closed injuries of the abdomen caused by acute flexion over the restraining strap. The duodenum is usually damaged because of its relative fixity to the posterior abdominal wall. An intramural haematoma may cause partial or complete obstruction, usually at the level of the second part of the duodenum. This usually resolves in the course of a few days. Laceration of the mesentery or the bowel may give rise to mucosal or extramucosal haematoma. Rupture of the small bowel resulting in the radiological features of perforation and peritonitis may occur in severe cases.

TUMOURS

Tumours occur less frequently in the small bowel than in other parts of the gastrointestinal tract. Many give rise to no symptoms and are commonly missed on conventional radiological examination. They may present clinically in a variety of ways, including bleeding, obstruction and occasionally perforation.

Benign tumours include leiomyomas, adenomas, lipomas, haemangiomas and fibromas. Those that present with bleeding may be demonstrated by small bowel enema but are frequently first shown by angiography. This applies particularly to leiomyomas (Fig. 31.22) and haemangiomas. Small tumours may give rise to intermittent obstruction by acting as the apex of an intussusceptum.

A diffuse polyposis of the gut, particularly the small bowel, may be associated with mucocutaneous pigmentation in the *Peutz-Jeghers syndrome* (Fig. 31.23). The condition shows dominant inheritance. The polyps are hamartomatous tumours, which are not themselves premalignant, but the condition may be associated with a higher incidence of carcinoma of the stomach, duodenum and ovaries. The *Cronkhite-Canada syndrome* gives rise to polyposis throughout the gastrointestinal tract and is associated with diarrhoea, alopecia, nail atrophy and skin pigmentation.

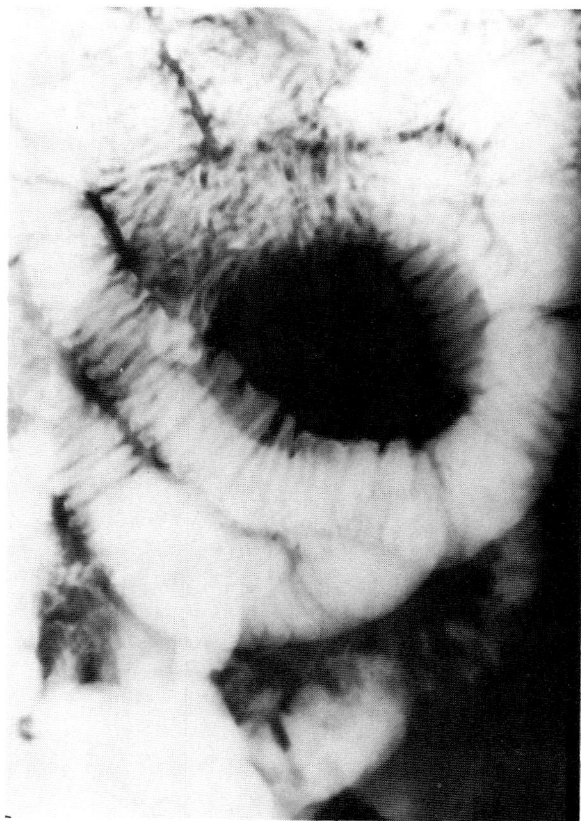

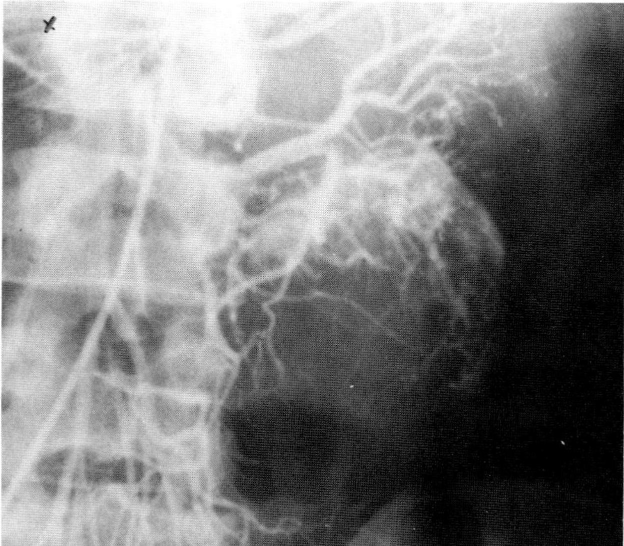

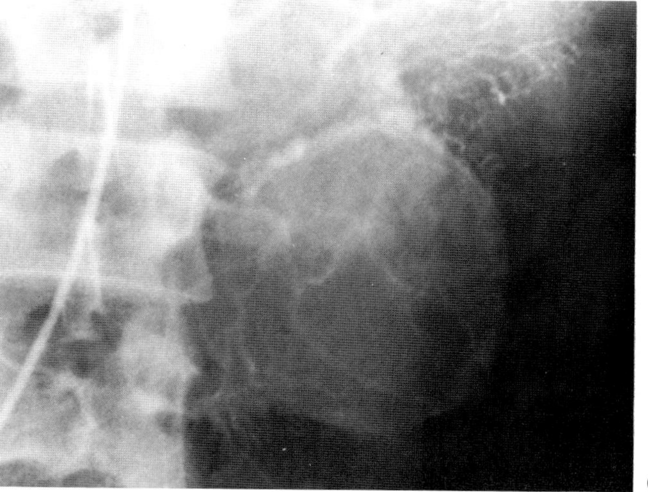

Fig. 31.22 Leiomyoma of jejunum. A young male with occasional colic, melaena and anemia. Endoscopy negative. **A.** Small bowel enema showing displacement of loops of jejunum around a soft tissue mass. **B.** Selective superior mesenteric arteriogram in the arterial phase showing the vascular supply to a smooth soft tissue tumour. **C.** Venous phase with no evidence of tumour circulation. (Courtesy Dr Louise Sheppard.)

Malignant tumours. Most malignant tumours of the small bowel give rise to pain and loss of weight is common; bleeding and a palpable mass occur less often. Carcinoid tumours are frequently very small and give rise to no local symptoms but present with the carcinoid syndrome.

Carcinoid. These tumours, which are twice as common in males as females, commonly occur in the distal ileum. If the tumour invades the mesentery it may give rise to a fibrous reaction causing intestinal obstruction (Fig. 31.39). The tumours may be multiple and may ulcerate and bleed. The carcinoid syndrome occurs only if there are massive metastases in the liver and its severity is related to the tumour mass.

Lymphoma. Lymphoma of the small bowel may occur as one aspect of a generalized disease, as a primary small bowel tumour, or as a complication of coeliac disease. A mass of enlarged lymph nodes in the mesentery or para-aortic region may displace the small bowel, smoothing or effacing the folds on the concave border (Fig. 31.24). Local mural invasion may result in the digestion of the mass with a formation of a large irregular cavity (Fig. 31.31). Primary lymphomas, particularly if they are cellular and have little fibrous stroma, may ulcerate deeply (Fig. 31.25) and give rise to a local dilatation, which is devoid of mucosa and may even perforate into the peritoneal cavity.

Carcinomas of the small bowel are uncommon, tend to occur in the proximal small bowel and usually give rise to obstruction with pain, loss of weight and malaena. Some may be associated with long-standing coeliac disease.

Metastatic tumours. Secondary neoplasms may involve the small bowel by direct invasion, by seeding across the peritoneum or by haematoganeous spread. Direct invasion may occur from any tumour within the abdomen but particularly the colon, stomach and uterus. Seeded deposits, commonly from the ovary or cervix, often occur in the right iliac fossa involving the terminal ileum and caecum. Haematoganeous metastases usually occur on the antimesenteric convex border and are often multiple. Melanoma (Fig. 31.26) breast and bronchus are the usual primary sites.

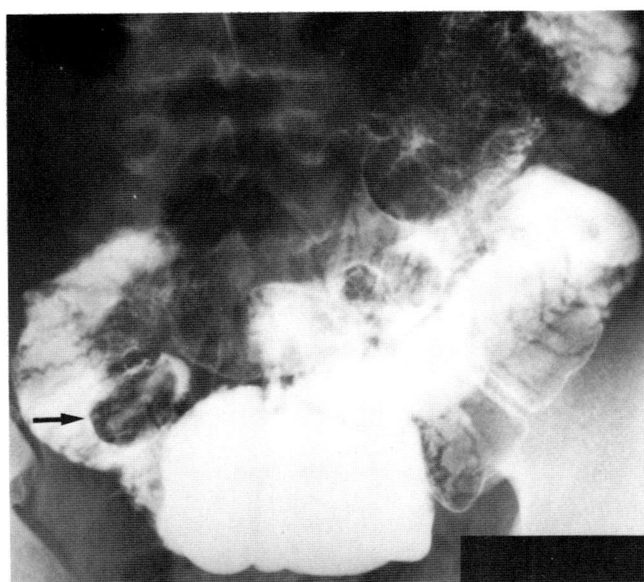

Fig. 31.23 Peutz-Jegher's syndrome. Male aged 22 years with typical buccal figmentation and recurrent colic. Many hamartomatous tumours (arrow) were excised (arrow). (Courtesy Dr Louise Sheppard.)

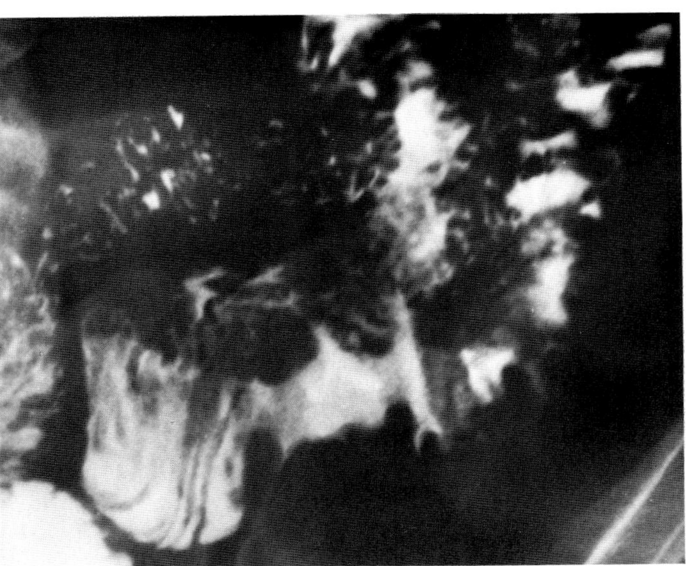

Fig. 31.25 Reticulosarcoma of jejunum. Female 45 years. Presented with intestinal haemorrhage. The tumour was resected and subsequently recurred with obstructive symptoms.

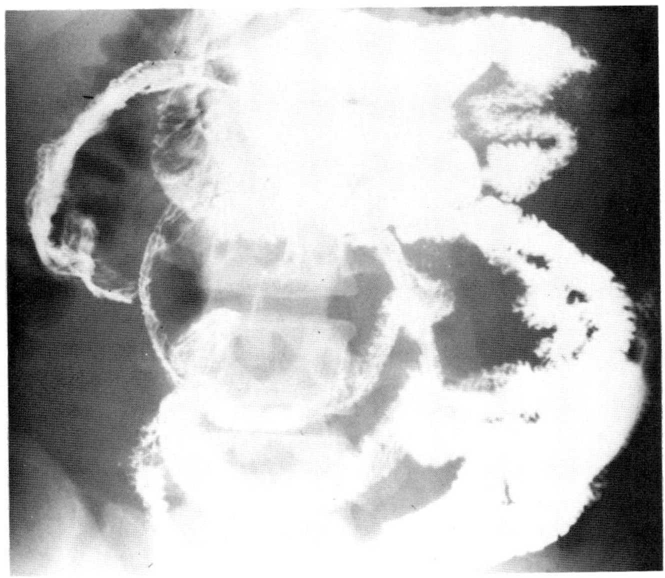

Fig. 31.24 Lymphoma. Small bowel meal showing displacement of loops of jejunum around masses of lymph nodes in the mesentery.

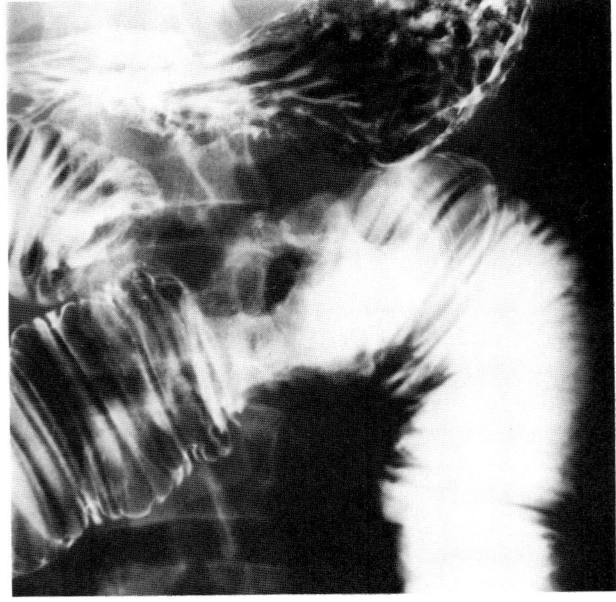

Fig. 31.26 Melanoma metastasis. Small bowel enema showing a localized tumour mass in the jejunum.

MALABSORPTION SYNDROMES

ABSORPTION AND MALABSORPTION

An understanding of the physiology of digestion and absorption is essential if patients with malabsorption are to be investigated by radiological means to the best effect. After homogenization and lubrication in the mouth, food is swallowed into the stomach, where further homogenization occurs and digestion begins. The chyme is then propelled through the pylorus into the small intestine where digestion and absorption are completed. The sites at which different substances are absorbed in the small intestine are illustrated in Figure 31.27. Substances which require no digestion, such as glucose, inorganic iron and folic acid appear to be absorbed as soon as they reach the small intestine. Fat and protein, however, require pre-

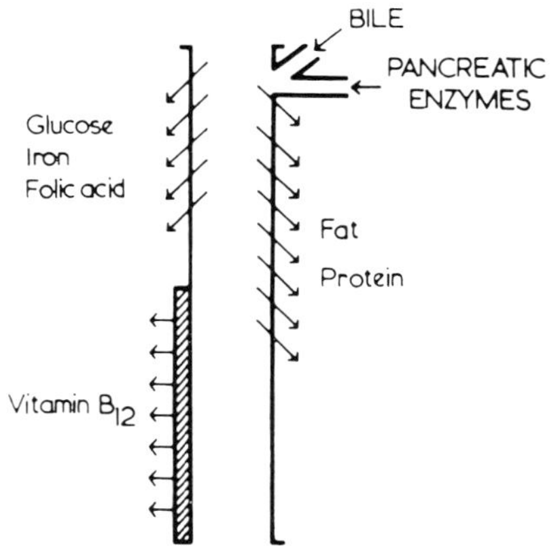

Fig. 31.27 Diagram of the sites at which different substances are absorbed in the small intestine.

liminary emulsification and digestion by the bile and pancreatic enzymes and are therefore absorbed more slowly. These substances may be absorbed in the upper jejunum, but it is probable that the motility of the upper intestine propels them more distally than glucose, before absorption is complete. The absorption of vitamin B_{12} is remarkable in that it is absorbed only from the distal ileum.

From this it will be seen that folic acid deficiency, or a flat glucose tolerance test usually indicates a diffuse abnormality of the small intestine, the cause of which is often more accurately diagnosed by a biopsy than by radiology. Steatorrhoea, on the other hand, may be due to a failure of emulsification and digestion caused by a lack of bile or pancreatic enzymes, or to failure of absorption caused by a widespread intestinal abnormality. Both radiology and biopsy are required in such cases. Pure B_{12} deficiency is occasionally due to disease or resection of the distal ileum, but may be due to bacterial contamination of the small bowel, the bacteria competing with the host for the vitamin. Radiology has an essential part to play in this group of patients, since clinical symptoms of small bowel disease may be minimal, or absent, as in jejunal diverticulosis.

Gastrectomy may cause malabsorption in a number of ways. Severe deficiencies are not common after the Bilroth type of operation; since there is frequently a large gastric remnant, some control of the rate of emptying of the stomach is retained and the continuity of the alimentary tract is not interrupted, so that normal mixing of chyme with bile and pancreatic enzymes occurs. After a *Polya* type of gastrectomy there are several potential reasons for severe malabsorption. There may be B_{12} deficiency due to lack of intrinsic factor, due to a small or atrophic gastric remnant. There is loss of the normal mixing and homogenization of food in the stomach, and this ill-prepared chyme may enter the small intestine at a rapid rate. Because of this, and the discontinuity of the alimentary tract, the chyme does not mix properly with bile and pancreatic enzymes so that digestion is impaired. A stagnant afferent loop may cause malabsorption by pooling bile and pancreatic enzymes so that they do not mix with chyme and perhaps enter the jejunum at times when there is no food present, causing a gastritis and oesophagitis. Infection of this stagnant afferent loop may cause bacterial

Table 31.2 The main mechanism involved in 'the malabsorption syndrome'

Cause	Mechanism	Example	
'Maldigestion'	a. Mechanical		Polya gastrectomy
	b. Lack of bile		Biliary atresia Obstructive jaundice Cholangitis Hepatic cell failure
	c. Lack of pancreatic enzymes		Fibrocystic disease of pancreas Chronic pancreatitis Pancreatic carcinoma/resection
'Malabsorption'	a. Lack of absorbing surface	Local	Resection Gastroileostomy
		General	Villous atrophy Whipple's disease
	b. Bacterial competition	Stagnation	Stagnant loop Jejunal diverticulosis Ileal stricture
		Fistula from colon to proximal gut	
'Excessive loss'	Loss of protein and electrolytes into lumen exceeds reabsorption		Protein-losing enteropathy Hypokalaemic ileus

contamination of the alimentary tract. Any form of gastrectomy may unmask previously subclinical malabsorption. For example, adult coelic disease or disaccharidase deficiency may become clinically important after gastrectomy, although not recognized before operation.

The main mechanisms involved in 'the malabsorption syndrome' are listed in Table 31.2.

RADIOLOGICAL INVESTIGATION

The term 'malabsorption syndrome' is sometimes used as though it was a firm diagnosis (sometimes even synonymous with adult coeliac disease) instead of a general statement about a condition for which one or more of many causes could be responsible. It is no more precise as a diagnosis than 'shortness of breath' and requires the same detailed investigation, in which radiology is important but must be correlated with all the other clinical data. Before a patient with malabsorption is examined radiologically it should be known what type of malabsorption or deficiency is suspected or proven, and what type of abdominal surgery, if any, has been performed. The examination can be planned accordingly and the findings subsequently fitted in to the whole clinical picture.

From the radiological point of view, the malabsorption syndromes may be divided into two main groups (Table 31.3). The *first* group contains those conditions in which the radiological features are mainly those associated with steatorrhoea. In this group the radiological features are usually non-specific and a firm diagnosis depends on other methods, usually small bowel biopsy. Even in this group, however, radiology is frequently indicated in order to rule out some local anatomical cause for malabsorption (listed in group 2). The *second* group contains conditions with specific radiological features. It is in this group, particularly when there is some anatomical lesion of the small bowel, that radiology may be of great value and is frequently the only method of arriving at a firm diagnosis.

Table 31.3 Radiological classification of malabsorption

Group 1. Radiological features mainly those of steatorrhoea
A. Diffuse lesions of the intestinal mucosa:
coeliac disease
idiopathic steatorrhoea (adult coeliac disease)
tropical sprue
infiltrations — Whipple's disease
— amyloidosis
B. Defects of digestion:
a. Deficiency of bile
obstructive jaundice
biliary cirrhosis
b. Deficiency of pancreatic enzymes
cystic fibrosis
chronic pancreatitis
pancreatectomy
C. Postgastrectomy steatorrhoea
Group 2. Conditions with specific radiological features
A. Localized (often multiple) lesions of the small intestine:
regional ileitis
Hodgkin's disease
lymphosarcoma
diffuse sclerosis (scleroderma)
B. Anatomical lesions of the small intestine:
a. Resection
proximal resection
distal resection
b. Bacterial contamination
jejunal diverticulosis
stagnant loop
ileal stricture
fistula
c. Mixed lesions (resection plus bacterial contamination)
C. Disaccharidase deficiency
hypolactasia
hyposucrasia

GROUP 1: RADIOLOGICAL FEATURES MAINLY THOSE OF STEATORRHOEA

A. DIFFUSE LESIONS OF THE INTESTINAL MUCOSA

In this group of conditions a firm diagnosis rests on intestinal biopsy, but at times suspicion may be raised and a presumptive diagnosis made on the radiological appearances, *dilatation* of the jejunum and *flocculation* of the barium sulphate preparation.

Most modern barium sulphate preparations contain suspending agents designed to prevent flocculation or clumping together of the barium particles in the presence of mucus, so that flocculation of undiluted barium sulphate preparation in the small intestine of an adult in the United Kingdom is abnormal, provided no gastric residue was present before the barium sulphate was administered and that food has not been taken after the barium. Steatorrhoea secondary to adult coeliac disease is the most likely cause, but biopsy would be needed for confirmation. However, it is an unreliable sign since many patients with steatorrhoea do not flocculate barium and there is no correlation between the amount of flocculation and the severity of the steatorrhoea or the degree of villous atrophy present. Moreover, when flocculation occurs, radiographs show only the barium particles clumped together in the sump of individual coils of bowel. Coating of the mucosa does not occur and no details of the intestinal anatomy can be made out. A repeat examination with a more flocculation-resistant barium preparation, or a small bowel enema, would then be necessary to exclude a localized lesion such as a stricture.

Dilatation of the jejunum results in the secondary folds being smoothed out, revealing the primary transverse folds, the valvulae conniventes. Normally, individual folds

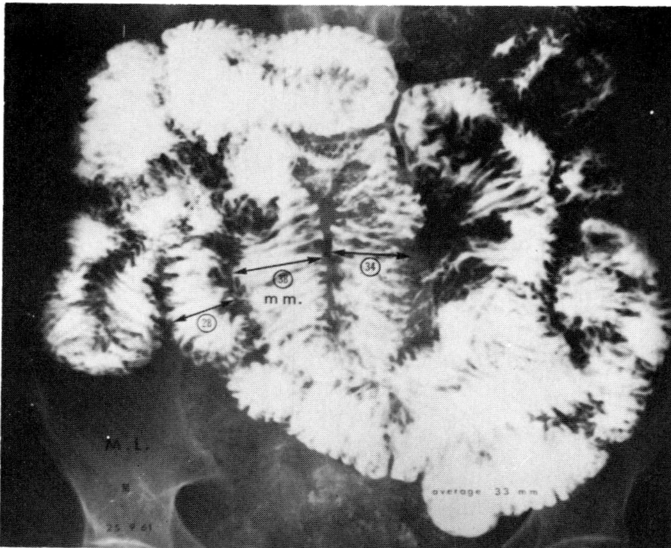

Fig. 31.28 Adult coeliac disease, moderate dilatation of the jejunum in a patient with diarrhoea due to steatorrhoea. Biopsy showed sub-total villos atrophy.

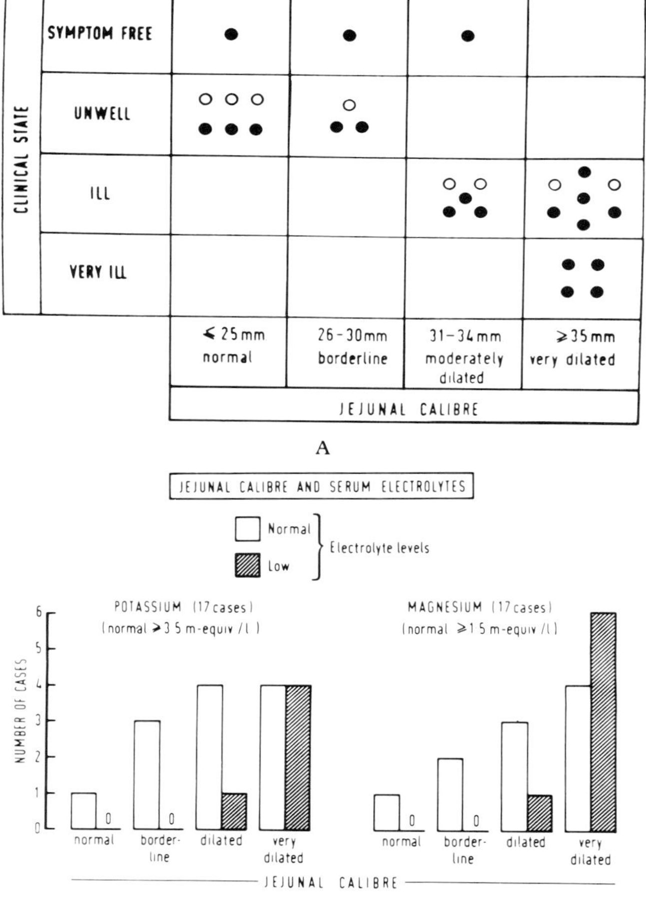

Fig. 31.29 Relationship between jejunal calibre and clinical state in 28 patients with adult coeliac disease. (Closed circles indicate sub-total villos atrophy. Open circles indicate partial villos atrophy.)

of mucosa cannot be traced completely across the lumen of the jejunum, except transiently during the passage of a bolus. If several coils of bowel on one film show this smoothing out of the secondary folds the appearances are abnormal (Fig. 31.28).

Coeliac disease

In adult coeliac disease there is a correlation between the calibre of the small bowel and the clinical state of the patient (Fig. 31.29). Those patients who are most severely ill show the most severe dilatation. All patients with hypokalaemia show moderate or severe dilatation but equal dilatation may be seen in those patients with normal serum potassium levels. Moreover, restoration of serum potassium to normal does not necessarily result in a reduction in the calibre of the small bowel. However, the calibre of the small bowel does mirror the clinical state quite closely, in that patients who respond to a gluten-free diet show a similar improvement in the radiological appearances of their small bowel (Fig. 31.30). On relapse the small bowel calibre increases. If a patient on a gluten-free diet shows a worsening radiological picture, one should suspect that either the diet is not being adhered to or that some complication has occurred, such as the development of a reticulosis or a carcinoma of the gastrointestinal tract (Fig. 31.31).

At the other end of the spectrum of coeliac disease, some patients with villous atrophy have few or no intestinal symptoms and present with a mild macrocytic megalo-

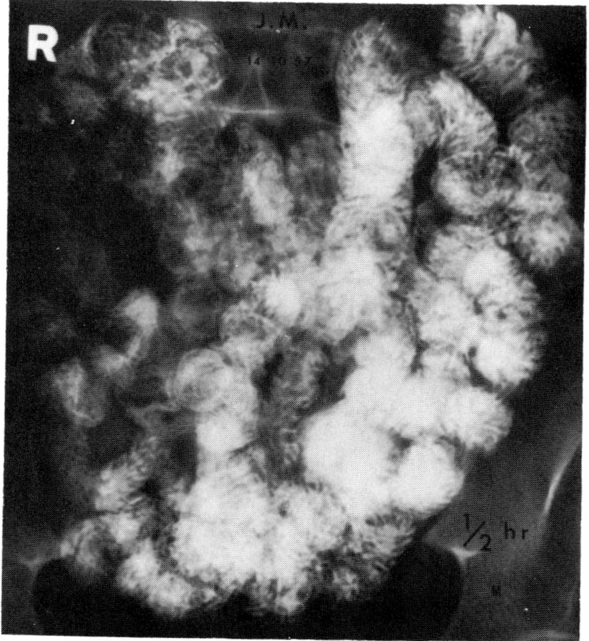

Fig. 31.30 Adult coeliac disease. Normal small bowel appearance in patient with megaloblastic anaemia but no intestinal symptoms. Biopsy showed partial villos atrophy.

blastic anaemia. Such patients usually have either a completely normal small bowel appearance or show minimal dilatation. A normal radiological appearance in no way excludes either partial or subtotal villous atrophy, but such patients are not clinically ill (Fig. 31.30). Transient small bowel intussusception may be seen.

Radiological appearance of the small bowel in *tropical sprue* is identical to that of gluten-induced enteropathy. The degree of dilatation correlates roughly with the severity of the clinical illness and improvement follows successful treatment with a broad spectrum antibiotic (Fig. 31.32).

In *intestinal lipodystrophy* (Whipple's disease), there may be the non-specific changes found in patients with steatorrhoea from any cause — dilatation and sometimes flocculation. In addition, that may be evidence of enlarged abdominal lymph nodes, bone changes, particularly in the spine and resembling rheumatoid arthritis, as well as sclerosis of the sacroiliac joints. The diagnosis, as in *amyloid infiltration*, depends on intestinal biopsy. *Giardiasis* may cause quite severe steatorrhoea with dilatation of the jejunum, thickening of folds and flocculation of barium (Fig. 31.6). The changes resolve when the condition is treated.

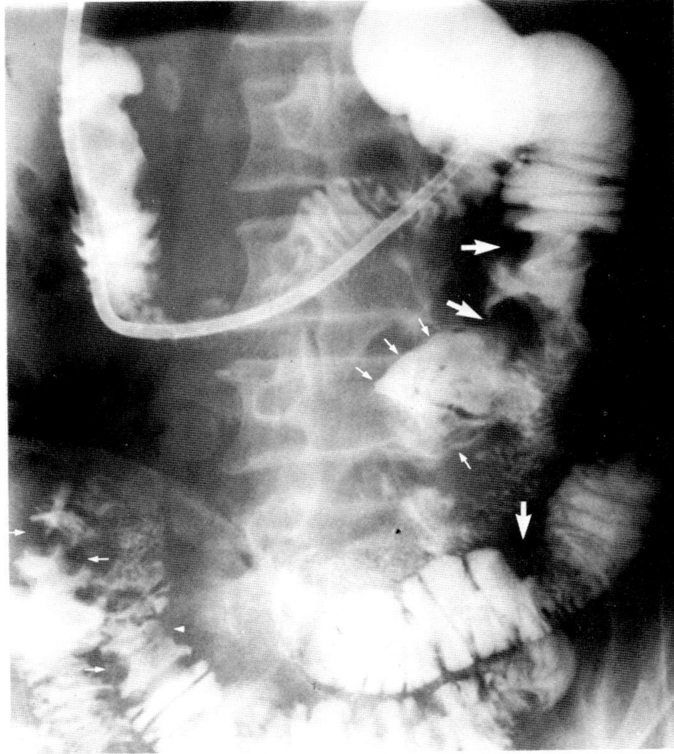

Fig. 31.31 Histiocytic lymphoma complicating adult coeliac disease. Small bowel enema showing numerous masses scattered throughout the small bowel (large arrows) one of which has excavated giving rise to a large cavity (small arrows).

B. DEFECTS OF DIGESTION

In this group of conditions there may be malabsorption of fat, but the radiological changes associated with the steatorrhoea are usually not as severe as when there is a generalized abnormality of the intestinal mucosa. The value of radiology is mainly in demonstrating the underlying cause of the digestive defect, such as the presence of gall stones or pancreatic carcinoma giving rise to obstructive jaundice, or pancreatic calcification indicating the presence of chronic pancreatitis.

C. POSTGASTRECTOMY STEATORRHOEA

In most cases, malabsorption following gastrectomy is a

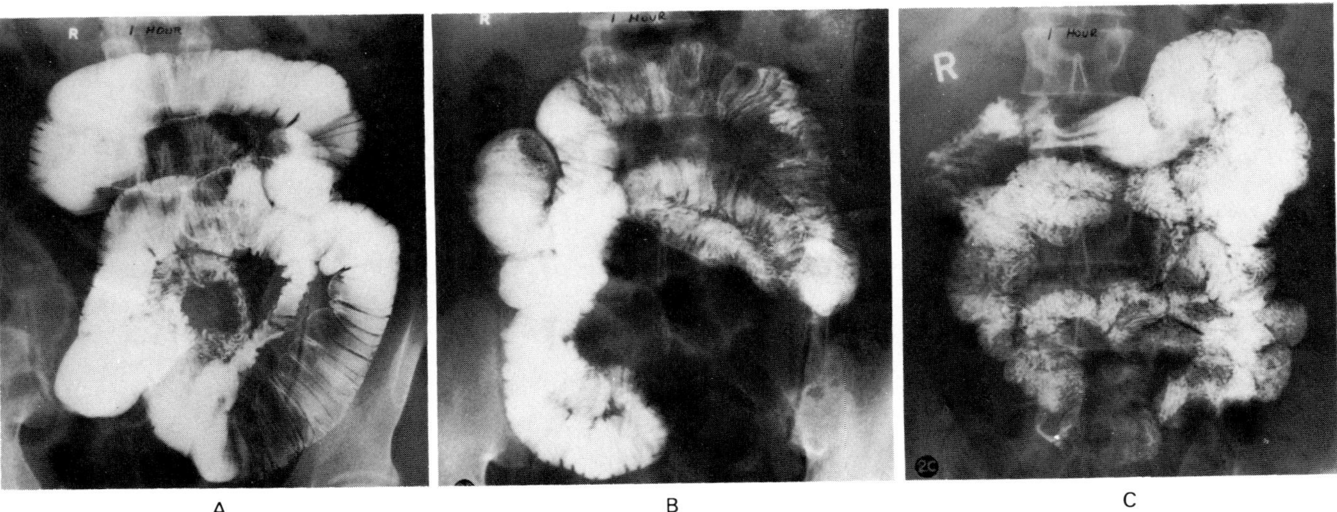

Fig. 31.32 Tropical sprue showing response to treatment with a broad spectrum antibiotic. **A.** Patient is severely ill with diarrhoea and megaloblastic anaemia. Moderate dilatation of the jejunum. **B.** One month after treatment patient recovering and small bowel returning to normal. **C.** Three months later. Patient has completely recovered and the small bowel appearances are normal.

defect of digestion, due to poor mixing of food with bile and pancreatic enzymes, and radiology has little part to play. *Stagnation in the afferent loop*, either due to kinking or undue length, is a rare cause. This dilated afferent loop may be demonstrated by barium meal but frequently fails to fill as peristalsis tends to prevent filling. Stagnation within the afferent loop may be demonstrated by *isotope studies* following injection of ^{99m}Tc-IDA.

Sideropenic webs may occur between 2 and 20 years after gastrectomy and be associated with iron deficiency anaemia, dysphagia, glossitis and angular stomatitis. Whereas the webs of the Plummer-Vinson syndrome are seen only in women, postgastrectomy webs also occur in men.

GROUP 2: CONDITIONS WITH SPECIFIC RADIOLOGICAL FEATURES

A. LOCALIZED (OFTEN MULTIPLE) LESIONS OF THE SMALL INTESTINE

Although some form of malabsorption is common in *Crohn's disease* it is rarely, if ever, caused simply by destruction of absorbing surface alone. When malabsorption is severe there are usually multiple lesions throughout the small bowel causing stagnation in individual loops and fistulae between loops may be present. There is often the added problem of previous surgical resection and the possibility of stagnant loops following surgery. Loss of protein from the ulcerated lesions of regional ileitis further contribute to the patient's malnutrition.

Demonstration of the areas of small bowel affected by Crohn's disease, the extent of stagnation in different loops and the presence of fistulous connections between different loops of small bowel require very detailed radiological examination. Paired erect and supine films should be taken and the examination continued until all the barium has left the small intestine, in order to assess the extent and demonstrate the site of stagnation. Small bowel enema examination may be necessary, particularly to demonstrate the fistulous communications.

Lymphoma of the small bowel is often associated with a villous atrophy and may complicate long-standing gluten-induced enteropathy (Fig. 31.31). Multiple ulcerated filling defects or rigid areas devoid of mucosa may be seen in the small bowel. These may cause partial but rarely complete obstruction; in fact the lumen of the small bowel may show irregular dilatation at the site of the lymphoma. Enlarged lymph nodes in the mesentery may displace the gut and an enlarged spleen may be present. The spleen is usually small in uncomplicated coeliac disease.

In *diffuse sclerosis* (scleroderma) the duodenum is often severely dilated together with other loops of proximal small bowel (Fig. 31.33). Although the loops may be very dilated, the folds are not thickened and there is no evidence of ulceration. There are in effect multiple sites of functional obstruction because of lack of effective peristalsis. Severe stagnation in dilated loops may be demonstrated by continuing the examination until nearly all the barium has left the small bowel, up to 24 or 48 hours if necessary.

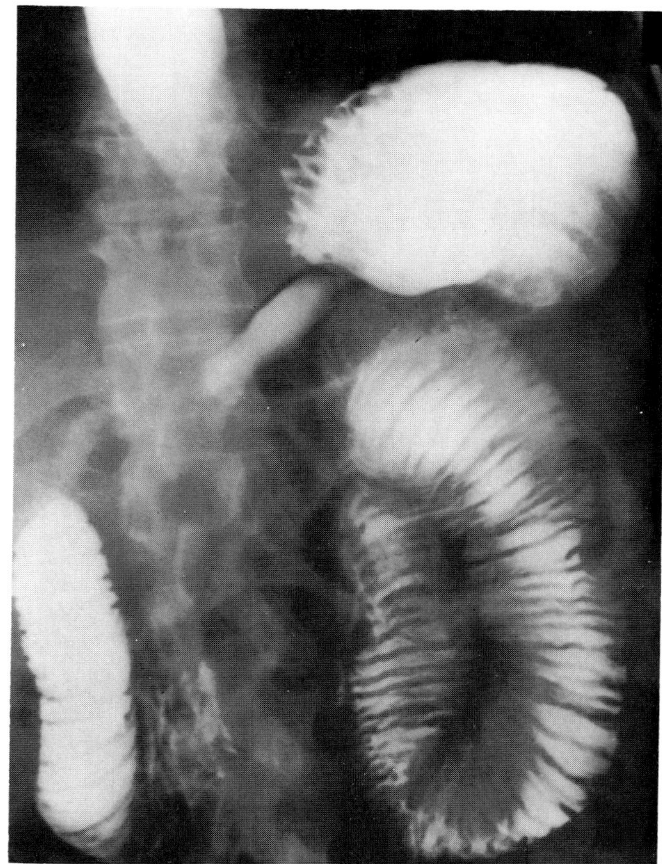

Fig. 31.33 Scleroderma affecting the oesophagus, duodenum and jejunum.

B. ANATOMICAL LESIONS OF THE SMALL BOWEL

1. Resection.

Examination of the small intestine after resection is carried out for the following reasons:

a. In order to assess the length and normality of the remaining small intestine. Massive resections are often carried out for infarction of bowel and surgical details of emergency operations are not always available. It is possible for up to one quarter of the small intestine to be resected without it being recognizable radiologically.

b. In order to exclude a recurrence of the disease or the formation of a stricture or a stagnant loop at the site of the anastomosis.

The radiological appearances will depend not only on the length of bowel resected but also on whether a proximal or distal resection has been carried out.

Peristalsis is more active in the jejunum than in the ileum so that chyme and hence barium, move through it relatively rapidly. After a massive resection of jejunum, usually following infarction, the overall transit time from stomach to caecum remains normal or is only slightly reduced, provided the slower moving ileum and ileocaecal valve has been retained (Fig. 31.34). Malabsorption is unlikely to occur since the ileum is capable of taking over most if not all of the functions of the jejunum. The small bowel examination is likely to appear normal except for some recognizable shortening of small bowel.

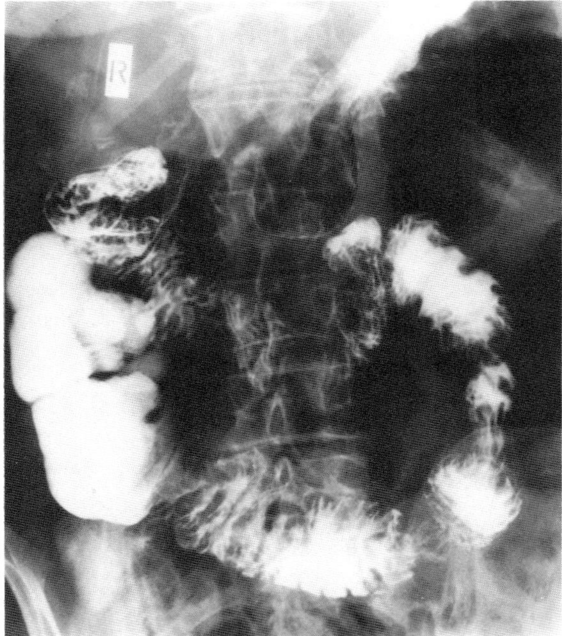

Fig. 31.34 Massive small bowel resection following mesenteric infarction. This elderly lady survived 1 year with less than 30 cm of jejunum.

The ileum is resected far more often than the jejunum, usually for Crohn's disease, sometimes for tumour, adhesions or infarction. Since the active jejunum is retained the transit time from stomach to caecum is much reduced, especially if the ileocaecal valve has been resected also. Malabsorption is more likely to occur and specific vitamin B_{12} deficiency develop if the distal ileum has been removed.

If less than a quarter of the jejunum has been resected and the ileocaecal valve remains intact, the radiological appearances may be entirely normal. With more massive jejunal resection the transit time is reduced and fluid levels may be seen in the ascending colon. These fluid levels are commonly seen after massive distal resections and should not by themselves be accepted as evidence of obstruction (Fig. 31.35). Normally, following distal resection there is no hypertrophy or dilatation of the remaining bowel unless only a metre or so of jejunum remain. Dilatation of the small bowel following a distal resection is almost invariably due to a recurrence of the disease, adhesions or a stricture at the site of the anastomosis.

2. Bacterial contamination

Bacterial contamination in the small intestine, of sufficient severity to cause malabsorption, is usually due to stag-

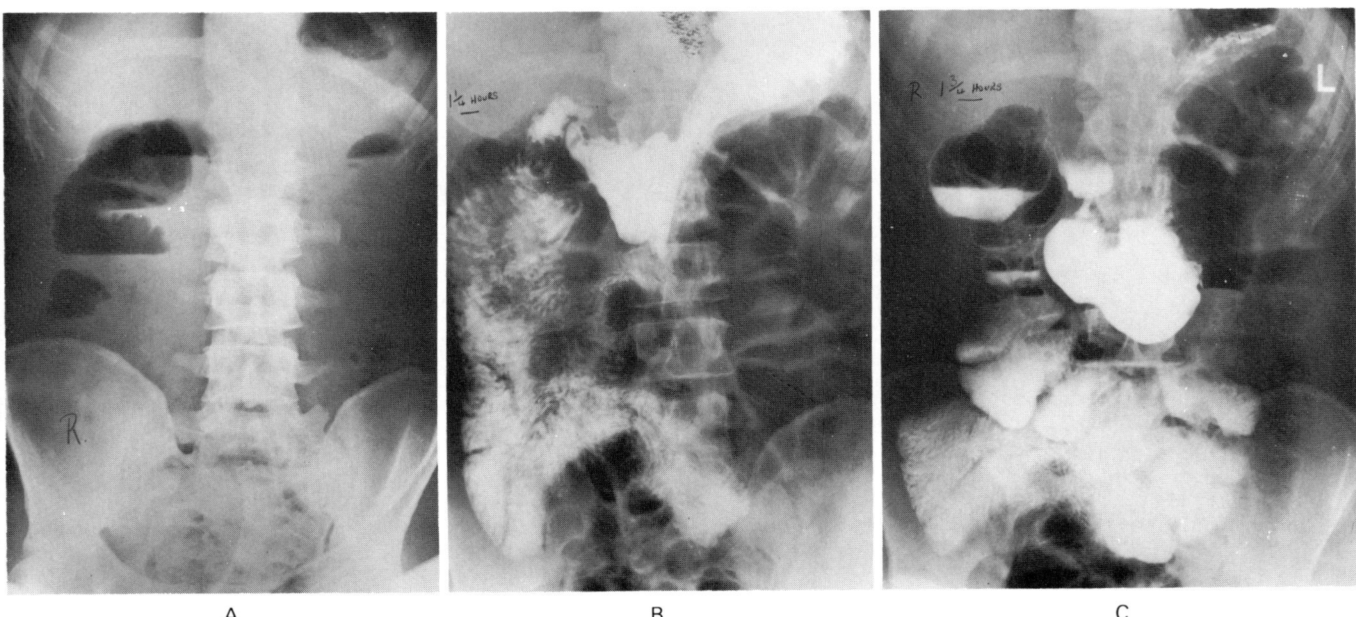

Fig. 31.35 Massive resection of distal small bowel without obstruction. All except 1.2 m of jejunum have been resected for volvulus. **A.** Straight radiograph, patient erect, showing fluid levels. These do not indicate obstruction. **B.** Small bowel examination. $1\frac{1}{4}$ hour film showing jejunum of normal calibre but to the right of the midline. **C.** $1\frac{3}{4}$ hour film. The fluid barium in the colon demonstrates the site of the fluid levels in **A.**

nation of intestinal contents, the extent of which can be estimated on the barium follow-through examination, provided the films are taken until most of the barium has passed into the colon. Films taken 24, 48 or even 72 hours after the ingestion of barium may be necessary. Much less commonly bacterial contamination may be due to a fistula from the colon to small bowel.

Jejunal diverticulosis. Diverticulosis sufficiently severe to cause malabsorption can be recognized on the small bowel examination. Erect films, with and without barium, will show fluid levels within the diverticula and may simulate small bowel obstruction, except that there tend to be numerous short fluid levels all of similar length and no dilated bowel is seen on the supine film (Fig. 31.36). The diverticula themselves are commonly seen as round, oval or flask-shaped structures leading from the mesenteric border of the small bowel. The most certain method of diagnosis is to demonstrate mucosa leading into the neck of individual diverticula (Fig. 31.37). Occasionally, accurate localization of the diverticula may be important because, if they are confined to one loop or a short segment of jejunum, resection with cure may be possible. In selected cases intubation of the lower jejunum or ileum may be useful by demonstrating the normality of the ileum before withdrawing the tube and showing segments of bowel affected by diverticulosis. However, since these patients are usually elderly and their anaemia can usually be controlled by antibiotics and replacement therapy, this localization is not required in most cases.

Stagnant loops. A distinction should be made between blind loops and stagnant loops. A blind loop is closed at one end. Only a small proportion of blind loops are stagnant and not all stagnant loops are blind. If peristalsis tends to keep the loop empty (isoperistaltic loop) there is no stagnation of contents and no malabsorption. The ascending colon following an end-to-end ileotransverse anastomosis is an example of such a loop and causes no disability. If peristalsis in the loop tends to keep it full (retroperistaltic loop) stasis of contents occurs and the loop may dilate to hold a large volume of stagnant intestinal contents. This type of blind loop occurs after a side-to-side enteroanastomosis, around an obstruction or other resection. Faecoliths may occur in these loops causing ulceration, haemorrhage and iron deficiency anaemia (Fig. 31.38). Fortunately, only a small proportion of people with blind loops get malabsorption, the important factor being stagnation. Of course, many stagnant loops are not 'blind' but are incompletely obstructed loops in the mainstream of the ileum.

Stricture. Strictures of the jejunum usually present as an acute or subacute surgical emergency calling for immediate treatment and so rarely cause malabsorption. Ileal strictures, on the other hand, often cause few symptoms and are therefore of sufficient chronicity to cause stagnation and malabsorption. Crohn's disease, tuberculosis and adhesions are the common causes. There may be surprisingly few intestinal symptoms, even though there is gross dilatation of the ileum (Fig. 31.39). Small bowel examination shows progressive dilution of the barium sulphate suspension as it enters the dilated ileum. Thickened walls due to muscular hypertrophy may be seen in the less dilated proximal loops. The presence of a stricture can

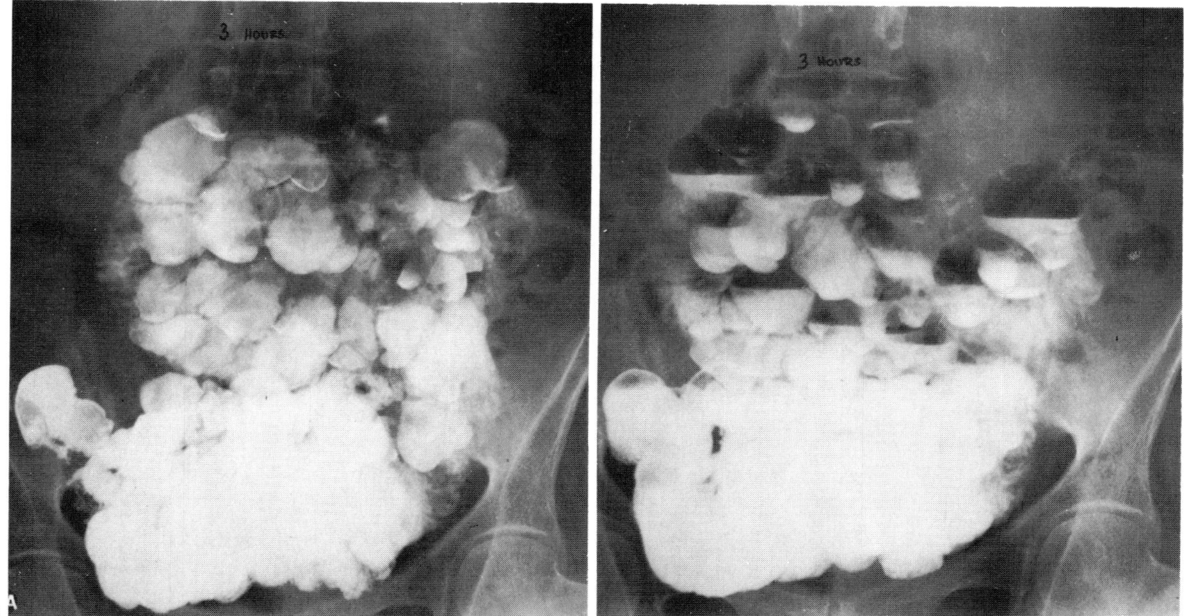

Fig. 31.36 Jejunum diverticulosis. **A.** Small bowel meal showing dilute barium in the diverticula resembling flocculation. **B.** Horizontal ray film taken at the same time demonstrates the diverticula containing fluid levels.

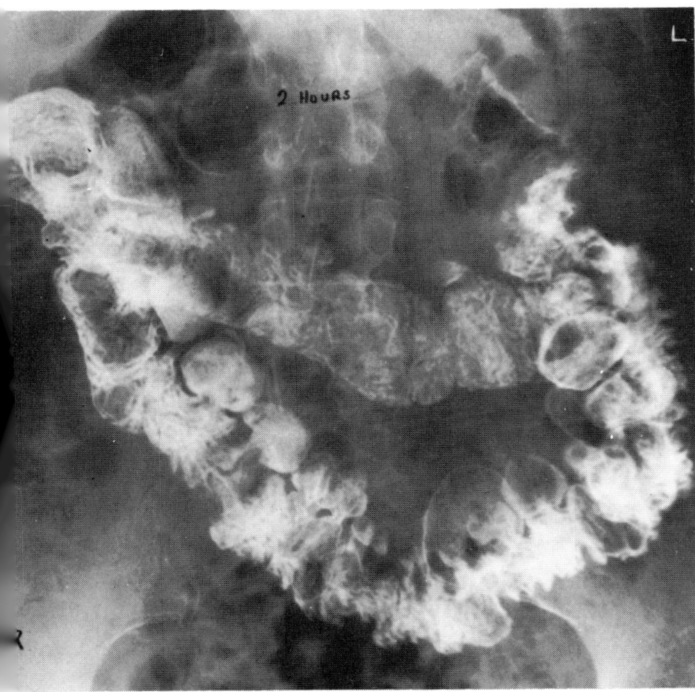

Fig. 31.37 Jejunal diverticulosis. Multiple diverticula are shown on the mesenteric border of a loop of jejunum. The mucosal folds entering the neck of the diverticula are well seen.

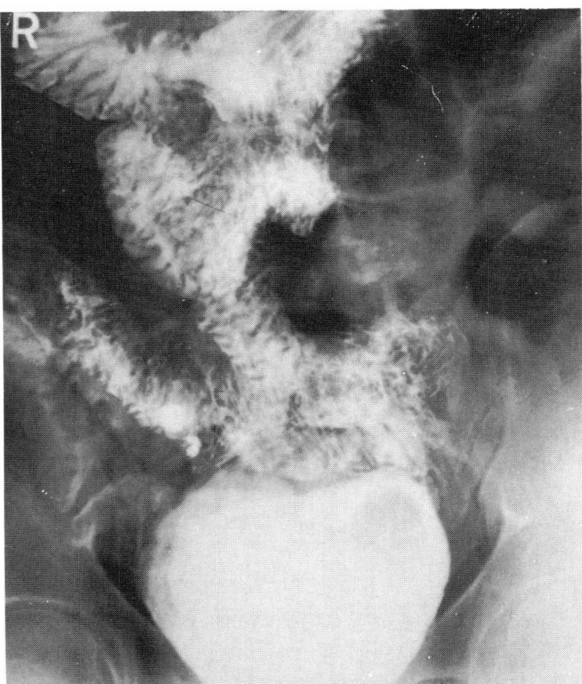

Fig. 31.38 Stagnant loop. Resection of distal ileum with side-to-side anastomosis following gun shot wound. A large stagnant loop of ileum has developed. A faecolith within this gave rise to ulceration and iron deficiency anaemia in addition to the megaloblastic anaemia caused by the bacterial contamination following stagnation.

often be demonstrated by careful fluoroscopy, with separation of the loops by compression and local views. The size and length of the stricture should be noted together with any evidence of ulceration, fistula formation or associated soft tissue mass. In severe and long-standing cases however, the actual site of the obstruction may be difficult or impossible to demonstrate, even after intubation of the ileum because of dilution and stagnation of barium. It may be possible to show the stricture by retrograde examination after barium enema.

Fistula. A large fistula may cause malabsorption by allowing contents of the gut to short circuit the absorbing mucosal area of the small intestine. On the other hand, even a small fistula between the colon and the proximal gut may cause malabsorption by bacterial contamination with colonic organisms (Fig. 31.14). The pressure in the colon is usually higher than in the stomach or small intestine, so that in gastrocolic or ileocolic fistulae the intestinal contents usually pass from the colon into the stomach or small bowel. Thus, these fistulae are more easily demonstrated by barium enema than by barium meal follow-through examination (Fig. 31.40). Unless the fistula is large, it may be impossible to demonstrate it conclusively on a follow-through examination, whereas it is usually obvious on barium enema. Occasionally intubation of the small bowel may be the only conclusive method of demonstrating an enterocolic fistula.

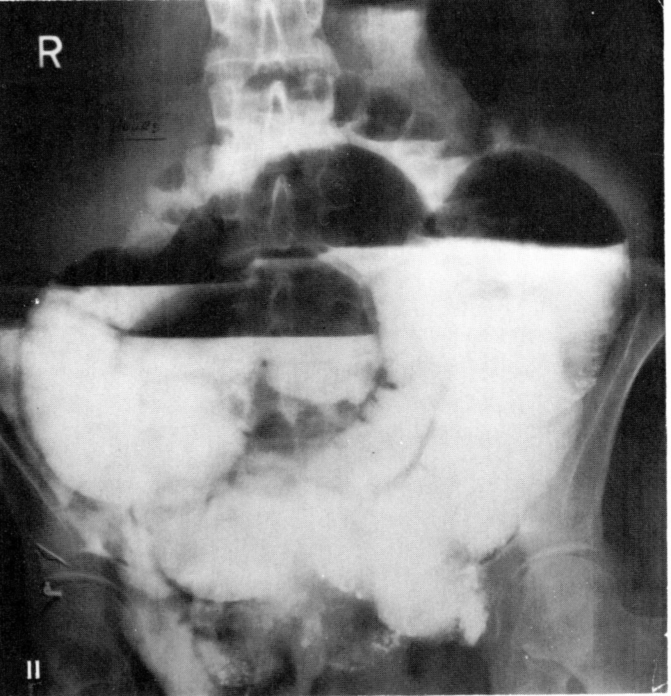

Fig. 31.39 Chronic ileal obstruction. The patient had a previous enteroenteric anastomosis for intestinal obstruction. Dilatation of this degree could not be due solely to a stagnant loop and must indicate mainstream obstruction. Laparotomy revealed a carcinoid tumour of lower ileum.

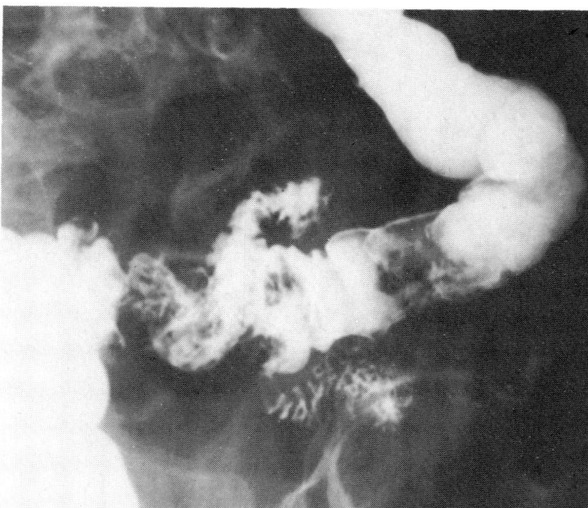

Fig. 31.40 Ileosigmoid fistula. A fistula formed spontaneously between the ileum and a diverticulum in the sigmoid. Barium follow-through examination was normal. Barium enema demonstrated the fistula.

Very rarely, malabsorption following gastrectomy may be due to an error of surgical technique, when a gastroileal instead of a gastrojejunal anastomosis has been performed, thus causing a short circuit of the jejunum.

3. Mixed lesions

Sometimes malabsorption is due to a combination of a number of factors. This is especially true of patients with Crohn's disease who have had surgical treatment. There may be loss of absorbing surface following resection as well as due to the primary disease. Bacterial contamination of intestinal contents may be due to the presence of fistulae as well as stagnant loops. Sinuses may be present.

Many forms of radiological investigation may be needed. A conventional follow-through examination gives an idea of the site of maximum stagnation within the gut. Small bowel enema may be needed to demonstrate a localized stricture or a fistula between adjacent loops. Barium enema may be needed to demonstrate the fistulae involving the colon. Sinography usually demonstrates the site or sites of leakage from the bowel. The radiological investigation of these patients leading to a full demonstration of the disordered anatomy can be very difficult and requires great patience. In no field is closer cooperation and understanding between radiologist and surgeon more important.

C. DISACCHARIDASE DEFICIENCY

The common disaccharides in our diet, *lactose, sucrose* and *maltose*, have to be split into monosaccharides by enzymes in the microvilli of the brush border of the small intestinal epithelial cell before they can be absorbed. Deficiency of one or other of these enzymes results in the large unsplit molecule remaining in the lumen of the small bowel where it causes an osmotic diarrhoea. Subsequently, the unabsorbed sugar passes into the large bowel where it is fermented by intestinal bacteria. The commonest disaccharidase deficiency is *hypolactasia*. In some, it appears to be genetically determined, being more common in some races (Greeks, Indians, Pakistanis) than others (white Caucasian). It is found in some cases of adult coeliac disease, where there is atrophy of the villi as well as the microvilli, and it may occur temporarily after severe infective enteritis. *Hyposucrasia* is rare and *hypomaltasia* does not occur, except as part of a multiple enzyme deficiency as seen in the kwashiorkor syndrome.

Adults with hypolactasia rarely present with a history of milk-induced diarrhoea, but often state they seldom drink milk. More frequently they have rather ill-defined complaints such as abdominal discomfort, distension, excess flatulence and occasional diarrhoea, which they do not relate to the ingestion of milk. Often they are subjected to many investigations, including barium studies of the whole intestine, without a firm diagnosis being made. Some of the them are regarded as suffering from 'spastic colon'; others are considered to be neurotic. The assurance that there is a rational explanation for their symptoms is one of the chief benefits of diagnosing hypolactasia.

Hyposucrasia is rare but may cause severe symptoms since it is difficult to avoid cane sugar in modern diets. Two teaspoonfuls of sugar or two segments of chocolate may cause abdominal discomfort, distension and diarrhoea.

The diagnosis of disaccharidase deficiency is made by estimating the enzyme activity in the biopsy of jejunal mucosa. Supporting evidence may be obtained by a sugar tolerance test, but the results of these may be difficult to interpret and occasionally misleading. A reliable diagnosis can be obtained by observing the radiological appearance of the small bowel after the ingestion of a barium preparation to which a test sugar has been added. This simple radiological method is useful as a screening test in patients with vague abdominal symptoms and in carrying out population surveys.

Method. 25 g of the test sugar is added to 110–170 g (4–6 oz) of barium sulphate preparation, which should contain no disaccharide and no hydroscopic agent, such as sodium carboxymethyl cellulose or sorbitol. Micropaque is suitable in this respect. A formal barium meal examination of the oesophagus, stomach and duodenum can be carried out if desired. The patient then lies on his right side and a film is taken after 60 minutes with the patient supine. If the transit time is expected to be shorter than usual, as after gastrectomy or resection of the distal small bowel, the film should be taken at 30–45 minutes, before all the barium has passed into the colon.

In normal patients the presence of the test sugar will not be detectable and the normal appearance of concentrated barium sulphate suspension will be seen. If dissaccharidase deficiency is present there will be dilution of the barium sulphate suspension and a large part of the small intestine will be filled with dilute contrast medium. At the end of 1 hour some barium is usually in the colon (Figs 31.41 and 31.42).

This combination of *dilution of contrast* together with relatively *rapid transit*, is easily recognized and is diagnostic. In some disorders, such as idiopathic steatorrhoea with severe intestinal symptoms, the intestine may be dilated and contrast medium may appear dilute, but the transit in these patients is slow, the radiographic appearances sometimes resembling an ileus (Fig. 31.43). In

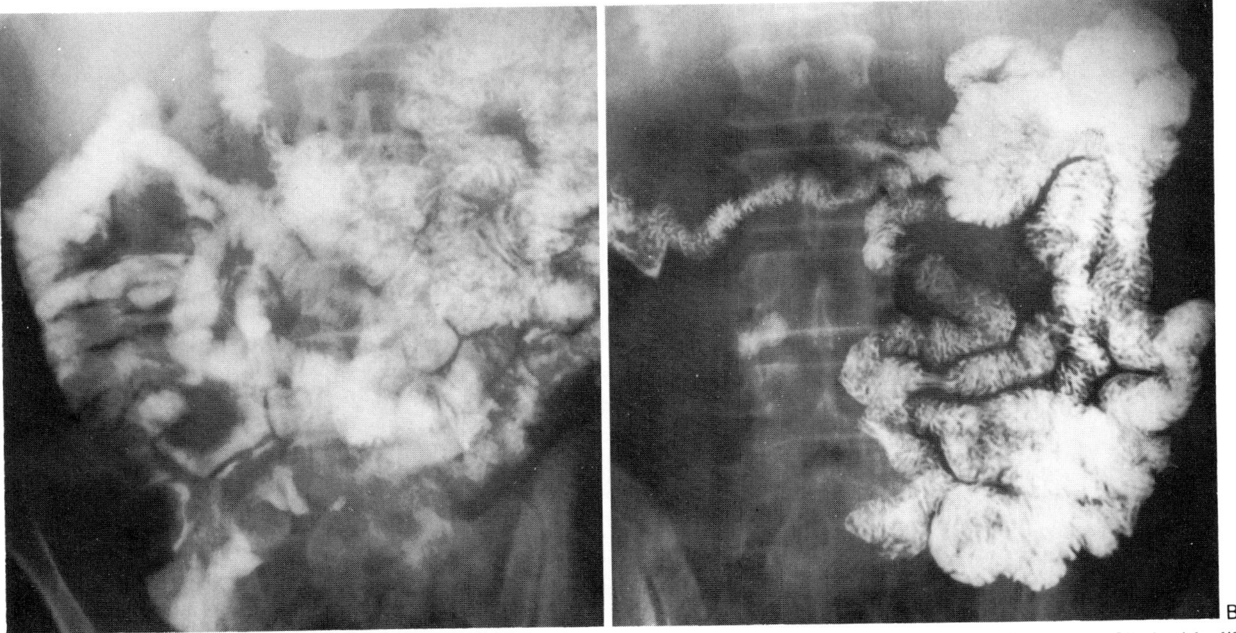

Fig. 31.41 Hypolactasia. **A.** Radiograph taken 1 hour after lactose-barium mixture, showing a large part of the small intestine filled with dilute contrast medium and some barium in the ascending colon (the lactase level 0.0 units). **B.** 1 hour after sucrose-barium mixture showing the normal appearance of concentrated barium in the small bowel (sucrose level 7.3 units).

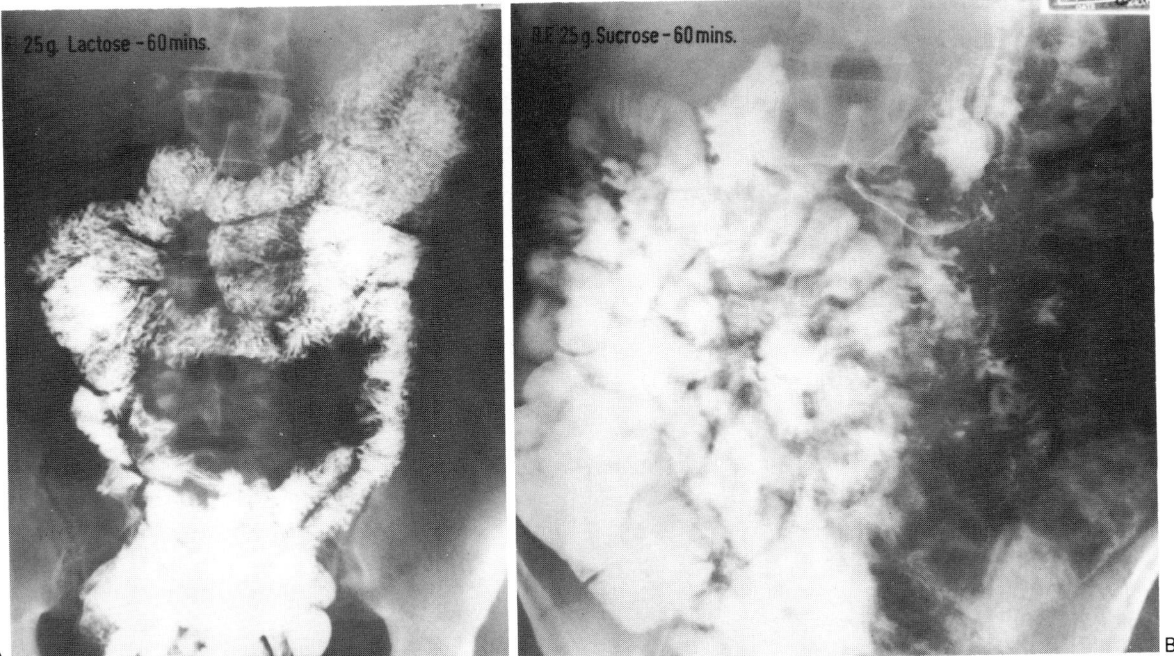

Fig. 31.42 Hyposucrasia. **A.** 1 hour after lactose-barium showing normal appearance of the small bowel (lactase 2.4 units). **B.** 1 hour after sucrose-barium showing dilute barium in the ileum and transverse colon (sucrase 0.0 units). 25 g of test sugar in 120 ml Micropaque.

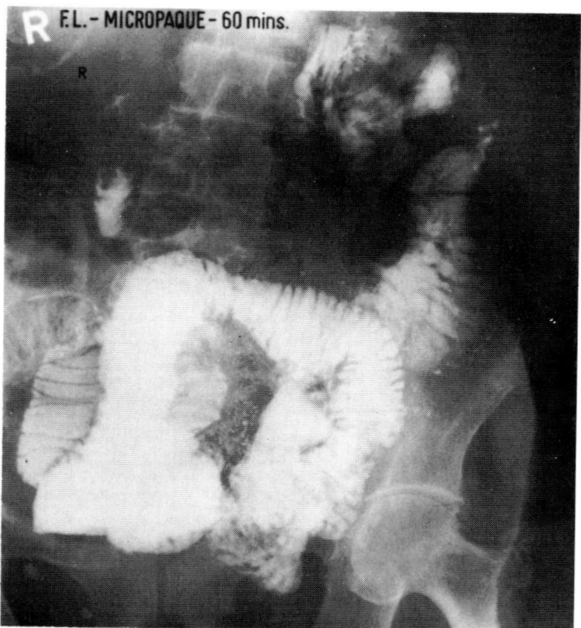

Fig. 31.43 Dilution but no hurry. Coeliac disease showing dilatation of the jejunum and dilution of barium with slow transit.

addition, in idiopathic steatorrhoea the mucosal folds are often thickened, a feature not seen in disaccharidase deficiency demonstrated by this method. Again, in subacute obstruction of the ileum there may be dilatation of the intestine with dilution of contrast medium but the rate of transit of barium in these patients is reduced. On the other hand, rapid transit is sometimes seen in healthy people, the contrast medium reaching the colon in well under an hour. When this happens the small intestine is not dilated and the contrast medium not diluted either in the small or large intestine (Fig. 31.44).

In patients with an anatomical normal small intestine this test gives a clear-cut result, although if the disaccharidase level is borderline the radiological appearances may be difficult to interpret. Comparison with films taken after using Micropaque alone or with another test sugar usually leads to a definite diagnosis. If transit of barium is so rapid that it is all in the colon at 60 minutes, the diagnosis can still be made because dilution of barium can be recognized in the colon just as readily as in the small intestine.

The addition of a disaccharide to Micropaque does not interfere with the examination of the small bowel (Fig. 31.45).

Hypolactasia occurs in some patients with subtotal villous atrophy due to gluten-induced enteropathy, presumably because of damage to the microvilli in the brush border of the small intestinal cell. When such a patient responds to a gluten-free diet the hypolactasia also improves (Fig. 31.47 A, B, C & D).

The radiological appearances in patients with hypolactasia following a lactose barium sulphate meal are similar to those seen when a similar osmolar load of magnesium sulphate and barium sulphate are given to a normal subject

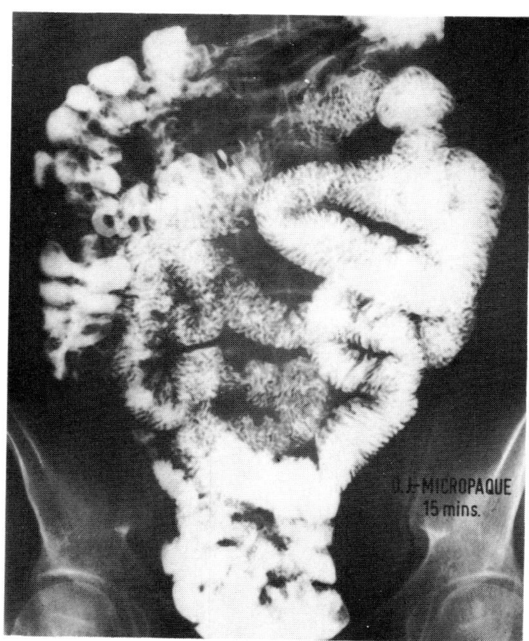

Fig. 31.44 Hurry but no dilution. Normal patient in whom the barium has reached the colon in 15 minutes but in whom no dilution has occurred. The mucosal pattern is normal.

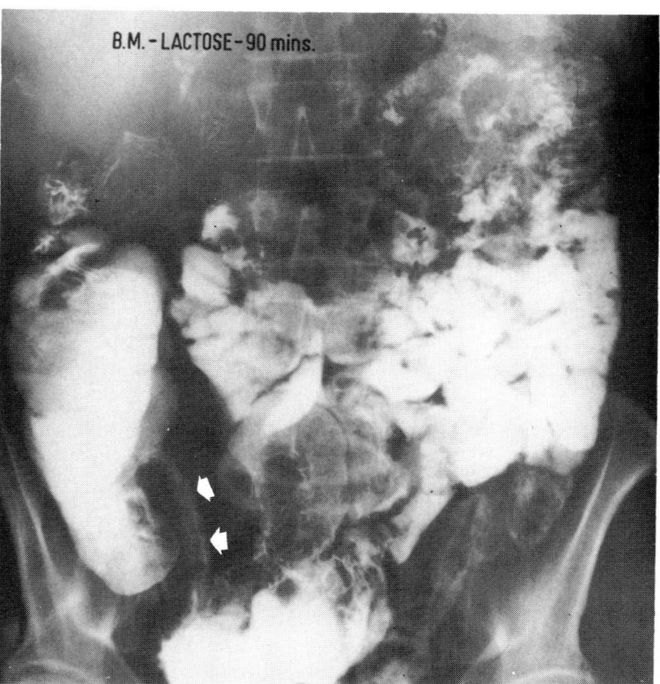

Fig. 31.45 Crohn's disease associated with hypolactasia. Dilution of contrast medium in the small bowel and colon has not prevented the demonstration of a narrow segment of terminal ileum due to Crohn's disease (arrows). Radiograph taken 90 minutes after ingestion of lactose barium.

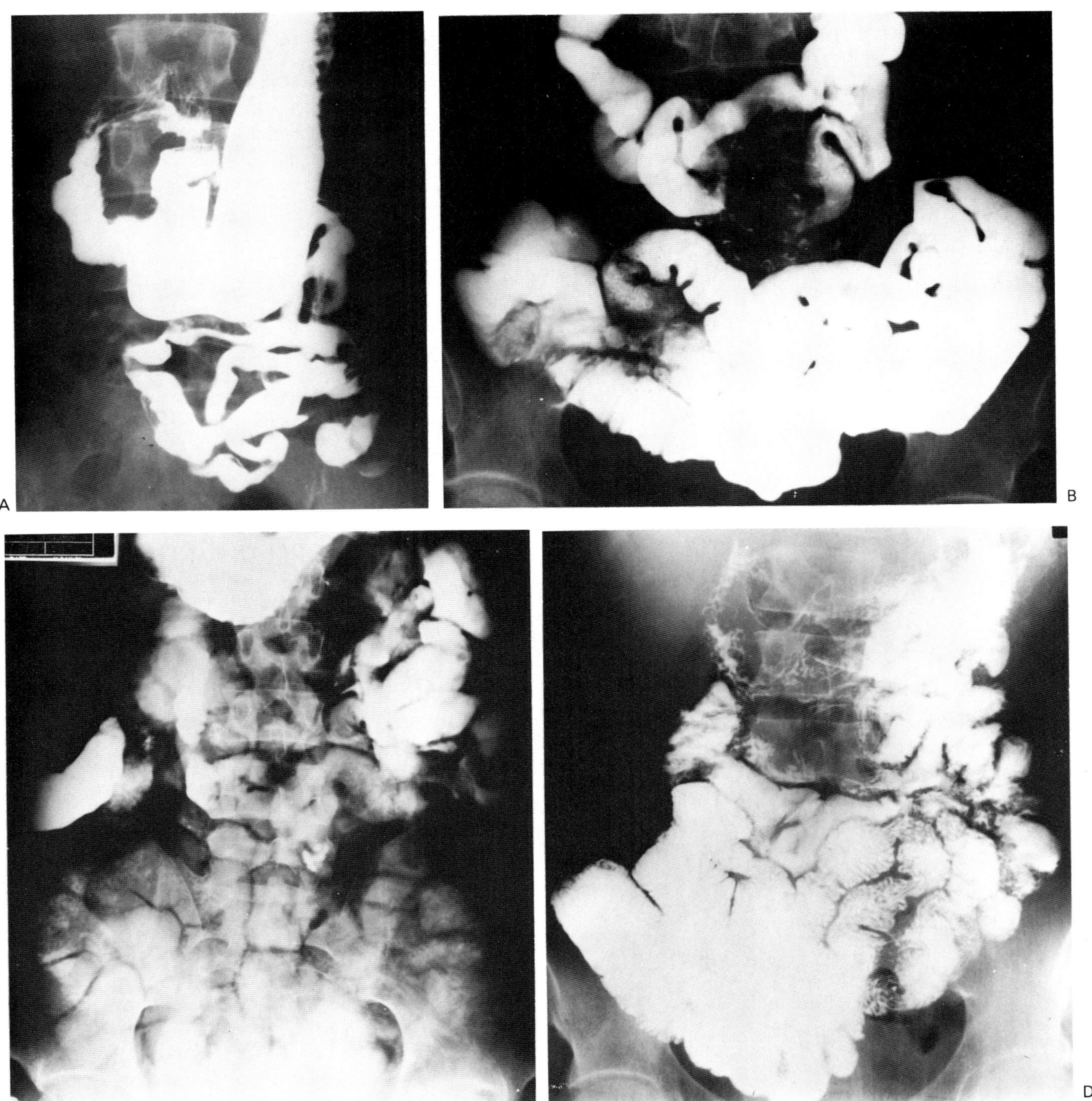

Fig. 31.46 Adult coeliac disease with hypolactasia responding to a gluten-free diet. **A.** and **B.** Small bowel meal showing a featureless jejunum and proximal ileum. Biopsy showed sub-total villus atrophy. **C.** Repeat examination with 25 g lactose in the barium shows dilution and hurry indicating hypolactasia. **D.** Examination after 6 months of a strict gluten-free diet. Lactose-barium examination showing a return to normal of the mucosal pattern. Biopsy showed regeneration of villi and improved lactase levels.

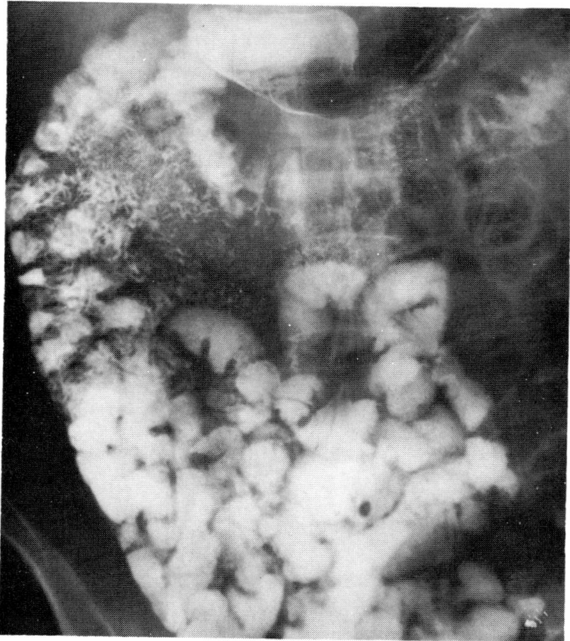

Fig. 31.46 Normal patient 1 hour after taking 120 ml of Micropaque and 16 g of magnesium sulphate. Dilution and hurry has occurred similar to that seen in patients with hypolactasia given 25 g of lactose in barium.

(Fig. 31.46). These appearances are at least in part due to the osmotic effect of the unsplit disaccharide within the lumen of the small intestine. The dose of lactose used in the test (25 g) seldom causes unpleasant symptoms and is only half that usually given for a lactose tolerance test.

PROTEIN-LOSING DISORDERS OF THE GASTROINTESTINAL TRACT

Protein is continually entering the lumen of the gut in the form of shed mucosal cells, lymph and other secretions. Normally most of it is reabsorbed. In a wide variety of conditions there may be excessive loss of protein so that the protein balance becomes negative. *Isotope* techniques particularly the use of ^{131}I-labelled polyvinylpyrrolindone, a synthetic polymer about the same molecular size as albumen, allows a quantitative assessment of the amount of protein leaking from the gastrointestinal tract to be made.

These patients usually present with oedema associated with a marked reduction in plasma protein, for which no obvious cause can be found. Some have no intestinal symptoms, while in others the protein loss complicates known organic disease of the gut. One classification is shown in Table 31.4.

Giant hypertrophy of the gastric rugae was first described by Ménétrièr (1888). The most striking radiological feature is the presence of giant rugal folds in the stomach, particularly on the greater curvature. There is no evidence of rigidity or ulceration, although the lumen may be narrowed by the enlarged folds. Peristaltic activity may be slightly diminished. The maximal gastric acid output may be low or nil; the folds weep protein, not acid.

Intestinal lymphangectasia chiefly affects children but may persist into adult life, or at least first present then. There is commonly oedema of the lower limbs associated with hypoalbuminaemia but the condition may present with rickets due to failure of absorption of vitamin D. The patients do not always have steatorrhoea. The lymphatic vessels in the mesentery and frequently in the lower limbs are hypoplastic. Biopsy of jejunal mucosa shows dilated lymph spaces in oedematous villi (Fig. 31.48). The barium follow-through examination shows thickening of rugal folds in the small intestine due to widespread oedema of the intestinal wall (Fig. 31.49 A & B). The thickened folds give the edge of the jejunum a 'cogwheel' appearance. *Lymphography* often shows hypoplastic lymphatics in the legs and occasionally contrast medium may be seen entering the lumen of the gut, possibly through ruptured lymph vessels, indicating the site of maximum protein loss. However, it is possible that lymphography may increase the protein loss by damaging the already inadequate lymphatic drainage of the gut and so should be used with circumspection.

Villous adenoma of the colon, usually situated in the caecum, sigmoid colon or rectum, may give rise to severe

Table 31.4 Diseases associated with protein-losing enteropathy

Lymphatic	Venous	Ulceration	Unknown mechanism

Intestinal lymphangectasia
Whipple's disease (intestinal lipodystrophy)
Mesenteric lymphatic obstruction
  reticulosis
  retroperitoneal fibrosis
  non-specific granuloma
Thoracic duct fistula, ligation or damage
	Congestive heart failure
	Constrictive pericarditis
	Tricuspid disease
	Thrombosis
	  superior mesenteric vein
	  portal vein
	  inferior vena cava
		Tumours, especially:
		  carcinoma of the stomach
		  carcinoma of the colon
		  villous adenoma
		Regional enteritis
		Ulcerative colitis
		Radiation enteropathy
			Ménétrier's disease (giant hypertrophy of gastric mucosal)
			Gluten-induced enteropathy, coeliac disease
			Tropical sprue
			Eosinophilic enteropathy
			Chronic intestinal ischaemia

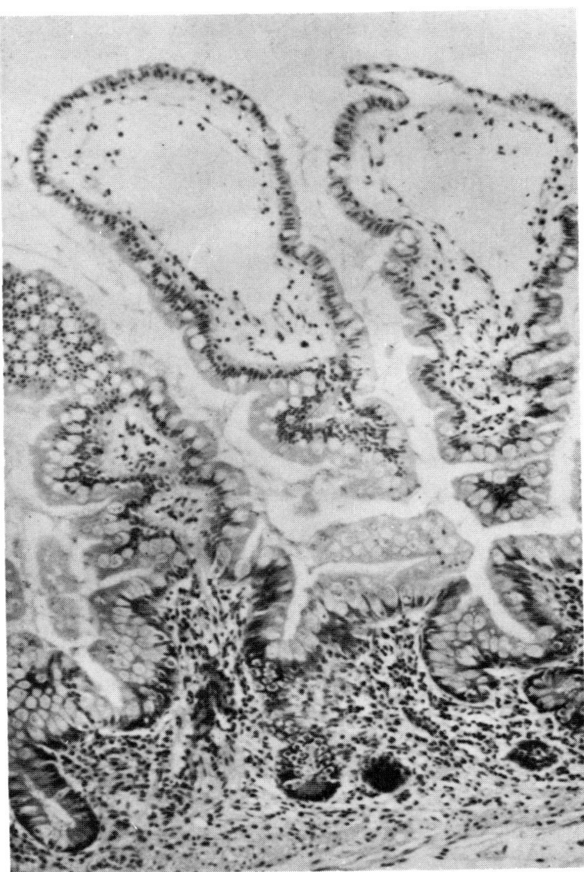

Fig. 31.48 Intestinal lymphangectasia. Biopsy showing villi containing grossly dilated lymph spaces.

hypoalbuminaemia or hypokalaemia. Because they weep protein, these tumours do not coat easily with barium and are easily mistaken for faecal residue on barium enema examination. They are very soft and may be impalpable even at laparotomy. Protein loss into the gut may be a prominent clinical feature of some cases of gut carcinoma and lymphosarcoma, especially when the stomach is involved.

In *regional enteritis* there is frequently severe loss of protein as well as malabsorption. In addition, protein loss may be a feature of certain patients with *coeliac disease, mesenteric vascular occlusion* and *ulcerative colitis*.

Table 31.5 Factors contributing to generalized oedema of the small bowel

Low plasma albumen (less than 2.0 g/100 ml)	as in: Nephrotic syndrome Cirrhosis of the liver Protein-losing gastroenteropathy Villous adenoma
Lymphatic	a. Hypoplasia — intestinal lymphangectasia b. Obstruction — reticulosis, tumour c. Obliteration — X-irradiation
Venous	a. Superior mesenteric vein thrombosis b. Portal hypertension c. Budd-Chiari syndrome d. Constrictive pericarditis e. Tricuspid insufficiency

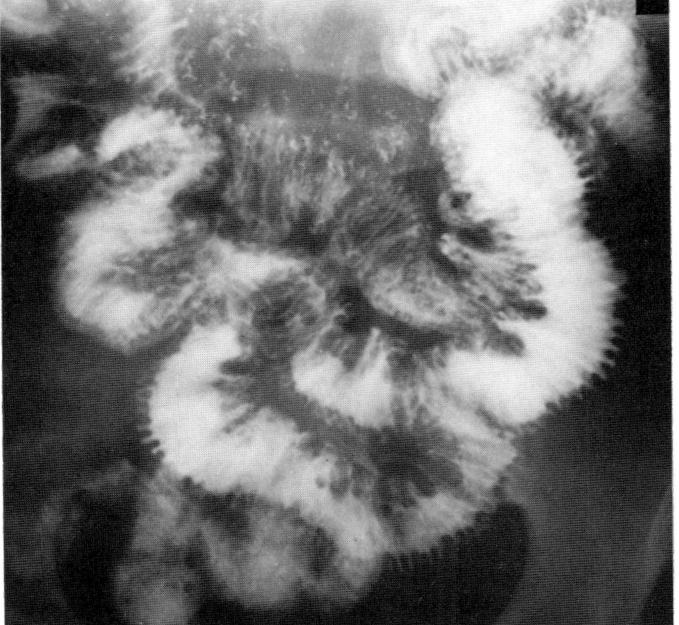

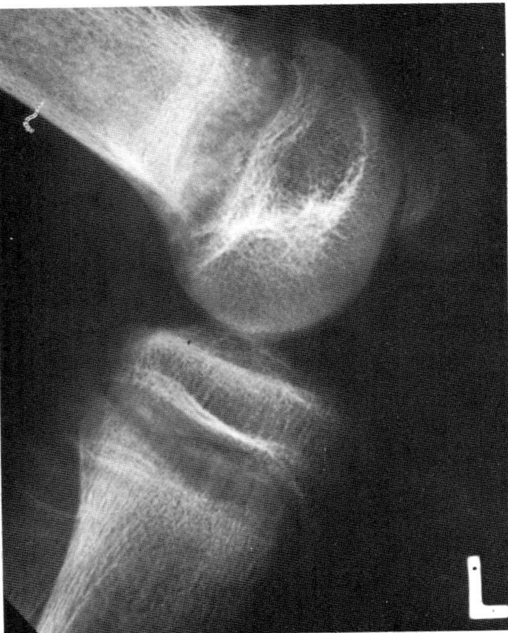

Fig. 31.49 Intestinal lymphangectasia in a boy aged 14 years who presented with hypoalbuminaemia and rickets due to vitamin D deficiency. **A.** Small bowel meal showing generalized oedema of the jejunum and proximal ileum. **B.** Knee showing severe rhachitic change. This responded to parenteral vitamin D therapy.

OEDEMA OF THE SMALL INTESTINE

Oedema of the wall of the small intestine may occur in a variety of conditions. The mechanisms are similar to those which cause oedema elsewhere; raised venous pressure, lymphatic insufficiency, lowered plasma osmotic pressure and altered capillary permeability. Sometimes more than one mechanism may be present in the same patient, as when a patient with intestinal lymphangectasia passes protein into the lumen of his gut so that the plasma albumen falls to a level at which oedema occurs in the gut and elsewhere in the body. Whenever the plasma albumen falls below 2.0 g per 100 ml, oedema of small bowel may occur, but it is usually not severe unless there is some complicating factor such as a raised portal venous pressure in a patient with cirrhosis of the liver. Thus, whenever widespread oedema of the small bowel is demonstrated radiologically, it is necessary to consider what mechanism or mechanisms may have operated to bring it about. Some of the factors contributing to generalized oedema of the small bowel are given in Table 31.5.

Lymphatic insufficiency

Intestinal lymphangectasia has been described above.

A secondary form of intestinal lymphangectasia may occur as a complication of inflammatory or neoplastic mesenteric lymphadenopathy. Local destruction of lymphatics may also occur as a result of X-irradiation.

Raised venous pressure

Venous oedema of the bowel may occur from a number of causes. There may be a localized mesenteric venous thrombosis due to extrinsic pressure from a tumour or enlarged lymph nodes or it may occur as part of some generalized thrombotic tendency such as chronic pancreatitis or the contraceptive pill.

Raised pressure in the superior mesenteric vein, with or without thrombosis, may occur in portal hypertension or as a result of the Budd Chiari syndrome, constrictive pericarditis or tricuspid insufficiency.

All these conditions may give rise to a generalized picture of small bowel oedema, which may vary in severity from time to time as the thrombosis extends, or collateral veins open up.

Altered capillary permeability

Angioneurotic oedema is an inherited condition in which there are recurrent episodes of oedematous swellings of the skin mucous membranes or viscera. The attacks are usually self-limiting and occur at irregular intervals. Visceral manifestations may be the first or the only presenting symptoms and may simulate an acute surgical emergency.

Small bowel examination during a visceral crisis may reveal oedema of the small bowel usually of a few adjacent loops which may be thickened and separated from each other (Fig. 31.20). The appearances revert to normal as soon as the attack subsides. This rapid return to normal, together with the family history, distinguishes angioneurotic oedema from other forms of small bowel oedema.

Localized oedema of the small bowel may be seen in the early stages *eosinophilic enteropathy*, but at a later stage there is irregular thickening and distortion of the small bowel wall as well as oedema (Fig. 31.50).

MISCELLANEOUS CONDITIONS

OBSTRUCTION

Obstruction is a prominent feature in many conditions affecting the small bowel such as *Crohn's disease*, *intestinal tuberculosis* and *stenosing tumours*. In some conditions, however, such as obstruction due to *adhesions*, *hernia* or *gallstone ileus* it may be virtually the only acute presenting symptom. Obstruction by bands or adhesions may be shown by small bowel enema (Fig. 31.51) but the primary lesion may be obscured if there is much dilatation of the proximal bowel. Contrast introduced by a Miller-Abbott tube low down in the small bowel may help in this respect. There is an abrupt change in calibre between the dilated and collapsed bowel distal to the obstruction. In gallstone ileus, the stone itself may be demonstrated within the lumen of the small bowel and, in addition, there may be air within the biliary tract. A gallstone large enough to cause intestinal obstruction has usually eroded straight from the gall bladder into the stomach or duodenum

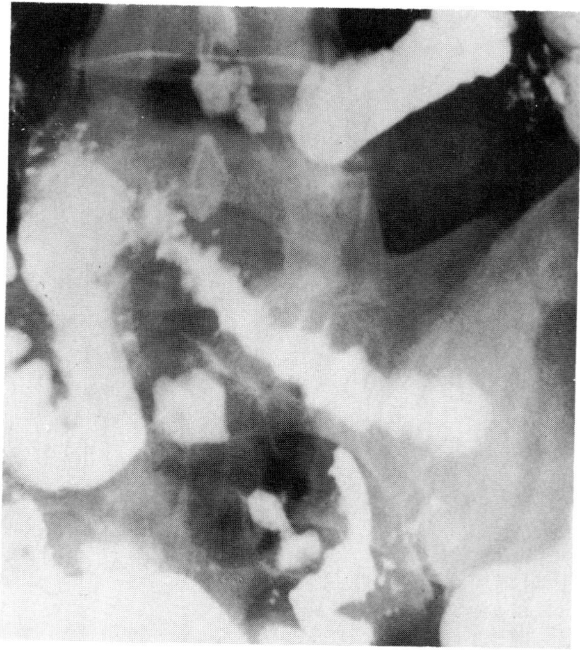

Fig. 31.50 Eosinophilic enteropathy showing a thickened irregular segment of jejunum with apparent ulceration similar to that seen in Crohn's disease. The appearance returned to normal with steroid therapy but relapsed when steroids were withdrawn.

following an empyema of the gall bladder. Since the cystic duct is usually occluded, it is common to see air within the gall bladder or gall bladder bed rather than in the bile duct (Fig. 31.52).

Internal hernias are rarely responsible for mechanical small bowel obstruction. They are most common in the paraduodenal area and are associated with abnormal small bowel fixation or some degree of malrotation. The history is of intermittent partial small bowel obstruction without previous surgery. Inguinal, femoral and incisional hernias may give rise to both obstruction and strangulation (Fig. 31.53 A & B). It should be remembered that it is possible to have strangulation of gut without evidence of intestinal obstruction when either the appendix, or a Meckel's diverticulum, enters a hernial sac, or one margin of the bowel only is in the sac without the main lumen being obstructed (Richter's hernia).

Occasionally fibrosis or tumour in the mesentery may cause a localized intestinal obstruction (Fig. 31.54).

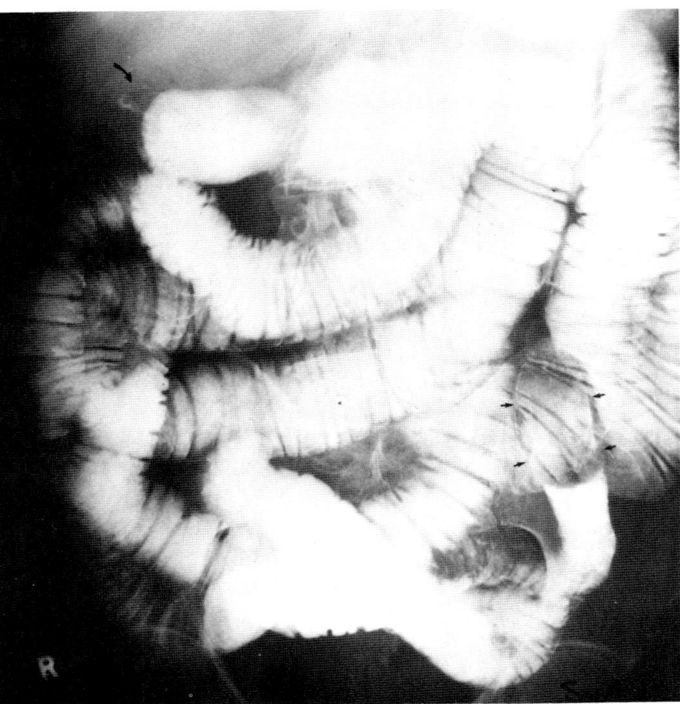

Fig. 31.52 Gallstone ileus. Small bowel meal showing a large intraluminal filling defect in the ileum causing gross obstruction (small arrows). A little barium has entered the bed of the gall bladder (arrow).

INTESTINAL BLEEDING

Bleeding from the small bowel may occur as the only symptom in *haemangioma, tumour, ulceration* or *Meckel's diverticulum*. Selective or superselective angiography is the best method of diagnosis and localization. Barium examination may be normal in haemangioma but phleboliths may be seen on the plain film. Angiography shows, in addition to the arterial malformation, a large draining vein (Fig. 31.55) and there may be pooling of contrast if bleeding is brisk at the time of the examination. Very small lesions require superselective examinations, both to demonstrate the lesion and to localize it within the small bowel (Fig. 31.56). Radioisotope scanning is a useful primary investigation (see p. 725).

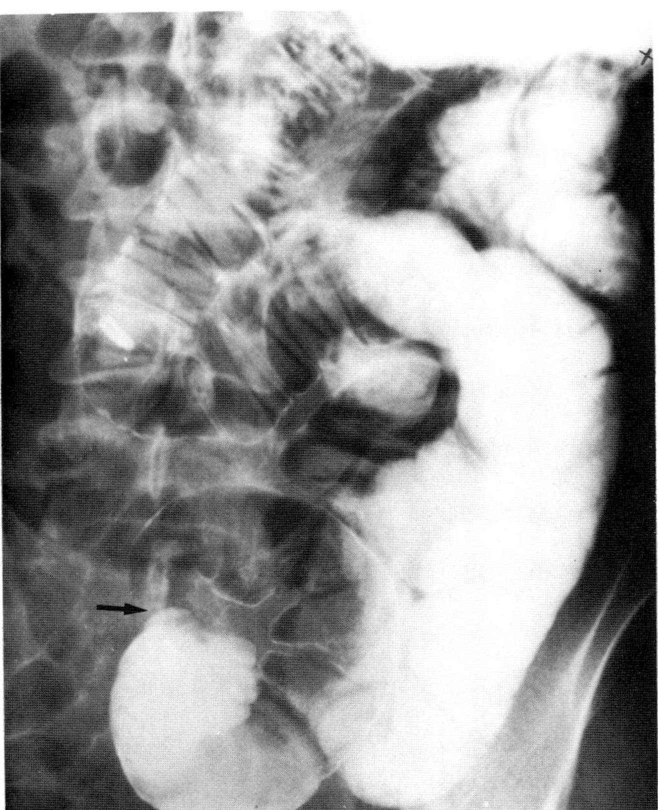

Fig. 31.51 Intestinal obstruction. Small bowel enema showing gross dilatation of the jejunum with an abrupt change of calibre (arrow). At laparotomy an obstructing band was found and freed.

RADIATION ENTEROPATHY

The small bowel is radiosensitive and is likely to suffer damage from dose in excess of 5000 rad. Radiation enteropathy is most commonly seen following irradiation of the pelvis for malignancy, either the body of the uterus, cervix or ovary. It is particularly likely to happen if the small bowel is stuck down in the pelvis and the same section becomes irradiated on each exposure. The ileum is usually involved and in the acute stages shows thickening, oedema and ulceration simulating extensive Crohn's disease (Fig. 31.57). This may heal by fibrosis when the loops become matted together with a narrow lumen. In the late stages there may be frank intestinal obstruction (Fig. 31.58).

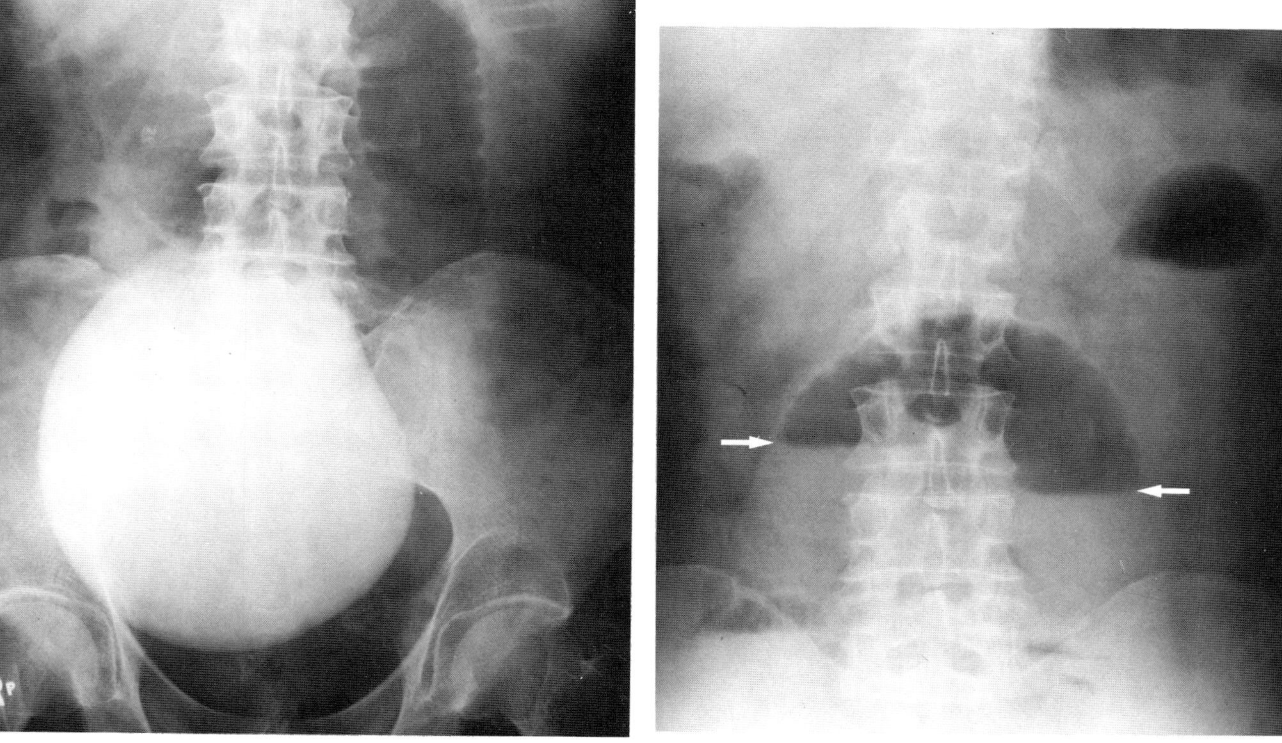

Fig. 31.53 Incisional hernia causing intestinal obstruction. **A.** Supine film showing a rounded opacity due to fluid in the incisional hernia. **B.** Horizontal ray film showing fluid levels within an obstructed loop.

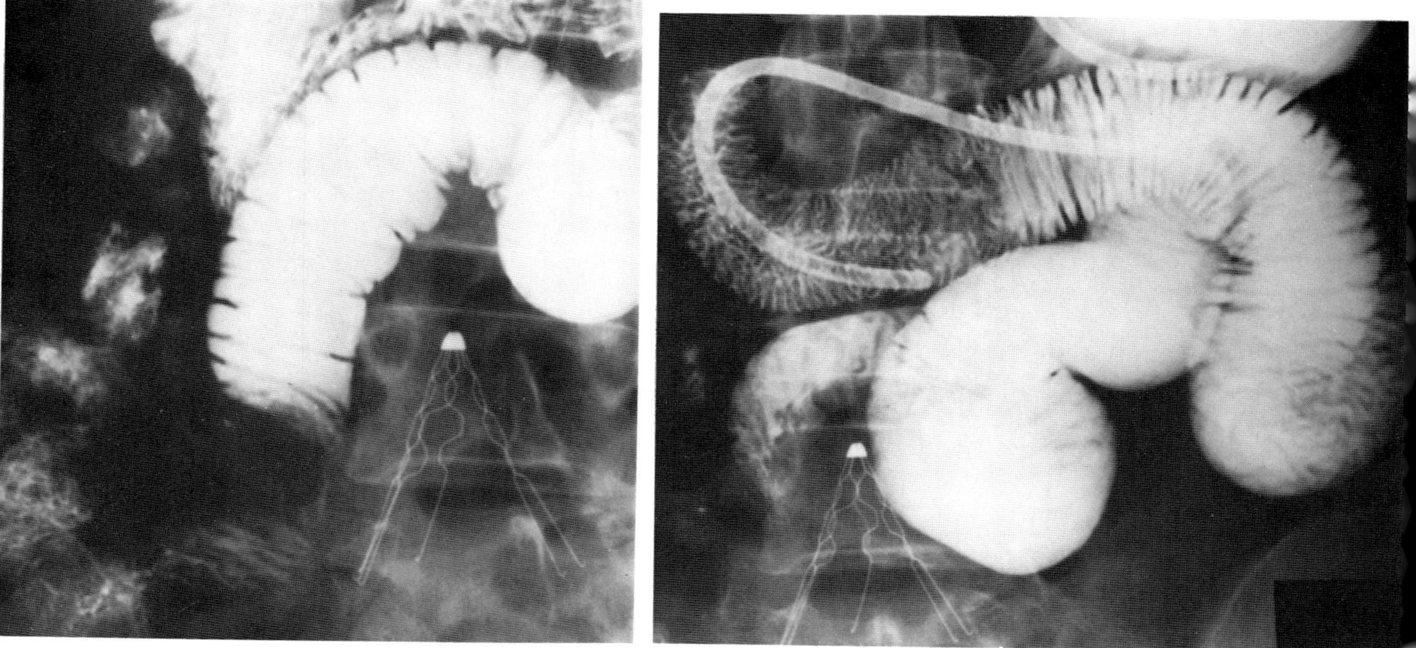

Fig. 31.54 Intestinal obstruction due to fibrosis in the mesentery. An umbrella has been inserted into the inferior vena cava but has perforated through the anterior wall with bleeding and consequent fibrosis. **A.** Barium examination showing faulty position of one part of the umbrella. **B.** Small bowel enema showing high jejunal obstruction. (Courtesy Dr Louise Sheppard.)

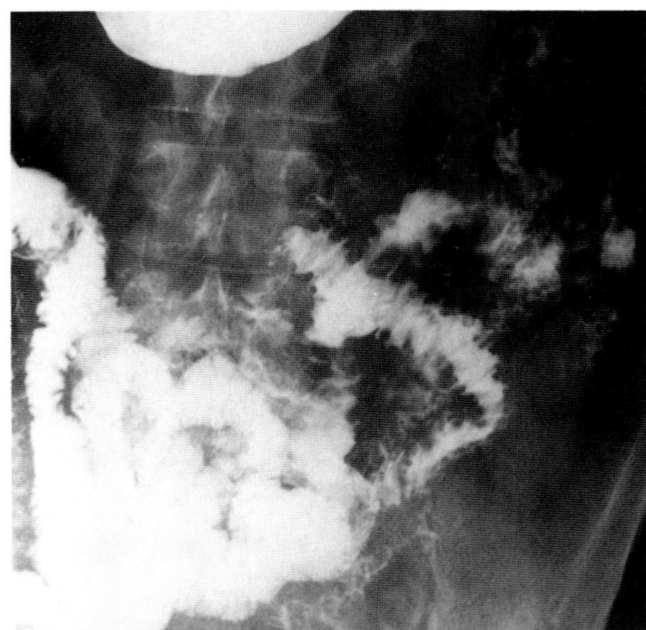

The space occupied by the abnormal bowel corresponds very closely to the irradiation field.

EOSINOPHILIC GASTROENTEROPATHY

In this uncommon condition there is a diffuse infiltration of eosinophils into one or more segments of the alimentary tract, usually the small bowel and gastric antrum. This is associated with oedema, thickening of the affected parts, sometimes with ascites. There is usually a blood eosinophilia. There may be a history of allergy but the causative agent is seldom discovered.

Patients present with recurrent attacks of abdominal pain, often colicky, with episodes of diarrhoea or vomiting or both. The condition responds to steroid therapy, but may run a course of several years, relapsing when steroids are withdrawn.

Radiologically, the affected loops of bowel are thickened, with widened and blunted mucosal folds (Fig. 31.50). The

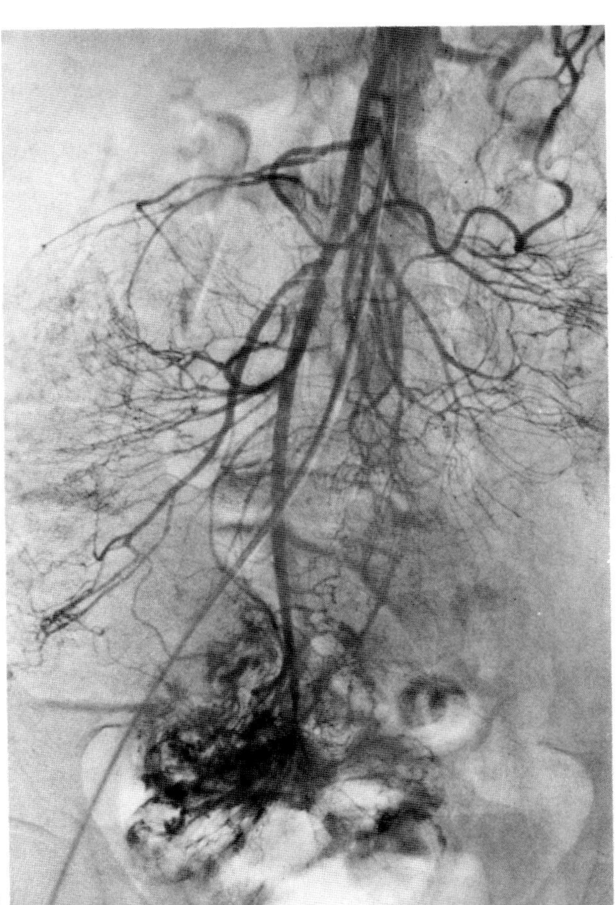

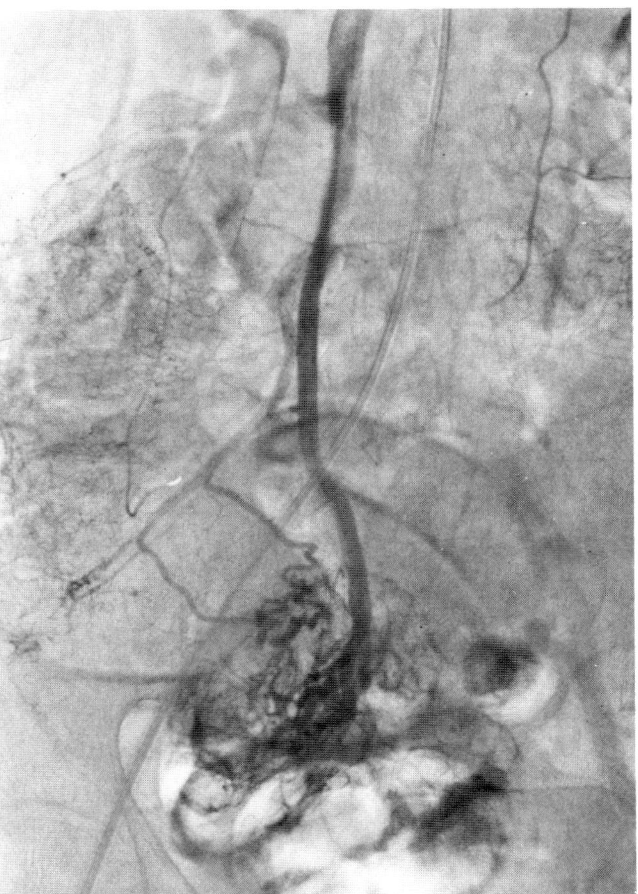

Fig. 31.55 Haemangioma. Young man with recurrent episodes of severe intestinal haemorrhage. Endoscopy normal. **A.** Small bowel meal showing localized jejunal abnormality with thickened folds. **B.** Superior mesenteric arteriogram showing extensive malformation. **C.** Venous phase showing large draining vein. Note the change of position of the haemangioma within the abdomen between the barium and arteriogram examinations. (Courtesy Dr H. L. Walters.)

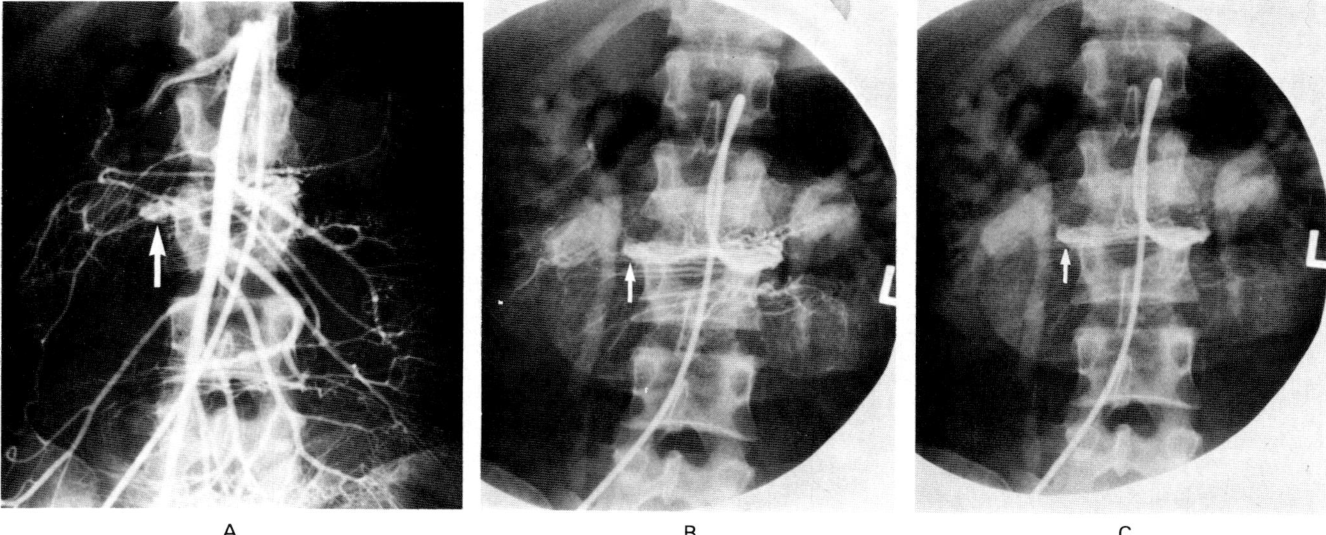

Fig. 31.56 Small haemangioma causing bleeding and severe anaemia. **A.** Superior mesenteric artery injection showing lesion (arrow). From this film it is not certain whether the lesion is in the duodenum, small bowel or hepatic flexure. **B.** Selective injection of first jejunal artery showing lesion (note back filling of pancreticoduodenal arcades). **C.** Late film showing mucosal blush in duodenal loop, lesion and draining veins. (Courtesy Prof. David Allison.)

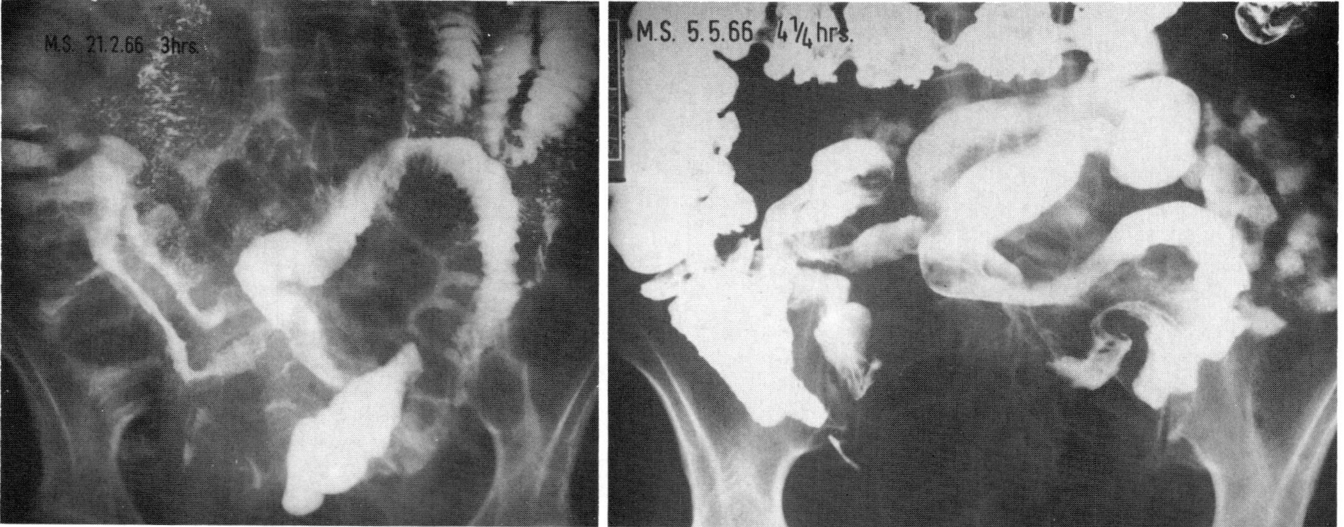

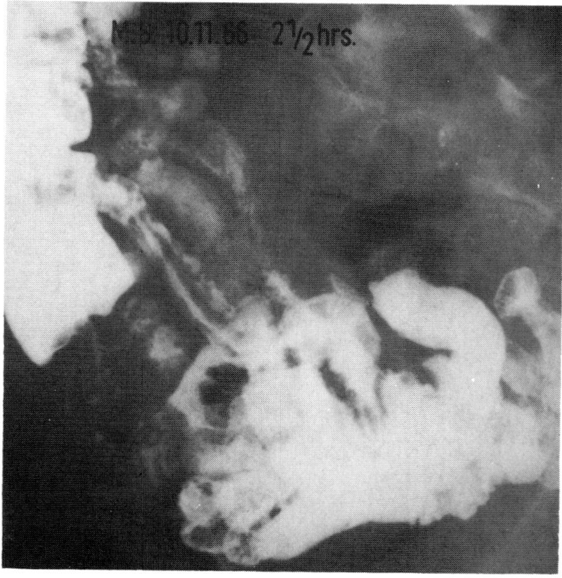

Fig. 31.57 Acute radiation ileitis following radiotherapy for carcinoma of the body of the uterus. Patient had severe diarrhoea, melaena, hypoproteinaemia and hypokalaemia. **A.** There are narrowed coils of distal small bowel and also thickened loops with prominent folds more proximally. **B.** Same case 10 weeks later with mucosal pattern destroyed and a featureless ileum. **C.** Some 6 months later the ileum has almost returned to normal but several loops are matted together.

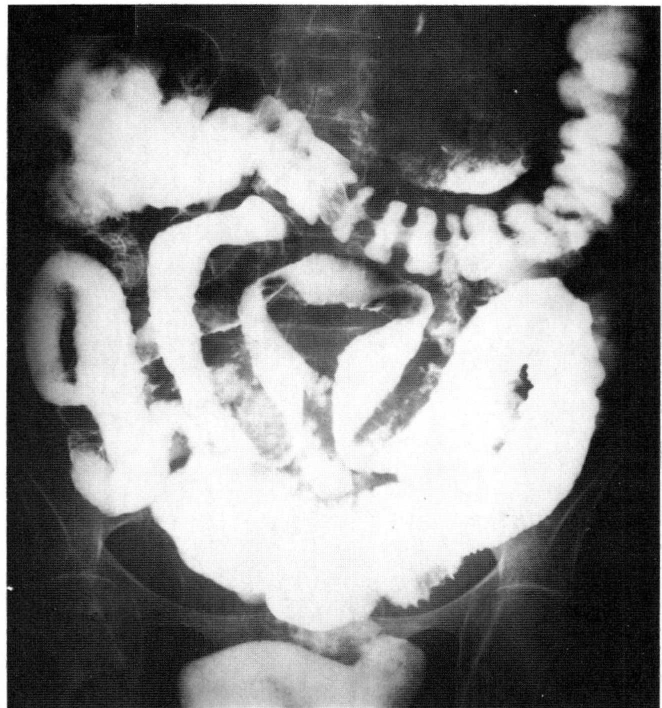

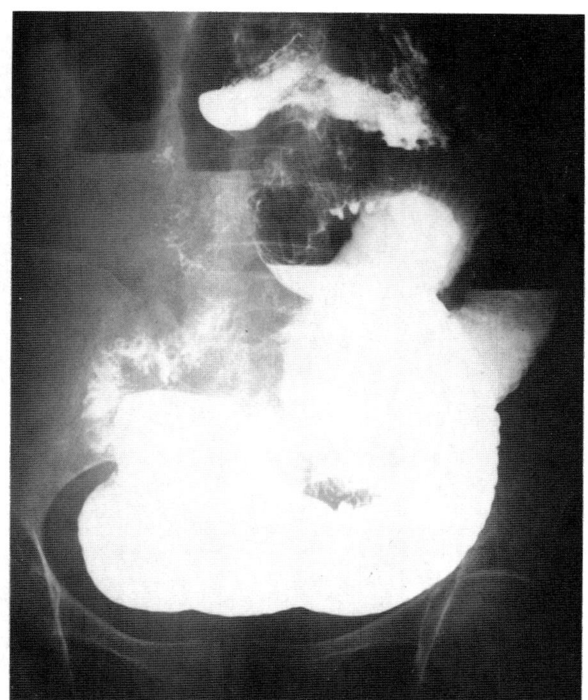

Fig. 31.58 Radiation enteropathy following radiotherapy for carcinoma of the body of the uterus. **A.** In the acute stage there is extensive ulceration and thickening of many coils of ileum. **B.** Some 9 months later there is severe ileal obstruction with proximal dilatation.

lumen becomes narrowed, causing some degree of obstruction. These appearances closely mimic regional enteritis but fistulae do not occur and ulceration is not a prominent feature, though it has been seen in resected specimens.

MASTOCYTOSIS

Urticaria pigmentosa is an uncommon skin condition in which there is infiltration of the dermis with mast cells. In some cases the mast cell proliferation involves the reticulo-endothelial system and many organs may be affected. Mast cells produce histamine which has the effect of producing local urticaria and stimulating fibrosis.

Involvement of the small intestine gives rise to nausea, vomiting and abdominal pain. There may be malabsorption associated with villous atrophy. The radiological changes are non-specific and include oedema of the mucosa, with thickening of the valvulae conniventes and the appearance of many mucosal nodules, 2–5 mm in diameter, throughout the jejunum. Sclerotic bone lesions simulating osteoblastic metastases may occur. The association of sclerotic bone lesions in a patient with diffuse small bowel abnormality raises the possibility of mastocytosis (Fig. 31.59).

PANCREATIC CYSTIC FIBROSIS

Pancreatic cystic fibrosis may show radiological changes in the large and small bowel in patients over 5 years of age. These include:

1. Loss of normal duodenal folds.
2. Hyperplasia and redundancy of folds affecting both large and small bowel.
3. In the large bowel, filling of dilated crypts and marginal nodularity associated with adherent indurated faecal masses at the lateral wall of the colon.
4. About 10% of patients develop hepatic fibrosis, portal hypertension and oesophageal varices.

ILEOCAECAL VALVE AND APPENDIX

The terminal ileum, ileocaecal valve and appendix are frequently the focus of radiological investigation owing to the relatively large number of diseases which may affect this area.

The terminal ileum is the commonest site in the small bowel to be affected by pathological processes and these have been considered above.

The ileocaecal valve presents more as a problem in radiological differential diagnosis of lesions occurring

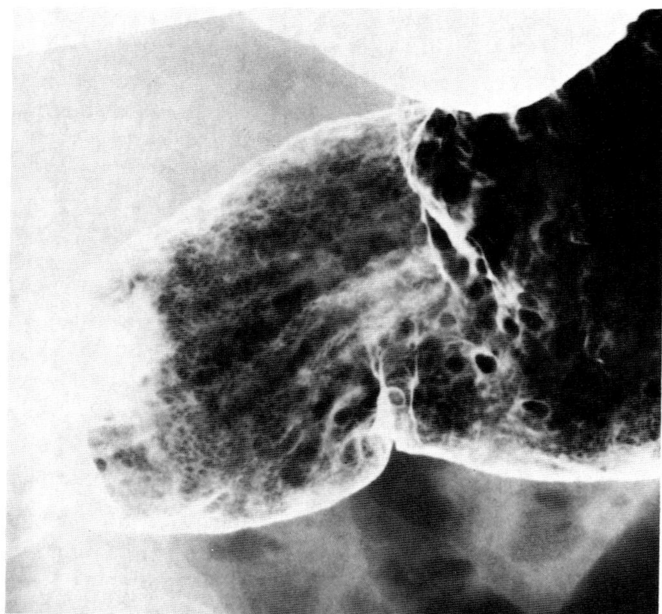

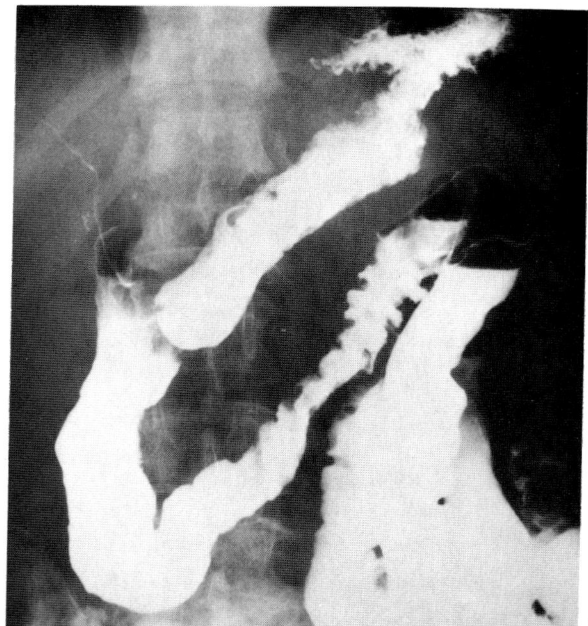

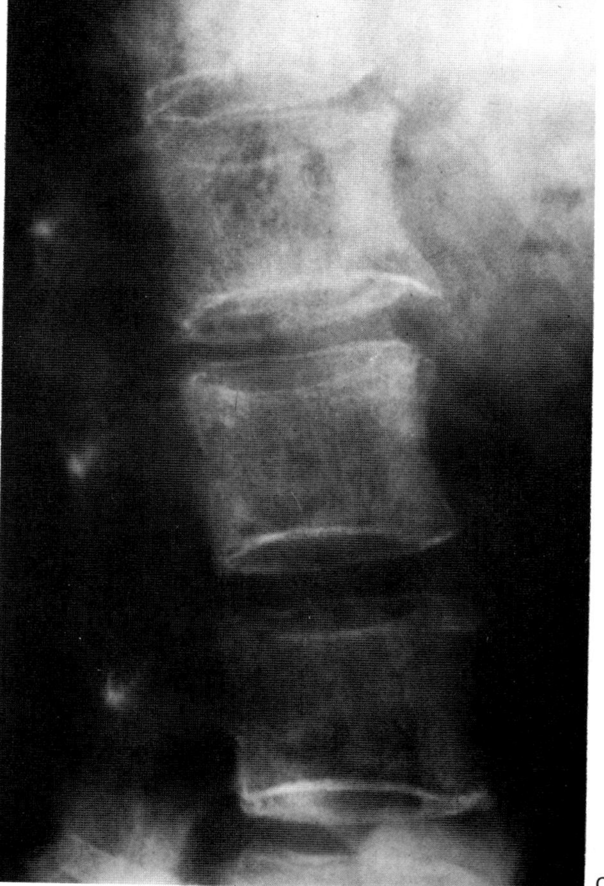

Fig. 31.59 Mastocytosis. A young woman with a long history of urticaria pigmentosa with intermittent abdominal pain. **A.** Barium meal showing polypoid lesions within the stomach. **B.** Small bowel meal showing nodularity of the duodenum and proximal jejunum. **C.** Lateral view of lumbar spine showing mainly sclerotic lesions in the vertebral bodies.

around the caecum rather than of disease affecting the valve itself.

The ileocaecal valve consists of an upper and well-developed lip covering a lower lip, both lips being continuous with mucosal frenulae which cross the posterior wall of the caecum in a horizontal direction.

The ileal opening appears as a transverse slit in the posterior wall of the caecum between these lips. The radiological appearances of the normal ileocaecal valve depend on whether the valve is seen in profile on the medial wall of the caecum, when it has been fancifully described as having a 'shark's mouth' appearance; or if it appears *en face* on the posterior wall when it appears as a round filling defect with a central stellate appearance due to mucosal folds (Fig. 31.60).

Enlargement of the lips of the ileocaecal valve may follow fatty deposits in the caecal lips or, rarely, oedematous changes, and the condition has been described as hypertrophy of the ileocaecal valve. This is a misnomer as no muscular hypertrophy is present and the condition is not associated with any obstruction of the terminal ileum.

The appearances have to be differentiated from 'appendicular stumps' and from polypoid lesions of the caecum. The identification of the mucosal folds in the ileocaecal valve enables this differentiation to be made.

The appendix

The place of radiology in the investigation of acute appendicitis and appendix abscess is considered in Chapter 33.

Chronic appendicitis or recurrent appendicitis is a complex problem from the standpoint of radiological diag-

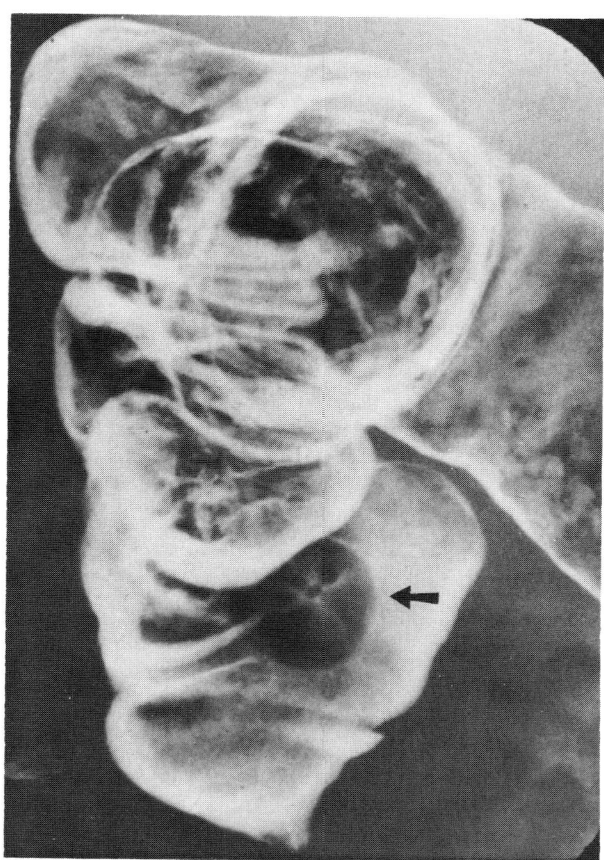

Fig. 31.60 Prominent ileocaecal valve seen *en face* with stellate radiation of folds towards the valve. These appearances are frequently described as hypertrophy of the ileocaecal valve but there is no thickening of the muscular wall and no obstruction is present.

nosis as the actual clinical status of these two syndromes is not clearly defined.

It is doubtful to what extent radiological signs of chronic inflammation of the appendix are valid. The radiological signs on which chronic inflammation has been diagnosed are:

1. Local tenderness over the barium-filled appendix — this feature varies considerably with patient's varying reactions to palpation and is a difficult sign to evaluate.
2. Fixity of the appendix as shown in a small bowel meal. Palpation under screen control confirms the fixity.
3. Kinking of appendix — the appendix when filled with barium can be shown to be angulated. Barium remaining in the appendix after a barium meal frequently appears as segmented clumps of barium.
4. Delay in emptying — delay in emptying of the barium from the appendix has been claimed as a radiological sign of chronic appendicitis. This sign is, however, so variable as to be worthless.

Mucocele of the appendix. Occasionally the appendix fills with mucus and forms a smooth round cyst-like structure, a mucocele. This may appear as a filling defect in the caecal pole. The outlines of the filling defect are smooth and rounded. On rare occasions it may show calcification in its wall.

In other instances the thickened omentum around an appendix which has been the seat of inflammation may produce a mass which indents the wall of the caecum when the caecum is distended by a barium enema.

Foreign bodies. Metallic foreign bodies lodged in the appendix and shotgun pellets in the appendix are not an infrequent finding in the game season.

Faecoliths in the appendix have to be differentiated from stones (enteroliths) in the alimentary canal, in diverticula or in a Meckel's diverticulum. The site may be confirmed by a follow-through barium meal. An intraperitoneal appendolith may be the cause of a persistent discharging sinus following a ruptured appendix or appendix abscess. Calcified appendoliths are usually oval and laminated.

COMPUTED TOMOGRAPHY AND THE SMALL BOWEL

One of the main problems in computed tomography of the abdomen is the distinguishing of fluid-filled loops of small bowel from abdominal masses and lymph nodes, especially when the small intestine is in an unusual site such as the renal fossa after nephrectomy where it may simulate a recurrence of tumour. Similarly small bowel may appear in the porta hepatis after an anastomosis between the biliary system and the gut, in the pelvis after a hysterectomy and in the left upper quadrant of the abdomen after a splenectomy. To avoid confusion, it is essential that the whole of the small bowel should be opacified with dilute contrast medium at the appropriate stage of the investigation. This may involve giving the patient repeated amounts of oral contrast medium and scanning a number of times with the patient in different positions. A normal loop of small bowel rarely exceeds 3 cm in diameter.

Computed tomography has comparatively little part to play in the primary diagnosis of small bowel disease. The common malignant tumours, adenocarcinoma, lymphosarcoma and carcinoid are demonstrated only if they are large. Computed tomography is, however, of value in demonstrating the spread of the tumour to the mesenteric or para-aortic lymph nodes or to the liver. It can also monitor the response to treatment. Metastatic disease is seldom recognized since they are usually small lesions scattered throughout the small bowel. Occasionally, however, a large mass with excavation may be seen.

Benign tumours of the small bowel are rare and cannot be distinguished from metastasis except for the lipoma which has a low attenuation value (−50 to −100 HU).

The changes in Crohn's disease are best demonstrated by barium studies but occasionally computed tomography may help in a complicated case in which fistulae, abscesses and other complications arise. In Whipple's disease, however, computed tomography has been of value in demonstrating the associated enlarged retroperitoneal and mesenteric lymph nodes, which are characteristically of low density presumably because of their high lipid content.

Computed tomography may also be of value in demonstrating the dilated afferent loop in the afferent loop syndrome. This loop, which lies to the right of the aorta, may simulate a cyst, but may on occasions be shown to pass behind the superior mesenteric artery into the duodenum.

REFERENCES AND SUGGESTIONS FOR FURTHER READING

Allison, D. J. (1980) Gastrointestinal diagnosis. Radiological diagnosis. *British Journal of Hospital Medicine*, **23**: 358–365

Berquist, T. H., Nolan, N. G., Stephens, D. H., Carlson, H. C. (1976) Specificity of ^{99}Tc^{m}-pertechnetate in scintigraphy diagnosis of Meckel's diverticulum: review of 100 cases. *Journal of Nulcear Medicine*, **17**: 465–469

Clemett, A. R., & Marshak, R. H. (1969) Whipple's disease: Roentgen features and differential diagnosis. *Radiologic Clinics of North America*, **7**: 105

Clemett, A. R., Fishbone, G., Levine, R. J. et al. (1975) Gastrointestinal lesions in mastocytosis. *American Journal of Roentgenology*, **103**: 405

Cohen, M. D. & Lintott, D. J. (1978) Transient small bowel intussusception in adult coeliac disease. *Clinical Radiology* **29**: 529–534

Collins, S. M., Hamilton, J. D., Lewis, T. D., & Laufer, I. (1978) Small bowel malabsorption and gastrointestinal malignancy (ab) *Radiology*, **126**:603

Conway, J. J., (1980) Radionuclide diagnosis of Meckel's diverticulum. *Gastrointestinal Radiology* **5**: 209–213

Cook, W. T., Cox, E. U., Fone, D. J. et al. (1963) The clinical and metabolic significance of jejunal diverticula. *Gut*, **4**:115

Crohn, B. B, Ginzburg, L., Oppenheimer, G. D. (1932) Regional ileitis. *Journal of the American Medical Association*, **99**: 1323–1329

Ekberg, O., Sjostrom, B., Brahme, F. J. (1977) Radiological findings in Yersinia ileitis. *Radiology*, **123**:15

Ekelund, L., Lunderquist, A., Dencker, H., & Akerman, M. (1977) Hepatic angiography in ulcerative colitis and Crohn's disease (ab) *Radiology*, **122**:853

Ghanremani, G. G., Meyers, M. A., Farman, J., & Port, R. B. (1978) Ischaemic disease of the small bowel and colon associated with oral contraceptives. *Radiology*, **127**:566

Herlinger, H. (1978) A modified technique for the double contrast small bowel enema. *Gastrointestinal Radiology*, **3**: 201–207

Herlinger, H. (1979) The small bowel. In: Laufer, I. (ed.) *Double Contrast Gastrointestinal Radiology with Endoscopic Correlation*. Philadelphia: W. B. Saunders

Herlinger, H. (1982) The small bowel enema and the diagnosis of Crohn's disease. *Radiological Clinics of North America*, **20**: 721–742

Hoffman, J. P., Taft, D. A., Wheelis, R. F., & Walker, J. H. (1977) Adenocarcinoma in regional enteritis of the small intestine. *Radiology*, **125**: 280

James, W. B., & Hume, R. (1968) Action of metoclopramide on gastric emptying and small bowel transit time. *Gut*, **9**: 203–205

Joffe, N., Goldman, H., Antonioli, D. A. (1977) Barium studies in small bowel infarction, radiological-pathological correlations. *Radiology*, **123**:303

Kellett, M. J., Boralske, F. F., & Margulis, A. R. (1979) Peroral pneumocolon examination of the ileocaecal region. *Gastrointestinal Radiology*, **1**: 361–365

Kreel, L. (1970) The use of oral metoclopramide in the barium meal and follow through examination. *British Journal of Radiology*, **43**: 31–35

Laufer, I. (1979) *Double Contrast Gastrointestinal Radiology with Endoscopic Correlation*. Philadelphia: W. B. Saunders

Laws, J. W., & Neale, G. (1966) Radiological diagnosis of disaccharidase deficiency. *Lancet*, **ii**: 139–143

Laws, J. W., & Pitman, R. G. (1960) The radiological investigation of the malabsorption syndromes. *British Journal of Radiology*, **33**: 211–222

Laws, J. W., Shandon, H., Stewart, J. S., & Booth, C. C. (1963) Correlation of radiological and histological findings in Idiopathic Steatorrhoea. *British Medical Journal*, **i**: 1310–1314

Lintott, D., & Herlinger, H. (1984) Radiology of the small intestine. In: Laws, J. W. (ed.) *Clinics in Gastroenterology, Non-invasive Radiology*. London: W. B. Saunders

Maglinte, D. D. T., Burney, B. T., & Miller, R. E. (1982) Lesions missed on small bowel follow-through: analysis and recommendations. *Radiology*, **144**: 737–739

Marshak, R. H., Hazzi, C., Lindner, A. E., & Marlansky, D. (1977) Small bowel in immunoglobulin deficiency syndromes (ab) *Radiology*, **124**: 569

Marshak, R. H., & Lindner, A. E. (1976) Intramural bleeding: carcinoid tumour and carcinoid syndrome. In: *Radiology of the Small Intestine*, 2nd edn. Philadelphia: W. B. Saunders

Mason, G. R., Dietrich, P., Friedland, G. W., & Hanks, G. E. (1970) The radiological findings in radiation-induced enteritis and colitis. A review of 30 cases. *Clinical Radiology*, **21**: 232–247

Meyers, M. A. (1976) Clinical involvement of mesenteric and anti mesenteric borders of small bowel loops. *Gastrointestinal Radiology*, **1(1)**: 41–48 and **1(1)**: 49–58

Meyers, M. A. (1976) The small bowel: normal and pathologic anatomy. In: *Dynamic Radiology of the Abdomen*, ch. 8. New York: Springer-Verlag

Miller, R. E., & Sellink, J. L. (1979) Enteroclysis: The small bowel enema. How to succeed and how to fail. *Gastrointestinal Radiology*, **4**: 269–283

Morson, B. C. (1971) Histopathology of regional enteritis (Crohn's disease). In: Engel, A., Larson, T. (eds) *Skandia International Symposia on Regional Enteritis (Crohn's Disease)*, pp. 15–33. Stockholm: Nordiska Bokhandelns Forlag

Nolan, D. J. (1983) The small bowel. In: Whitehouse, G. H., Worthington, B. S. (eds) *Techniques in Diagnostic Radiology*. Blackwell Scientific Publications

Ratcliffe, J. F. (1983) The small bowel enema in children, a description of a technique. *Clinical Radiology*, **34**: 287–289

Rohrmann, C. A., Ansel, H. J., Freeny, P. C., Silverstein, F. E., Protell, R. L., Fenster, F. L., Fenster, L. F., Ball, T., Vennes, J. A., & Silvis, S. E. (1978) Cholangiographic abnormalities in patients with inflammatory bowel disease. *Radiology*, **127**: 635

Santulli, T. V., Schullinger, J. N., Heird, W. C., Gongaware, R. D., Wigger, J., Barlow, B., Blan, C. W. A., Berdon, W. E. (1976) Acute necrotising enterocolitis in infancy, a review of 64 cases. *Radiology*, **118**: 245

Scott, B. B., Hardy, G. J., & Losowsky, M. S. (1975) Involvement of the small intestine in systemic mast-cell disease. *Gut*, **16**: 918

Sellink, J. L. (1976) *Radiological Atlas of Common Diseases of the Small Intestine*, pp. 377. Leiden, H. E., Stenfert Kroese, B. V.
Sellink, J. L. (1983) Enteroclysis. In: Margulis, A. R., Burhenne, H. J. (eds) *Alimentary Tract Radiology*, ch. 31. pp. 871–902. St Louis: C. V. Mosby Co.
Stevens, J. M., Northover, J. M. A., Raphael, M. J., & Slack, W. W. (1981) The localisation of bleeding small bowel lesions for conservative resection: a simple radiographic technique. *British Journal of Radiology*, 909–911

CHAPTER 32

THE COLON

IMAGING INVESTIGATION

The value of *plain abdominal films* in the supine and erect positions in the detection of lesions of the colon is described in Chapter 33. It must be emphasized that when such films are taken soon after an enema or bowel washout, fluid levels in the colon are not uncommon and may mimic pathological changes. It must also be remembered that sigmoidoscopic examination usually introduces air into the distal colon; this may confuse the appearances produced by a large bowel obstruction, since a variable amount of air can then appear in the colon distal to the obstructing lesion.

Barium enema

The barium enema is the routine method of examination of the colon. This was universally a single contrast study until Welin at Malmö, in the early 1950s, introduced the *double contrast* method. There is still lingering argument in the world literature as to the relative merits of the single or double contrast enema. 20 years ago the single contrast enema was the rule and the double contrast enema the exception, but over the past two decades the superiority of the double contrast method has slowly become established and this should now be the standard method of examination.

Adequate preliminary preparation of the colon is vital to remove faecal material prior to the administration of the barium enema. Careful cleansing of the colon by the administration of an aperient within the previous 24 hours, and a low residue diet for 48 hours prior to the examination, assists in clearing the colon of faecal material. An increased fluid intake during this period is also recommended. In addition, cleansing enemas with tap water are usually necessary to achieve optimum results.

Colon activators, so-called because they cause colonic muscular contraction, include *tannic acid* and *Veripaque* (oxyphenisitin). The former is no longer used because of its occasional hepatotoxic effect but the latter is safe and 3 g of Veripaque added to the second of two water enemas certainly assists in efficient cleansing. The use of *oral aperients* alone is always under review and good results may be achieved by using a combination of drugs such as Picolax and castor oil or Dulcolax and magnesium citrate. Clearly, if a satisfactory oral method of preparation is found which produces *consistently* good results, this obviates the need for cleansing enemas and is an advantage on all counts.

A barium sulphate and water mixture (80–95% w/v) is administered through a rectal catheter by gravity. In the double contrast enema, barium is run in as far as the mid-transverse colon, at which stage the tube is clamped and the rectum drained. Air is then insufflated with rotation of the patient as necessary until the whole colon is coated with barium and air. It is worth noting that turning the patient supine when the caecum is full of barium encourages ileal reflux because of the dependant position of the ileocaecal valve in this position. If, at this stage, ileal filling is seen to occur, a spot film of the sigmoid colon may be worthwhile in case this region becomes further obscured.

In elderly patients or others who have difficulty in retaining the barium, the use of a balloon rectal catheter has been recommended. This, however, is potentially hazardous. Whenever difficulty is encountered, the most important aid to success is to allow only a slow and intermittent inflow of barium. An uncontrolled flow of barium into the bowel of these patients almost always produces an uncontrolled flood of barium onto the X-ray table. Intravenous *Buscopan*, or *glucagon*, may also help. An antispasmodic is also indicated in any patient if marked or repeated spasm occurs during the filling phase.

The following films are then taken with the overcouch tube:

1. Prone PA film
2. Left lateral of rectum
3. Right 35° supine oblique
4. Left 35° supine oblique
5. R. lateral decubitus with horizontal beam
6. L. lateral decubitus with horizontal beam
7. Erect AP film

Occasionally additional views may be necessary to confirm a suspected abnormality on the routine films. If an additional view of the sigmoid is required, a supine film with the tube angled upwards is probably the most practical.

Colostomy enema

This examination requires effective occlusion of the stoma, either externally, or internally with careful insertion of a Foley catheter. An antispasmodic is given i.v. prior to administration of the barium. Supine, supine oblique, decubitus and erect films are taken after air insufflation in the usual way.

Gastrografin enema

A Gastrografin enema (diluted 1 in 3 with water) is used to check the patency and integrity of a recent surgical anastomosis. Gastrografin is also recommended in the investigation of adult patients with idiopathic megacolon or possible Hirschsprung's disease, since in these conditions there is likely to be difficulty in evacuating barium.

Arteriography

Arteriography has a limited value in colonic disease. It has little part to play in the diagnosis and management of ischaemic disease of the colon and is of no practical value in the differentiation of ulcerative colitis and Crohn's disease. Its application is restricted to the investigation of patients with acute bleeding of apparent colonic origin where the bleeding site may be demonstrated and in patients with chronic low-grade blood loss where lesions such as angiodysplasia may be detected.

Isotope scanning, ultrasound and CT scanning

In disease of the colon, isotope scanning and the newer imaging techniques have a relatively restricted application. All three modalities are of value in detecting hepatic metastases in carcinoma of the colon. Since the accuracy of each method in this respect is roughly comparable, the choice may depend upon local preference and service availability. Ultrasound examination has the advantage of being widely available and is rapid and non-invasive. CT scanning is used in the staging of tumours and may thus show extension of tumour into the pericolonic fat, invasion of adjacent structures and lymphadenopathy. CT scanning is also of particular value in the demonstration of pelvic recurrence following previous excision of a rectal carcinoma with an end colostomy. This is discussed further in the section on the rectum. Both ultrasound and CT help in the general management of patients with abdominal disease for instance in the demonstration of intra-abdominal abscesses and other pathology.

Colonoscopy

The advent of colonoscopy, which allows both visual inspection and, with biopsy, histological examination of the entire colon, represents a most important advance in the diagnosis of colonic disease. From the radiological point of view, colonoscopy is particularly useful when the radiological diagnosis is uncertain and in patients with rectal bleeding where the barium enema is normal. Similarly, limited endoscopy with the flexible sigmoidoscope is a significant advance in diagnosis. The rigid sigmoidoscope allows examination of the colon to about 25 cm at most and because of stretching of the bowel the measurement of the distance of a lesion from the anal margin on sigmoidoscopy may not always correspond with the radiological measurement. Such discrepancy can cause confusion if more than one lesion is present.

RADIOLOGICAL ANATOMY

The hepatic and splenic flexures of the colon are relatively constant in position and displacements are usually evidence of enlargement of the adjoining solid viscera. At the hepatic flexure displacements are usually from liver or gall bladder enlargement; the splenic flexure may be displaced by an enlarged spleen or a space-occupying lesion of the tail of the pancreas or kidney. A long and redundant colon

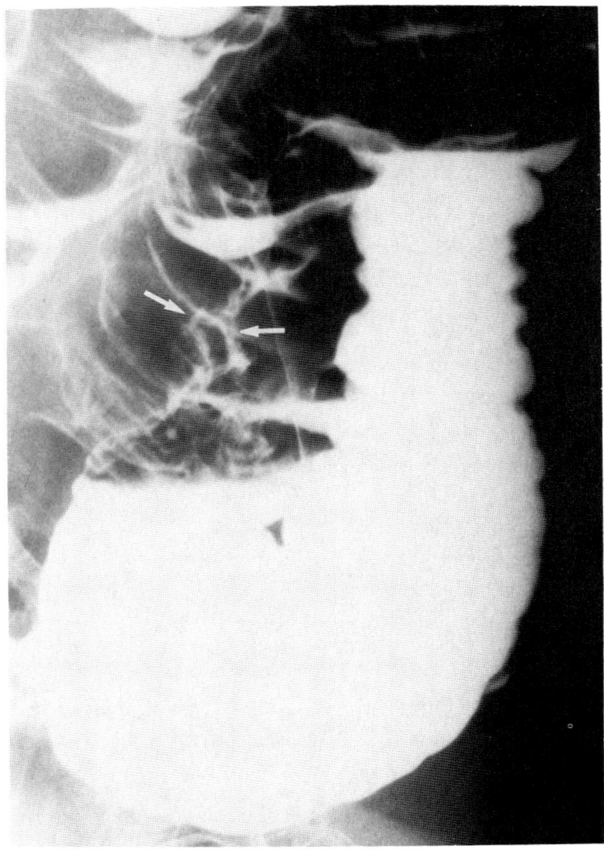

Fig. 32.1 An annular carcinoma of the colon (arrows) largely obscured by overlapping loops of bowel.

produces overlapping loops so that pathological lesions such as a carcinoma may be obscured (Fig. 32.1).

The recto-sigmoid junction is poorly shown in AP or PA projections and a lateral view is vital to show this region.

Certain areas of physiological narrowing, at times resembling sphincters, may be seen during filling of the colon by barium enema. They are all transient and show a normal mucosal pattern which enable them to be differentiated from true strictures.

Rotational anomalies are uncommon. The most frequently seen anatomical abnormality is failure of normal descent of the caecum, which may be sub-hepatic. In *situs inversus* there is a failure of rotation of the midgut loop and the right colon is displaced to the left and anteriorly with the caecum near the left iliac fossa. A lesser degree of displacement of the right colon is seen in *malrotation*.

The caecum occasionally has its own mesentery and is displaced medially and upwards with its tip beneath the transverse colon (*mobile caecum*). Another anomaly sometimes seen is a caecum reflected straight upwards to lie anterior to the ascending colon (*caecal bascule*). This is well shown by an oblique view.

Transposition of the abdominal viscera is readily recognized at barium enema, but can be missed on an X-ray unless the film is correctly labelled.

may only become apparent after some months have elapsed.

Radiological examination must not be carried out immediately after birth but should be delayed for 12 to 18 hours to allow sufficient swallowed air to reach and adequately fill the terminal rectal segment. The anal dimple is identified by a metallic marker and in the past the infant was held inverted for a few minutes to allow air to distend the rectal segment completely. A lateral film was then taken (Fig. 32.2). This is in addition to conventional supine and erect abdominal views which show the degree of distension proximal to the anomaly. The distance between the metal marker and the air-filled rectal segment is less than 1.5 cm in cases of low atresia, whilst in the intermediate and high groups the distance is considerably greater. An anatomic marker is provided by a line drawn between the terminal portion of the sacrum and the pubis on the lateral film and gas held up above this line indicates a high lesion.

The presence of air in the urogenital tract indicates a rectovesical, rectourethral or rectovaginal fistula and also shows that the atresia is high.

Certain limitations of the inverted lateral X-ray have long been appreciated: the distal blind pouch may not always fill with gas — if air escapes through a fistula — or may be plugged with meconium. In addition there may be slight distortion due to the effect of gravity.

CONGENITAL LESIONS

Anorectal anomalies

These are of varying anatomy ranging from relatively simple lesions, such as anal stenosis or a thin obstructing membrane (bulging with meconium), to complex abnormalities where atresia of the rectum may be associated with fistulae into the urogenital tract and bony defects in the sacrum. The abnormalities are divided into three main groups — low, intermediate and high — depending on the siting of the bowel anomaly below, at the level of, or above the levator ani respectively. Intermediate and high anomalies in particular may be associated with fistulae into the vagina or the urinary system, the latter being much commoner in males than females.

As the surgical management of anorectal anomalies is dependant on the type of defect and the extent of rectal atresia and associated anomalies, radiological demonstration of the exact anatomy of the defect should always be attempted.

Low defects of the rectum where the gap between the anal dimple and rectal stump is short may be dealt with surgically by the perineal approach, whilst those cases with more severe degrees of rectal atresia require an abdominal approach, involving a preliminary defunctioning colostomy.

Atresia and agenesis present with obstruction in the neonate; anal stenosis may not be recognized initially and

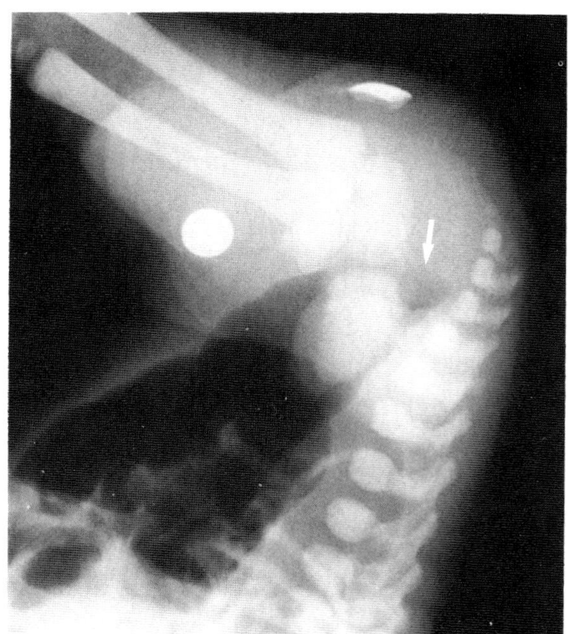

Fig. 32.2 Erect inverted lateral view showing a high rectal atresia. The anal dimple is labelled with a metallic marker. The arrow points to the uppermost air shadow and the site of the atresia. (Courtesy of Dr Christine Hall.)

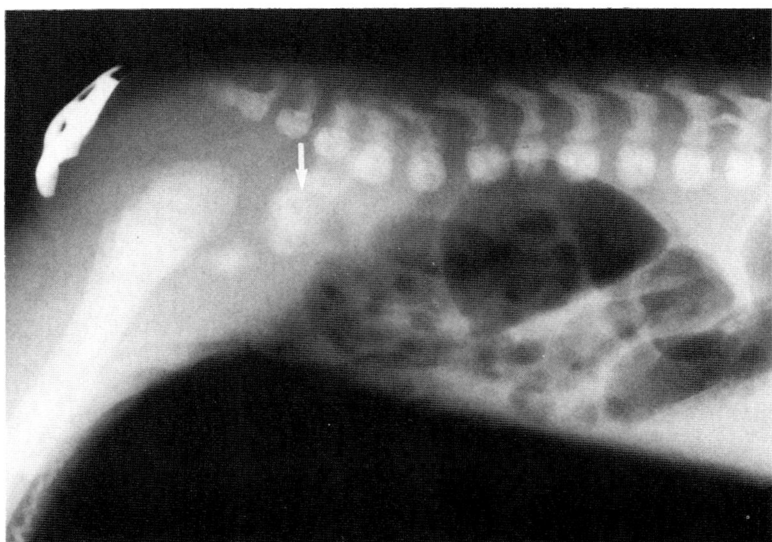

Fig. 32.3 Prone cross table lateral view showing a high rectal atresia (similar labelling to the previous figure). (Courtesy of Dr Christine Hall.)

The prone lateral shoot-through radiograph has recently been shown to provide equal or even more accurate information in demonstration of the level of rectal atresia in neonates (Narasimharao et al 1983). Its advantages are ease of positioning, less distress to the infant, elimination of the effect of gravity and better definition of the rectal gas shadow (Fig. 32.3). In the prone lateral position the rectum is the highest point of the bowel and in this position a fistula, if present, is dependent, as opposed to being highest in position with an inverted X-ray, so escape of gas through the fistula which may confuse the appearances does not occur.

As pointed out above, the initial treatment of high rectal atresia involves the formation of a defunctioning loop colostomy. Subsequent contrast injection into the distal loop will then give precise information about the state of the distal bowel and the anatomy of any fistulous tracks to the genitourinary system or perineum.

Microcolon

A small colon may be seen below a segment of colonic atresia, which is rare, or may be due to functional causes. In such atresia of the colon plain films reveal either small or large bowel obstruction. Barium enema examination reveals a microcolon extending to the lower level of the atretic segment.

Functional ileocaecal obstruction may occur with retention of meconium in premature infants and the colon in these cases, when a barium enema is done, may appear small in size. The distal colon may also appear small in the '*meconium plug syndrome*' in full-term infants. Microcolon necessarily occurs below higher gut lesions, such as partial duodenal atresia or obstruction from peritoneal bands, due to lack of distension by normal quantities of meconium and air. These small colons readily revert to a normal size when the obstruction is relieved.

Hirschsprung's disease

This disorder is due to an absence of ganglion cells in the myenteric plexus of the involved segment, which typically occurs in the distal large bowel but rarely extends more proximally, sometimes even throughout the colon. In over 70% the affected segment lies in the rectum or sigmoid, in which group the disease is 4 or 5 times more common in males.

The disease either presents with intestinal obstruction in the first months of life, or symptoms may be delayed until later in childhood or even adult life, when constipation is the main symptom.

Plain films commonly reveal distension with air-fluid levels in infancy and the characteristic mottled appearance caused by faeces admixed with gas in the adult. A contrast enema examination defines the anatomy of the disease and helps in excluding other forms of megacolon; barium is used in infants but Gastrografin is recommended in the adult to avoid the complication of faecal impaction. The distal aganglionic segment is narrow and the proximal normal colon is dilated. Care must be taken during rectal filling as the narrowed segment may be rapidly obscured by overlapping distended colonic loops. A lateral view is particularly important and the enema is stopped as soon as the full length of the narrowed segment is demonstrated.

In the neonate, failure to expel meconium may be an indication of aganglionosis. Since there is little colonic distension at this early stage it may be impossible to demonstrate the transition zone between the aganglionic and normal colon and lack of normal evacuation of barium is an important sign.

Anorectal physiology studies are abnormal in Hirschsprung's disease and definitive diagnosis depends upon the demonstration of characteristic pressure wave changes on pressure studies and the absence of ganglion cells on full thickness rectal biopsy.

Idiopathic megacolon

In this condition, which may be seen in the older child or adult, there is a varying degree of distension of the rectum, rectum and sigmoid or sometimes more proximal large bowel. Contrast studies show that the rectal dilatation extends to the anorectal junction with no evidence of a distal narrowed segment.

INFLAMMATORY LESIONS OF THE COLON

Inflammatory disease of the colon producing hyperaemia, cellular infiltration, increased mucus secretion and ulceration may be due to many causes.

These may be broadly subdivided into:

1. Colitis due to known organisms
2. Ulcerative colitis (idiopathic proctocolitis)
3. Crohn's disease (granulomatous colitis)
4. Ischaemic colitis

COLITIS DUE TO KNOWN ORGANISMS

Infection of the colon with specific bacterial organisms, e.g. those of the *Shigella* genus, results in *bacillary* dysentery, with inflammatory changes and an outpouring of fluid into the bowel lumen. The disease begins acutely with fever, followed by diarrhoea, abdominal cramps and sometimes vomiting. Clinical assessment with stool culture normally leads to the correct diagnosis before radiological examination is sought. In the acute stage, however, plain films may be requested to exclude other causes of the acute abdomen. These — as in any acute diarrhoeal illness — merely show gas-distended loops with short fluid levels.

Barium enema examination should not, therefore, be performed in the acute stage and even if the occasional chronic state results the diagnosis still essentially depends on bacteriological examination. In cases where a barium enema is performed the findings consist of haustral fold blunting and a segmental or pancolitis with ulceration which may be superficial or deep.

Pseudomembranous enterocolitis

This condition usually follows antibiotic administration, particularly clindamycin and lincomycin. It is caused by a mucosal toxin produced by overgrowth of *Clostridium difficile*. Plain films may show haustral blunting and marginal irregularity with varying degrees of colonic dilatation. Barium enema examination is seldom indicated since the diagnosis is usually readily made from the history and endoscopic examination. In cases where a barium study has been performed the appearances are usually those of a pancolitis in which the mucosal plaque-like lesions, characteristically seen on sigmoidoscopy, resemble severe ulcerative disease.

Amoebiasis

This disease is caused by the protozoon *Entamoeba histolytica*. Diagnosis depends upon isolation of amoebae in pus or stool specimens and on serology. Radiological changes in the colon consist of mucosal oedema, haustral blunting and ulceration which may be superficial or deep. Fulminating cases may show toxic dilatation. The so-called *amoeboma* is a focal lesion which manifests as an intraluminal mass, an annular lesion or irregularity with lack of normal distensibility (Fig. 32.4), all of which may mimic a carcinoma. Rapid disappearance of the lesion or lesions with appropriate antiamoebic therapy is seen in this disease which may help in confirming the diagnosis.

Amoebic infection of the colon is frequently associated with a spread of the parasite to the liver giving rise to amoebic hepatitis or an amoebic abscess. Elevation of the right diaphragm associated with restriction of movement and a pleural reaction obscuring the right costophrenic angle, are radiological signs associated with amoebic hepatitis. Isotope, ultrasound and CT scans are all useful in the diagnosis of hepatic abscess.

Schistosomiasis

Three species of schistosomes (blood flukes) commonly cause intestinal disease, *S. mansoni*, *S. japonicum* and *S. haematobium*. Colonic changes consist of spasm, blunting of haustral folds and superficial ulceration. Fibrosis and

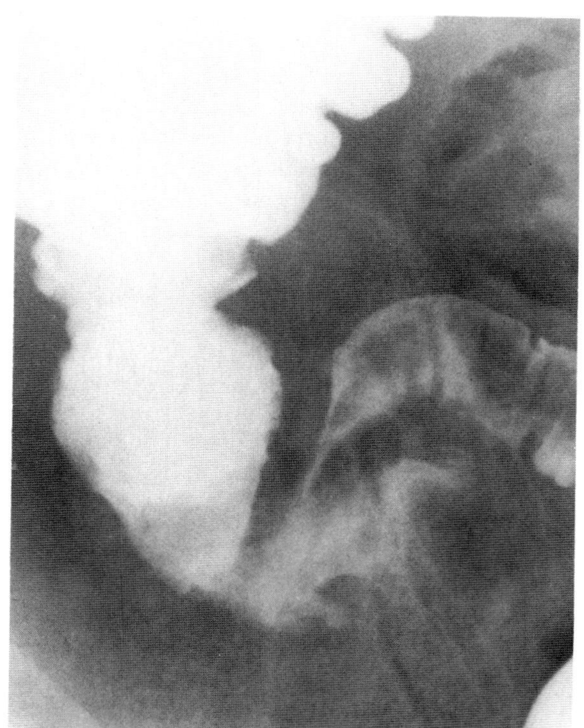

Fig. 32.4 Irregular narrowing of the caecum due to amoebiasis.

stricture formation are common, as is postinflammatory polyposis.

Lymphogranuloma venereum

The causative agent is a virus-like bacterium of the chlamydial group. Acute disease may cause a proctitis with a blood-stained discharge and ulceration. Chronic disease induces a lymphangitis which leads to fibrosis with stricturing and fistula formation (Fig. 32.5) in addition to oedema and ulceration. The diagnosis is confirmed by complement fixation tests.

Tuberculosis

Tuberculosis of the colon is described as predominantly hypertrophic, ulcerative or stricturing. The disease commonly involves the ileocaecal region, producing rigidity, shortening and distortion of the caecum. Marked thickening of the bowel wall occurs due to a combination of granulomatous infiltration, caseation and fibrosis. As a result, the bowel lumen becomes considerably narrowed with associated mucosal irregularity. Ulceration when it occurs tends to be circumferential. If in addition there is narrowing or ulceration of the terminal ileum these changes are easily mistaken for Crohn's disease. In a proportion of cases ileocaecal tuberculosis is associated with one or more small bowel strictures, usually in the terminal ileum. (see Figs 31.15 and 31.16, p. 874).

Tuberculosis of the more distal colon tends to produce segmental narrowing or stricture formation of varying length (Fig. 32.6).

This disease is now very rare in the indigenous population, but should always be considered whenever an ileocaecal inflammatory lesion or an unusual stricture of the colon is found in immigrants from Africa or Asia. It is worth noting that a right iliac fossa mass is palpable in the majority of patients with ileocaecal tuberculosis.

The differential diagnosis is from Crohn's disease, carcinoma, ischaemia and amoebiasis in particular.

Actinomycosis

This is a chronic suppurative and granulomatous disease caused by the anaerobic fungus *Actinomyces israelii*. It is of world wide distribution but is now exceedingly rare in the UK, only an average of four cases per year having been notified in England, Wales and Ireland over the period 1976 to 1983. The organism is often found as a harmless saprophyte in the oral cavity and gastrointestinal tract. It seems

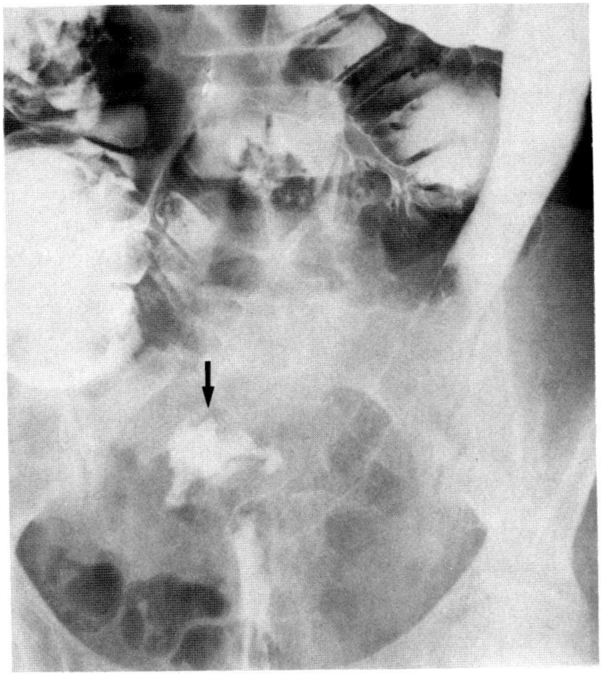

Fig. 32.5 Lymphogranuloma venereum. Diffuse narrowing of the rectum and sigmoid with pericolic leakage of contrast (arrow).

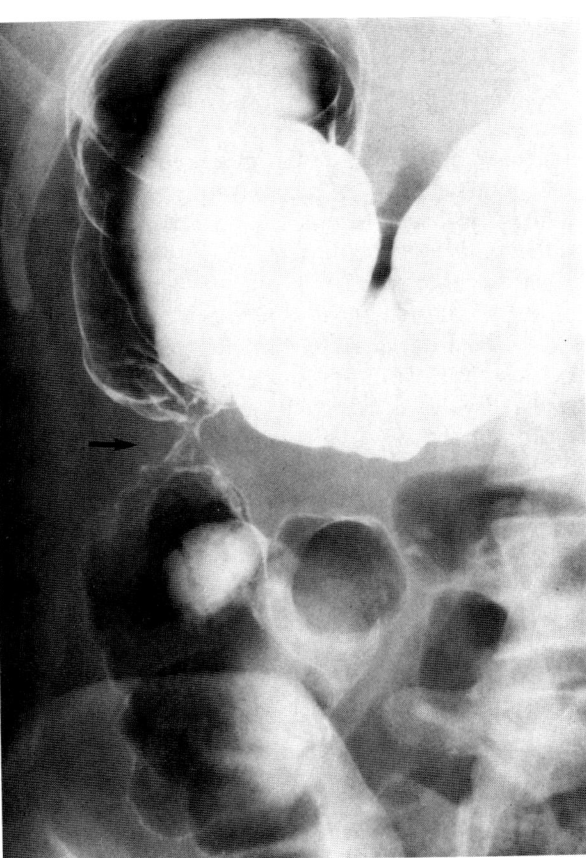

Fig. 32.6 Tuberculosis. There is a short irregular stricture in the ascending colon (arrow).

that infection occurs only after the mucosal surface is breached by disease, perforation or trauma.

Abdominal actinomycosis most frequently develops after an acute episode of perforative gastrointestinal disease and *appendicitis* in particular. In one series of 122 cases the preceding episode was acute appendicitis, with perforation in 88. Less commonly, the disease follows perforation of a peptic ulcer or colonic diverticulum; other occasional cases follow trauma or occur as a complication of long standing fistula-in-ano or ischio-rectal abscess.

The disease is characterised by the formation of multiple abscesses, internal and external fistulae, florid granulation tissue and dense fibrous scar tissue. The lesions arise in structures in contact with the site of perforation, particularly connective tissue and muscle. Usually the intestinal mucosa itself is not involved. In the common form of *right iliac fossa actinomycosis*, a hard mass develops followed by the formation of cutaneous draining sinuses some time after operation for acute appendicitis.

The **radiological findings** are non specific but signs of an extrinsic mass predominate with considerable deformity of the ileo-caecal region. The bowel lumen may become narrowed through involvement in the surrounding inflammatory and fibrous tissue. The sinus discharge contains the so-called 'sulphur granules' produced by the tangled mycelial masses.

Involvement of the colon in sites other than the right iliac fossa is very rare but when it does occur a hard mass develops in and around the bowel wall and mesentery. Spread of the disease is as a rule by direct continuity and wide extension through the abdominal cavity may occur with invasion of the abdominal wall, involvement of the liver via a sub-hepatic abscess, the kidney via a perinephric abscess and tubo-ovarian structures from downward spread into the pelvis. Spread to the liver may also occur through the portal vein. The diagnosis may be suggested by the clinical features and course of the disease but depends for confirmation on isolation of the causative fungus. The differential diagnosis is primarily from Crohn's disease, tuberculosis and carcinoma. In the past 20 years there have been increasing reports of pelvic actinomycosis in females associated with the use of intrauterine contraceptive devices.

NON-SPECIFIC COLITIS

In the United Kingdom the vast majority of cases of colitis are due either to ulcerative colitis or Crohn's disease. These diseases tend to show well-marked differences, although there is an overlap radiologically and at times an identical appearance may be produced by both. The distinction between them depends not only on the radiological findings but also on the clinical pattern, endoscopic appearances and histology. The first duty of the radiologist is to establish whether inflammatory disease exists, thereafter an attempt is made to distinguish between them.

ULCERATIVE COLITIS

The cause of ulcerative colitis remains obscure, although stress and an immunological response to unknown antigens have been suggested as possible causative factors.

Ulcerative colitis is essentially a mucosal disease which almost always involves the rectum and which may then spread proximally through the colon for a variable distance. On endoscopy the mucosa appears hyperaemic, granular and friable, bleeding readily to the touch. A varying degree of ulceration may be seen which as a rule is limited to the mucosa.

Pathologically there is a cellular inflammatory infiltrate which is confined to the mucosa with distortion of the glandular pattern, goblet cell depletion and numerous crypt abscesses. Subsequently loss of haustration with shortening and narrowing of the bowel occurs.

Inflammation may extend beyond the mucosa in an acute severe colitis. If patients present for the first time with such an acute episode, examination of biopsy material at this stage frequently reveals equivocal results so that it may not be possible to classify the colitis. A definitive diagnosis may not then be made until the operative specimen is examined, or further biopsies are taken from unresected bowel at follow up.

Disease may be confined to the rectum (idopathic proctitis) and, when proximal spread occurs, involvement is characteristically *in continuity*. Exceptions to this rule occur in patients where the distal disease heals as a response to local steroid enema therapy and in the very rare group where the rectum is spared, or where there is a so-called right-sided ulcerative colitis.

Double contrast studies correlate well with the sigmoidoscopic and endoscopic findings and so are used initially to determine the degree and extent of involvement and thereafter to follow the course of the disease. Comparison with colonoscopy shows that the barium enema tends slightly to underestimate the extent of disease, which means that all patients who appear on X-ray to have disease extending to the hepatic flexure must be regarded as having a total colitis and therefore require long-term follow up in respect of the carcinoma risk.

If active disease is shown on sigmoidoscopy without a defined upper limit, a satisfactory and diagnostic examination can be achieved by a limited double contrast enema without bowel preparation, the so-called *instant* or *unprepared enema*. This is because the actively inflamed colon is usually free of significant faecal content. A patient referred for X-ray with a diagnosis of proctitis, where the upper limit of disease is seen on sigmoidoscopy, should be given full preparation. Whenever there is doubt, a plain film of the abdomen should be inspected since there is a close correlation between the absence of faeces and the presence of abnormal gas shadows on a plain film, and mucosal lesions on the double contrast films. On a plain abdominal film the involved segment of colon is usually free of detectable residue. In addition the inflamed bowel may contain gas, showing either as a tubular shadow devoid of haustration or as a gas shadow with thickened blunted haustra or distinct marginal irregularity; the latter implies more severe disease with ulceration. Since a faecal residue is normally present in the caecum, a totally empty colon in a patient with known inflammatory bowel disease indicates a total colitis.

The instant enema. A preliminary plain film is taken and inspected prior to the contrast study to exclude toxic dilatation, which is an absolute contraindication to any form of contrast examination. Also, if a biopsy has been taken it is recommended that the examination be deferred for 10 days. Otherwise the barium study is conducted in the usual way except that the flow of barium is stopped if the patient complains of pain or when formed faecal content is reached. The rectum is then drained and air insufflated. Prone, lateral and erect films are then usually sufficient to show the extent and degree of disease. The prone film shows the overall pattern of involvement, the lateral view shows the rectosigmoid junction and the presacral space and the erect film gives more detailed information about the transverse colon and flexures.

Patients with long-standing ulcerative colitis in a quiescent phase require full preparation prior to barium enema examination.

Radiological appearances. Early changes consist of an alteration of the normal sharp mucosal line — the tangential view of the mucosal surface — which becomes blurred and slightly thickened; this is accompanied by a fine granular appearance in the *en face* view (Fig. 32.7). As the disease progresses, a more coarse granular appearance is seen and the mucosal line becomes frankly beaded (Fig. 32.8). If and when ulceration develops, it is usually restricted to the mucosa and therefore appears shallow: it is both part of and an accentuation of the coarse granular beaded appearance. Overt ulceration is shown by projections of barium outside the mucosal line and pools of barium in the *en face* view (Fig. 32.9). Deep ulceration, in contrast to Crohn's disease, is distinctly uncommon, but when it does occur the ulcers tend to assume a *collar-stud* configuration and may coalesce. Deep ulceration and penetration into the external muscle layers is associated with loss of large areas of mucosa. Such extensive mucosal stripping, with exposure of the circular muscle fibres, is seen quite frequently in resected specimens, where operation has been required for unrelenting acute disease. It should be remembered that deep ulcers in this disease may not necessarily be penetrating; the presence of significant mucosal oedema gives an impression of greater depth even though the ulcer may still be limited to the mucosa. Also it is worth pointing out that florid ulceration in ulcerative colitis always occurs on a background of a diffusely abnormal mucosa and that discrete ulceration with intervening normal mucosa, as may occur in Crohn's disease, is never seen.

The width of the *presacral space* tends to increase with active proctitis above the upper limit of normal of 1 cm. As the presacral space increases, the calibre of the rectum narrows and such increase and decrease in the width of the presacral space may parallel exacerbations and remissions of disease.

In one group of patients, however, the space remains persistently wide and the rectum narrow. These patients may have unusually severe symptoms, even with a limited

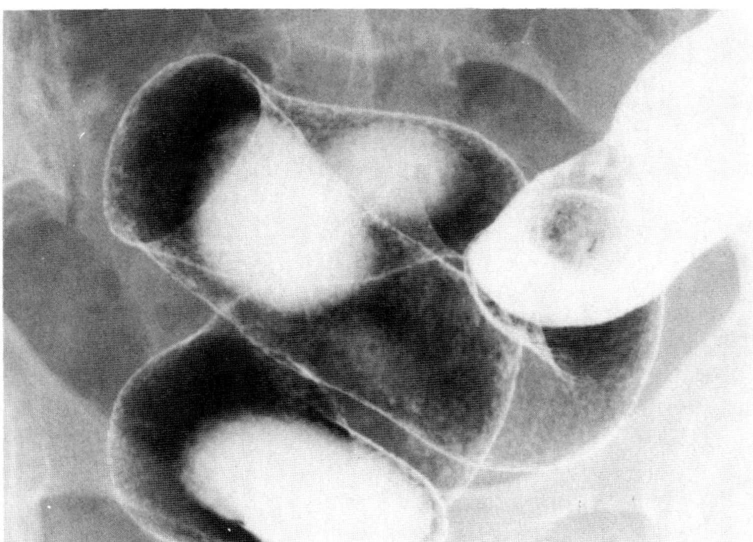

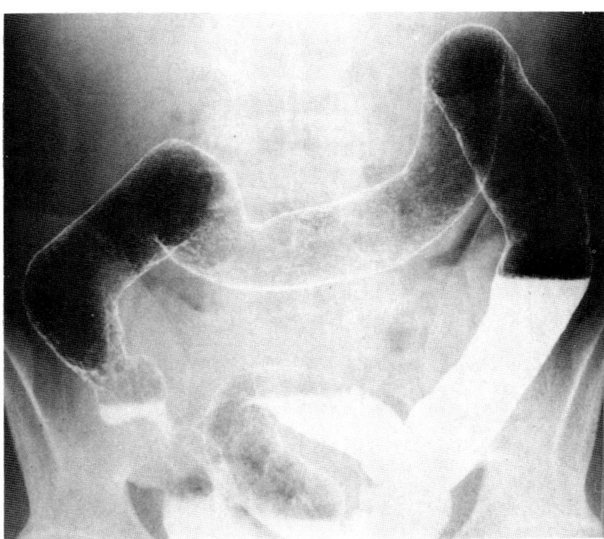

Fig. 32.7 Ulcerative colitis. **A.** Fine granularity in the rectum and sigmoid colon. **B.** Fine granularity throughout the colon which is shortened and totally devoid of haustration.

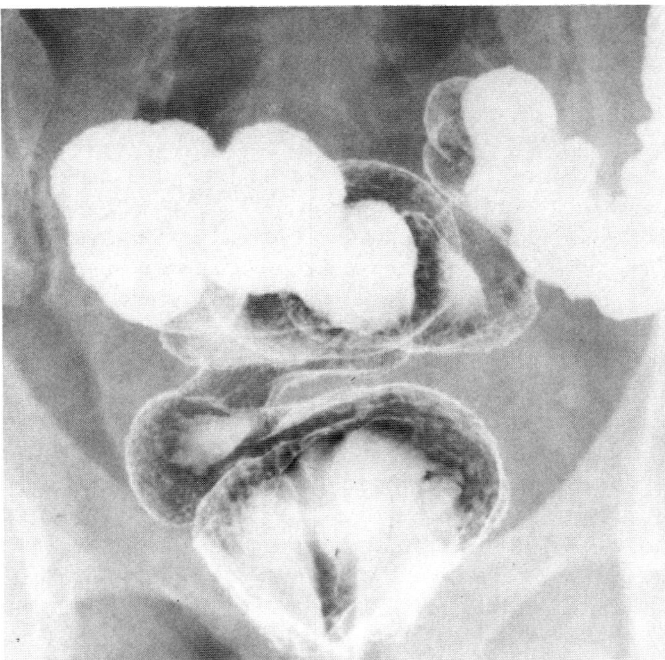

Fig. 32.8 Ulcerative colitis. Coarse granularity.

distal colitis and, in particular, tend to complain of disproportionate urgency and frequency of bowel actions due to lack of the normal rectal reservoir. Widening of the presacral space without evidence of past or present inflammatory disease and with a normally distensible rectum is usually a normal anatomical variant due to an increase in presacral adipose tissue.

Varying degrees of *postinflammatory polyposis* may occur; the postinflammatory polyp — previously known as the *pseudopolyp* — consists of granulation or fibrous tissue with an epithelial covering. Polypoidal change seen in the course of acute disease represents a combination of postinflammatory polyps and mucosal tags which, together with acutely active and ulcerating disease, produces gross and florid mucosal changes (Fig. 32.10). Postinflammatory polyposis follows healing of acute disease. Once developed, it persists after the acute phase has settled and may be generalized or segmental. These inflammatory polyps are usually frond-like and sometimes likened to seaweed (Fig. 32.11), but may be quite smooth and resemble adenomas. True adenomatous polyps in ulcerative colitis are uncommon.

The mucosal changes are accompanied by haustral blunting or effacement and, as the disease progresses, the

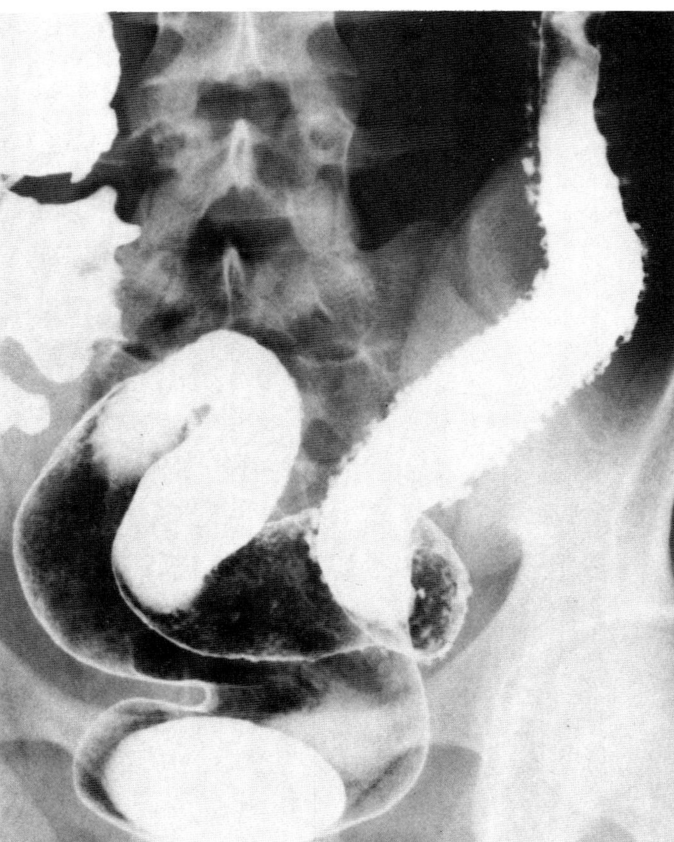

Fig. 32.9 Ulcerative colitis. Shallow ulceration superimposed on coarse granularity.

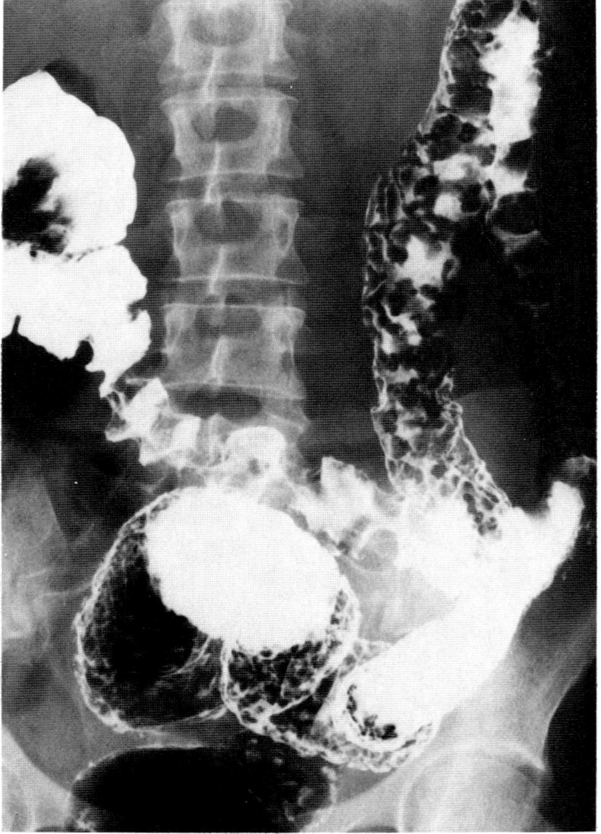

Fig. 32.10 Ulcerative colitis. Ulceration together with polypoid change due to mucosal tags and postinflammatory polyposis.

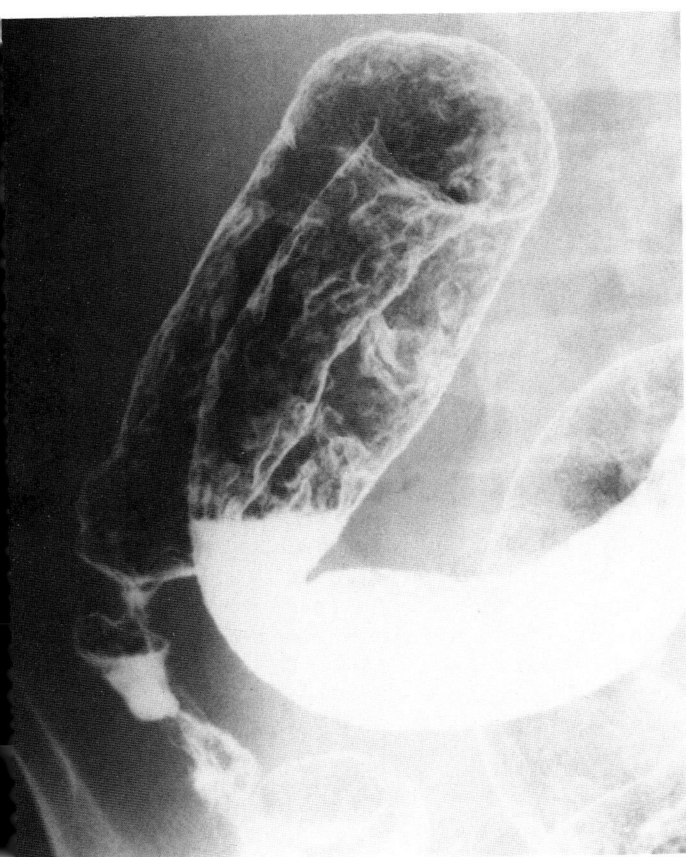

Fig. 32.11 Ulcerative colitis. Filiform or seaweed-like postinflammatory polyps.

colon tends to shorten and the lumen becomes narrowed. This is due to a muscular abnormality rather than fibrosis, which is not a feature of ulcerative colitis: in the fully developed state it produces the tubular *'pipe-stem'* colon of late ulcerative colitis. Haustral abnormalities may be reversible or may persist despite healing of the mucosal lesion. It should be noted that the left colon frequently shows absence of haustration as a normal variant.

In an acute total colitis there may be spread of mild inflammation into the terminal ileum, which then appears slightly dilated with a dilated and incompetent ileocaecal valve. The mucosa sometimes shows faint granularity over a length of 5–15 cm. This is referred to as *'backwash ileitis'* and is quite unlike the appearances seen in Crohn's disease.

Acute toxic dilatation. Toxic dilatation of the colon occurs in a small proportion of patients with ulcerative colitis who are acutely ill. It may be the presenting syndrome heralding the onset of the disease or may develop in cases of established ulcerative colitis during an exacerbation. Toxic dilatation may also occur in Crohn's disease and occasionally in other conditions such as ischaemia and amoebiasis. The patient is acutely ill with tachycardia, fever, diarrhoea and sometimes hypokalaemia.

Plain radiographs of the abdomen show a gas-filled colon, dilated either in whole or in part. The transverse colon is particularly affected and a measurement of width of more than 5.5 cm in association with haustral blunting or effacement indicate that toxic dilatation is present (Fig. 32.12).

Irregular soft tissue shadows are often seen at the margins of the bowel: these so-called mucosal islands project into the lumen and represent a combination of mucosal tags, where the surrounding epithelial surface has stripped, and postinflammatory polyps. *Perforation* of the affected oedematous segment or of the overdistended caecum is a very serious risk.

Carcinoma of the colon. Ulcerative colitis predisposes to malignancy, the frequency of malignant change being related to the duration of disease (more than 10 years) and appears confined to those patients who have total colonic involvement. The incidence of malignant change is approximately 5–10% in patients who have suffered from ulcerative colitis for more than 20 years. This figure is less than in earlier reported series and it is likely that the incidence will continue to fall due to changing patterns in treatment and management and an increased awareness of the cancer risk.

Carcinomatous change in this disease tends to arise diffusely in a flat mucosa; the common radiological appearance is therefore of a stricture or occasionally a marginal flattening and rigidity of the bowel wall. The majority of strictures seen in ulcerative colitis are in fact benign and due to hypertrophy of the muscularis mucosae. Theoretically, benign strictures are entirely smooth with no mucosal irregularity and with even tapering ends, whereas malignant strictures may show mucosal irregularity and uneven

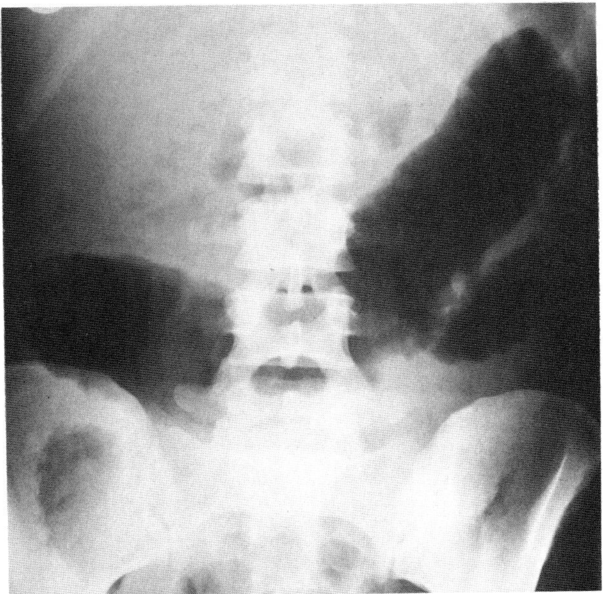

Fig. 32.12 Toxic dilatation in ulcerative colitis. The colon is dilated and the haustral pattern blunted.

narrowing, but in practice any stricture demonstrated radiologically requires endoscopic examination and biopsy. Epithelial dysplasia on histological examination of biopsy material is a sign of precancer in the 'at risk' colon and the evaluation of biopsy results in this group of patients is an important aid to management.

When surgery is indicated, the usual operation is total proctocolectomy and ileostomy. If there is relative rectal sparing, some patients may be suitable for a sub-total colectomy and ileorectal anastomosis. With this procedure, however, there is a constant risk both of further active disease, or malignant change, in the retained rectum.

More recent alternatives are the Kock continent ileostomy and the pelvic pouch procedure developed by Parks.

With the *Kock ileostomy* an ileal pouch is formed to act as a reservoir behind the stomal opening on the abdominal wall; fashioning of a nipple valve prevents efflux of the pouch contents through the stoma. The pouch is periodically emptied though a catheter inserted through the stomal opening.

In the *Parks operation* a pelvic ileal pouch is fashioned after a sphincter-saving proctocolectomy; the efferent ileal loop passes through the normal anal canal (Fig. 32.13). Continence may, therefore, be retained with a normal anal anatomy; some patients, however, may not be able to evacuate spontaneously and need to empty the pouch by catheter.

CROHN'S DISEASE

First described in 1932, this disease can involve any part of the gastrointestinal tract but tends to affect the terminal ileum and anal region in particular. Its cause is unknown and evidence of a transmissible agent is unproven. The colon is involved alone in about 20% of cases; in 60% there is both colonic and small bowel, usually distal ileal, disease. Generally the colonic disease is right sided; involvement may, however, be total or may be restricted to the left side, particularly in the elderly. It is generally agreed that colonic Crohn's disease has become gradually more common and that this increased incidence cannot be explained solely on the basis of more accurate diagnosis.

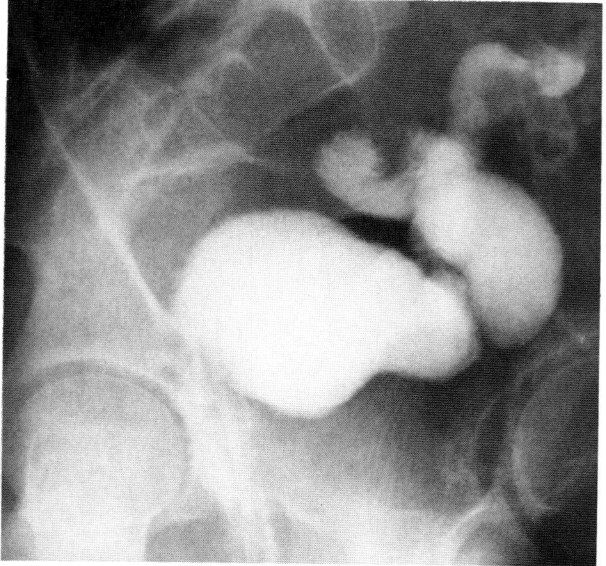

Fig. 32.13 Contrast study of a pelvic pouch (oblique view) showing the afferent loop entering the pouch and the efferent loop passing through the anal canal. Enema catheter in situ.

Pathologically, Crohn's disease is a transmural inflammatory lesion, usually discontinuous, with thickening of the bowel wall, transmural inflammatory cellular infiltration, deep ulceration and fissuring; subsequently fibrosis is common. The presence of non-caseating granulomas with giant cell infiltration is diagnostic but not seen in all cases. The mucosa is oedematous and linear ulceration, both longitudinal and transverse, is common, imparting a 'cobblestone' appearance to the surface. The mesenteric and pericolic lymph nodes become enlarged, the fibrosis which occurs leads to stricture formation, and the transmural inflammation may lead to adherence of bowel loops and fistula formation. The disease tends to be discontinuous both along and around the bowel with *skip lesions* separated by normal segments of bowel. This pattern is therefore quite unlike the even continuous lesion seen in ulcerative colitis.

Anal Crohn's disease may cause oedematous skin tags, fissuring, ulceration of the anal canal, recurrent abscesses, fistulae and occasionally anorectal stenosis.

Although the risk of cancer is far less than with chronic total ulcerative colitis, there does appear to be a slight but significant increase in the risk of cancer developing in both the small and large bowel in this disease.

Radiological appearances. The instant enema is of relatively limited use in this condition due to the patchy nature of the disease process and full bowel preparation is usually required. In Crohn's disease the changes found differ from those in ulcerative colitis in degree and distribution, although in individual cases radiological differentiation is not always readily made.

As has been noted, the disease process is characteristically discontinuous, both along the length of the bowel and circumferentially. Mucosal involvement tends to be patchy and the even granularity seen in ulcerative colitis is distinctly uncommon. Probably the earliest manifestation of Crohn's disease anywhere in the gut is the *apthoid ulcer*. This appears as a small central collection of barium surrounded by a radiolucent halo, producing a 'bull's eye' or target lesion (Fig. 32.14). Larger ulcers may in themselves be indistinguishable from those in ulcerative colitis, but in Crohn's disease these often occur within an otherwise normal mucosa which is an important distinguishing feature (Fig. 32.14). Pathologically, ulceration tends to be deeper and *linear ulcers* are common. The presence of linear

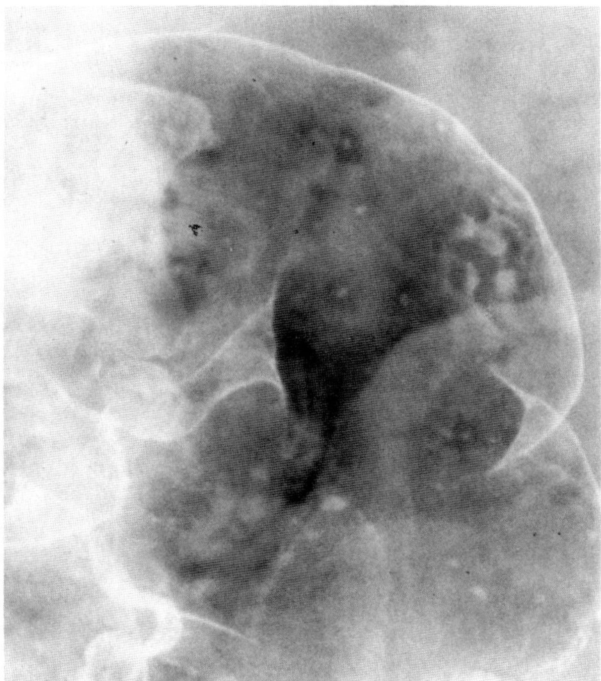

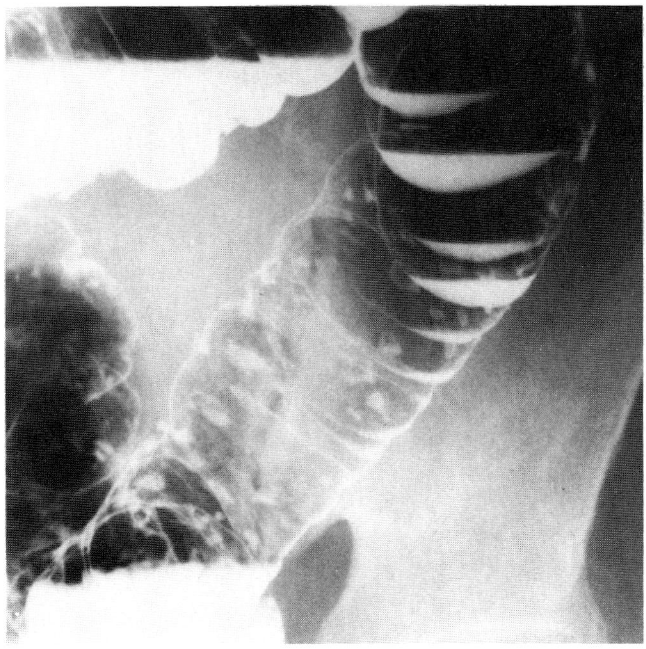

Fig. 32.14 Crohn's disease. **A.** Apthoid ulcers with a central target surrounded by a halo. **B.** Larger discrete ulcers within an otherwise normal mucosa.

ulceration contributes, as has been stated, to the 'cobblestone' appearance of the mucosa. Even in the absence of true cobblestoning, linear ulcers show as linear streaks of barium traversing the mucosal surface; this appearance has been described as an 'extra' line of barium by Young and as a linear 'stripe' by Welin.

As well as deep ulceration, fissuring is a characteristic feature with thorn-like projections of barium which may be coarse (*rose thorn*) or fine (*raspberry thorn*) extending outwards into the wall of the colon. Deep ulcers and fissures may penetrate to the serosal surface; acute perforation is rare but localized perforation with the formation of a *pericolic abscess* is not uncommon. Paracolonic tracking may be demonstrated, particularly in patients with associated diverticular disease.

Asymmetric involvement is common with one wall of the bowel affected while the opposite wall is spared. Fibrosis also frequently occurs; this produces stricture formation if circumferential, while if the fibrotic scarring is marginal and eccentric, stiffening and loss of haustration occurs on one wall with preservation of the haustral folds on the opposite wall (Fig. 32.15). Such eccentric fibrotic scarring may cause exaggeration of the remaining haustra to produce sacculation. Skip lesions with intervening areas of normal mucosa are classically seen, although it must be remembered that the whole colon may be affected.

The rectum is spared in some 50% of patients with colonic Crohn's disease as judged by endoscopic and histological studies. Radiological evidence of rectal involvement is in fact seen considerably less often and the demonstration of an apparently normal rectal mucosa in the presence of colonic inflammatory disease is a strong pointer towards Crohn's disease as opposed to ulcerative colitis. If the rectum is involved deep ulcers and fissures are often seen (Fig. 32.16) and anorectal sinus tracks are common.

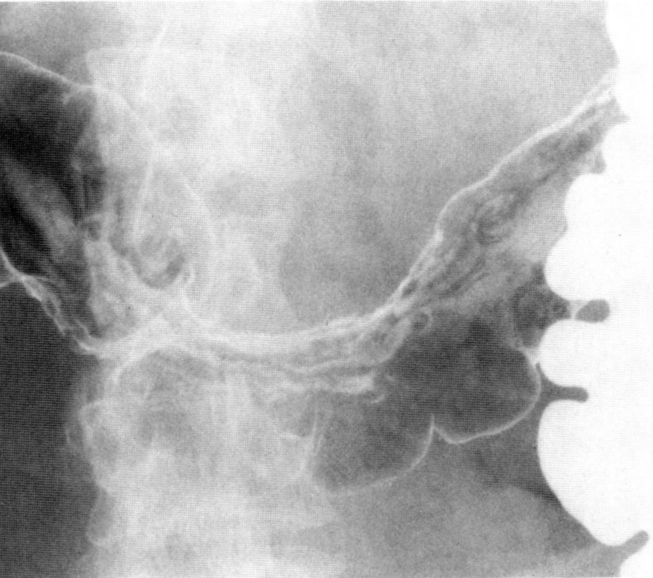

Fig. 32.15 Crohn's disease. Irregular and eccentric haustral effacement and linear ulceration.

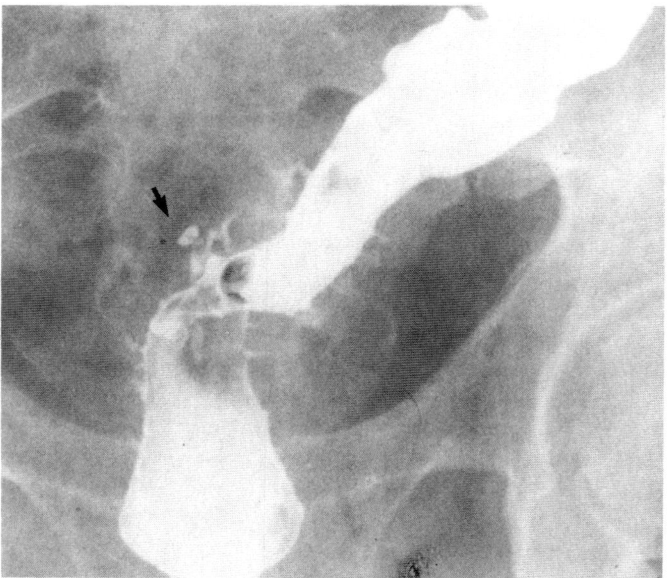

Fig. 32.16 Crohn's disease. Deep ulceration (arrow) and fissuring in the rectum.

Anorectal disease may spread to involve the external genitalia or produce a rectovaginal fistula.

In colonic Crohn's disease the sigmoid colon may become adherent to the bladder which sometimes leads to a colovesical fistula. In addition, the fallopian tube or ureter may be affected and a chronic retroperitoneal abscess occasionally spreads to the psoas sheath.

A defect in the medial wall of the caecum has been described due to thickening of the wall of the terminal ileum and mesentery. Matted loops of terminal ileum occasionally become adherent to the sigmoid colon to produce so-called disease in continuity, in which the sigmoid shows only a non-specific inflammatory response; a proportion of these cases progress to form an ileosigmoid fistula.

Postinflammatory polyposis occurs as in ulcerative colitis, but in Crohn's disease this is more often segmental in distribution, reflecting the healing stage of the patchy disease process.

A most important hallmark of Crohn's disease is, of course, evidence of small bowel disease, particularly in the terminal ileum.

Crohn's disease, in association with diverticular disease, is described in the section on diverticular disease.

Differentiation in particular must be made from ulcerative colitis; this presents no problem when classical features of Crohn's disease are present, such as severe right-sided colitis with deep ulceration and fissuring with a normal distal bowel. Inevitably there is, however, an overlap in appearances in certain cases and it should be remembered that radiology is only one of the parameters by which distinction is made between the two diseases. Crohn's disease must also be distinguished from ileocaecal tuberculosis — which is now very uncommon in this country — and also occasionally from ischaemia and secondary carcinoma.

ISCHAEMIC COLITIS

It may seem paradoxical to include ischaemic colitis in the group of inflammatory disorders but failure of the blood supply of the colon induces rapid damage of the mucosa and wall of the colon due to the normal bacterial content of the large bowel which produces an inflammatory response in the ischaemic area.

Pathologically the effects may be mild, moderate or severe and these changes are reflected in the clinical state of the affected patient. In severe ischaemia, progressive destruction of the colonic wall occurs leading to full thickness necrosis, sloughing and possible rupture. With minimal disease, superficial congestion and inflammation occur which usually resolve completely as the collateral supply dilates. Between these two groups an initial marked inflammatory reaction with mucosal oedema is followed by mucosal ulceration and gradual replacement of the muscle layers by fibrous tissue which may result in a permanent stricture of the bowel wall.

Interference with the arterial or venous supply of the colon may thus result in varying degrees of damage to the affected segment of colon. Depending upon the extent and rapidity of development of a collateral circulation and revascularization, the effects may vary from a relatively minor and transient incident to the development of an established ischaemic colitis or may, in the severest form, cause gangrene of the colon with necrosis of the wall. With slow and insidious mesenteric arterial occlusion, as in atheromatous aortic thrombosis or abdominal aortic aneurysm, the collateral circulation usually proves adequate to maintain the vitality of the bowel and clinical ischaemia does not develop.

Causes of colonic ischaemia may be *arterial*, due to thrombosis, embolism, aneurysm or surgical trauma; *venous*, due to thrombosis, *small vessel disease* as in diabetes and polyarteritis; or *non-occlusive lesions*, which include cardiac failure, other low flow states and disseminated intravascular coagulation. Venous occlusion is usually less dramatic in its effects than interruption of the arterial supply of the colon, but major venous thrombosis produces a lesion which resembles the late results of arterial occlusion.

Clinically the disease may be divided into two main groups, acute infarction with gangrene of the colon and ischaemic (non-gangrenous) colitis.

Acute infarction with gangrene. This presents with the sudden onset of abdominal pain often with vomiting and diarrhoea, followed by shock, occurring characteristically in a middle-aged or elderly patient. The condition cannot clinically be distinguished from various other causes of the acute abdomen and usually requires emergency laparotomy. Some hours after the onset plain abdominal films usually show progressive dilatation of the large and subsequently the small bowel. Barium enema examination is contraindicated since the patient is too ill and arteriography is of little value.

Ischaemic colitis. Less severe arterial lesions, or extensive venous thrombosis which may be the sequel of intraperitoneal infection or strangulation of the bowel and which behaves in a similar fashion, usually also present acutely with pain and bleeding in the older age groups. A plain abdominal film may reveal a segment of colon where the intraluminal gas shadow shows evidence of severe mucosal oedema in the form of '*thumb-printing*'. Barium enema examination is particularly helpful and shows an abnormal segment of colon often with an abrupt demarcation from the adjacent normal bowel. The involved segment is always narrowed with loss of normal haustration, spasm and rigidity, with 'thumb-printing' in the early stages due to mucosal oedema and haemorrhage into the colonic wall (Fig. 32.17). The majority of cases show complete resolution; occasionally florid ulceration is seen during the course of the disease and in perhaps one third of all cases a smooth permanent fibrous stricture develops. It is generally agreed that arteriography is also of little value in this group.

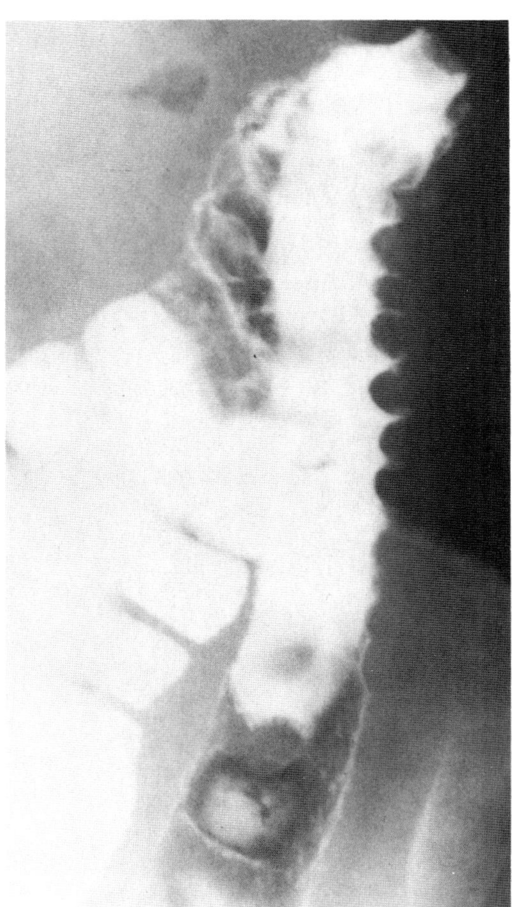

ig. 32.17 Ischaemia. Narrowing and 'thumb-printing' around the plenic flexure.

CATHARTIC COLON

Prolonged purgative ingestion may cause neural damage and radiologically demonstrable changes in the colon. Laxative abuse is not uncommon but the fully developed condition of cathartic colon is rarely seen. Patients may complain of diarrhoea from the purgative intake and because the colon has become virtually functionless, but the main presenting features are weakness due to hypokalaemia and thirst due to dehydration. Symptoms may be confused with renal disease or Addison's disease, particularly as a high purgative intake may be denied.

The *radiological changes* always involve, and first occur on, the right side of the colon and consist in loss of normal haustration and the development of a smooth bowel wall. Smooth tapering contractions of the colon are described mimicking strictures (*pseudostrictures*) which are inconstant. In more advanced cases the whole of the colon may be involved and the appearances of general atony are the result of gross neuromuscular dysfunction.

The main differential diagnosis is from chronic ulcerative colitis: in the cathartic colon there is never evidence of mucosal inflammation and the widespread haustral loss is not accompanied by uniform narrowing of the bowel lumen or polypoid change.

DIVERTICULAR DISEASE OF THE COLON

Diverticular disease is a common disorder of Western civilization, affecting about one third of the population by the fifth decade. The two components of uncomplicated diverticular disease consist of the diverticula themselves and the associated and causative muscular abnormality within the sigmoid colon.

The work of Morson (1963), Williams (1963) and others has drawn attention to the gross muscle changes which occur in the sigmoid colon in this disease. Thickening of both the longitudinal and circular muscle fibres occurs. In addition the thickened taeniae are contracted and the combination of these changes produces contraction and pleating of the sigmoid with the formation of folds of mucosa and hence the characteristic accordion-like or irregularly serrated pattern on X-ray.

Most diverticula arise from the side walls of the colon between the mesenteric and the two antimesenteric taeniae. Herniation occurs between the muscle bundles at the site of entry of blood vessels and the herniated diverticula project into the pericolic fat. They therefore have an inner mucosal and an outer serosal coat. Less commonly, small protrusions of mucosa occur in the antimesenteric intertaenial area; frequently these protrusions are too small to reach the serosa (intramural diverticula) but sometimes they do reach the serosa to produce small transverse ridges and an appearance of fine mucosal pleating (ridge diverticula).

Gross distortion of the sigmoid colon in fully developed cases used to be regarded as evidence of past or present inflammation but is now known to be purely a reflection of the severe muscular component.

Intracolonic pressure studies and cineradiography have shown that considerable muscular dysfunction of the colon is present and that the diverticula are formed, not from inherent weakness of the colonic wall, but by the generation of abnormally high intracolonic pressures. The racial and geographical pattern of the disease suggests that it is directly related to modern methods of food processing and refinement in Western industrialized countries.

The sigmoid colon is most commonly involved, showing both diverticula and the muscle change; extension of diverticula through the remainder of the left colon is the next most common type. Sometimes diverticula occur throughout the colon and occasionally they are confined to the right side. Radiologically demonstrable muscular hypertrophy is confined to the sigmoid colon and the occurrence of diverticula more proximally is presumed to be due to a summation back pressure effect.

The presence in the sigmoid colon of a minor but characteristic muscular abnormality without diverticula is best described as sigmoid muscular hypertrophy, rather than prediverticular disease.

The rare large *solitary caecal diverticulum* is probably of congenital origin and the even rarer *giant sigmoid diverticulum* is believed, to be due to a previous walled-off perforation occurring in an episode of diverticulitis, or to a 'ball-valve' effect at the orifice of the diverticulum.

The task of the radiologist in this disease is threefold:

1. Documentation of the degree and extent of disease
2. Diagnosis of complications
3. Detection of any other pathology.

It is probable that up to 80% of patients with colonic diverticula are asymptomatic, the disease being an incidental finding. Some patients may have symptoms such as abdominal pain consequent upon abnormal muscle motility. Otherwise symptoms are usually due to the complications of the disease.

Radiological investigation. On barium enema examination the radiological appearances are:

1. Diverticula. These appear as flask-like outpouchings from the bowel wall. When seen *en face* they are ring shadows; a narrower neck may be visible producing a smaller and usually eccentrically placed ring shadow within the larger circle of the diverticulum itself. Other definitive signs of a diverticulum are projection beyond the bowel wall and the presence, in erect or decubitus views, of a fluid level. A round pool of barium is seen if the diverticulum is totally filled with barium in an air-filled segment of colon, but the appearances may alter depending on the amount of faecal content within the diverticulum.

2. The muscle change. This, in the sigmoid colon, produces the accordion-like pleating or serrated appearance of the affected area. Localized muscular hypertrophy may mimic a neoplastic stricture. Patients with marked diverticular disease often sustain severe and persistent spasm during the filling stage of the barium enema which requires the administration of an intravenous antispasmodic.

Complications

Diverticulitis. When a diverticulum becomes inflamed, the infection initially affects and is localized to the pericolic tissue into which it projects. Pericolic abscess formation and localized peritonitis ensues producing a clinical picture which resembles a 'left-sided appendicitis'. Rupture into the peritoneal cavity may occur at any time to cause generalized peritonitis, so barium enema examination is contraindicated in the acute phase. When this acute inflammation has settled, radiological examination may then show an area of narrowing and often irritability. A pericolic abscess produces an extrinsic filling defect which is usually eccentric. A leak of barium outside the lumen may also be seen (Fig. 32.18). Careful examination shows that the mucosa, although distorted, is not invaded or destroyed as would occur with a malignant tumour, but differentiation may be difficult and is further discussed under 'malignant change'.

Perforation of the colon may be associated with the spread of gas into the retroperitoneal tissues, recognized by a 'soap bubble' appearance on the plain film.

Fistula. Once an abscess forms, extension of the inflammation to a neighbouring viscus or the abdominal wall may lead to the development of a fistula.

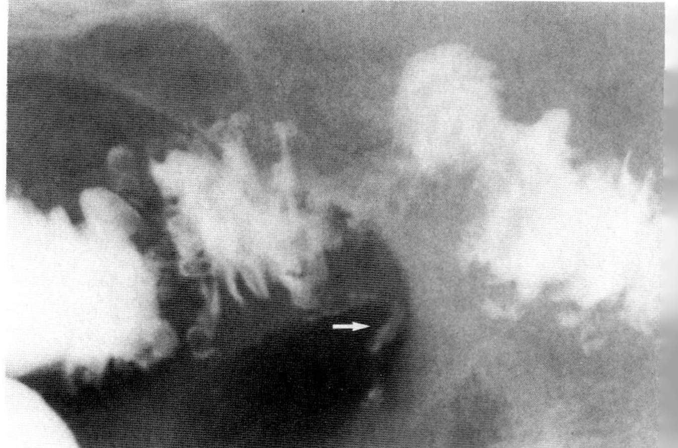

Fig. 32.18 Diverticular disease with leakage of contrast (arrow) into the pericolic tissues indicating diverticulitis.

The commonest fistula is between the sigmoid colon and the bladder; this occurs more often in males due to the interposition of the uterus between the colon and bladder in the female. A *colovesical fistula* produces pneumaturia and possibly even the passage of faeces per urethram. A plain film occasionally shows air in the bladder and the fistula itself may be demonstrated by contrast studies in about 30% of cases (Fig. 32.19). Fistulae may also occur between the colon and vagina, colon and bowel — usually ileum — or to the skin of the abdominal wall or buttock.

Obstruction. Subacute large bowel obstruction may occur with an episode of diverticulitis, or less often small bowel obstruction results from adhesion of ileal loops to the inflamed sigmoid colon.

Malignant change. There is no evidence that diverticular disease predisposes to malignancy but, inevitably, since diverticular disease is so common in the older age groups, the two conditions not infrequently coexist. Detection of malignant change is more difficult in these circumstances due to the distortion of the bowel wall and mucosa by the diverticular disease itself. It is important, whenever stricturing is demonstrated, to try to establish whether there is mucosal destruction and shouldering which indicates neoplastic change (Fig. 32.20) but endoscopy and biopsy is indicated whenever there is doubt.

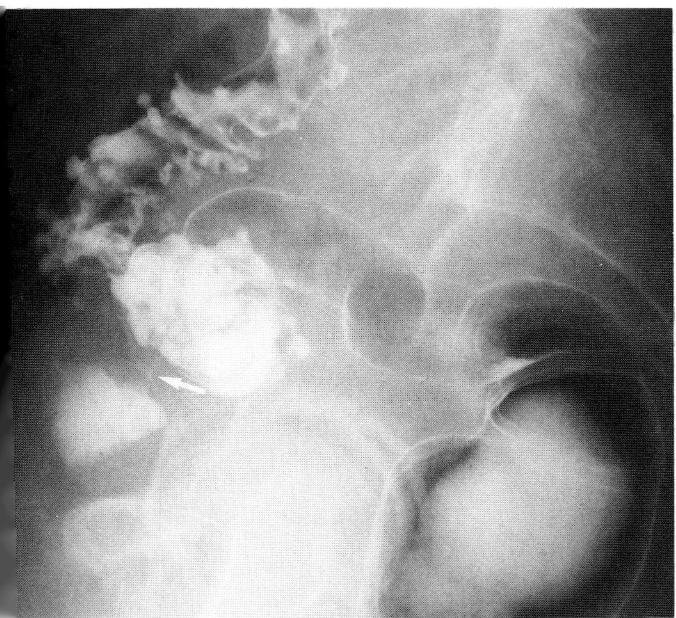

Fig. 32.19 A colovesical fistula in diverticular disease (arrowed).

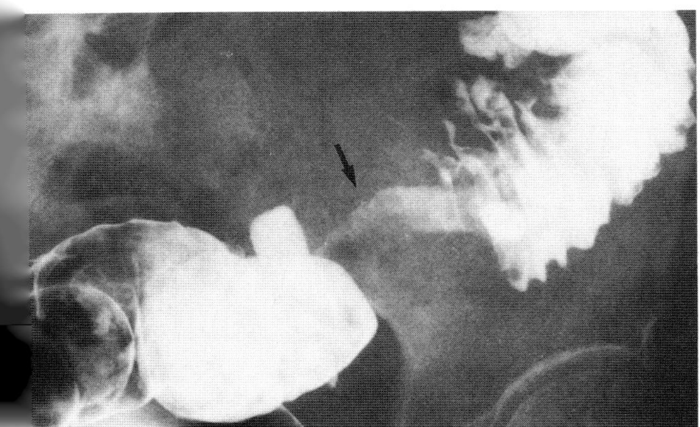

Fig. 32.20 Carcinoma (arrow) in diverticular disease.

Polyps. Polyps are similarly difficult to detect due to the distortion of the mucosa and the confusing shadows of the diverticula themselves. The aim is to look for positive signs of either a polyp or diverticulum but in gross diverticular disease this is far from easy and endoscopic examination may again be necessary.

Haemorrhage. It seems that there is an increased incidence of minor bleeding in diverticular disease but this symptom is an indication for colonoscopy or, at least, flexible sigmoidoscopy to exclude other causes if no other lesion is detected on the barium enema. Massive haemorrhage in the elderly certainly occurs and a number of reports (Caserella et al 1972, Parsa et al 1975) indicate that such bleeding occurs more often from right-sided diverticula, even allowing for possible confusion in certain cases with the lesions of angiodysplasia. Selective mesenteric angiography may show the bleeding site if carried out while brisk bleeding is occurring.

Inflammatory bowel disease. Ulcerative colitis is uncommon in patients with diverticular disease partly because a significant number of patients with colitis will have had a colectomy by the 5th decade, and also because longstanding colitis tends to prevent the natural mechanism of development of diverticular disease. When it does occur, which is usually therefore as a late onset in patients who

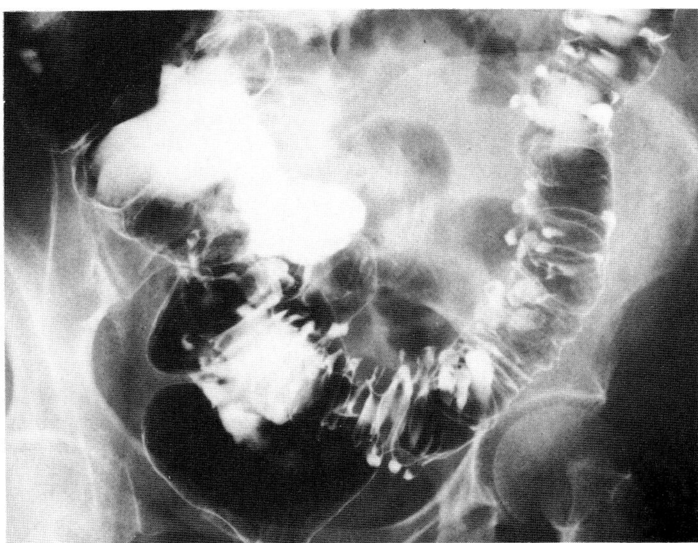

Fig. 32.21 Uncomplicated diverticular disease.

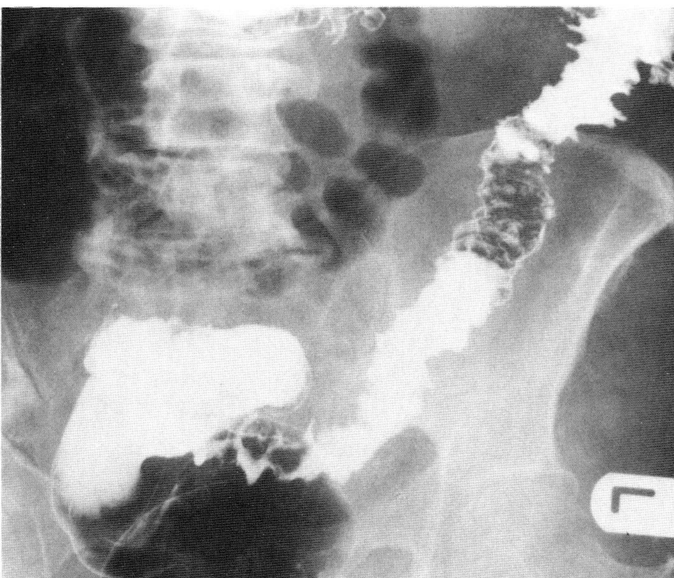

Fig. 32.22 The same patient 3 years later with superimposed Crohn's disease. Note the partial effacement of the diverticula due to mucosal oedema and inflammation and the presence of ulceration.

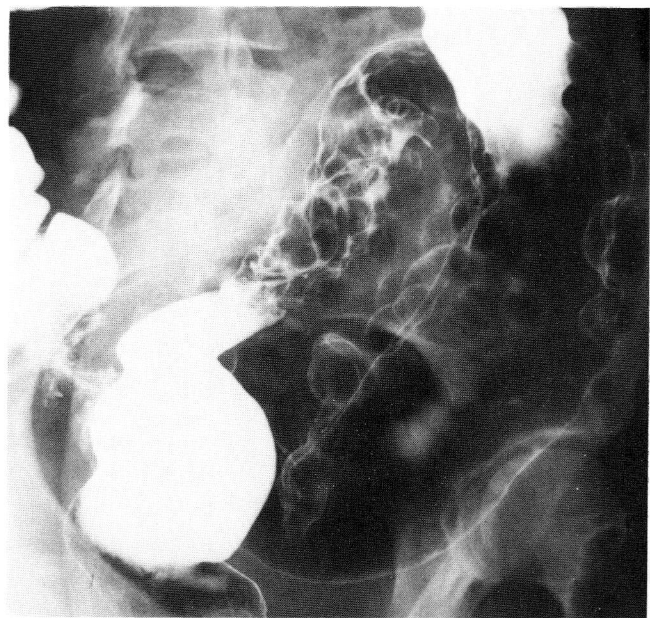

Fig. 32.23 Pneumatosis coli with the characteristic serpiginous margin of the lumen due to the presence of multiple submucosal cysts of varying size.

already have diverticular disease, it usually shows as superimposed mucosal granularity. An association with Crohn's disease is more common since there is an increased incidence of Crohn's disease involving the distal colon in the older age groups in whom, of course, a significant number will already have established diverticular disease. When Crohn's disease does develop, the diverticula become much less obvious due to mucosal oedema, the mucosal line becomes thickened and blurred and ulceration becomes obvious (Figs 32.21 and 32.22).

PNEUMATOSIS COLI

Pneumatosis cystoides intestinalis is a rare condition which may affect the small or large bowel. Gas-filled cysts occur in the submucosa or less commonly the subserosa of the bowel. Earlier reports stressed predominant involvement of the small bowel, but in more recent years the majority of cases of pneumatosis reported in the literature have been confined to the colon.

Many of the reported series describe a significant association with obstructive airways disease. In this group it is postulated that alveolar rupture allows air to track from the mediastinum into the retroperitoneal space and thence through the mesentery into the bowel wall. A much smaller number of cases appear to be associated with gastric or duodenal ulceration and pyloric stenosis but many remain of unknown aetiology.

The commoner submucosal cysts are visible both on a plain film — showing as a clustered chain of bubble-like translucencies — and on a barium enema, where they characteristically produce a wavy serpiginous border to the bowel lumen (Fig. 32.23). Subserosal cysts tend to be smaller, usually show no mucosal abnormality on contrast examination and appear as smaller beaded radiolucent shadows on a plain film.

The cysts are commonest in the sigmoid and descending colon. Perforation with pneumoperitoneum is uncommon. Symptoms, if they occur, are usually of pain, diarrhoea and occasionally bleeding.

It has recently been shown that the condition can be treated by high-dose oxygen therapy and that response to treatment can be monitored by plain films.

THE IRRITABLE BOWEL SYNDROME

This is a common condition in Western civilization, the diagnosis being made on the characteristic clinical features although other disease processes may need to be excluded. Earlier reports in the literature stressed the significance of segmental spasm occurring during a barium enema examination and the presence of increased haustral markings. Whether or not this was true in relation to the single contrast enema, which was at the time the standard method of examination, these changes are certainly not found with the double contrast enema. The place of radiology in this condition is primarily to exclude other lesions if there is any clinical doubt, and the only positive finding is the production of the patient's characteristic pain by air insufflation.

It must also be remembered that a number of patients with the irritable bowel syndrome will in later life develop other unrelated bowel pathology and in particular a neoplasm. Any change in symptoms which leads to clinical suspicion is therefore an indication for reinvestigation rather than to assume that they are part of the known disease.

TUMOURS OF THE COLON

POLYPOID LESIONS OF THE COLON

An abbreviated list of polypoid lesions which may occur in the large bowel is shown in Table 32.1. It must be realized that, with the exception of overt carcinomas, the various histological types of polyp cannot be differentiated on radiological grounds alone.

Table 32.1 Classification of polyps of the large intestine

Class	Types
Inflammatory	Inflammatory polyp
Metaplastic	Metaplastic polyp
Hamartomatous	Juvenile polyp Peutz-Jegher's polyp
Neoplastic	Adenoma — tubular — tubulovillous — villous Lipoma Adenocarcinoma Colloid and signet ring cell carcinoma Carcinoid Lymphoma

Whenever any polypoid lesion is identified in the colon a careful search must be made for other lesions since they are often multiple.

Metaplastic polyps are common and occur particularly in the rectum. They are usually small in size, around 5 mm in diameter, and are identical in appearance to small sessile adenomas from which they can be distinguished only by biopsy. They have no malignant potential.

Inflammatory polyps may follow any severe ulceration in the large bowel and are particularly seen in ulcerative colitis, Crohn's disease, schistosomiasis and the dysenteries. They can resemble adenomas but usually appear slightly irregular in shape like fragments of seaweed. Postinflammatory polyps have no malignant potential even in ulcerative colitis where there is a well-known cancer risk; carcinoma, if it occurs in this disease, arises in an area of flat mucosa.

Adenomatous polyps are subdivided into the tubular adenoma, intermediate type (tubulovillous adenoma) and villous adenoma according to the histological arrangement of the stroma and epithelium. The first type is much the commonest, the latter has the greatest malignant potential. The incidence of carcinomatous change varies with the histological type (Table 32.2).

Table 32.2 Frequency of malignant invasion in polyps and villous adenomas

Histological type	Size *Under 1 cm*	*1–2 cm*	*Over 2 cm*
Tubular adenoma	1.0%	10.2%	34.7%
Intermediate type	3.9%	7.4%	45.8%
Villous adenoma	9.5%	10.3%	52.9%

Tubular adenomas are by far the commonest; they may be single or multiple and sessile or pedunculated. They occur in large numbers in *familial polyposis of the colon* and in *Gardner's syndrome*.

A sessile adenomatous polyp depending on its size shows either as an obvious large rounded mass projecting into the colonic lumen (Fig. 32.24), or a small shadow which projects as a ring, an oval shadow or an ellipse depending on the projection of the lesion. Barium coating the base of the polyp often produces a basal rim or ellipse separate from the dome of the polyp itself (Fig. 32.25). A cardinal feature of the pedunculated polyp is its stalk or pedicle (Fig. 32.26).

The *villous adenoma* is much less common than the simple adenoma, comprising about 10% of colonic neoplastic polyps. Villous tumours may occur anywhere in the colon but are much more common in the lower bowel, particularly the rectum and sigmoid colon. Most are broad-based and large in size, averaging between 3–8 cm in diameter, with a frond-like surface. Radiologically they appear as flat sessile masses with the interstices of the villous fronds filled with barium; thus they present a fairly characteristic appearance of a tumour composed of frond-like stalks (Fig. 32.27) or a lace-work pattern (Fig. 32.28). They may occasionally be associated with a protein-losing

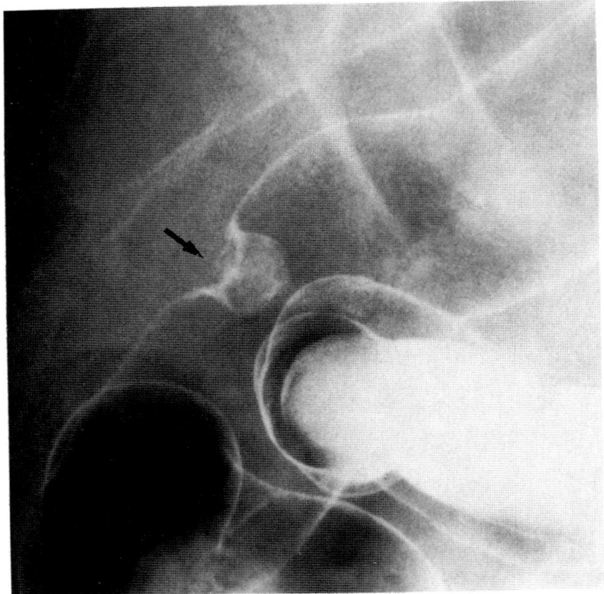

Fig. 32.24 A large polyp arising from the posterior rectal wall (arrow). The irregular indrawn base suggests malignant change.

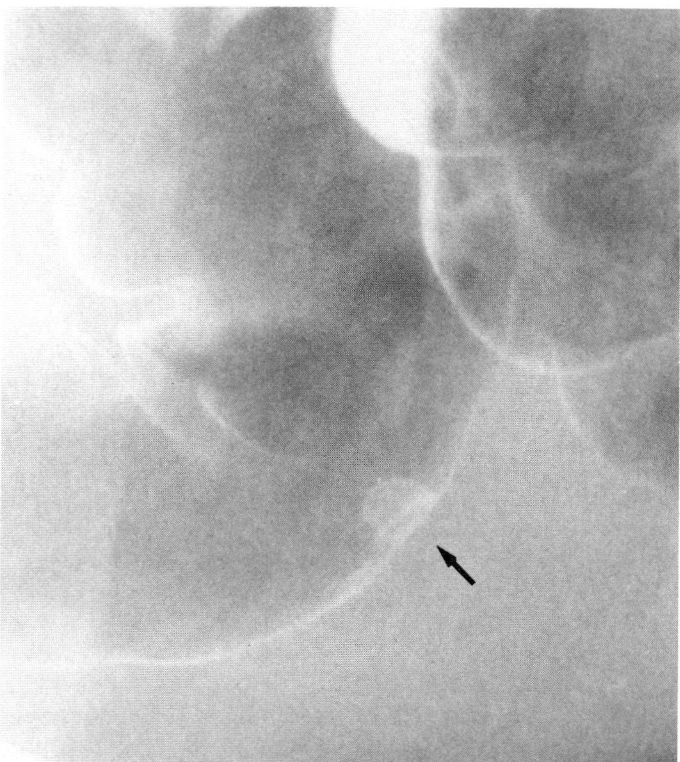

Fig. 32.25 A sessile polyp (arrow) showing a rim of barium coating the base of the polyp and the dome of the polyp itself.

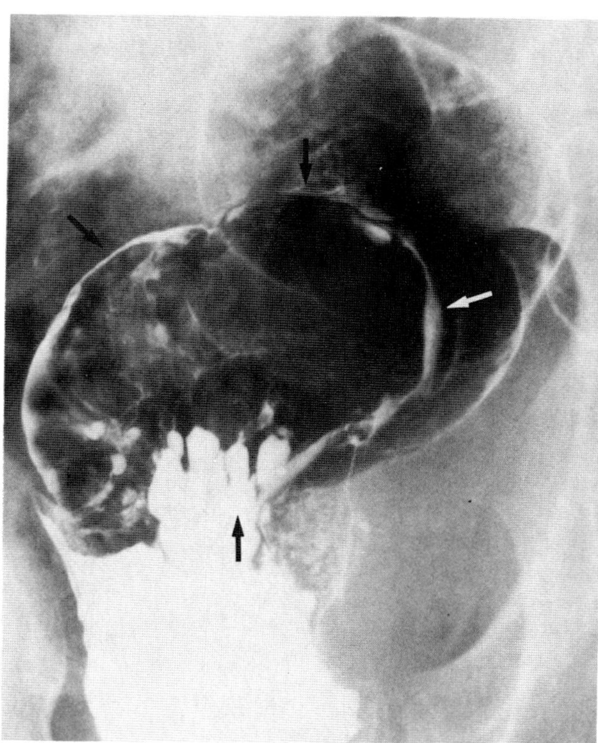

Fig. 32.27 A large villous adenoma of the rectum (arrows) showing a frond-like pattern at lower margin due to barium trapped between the folds of the tumour (↑).

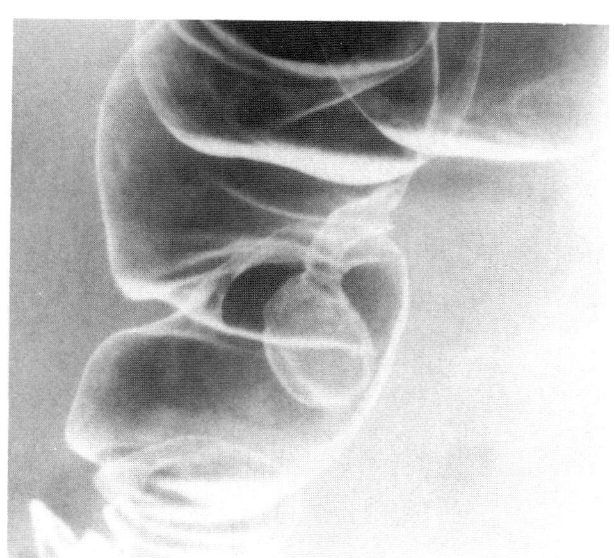

Fig. 32.26 A pedunculated polyp in the erect position.

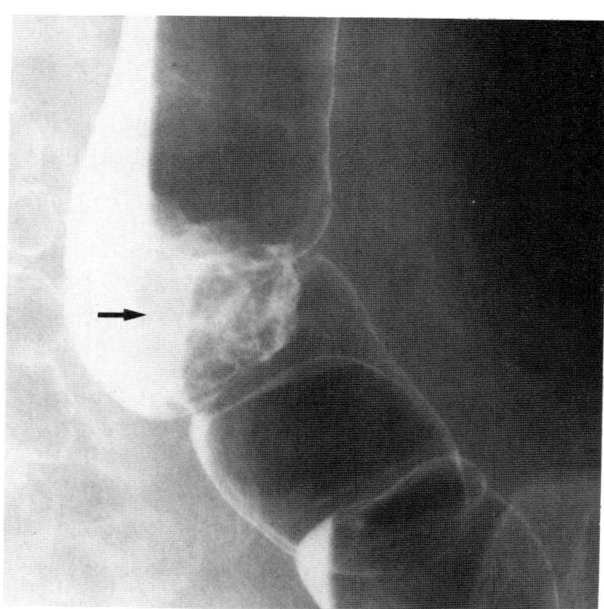

Fig. 32.28 A small villous adenoma of the descending colon (arrow) showing a lace-like pattern.

enteropathy or hypokalaemia. The incidence of malignant change is high with this tumour, but basal irregularity or indentation, which normally suggests malignancy, is not infrequently seen with a benign lesion. In itself it is almost always a solitary lesion but it has a particular tendency to be associated with other neoplasms in the colon, including carcinoma.

Whenever a polypoid lesion is demonstrated radiologically, an attempt to assess whether the lesion is benign or malignant should be made (Table 32.3) but it should be noted that the management of the polyp patient has changed since the advent of colonoscopy.

Table 32.3 Radiological differentiation of benign and malignant polyps

Benign	Malignant
Diameter less than 1 cm	Incidence increases significantly with size above 1 cm
Pedunculated polyp with a long stalk	Sessile polyp with a broad base
Smooth surface	Irregular surface
Colon contour and wall unaffected by polyp	Indentation of colonic wall at the base of the polyp

Prior to the development of flexible endoscopy, polyps above the reach of the rigid sigmoidoscope required laparotomy for removal. Since about 80% of polyps prove to be adenomas, which are potentially malignant, current practice favours removal, for histological assessment, of all lesions which are demonstrated on X-ray. This certainly applies to polyps of 1.0 cm or more in diameter. Endoscopic biopsy and removal of smaller lesions depends on consideration of various factors such as the age and general health of the patient and the availability of a colonoscopic service. The correct management of a patient with an adenomatous polyp requires close liaison between the radiologist, the clinician and the endoscopist. In certain instances it is certainly justified to repeat the barium enema for confirmation if the original radiological findings are equivocal.

Once an adenoma is found and removed, patients require regular follow up, either with a double contrast barium enema or colonoscopy probably every 3–5 years since there is an increased risk of the development of further adenomas or a carcinoma in this group. Earlier examination is, of course, indicated if the patient presents with bowel symptoms, particularly bleeding.

Lipoma. Lipomas most commonly occur in the right colon, sometimes as fatty infiltration of the ileocaecal valve. The radiological appearance is of a perfectly smooth polypoid lesion with a sharp outline which may appear relatively radiolucent.

POLYPOSIS SYNDROMES

Familial polyposis of the colon. This disease is inherited as a Mendelian dominant; all cases develop a carcinoma if untreated. In affected families it is distinctly rare for polyps to occur before 10 years of age and symptoms are uncommon before the age of 15, so periodic examination by sigmoidoscopy is commenced at about the age of 14. The onset of the disease may, however, be delayed: in the St Mark's series 50% were over 35 years of age at the time of diagnosis and 12% were over 50. It is therefore necessary to continue regular follow up throughout life in those persons at risk.

In the fully established case the polyps are usually evenly scattered from the rectum to the caecum and number at least 100. The double contrast barium enema shows multiple polyps throughout the colon (Fig. 32.29). Most of the polyps are from 0.5 cm to 1.0 cm in size; larger polyps suggest that malignant change may have supervened and occasionally an overt carcinoma is already present when the patient is first seen.

Sometime after treatment of the colonic lesion, a number of patients develop polyps in the stomach, duodenum or small intestine; occasionally a periampullary carcinoma occurs.

Gardner's syndrome. This consists of adenomatous polyposis of the colon, multiple osteomata of the mandible and skull, multiple epidermoid cysts and soft tissue tumours of the skin. The risk of malignant change is the

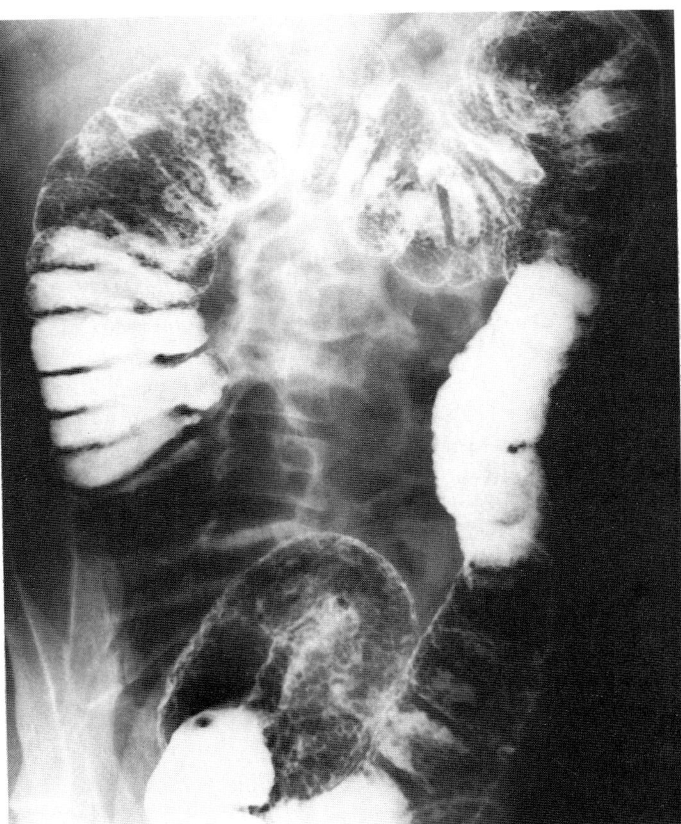

Fig. 32.29 Familial adenomatous polyposis. There are sessile polyps of varying size throughout the colon and rectum.

same as in familial polyposis of the colon. Certain other lesions may be found with this syndrome, including small bowel adenomas, carcinoma of the thyroid, adrenal cancer and carcinoid tumours. The two most important lesions, however, are periampullary carcinoma, as in familial adenomatous polyposis, and desmoid tumours. The latter tend to arise 1–3 years after surgery, appearing either in the abdominal wall or in the mesentery of the small bowel. Intra-abdominal desmoid tumours produce symptoms of obstruction of either the gastrointestinal or urinary tract.

The treatment of both familial adenomatous polyposis and Gardner's syndrome is the same, namely total colectomy with ileorectal anastomosis. Thereafter regular follow up is needed to deal with polyps which subsequently occur in the retained rectum. In addition the family must be screened.

Minor or recessive adenomatous polyposis. As opposed to the dominant gene of familial adenomatous polyposis it is postulated that there may be a recessive gene which is associated with the presence of multiple but fewer adenomas. There is no doubt that a number of patients present in adult life with multiple adenomas of the colon who do not have familial polyposis, either as inherited disease or as a genetic mutation. If given a name at all this condition at present is best called *multiple adenomatous polyposis*. In these patients it seems that the colonic epithelium has suddenly undergone a change which predisposes to multiple neoplastic transformation. This is, therefore, a high-risk group, since the chance of developing a carcinoma is high and radical surgery, rather than endoscopic removal of the polyps, may need to be considered.

Juvenile polyposis. The juvenile polyp can occur as a solitary lesion or may in juvenile polyposis present with multiple polyps either few or large in number. The juvenile polyp may occur anywhere in the gastrointestinal tract but is more commonly found in the colon. The main symptoms are rectal bleeding and, in childhood, prolapse of polyps out of the rectum. The average age of presentation is 6 years, which is considerably younger than in familial polyposis and there may be a familial factor. Congenital abnormalities such as heart lesions, malrotation of the bowel and hydrocephalus sometimes occur in the non-familial cases. The polyps are often pedunculated and histologically they are hamartomas with virtually no malignant potential. In patients with juvenile polyposis there are, however, a few reported cases of intestinal carcinoma developing in later life, usually involving the upper gastrointestinal tract.

Peutz-Jegher's syndrome. This consists of pigmentation of the skin and buccal mucosa and gastrointestinal polyposis. Polyps may occur anywhere in the alimentary tract but are more often found in the small bowel. The colon is involved in 30–50% of cases and colonic polyps, when they occur, tend to be relatively few in number. As with juvenile polyposis, the disease usually presents earlier in life than familial adenomatous polyposis. The Peutz-Jegher polyp is also a hamartoma and in itself has no malignant potential. There is, however, again a small risk of development of a carcinoma of the upper gastrointestinal tract at an early age. There is also an association between this syndrome and tumours of the ovary.

Other rare types of polyposis

Lymphoid hyperplasia occasionally occurs, usually in children or young adults. The polyps are due to non-neoplastic hypertrophy of lymphoid follicles, possibly secondary to inflammation or the result of an abnormal immunological response.

In the **Cronkhite-Canada syndrome**, which is exceedingly rare, there is diarrhoea, alopecia, atrophy of the nails and pigmentation of the skin. Radiological examination reveals diffuse gastrointestinal polyposis, the polyps resembling inflammatory polyps in structure with cystic changes within them. The disease is of unknown aetiology, is more common in females beyond middle age and carries a very poor prognosis due to the associated nutritional and metabolic problems.

Colitis cystica profunda is another rare condition in which nodular plaque-like or polypoid lesions occur particularly in the rectum and sigmoid colon, but occasionally more diffusely in the large bowel. Histologically cystic degeneration is seen in the mucous glands. There appears to be some association with previous proctocolitis.

MALIGNANT TUMOURS

The vast majority of malignant tumours of the large bowel are **adenocarcinomas**; 60% occur in the rectum and sigmoid colon and about 20% in the right colon. Pathologically the tumour may assume one of four types — polypoid (encephaloid), ulcerative, annular or diffusely infiltrating forms.

The two other forms of malignant tumour which are of particular importance are the **malignant carcinoid** and the **mucinous (colloid) carcinoma**. The appearance of the former varies from a small polypoid lesion to a large tumour indistinguishable from a villous adenoma or carcinoma. The latter shows no particular radiological differences from an adenocarcinoma, except for a tendency to develop *calcification* either in the primary tumour itself or more particularly in hepatic or peritoneal deposits.

Local spread of the growth occurs along the bowel and circumferentially; ulceration of the tumour may occur with perforation, whilst in other instances a scirrhous reaction may produce stricture formation.

Further spread of growths of the colon occurs through four pathways:

1. Through the bowel wall.
2. Through the peritoneal cavity; this may initially take the form of localized plaques in the adjacent peritoneum,

but subsequently there may be widespread involvement of the peritoneum and adjacent viscera.

3. Lymphatic spread to involve the adjacent glands.

4. Blood-borne spread particularly to the liver, occasionally to the lungs and less often to the skeleton, brain or ovary.

The **radiological appearances** are those of:

1. A filling defect projecting into the colonic lumen, separated from normal mucosa by a sharp margin. This is sometimes referred to as a '*saddle*' cancer (Fig. 32.30).
2. Destruction of the mucosal pattern again with a sharp margin separating the growth from normal mucosa (Fig. 32.31).
3. A tumour mass projecting into the colon having the classical half shadows and irregular deformities (Fig. 32.32).
4. A classical annular carcinoma (Fig. 32.33).
5. Long segment stricturing (*linitis plastica*) which is indistinguishable from secondary carcinoma (Fig. 32.34).

A short constricting lesion may be difficult to demonstrate due to overlapping loops of bowel, the colon proximal to the lesion often being distended.

Occasionally and especially with encephaloid tumours, *intussusception* may occur.

A predominantly ulcerating tumour is the most difficult to demonstrate radiologically since there is little soft tissue protrusion from the raised edge of the ulcer and the lesion usually shows only as a circular rim of barium coating the edge of the lesion: careful inspection, however, should reveal a circular shadow which cannot be accounted for by a normal anatomical structure.

Multiple (synchronous) carcinomas occur in 3–4% of cases, while, with a solitary carcinoma, one or more adenomatous polyps may be seen in the adjacent part of the bowel or elsewhere in the colon.

In recent years there have been a number of published reports of the occurrence of colonic cancer within the sigmoid colon many years after *ureterosigmoidostomy*.

Metastatic spread to the liver may be demonstrated by isotope, ultrasound or CT scans.

Differential diagnosis. Conditions to be considered are:

1. Secondary carcinoma
2. Local spread from a primary tumour elsewhere
3. Adhesions
4. Amoebiasis, tuberculosis and other inflammatory disorders
5. Spasm
6. Muscular hypertrophy in diverticular disease
7. Crohn's disease or ischaemic colitis.

Malignant deposits in the bowel may produce localized nodular defects in the wall of the colon, or, alternatively, may be extensive where infiltration of the wall produces long segment stricturing. An identical appearance can be

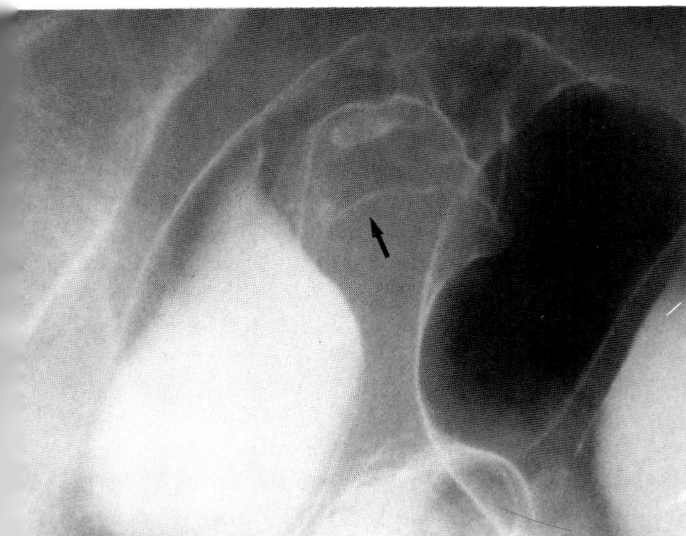

Fig. 32.30 A marginal or 'saddle' carcinoma arising anteriorly close to the rectosigmoid junction (arrow).

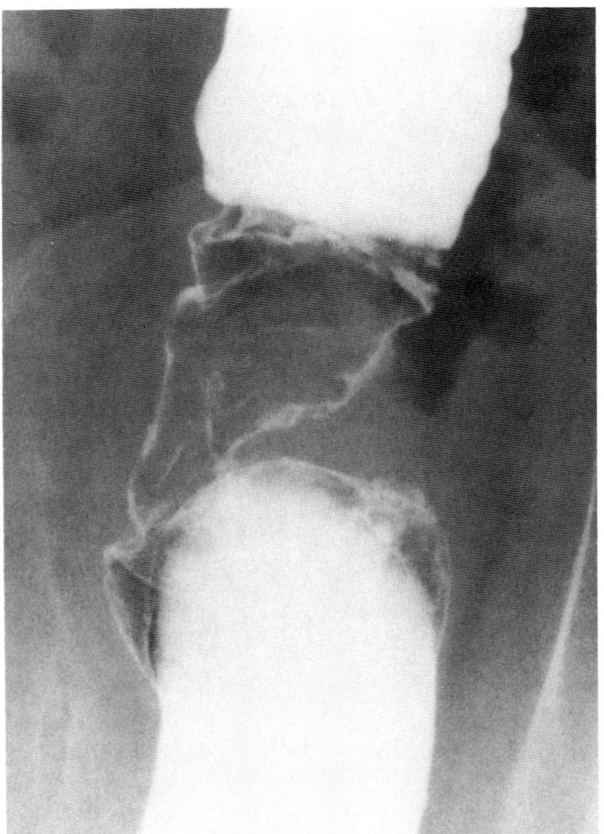

Fig. 32.31 Carcinoma of the descending colon showing an irregular filling defect, distal narrowing and loss of normal mucosa.

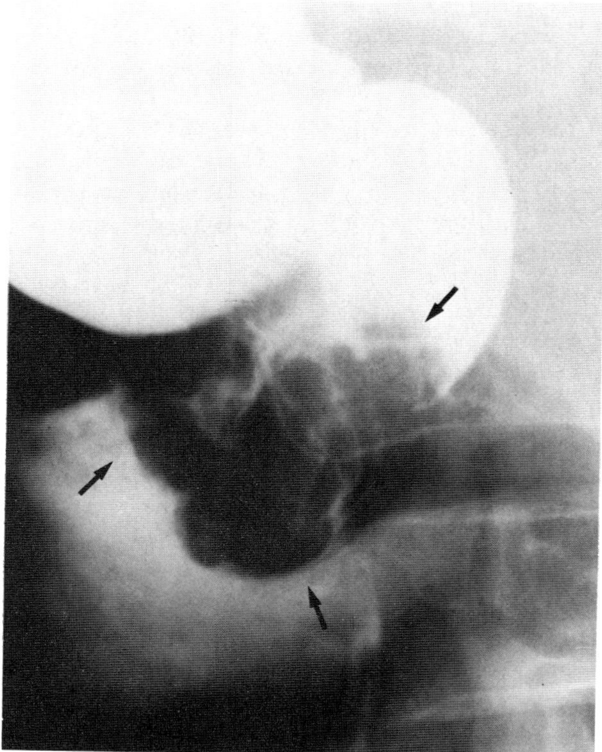

Fig. 32.32 A large proliferative carcinoma of the ascending colon (arrows).

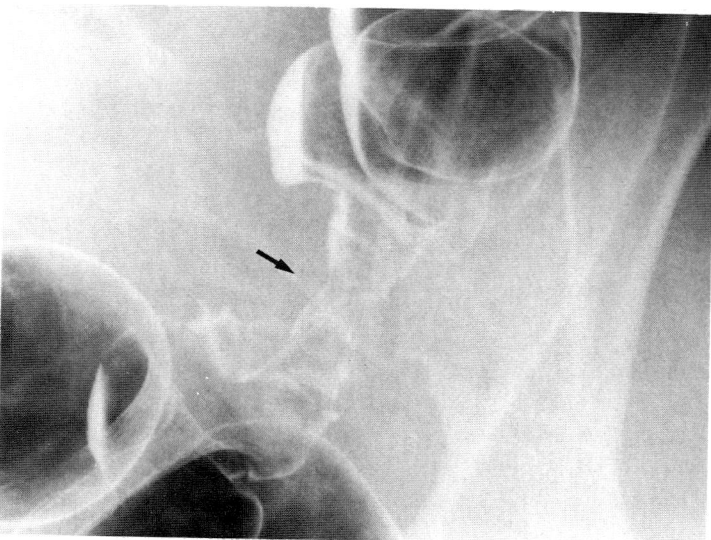

Fig. 32.33 A classical annular carcinoma (arrow).

produced by the unusual linitis plastica type of primary colonic tumour.

Local spread from an adjacent primary tumour is usually associated with a large extracolonic component; the mucosal folds become fixed and subsequently nodular defects and mucosal ulceration may be seen.

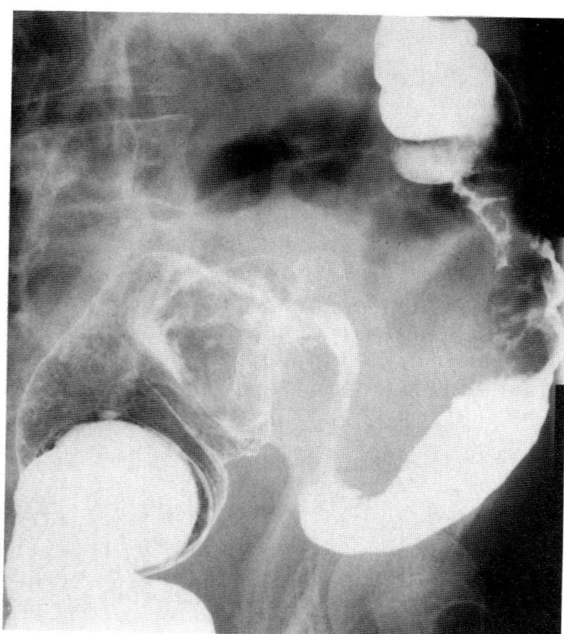

Fig. 32.34 Long segment narrowing from secondary carcinoma.

Adhesions may occur at any site but are particularly common around the transverse colon following cholecystitis or pancreatitis. The involved segment of colon becomes fixed and rigid and variable narrowing occurs, but the mucosa remains intact.

Carcinoma may mimic *amoebiasis* and *tuberculosis* but other features of these diseases usually aid in differentiation. Strictures in *schistosomiasis* and *lymphogranuloma venereum* are also as a rule readily distinguishable.

Local segmental spasm is common and produces an area of narrowing which may be remarkably constant but the mucosal pattern is always intact and traceable through the centre of the involved area.

Muscular hypertrophy in diverticular disease has already been discussed.

Both *Crohn's disease* and *ischaemic colitis* may produce narrowing over a variable length of the colon. The characteristic radiological signs of these conditions together with absence of the cardinal signs of malignancy usually allow ready differentiation, although secondary carcinoma can certainly at times resemble Crohn's disease quite closely.

Lymphoma. *Primary lymphoma* of the colon is rare, comprising less than 1% of malignant tumours of the large bowel. In this group the caecum and rectum are most frequently involved.

Secondary lymphoma of the colon in patients with known advanced lymphoma is more common although it must be noted that even in this group the stomach and small bowel are more often involved. With secondary disease the lesions are often widespread. The manifestations range from diffuse nodularity and mural infiltration to large polypoid masses indistinguishable from a carcinoma.

THE POSTOPERATIVE COLON

Growths of the caecum and ascending colon are treated by a standard *right hemicolectomy* with anastomosis of the ileum to the remaining transverse colon. More distal growths are treated by *resection with end-to-end anastomosis*.

Low rectal tumours which are unsuitable for an anterior resection with end-to-end anastomosis require an abdomino-perineal resection or a synchronous combined excision, with formation of a terminal colostomy. Radiology in these patients presents a difficult problem both in terms of bowel cleansing and because of absence of sphincteric control at the colostomy site. The technique of a colostomy enema has already been described.

Following resection of a segment of the colon, with end-to-end anastomosis, the site of anastomosis may not be detectable. Occasionally a degree of narrowing occurs with smooth funnelled ends. However, nodular, irregular or eccentric filling defects at the site of anastomosis raise the suspicion of tumour recurrence and require endoscopic examination with biopsy.

Investigation of a recent surgical anastomosis is undertaken with a Gastrografin enema (Gastrografin diluted 1 in 3 with water). Films are taken in the AP and lateral planes and leakage into the pericolic tissues or into a cavity is readily demonstrated.

RADIATION DAMAGE

About 10% of patients who have received 5000 rads or more of abdominal or pelvic irradiation develop gastrointestinal symptoms due to damage of either the small or large intestine. Symptoms, which may be early or delayed, consist of pain, diarrhoea and the passage of blood and mucus. Irradiation disease is primarily due to small vessel damage and obliteration, with secondary ischaemic fibrosis.

The radiological signs in the colon are those of *stricture* formation, usually over a relatively long segment with tapering ends; a degree of ulceration or fissuring may be seen. The rectosigmoid region and sigmoid colon are commonly involved and the diagnosis is usually readily made from the site and features of the lesion and the appropriate history.

THE RECTUM

Although the rectum is readily available to endoscopic examination by proctoscopy and sigmoidoscopy, radiology is an important complementary investigation. For this reason the rectum is always included on the standard double contrast barium enema films. The *lateral* view of the rectum is particularly important for the detection of tumours around the rectosigmoid junction.

Haemorrhoids are of no direct concern to the radiologist but it should be noted that internal haemorrhoids not infrequently produce polypoid filling defects in the distal rectum extending to the anal margin. *Polyps, carcinoma* and *inflammatory lesions* in the rectum are common and do not differ in appearances from similar lesions elsewhere in the colon.

CT scanning is of particular value in the diagnosis of tumour recurrence following previous excision of a rectal carcinoma by abdominoperineal resection or synchronous combined excision. Regrowth of tumour shows on CT as a rounded soft tissue mass which is usually homogeneous but which sometimes undergoes central necrosis with a low density centre (Fig. 32.35). Differentiation must be made from an abscess, loops of small bowel, postoperative granulation and fibrous tissue and resited pelvic organs.

The presacral space. The posterior peritoneal reflection usually lies at the pelvic brim. Occasionally the reflection is sited at a lower level, resulting in a forward sweep of the upper rectum and a corresponding increase in the width of the upper part of the presacral space.

In the majority of subjects the whole of the rectum is closely applied to the anterior wall of the sacrum. Enlargement of this space above a width of 1 cm is most often due to a normal anatomical variant. The commonest pathological cause of widening is inflammatory proctitis, especially in ulcerative colitis. In this disease the space may widen in relapse and return to normal size on remission, although more often enlargement is seen to persist. Other inflammatory causes include Crohn's disease, ischaemia and tuberculosis.

Additional causes of widening of the presacral space include rectal carcinoma, prostatic carcinoma, tumours within the space itself which are commonly developmental in origin, particularly dermoid cysts, and primary and secondary bone tumours.

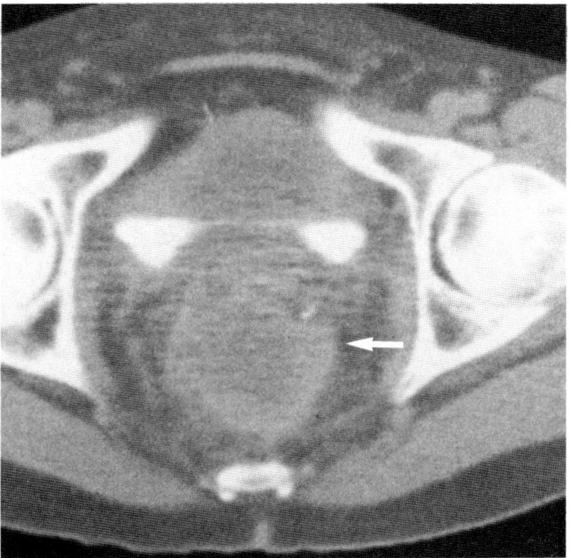

Fig. 32.35 CT demonstration of recurrent rectal tumour (arrow) following previous AP resection.

Anterior compression of the rectosigmoid region may be produced by large pelvic masses, commonly ovarian or occasionally uterine tumours.

Endometriosis not infrequently produces an anterior indentation on the bowel wall at the rectosigmoid junction and a similar deformity may be seen with secondary deposits in the pouch of Douglas. Endometriosis elsewhere in the colon produces an area of narrowing with an intact mucosa.

Pelvic lipomatosis is a rare benign disorder characterized by an overgrowth of fatty tissue in the pelvis. This can produce elongation of the rectosigmoid which is straightened and narrowed. The bladder is also elevated and compressed (pear-shaped bladder). The excess of fatty tissue causes increased radiolucency in the pelvis, and shows a characteristic appearance at CT.

REFERENCES AND SUGGESTIONS FOR FURTHER READING

Bartram, C. I. (1977) Radiology in the current assessment of ulcerative colitis. *Gastrointestinal Radiology*, **1**: 383–392

Bartram, C. I., & Hale, J. E. (1970) Radiological diagnosis of recurrent carcinoma at the anastomosis. *Gut*, **11**: 778–781

Bresnihan, E. R., & Simpkins, K. C. (1975) Villous adenoma of the large bowel; benign and malignant. *British Journal of Radiology*, **48**: 801–806

Bussey, H. J. R. (1975) *Familial Polyposis Coli*: family studies, histopathology, differential diagnosis and results of treatment. Baltimore: Johns Hopkins Press

Caserella, W. J., Kantor, I. E., & Seaman, W. B. (1972) Right-sided colonic diverticula as a cause of acute rectal haemorrhage. *New England Journal of Medicine*, **286**: 450–453

Cremin, B. J. (1971) Radiological assessment of anorectal anomalies. *Clinical Radiology*, **22**: 239–250

Dodds, W. J. (1976) Clinical and roentgen features of the intestinal polyposis syndromes. *Gastrointestinal Radiology*, **1**: 127–142

Fork, F. T. (1981) Double contrast enema and colonoscopy in polyp detection. *Gut*, **22**: 971–977

Fraser, G. M., & Findley, J. M. (1976) The double contrast enema in ulcerative and Crohn's colitis. *Clinical Radiology*, **27**: 103–112

Gohel, V. K., Kressel, H. Y., & Laufer, I. (1978) Double contrast artefacts. *Gastrointestinal Radiology*, **3**: 139–146

Laufer, I. (1979) *Double Contrast Gastrointestinal Radiology with Endoscopic Correlation*. London: Saunders

Laufer, I. Mullens, J. E., & Hamilton, J. (1976) Correlation of endoscopy and double contrast radiography in the early stages of ulcerative and granulomatous colitis. *Radiology*, **118**: 1–5

Lennard-Jones, J. E., Lockhart-Mummery, H. E., & Morson, B. C. (1968) Clinical and pathological differentiation of Crohn's disease and proctocolitis. *Gastroenterology*, **54**: 1162–1170

Marshak, R. H., Lindner, A. E., & Maklansky, D. (1977) Pneumatosis cystoides coli. *Gastrointestinal Radiology*, **2**: 85–89

Meyers, M. A., Alonso, D. R. & Baer, J. W. (1976) Pathogenesis of massively bleeding colonic diverticulosis: new observations. *American Journal of Roentgenology*, **127**: 901–908

Morson, B. C. (1963) The muscle abnormality in diverticular disease of the sigmoid colon. *British Journal of Radiology*, **36**: 385–392

Muto, T., Bussey, H. J. R., & Morson, B. C. (1975) The evolution of cancer of the colon and rectum. *Cancer*, **36**: 6, 2251–2270

Narasimharao, K. L., Prasad, G. R., Katariya, S., Yadav, K., Mitra, S. K., & Pathak, I. C. (1983) Prone cross-table lateral view: an alternative to the invertogram in imperforate anus. *American Journal of Roentgenology*, **140**: 227–229

O'Connell, D. J., & Thompson, A. J. (1978) Lymphoma of the colon — the spectrum of radiological changes. *Gastrointestinal Radiology*, **2**(4): 377–387

Parsa, F., Gordon, H. E., & Wilson, S. E. (1975) Bleeding diverticulosis of the colon: a review of 83 cases. *Diseases of the Colon and Rectum*, **18**(1): 37–41

Reuter, S. R., & Redman, H. C. (1977) *Gastrointestinal Angiography*. Philadelphia: W. B. Saunders Co.

Seminars in Roentgenology (1976) **2**: 1–137. Seven articles dealing with colonic lesions.

Simpkins, K. C., & Stevenson, G. W. (1972) The modified Malmo double contrast barium enema in colitis. An assessment of its accuracy in reflecting sigmoidoscopic findings. *British Journal of Radiology*, **45**: 486–492

Simpkins, K. C., & Young, A. C. (1971) The differential diagnosis of large bowel strictures. *Clinical Radiology*, **22**: 449–457

Teplick, S. K., Stark, P., Clark, R. E., Metz, J. R., & Shapiro, J. H. (1978) The retrorectal space. *Clinical Radiology*, **29**: 177–184

Thomas, B. M. (1979) The 'instant enema' in inflammatory disease of the colon. *Clinical Radiology*, **30**, 165–173

Werbeloff, L., Novis, B. H., Bank, S., & Marks, I. N. (1973) The radiology of tuberculosis of the gastrointestinal tract. *British Journal of Radiology*, **46**: 329–336

Williams, I. (1963) Changing emphasis in diverticular disease of the colon. *British Journal of Radiology*, **36**: 393–406

Williams, I. (1965) Mucosa innominate grooves in the surface of the colonic mucosa. *Radiology*, **84**: 877–880

CHAPTER 33

THE ACUTE ABDOMEN

Patients with an acute abdomen comprise the largest group of people presenting as a general surgical emergency. Following the history and clinical examination, plain film radiographs have traditionally been one of the first and most useful methods of further investigation. In spite of the recent increase in other imaging techniques, plain films still retain this position as one of the most useful initial investigations.

In most acute abdominal conditions, the radiological diagnosis depends on *gas patterns*; for example the distribution of gas in dilated and non-dilated bowel and the presence of gas inside or outside the bowel lumen. Plain films are likely to remain the best method of imaging these gas shadows for many years to come and *isotope studies*, *computed tomography* and *nuclear magnetic resonance*, are unlikely to play any major role in the initial investigation of the acute abdomen.

In certain specific conditions, however, where gas shadows play a relatively minor role, for example leaking abdominal aortic aneurysm or acute cholecystitis, *ultrasound* has become the imaging technique of choice. However the presence of moderate or large amounts of intra-abdominal gas, which acts as a barrier to ultrasound waves, can make the ultrasound examination of an acute abdomen difficult or sometimes impossible.

Interpretation of plain films in the acute abdomen may present a formidable challenge to the radiologist for, while in many cases a specific diagnosis can be made, not infrequently the appearances are non-specific or even positively misleading and further investigations using contrast media, ultrasound or isotopes may be required. When the radiological diagnosis is specific or supports the clinical findings, surgery is often indicated without further investigation. However, if there are clinical signs to indicate that surgery should be performed, negative or equivocal radiology should be ignored.

The radiologist has one major role, to help the surgeon decide whether or not a patient with acute abdominal pain needs to have an operation. He should then try and indicate to his surgical colleague whether the operation should be performed immediately or whether time can be spent in resuscitating the patient or undergoing further investigation.

It is often of value to initially view the radiographs in the absence of any clinical information. In this way an objective evaluation of the radiological signs can be made and a full differential diagnosis considered without being biased by the clinical findings. It is absolutely essential, however, that before a final opinion is given, the radiologist should be aware of the full clinical history so that minor abnormalities are not overlooked or the wrong interpretation placed on certain signs.

RADIOGRAPHIC TECHNIQUE

A supine abdomen and an erect chest can be regarded as the basic standard radiographs. A horizontal ray abdominal radiograph, either erect or left lateral decubitus, is frequently taken to add more information and to demonstrate fluid levels.

The clinical condition of the patient will determine whether he can sit or stand for the erect radiograph. Sometimes it is only possible to obtain a lateral decubitus or even a supine radiograph with a horizontal ray in patients who are too ill to be moved. It is essential that patients should be in position for 10 minutes prior to the horizontal ray radiograph to allow free gas time to rise to the highest point. Wherever possible, the bladder should be emptied prior to the supine radiograph and this should always include the area from the diaphragm to the hernial orifices.

Chest X-ray

A chest radiograph can be regarded as an essential examination for any patient presenting with an acute abdomen. The reasons are as follows:

1. The erect chest is the best radiograph to show the presence of a small pneumoperitoneum, particularly on the right side between the liver and the diaphragm. It is superior to the erect abdominal film because in the latter the divergent X-ray beam penetrates the gas at the top of the diaphragm obliquely and this area is also relatively dark

due to overexposure. In the erect chest film however, the top of the diaphragm and the gas beneath are penetrated almost tangentially by the X-ray beam, and the exposure of the diaphragm is optimal to show small amounts of gas.

2. A number of chest conditions may present as acute abdominal pain and mimic an acute abdomen exactly (Table 33.1). They may be suspected on the chest radiograph.

Table 33.1 Chest conditions which may mimic an acute abdomen

Pneumonia — particularly lower lobe
Myocardial infarction
Pulmonary infarction
Congestive cardiac failure
Pericarditis
Leaking or dissecting thoracic aortic aneurysm

3. Acute abdominal conditions may be complicated by chest pathology. For example, pleural effusions frequently complicate acute pancreatitis, elderly patients may have heart failure, or aspiration pneumonia may follow prolonged vomiting in intestinal obstruction.

4. Even when the chest radiograph is normal it acts as a most valuable baseline. Postoperative chest complications and subphrenic abscesses are relatively common following emergency surgery for an acute abdomen. A previously normal film may allow subtle new changes to be detected, and so enable an early diagnosis of complications to be made.

ABDOMINAL RADIOGRAPHS

The *supine abdominal radiograph* is probably the single most useful film. It allows the distribution of gas and the calibre of bowel to be determined and may show displacement of bowel by soft tissue masses. Furthermore obliteration of fat lines normally visualized, for example psoas outlines, may indicate fluid or inflammatory exudate in these regions.

Traditionally an erect abdominal radiograph is taken 'to show fluid levels and free gas'. As discussed already, the *erect chest radiograph* is superior to the erect abdominal film for the demonstration of a pneumoperitoneum. Furthermore, the presence of fluid levels in bowel rarely contributes to the overall diagnosis in an acute abdomen. This is because there are numerous causes of small bowel fluid levels and the number, distribution and length will not usually help to distinguish between the two commonest causes, obstruction and paralytic ileus or any of the others (Table 33.2). Gammill and Nice (1972) have demonstrated that small numbers of short fluid levels are present frequently and sometimes as many as 26 fluid levels up to 10 cm in length may be seen in normal patients. However, although most of these fluid levels lie within the colon, they may be difficult to differentiate from small bowel fluid levels. They also concluded that three or more *small bowel* fluid levels greater than 2.5 cm in length were abnormal, and indicated dilated small bowel with stasis.

Table 33.2 Some of the variety of causes of small bowel fluid levels

Small bowel obstruction
Large bowel obstruction
Paralytic ileus
Gastroenteritis
Mesenteric thrombosis
Jejunal diverticulosis
Uraemia
Hypokalaemia
Cleansing enemas
Congestive cardiac failure
Serosal metastases
Normal

Horizontal ray films, either *erect* or *lateral decubitus*, by allowing redistribution of gas within distended bowel, may enable its exact location and identity to be determined. If gas shadows are demonstrated which are suspected as lying outside the bowel, then horizontal ray films in this situation are often particularly helpful by demonstrating that air/fluid levels lie within a confined space and are thus likely to represent an abscess cavity.

A left lateral decubitus abdominal radiograph is one taken with the patient lying on their left side but with the X-ray beam horizontal. In patients who are unfit to sit or stand for an erect film, it is the projection of choice to show a small pneumoperitoneum. Miller and Nelson (1971) have suggested that it should be the first film taken when searching for a pneumoperitoneum. In this projection, free gas may be trapped between the edge of the liver and the lateral abdominal wall or sometimes over the pelvis when this is the highest point, which is more likely to occur in females. In this position, air will preferentially leave a perforated duodenal or antral ulcer while fluid is more likely to leak when the patient is erect. Furthermore, if air is present in the lesser sac of the peritoneum following a perforated posterior gastric ulcer, it will enter the main abdominal cavity and be more readily identified. A gas-filled dilated duodenal loop, one of the commonest signs of acute pancreatitis, is best shown in this projection.

A lateral abdominal view may demonstrate calcification in an aortic aneurysm which has not been detected on the supine view and this projection should always be taken if the diagnosis is suspected, and ultrasound is not available.

It has been suggested that as many as six standard films are the minimum requirement for an acute abdomen (Miller 1973). However, there is considerable merit and saving in time and film costs in taking an erect chest and a supine abdominal radiograph and only proceeding if these films do not confirm the clinical diagnosis or if abnormalities are detected which need further elucidation.

To obtain good radiographic contrast between the water density of the soft tissues and the relative transradiancy of fat, the kilovoltage used should be kept low, ideally in the range 60–65 kV, and the output of the set must be sufficient to keep the exposure time short. Blurring, due to even slight respiratory movement, may obscure details of fat lines, small gas bubbles and calcification.

NORMAL APPEARANCES

Organ identification on plain radiographs depends on anatomical position, helped by the tissue/fat interface, and the presence of gas, fluid or food residue within the bowel.

Relatively large amounts of gas are usually present in the stomach, which can be identified by its position and the gastric rugae on supine radiographs, and it is common to see a long air/fluid level in the stomach when erect. The duodenal cap is often gas filled and frequently contains a fluid level on erect films.

Small bowel gas is extremely variable; usually relatively small amounts of gas are present and insufficient for more than a short length to be demonstrated. Sometimes, however, with air swallowing, such as is seen in breathless patients or those with abdominal pain, sufficient air may be swallowed for longer lengths of small bowel to be outlined and the valvulae conniventes identified (Fig. 33.1). However, in the non-obstructed patient it is rare to see the thin bands of valvulae conniventes stretching over more than a short segment of small bowel. Fluid is a normal constituent of small bowel, and short fluid levels are not abnormal. A small bowel calibre exceeding 2.5 cm is abnormal and indicates dilated small bowel.

Enough gas is usually present in the colon for it to be readily identified by its haustra and position. However, the calibre of the colon is more extremely variable than any other viscus and no satisfactory measurement of the upper limit of normal diameter is possible. Old, mentally subnormal, psychiatric or institutionalized patients may have enormous colons measuring 10–15 cm in diameter and yet apparently be without symptoms. Their colonic diameters frequently exceed those of younger patients with clear-cut large bowel obstruction. In inflammatory bowel disease, however, a transverse colonic diameter exceeding 5.5 cm has been suggested as the upper limit of normal and above this megacolon should be diagnosed. In patients with large bowel obstruction, a transverse caecal diameter exceeding 9 cm is the level above which a state of 'impending perforation' exists.

Colonic fluid levels are a normal finding, and some several centimetres in length may be seen. 18% of normal people also have a caecal fluid level.

Most of the gas in the bowel has been swallowed and it normally reaches the colon within 30 minutes (Magnusson 1931). People in severe pain, or when respiration is laboured such as in pneumonia or asthma, increase the amount of air swallowed, often producing a dramatic plain abdominal radiograph. The gas-filled, slightly dilated loops of bowel so produced contain relatively little fluid; the term *meteorism* is applied to this appearance. It is sometimes difficult to distinguish meteorism produced, for example, by renal colic, from intestinal obstruction. A clinical history and examination frequently allow the correct interpretation of the radiological findings to be made.

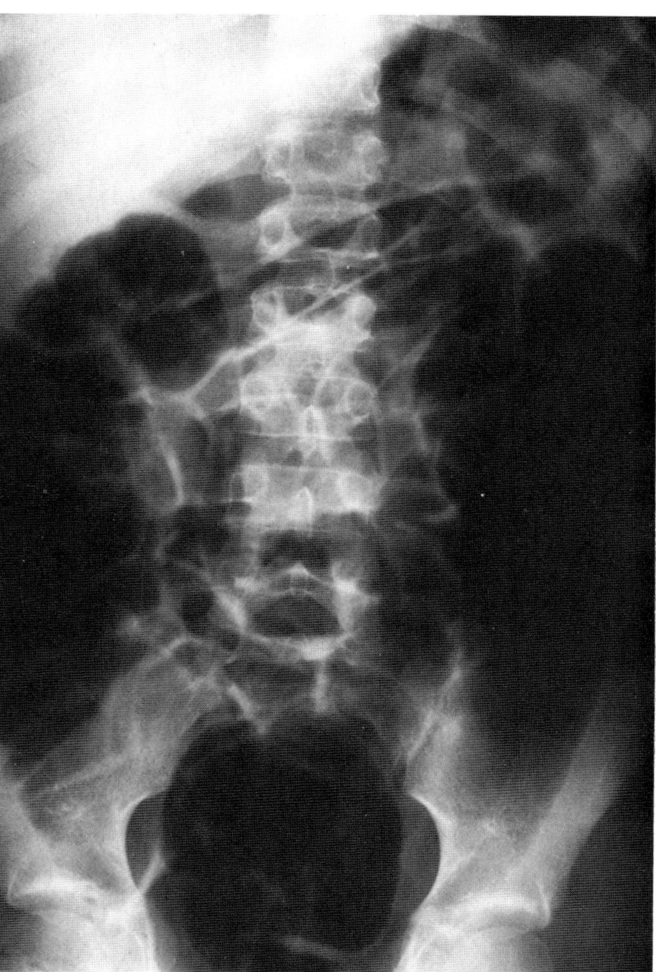

Fig. 33.1 Air swallowing. There is slight gaseous distension of both small and large bowel, but this extends down to the rectum. A 7-year-old girl admitted to hospital with abdominal pain and distension following a single episode of vomiting. At the time of admission she was noted to be distressed and crying. Shortly after admission her bowels were opened normally and the abdominal distension and pain disappeared.

The posterior extraperitoneal fat pad which completely surrounds the kidneys, psoas muscles and the posterior borders of the liver and spleen, extends anteriorly and laterally to surround the parietal peritoneum and so is also intimately related to intraperitoneal organs. The fat lines produced are responsible for the visualization of most of these intra-abdominal organs. These fat lines can be displaced by organ enlargement and may be blurred or effaced by inflammation or fluid. However, visualization of these structures by fat lines is not universal. The right psoas outline is blurred in 19% of normals and the lower border of the spleen can only be visualized in 58% of normal people. This is particularly important in children, where loss of the psoas outlines occurred in 52% and loss of the properitoneal fat lines in 18% of normals (Bakhda & McNair 1977). These factors must therefore be considered carefully before undue emphasis is placed on these signs in the abnormal patient.

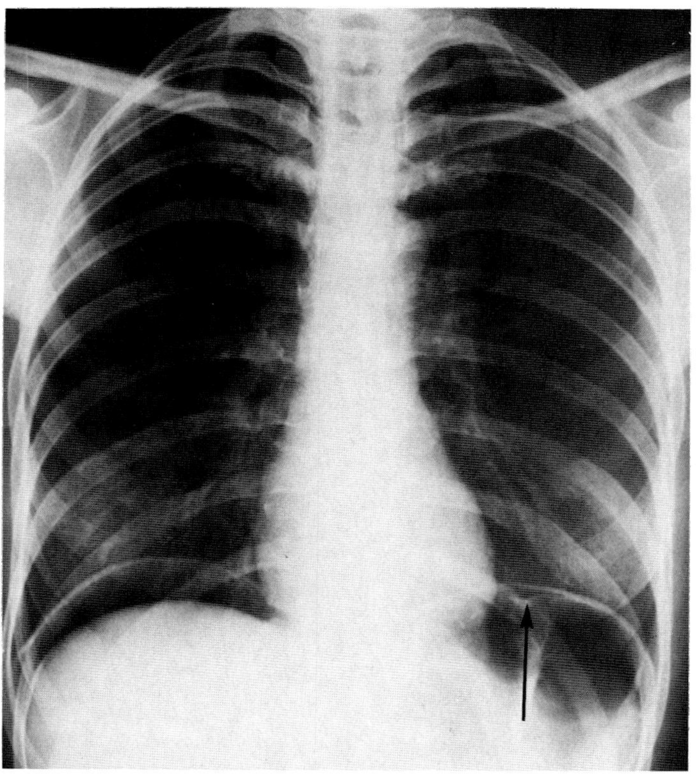

Fig. 33.2 Pneumoperitoneum. Erect chest. Free intra-abdominal gas is clearly demonstrated under the right hemidiaphragm. Under the left hemidiaphragm a small triangular collection of free gas can be identified between loops of gas-filled bowel (↑).

PNEUMOPERITONEUM

The demonstration of a small pneumoperitoneum in a patient presenting with acute abdominal pain is one of the most significant signs in medicine. In over 90% of cases the cause of the pneumoperitoneum will require emergency surgery.

Miller and Nelson (1971), in experiments on themselves, have demonstrated that it is possible, by careful radiographic technique, to demonstrate as little as 1 ml of free gas on *erect chest* or *left lateral decubitus* abdominal films. However, radiographic technique and positioning are important and a patient should be in position for 10 minutes prior to the film being taken for it takes this time for free gas to rise to the highest point in the abdomen (Figs 33.2, 33.3).

The demonstration of a pneumoperitoneum following a perforated viscus, is, however, not invariable and most series show that only 75–80% of perforations will show demonstrable free gas. A number of reasons for this have been suggested, including sealing of the perforation, lack of gas at the site of perforation, or adhesions around the site of the perforation. However, radiographic technique is also important and Williams and Hartzell (1940) demonstrated that a pneumoperitoneum could be detected in 76% of cases using an erect film only, but when a left lateral decubitus projection was included, a pneumoperitoneum was demonstrated in nearly 90% of cases.

If a perforated viscus is suspected, then a horizontal ray radiograph, either in an erect chest or decubitus abdomen, is mandatory. However, in many patients, particularly following trauma, the elderly or critically ill, and those who are unconscious, perforation may be clinically silent or is overshadowed by another serious medical or surgical condition. A supine, abdominal radiograph, frequently taken using a mobile unit, may be the only radiograph that has been obtained. It is therefore important to recognize the signs of pneumoperitoneum on these.

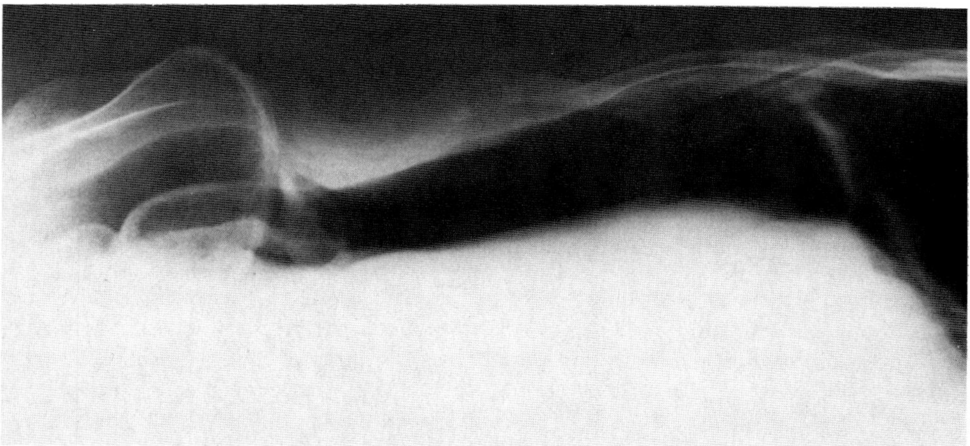

Fig. 33.3 Pneumoperitoneum. Left lateral decubitus abdominal film. A large collection of free intra-abdominal gas is demonstrated between the liver and the lateral abdominal wall.

About 56% of patients with a pneumoperitoneum may have free gas detectable on a supine radiograph (Menuck & Siemers 1976). Almost half the patients will have a collection in the right upper quadrant adjacent to the liver and lying mainly in the subhepatic space and the hepatorenal fossa (Morrison's pouch), and visible as an oval or linear collection of gas (Fig. 33.4). Visualization of the inner as well as the outer wall of a loop of bowel, Rigler's sign (1941), is a valuable indication of a pneumoperitoneum (Fig. 33.5). However, De Lacey and others (1977) have pointed out that this sign may be misleading by the apposition of gas-distended loops of bowel with apparent visualization of outer and inner walls, when in fact the inner walls of two loops of bowel are seen. Small triangular collections of gas between loops of bowel may sometimes be identified and are a valuable sign of pneumoperitoneum in supine radiographs.

Reflections of the peritoneum normally present on the inner surface of the anterior abdominal wall and are not usually identified, but may be visualized by free gas when it lies on either side. Thus the falciform ligament (Fig. 33.6), umbilical ligaments and the urachus can occasionally be identified when relatively large amounts of gas are present.

Relatively large amounts of gas may accumulate beneath the diaphragm (the '*cupola sign*') or in the centre of the abdomen over a fluid collection (the '*football sign*').

PSEUDOPNEUMOPERITONEUM

A number of conditions have been described which simulate free air in the peritoneal cavity — pseudopneumoperitoneum (Table 33.3). These are important because failing to recognize them may lead to an unnecessary laparotomy in search of a perforated viscus. One of the commonest of these is distended bowel, usually hepatic flexure of the colon, interposed between the liver and the diaphragm — Chilaiditi's syndrome (1910). Although this is relatively uncommon in Western countries, it is more often seen in Iran, pregnant women, chronic lung disease and patients

Table 33.3 Causes of pseudopneumoperitoneum

Chilaiditi's syndrome
Subdiaphragmatic fat
Curvilinear pulmonary collapse
Uneven diaphragm
Distended viscus
Omental fat
Subphrenic abscess

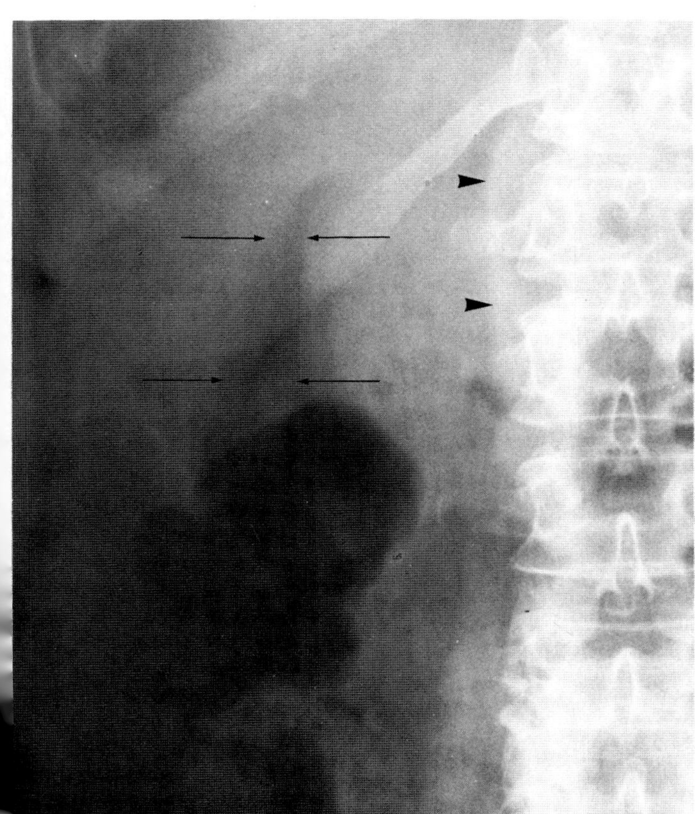

Fig. 33.4 Pneumoperitoneum. Abdomen supine. A triangular collection of free gas is demonstrated in the subhepatic region (→←). The falciform ligament is also outlined (►).

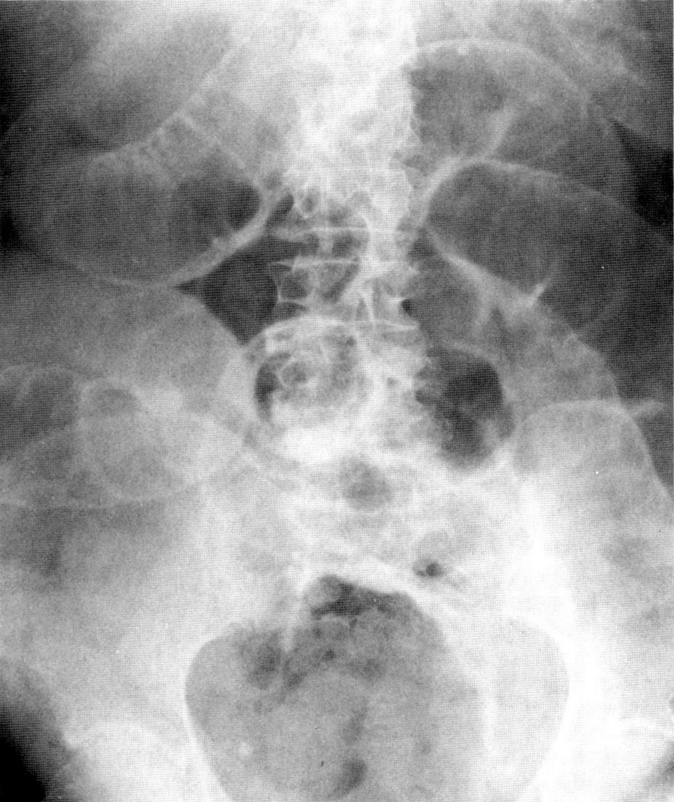

Fig. 33.5 Pneumoperitoneum. Abdomen supine. Visualization of both sides of the bowel wall (Rigler's sign). Both the inside and outside wall of multiple loops of small bowel can clearly be identified.

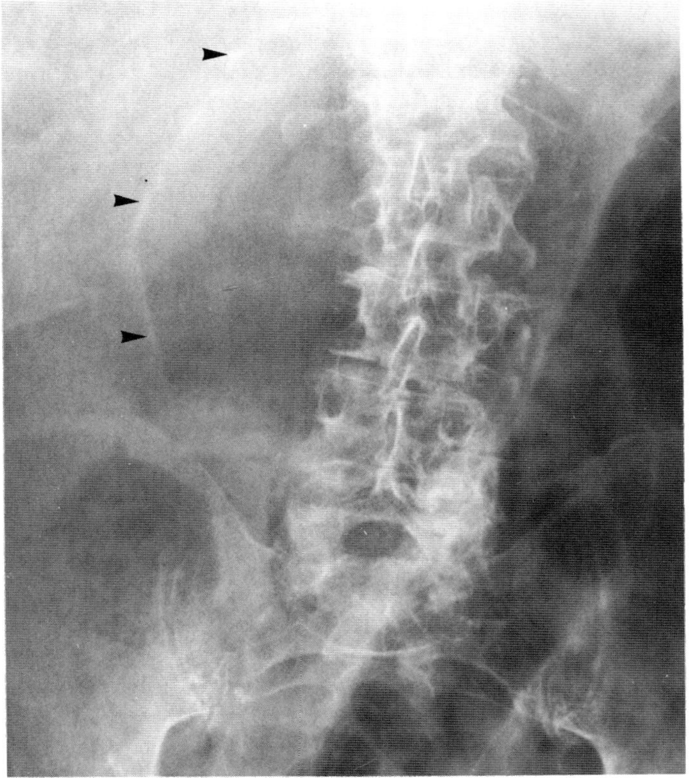

Fig. 33.6 Pneumoperitoneum. Abdomen supine. Visualization of the falciform ligament is caused by free gas lying on either side of it (▶).

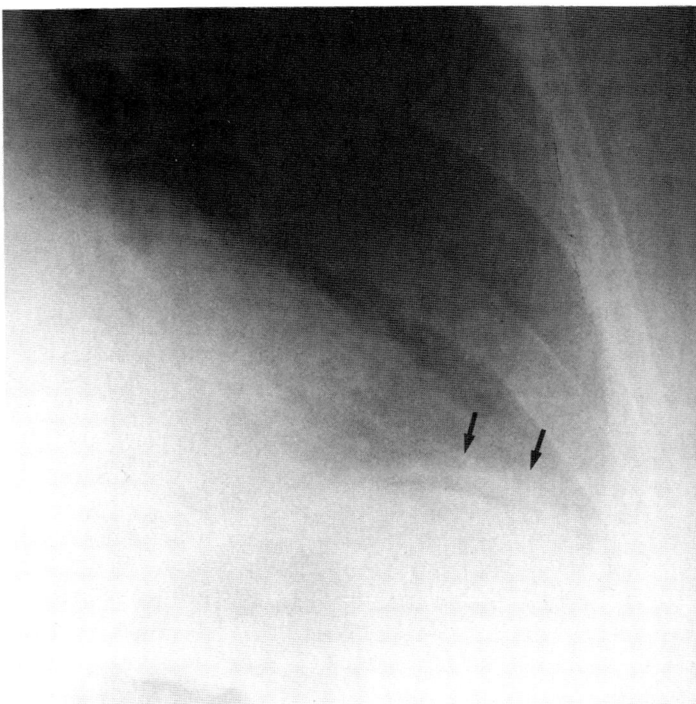

Fig. 33.7 Pseudopneumoperitoneum. A band of curvilinear pulmonary collapse with a crescent of normal lung beneath it simulates a pneumoperitoneum almost exactly.

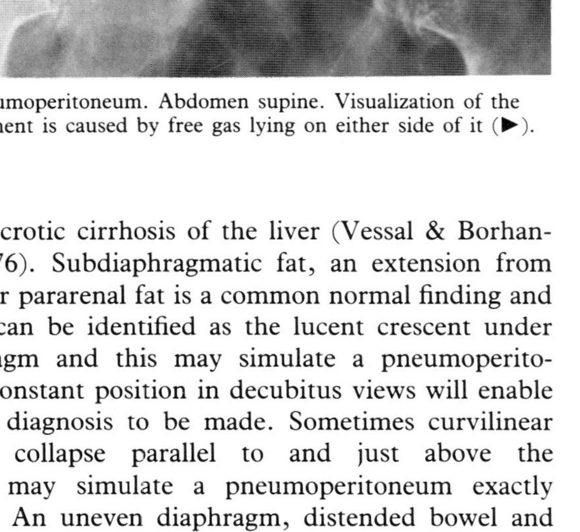

with postnecrotic cirrhosis of the liver (Vessal & Borhanmanesh 1976). Subdiaphragmatic fat, an extension from the posterior pararenal fat is a common normal finding and frequently can be identified as the lucent crescent under the diaphragm and this may simulate a pneumoperitoneum. Its constant position in decubitus views will enable the correct diagnosis to be made. Sometimes curvilinear pulmonary collapse parallel to and just above the diaphragm may simulate a pneumoperitoneum exactly (Fig. 33.7). An uneven diaphragm, distended bowel and omental fat between the liver and the diaphragm may also simulate free gas on occasions.

PNEUMOPERITONEUM WITHOUT PERITONITIS

Occasionally, asymptomatic patients or those with very minimal signs and symptoms, are found to have a pneumoperitoneum. The largest group of these patients will subsequently be found to have perforated an ulcer which has sealed itself, or are those in whom the signs of peritonitis have not yet developed. Numerous other conditions which may produce a spontaneous pneumoperitoneum without peritonitis have been described. They are summarized in Table 33.4, and have been reviewed by Felson and Wiot (1973) (Fig. 33.8).

Table 33.4 Causes of a pneumoperitoneum without peritonitis

Silent perforation of a viscus:
Which has sealed
Related to steroid therapy
In the elderly
In coma
In the presence of other serious medical conditions
Postoperative
Peritoneal dialysis
Perforated jejunal diverticulosis
Intra-abdominal therapeutic embolization
Leakage through distended bowel (e.g. stomach at endoscopy)
Entry through the female genital tract
Associated chest conditions:
Pneumonia
Emphysema
Carcinoma of the lung
Pneumomediastinum
Intermittent positive pressure ventilation

POSTOPERATIVE PNEUMOPERITONEUM

About 60% of all postlaparotomy patients will have evidence of a pneumoperitoneum. Although, in most patients, the air will have been absorbed within a few days, it has been reported that it may take up to 24 days before

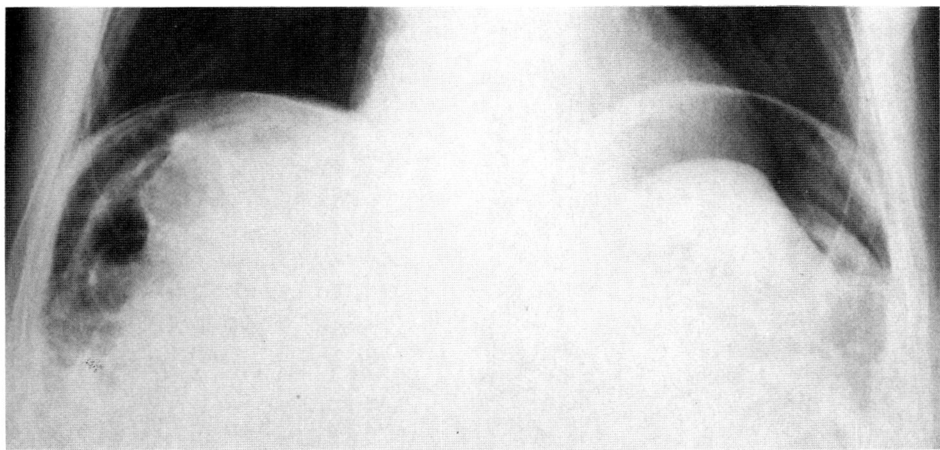

Fig. 33.8 Pneumoperitoneum without peritonitis. Small bowel pneumatosis. Free gas is readily identified under the left hemidiaphragm and there is a thin crescent of gas under the right hemidiaphragm. The typical cysts of pneumatosis can be identified in the small bowel under the right hemidiaphragm. A 69-year-old man admitted with haematemesis. (Courtesy Dr A.R. Carter.)

all the air has disappeared. A pneumoperitoneum occurs in the postoperative period more commonly in thin patients than in obese ones, and the rate of absorption is faster in the obese — in these, the air has usually all been absorbed by the third postoperative day. Providing identical radiographic technique is used, and adequate time spent in positioning the horizontal ray radiograph, any increase in the volume of gas postoperatively indicates an anastomotic leak or a perforation.

USE OF CONTRAST MEDIA IN SUSPECTED PERFORATION

If a patient with severe upper abdominal pain has equivocal clinical signs and no free gas on plain films, further investigations may be needed to exclude a perforation. A nasogastric tube is normally in position and 100 ml of air can be injected down the tube and a further film taken after the patient has been lying in the left lateral decubitus position for 10 minutes. More than 80% of perforations occur in the duodenum or pyloric antrum and this technique will facilitate the passage of air into the peritoneal cavity. Alternatively, 50 ml of Gastrografin can be given orally, the patient placed on their right side and a further abdominal film taken after 5 minutes. A leak of Gastrografin may occur in ulcers which have perforated but which do not show free gas. Furthermore, an oedematous stretched duodenal loop may be seen in patients with acute pancreatitis.

INTESTINAL OBSTRUCTION

Dilatation of bowel occurs in mechanical intestinal obstruction, pseudo-obstruction, paralytic ileus, air swallowing and several other conditions. The radiological differentiation depends mainly on the size, mucosal appearance, and the distribution of the loops of bowel. The diagnosis of intestinal obstruction depends on the demonstration of dilated loops of bowel proximally with non-dilated or collapsed bowel distal to the presumed point of obstruction.

GASTRIC DILATATION

Dilatation of the stomach can be caused by four main groups of conditions; mechanical gastric outlet obstruction, paralytic ileus, gastric volvulus and air swallowing. These are summarized in Table 33.5.

Table 33.5 Causes of a massively dilated stomach

Paralytic ileus:
Postoperative
Trauma
Peritonitis
Pancreatitis
Cholecystitis
Diabetic coma
Hepatic coma
Mechanical gastric outlet obstruction:
Duodenal ulceration
Antral carcinoma
Extrinsic duodenal compression
Gastric volvulus
Air swallowing. Intubation
Secondary to intestinal obstruction
Drugs

The '*paralytic ileus*' group of conditions is frequently referred to as '*acute gastric dilatation*', often occurs in old people and is associated with considerable fluid and electrolyte disturbance and as a result carries a high mortality (Fig. 33.9).

Mechanical gastric outlet obstruction, caused by peptic ulceration or a carcinoma of the pyloric antrum, often leads

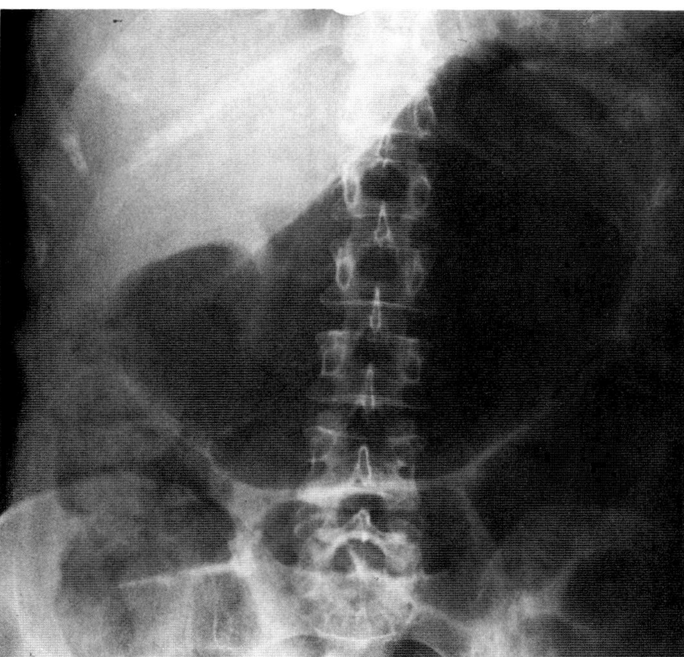

Fig. 33.9 Acute gastric dilatation. Abdomen supine. A 38-year-old woman admitted in diabetic precoma.

to a massive fluid-filled stomach which occupies most of the upper abdomen and is demonstrable as a large soft tissue mass with little or no bowel gas beyond. Fortunately, a little gas is usually present within the stomach and this can be identified on horizontal ray films, which allows the organ to be identified.

Volvulus of the stomach is a relatively uncommon condition and may result from the stomach twisting around the longitudinal or mesenteric axis. In a gastric volvulus the dilated stomach usually contains both air and fluid, is identified as a spherical viscus, displaced upwards and to the left, and is associated with elevation of the left hemidiaphragm. It is usual for the small bowel to be collapsed and it is uncommon to see any gas shadows beyond the stomach. It is important to differentiate a volvulus of the stomach from a caecal volvulus; both may produce a distended viscus containing fluid and air lying beneath the left hemidiaphragm. If barium is given in a suspected gastric volvulus, there may be complete obstruction at the lower end of the oesophagus, or if barium does enter the stomach, it may not pass beyond the obstructed pylorus.

Frequently after resuscitation and *intubation* large amounts of gas enter the stomach and may lead to massive dilatation. This may sometimes occur after *air swallowing* alone, for example, in hysteria or in near drowning.

When supine, the gas-filled stomach can usually be identified with the wall of the greater curvature convex caudally and the pyloric antrum pointing cranially. It is very important to differentiate a distended stomach from a caecal volvulus, which may also be positioned beneath an elevated left hemidiaphragm as noted above. However, with caecal volvulus, one or two haustra can frequently be identified and the inferior part of the caecum usually points caudally.

THE DISTINCTION BETWEEN SMALL AND LARGE BOWEL DILATATION

When a radiograph shows dilated bowel it is important to try to determine whether it is small or large bowel, or both. Useful differentiating features depend on the size, distribution and markings of the loops and are summarized in Table 33.6.

Table 33.6 The distinction between small and large bowel dilatation

	Small bowel	Large bowel
Valvulae conniventes	Present in jejunum	Absent
Number of loops	Many	Few
Distribution of loops	Central	Peripheral
Haustra	Absent	Present
Diameter	3–5 cm	5 cm +
Radius of curvature	Small	Large
Solid faeces	Absent	Present

Although the features listed in the table are useful, there is often considerable overlap of these signs. For example, problems in distinguishing the lower ileum from the sigmoid colon are relatively frequent as both may be smooth in outline and occupy a similar position low in the mid-line in the abdomen. Haustra usually form thick, incomplete bands across the colonic gas shadow; however, sometimes they may form complete transverse bands. Usually these can still be distinguished from valvulae conniventes because they are thicker and further apart than the small bowel folds. Haustra may be completely absent from the descending and sigmoid colon although they can usually still be identified in other parts of the colon even when it is massively distended.

The small bowel folds, or valvulae conniventes, usually form thin complete lines across the dilated small bowel. They are prominent in the jejunum but become less marked as the ileum is reached. The valvulae conniventes are situated much closer together than colonic haustra and become thinner when stretched, but still remain relatively close to each other even as the small bowel calibre increases. However, if the small bowel blood supply becomes compromised and the bowel becomes oedematous or gangrenous, the valvulae conniventes may become greatly thickened and then become extremely difficult to distinguish from colonic haustra.

When numerous loops of dilated bowel are present, this almost invariably indicates that small bowel is dilated. However, in large bowel obstruction, both dilated large and small bowel may be present.

Although bowel calibre may be extremely variable in intestinal obstruction, in small bowel obstruction it is unusual for the diameter to greatly exceed 5 cm except in cases of long-standing obstruction. Equally, it is unusual in large bowel obstruction for the calibre of the large bowel to be less than 5 cm; indeed it usually greatly exceeds this.

The causes and management of small bowel obstruction are very different from those of large bowel obstruction and so it is essential to differentiate wherever possible between them. In most patients, this is relatively easy but some can present a major diagnostic problem, and in these further investigation may be needed.

SMALL BOWEL OBSTRUCTION

Due to the high incidence of elective surgery the commonest cause of small bowel obstruction in the USA and the UK is *adhesions* due to previous surgery and comprises 75% of all cases (Ellis 1981). *Strangulated hernias*, which were once the commonest cause now comprise only 8%, although in underdeveloped parts of the world, they still remain the commonest cause. Complete obstruction of the small bowel usually causes small bowel dilatation with accumulation of both gas and fluid and a reduction in calibre of the large bowel. The amount of gas present in the large bowel depends on the duration and completeness or otherwise of the small bowel obstruction. It frequently takes several bowel movements to entirely empty the large bowel of gas and faeces. Plain film changes in small bowel obstruction may appear after 3–5 hours if there is complete small bowel obstruction and is usually marked after 12 hours. With incomplete obstruction, or if films are taken very shortly after the onset of symptoms, plain films may be normal and barium studies may have to be done to establish a diagnosis.

In most cases of small bowel obstruction, however, dilated gas-filled loops of small bowel are readily identified on the supine radiograph, multiple fluid levels are present on erect films and in most cases there is little diagnostic difficulty (Fig. 33.10). However, one must resist the temptation to diagnose obstruction by the presence of fluid levels alone, as there are many other causes of these. Dilated fluid-filled loops of small bowel may be identified as sausage-shaped, oval or round soft tissue densities that change in position in different views. In dilated small bowel which is almost completely filled with fluid, small

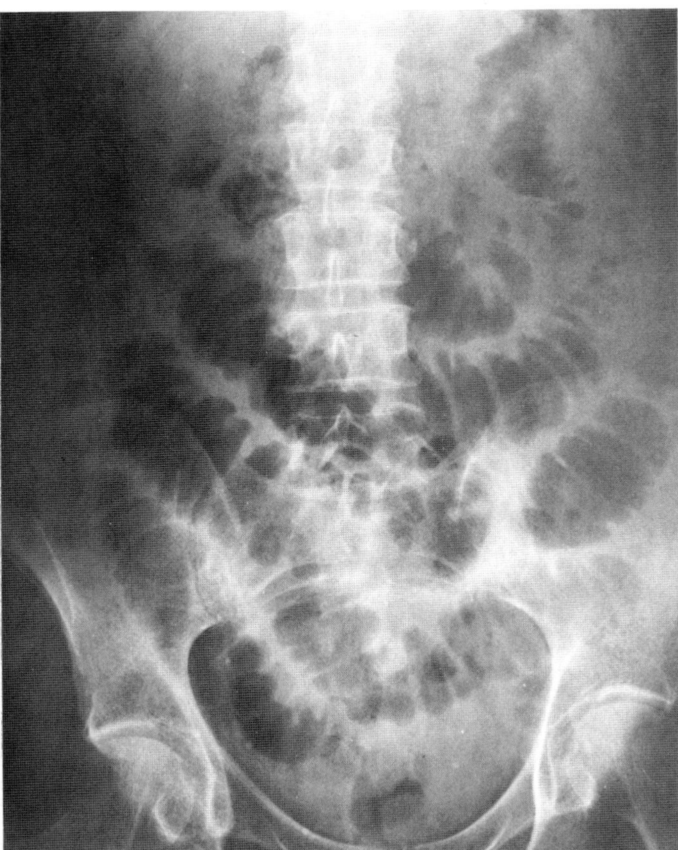

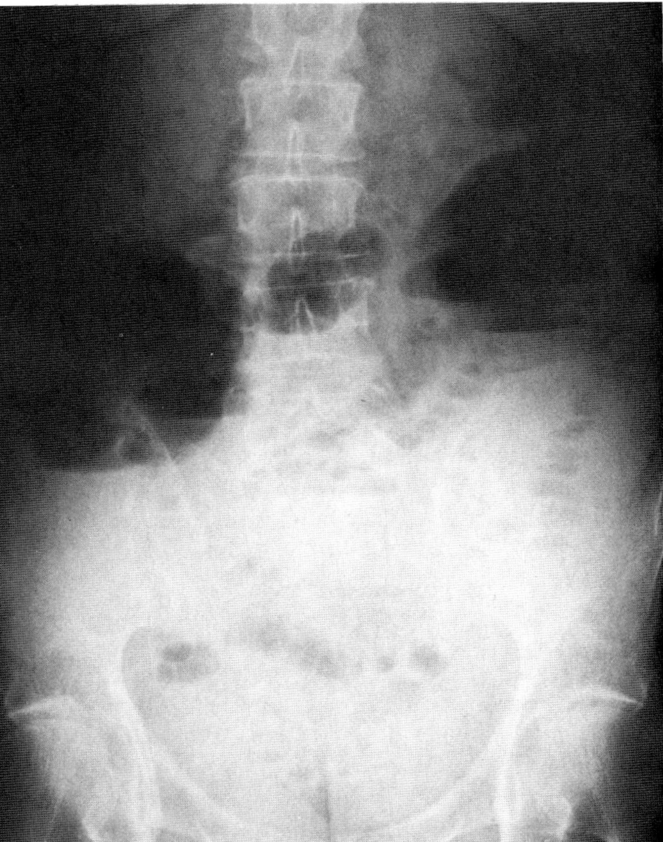

Fig. 33.10 Small bowel obstruction. **A.** Supine. **B.** Erect. Multiple dilated loops of both gas-filled and fluid-filled small bowel are readily identified. There is little or no gas in large bowel. Multiple fluid levels are noted on erect film. A 77-year-old woman with a past history of several abdominal operations. The small bowel obstruction was presumed to be due to adhesions and resolved with conservative management.

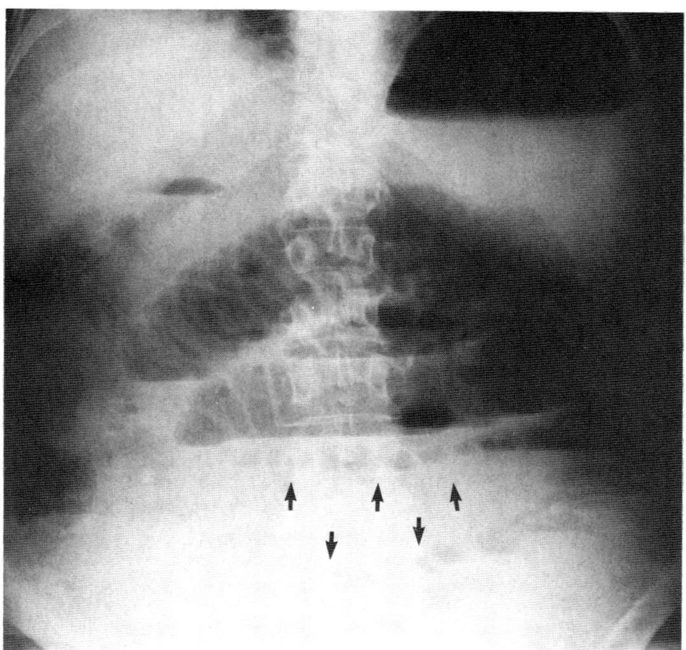

Fig. 33.11 Small bowel obstruction — string of beads sign. Erect. The dilated proximal small bowel is predominantly gas-filled with a few long fluid levels. More distally the small bowel is fluid filled and bubbles of gas are trapped between the valvulae conniventes producing a chain of bubbles.

bubbles of gas may be trapped in rows between the valvulae conniventes on horizontal ray films — this is known as the 'string of beads' sign (Fig. 33.11). This sign, if present, is virtually diagnostic of small bowel obstruction and does not occur in normal people.

In about 6% of small bowel obstructions, small bowel loops may be predominantly fluid-filled with little or no gas visible. Fluid-filled loops should be carefully searched for in patients who are clinically suspected of having intestinal obstruction, otherwise diagnosis may be delayed and, as a result, the mortality and morbidity of the condition increased. The normal tinkling obstructive bowel sounds, which are so characteristic of small bowel obstruction, are caused by fluid moving in predominantly gas-filled dilated bowel. When little or no gas is present and the dilated loops are predominantly fluid-filled, the classical obstructive bowel sounds may be absent, and so it is even more important for the radiologist to consider fluid-filled loops in small bowel obstruction.

If the initial radiographs are considered normal, there is frequently a delay in making the diagnosis of small bowel obstruction. If there is persistent diagnostic difficulty, repeat films taken within a few hours of the first will often solve the problem; if not, oral barium should be given. Giving barium in suspected small bowel obstruction is not harmful, due to the large amounts of fluid present and it will not complete an otherwise incomplete obstruction (Fig. 33.12).

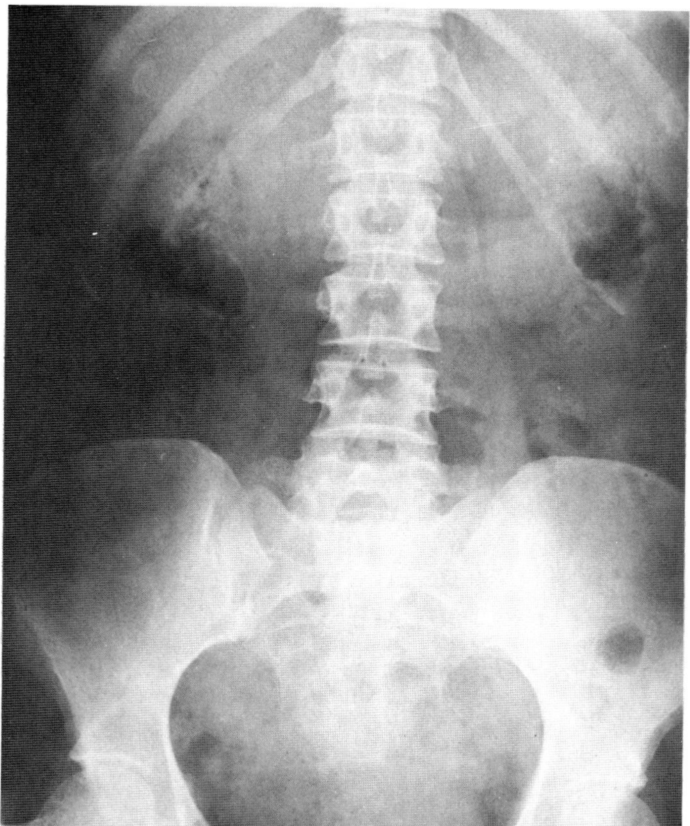

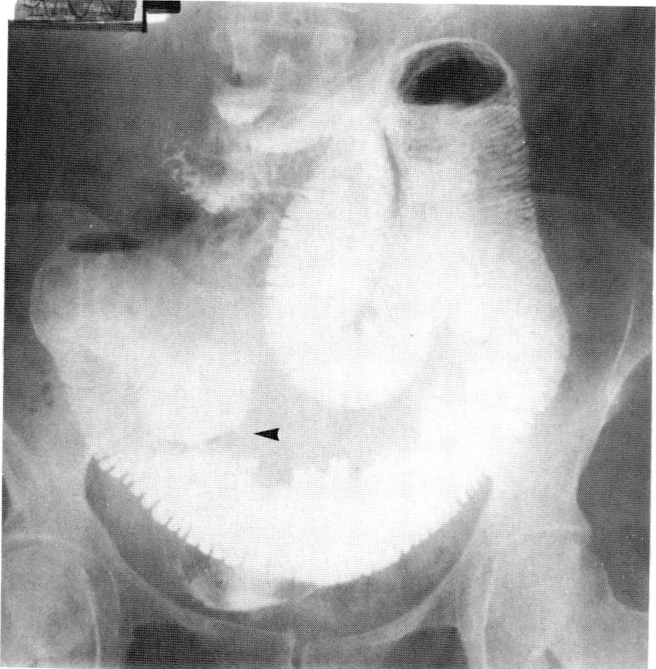

Fig. 33.12 Small bowel obstruction in the proximal jejunum. **A.** Supine abdomen. **B.** Small bowel examination. In the plain abdominal film the dilated small bowel is easily missed because there is only a short segment of gas-filled bowel — the remainder is fluid-filled and almost impossible to identify. The barium study demonstrates dilated small bowel with complete occlusion of the proximal jejunum (◄) caused by a tumour. Note that even on the barium study most of the small bowel is fluid-filled and there are only two small collections of gas. The tumour was lymphoma.

The initial management of a patient who has small bowel obstruction due to presumed adhesions is usually conservative, using a 'drip and suck' regime. Prolonged conservative management warrants repeat supine radiographs to assess the bowel diameter, thickness of the bowel wall and valvulae conniventes, so that radiological progress can also be monitored. Failure to respond radiologically, or evidence of increasing obstruction or of bowel necrosis, are indications for surgery.

Strangulating obstruction

Strangulating obstruction is mechanical small bowel obstruction caused when two limbs of a loop are incarcerated by a band or in a hernia, frequently compromising the blood supply due to compression of the mesenteric vessels. The closed loop may fill with fluid and be palpable, or it may be visible on the radiograph as a soft tissue mass or 'pseudotumour'. The strangulated loop rarely contains gas and the limbs of the loop, separated only by the thickened intestinal walls, may resemble a large coffee bean. If gangrene occurs, linear gas may be seen in the wall of small bowel. However, the appearance in strangulating obstruction, with all its lethal potential, may be indistinguishable from simple small bowel obstruction.

Volvulus of the small intestine

Volvulus of the small bowel may occur as an isolated lesion or combined with obstruction due to adhesive bands. It is often associated with congenital abnormalities of the mesentery and there is frequently malrotation. In children, incomplete rotation, malrotation or non-rotation of the gut may be associated with a massive small bowel volvulus which may occur in the neonatal period or months or even years after birth. There is frequently an impaired blood supply in the small bowel so that intramural gas or thumb printing may be seen. However, it is not usually possible to distinguish simple obstruction, strangulating obstruction or small bowel volvulus on plain radiographs alone.

When a **strangulated external hernia** is the cause of obstruction, it is usually detected clinically. However, sometimes due to obesity this is overlooked and so it is important to search the radiograph for evidence of a hernia. Many strangulated hernias will be fluid filled and not visible on a plain film and furthermore, the mere presence of a hernia does not mean this is the cause of obstruction. However, if dilated bowel is identified ending at a hernial orifice, then the hernia is probably the cause of obstruction.

An **appendix abscess**, particularly in the elderly, may present as small bowel obstruction due to small bowel becoming adherent to the wall of the abscess. The appendix abscess may be identified as a soft tissue mass which may contain gas and indent the caecum (Fig. 33.13).

Crohn's disease sometimes presents as small bowel obstruction. When this occurs the abnormal segment of

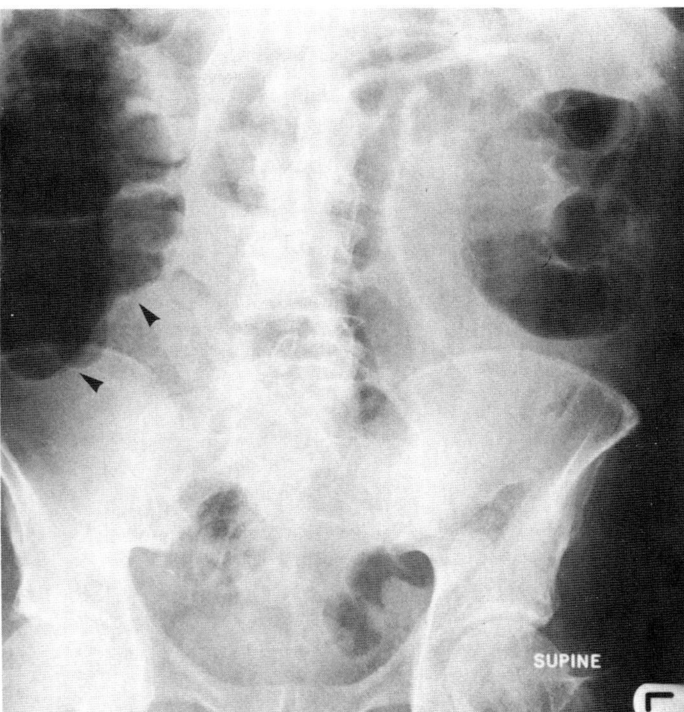

Fig. 33.13 Small bowel obstruction — appendix abscess. Supine. Multiple dilated loops of small bowel can be identified but there is also some gas in the ascending colon and caecum. Note the mass in the right iliac fossa which is indenting the caecum (◄).

small bowel causing the obstruction is never identified — the appearances are those of non-specific small bowel obstruction.

The presence of a *distended caecum* in someone with small bowel obstruction suggests a carcinoma of the ascending colon or a caecal volvulus.

The majority of patients who present with small bowel obstruction, have adhesions and the cause cannot be identified on plain films. The main value of plain films is in assessing the degree and severity of the obstruction.

GALLSTONE ILEUS

Gallstone ileus is mechanical intestinal obstruction caused by the impaction of one or more gallstones in the intestine, usually in the terminal ileum, but rarely in the duodenum or colon. The patient, most commonly a middle-aged or elderly woman, will often have had recurrent episodes of right hypochondrial pain characteristic of cholecystitis. The most recent attack may have been more severe and associated with prolonged vomiting. The gallstones pass into the duodenum or rarely into the colon, by eroding through the inflamed gall bladder wall.

Gallstone ileus comprises about 2% of all small bowel obstruction, but in elderly females who have not had a previous laparotomy, it is much more common. Gallstone ileus is an important condition, because the operative mortality is high, and the diagnosis is frequently delayed or missed even though specific radiological signs may be present in 38% of cases. Over half the patients will have evidence of intestinal obstruction and about one third will have gas present in the biliary tree (Fig. 33.14).

Gas in the biliary tree can be recognized by its branching pattern, but with the gas more prominent centrally. Gas in the portal vein from which it must be distinguished, tends to be more peripherally located in small veins around the edge of the liver. The obstructing gallstone which is frequently located in the pelvic loops of ileum overlying the sacrum, will be identified in about one third of patients either on plain radiographs or barium examinations. However, visualization of the obstructing gallstone on plain films is frequently difficult, because it is often composed almost entirely of cholesterol with only a thin rim of calcium within it. Furthermore, the gallstone is often located over the sacrum and further obscured by dilated small bowel. Change in position of a previously observed gallstone is uncommon, and only occurs in 6% of cases. Signs of gallstone ileus are summarized in Table 33.7.

Table 33.7 Signs of gallstone ileus

Gas within the bile ducts and/or the gall bladder
Complete or incomplete small bowel obstruction
Abnormal location of gallstone
Change in position of gallstone

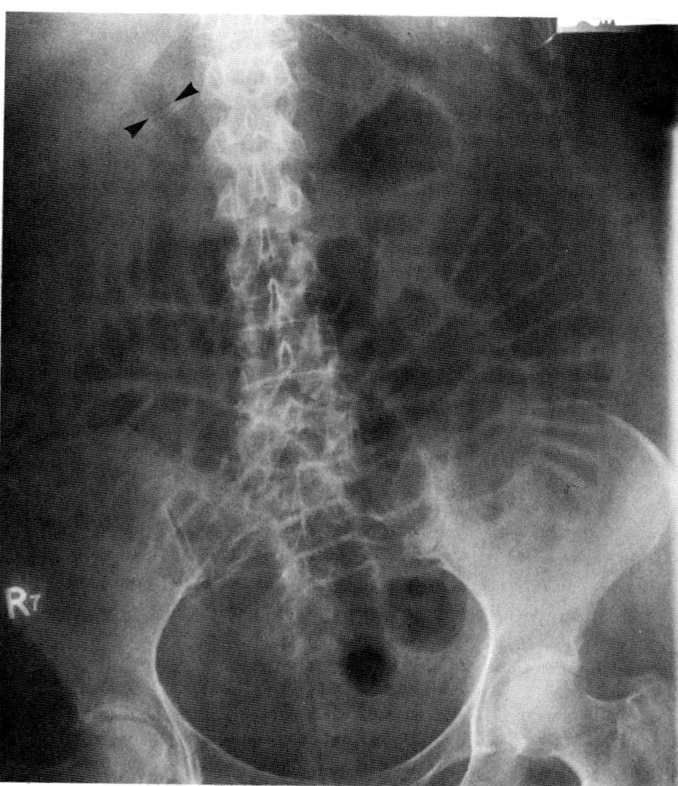

Fig. 33.14 Gallstone ileus. Supine. Multiple dilated loops of small bowel are seen. A band of gas in the right hypochondrium (▶ ◀) lies within the common bile duct. The obstructing gallstone cannot be identified.

GAS IN THE BILIARY TREE

Gas in the biliary tree is most commonly seen following biliary surgery. Anastomoses between the gall bladder or bile duct and the duodenum or jejunum, or the performance of sphincterotomy, will almost invariably result in gas in the biliary tree, and it is therefore essential to know of these operations prior to interpretation of plain films. On occasions, malignant disease of the duodenum or colon may involve the gall bladder or bile ducts, resulting in a fistula. A posterior perforation of a peptic ulcer into the bile duct is a further cause of communication between the bowel and a bile duct. Emphysematous cholecystitis or cholangitis may result in gas filling of the gall bladder and bile ducts but in this situation the gall bladder is usually enlarged. Sometimes gas in the biliary tree may be identified in small bowel obstruction which is not due to gallstone ileus. In these cases it is presumed gas has entered through a physiologically lax sphincter. Causes of gas in the biliary tree are summarized in Table 33.8.

Table 33.8 Causes of gas in the biliary tree

Following biliary surgery
Gallstone fistula — gall bladder usually small
Emphysematous cholecystitis — gall bladder usually enlarged
Malignant fistula
Perforated peptic ulcer into bile duct
Physiological — due to lax sphincter

INTUSSUSCEPTION

The incidence of intussusception varies considerably in different countries but in general it is most frequently seen in children under 2 years of age. In children, it usually commences in the ileum as the result of inflammation of the lymphoid tissue and is usually associated with mesenteric adenitis. The enlarged lymphatic patches are forced into the ileum by peristaltic movement and, acting as a tumour, one part of the ileum is pulled into the other and finally pulled into the colon. Although the condition is usually recognized clinically by pain, vomiting, blood in the stool and a palpable tumour, the diagnosis may not be apparent initially and further investigations may be needed.

Plain films may show evidence of small bowel obstruction or the intussusception itself may be identified as a soft tissue mass, sometimes surrounded by a crescent of gas and most frequently identified in the right hypochondrium (Fig. 33.15). However, a barium enema is frequently

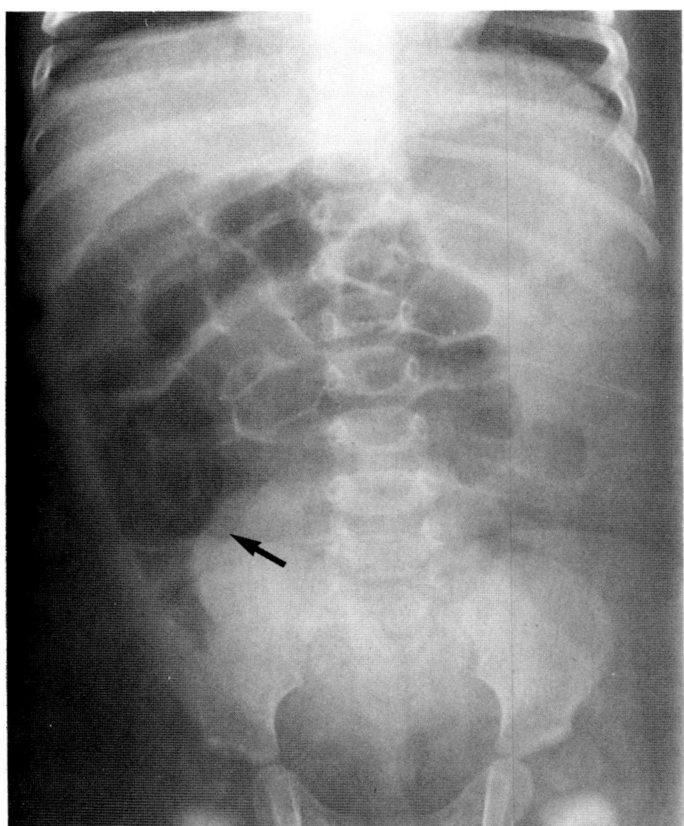

Fig. 33.15 Intussusception. Supine. There are multiple gas-filled loops of slightly dilated small bowel. In addition, there is soft tissue mass in the right iliac fossa (arrowed). A 5-month-old child with mesenteric adenitis.

required to establish a definite diagnosis and, providing certain precautions are taken, can also be used to reduce it (see Ch 37).

MESENTERIC THROMBOSIS — SMALL INTESTINAL INFARCTION

Necrosis of the small bowel is the most serious abdominal condition caused by thrombosis or embolism of the superior mesenteric artery. The clinical diagnosis is often uncertain until laparotomy, but the sudden onset of abdominal pain, often associated with bloody diarrhoea, in an elderly person, is very suggestive of this condition. Gas-filled, slightly dilated loops of small bowel with multiple fluid levels or fluid-filled loops of small bowel are frequent plain film findings. The walls of the small bowel may be thickened due to submucosal haemorrhage and oedema. Linear gas streaks may be seen if there is gangrene and free gas may be present if perforation has occurred. Colonic distension may also be present if there is a generalized paralytic ileus. Gas in the portal vein may occur secondary to bowel necrosis and is a grave prognostic sign.

LARGE BOWEL OBSTRUCTION

The commonest cause of large bowel obstruction is carcinoma and about 60% of these are situated in the sigmoid colon. Diverticular disease as a cause of obstruction has decreased in frequency since the introduction of high-fibre diets. Volvulus of the colon comprises about 10% of large bowel obstruction in the USA and UK but in underdeveloped parts of the world, such as Iran or Africa, volvulus accounts for 85%.

The key to the radiological appearances of large bowel obstruction depends on the state of competence of the ileocaecal valve. Love (1960, 1973) describes three patterns of obstruction (Fig. 33.16). In type 1A the ileocaecal valve is competent and the radiological appearance is one of dilated colon with a distended thin-walled caecum but no

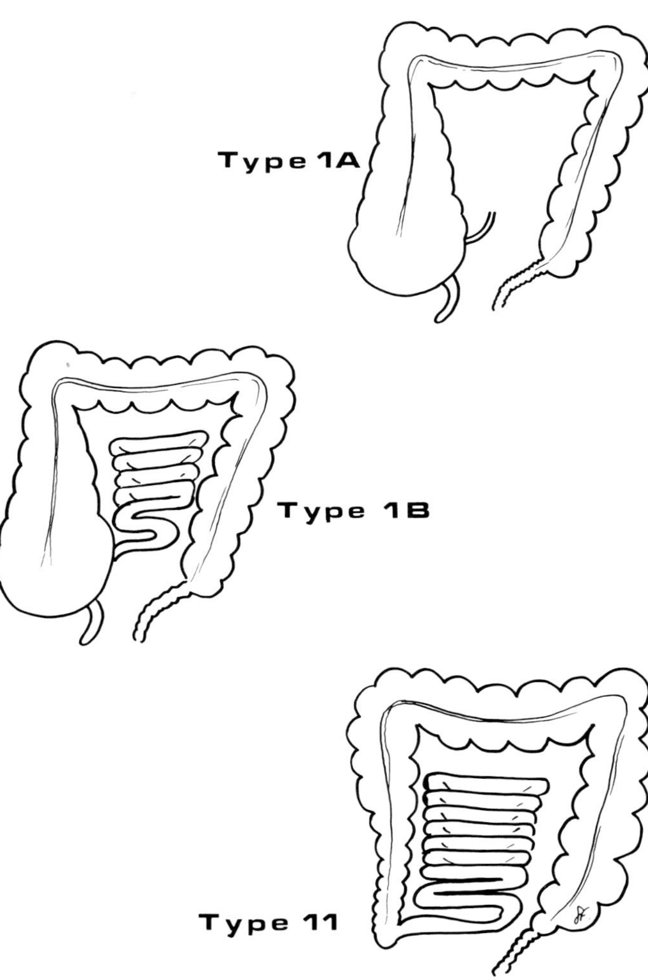

Fig. 33.16 Large bowel obstruction. Diagram demonstrating the different types of large bowel obstruction (after Love 1960, 1973). Type 1A — competent ileocaecal valve. Distended large bowel particularly ascending colon and caecum. No distension of small bowel. Type 1B — competent ileocaecal valve. Caecal distension and small bowel distension. Type II — incompetent ileocaecal valve. No distension of caecum and ascending colon but distension of small bowel. Caecal perforation is much more likely to occur in type 1 large bowel obstruction.

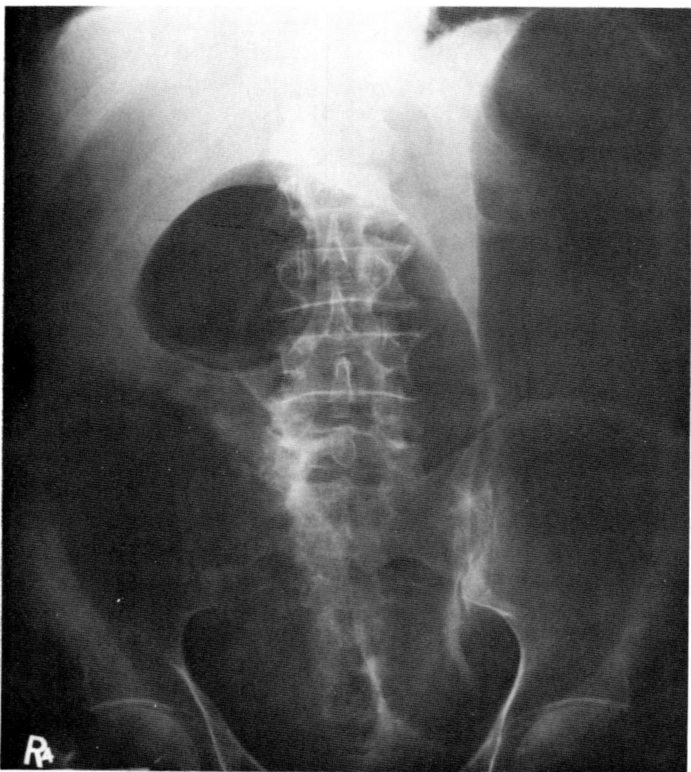

Fig. 33.17 Large bowel obstruction — type 1A competent ileocaecal valve. Supine. There is gaseous distension of the large bowel from the sigmoid backwards including the ascending colon and caecum. The dilated caecum lies in the pelvis. There is no visible small bowel distension. Carcinoma of the sigmoid.

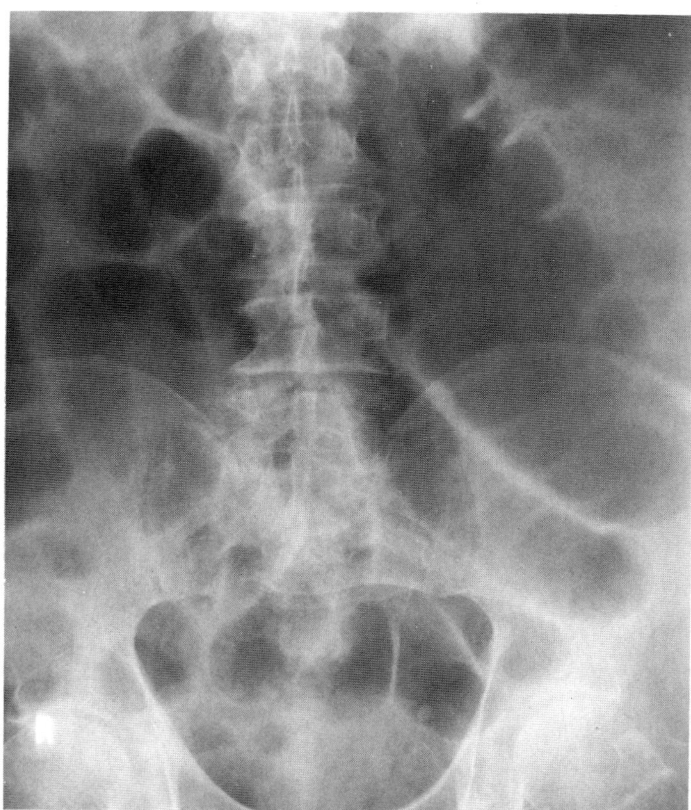

Fig. 33.18 Large bowel obstruction — type II incompetent ileocaecal valve. There is small and large bowel dilatation but caecal distension is not visualized. Carcinoma of the sigmoid.

distension of small bowel (Fig. 33.17). As this type progresses small bowel distension occurs (type 1B), probably secondary to the tightly closed ileocaecal valve. Both type 1 obstructions can lead to massive caecal distension, which is then at risk of perforation secondary to ischaemia. A transverse caecal diameter of 9 cm has been suggested as the critical point above which the danger of perforation exists. In type 2 obstruction, the ileocaecal valve is incompetent and the caecum and ascending colon are not distended, but the back pressure from the colon extends into the small bowel and there are numerous dilated loops of small bowel present (Fig. 33.18).

The obstructed colon almost invariably contains large amounts of air and can usually be identified by its haustral margin around the periphery of the abdomen. However, on occasions the right half of the colon may be fluid filled and massive caecal distension may be overlooked. Even more rarely, the whole colon up to the point of obstruction may be filled with fluid and so the diagnosis may be overlooked initially.

When both small and large bowel dilatation are present in large bowel obstruction, the radiographic appearances may be identical to a paralytic ileus. However, the clinical signs will usually help to differentiate. If problems in interpretation still occur, however, a left lateral radiograph by demonstrating air in the rectum may differentiate low large bowel obstruction from paralytic ileus.

There are numerous causes of colonic distension without obstruction. These include all forms of paralytic ileus and pseudo-obstruction. It is extremely important, therefore, that prior to surgery a single contrast barium enema examination is performed as an emergency to confirm mechanical obstruction and to exclude pseudo-obstruction or colonic ileus.

The cause of simple large bowel obstruction cannot usually be determined from plain radiographs alone, although sometimes a pericolic abscess secondary to diverticular disease may be identified.

PSEUDO-OBSTRUCTION

Pseudo-obstruction is a disorder of bowel which, symptomatically, clinically and radiologically, may mimic intestinal obstruction (Snape 1982). It may be acute and self-limiting and associated with pneumonia, septicaemia or certain drugs, or chronic with acute flare-ups, as seen in diabetes mellitis, collagen disorders, neurological disorders and amyloid disease.

A large proportion of patients, however, have no associated medical condition and these are called *idiopathic intestinal pseudo-obstruction* (Fig. 33.19). A large quantity of bowel gas is usually present and there may be gastric, small or large bowel distension with associated fluid levels to a degree that mimics true obstruction exactly. If an unnecessary operation is to be avoided it is essential that barium studies are performed to exclude true organic obstruction.

LARGE BOWEL VOLVULUS

A prerequisite for the formation of a volvulus is that a long and freely mobile mesentery must be present. This occurs normally in the sigmoid which is the commonest organ involved. Occasionally the caecum and ascending colon are on a mesentery, which is often associated with a degree of malrotation, and they comprise the second commonest organs. Volvuli of the transverse colon or flexures do occur, but they are exceedingly rare in the UK and USA. A compound volvulus involving the intertwining of two loops of bowel such as an ileosigmoid knot is very rare in developed countries, but not uncommon in Africa. Large bowel volvulus is the commonest cause of large bowel obstruction in certain underdeveloped parts of the world.

CAECAL VOLVULUS (Right Colon Volvulus)

Caecal or right colon volvulus can only occur when the caecum and ascending colon are on a mesentery and this is often associated with a degree of malrotation; it has been estimated that this occurs in about 11% of the population. Caecal volvulus accounts for less than 2% of all cases of adult intestinal obstruction. It usually occurs in a relatively young age group, 30–60 years. Gangrene may occur early in the course of the condition, and it is therefore vital that an accurate diagnosis be made promptly. The diagnosis of acute caecal volvulus is rarely made on clinical grounds alone and so the radiological diagnosis becomes much more important (Anderson & Mills 1984). In about half the patients the caecum twists and inverts so that the pole of the caecum and appendix occupy the left upper quadrant. In the other half it twists in an axial plane without inversion and then the caecum still occupies the right half or the central part of the abdomen. Even though there is considerable distension of the volved caecum, one or two

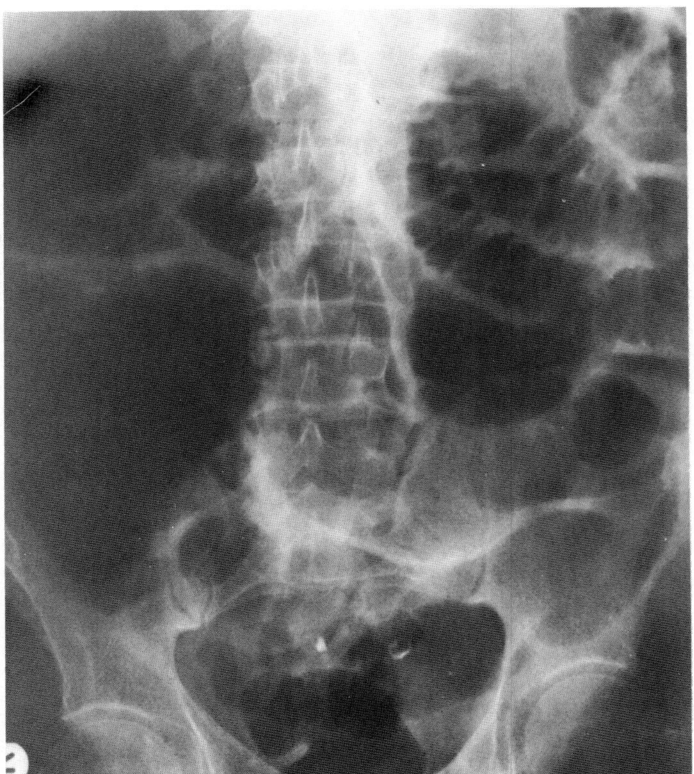

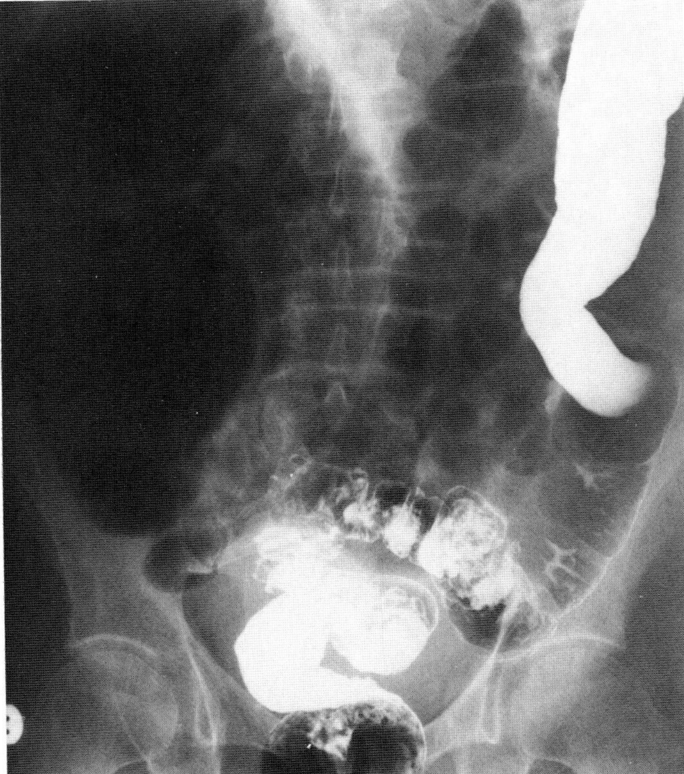

B

Fig. 33.19 Pseudo-obstruction. **A.** Supine abdomen. **B.** Barium enema. On the plain film gas-filled loops of both small and large bowel can be identified with gas extending down to the rectum. The barium examination demonstrates diverticular disease in the sigmoid but this is not obstructing and barium flows freely into the dilated descending colon. Conservative management, using a flatus tube, failed and a laparotomy had to be undertaken. Dilated small and large bowel were found but there was no obstructing lesion. A caecostomy was performed.

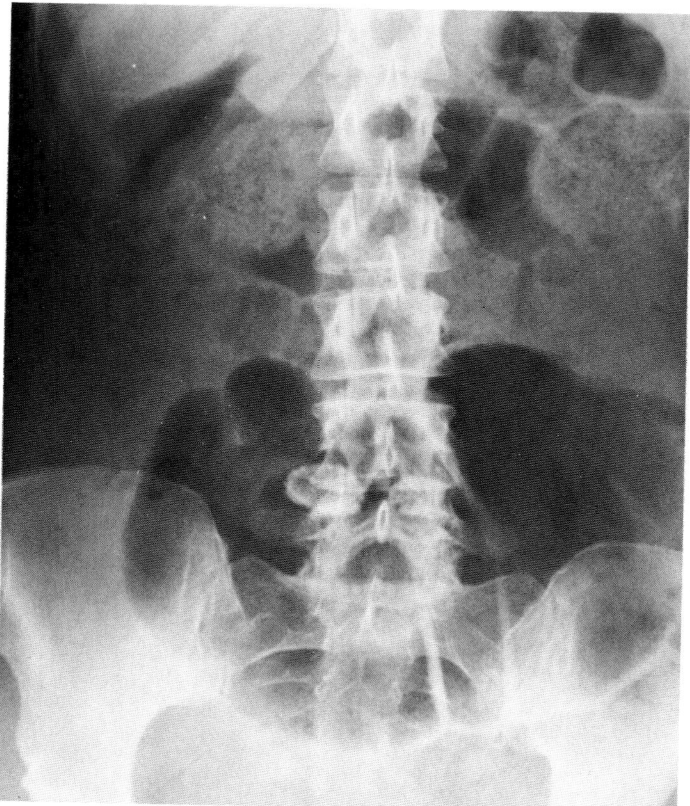

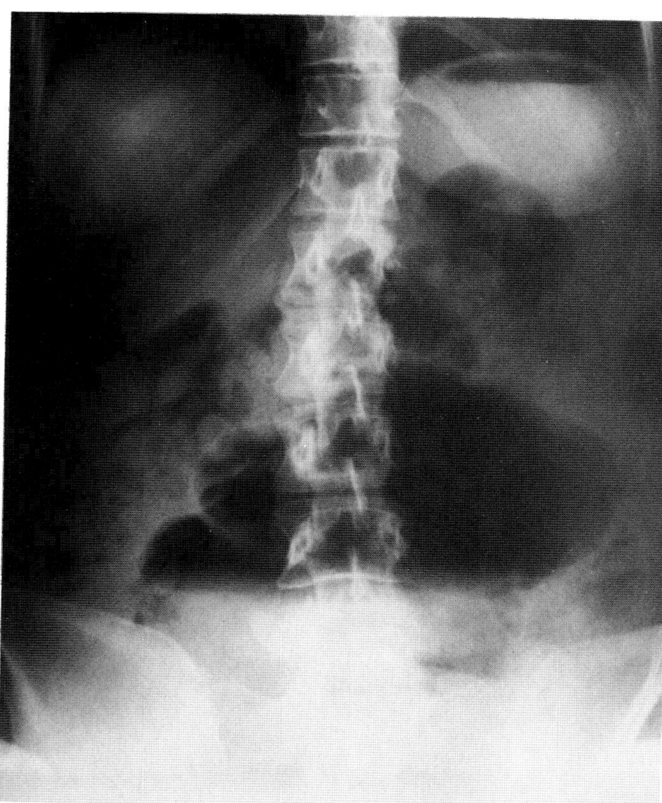

Fig. 33.20 Caecal volvulus. **A.** Supine. **B.** Erect. The considerably distended caecum with its haustral markings is readily identified lying low in the central abdomen. There is no significant small bowel distension.

haustral, markings can usually be identified, which is unlike sigmoid volvulus, where haustral markings are usually absent. The distended caecum can frequently be identified as a large gas- and fluid-filled viscus situated almost anywhere in the abdomen. Identification of an attached gas-filled appendix confirms the diagnosis. Moderate or severe small bowel distension is present in about half the cases, but the remainder only show minimal small bowel distension. The left half of the colon is usually collapsed (Fig. 33.20).

Table 33.9 Identification of the loop in sigmoid volvulus

Ahaustral margin
Left flank overlap sign
Liver overlap sign
Apex above D.10
Apex under the left hemidiaphragm
Inferior convergence on the left
Air/fluid level greater than 2:1

From Young, Engelbrecht and Stoker (1978)

SIGMOID VOLVULUS

This is the classical volvulus, occurring in old, mentally subnormal, psychiatric or institutionalized people. The usual mechanism is twisting of the sigmoid loop around the mesenteric axis; only rarely does one limb twist in an axial torsion. Sigmoid volvulus is usually chronic with intermittent acute attacks or less commonly, a true acute torsion occurs. Although plain film diagnosis is often easy, up to one third of cases can present diagnostic difficulty, the main problem being to differentiate the sigmoid volvulus from distended but non-twisted sigmoid, or distended transverse colon looping down into the pelvis (pseudovolvulus). Young et al (1978) have analysed the frequency of the features present and these are summarized in Table 33.9. The essential feature present to make the diagnosis is to identify the wall of the twisted sigmoid loop separate from the remaining distended colon. When a sigmoid volvulus occurs, the inverted U-shaped loop is usually massively distended and it is commonly devoid of haustra. This is a most important diagnostic point. The ahaustral margin can often be identified overlapping the lower border of the liver shadow — the 'liver overlap' sign. Where the ahaustral margin of the volvulus overlies the haustrated and dilated descending colon, the term 'left flank overlap' sign has been used. The apex of the sigmoid volvulus usually lies high in the abdomen, under the left hemidiaphragm with its apex at or above the level of D.10.

Inferiorly, where the two limbs of the loop converge, three white lines representing the outer walls and the two adjacent inner walls of the volved loop, meet. This is called the inferior convergence; it is usually on the left side of the pelvis at the level of the upper sacral segments. Frequently a huge amount of air is present in a sigmoid volvulus and an air/fluid ratio greater than 2:1, is usual (Fig. 33.21).

The initial treatment of a sigmoid volvulus frequently involves the insertion of a flatus tube per rectum. However, if there is a doubt about the diagnosis on the plain films, a barium enema should be performed. Features seen at the point of torsion include a smooth tapered narrowing — the '*bird of prey*' sign — and the mucosal folds often show a screw pattern at the point of twist. In chronic sigmoid volvulus, shouldering may be seen at the point of torsion and this corresponds to the localized thickening, which is frequently found in the wall of the sigmoid at the site of the chronic volvulus.

ILEOSIGMOID KNOT

An ileosigmoid knot is a compound volvulus involving the small bowel and the pelvic colon. It is not uncommon in developing countries, but it is rare elsewhere. An abnormally mobile loop of small bowel passes round the base of the pelvic colon below the attachment of the pelvic mesocolon and forms a knot. The clinical onset is frequently abrupt with a fulminating course and intense pain in the abdomen and back. The key radiological features are a dilated loop of pelvic colon, evidence of small bowel obstruction and retained faeces in an undistended proximal colon. The dilated loop usually lies in the right side of the abdomen.

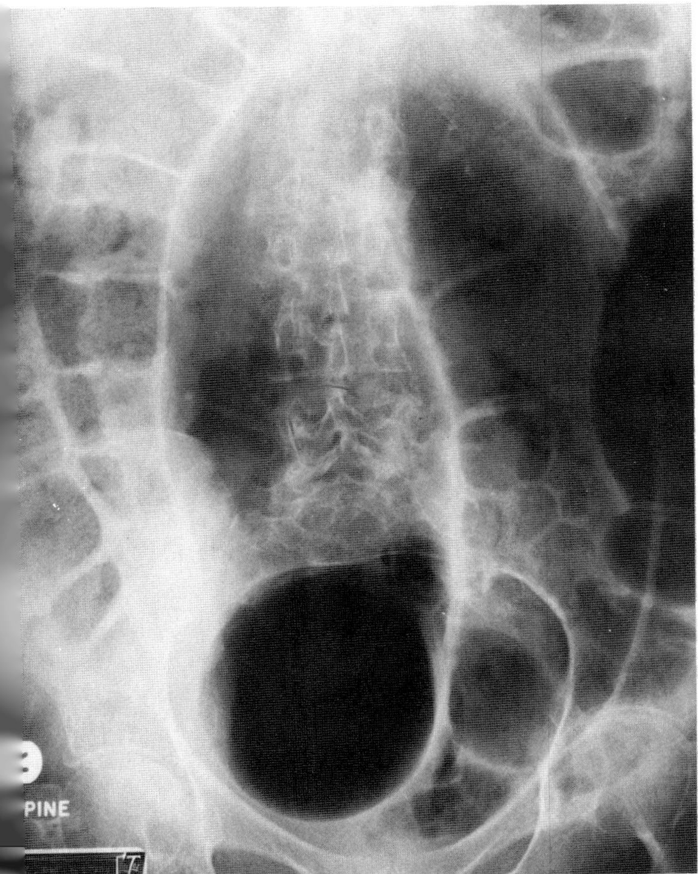

Fig. 33.21 Sigmoid volvulus. Supine. The hugely dilated ahaustral loop of sigmoid can be seen rising out of the pelvis in the shape of an inverted 'U'. Haustrated ascending and descending colon can be identified separate from the volved sigmoid loop.

PARALYTIC ILEUS

Paralytic ileus occurs when intestinal peristalsis ceases and, as a result, fluid and gas accumulate in the dilated bowel. It is very common but most frequently occurs in *peritonitis* and in the *postoperative* period. When it is generalized, it results in both small and large bowel dilatation and, on horizontal ray films, multiple fluid levels will be seen. Sometimes it can be very difficult to distinguish paralytic ileus from some types of large bowel obstruction (Fig. 33.22). There are numerous causes of a generalized paralytic ileus and these are summarized in Table 33.10.

Sometimes local inflammatory processes such as pancreatitis, cholecystitis or appendicitis may result in a localized

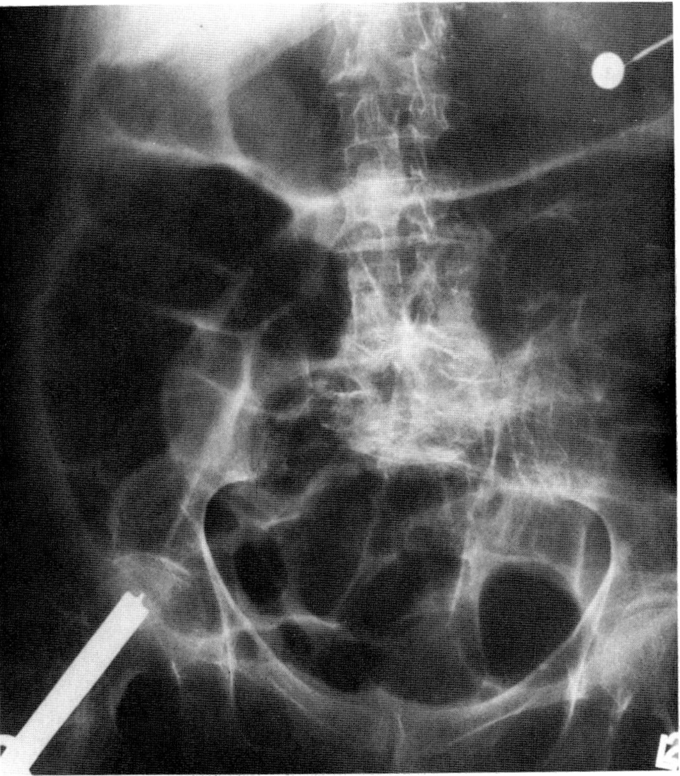

Fig. 33.22 Paralytic ileus. Supine. There is generalized dilatation of both small and large bowel. An 84-year-old woman with generalized peritonitis following perforation of a gastric ulcer.

Table 33.10 Some of the variety of causes of a paralytic ileus

Postoperative
Peritonitis
Inflammation:
Appendicitis
Pancreatitis
Cholecystitis
Salpingitis
Trauma
Spine
Ribs
Retroperitoneum
Congestive cardiac failure
Pneumonia
Renal failure
Renal colic
Leaking abdominal aortic aneurysm
Hypokalaemia
Drugs, e.g. morphine
General debility or infection
Vascular occlusion

ileus leading to dilatation of one or two adjacent loops of bowel only. These appearances are not specific and they sometimes mimic small or even large bowel obstruction.

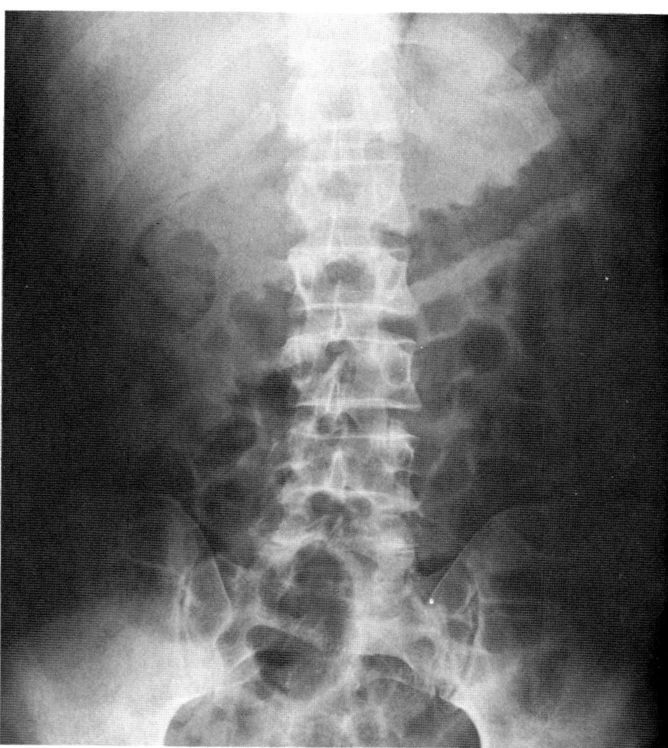

Fig. 33.23 Acute inflammatory bowel disease. Supine. Loss of haustration and irregular mucosa with mucosal island formation is most readily identified in the transverse colon. A 35-year-old man with progressive severe bloody diarrhoea subsequently proven to have ulcerative colitis.

POSTOPERATIVE ABDOMEN

The same general principles of interpretation which apply to preoperative radiographs apply to the postoperative films. However, the features are frequently complicated by paralytic ileus and a postoperative pneumoperitoneum. Sometimes abdominal films are requested in the postoperative period in patients who remain distended and who continue to vomit. If both large and small bowel are gas filled, it is usually impossible to distinguish incomplete small bowel obstruction from paralytic ileus.

ACUTE COLITIS

ACUTE INFLAMMATORY COLITIS

The plain abdominal radiograph can usually predict the extent of mucosal lesions in acute inflammatory disease of the colon. An assessment of the extent of the colitis, the state of the mucosa, the depth of the ulceration and the presence or absence of megacolon and/or perforation can be made. The assessment of the state of the colonic mucosa can be made from the faecal residue, the width of the bowel lumen, the mucosal edge and the haustral pattern. In left-sided disease the proximal limit of faecal residue will usually indicate the extent of active mucosal lesions and where the mucosal edge is smooth and the haustral clefts are sharp, there is unlikely to be any mucosal change. Fuzzy mucosal edges, widened clefts or absent haustrations indicate active disease. Coarse irregularity of the mucosal edge and absent haustrations are associated with marked ulceration (Fig. 33.23). Where extensive mucosal destruction has taken place 'mucosal islands' or 'pseudopolyps' may be seen which may precede 'toxic dilatation' and in itself has been suggested as an indication for surgery. When there are signs of left-sided disease, the presence of large amounts of faeces in the caecum and ascending colon is always associated with a disease process of marked severity.

When intracolonic air is present, the mucosal state can be accurately assessed. However, severe mucosal changes can be missed on the plain radiograph if there is no air to outline the mucosa. A '*gasless colon*' in someone with known inflammatory bowel disease is strongly suggestive of severe disease.

The absence of ulceration or dilatation means that a patient is not in any immediate danger and may be managed medically. Ulceration is responsible for the major complications and so places the patient at risk. When the bowel becomes dilated to above 5.5 cm, the ulceration has penetrated the muscle layer and the patient moves into a higher risk group where urgent surgery must be considered and the patient monitored by daily plain abdominal radiographs. These daily films should be assessed to monitor changing colonic diameter, detect early megacolon or to identify a perforation which may be masked clinically when a patient is taking steroids. Radiological evidence of failing medical treatment is a strong indication for surgery.

TOXIC MEGACOLON

Toxic megacolon is a fulminating form of colitis with transmural inflammation extensive and deep ulceration and neuromuscular degeneration. *Perforation* and *peritonitis* are common complications with a mortality as high as 30%. The most important radiological signs are mucosal islands and dilatation; both are usually seen together. In severe cases, a mean dilatation of 8 cm may be seen (Fig. 33.24). Changes are most frequently seen in the transverse colon as gas collects here because it is the highest part in the supine position.

Perforation of the colon may occur during an acute attack of ulcerative colitis and the sigmoid is the most common site. Perforation results from deep ulceration, which may be localized or associated with a toxic megacolon. Perforations may be free, when a pneumoperitoneum will usually be detected, but sealed perforations occur which cannot be detected reliably on plain radiographs.

PSEUDOMEMBRANOUS COLITIS

Pseudomembranous colitis may follow the administration of antibiotics, particularly the Clindamycin and Lincomycin groups, and *Clostridium difficile* is frequently cultured in the stools. Thumb printing, thickened haustra and abnormal mucosa may be identified on plain films and involvement of the whole of the colon differentiates from ischaemic colitis. Associated small bowel dilatation is frequently seen and the presence of ascites is a further pointer to the diagnosis. Appearances may mimic acute inflammatory bowel disease.

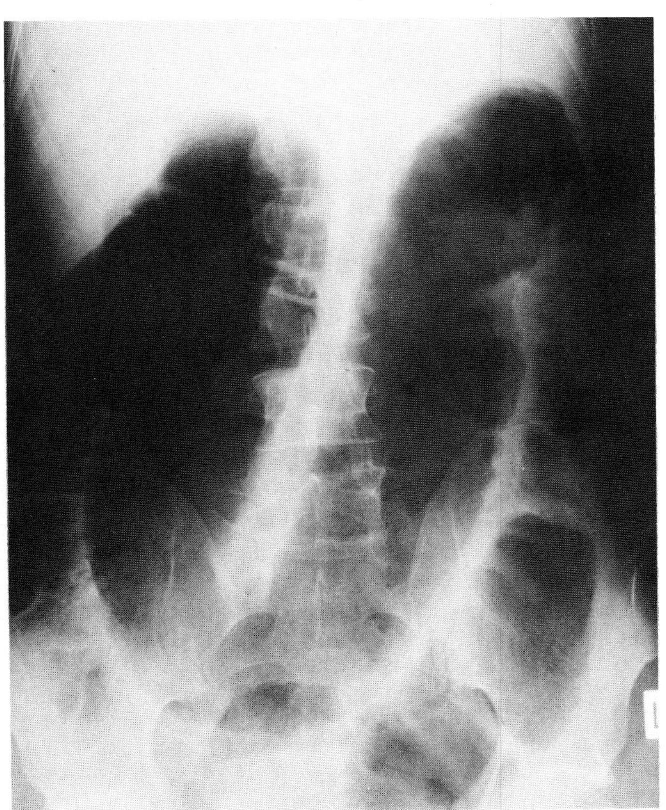

Fig. 33.24 Toxic megacolon. Supine. A 37-year-old woman with progressively severe diarrhoea over a period of 3 weeks, which failed to respond to medical treatment, subsequently requiring a total colectomy. Final diagnosis Crohn's disease.

ISCHAEMIC COLITIS

Ischaemic colitis is a disorder caused by vascular insufficiency and bleeding into the wall of the colon. It is characterized by the sudden onset of severe abdominal pain, often occurring in the early hours of the morning, followed by bloody diarrhoea. It most commonly occurs in middle-aged and elderly patients, and affects the *splenic flexure* and *descending colon* preferentially. The affected wall of the colon is greatly thickened due to submucosal haemorrhage and oedema. This may be identified on plain films as 'thumb printing' although barium studies are frequently required to demonstrate this. The involved area of the colon usually acts as an area of functional obstruction so that the right side of the colon is frequently distended.

INTRAPERITONEAL FLUID

Fluid within the peritoneal cavity is commonly present in acute abdominal conditions but even moderate amounts can be quite difficult to diagnose from plain films alone. The pelvis is the most dependent part of the peritoneal cavity, in both the erect and supine positions, and fluid preferentially accumulates here. As more fluid collects it passes into the paracolic gutters and on the right side reaches the subhepatic and subphrenic spaces. The earliest signs are fluid densities within the pelvis, visualized superiorly and laterally to the bladder or rectal gas shadows. As more fluid accumulates it displaces the bowel out of the pelvis and, as the fluid enters the paracolic gutters, it displaces colon medially from the flank fat stripes. Fluid in Morrison's pouch can obscure the fat interface with the posterior inferior border of the liver and results in failure of visualization of its lower border.

Ascitic fluid between the liver and the lateral abdominal wall may result in the visualization of a lucent band, the fluid being slightly less dense than liver tissue — Hellmer's sign (1942). Blood has a similar density to liver and a haemoperitoneum does not demonstrate this sign.

When huge amounts of fluid are present within the abdomen, it causes separation of bowel loops and the general distension of the abdomen causes thinning of the flank stripes laterally. Large amounts of fluid cause a generalized haze over the abdomen and the scattered radiation produced results in poor visualization of normal structures, such as psoas and renal outlines.

In the pelvis, tumours, particularly when bilateral and of gynaecological origin, can simulate free fluid. In addition, fluid-filled loops of small bowel in the pelvis and in the flanks can also mimic free fluid exactly.

INFLAMMATORY CONDITIONS

INTRA-ABDOMINAL ABSCESSES

Abscesses are mass lesions, usually of soft tissue density, which may be identified by displacement of adjacent structures or by causing loss of visualization of normal fat lines following their involvement by the inflammatory process. Many abscesses contain gas which can be identified as one, several or multiple tiny bubble-like lucencies, which on first appearance may look like faeces. Others may contain much larger quantities of gas, exhibit long air/fluid levels on horizontal ray films, and may mimic gas in normal or dilated bowel. Others may fill anatomical spaces.

Most *subphrenic abscesses* appear in the postoperative period, following elective or emergency surgery, and many are related to anastomotic leaks. Most of the remainder are caused by perforated peptic ulcers, appendicitis and diverticulitis or follow other perforations of the gastrointestinal tract or penetrating abdominal injuries.

Knowledge of the basic anatomy of the peritoneum and its reflections, together with an understanding of the spread of intraperitoneal infections is a prerequisite for radiological diagnosis and localization. A brief summary will follow, but Myers (1982) and Whalen (1976) have made a comprehensive study of this topic.

The abdominal cavity is divided into *supramesocolic* and *inframesocolic compartments* by the transverse mesocolon. The root of the small bowel mesentery divides the infracolic compartment into the *right infracolic space* and a larger *left infracolic space*, which is anatomically open towards the pelvis (Fig. 33.25).

The pelvis is the most dependent part of the peritoneal cavity and is continuous with both *paracolic gutters*. On the right, the gutter extends superiorly to the *subhepatic space* where an extension deep to the liver is known as *Morrison's pouch*. The right subhepatic space is continuous with the

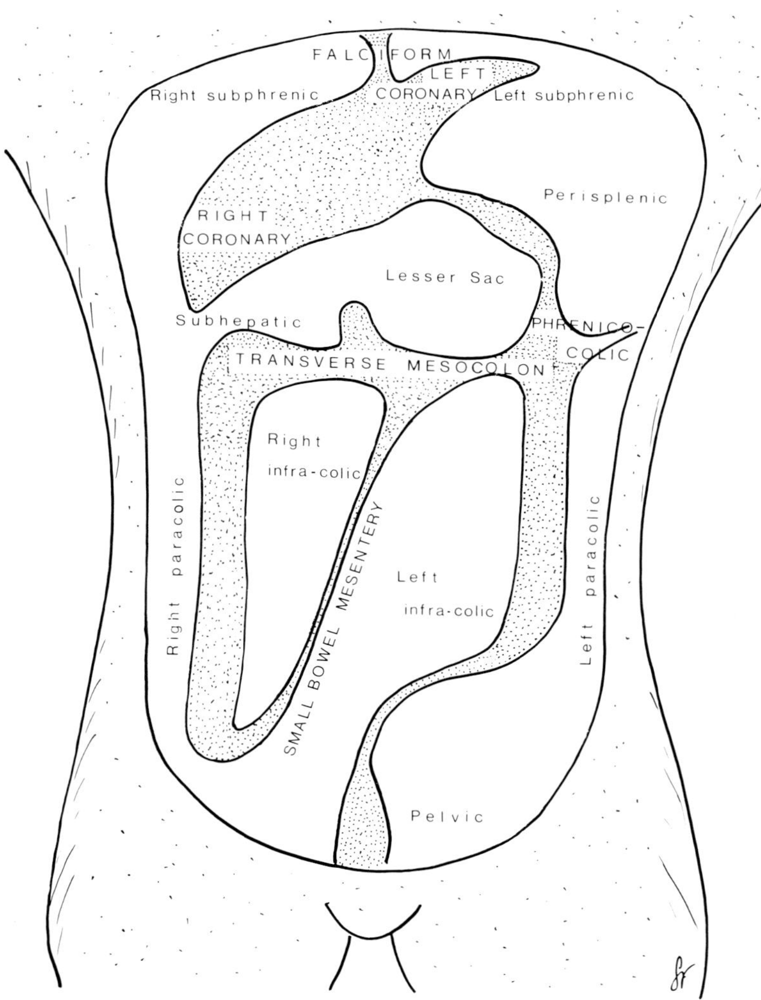

Fig. 33.25 Peritoneal reflections. Diagram demonstrating the peritoneal spaces and the reflections of the peritoneum.

right subphrenic space. The left paracolic gutter is smaller and does not communicate with the subphrenic space being prevented by the phrenicocolic ligament.

The subphrenic area can be divided into four spaces, two on each side. The *falciform ligament* separates the left and right subphrenic space.

The key to the right upper quadrant is the *right coronary ligament*, which suspends the right lobe of the liver from the parietes posteriorly, and which divides the peritoneal recess into the subphrenic and subhepatic spaces.

On the left side the two spaces are the left subphrenic space and the *lesser sac* of the peritoneum. The *left coronary ligament* unlike the right, is attached superiorly but is fairly small and insufficient for the separation of an abscess cavity. Infero-laterally the *phrenicocolic ligament* limits the communication with the left paracolic gutter and so helps to prevent infection spreading up from the left paracolic gutter into the subphrenic space.

The spread and localization of infection within the peritoneal cavity is governed by a number of factors. The site, nature and rapidity of outflow of the escaping visceral contents, together with the prevalence of the disease processes which lead to the escape are clearly of major importance.

The pelvis being the most dependent part of the peritoneal cavity is the most common site of residual abscess formation following generalized peritonitis. Furthermore, spreading infection from two common inflammatory conditions, appendicitis and diverticulitis, will readily enter the pelvis. Displacement and compression of the bladder and pelvic colon frequently occur and can be observed on plain films. However, both *ultrasound* and *computed tomography* will usually provide greater sensitivity and specificity in diagnosis and are usually of considerable help in further evaluation.

SUBPHRENIC AND SUBHEPATIC ABSCESSES

Upper abdominal abscesses continue to have a bad prognosis and in spite of modern antibiotics and surgical techniques, the mortality remains at nearly 30%. A negative upper abdominal pressure in both erect and supine positions, secondary to diaphragmatic movement, favours the passage of fluid out of the pelvis into the right paracolic gutter. Here it drains into the most dependant part, which is Morrison's pouch. Once in the subhepatic space, fluid may readily enter the right subphrenic space, but is usually prevented from passing to the left side by the falciform ligament. Left subphrenic abscesses do not frequently follow pelvic disease, but more commonly arise locally from anterior perforation of the stomach or duodenum or, more frequently, following gastric or colonic surgery or splenectomy.

In addition to the primary signs of an abscess, secondary manifestations of subphrenic and subhepatic abscesses frequently occur. A chest X-ray taken in a patient who has a postoperative pyrexia often provides vital clues to the presence of a subphrenic or subhepatic abscess. Over 80% of subphrenic abscesses will show a *raised hemidiaphragm*, 70% evidence of *basal consolidation* and 60% will have a *pleural effusion*. In a postlaparotomy patient, a subphrenic abscess is the commonest cause of a pleural effusion. Other signs are decreased diaphragmatic movement, generalized or localized paralytic ileus, scoliosis towards the lesion and decreased organ mobility (Fig. 33.26).

The localization of an abnormal gas collection to a subphrenic position can be quite difficult, since the commonly associated pleural effusion will mask the diaphragmatic contour. Penetrated PA, lateral and both decubiti projections centred over the area of interest, give useful information. Not all abnormal gas and air/fluid collections in the upper abdomen lie in abscesses, and bowel may become adherent to operation sites, e.g. the gall bladder bed following cholecystectomy, and simulate an abscess. Barium studies may yield further diagnostic information and can be extremely accurate for diagnosis and localization, although they are often underutilized. Screening of the diaphragms, although formerly popular, rarely adds to plain film findings.

On the right it is important to determine if the abnormal gas collections are inside or outside the liver. This is usually difficult from plain films alone, so *ultrasound*, *computed tomography* or *isotope scanning* of the liver may be required.

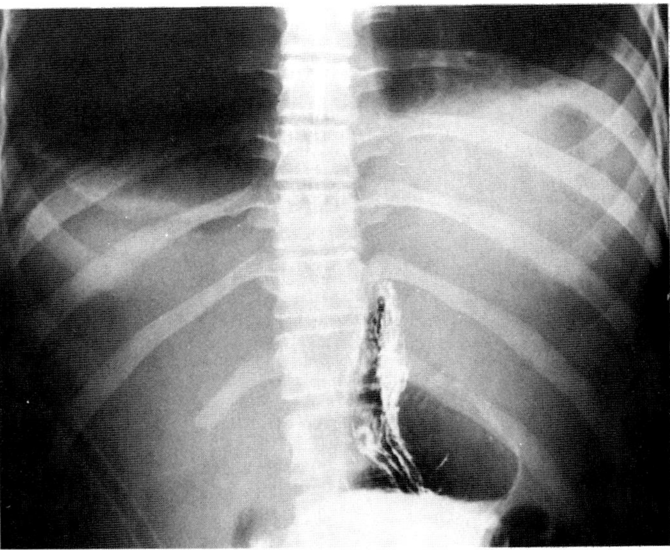

Fig. 33.26 Subphrenic abscess. Barium meal. Erect. The left hemidiaphragm is obscured by a left pleural effusion and some collapse in the left lower lobe. There is a large mass in the left hypochondrium which is causing displacement and indentation of the fundus of the stomach. On the right side the 12th rib has been partly resected and there is a drain in the right subphrenic space. There is a small right-sided pleural effusion. A 15-year-old girl who developed a right subphrenic abscess 5 days, and a left subphrenic 10 days following acute appendicitis.

Right paracolic abscess

Abscesses in the right paracolic gutter are most likely to originate from *appendicitis*, although they may be secondary to a *subphrenic abscess* tracking down towards the pelvis. The ascending colon would be displaced medially.

Left paracolic abscess

The left paracolic gutter is limited superiorly by the phrenicocolic ligament, but it communicates freely with the pelvis inferiorly. Abscesses here are most commonly caused by *perforated diverticular disease*, although they may be caused by *ascending infection from the pelvis*.

Plain film diagnosis of abscesses requires a high degree of suspicion combined with meticulous perusal of the radiographs in search of *small gas bubbles*, usually unchanged in position on consecutive films, *displacement of organs and bowel* from their usual anatomical position and *effacement of fat lines* normally present. Plain film changes are present in nearly 70% of subphrenic abscesses, but very frequently *ultrasound, isotope studies* or *computed tomography* are required to make a definite diagnosis.

CT scanning is a highly accurate method of detecting intra-abdominal abscesses and the technique may also be used for *percutaneous abscess drainage*. The latter technique has revolutionized the treatment of intra-abdominal abscesses and now provides a safer and simpler alternative to laparotomy in seriously ill patients. It can be performed by the radiologist in the imaging department after localization of the abscess using ultrasound or CT control (Fig. 33.27).

APPENDICITIS

Acute appendicitis is the commonest acute surgical condition in the developed world and it carries an overall mortality of about 1%. When clinical findings are typical, a prompt diagnosis is usually made and there is no indication for taking abdominal radiographs. In older patients, who present with typical findings, a chest X-ray should be taken, predominantly to act as a baseline in case of postoperative complications.

In a significant minority of patients, particularly the young and old, clinical features of appendicitis are obscure, the diagnosis is difficult and plain films are frequently taken to elucidate the cause of abdominal pain and may subsequently play a significant role in making the diagnosis. The radiological signs result from the localized

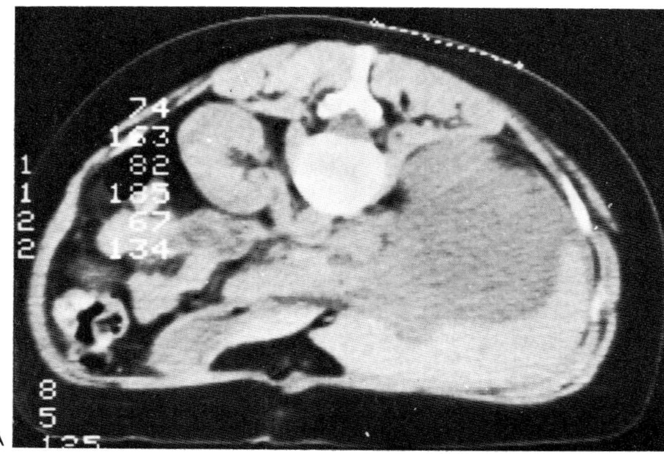

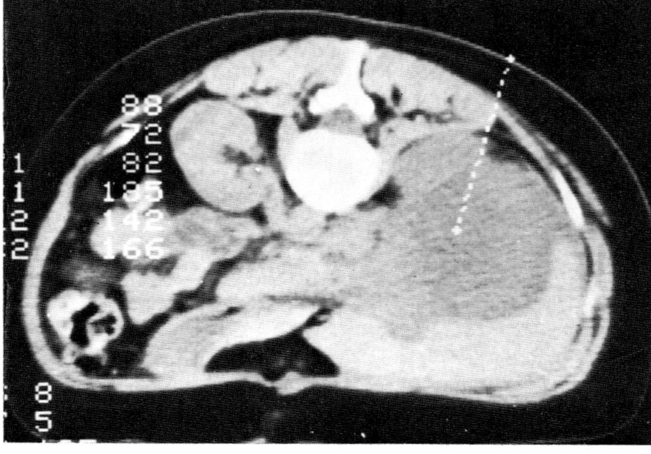

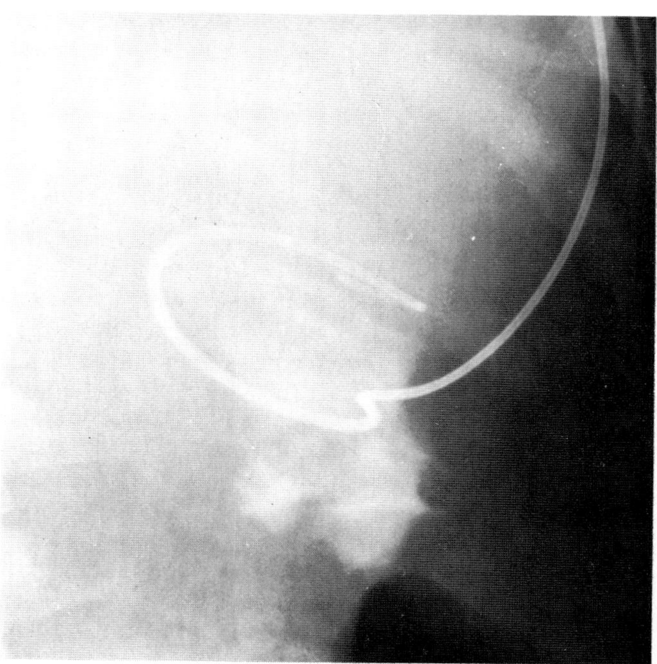

Fig. 33.27 A. and **B.** CT scans of prone patient showing a large Rt subhepatic abscess, secondary to GB surgery. Electronic cursors are used to measure (**A**) distance from midline to avoid kidney (**B**) distance to centre of abscess. **C.** Prone x-ray showing catheter in situ after insertion from posterior approach. A small amount of contrast has been injected. (Courtesy of Dr David Sutton.)

inflammatory change, which may then progress to perforation and abscess formation with an associated paralytic ileus. *Abscess formation* results in indentation of the caecum on its medial border and when inflammation permeates into the adjacent fat, it leads to loss of the lower part of the properitoneal fat line and the right psoas muscle shadow. *Intestinal obstruction* may occur as several loops of small bowel become matted together or stuck to the inflamed appendix. There is a high correlation between the presence of a *calcified appendolith* and appendicitis, and these can be identified in about 13% of cases. About 90% of patients with right lower quadrant pain and ring-shaped calcification in the same area are found to have acute appendicitis and a gangrenous appendix is found in about three-quarters of these (Fig. 33.28).

Ileal and caecal fluid levels can be seen in nearly 50% of cases. It should be remembered, however, that a number of the signs of appendicitis are non-specific and caecal fluid levels and loss of the right psoas outline may occur in about one-fifth of normal people. Air in the appendix may be seen in acute appendicitis, but this also occurs in normals, large bowel obstruction and paralytic ileus, particularly if the appendix is high and retrocaecal. The signs of acute appendicitis are summarized in Table 33.11.

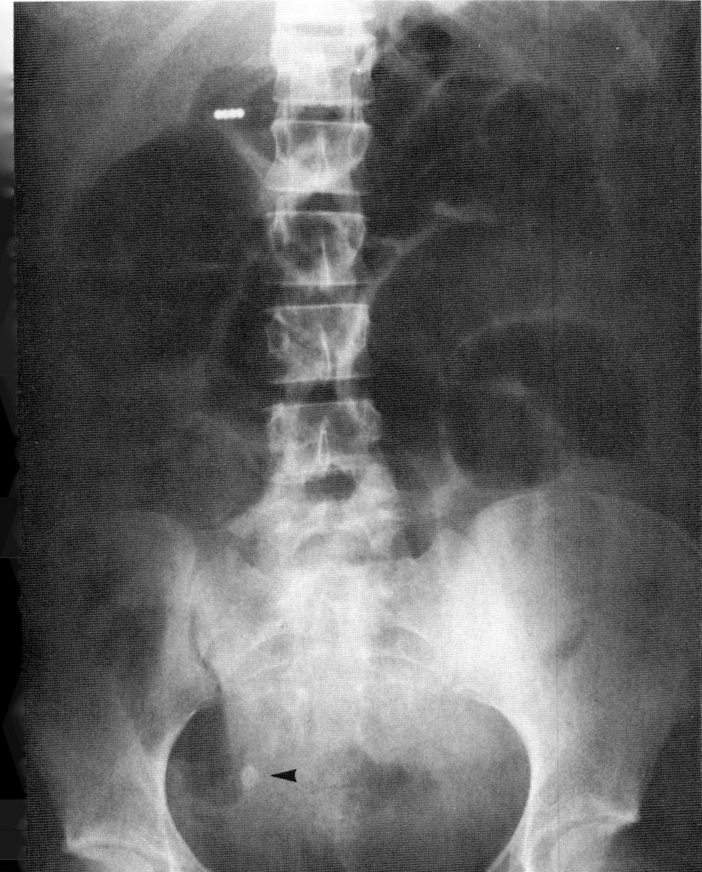

Fig. 33.28 Acute appendicitis. Supine. Dilated loops of small and large bowel result from a paralytic ileus secondary to peritonitis. A calcified appendolith can be identified (◀) in the right side of the pelvis.

Table 33.11 Signs of acute appendicitis

Appendix calculus (0.5–6 cm)
Sentinel loop — dilated atonic ileum containing a fluid level
Dilated caecum
Widening of the properitoneal fat line
Blurring of the properitoneal fat line
Right lower quadrant haze due to fluid and oedema
Scoliosis concave to the right
Right lower quadrant mass indenting the caecum
Blurring of the right psoas outline — unreliable
Gas in the appendix — rare, unreliable

ACUTE CHOLECYSTITIS

Almost all cases of acute cholecystitis are associated with gallstones and most are caused by obstruction of the cystic duct. However, only about 20% of gallstones contain sufficient calcium to be visible on plain radiographs; only rarely does the wall of the gall bladder itself calcify. It is uncommon to identify a normal-sized gall bladder on plain films because it is not surrounded by fat. However, in cholecystitis the gall bladder may enlarge due to obstruction and a mass may be visualized by displacement of adjacent gas-filled structures. The duodenum and hepatic flexure of the colon may show an ileus secondary to the inflamed gall bladder and rarely gas may be seen in the lumen and wall of the gall bladder itself. However, in two thirds of cases, the plain radiographs will be completely normal or show only borderline dilatation of small or large bowel. Signs of acute cholecystitis are summarized in Table 33.12 but many of these are noted to be non-specific.

Table 33.12 Signs of acute cholecystitis

Gallstones — seen in 20%
Duodenal ileus
Ileus of hepatic flexure of colon
Right hypochondrial mass due to enlarged gall bladder
Gas within the biliary system

Ultrasound is widely used for the diagnosis of acute cholecystitis because gallstones, gall bladder size and gall bladder wall thickness can all be determined (Fig. 33.29). Tenderness of the gall bladder, as it lies immediately beneath the ultrasound transducer, is also a very reliable sign that the gall bladder is acutely inflamed. Contrast examinations in acute cholecystitis have now been superceded by ultrasound (see Ch. 34).

Scintigraphy, using ^{99m}Tc-labelled derivatives of aminodiacetic acid (HIDA. PIPIDA) and pyridoxylidene glutamate, is a simple and highly accurate method of diagnosing acute cholecystitis. The technique depends on the fact that acute cholecystitis occurs in association with a blocked

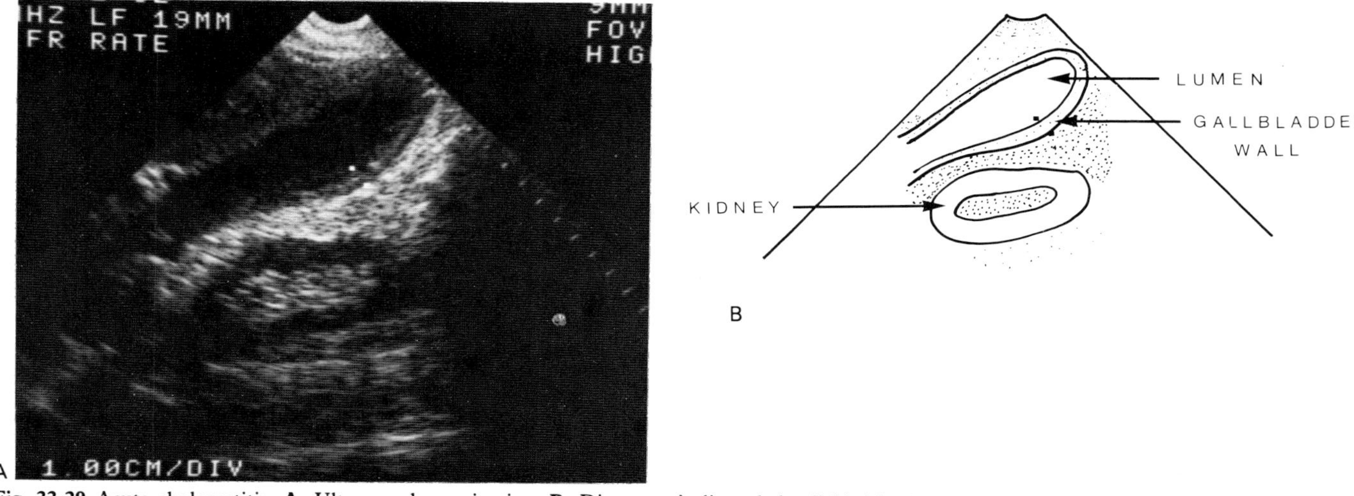

Fig. 33.29 Acute cholecystitis. **A.** Ultrasound examination. **B.** Diagram. A distended gall bladder has been identified with a considerably thickened gall bladder wall. Markers placed across the gall bladder wall indicate a thickness of 9 mm. No gallstones have been identified. (Courtesy Dr M.O. Downes.)

cystic duct. A positive scan occurs when there is non-visualization of the gall bladder but prompt visualization of the bile duct and duodenum. Although highly accurate, enthusiasm for radionuclides is very variable and false positive scans occur in alcoholic liver disease and in patients receiving parenteral nutrition.

Obstruction of the common bile duct, producing biliary colic, may present as an acute abdomen and is usually indistinguishable clinically from cholecystitis. Plain film findings in acute bile duct obstruction are usually absent although occasionally the obstructing stone may be seen on the right, adjacent to the transverse process of L.1 or L.2.

An *empyema of the gall bladder* may be identified on plain films, when a distended gall bladder is seen as a large soft tissue mass. Sometimes the obstructing stone may be identified in the cystic duct or Hartman's pouch.

EMPHYSEMATOUS CHOLECYSTITIS

Emphysematous cholecystitis is characterized by gas in either the wall or the lumen of the gall bladder, and in 20% of cases gas will also be present in the bile ducts. There is usually obstruction of the cystic duct followed by ischaemia and proliferation of gas-forming organisms — *Clostridium welchii* is the most common infecting organism. About 30% of cases are *diabetic* and, unlike ordinary cholecystitis, it is much more common in men. A substantial number of patients will have no evidence of stones in the gall bladder (Fig. 34.8, p. 960).

Clinically, patients present with cholecystitis, but plain films will usually reveal a gas collection, constant in position in the right hypochondrium, which will demonstrate either linear gas bubbles paralleling the wall, or an oval collection of gas within the gall bladder lumen. Air in the gall bladder from a gallstone ileus, or enteric fistula, may simulate emphysematous cholecystitis, but will usually demonstrate a small, or normal-sized gall bladder, while in emphysematous cholecystitis, the gall bladder is usually enlarged. Small bowel fluid levels may be seen in both conditions.

Patients frequently undergo ultrasound examination and air within the gall bladder wall and in the lumen of the gall bladder has a characteristic appearance.

Although rare, diagnosis is important because gangrene of the gall bladder is common and the mortality is higher than in conventional cholecystitis. Most authorities, therefore, advise early surgery in this condition.

ACUTE PANCREATITIS

The clinical diagnosis of acute pancreatitis can be extremely difficult and, in the initial stages, other acute abdominal conditions such as perforated peptic ulcer or acute cholecystitis have to be included in the differential diagnosis. Plain abdominal radiographs are frequently taken as part of the initial investigation and a multitude of plain film signs have been described. The pathological changes of acute pancreatitis include oedema, haemorrhage, fat necrosis and infarction, which is sometimes followed by acute suppuration. The inflammatory process may extend into the gastrocolic ligament, the duodenal area, and follow the root of the mesentery or extend out of the peritoneum into the pararenal space. The clinical diagnosis is usually confirmed by a markedly elevated *serum amylase* level. However, this test has a number of well-recognized limitations, and the amylase levels may also be raised in perforated peptic ulcers, acute cholecystitis and intestinal obstruction.

A large number of radiological signs have been described in acute pancreatitis (Table 33.13); many of these are

Table 33.13 Signs of acute pancreatitis

Common and sometimes useful:
Gas-filled duodenal cap and loop
Gas-filled dilated stomach
Single dilated small bowel loop (Sentinel loop)
Small bowel ileus
Dilated colon, particularly transverse and ascending
Dilated terminal ileum
Loss of the left psoas outline
Uncommon and/or non-specific and so unhelpful:
Opaque gallstones
Gasless abdomen (due to persistent vomiting)
Pancreatic calcification
Pancreatic enlargement
Gastrocolic separation
Absent right psoas shadow
Elevated left hemidiaphragm
Colon 'cut-off' signs
Rare but diagnostic:
Gas within the pancreas
Faint mottling due to fat necrosis

uncommon, most are non-specific, and in two thirds of cases plain films may be normal or show only borderline dilatation of bowel. As a result, most of the signs are of little or no value in the diagnosis of acute pancreatitis in individual cases. *Gas in a dilated duodenal loop* is optimally demonstrated in the left lateral decubitus position and this view should be included in all patients with suspected pancreatitis. Demonstration of *gas within the pancreas*, usually as multiple small bubbles giving a mottled appearance, is diagnostic of a pancreatic abscess and the prognosis is grave. Other frequently seen signs are dilated loops of bowel — small bowel, terminal ileum, ascending and transverse colon — as well as a generalized paralytic ileus. Loss of the left psoas outline may also occur. Other signs which may occur relatively frequently are, however, non-specific and so are unlikely to distinguish between pancreatitis and other acute abdominal conditions. These include opaque gallstones, pancreatic calcification, pancreatic enlargement, gastrocolic separation, absent right psoas shadow, elevated left hemidiaphragm and the 'renal halo' sign.

Four different types of colon 'cut-off' sign have been described; this can lead to great confusion and so this term is best avoided and a description of the colonic dilatation used instead. A very rare but diagnostic sign is faint mottling over the pancreas due to fat necrosis.

A recent series comparing plain film findings in acute pancreatitis, cholecystitis and perforated duodenal ulcer concluded that the only abdominal signs seen more frequently in pancreatitis were fluid levels in dilated stomach and duodenum (Millward et al 1983). However, these signs were also seen in a smaller number of the other patients. This study also concluded that a left-sided pleural effusion was seen significantly more often in severe pancreatitis, as compared with mild pancreatitis or the control group.

Plain films will only occasionally enable a specific diagnosis of acute pancreatitis to be made, although it will be included in the differential diagnosis frequently. Their main value is to exclude other acute abdominal conditions. In the acute stage, *ultrasound* and *CT scanning*, by demonstrating an enlarged and oedematous pancreas, will often help towards the diagnosis. However, even these imaging techniques may be completely normal in the early stages of acute pancreatitis.

A pancreatic pseudocyst may complicate the later stages of acute pancreatitis. This may be identified on plain films as a large soft tissue mass, on barium studies as causing displacement of the stomach or duodenum, or on ultrasound examination as a transonic mass (Fig. 33.30). CT is also useful for assessing patients with complications of

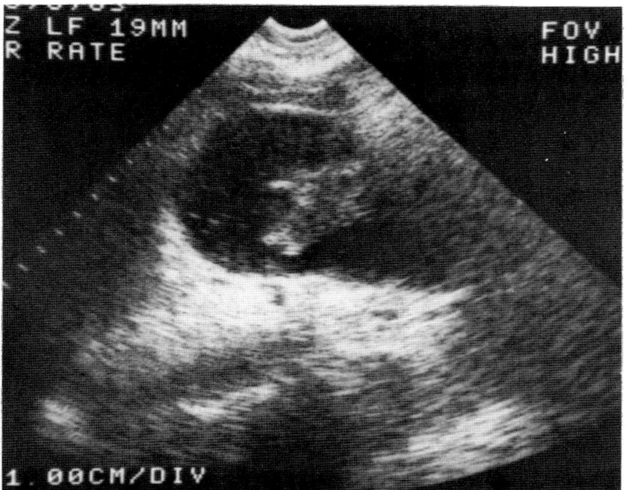

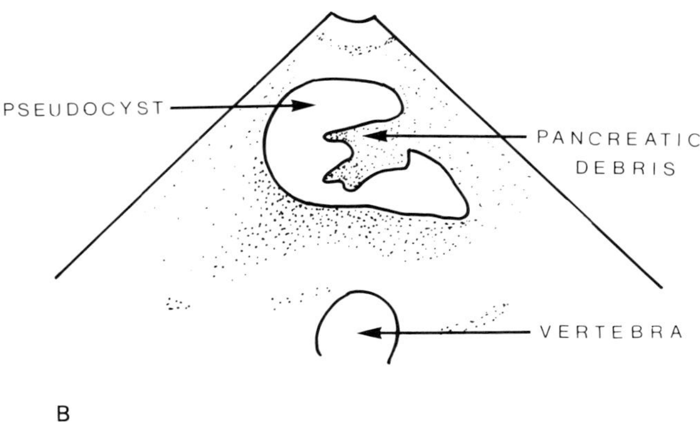

Fig. 33.30 Acute pancreatitis — pancreatic pseudocyst. **A.** Ultrasound. **B.** Diagram. A large transonic area is demonstrated in the region of the head of the pancreas and within it irregular echoes represent pancreatic debris. 10 days following an attack of acute pancreatitis. (Courtesy Dr M.O. Downes.)

acute pancreatitis, because pseudocysts, abscess, haemorrhage and ascites are all readily detected. A patient with acute pancreatitis, who is not improving clinically, should undergo regular ultrasound examinations to detect pseudocyst formation and other complications at the earliest possible time (see Ch. 35).

ACUTE GYNAECOLOGICAL DISORDERS

The primary disorder may produce specific signs within the pelvis, while secondary signs within the peritoneal cavity may result from free fluid or a paralytic ileus. Torsion of an ovarian cyst may produce a pelvic mass and an ovarian dermoid can be diagnosed if it contains calcification, teeth or fat. Salpingitis often produces a localized paralytic ileus but it cannot usually be distinguished from appendicitis or diverticulitis on plain films. A ruptured ectopic pregnancy may produce a pelvic mass, free fluid and a paralytic ileus, but *ultrasound* is usually of particular value in these patients.

INTRAMURAL GAS

Sometimes gas is found within the walls of a hollow viscus. This can be easily recognized radiologically and different varieties are distinguishable. Colquhoun (1965) has suggested classification into 'cystic pneumatosis', 'interstitial emphysema' and 'gas-forming infections'. Cystic pneumatosis is usually a relatively benign condition, but the identification of linear gas shadows in the bowel wall is usually a sign of bowel necrosis.

CYSTIC PNEUMATOSIS (Pneumatosis Cystoides Intestinalis)

This is an uncommon condition comprising cyst-like collections of gas in the walls of hollow viscera, most frequently seen in the gastrointestinal tract where it is called pneumatosis cystoides intestinalis. Although it may occur anywhere in the gastrointestinal tract, the left half of the colon is the site most commonly affected and this is termed *pneumatosis coli*. Most patients are past middle-age and the symptoms include vague abdominal pain, diarrhoea and mucous discharge. However, in some patients air cysts are discovered by chance during the investigation of other symptoms. The cysts vary in size from 0.5 to 3 cm in diameter and they lie both subserosally and submucosally. Plain film findings are typical, with the gas-containing cysts producing a characteristic appearance easily distinguishable from normal bowel gas shadows. Occasionally these cysts rupture, producing a pneumoperitoneum without evidence of peritonitis, but it is extremely important to recognize that pneumatosis is the cause of the pneumoperitoneum and so avoid an unnecessary laparotomy (Fig. 33.8). The condition is also discussed in Chapter 32.

INTERSTITIAL EMPHYSEMA

This is a rare condition where linear gas, in single or double streaks, is found in the bowel wall and is not associated with infection. The commonest sites are the stomach and the colon. A breach in the mucosa, with an increase in the intraluminal pressure, would seem to be important aetiologically. In the stomach, gastroscopy and pyloric stenosis have been implicated as a cause. In the colon it is associated with toxic megacolon and is a sign of impending perforation.

GAS-FORMING INFECTIONS

Numerous bacteria are capable of producing gas, but those most commonly involved in humans are *Escherichia coli*, *Clostridium welchii* and *Klebsiella aerogenes*. Such infections usually give rise to severe constitutional disturbance and toxaemia with a high mortality. However, over half of all gas-forming infections occur in diabetics; the infecting organism is frequently *E. coli*, and in this group the constitutional disturbance is usually much less.

Emphysematous gastritis

This results from a severe infection in the wall of the stomach, resulting in a contracted stomach, with a frothy or mottled radiolucency visible in the left upper abdomen due to gas within the stomach wall. It has a high mortality.

Emphysematous cholecystitis

This occurs most frequently in elderly male diabetics and is frequently associated with an absence of gallstones. The clinical findings are suggestive of acute cholecystitis and this has been previously discussed.

Emphysematous enterocolitis

This occurs predominantly in premature babies, and is covered in Chapter 37. In adults, it is associated with profound constitutional disturbance and usually indicates necrotic bowel. It may be associated with gas in the portal vein; a sign which, in an adult, has a grave prognosis.

Emphysematous cystitis

Emphysematous cystitis causes linear gas streaks and gas cysts within the wall of the urinary bladder and is frequently associated with gas within the lumen of the bladder itself. *E. coli* and *Klebsiella aerogenes* are the usual infecting organisms and the condition is much more common in diabetics. Emphysematous cystitis must be distinguished from gas within the lumen of the bladder and due to a vesicocolic fistula. The latter is not usually associated with gas within the wall of the bladder.

RENAL COLIC

A large number of patients with acute ureteric obstruction due to a stone present as an acute abdomen. Although most ureteric calculi are opaque, they are frequently small and difficult to identify on plain films alone, or, if identified, impossible to place within the ureter with certainty. Phleboliths within the pelvis are a frequent source of potential confusion but their smooth outline and radiolucent centre, are quite different from stones which are frequently less calcified, oval and with no radiolucent centre.

The severe pain which accompanies renal colic frequently leads to air swallowing and this, together with an associated paralytic ileus which is common, frequently results in gas-filled small and large bowel which is often slightly distended and may contain fluid levels. Sometimes colonic distension may be so great as to mimic large bowel obstruction (Fig. 33.31). An intravenous urogram is required to confirm the diagnosis and to identify the degree and site of obstruction. It is important to confirm the diagnosis for many patients who are initially thought to have ureteric colic, have a normal emergency i.v.u and are eventually found to have another abnormality. A normal intravenous urogram, done while the pain is still present, excludes the diagnosis of renal colic; a normal urogram done once the pain has ceased is much less helpful. The author believes that the i.v.u. should be done as an emergency and at the earliest convenience.

Sometimes ureteric colic is complicated by the spontaneous rupture of the renal pelvis or the calyces. This can lead to a retroperitoneal collection of urine — a *urinoma*. A urinoma may be identified on plain films as a soft tissue mass causing loss of the renal and psoas outlines. It is frequently associated with a marked paralytic ileus. Diagnosis is confirmed by emergency urography.

Emphysematous pyelonephritis may be recognized by gas bubbles within the kidney or linear gas beneath the renal capsule. It occurs most commonly with uncontrolled diabetics or associated with obstructive uropathy.

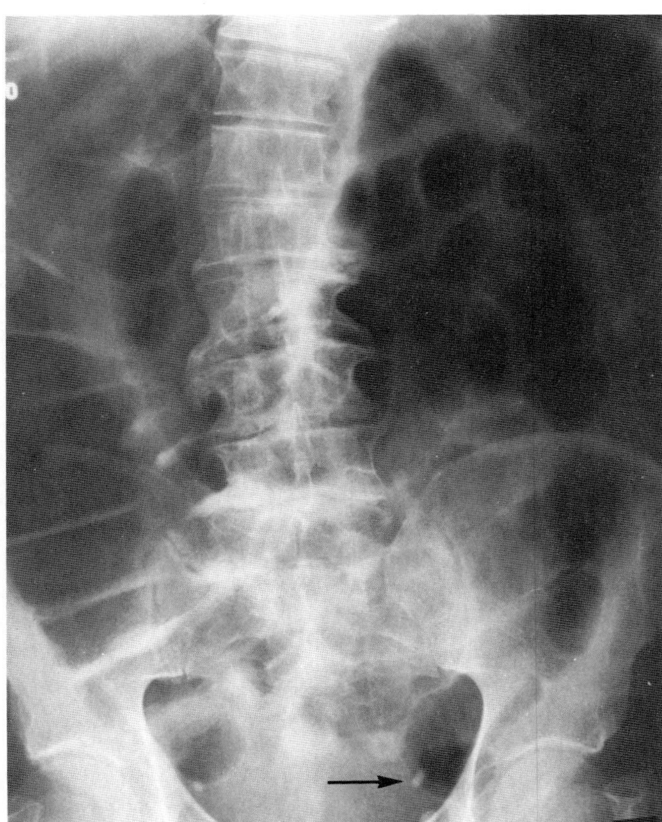

Fig. 33.31 Ureteric colic. Plain abdomen supine. There is considerable gaseous distension of large bowel and multiple loops of gas-filled small bowel. On the left side of the pelvis an oval opacity (→) represents a calculus impacted at the lower end of the left ureter. (Reproduced with permission, see Field 1984).

LEAKING ABDOMINAL AORTIC ANEURYSM

A leaking aortic aneurysm frequently presents as an acute abdomen and sometimes may simulate renal colic. Although clinical diagnosis may be obvious and urgent

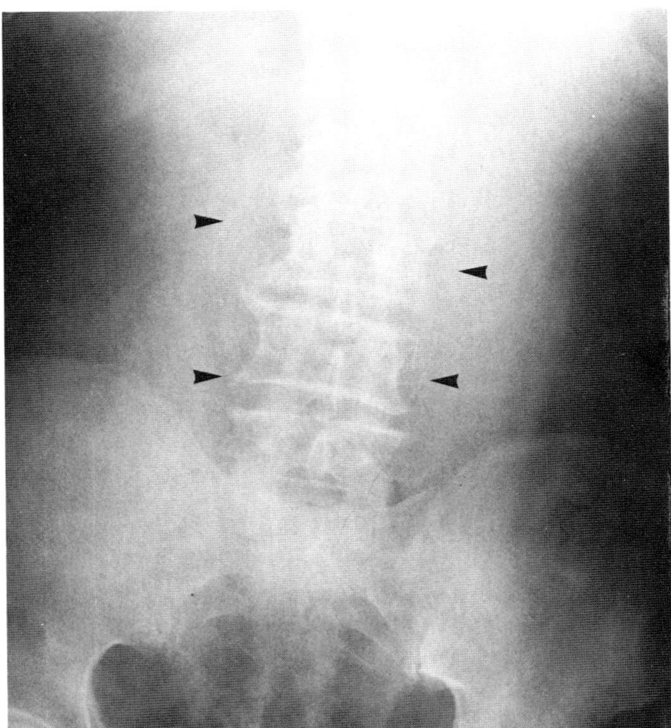

Fig. 33.32 Leaking aortic aneurysm. Supine. The faintly calcified rim of aortic aneurysm is identified (► ◄). In addition there is a large soft tissue mass outside the aneurysm indicating a retroperitoneal haematoma.

surgery indicated without any further investigations, in only one third of one series was the correct diagnosis made on admission (Prior 1972). If confirmation is required, ultrasound will establish the diagnosis of an aortic aneurysm but a leak or a retroperitoneal haematoma may be difficult to diagnose except by CT. Frequently, however, a leaking aneurysm is not suspected clinically and plain films are taken to investigate the cause of the abdominal pain. An aneurysm may be detected as a central soft tissue mass which may obscure the psoas outline on the left. Frequently curvilinear calcification may be seen on the antero-posterior view but if confirmation is required it is usually better demonstrated on a lateral film. The mere demonstration of an aortic aneurysm does not necessarily indicate that leaking has occurred. If, however, a soft tissue mass can be identified outside the calcified wall of the aneurysm, or bowel gas is displaced anteriorly, this is usually strong confirmation of a leak (Fig. 33.32).

On occasions an aneurysm is only suspected when laterally displaced and slightly obstructed ureters are detected on an emergency intravenous urogram done to investigate suspected renal colic.

A secondary paralytic ileus with associated air swallowing is frequently present, producing much gas-filled bowel and this may completely obscure the aneurysm itself.

Table 33.14 Abdominal calcification associated with an acute abdomen

Calcification	Acute condition
Appendix calculus	Appendicitis
Gallstones	Acute cholecystitis Acute pancreatitis Biliary colic Empyema of gall bladder Gallstone ileus
Calcified gall bladder wall	Cholecystitis
Limy bile	Cholecystitis
Calculus in Meckel's diverticulum or jejunal diverticulum	Acute inflammation or perforation
Pancreatic calculi	Pancreatitis — chronic and acute
Calcified aneurysms: aortic splenic hepatic	Rupture
Teeth or bone in ovarian dermoid	Torsion
Ureteric calculus	Ureteric colic

CALCIFICATION ASSOCIATED WITH ACUTE ABDOMINAL CONDITIONS

There are numerous causes of calcification within the abdomen. However, only a very few of these are associated with conditions which may give rise to an acute abdomen. These are summarized in Table 33.14.

REFERENCES AND SUGGESTIONS FOR FURTHER READING

Monographs

Field, S. (in press) *The Acute Abdomen — An Atlas of Plain Abdominal Radiography*. Chichester: John Wiley.

Frimann-Dahl, J. (1974) *Roentgen Examinations in Acute Abdominal Diseases*. Springfield, Ill.: Charles C. Thomas.

McCortt, J. J. (1981) *Abdominal Radiology*. Baltimore/London: Williams and Wilkins.

Myers, M. A. (1982) *Dynamic Radiology of the Abdomen*. New York: Springer-Verlag.

References

Anderson, J. R. & Lee, D. (1980) Acute caecal volvulus. *British Journal of Surgery*, **67**, 39–41.

Anderson, J. R. & Mills, J. O. M. (1984) Caecal volvulus; a frequently missed diagnosis? *Clinical Radiology*, **35**, 65–69.

Bakhda, R. K. & McNair, M. M. (1977) Appendicitis in children. *Clinical Radiology*, **28**, 193–196.

Bartram, C. I. (1976) Plain abdominal X-ray in acute colitis. *Proceedings of the Royal Society of Medicine*, **69**, 617–618.

Brockis, J. G. & Gilbert, M. C. (1957) Intestinal obstruction by gallstones. *British Journal of Surgery*, **44**, 461–466.

Brooke, B. N. & Sampson, P. A. (1964) An indication for surgery in acute ulcerative colitis. *Lancet*, **ii**, 1272–1273.

Bryant, L. R., Wiot, J. F. & Kloecker, R. J. (1963) A study of the factors affecting the incidence and duration of postoperative pneumoperitoneum. *Surgery, Gynecology and Obstetrics*, **117**, 145–150.

Chilaiditi, D. (1910) Zur frage der hepatoptose und ptose im allgemeinen im Anschluss an drei falle von temporarae partiellar leberverlagerung. *Fortschritte auf dem Gebiete der Roentgenstrahlen*, **16**, 173–208.

Colquhoun, J. (1965) Intramural gas in hollow viscera. *Clinical Radiology*, **16**, 71–85.

Connell, T. R., Stephens, D. H., Carlson, H. C. & Brown, M. I. (1980) Upper abdominal abscess; a continuing and deadly problem. *American Journal of Roentgenology*, **134**, 759–765.

Davis, L. & Lowman, R. M. (1957) Roentgen criteria of impending perforation of the caecum. *Radiology*, **68**, 542–548.

Day, E. A. & Marks, C. (1975) Gallstone ileus. *American Journal of Surgery*, **129**, 552–558.

De Lacey, G., Bloomberg, T. & Wignall, B. K. (1977) Pneumoperitoneum: the misleading double wall sign. *Clinical Radiology*, **28**, 445–448.

Ellis, H. (1981) Mechanical intestinal obstruction. *British Medical Journal*, **283**, 1203–1204.

Fagenberg, D. (1963) Fecaliths of the appendix, incidence and significance. *American Journal of Roentgenology*, **89**, 572–579.

Fataar, S. & Schulman, A. (1981) Subphrenic abscess: the radiological approach. *Clinical Radiology*, **32**, 147–156.

Field, S. (1984) Plain films: the acute abdomen. *Clinics in Gastroenterology*, **13**, 3–40.

Felson, B. & Wiot, J. F. (1973) Another look at pneumoperitoneum. *Seminars in Roentgenology VIII*, **4**, 437–443.

Fraser, F. M. & Fraser, I. D. (1974) Gastrografin in perforated duodenal ulcer and acute pancreatitis. *Clinical Radiology*, **25**, 397–402.

Gammill, S. L. & Nice, C. M. (1972) Air fluid levels: their occurrence in normal patients and their role in the analysis of ileus. *Surgery*, **71**, 771–780.

Gerzof, S. G., Robbins, A. H., Birkett, D. H., Johnson, W. C., Pugatch, R. D. & Vincent, M. E. (1979) Percutaneous catheter drainage of abdominal abscesses guided by ultrasound and computed tomography. *American Journal of Roentgenology*, **133**, 1–8.

Gough, N. R. (1978) Strangulating adhesive small bowel obstruction with normal radiographs. *British Journal of Surgery*, **65**, 431–434.

Graham, D. A. & Johnson, F. H. (1966) The incidence of radiographic findings in acute appendicitis compared to two hundred normals. *Military Medicine*, **131**, 272–276.

Halls, J. & Young, A. C. (1964) Plain abdominal films in colonic disease. *Proceedings of the Royal Society of Medicine*, **57**, 893–894.

Hellmer, H. (1942) Die konturen des rechten leberlappens beim ascites. *Acta Radiologica*, **23**, 533–540.

Jones, H. L. & Chapman, M. (1969) Definition of megacolon in colitis. *Gut*, **10**, 562–564.

Kerry, R. L. & Ransom, K. (1969) Volvulus of the colon. *Archives of Surgery*, **99**, 215–222.

Kolmannskog, F., Kolbenstvedt, A. & Aakhus, T. (1981) Computed tomography in inflammatory mass lesions following acute pancreatitis. *Journal of Computer Assisted Tomography*, **5**, 169–172.

Kramer, P. & Wittenberg, J. (1981) Colonic gas distribution in toxic megacolon. *Gastroenterology*, **80**, 433–437.

Lee, J. K. T., Stanley, R. J., Melson, G. L. & Sagel, S. A. (1979) Pancreatic imaging by ultrasound and computed tomography. *Radiologic Clinics of North America*, **16**, 105–117.

Loughran, C. F., Tappin, J. A. & Whitehouse, G. H. (1982) The plain abdominal radiograph in pseudomembranous colitis due to *Clostridium difficile*. *Clinical Radiology*, **33**, 277–281.

Love, L. (1960) The role of the ileocaecal valve in large bowel obstruction; a preliminary report. *Radiology*, **75**, 391–398.

Love, L. (1973) Large bowel obstruction. *Seminars in Roentgenology*, **8**, 299–322.

Magnusson, W. (1931) On meteorism in pyelography and on the passage of gas through the small intestine. *Acta Radiologica*, **12**, 552–561.

Mentzer, R. M., Golden, G. T., Chandler, J. G. & Horsley, J. S. (1975) A comparative appraisal of emphysematous cholecystitis. *American Journal of Surgery*, **129**, 10–15.

Menuck, L. & Siemers, P. T. (1976) Pneumoperitoneum: importance of right upper quadrant features. *American Journal of Roentgenology*, **127**,753–756.

Miller, R. E. (1973) The technical approach to the acute abdomen. *Seminars in Roentgenology VIII*, **3**, 267–279.

Miller, R. E. (1973) The radiological evaluation of intraperitoneal gas (pneumoperitoneum) CRC. *Critical Reviews in Radiological Sciences*, **4**, 61–84.

Miller, R. E. & Nelson, S. W. (1971) The roentgenologic demonstration of tiny amounts of free intraperitoneal gas; experimental and clinical studies. *American Journal of Roentgenology*, **112**, 574–585.

Millward, S. F., Breatnach, E., Simpkins, K. C. & Mahon, M. J. (1983) Do plain films of the chest and abdomen have a role in the diagnosis of acute pancreatitis? *Clinical Radiology*, **34**, 133–137.

Myers, M. A. (1982) *Dynamic Radiology of the Abdomen*. New York: Springer Verlag.

Prior, J. P. (1972) Diagnosis of ruptured aneurysm of abdominal aorta. *British Medical Journal*, **3**, 735–736.

Reeder, M. M. & Felson, B. (1975) *Gamuts in Radiology*. Oxford: Pergamon Press.

Rigler, L. G. (1941) Spontaneous pneumoperitoneum. A roentgen sign found in the supine patient. *Radiology*, **37**, 604–607.

Sander, R. C. (1970) Postoperative pleural effusion and subphrenic abscess. *Clinical Radiology*, **21**, 308–312.

Shaw, R. E. (1965) Appendix calculi and acute appendicitis. *British Journal of Surgery*, **52**, 451–459.

Snape, W. J. Jnr (1982) Pseudo-obstruction and other obstructive disorders. *Clinics in Gastroenterology*, **11**, (3), 593–608.

Vessal, K. & Borhanmanesh, F. (1976) Hepatodiaphragmatic interposition of the intestine (Chilaiditi's syndrome). *Clinical Radiology*, **27**, 113–116.

Weens, H. S. & Walker, L. A. (1964) The radiologic diagnosis of acute cholecystitis and pancreatitis. *Radiologic Clinics of North America*, **2**, 89–106.

Williams, J. L. (1962) Fluid-filled loops in intestinal obstruction. *American Journal of Roentgenology*, **88**, 667–686.

Williams, A. J. & Hartzell, H. V. (1940) Perforated peptic ulcer. *Surgery, Gynecology and Obstetrics*, **71**, 606–614.

Whalen, J. P. (1976) *Radiology of the Abdomen, Anatomic Basis*. Philadelphia: Lea and Febiger.

Wolfer, J. A., Beaton, L. E. & Anson, B. J. (1942) Volvulus of the caecum. *Surgery, Gynecology and Obstetrics*, **74**, 882–894.

Wolverson, M. K., Jaganna, I. B., Sundaram, M., Joyce, P. F., Riaz, M. A. & Shields, J. B. (1979) CT as a primary diagnostic method in evaluating abdominal abscesses. *American Journal of Roentgenology*, **133**, 1089–1095.

Wyman, A. C. (1954) Traumatic rupture of the spleen. *American Journal of Roentgenology*, **72**, 51–63.

Young, W. S., Englebrecht, H. E., Stoker, A. (1978) Plain film analysis of sigmoid volvulus. *Clinical Radiology*, **29**, 553–560.

Young, W. S., White, A. & Grave, G. F. (1978) The radiology of ileosigmoid knot. *Clinical Radiology*, **29**, 211–216.

CHAPTER 34

THE BILIARY TRACT

The biliary tract will be discussed under the following headings:

1. IMAGING INVESTIGATIONS
   a. Plain radiography
   b. Indirect contrast studies
      (i) Oral cholecystography
      (ii) Intravenous cholangiography
   c. Direct cholangiography
      (i) Operative
      (ii) T-tube (postoperative)
      (iii) PTC (percutaneous transhepatic cholangiography)
      (iv) ERCP (endoscopic retrograde cholangio-pancreatography)
   d. Ultrasound
   e. CT (computed tomography)
   f. Isotope scanning
   g. MRI (magnetic resonance imaging)
2. THE ABNORMAL GALL BLADDER
3. THE ABNORMAL BILIARY TREE
4. INTERVENTIONAL RADIOLOGY IN THE BILIARY TREE
5. THE INVESTIGATION OF JAUNDICE

IMAGING INVESTIGATIONS

PLAIN RADIOGRAPHY

It is essential that a control film is taken before any radiological examination of the biliary tract as the complete diagnosis in biliary tract disease may be available on the plain film. Further, vital information may be undetected if the plain film is not taken or examined before contrast obscures opaque stones.

Gallstones are a mixture of cholesterol, pigment, protein and calcium, the content of calcium determining their radiodensity. The densest gallstones are almost pure calcium carbonate, often of mulberry shape (Figs 34.1 and 34.2). The most common opaque stones however are mixed stones. These are characterized by lamination and they are often faceted (Fig. 34.3). Opaque gallstones may be missed either because their radiodensity is very low, or because they overlie the spine, especially when attention is distracted at barium meal or barium enema examination.

Calcium carbonate deposits may occur in the gall bladder as '*biliary sand*' or '*limy bile*'. A 'level' is usually seen on

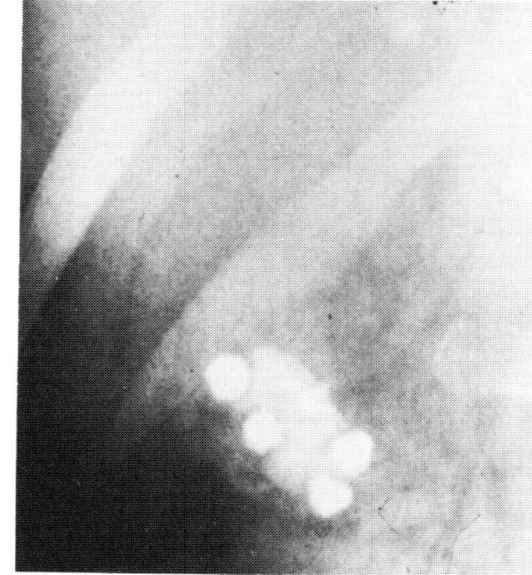

Fig. 34.1 Calcium carbonate ('mulberry') stones.

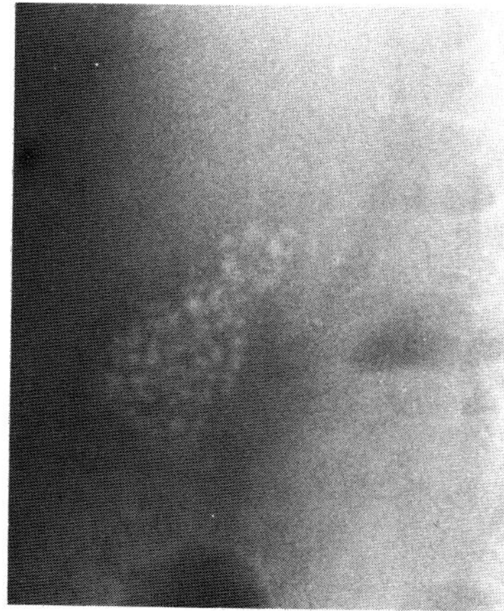

Fig. 34.2 Small, very dense stones, probably calcium carbonate.

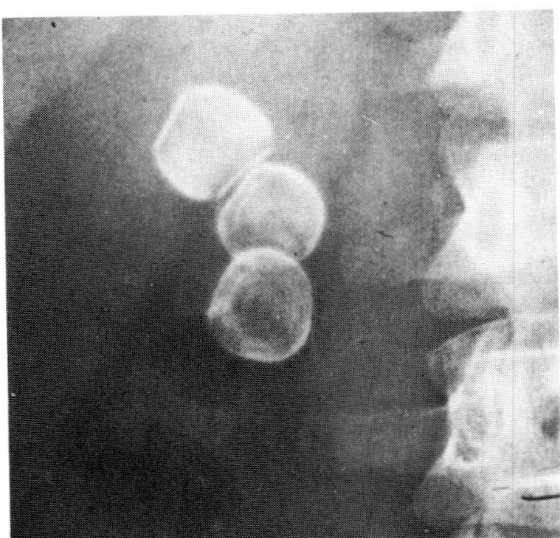

Fig. 34.3 'Mixed stones' showing lamination and facets.

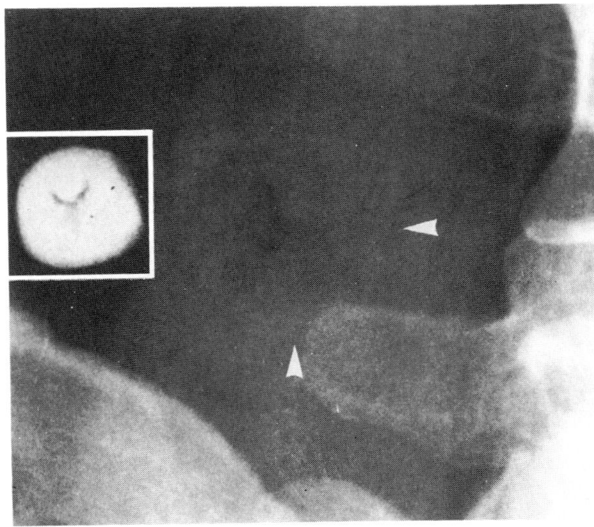

Fig. 34.5 'Mercedes Benz' stone; characteristic appearance on the plain radiograph (arrows) and after removal (insert).

the erect film (Fig. 34.4). Mulberry stones may be present in addition and the cystic duct is usually blocked. Caution should be exercised in making this plain film diagnosis as similar appearances may occur with opaque 'sand' and tiny stones in the right renal pelvis.

Rarely, a non-opaque gallstone can be diagnosed on plain radiography by the presence of gas-containing clefts within it (Fig. 34.5). The clefts are said to result from gas-forming organisms trapped within the stone.

About 20% of patients with multiple gall bladder stones also harbour stones within the common bile duct (Fig. 34.6). The incidence of bile duct stones is strongly age-related. However, the incidence of calcification in bile duct stones is very much less than that of gall bladder stones (about 1% compared with 25%). The reasons for this disparity are not known.

Very rarely, the wall of the gall bladder affected by chronic inflammatory disease may undergo calcification, resulting in '*porcelain gall bladder*' (Fig. 34.7). The cystic duct is usually blocked. The porcelain gall bladder has an even stronger predisposition towards malignant change than the gall bladder which contains stones.

When radiopaque gallstones are widely separated from each other, a confident diagnosis of obstructed and distended gall bladder may be made. The obstructing stone may be seen separately in Hartmann's pouch. If there is evidence of dilated intestinal loops, the diagnosis is almost certainly an *empyema* rather than a simple *mucocele* of the gall bladder.

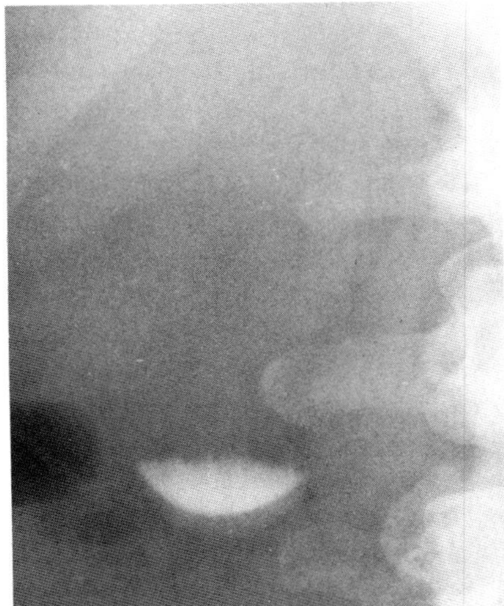

Fig. 34.4 'Limy bile' (calcium carbonate sand) on erect film.

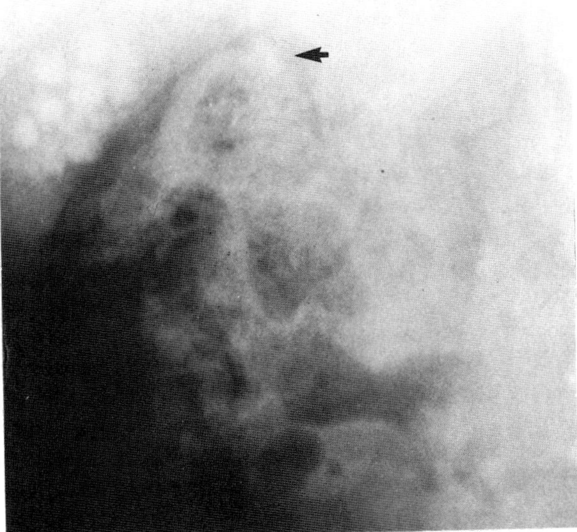

Fig. 34.6 'Mulberry stones' in gall bladder and bile duct (arrow).

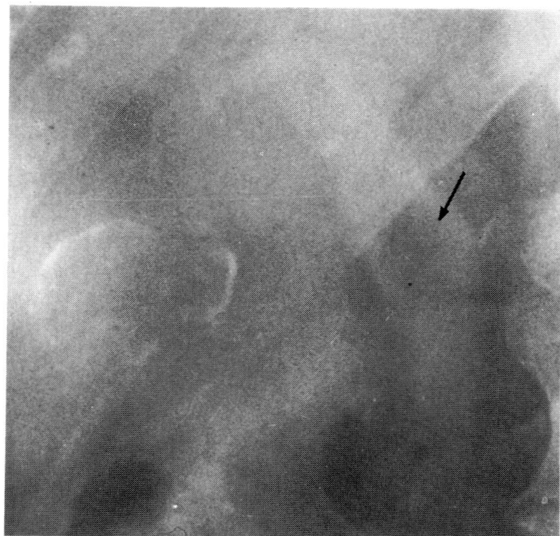

Fig. 34.7 Calcified ('porcelain') gall bladder; the common duct is dilated and contains a large stone (i.v.c.).

Gas in the biliary tract

Gas may be seen in the biliary tract on plain films in two separate circumstances:

1. *Emphysematous cholecystitis*. The patient is usually diabetic and desperately ill. Gas, produced by organisms, is seen both within the lumen of the gall bladder and in the gall bladder wall (Fig. 34.8A and B).

2. *Abnormal communication between the biliary tract and the intestine*. This is most commonly seen following endoscopic sphincterotomy (Fig. 34.9). Gas is also seen in the bile ducts after surgical sphincterotomy or sphincteroplasty, cholecyst-duodenostomy or choledocho-enterostomy. Indeed, if gas is absent from the biliary tree after these surgical procedures, there is strong evidence that the surgical anastomosis has become strictured.

Rare causes of gas in the biliary tree are:

1. *Penetration of a benign peptic ulcer* into the bile duct or gall bladder.

2. Sphincter dysfunction in *tumours of the ampulla* and when the sphincter remains patulous after the *recent passage of a stone*.

Gall stone ileus (Fig. 33.14, p. 940) is a rare condition much loved by examiners because the diagnosis can be made on the basis of the constellation of the following radiological signs: gas in the gall bladder (and perhaps in the biliary tree), distended small intestine and an obstructing faintly calcified gallstone (see also Fig. 31.52).

Chronic Ascaris abscesses, a rare complication in the liver, may be diagnosed on the plain film when the worms are seen as opacities against the background of gas in the cavity (Fig. 34.10).

Barium may reflux into the biliary tree through any abnormal communication (Fig. 34.11).

INDIRECT CONTRAST STUDIES

Oral cholecystography

Despite the increasing availability and popularity of ultrasound, the oral cholecystogram remains the most common first-line investigation for suspected disease of the gall bladder.

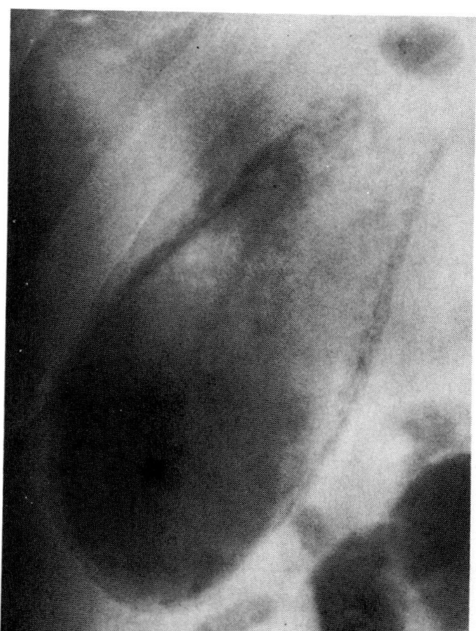

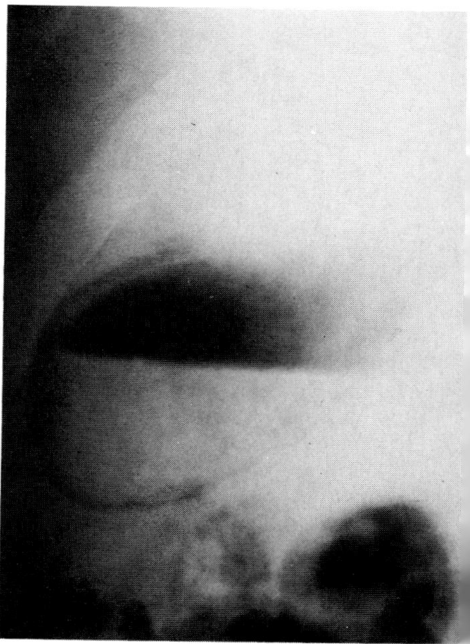

Fig. 34.8 Emphysematous cholecystitis showing (**A**) gas in the lumen and wall of the gall bladder, (**B**) a gas-fluid level in the erect posture.

A

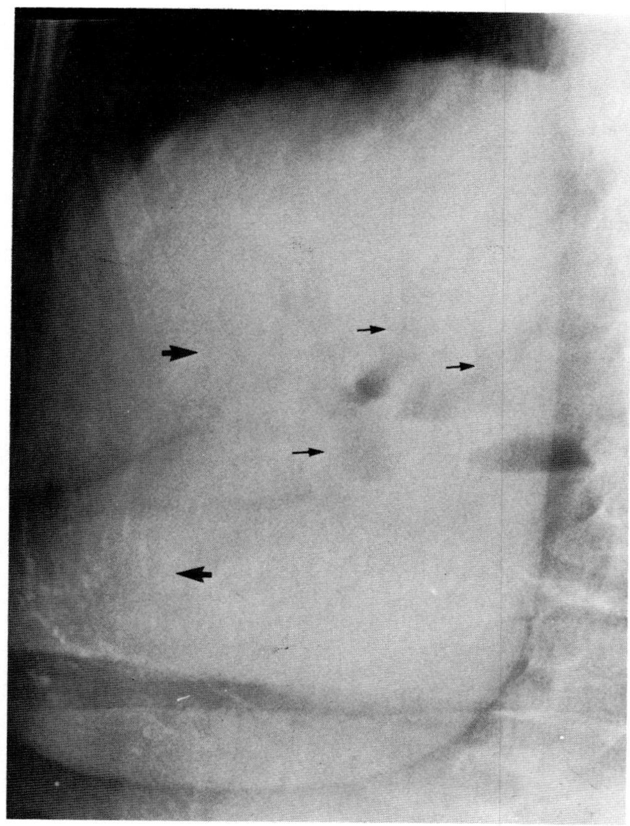

Fig. 34.9 Gas in biliary tree following endoscopic sphincterotomy (→). Note overlying benign calcifying breast disease (←).

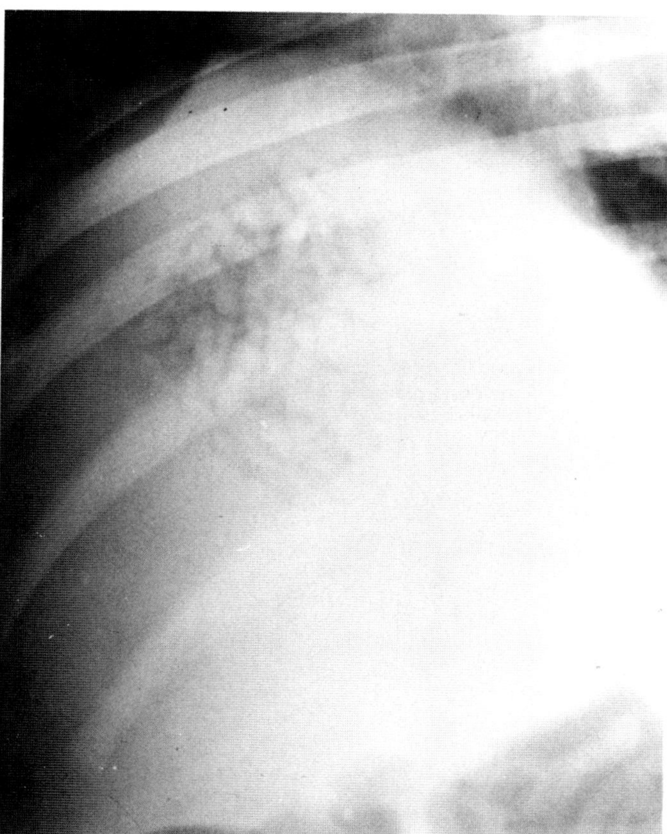

Fig. 34.10 Chronic *Ascaris* abscess of liver. The worms are seen in contrast against gas in the cavity.

Appearance of contrast in the gall bladder depends upon the following sequence of steps:

1. Ingestion of the contrast agent by the patient.
2. Adequate absorption of the contrast agent from the gut. Absorption may be delayed if the patient has achalasia of the oesophagus or pyloric stenosis, and adequate absorption may fail to occur in the presence of vomiting, diarrhoea or small intestinal disease.
3. Hepatic excretion of contrast in the bile. Excretion may be inadequate in the presence of significant hepatocellular disease. The examination is contraindicated in the presence of jaundice.
4. Patency of the cystic duct. Contrast cannot reach the gall bladder if the cystic duct is blocked.
5. Concentration of the contrast agent in the gall bladder. This requires both time and a normal gall bladder mucosa. All oral contrast agents also undergo enterohepatic recirculation.

Modern oral contrast media. The media in common use today are Biloptin (sodium ipodate) and Solu-Biloptin (calcium ipodate). As may be seen in Figure 34.12, they are tri-iodinated benzene rings. They differ from conventional urographic agents by virtue of incomplete substi-

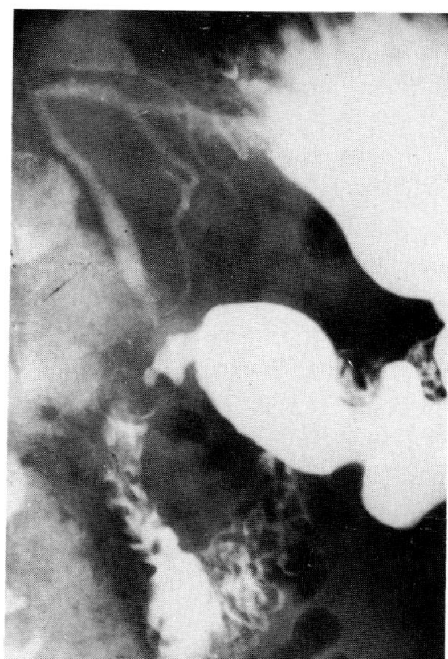

Fig. 34.11 Barium entering the common duct from a penetrating duodenal ulcer.

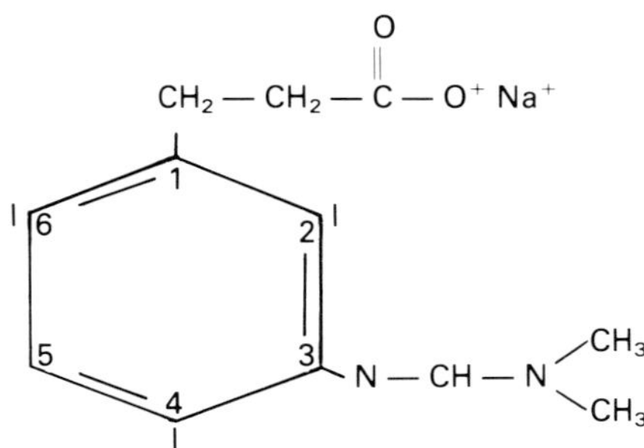

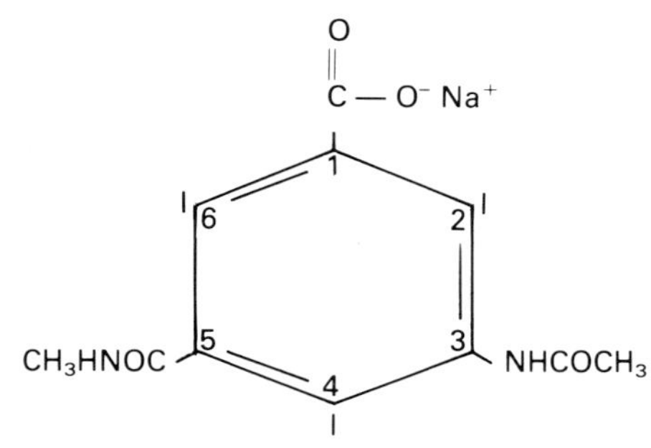

Fig. 34.12 Chemical structure of a typical oral contrast medium (**A**) and a typical urographic medium (**B**) for comparison.

tution at position 5 on the nucleus. These agents have the advantage over older oral contrast agents that they are excreted in sufficient concentration in hepatic bile to enable visualization of the extrahepatic bile ducts (Fig. 34.13).

Unwanted side effects consist of headache, nausea, diarrhoea and dysuria and, while usually of mild degree, they occur with an incidence of up to 50%. Hypersensitivity reactions (urticaria and oedema) have also been reported.

Technique. The control film is first obtained. If this shows opacities characteristic of gall bladder stones, the examination is concluded and the diagnosis is made. Otherwise, the patient is asked to take 3 g of the contrast medium (according to the manufacturer's instruction) after the evening meal. Nothing further is taken by mouth until 7.00 a.m. the next day when a further dose of contrast medium is taken. Again, nothing further is taken by mouth and the patient reports for the second part of the examination at 9.00 a.m. The rationale of evening and morning doses is as follows. The 12–15-hour interval between evening dose and 2nd day films is sufficient to allow adequate concentration of contrast in the gall bladder. The additional morning dose (2–3 hours before films) theoretically allows maximal bile duct opacification with oral media.

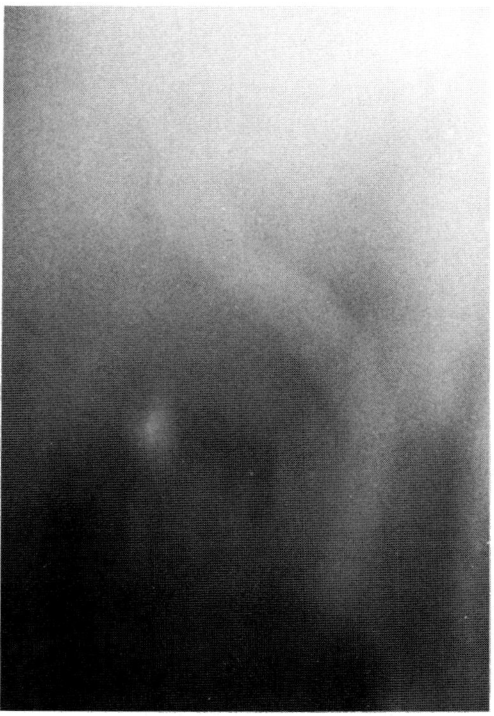

Fig. 34.13 Bile ducts well visualized after oral (not intravenous) contrast.

Coned films (low kV) are taken in the prone oblique, supine oblique and erect (or decubitus) positions. The various projections help to distinguish mobile stones (which sink or occasionally float) from fixed mural filling defects and extraneous shadows.

When these films have been seen by the radiologist, a fatty meal (usually a proprietary preparation) is given and a further single film is taken 30–60 minutes later. The AFM (after fatty meal) film is not obtained primarily to determine whether the gall bladder contracts. Contraction itself is of very doubtful importance, but, if the gall bladder does contract, it may allow an abnormality to be more confidently diagnosed and may improve visualization of the bile duct (Fig. 34.14).

Non-opacifying gall bladder (no opaque calculi). When the gall bladder is not visualized on the second day films, the following steps should be taken:

1. The patient is asked whether the medium was in fact ingested. Traces of contrast seen in the intestine will confirm that the medium has been taken by the patient.
2. The patient is asked whether diarrhoea or vomiting occurred.
3. A film of the whole abdomen is taken to exclude the possibility of grossly ptosed or ectopic gall bladder.

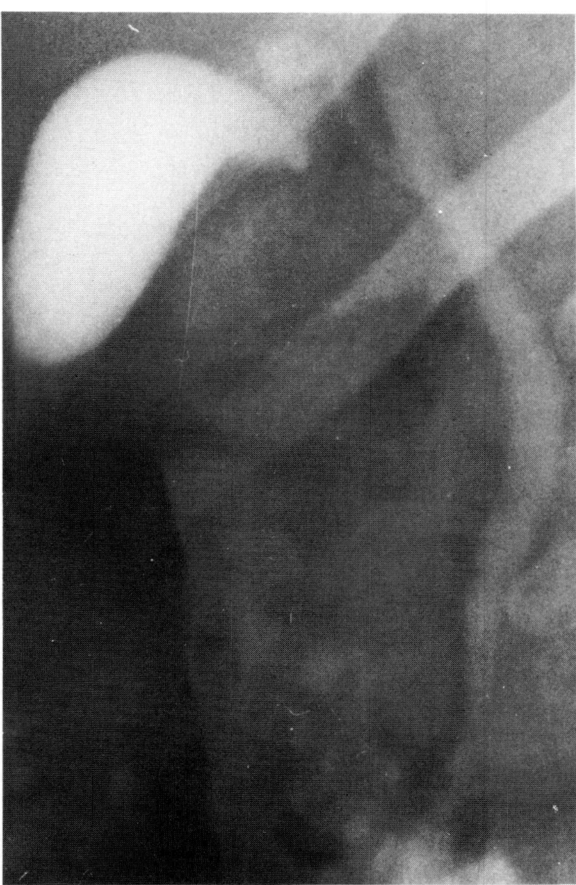

Fig. 34.14 Common bile duct well visualized at oral cholecystography after fatty meal.

4. The films are closely inspected for evidence of bile duct opacification. It is even worth taking tomograms of the bile duct at this stage. If the bile duct has opacified and the gall bladder has not, the gall bladder is unquestionably abnormal. There are three possibilities:

a. The gall bladder has been removed surgically.
b. The cystic duct is blocked, usually by a stone.
c. The gall bladder mucosa is abnormal, preventing concentration of the medium.

5. Further doses of contrast medium are given (evening and morning) and the examination repeated ('double dose' technique).

6. Alternatively, if facilities are available, an ultrasound examination is performed.

Accuracy. The reliability of oral cholecystography in detection of gall bladder calculi is greater than 95% and it is therefore one of the most accurate diagnostic examinations of any kind.

Intravenous cholangiography

The indications for intravenous cholangiography are diminishing rapidly because:

1. If cholecystectomy is contemplated, the bile ducts will usually be investigated by operative cholangiography.
2. In the symptomatic postcholecystectomy patient (the traditional indication for i.v.c.) the examination is simply not reliable enough for stone or stricture of the duct to be confidently excluded. I.v.c. in these circumstances is being replaced by ERCP (because of the therapeutic possibilities described below) or by PTC.
3. The extrahepatic bile ducts are frequently well visualized at oral cholecystography, especially after gall bladder contraction or if tomography is performed.

Contrast agents. The chemical structure of a typical intravenous cholangiographic agent Biligram (meglumine ioglycamate) is shown in Figure 34.15. Intravenous agents have a high aqueous solubility rendering them suitable for intravenous, but not for oral, administration. They become even more highly bound to albumin than the oral agents, a source of their high toxicity. Unlike the oral agents, they do not undergo glucuronization on passage through the liver and do not undergo significant enterohepatic recirculation.

Technique. A control film is taken to exclude air or opaque stone in the ducts. The contrast agent (typically 30 ml Biligram)is given by slow intravenous injection (5 minutes) or by infusion (10–15 minutes). The medium appears in the duct about 20 minutes after commencement of injection and a coned, low kV film should be taken at

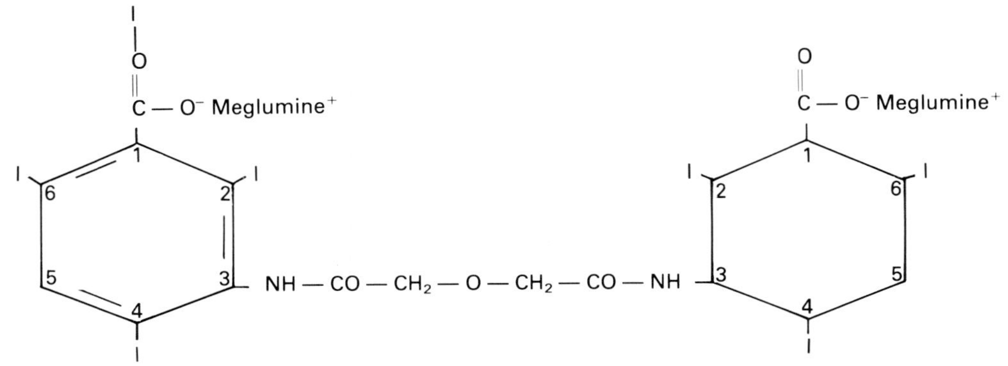

C — O⁻ Meglumine⁺   C — O⁻ Meglumine⁺

NH — CO — CH_2 — O — CH_2 — CO — NH

Fig. 34.15 Chemical structure of the intravenous cholangiographic agent Biligram (ioglycamide). Protein binding results from the two unsubstituted 5 positions and, to a lesser extent, from the long linking chain.

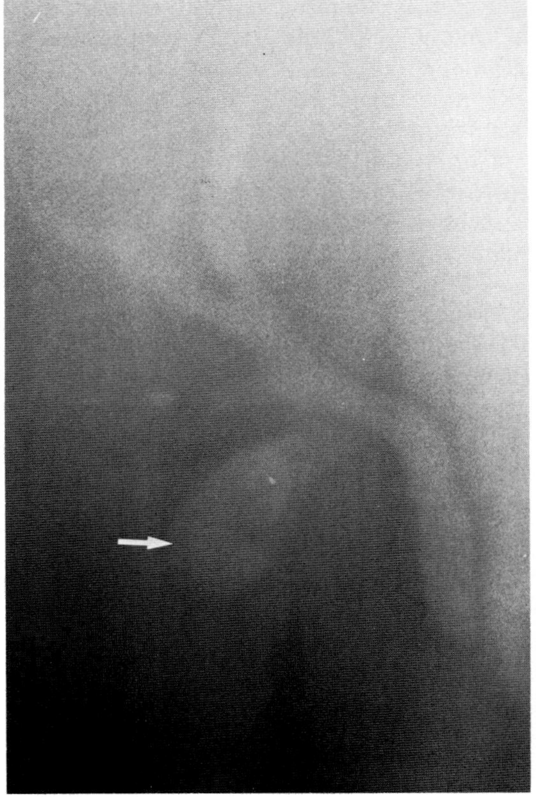

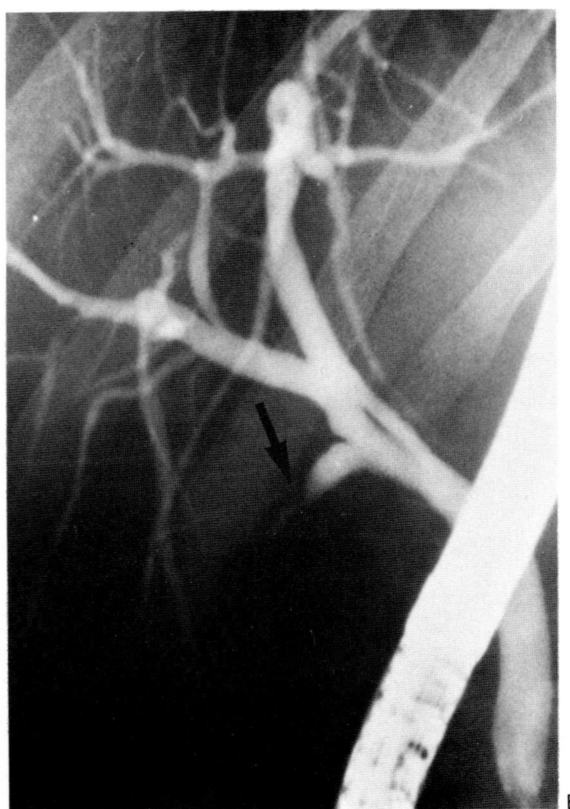

Fig. 34.16 A. Contrast pooling in duodenal cap (arrow) mimics gall bladder containing stones in patient alleged to have had cholecystectomy. **B.** ERC in same patient shows occluded cystic duct (arrow) confirming the history given.

this time with the patient slightly prone oblique to throw the duct clear of the spine. Tomography is almost always required for adequate visualization.

Interpretation. The examination is normal if the following conditions are satisfied:

1. The duct calibre is less than 1 cm.
2. No filling defects are seen within it.
3. Contrast appears in the duodenum.
4. Contrast density in the duct is less on a film taken after 1 hour than on the 20-minute film.

Injunctions to obtain 24 or 48 hour films 'for the gall bladder' should be resisted strongly. The i.v.c. is not an examination for the gall bladder. It is an investigation and an unsatisfactory one at that, of the bile duct. The i.v.c. has no place in investigating patients who have had surgical anastomoses of the bile duct to the intestine. If the anastomosis is patent, the bile duct will not be visualized. If there is a strictured anastomosis, the i.v.c. is likely to be unhelpful or misleading.

Complications. Hypersensitivity reactions are much more common than at intravenous urography and the mortality rate is possibly as high as 1 in 3000.

In the postcholecystecomy patient, contrast at i.v.c. may pool in the duodenal cap mimicking the gall bladder. Direct cholangiography reveals the true state of affairs (Fig. 34.16A and B).

DIRECT CHOLANGIOGRAPHY

By this term is meant the injection of contrast direct into the biliary tree by needle or catheter. In general terms, direct contrast studies are more accurate than indirect studies because a higher contrast density can be achieved and the volume and concentration of contrast can be varied at will.

Operative cholangiography (Fig. 34.17A and B). Most surgeons routinely employ cholangiography to examine the extrahepatic bile ducts at the time of cholecystectomy. A catheter is usually inserted through an incision into the cystic duct and advanced into the common duct. Films are exposed after three increments of contrast injection. As for all cholangiography, the criteria of normality are:

1. Non-dilated duct.
2. Absence of filling defects.
3. Free flow of contrast into the duodenum.

Ideally the films should be examined by a radiologist as

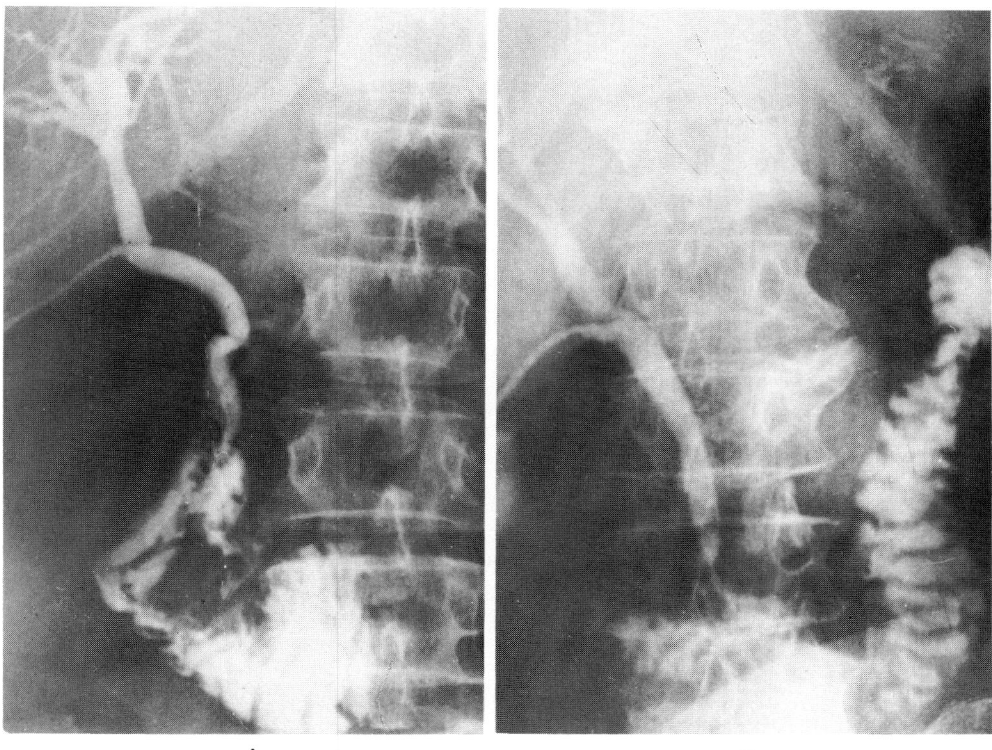

Fig. 34.17 A. and **B.** Normal pre-exploratory operative cholangiograms in two patients showing the limits of variation in the position of the ampulla of Vater.

soon as they are processed. Abnormalities can then be reported immediately to the surgeon. If the films are technically inadequate, the examination may be repeated on the spot.

If stones are present and the duct is explored surgically, a 'completion' cholangiogram is sometimes performed. The aim of this study is to confirm that all stones have been removed. However, the completion examination is technically inferior to the initial operative cholangiogram because air bubbles and blood clots have usually been introduced.

T-tube cholangiography

After surgical exploration, the duct is usually closed around a T-tube. After 7–10 days, when any air introduced at surgery has been absorbed and any blood clots lysed, a T-tube cholangiogram is performed. The specific purpose of this examination is to exclude residual stones or other abnormality. The criteria for a normal examination are the same as those listed for operative cholangiography.

A number of technical aspects need attention. A preliminary film should be obtained. The concentration of contrast medium should initially be around 150 mg I/ml in order that small stones are not obscured (Fig. 34.18A and B). If the duct is considerably dilated, the contrast should be diluted further (as a rough guide, the contrast should be diluted 50% with saline for every 5 mm increase in duct diameter). The whole of the biliary tree must be visualized and this may necessitate turning the patient on the left side, and even head down, in order to opacify the ducts within the left lobe of the liver (Fig. 34.19). A delay of a few seconds should be allowed between injection of contrast and exposure of film to ensure that any stones are at rest during exposure. A moving stone may not be seen on the film. If sphincteroplasty has been performed, there may be such rapid flow of contrast into the duodenum that a steep head down tilt is required to opacify the intrahepatic ducts.

Percutaneous transhepatic cholangiography (PTC)

In this examination, a needle is passed percutaneously into the liver under local or general anaesthesia. Contrast is continuously injected while the needle is slowly withdrawn. When the biliary tree begins to fill, needle withdrawal is stopped and further injection outlines the intrahepatic and extrahepatic biliary tract. If the bile duct is seen to be dilated, the concentration of contrast is immediately reduced for the reason given above. When the bile ducts have been filled with contrast, the needle is withdrawn and films are exposed. As with any direct cholangiogram, erect or decubitus films may be required to complete the examination.

The prothrombin time should not be more than 3 seconds prolonged; antibiotic cover should be used to

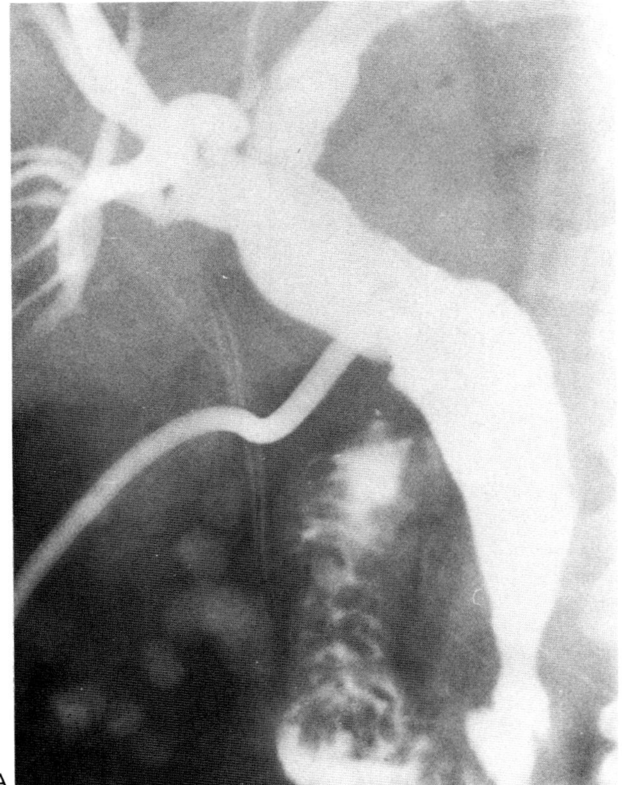

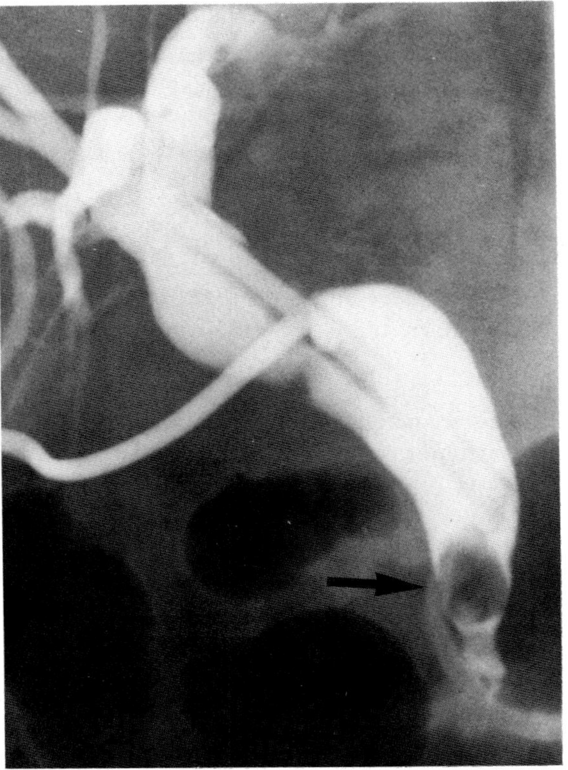

Fig. 34.18 T-tube cholangiogram. **A.** Dilated duct but no stones seen with contrast concentration 280 mg I/ml. **B.** Contrast diluted 50% with saline. Large stone now visible (arrow), as is previously obscured T-tube.

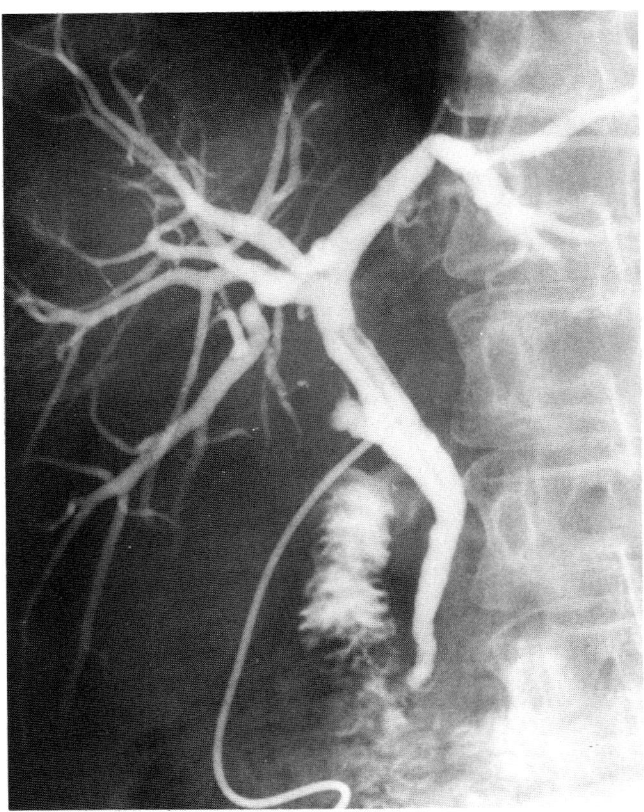

Fig. 34.19 'Complete' cholangiogram. Opacification of all the intrahepatic ducts at direct cholangiography is essential. This may require head down or left lateral decubitus positions.

minimize the risk of septicaemia; and preparation should be made for decompression (transhepatic or surgical) if the bile duct is obstructed.

The main indications for diagnostic PTC are:

1. *Jaundice*. If the jaundice is obstructive, the intrahepatic ducts are usually dilated and the level of obstruction, and usually the cause of obstruction, can be diagnosed. Failure to obtain a percutaneous cholangiogram, in the hands of an experienced operator, is a highly reliable indication that the intrahepatic ducts are not dilated and that the cause of the jaundice is not obstruction.

2. *Postcholecystectomy syndrome*. A significant proportion of patients who have cholecystectomy for pain do not have permanent relief of their symptoms. If cholangitis or intermittent jaundice has occurred since cholecystectomy, PTC will usually show a stone or duct stricture. If pain has been the only symptom since surgery, the examination is usually normal (Fig. 34.20).

Portal vein branches and hepatic veins are frequently demonstrated at PTC. Occasionally lymphatic vessels coursing through the lesser omentum are opacified if a parenchymal injection is inadvertently made (Fig. 34.21).

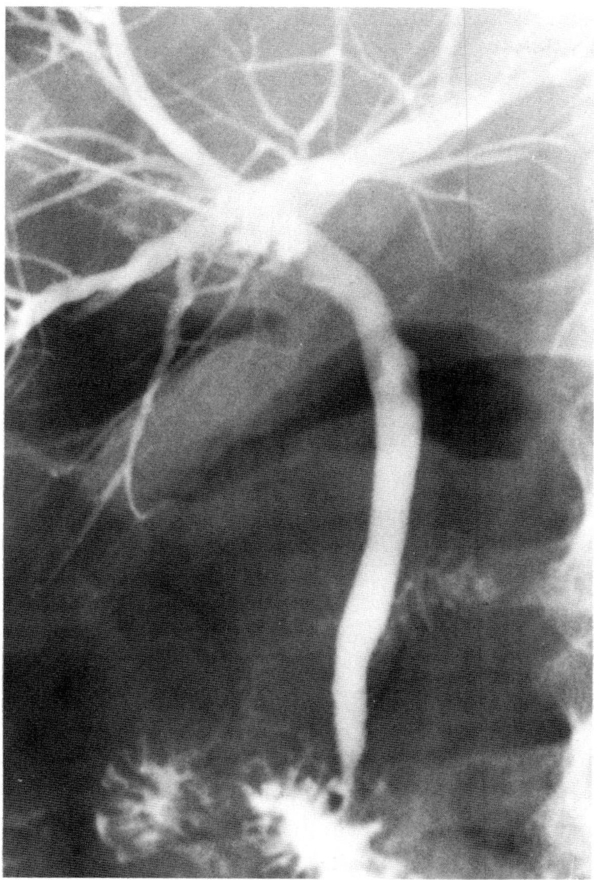

Fig. 34.20 Normal PTC. Postcholecystectomy (22-gauge transhepatic needle shown). Procedure complete when entire extrahepatic duct is filled and contrast has entered duodenum.

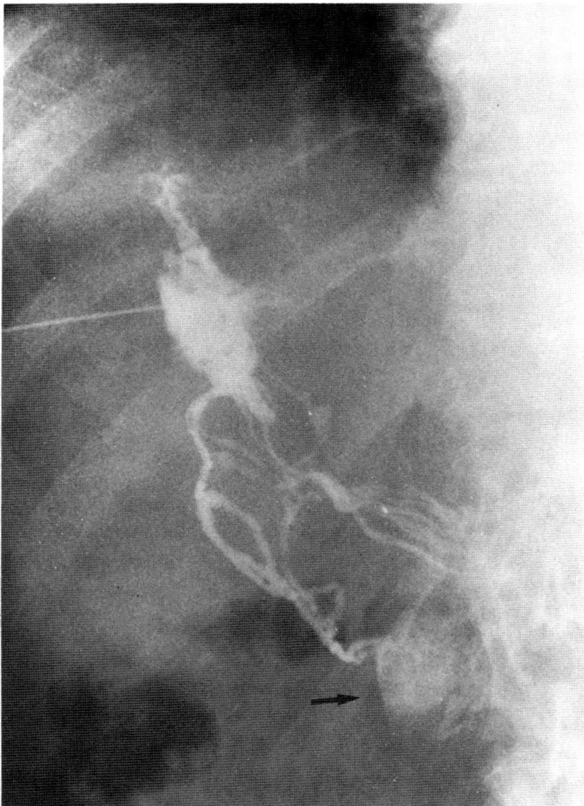

Fig. 34.21 Parenchymal injection at PTC. Lymphatic vessels draining to lymph node (arrow).

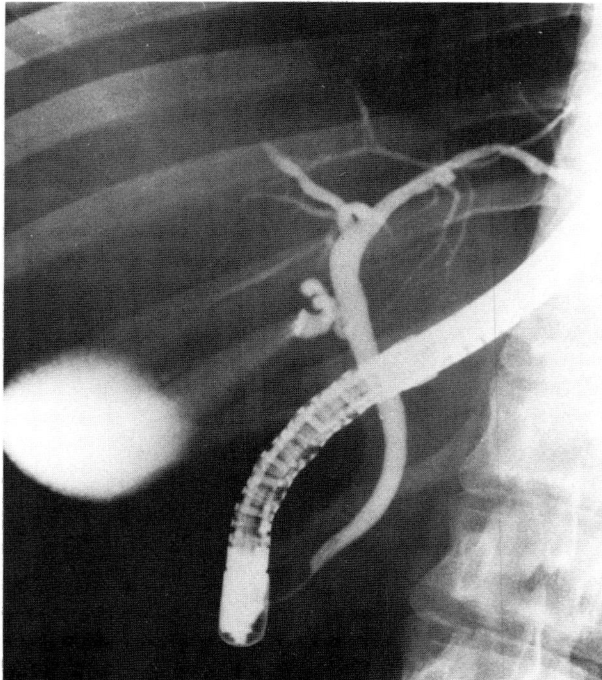

Fig. 34.22 Normal ERC.

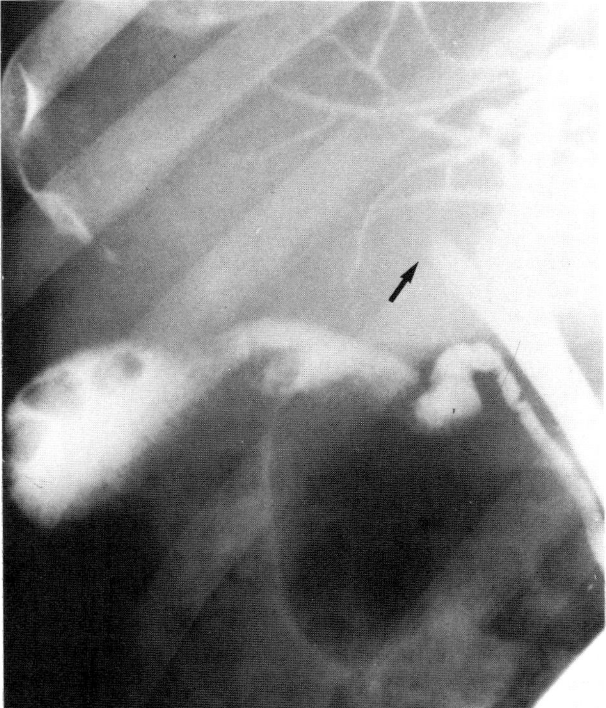

Fig. 34.23 ERCP showing stones in gall bladder. The ill-defined cut-off of the right hepatic duct (arrow) results from the patient's prone oblique position and not from an organic lesion.

Endoscopic retrograde cholangiography (ERC)

This technique is rapidly replacing PTC, the indications being broadly similar. It may be safely performed when the prothrombin time is significantly prolonged but is contra-indicated when endoscopic access to the papilla of Vater is restricted as a result of pyloric or duodenal stenosis, Polya gastrectomy or choledocho-enterostomy. A side-viewing duodenoscope is passed and a fine catheter is introduced through it into the bile duct. Contrast is injected and films are exposed. Consistently good quality films can only be obtained if a radiologist supervises the examination (Fig. 34.22).

Because the films are exposed in the prone oblique position (left side down) there is commonly underfilling of the right lobe. An ill-defined cut-off of the right hepatic duct (Fig. 34.23) should not be interpreted as obstruction.

ULTRASOUND
(by W. R. Lees)

Gall bladder

A 6-hour fast ensures an uncontracted gall bladder, the optimal condition for diagnosis of intraluminal abnormalities. Good visualization of the entire gall bladder can be obtained by scanning in at least two planes and two positions. Movement of calculi within the lumen may then be observed and the dependent walls of the organ may be visualized with the beam orientated vertically. The left lateral decubitus is the single most reliable position for scanning the gall bladder or porta hepatis region.

Contraction of the gall bladder in response to a fatty meal or cholecystokinin may be observed but rarely assists diagnosis. It does, however, allow ultrasonic separation of the gall bladder wall into mucosa, muscularis and serosa. These layers are best seen at high frequencies (5 MHz and above). The normal contracted gall bladder has a wall up to 3 mm thick (Fig. 34.24).

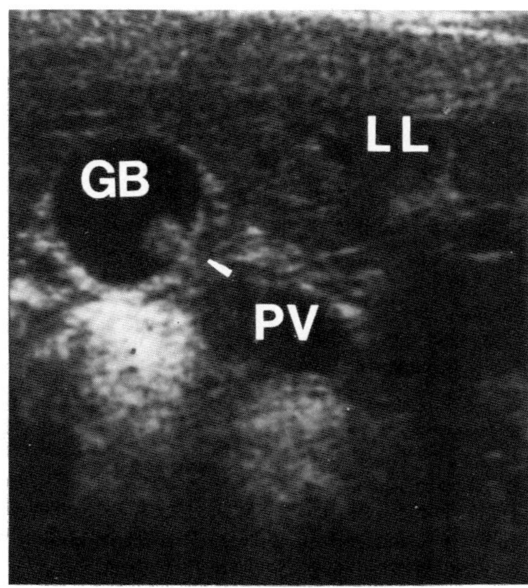

Fig. 34.24 Transverse section. Normal gall bladder with small mucosal polyp (small arrow head) (GB = gall bladder, PV = portal vein, LL = left lobe of liver).

The biliary tree

The normal intrahepatic ducts are seen to their third or fourth divisions with modern ultrasound. Assessment of calibre is largely subjective but comparison with the associated portal vein branch allows use of the 'sign of four'. A ratio (biliary: portal) of 1:4 is definitely normal, 2:4 indicates minimal dilatation and greater than 3:4 significant dilatation.

The calibre of the extrahepatic bile duct is directly measured and compared with standard nomograms.

Visualization of the lower part of the common bile duct is best in the erect position with the duodenum distended with water. Figure 34.25 shows dilated intrahepatic bile ducts, and Figure 34.26 (A and B) shows obstructed and dilated common bile ducts in patients with stone and malignant obstruction respectively.

CT SCANNING

Although gall bladder stones, which are too poorly calcified to be seen on plain X-rays, may be visualized on CT, CT has no primary role in the investigation of non-acute gall bladder disease. CT, however, plays a vital role in the investigation of jaundice as an alternative to ultrasound examination (see below).

ISOTOPE SCANNING (see Ch. 66)

Isotope scanning has a limited role in biliary, as opposed to parenchymal hepatic disease. Although dynamic scans with HIDA (and newer modifications of this agent) allow functional studies of excretion, even when the patient is

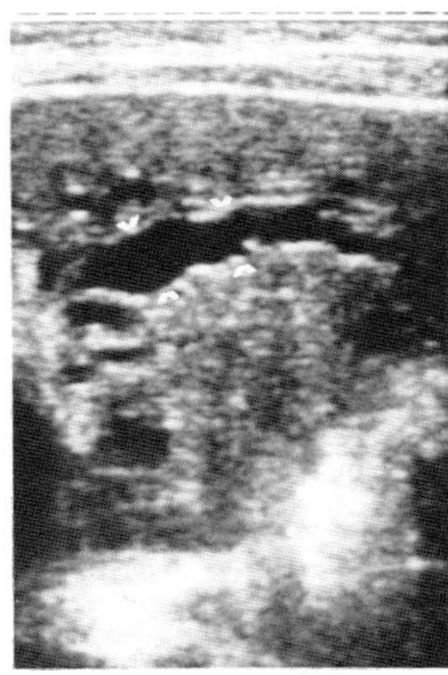

Fig. 34.25 Transverse section. Dilated intrahepatic bile ducts (small arrow heads) in the left lobe of the liver. Note the sharp but irregular margins, echo-free contents and distal acoustic enhancement.

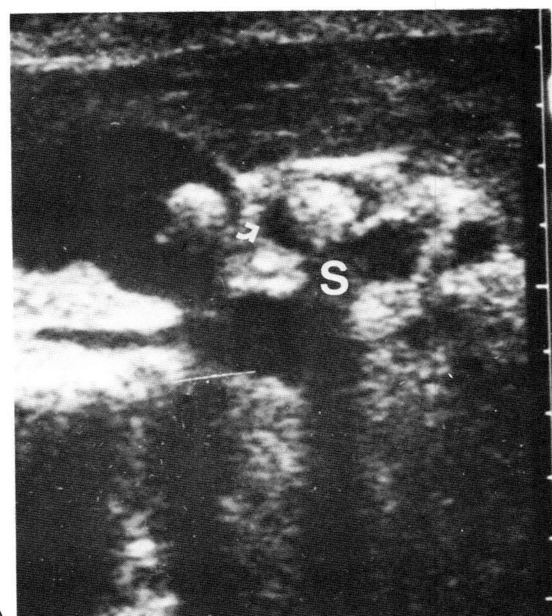

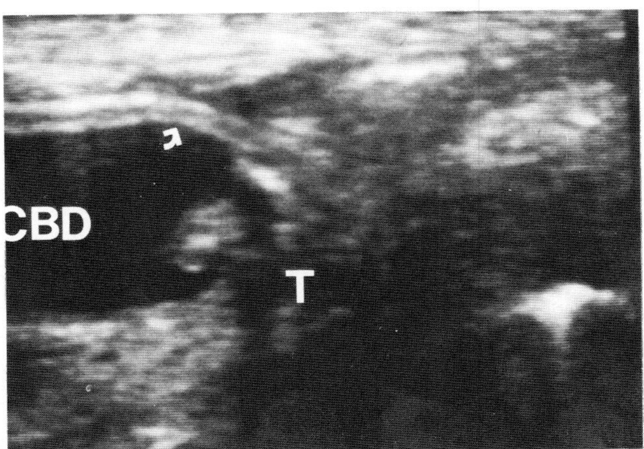

Fig. 34.26 A. Transverse section. Choledochal stone. Note the double crescent of fluid-filled lumen surrounding the strongly echogenic and shadowing stone (arrow head points to crescent of fluid, S indicates stone and acoustic shadow). **B.** Longitudinal section. Malignant obstruction of the lower common bile duct (CBD). The letter T indicates tumour mass in the head of the pancreas with polypoid extension into the lumen of the distal common bile duct. Curved arrow head indicates percutaneously placed drainage catheter.

mildly jaundiced, their use in clinical practice is limited.

The main value of the technique lies in the diagnosis of acute cholecystitis (see below).

MRI

Magnetic resonance will image the gall bladder and biliary tract, but as yet offers no advantage over cheaper conventional techniques by X-rays and ultrasound.

THE ABNORMAL GALL BLADDER

GALLSTONES

Non-calcified gallstones appear in the functioning gall bladder on oral cholecystography as single or multiple mobile filling defects. The diagnosis is usually easy to make but difficulties arise in three circumstances:

1. *Small gallstones.* These can sometimes only be diagnosed confidently on the erect or lateral decubitus film where they either aggregate in the dependent part of the gall bladder (Fig. 34.27A and B) or form a layer (Fig. 34.28) according to their specific gravity relative to that of the contrast/bile mixture in the gall bladder.
2. *Poorly calcified stones.* Stones which are very poorly calcified may be missed on the control film and missed again if the gall bladder has concentrated the medium poorly.
3. *Overlying gas shadows.* It may be impossible to separate the gall bladder from overlying bowel shadows, even with compression and spot films.

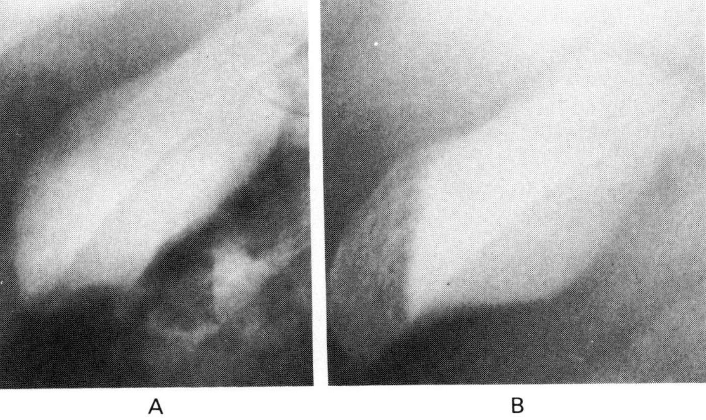

Fig. 34.27 Multiple small translucent calculi invisible in prone film (**A**), but easily seen in lateral decubitus film (**B**).

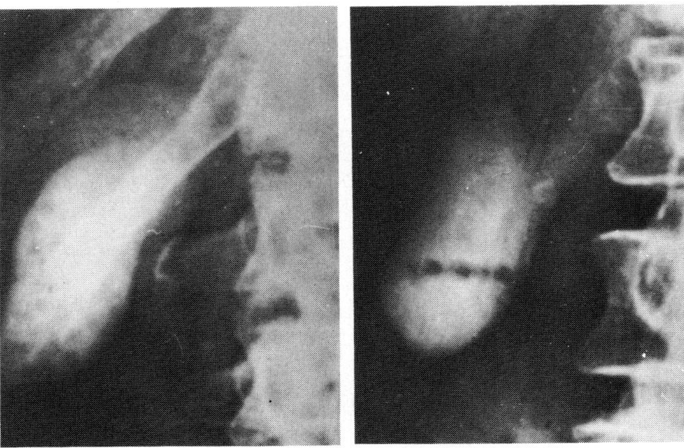

Fig. 34.28 Small cholesterol calculi which float in the erect posture. **A.** Prone. **B.** Erect.

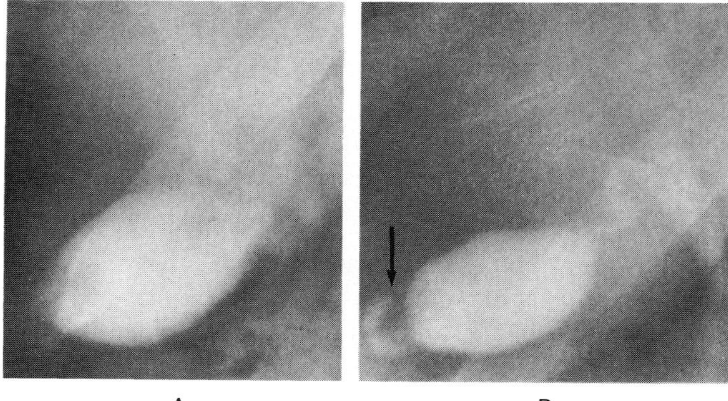

Fig. 34.29 A. Prone film (oral cholecystography); the gall bladder appears normal. **B.** After contraction, a stone confined by a stricture in the fundus is revealed (↓).

The importance of the AFM film has been stressed above (Fig. 34.29A and B).

The diagnosis of gallstones by ultrasound is discussed below.

THE CHOLECYSTOSES

The 'hyperplastic' cholecystoses, of which cholesterosis and adenomyomatosis are the most common, are curious entities in which the various components of the normal gall bladder are present in excessive quantity.

Cholesterosis ('strawberry gall bladder')

The common form of this condition consists of 1–2 mm cholesterol deposits evenly scattered over the gall bladder mucosa. These tiny yellow nodules on the slightly inflamed reddened background mucosa give the appearance of the surface of the strawberry. It is very doubtful whether this common variety of cholesterosis can be diagnosed radiologically. Although it is claimed that cholesterosis produces a fuzzy outline of the gall bladder, such an appearance is far more likely to be due to the more familiar causes of radiographic unsharpness.

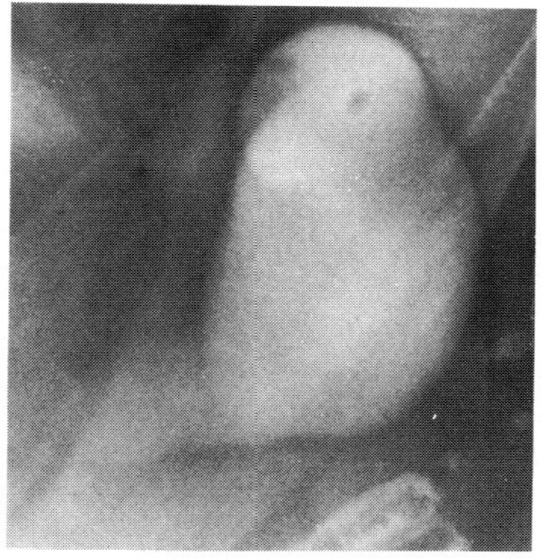

Fig. 34.30 Cholesterosis, showing fixed mural defects.

Occasionally the cholesterol deposits are slightly larger and fewer in number. Multiple fixed mural deposits up to 4 mm or so in size are diagnostic of cholesterosis (Fig. 34.30).

Adenomyomatosis

This condition of unknown aetiology (also known as *cholecystitis glandularis proliferans*) is more frequently encountered radiologically than cholesterosis. The pathological features are muscle hypertrophy and the formation of mucosal pockets (*Rokitansky-Aschoff sinuses*).

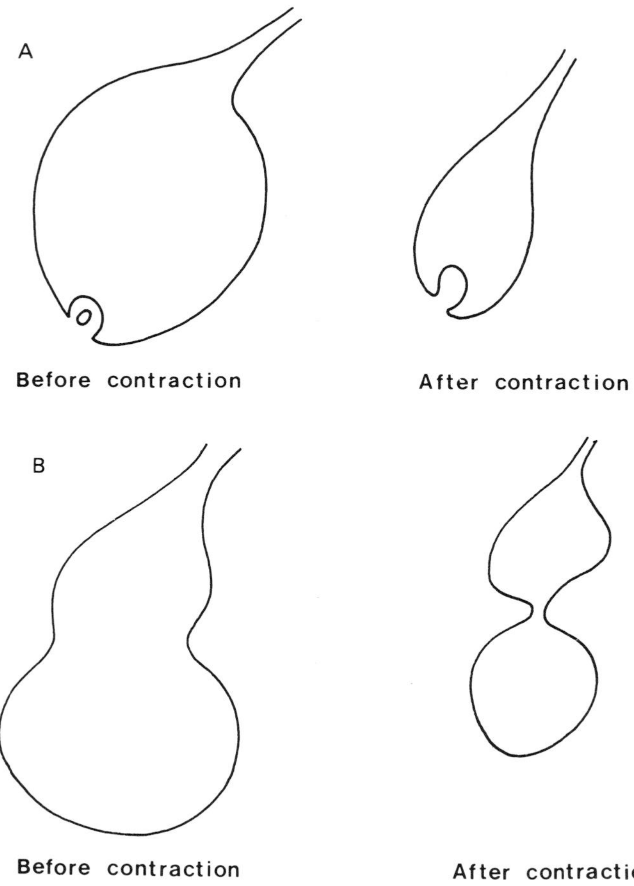

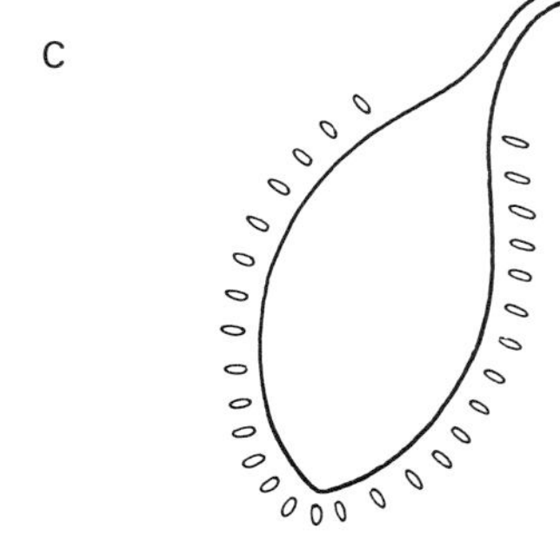

Fig. 34.31 Schematic representation of types of adenomyomatosis. **A.** A fundal nodule before and after contraction. **B.** Stricture before and after contraction. **C.** Rokitansky-Aschoff sinuses.

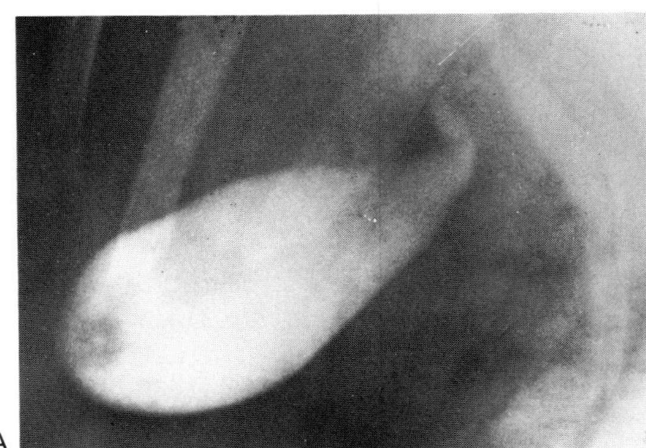
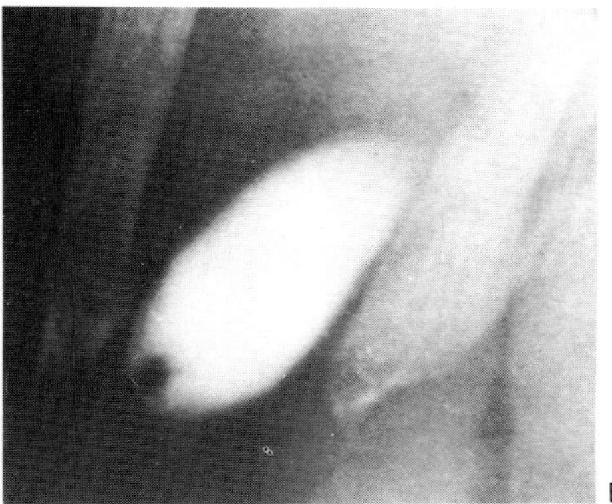

Fig. 34.32 (**A.** and **B.**) Fundal nodule of adenomyomatosis before and after gall bladder contraction. Note long cystic duct medial to common bile duct, a congenital anomaly.

Radiologically the condition occurs in three distinct forms (Fig. 34.31) although mixed types are common:

1. A fixed *fundal nodular filling defect*, sometimes umbilicated (Fig. 34.32).

2. A *stricture* (Fig. 34.33). The stricture may be situated anywhere in the gall bladder and may be sharply localized or a more diffuse narrowing. Because the stricture results from muscle hypertrophy, on contraction it characteristically becomes both tighter and wider, often with non-parallel sides. This appearance on contraction helps to distinguish the stricture of adenomyosis from the presence of a septum across the gall bladder fundus (Fig. 34.34) (a normal variant producing the so-called Phrygian cap) and from simple folds or postural kinks in the gall bladder.

3. *Rokitansky-Aschoff sinuses* (Figs 34.35 and 34.36). These may only fill and become visible after gall bladder contraction. A stricture is commonly also present. Sinuses are often seen histologically when they have not been demonstrated at cholecystography.

Carcinoma of the gall bladder

Carcinoma of the gall bladder is an uncommon tumour. Although is is almost always associated with gallstones, and therefore more frequent in women, the incidence is

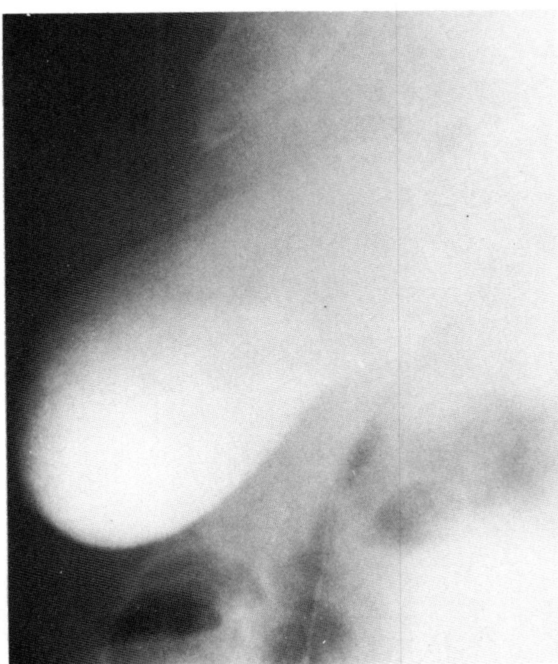
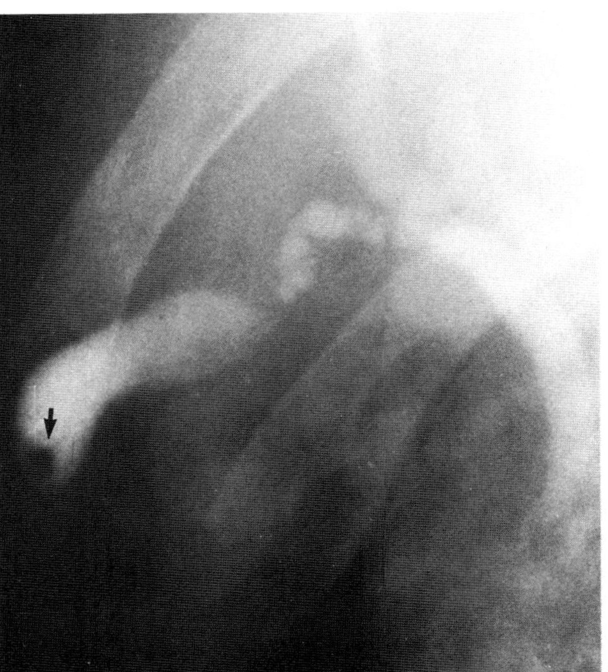

Fig. 34.33 A. The erect film appears normal. **B.** After contraction, a stricture is shown in the neck of the gall bladder. A fundal nodule is now also apparent (arrow).

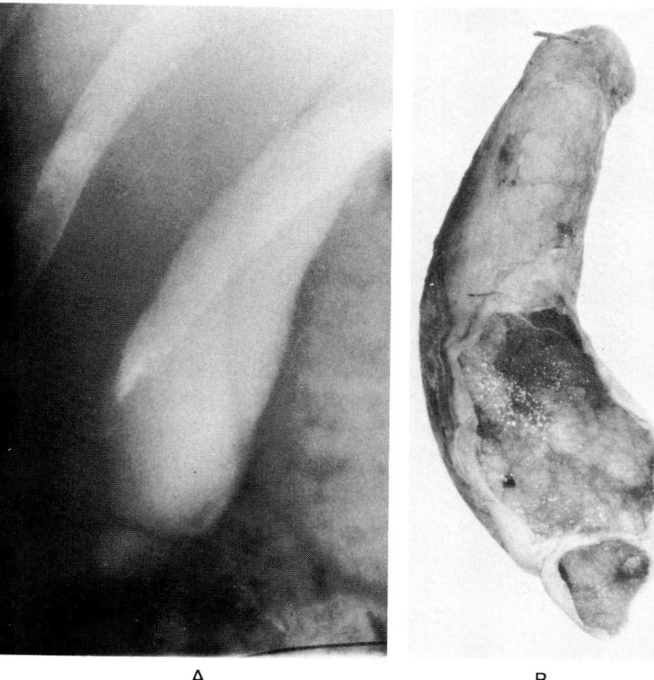

Fig. 34.34 Phrygian cap resulting from partial septum across the fundus of an otherwise normal gall bladder. This is a normal variant. **A.** Cholecystogram. **B.** Specimen.

low. The condition is very rarely diagnosed at oral cholecystography, the usual presentations being:

1. An unpleasant surprise at cholecystectomy, or on histological examination of the gall bladder following cholecystectomy.

2. As obstructive jaundice, when the tumour has occluded the common hepatic duct by direct extension. Compression or displacement of the dorsocaudal ducts of the right lobe of the liver on direct cholangiography are typical.

Acute cholecystitis

When conservative management of suspected acute cholecystitis is practised, oral cholecystography is performed after an interval of a few weeks. If surgery is to be performed in the acute phase, either because the condition is not resolving or because of local policy, it is helpful to confirm the diagnosis preoperatively.

Isotope scanning (see p. 951 and Ch. 66) is the most valuable investigation. The diagnosis of acute cholecystitis is made if bile duct and duodenum are visualized in the absence of gall bladder visualization in a patient with appropriate clinical symptoms.

Emergency intravenous cholangiography may be helpful if emergency isotope scanning is unavailable. Again, diagnosis depends on bile duct visualization in the absence of gall bladder visualization. The i.v.c. is less valuable than isotope scanning since the bile duct is not reliably imaged.

Ultrasound. Both i.v.c. and isotope scanning in acute cholecystitis rely on the inference of cystic duct obstruction for a positive diagnosis. The ultrasound diagnosis of acute cholecystitis relies on positive rather than negative findings: wall thickening, separation of the wall layers (particularly oedema of the submucosa producing a hypoechoic zone within the wall), an irregular mucosal thickness, fine echoes within the gall bladder lumen and pericholecystic fluid. Gall stones of course are usually present. Even if they

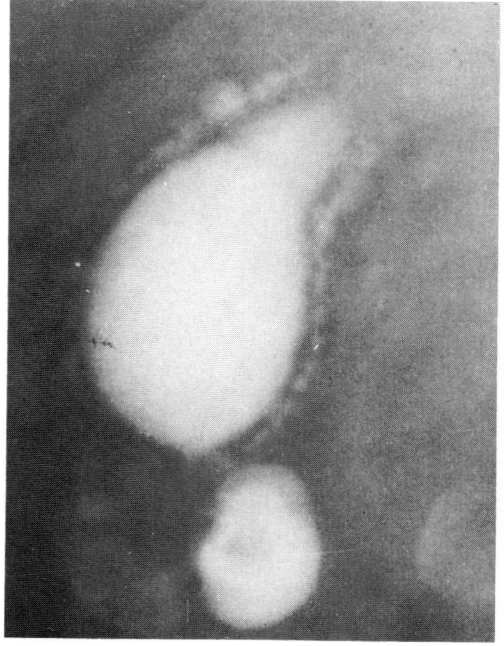

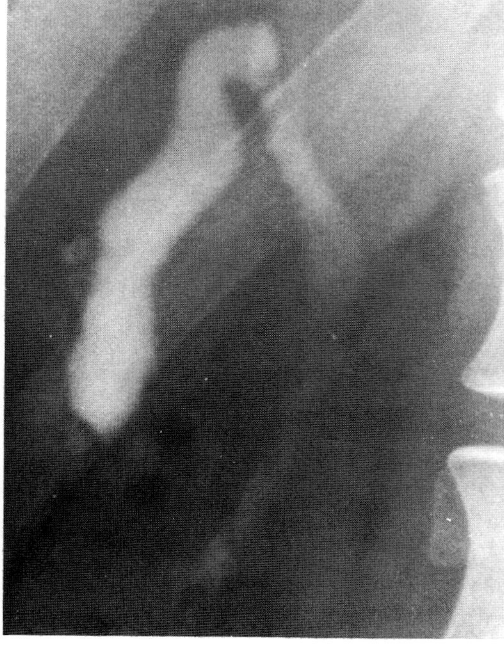

Fig. 34.35 (**A.** and **B.**) Two examples of Rokitansky-Aschoff sinuses shown on AFM films at cholecystography. Stricture is also present in (**A**).

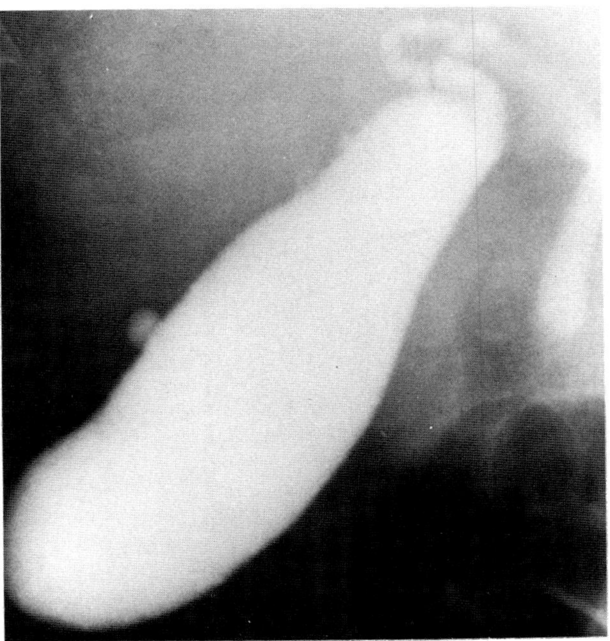

Fig. 34.36 Rokitansky-Aschoff sinuses shown on delayed gall bladder film following ERC.

are absent, a confident diagnosis of acute cholecystitis can be made on the above findings (Fig. 34.37). With a skilled operator the diagnosis is correct in about 80% of cases, but this is less than the accuracy achieved with isotope scanning (95% or more).

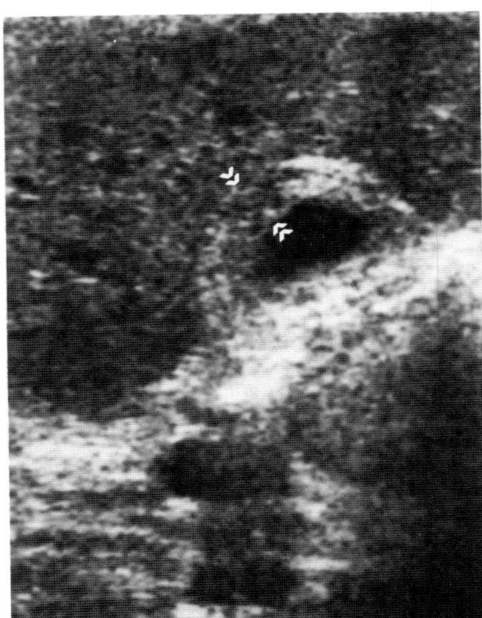

Fig. 34.37 Transverse section. Acute acalculous cholecystitis. The gall bladder wall is markedly thickened and separated into layers with oedema in the subserosal plane. The gall bladder wall thickening is indicated by the double arrow heads.

Congenital abnormalities of the gall bladder

1. *Absence of the gall bladder* in the presence of an otherwise normal biliary tree is extremely rare. Although the presence of other congenital abnormalities, particularly of the digestive tract, may alert the wary radiologist, the diagnosis is usually made only after a fruitless search at laparotomy.

2. *Double gall bladder* has an incidence of about 1 in 4000. There may be a longitudinally septate viscus with a single cystic duct or, very rarely, two separate gall bladders each with a separate cystic duct (Fig. 34.38). In the latter case, one cystic duct may drain anomalously into a hepatic duct.

3. *Intrahepatic gall bladder*. This may be diagnosed on ultrasound but not on cholecystography. A solitary central defect on isotope liver scan is characteristic.

4. *Partial transverse septa* may occur in either the neck or near the fundus, when they produce the Phrygian cap deformity (Fig. 34.34). They are only important in that they must be distinguished from the strictures of adenomyosis.

THE ABNORMAL GALL BLADDER AT ULTRASOUND (by W.R. Lees)

Gall stones (Fig. 34.39).

In a fluid-filled gall bladder, a specific diagnosis of gall-stone can be made if the intraluminal opacity:

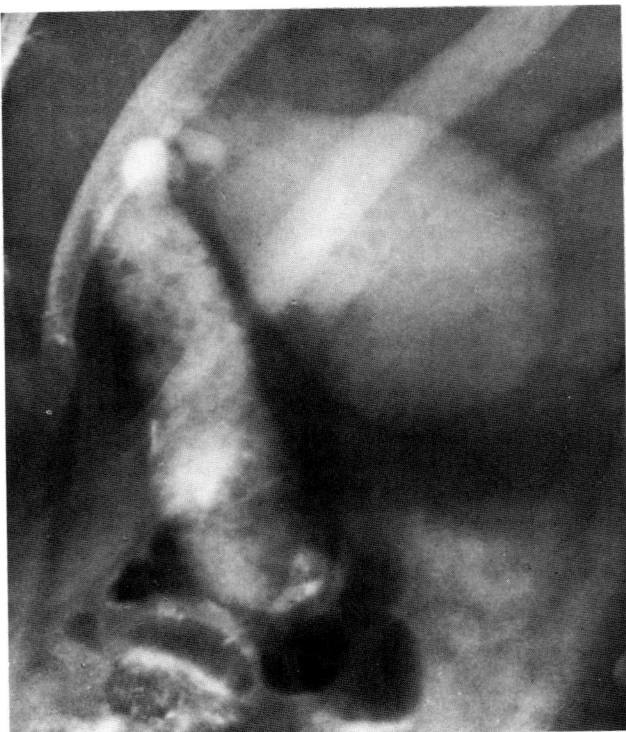

Fig. 34.38 Double gall bladder, both containing stones.

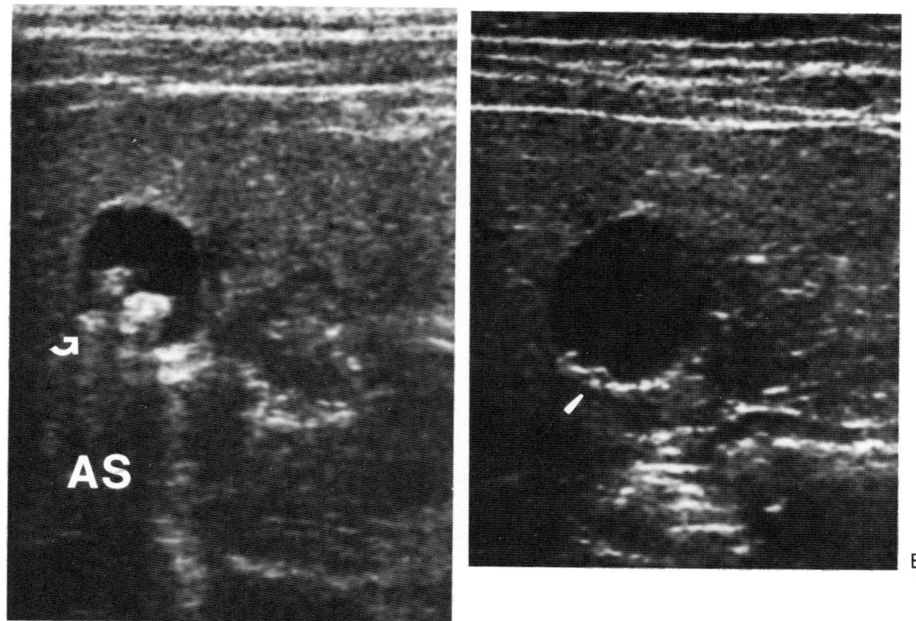

Fig. 34.39 **A.** Transverse section. Gall bladder stones (curved arrow) (AS = acoustic shadow). **B.** Transverse section. Microlithiasis. Small strongly echogenic, mobile intraluminal densities are seen in the dependent part of the gall bladder (small arrow head). Note the lack of acoustic shadow.

1. Is strongly echogenic
2. Casts an acoustic shadow
3. Moves with changes in posture.

Acoustic shadowing is the most difficult sign to demonstrate. It depends on:

1. Optimal beam focussing on to the stone.
2. High transducer frequency.
3. Size of stone (small stones produce small shadows).
4. Careful scanning technique.

Even if shadowing cannot be demonstrated, strongly echogenic mobile opacities are nearly always stones. Small stones do not produce shadows but are seen as small echogenic heaps on the dependent wall. Differentiation from biliary sludge may be difficult. Sludge is a physiological phenomenon seen in any long-standing cholestasis and particularly with total parenteral nutrition (Fig. 34.40).

When the gall bladder is contracted, demonstration of the 'WES' triad is specific for calculi:

W = wall echo
E = stone echo
S = acoustic shadow.

Cholecystitis

The ultrasonographic features of *chronic cholecystitis* are as follows: gallstones, wall thickening, increased reflectivity of the wall, a contracted gall bladder with no demonstrable lumen and marked acoustic shadowing behind the gall bladder fossa. *Acute cholecystitis* is discussed above.

Mucosal lesions (Fig. 34.24)

Fixed non-shadowing mucosal lesions are very frequent findings at ultrasound. The causes of such a fixed mucosal lesion include common and rare lesions (Table 34.1).

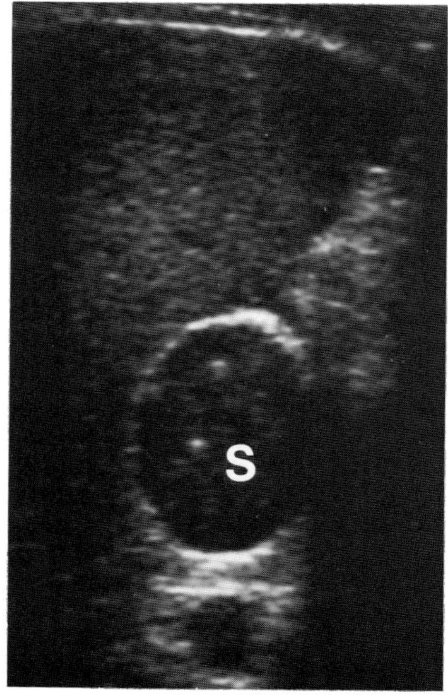

Fig. 34.40 Gall bladder sludge (S) resulting from long-standing total parenteral nutrition. Transverse section.

Table 34.1

Common mucosal lesions	*Rare mucosal lesions*
Junctional fold	Inflammatory polyp
Adherent gallstone	Epithelial cyst
Cholesterosis	Mucous retention cyst
Adenomyomatosis	Parasites
Mucosal hyperplasia	Heterotopic pancreatic tissue
	Tumours:
	Adenoma
	Papilloma
	Carcinoid
	Carcinoma
	Metastases

COMPARISON OF ULTRASONOGRAPHY AND ORAL CHOLECYSTOGRAPHY IN GALL BLADDER DISEASE

The accuracy of the two diagnostic techniques in detection of gall bladder stones is similar. Ultrasound may be more accurate in the diagnosis of mural abnormalities (such as cholesterosis) but these findings are of doubtful clinical significance. The choice between ultrasonography and oral cholecystography will depend greatly on local availability of these diagnostic modalities. Ultrasound is operator dependent, but the advantages of ultrasound should be kept in mind:

1. The patient attends for a single visit and the examination rarely takes more than 10 minutes.
2. Information may be obtained relating to the thickness of the mucosa and other layers of the gall bladder wall.
3. Accurate measurement of the common bile duct and intrahepatic ducts is possible.
4. The study may be extended to include examination of the liver, spleen, pancreas, kidneys and upper retroperitoneum. Non-biliary causes for the right upper quadrant symptoms are frequently found.

Because of inconclusive results, both ultrasonography and oral cholecystography may occasionally be required in the same patient. The number of attendances of the patient may be reduced by the following technique. The patient ingests an oral cholecystographic contrast medium and attends for an ultrasound examination. If this examination is confidently normal or abnormal, the patient may leave the department. However, if ultrasound is inconclusive, cholecystogram films may be taken immediately.

THE ABNORMAL BILIARY TREE

The most common abnormalities of the biliary tree demonstrated at cholangiography are stones and strictures.

BILE DUCT STONES

The diagnostic features are radiolucent, mobile, single or multiple filling defects within the extrahepatic or intrahepatic ducts or both (Fig. 34.41A, B and C). Stones may reach enormous proportions and produce gross dilatation of the bile duct before symptoms call attention to them (Fig. 34.42).

When impacted, a stone causes complete obstruction and may produce the 'meniscus sign' (Fig. 34.43). Malignant tumours invading the duct may rarely cause an identical appearance.

When PTC is performed before surgical exploration or re-exploration of the duct, it may be helpful for the surgeon to know precisely how many stones to seek (Fig. 34.44).

Spontaneous passage of bile duct stones, even up to 1 cm in size, is well recognized and is the usual explanation for normal direct cholangiography following an episode of obstructive jaundice. Stones may also pass during cholangiography, especially if sphincterotomy has been performed (Fig. 34.45).

Lateral films are often essential for defining intrahepatic duct calculi (Fig. 34.46).

Multiple intrahepatic stones are the hallmark of *oriental cholangiohepatitis* (Fig. 34.47). This condition of uncertain aetiology is common in the East and is extremely refractory to treatment. The association with *Clonorchis sinensis* is probably only fortuitous.

Gas bubbles may be inadvertently introduced into the bile duct on direct cholangiography. They can usually be differentiated from stones because they are multiple, perfectly spherical and tend to shift to the lower end of the duct when the table is tilted head-down (Fig. 34.48).

BILE DUCT STRICTURES (Fig. 34.49)

Malignant strictures

The vast majority of bile duct strictures are malignant. They may result from primary growths of the pancreas, ampulla, bile ducts or gall bladder or from secondary growths in nodes in the porta hepatis. The stricture is usually complete at diagnosis, the characteristic appearance being a convex cut-off with moderate to gross dilatation of the extrahepatic and intrahepatic ducts (Fig. 34.50). Less commonly, the stricture is incomplete and cholangiography demonstrates its entire length (Fig. 34.51).

Cholangiography may be combined with *fine needle aspiration biopsy* (FNAB), providing cytological confirmation of the diagnosis.

Concomitant strictures of the bile duct and pancreatic duct may be demonstrated at ERCP (Fig. 34.52). This 'double duct sign' is virtually pathognomonic of malignancy.

Benign strictures

Primary benign strictures of the bile duct are exceedingly

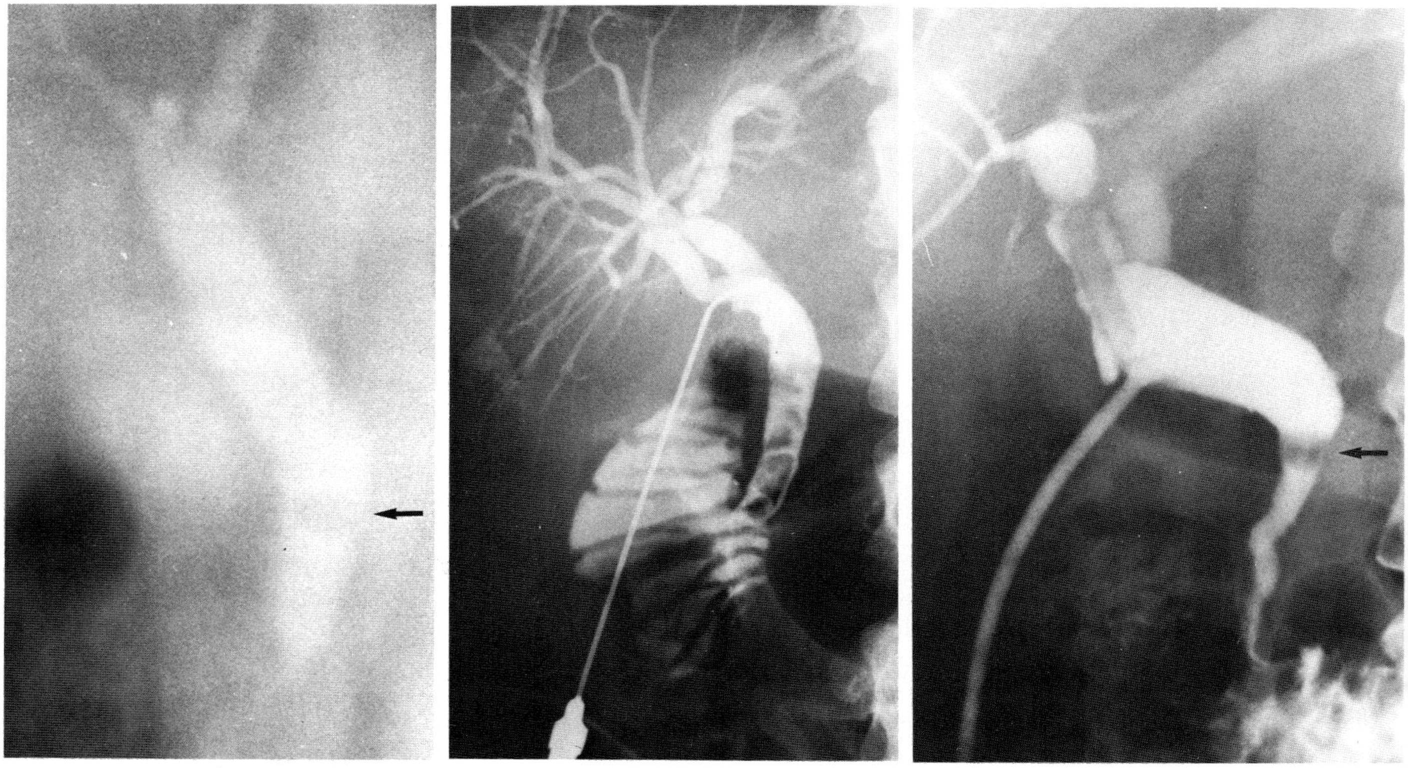

A

B

C

Fig. 34.41 Bile duct stones shown on: (**A**) IVC, (**B**) peroperative cholangiogram, (**C**) T-tube cholangiogram.

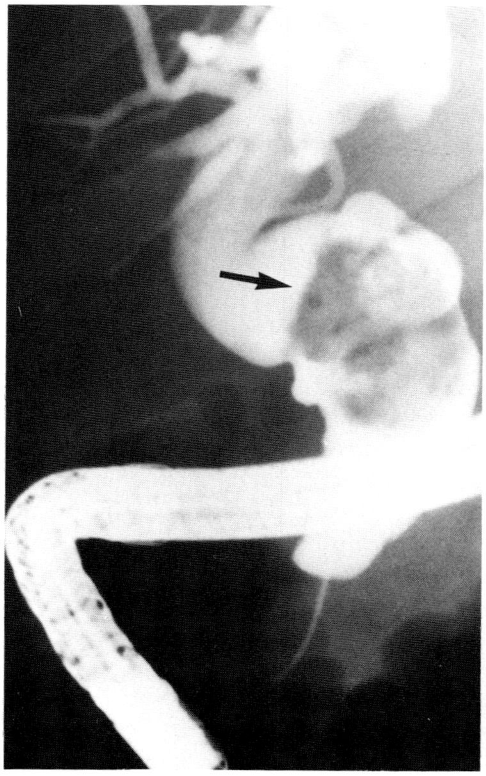

Fig. 34.42

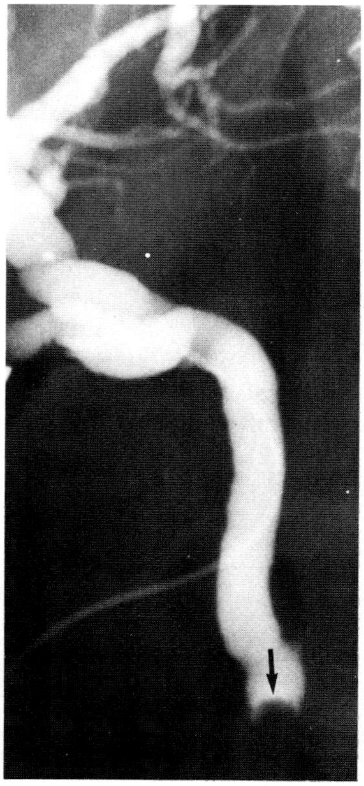

Fig. 34.43

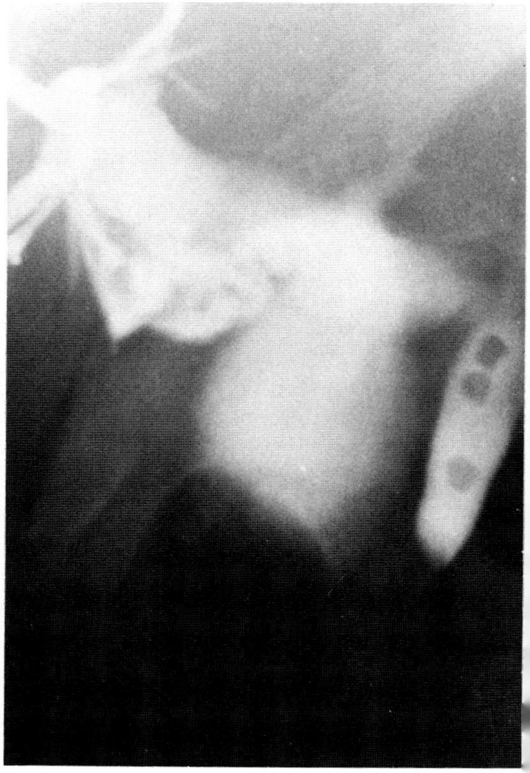

Fig. 34.44

Fig. 34.42 Very large gallstone (arrow) in dilated bile duct shown at ERC.

Fig. 34.43 'Meniscus' sign of impacted stone (↓) in bile duct.

Fig. 34.44 PTC clearly shows three small stones in the common bile duct. There is, however, a fourth stone producing the complete obstruction. Note unusual absence of stones from gall bladder.

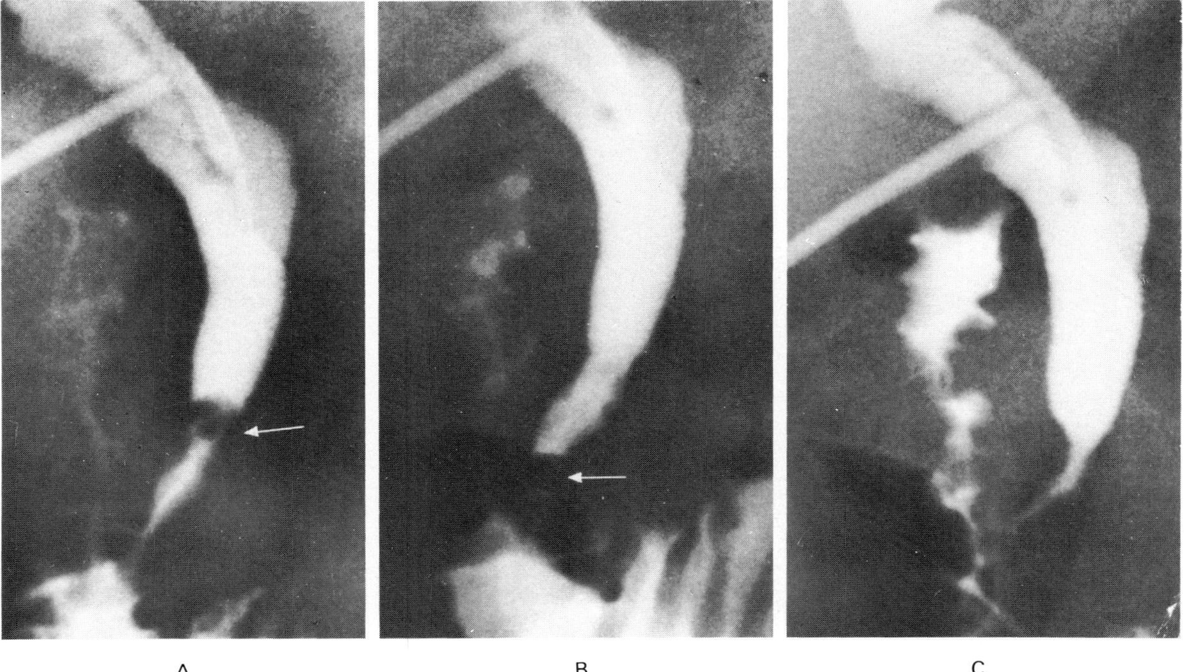

Fig. 34.45 Postoperative T-tube cholangiogram showing a stone being passed during the examination (**A.** and **B.** arrows). A sphincterotomy had been performed.

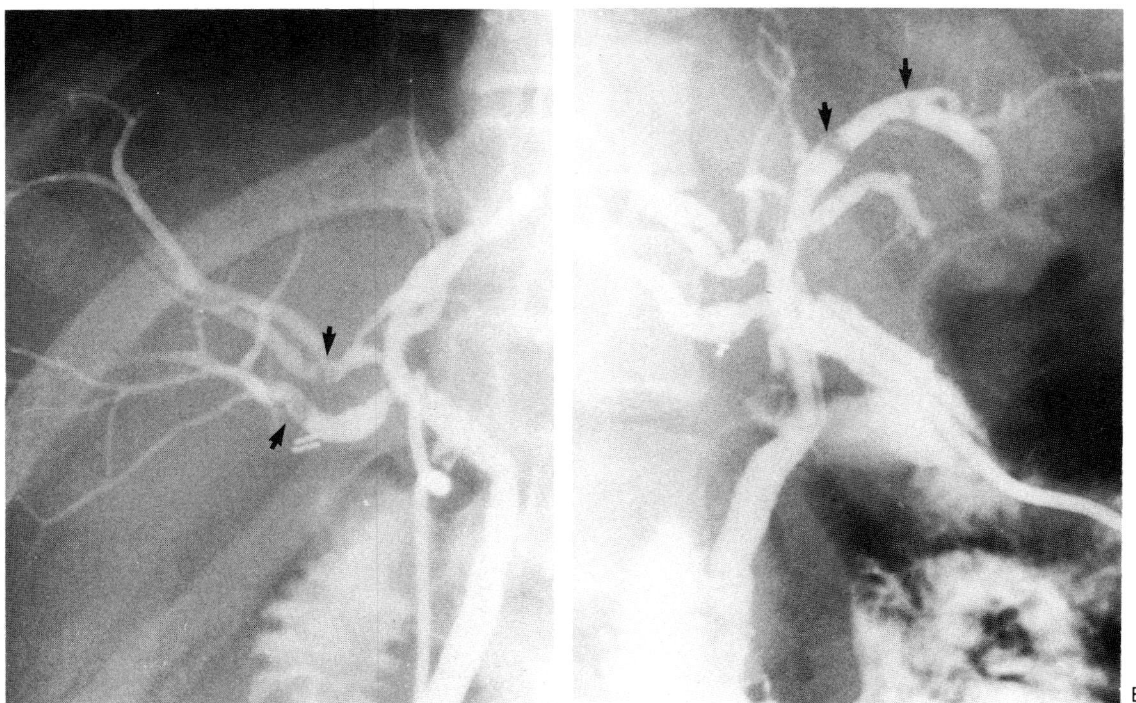

Fig. 34.46 **A.** Two stones are identified in the right lobe duct on the AP projection (arrows). **B.** The patient has been turned about 60% to the left side. Two further stones are identified in the left lobe (arrows).

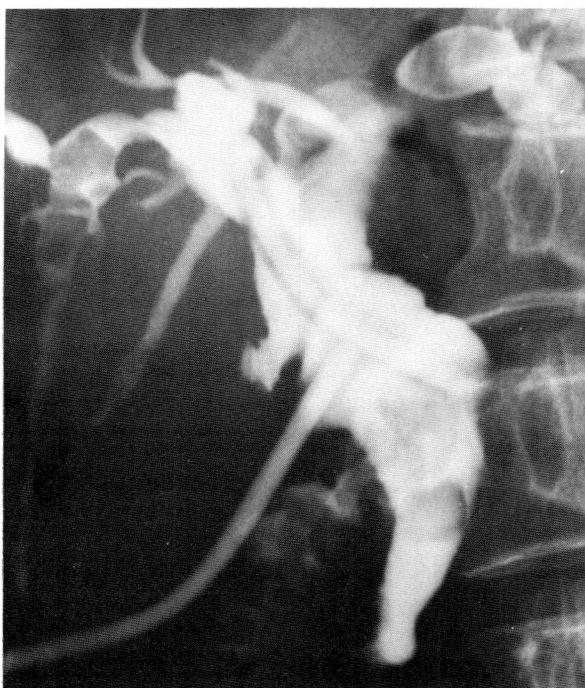

Fig. 34.47 Multiple intra- and extra-hepatic stones in oriental cholangiohepatitis.

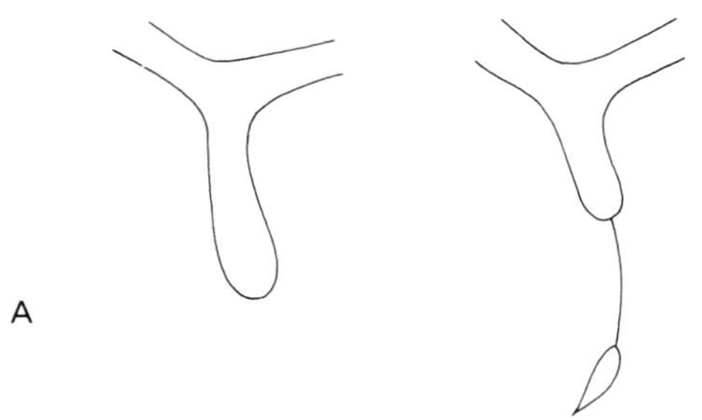

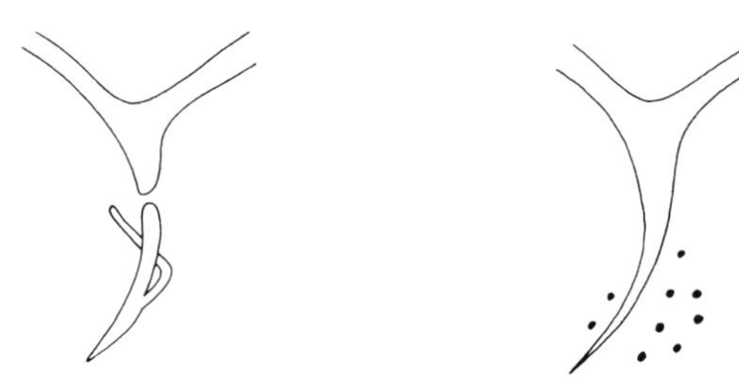

Fig. 34.49 Schematic appearances of bile duct strictures. **A.** Malignant. **B.** Benign.

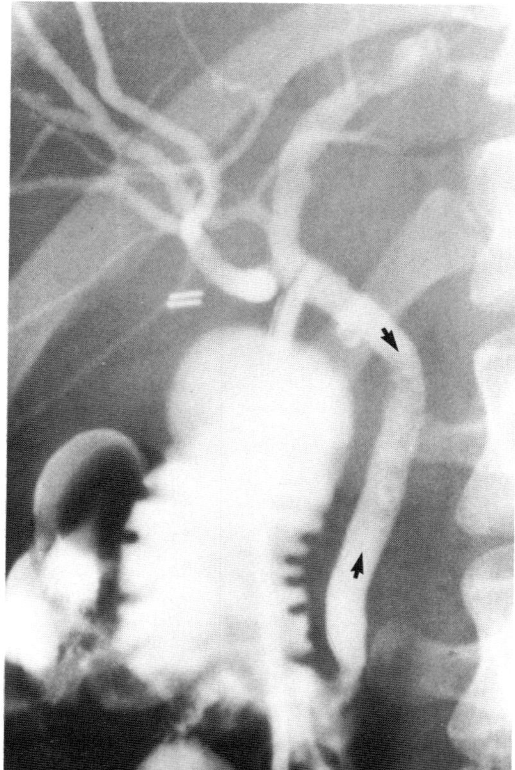

Fig. 34.48 Gas bubbles in common bile duct (between arrows). They are multiple, spherical and of varying sizes and may be observed either to coalesce or break up during cholangiography.

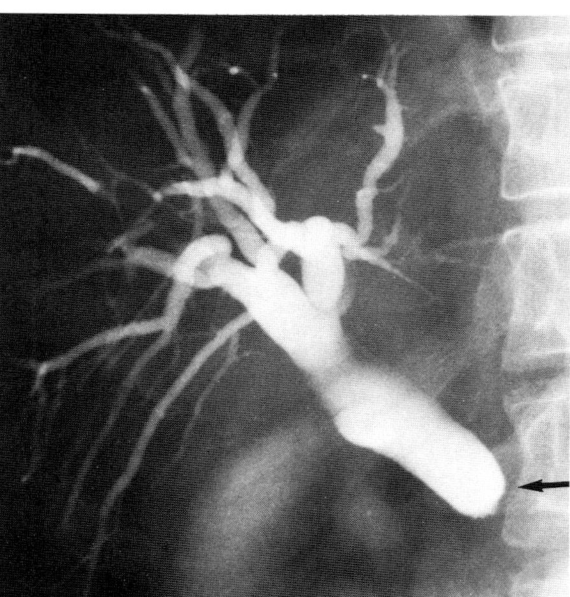

Fig. 34.50 Typical convex margin (←) of malignant stricture of bile duct (carcinoma of pancreas).

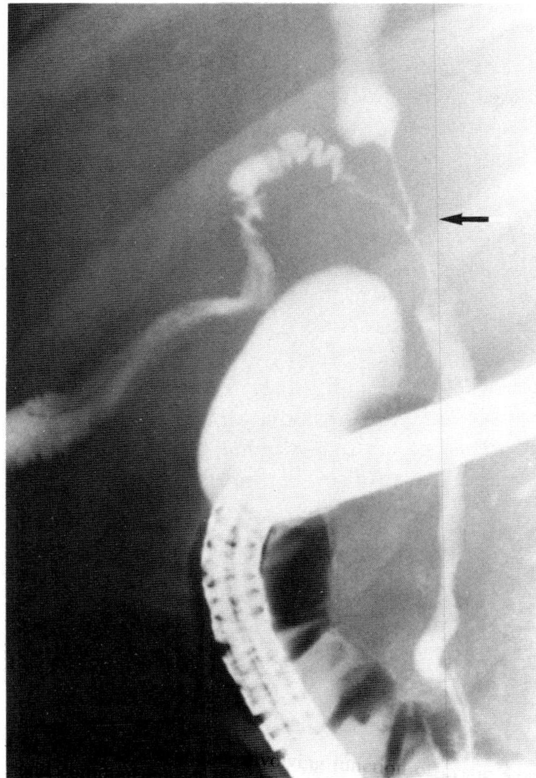

Fig. 34.51 Cholangiocarcinoma involving junction of cystic, common hepatic and common bile ducts, shown by ERC (←).

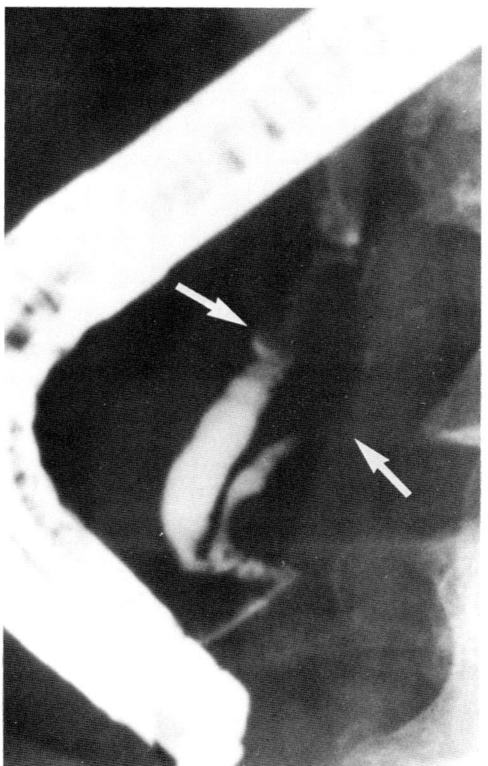

Fig. 34.52 'Double duct' sign. Concomitant strictures of pancreatic duct and bile duct (arrows) diagnostic of carcinoma of head of pancreas.

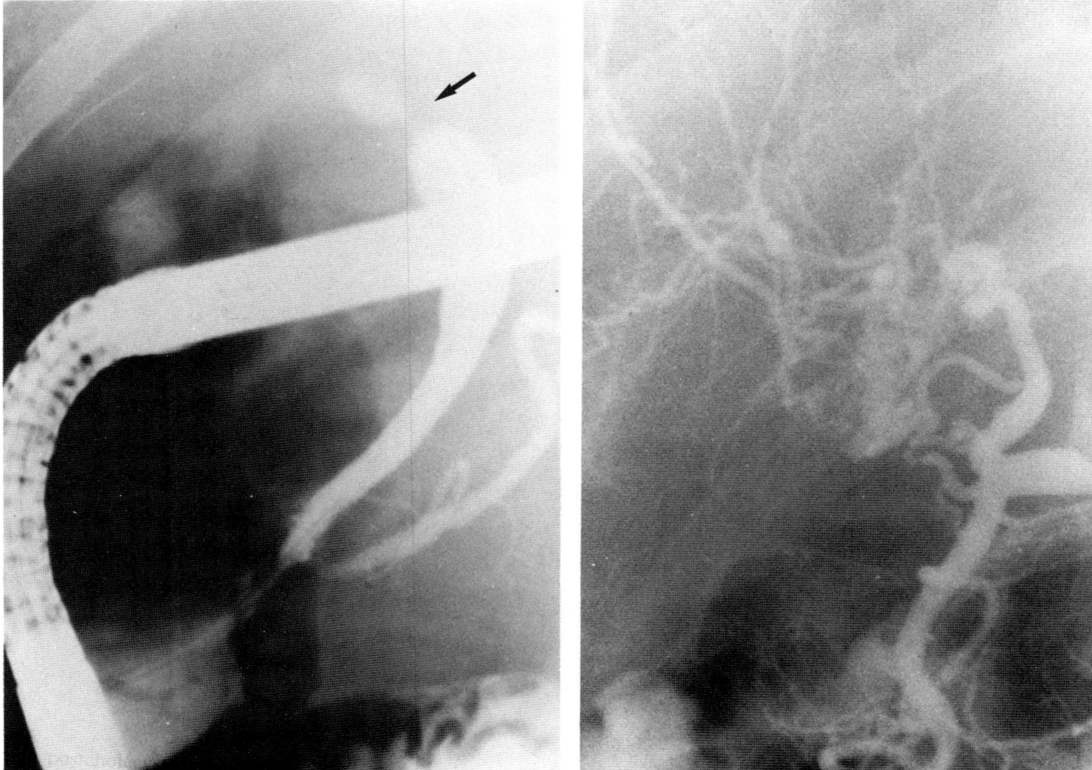

Fig. 34.53 A. Benign postcholecystectomy stricture of common duct (arrow). Typical site at level of ligation of cystic duct. **B.** Arteriogram showing collateral circulation resulting from traumatic interruption of branch of right hepatic artery at the same time as surgical trauma to the bile duct.

rare. Secondary benign strictures occur following cholecystectomy or in association with chronic pancreatitis.

Postcholecystectomy strictures are very short, very tight and typically occur at the level at which the cystic duct has been ligated (Fig. 34.53). Dilatation of the duct above the stricture is rarely impressive. This absence of upstream dilatation is probably due to fibrosis in the walls of the ducts following the recurrent episodes of ascending cholangitis with which these patients usually present.

Chronic pancreatitis produces a 'rat-tail' stricture, which rarely causes complete obstruction. The stricture is usually several centimetres long and the finding of calcification in the head of the pancreas enables a confident diagnosis to be made (Fig. 34.54A and B).

SCLEROSING CHOLANGITIS

Multiple extra- and intra-hepatic duct strictures are the hallmark of this condition and there is usually slight to moderate dilatation of the intervening duct segments (Fig. 34.55A and B). About one third of cases have inflammatory bowel disease (usually ulcerative colitis) and there are much less common associations with retroperitoneal fibrosis, fibrosing mediastinitis and Riedel's thyroiditis.

Sclerosing cholangitis is a premalignant condition, the resulting cholangiocarcinomas often being multiple or diffuse growths.

PARASITES

Hydatid cysts may produce compression or displacement effects on the biliary tree. Unless the wall of the cyst is calcified, an intrahepatic hydatid cyst is indistinguishable on cholangiography from other mass lesions such as secondary tumours (Fig. 34.56A and B). Hydatid cysts rarely communicate with the biliary tree.

The *roundworm*, *Ascaris lumbricoides*, may migrate from the duodenum into the bile duct and produce intermittent biliary obstruction. The worms produce characteristic filling defects, just as they do in the intestine, and may be multiple (Fig. 34.57A, B and C). Passage up into the liver may produce liver abscesses (Figs 34.10 and 34.57C).

The *Chinese liver fluke*, *Clonorchis sinensis*, produces small crescentic and linear filling defects usually of the

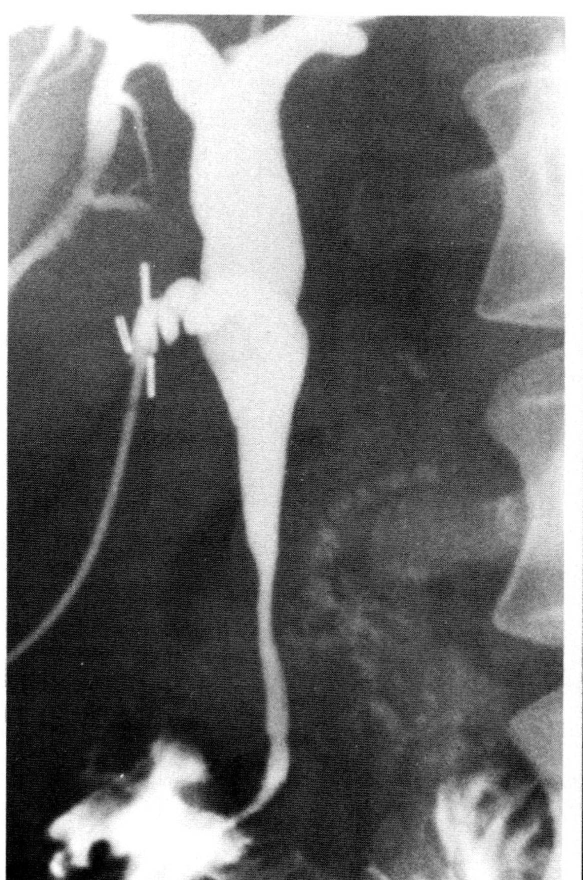

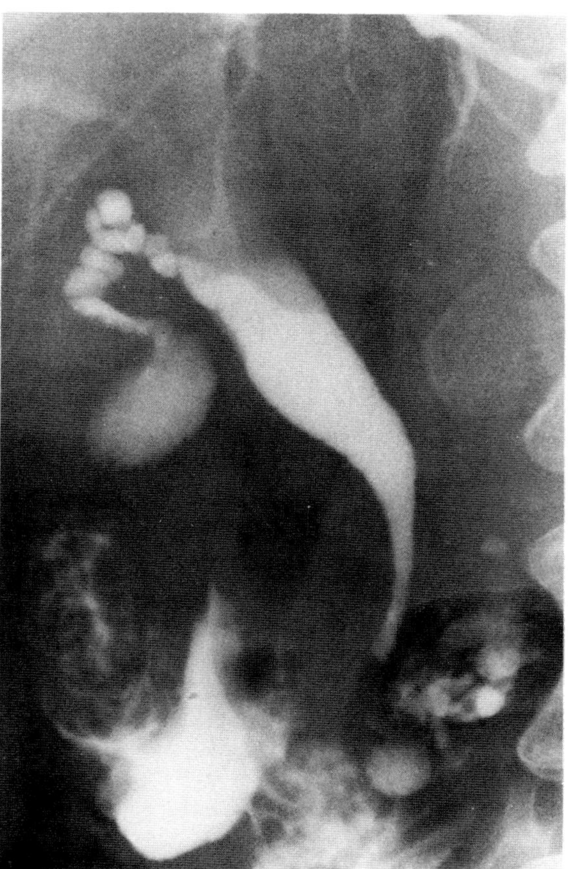

Fig. 34.54 A. and **B.** 'Rat-tail' stricture of common bile duct due to chronic pancreatitis. Note calcification in pancreatic head in both examples.

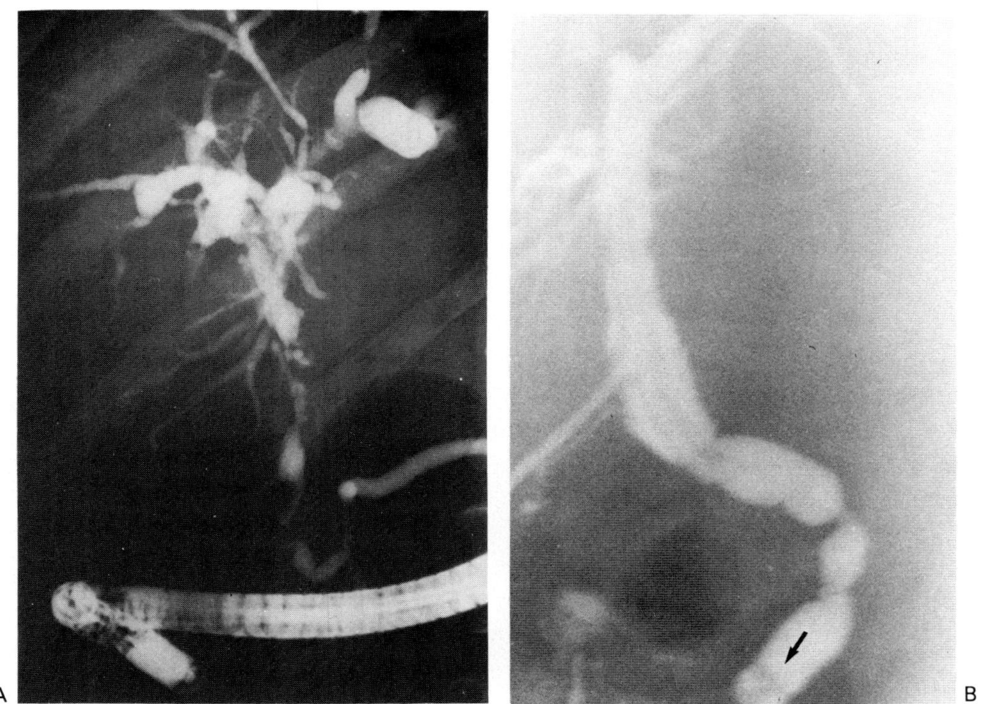

Fig. 34.55 Sclerosing cholangitis. **A.** Multiple strictures of intra- and extrahepatic ducts with dilatation of intervening segments (ERC). **B.** Predominantly extrahepatic manifestations. Stones (↓) also present at lower end of duct (T-tube cholangiogram).

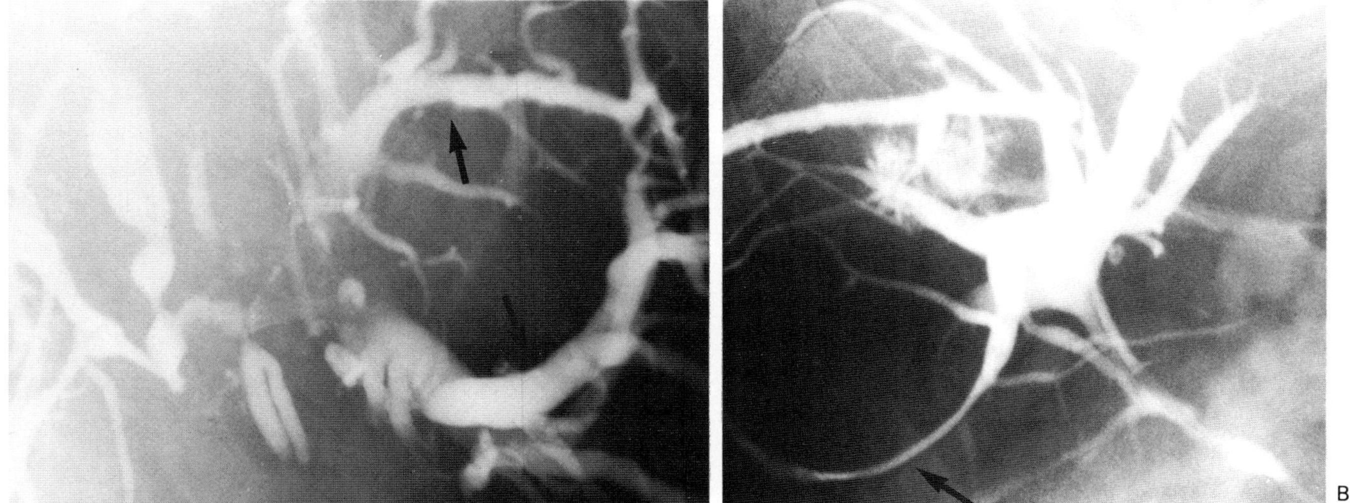

Fig. 34.56 Appearances of mass lesions in liver on cholangiography. **A.** Separation of tributaries of left hepatic duct (arrows). **B.** Dorsocaudal duct of right lobe swept around mass lesion (arrow).

intrahepatic ducts, but occasionally in the extrahepatic ducts as well (Fig. 34.58).

ACUTE SUPPURATIVE CHOLANGITIS

Bile duct obstruction predisposes to infection, known as ascending cholangitis. If the obstruction is not relieved, suppuration occurs and multiple abscess cavities communicate with the intrahepatic ducts (Figs 34.59 and 34.60A and B). The obstructing agent is almost always a calculus, much less commonly a benign structure of the bile duct (following cholecystectomy) or of a surgical anastomosis between the bile duct and the intestine. The finding of multiple communicating intrahepatic abscesses virtually excludes a malignant cause for the obstruction provided there has been no prior intervention (surgery, PTC or ERC).

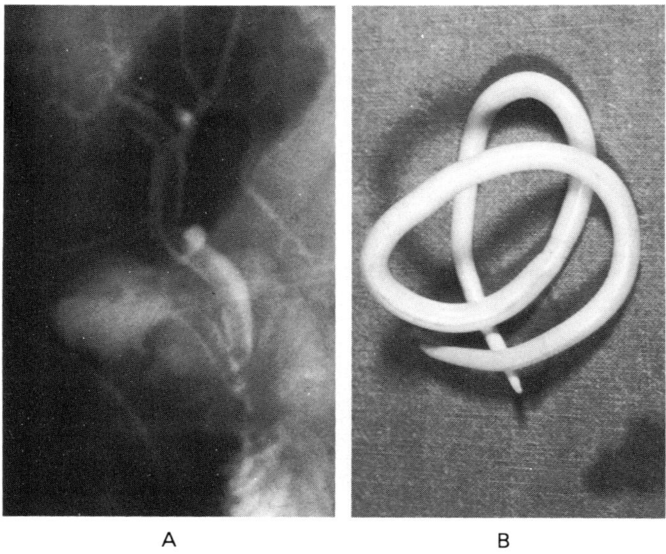

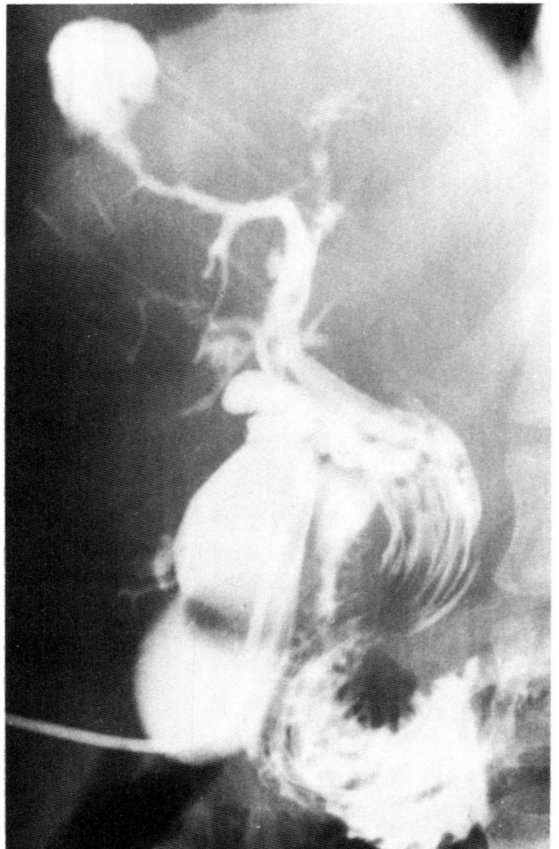

Fig. 34.57 *Ascaris lumbricoides*. **A.** *Ascaris* worm in the biliary ducts. **B.** Specimen after surgical removal. **C.** Cholecystostomy tube study showing multiple worms extending from common bile duct into duodenum. Note associated abscess in right lobe of liver.

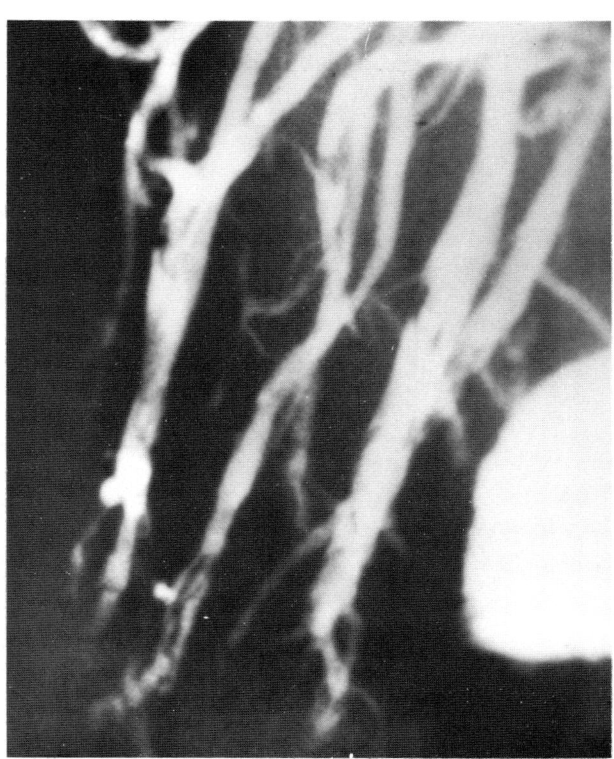

Fig. 34.58 Filling defects due to *Clonorchis sinensis* in intrahepatic ducts.

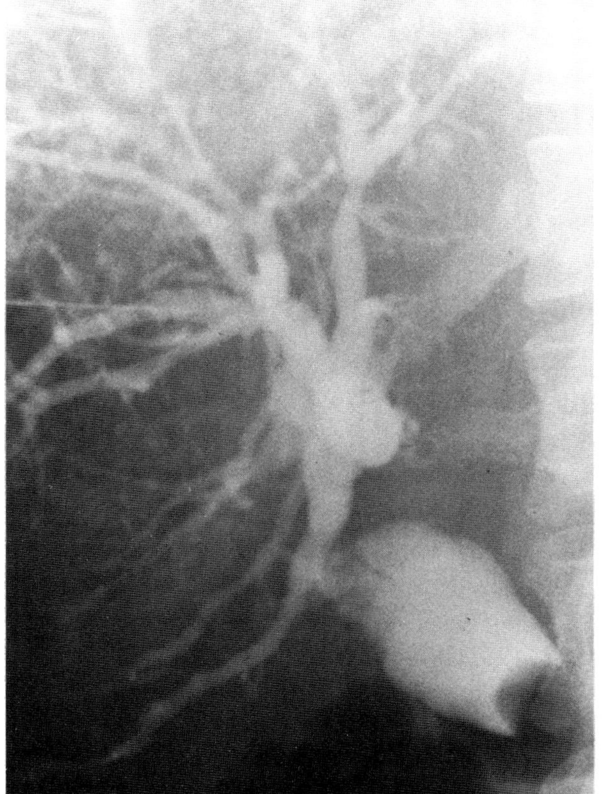

Fig. 34.59 PTC showing multiple abscess cavities communicating with intrahepatic bile ducts secondary to calculous obstruction of common hepatic duct.

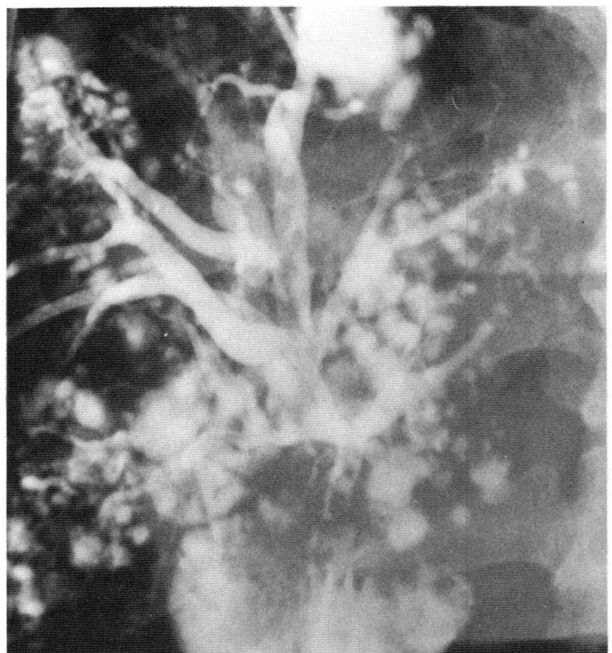

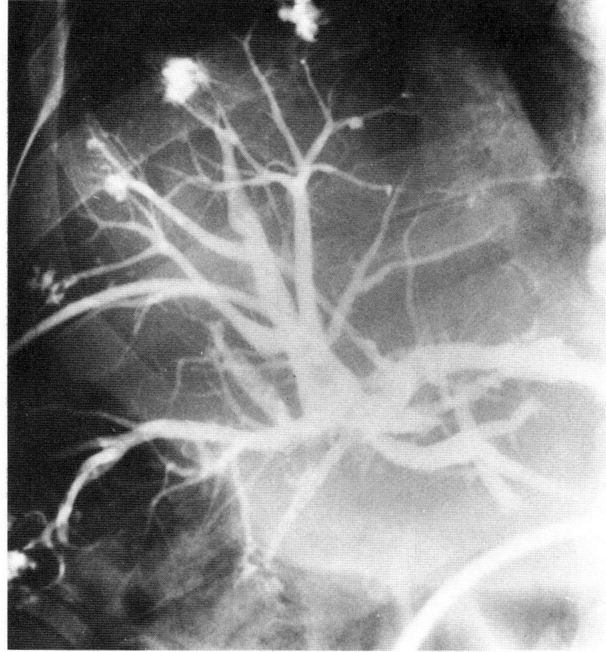

Fig. 34.60 Acute suppurative cholangitis. **A.** Abscess cavities communicating with dilated ducts following stricture of choledocho-enterostomy for malignant disease. **B.** After 5 days external drainage via transhepatic tubes, most of the abscess cavities have healed and the ducts are less distended. Biliary sepsis rarely occurs in association with malignant obstruction unless there has been previous intervention.

CONGENITAL ABNORMALITIES OF THE BILE DUCT

Choledochal cyst (Fig. 34.61)
Smooth, saccular, usually gross dilatation of the whole of the extrahepatic duct is the typical appearance of choledochal cyst, and the dilatation may extend to a varying degree into the terminations of the major intrahepatic ducts. Presentation is classically in childhood with the triad of recurrent jaundice, fever and a mass, but presentation in later life with recurrent cholangitis mimicking calculus obstruction also occurs. ERC may demonstrate an abnormal connection between the pancreatic duct and the bile duct.

Caroli's disease
This condition may be considered the intrahepatic counterpart of choledochal cyst. There are multiple saccular dilatations of the intrahepatic ducts usually situated peripherally in the liver. Infection and stone formation occur within the sacs (Fig. 34.62).

Choledochocele (Fig. 34.63)
Usually an incidental finding, like the ureterocoele which it resembles morphologically, this rare dilatation of the terminal bile duct may be diagnosed definitively by cholangiography. It may also produce a filling defect on the medial wall of the duodenum at barium meal examination.

Choledochal diverticulum (Fig. 34.64)
This presumed congenital variant has the appearance of a tiny cherry on a stalk extending from the medial side of the extreme lower end of the bile duct. It has no known clinical

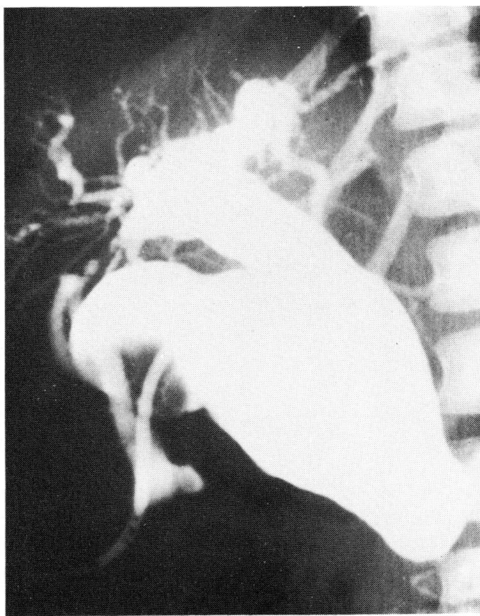

Fig. 34.61 Choledochal cyst (operative cholangiogram).

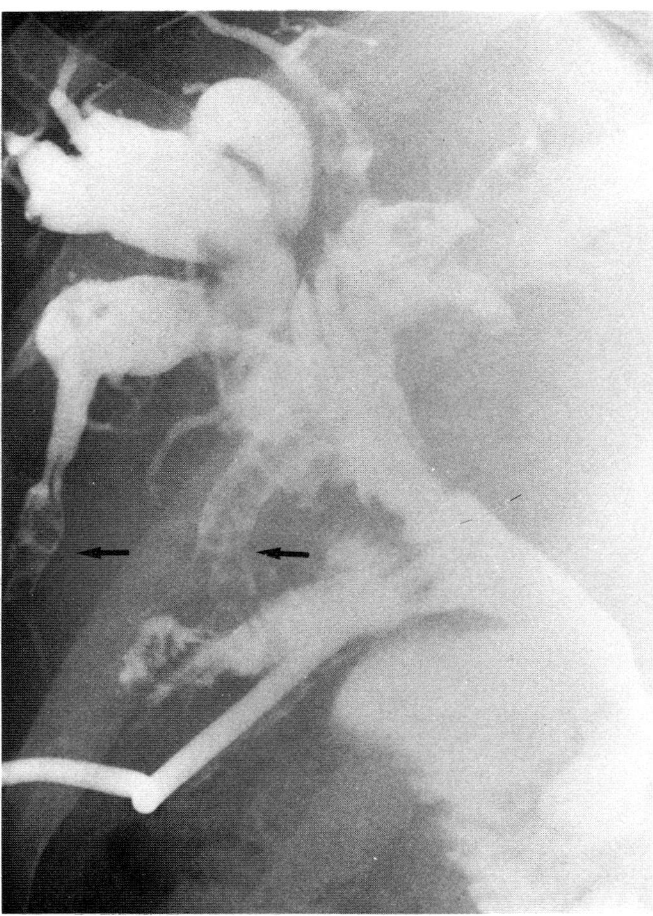

Fig. 34.62 Caroli's disease. Fusiform and saccular dilatations of intrahepatic ducts, some containing stones (arrows). Normal terminations of bile duct and pancreatic duct.

significance but must be distinguished from fistula and sinus which may result from surgical instrumentation (Fig. 34.65 and 34.66).

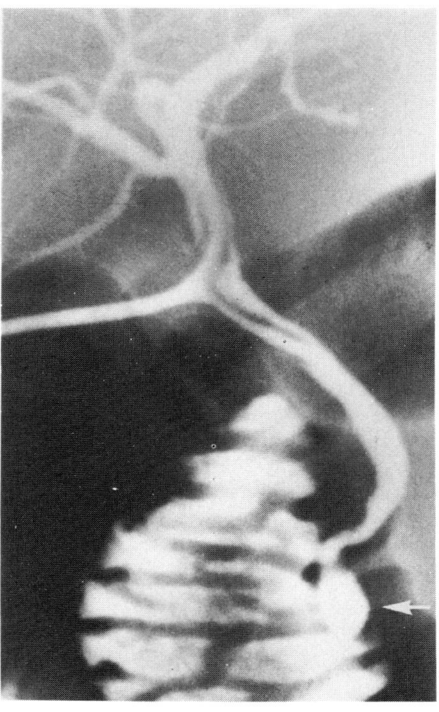

Fig. 34.63 Choledochocele (arrow). Incidental finding on postoperative T-tube examination.

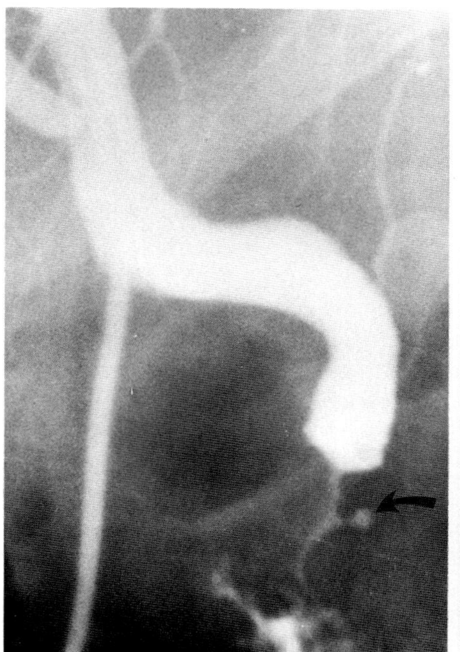

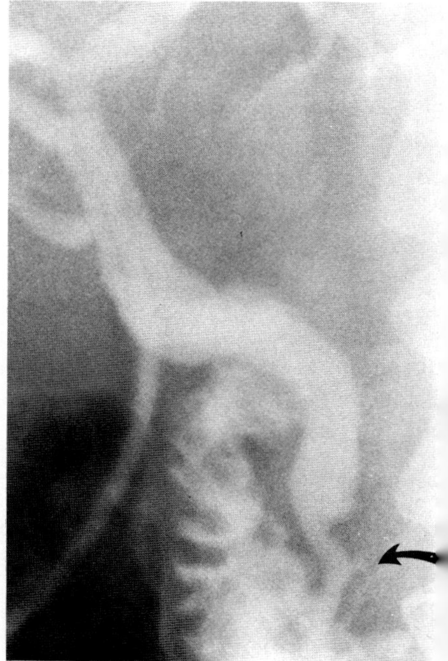

Fig. 34.64 Choledochal diverticulum (arrow) during contraction (**A**) and relaxation (**B**) of sphincter.

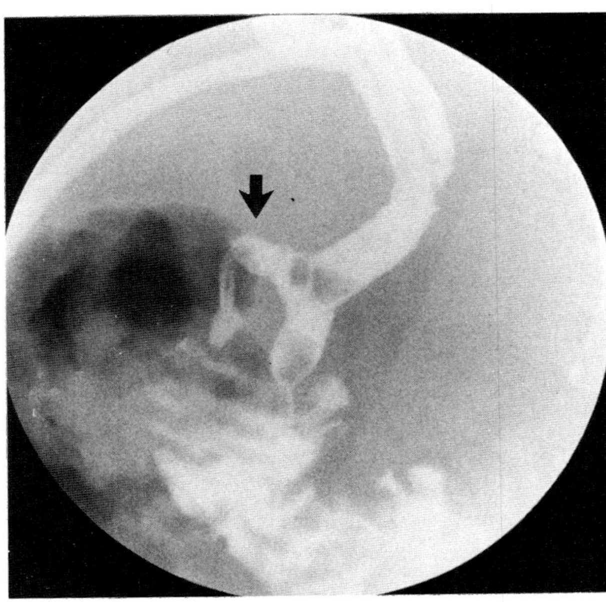

Fig. 34.65 Postoperative T-tube cholangiogram showing sinus track (arrow) produced by surgical instrumentation of the duct. Note residual stones.

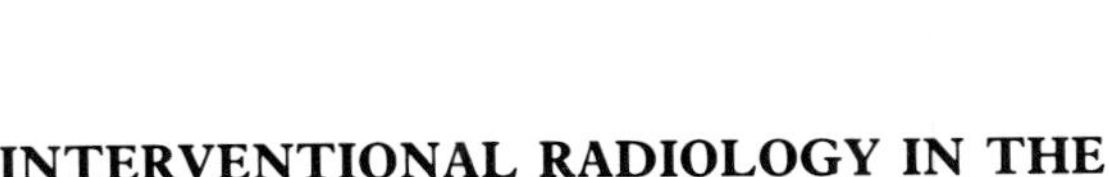

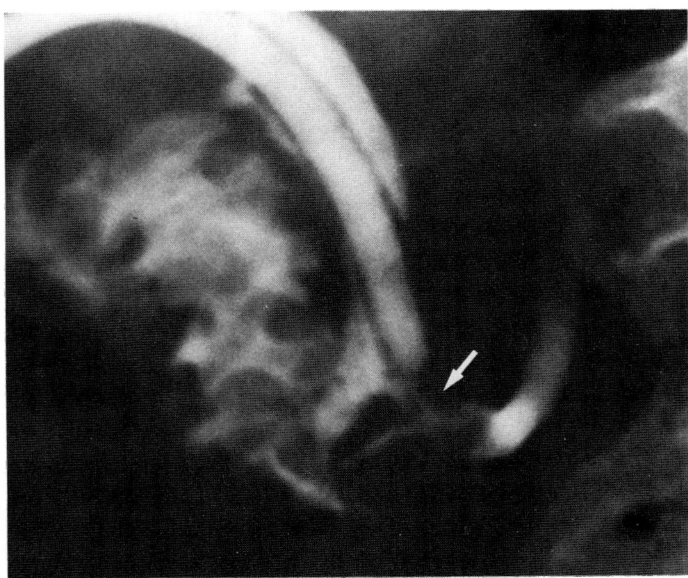

Fig. 34.66 Postoperative cholangiogram showing fistula between bile duct and pancreatic duct (arrow) produced during surgical instrumentation.

INTERVENTIONAL RADIOLOGY IN THE BILIARY TREE

Since the opacification of the gall bladder by Graham and Cole in 1924 (using intravenous sodium tetrabromphenolphthalein), the development of radiology of the biliary tract has been punctuated at intervals by a number of significant advances. The most recent of these has been the development of interventional procedures which have enabled either confirmation of diagnosis by cytology or have added a therapeutic modality to the traditional diagnostic procedures. Aspiration biopsy and the management of bile duct stones and strictures will be considered separately.

FINE NEEDLE ASPIRATION BIOPSY

Aspiration of cells through needles as fine as 22-gauge may permit the confirmation of malignancy of extrahepatic obstructing lesions or intrahepatic masses. Aspiration may be performed under ultrasound, screening or CT control and a variety of shaped cutting tips on the needles has increased the diagnostic yield. The procedure may be performed safely under local anaesthesia, but is conveniently combined with endoprosthesis insertion when general anaesthesia or intravenous sedation is likely to be employed. False-negative results are most likely in the case of scirrhous tumours which are cell-poor.

An experienced cytopathologist is an indispensable member of the interventional radiology team.

BILE DUCT STONE EXTRACTION

Percutaneous stone extraction

Following surgical exploration of the common duct for stone, the T-tube cholangiogram shows residual stone or stones in about 5% of cases. Provided a T-tube of calibre at least the size of the stone has been brought out to the right flank, the residual stones can almost always be removed via the T-tube track. After a delay of 5 weeks from operation to allow the track to mature, the T-tube is removed and under fluoroscopic control a steerable catheter is directed down the track and into the duct. The stone is engaged in a basket introduced through the steerable catheter and is removed with it. The procedure is simply repeated if there are multiple retained stones (Figs 34.67 and 34.68).

This technique is the procedure of choice for postoperative retained stones which have not responded to dissolution therapy via the T-tube. Complications are minor and occur in less than 10% of cases. Deaths have occurred from acute pancreatitis following this procedure but the mortality rate is much less than for endoscopic sphincterotomy.

When the nature of an abnormality on postoperative cholangiography is uncertain, it may be inspected endoscopically (Fig. 34.69).

Endoscopic sphincterotomy

This is the therapeutic procedure of choice for most common duct stones in middle life and beyond. It does not require the presence of a T-tube and is being increasingly

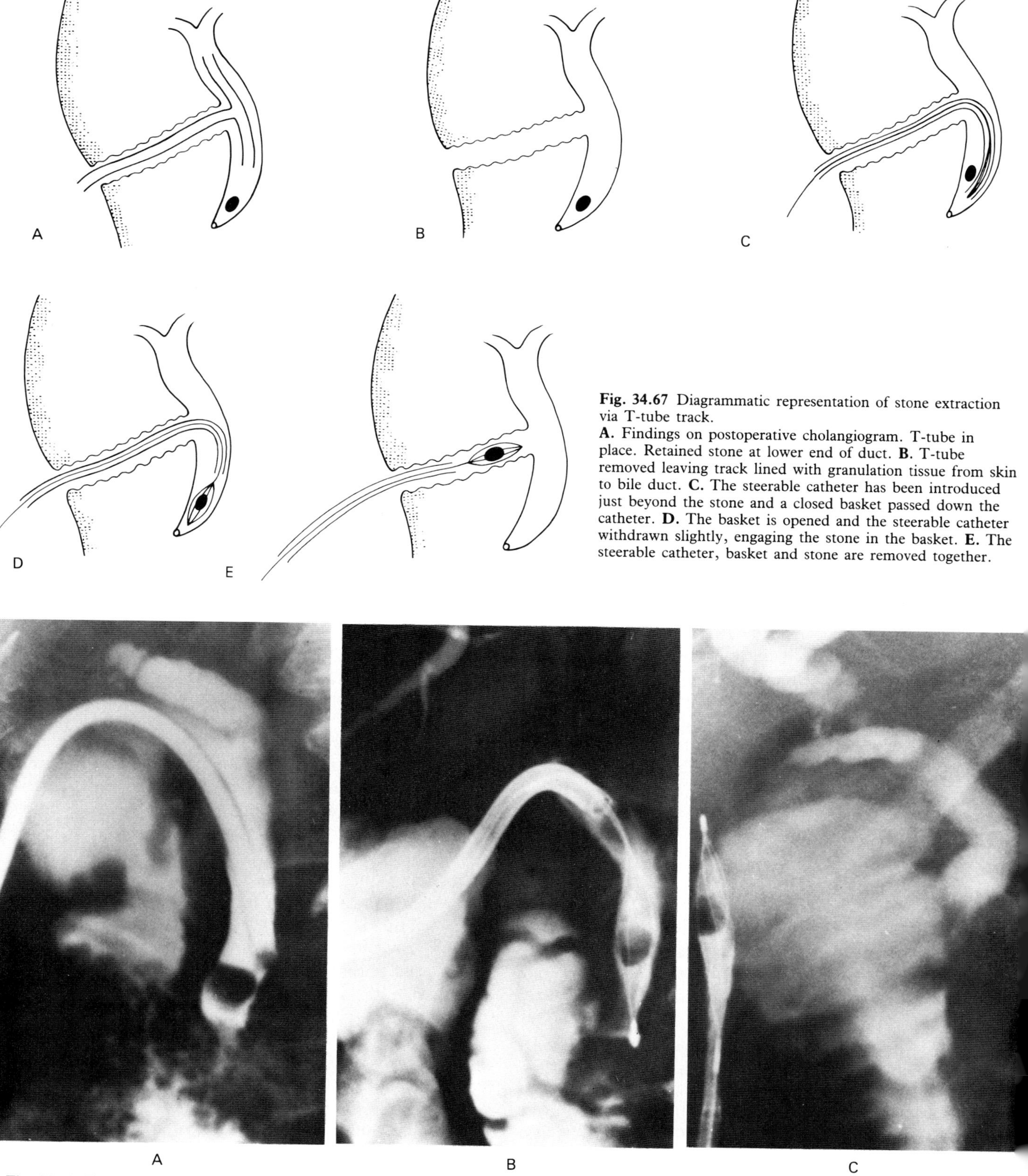

Fig. 34.67 Diagrammatic representation of stone extraction via T-tube track.
A. Findings on postoperative cholangiogram. T-tube in place. Retained stone at lower end of duct. **B.** T-tube removed leaving track lined with granulation tissue from skin to bile duct. **C.** The steerable catheter has been introduced just beyond the stone and a closed basket passed down the catheter. **D.** The basket is opened and the steerable catheter withdrawn slightly, engaging the stone in the basket. **E.** The steerable catheter, basket and stone are removed together.

Fig. 34.68 Films taken during extraction procedure. **A.** The steerable catheter has been positioned with its tip just above the stone. **B.** The stone is engaged in the basket. **C.** Steerable catheter, basket and stone during extraction through T-tube track.

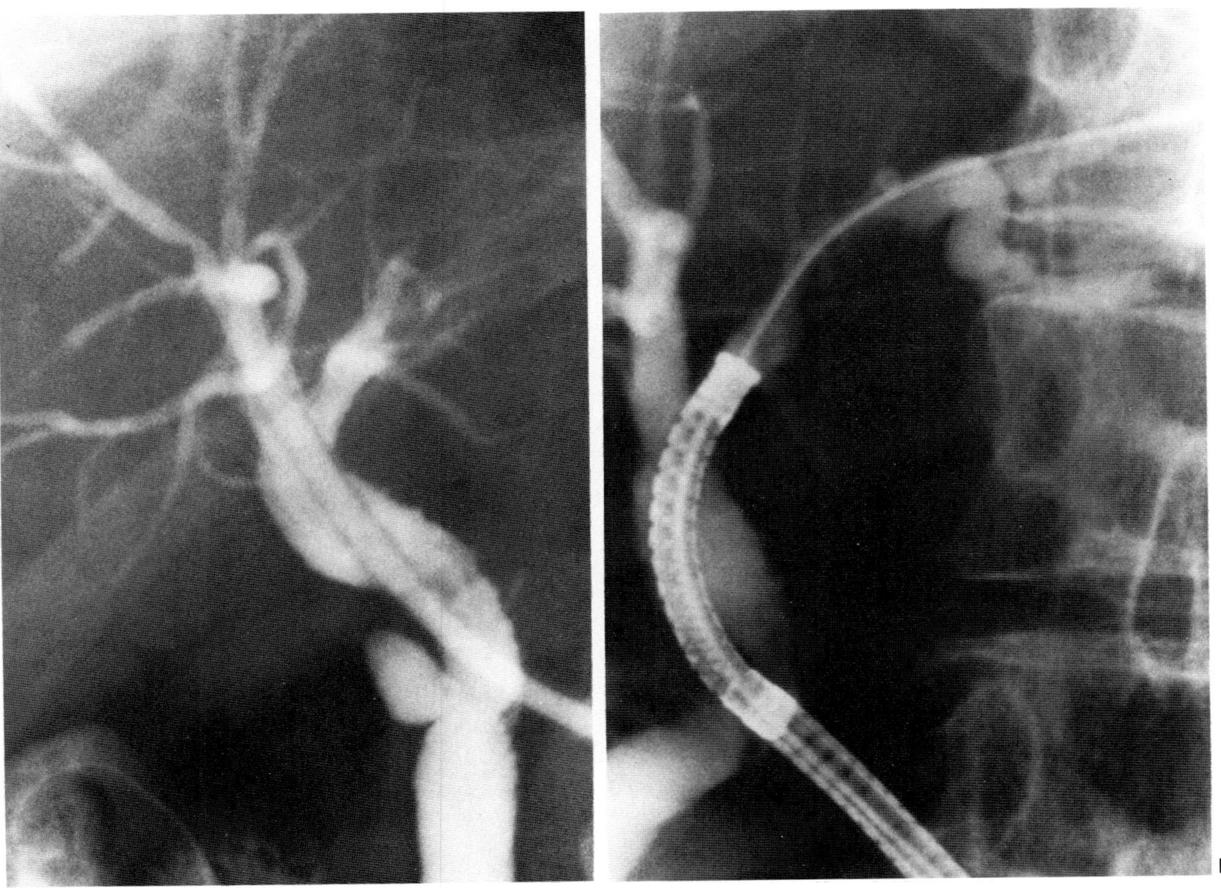

Fig. 34.69 A. Postoperative cholangiogram. The left hepatic duct is occluded (? stone ? tumour). **B.** A guide-wire has been passed beyond the obstruction with the aid of a steerable catheter. A flexible fibreoptic choledochoscope is passed down the T-tube track over the guide-wire to determine the nature of the obstructing lesion. Diagnosis: stone.

performed for symptomatic duct stones in the elderly even in the presence of gall bladder stones. Immediately following endoscopic retrograde cholangiography to demonstrate the stones, a diathermy wire is introduced through the operating channel of the endoscope and passed into the bile duct. After accurate positioning, current is applied to the wire and the sphincter is divided. Stones may be removed immediately by means of a balloon or basket or, alternatively, spontaneous passage may be awaited (Fig. 34.70).

STRICTURES

As an alternative to surgical bypass in order to restore drainage, stents (or endoprostheses) may be introduced through a bile duct stricture, either percutaneously or endoscopically. In either case, a guide-wire is first passed through the stricture and the stricture is dilated to the calibre of the endoprosthesis to be introduced. The endoprosthesis is then loaded on to the guide-wire and impacted into position with a pushing catheter (Figs 34.71, 34.72 and 34.73). This is clearly a palliative procedure which has no effect on the growth of the tumour. Endoprostheses commonly remain patent and functioning for periods up to 1 year. If the patient survives long enough for jaundice to recur as a result of tumour extension, or encrustation of the endoprosthesis, the implant can often be changed or bypassed with another introduced alongside it.

The morbidity and mortality of percutaneous endoprosthesis insertion are probably greater than those of endoscopic insertion. As more centres are gaining the expertise for the latter technique, it is expected to become the procedure of choice for malignant obstructive jaundice in all patients except those fit for major resection, under the age of 60, and in whom no metastases or involvement of major vessels have been demonstrated.

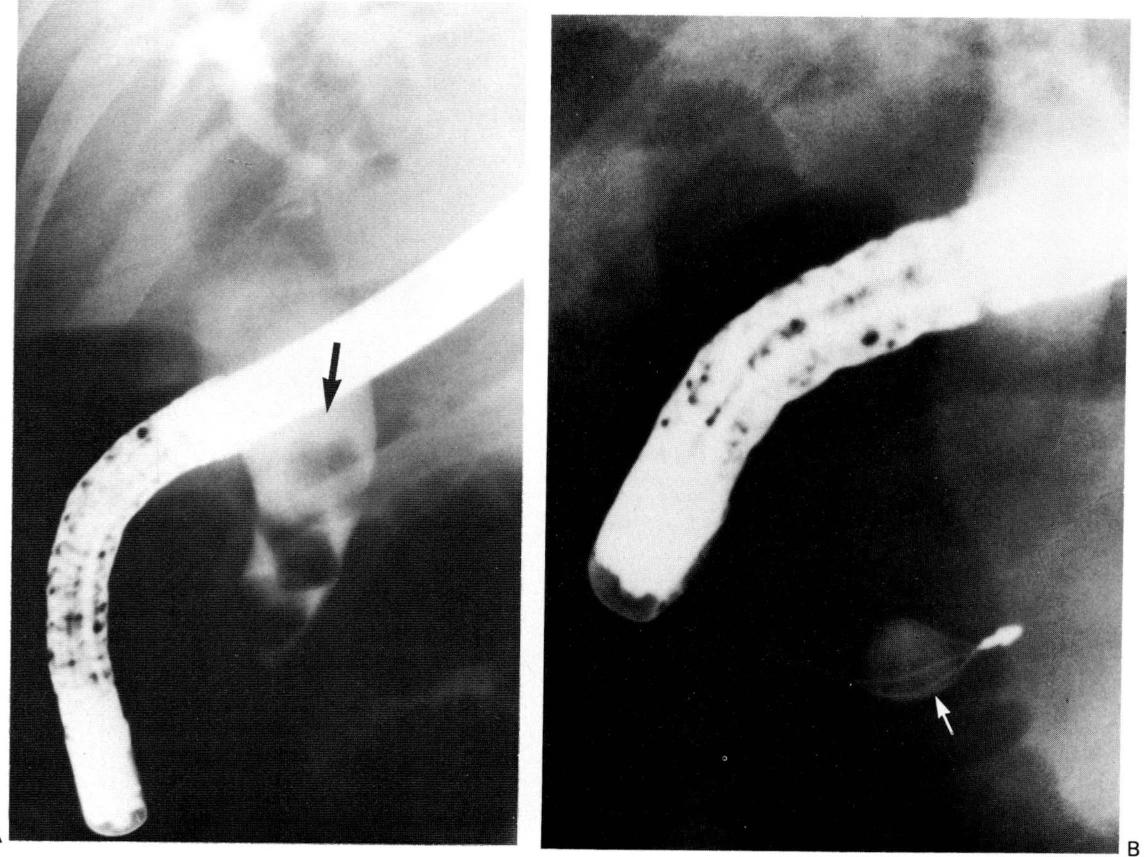

Fig. 34.70 A. Following endoscopic sphincterotomy, a balloon-tipped catheter has been passed down the endoscope and into the duct. The balloon is inflated (arrow) above the stones and traction delivers the stones into the duodenum. **B.** A stone coated with contrast (arrow) lies in the duodenum after endoscopic basket extraction.

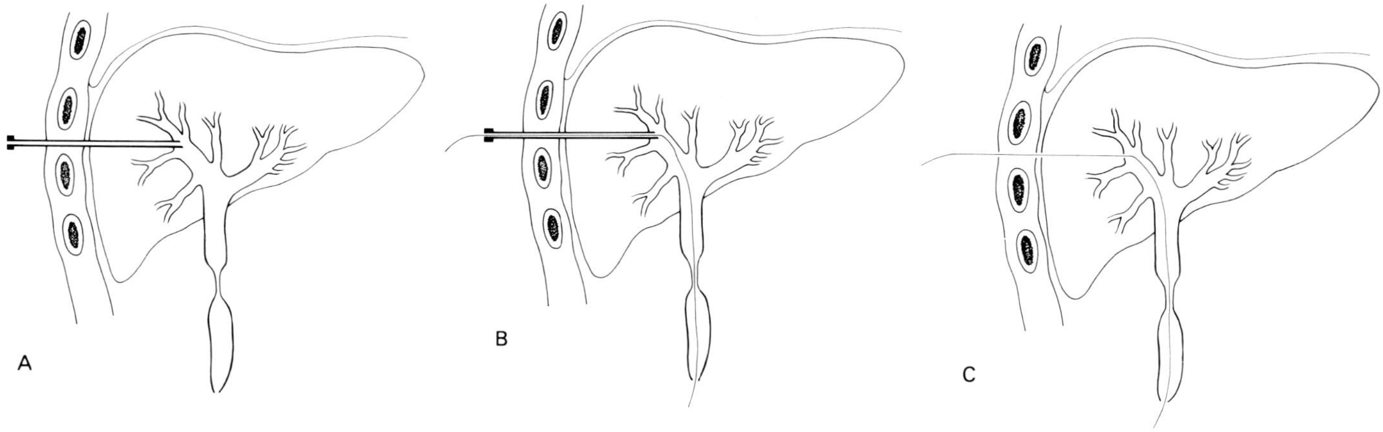

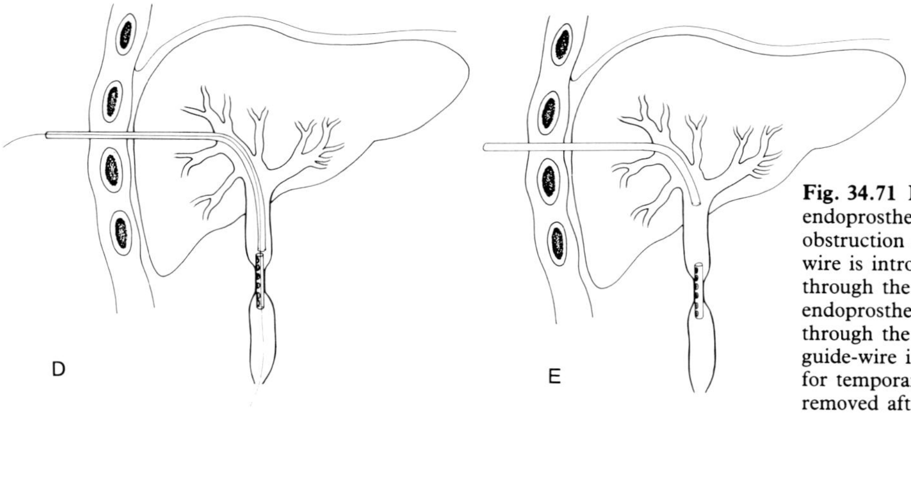

Fig. 34.71 Diagrammatic representation of transhepatic endoprosthesis insertion. **A.** The dilated biliary tree above an obstruction is tapped with a sheathed needle. **B.** A guide-wire is introduced through the sheath and manipulated through the stricture. **C.** The sheath is removed. **D.** The endoprosthesis is passed over the guide wire and impacted through the stricture by means of a pushing catheter. **E.** The guide-wire is removed and the pushing catheter withdrawn for temporary external drainage. The external drain is removed after two days.

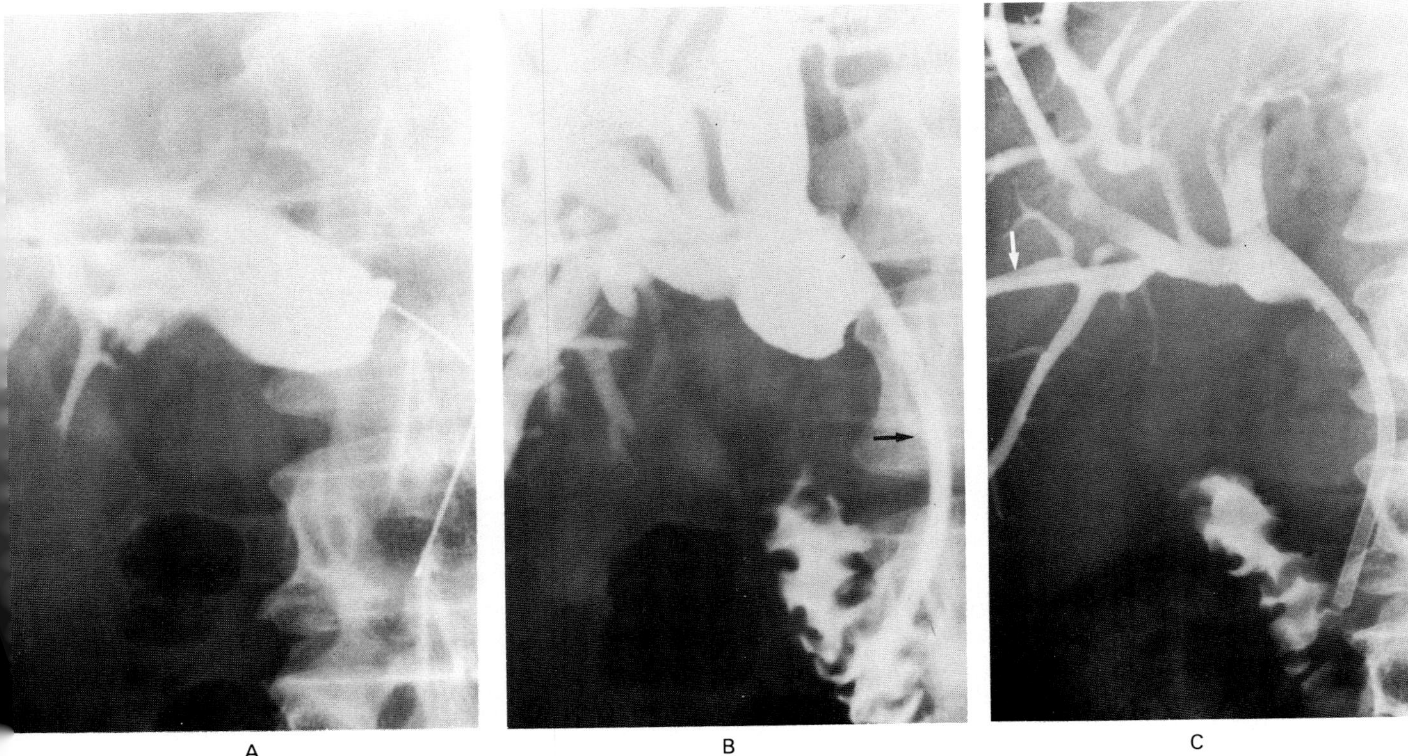

Fig. 34.72 Transhepatic endoprosthesis. **A.** A guide-wire has been manipulated through the completely obstructing lesion of the common hepatic duct. **B.** An endoprosthesis (arrow) has been positioned through the stricture. **C.** 2 days later, cholangiography through the external drain (arrow) shows that the prosthesis is functioning (contrast in duodenum) and that the intrahepatic ducts have been decompressed. The external drain is now removed.

THE INVESTIGATION OF JAUNDICE

Jaundice may be *obstructive* (surgical) or *non-obstructive* (medical). This basic distinction can usually be made on the basis of the history, physical findings and liver function tests. Further investigation of assumed or suspected obstructive jaundice begins ideally with an *ultrasound* examination. The demonstration of dilated intrahepatic ducts is pathognomonic of obstructive jaundice and ultrasound may give the additional information of the level of obstruction and the nature of the obstructing lesion (Figs 34.25 and 34.26). The finding of hepatic secondary deposits, perhaps with ascites, is an important one because no further diagnostic or therapeutic procedures may be required. The ultrasound examination may be combined with fine needle aspiration biopsy of an intrahepatic lesion or of an extrahepatic obstructing mass.

Alternatively, *CT* can often provide the same information: presence or absence of dilated ducts, intrahepatic mass lesions and an extrahepatic mass (see Ch. 65). It will also show glandular masses and involvement of other abdominal organs.

Even when obstruction is shown to be the cause of the jaundice by ultrasound or CT, *direct cholangiography* is usually required for planning the appropriate treatment. If the treatment is to be surgical, PTC or ERCP will be chosen according to local availability. The complication rates of these two diagnostic procedures are broadly similar. PTC has the slight advantage that if the obstruction is complete, the upper end of the stricture (rather than the lower) will be demonstrated. It is the level of the upper end of the stricture which is important for surgical planning.

The advent of non-surgical therapeutic procedures for biliary obstruction has had a considerable influence on selection of diagnostic modalities. If endoscopic sphincterotomy is available and calculous obstruction is strongly suspected, then ERC is the appropriate direct cholangiogram to perform as it may be followed immediately by sphincterotomy. Endoscopic diathermy incision is also appropriate treatment for small tumours of the ampulla/papilla if, as is usual, the patient is unfit for a major surgical resection.

As an alternative to surgery, stents (or endoprostheses) may be inserted through malignant obstructions in order to restore drainage. Stents may be inserted transhepatically or endoscopically (as described above) and the appropriate

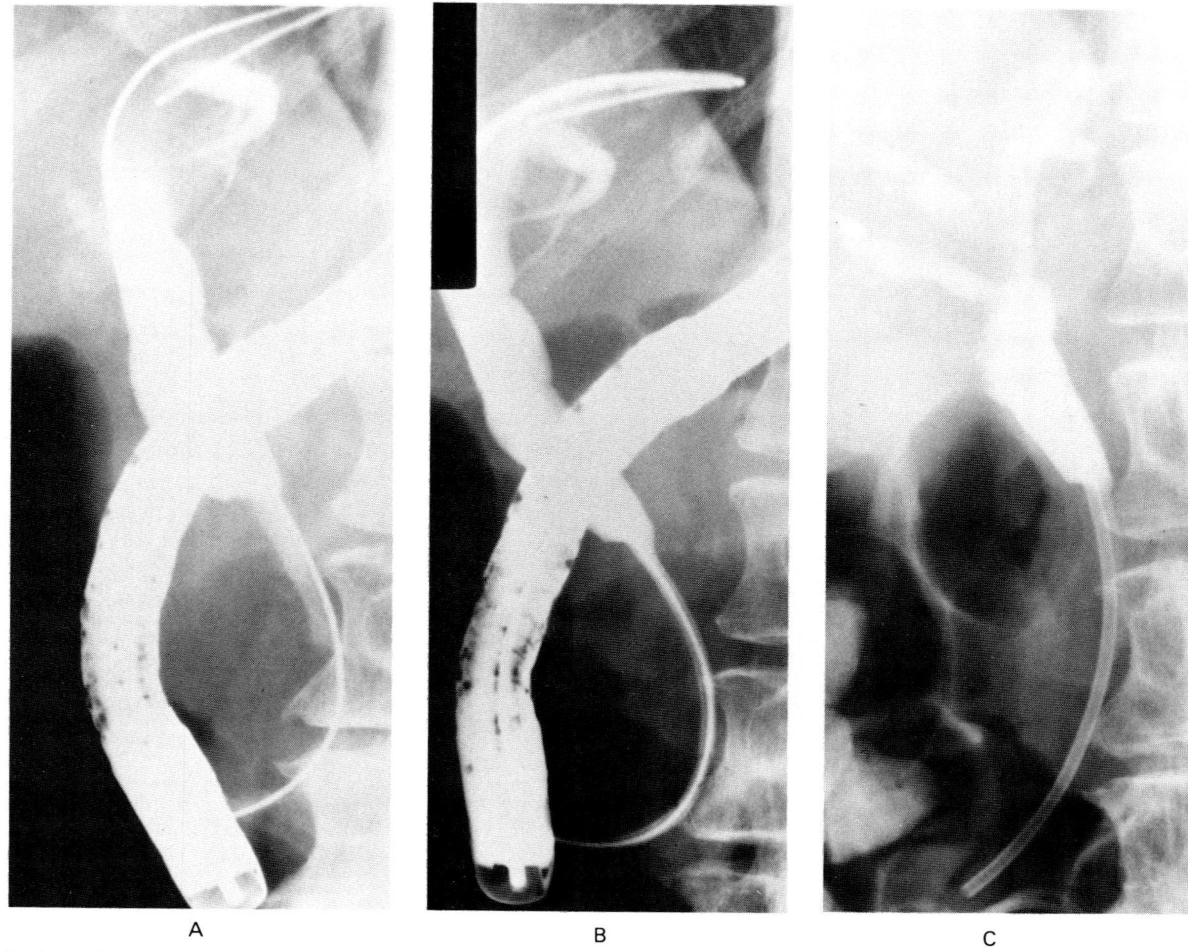

Fig. 34.73 Endoscopic endoprosthesis insertion. **A.** Guide-wire passed endoscopically through malignant bile duct stricture. **B.** Endoprosthesis inserted over guide-wire. **C.** Guide-wire and endoscope removed leaving endoprosthesis in permanent position stenting the stricture.

direct cholangiogram is that which accompanies whichever method of stent insertion is locally available.

There remains the problem of the jaundiced patient with a normal ultrasound or CT scan. Obstructive jaundice may occur in the absence of demonstrable duct dilatation and strong suspicion of an obstructive cause of the jaundice is an indication for direct cholangiography. ERC in experienced hands has a higher success rate than PTC when the ducts are not dilated.

REFERENCES AND SUGGESTIONS FOR FURTHER READING

Baddeley, H., Nolan, D. J. & Salmon, P. R. (1978) *Radiological Atlas of Biliary and Pancreatic Disease*. HM & M.

Berk, R. M. & Clemett, A. R. (1977) *Radiology of the Gallbladder and Bile Ducts*. Philadelphia: W. B. Saunders Company.

Ferruci, J. T. et al. (1985) *Interventional Radiology of the Abdomen*, Chs. 11–18, 2nd edn. Baltimore: Williams and Wilkins.

Margulis, A. R. & Burhenne, H. J. (eds) (1983) *Alimentary Tract Radiology*, chs 53 & 90. St Louis: The C. V. Mosby Company.

Mason, R. R. (1985) Percutaneous extraction of retained gallstones. *Clinics in Gastroenterology*, **14(2)**, 403–419

Motson, R. W. (ed.) (1985) *Retained Common Duct Stones — Prevention & Treatment*. New York: Grune and Stratton Ltd.

Owen, J. P. (1983) The Biliary Tract. In: Whitehouse, G. H. & Worthington, B. S. *Techniques in Diagnostic Radiology*, ch. 6. London: Blackwell Scientific Publications.

Teplick, J. G. & Haskin, M. E. (eds) (1981) *Surgical Radiology*, ch. 16, 3rd edn. Philadelphia: W. B. Saunders Company.

CHAPTER 35

THE LIVER, SPLEEN AND PANCREAS

THE LIVER

Imaging of the liver is required for three main purposes. First to assess the cause of hepatomegaly or of a localized liver mass. Secondly to confirm or exclude the presence of neoplasm, primary or secondary. Thirdly to confirm or exclude suspected inflammatory or parasitic disease.

Many different techniques are now available for imaging the liver. They include the long-established techniques of simple X-ray and arteriography as well as the later techniques of radionuclide scanning, ultrasound, CT and MRI. Simple X-ray is the usual first investigation, followed by radioisotope scan or ultrasound as the most cost-effective further investigations. CT can provide more information but is more expensive, and its use may be avoided if the other techniques prove diagnostic. Some workers, however, prefer it as the special investigation of choice rather than as a supplementary or back-up procedure. Arteriography, once widely used for diagnostic purposes, is now used less for this purpose but more for interventional techniques and therapy. MRI is still being assessed and is not yet generally available, but holds out great promise for the future.

Table 35.1 Causes of generalized liver enlargement

1. Vascular
   - Congestive heart failure
   - Constrictive pericarditis
2. Cirrhosis
   - Hypertrophic nodular
   - Congenital cystic disease with hepatic fibrosis
3. Infiltrative
   - Fatty infiltration
   - Reticulosis
   - Storage diseases (histiocytosis, amyloid)
4. Biliary
   - Obstructive jaundice
5. Blood disorders
   - Myelofibrosis
   - Thalassaemia
6. Infection and infestation
   - Portal pyaemia
   - Pyogenic and amoebic abscess
   - Hydatid disease
7. Neoplasm
   - Primary hepatoma
   - Cholangiocarcinoma
   - Adenoma
   - Metastases

Hepatomegaly is a common clinical finding with numerous and varied causes which are classified in Table 35.1.

Simple X-ray

Being the bulkiest organ in the body, the liver casts an appreciable shadow on a radiograph, though modified by individual variations of shape and orientation. Its outline is deduced because of contrast differences between the right lobe and adjacent tissues, namely the right lung and hemidiaphragm above, the properitoneal fat line along its lateral border and the right kidney and extraperitoneal fat below the sloping posterior border. The lower anterior edge of liver, the surface palpated clinically, is not directly visualized on a plain film, though gas in the hepatic flexure of the colon may indicate its position.

The left lobe of liver is seen less easily radiographically because of its smaller size and central position over the spine. However, it may be indirectly outlined due to air in the stomach (Fig. 35.1). *Riedel's lobe* is an inferior tongue-like extension from the lateral margin of the right lobe of liver, and is found most often in adult females (Fig. 35.2).

Plain radiographs to assess hepatomegaly should include both the diaphragm and pubic symphysis on the same film. Gross enlargement is usually obvious (Fig. 35.3). Clinical and radiological assessment of liver size may not tally. Early enlargement may be palpable yet a supine radiograph appear normal. Should the liver enlarge in a purely upwards direction then a sequential chest film may

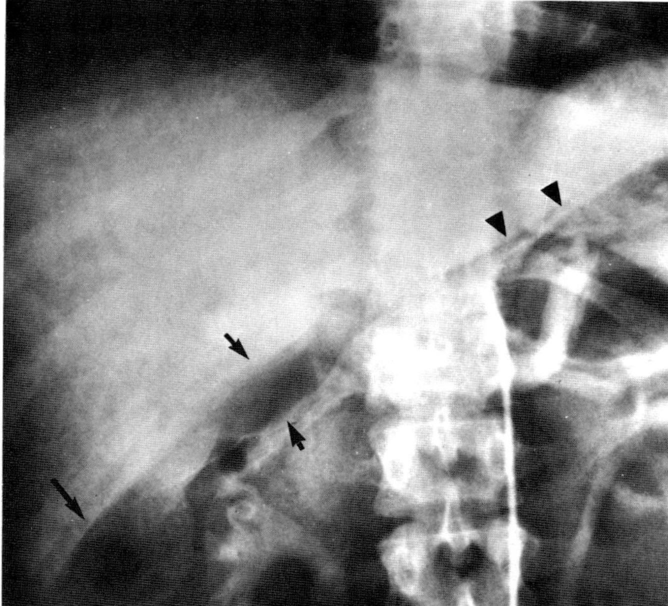

Fig. 35.1 Liver of 'normal' size and shape. Hepatogram following coeliac angiogram. Lower R lobe related to hepatic flexure (single arrow), caudate lobe to duodenum (facing arrows), left lobe to gastric fundus (arrowheads).

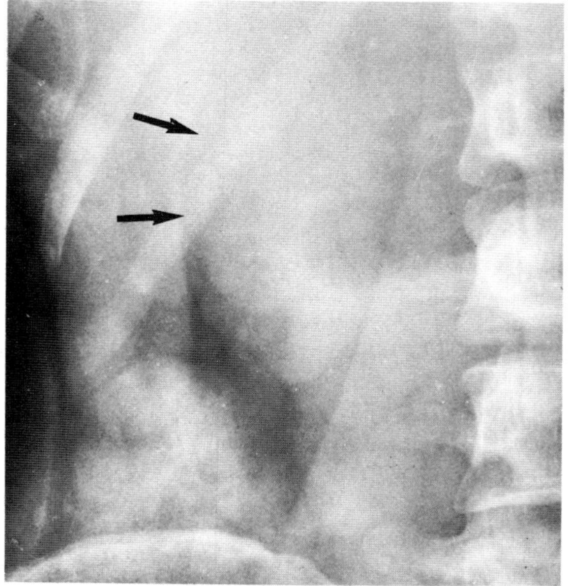

Fig. 35.2 Riedel's lobe extending down towards right iliac fossa. Note fat plane between lower border right lobe liver and right kidney (arrowed).

be invaluable in demonstrating changes in the height or contour of the diaphragm (Fig. 35.4). On the other hand, an enlarging left lobe can usually be palpated anteriorly, even though not yet apparent on film, whilst a large caudate lobe, which occurs in many cirrhoses, can be suspected by anterior displacement of gas or barium in the duodenal cap.

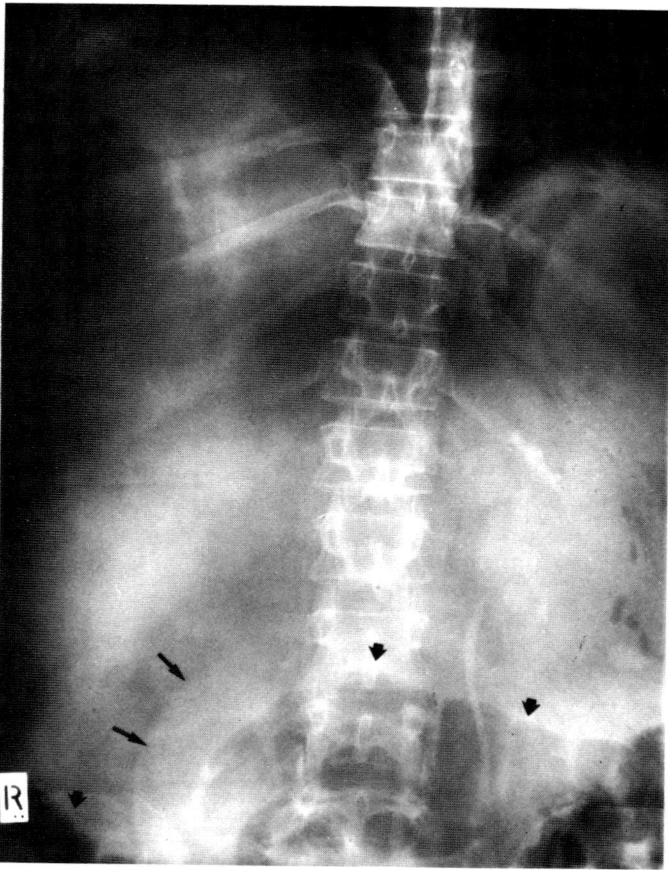

Fig. 35.3 Multiple large bowel metastases causing gross hepatomegaly. Elevated R. hemidiaphragm, depressed R. kidney (thin arrows) and transverse colon (thick arrows).

Radiological signs of liver enlargement are;

1. *Right lobe*:
   a. elevated right hemidiaphragm
   b. depressed hepatic flexure
   c. depressed right kidney (occasionally it remains high)
   d. bulging of the right lateral properitoneal fat line
   e. occasionally, splaying of the lower R ribs posteriorly.
2. *Left lobe*:
   a. gastric fundus displaced downwards and laterally
   b. intra-abdominal oesophagus elongated
   c. extrinsic pressure on lesser curvature of stomach
   d. sometimes, posterior displacement of stomach noted on lateral film.

Other imaging modalities, such as angiography, ultrasound, nuclear medicine and CT will readily demonstrate enlargement of one or both lobes and may characterize the pathology in some (Figs 35.5, 35.6).

Before true hepatomegaly is diagnosed clinically *or* radiologically it is essential to check on the diaphragm

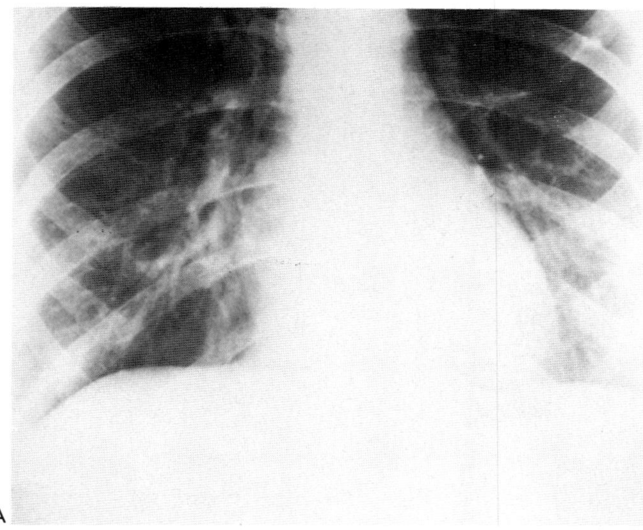

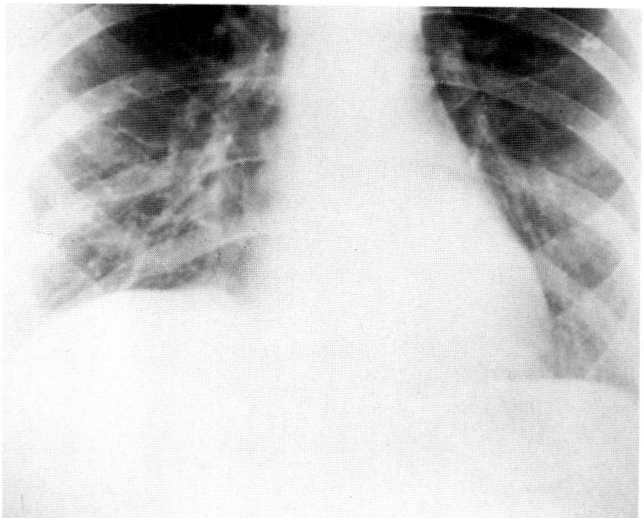

Fig. 35.4 A. Patient with carcinoma stomach. R. hemidiaphragm normal preoperatively. **B.** Same patient 3 months postoperative. Elevation of R. hemidiaphragm with slight humping medially. Liver biopsy = metastatic adenocarcinoma.

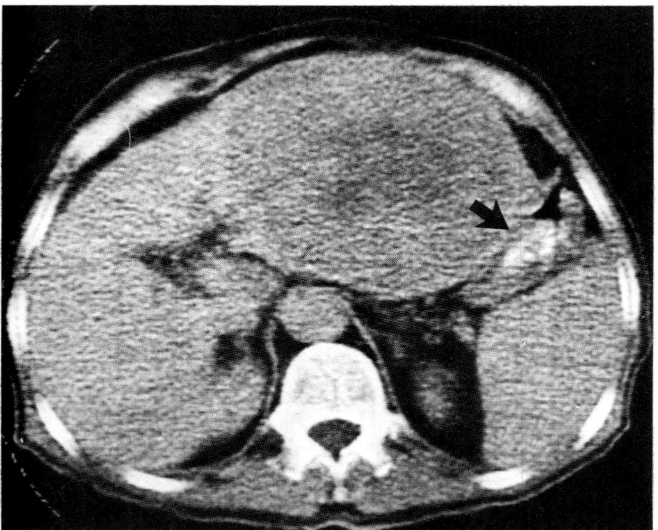

Fig. 35.5 CT scan. Left lobe expanded anteriorly and to left (compressed stomach arrowed) by low density mass with necrotic centre. Hepatoma.

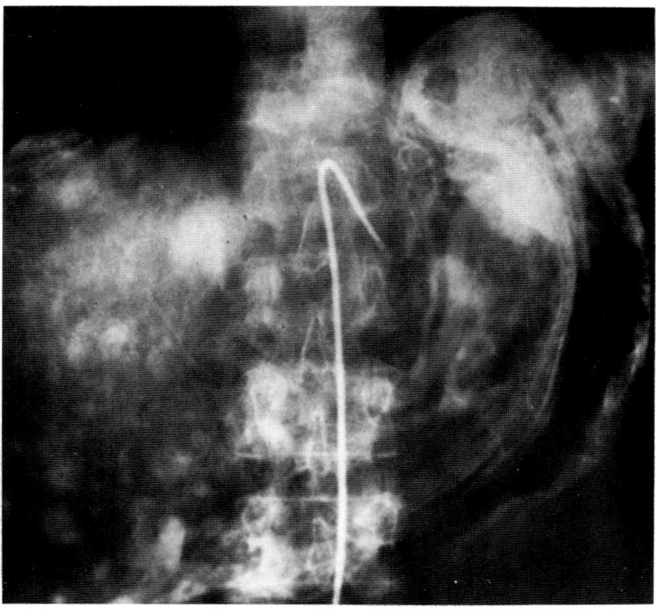

Fig. 35.6 Hepatic angiogram-capillary phase. Multiple vascular metastases (carcinoid). Enlarged left lobe indents and displaces lesser curve stomach.

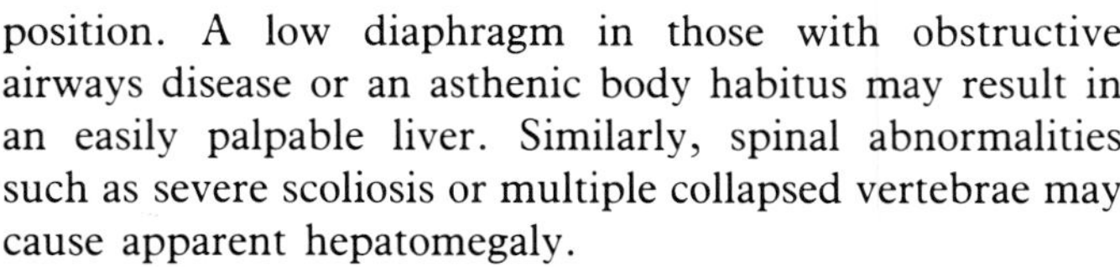

position. A low diaphragm in those with obstructive airways disease or an asthenic body habitus may result in an easily palpable liver. Similarly, spinal abnormalities such as severe scoliosis or multiple collapsed vertebrae may cause apparent hepatomegaly.

Localized masses in the liver are only detectable on plain X-rays if they lie adjacent to or deform one of the visible linear borders, or cause a change in an adjacent structure such as the diaphragm (Fig. 35.7). Masses invisible at simple X-ray may be readily shown by ultrasound, scintigraphy or CT.

Subphrenic abscess. Early in the course, the affected diaphragm will show diminished excursion during *fluoroscopy*, and later becomes raised and immobile, or show paradoxical movement with sniffing. The important differential diagnosis is postoperative gas, which may persist under the diaphragm for 10 days after a laparotomy. Hence the value of repeated screening, since any *increase* in gas, or formation of a fluid level indicates subphrenic abscess. A pleural effusion is common, and results from irritation

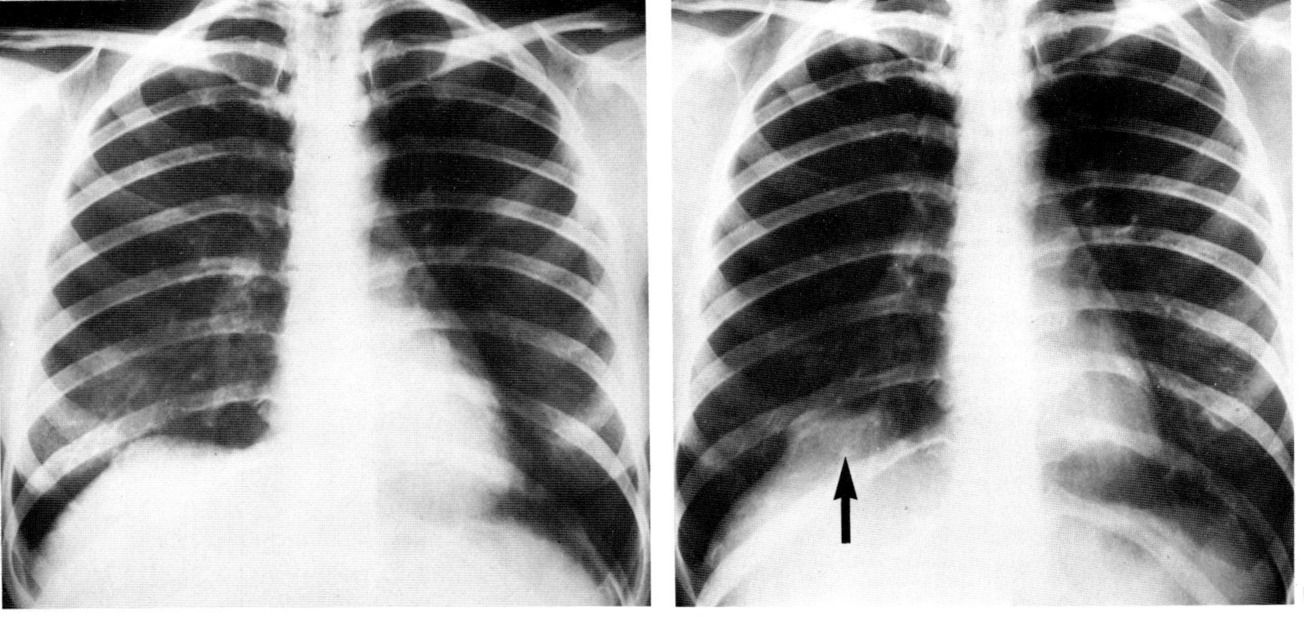

Fig. 35.7 **A.** Chest film on 28-year-old female with fever, reported as normal. **B.** Repeat film after 1 week shows marked localized hump of diaphragm (↑). Aspiration = amoebic abscess.

of the parietal pleura by the inflammatory process. On the left the abscess lies between the gastric fundus, spleen and diaphragm (Fig. 35.8). Postoperative pulmonary collapse with effusion and pulmonary infarction may mimic the diaphragmatic and supradiaphragmatic signs of subphrenic abscess. Collapse usually occurs very early in the post-operative period and infarction often in the first week, and possibly accompanied by haemoptysis.

Ultrasound is the most cost-effective investigation for subphrenic, hepatic and subhepatic abscesses, though isotope scanning and CT may also be very useful (Fig. 35.9).

Calcification in the liver, whether localized or diffuse,

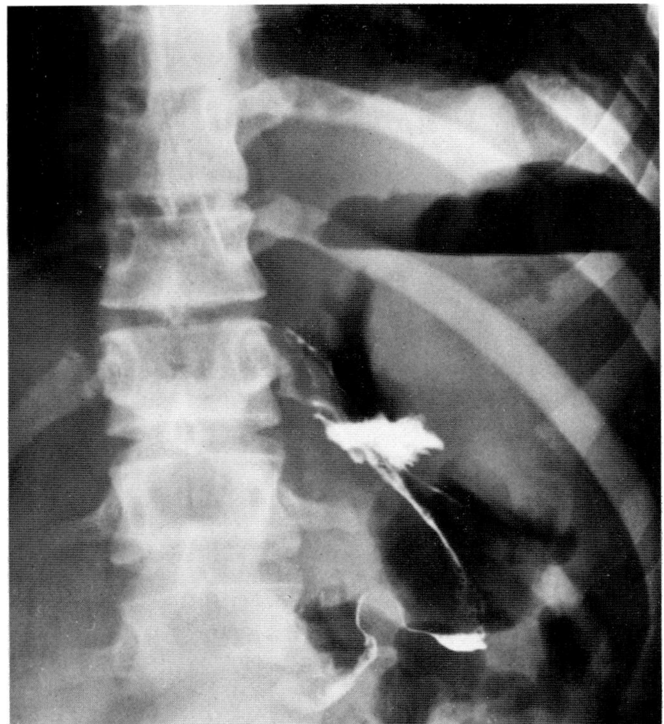

Fig. 35.8 Left subphrenic abscess 12 days after perforated gastric ulcer. Barium has shown stomach to be compressed and displaced medially by the abscess, with fluid level. High hemidiaphragm with fluid above.

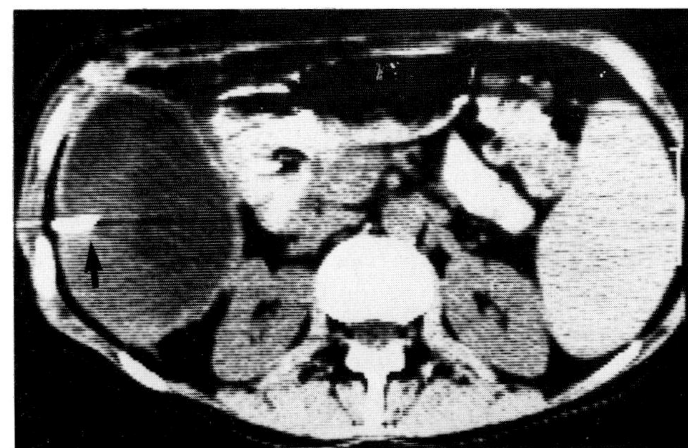

Fig. 35.9 High fever 6 weeks after successful liver transplantation. CT scan shows large R. subhepatic fluid collection. Note catheter drain inserted under CT control (arrow).

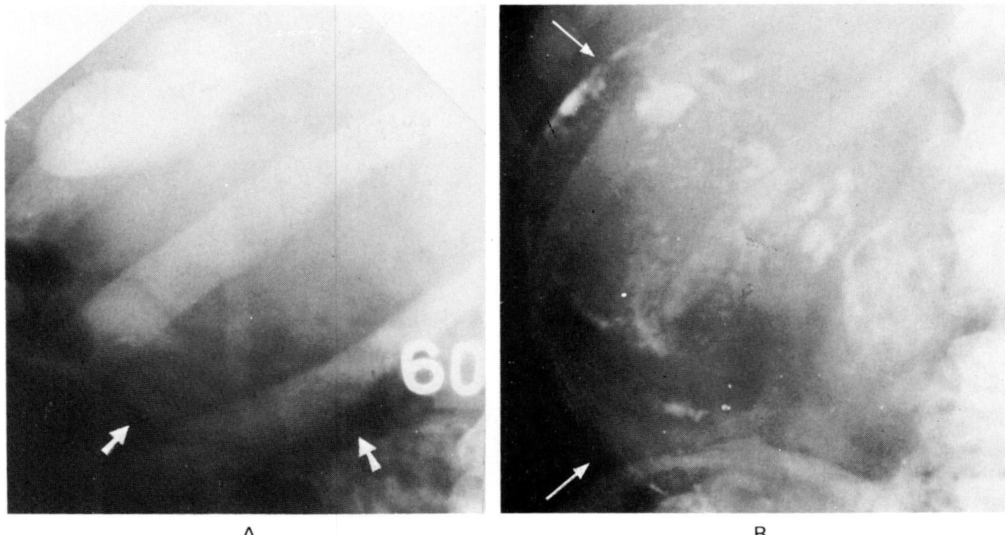

Fig. 35.10 Hydatid cysts of the liver (arrows). **A.** Stretching of the common duct and displacing the gallbladder upwards. **B.** Showing cystic calcification (arrows).

can often be detected on plain radiographs. Its pattern may characterize the pathology. Many *hydatids* calcify, the appearance resembling a crumpling eggshell (Fig. 35.10). In an expanding cyst, the ectocyst itself may be radio-opaque.

Primary liver carcinoma may occasionally be manifest by either faint stippled calcification (Fig. 35.11) or very rarely by 'sunburst' type calcification. *Mucus-secreting adenocarcinoma* deposits from the large bowel commonly contain multiple areas of faint granular calcification, as may calcitonin-secreting metastases from *medullary carcinoma of the thyroid* (Fig. 35.12).

Old *abscesses* and *granulomata* may also calcify and may be multiple. It is often the nature of the liver *adjacent* to calcification which gives a clue as to the pathology and to assess this plain radiography may be supplemented by CT (Fig. 35.13).

Generalized increased radiodensity of the liver occurs in haemochromatosis, or following previous thorotrast injection. It may not be recognized at simple X-ray but is readily shown by CT (Fig. 35.14).

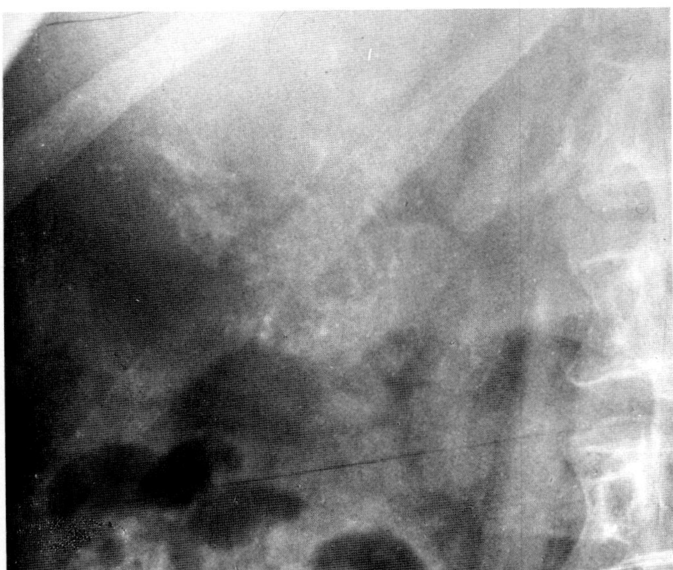

Fig. 35.11 Faint amorphous calcification within liver. Biopsy primary liver cancer.

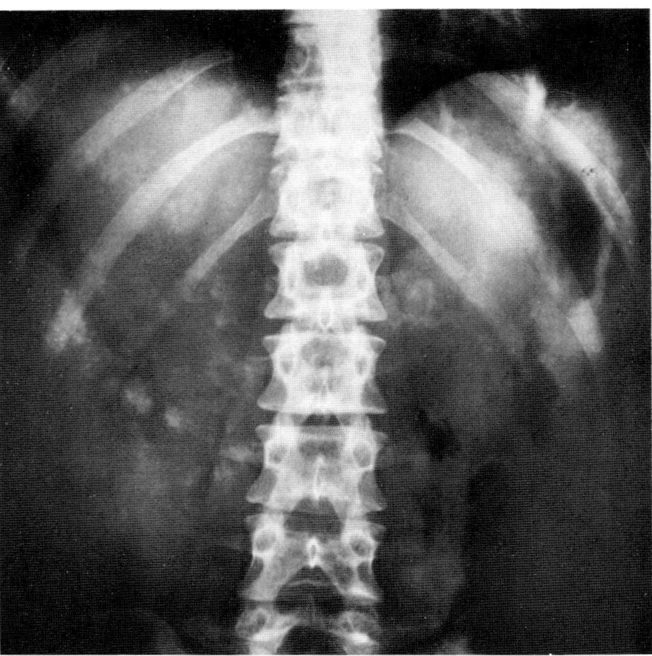

Fig. 35.12 Multiple areas of fluffy calcification in patient with metastases from carcinoma thyroid. All of the signs of hepatomegaly are present.

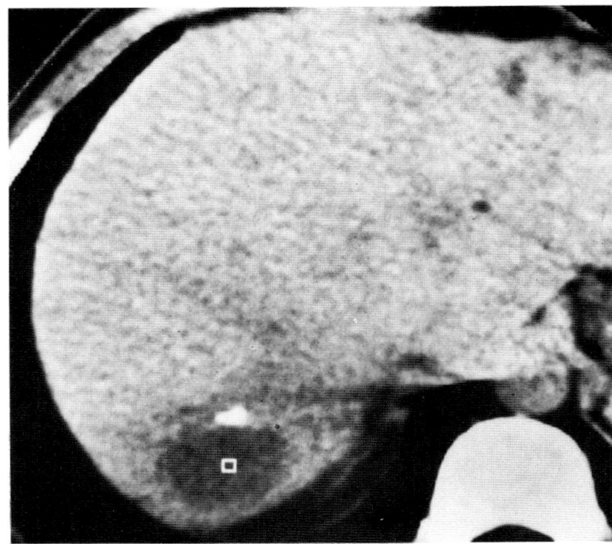

Fig. 35.13 CT scan high right lobe of liver. A small speck of calcium lies adjacent to a cyst, suggesting it to be hydatid. Strongly positive hydatid serology.

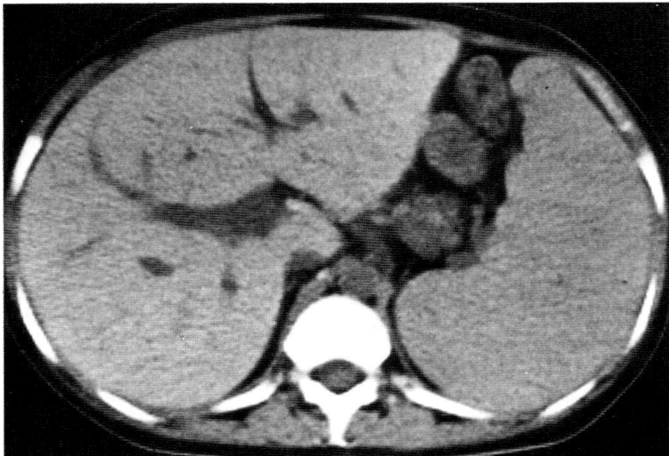

Fig. 35.14 CT non-enhanced liver scan in haemochromatosis. Portal vessels appear as striking low density channels within the dense iron loaded liver. Splenomegaly.

Increased transradiancy of the liver due to gas may be localized within an abscess. Gas may also be present in a vascular or ductal structure, when it is linear in distribution. Gas in the biliary tree generally accumulates in the common hepatic or major bile ducts (Fig. 34.9). The clinically ominous gas in portal vessels takes a branching pattern extending to the periphery of the liver (Fig. 35.15).

A degree of hepatodiaphragmatic interposition of colon is a not uncommon finding (Fig. 35.16), though gross forms of 'Chilaiditi's syndrome' are commonest in elderly patients. To the unwary this may simulate free gas under the diaphragm or a gas-containing right subphrenic abscess. Diagnosis of a fatty liver is not possible on plain radiographs though again the condition is strikingly obvious on CT (Fig. 35.17).

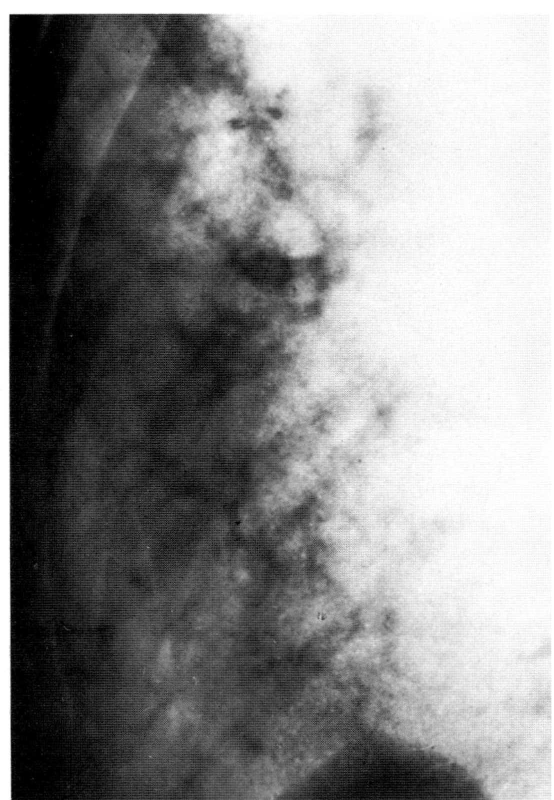

Fig. 35.15 Portal pyaemia following mesenteric artery infarction. Gas is present in peripheral branches of the portal vein.

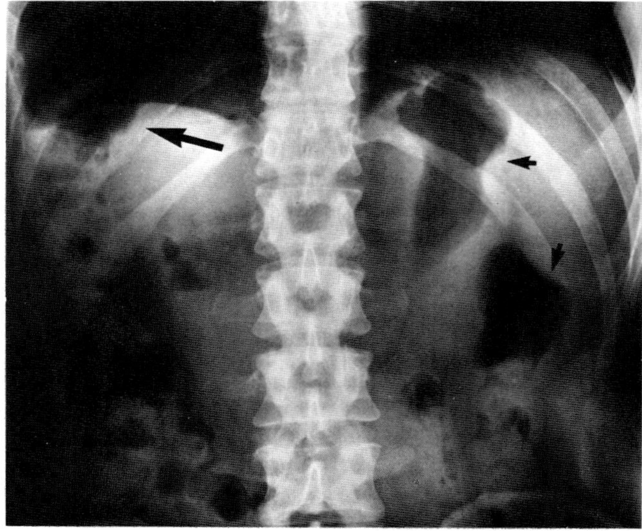

Fig. 35.16 Male aged 46. There is partial interposition of colon between the liver and right hemidiaphragm (large arrow). Note normal spleen size and its relationships to stomach and colon (arrowheads).

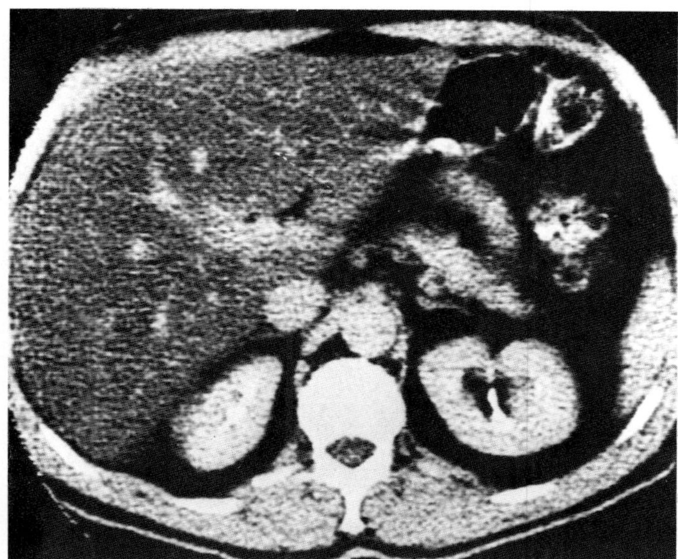

Fig. 35.17 Enhanced CT scan. Liver of very low density (fat) surrounding portal veins.

Angiography of the liver

Angiography of the liver was originally used mainly for the assessment and differential diagnosis of liver masses. With the development of other imaging techniques, particularly ultrasound and CT, this role has diminished. At the same time its use in interventional procedures such as embolization had expanded greatly.

Whether being performed as a diagnostic or therapeutic procedure, it is important to demonstrate fully both the arterial and venous (portal and hepatic) vascular supply to the liver.

Arteriography requires selective catheterization of the coeliac axis followed by the superior mesenteric artery, ensuring that the total hepatic arterial supply has been accounted for, since there are many variations in anatomy (see Ch. 26). In an adult, 50–80 ml of low-osmolality contrast are injected over a 7–10 second period, so as to ensure a rich portogram when the contrast returns from either the spleen or the bowel. If digital subtraction angiography is available, smaller catheters and smaller volumes of contrast may be used. Figure 35.18 shows the ordered division and distribution of hepatic artery branches in the normal liver. Compare this with the irregular pattern in cirrhosis (Fig. 35.19), a tumour circulation with varying degrees of venous shunt (Figs 26.61 and 35.27), the typical appearance of benign haemangiomas (Figs 35.21 and 26.63), and the grossly abnormal angiogram in hereditary haemorrhagic telangiectasia (Fig. 35.22). Pharmacoangiography has been used to show poorly vascularized neoplasms (Fig. 35.23), though the main requisite for successful diagnostic angiography is a large

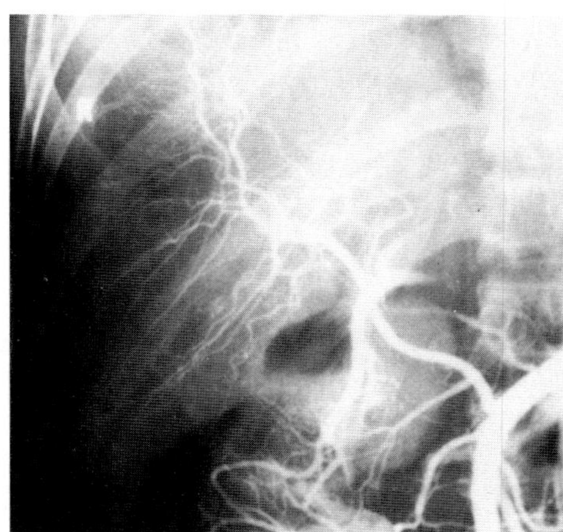

Fig. 35.18 Normal intrahepatic branches of right hepatic artery (which arises from superior mesenteric artery).

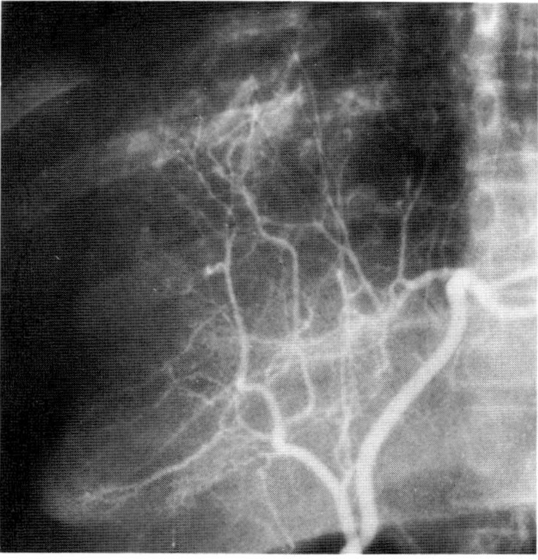

Fig. 35.19 Selective hepatic arteriogram. Intrahepatic arteries displaced around nodules. Irregular liver outline (cirrhosis) with surrounding ascites.

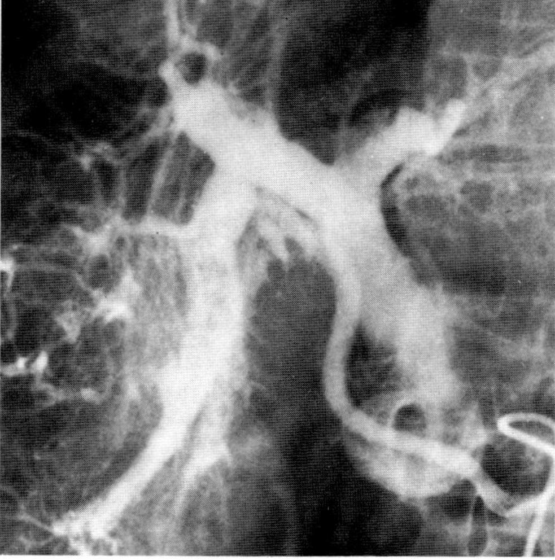

Fig. 35.20 Selective hepatic arteriogram. Bizarre tumour vessels right lobe liver with immediate shunting to large portal vein branches. Hepatoma.

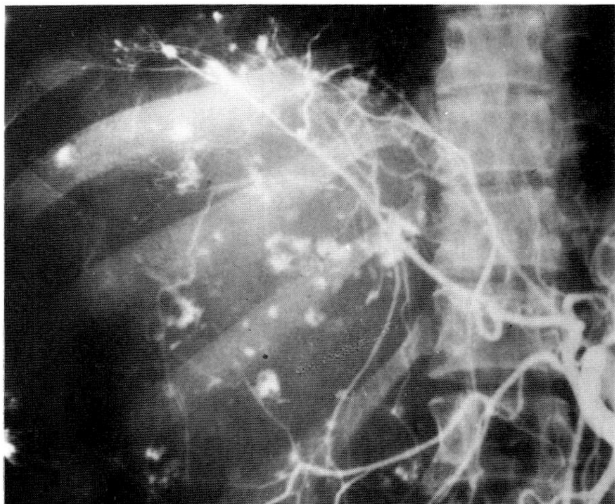

Fig. 35.21 Selective hepatic arteriogram. Multiple small, dense, well-defined stains arise from normal-sized hepatic arteries, and persist over 26 seconds. Haemangiomata.

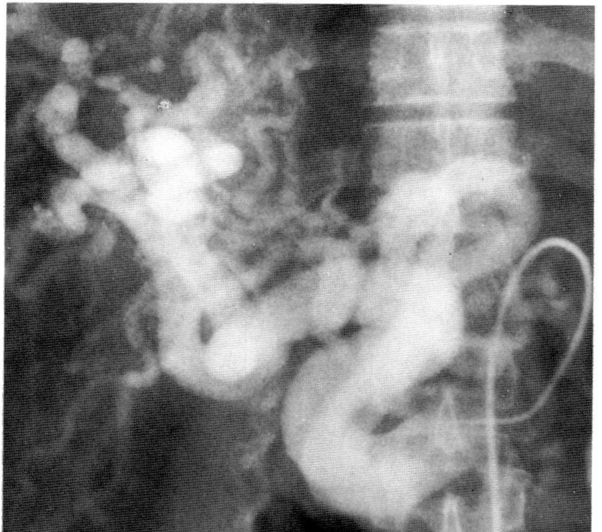

Fig. 35.22 Osler-Rendu-Weber syndrome (hereditary haemorrhagic telangiectasia). Selective hepatic arteriogram. Grossly dilated hepatic arteries, which shunted early to hepatic veins. No tumour circulation.

dose of contrast selectively delivered to the liver, coupled with high quality radiography. Portal phlebography is discussed below (p. 1003), as is hepatic phlebography (p. 1004).

Interventional angiography procedures in the liver, as in other body regions, aim to provide therapeutic alternatives to surgery, or sometimes adjuncts to it. Embolization has been performed both for vascular lesions and for tumours. Embolization of a traumatic blood-bile fistula or an aneurysm is usually successful at a single session and prevents a major operation (Fig. 35.24).

In some metastatic liver tumours chemotherapy can be

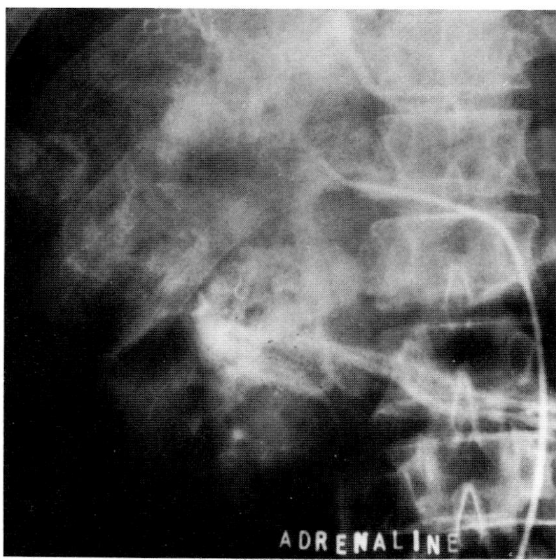

Fig. 35.23 Highly selective hepatic arteriogram after 20 μg adrenaline injected into hepatic artery. Poorly vascularized ring shadows. Biopsy = metastatic mucin-secreting adenocarcinoma.

delivered via arterial catheter, in others arteriography may indicate response to systemic therapy (Fig. 35.25).

Embolization alone may be curative in treating benign liver tumours such as the 'adenoma' associated with the contraceptive pill (Fig. 35.26), whilst, for very vascular masses, embolization may be used preoperatively to attempt reduction in bulk or to devascularize (Fig. 35.27). The place for embolization in hepatoma is controversial. It may reduce liver size as well as pain, but the patient should have a patent portal vein and not have liver decompensation. Apart from this proviso, patients usually tolerate liver embolization very well.

Biopsy

Biopsies under imaging control are becoming a common interventional procedure. One common indication is the small liver 'missed' on ward biopsy, though the more usual indication is to accurately biopsy a localized region of pathology (Fig. 35.28).

Radionuclide scanning

Isotope scanning was the first of the newer imaging techniques to be widely used in liver examinations. The technique and indications are discussed in detail in Chapter 66.

The technique will confirm the presence of an enlarged or small liver, and will demonstrate focal areas of diminished uptake. Unfortunately these are non-specific, and can be due to neoplasm, primary or secondary, to abscess, cyst, haematoma or haemangioma.

Isotope scanning was perhaps most widely used in the confirmation or exclusion of metastases where it still plays a major role.

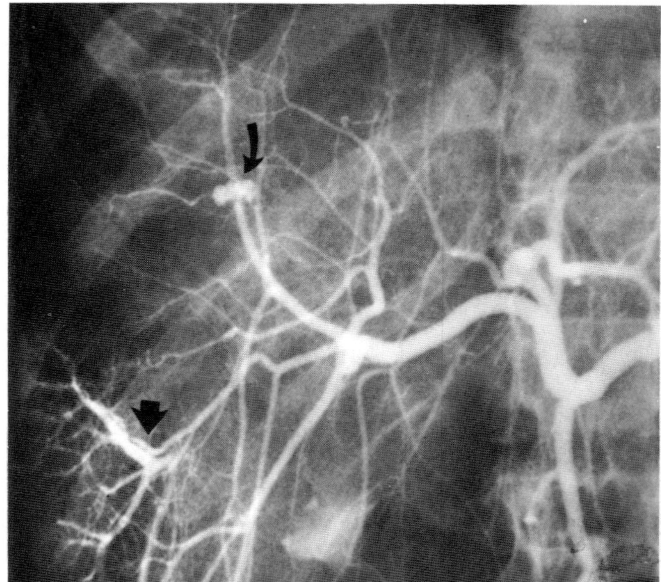

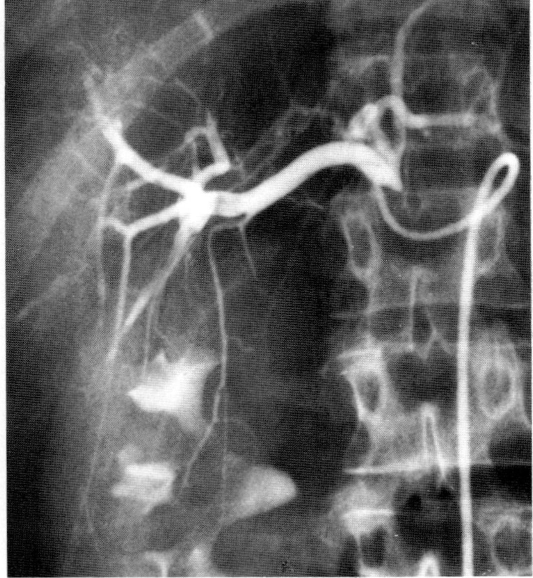

Fig. 35.24 A. Haemobilia following liver biopsy. Arteriogram shows (traumatic) hepatic artery-portal vein fistula (straight arrow) and pseudoaneurysm (curved arrow). **B.** Fistula embolized with gelfoam fragments alone. Haemobilia ceased.

Fig. 35.25 Female aged 42. Hepatomegaly due to multiple metastases from carcinoma of the breast. Large liver with large feeding arteries and tumour blushes. Catheter left in situ for 5 fluorouracil infusion over 48 hours.

Ultrasound

Ultrasound is now considered by many to be the most cost-effective primary investigation of choice in the elucidation of liver masses and other problems since its use can be combined with examination of the gall bladder, biliary tract and pancreas.

The abnormalities demonstrated by ultrasound of the liver are described in detail in Chapter 67. They include neoplasms — primary and secondary, cysts, abscesses and dilated ducts. Ultrasound is more specific than scintiscanning since it will differentiate solid from cystic lesions.

Computed tomography

CT rapidly established itself as a valuable technique for demonstrating abnormalities of the liver whether diffuse or focal. Specific diagnosis can be made immediately in such diffuse lesions as fatty infiltration and haemochromatosis (Figs 35.14, 35.17). Focal lesions in the liver are usually well demonstrated, and contrast enhancement may aid diagnosis where the findings are equivocal or non-specific. There is a high degree of accuracy in the demonstration of malignant tumours, primary or secondary, and in showing such lesions as adenoma, focal nodular hyperplasia, haemangioma, cyst and abscess (Figs 35.5, 35.9, 35.13, 35.28, 37.50 and 37.51).

CT also has the advantage of showing, at the same time as the liver, other adjacent organs and will demonstrate masses in the porta hepatis, adrenals or para-aortic glands. It will also demonstrate ascites and subphrenic or other focal fluid or pus collections (Fig. 35.9).

A more detailed discussion of CT appearances will be found in Chapter 65.

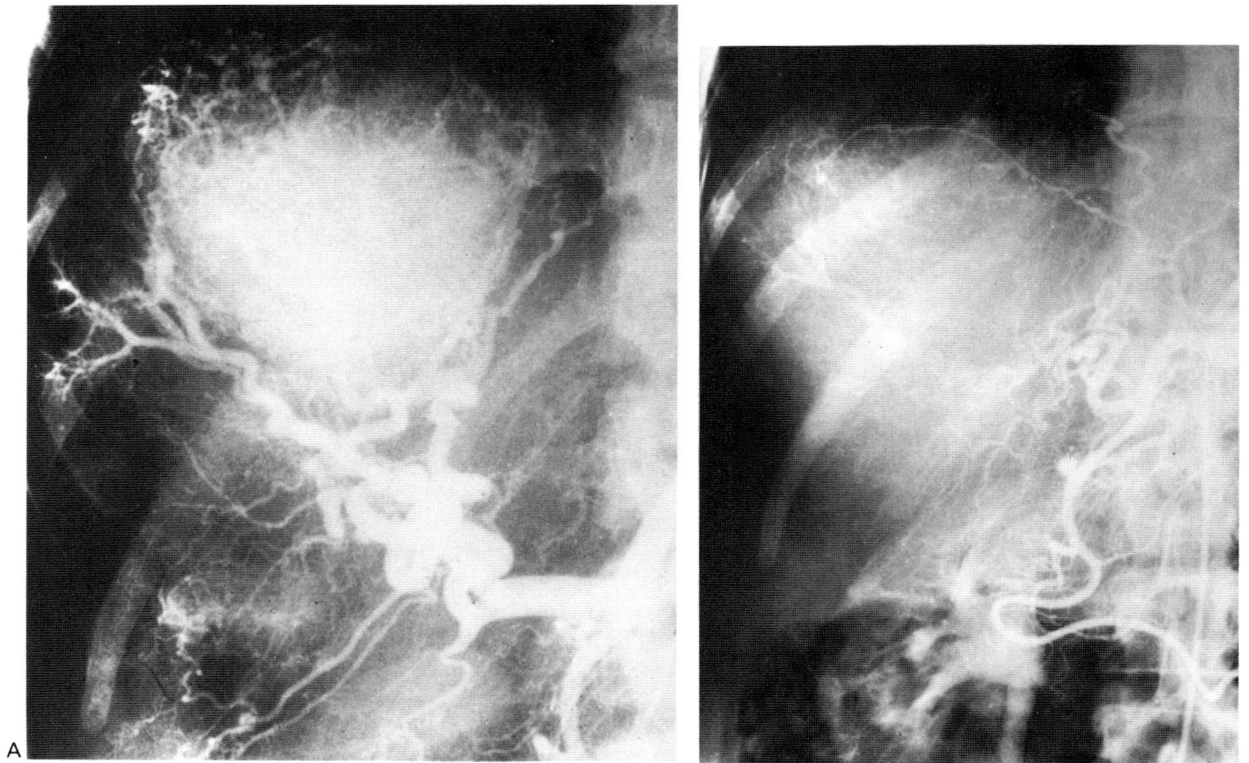

Fig. 35.26 A. Female 45. Contraceptive 'pill' for 16 years. Vascular adenomata liver (biopsy proof). **B.** Angiogram postembolization with dextrose, Gelfoam, absolute alcohol. No tumour circulation. No further therapy. Asymptomatic 14 months later.

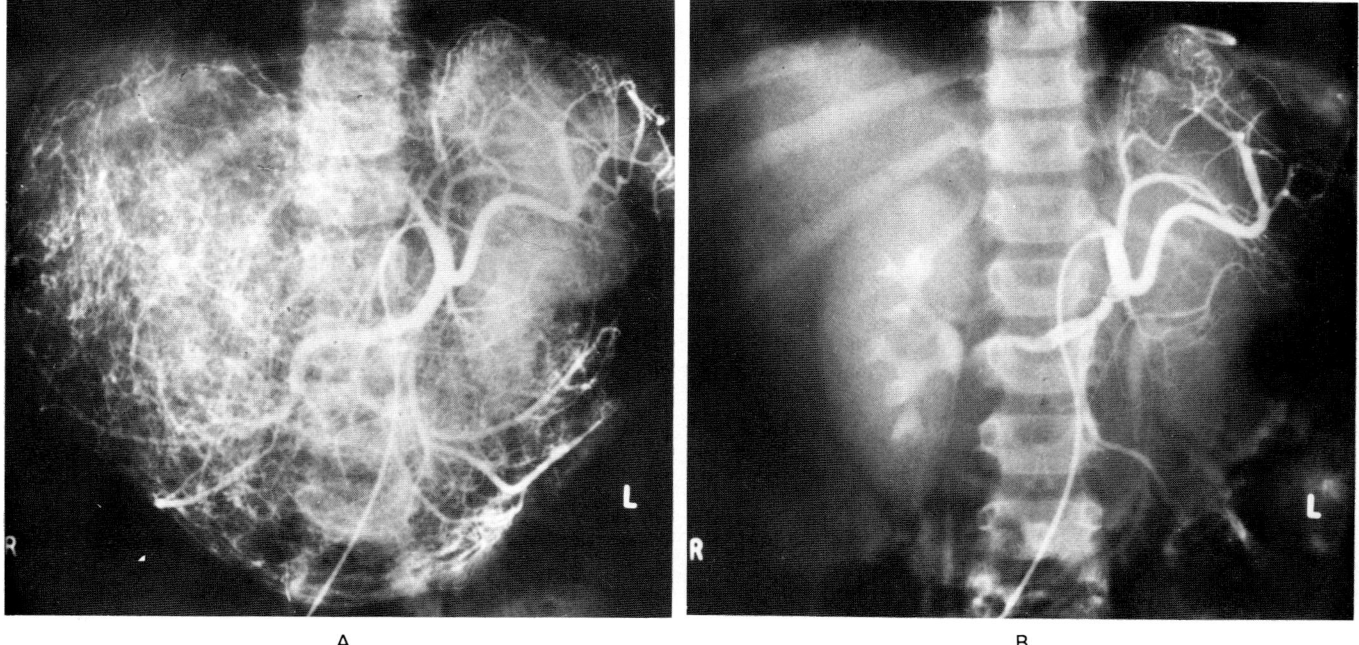

Fig. 35.27 A. Boy of 5 with rapidly enlarging liver and highly vascular unusual 'tumour', left lobe of liver. Embolized prior to surgery. **B.** Postembolization angiogram. Note wire coil in mouth of left hepatic artery (right hepatic originated from superior mesenteric).

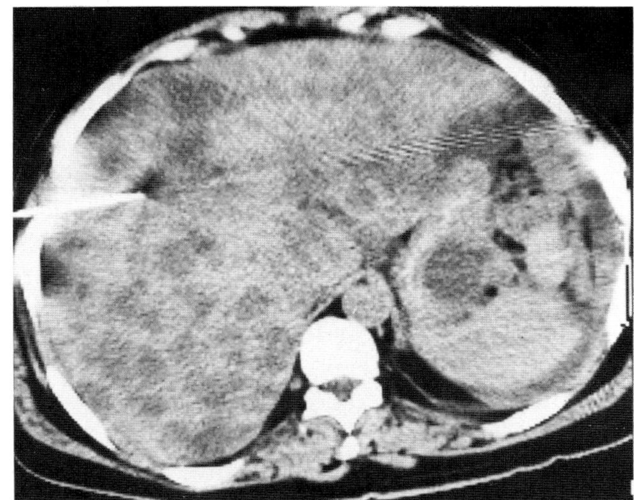

Fig. 35.28 CT scan showing guided biopsy of one of numerous low-density lesions in large liver. Metastatic carcinoma — primary unknown. Previous ward biopsy — normal liver!

THE SPLEEN

MRI

MRI in the investigation of liver disease is currently being evaluated (see Ch. 68).

As with the liver, images of the spleen can be obtained by simple X-rays and arteriography, and by the various newer imaging techniques of isotope scanning, ultrasound, CT and MRI. Since the diagnosis of splenic enlargement is easily made by clinical examination or simple X-ray, expensive or time-consuming imaging methods are rarely used for this purpose.

Simple X-ray

The spleen must be moderately enlarged to be palpated clinically, but even a normal-sized spleen is usually visible on good quality radiographs. Thus the radiologist may alert an unsuspecting physician to an early splenomegaly.

Good quality abdominal films show the spleen to lie in the concavity of the left 9th, 10th and 11th ribs, with the left hemidiaphragm above, the stomach medially and the splenic flexure of the colon inferiorly (Fig. 35.16). In the adult, the long axis of the spleen does not usually exceed 11 cm in length. A length exceeding 15 cm is regarded as evidence of splenomegaly.

Accessory spleens are not uncommon, lying along the splenic artery, near the hilum, or in the omental ligaments around the spleen. Such 'splenunculi' occur in normal people and sometimes enlarge following splenectomy. Though rarely diagnosed on plain X-ray films, they may appear as an extrinsic mass indenting the stomach (Fig. 35.29), and have been mistaken for pancreatic or adrenal masses. They can be readily identified by isotopes or CT and should not be mistaken for tumours.

Table 35.2 Causes of splenomegaly

1. *Blood disorders*: leukaemias; haemolytic anaemias, congenital or acquired; myelosclerosis; polycythaemia
2. *Lymphomas*: Hodgkins; non-Hodgkins
3. *Reticulo-endothelial disorders*: histiocytosis; Gaucher's disease; Niemann Pick
4. *Infections and infestations*: Acute and subacute bacterial and viral infections (e.g. subacute bacterial endocarditis and infectious mononucleosis); chronic bacterial infections (e.g. tuberculosis and brucellosis); malaria; kala-azar; schistosomiasis; hydatid
5. *Vascular*: congestive; portal hypertension
6. *Trauma*: rupture; subcapsular haematoma
7. *Cysts*: pseudocysts (posthaemorrhagic); epidermoid; hydatid
8. *Metastases*: breast, bronchus, gastrointestinal, etc.
9. *Miscellaneous*: sarcoid; amyloid; SLE; Felty's syndrome

Splenomegaly. There are numerous causes of splenic enlargement, and these can be classified as in Table 35.2.

Plain films will sometimes provide a clue as to the cause of splenomegaly. For example, small pigment stones in the gall bladder and abnormal bony trabeculae affecting all bones suggests *thalassaemia*; overlying rib fracture may occur with traumatic splenic *haematoma*; a miliary lung pattern is seen in *miliary tuberculosis*; with *myelosclerosis* all of the bones may be dense.

An enlarged spleen extends downwards and to the right. The stomach is displaced forwards and medially and the left diaphragm may rise. Loss of the left psoas margin and depression of the left kidney are variable signs, the kidney perhaps staying high (Fig. 35.30). Though a depressed splenic flexure is a seminal sign of splenomegaly, the large spleen occasionally lies totally below the flexure.

Calcification in or adjacent to the spleen is common, especially beyond the 5th decade. Calcification of the splenic

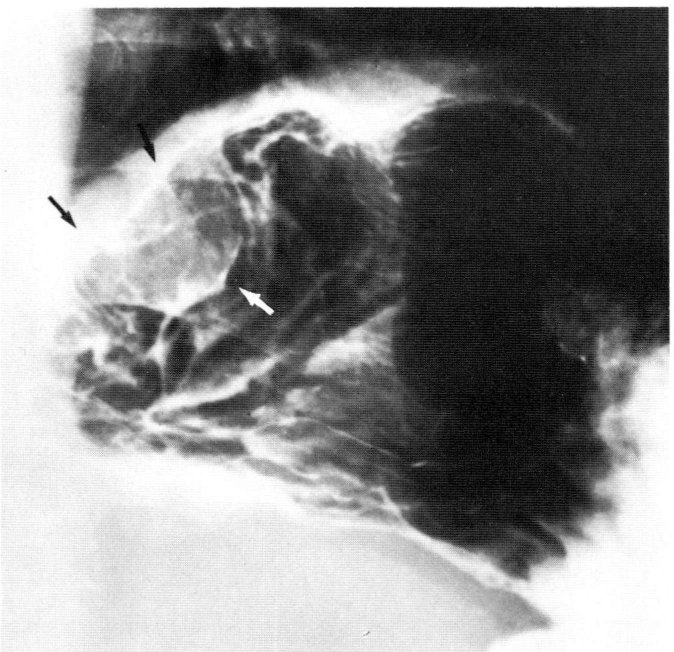

Fig. 35.29 Barium meal. Indentation on gastric mucosa (arrowed) was due to a splenunculus. (Courtesy of Dr A. Broadbridge.)

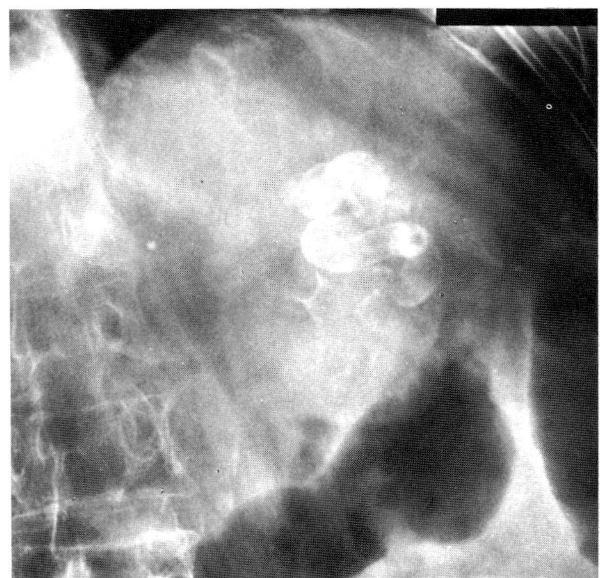

Fig. 35.31 Female aged 89. Plain abdomen. Tortuous parallel line calcification in splenic artery.

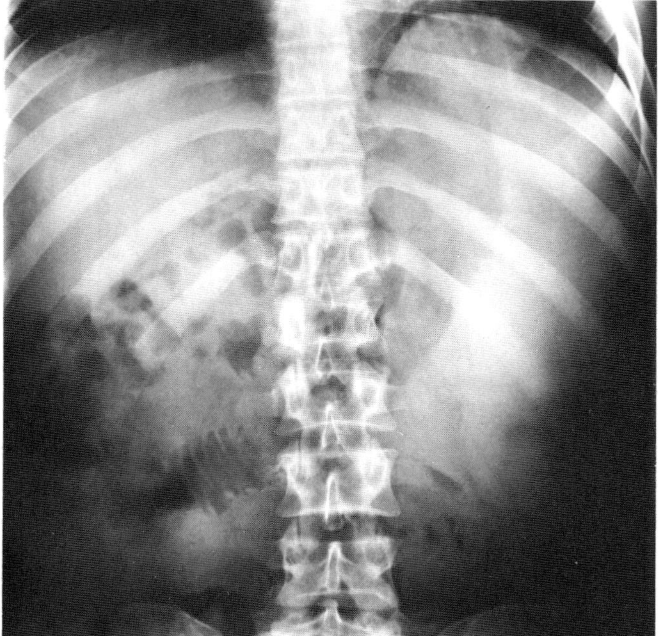

Fig. 35.30 Gross splenomegaly in Banti's syndrome. Note elevation of left hemidiaphragm.

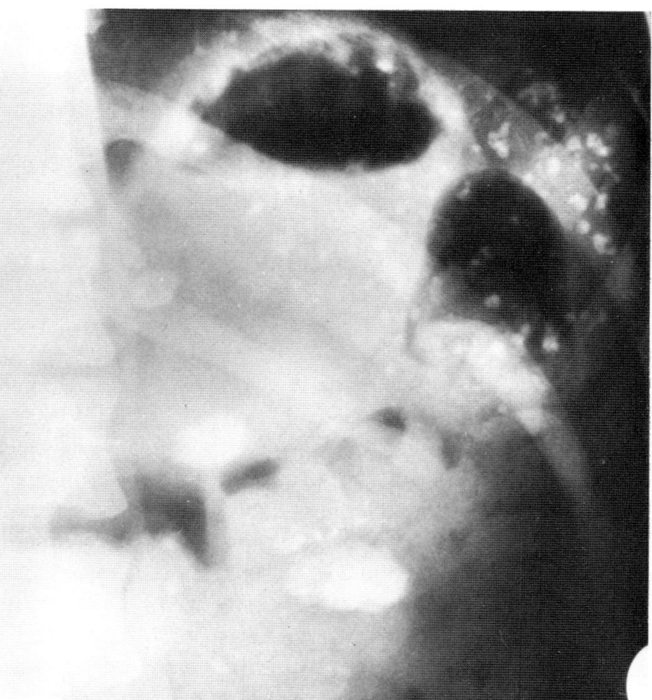

Fig. 35.32 Arab male aged 31. Known previous tuberculosis affecting spleen and left kidney. Both show areas of calcification.

artery (or aneurysms of it) are frequent chance findings on abdominal radiographs (Fig. 35.31). Splenic vein calcification in uncommon, as are phleboliths in the spleen. When present, these have the typical appearance of those seen in the pelvis. Granulomas, such as tuberculosis, produce single or multiple well-defined calcifications in the parenchyma (Fig. 35.32). Rarely, old splenic abscesses and haematomas calcify. Splenic cysts may show characteristic curvilinear or oval calcification (Fig. 35.33). A completely infarcted spleen such as occurs in sickle cell anaemia may, late in the course of the disease, appear as a small curved calcified structure below the left hemidiaphragm.

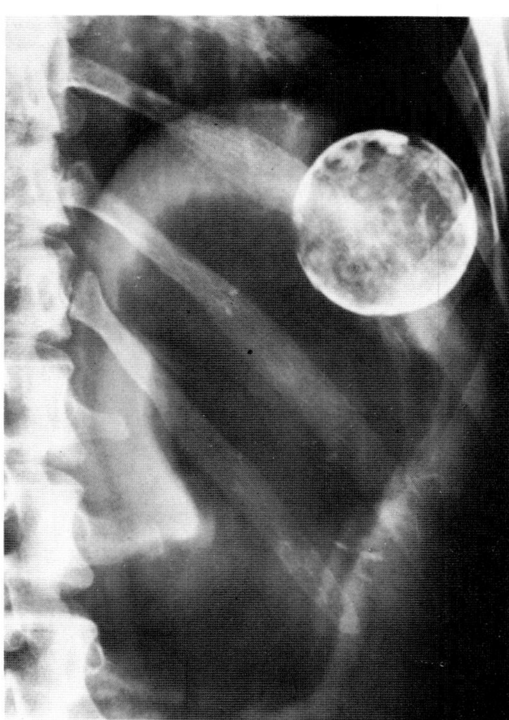

Fig. 35.33 Female aged 39. Calcified non-parasitic cyst in spleen.

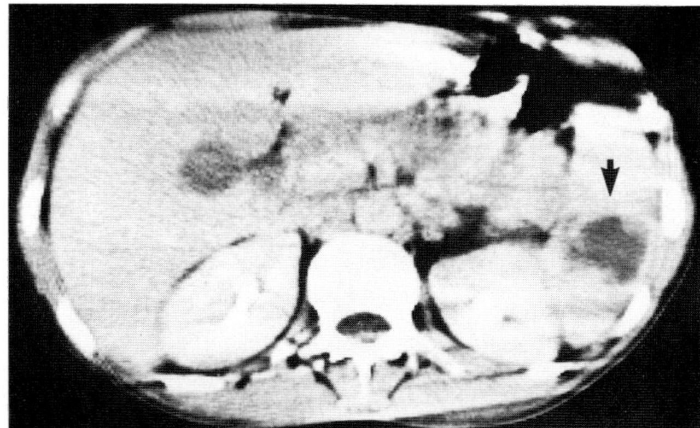

Fig. 35.34 CT scan (enhanced) following embolization for vascular abnormality. Low density area in spleen is area of infarction (arrow). Asymptomatic.

Thorotrast spleen should not be mistaken for multiple calcifications in the spleen. Thorium dioxide was widely used for angiography prior to 1950, and was finally deposited in the spleen where it is seen as multiple punctate opacities (Fig. 26.4).

Gas translucency is seen in the spleen with **splenic abscess**. Though very rare, it is important to diagnose as the patient is gravely ill. As noted above, the condition may follow embolization of the splenic artery. It is usually associated with decreased movement of the left diaphragm, and there may be a pleural effusion above. The mottled appearance of the gas must not be mistaken for faeces in the splenic flexure. A fluid level in the erect radiograph may clinch the diagnosis. If no gas is present, an abscess may be suggested by radioisotope scanning, though the area of reduced uptake is not specific. The same applies to the cystic area seen at ultrasound or CT, though the finding may clinch a clinical suspicion of abscess.

Splenic infarcts such as occur in sickle cell disease can also be shown as localized defects by radionuclide scanning. They can also be demonstrated by CT.

Floating spleen (wandering spleen). This rare condition is occasionally found in adult females with large spleens, and can mimic an abdominal tumour. The diagnosis can be confirmed by radioisotope scanning or by CT.

Splenic cysts are usually *pseudocysts* following old haematomas or infarcts. Other rarer cysts are *epidermoid*, presumably congenital and usually presenting in children, or *hydatids* which are seen in adults. All three types, but especially the latter two, may show marginal calcification on simple X-ray examination. If this is absent, as with most pseudocysts, ultrasound or CT will be necessary to confirm the diagnosis of cyst. Radioisotope scanning will show the lesion as a defect in the opacified spleen, but this is not specific, being present with abscess and haematoma also.

Splenic rupture may follow a direct penetrating wound, or may follow closed abdominal trauma. Simple X-ray may show splenomegaly with indistinct margins to the spleen, kidney or psoas, and fracture of one or more of the left lower ribs may be seen, as noted above. Scintiscanning may show a defect due to the haematoma as may ultrasound, but CT should prove diagnostic with its ability to resolve recent haemorrhage.

Splenectomy is normally indicated if there is significant splenic haemorrhage, but suture or partial splenectomy may be attempted in small children as severe sepsis can follow splenectomy in this age group.

PORTAL HYPERTENSION

Liver *cirrhosis* is the commonest cause of portal hypertension. Radioisotope scanning remains the most useful imaging technique in detecting diffuse liver disease. Many patients will present with bleeding oesophageal varices and require angiography if active treatment is proposed. This is either *direct*, performed via the trans-splenic or trans-hepatic route, or *indirect*, whereby the portal venous system and any gastro-oesophageal collaterals are visualized from the venous return of contrast injected selectively into the splenic or superior mesenteric arteries (see Ch. 27).

The appearance of a normal splenic artery, spleen, splenic and portal veins is shown in Figure 35.35. In portal hypertension, the splenic artery dilates, and aneurysms may form on its extra or intrasplenic portions (Fig. 35.36). Due to dilution of contrast in an enlarged spleen, the best indirect portograms in patients with portal hyperten-

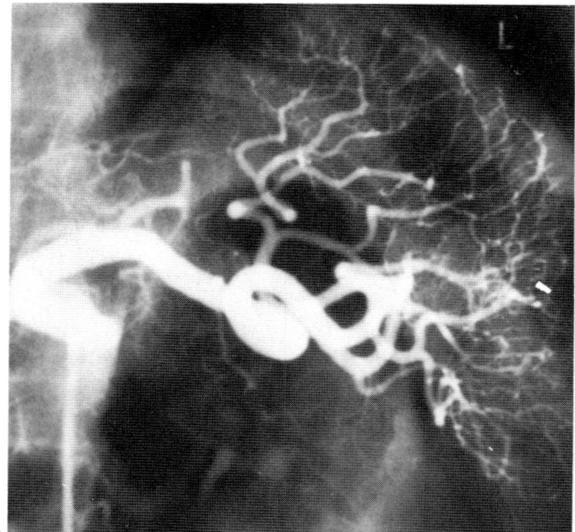

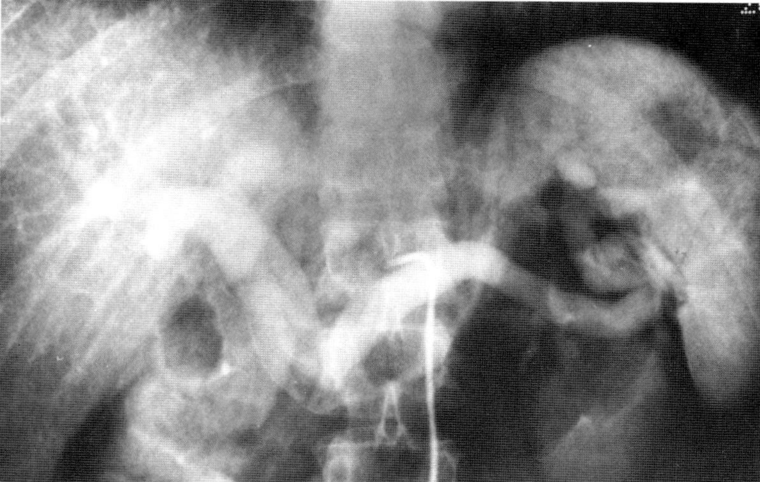

Fig. 35.35 A. Normal selective splenic arteriogram. Normal size spleen. **B.** Venous phase. Normal splenic and portal veins. No filling of collateral veins. Relations of spleen to stomach and left kidney shown.

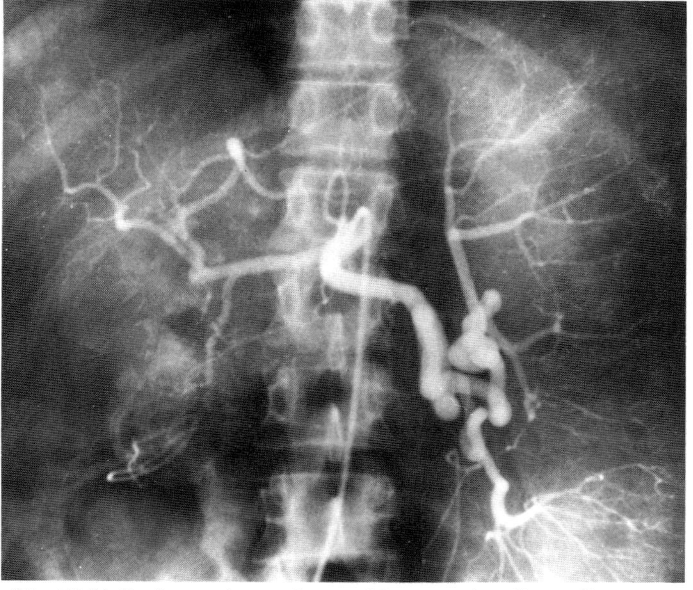

Fig. 35.36 Coeliac angiogram in portal hypertension. Sparse liver arteries. Enlarged tortuous splenic artery with aneurysms on main trunk and divisions. Intrasplenic branches stretched within grossly enlarged spleen which has a vertical axis (cf. Fig. 35.35A).

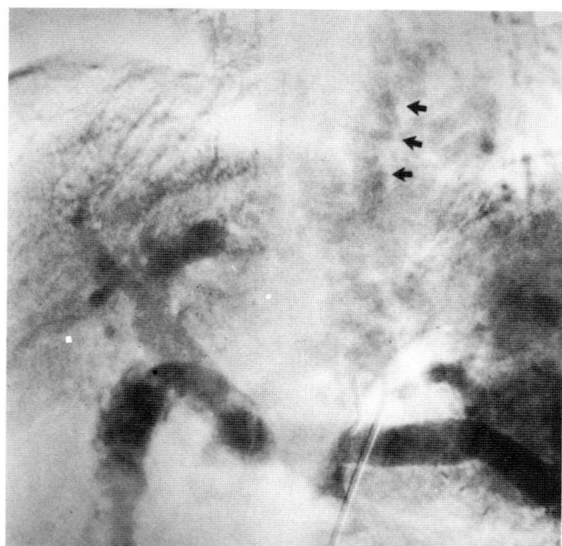

Fig. 35.37 Venous phase coeliac angiogram. Subtraction film demonstrates oesophageal collaterals (arrows).

sion often follow superior mesenteric rather than splenic arteriograms. With either, subtraction studies, particularly DSA, are recommended to show the state of major veins and any varices (Fig. 35.37). Angiograms are used as a road map for planning portosystemic shunts (or deferring them) as well as being an absolute requirement if the patient is being considered for liver transplantation.

Direct portography via a *splenic pulp injection* is a safe procedure providing the patients' clotting is not too abnormal. A platelet infusion should also be available since thrombocytopaenia is invariably present. Portal vein block is clearly seen on portography (Fig. 35.38). It may also be shown by ultrasound (Fig. 35.39).

Portal pressure may be registered from the splenic pulp. During cannula removal, the tract in the spleen is advisedly plugged with gelfoam fragments to prevent the complication of haemorrhage.

CT scanning in portal hypertension is of limited value in showing varices, though it can demonstrate patent major veins and a patent shunt (Fig. 35.40). Ultrasound may show dilated collaterals around the spleen (Fig. 35.41) as well as portal vein block.

Hepatic vein catheterization, using an occlusal-balloon catheter, is a useful procedure which will provide hepatic venograms and sinusoidograms as well as pressure meas-

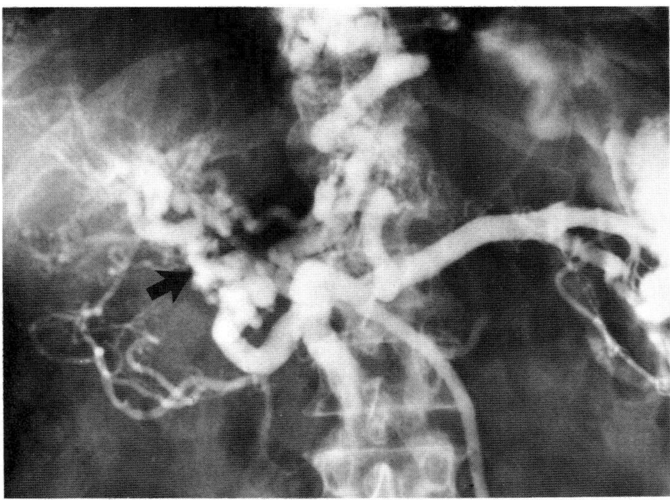

Fig. 35.38 Trans-splenic portogram. Block of portal vein with bridging collaterals (arrowed). Large left gastric, varices and bimesenteric collaterals.

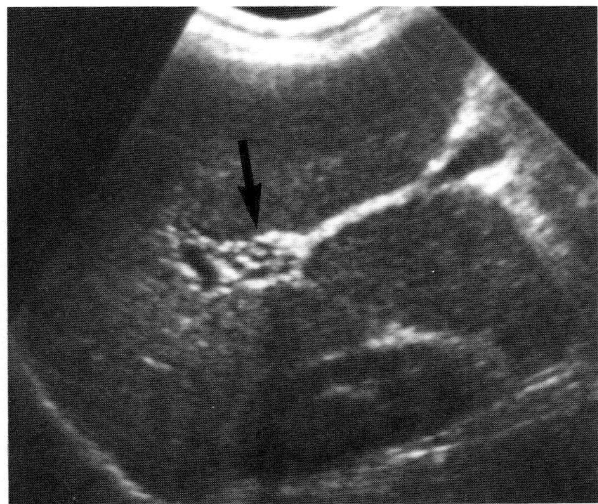

Fig. 35.39 Ultrasound (longitudinal scan) showing porta hepatis. Partially thrombosed portal vein with surrounding varices (arrow). (Courtesy Dr L. Berger.)

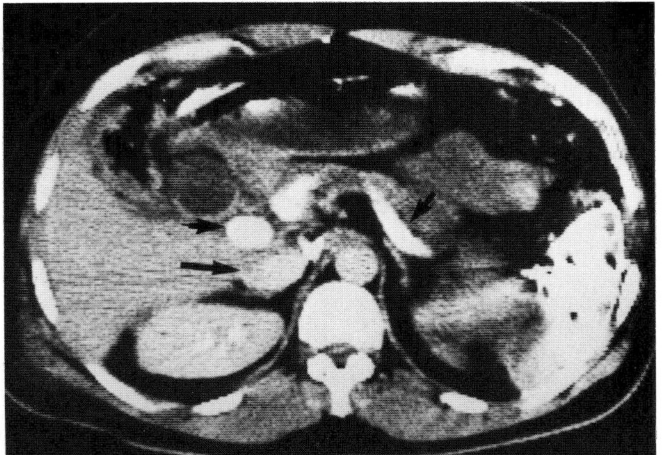

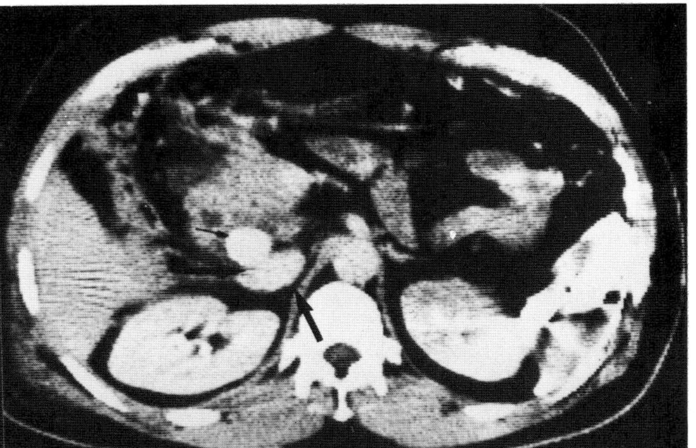

Fig. 35.40 A. CT scan with 10 ml contrast injected into splenic pulp. Patent splenic and portal veins seen behind pancreas (small arrows). IVC (large arrow). **B.** Same patient, lower cut. Contrast is seen going from portal vein via shunt to cava. (Small arrow portal vein, large arrow IVC.)

urements. The vascular pattern varies between normal (Fig. 35.42) and grossly abnormal (Fig. 35.43), whilst corrected pressure measurements, especially when performed serially, can localize the site of cirrhosis as well as indicate its progress.

Interventional procedures in portal hypertension

Liver biopsy is usually performed *percutaneously* with sealing of the needle track by gelfoam. It can also be performed via a catheter following *transjugular catheterization*.

Embolization of varices. This procedure is performed by *percutaneous transhepatic portography*. The aim is to catheterize all the gastro-oesophageal collaterals arising from the splenic and portal veins and to embolize the varices.

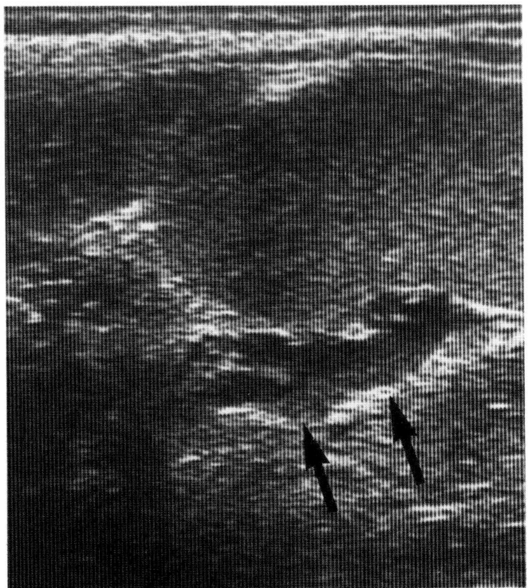

Fig. 35.41 Ultrasound scan spleen (longitudinal). Dilated collateral veins around splenic hilum (arrows). (Courtesy Dr R. Num.)

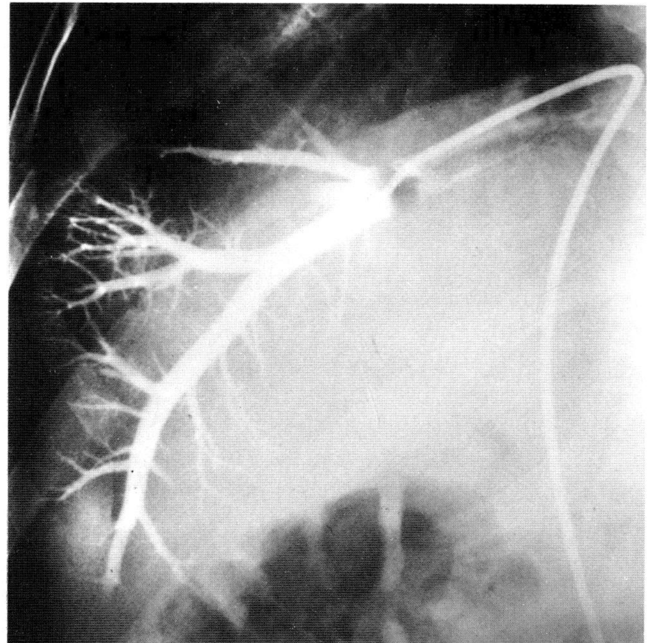

Fig. 35.42 Hepatic venogram. Occlusal balloon method. Normal major and minor veins. Occlusion pressure 6 mmHg.

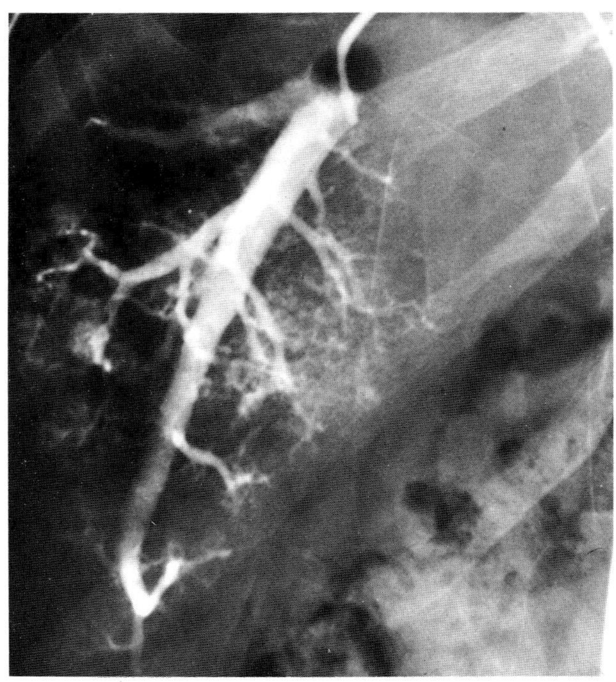

Fig. 35.43 Hepatic venogram. Occlusal balloon method. Irregular hepatic vein tributaries and bizarre sinusoidogram. Corrected pressure 16 mmHg. Cirrhosis.

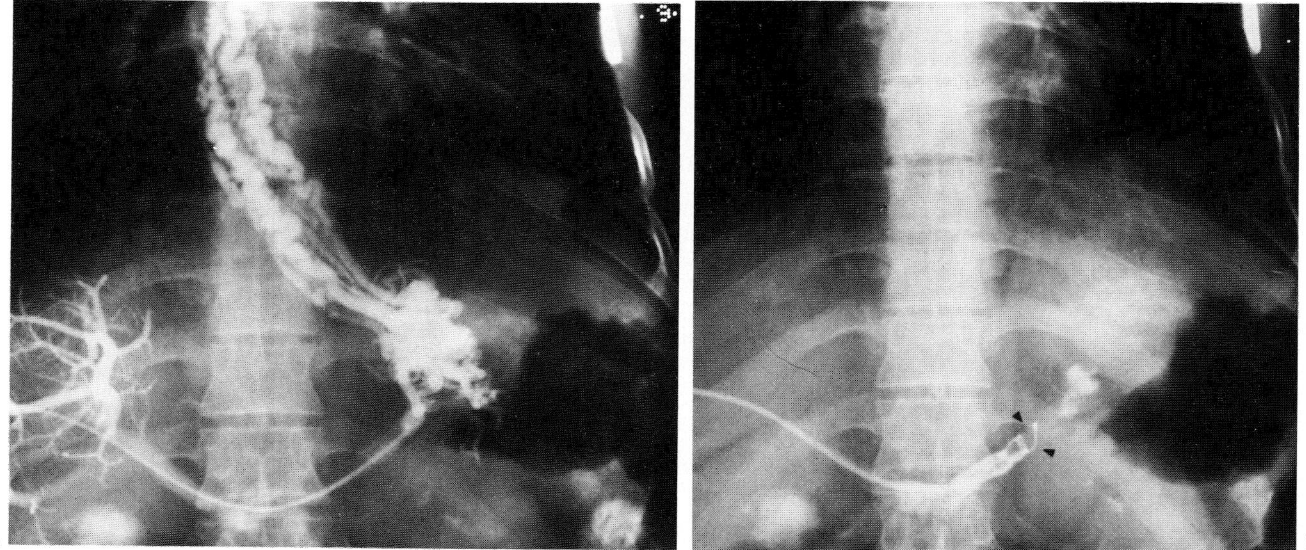

Fig. 35.44 A. Transhepatic portogram. Selective catheterization of left gastric vein using tip-deflecting wire and catheter. Huge gastric and oesophageal varices demonstrated. **B.** Postembolization study. Varices and feeding vein have been embolized and occluded with 100% alcohol, Gelfoam and finally a wire coil (arrowed at root of left gastric vein). No varices fill. Patient later had successful portocaval shunt.

A variety of agents have been used for this purpose (see Ch. 26). They include gelfoam, lyodura, dextrose, 100% alcohol and wire coils. The procedure is technically difficult but it will stop *acute* variceal bleeding in 70% of patients. Recurrence, unfortunately, is common in the subsequent weeks, so that aggressive follow-up treatment is required, including direct injection sclerotherapy of varices at multiple sessions (Fig. 35.44).

Embolization of the splenic artery has been used in the treatment of hypersplenism. The procedure is not without hazard and has resulted in splenic infection and abscess formation.

THE PANCREAS

In the last decade advances in ultrasound and CT have, together with the development of ERCP, revolutionized the diagnosis and treatment of pancreatic disease.

The methods of examination now available include:

1. Simple X-ray
2. Contrast X-ray
   a. Barium meal
   b. Angiography
   c. ERCP
   d. Transhepatic portal catheterization and pancreatic venous sampling
3. Radio-isotope scanning
4. Ultrasound
5. CT
6. MRI
7. Fine-needle biopsy (with ultrasound or CT control).

Isotope scanning has never been a reliable means of diagnosing pancreatic lesions and has now been displaced by ultrasound and CT. MRI has so far proved less reliable than CT in demonstrating solid pancreatic lesions, though it shows cystic lesions well. It seems unlikely, therefore, to supplant CT in this field in the near future.

Barium meals have also diminished in importance, as has angiography, though both are still occasionally useful. Pancreatic lesions may still occasionally be demonstrated at barium meal when unsuspected clinically. ERCP has become a very useful contrast method for evaluating internal duct structure and the state of the adjacent biliary system.

CT of the pancreas is now generally accepted as the most reliable method for imaging pancreatic anatomy and major lesions, and it will clearly show the size and shape of the pancreas in all but the occasional patient. However, it cannot, by itself, differentiate between the swelling of tumour and that of chronic pancreatitis or oedema. It is also of little value with small lesions like islet cell tumours.

Individual pancreatic diseases are discussed in this section using an integrated approach. This is followed by more detailed individual discussions of the techniques of ERP and ultrasound, whilst pancreatic CT is dealt with in detail in Chapter 65 and MRI in Chapter 68.

Barium studies

Depending on its situation within the gland, any sizable pancreatic mass may affect the upper gastrointestinal tract. A barium meal should include views of lower oesophagus in addition to those of stomach, duodenum and upper jejunal loops. Surprisingly, the lower oesophagus has, on rare occasions, been invaded by a carcinoma of the pancreatic tail, but in most patients this indents the body of the stomach (Fig. 35.45). Tumours in the body or head of pancreas may cause abnormalities in the pyloric antrum and duodenal loop (Fig. 35.46). Large cysts or neoplasms of the pancreas do not cause specific displacements of either stomach or duodenal flexure; the changes can be mimicked by large swellings of the left kidney or adrenal, by enlarged retroperitoneal lymph nodes, a large spleen, or by an abscess or cyst in the lesser sac. Clearly, more specific imaging than the indirect abnormalities shown on barium-filled upper gut are required to show the true nature of the lesion, and this is supplied by ultrasound or CT.

In the congenital abnormality *'annular pancreas'*, the descending loop or second part of the duodenum is narrowed or occluded by the pressure of an encircling band of normal pancreatic tissue. Some patients present in adult life, though the condition more usually presents in infancy as vomiting of bile. As with infantile pyloric stenosis, males predominate. Plain radiography shows a gas-distended stomach and duodenal bulb, with little gas in the remainder of the bowel. Barium studies will confirm the diagnosis (Fig. 35.47). About 50% of cases manifest other anomalies such as malrotation of gut, oesophageal atresia or congenital heart disease. There is also an association with Down's syndrome. In adults, a neoplasm of the

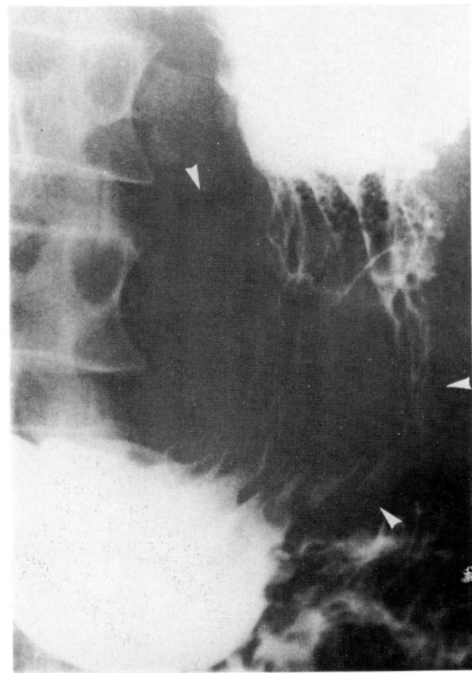

Fig. 35.45 Soft tissue mass in the tail of the pancreas, indenting the body of the stomach (arrows). This proved to be an adenocarcinoma at surgery.

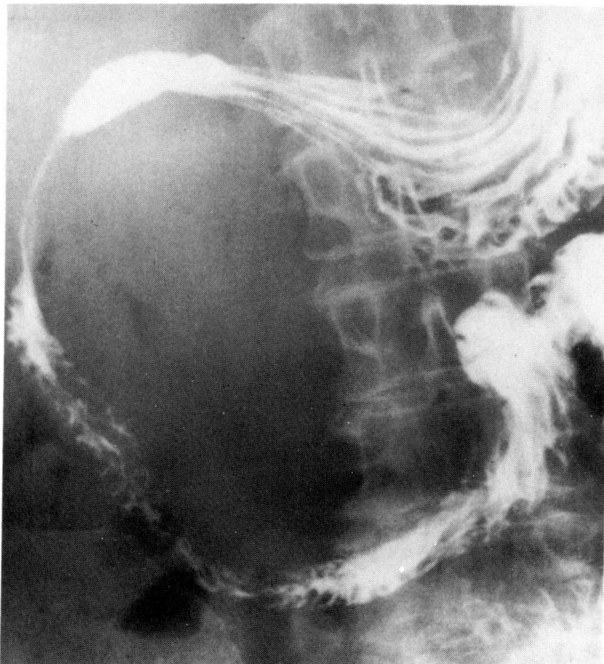

Fig. 35.46 Large carcinoma of the head of the pancreas displacing and compressing the pyloric antrum and duodenal circle.

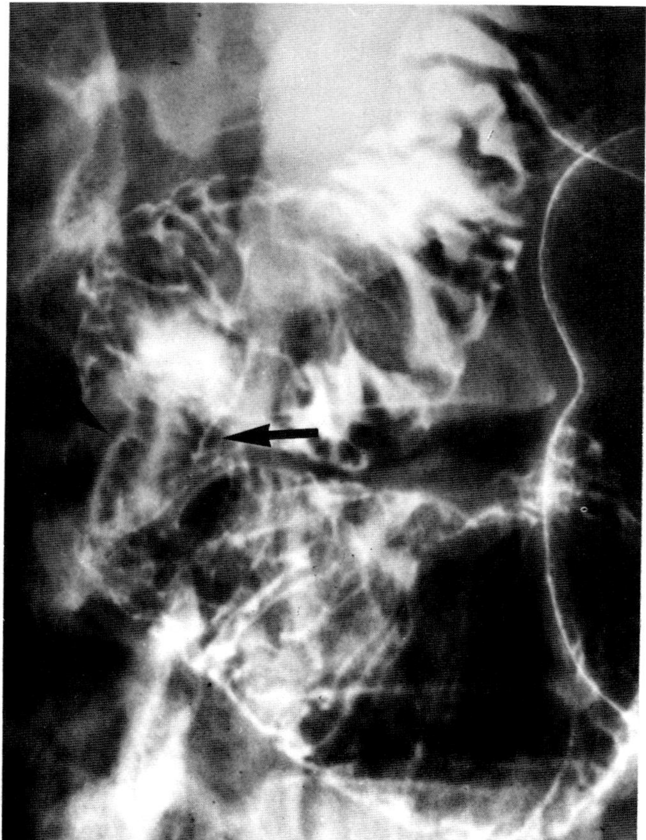

Fig. 35.47 Hypotonic duodenogram. Annular constriction of 2nd part duodenum with preservation of folds (arrows). Proven annular pancreas.

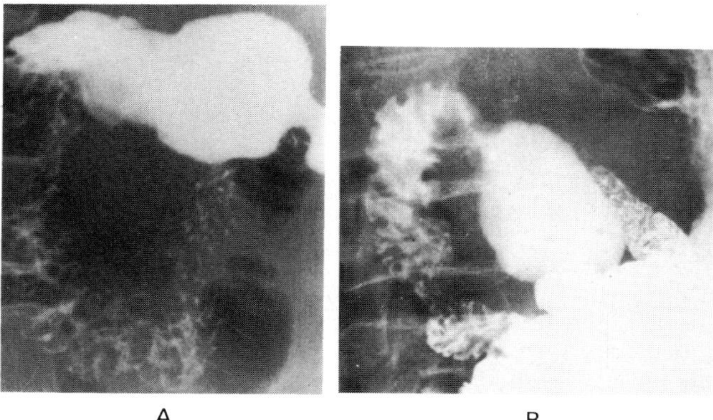

Fig. 35.48 Narrowing of the postbulbar portion of the duodenum: (**A**) by an encircling new growth of the pancreas; (**B**) by an otherwise silent carcinoma of the right kidney.

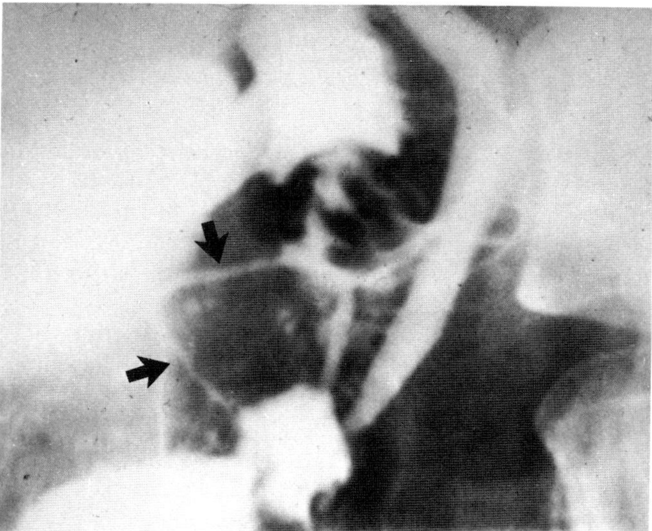

Fig. 35.49 ERCP indicated pancreatic duct of Wirsung encircling (arrows) gas-filled 2nd part of duodenum. Annular pancreas. Duct of Santorini not filled. (See also Fig. 35.79.)

pancreatic head may encircle the postbulbar portion of duodenum in a similar way (Fig. 35.48). ERCP will be definitive in annular pancreas (Fig. 35.49).

Acute pancreatitis

Whilst the majority of patients have an elevated serum amylase, about 5% do not, and imaging is required to clinch a clinical diagnosis. Plain radiography may appear normal, though subtle abnormalities may sometimes be elicited by careful examination. An important sign is that of a selective ileus of the 2nd part of the duodenum. Other patients may have a 'gasless' abdomen, or ileus of an upper abdominal small bowel loop or of the transverse colon (Fig. 35.50). Plain films will also exclude a bowel obstruction or a perforation. Other features of pancreatitis include retroperitoneal oedema with obliteration of psoas shadows,

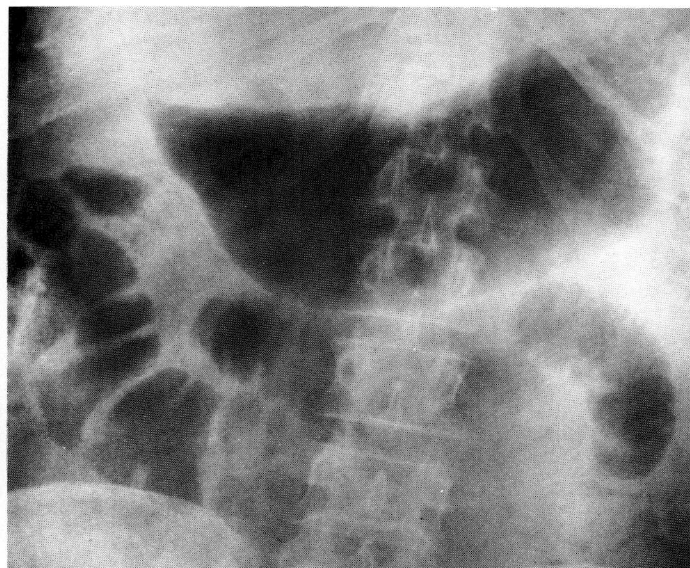

Fig. 35.50 Plain abdomen in acute pancreatitis. Ileus affects stomach, 3rd part of duodenum, early jejunal loop and proximal transverse colon. Alcoholic.

gallstones (present in 50%) and fluid in the left costophrenic angle.

Oral Gastrografin may outline obvious swelling of the pancreatic head within the duodenal loop (Fig. 35.51).

Ultrasound and computed tomography (Fig. 35.52) are

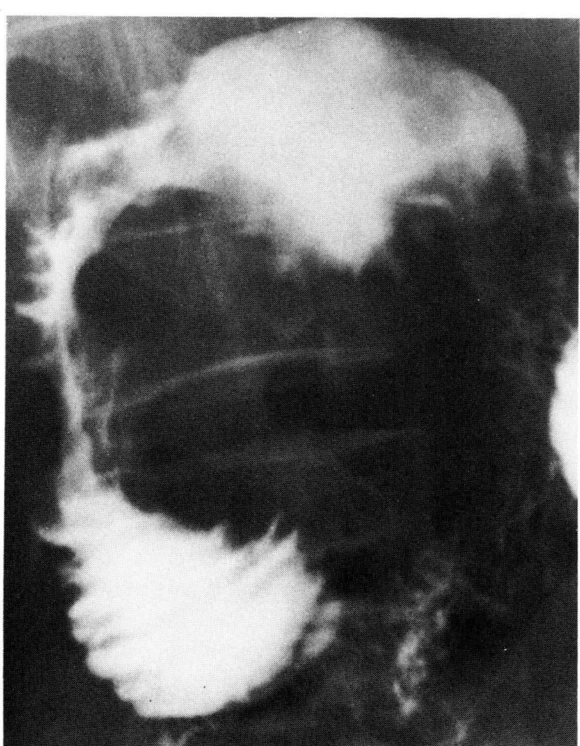

Fig. 35.51 Swelling of the head of the pancreas due to subacute pancreatitis

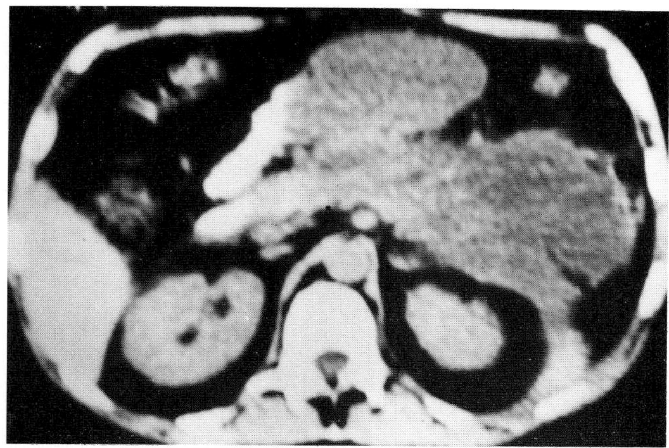

Fig. 35.52 Acute pancreatitis becoming subacute (CT). Note swelling of body of gland, with ill-defined borders, also phlegmonous fluid collections extending towards anterior abdominal wall and posterolaterally to invade retroperitoneal fascia lateral to left kidney.

discussed below and in Chapter 65. They are immeasureably more valuable than plain and oral contrast films both in the acute and subacute phase, and in the detection of pseudocysts. Alcoholism is now an important aetiological agent in the UK and pseudocysts occur with more frequency in such patients than in those with biliary disease.

Vascular complications of acute pancreatitis include vascular erosion leading to retroperitoneal or gastrointestinal haemorrhage, or to pseudoaneurysm formation. Angiography may be required for confirmation or embolization (Fig. 26.36).

Chronic pancreatitis

Calcification occurs late and infrequently in chronic pancreatitis. When present on a plain film its appearance may be dramatic (Fig. 35.53). Such a film may also demonstrate calcified gallstones, or bulky foamy faeces in the large bowel resulting from pancreatic steatorrhoea. Ultrasound will show a highly echogenic gland and CT may demonstrate a dilated pancreatic duct (Fig. 35.54) or calcification not visible on plain radiographs. ERCP is the most definitive test, showing a characteristic long, smooth stricture affecting the intrapancreatic portion of the common bile duct, adjacent to a dilated main pancreatic duct with 'nipped' side branch origins. PTC may be required if ERCP has failed.

Pancreatic cysts

The retention cyst is the result of obstruction following pancreatitis and is variable in size. 'Pseudocysts' follow acute pancreatitis or trauma, occur in the lesser sac and may grow rapidly (Fig. 35.55). They may migrate widely from their point of origin and sometimes appear in the mediastinum, posterior lower abdomen (Fig. 35.56) or

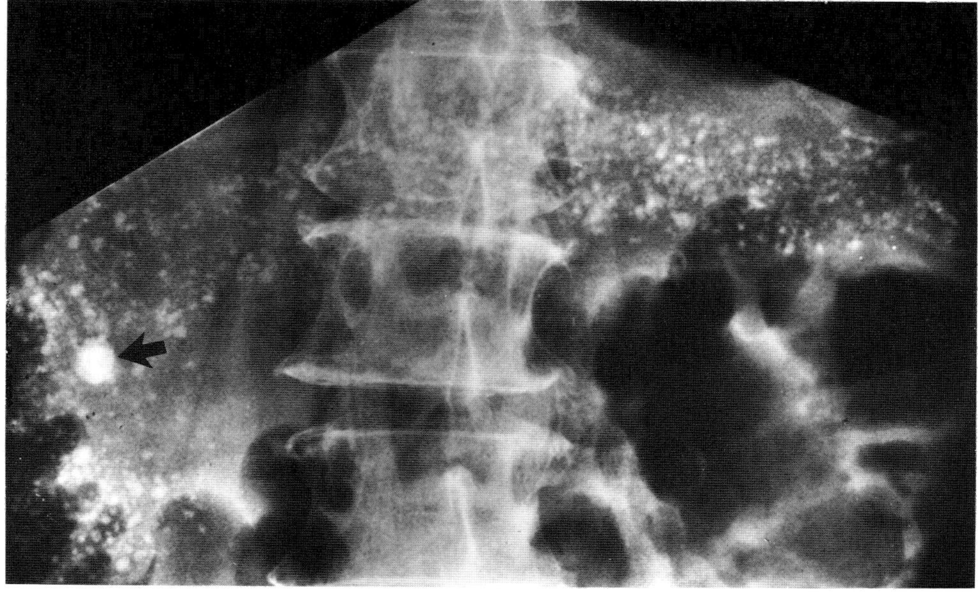

Fig. 35.53 Plain abdominal film demonstrating extensive chronic calcific pancreatitis. There is a gallstone in the lower end of common bile duct (←).

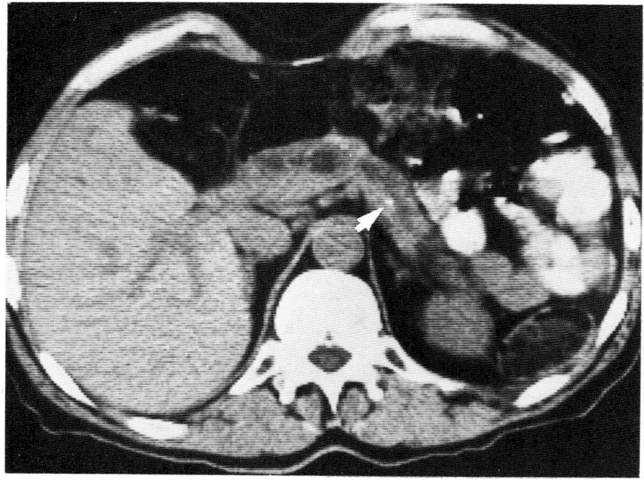

Fig. 35.54 CT abdomen demonstrating dilated pancreatic duct within chronically inflamed pancreas. (Note speck of calcium at junction of body and tail — arrow.)

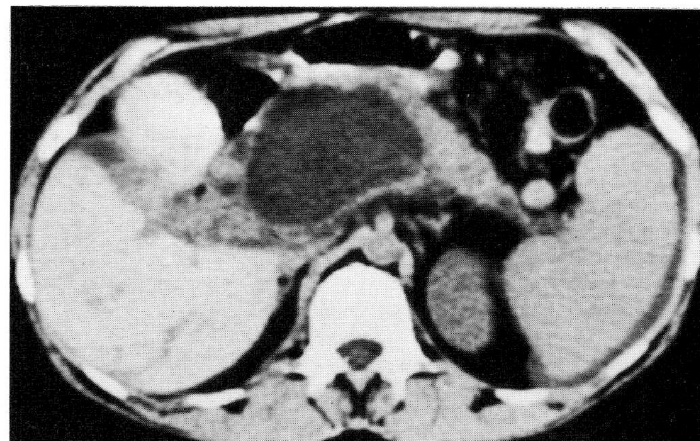

Fig. 35.55 CT shows pancreatic 'pseudocyst' in lesser sac.

even inguinal region! Cysts may be palpable and, when sizable, may displace portions of the upper or lower gastrointestinal tract around them, causing smooth indentations of the wall of stomach or bowel, without signs of invasion. Ultrasound is the most effective method for demonstrating cysts, whereas CT can probably best show their foreign extensions and relationships. 'Interventional' drainage of such cysts may be undertaken under conventional fluoroscopy (Fig. 35.57), or either ultrasound or CT scanning (Fig. 35.58).

Computed tomography may show scattered small cysts in the pancreas in patients with fibropolycystic disease affecting the liver and kidneys. Hydatid cysts of the pancreas are extremely rare.

NEOPLASMS OF THE PANCREAS

The majority of pancreatic neoplasms arise from ductal epithelium (*adenocarcinomas*) or from islet cells (*endocrine tumours*). Tumours arising from other tissues are very rare, though all types have been described including malignant sarcoma and benign fibroma, lymphangioma and neurofibroma. Metastases to the pancreas have also been described and are also very rare.

Cystic neoplasms of the pancreas are also uncommon. They include serous cystadenomas (microcystic adenoma, glycogen-rich adenoma), which are benign, and mucinous

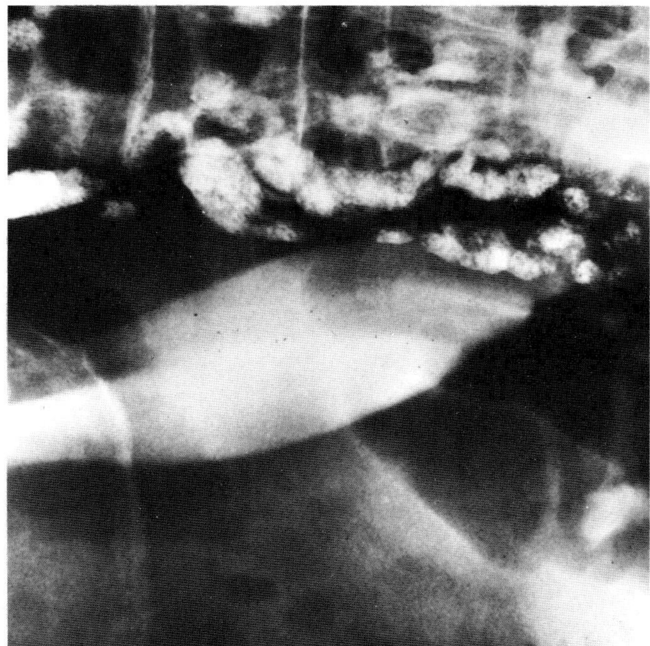

Fig. 35.56 Injection of contrast into a fluid-filled space in the left inguinal region of this patient showed communication with left psoas space (retroperitoneum). Exploration showed this to be a migrating pancreatic pseudocyst. Note recent lymphogram. (Courtesy Prof. J. Rosenquist.)

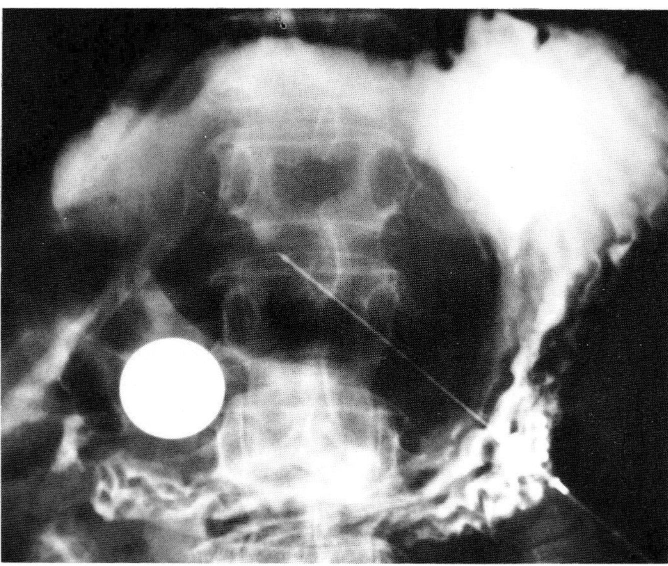

Fig. 35.57 Pseudocyst being outlined with contrast prior to its aspiration under fluoroscopy. Gastrografin introduced into stomach via nasogastric tube. Metal marker on anterior abdominal wall. A fine Chiba needle was passed through the anterior abdominal wall and contents finally drained with a sheathed catheter.

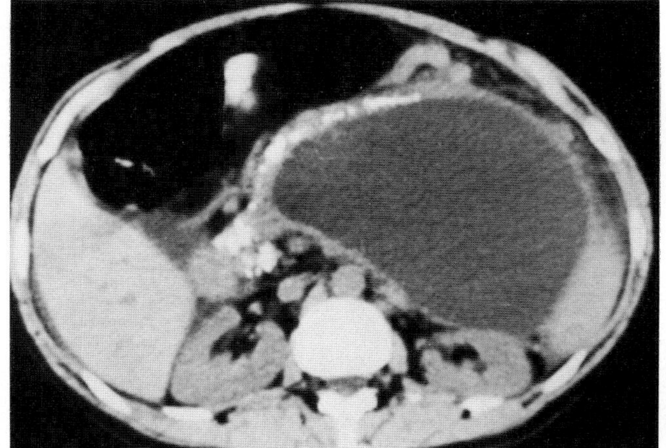

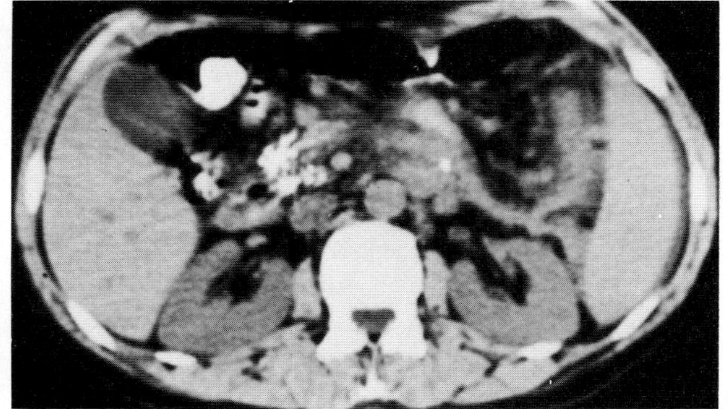

Fig. 35.58 A. Large pancreatic pseudocyst demonstrated on CT. **B.** CT scan repeated after complete aspiration under CT control.

cystadenomas, which are potentially malignant. Freeny and Lawson believe it is now possible to differentiate the two types, and that evidence of malignancy may be shown at ERCP by duct encasement, or at angiography by vessel encasement or blockage.

These cystic neoplasms of the pancreas can form quite large masses and in both types calcification may be shown at simple radiography. The mucinous type can reach over 20 cm in diameter and shows more central calcification which may be stellate in pattern. In both types the tumours can be hypervascular at angiography (Fig. 26.60, p. 729).

Carcinoma of the ampulla of Vater

The diagnosis is often endoscopic. Alternatively, because of their site, these tumours, even when small, can be detected by duodenography (Fig. 35.59). If technique is less than meticulous, the tumour may be missed. With the patient supine and in the right anterior oblique position, a barium and air contrast coating of the duodenal folds is achieved. Tiny lesions may be shown, particularly if hypotonic duodenography using either Buscopan or glucagon intravenously is a standard part of the upper GI examination. Spot films may show an extrinsic filling defect constantly present at the site of the ampulla, actual

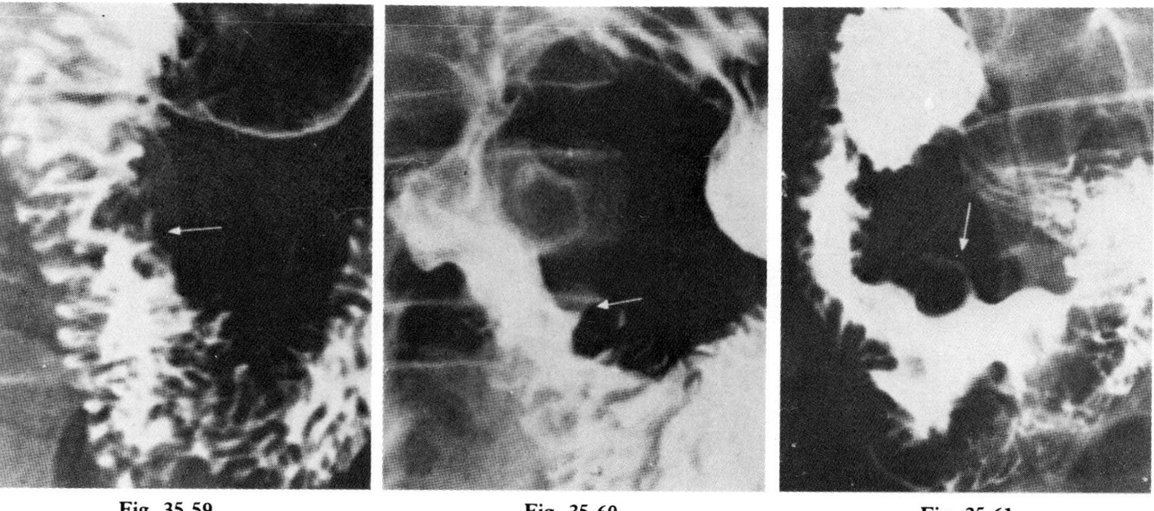

Fig. 35.59 Fig. 35.60 Fig. 35.61

Figs 35.59, 35.60, 35.61 Three cases of ampullary carcinoma. Note the position of one tumour (Fig. 35.61) in the horizontal portion of the duodenum.

duodenal invasion (Fig. 35.60;) or infrequently barium entering the ampulla. Occasionally the ampulla is abnormally sited in the duodenum, including the lateral wall of the 2nd part or the inner wall of the 3rd part (Fig. 35.61).

Obstructive jaundice, sometimes intermittent, is an invariable association of an ampullary tumour. Other causes of jaundice from pathology in this area must be considered, namely a stone or stones in the lower end of a common bile duct (for which ERCP with papillotomy may be both a diagnostic and therapeutic procedure) and carcinoma of the head of the pancreas. Both of these conditions are common and further imaging with ultrasound, computed tomography or even angiography may be necessary to distinguish the localized ampullary carcinoma from the more extensive carcinoma of the pancreatic head. This is important, as ampullary tumours, when detected early, may be resected by pancreatico-duodenectomy (Whipple's operation), whereas curative resection of a carcinoma in the head, body or tail of pancreas is frequently impossible.

Carcinoma of the pancreas

This is a malignant tumour of increasing frequency which is most often in the head of the gland where the pancreatic portion of the common bile duct becomes obstructed. Duodenography is abnormal in only 66% of cases, the tumour encroaching upon the duodenal wall and causing 'spiculation' of adjacent folds (Fig. 35.62), or even destruction of mucosa (Fig. 35.63). Eccentric tumours may encroach upon or destroy mucosa in the pyloric antrum. Widening of the 'C' loop of duodenum by itself is an unreliable sign of a pancreatic mass, as some normal patients have an exaggerated loop. Gross widening, however, is always significant (Fig. 35.64), though it may not always be possible to differentiate cyst or tumour as the cause on simple studies (Fig. 35.46). Sometimes a penetrating chronic duodenal ulcer may result in oedema of the pancreatic head (Fig. 35.65), more rarely distortion of the duodenal loop may be consequent to its involvement by gall-bladder tumours, or from invasive tumours of the right kidney.

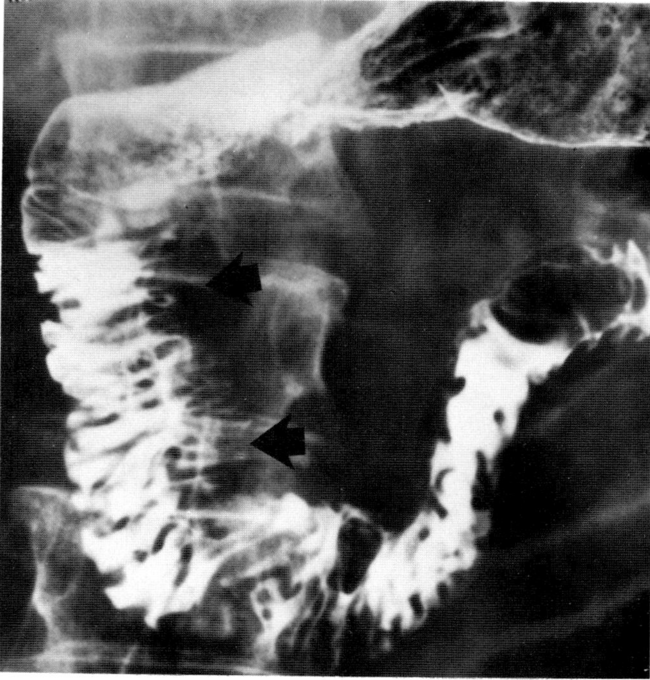

Fig. 35.62 Hypotonic duodenogram. Spiculation of medial wall of 2nd part duodenum (arrows) is characteristic of malignancy in the pancreatic head.

ERCP or PTC will show narrowing, or more often total obstruction of the intrapancreatic common bile duct (Fig. 35.64).

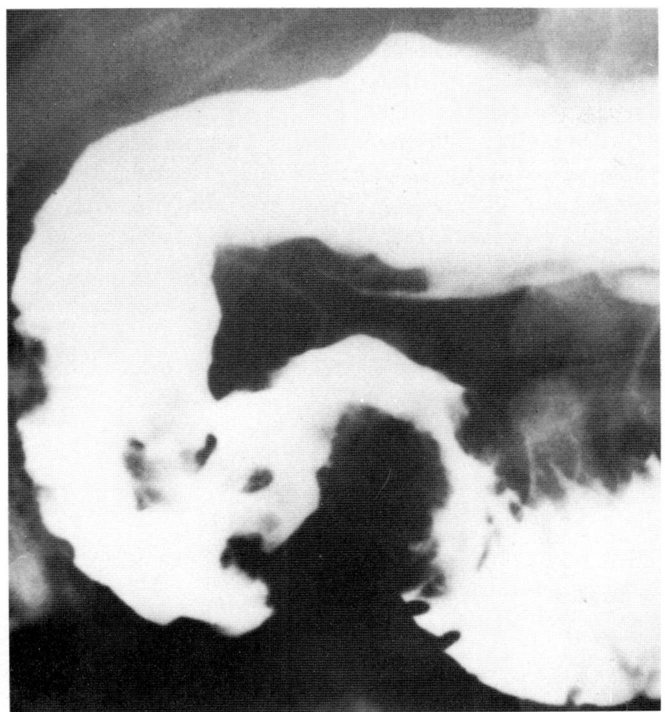

Fig. 35.63 Proven carcinoma head of pancreas. Destruction of mucosa third part duodenum.

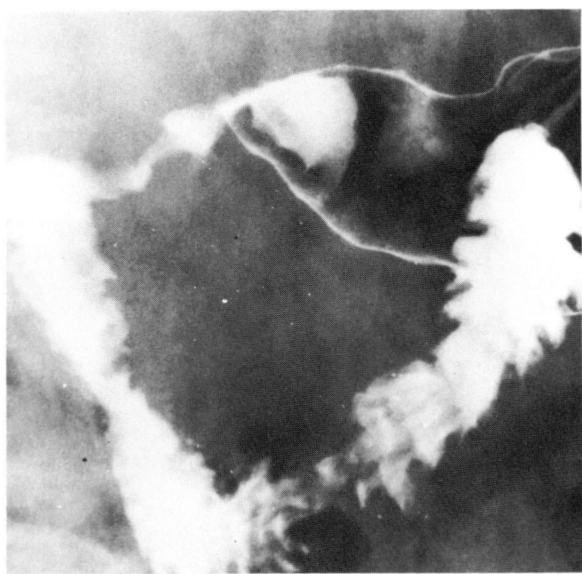

Fig. 35.65 Penetrating chronic duodenal ulcer causing oedematous swelling of the pancreatic head and obstructive jaundice.

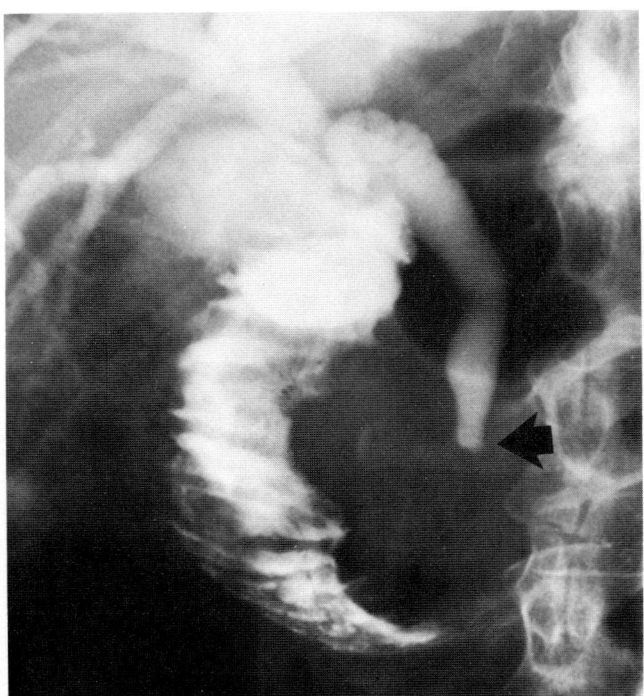

Fig. 35.64 Enlarged duodenal loop with reversed '3' sign of Frostberg. Earlier PTC shows characteristic 'gloved finger' obstruction of intrapancreatic common bile duct pathognomonic of carcinoma pancreatic head (arrow).

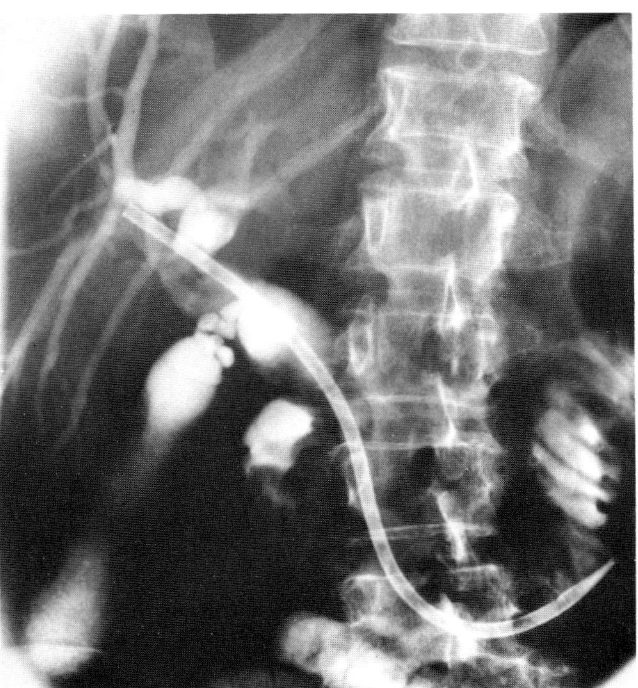

Fig. 35.66 A biliary endoprosthesis has been passed percutaneously through the liver and carcinoma in head of pancreas to the duodenum. Good early response, with relief of jaundice on 3-month follow up.

Interventional procedures include either endoscopic or percutaneous passage of an endoprosthesis through the obstruction, thus establishing internal bile drainage (Fig. 35.66). Some patients develop gastric outflow obstruction and here a surgical bypass is indicated. At the same time the surgeon may create a choledochoduodenostomy. Certainly, any prosthesis introduced under imaging control should have its lower end through the ampulla, so that should siltage of the plastic tubing occur, it may be removed endoscopically and replaced with another.

Techniques such as ultrasound or CT have revolutionized pancreatic imaging. In addition to demonstrating the normal organ, they show neoplasms in head, body or tail in a high percentage of patients. Gas around the pancreatic head can cause difficulties with ultrasonography and CT is currently thought to be the superior technique, and may show the entire extent of the tumour (Fig. 35.67 A,B). It is now possible to make a cytological diagnosis under imaging control by percutaneous needle biopsy.

Intravenous enhancement under CT or pancreatic arteriography give useful information about vascular involvement by the tumour (Fig. 35.68 A,B), but angiography is now rarely indicated, many carcinomata being obviously inoperable on less invasive imaging techniques.

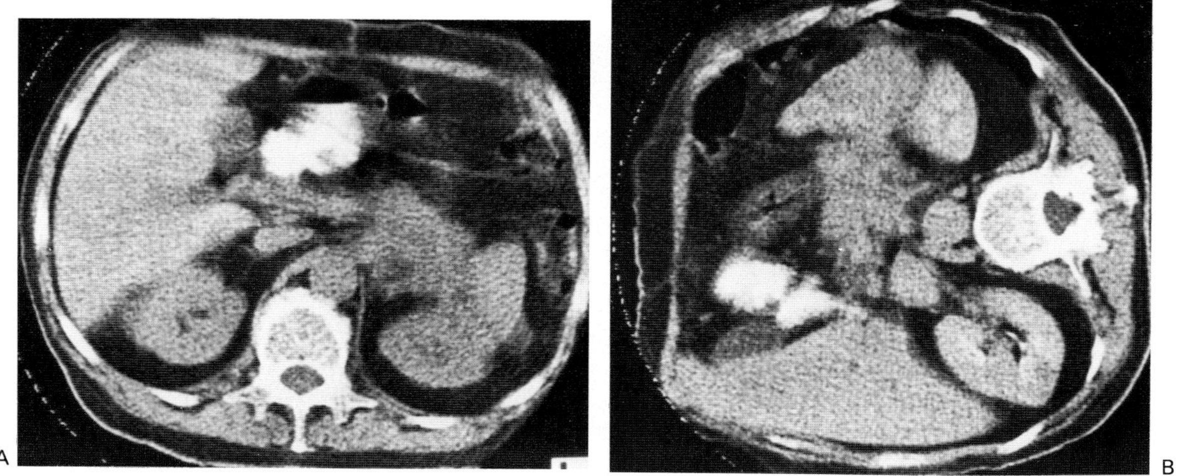

Fig. 35.67 A. CT in patient with severe abdominal pain shows an irregular mass of tail of pancreas containing a necrotic area posteriorly. Diagnosis: carcinoma. **B.** CT scan repeated with patient lying right side down confirms fixity of mass to spleen (i.e. inoperable), though it has been cleared from the aorta.

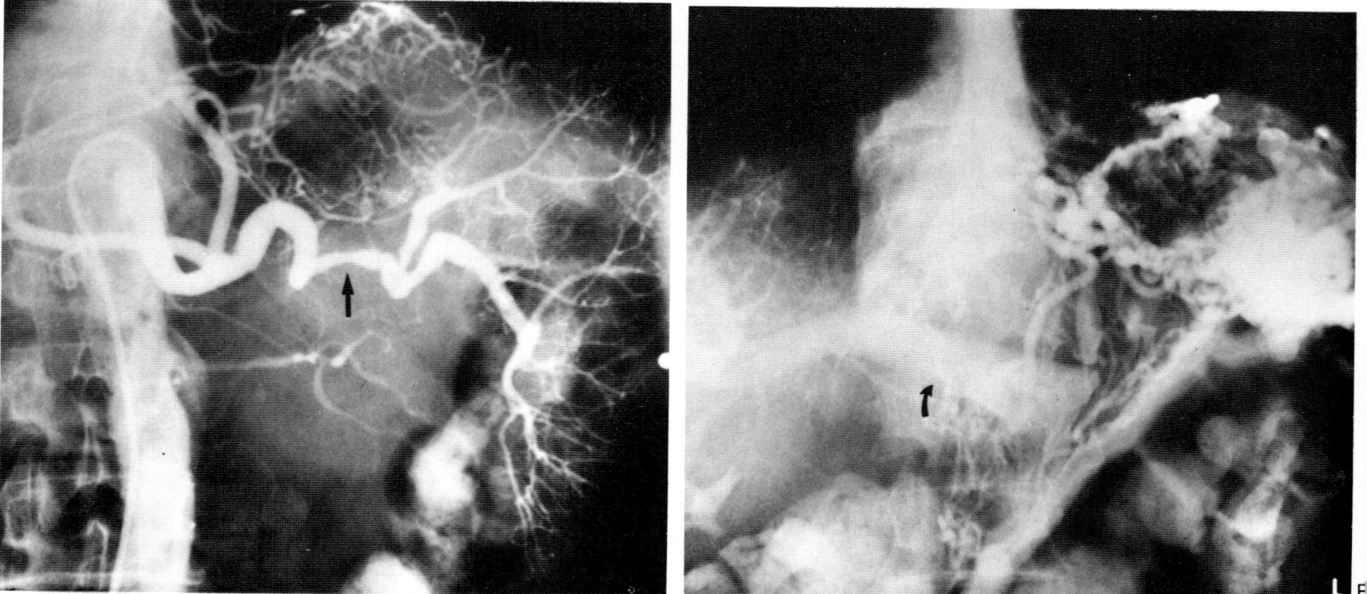

Fig. 35.68 Coeliac axis arteriography in patient with known carcinoma body of pancreas. Arterial phase (**A**) confirms encasement of middle third splenic artery (arrow). Reflux into aorta has shown similar encasement of left renal artery. Venous phase (**B**) shows blocked splenic vein with bridging collaterals (varices). Curved arrow = portal vein.

Endocrine tumours of the pancreas

Islet cells were described in 1869 (Langerhans). Insulin was discovered by Banting and Best in 1922 when they produced diabetes mellitus in dogs by removing the pancreas. Islet cells are now recognized as the source of many important hormones besides insulin, and are responsible for various endocrine neoplasms and clinical syndromes.

The APUD cell concept was developed by Everson Pearse (1974), who considered that the polypeptide hormone-producing cells of the pancreatic islet have a common embryological origin in the neural crest and emigrate to the foregut anlage of the pancreas. These pluripotential cells differentiate into islet cells capable of producing specific hormones. The cytochemical properties are characterized as Amine Precursor Uptake and Decarboxylation (APUD). These cells are also found in the pituitary (ACTH and MSH — melanin stimulating hormone — cells); thyroid (calcitonin); gastric wall (gastrin and enteroglucagon); duodenal wall (gastric inhibitory polypeptide); and small bowel (enteroglucagon).

The pancreatic islet cells and their products are listed as:

B — insulin	D — somatostatin
A — glucagon	D — VIP (vasoactive intestinal polypeptide)
G — gastrin	PP — pancreatic polypeptide.

Islet cell tumours can be classified as endocrine active or endocrine quiescent:

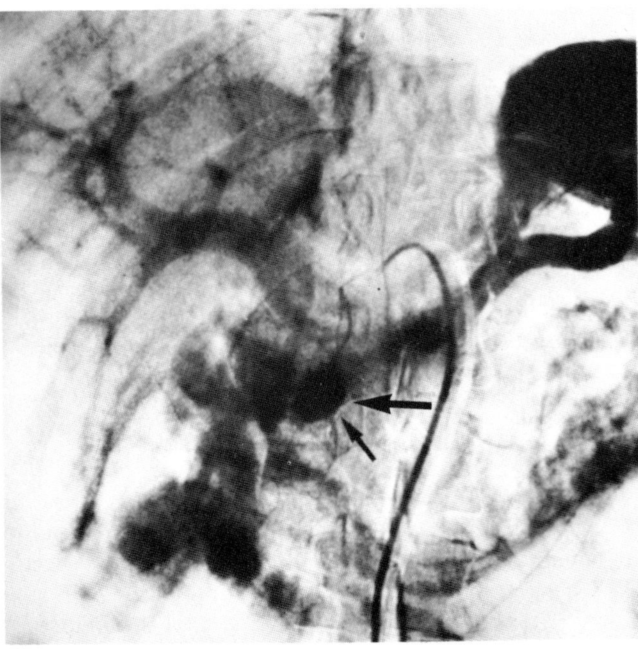

Fig. 35.69 Coeliac axis angiogram capillary and venous phase. Subtraction film. The well-defined blush in the pancreatic head (arrowed) was an insulinoma.

A. *Endocrine active*

APUDOMA: insulinoma
glucagonoma
gastrinoma (Zollinger-Ellison)
somatostatinoma
VIPoma (Verner-Morrison)

B. *Endocrine quiescent*

Most endocrine tumours are quite small, being only 1 or 2 cm in diameter. Because of this, and the fact that they may be multiple or in ectopic pancreatic tissue, they are difficult to localize, except by invasive investigations such as selective angiography or transhepatic portal vein catheterization with venous sampling. They are generally benign, but some may become malignant, particularly the gastrinoma giving rise to Zollinger-Ellison syndrome. In this case CT is particularly useful in showing both the primary tumour and deposits. VIPomas may give rise to the WDHH syndrome (watery diarrhoea, hypokalaemia and hypovolaemia).

Insulinoma is the commonest endocrine neoplasm of the pancreas. Although it may occupy any portion of the gland, the tumour is commonest in the head, and multiple lesions may occur. Fortunately most tumours are vascular and 'blush' on either enhanced CT scans or at coeliac axis arteriography (Fig. 35.69). Gastrinoma, glucagonoma and other polypeptide-secreting neoplasms have variable vascularity and if small may be best detected by *transhepatic pancreatic venous sampling*. In this technique, the portal vein is entered via a transhepatic approach under local anaesthesia. Selective samples from small veins in each region of the pancreas are obtained and sent for hormone assay (Fig. 35.70). Unfortunately results may be confusing, since some tumours are multiple or exhibit aberrant venous drainage. In addition, the technique can be difficult and time-consuming and is therefore reserved for individual problem cases.

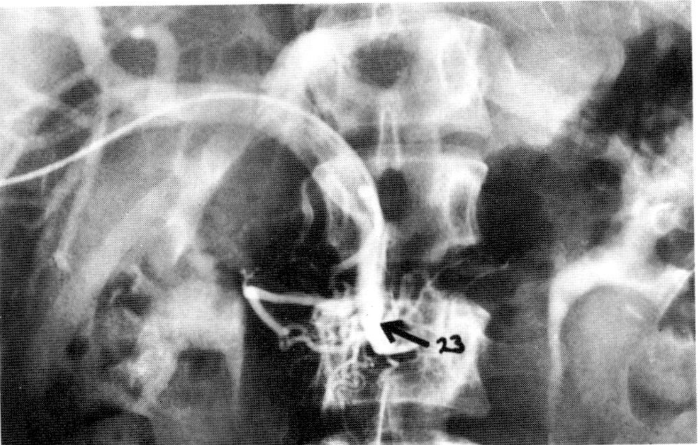

Fig. 35.70 Transhepatic venous sampling of pancreatic head vein in patient with suspected glucagonoma. '23' is the sample number.

ENDOSCOPIC RETROGRADE PANCREATOGRAPHY (ERP)

(by Richard Mason)

The present uses of ERCP or ERP in pancreatic disease include the following:

1. Further assessment of pancreatic abnormality demonstrated on ultrasound and CT, which has not been clarified by these diagnostic techniques or by fine-needle aspiration biopsy where clinically appropriate.
2. Further investigation of suspected pancreatic disease where ultrasound and CT are normal or technically unsatisfactory.
3. Definition of ductal anatomy in chronic pancreatitis for planning surgery (resection or drainage).
4. Assessment of complications of acute pancreatitis (abscess and pseudocyst).
5. Interventional — gallstone disimpaction in acute pancreatitis, pancreatic duct stone extraction, balloon dilatation of minor papilla in pancreas divisum.

The technique has a very high sensitivity for pancreatic disease but a normal ERP does not exclude either chronic pancreatitis or carcinoma.

The normal ERP

This shows a smoothly tapering main duct. There may be a slight constriction in the duct at the junction of the head and neck as a normal variant. There are also smoothly tapered side branches distributed throughout the gland, and there is complete filling of the main duct right to the tail, which may be bifid (Fig. 35.71).

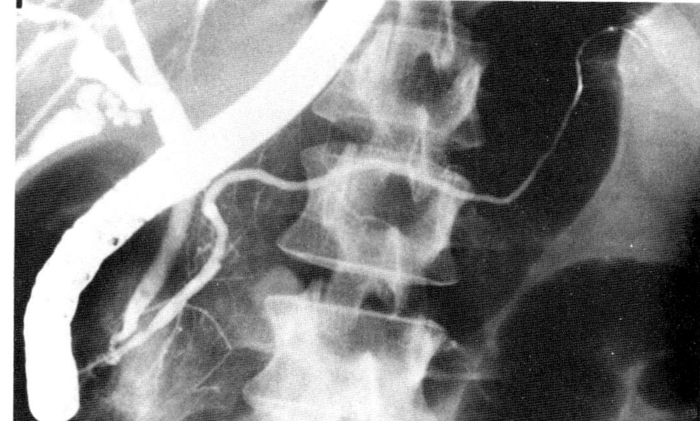

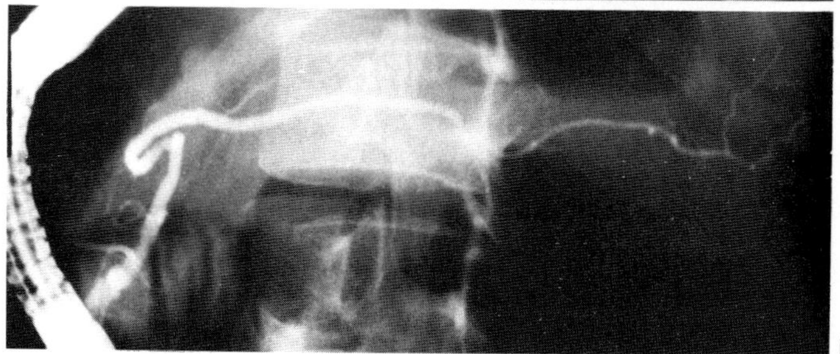

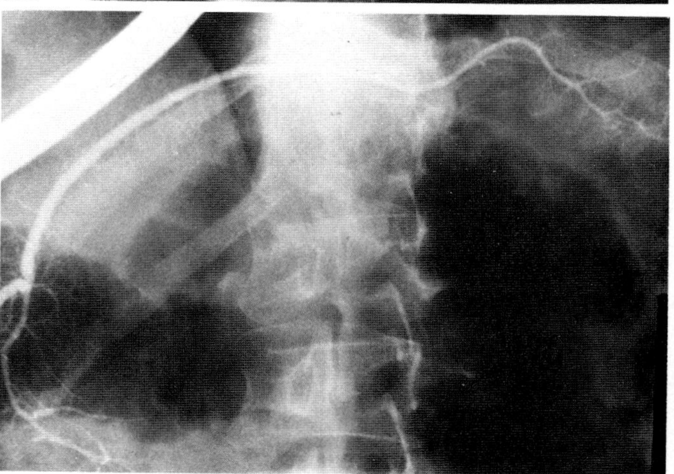

Fig. 35.71 A. B. and **C.** Normal variations in the shape of the pancreatic duct. Note complete filling of the duct system, both main and side ducts.

THE ABNORMAL ERP

Carcinoma

The signs of pancreatic carcinoma on the pancreatogram are in order of frequency (1) main pancreatic duct abnormality, (2) cavities and (3) field defects.

Main pancreatic duct abnormality

1. *Pancreatic duct occlusion.* A complete block of the pancreatic duct is the commonest finding in pancreatic carcinoma (Fig. 35.72). When this occurs in the head of the gland, it is commonly accompanied by complete block of the common bile duct.

Diagnostic difficulty may arise since chronic pancreatitis may similarly produce a complete block. Reported differences in the contour of the duct stump have not proved helpful in making the distinction. Most useful is the state of the side branches downstream from the block. In pancreatic carcinoma, these are usually normal and in chronic pancreatitis, usually abnormal (see below).

2. *Pancreatic duct stricture.* This is an uncommon finding in carcinoma and is seen when clinical presentation occurs before the main pancreatic duct becomes completely blocked. The stricture may be from several millimetres to several centimetres in length and there may be accompanying displacement of the main and side ducts around the tumour mass.

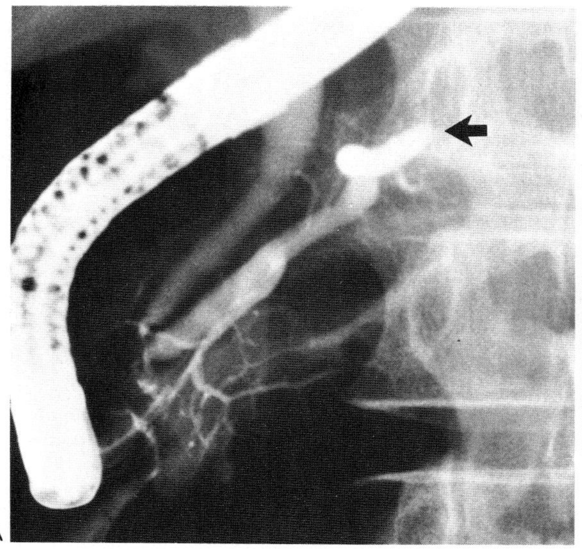

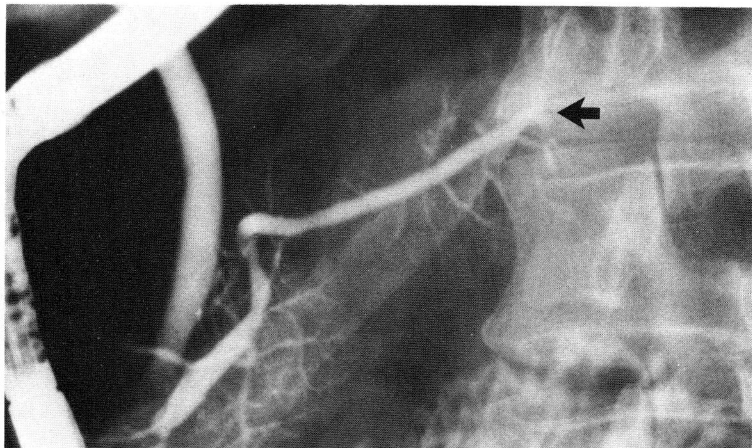

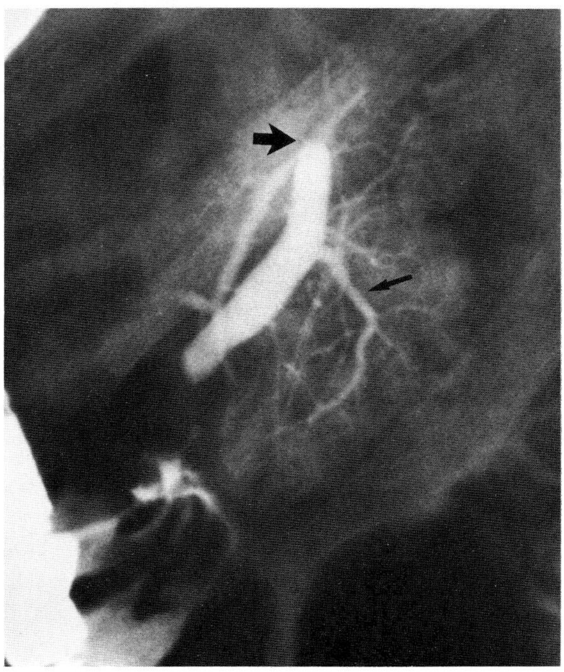

Fig. 35.72 A. B. and **C.** Pancreatic carcinoma producing complete occlusion of the main pancreatic duct (arrows). Note that the side branches downstream from the block are of normal calibre, aiding the differential diagnosis from main duct obstruction in chronic pancreatitis. In **C**, 'acinarization' has occurred because of excessive injection of contrast. This appearance of a block in the head of the gland must be distinguished from the ventral pancreas of pancreas divisum. The distinction can be made in this case because the main pancreatic duct is of normal calibire.

Cavities

When the tumour is necrotic, contrast may enter cavities within the tumour. When irregular and multiple, this gives the pancreatogram a 'scrambled egg' appearance (Fig. 35.73).

Field defect

Destruction of part of the normal pancreas by carcinoma may simply lead to non-filling of several adjacent side branches, leaving the main pancreatic duct intact.

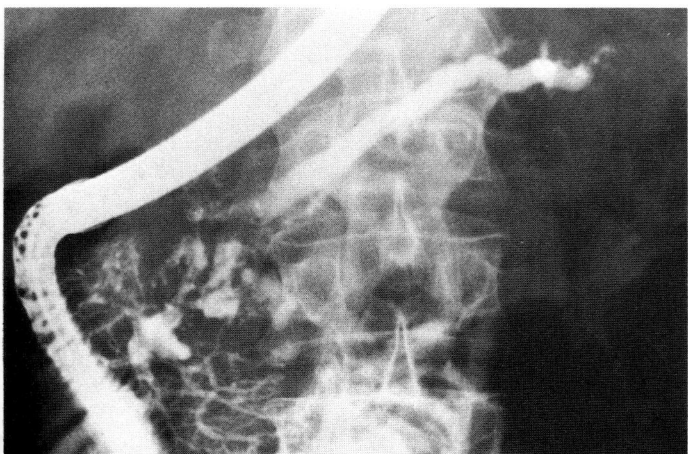

Fig. 35.73 'Scrambled egg' appearance in pancreatic carcinoma. Numerous necrotic cavities within the tumour in the head of the gland have filled with contrast. Note upstream dilatation of main duct and side branches resulting from obstruction.

Chronic pancreatitis

The hallmarks of chronic pancreatitis are:

1. Dilatation and beading of the pancreatic duct and its branches (Fig. 35.75). In early chronic pancreatitis (so-called 'minimal change'), the main pancreatic duct remains normal and there is subtle dilatation and perhaps irregularity of some or all of the side branches (Fig. 35.74).
2. Block. As in carcinoma, the block in the main pancreatic duct may be complete or incomplete.
3. Cavities. These are variable in size but usually small and communicate with the main duct or branch ducts (Fig. 35.76).
4. Calculi. Calculi are virtually pathognomonic of chronic pancreatitis. They may be single or multiple and are usually, but not always (Fig. 35.77) calcified. They may be found in a non-dilated duct system.

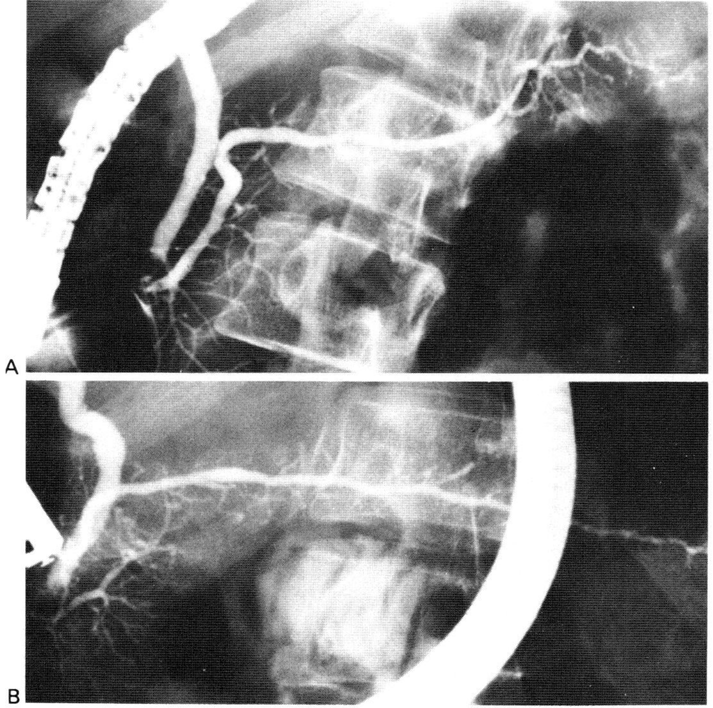

Fig. 35.74 A, B 'Minimal change' chronic pancreatitis. The main pancreatic duct is normal but there are subtle dilatations of some of the side branches. Note the slight narrowing of the main duct at junction of head and body in **A**. This is a normal variant.

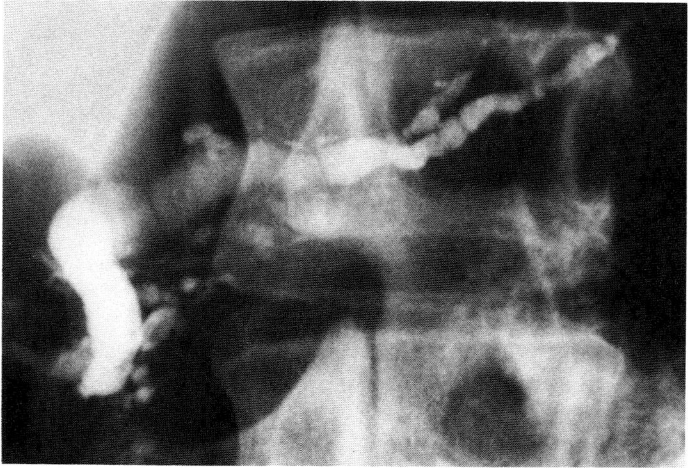

Fig. 35.75 Advanced chronic pancreatitis. The main duct and the side branches are dilated and beaded.

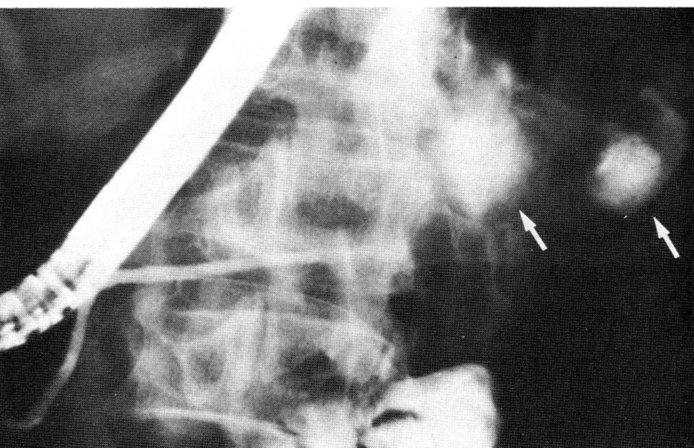

Fig. 35.76 Cavities have filled from the main duct in the tail of the gland (arrows). Chronic or recurrent pancreatitis.

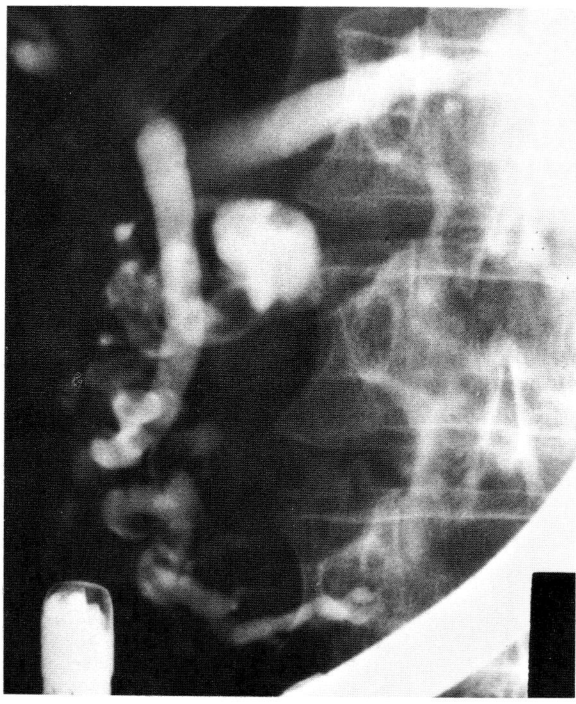

Fig. 35.77 The main pancreatic duct is dilated and contains numerous lucent stones. These findings are pathognomonic of chronic pancreatitis.

Pancreas divisum (Figs 35.78, 35.79)

In the embryo, separate dorsal and ventral pancreatic segments bud from the duodenum. The ventral segment develops in association with the bile duct, the two structures draining together through the major papilla. The ventral segment rotates around the duodenum to lie below the dorsal segment and carries the bile duct with it. A communication develops between the dorsal and ventral ducts resulting in the dorsal pancreas draining principally through the duct of the ventral pancreas. The duct of the dorsal pancreas downstream from the communication becomes relatively smaller in size and may disappear completely.

Sometimes the communication between the two pancreatic duct systems is not established and the embryonic state of divided pancreas persists into adult life ('pancreas divisum').

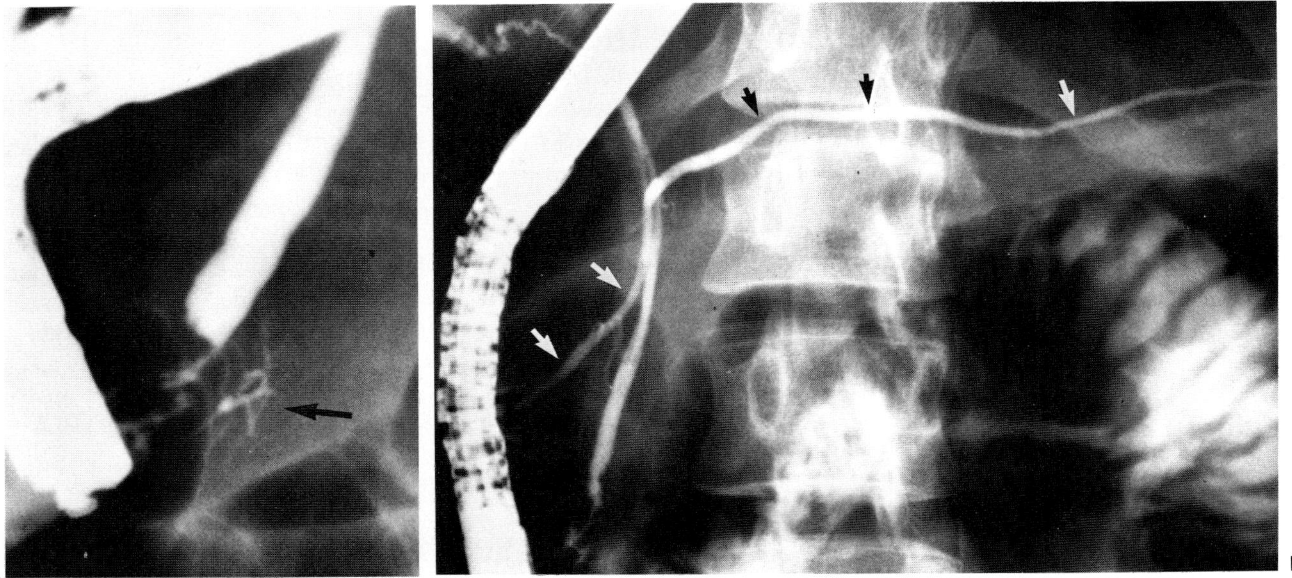

Fig. 35.78 A. Tiny ventral component (arrow). The bile duct is also opacified. **B.** The dorsal component (in a different patient) has been filled (arrows) from the minor papilla. The bile duct terminates at the major papilla, below the minor.

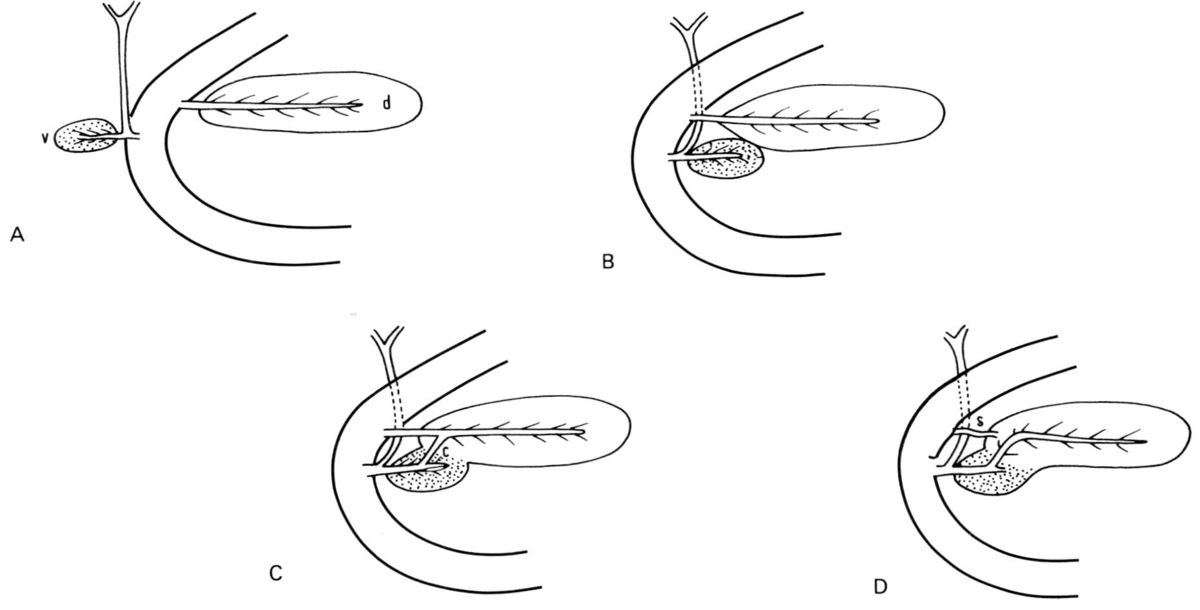

Fig. 35.79 Embryological development of the pancreas. **A.** Dorsal segment (d) draining through duct of Santorini and minor papilla. Ventral segment (v) developing in association with bile duct and draining through duct of Wirsung and major papilla. **B.** The ventral segment has rotated with the bile duct to occupy its definitive position. This is the arrested embryological position of the adult pancreas divisum. Failure to rotate can give rise to annular pancreas (Fig. 35.49). **C.** A wide communication (c) has developed between the dorsal and ventral ducts. **D.** The terminal portion of the dorsal duct or duct of Santorini (s) becomes relatively smaller and may disappear completely. This is the normal adult arrangement.

The clinical significance of pancreas divisum is not yet established. Changes of chronic pancreatitis have however been reported in the dorsal segment. In such cases, the dorsal duct is dilated and it is postulated the orifice of the minor papilla is not wide enough for adequate drainage.

The pancreas divisum abnormality is diagnosed when cannulation of the major papilla at ERP outlines only a small branching duct system without communication with the main pancreatic duct.

PANCREATIC ULTRASOUND

(by W. R. Lees)

Techniques of pancreatic ultrasonography

Using high resolution real-time equipment of frequencies up to 7.5 MHz, the major part of the pancreas can be visualized in up to 95% of patients, but despite the improvements in technique visualization is rarely complete. This remains the major cause of failure of the method.

Visualization in the difficult patient can be improved in two ways.

Fluid loads to the stomach provide an acoustic window through to the pancreas. The fluid can be manipulated from the gastric fundus, to body and antrum, and then into the duodenum in the same way as in a barium meal, visualizing different parts of the pancreas with each change in position.

The pancreas is less mobile than the liver, stomach and colon. Changing from the supine to the erect posture changes the relative position of these structures considerably. The liver rides down over the head and body of the pancreas giving an acoustic window. The fluid-filled stomach provides a window to the body and tail and gives the extra benefit of displacing the colon caudally.

Gastric paralysis may improve visualization of the head and the distal common bile duct by holding the fluid in the duodenum and antrum.

NORMAL PANCREATIC ANATOMY AND DIAGNOSTIC FEATURES

Gland size. Normal values for pancreatic size have been repeatedly published for ultrasound and CT scanning. Maximum antero-posterior dimensions of 25 mm, 15 mm and 20 mm for the head, body and tail respectively are usually quoted, but shape variations make measurements unreliable. With failure of fusion between the dorsal and ventral anlages the size of the ventral segment may vary from very small to very large with cranial extension; this variant often produces a mass effect simulating a tumour. A size of 1–2 times normal is significant, but not as an isolated sign. Similarly changes in posture can cause considerable movement of the pancreas within the retroperitoneum, with corresponding thickening of the dependent part.

Pancreatic duct (MPD). Demonstration of the duct is the single most important criterion of adequate visualization. The calibre of the duct increases with age, but 2–4 mm is abnormal in a patient of less than 60. Measurement is easiest in the midline where the duct follows a straight course.

The duct is seen as two strong parallel linear echoes separated by the anechoic lumen. The strong echoes come from the wall, and are increased in amplitude by periductal fibrosis (Fig. 35.80). The ductal anatomy can be demonstrated at least in part, in 90% or more of patients examined. The normal duct is seen in only 50–70% by CT scanning.

Parenchyma. The normal parenchyma is homogeneous with an echogenicity slightly greater than that of the liver. In the obese or the elderly there can be considerable fatty replacement which increases parenchymal echogenicity, often to the level of retroperitoneal fat. The boundaries of the gland are then difficult to determine (Fig. 35.81).

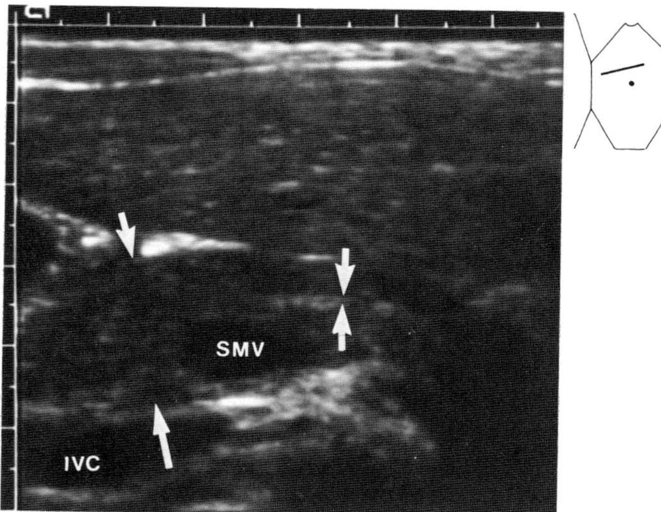

Fig. 35.80 Normal pancreas. Horizontal section. Head of pancreas = long arrows; pancreatic duct = short arrows; SMV = superior mesenteric vein; IVC = inferior vena cava.

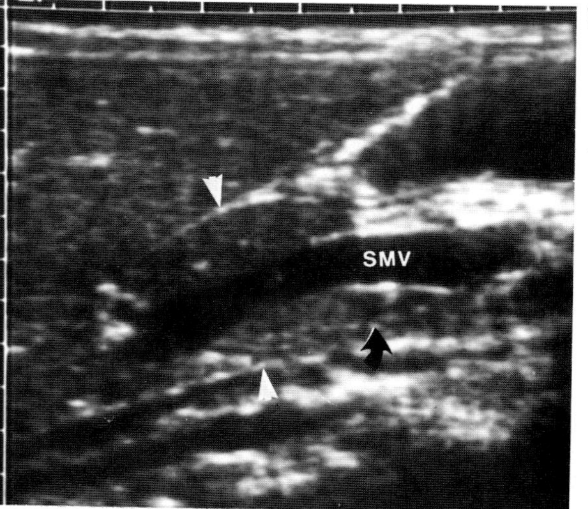

Fig. 35.81 Normal pancreas. Sagittal section (arrowheads); long arrow = draining pancreatic vein; MPD (main pancreatic duct) lies above lower arrowhead; stomach lies above SMV on right.

A uniform increase in echogenicity throughout the whole gland is almost always due to fatty infiltration, and is unusual in chronic pancreatitis, where focal changes predominate.

Acute inflammation causes reduced echogenicity, with fluid formation in all but mild acute pancreatitis. The echogenicity of the duct walls may then be enhanced relative to the parenchyma.

The texture of the parenchyma depends on the transducer frequency used as much as the character of the tissue itself.

Acute inflammation reduces the amplitude of the echoes which form the textural pattern, whereas chronic inflammation makes the tissue more heterogeneous with strongly echogenic foci, and frequent areas of cyst formation. It is difficult objectively to measure the inherent reflectivity of the pancreatic tissue. Reference should always be made to internal standards, which can be visualized under comparable conditions. The usual references are the liver, spleen and renal cortex. Each of these must first be tested against one another in case they themselves are diseased, and finally against the pancreas.

Fluid loads in the stomach complicate this process. Visualization is improved in the difficult areas, but the fluid pathway makes it impossible to comment on the echogenicity of the tissue beyond. However, in the erect posture, the weight of the stomach and the liver pulls both caudad, and the head and body are clearly seen through the overlying liver, which will provide the reference tissue.

Vascular anatomy. The arteries directly supplying the pancreas are too small to be visualized, although it is occasionally possible to identify a large draining vein. The predeliction of ultrasonography for displaying fluid-filled structures makes the superior mesenteric, splenic and gastroduodenal arteries important anatomical references in identification of the gland.

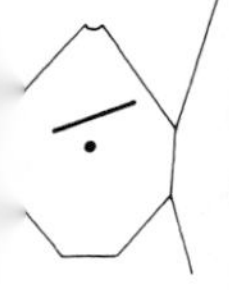

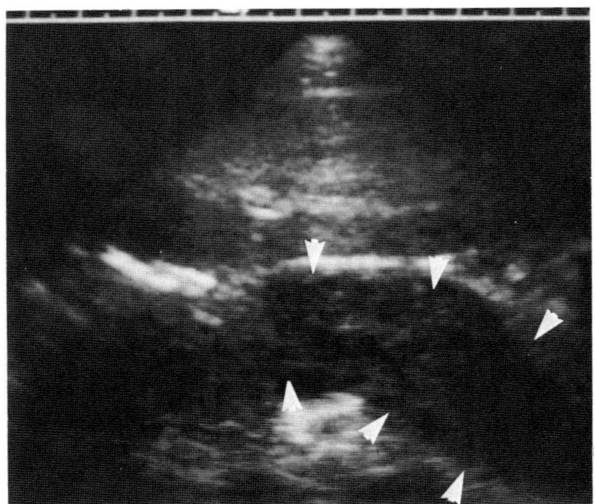

Fig. 35.82 Mild acute pancreatitis showing reduction in parenchymal echogenicity and enlargement (arrowheads).

Associated structures. Retroperitoneal fat is strongly echogenic with a fine texture. Fat which infiltrates into the gland will do so predominantly in the tail, spreading between the lobules of acinar tissue and separating them. The tail may then show slight enlargement with loss of the normal smooth contour.

CT demonstrates the retroperitoneal fat and the peritoneum itself with great clarity. The borders of the pancreas are not as well seen ultrasonographically and contour changes are not as obvious. Acute inflammation disturbs the echo pattern of retroperitoneal fat, making it heterogeneous, more echogenic, and produces associated peripancreatic fluid collections.

Thickening of the peritoneum and of the retroperitoneal fascial planes is seen more easily with CT.

ACUTE PANCREATITIS

The ultrasonographic appearances of acute pancreatitis vary with the severity and the stage of the disease, and can change significantly over a period of a few hours.

The changes can be focal or global, and with severe disease spread far beyond the confines of the pancreas. The affected pancreas can be oedematous, necrotic, haemorrhagic or even infected.

Oedema enlarges and reduces the echogenicity of the affected segment (Fig. 35.82). In the earliest stages of interstitial pancreatitis the gland may appear acoustically normal, with the typical changes not seen for 12–24 hours. Approximately one-third of patients with mild acute pancreatitis (amylase over 1000) will have no changes seen at all ultrasonographically, although careful scanning and serial measurement may demonstrate a small area of focal swelling.

Necrosis is usually associated with a fluid collection and will produce interfaces which are inherently echogenic.

Haemorrhage is echogenic, and inflammation of retroperitoneal fat can produce very strong echoes with loss of the normal anatomical detail. Under these circumstances it is unusual to demonstrate the pancreatic duct (Figs 35.83, 35.84).

The diagnosis of acute pancreatitis can be extremely accurate, provided that adequate visualization can be obtained, and is of great assistance in those cases in whom the clinical diagnosis is not clear. CT is the best tool for demonstrating the full extent of the inflammation both within and around the pancreas but is often not specific, particularly in mild or focal inflammatory processes. In these patients serial scanning can be performed, if necessary every few hours, although in practice every other day is sufficient. Virtually all the complications of acute pancreatitis can be observed developing; the pseudocyst, pancreatic phlegmon, haemorrhage and abscess formation are well seen and their nature can be proved by fine-needle aspiration. Although peri- or intrapancreatic fluid collec-

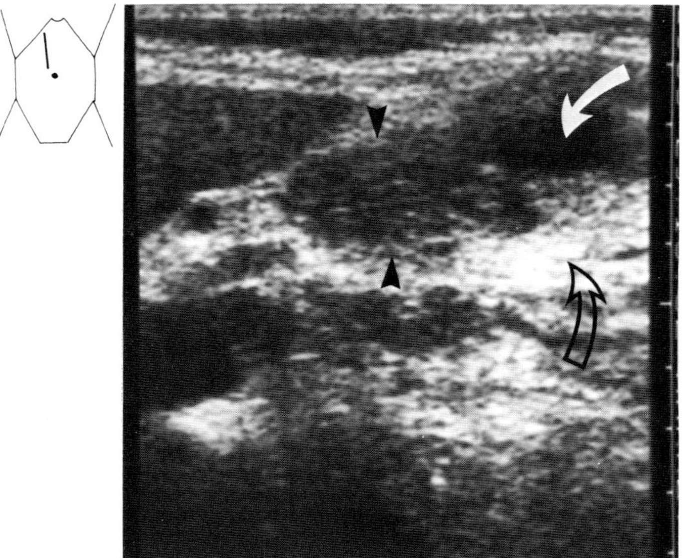

Fig. 35.83 Severe acute pancreatitis. Short arrowheads = inflamed pancreas; long white arrow = focal necrosis with fluid collection; hollow arrow = abnormal retroperitoneal fat.

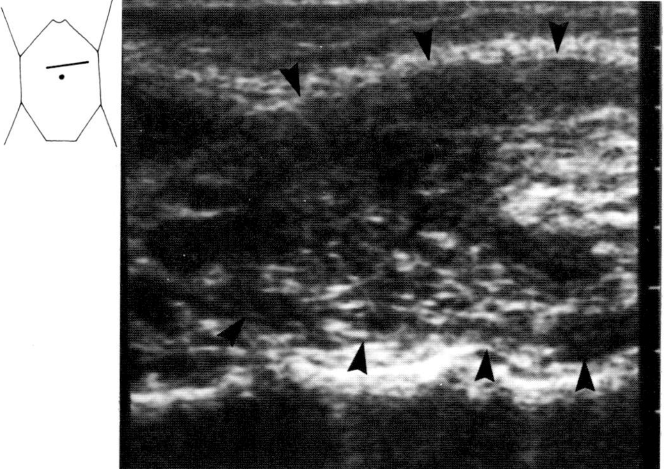

Fig. 35.84 Severe acute pancreatitis. Horizontal section. Arrows denote contour. Markedly heterogeneous parenchyma.

tions are almost always seen at some stage of any severe inflammation, the late complication of the pseudocyst will always be preceded by a peripancreatic fluid collection in the acute phase. No patient should be discharged from hospital without check ultrasonography or CT.

To perform ERCP in AP has traditionally been regarded as dangerous, even though there is little direct evidence of this. Ultrasonography can select those patients who may be suitable for these procedures. A combination of gall-bladder stones and a dilated CBD (Fig. 35.85) is very strong evidence for a gallstone aetiology. Either is probably sufficient to indicate endoscopy.

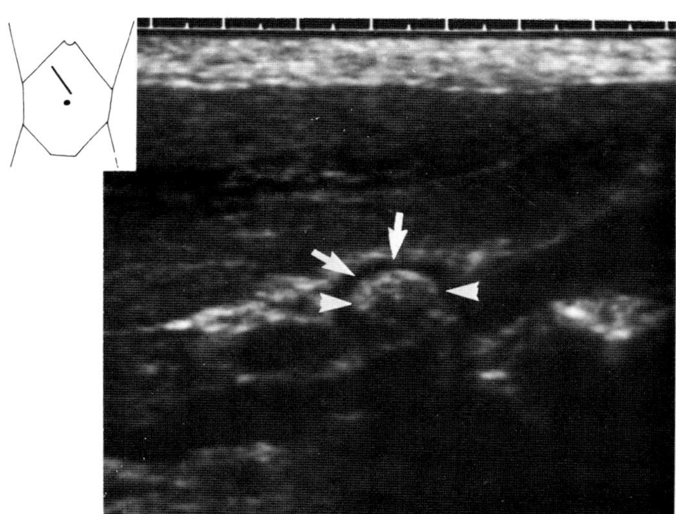

Fig. 35.85 CBD stone (arrowheads). Note crescent of bile around the contour of the stone (arrows).

The stones that are responsible for the acute attack are usually small, and a very careful scanning technique is necessary (Fig. 35.86). Although ultrasonography is the most sensitive method of detecting gallstones in the gall bladder, very small stones may be missed.

Correlation with clinical findings. Separation of patients into mild and severe acute pancreatitis on clinical criteria has proved useful prognostically, but no equivalent imaging criteria for grading have yet been developed. Hill

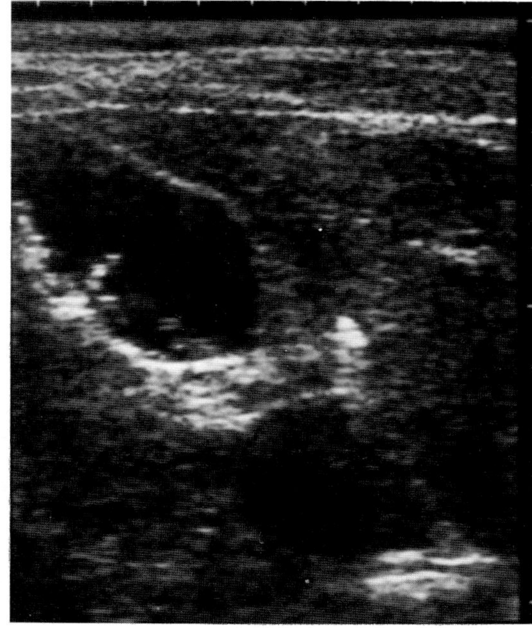

Fig. 35.86 Gall-bladder microlithiasis.

and colleagues showed that in mild AP the pancreas may appear normal in 28%, show focal or diffuse enlargement in 61% or develop a phlegmon in 11%.

In severe AP the pancreas will always be abnormal after the first few hours. Phlegmon formation (tissue necrosis) will be seen in the majority, up to 89% in the cases of Hill.

Abscess formation occurs in about 3%. Haemorrhagic pancreatitis as a clinical entity occurs with roughly the same frequency, but some haemorrhagic effects are seen in nearly all cases of severe AP.

Recurrent acute pancreatitis. There is no doubt that there is a group of patients who have repeated attacks of acute pancreatitis. Ultrasonography has shown changes of CP in almost 80% of patients with more than one attack, although almost all will have focal fibrosis histologically. There are also patients with definite chronic pancreatitis who have repeated attacks of AP as a feature of their disease process. These attacks are usually, but not invariably, associated with bouts of severe pain, and present focal swelling on ultrasonography with the characteristic reduction in echogenicity. In severe CP the acute episodes are predominantly focal and are often associated with cyst formation.

A diagnosis of relapsing pancreatitis is wholly clinical and cannot be made on imaging criteria, where the only possible diagnoses are acute or chronic pancreatitis.

Clinically this is an extremely difficult group of patients to manage. Pain may be very severe and, despite extensive investigation over a period of years, narcotic consumption may be high. Less than 20% of those with more than one previously abnormal amylase will have normal ultrasonography by our criteria and few of these patients will have any changes on pancreatography. The response to therapy in this fringe group is invariably poor and, despite abnormal amylase levels, a confident ultrasonographic diagnosis of a normal gland can be considered a strong indication for conservative therapy.

If ultrasonographic visualization is adequate then neither CT nor ERCP is of demonstrable value. This situation is an indication for endoscopic ultrasonography, where a high frequency ultrasound probe mounted on a duodenoscope is applied directly to the surface of the pancreas through the gastric or duodenal wall.

In this way the problems caused by intestinal gas or obesity are circumvented. Very high resolution scans can be obtained, but at the cost of an invasive technique which produces images which are difficult to interpret.

CHRONIC PANCREATITIS

Aetiology. Most cases of chronic pancreatitis seen in this country are secondary to ethanol consumption, but less than 2% of alcoholics will develop the disease. There is no threshold level of alcohol intake, and even moderate drinking carries an increased risk. Chronic pancreatitis can occur in children or young adults, and is seen as a calcifying pancreatitis. A pure obstructive pancreatopathy, without calcification, can occur secondary to neoplastic duct obstruction or to congenital anomalies of duct anatomy with faulty drainage.

Chronic pancreatitis has always been a difficult diagnosis to make. Definitive features such as strictures and dilatation of the MPD, cyst formation and calculi are by definition features of severe disease, and for mild and moderate disease there is a poor correlation between symptoms, morphology and functional disturbance.

Gland size. In mild CP, enlargement is unusual and, if present, is likely to be focal as the result of a localized acute inflammation. Moderate changes of chronic pancreatitis will usually include enlargement which is less than twice normal. This is a non-specific finding found in almost all pancreatic disease. Severe changes of chronic pancreatitis are associated with focal enlargement in approximately 25%, atrophy in 10% and global enlargement in 40%.

Contour change. The intralobular fibrosis of chronic pancreatitis distorts the outline of the gland. This should be easy to see by ultrasonography but in practice the fibrous tissue increases the echogenicity of the parenchyma to the point where the outline is no longer clearly visible. Thus only the gross changes of contour can be precisely evaluated.

Parenchyma. Overall changes of parenchymal echogenicity are of no importance; the fatty pancreas is common and is rarely pathological except in cystic fibrosis. Heterogeneity of parenchymal pattern is far more significant, and a valuable single sign. The fibrosis in the earlier stages of CP is periductal and very localized resulting in strongly echogenic foci centrally placed within the gland (Fig. 35.87).

Duct changes. In moderate or mild disease, there is usually an increase in the echogenicity of the walls of the MPD relative to the parenchyma. This is a relatively subjective sign and only lends support to a diagnosis of CP.

The normal calibre of the duct varies as a function of age and possibly of race. In a patient of less than 60 years a duct calibre of greater than 2 mm is significant (Fig. 35.88). Irregularities in a duct of this calibre are not visible, but will be seen in larger ducts. Strictures are usually observed as abrupt changes in calibre, but without the fine detail afforded by direct pancreatography. Ectatic branch ducts present the appearance of very small intrapancreatic cysts.

An accurate assessment of the state of the duct system is essential for any objective pancreatic diagnosis.

Severe CP is almost always associated with distension of some part of the duct system. The surrounding parenchyma is either normal in thickness or more usually bulky.

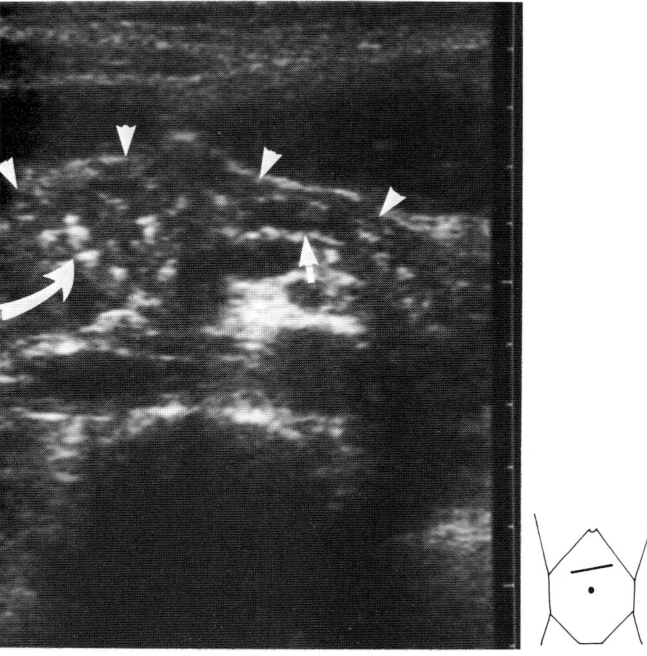

Fig. 35.87 Chronic pancreatitis. Horizontal section. Irregular contour (arrowheads); strongly echogenic foci (long curved arrow) and dilated section of main pancreatic duct (straight arrow).

Pure obstructive atrophy, which is typical of pancreatic carcinoma, is uncommon in CP.

Complete obstruction leads to an increase in the duct pressure above 30 cm of water, with duct dilatation and parenchymal atrophy. Other features of chronic pancreatitis are not seen. Partial duct obstruction may lead to an obstructive pancreatopathy with all of the features of CP except calculi.

Calculi. Calculi are seen as strongly echogenic foci within the parenchyma or the duct system. As in the kidney, only the larger stones will produce acoustic shadows which are diagnostic of calcification (Fig. 35.89). Calcifications in the tail or in the surrounding retroperitoneum are more difficult to detect than with CT.

Almost all pancreatic calculi occur within the duct system; predominantly within ectatic branch ducts. Not all intraluminal filling defects are calculi. Protein plugs are more common, but are not readily visualized by US.

Cysts. Cysts of less than 5 mm in diameter are common in moderate CP, and usually represent ectatic ducts. Cysts over 10 mm in diameter imply severe CP, and will be seen in approximately 10%. The cystic lesions seen in CP are usually intra- or peripancreatic, and smaller and more spherical than in AP (Fig. 35.90).

Pseudoaneurysms. These have not been described ultrasonographically.

Correlations with other imaging methods

The Cambridge classification of chronic pancreatitis (1983) proposes for ERCP a system with three levels. Mild changes were those affecting at least three side branches. Moderate changes were to be those which in addition affected the main pancreatic duct. Severe changes were those producing severe irregularity of the MPD with dilatation, calculi or cysts of greater than 10 mm.

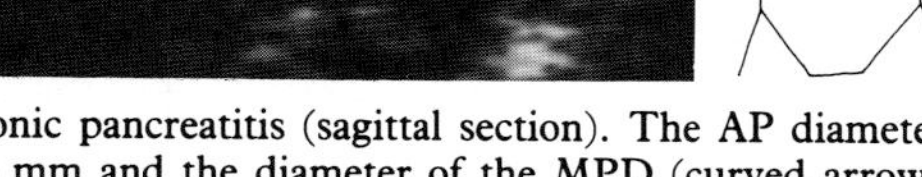

Fig. 35.88 Mild chronic pancreatitis (sagittal section). The AP diameter of the pancreas is 28 mm and the diameter of the MPD (curved arrow) is 4 mm.

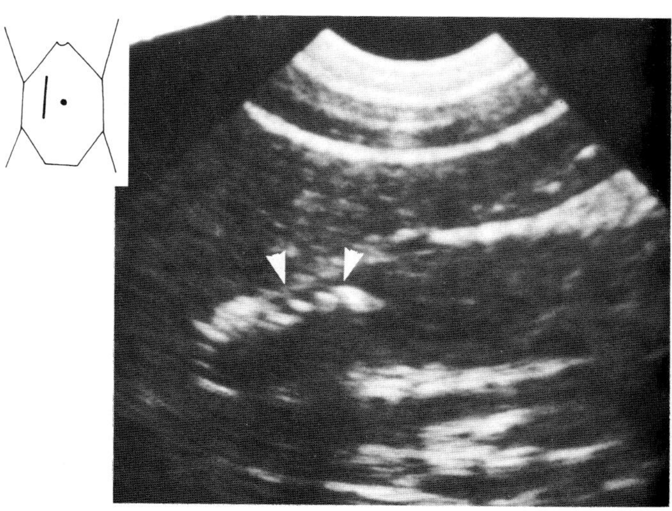

Fig. 35.89 Focal chronic pancreatitis (sagittal section). Focal calcification (arrowheads) in an otherwise normal pancreas.

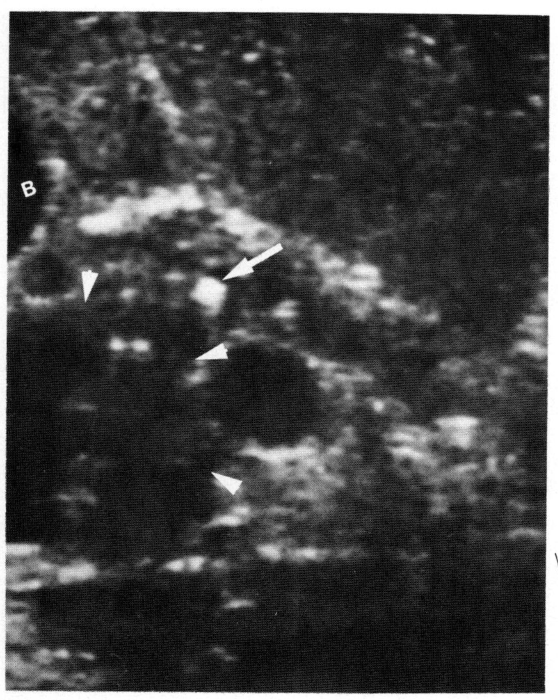

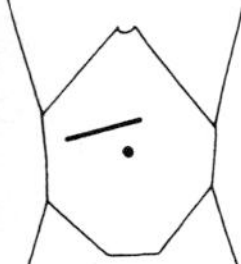

Fig. 35.90 Chronic pancreatitis with cyst formation (arrowheads) and intraduct calculus (long arrow). B = gall-bladder.

It is easy to relate these features to those seen by ultrasonography or CT.

For ultrasonography, none of the mild changes seen are specific by themselves, but with due allowance for age, two or more features allow a diagnosis of mild CP. A typical feature complex would be; size 1.5 times normal, MPD 2–4 mm and a slightly heterogeneous parenchyma with increase in the reflectivity of the duct walls relative to an internal reference tissue. The more abnormal features recorded, the more confident is the diagnosis.

Because of the inferior spatial resolution of ultrasonography and CT, minor irregularities of the MPD cannot be visualized, only major changes in calibre. There is, therefore, no clear discrimination point between mild and moderate changes.

Severe change — cysts, calculi, severe irregularity of the MPD with dilatation — are well seen with all the techniques.

PANCREATIC NEOPLASMS

Benign tumours

Papillomas of the pancreas have not been described ultrasonographically, but any associated duct dilatation should be recognized.

Adenomas are very rarely solid, but *cystadenomas*, and their malignant counterparts, are well described. These lesions are slow-growing, predominantly multilocular, possess fine septae and either an eccentric solid component or a thick wall. The cystic components are often blood pools or mucus, and high gain scans will reveal the characteristic fine echo pattern. Calcifications are common (>10%), but do not discriminate either benign from malignant, or inflammatory from neoplastic.

Cystadenomas may reach 20 cm in size, but the likelihood of malignancy increases with age of patient, size of the tumour and extent of the solid component.

Most cystic tumours are vascular, and fine-needle puncture yields copious blood.

The differential diagnosis includes inflammatory pseudocysts, congenital cysts, ductal adenocarcinoma with obstruction or necrosis, mucinous adenocarcinoma, cystic islet cell tumours, and peripancreatic cysts of other origin. The main differential is from a pancreatic pseudocyst. Estimation of the amylase content of the cyst fluid is the simplest discriminator, but a characteristic vascular pattern may be seen on dynamic CT or angiography (see above).

Benign islet cell tumours are infrequently seen by ultrasonography. This is not just because these tumours are usually very small, but because they have a composition very similar to that of normal pancreatic tissue. Even where an apudoma is found, it is not possible to exclude the possibility of multiple lesions.

Insulinomas are rarely more than 10 mm in diameter. 70% are solitary, 10% multiple and 10% metastasize and ultimately behave in a malignant fashion. Metastases in the liver produce a unique pattern; very high insulin levels around the micrometastases induce marked and very circumscribed fatty change, which is intensely echogenic. The liver becomes studded with innumerable bright foci at ultrasound.

Gastrinomas are more often multiple and malignant, but are usually even smaller. Approximately 10% occur in the duodenal wall.

Very high resolution scanning within the abdomen at operation has been successful, and may well become a standard technique to help the surgeon locate the nonpalpable lesion.

Pancreatic carcinoma

Virtually all pancreatic carcinomas arise from ductal epithelium. There is a strong male preponderance. 60–70% arise in the head, 20–30% in the body and less than 10% in the tail.

Carcinoma of the head of the pancreas causes *obstructive jaundice* in over 80% of cases, and the majority of pancreatic carcinomas will be diagnosed as part of the evaluation of the jaundiced patient, a role ultrasonography plays well.

Other pancreatic carcinomas are more difficult to find, but where the criteria for adequate visualization have been achieved, a normal study will only rarely be in error.

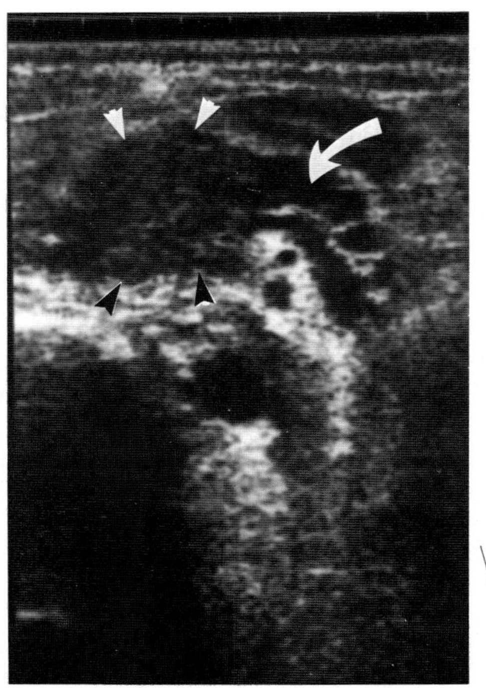

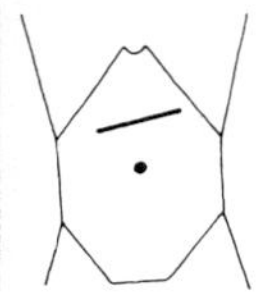

Fig. 35.91 Small pancreatic carcinoma in the head with dilatation of the main pancreatic duct (curved arrow). There is a very uniform echo pattern within this small tumour.

Size. Lesions producing obstruction to either the bile or pancreatic ducts are easily seen by ultrasonography. It is a simple task to identify the dilated duct which acts as a pointer to the obstructing lesion. Tumours as small as 10 mm can be regularly identified in this way (Fig. 35.91).

Where neither duct is obstructed then it is nearly always necessary to demonstrate changes in the pancreatic contour. Small tumours of the tail are the most difficult to visualize, but most are larger than 5 cm at the time of presentation.

Minor deformities of the contour can be confused with normal variations in shape unless supporting signs are present.

As many as 20% of ductal adenocarcinomas are either diffuse or multifocal. These are difficult to differentiate from the more frequent diffuse inflammatory changes associated with slow-growing carcinomas.

Parenchymal features. The echogenicity of a pancreatic adenocarcinoma is predominantly a function of its size. Small cancers which have not outgrown their blood supply have a uniform internal structure, and present few interfaces to the interrogating ultrasound beam. This, together with the high connective tissue content of most of these lesions, presents a poorly echogenic mass. With increasing disorganization of the internal structure more echoes are produced in the centre. However, it is rare for an adenocarcinoma to be uniformly strongly echogenic.

Marginal definition. The most characteristic feature of a pancreatic cancer is that the margins are well defined

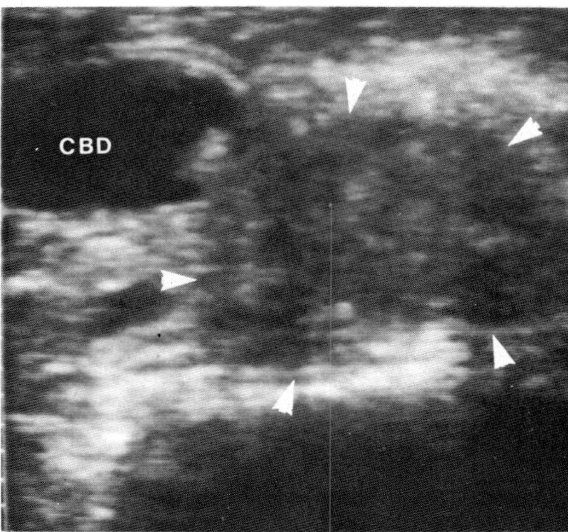

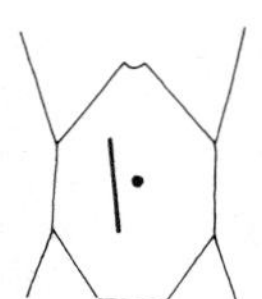

Fig. 35.92 30 mm carcinoma in the head of the pancreas with associated CBD dilatation. This tumour has a more heterogeneous echo pattern.

(Fig. 35.92); associated irregularity makes the diagnosis virtually certain. The causes of poor definition are pre-existing chronic pancreatitis, inflammation induced by the tumour (usually obstructive), a multifocal carcinoma or an echogenicity similar to that of the surrounding parenchyma. Less than 10% will be poorly defined if the viewing conditions are reasonable.

Duct signs. Dilatation of both the CBD and the MPD (Fig. 35.93) is found in over 80% of those cancers responsible for jaundice, and jaundice will feature at some stage of the disease process in 70%. Even small intraduct cancers may reveal themselves in this way. The pancreatic duct is smoothly dilated, and the surrounding parenchyma atrophic; however, a combination of duct elongation secondary to obstruction and shortening of the pancreas secondary to atrophy may cause the duct to become tortuous, with kinks simulating strictures. The 'double

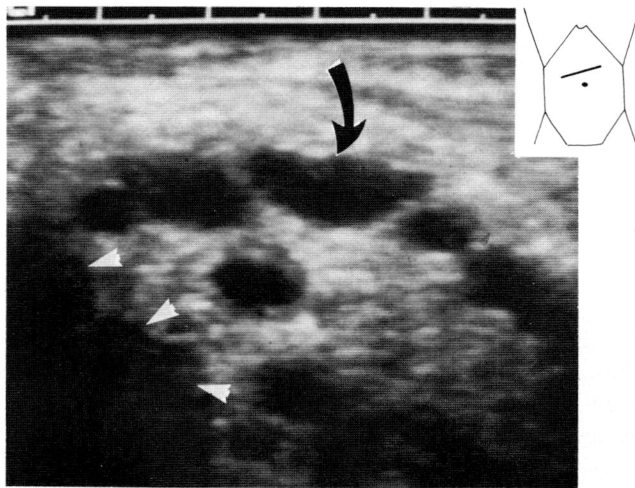

Fig. 35.93 Pancreatic duct dilatation (arrow) secondary to obstructing carcinoma (arrowheads).

duct sign' is a very reliable indicator of a pancreatic malignant tumour.

Retention cysts secondary to duct obstruction are found in less than 2% of carcinomas; calcifications are similarly uncommon.

Staging. Ultrasonography is at least 90% sensitive in the detection of liver metastases, which are present in almost half the patients with pancreatic cancer. The accuracy falls considerably in the patient with obstructive jaundice, when it is more difficult to assess the liver parenchyma.

Involvement of the draining lymph nodes (Fig. 35.94) is infrequently seen, but encroachment on the portal venous system can be demonstrated.

CT with contrast enhancement or angiography will often provide more precise staging data.

Differential diagnosis. The differential diagnosis of a solid pancreatic mass is adenocarcinoma, malignant islet cell tumour, metastatic tumour, focal inflammation and benign pancreatic tumours.

Focal inflammations are often seen in the head of the pancreas in patients with a gallstone jaundice of acute origin. The swelling is almost always poorly marginated, and the involved parenchyma although poorly echogenic retains the normal spatial distribution of echoes.

Acute inflammatory processes, particularly those secondary to chronic pancreatitis, are very difficult to distinguish from malignancy without biopsy. Focal chronic pancreatitis is a definite entity, and is most commonly seen as 'groove pancreatitis' in that segment of pancreas surrounding the CBD. In some patients with the divisum anomaly a pure dorsal pancreatitis may occur.

The presence of cysts, calcifications and irregular dilatation of the duct system strongly favour an inflammatory origin, but are not specific. Fine-needle aspiration biopsy is the only specific diagnostic test presently available.

Between 5 and 10% of pancreatic malignancies prove difficult to diagnose. The most common cause of difficulty is coexisting disease, either choledochal stones, disseminated malignancy of other origin or pancreatitis either preceding or consequent on the pancreatic carcinoma. Only a complete morphological description, gathered by ultrasonography, CT, ERCP and even arteriography, coupled with biopsy proof of diagnosis is adequate in these cases.

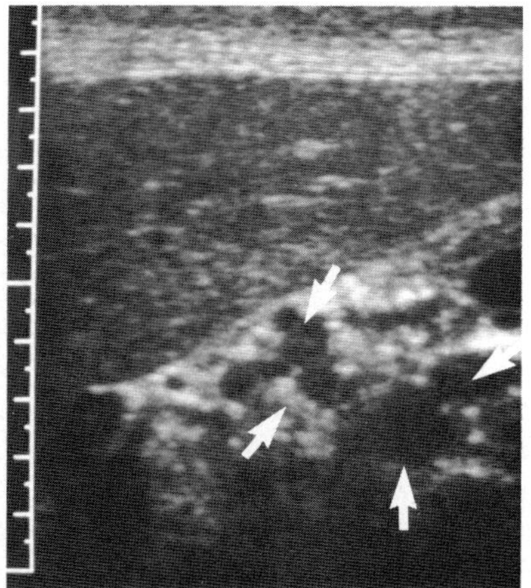

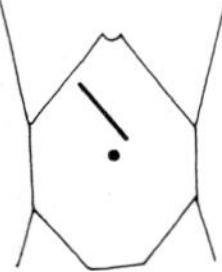

Fig. 35.94 Local nodal metastases (arrows) secondary to a pancreatic carcinoma.

Diagnostic accuracy. ERCP has a sensitivity of over 95% in the best hands for the detection of pancreatic carcinoma. Both ultrasonography and CT are comparable if the higher technical failure rate of ultrasonography is taken into account, with ultrasonography being more specific in differentiating small lesions. Excluding technical failures, the accuracy of ultrasonography varies between 80 and 95% in a number of large series, with a predictive value of both a positive and a negative examination as high as 98% and 99% respectively.

PSEUDOCYSTS

The appearance, natural history and response to treatment of a pseudocyst is very dependent on its aetiology. The majority arise as a result of **acute pancreatitis** and, since the introduction of ultrasonography and CT scanning, the reported incidence of this complication has risen from 2–3% to over 50% in some series. Areas of inflamed pancreatic tissue are nearly always associated with a local peripancreatic collection, which may shift in position over the space of a few days as the state of the pancreas itself changes. These are not pseudocysts as recognized by the pathologist.

Focal pancreatic necrosis is more likely to lead to the development of a pseudocyst, with the process of maturation taking from 2 to 6 weeks. This evolution can be followed by sequential ultrasound scanning, and it is unusual for a pseudocyst, seen as a complication of acute pancreatitis, not to have been forming since the acute phase. Development and regression can both be very rapid.

The most common site for pseudocysts to form is anterior to the body and tail of the pancreas, extending into the lesser sac (Fig. 35.95). With severe pancreatitis the initial inflammation may spread widely into the anterior pararenal spaces and the root of the mesentery, and the pseudocyst may be left at the high water mark as the pancreas returns to normal.

If disruption of the duct system occurs with spillage of pancreatic juice, then the cyst may dissect its way between the tissue planes, and many exotic locations have been described both in the abdomen and thorax.

Haemorrhage into, and superimposed infection of, the pseudocyst are more likely with acute pancreatitis as an aetiology, and will show by the formation of echogenic debris in the dependent part of the collection. Septation is rare, but has been described, as has the acoustically

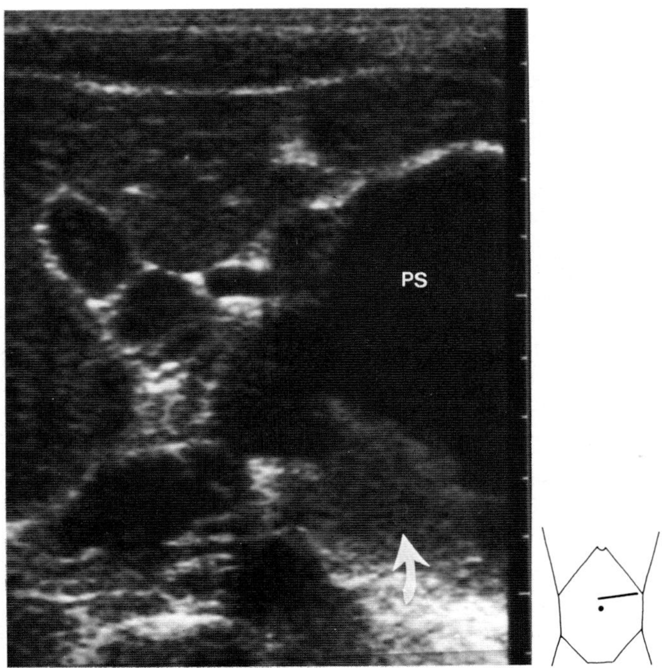

Fig. 35.95 Lesser sac pseudocyst (PS). Residual tissue of the tail of the pancreas is marked by the curved arrow.

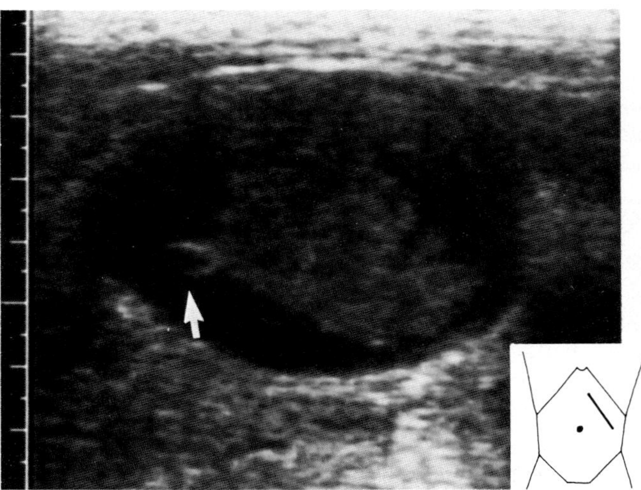

Fig. 35.96 Small pseudocyst enveloping the tail of the pancreas. Note the splenic artery is exposed to the pseudocyst contents (arrow).

'solid' pseudocyst. This latter is then likely to be misdiagnosed as a tumour or a cystadenoma.

After the process of maturation is complete then the majority of pseudocysts will be echo free and intimately related to the underlying pancreatric tissue (Fig. 35.96). At this stage the characteristic feature is a projection of a segment of pancreas of normal appearance into the lumen of the cyst.

Acute inflammatory pseudocysts vary markedly in size, and can contain as much as 5 litres of fluid.

The cysts which form as a complication of **chronic pancreatitis** are usually much smaller, frequently multiple, and are found within the pancreatic substance. The presence of a cyst defines the CP as severe, and it is not surprising that these are commonly associated with intraduct calculi. These are nearly always *retention cysts*, rather than pseudocysts, but the terminology is often very loosely applied. The distinction is, however, purely academic.

Serial scans are particularly valuable for initial diagnosis, follow up, and for assessment of the most appropriate treatment. Although ultrasonographic criteria for the diagnosis of pseudocysts have been described, fine-needle aspiration and chemical analysis of the fluid will usually provide a definitive diagnosis.

Trauma to the pancreas which results in disruption of the MPD is strongly associated with pseudocyst formation. These are large and, if resulting from blunt trauma, usually arise from the point at which the body of the pancreas is stretched over the aorta. Debridinous contents have not been described in traumatic pseudocysts, but fistula formation may follow penetrating injury.

The fluid collections which occur secondary to *pancreatic malignancy* are the result of obstruction, are rare and are unlikely to be diagnosed by retrograde pancreatography. If underlying malignancy is suspected, then direct puncture of the cyst with a radiographic contrast study and aspiration biopsy is practically the only way to establish the diagnosis preoperatively.

The **differential diagnosis** of pseudocysts includes true cysts of the pancreas, which are extremely rare, and cysts of contiguous organs. With very large cysts (or even a massive hydronephrosis), the anatomy is so distorted that even the organ of origin may be in doubt. A rapid ingestion of fluid into the stomach will outline that organ and a careful check of each organ in turn will exclude other origins. CT is more accurate under these circumstances but is often not definitive. Direct fine-needle puncture with biochemical and cytological analysis of the cyst fluid is a rapid and simple way of discriminating virtually all the diagnostic possibilities. A simultaneous study of the morphology of the cyst with a radiographic contrast agent is valuable in planning treatment, and appears much safer than a retrograde pancreatogram.

Percutaneous drainage of a pseudocyst is technically easy, and can be performed in stages. Small collections can be aspirated to dryness as part of a diagnostic aspiration, and may resolve completely following this. This is particularly true of collections which are the residuum of an attack of acute pancreatitis. Larger or more persistent pseudocysts can be drained by catheter using any one of many different methods of catheter insertion, all performed under local anaesthesia. There is an immediate response in the general status of the patient, and indwelling catheters have been left in for many months without any significant complications.

The most serious complication of surgical pseudocyst drainage is haemorrhage. This has not yet been recorded following a catheter procedure, but a death has occurred following fine-needle aspiration of a pancreatic abscess.

These therapeutic drainage procedures are very rarely successful, except in the short term, for reasons relating to the underlying cause of the pseudocyst. If there is disruption of the duct system then a surgical resection is the only likely successful procedure. The cysts of chronic pancreatitis can usually be adequately drained, but the underlying disease is unaffected, and the patient will represent with more pseudocysts or pain.

In acute pancreatitis, many of the fluid collections will spontaneously resolve. It is possible that a simple aspiration of a fluid collection in the recovery phase may prevent formation of a pseudocyst as a late complication, but this supposition is impossible to prove.

These considerations explain why the quoted success rate of percutaneous drainage varies from 16 to 80%.

The role of catheter drainage is in the acute and temporary management of pseudocysts, where the place of definitive surgery has not yet become clear.

ULTRASOUND-GUIDED FINE-NEEDLE ASPIRATION BIOPSY

Extensive worldwide experience has shown that this is a technique that is almost 100% specific in the diagnosis of abdominal malignancy, and has an extremely low complication rate. A true positive rate of 95% has been reported by more than one author in large series. The world average is somewhat lower but, with experience on the part of both the radiologist and cytologist, it lies between 80 and 90%. Only a handful of false positives have been reported, and most have occurred early within the experience of a particular institution.

Complications. There are two reported deaths from acute pancreatitis following fine-needle biopsy, and two cases of severe but non-fatal acute pancreatitis. All other complications have been minor. An estimate of total world experience and these cases give a mortality rate of approximately 1 in 50 000, and a significant morbidity of less than 1 in 5000. We have recorded no significant complication in over 1000 retroperitoneal puncture procedures.

Technique. Many patients experience severe pain during or after pancreatic FNAB. Pain is a feature of both pancreatic cancer and chronic pancreatitis, and is related to duct obstruction and perineural infiltration. These patients require regular opiates for pain relief. Moving the pancreatic mass and puncturing multiple layers of peritoneum causes much greater discomfort than is encountered with renal or liver biopsies. An intravenous benzodiazepine and pethidine gives good control for the 15 minutes or more needed for the procedure, with excellent retrograde amnesia.

The excellent safety record of this method means that there are few contraindications to the use of needles of 0.8 mm or less diameter; even vascular lesions can be punctured without hazard. There are only two reports of needle track seeding, or of infective complications, with needles of less than 20 s.w.g.

The simplest method involves inserting a 10 cm needle through the cleansed skin alongside a real-time transducer (Fig. 35.97), observing the passage of the needle through the image plane until the tip is seen to interact with the target. A short needle is easily controlled with minimal deflection and tracking through the tissue planes. This 'no touch' method is quick, simple, sterile and needs no special apparatus. Any type of ultrasound machine can be used.

Many different types of special biopsy transducer have been devised; all require stabilization of a much longer needle, with a greater requirement for asepsis, and an increase in time and cost.

The greatest difficulty encountered is adequately to visualize the tip of the needle. This becomes easier with practice, but visualization is often poor in the obese or gassy patient. The simplest way around this problem is to combine ultrasound and conventional radiography.

Our early experience with ultrasound guidance alone yielded no more than 76% positives in pancreatic malignancy, with most of the failures in tumours of less than 3 cm in diameter, although our yield in liver lesions exceeded 90%.

It is now our practice to biopsy large lesions at the time of the diagnostic scan and to defer biopsy of the small lesions until after ERCP and endoprosthesis insertion. Biopsies taken at ERCP may well prove positive, and the prosthesis serves as an excellent radiographic marker.

Further diagnostic information and help with guidance can be obtained from an ultrasound-guided transhepatic

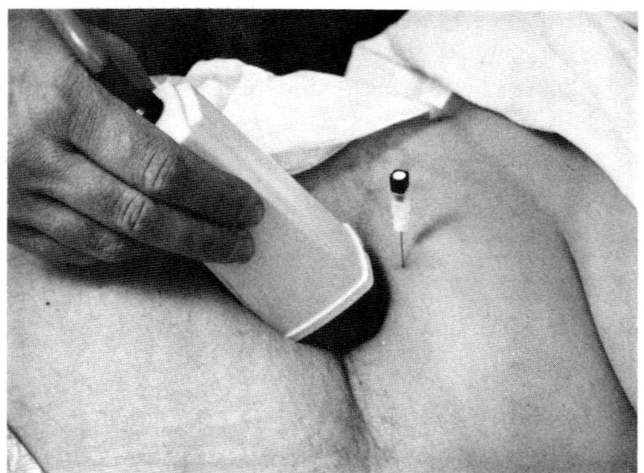

Fig. 35.97 Fine-needle aspiration biopsy.

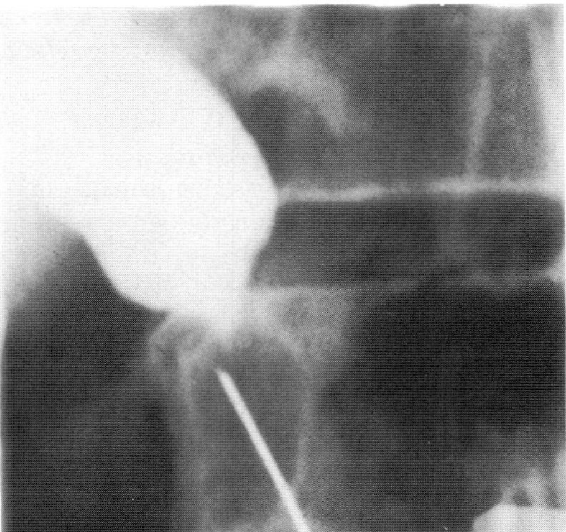

Fig. 35.98 Fine-needle biopsy of biliary stricture.

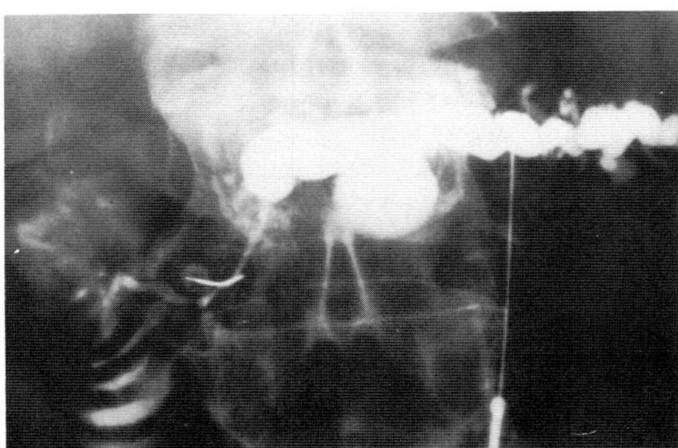

Fig. 35.99 Fine-needle biopsy of pancreatic duct stricture following percutaneous pancreatogram. Biopsy needle to Rt of spine.

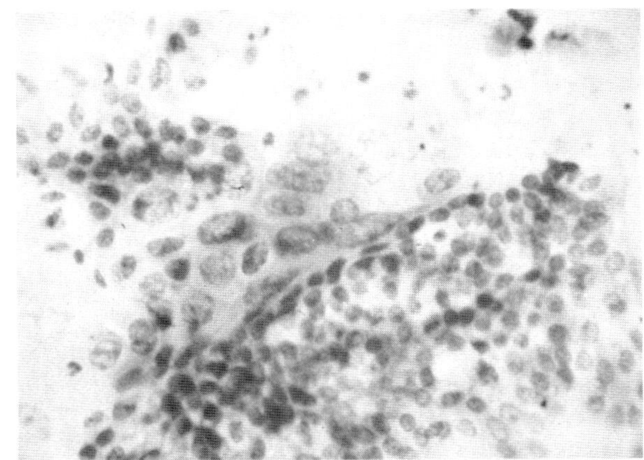

Fig. 35.100 Cytology. Pancreatic ductal adenocarcinoma.

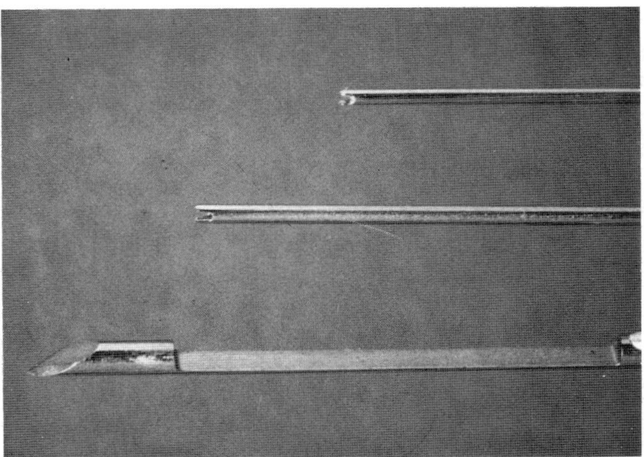

Fig. 35.101 Small calibre core cut needles (Otto type) with Tru-cut needle below for comparison.

cholangiogram or percutaneous pancreatogram (Figs 35.98, 35.99).

CT-guided biopsy is always more time consuming and is held in reserve for those cases in whom ultrasonographic visualization is inadequate.

Ferrucci has shown that there is a definite improvement in yield with every subsequent pass of the needle through the tumour, and it is recommended to achieve at least three adequate samples as defined by close visual inspection of the aspirate. The samples are best taken from the periphery of the tumour mass, rather than the often necrotic or fibrous centre, with best results being obtained if a skilled cytologist examines the samples by phase contrast microscopy during the procedure (Fig. 35.100).

There are now many different needle types available, including those which are capable of retrieving a coherent core of tissue, on which histological methods can be used (Fig. 35.101). These core biopsies have been shown to increase slightly the sensitivity of the technique in diagnosing malignancy, but are also capable of giving a true 'histological' diagnosis in over half.

The cores that are produced are also ideal for electron microscopy and for preparation for staining for surface antigens with labelled monoclonal antibodies. Both are new techniques which will expand the role of the cytologist.

ULTRASOUND-GUIDED PERCUTANEOUS PANCREATOGRAPHY

A dilated pancreatic duct provides an easy target for ultrasound-guided puncture, and hence an alternative route for pancreatography (Fig. 35.102). This may be used when ERCP has failed and where the surgeon needs a preoperative map of the ductal anatomy.

Technically the procedure is no more difficult than transhepatic cholangiography, and there have been as yet no reported complications.

Fine-needle puncture of the spleen or of the portal veins is also safe and easy to perform, and with hand injection of radiographic contrast, digital subtraction methods yield

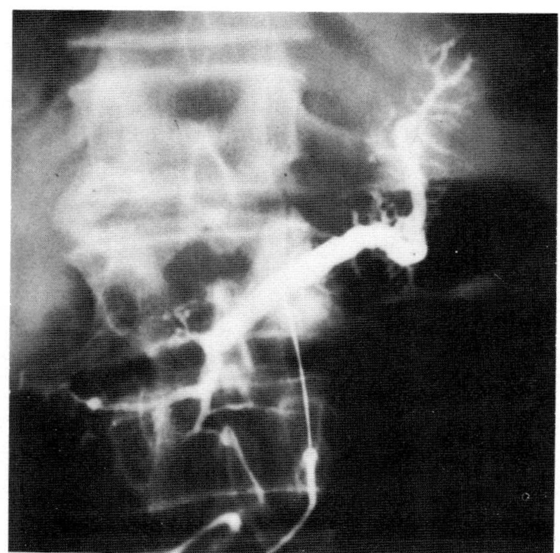

Fig. 35.102 Diagnostic percutaneous pancreatogram in patient with the pancreas divisum anomaly.

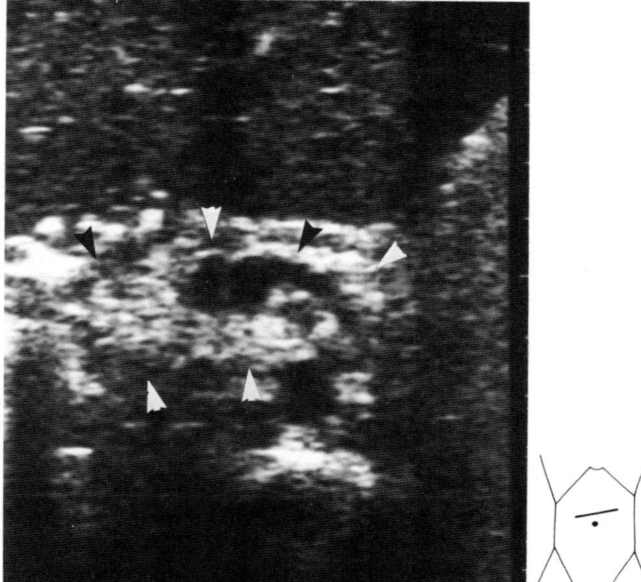

Fig. 35.103 Cystic fibrosis. Increased parenchymal echogenicity and atrophy.

excellent portograms, which can be directly related to pressure measurements.

CYSTIC FIBROSIS

Cystic fibrosis is unlike adult chronic pancreatitis in both behaviour and ultrasonographic appearance. The predominant pancreatic damage occurs in the early years and, by adolescence, almost all will have pancreatic exocrine insufficiency. Mucus plugging of tiny branch ducts and acini leads to atrophy with fibrosis and fatty replacement.

Ultrasonographically, the gland will invariably be strongly echogenic (Fig. 35.103) (both fat and fibrosis are responsible for this) and the duct, if visible, will be extremely small. Cysts and calcifications can occur but are very uncommon.

Other common findings are diffuse liver parenchymal changes, microgallbladder, gallstones and splenomegaly. The splenic enlargement appears to be related to pulmonary infections rather than the result of portal hypertension.

REFERENCES AND SUGGESTIONS FOR FURTHER READING

Books

Freeny, P. C. & Lawson, T. L. (1982) *Radiology of the Pancreas*. New York: Springer Verlag.

Ring, E. J. & McLean, G. K. (1981) *Interventional Radiology: Principles and Techniques*. Boston: Little Brown & Co.

Articles

Axon, A. T. R., Classen, M., Cotton, P. B., et al. (1984) Pancreatography in chronic pancreatitis: international definitions. *Gut* (in press).

Cotton, P. B., Lees, W. R., Vallon, A. G., et al. (1980) Grey-scale ultrasonography and endoscopic pancreatography in pancreatic diagnosis. *Radiology*, **134**, 453–459.

Cubilla, A. & Fitzgerald, P. J. (1978) Pancreas cancer. 1 Duct carcinoma. A clinico-pathological study of 380 patients. *Pathological Annual*, 241–287.

Freeny, P. C., Marks, W. M. & Ball, T. J. (1982) Impact of high resolution CT of the pancreas on utilization of ERCP and angiography. *Radiology*, **142**, 35–39.

Hill, M. C., Barkin, J., Isikoff, M. B., et al. (1982) Acute pancreatitis: clinical vs CT findings. *American Journal of Roentgenology*, **139**, 263–269.

Haaga, J. R. & Alfidi, R. J. (1977) CT scanning of the pancreas. *Radiologic Clinics of North America*, **15**, 367–376.

Kamin, P. D., Bernardino, M. E., Wallace, S. & Bao-Shan, Jing (1980) Comparison of ultrasound and CT in detection of pancreatic malignancy. *Cancer*, **46**, 2410–2412.

Kattan, K. R. (1980) Non-invasive radiology of the liver. *Radiologic Clinics of North America*, **18**, 177–341.

Kolmannskog, F., Swenson, T., Vatn, M. H., et al. (1982) CT and ultrasound of the normal pancreas. *Acta Radiologica*, **23** (5), 443–451.

Livraghi, T., et al. (1983) Risk in fine-needle abdominal biopsy. *Journal of Clinical Ultrasound*, **11**, 77–81.

Montali, G., et al. (1982) Fine-needle aspiration biopsy of liver focal lesions, ultrasonically guided with a real time probe. Report on 126 cases. *British Journal of Radiology*, **55**, 717–723.

O'Halpin, D., Legge, D. & MacErlean, D. P. (1984) Therapeutic arterial embolisation. Report of five years experience. *Clinical Radiology*, **35**, 85–93.

Parulekar, S. G. (1980) Ultrasonic evaluation of the pancreatic duct. *Journal of Clinical Ultrasound*, **4**, 457–463.

Pearse, A. G. E. & Polak, J. M. (1978) The diffuse neuroendocrine system and the APUD concept. In Bloom, S. R. (ed.) *Gut Hormones*. Edinburgh: Churchill Livingstone.

Plumley, T. F., Rohrmann, C. A., Freeny, P. C., et al. (1983) The double duct sign: reassessed significance in ERCP. *American Journal of Roentgenology*, **138** (1), 31–36.

Sankaran, S. & Walt, A. J. (1979) The natural and unnatural history of pancreatic pseudocyst. *British Journal of Surgery*, **62**, 37–44.

Silverstein, W., et al. (1981) Diagnostic imaging of acute pancreatitis: prospective study using CT and sonography. *American Journal of Roentgenology*, **137**, 497–502.

Turner, R. C., et al. (1978) Localization of insulinomas. *Lancet*, **ii**, 515–518.

Warren, P. S., Garret, W. J. & Kossof, G. (1978) The liquid-filled stomach: an ultrasonic window to the upper abdomen. *Journal of Clinical Ultrasound*, **6**, 295.

Weinstein, B. J., Weinstein, D. P. & Brodmerkel, G. J. (1980) Ultrasonography of pancreatic lithiasis. *Radiology*, **134**, 185–189.

Weinstein, D. P., Wolfman, N. T. & Weinstein, B. J. (1979) Ultrasonic characteristics of pancreatic tumours. *Gastrointestinal Radiology*, **4**, 245–251.

CHAPTER 36

THE ADRENAL GLANDS

The adrenal glands are, for their size, among the most important structures in the body. The function was quite unknown until 1855, when Addison first described the syndrome resulting from their destruction. In 1856 Brown-Séquard showed that their removal led to death in animals.

The adrenal glands lie just above the kidneys and are composed of a *cortex* and a *medulla*. The medulla has a totally different origin to the cortex, and arises with the sympathetic nervous system. Both cortex and medulla secrete hormones.

Three main groups of hormones are secreted by the adrenal *cortex*. These are all chemically related and have a similar basic chemical structure. They are:

1. *Glucocorticoids*. The secretion of these is controlled by the pituitary gland through its adrenocorticotrophic hormone (ACTH). The most important glucocorticoid is hydrocortisone (cortisol) and this is normally secreted at the rate of about 20 mg per day. The glucocorticoids have many actions such as stimulation of protein breakdown, antagonism to the action of insulin, and the inhibition of tissue response in injury.

2. *Mineralocorticoids*. Aldosterone is the most important of these. Its secretion is mainly controlled by the renin-angiotensin system and by the level of plasma potassium. Aldosterone stimulates the reabsorption of sodium in the distal renal tubules of the kidney in exchange for potassium.

3. *Androgens*. Though they are produced in relatively large amounts, the adrenal androgens are very weak compared with testosterone.

The *medulla* also secretes hormones, mainly adrenalin and noradrenalin.

ANATOMY

The right adrenal gland is triangular and is closely related to the upper pole of the right kidney. The left adrenal is crescent shaped and is related to the upper and medial part of the left kidney. The average size of the adrenals varies from 3 to 5 cm in length by 2–3 cm in width and their average thickness is only about 5 mm. The average weight is 3–5 g, of which 90% is contributed by the cortex.

The blood supply has been of considerable importance in radiology and it is therefore important to know the vascular anatomy. Anatomists describe three main arteries of supply (Fig. 36.1):

1. An inferior adrenal artery arising from the renal artery
2. A middle adrenal artery arising from the aorta
3. A superior adrenal artery arising from the inferior phrenic artery.

However, this anatomy is subject to considerable variation. Thus, the inferior phrenic artery can arise direct from the aorta or from the coeliac axis, or from other vessels. There may be arteries of supply from other adjacent large arteries. The major arteries of supply break up into numerous smaller branches before entering the gland, which thus has multiple small vessels of supply.

The venous drainage of the adrenal (Fig. 36.2) is also of considerable importance since adrenal phlebography and adrenal hormone assay became established radiological

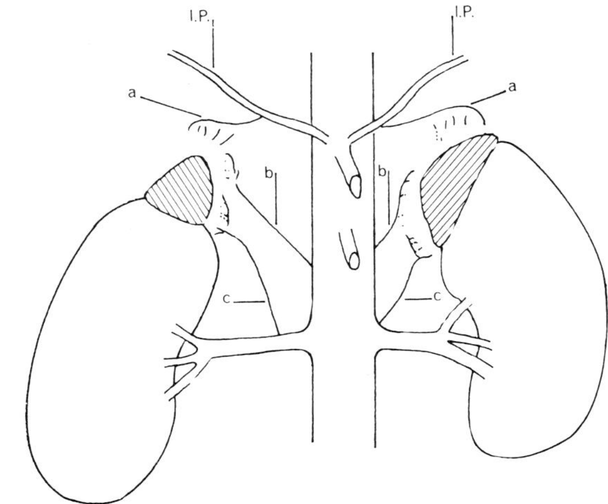

Fig. 36.1 Arterial supply of the adrenals. I.P. = inferior phrenic artery; a = superior adrenal artery; b = middle adrenal artery; c = inferior adrenal artery.

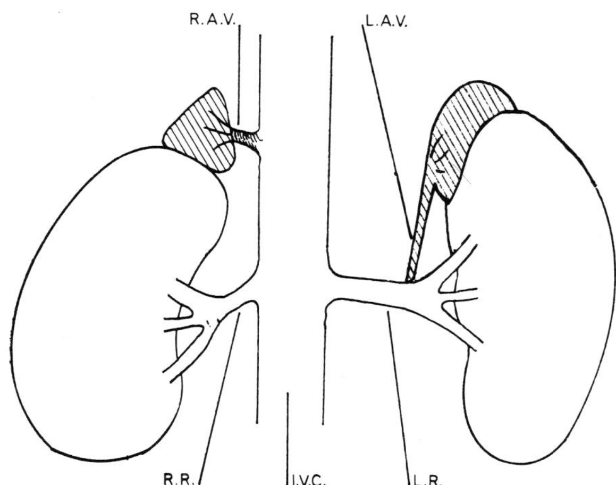

Fig. 36.2 Venous drainage of the adrenal gland. R.A.V. = right adrenal vein; L.A.V. = left adrenal vein; L.R. = left renal vein; I.V.C. = inferior vena cava.

techniques. There is usually a fairly large adrenal vein on the *left* which passes downwards medial to the upper part of the kidney to join the main renal vein, and lies just lateral to the left vertebral border. This vein may also have connections with the inferior phrenic vein and veins from the kidney.

On the *right* side, the anatomy is quite different since the adrenal vein has only a very short trunk which passes straight from the right adrenal into the postero-lateral aspect of the inferior vena cava at a level just above the upper pole of the right kidney. Occasionally it may pass to an accessory hepatic vein before entering the inferior vena cava and, in rare cases, to the right renal vein.

The normal adrenal glands at CT. With modern body scanners the normal adrenal glands can be demonstrated by CT in all but the occasional case, usually a thin person, or child with a paucity of retroperitoneal fat. In these axial cross-sections the glands appear quite different from their conventional anatomical description.

The right gland lies directly above the level of the kidney and directly behind the inferior vena cava just below its point of entry into the liver. The right lobe of the liver lies on its right lateral aspect and the right crus of the diaphragm on its medial aspect (Fig. 36.3).

The left adrenal gland is a little lower in position, its lower pole lying antero-medial to the upper pole of the left kidney. The left crus of the diaphragm is medial to it and

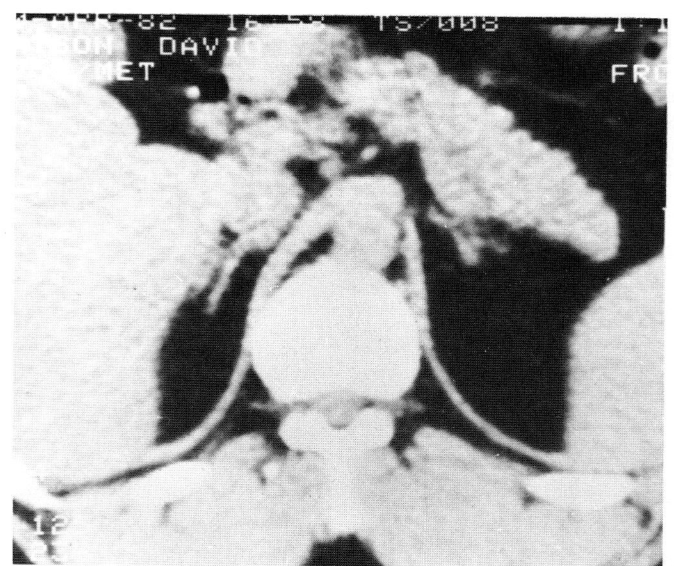

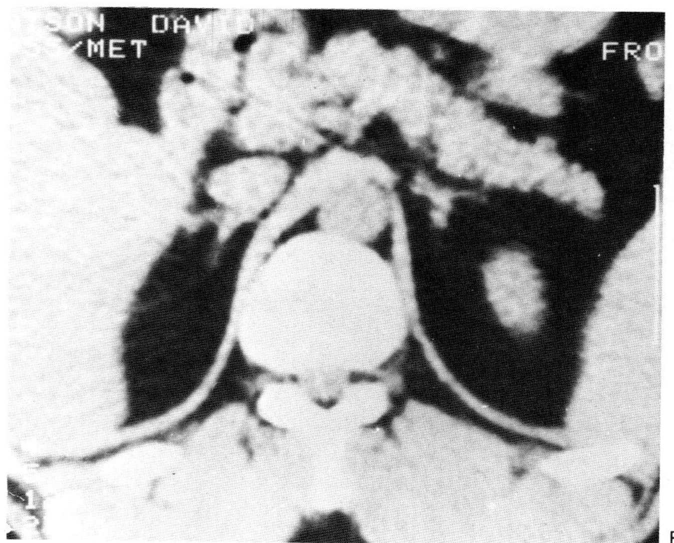

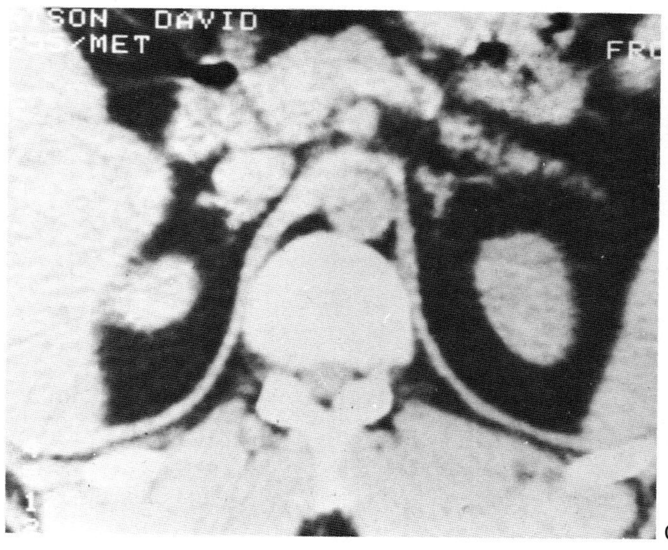

Fig. 36.3 Normal adrenals as shown by CT (see text) **A.** Section just above right kidney. In this example the right adrenal has well-marked lateral and medial limbs. The top of the left adrenal is also shown behind the pancreas, though frequently it is not seen at this level (L 43 W 512). **B.** Section including top of left kidney. The left adrenal resembling an arrowhead is well seen, as is the right adrenal, though the limbs now appear shorter (L43 W572). **C.** Section at slightly lower level, including tops of both kidneys (L43 W572).

the spleen lateral to its upper pole. Anteriorly lie the tail of the pancreas and the splenic vessels.

The right gland appears as an elongated, slightly curved structure pointing backwards and laterally. It is sometimes described as having a body and two limbs. The medial elongated limb is the one easily recognizable at CT but the smaller body and lateral limb may be difficult to identify, the latter often merging with the liver shadow. The left gland is more easily identified, resembling an arrow head pointing antero-medially (Fig. 36.3). It should be noted that, unlike the conventional anatomical descriptions, both glands are not in direct apposition to the kidneys, but may be separated by a centimetre or more of fatty or areolar tissue. As the glands are 3–5 cm in height, they are usually seen on more than one section, particularly where contiguous narrow cuts are made. The left gland in particular may extend well down the medial surface of the kidney to just above the hilum.

PATHOLOGY

Disorders of the adrenal gland may be due to *infections*, either acute, as in meningococcal or other fulminating septicaemia, or chronic, as in tuberculosis or histoplasmosis.

Adrenal haemorrhage (adrenal apoplexy) is usually associated with overwhelming septicaemia, and characterized by acute adrenal insufficiency. This may also occur without infection, as in neonatal birth trauma. It can also occur in pregnancy and in severe hypertension, or following adrenal vein thrombosis or severe convulsions in epilepsy.

Most of the above conditions are of little radiological interest with the exception of the chronic infections, which may give rise to granulomatous masses or to adrenal calcification and Addison's syndrome. The latter, however, is nowadays more commonly associated with *autoimmune disease*.

Of greater radiological interest are *tumours* of the adrenal gland and *bilateral hyperplasia* (Table 36.1).

Table 36.1 Adrenal tumours

A. Neoplasms	B. Other mass lesions
1. *Cortical*	1. *Granulomas*
Carcinoma	Tuberculosis
Adenoma	Histoplasmosis
2. *Medullary*	Blastomycosis
Neuroblastoma	2. *Bilateral hyperplasia*
Phaeochromocytoma	3. *Cysts*
Ganglioneuroma	4. *Haematoma*
3. *Stromal*	
Lipoma	
Myolipoma	
4. *Metastases*	

Clinical presentation. Adrenal lesions may present with a wide variety of clinical syndromes including:

1. Addison's disease
2. Cushing's syndrome
3. Conn's syndrome (hyperaldosteronism)
4. The adrenogenital syndrome
5. Adrenalism and noradrenalism (pheochromocytoma)
6. Abdominal tumour
7. Metastases to bone or liver in childhood
8. Wolman's disease.

Most patients with suspected adrenal disorder present with one or other of the syndromes or clinical manifestations listed above.

Imaging investigation is aimed mainly at those cases thought to be suffering from adrenal tumours in the hope of demonstrating and localizing the lesion.

IMAGING INVESTIGATION

The methods available in the past and at present include:

1. Simple X-ray and tomography
2. IVP and high-dose IVP with tomography
3. Retroperitoneal air insufflation
4. Arteriography
5. Phlebography
6. Vena caval and adrenal vein blood sampling
7. Isotope scanning
8. Ultrasound
9. CT
10. MRI
11. Needle biopsy.

Apart from simple X-ray and tomography, the techniques listed above are, or have been, used largely for the assessment of suspected adrenal tumours.

Simple X-ray. In a suspected adrenal lesion plain radiology of the abdomen with or without tomography may help in two ways.

First, a **mass** in the adrenal area may be obvious and may be seen to be displacing the kidney. This is particularly evident with large tumours, but can occasionally be seen even with relatively small lesions provided there is a fair amount of perinephric fat present to help contrast. In general, however, masses smaller than 5 cm in diameter are not likely to be visualized. There are several important aspects of differential diagnosis; thus, all the following structures have been known to simulate a mass in the adrenal areas and must be borne in mind:

1. Renal cysts or tumours
2. Spleen and accessory spleen
3. Pancreatic cyst or tumour
4. Liver mass
5. Para-aortic glands
6. Retroperitoneal tumour
7. Stomach mass.

Of considerable importance are the normal fluid-filled gastric fundus in the supine position, which can simulate a mass over the left kidney, and the fluid-filled antrum or duodenal bulb which can simulate a mass over the right kidney. As long as these possibilities are borne in mind there is usually little difficulty in differential diagnosis, though occasionally erect films or even barium contrast will have to be used to exclude fluid in the stomach simulating a mass.

The second abnormality which may be seen on plain X-ray is **calcification** in the adrenal area. This may be seen both in tumours and in non-tumourous conditions (Table 36.2).

Table 36.2 Adrenal calcification

1. Idiopathic
2. Neoplasm
3. Granuloma
4. Cystic disease
5. Old haemorrhage
6. Wolman's disease

So-called *idiopathic calcification* may be found as a chance finding on routine abdominal examination of patients with no relevant symptoms of adrenal disease. It is possible that such calcification may be the result of old haemorrhage or infection in infancy or childhood which has healed with no effect on function (Fig. 36.4). When tuberculosis was common in Britain, involvement of the adrenals was said to be the commonest cause of *Addison's disease* and to be frequently followed by adrenal calcification. However, tuberculosis is now rare in our indigenous population and most of the cases seen today are due to 'atrophy'. This is now considered to be an *autoimmune disease*, since it may occur in association with such conditions as Hashimoto's thyroiditis and pernicious anaemia. Circulating antibodies to the adrenocortical tissue have been shown in the serum of such patients.

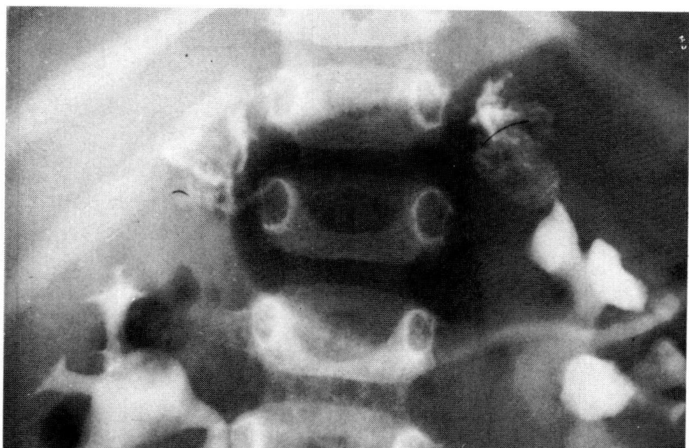

Fig. 36.4 Calcified adrenals in a child. These were a chance finding, the IVP being performed for urinary infection.

Addison's disease is not caused by primary tumours but it can very rarely be due to secondary carcinomatosis. Addison's disease may also occur with bilateral mass lesions such as granulomas or amyloidosis. The clinical features are largely due to the resulting deficiency of glucocorticoids and mineralocorticoids. The former leads to anorexia, nausea, vomiting and later to pyrexia, hypotension and hyperglycaemia. The latter causes sodium depletion with dehydration and hypotension. Abnormal brown pigmentation of the skin, involving in particular parts exposed to the sun and pressure areas, occurs. In addition, there are deposits of pigment in the mouth and conjunctival mucous membrane.

Wolman's disease (Abramov-Wolman's disease) is a lipoidosis which was formerly confused with Neiman Pick disease. It is associated with hepatomegaly, splenomegaly and a characteristic calcification of the adrenal glands which are enlarged. It was first defined in 1961 and many well-documented cases have since been reported. Most of the affected infants died in the first 6 months of life. Abdominal X-ray in these infants show large adrenals with diffuse stippled calcification which is virtually diagnostic.

Benign cysts of the adrenal, possibly of haemorrhagic origin, and in patients with no symptoms of adrenal pathology, may show arc-like marginal calcification. Similar calcification has been described in patients with phaeochromocytomas but is very rare.

Irregular calcification has been described in most adrenal tumours but is very uncommon except in malignant tumours. It is said to occur in about one-third of *carcinomas*, usually as faint irregular calcification. It also occurs in *neuroblastomas* in over one-third of cases. The calcification is usually stippled and non-homogeneous (Fig. 36.5), but can occasionally be linear or curvilinear. In this respect, it is interesting that liver metastases from neuroblastomas may also calcify.

Ganglioneuromas, which may be regarded as a mature type of neurogenic tumour, also calcify frequently, the calcification being similar to that in neuroblastomas (see Fig. 36.6). The majority of ganglioneuromas are extra-adrenal in origin, arising from sympathetic ganglia along the sympathetic chain.

Intravenous urography. In the investigation of suspected adrenal tumours intravenous urography is often very helpful by differentiating between a mass in the upper pole of the kidney and one in the adrenal. In this respect *high-dose urography with tomography* will frequently define the kidney quite clearly and show whether it is normal. Occasionally it will accentuate a mass in the adrenal and show it more clearly. Downward displacement of an intact kidney by a large suprarenal mass is usually well shown.

Retroperitoneal air insufflation. This technique was widely practised in the 1950s for the demonstration of adrenal masses, but was replaced in the 1960s with arteriography and phlebography. The technique of air insuf-

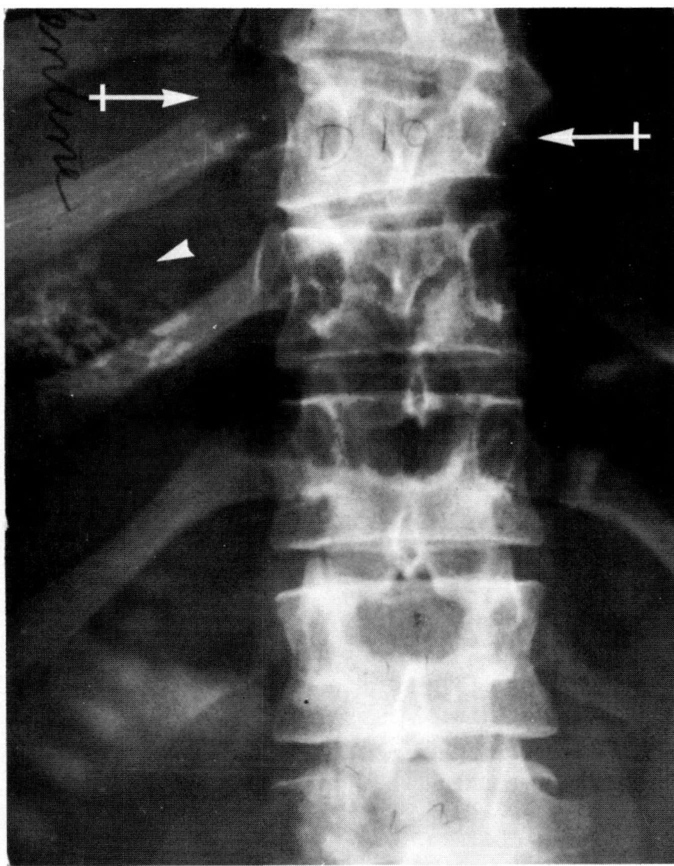

Fig. 36.5 Calcification in a neuroblastoma presenting in pregnancy (arrowhead). There is a secondary deposit in the 10th dorsal vertebra, extending into the transverse process of the 10th right rib (crossed arrows). (Courtesy of Dr J. Haggar.)

flation gave rise to occasional fatalities from air embolus and was not very accurate with small tumours. Some of the series reported showed a high incidence both of false positive and false negative results.

Arteriography. Simple flush aortography will readily show large or highly vascular adrenal masses. Small or non-vascular tumours, however, will usually require selective techniques for their demonstration as will ectopic tumours. The method was widely used for some 20 years before the advent of the newer imaging techniques in the 1970s.

Phlebography. Selective adrenal vein phlebography can be performed on both sides and proved a most reliable method for demonstrating small tumours such as occur in primary hyperaldosteronism. The adrenal veins are selectively catheterized percutaneously from the femoral vein. The right adrenal vein is the more difficult to catheterize, but, using specially designed catheters, a high success rate can be achieved on both sides. Care must be taken not to overfill the glands by using excessive doses of contrast media or excessive injection pressures and hand injections only are used. On the left side 5 ml of a water soluble

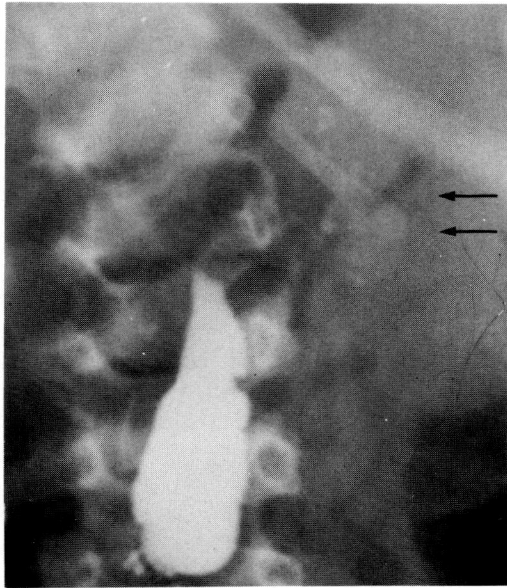

Fig. 36.6 Calcification in a dumbbell ganglioneuroma (arrows). The child presented with evidence of a spinal tumour and showed an almost complete block at myelography.

medium were used, and on the right side 2 ml. On both sides the volume necessary was first judged by small test doses observed whilst screening, since adrenal infarction has resulted from using excessive doses.

The method has also been used for deliberate infarction of the adrenal or of small adrenal tumours.

Inferior vena cavography. This procedure has occasionally proved useful in showing the relationship of large ectopic phaeochromocytomas (Fig. 36.25).

Hormone assay. Catheterization of the vena cava can be performed for blood sampling at different sites and levels in suspected *phaeochromocytomas*. This is usually done when other techniques have failed to localize a suspected tumour. Samples are taken from the renal veins, and high and low in the inferior vena cava. Since these tumours can be intrathoracic or in the pelvis samples may also be taken from the superior vena cava and the iliac veins.

The techniques of blood sampling and hormone assay are also used in suspected *Conn's tumours*. Samples are taken from the adrenal veins or as near to their mouths as possible. Some consider that adrenal vein aldosterone is diagnostic in cases of Conn's tumour, even without phlebography, the value being abnormally high on the tumour side and normal on the other. In cases of bilateral hyperplasia the aldosterone level is elevated on both sides.

Isotope scanning. Conn et al (1972) first reported the successful demonstration of Conn's tumours by radioisotope scanning. Unfortunately the isotope then used gave a rather high radiation dose, but later radiopharmaceuticals have been produced which give more acceptable doses. Where the technique is available it is a useful non-invasive method of investigating Conn's tumours (Fig. 36.23).

However, there are pitfalls and we have seen a tumour wrongly diagnosed in a patient with a normal gland and a non-functioning gland on the opposite side. Using the same isotope, scanning can also be used to demonstrate adrenal adenomas in Cushing's disease, but the drug is of no use with the commoner phaeochromocytoma. More recently an isotope has been developed (MIGB) which will demonstrate phaeochromocytomas (see below and Fig. 36.35A).

Ultrasound. Large adrenal masses are readily demonstrable by ultrasound (Fig. 36.29), but small tumours, as with Conn's syndrome, are not easily identified by this method and can be missed. Ectopic tumours can also be easily missed. However, ultrasound should always be the investigation of first choice in infants and children and in pregnant women.

CT scanning. The advent of high resolution body scanners in the late 1970s revolutionized the diagnosis of adrenal tumours. A modern body scanner will demonstrate the normal adrenal glands in all but exceptional cases, and tumours of 1 cm diameter or less can be identified. CT will also demonstrate ectopic tumours such as phaeochromocytomas in the majority of cases where the lesion is locally ectopic in the region of the kidney. Even when the tumour lies in the pelvis or the thorax CT can identify the lesion, provided the correct area is scanned.

MRI Adrenal tumours have already been identified by this revolutionary new technique. Since the method is not only non-invasive but also involves no radiation or known hazard it may eventually become the method of choice. However, the technique is not yet widely available, nor is resolution of abdominal structures yet as good as that achieved by CT. When these defects have been overcome, the future will undoubtedly lie with MRI.

Needle biopsy. This can be performed on adrenal masses, either with X-ray or ultrasound control, when the mass is large, or under CT control with smaller lesions. The procedure is useful when an adrenal mass has been demonstrated and its nature is not yet clinically clear. This may occur when an adrenal mass is found unexpectedly during CT of the abdomen for other causes, or when an abdominal mass in the adrenal area, but without other clinical manifestation, is under investigation. Figure 36.7 shows needling of a mass which proved positive for secondary carcinoma. Primary adrenal carcinoma frequently presents as a large mass with no other physical signs.

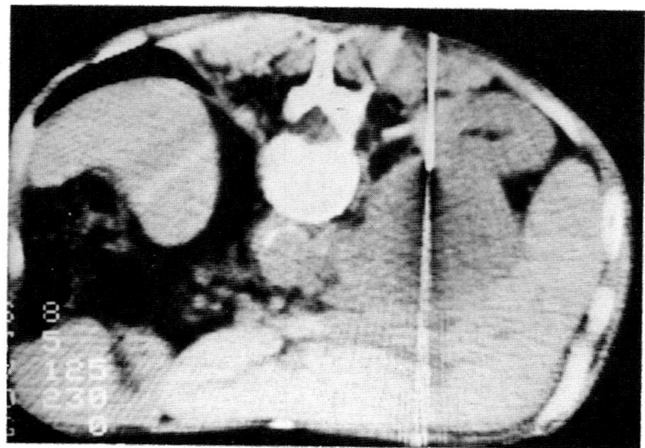

Fig. 36.7 Needle biopsy of right adrenal tumour under CT control with patient prone. Histology adenocarcinoma from bowel (L36 W256).

CHOICE OF INVESTIGATION

It is clear from the above discussion that there are now a large battery of tests available using radiology or imaging to show adrenal tumours. On general principles, the least invasive techniques will be used first.

Simple X-rays, or tomography with high-dose IVP, are relatively cheap and easily available.

Of the newer imaging techniques ultrasound is cheapest and most widely available. It is certainly the method of choice in infants and children. However, it is unlikely to be helpful with very small or ectopic lesions, and is less useful in adults where such tumours are common.

Isotope scanning is useful with the small Conn's tumour and with Cushing's syndrome, but the technique is time consuming and expensive, and does not yield the immediate results possible with other techniques. The recent introduction of an isotope which will demonstrate phaeochromocytomas has extended the value of the method and has the advantage of including ectopic tumours (see below).

CT scanning has proved the most useful and most widely accepted of the newer imaging techniques, since it provides immediate and accurate diagnosis in all but the tiniest of adrenal tumours and the occasional ectopic phaeochromocytoma. This is likely to remain the case until MRI becomes more widely available.

The invasive techniques of arteriography and phlebography are now rarely necessary where access to modern imaging techniques is freely available. However, there are still large areas of the world where this is not the case, and where invasive methods remain the only means of diagnosis. Otherwise they will be reserved for the occasional problem case, such as the suspected phaeochromocytoma which other methods have failed to demonstrate.

NEUROBLASTOMA

Characteristically these tumours occur in children and present either with an abdominal mass or with manifestations of secondary deposit. Over half of them arise in the adrenals, but they can arise from sympathetic tissue anywhere in the body.

Radiological investigation by plain X-rays can be very helpful. They may show an abdominal mass visible by virtue of its size, or by downward displacement of the kidney, or by the presence of calcification. The latter has been noted to occur in over one-third of cases. An IVP

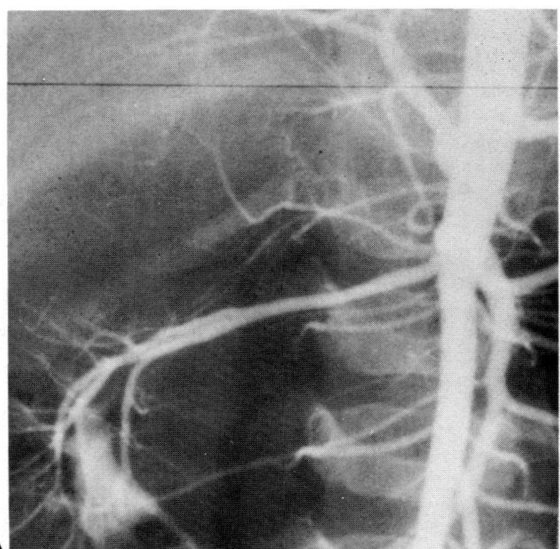

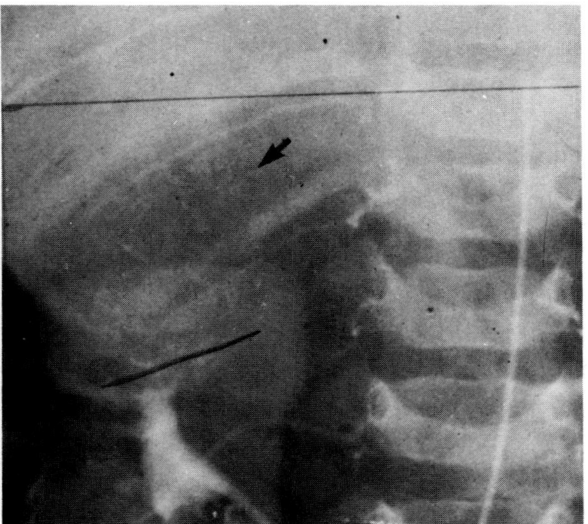

Fig. 36.8 A and **B.** Renal arteriogram in a child with neuroblastoma. The nephrogram shows clearly that the mass lies above the kidney. There is limited pathological circulation supplied by a hypertrophied middle adrenal artery. (Courtesy of Dr F. Starer.)

may be helpful in confirming the kidney displacement, with downward drooping of the pelvis and calyces.

Sometimes it is very difficult to differentiate between a renal mass, such as Wilm's tumour, and a suprarenal mass on simple X-ray and even on IVP. Calcification, if present, is an important point in favour of neuroblastoma since it is less common in Wilm's tumour. In the past, angiography has been helpful and has been used to settle the differential point (Fig. 36.8). Both Wilm's tumour and neuroblastoma can be quite vascular but are sometimes very poorly vascularized. However, a Wilm's tumour is more likely to show a florid pathological circulation than a neuroblastoma. The latter usually displaces the kidney downwards and produces extrinsic distortion of its outline, but the renal substance, as shown in the nephrogram is seen to be intact.

Ultrasound is now most widely used in the investigation of abdominal masses in children (see Ch. 37). CT may be more specific but has the disadvantage of using ionizing radiation. MRI may prove a safer and better imaging method, but is not yet widely available or fully evaluated.

GANGLIONEUROMA

This is a mature form of neurogenic tumour. Apart from arising in the adrenal, these tumours can, like neuroblastoma, arise from the parasympathetic system elsewhere along the spine, particularly in the thorax.

Like neuroblastomas they are commoner in children but although 60% occur before the age of 20 a good proportion present in adults.

Ganglioneuromas occurring in children may also show calcification, which can help in suggesting a diagnosis of neurogenic tumour (Fig. 36.6). Occasionally, as in this case, ganglioneuromata invade the spinal canal. In these cases there is not only an extraspinal mass but also an intraspinal component causing neurological symptoms either from cord compression or from involvement of the cauda equina. These rare cases are usually mistaken for dumb-bell neurofibromata.

If the lesion presents in a child, and calcification is present in the paraspinal mass, the diagnosis of ganglioneuroma should always be considered. It is interesting that some of the recorded cases were first reported histologically as neuroblastomas but a second and later biopsy showed ganglioneuroma. It is now well recognized that neuroblastomas can sometimes mature into the more benign and well-differentiated tumour.

ADRENAL CORTICAL ADENOMA

Cortical adenomas, usually small, are said to be present in 5% of routine necropsies. The vast majority of these are presumably non-functional and symptomless during life, but the figure implies that such adenomas will occasionally be seen as purely chance findings at CT.

Functioning adenomas may give rise to Cushing's syndrome (cortisol secreting), Conn's syndrome (mineralocorticoid secreting) or very rarely a virilizing syndrome (androgen secreting). These are discussed in more detail below.

ADRENAL CORTICAL CARCINOMA

As with adenomas, these tumours may be non-functional. Such tumours eventually present either with metastases or with a mass in the abdomen. Like adenomas, the functioning tumours can present in different ways. Depending

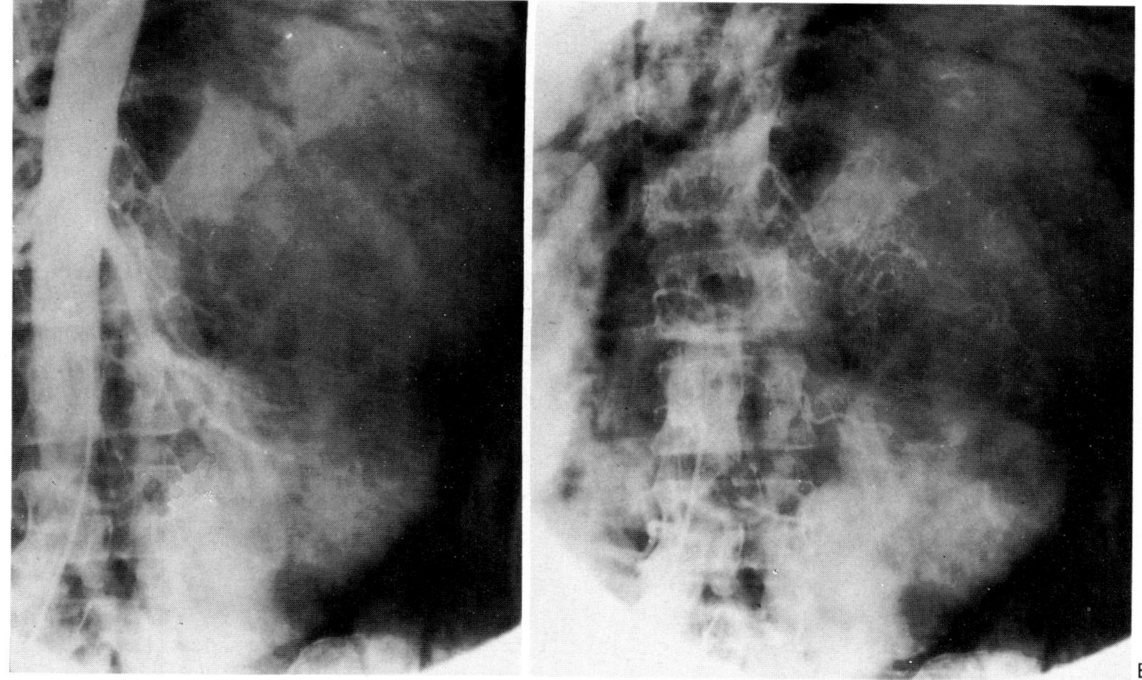

Fig. 36.9 A. and **B.** Adrenal carcinoma shown by flush aortogram. There is a pathological circulation supplied by hypertrophied adrenal arteries. The nephrogram of the kidney is displaced downwards.

on the type of secretion, Cushing's syndrome, a virilizing syndrome or Conn's syndrome may all occur. Though commoner in adults — the average age of diagnosis is 45 years — they are occasionally seen in children.

Adrenal carcinomas are often quite large at discovery. In one series the average size was about 15 cm in diameter. With such large masses, simple X-ray or IVU with tomography will often show the lesion well and there will be downward displacement of the kidney. About one-third of such carcinomas show calcification at simple X-ray and even more do so at CT (Fig. 36.11). This is usually patchy and irregular.

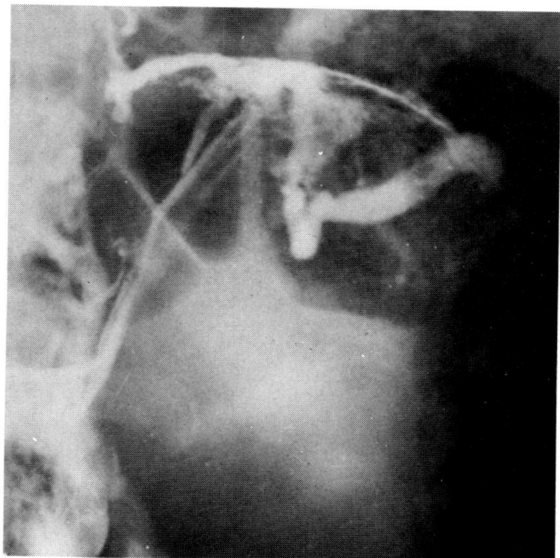

Fig. 36.10 Left adrenal phlebogram. This shows a large adrenal mass which has drainage veins communicating with other retroperitoneal veins. The patient presented with Conn's syndrome due to an adrenal carcinoma.

Invasive methods have been used in the past in the investigation of suspected cases but should rarely be required now except in problem cases, e.g. in helping to differentiate a non-functional adrenal carcinoma from an upper pole renal carcinoma (Fig. 36.9), or a functional adenoma from a carcinoma (Fig. 36.10).

Ultrasound will demonstrate large adrenal masses well, but CT is preferable, except in children, since it will show spread to adjacent structures better and will define involvement of glands and liver (Figs 36.11, 36.12). This is found in 50% of cases and the peritoneum and the opposite adrenal become involved in 10% of patients.

The prognosis in these cases is poor. Few patients survive 5 years and most die within 2 years of diagnosis.

METASTASES

The adrenal glands may be involved on one or both sides by metastases from primary carcinoma elsewhere in the body and are commonly involved in patients with bronchial and breast carcinoma. CT surveys of the liver and abdomen are frequently made in these patients, and the adrenals should always be carefully checked at such examinations (Fig. 36.13).

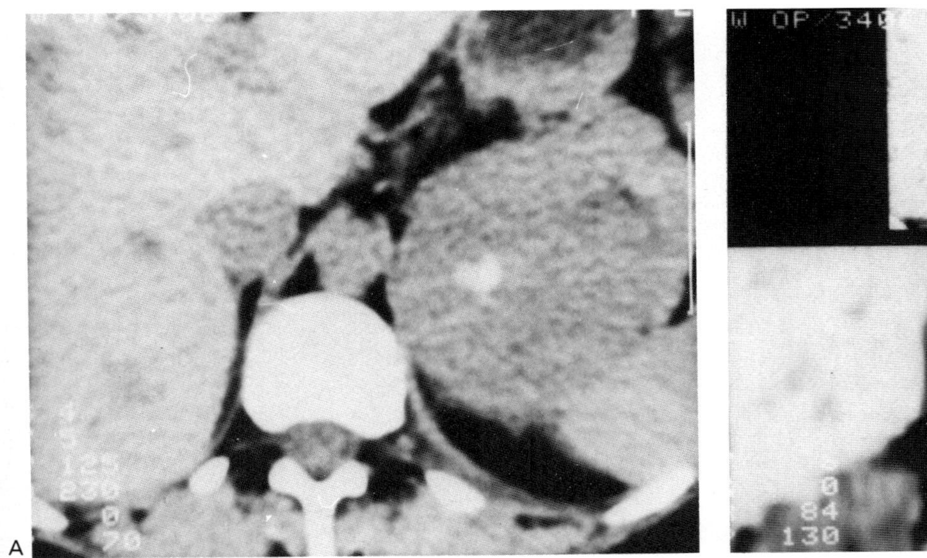

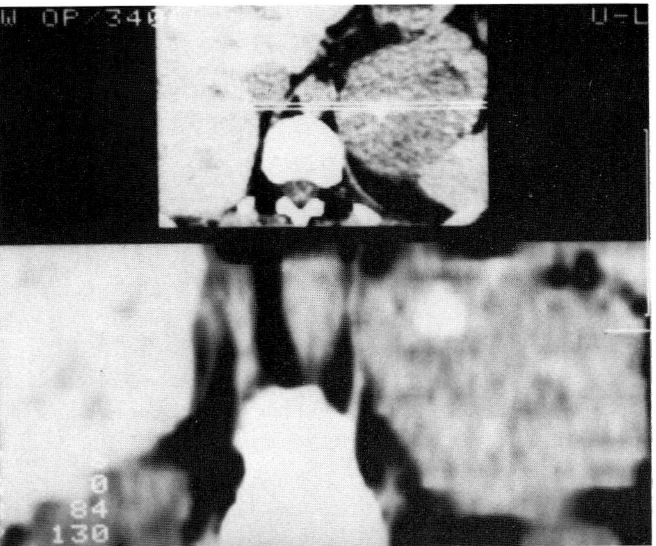

Fig. 36.11 A. Large mass in left adrenal. Note the nodular calcification in the tumour and low density areas in the liver. Adrenal carcinoma presenting with Cushing's syndrome (L36 W256). **B.** Coronal reconstruction of tumour (L38 W128).

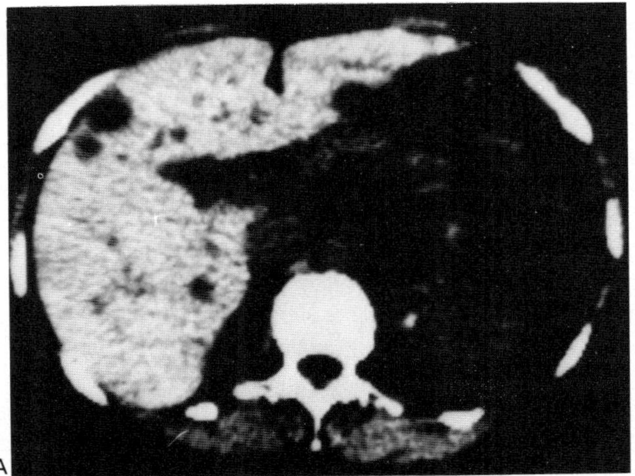

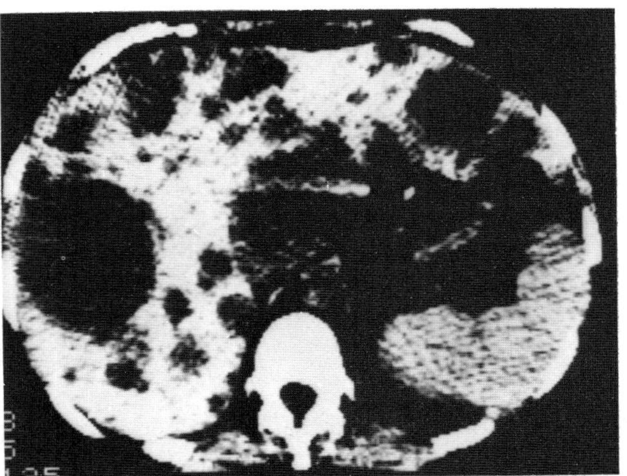

Fig. 36.12 A. Same patient as Figure 36.11, showing deposits in liver at narrow window (L63 W64). **B.** Six months later, and following removal of adrenal tumour, deposits have increased in size (L50 W64).

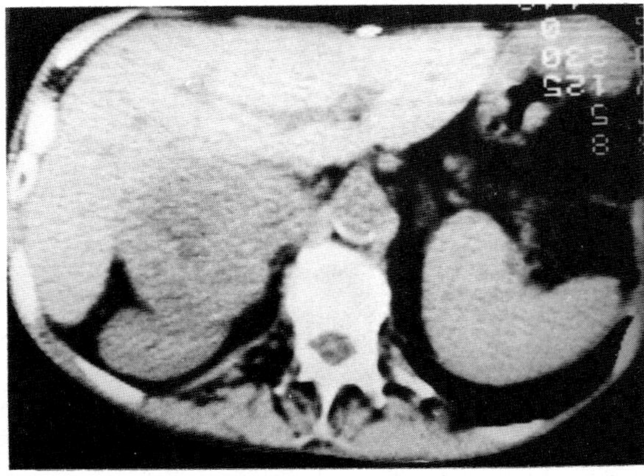

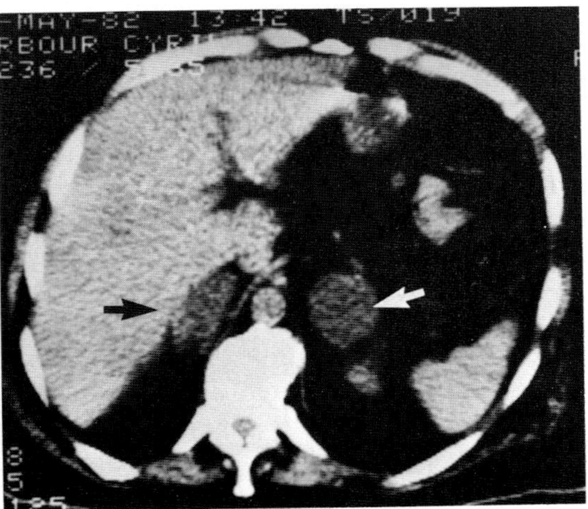

Fig. 36.13 A. Large metastasis in right adrenal (L36 W256). **B.** Bilateral metastases (arrows) in the adrenals from bronchial carcinoma (L45 W256).

Sometimes a mass is found in the adrenal in the presence of secondaries elsewhere and no apparent primary. In such cases, or with a solitary mass in the adrenal and no clinical clue as to its nature, needle biopsy may help to establish a diagnosis (Fig. 36.7).

LIPOMA AND MYELOLIPOMA

These are rare tumours of the adrenal which have been reported at autopsy in the past. Though usually small, they have been recorded up to 12 cm in diameter. They are composed mainly of fat cells, but may contain focal areas of myeloid tissue. With the increasing use of CT they are now being encountered as chance findings (Fig. 36.14), when they are of fatty density, or occasionally of density suggesting mixed tissue.

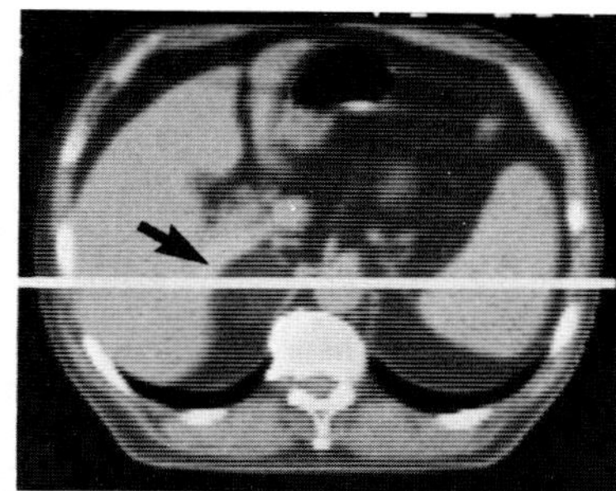

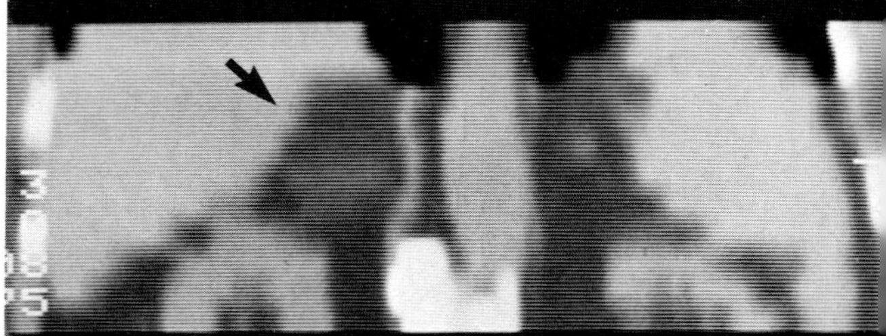

Fig. 36.14 Rt adrenal lipoma (↘). Coronal reconstruction of low-density mass (-67 HU) (L46 41024).

ADRENAL CYSTS

Kearney and Mahoney (1977) have classified adrenal cysts as:

1. Endothelial (45%)
2. Pseudocyst (39%)
3. Epithelial (9%)
4. Parasitic (hydatid)

Pseudocysts are the type clinically encountered most commonly, though endothelial cysts are commoner at autopsy. Pseudocysts result from haemorrhage or necrosis and are seen in both normal glands and in tumours, varying in diameter from a few millimetres to many centimetres. Calcification may ensue in the wall of the haemorrhagic or necrotic cyst. Presentation is either in neonates or in adults.

Neonatal adrenal haemorrhage is not uncommon in association with birth trauma or infection and often goes undiagnosed with recovery of the child. The neonate adrenal gland is relatively huge weighing 8 g against the adult weight of 5 g. The haemorrhage may present as an abdominal mass or as bilateral masses which can develop marginal calcification as they regress over several weeks. If clinically suspected, the diagnosis can best be confirmed by ultrasound, which should differentiate from the more solid neuroblastoma (see Ch. 37 p. 1084).

Adult adrenal cysts can occur as benign pseudocysts following haemorrhage. They may also occur following haemorrhage or necrosis in large tumours (Fig. 36.28), either benign or malignant. They are best shown by ultrasound or CT, the latter being preferred as usually providing more information, particularly with neoplasms. Asymptomatic adrenal cysts observed as chance findings at CT and with no apparent tumour present can be treated conservatively. Marginal curvilinear or eggshell calcification may be noted in some 20% of cases. In doubtful cases, needle aspiration of the fluid may help by cytology for malignant cells or confirming evidence of old haemorrhage.

ANDROGEN EXCESS

The term 'adrenogenital syndrome' is no longer favoured by endocrinologists. Several different adrenal lesions may give rise to excess of androgen production including *congenital adrenal hyperplasis (CAH)*, adrenal adenoma and adrenal carcinoma.

CAH is a complex group of congenital disorders of adrenal steroid synthesizing enzymes with a wide spectrum of clinical presentation. These range from neonatal collapse, through intersex to adult presentation with sex hormone disorders.

Neonates may present with ambiguous genitalia, and older children with a virilizing syndrome in the female, or isosexual precocity in the male. In the adult, hirsuties or masculinizing features may be the presenting features.

Biochemical tests will usually establish the diagnosis and CT will clearly demonstrate CAH or an adrenal mass. In infants and children, ultrasound should be used as the primary investigation.

CUSHING'S SYNDROME

The following table summarizes the different types of spontaneous Cushing's syndrome and their approximate incidence.

Imaging findings. There are many interesting simple radiological features in Cushing's syndrome. These are discussed in Chapter 8 and depend on the catabolic effect

Table 36.3 Spontaneous Cushing's syndrome

	Approximate incidence
A. Due to excess ACTH production	
1. Pituitary dependent	
a. Pituitary microadenoma	very common 80%
b. Alcoholic	common
c. Depressive psychosis	very rare
2. Ectopic ACTH production	
a. Malignant tumours	common
b. Benign tumours	rare
B. Due to primary adrenal lesions	
1. Adrenal cortical adenoma	common (5–10%)
2. Adrenal cortical carcinoma	rare (1%)
3. Micronodular dysplasia	very rare

resulting in osteoporosis affecting mainly the axial skeleton. *Vertebral collapse* is common, as are *spontaneous rib fractures*, often painless and with excessive callus formation. *Ischaemic necrosis of the femoral heads* may also occur.

In patients with suspected adrenal tumours simple X-ray may sometimes demonstrate an adrenal mass. An adenoma may be shown by high-dose IVP with tomography. Carcinomas may contain calcification and are usually quite large in size at presentation. In children ultrasound should be used as the first imaging procedure, but in adults the presence of suspected adrenal tumours is best confirmed by CT. Cortical adenomas are readily identified being usually 3–8 cm in diameter. Carcinomas are usually larger in size and often contain calcification (Fig. 36.11). CT may also show evidence of secondaries in the liver or glandular involvement (Fig. 36.12). Fatty infiltration of the liver, a recognized feature of Cushing's syndrome, may be identified at CT in some cases.

Pituitary-dependent cases may show clear evidence of bilateral adrenal hyperplasia (Fig. 36.15) as may cases due to ectopic ACTH production, but the adrenals frequently seem normal at CT in these cases. Some of these cases with apparently normal adrenals have been operated on and moderate enlargement of the adrenals proved. It appears therefore that mild enlargement can be missed by CT.

The radiologist is frequently asked to X-ray the skull in patients presenting with Cushing's syndrome, but this is rarely necessary since pituitary tumours in this condition are usually microscopic and do not produce enlargement of the sella. There are occasional exceptions to this rule. In particular, patients who have been treated by adrenalectomy may develop large adenomas which enlarge the sella (Nelson's syndrome).

Petrosal vein sampling for raised ACTH levels has been used to identify pituitary microadenomas. These lesions

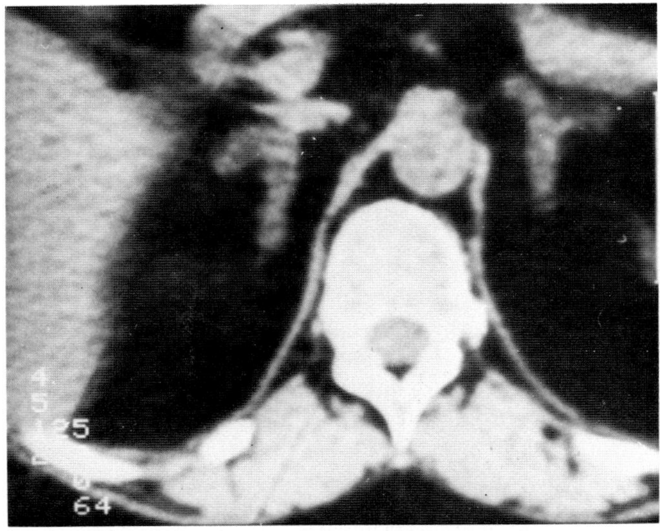

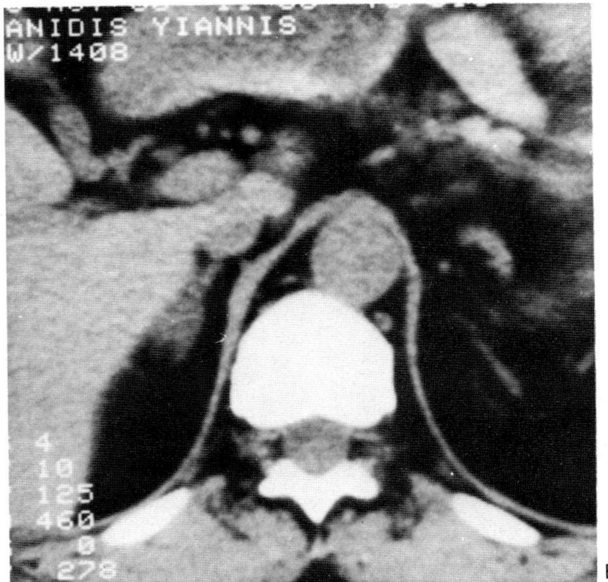

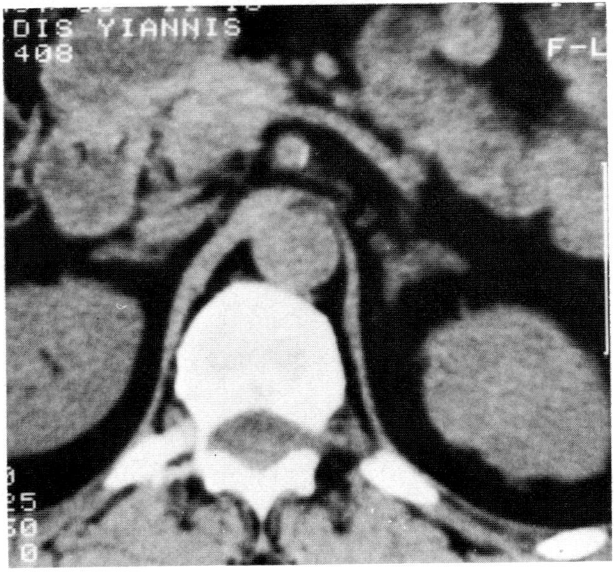

Fig. 36.15 A. Bilateral adrenal hyperplasia (L36 W512). **B.** and **C.** Hypertrophied R and L adrenals in another patient (L36 W512).

may be small and unilateral. Thus, it is vital that sampling should be bilateral, since an abnormal value may be present on one side only (Doppman et al., 1984). Lateralization will also be invaluable in aiding trans-sphenoidal surgery.

Patients with *ectopic ACTH production* are most commonly suffering from malignant tumours. This is most likely to be a lung carcinoma, which is the cause in 60% of such cases. Pancreatic carcinoma, malignant thymoma and medullary carcinoma of the thyroid are also well-documented causes, whilst isolated cases have been described with other forms of primary carcinoma. Benign tumours involved include carcinoids, benign thymomas and very rarely phaeochromocytomas and ganglioneuromas. In some patients with ectopic ACTH production the clinical features may give some clue as to the primary tumour. Simple X-ray of the chest may demonstrate the lesion. If not, CT may be helpful with particular attention to the lungs, mediastinum, pancreas and upper abdomen.

Micronodular adrenal dysplasia is a rare cause of Cushing's syndrome in children. The aetiology is unknown. The adrenals are enlarged and contain multiple tiny adenomas a millimetre or so in diameter. Excess cortical production in *alcoholism* is well recognized and, like that seen occasionally in severe *depressive psychosis*, is ACTH dependent. However, the mechanism remains uncertain.

PRIMARY ALDOSTERONISM (CONN'S SYNDROME)

Primary hyperaldosteronism, or Conn's syndrome, is characterized by hypokalaemia, weakness and hypertension. It is known that in most cases the cause is a small adenoma of the adrenal. The demonstration of such a small lesion by radiological methods was, until recent years, not possible. Certainly, plain X-ray or even arteriography could hardly hope to show lesions 1 cm or less in size. Historically, it was the development of adrenal phlebography which first made it possible to demonstrate these small adenomas in Conn's syndrome (Sutton 1968). The characteristic feature is usually an arc-like vein in the circumference of the tumour, which is relatively avascular (Figs 36.16, 36.17).

Larger Conn's tumours were occasionally seen as in Figure 36.18. Calcification has not been recorded in the literature in these small tumours, but was present in the case illustrated, and it was thought that this was in a haemorrhagic cyst in an unusually large tumour. When adrenal phlebography was more widely used, occasional cases of adrenal infarction were reported. However, this was probably associated with the use of excessive doses of contrast or excessive injection pressures (see above).

Adrenal vein sampling can be carried out at the same time and was practised by some workers without phlebography because of the fear of infarction. Aldosterone concentrations in relation to cortisol are measured on the two sides. In adenoma patients the concentration is increased on the affected side and suppressed on the other. In patients with hyperplasia the raised concentrations are similar on the two sides.

With the advent of CT it has become clear that even small adenomas can be identified without the need for invasive techniques. Figures 36.19–36.22 illustrate the appearance of Conn's tumours at CT. Since the tumours are usually small and may be under 1 cm in diameter, it is vital that the CT examination should cover the whole of the gland by continuous cuts and be undertaken with 4 mm or 5 mm collimators. Narrower collimators, i.e. 2 mm or less are at a disadvantage in the abdomen, since it is difficult to stop expiration at exactly the same point for each section. Conn's tumours are of relatively low density averaging (about 20 H). Presumably this is due to

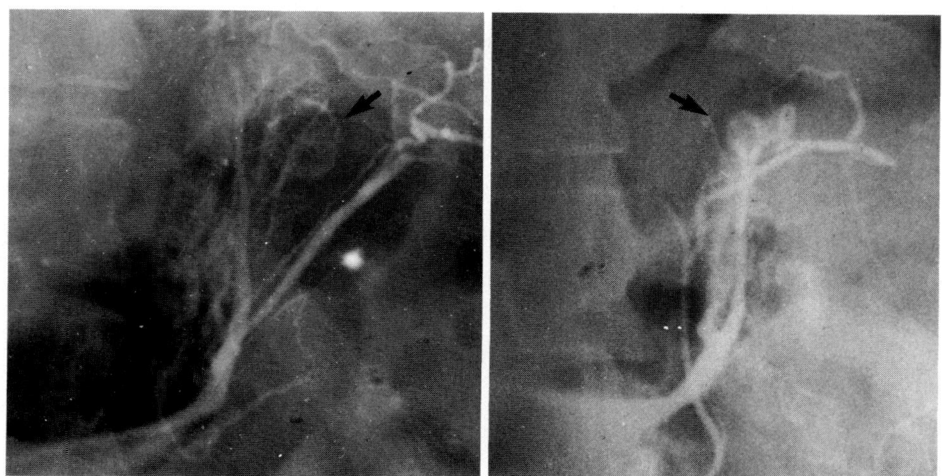

Fig. 36.16 A. and **B.** Left adrenal phlebogram showing small Conn's tumours (arrows) in two different cases.

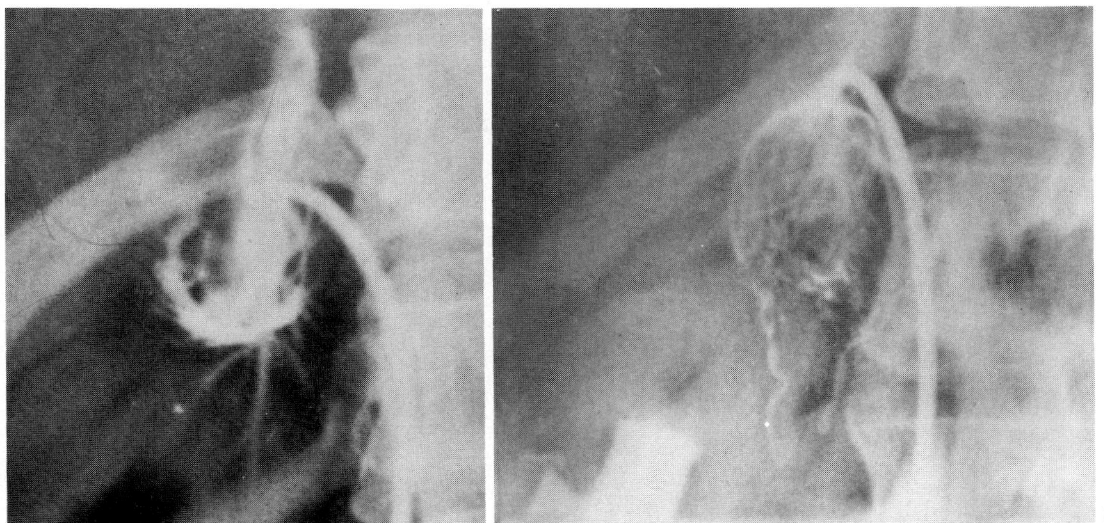

Fig. 36.17 A. and **B.** Right adrenal phlebograms showing Conn's tumours. Two different patients.

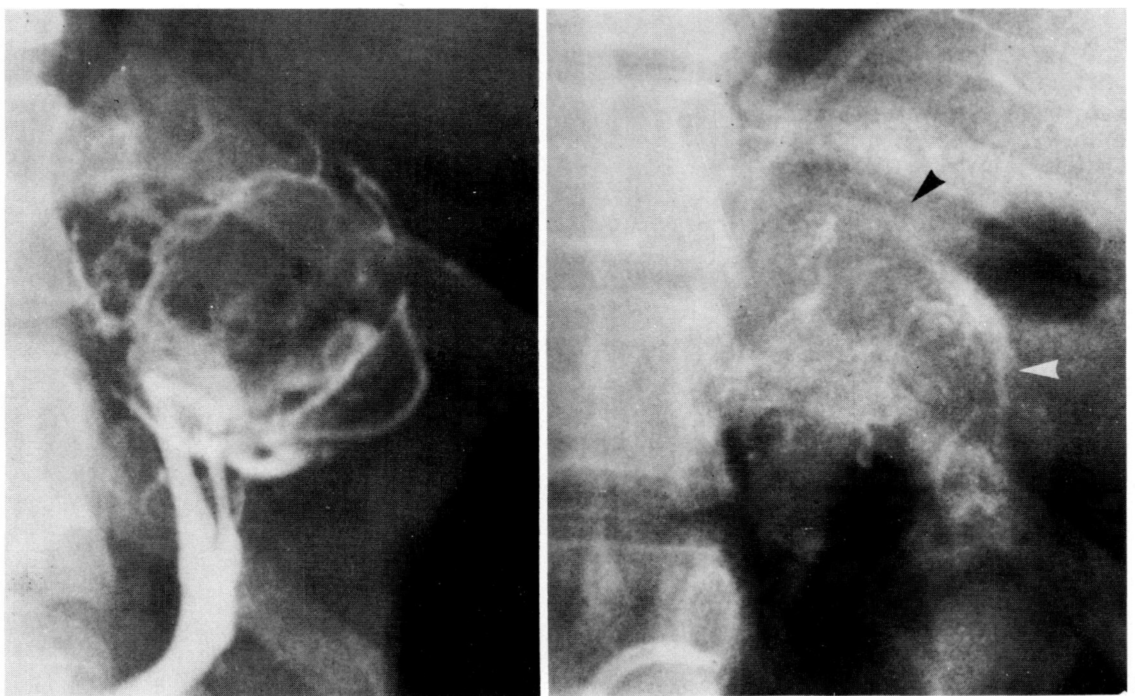

Fig. 36.18 A. Left adrenal phlebogram showing large Conn's tumour. **B.** Selective inferior phrenic arteriogram showing the same tumour (arrows) as in **A.**

their high cholesterol content. These tumours are unusual in children, but it would theoretically be desirable to use ultrasound before CT in a child. However, ultrasound has been of little use so far in diagnosing these small lesions in adults.

Scintigraphy has been successfully used to demonstrate Conn's tumours using labelled cholesterol during dexamethasone suppression (2 mg 6-hourly for 2 days previously) (Fig. 36.23). However, CT is now generally accepted as the primary investigation of choice.

Excessive production of aldosterone from an adenoma of the zona glomerulosa of the adrenal cortex is the cause of the syndrome in up to 80% of cases. A smaller proportion are due to bilateral micronodular hyperplasia and, in a few mysterious cases, the adrenals are found to be normal both macroscopically and microscopically.

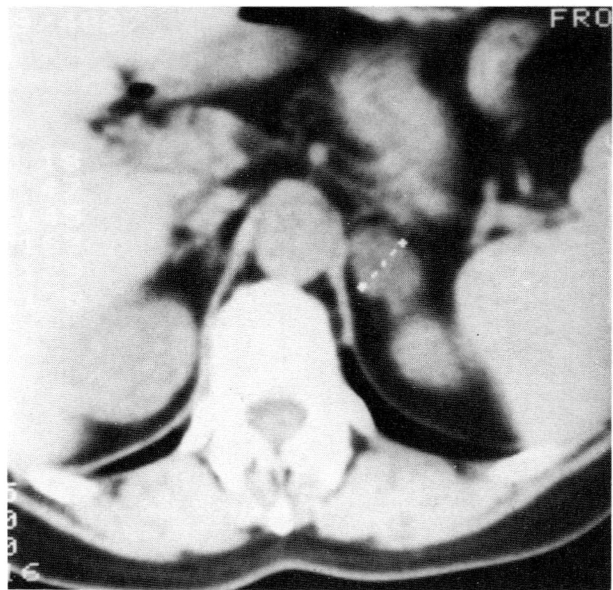

Fig. 36.19

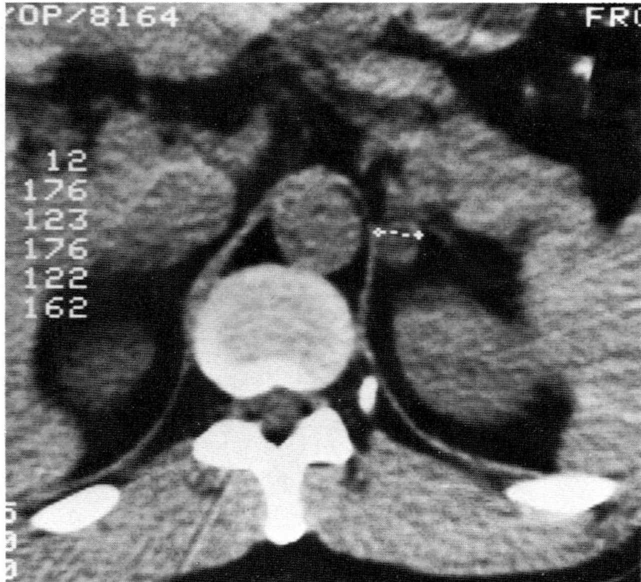

Fig. 36.20

Figs 36.19 and 36.20 Left-sided Conn's tumours in different patients. They measure 1.8 and 1.2 cm in diameter respectively (L36 and L45 W512).

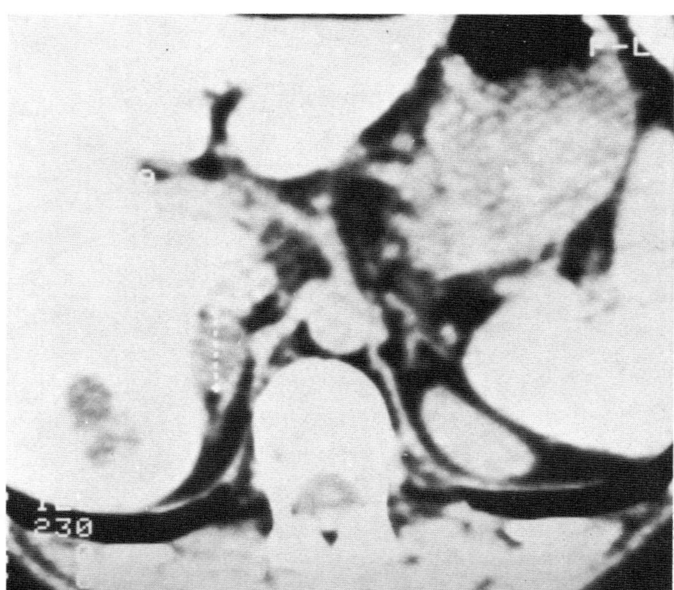

Fig. 36.21 Right-sided Conn's tumour 1.9 cm in diameter. Normal L. adrenal also well shown. (L36 W256).

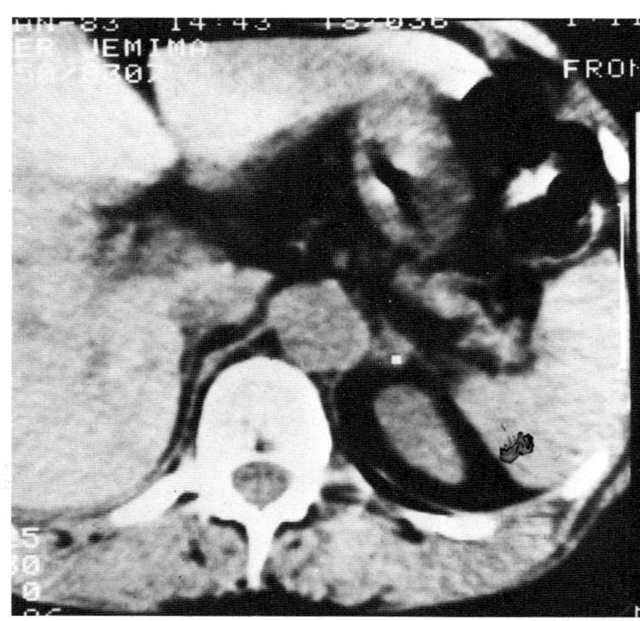

Fig. 36.22 Small L Conn's tumour 0.8 cm in diameter (Density 20 H) (L43 W512).

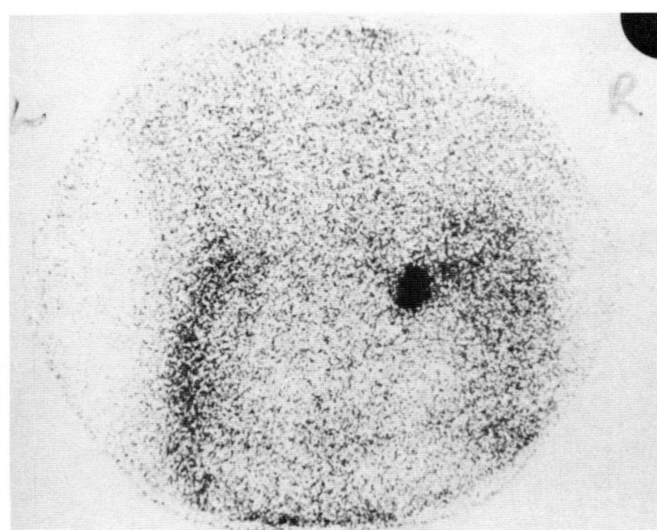

Fig. 36.23 Right-sided Conn's tumour shown by scintigraphy 7 days postinjection.

PHAEOCHROMOCYTOMA

This has proved to be the commonest adrenal tumour observed in our clinical practice. The classical clinical presentation is with attacks of paroxysmal hypertension accompanied by headache, sweating, palpitation, anxiety and tremor. The attacks may last from 15 minutes to an hour and may occur several times a week or even a day. However, many cases are less typical and 50% of adult cases present with sustained hypertension.

90% of these tumours arise in the adrenals but the remaining 10% may be found anywhere in the sympathetic system from the neck to the pelvis. The majority of these *ectopic tumours* are adjacent to the kidneys and we have seen such tumours at the hilum of the kidney (Figs 36.24, 36.34), medial to the inferior vena cava (Fig. 36.25) and below the kidney (Fig. 36.26). The organs of Zuckerkandl adjacent to the aortic bifurcation is also a common extra-adrenal site. Other tumours have been found in the bladder wall, and such patients have sometimes presented with attacks of hypertension brought on by micturition. Thoracic tumours are usually paravertebral (Fig. 36.39) but have been found in the mediastinum (Fig. 36.27).

Some 10% of these tumours appear to be familial, and a similar proportion occur in children. Multiple tumours also occur in a similar percentage, as do bilateral adrenal tumours and malignant tumours. The so-called 'rule of ten' summarizes this by postulating that 10% of cases are:

1. Familial
2. Bilateral adrenal
3. Multiple (other than above)
4. Extra-adrenal
5. Children
6. Malignant

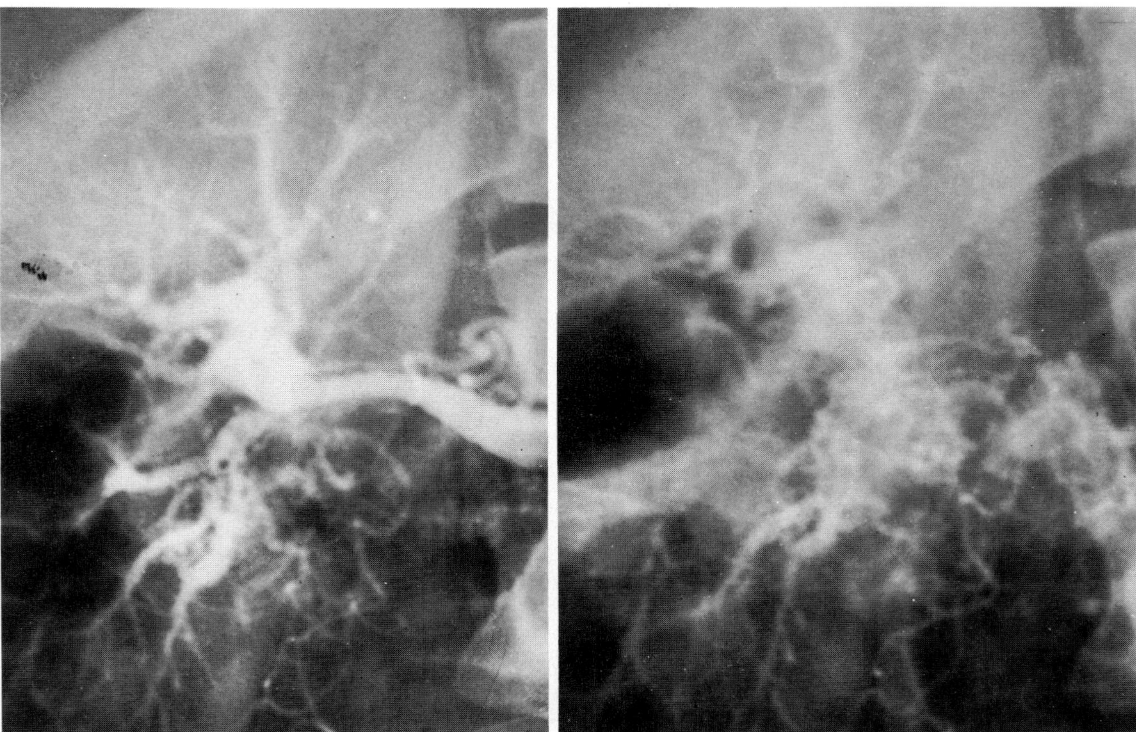

Fig. 36.24 A. and **B.** Vascular phaeochromocytoma below right renal artery, which is stretched over the tumour.

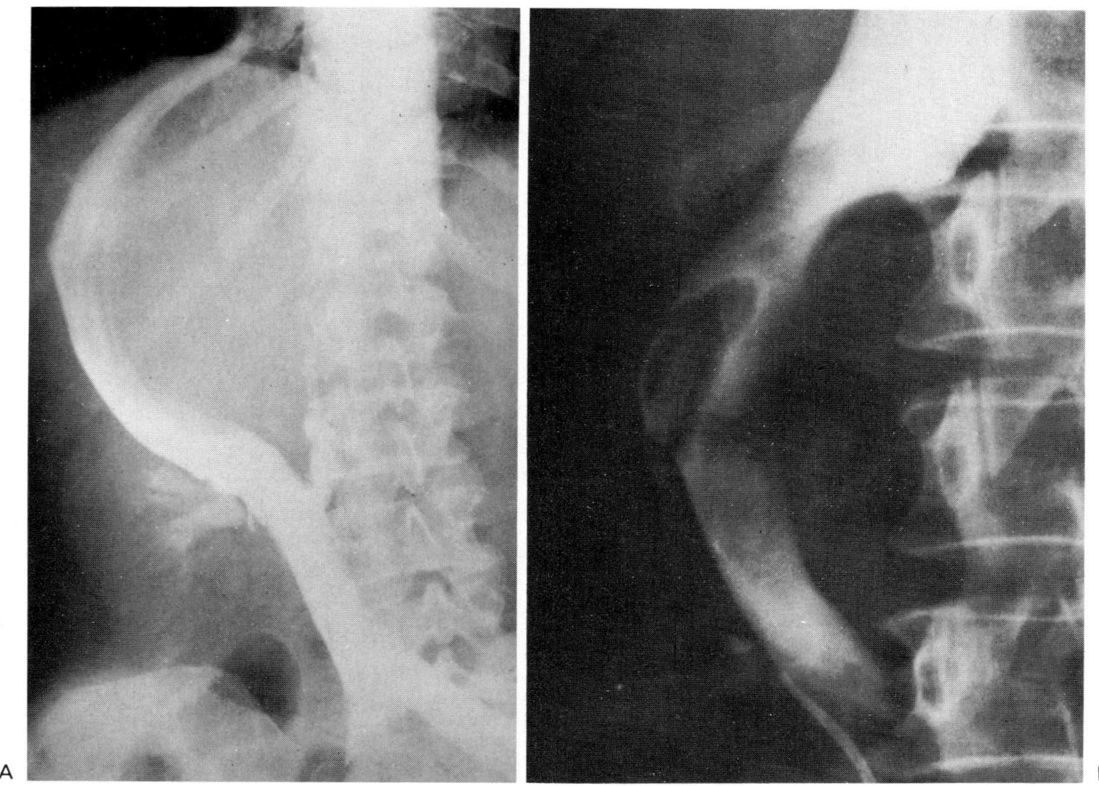

Fig. 36.25 A. and **B.** Inferior vena cavography in two different patients, each with phaeochromocytomas lying medial to the inferior vena cava.

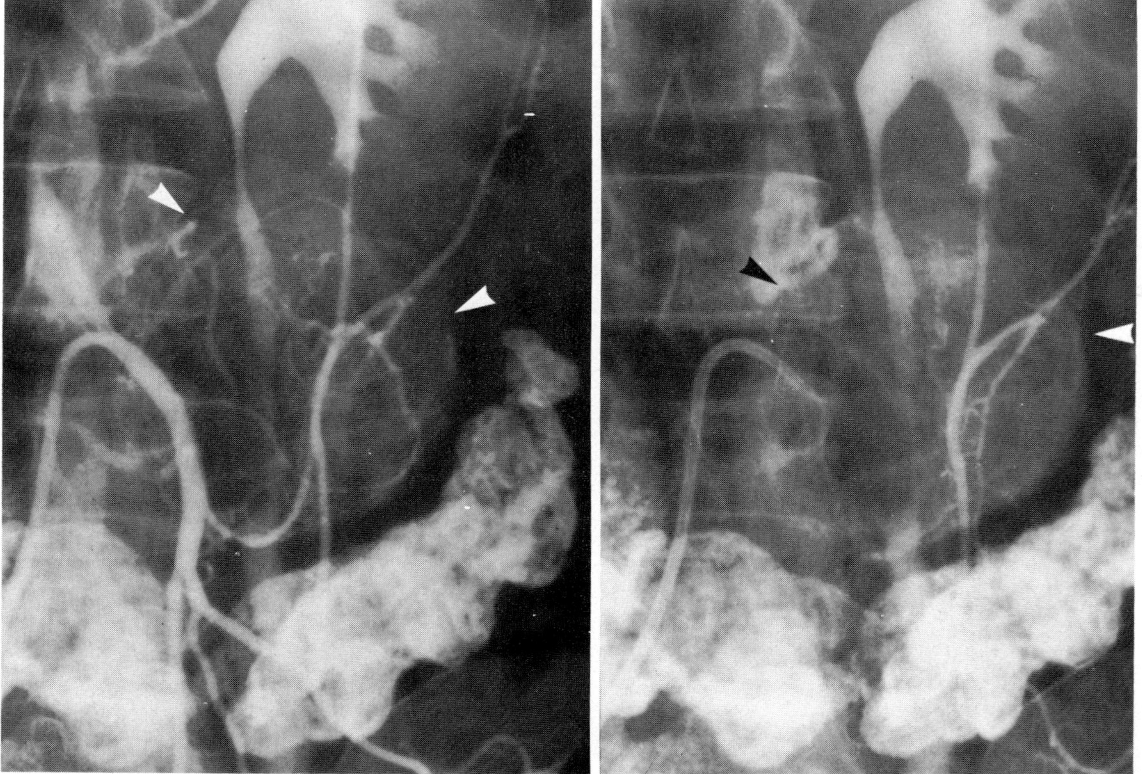

Fig. 36.26 A. and **B.** Phaeochromocytoma lying below the left kidney and shown by selective inferior mesenteric arteriography. It had no other artery of supply.

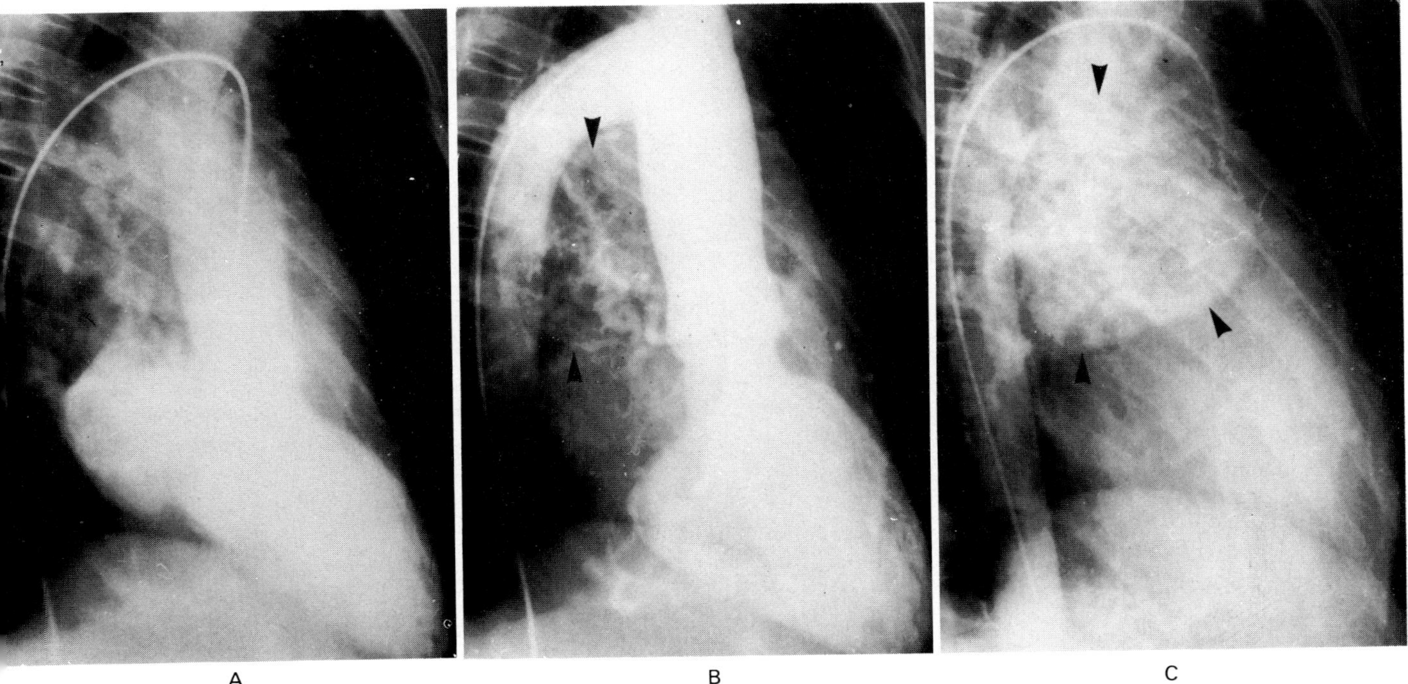

Fig. 36.27 Left ventricular angiocardiogram. **A.** There is evidence of marked mitral incompetence. **B.** and **C.** Pathological vessels are shown arising from the aorta to supply a large vascular mass above the left auricle. Phaeochromocytoma removed by surgery.

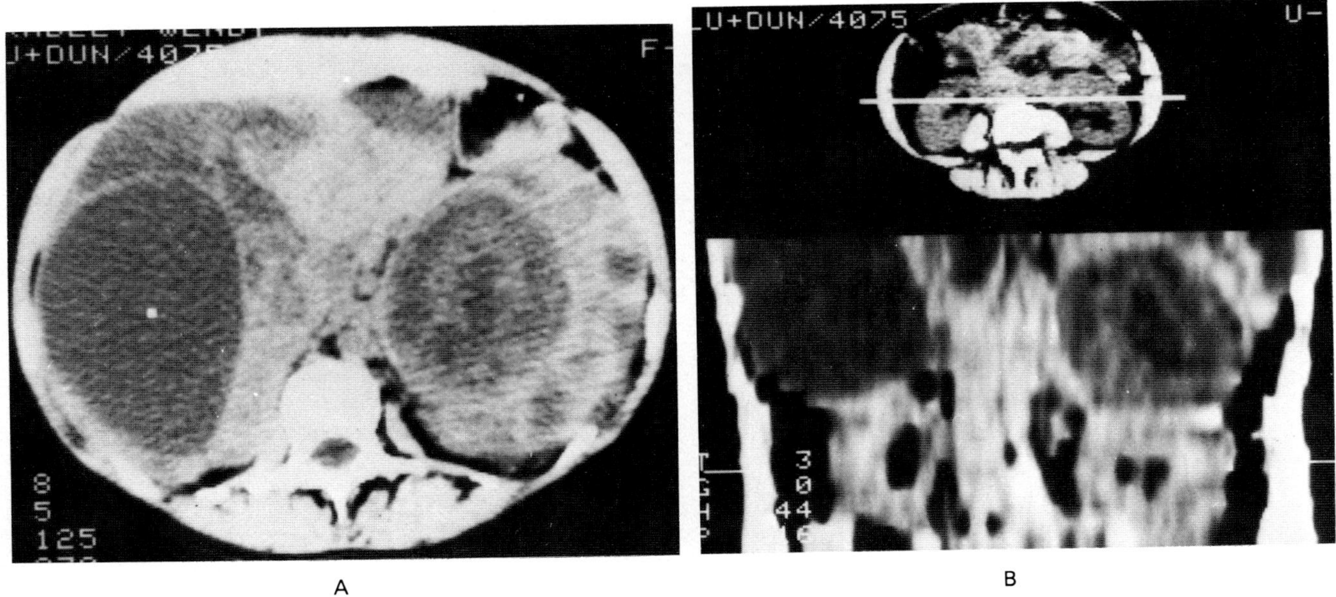

Fig. 36.28 A. Giant bilateral cystic phaeochromocytomas displacing the kidneys down and liver upwards (L36 W128). **B.** Coronal reconstruction through tumours and downward displaced kidneys (L36 W64).

Some 5% of cases are associated with *neurofibromatosis*, but the reverse is less common, since only 1% of patients with neurofibromatosis develop phaeochromocytoma.

There is also a less common, but well-recognized, association with medullary carcinoma of the thyroid and hyperparathyroidism which may be familial. This is usually referred to as multiple endocrine neoplasia (MEN type 2) or Sipple's syndrome. When the medullary carcinoma of the thyroid and phaeochromocytoma are associated with mucosal neuromata involving conjunctiva, eyelid, mouth and sometimes gut, and with a Marfanoid habitus it is referred to as MEN type 3.

Apart from the clinical aspects, the firm diagnosis of phaeochromocytoma depends on the biochemical assays of catecholamines in urine or blood or both; repeated assays may be necessary as hypersecretion may be paroxysmal.

Imaging investigation. The size of the adrenal tumour at diagnosis has varied in our material from 2 or 3 cm to 20 cm in diameter, with an average of some 7 cm.

Simple abdominal X-ray or *IVU with tomography* is reasonable as the primary investigation, and may reveal a mass above the kidney with associated renal displacement.

Large adrenal masses will also be quite well shown by *ultrasound*(Fig. 36.29). However, smaller and ectopic tumours will be more difficult to demonstrate by these means. Very large tumours may undergo central necrosis and become cystic, a feature which is well seen at ultrasound or CT (Fig. 36.28).

Calcification is in our experience very rare and has only been seen once in 60 cases. In this case, as in others described in the literature, it was curvilinear and probably in the wall of a haemorrhagic cyst.

Retroperitoneal air insufflation was once widely used for the localization of phaeochromocytomas but is now obsolete. *Angiography*, after initial worries about its safety because of reports of fatalities from hypertensive crises, became widely used during the 1960s and 1970s, and proved highly successful. Some 20 cases in our material were demonstrated by angiographic techniques. Flush aortography with injection direct into the aorta showed large or vascular adrenal tumours well but could miss small and poorly vascularized tumours. Selective adrenal arteriography, if possible, would show such tumours, but it was often simpler and quicker to perform selective renal angiography. Even when the inferior adrenal artery was small it would show well by this technique; if it was enlarged it would show very well and could often be entered selectively (Fig. 36.30).

CT body scanners first begun to be used in the late 1970s and it soon became apparent that they provided an excellent non-invasive method for diagnosing phaeochromocytoma. Tumours lying in the adrenal gland are easily identified (Figs 36.31–36.33) as are bilateral adrenal tumours (Fig. 36.28). Locally, ectopic tumours are also easily identified if the examination covers the whole of

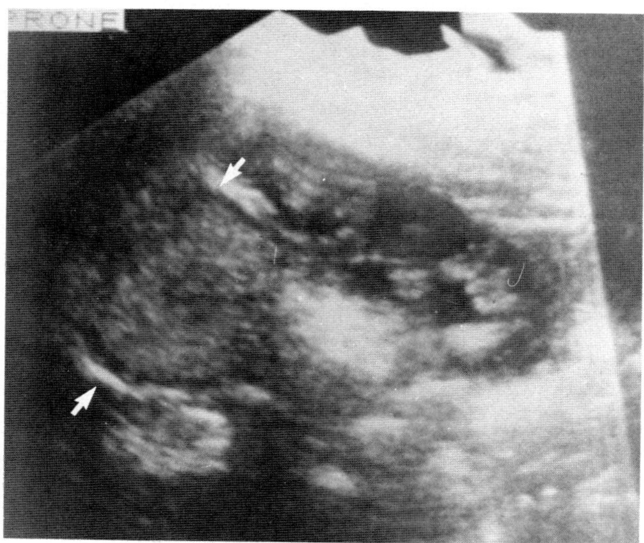

Fig. 36.29 Ultrasound scan shows large rounded tumour (arrows) above upper pole of right kidney (arrow). (Same case as Fig. 36.35.)

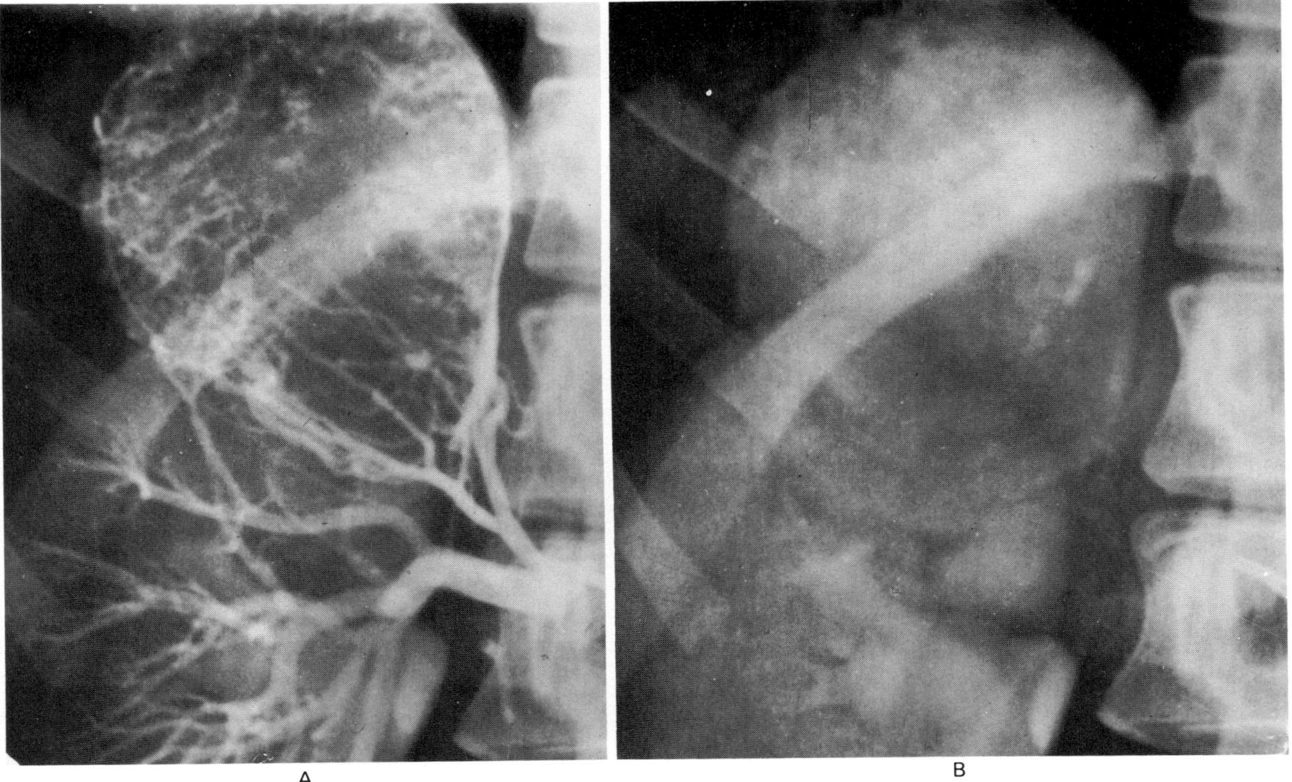

Fig. 36.30 A. and **B.** Large vascular phaeochromocytoma shown by selective right renal angiography with the catheter tip in the hypertrophied right inferior adrenal artery.

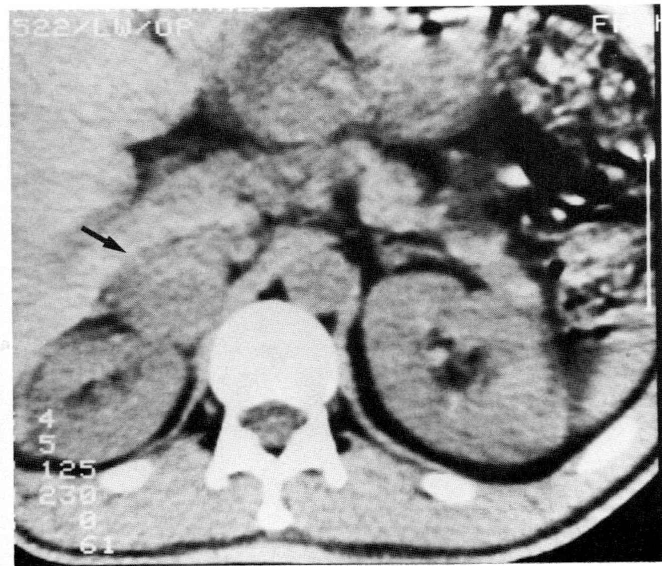

Fig. 36.31 Small phaeochromocytoma (↘) (3 cm diameter) anterior to upper pole of right kidney (L45 W512).

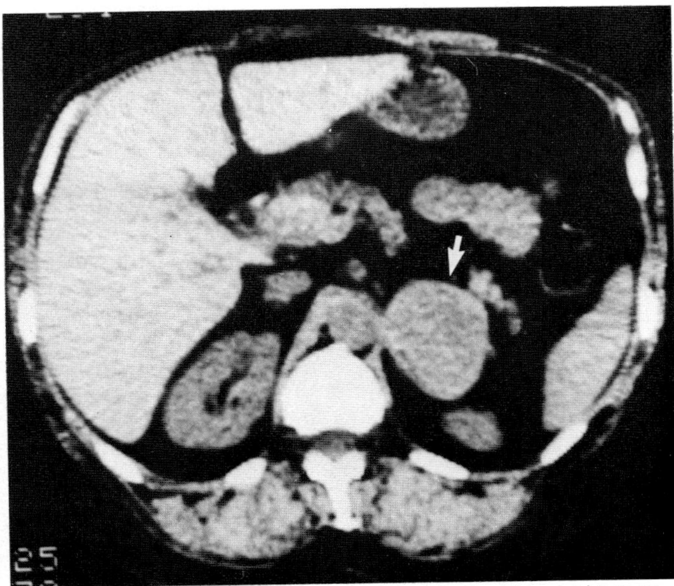

Fig. 36.32 Phaeochromocytoma (5 × 3.5 cm) in L. adrenal (↓) (L41 W256).

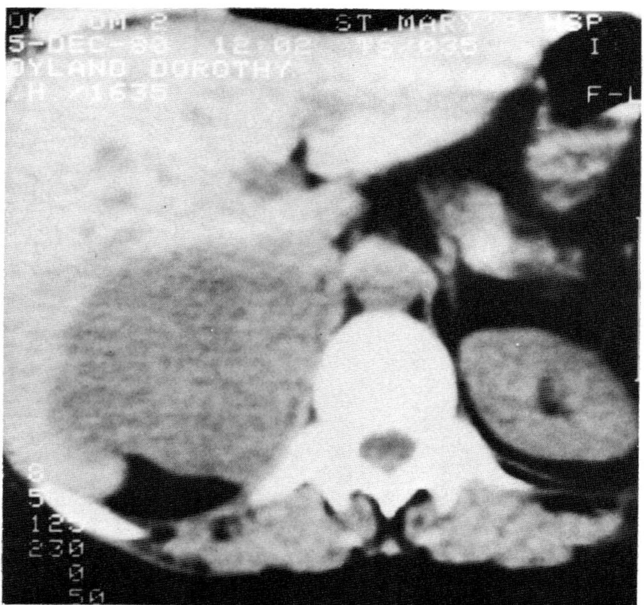

Fig. 36.33 Large R. phaeochromocytoma (7 × 8 cm) in R. adrenal and displacing liver (L36 W256).

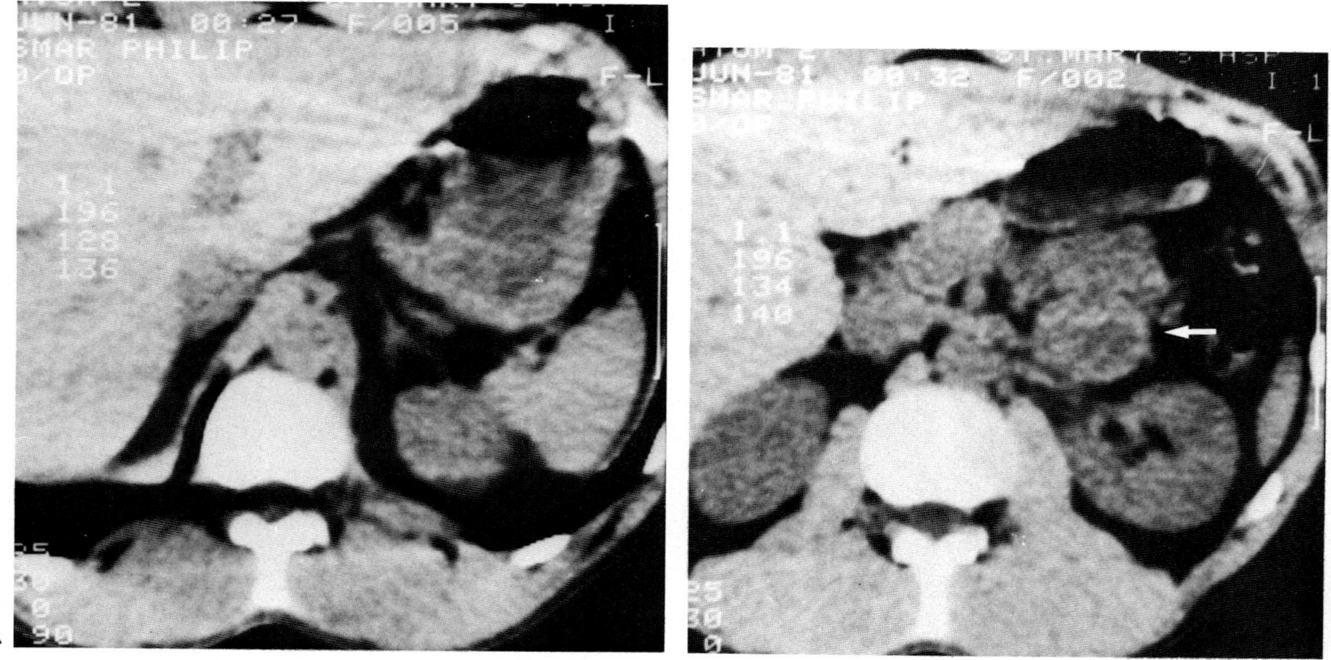

Fig. 36.34 A. Normal L and R adrenals. **B.** Ectopic small phaeochromocytoma (←) (3 cm diameter) anterior to L. hilum in same patient (L36 W256).

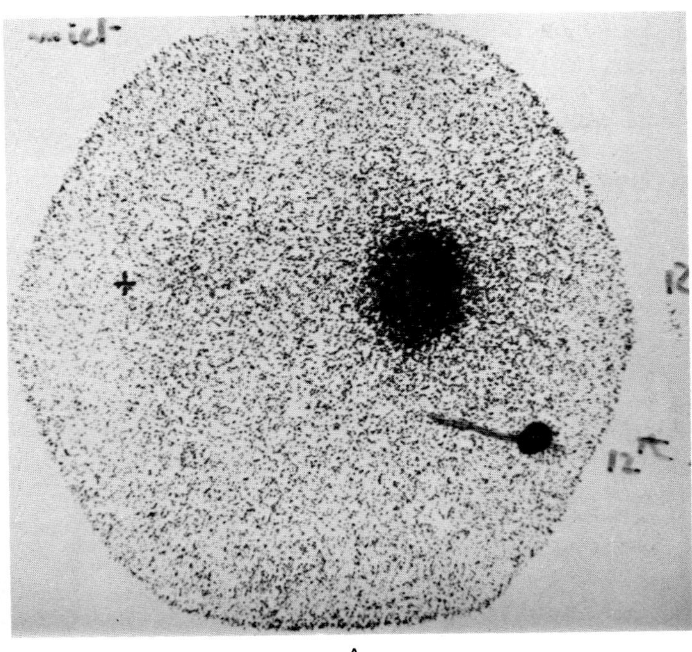

A

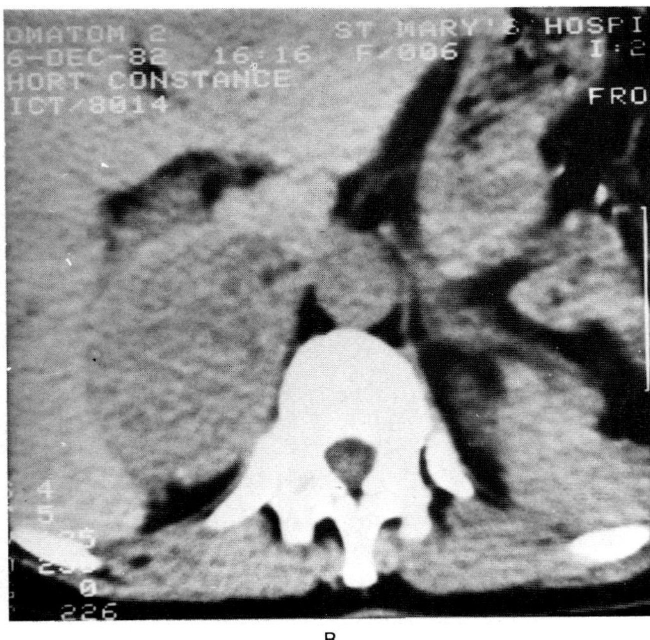

B

Fig. 36.35 A. Scintiscan using MIBG shows large right phaeochromocytoma (12th rib marked). **B.** CT of same patient confirms a large phaeochromocytoma (7 cm) (L45 W512). The tumour was also shown by ultrasound (Fig. 36.29).

both kidneys (Fig. 36.34). If the biochemical evidence of phaeochromocytoma is established, the demonstration of normal adrenal glands indicates that an ectopic tumour is present. If there is no evidence of this in the region of the kidneys the lower abdomen and pelvis should also be examined by CT and simple X-rays of the thorax (Fig. 36.39) should be carefully scrutinized.

If these are negative *scintiscanning* using MIBG (^{131}I meta-Iodo-benzylguanidine) should be tried. Although time consuming and expensive this test has been shown to demonstrate functioning phaeochromocytomas with a high degree of accuracy (Fig. 36.35), though false positive and false negative results have both been recorded. It is important of course to cover all possible sites of ectopia, including pelvis, thorax and neck. Only in rare cases should it be necessary to proceed to other investigations.

In such cases resort will be had to *venous sampling* in an attempt to localize the lesion. Samples should be obtained from the internal jugular and innominate veins on both sides, from the superior vena cava and right auricle, from the high inferior vena cava and both renal veins, from the low inferior vena cava and from both iliac veins. This should result in a localization of the tumour to a confined area, which can be further assessed by CT, ultrasound or scintiscanning. Venous sampling and assay of all areas is normally possible by simple percutaneous catheterization of a femoral vein.

It is clear from the above discussion that CT is now the investigation of choice for diagnosing phaeochromocytomas, though there is a place for ultrasound in assessing children and large tumours. Other methods (venous sampling, scintigraphy and arteriography) will occasionally be used in the search for the occasional problem ectopic tumour.

MRI has been successfully used to demonstrate adrenal masses and may eventually replace CT as the investigation of choice, since it involves no radiation and appears to be completely innocuous. To date its use has been limited by cost and availability.

Ectopic tumours at the renal hilum sometimes displace

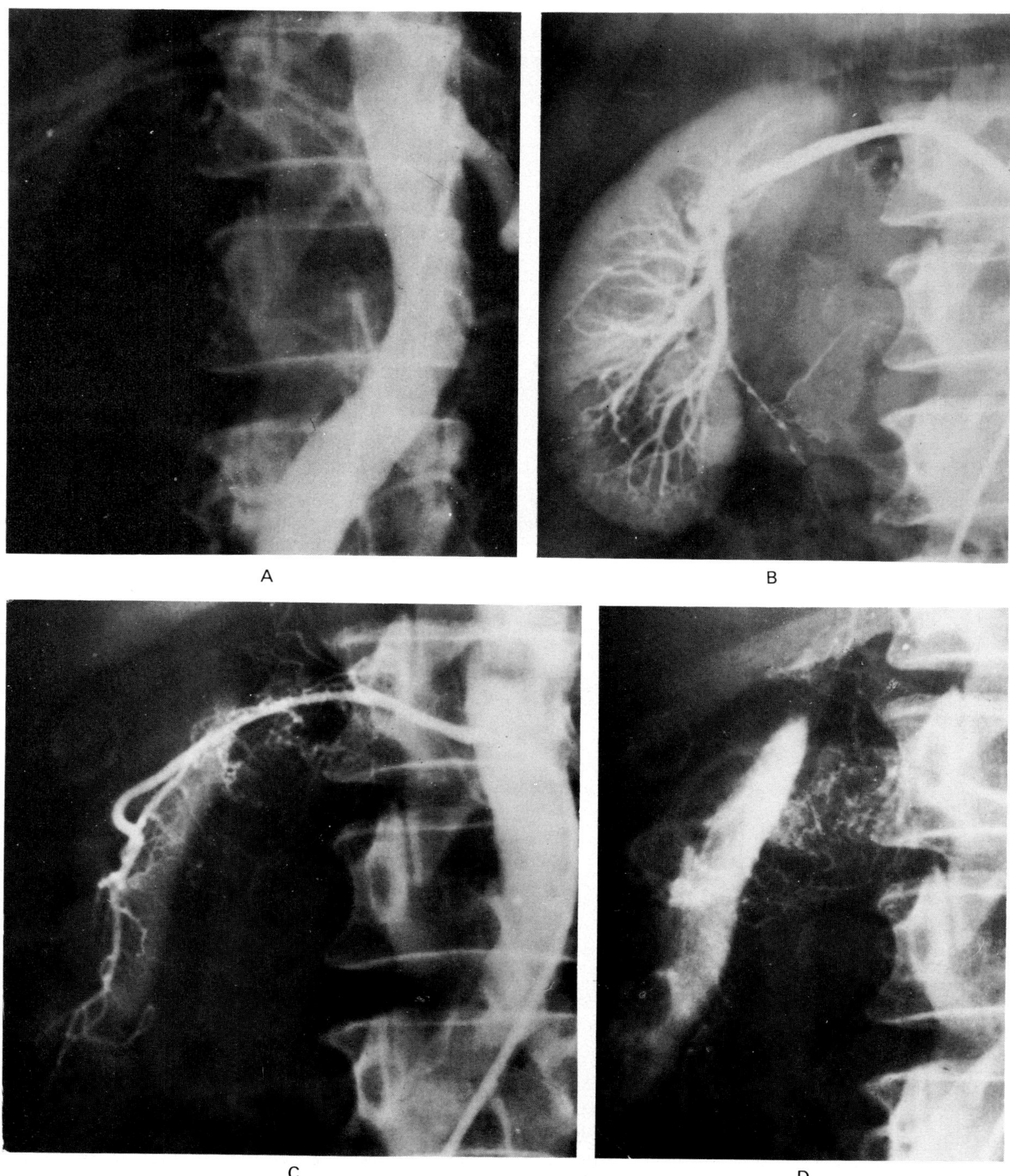

Fig. 36.36 A. Flush aortogram. **B.** selective arteriogram of main right renal artery. **C.** and **D.** Selective arteriogram of accessory right renal artery. The tumour is mainly supplied by the accessory artery. A pathological circulation is evident which was not seen on flush aortography.

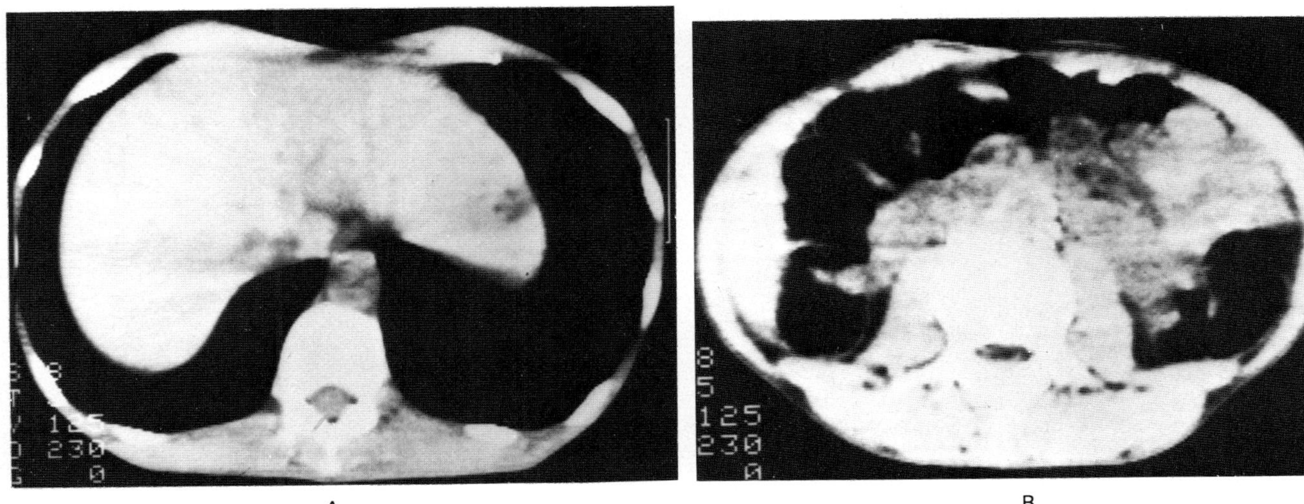

Fig. 36.37 A. Deposits in liver (L36 W128). B. Glandular masses around the aorta (L36 W256). The patient had a malignant phaeochromocytoma removed 6 months previously.

and stretch the renal arteries, giving rise to *renal artery stenosis* (Figs 36.24, 36.36). In these cases arteriography will be helpful in confirming the stenosis and planning surgical intervention.

Malignant phaeochromocytomas are probably less frequent than the 10% figure given in the older literature, since the diagnosis was then rarely confirmed in the atypical cases with small benign or ectopic tumours. Metastases from malignant tumours can involve lymph glands, bone, liver and chest (Figs 36.37, 36.38), but the tumours are usually slow growing and patients can survive several years after surgery and careful medical treatment. Isotope scanning is particularly valuable in assessing bone and other deposits.

Phaeochromocytomas presenting in childhood are often both multiple and familial (Fig. 36.39).

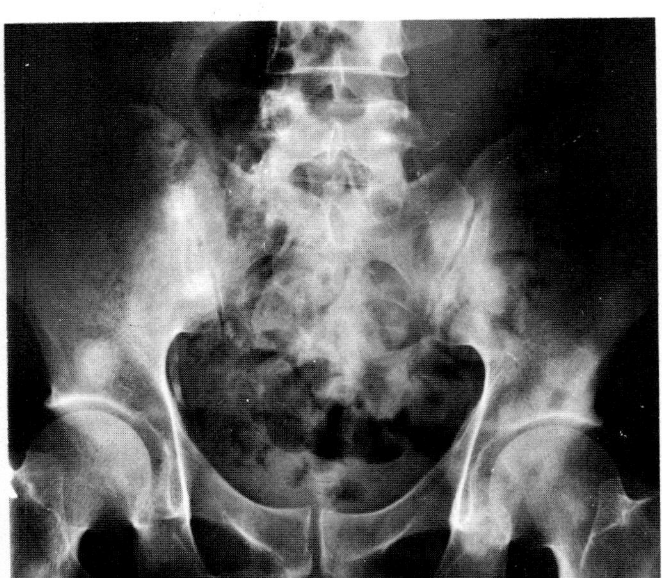

Fig. 36.38 Sclerotic bone deposits in same patient as Figure 36.37.

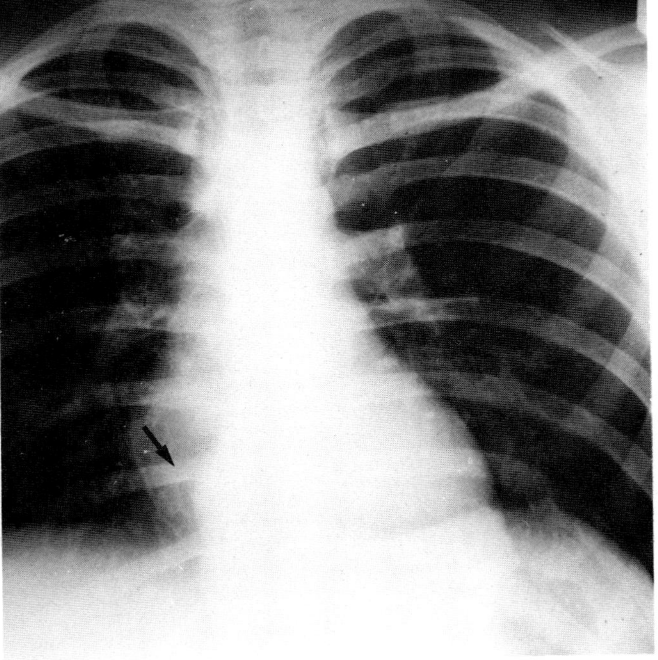

Fig. 36.39 Intrathoracic paravertebral tumour in a 12-year-old boy shown to right of lower spine (arrow). Further intra-abdominal tumours were shown by angiography. There was a familial history. (Courtesy of Dr F. Starer.)

REFERENCES AND SUGGESTIONS FOR FURTHER READING

Ackery, D. M. et al. (1984) New approach to the localization of phaeochromocytoma: imaging with iodine-131-meta-indobenzylguanidine. *British Medical Journal*, **288**, 1587–1591.

Adams, J. E. et al. (1983) Computed tomography in adrenal disease. *Clinical Radiology*, **34**, 39–49.

Bernardino, M. E., Goldstein, H. M. & Green, B. (1978) Grey scale ultrasonography of adrenal neoplasms. *American Journal of Roentgenology*, **130**, 741–744.

Conn, J. W., Morita, R., Cohen, E. L. et al. (1972) Primary aldosteronism. Photoscanning of tumours after administration of ^{131}I-19-iodocholesterol. *Archives of Internal Medicine*, **129**, 417–425.

Hartmann, C. W., Witton, D. M. & Weeks, R. E. (1966) The role of nephrotomography in diagnosis of adrenal tumours. *Radiology*, **86**, 1030–1034.

Hattery, R. R., Sheedy, P. F., Stephens, D. H. et al. (1981) Computed tomography of the adrenal gland. *Seminars in Roentgenology*, **16**, 290–300.

Huebener, K. H. & Treugut, H. (1984) Adrenal cortex dysfunction. CT findings. *Radiology*, **150**, 195–199.

Doppman, J. L. et al. (1984) Petrosal sinus sampling for Cushing syndrome: anatomical and technical considerations. *Radiology*, **150**, 99–103.

Dunnick, N. R. et al. (1982) CT appearance of adrenal cortical carcinoma. *Journal of Computer Assisted Tomography*, **6**, 978–982.

El-Sherief, M. A. & Hemmingson, A. (1982) Computed tomography of the normal adrenal gland. *Acta Radiologica Diagnosis*, **23**, 433–442.

Eghrari, M., McLoughlin, M. J. & Rosen, I. E. et al. (1980) The role of computed tomography in assessment of tumour pathology of the adrenal glands. *Journal of Computer Assisted Tomography*, **4**, 71–77.

Glazer, H. S. et al. (1982) Non-functioning adrenal masses: incidental discovery on computed tomography. *American Journal of Roentgenology*, **139**, 81–85.

Ishikawa, H. et al. (1981) Myelolipoma of the adrenal gland. *Journal of Urology*, **126**, 777–779.

Kearney, G. P. & Mahoney, E. M. (1977) Adrenal cysts. *Urologic Clinics of North America*, **4(2)**, 305–318.

Korobkin, M. et al. (1979) Computed tomography in the diagnosis of adrenal disease. *American Journal of Roentgenology*, **132**, 231–238.

Queloz, J. M., Capitanio, M. A. & Kirkpatrick, I. A. (1972) Wolman's disease. Roentgen observations in three siblings. *Radiology*, **104**, 357–359.

Seigel, M. J. & Sagel, S. S. (1982) Computed tomography as a supplement to urography in the evaluation of suspected neuroblastoma. *Radiology*, **142**, 435–438.

Sutton, D. (1968) Diagnosis of Conn's and other adrenal tumours by left adrenal phlebography. *Lancet*, **i**, 453–455.

CHAPTER 37

THE PAEDIATRIC ABDOMEN

THE GASTROINTESTINAL TRACT

(by F. Starer)

THE GASTROINTESTINAL TRACT IN THE NEONATE

INTRODUCTION

Paediatricians are apt to say that children are not just small adults. Radiologists dealing with very young babies will quickly appreciate the truth of this statement. The diseases one meets are different from those found in an older age group. Moreover, the infant is in the process of adapting its physiology to a completely new set of circumstances after birth, and is therefore in a most vulnerable situation. Speidel (1978) has shown that even minor interference with the neonate, such as handling it, causes a drop in blood oxygen levels. This is accompanied by an increased heart and respiratory rate. These are highly undesirable changes and it follows that neonates should be handled as little and as gently as possible while they are being X-rayed. For instance, 'erect' films are rarely necessary and more information with less stress is usually obtainable from decubitus horizontal-ray projections (Gyll 1984). Examinations with the baby inverted are an abomination, as are many of the restraining devices one sees illustrated in some textbooks. Sedation is sometimes indicated but it is impossible to give general advice on this as each case will have to be considered individually in conjunction with the referring paediatrician. The frequency with which sedation will be found necessary will vary inversely with the patience and skill of the radiographer.

Neonates are peculiarly liable to lose heat and become hypothermic. Once this has happened it is not easy to warm them again. Hypothermia leads to cardiac arrhythmias and is a dangerous condition. The radiologist must be very careful to ensure that body temperature is not allowed to drop. A warm room alone may not be enough and sheets of cotton wool and aluminium foil are helpful in keeping the baby warm without overheating it. It is often wiser to abandon a lengthy examination and return the baby to the incubator rather than run the risk of hypothermia.

Contrast studies

Special thought should be given to the choice of contrast material for neonates. In general, *barium* is satisfactory and safe for most purposes. Even in the lungs, small amounts of barium do little harm and are cleared quickly. Cases of water intoxication from the use of large volumes of barium suspensions in the investigation of congenital megacolon have been reported and it is wise to make up the suspension in normal saline for this purpose. On the other hand, the occasional stories of barium converting a partial to a complete obstruction are difficult to substantiate. Barium is, however, contraindicated if there is a risk of a leak into the peritoneal cavity. In this connection, one should remember that it is unwise to carry out a contrast enema for about 10 days after a rectal biopsy, even if the surgeon claims only to have taken a mucosal sample.

In recent years there has been a vogue for *water-soluble contrast agents*, but the older hypertonic types had many disadvantages. Their hyperosmolarity caused water to be drawn into the gut, diluting contrast in the small bowel and leading to loss of information. The loss of fluid into the gut may cause serious dehydration of the infant and hypertonic contrast media should not be used orally unless it is possible to rehydrate the baby quickly if necessary. These contrast media are also liable to cause pulmonary oedema if they reach the lungs and they should never be used if there is any possibility of this happening, as for instance in the investigation for tracheo-oesophageal fistula. Hypertonic contrast media do, however, retain one very useful function in the treatment of meconium ileus. Here their hypertonicity becomes a desirable feature and there is a great deal to be said for using hypertonic contrast enemas in the investigation of suspected distal small bowel obstructions. Fortunately, the newer isotonic contrast media do not suffer from the disadvantages mentioned above. Iopamidol 370 (Niopam) diluted with twice its volume of normal saline, or ioxaglate 320 (Hexabrix) diluted with an equal volume of water produces an osmolarity which is almost identical with that of plasma and these should be ideal for many studies in the neonatal period (Ratcliffe 1984).

The radiologist should also be particularly concerned to reduce the amount of radiation to a minimum. Because of the small size of the patient and, consequently, the small amount of scatter it is often possible to do without a grid, both for fluoroscopy and radiography. Here the radiographer's skill becomes crucial. However, it is a mistake to accept films which are diagnostically inadequate for the sake of saving a small amount of radiation.

An additional problem which often arises when dealing with young children is the parents' desire to be present during the examination. This may be inconvenient and sometimes undesirable, but one must bear in mind the parents' natural distress at having an ill or abnormal baby. Each radiologist will have to formulate his own attitudes towards this particular problem.

In this section it is intended to deal only with the major abnormalities of the neonatal gastrointestinal tract.

OESOPHAGEAL ATRESIA

The diagnosis is suggested soon after birth by the infant's inability to feed and by choking during swallowing. Maternal hydramnios may be an early warning. The atresia is frequently associated with a tracheo-oesophageal fistula; four types are recognized (Fig. 37.1A).

Radiology. Only the first two types need to be considered. The upper oesophageal pouch is dilated and can often be seen as a structure of air density in the lower neck or upper thorax. *In the absence of a fistula*, gas cannot reach the stomach and the gut remains airless. In a normal neonate, swallowing of air begins almost immediately after birth and gas should be present in the stomach within 15 minutes. Absence of intestinal gas later than this is therefore significant and suggests oesophageal obstruction. Occasionally, absence of gas is found in brain-damaged children who have no swallowing reflex. This type of atresia is associated with maternal hydramnios and there is also a high incidence of other congenital abnormalities, including Down's syndrome, duodenal and anal atresia, and abnormalities in the cardiovascular and urinary systems and in the skeleton.

In the second, more common type, air can reach the stomach and these children often have a distended abdomen. Hydramnios and other congenital anomalies also occur but not with quite such a high frequency as in the first type. One curious abnormality is the presence of 13 pairs of ribs in almost half the cases. All patients with oesophageal atresia tend to develop pneumonias due to aspiration from the pouch. They also tend to show narrowing of the trachea, either from pressure from the distended pouch or from an associated weakness of the tracheal cartilage.

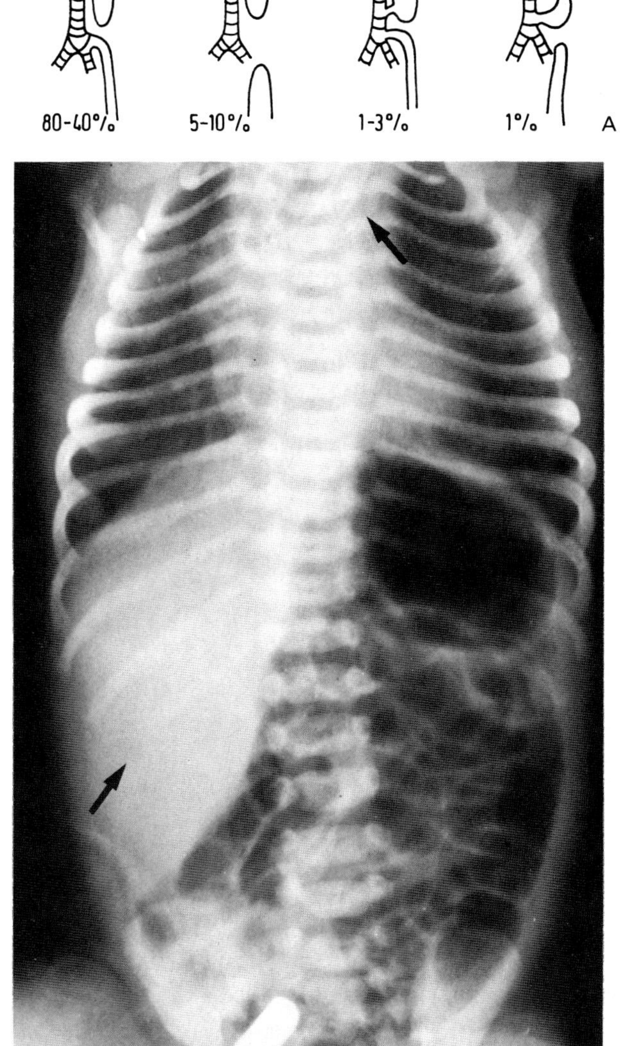

Fig. 37.1 A. Types of oesophageal atresia. and their frequency. **B.** Oesophageal atresia with tracheo-oesophageal fistula. Note: a) tube coiled in the oesophageal pouch (↖), b) gaseous distension of the bowel, c) thirteen pairs of ribs (↗).

The diagnosis should be established by passing a fairly stiff nasogastric tube to the bottom of the pouch and taking a radiograph to include the neck, chest and abdomen (Fig. 37.1B). It is essential to confirm that the tube is not curled up in the pouch, thereby giving a misleading impression of the length of tube that has been passed. It cannot be stressed too much that in the great majority of these patients contrast studies should be avoided. They provide little additional information and the risk of flooding the lungs with contrast is considerable. Several published series indicate that operative mortality rises sharply in infants with contrast in the lungs. If special circumstances dictate the use of contrast, the smallest possible amount of barium should be introduced into the pouch through a nasogastric tube with the baby lying on its side. A film is obtained and the barium sucked out as quickly as possible.

The first stage in treatment is often the establishment of a gastrostomy. The radiologist can play a useful part at this stage by excluding a distal obstruction such as pyloric or duodenal stenosis as a coexisting lesion. It is often also useful to try and reflux barium into the lower oesophagus in order to show the length of the atretic segment. It goes without saying that barium should be introduced into the stomach only under direct visual control (Fig. 37.2).

Following repair of the atresia the upper pouch remains dilated for months and the anastomosis often looks very narrow, even though the patient can swallow quite well. At this stage another problem may become apparent. Patients with repaired oesophageal atresia show a high incidence of abnormal peristalsis in the lower oesophagus, which may cause dysphagia. Hiatus hernias are not uncommon and reflux into the oesophagus may occur even in the absence of an hiatus hernia.

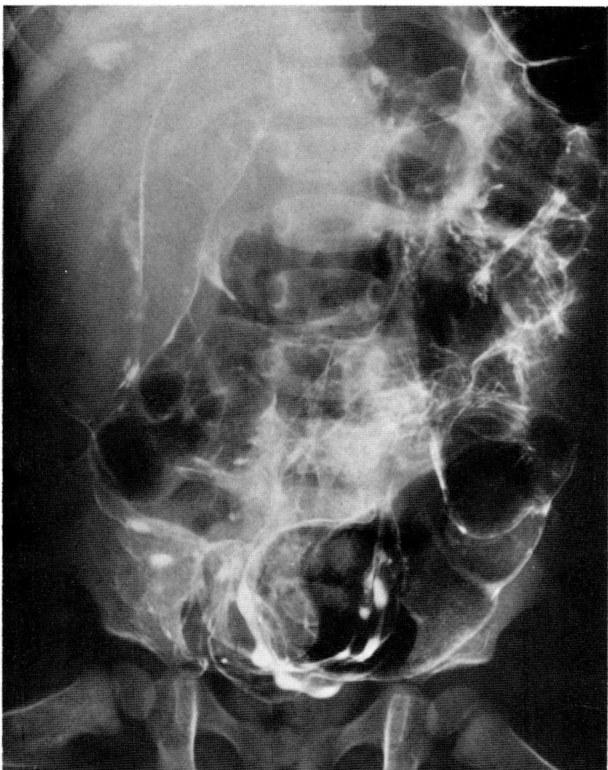

Fig. 37.2 Barium in peritoneum. The patient had an oesophageal atresia and a gastrostomy had been performed. Barium was introduced without screening and the radiologist did not realize that the gastrostomy tube had come out of the stomach. There were no immediate serious consequences from this procedure, although dense adhesions were found at a subsequent laparotomy.

ISOLATED TRACHEO-OESOPHAGEAL FISTULA

It has unfortunately become common to confuse oesophageal atresias and isolated tracheo-oesophageal (or H) fistulas. They should be clearly separated. Isolated fistulas produce coughing during swallowing and frequent chest infections. They are often difficult to demonstrate and may not be discovered for some time. The fistula usually takes an oblique course and the description of an H-fistula is not really very apt. There are two main reasons why these lesions are often missed. They may be very narrow and have muscular walls which may close the fistula; moreover, many occur in a high position in the neck. One frequently sees examinations which were not taken high enough to show the fistula (Fig. 37.3).

Sometimes a simple barium swallow will show the connection between the trachea and oesophagus. More often than not this fails and a special technique must be used. The baby is placed in the prone oblique position with the left shoulder raised after a nasogastric tube has been passed into the stomach. Barium is injected rapidly through the tube by a syringe and the tube is withdrawn. It needs to be emphasized again that hypertonic water-soluble contrast media should not be used. The barium distends the oesophagus and then passes through the fistula. It will be apparent, from what has been said

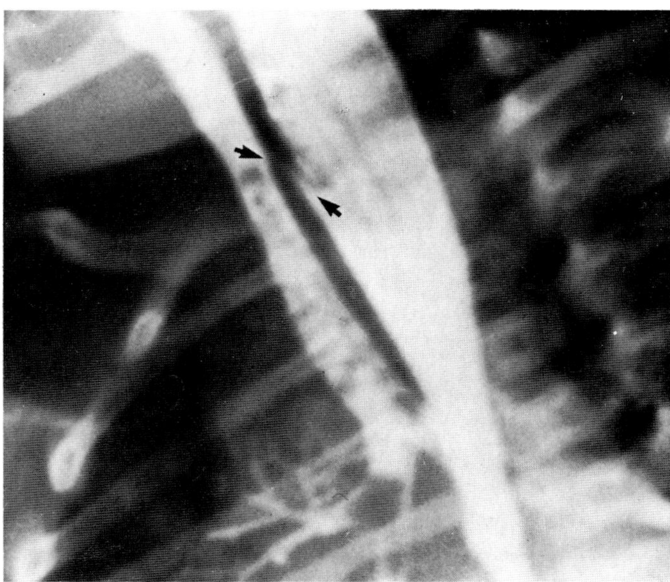

Fig. 37.3 Tracheo-oesophageal fistula. Note thin barium track just above the level of the first ribs (arrows) and contrast in the trachea and bronchi.

already, that it is necessary to withdraw the tube right up into the oesophagus in the neck. It will also be apparent that there is a very real risk of causing aspiration and flooding of the lungs by this technique which is not without risk. It is absolutely essential that there are trained personnel at hand to suck out the bronchial tree and even resuscitate the patient if it should become necessary. Oxygen and a sucker which is actually running should be immediately available. Finally, since one clearly does not wish to repeat the procedure more often than necessary, the examination should be recorded on videotape for repeated study if necessary.

OTHER CAUSES OF SWALLOWING DIFFICULTIES IN NEONATES

Bilateral *choanal atresia* prevents the infant from sucking and breathing at the same time, whereas choanal atresia on one side only has little noticeable effect at this age (Fig. 37.4).

In very *premature* infants the swallowing reflex may be defective and it may take several days for normal swallowing to be initiated. *Neuromuscular disturbances* may be caused by a variety of neurological disorders and occur after anoxia during birth and also in the Riley-Day syndrome. Barium spills over into the larynx or may regurgitate into the nose or even into the Eustachian tubes, to be aspirated into the larynx subsequently (Fig. 37.5). It is essential to examine the oro- and nasopharynx in all babies with swallowing difficulties during the course of a barium meal.

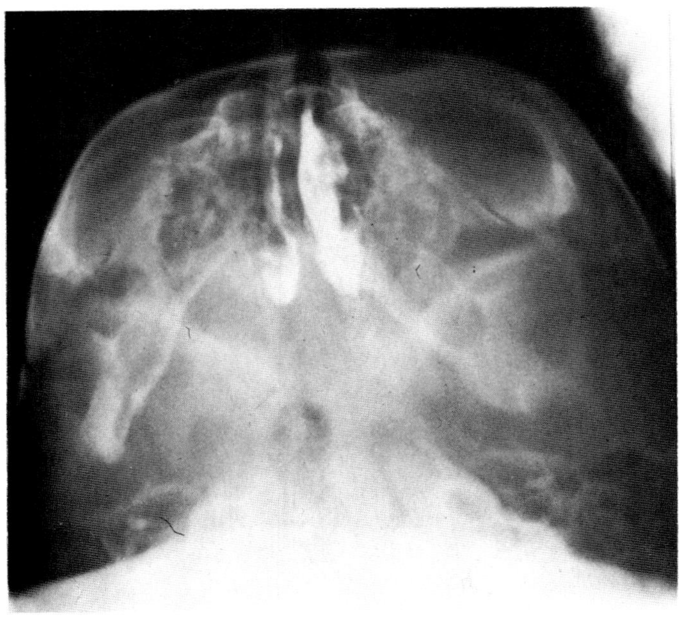

Fig. 37.4 Bilateral choanal atresia.

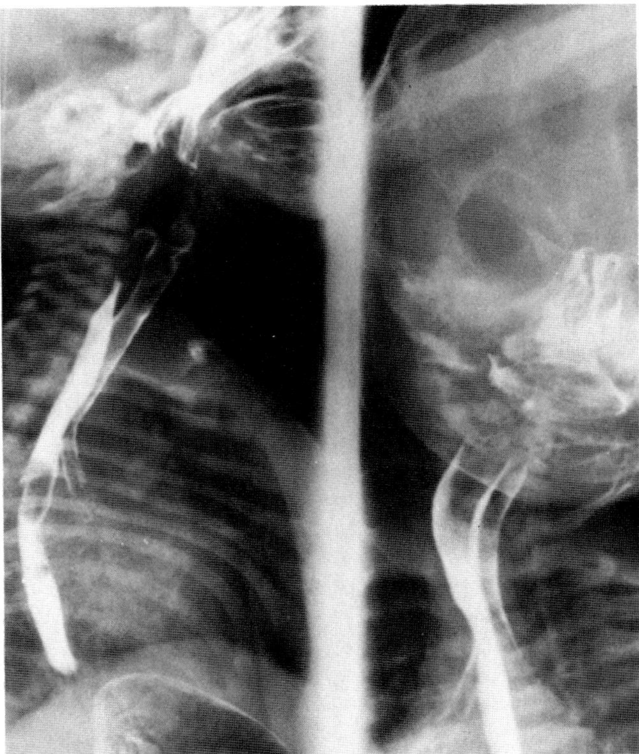

Fig. 37.5 Barium spill into the trachea during swallowing. Note barium in the nose as well as in the trachea. Brain-damaged child due to cerebral anoxia during birth.

An unusual situation is overactivity of the *cricopharyngeus*, producing a muscular 'bar' across the posterior aspect of the pharynx. This may give rise to dysphagia. Attempted oesophageal intubation in such cases has led to mediastinal perforation by the nasogastric tube in a number of cases. The position of the tube may then simulate oesophageal atresia.

OBSTRUCTIONS AT THE LOWER END OF THE OESOPHAGUS

Various congenital obstructive lesions at the lower end of the oesophagus have been described, such as a cartilagenous ring. All are very rare. Achalasia is also exceedingly rare in this age group and one should be quite certain, before making this diagnosis, that one is not looking at a stricture from peptic oesophagitis. Surprisingly, neonates have a highly acid gastric secretion and gastro-oesophageal reflux in this age group does occasionally cause strictures.

HIATUS HERNIA AND GASTRO-OESOPHAGEAL REFLUX

One of the intriguing problems in neonatal radiology is the difference in the reported incidence of hiatus hernias on the two sides of the Atlantic. This is much higher in Europe and the UK than in the United States. It has been suggested that this reflects a genuine difference due to different habits of nursing babies, but perhaps it is more likely the result of different habits of radiologists. Vomiting in a baby beginning shortly after birth is very suggestive of an hiatus hernia with reflux. There is still no unanimity concerning the best method for demonstrating this. Some hernias show on a simple barium swallow. Often it is helpful to turn the patient semiprone and let him cry. The changes in intra-abdominal and intrathoracic pressure relationships may show an otherwise invisible hernia. Sometimes it is helpful to rock the baby from side to side in the supine position. Many radiologists no longer favour the Trendelenburg position nor abdominal compression as being unphysiological. The hiatus hernia may be intermittent and is therefore easily missed on a single examination.

As regards reflux, it must be remembered that many babies regurgitate small amounts of fluid if their stomachs are full. A variety of techniques have been introduced to look for reflux, none entirely satisfactory. In addition to simple screening, the baby may be given barium followed by water, the so-called 'syphon test'. During the initiation of swallowing the water, the lower oesophageal sphincter relaxes and reflux may occur. In addition, reflux can be sought by introducing radioactive material into the stomach and scanning over the oesophagus or by oesophageal pH monitoring. None of these methods appears to have any great advantages over standard radiological procedures. Whenever a hiatus hernia or reflux is found it is necessary to make certain that this is not associated with gastric outlet obstruction. Many children with hiatus hernias in infancy still show evidence of a hernia in adult life although they may be symptom free.

SPONTANEOUS PERFORATION OF THE OESOPHAGUS

This is a rare event of unknown aetiology. Perforation usually occurs on the right lower aspect of the oesophagus, unlike adult perforations. It results in a right-sided pneumothorax, sometimes under tension, or a hydropneumothorax.

SPONTANEOUS PERFORATION OF THE STOMACH

This is another rare but catastrophic event. It may be due to acute gastric ulceration or focal hypoxia and leads to massive pneumoperitoneum associated, sometimes, with absence of gas in the stomach itself.

INTESTINAL OBSTRUCTION

Numerous congenital abnormalities may give rise to intestinal obstruction in the neonate. Hernias and postoperative adhesions are rare causes and will not be considered further. As in adults, the radiological features consist of distended loops and fluid levels above the obstruction. A number of problems specific to this age group should be borne in mind, however. In infants it is much more difficult to distinguish large from small bowel and sometimes this may be impossible on plain films. Dilated loops and fluid levels may be due to gastroenteritis, which may simulate obstruction. In the very young child an exact knowledge of the age, even to the nearest half-hour, is essential. At birth the gut contains no air and before a diagnosis of obstruction can be made it is necessary to know how far air should have reached. The time taken for air to reach various parts of the gastrointestinal tract is shown below:

Stomach	within minutes
Upper small bowel	5–30 minutes
Entire small bowel	3 hours
Caecum	3–4 hours
Descending colon	5–6 hours
Sigmoid colon	8–9 hours
Rectum	variable, up to all hours

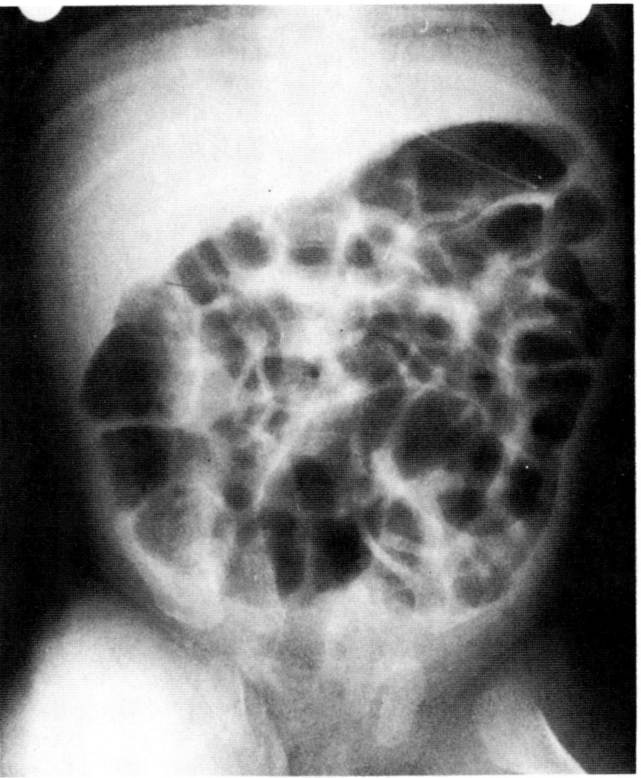

Fig. 37.6 Dilatation of immature gut in a premature baby during the first 24 hours of life. This resolved spontaneously.

In a collapsed or brain-damaged child the abdomen may remain airless because swallowing is inhibited.

An interesting but confusing form of intestinal obstruction is **functional ileus** in the newborn. It can be due to generalized sepsis, adrenal insufficiency, hypothyroidism, neurological abnormalities or hypermagnesaemia. Most commonly, however, it is due to immaturity of the gut and particularly of the left half of the colon (Fig. 37.6). Most of these infants are premature and of low birth weight and there is a high incidence of diabetic mothers. Normally, meconium is passed in the first 24 hours but this is delayed in these premature children. The bowel becomes uniformly distended but peristalsis commences after 2 or 3 days and no treatment is required. A contrast enema during this time may show a narrow colon beyond the splenic flexure. Distinction from Hirschsprung's disease is difficult, but the problem is resolved if the examination is repeated in 48 hours. It is suggested that this is also responsible for the meconium plug syndrome in which pellets of normal meconium are held up in the left side of the colon. It is important to recognize the syndrome of functional immaturity in order to avoid fruitless and unnecessary laparotomy.

The causes of neonatal intestinal obstruction can now be discussed in anatomical sequence.

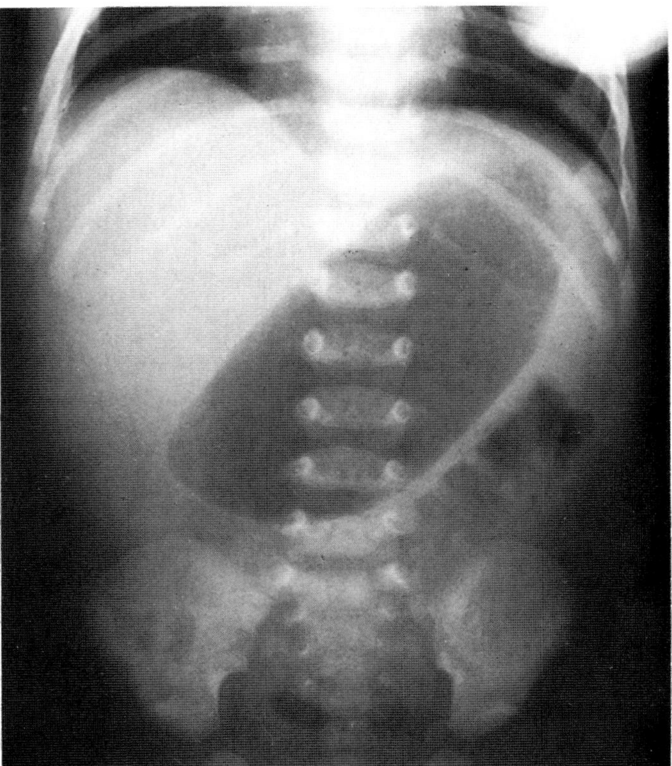

Fig. 37.7 Large gastric air bubble due to congenital pyloric stenosis.

HYPERTROPHIC PYLORIC STENOSIS

This condition is more common in boys than in girls and usually manifests itself between 2 and 8 weeks of age. An earlier onset is rare and one should then be careful not to miss an underlying lesion such as a peptic ulcer. Coexistent gastro-oesophageal reflux is not uncommon. Pyloric stenosis is no longer thought to be of congenital origin but to arise as the result of prolonged pyloric spasm. The symptoms of projectile vomiting and visible peristalsis are well known and the children quickly develop alkalosis and dehydration. Palpation often reveals an abdominal tumour due to the hypertrophied pyloric muscle. If these symptoms and signs are found, radiological examination may be considered to be superfluous. However, mistakes are occasionally made on clinical grounds alone. Radiology becomes important if the clinical features are indefinite. Unfortunately, experience has shown that in these babies the radiological findings may also be difficult to interpret. Plain films often show a distended stomach and little gas in the small bowel (Fig. 37.7). They are not reliable for making or excluding the diagnosis. This depends traditionally on a barium meal. Barium is best given orally by means of a teat and bottle. Injection into the mouth by a syringe is not without danger as it may cause aspiration into the lungs if the barium is administered too rapidly. Some radiologists prefer to introduce barium through a nasogastric tube, but this prevents examination of the pharynx and oesophagus and may hide reflux. In any case, it is important not to give too much barium. The infant's stomach lies horizontally and an excess of barium may obscure the pyloric canal.

In the early stages of the disease there is usually vigorous gastric peristalsis. In the later stages peristalsis may cease altogether. Generally, pyloric opening is delayed, often for a very long time. In that case the examination may be speeded up by an intravenous injection of metoclopramide hydrochloride (1 mg). Occasionally there is no marked delay and the time interval is, in itself, not diagnostic. Characteristically, the pylorus is elongated and curves upwards and there is 'shouldering' of the antrum due to the hypertrophied muscle (Fig. 37.8). In atypical cases the pyloric canal may be band-like or irregular. In the absence of peristalsis the pyloric canal may not fill at all; these patients require surgery.

Treatment is by the well-known Ramsted's myotomy. The appearances following surgery persist unchanged for weeks, months or even years but after successful surgery there is no hold up. Other causes of gastric outlet obstruction which may need to be differentiated from hypertrophic pyloric stenosis are pylorospasm (with or without peptic ulceration), antral diaphragms and obstruction from gastric duplications.

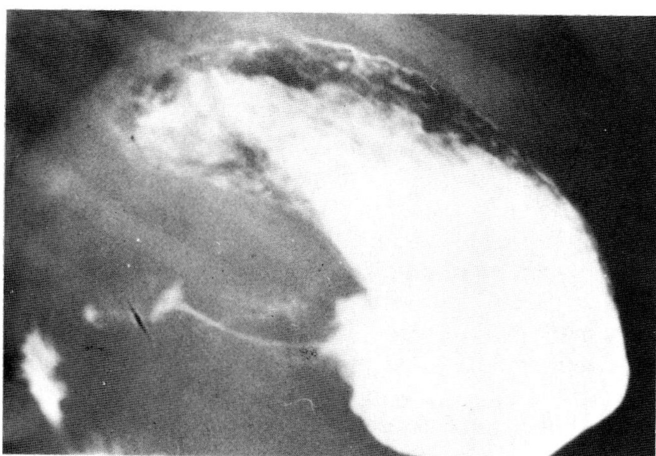

Fig. 37.8 Congenital pyloric stenosis. Note greatly elongated pyloric canal and 'shouldering' of the antrum due to the hypertrophied pyloric muscle.

More recently it has been shown that the hypertrophied pyloric muscle can be well demonstrated by *ultrasound.* It may be that this will replace conventional radiology in the future.

DUODENAL OBSTRUCTIONS

The majority of lesions causing obstruction to the duodenum occur in the second part. They then produce the well-known 'double bubble', with some distal gas if the obstruction is incomplete (Fig. 37.9). It has become customary to diagnose *duodenal atresia* as soon as this appearance is seen but this is unjustified since other lesions may be responsible and it is important to differentiate these. It is, however, true that duodenal atresia or stenosis is the most common cause. 25% of these patients will have Down's syndrome, with all the possible anomalies associated with that condition. It is often useful to count the ribs in babies with duodenal atresia. The presence of 11 pairs of ribs will tend to support the diagnosis of Down's syndrome, which may have been missed clinically up to this point. The obstruction usually occurs below the ampulla of Vater.

Another cause of obstruction is Ladd's bands, *peritoneal bands* which occur either with malrotation or sometimes on their own (Fig. 37.10). Malrotation may result in a *small bowel volvulus*, an extremely serious condition with a high mortality. Usually there is no need, nor opportunity, to undertake contrast studies in babies with complete duodenal obstruction since they require immediate surgery. If, for any reason, surgical treatment is deferred, a barium enema is advisable to exclude the presence of a malrotation.

Diaphragms may be encountered in the duodenum. By stretching, they form 'intraduodenal diverticula', *Annular pancreas* is associated with duodenal obstruction, but it is debatable whether it is the pancreas that actually causes

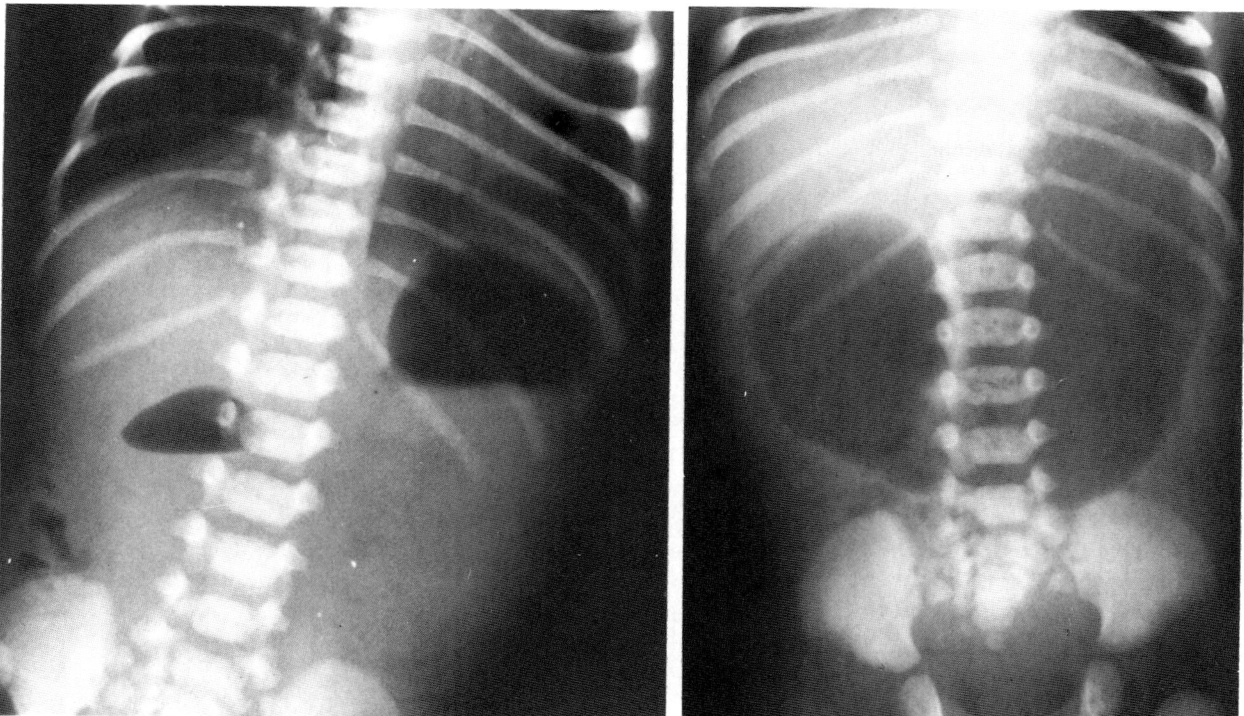

Fig. 37.9 A. and **B**. Erect and supine abdomen showing the so-called 'double bubble' appearance of duodenal obstruction. A little gas is present in the small bowel.

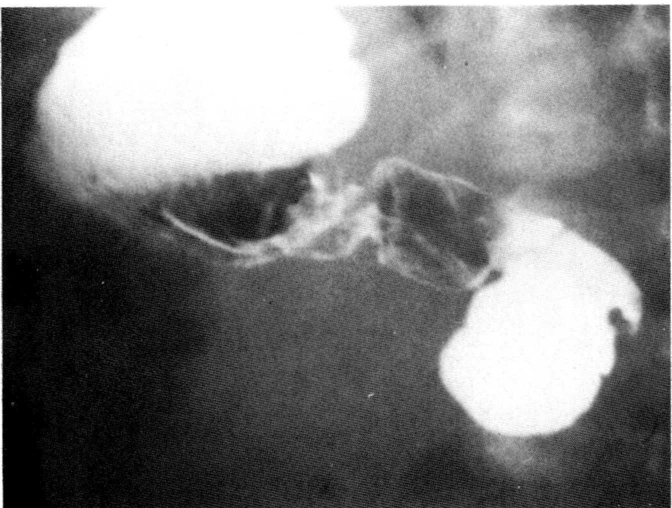

Fig. 37.10 Prone view of stomach and duodenum in neonate, showing obstruction in the second part of the duodenum due to Ladd's bands in a child with malrotation.

the obstruction since diaphragms are also frequently present. Finally, on rare occasions, the portal vein may take a preduodenal course, a lesion often associated with other congenital anomalies involving the pancreas, bile ducts and gall bladder and which may be associated with obstruction of the duodenum.

SMALL BOWEL ATRESIA AND STENOSIS

Obstruction of the small bowel may occur at any level; it may be complete or incomplete, single or multiple. The cause is believed to be an intrauterine ischaemic episode affecting the gut (unlike duodenal atresia, which is a true developmental abnormality) and small bowel atresias therefore occur as isolated lesions without associated abnormalities. Radiologically, one finds dilated loops and fluid levels, their extent depending on the level of the obstruction. Occasionally, calcification can be recognized in relation to the obstructed segment. Similar lesions in the colon are rare.

MECONIUM ILEUS

Meconium ileus is a manifestation of *cystic fibrosis*, although rare cases due to *pancreatic duct atresia* have been recorded. The absence of pancreatic secretions and abnormal intestinal mucus found in cystic fibrosis result in the development of thick, sticky meconium which has difficulty passing through the terminal ileum. There it becomes further inspissated to form dry pellets said to resemble deer droppings (a description no doubt helpful to those familiar with deer droppings). These changes result in low small bowel obstruction. There is a high incidence of perforation. This may occur before or after birth. Prenatal intestinal perforation results in a chemical but sterile peritonitis which leads to adhesions and may produce peritoneal or mural calcification (Fig. 37.11). Since the processus vaginalis is still open at this age, calcification may also be produced in the scrotum. Perforation after birth results in peritonitis with a pneumoperitoneum. Segmental small bowel volvulus is not uncommon; there may be secondary ileal atresia and pseudocysts may develop. These children do not usually show evidence of pulmonary involvement by cystic fibrosis at this age, but are liable to develop respiratory problems later, particularly following surgery.

The radiological findings provide evidence of low small bowel obstruction. There is often remarkable variation in the size of the loops and the distal ileum may closely simulate the colon. Because of the sticky nature of the meconium, fluid levels are often absent or sparse. Air mixed with the meconium produces a bubbly appearance, particularly in the right iliac fossa (Fig. 37.12). None of these changes is pathognomonic, but their combination in a child who has not passed meconium after 24 hours is suggestive. The sweat test is difficult to carry out and unreliable at this age; provided there is no evidence of perforation it is up to the radiologist to confirm the diagnosis. There is a high mortality amongst babies with meconium ileus treated surgically and operation should, if possible, be avoided. Fortunately, the radiologist can often help by carrying out an enema using hypertonic water-soluble contrast media. The hypertonic solution should, if possible, be run into the small bowel but experience has shown that even when this is not possible the enema may produce the passage of meconium. The hypertonic solution draws water into the gut and softens the meconium and stimulates the bowel. There is some uncertainty regarding the best contrast agent to use. Gastrografin contains Tween 80; this is a wetting agent and it is claimed that it produces better results. On the other hand, there is some experimental evidence to suggest that it may damage the colonic mucosa and therefore many radiologists prefer to use ordinary urographic contrast media, often at half strength. It is essential during this procedure to make sure that the infant is well hydrated, and therefore an intravenous drip is advisable.

The colon in babies with meconium ileus will invariably be found to be very narrow (Fig. 37.13). This is not a true microcolon but is the result of disuse. A small colon also occurs in children with ileal atresia but not with high small bowel obstructions. The colon rapidly returns to normal size when it is brought into use.

ANOMALIES OF MID-GUT ROTATION

The events by which the mid-gut rotates as it returns into the abdominal cavity during fetal life are well known.

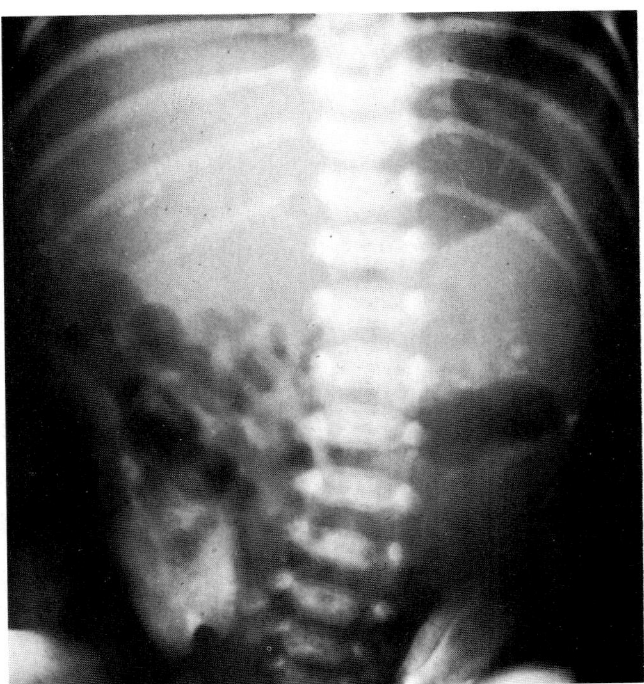

Fig. 37.11 Peritoneal calcification in an infant with meconium ileus due to prenatal perforation.

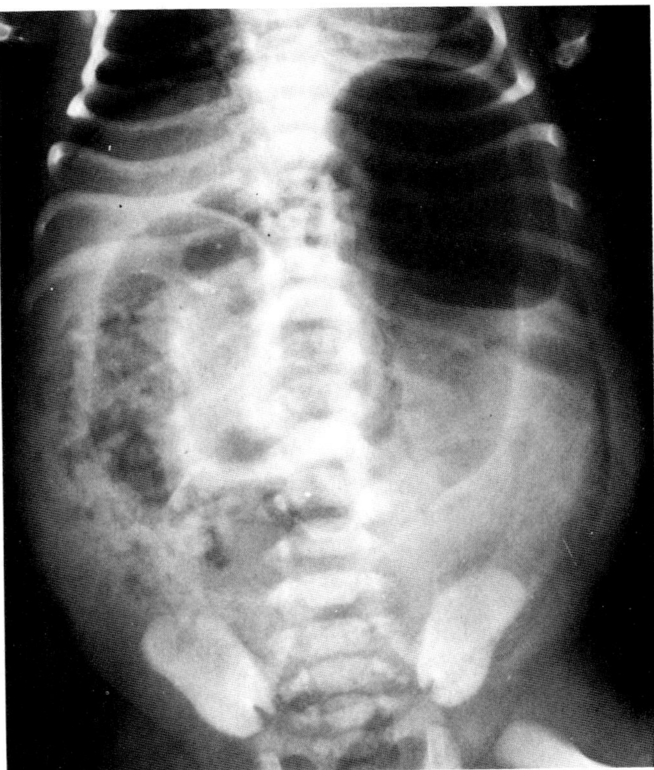

Fig. 37.12 Meconium ileus. Note the dilated loops of small bowel, the 'bubbly' appearance of the meconium in the right side of the abdomen and gas free in the peritoneal cavity, indicating a perforation.

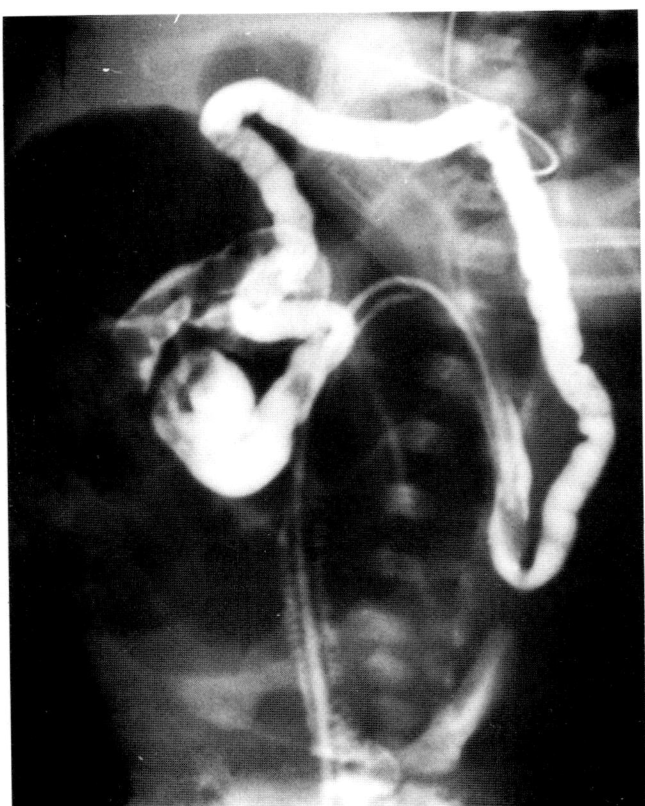

Fig. 37.13 Meconium ileus. Water-soluble contrast enema showing a small colon. Contrast has refluxed into the terminal ileum showing the filling defects due to meconium.

Errors in rotation give rise to a series of abnormalities, some of which may have serious consequences.

'Non-rotation' is a misnomer, since it describes a condition resulting from a 90° rotation instead of the normal 270° anticlockwise rotation. In this condition the entire small bowel comes to lie on the right and the colon on the left of the abdomen. It is not usually associated with symptoms.

Reversed rotation results from a 90° clockwise rotation which brings the transverse colon behind the duodenum; it is rare and may produce symptoms.

The really important situation, however, is malrotation. This implies incomplete rotation, the gut assuming a position somewhere between non-rotation and the normal. This in itself would not give rise to symptoms but for two factors: the presence of Ladd's bands and shortening of the attachment of the mesentery. Ladd's bands have been mentioned already in connection with duodenal obstruction. The mesenteric attachment runs from the duodenojejunal junction to the caecum. Normally, this is the maximum diagonal across the abdomen and this wide attachment ensures that the mesentery cannot twist. In patients with malrotation the duodenojejunal junction is displaced medially and downwards and the caecum medially and upwards. The mesenteric attachment is correspondingly shortened and twisting is liable to occur, leading to small bowel volvulus.

The symptoms of malrotation, therefore, may be partial or complete high obstruction due to bands; this may be intermittent. If volvulus develops, the consequences tend to be a catastrophic and there is a high mortality. Some of these children, without acute episodes, develop malabsorption resembling coeliac disease.

Radiologists used to dealing mainly with adults are prone to forget malrotation as a common and serious cause of obstruction and should deliberately remind themselves of this possibility when dealing with an incomplete or intermittent obstruction in a baby. At this stage the diagnosis can be made by contrast studies, either an enema or meal. Traditionally a barium enema has been used to show displacement of the caecum. However, the caecum in small babies can be quite mobile and must be displaced well above the level of the iliac crest or well medially before one can be sure of the diagnosis. There are considerable advantages in performing a barium meal instead, particularly now that isotonic aqueous media are available. In this way, displacement of the duodenojejunal junction can be determined (Fig. 37.14). This normally lies to the left of the body of the first or second lumbar vertebra. Duodenal bands can be visualized. The contrast is then followed through the small bowel (Fig. 37.15) and eventually the position of the caecum can be defined (Fig. 37.16). The degree of shortening between the ligament of Treitz and the caecum gives some indication of the likelihood of a volvulus occurring.

With the development of a small bowel volvulus one of three radiological patterns may be seen. The appearances may be deceptively normal. On the other hand, the abdomen may be unusually free of gas. This is thought to be due to the presence of fluid in loops closed at both ends but with absorption of gas from the gut, the latter implying a normal venous drainage. Finally, the gut may be distended by gas as well as fluid. It is believed that, under these circumstances, the presence of gas indicates that the venous return from the bowel has been cut off by the volvulus and that the gas is therefore no longer being absorbed.

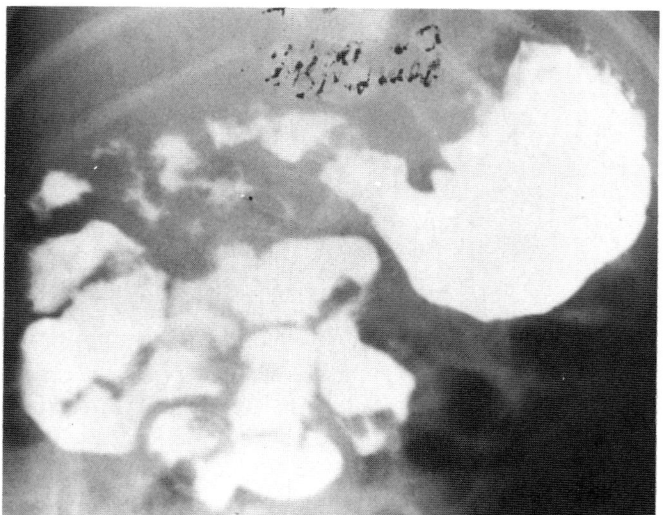

Fig. 37.14 Malrotation. Note that the duodenojejunal junction is to the right of L.2.

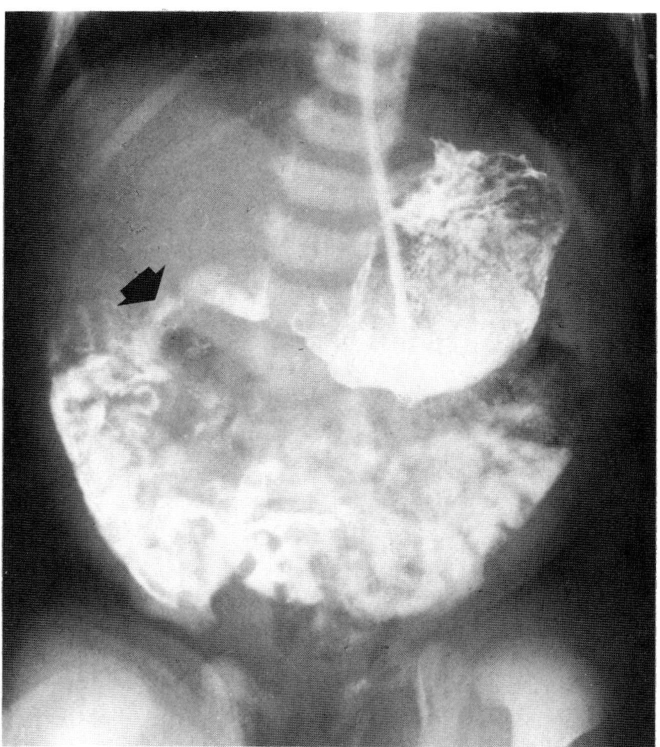

Fig. 37.15 Malrotation. The duodenojejunal junction (↘) lies to the right of the spine.

It remains to add that omphalocoeles and gastroschisis are invariably associated with malrotation.

INTUSSUSCEPTION

Intussusception is a rare event in the neonate, its incidence rising after the age of 6–9 months when mixed feeding is being introduced. When it occurs in the very young, it is often due to the presence of a Meckel's diverticulum, polyp or hamartoma.

The plain film often shows moderately severe small bowel distension, but often with an 'empty' right iliac fossa. Sometimes the terminal ileum can be seen passing upwards and to the right, dragged up by the intussuscepting gut. Occasionally the head of the intussusceptum is outlined by a little gas remaining distal to it in the colon. In general, the diagnosis should be confirmed by a contrast

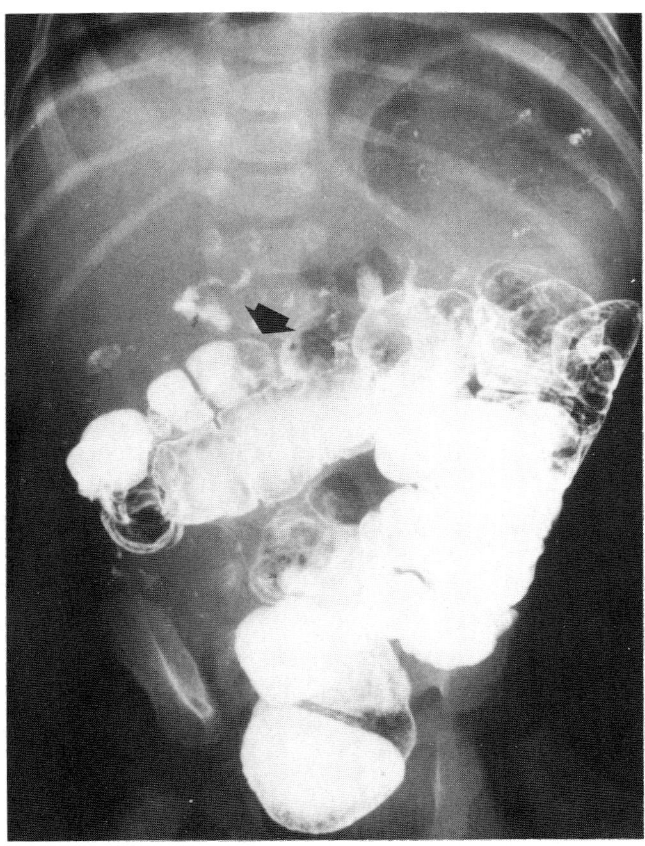

Fig. 37.16 Malrotation. The caecum (↙) lies in the midline opposite L.3!

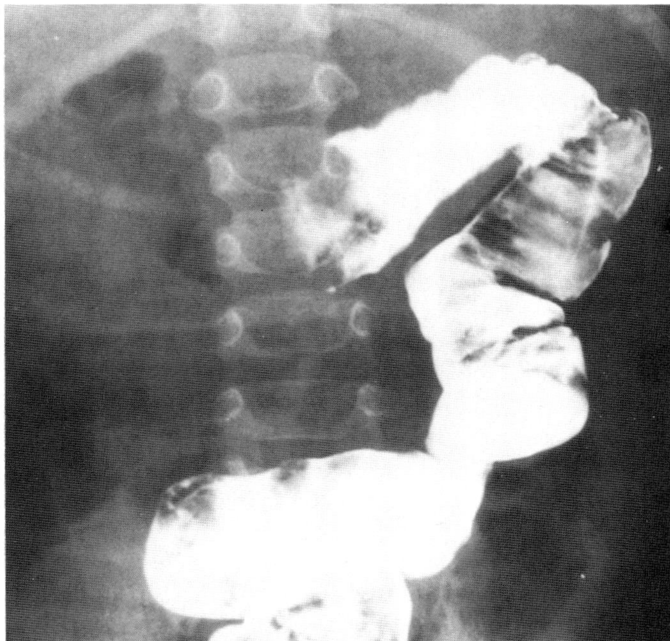

Fig. 37.17 Intussusception. The barium has demonstrated the head of the intussusception just to the left of spine.

enema. This, however, is contraindicated if there is any clinical evidence of peritonitis or peritoneal irritation. The findings on the enema are quite characteristic. The intussusceptum produces a concave defect in the head of the contrast column (Fig. 37.17), but contrast may pass beyond this, causing the well-known 'coiled spring' appearance.

At this stage the question of hydrostatic reduction will arise. While it is tempting to proceed with this, one should bear in mind the possible aetiologic factors at this age and one would therefore, in general, be less enthusiastic than in an older age group. Reduction becomes more difficult the longer the condition has been present and where there is evidence of significant small bowel obstruction. The technique of reduction is the same as for older infants. The use of balloon catheters has been condemned by some radiologists because of the risk of rupturing the rectum; moreover, the balloon may stimulate the rectum to contract and expel it. Nevertheless, the use of small unlubricated Foley catheters is permissible if the balloon is blown up gently under direct fluoroscopic observation. The baby's buttocks are then tightly taped together and barium at body temperature is run in keeping the barium reservoir at less than a metre above table height. In spite of all precautions, barium and balloon are often expelled several times and their insertion has to be repeated. When the head of the intussusception is reached, pressure is maintained as long as progress is being made. If no further progress has occurred for about 20 minutes it is usually useless to persist. Palpation and external pressure are rarely helpful, but sometimes a relaxant such as Buscopan or glucagon may be useful, although this is somewhat controversial.

Ideally, barium should reach the small bowel and enter it. Frequently this cannot be achieved. If a small filling defect persists in the caecum it may be difficult to know whether a small intussusception persists or whether one is looking merely at an oedematous ileocaecal valve. In such cases it is worthwhile waiting for about 2 hours; further events will make the situation clear and very often one has in fact reduced the intussusception. Even partial reduction helps the surgeon.

Prolonged attempts at reduction may result in an infant lying in a pool of cold barium and becoming progressively colder. All precautions should be taken to avoid this. If, after reduction, the intussusception recurs, a further attempt at reduction may be made. Recurrences are not unknown after surgical reduction.

HIRSCHSPRUNG'S DISEASE

During fetal life, migration of neuroblasts occurs in the gut in a craniocaudal direction. These form the myenteric plexuses. If the migration is incomplete, the distal gut remains aganglionic and this results in failure of relaxation and of coordinated peristaltic activity in the distal gut. The bowel proximal to the aganglionic segment becomes dilated, whereas the aganglionic portion itself remains relatively narrow.

Hirschsprung's disease (colonic aganglionosis) is more common in boys. Symptoms often become apparent in the neonatal period, with constipation but occasional violent bouts of diarrhoea. Serious complications are not uncommon, consisting of enterocolitis and bowel perforation. The diagnosis should therefore be confirmed as quickly as possible.

Plain abdominal films show generalized dilatation of the intestine, often with absence of gas in the rectum. An upside down lateral view has been advocated to demonstrate the rectum, but this can be achieved more easily and with less stress by placing the baby prone across a pad and obtaining a lateral film with a horizontal ray. The radiological diagnosis, however, depends on the barium enema. It is important that no attempt be made to clear the colon first, since this may obscure the diagnostic features. Barium in saline should be introduced through a soft rubber catheter without a balloon and the introduction of barium should be stopped as soon as a definite diagnosis can be made. There are three signs which help to establish the diagnosis. The most important is the demonstration of a change of calibre between the relatively narrow distal aganglionic segment and the more dilated proximal segment (Fig. 37.18). This is found commonly in the rectosigmoid region, but may occur in any part of the colon or in the small bowel. The transition may be abrupt or tapering. It is important to realize that the term 'narrow' is relative. The rectum may at first sight look normal; it is the transition to a wider calibre which matters. Unfortunately, in the neonate there may not have been enough time for the colon to dilate and it may not be possible to show a transition zone.

Another helpful sign, but one which is not always present, is an irregular serrated outline of the aganglionic segment. Finally, if the diagnosis is in doubt, a delayed film should be obtained after 24 hours. A normal baby will have expelled nearly all the barium, whereas much of it will be retained in a child with Hirschsprung's disease.

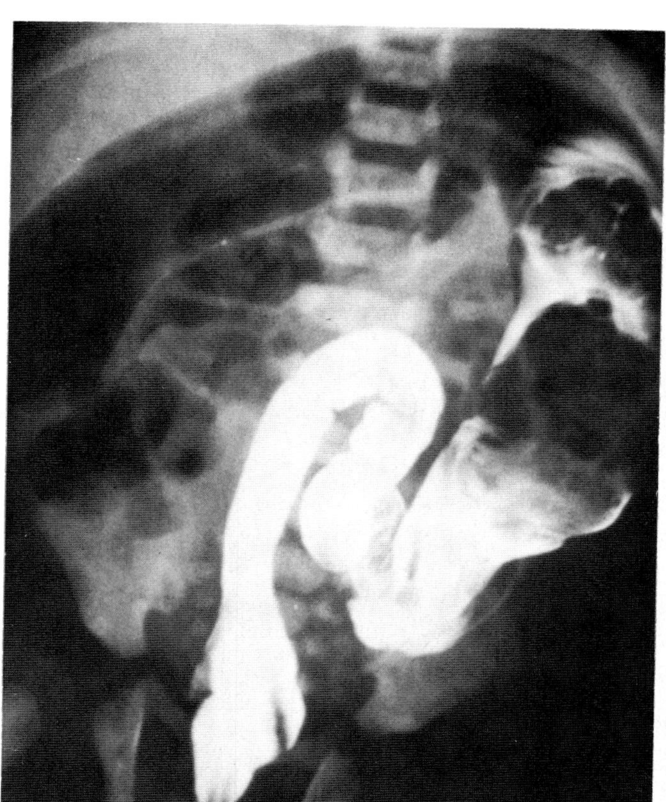

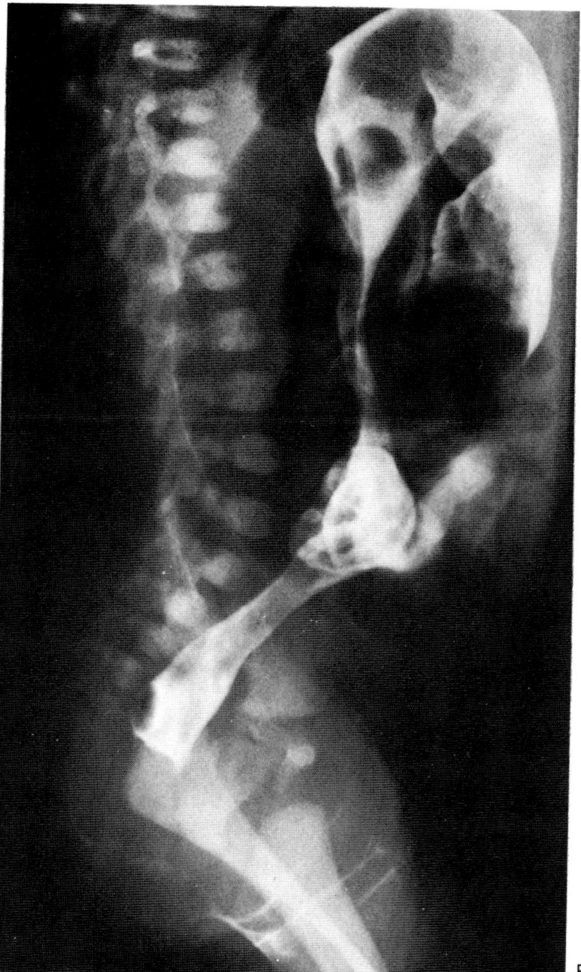

Fig. 37.18 A. and **B.** Hirschsprung's disease. There is a fairly long aganglionic segment. Note the transition zone, which is shown particularly well on the lateral view.

The transition zone is often best seen on a lateral view but should not be confused with the posterior identation on the rectum which is often found in babies due to the effect of the puborectalis sling. Difficulty may arise if the aganglionic segment is very short. It may then be impossible to demonstrate it radiologically and the diagnosis will have to depend on anorectal pressure studies and on biopsy. At the opposite extreme the diagnosis may be difficult if the entire colon and part of the small bowel are affected. Under these circumstances, the colon is often rather short and there is massive reflux into the ileum. Again, a 24-hour film will show much retained barium.

The problem of skip lesions is sometimes raised. Embryological considerations make it unlikely that these can occur, and it is probable that reported skip lesions were due to forms of ganglion cell degeneration and not to true congenital aganglionosis. A number of such conditions, termed neonatal colonic dysplasia, have been described. These may imitate Hirschsprung's disease. Another rare differential diagnosis is plexiform neurofibromatosis of the colon. The problem of meconium plug and small left colon syndrome in very small babies has already been discussed.

ANORECTAL MALFORMATIONS

The complexity of embryological development of the rectum, anus and urogenital systems leads to a large number of anomalies in this region. This has resulted in many confusing and complex classifications. That adopted at the International Paediatric Congress in Melbourne in 1970 is the most practical. This divides the lesions into three types: high, intermediate and low, depending whether the distal bowel terminates above, at, or below the puborectalis sling of the levator ani group of muscles. In these conditions, hope for rectal continence depends on the functional adequacy of the puborectalis. With high termination of the bowel, the puborectalis is nearly always functionally inadequate and it is this fact which largely determines the surgical approach. Failure of proper descent of the hindgut almost invariably causes the most distal portion to join the urogenital system, leading to a fistula. In the male this is usually a rectourethral fistula, less commonly it is rectovesical or rectoperineal; in the female it is usually rectovaginal, less commonly rectoperineal and rarely rectovesical. If the urethra in a female also enters the vagina, a cloacal anomaly results. With low lesions, there may be a dimple or an anocutaneous or anovulvar fistula.

Anorectal malformations are associated in a high proportion of patients with other anomalies. The acronym VATER has become popular to remind one that vertebral (V), anorectal (A), tracheal (T), oesophageal (E) and renal (R) abnormalities are frequently found together. Amongst vertebral defects, those in the sacrum are particularly common and worth noting since the absence of the third and fourth sacral segments tends to indicate that the puborectalis is underdeveloped. Malformation of the colon with ganglion cell dysplasia is another complication which can lead to gross colonic distension.

The choice of the surgical approach at this stage is crucial in deciding whether faecal continence can be attained. It is determined to a large extent by clinical evaluation and the radiologist's contribution is important but limited. A plain film of the abdomen shows evidence of a low intestinal obstruction (Fig. 37.19). Rarely, calcification can be seen within the meconium. Attention should be paid to any skeletal abnormalities, particularly of the sacrum. In the presence of a fistula, air may be seen in the bladder. Air rarely stays in the vagina unless its outlet is obstructed.

At one time the mainstay of diagnosis was the upside down lateral view, often with a marker on the position of the anus. This view has fallen into disrepute and should be discouraged. Not only does it cause unnecessary stress, but it is also quite unreliable. It is often taken too soon (Fig. 37.20), before air has reached the extreme end of the bowel (Fig. 37.21), or air may not be able to reach the end of the bowel because of impacted meconium. A high lesion

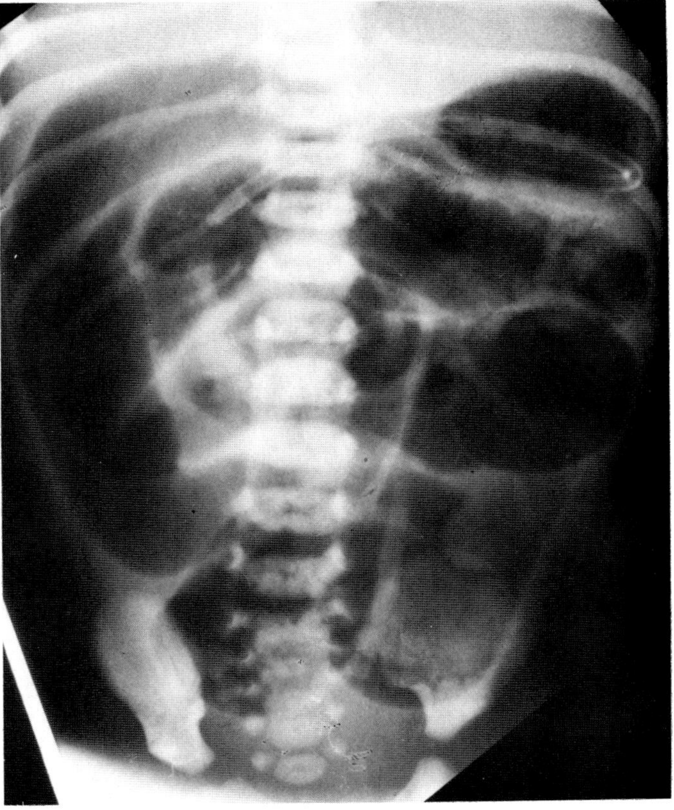

Fig. 37.19 Low intestinal obstruction, due to imperforate anus.

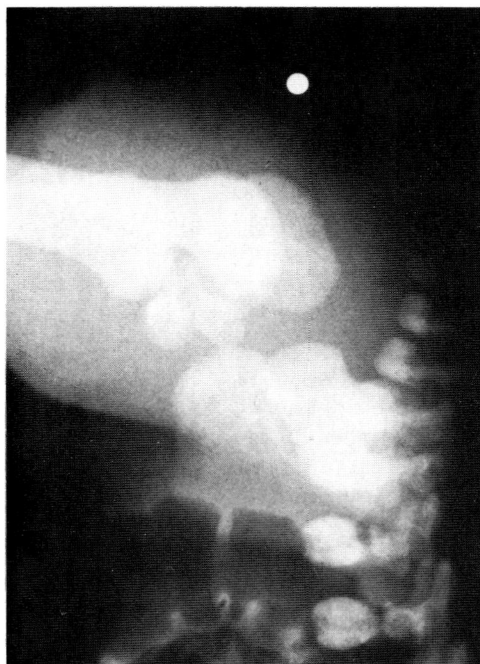

Fig. 37.20 Suspected imperforate anus. Film taken at 4 hours of age suggests a high obstruction.

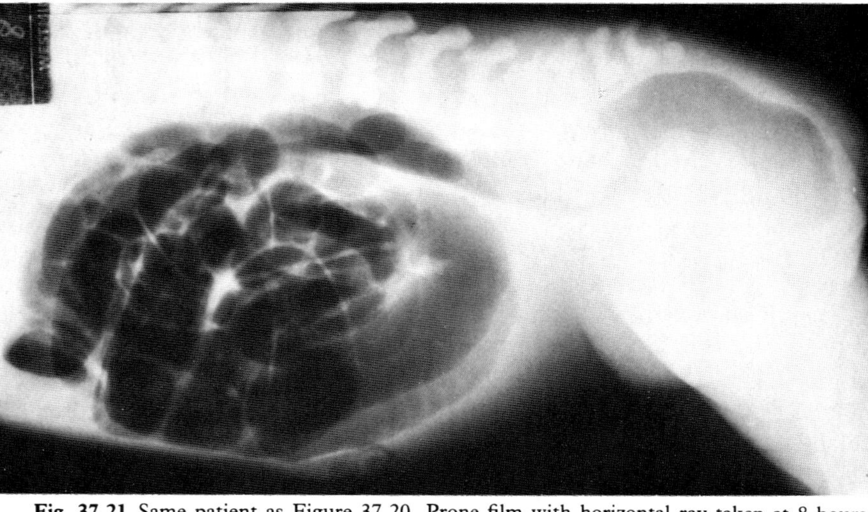

Fig. 37.21 Same patient as Figure 37.20. Prone film with horizontal ray taken at 8 hours shows that the obstruction is, in fact, quite low. The first film had been taken much too early.

may look low if the baby is crying and increasing intra-abdominal pressure. An error in classification at this stage leading to inappropriate surgery would destroy any hope of continence. However, a shoot through lateral with the baby prone can be attempted and the findings interpreted with caution. Direct injection of contrast into the distal bowel by means of a needle passed through the perineum is used in some clinics but this has not gained universal acceptance and is subject to some of the criticisms mentioned above. Surgeons no longer place much reliance on the various lines that have been described for defining the level of the puborectalis sling. These are the pubococcygeal line (from the upper border of the symphysis to the sacrococcygeal junction, or, if the sacrum is absent, from the upper border of the symphysis through the upper fourth of the ischium) and the 'M' line which runs through the junction of the upper two-thirds and lower one-third of the lower ischium seen on the lateral view.

The demonstration of fistulas is of considerable importance and the technique will depend on individual circumstances. Retrograde urethrograms in boys and vaginograms in girls may show them. Sometimes it is better to introduce contrast into the distal bowel through a colostomy but often fistulae are difficult to demonstrate. In addition, intravenous urograms and micturating cystograms should be performed to exclude abnormalities of the urinary tract.

GASTROINTESTINAL BLEEDING IN THE NEWBORN

This is rather uncommon and the causes differ considerably from those found in a later age group. In at least half of these patients no cause is ever found. Maternal blood may have been swallowed during birth, or bleeding may be due to hypoprothrombinaemia, neither of radiological importance. Bleeding at this age can also be due to reflux oesophagitis or acute peptic ulceration. Henoch-Schönlein purpura, polyps and tumours are rare at this age and intussusceptions are also uncommon. Duplication cysts of any part of the gut may bleed.

MECKEL'S DIVERTICULUM

This may contain ectopic gastric mucosa which may ulcerate and give rise to serious bleeding. It is rare to be able to demonstrate a Meckel's diverticulum by barium studies since the diverticulum does not retain the barium. If gastric mucosa is present it may be possible to identify the diverticulum by a technetium scan. Angiographically one can identify the artery supplying the diverticulum or the contrast leak if bleeding is brisk enough, but the opportunity to perform this examination in a neonate is rare. These diverticula may perforate, obstruct the bowel or produce a volvulus if they are adherent to the anterior abdominal wall. Later in life, faecoliths may form in a diverticulum.

NECROTIZING ENTEROCOLITIS

This condition is found most frequently in premature infants who have been subjected to some additional stress.

It is associated with respiratory distress, the passage of umbilical catheters, with any form of intestinal obstruction (particularly Hirschsprung's disease) or it may follow surgery. Breast feeding seems to give some protection from necrotizing enterocolitis. It is believed that the stress is responsible for ischaemia of the bowel produced by a reflex mechanism. This leads to mucosal necrosis and the proliferation of pathogenic organisms in the wall of the gut.

The onset is usually between 2 and 5 days. The baby becomes toxic, distended and vomits and there is frequently rectal bleeding.

Plain abdominal radiographs show intestinal distension: in the earliest stages this is mostly in the right lower quadrant. Later, a bubbly appearance may be found in the colon, particularly in the region of the caecum. This appearance should be regarded with suspicion at this age but needs to be distinguished from similar appearances due to meconium ileus. The clinical background and age of the child help in the distinction between these conditions. Later still, gas appears in the bowel wall and can be recognized as longitudinal translucent streaks or as ring translucencies if the bowel is seen end on (Fig. 37.22). Necrotizing enterocolitis can involve any part of the intestine but it most commonly affects the terminal ileum and colon and gas is seen most easily in the wall of the colon. It is, of course, important to differentiate this appearance from the well-known properitoneal fat line. A definitive diagnosis can be made at this stage, but it cannot be stressed too strongly that the diagnosis should be considered at a much earlier stage if mortality is to be reduced. Later in the disease gas may be found in the portal system (Fig. 37.23). While this is no longer considered as a sign that the condition is inevitably fatal, it is nevertheless of serious import. Other ominous signs are the presence of an unchanging loop since this implies gangrene, ascites, abdominal wall oedema and intestinal perforation. The latter may be asymptomatic in a baby and it is therefore accepted practice to obtain supine and lateral shoot through films every 6 hours during the acute phase.

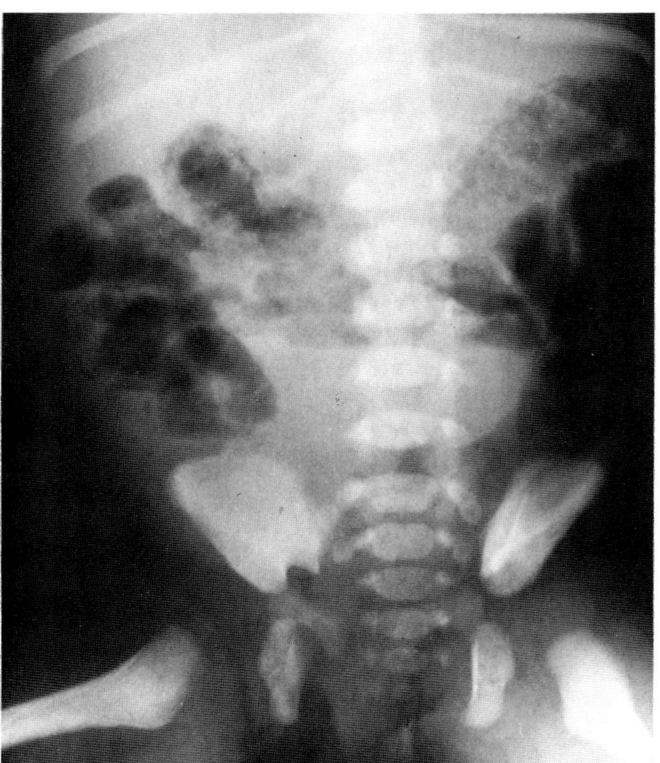

Fig. 37.22 Necrotizing enterocolitis. Note the appearance of the faeces in the gut and air in the bowel wall.

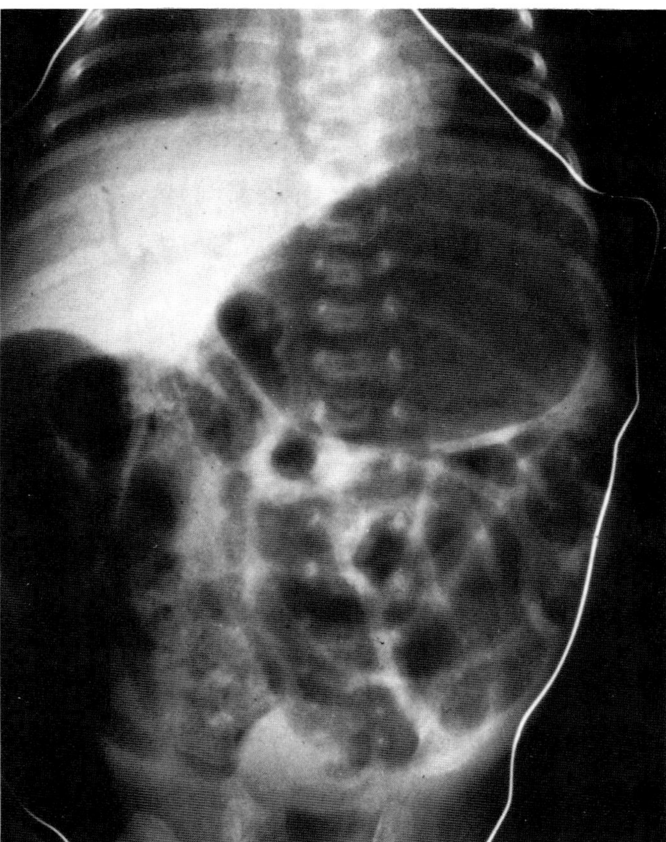

Fig. 37.23 Necrotizing enterocolitis. There is gas in the portal tracts in the liver.

Contrast examinations should be avoided during this period unless there is some very specific indication because there is a very real danger of colonic perforation. Strictures often develop in the ileum or colon as a sequel to necrotizing enterocolitis, often after only 3 or 4 weeks. At this stage contrast studies will be necessary and safe (Fig. 37.24). One should remember that some narrow segments may be due to temporary spasm and not necessarily due to permanent fibrous strictures (Fig. 37.25).

Barium enemas at this age can, with advantage, be carried out using a double contrast technique. One

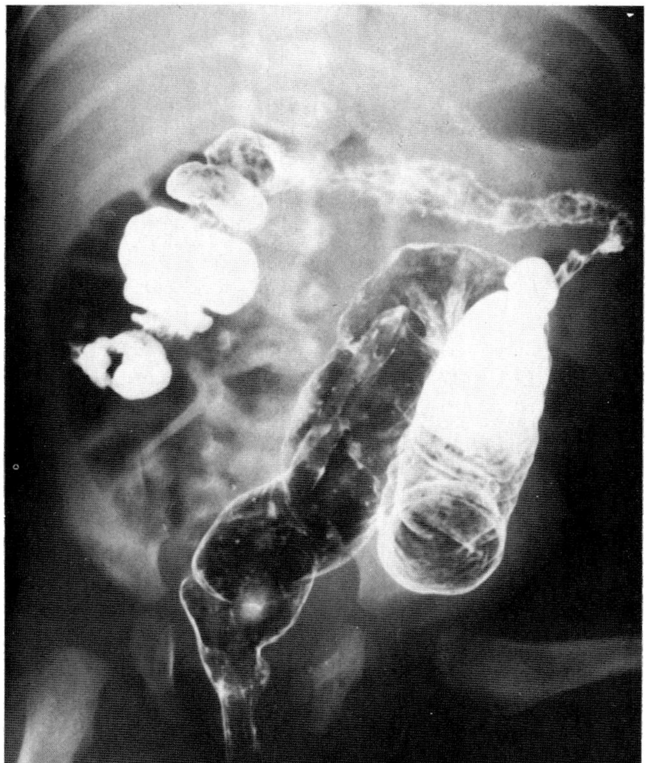

Fig. 37.24 Necrotizing enterocolitis. Same patient as Figure 37.22. A long stricture has developed in that part of the colon affected by the necrotizing enterocolitis.

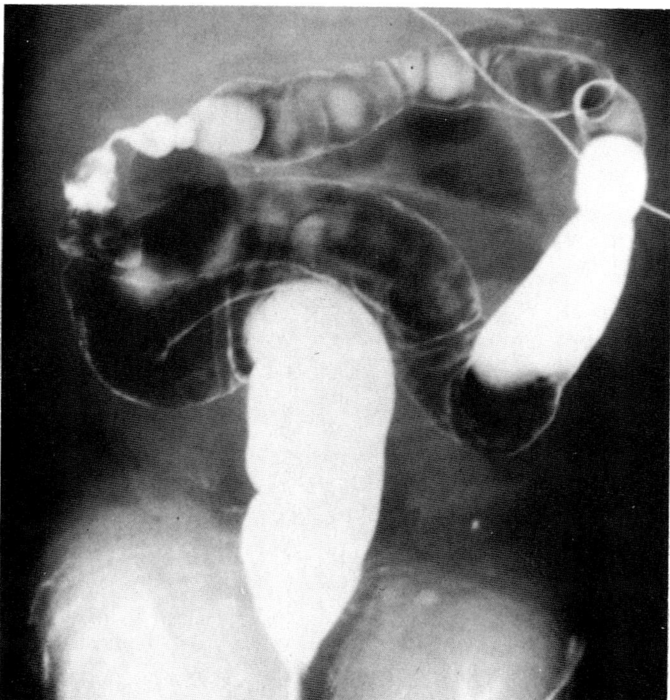

Fig. 37.25 Barium enema following necrotizing enterocolitis. The narrowing at the hepatic flexure was not permanent and did not require resection.

frequently sees a large number of small translucencies in the distal colon due to lymphatic nodules. This should be regarded as a normal appearance at this age.

LIVER AND BILIARY TRACT

BILIARY ATRESIA

Jaundice is common in newborn babies, but if this has not cleared after 2 or 3 weeks the possibility of biliary atresia must be considered. Atresia may be intrahepatic, with absence of the bile ducts, or extrahepatic. In the latter case, the whole of the common bile duct may be atretic or there may be a localized obstruction. The extrahepatic variety may be amenable to surgical treatment but must be distinguished from neonatal hepatitis. Surgery in the latter condition carries a high mortality. Preoperative diagnosis is difficult. A few attempts at performing percutaneous cholangiography have been made, but this technique at this age has obvious difficulties. ^{131}I-rose bengal excretion studies may be useful, recovery of less than 10% from the faeces suggesting biliary obstruction. The test is not entirely reliable, however, and laparotomy and operative cholangiography may be required.

CHOLEDOCHAL CYST

This lesion may be present at birth and it may cause jaundice, fever and pain. It is best demonstrated by ultrasound or computed tomography.

LIVER TUMOURS

These may be benign or malignant. The liver is usually enlarged and occasionally shows calcification. Hepatic haemangiomas or haemangioblastomas may shunt an enormous amount of blood and cause cardiac failure as well as platelet sequestration.

ABNORMALITIES OF THE ABDOMINAL WALL

Only the most important abnormalities in the development of the anterior abdominal wall will be mentioned.

Omphalocele

This is due to a deficiency of the abdominal wall at the umbilicus. A variable amount of gut herniates through the defect. The sac is covered by peritoneum and amnion, with the umbilical cord entering it. Most patients also show other gut abnormalities and the genitourinary system may be abnormal. There may also be exstrophy of the bladder.

Gastroschisis

Bowel passes through a defect of the abdominal wall lateral

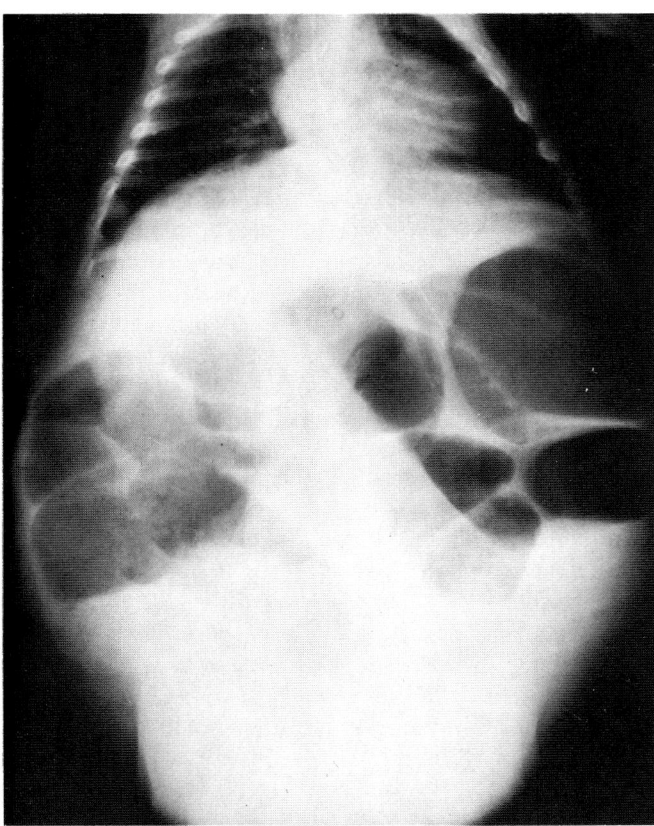

Fig. 37.26 'Prune belly' syndrome. Note splaying of the abdominal wall and lower ribs.

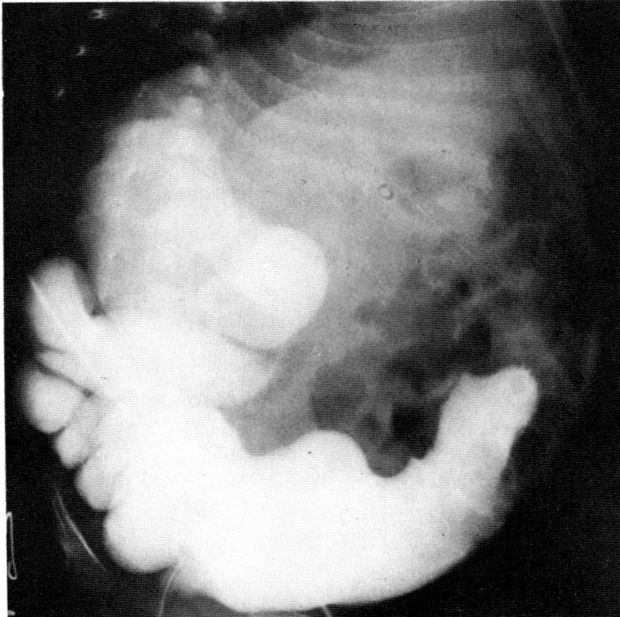

Fig. 37.27 'Prune belly' syndrome. Micturating cystogram. Note the abnormal and grossly dilated ureters.

to the umbilicus, which itself is normal. There is no peritoneal cover. Fixation of the gut is often incomplete but there are no other abnormalities.

Prune belly syndrome

In this condition the muscles in the lower abdomen are defective and the recti muscles are absent (Fig. 37.26). It occurs almost exclusively in boys and is associated with undescended testes and gross hydronephrosis with dilated and elongated ureters (Fig. 37.27). The ureteric abnormality is due to a defect in smooth muscle development in the urinary tract. The urethra is frequently abnormal and may be obstructed, sometimes by a valve. The condition takes its name from the wrinkled appearance of the skin on the abdominal wall which is said to resemble a dried prune.

THE GASTROINTESTINAL TRACT IN CHILDREN

After the first few months of life, radiological changes in the gastrointestinal tract in general resemble those found in adults. In this section only those features will be described which are peculiar to, or are particularly frequent during, childhood.

THE OESOPHAGUS, STOMACH AND DUODENUM

Foreign bodies are a common cause of concern when they have been swallowed by a child. Even babies still in their cots may be fed foreign objects by older sibs. It is important to realize that impaction of a foreign body in the oesophagus need not be associated with localizing symptoms.

Coins are amongst the most common swallowed foreign bodies. On a radiograph of the chest, coins in the oesophagus are seen to lie transversely whereas coins in the trachea are seen end-on. While coins usually traverse the gut without difficulty, other objects, because of their shape, tend to become impacted. *Hair grips* and *open safety pins* are notorious in this respect. The *ring-pulls* used on drink cans also tend to become arrested in the oesophagus. Since they are made of metal of low radio-opacity, they are difficult to see and often remain unrecognized. They have been known to perforate the oesophagus and cause a mediastinal abscess.

A new and increasingly common hazard is caused by swallowing the tiny *mercury batteries* used in cameras, quartz watches and calculators. The batteries disintegrate in the stomach, releasing highly toxic and corrosive mercuric chloride. They are easily recognized by their small size; sometimes a rim is visible round them. When they begin to disintegrate a cloud caused by the mercury salt may become apparent. These foreign bodies must be removed immediately.

If a foreign body is arrested in its course, this occurs usually either in the oesophagus or in the terminal ileum. A child suspected of having swallowed a foreign body should be X-rayed in order to make certain that the object is beyond the oesophagus and not in the oesophagus or lungs. It is usually not necessary to re-X-ray the patient once the object is in the stomach, although one is frequently asked to do so and the decision whether to re-X-ray must be assessed in each case.

The removal of foreign bodies from the oesophagus by means of an inflated Foley catheter is a simple technique which, nevertheless, is best left to the experienced operator.

Another type of foreign body in the stomach not generally found in the adult is a **bezoar**. They usually consist of hair (trichobezoar) or vegetable fibres (phytobezoar). A plain film of the left upper quadrant may show a mass in the stomach but this is more clearly seen on a barium meal as a more or less perfect cast of the stomach.

Corrosive poisoning affecting the oesophagus and stomach is more common in children, but the course of events and the radiological appearances do not differ from those found in adults and are described in the section on the adult oesophagus.

Peptic ulcers. Acute stress ulcers may occur at any age but chronic peptic ulceration is rare in childhood, particularly affecting the stomach. The appearances, however, do not differ from those seen in adults. Children with chronic duodenal ulcers very often have a strong family history of peptic ulcer disease.

THE SMALL BOWEL

Intramural haematoma. Although this may occur in any part of the bowel, it is most common in the *duodenum*. During childhood it occurs as a manifestation of Henoch-Schönlein purpura, and may precede other changes of that disease. Haematomas may also result from other bleeding diatheses although the cause which is most common in adults, anticoagulant therapy, is of little importance in childhood.

The involved portion of gut is rigid and its lumen is narrow. There is thickening of the valvulae conniventes causing a 'stacked coin' appearance, or there may be 'thumb printing' of the margin of the bowel. These changes are transient but give rise to abdominal pain and malaena.

Parasites. Round worms are more common in children than in adults but their radiological appearances are the same. Tapeworms are not recognized radiologically.

Regional enteritis (Crohn's disease). There is a general impression that this condition is becoming more common during childhood. Atypical symptoms are seen more frequently than in adults; the patient may present with pyrexia of unknown origin, anorexia nervosa, erythema nodosum, malabsorption, protein-losing enteropathy, arthritis or hydronephrosis. Abdominal symptoms may be slight and could be overlooked. There is said to be a higher incidence of colonic involvement than in adults, but apart from this the radiological appearances are the same.

Tumours. Benign tumours are exceedingly rare. The lesions of the Peutz-Jeghers syndrome, although they may occur in any portion of the bowel, are particularly common in the small gut.

Malignant tumours of the small bowel in childhood are most commonly *lymphosarcomas* and this is said to be the most common manifestation of lymphosarcoma in the child. The prognosis following resection of an isolated piece of sarcomatous bowel is surprisingly good. All tumours of the small bowel may give rise to an *intussusception*.

Malabsorption. This subject is extensively covered in the adult section (Ch. 31), to which the reader is referred. During childhood the most common cause of malabsorption is *cystic fibrosis*, followed by *coeliac disease*. The comments on the limitations of the barium meal in the diagnosis of malabsorption states apply in equal measure in the paediatric age group, particularly as there is a considerable tendency for many types of barium to flocculate in the intestines of very young babies. Moreover, the appearance of the normal small bowel depends to some extent on the type of barium used; it is advisable to use only one type of barium and become accustomed to the appearances with that particular product. Barium examinations are useful in excluding some specific causes of malabsorption, such as malrotation or jejunal diverticulosis, and to some extent to monitor progress.

Immune defects. Various types of congenital immunological defects are being recognized with increasing frequency during childhood. These may be reflected by complex changes in the gut. Intestinal *candidiasis* is a common complication. *IgA deficiency* is frequently accompanied by *giardiasis*, but also bears a complex relationship to *coeliac disease*; these two conditions may be found together. At present it is not clear which is the primary event. It is well known that IgA deficiency is associated with an increased incidence of small bowel sarcomas, as is coeliac disease. It is tempting to assume that there is some fundamental association between these conditions.

The radiological appearances found in IgA deficiency may be identical with those seen in coeliac disease, or there may be nodular filling defects throughout the gut due to nodular lymphoid hyperplasia (Figs 37.28, 37.29).

Dilatation of the small bowel with absence of the normal mucosal pattern (the so-called 'moulage' appearance) may also be seen in *chronic granulomatous disease*. In this

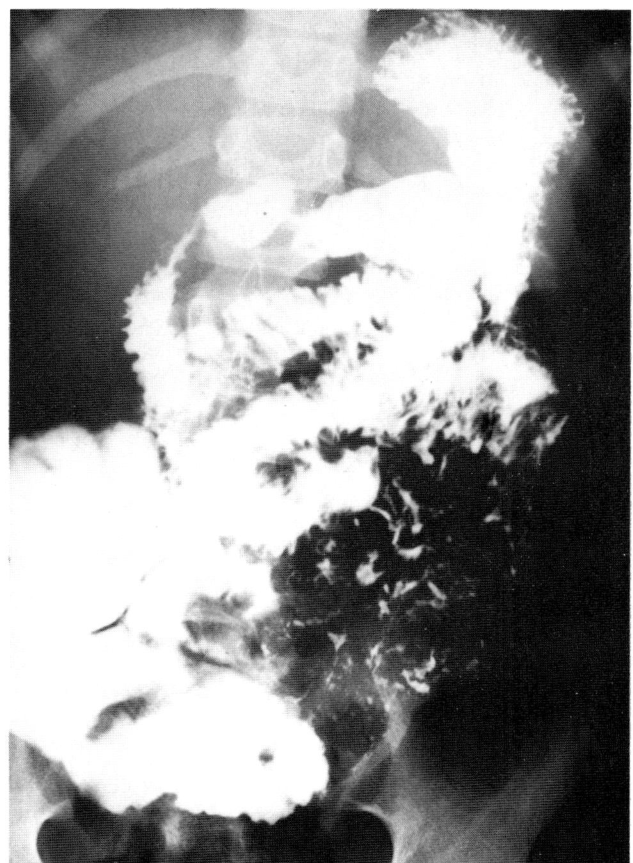

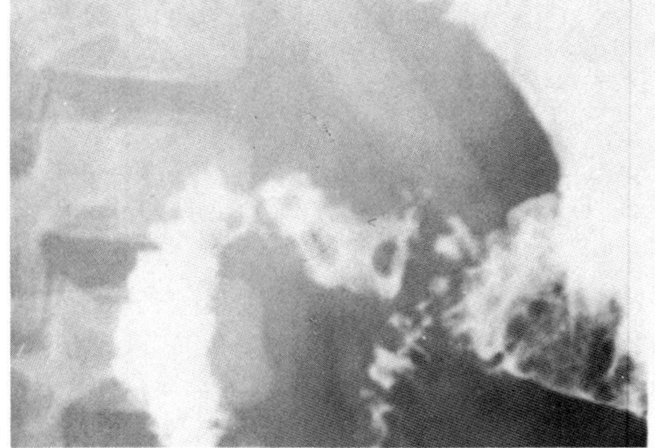

Fig. 37.28 **A.** Barium meal of child with IgA deficiency. Note coarse mucosa in the duodenum and appearances in the lower small bowel resembling those of coeliac disease. **B.** Same patient. There are filling defects in the duodenum due to nodular lymphoid hyperplasia.

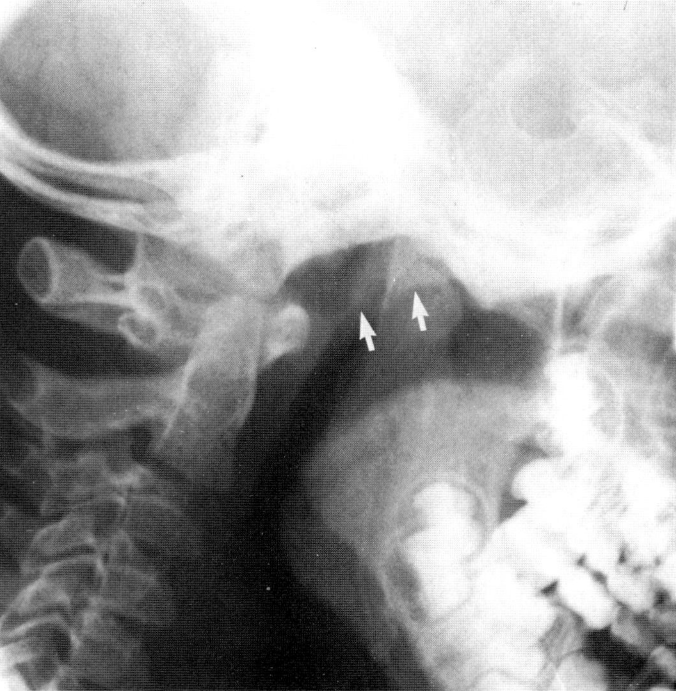

Fig. 37.29 Same patient. Postnasal space showing absence of adenoidal soft tissue pad (arrows), a common feature in immune deficiency states.

condition there is also a high incidence of calcified liver abscesses.

A new set of problems has been created by organ, and particularly bone marrow, transplantation giving rise to *graft-versus-host reactions*. This may affect the gut by producing generalized ileus. Pneumatosis intestinale has been observed on a number of occasions and in the most severe cases changes closely resembling those of Crohn's disease are found (Fig. 37.30).

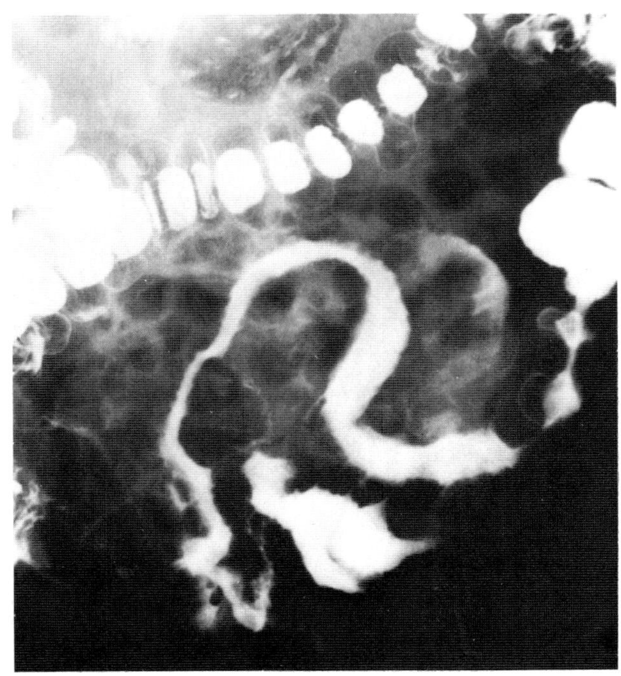

Fig. 37.30 Rectum and sigmoid in a child, following a bone marrow graft for Hunter's syndrome, who developed severe graft-host-reaction.

THE COLON

Idiopathic megacolon has its onset after the age of 2 or 3 years, when it needs to be differentiated from Hirschsprung's disease. The entire distal colon and rectum right down to the anal canal is grossly dilated and full of faeces. Unlike Hirschsprung's disease there is no narrow distal segment but the differentiation is not always easy and may have to depend on anal pressure studies or mucosal biopsy.

Appendicitis is rare in infants, becoming increasingly more common in older age groups. An appendicolith may be present and the diagnosis may be made if this is associated with dilated terminal ileum and caecum. The absence of these signs, however, does not rule out a diagnosis of appendicitis.

Ulcerative colitis is very rare in the youngest age group, becoming more common as adolescence is approached. The radiological appearances are the same as in adults.

Polyps of the colon. About 90% of polyps in the age group 1–10 years are the so-called *juvenile polyps* (Fig. 37.31). These are benign hamartomatous lesions. They tend to be large, often have a stalk and are most frequently single. They nearly always occur in the distal part of the colon and cause rectal bleeding. Sometimes they slough off, causing a spontaneous cure. These lesions are readily diagnosed by a double contrast enema, provided the colon has been adequately cleared beforehand.

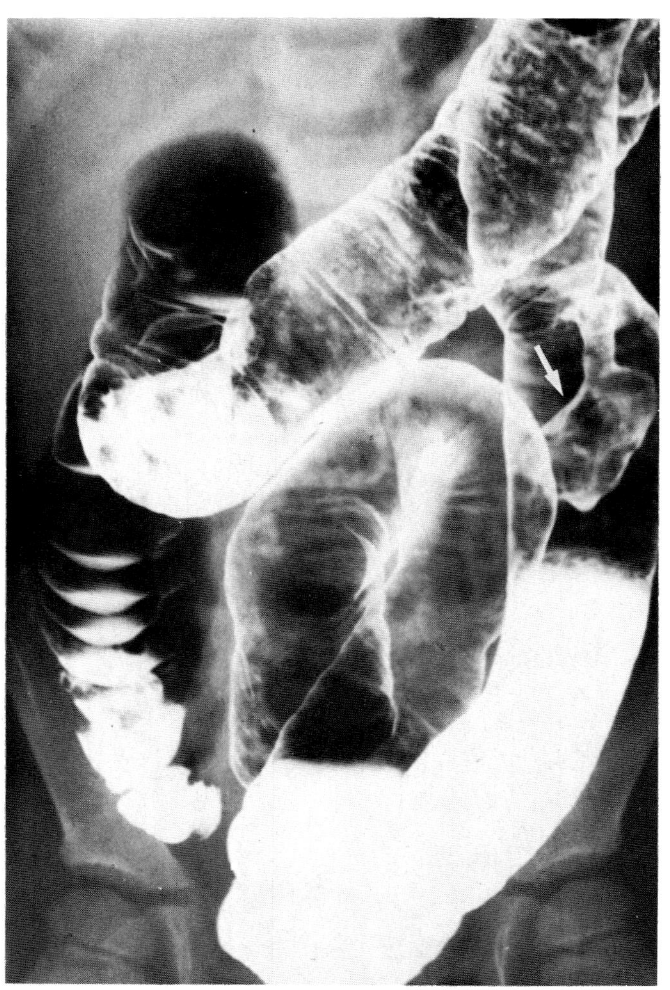

Fig. 37.31 Juvenile polyp in descending colon (↘).

Juvenile polyposis of the colon is characterized by numerous, often hundreds of, tiny polyps. These are hamartomatous and not premalignant and occur quite early in life. The disease is an autosomal dominant.

The above condition must be distinguished from *familial polyposis*. This is also an autosomal dominant but the lesions are adenomas with a 90% incidence of malignancy by the fifth decade. The polyps are often not visible in young children and a normal barium enema during infancy should not create a false sense of security.

Other rare conditions associated with colonic polyps which may be found in childhood are summarized below:

1. *Peutz-Jeghers syndrome*: autosomal dominant, slight risk of malignancy. Characterized by mucocutaneous pigmentation.
2. *Gardener syndrome*: autosomal dominant, strong tendency to malignancy. Associated with osteomas of bone, especially of the skull and mandible and with soft tissue tumours.
3. *Cronkhite-Canada syndrome*: non-genetic, associated with alopecia, skin hyperpigmentation and nail changes.
4. *Turcot syndrome*: autosomal recessive, colonic polyps associated with c.n.s. tumours.
5. *Neurofibromatosis*: autosomal dominant. May produce neurofibromata in the gut.

THE GALL BLADDER

Gallstones in children are very rare. Both oral and intravenous cholangiograms may be carried out as in adults, reducing the dose of contrast on a proportional weight basis. However, gallstones will be diagnosed most by ultrasound. It is essential to exclude *haemolytic anaemia* as the cause of biliary stones in the paediatric age group, although by no means all stones in children are due to this cause.

THE PANCREAS

Acute pancreatitis sometimes follows mumps, but may also be due to steroids or immunosuppressive drugs, hyperparathyroidism or ascaris. An hereditary form transmitted as an autosomal dominant has been described and may cause recurrent attacks of pancreatitis. The radiological appearances and complications do not differ from those of the adult disease.

Pancreatic tumours. Malignant tumours have been described but are exceedingly rare. Benign tumours are also uncommon. *Beta-cell tumours* cause hypoglycaemia as in adults but may manifest themselves by bizarre behaviour patterns as well as by the other better known features of hypoglycaemia. These tumours are usually single but may be multiple. *Non-beta cell tumours* are responsible for the Zollinger-Ellison syndrome as in adults. They are very rare in childhood, as are *glucagon-secreting tumours*. The radiological investigations are identical with those undertaken in adults.

ABDOMINAL MASSES IN CHILDHOOD

(by C. E. Dicks-Mireaux)

In the neonate (less than 1 month of age) hydronephrosis and multicystic kidney disease together account for almost 40% of the cases and the prognosis is good. However, the incidence of malignant disease increases with increasing age and in older children (2–12 years) malignant neoplasms account for 60% of all abdominal masses, the most common being nephroblastoma and neuroblastoma.

The presentation of a child with an abdominal mass is a source of concern to the paediatrician and parent. The investigation of this problem presents a diagnostic challenge in which the radiologist can be of great help. The approach to the problem cannot be the same as in adult patients, because of different constraints on the choice of imaging methods, and a different range of presenting pathologies. Within the paediatric age group there is a greater emphasis on congenital abnormalities. More than half of the abdominal masses will be renal in origin with a large proportion of these being congenital abnormalities.

Diagnostic imaging methods must be selected with care and exposure to radiation kept to a minimum in children. Certain imaging modalities are more suitable than others; for example, the paucity of abdominal fat in children results in good quality images on ultrasound, but reduces the quality of images produced by computerized tomography. Sedation or general anaesthesia is required in children if procedures are painful, or if the patient has to remain immobile for any length of time. All these factors must be taken into consideration in the investigation of a child with an abdominal mass.

Plain radiographs

Plain abdominal films are limited in their diagnostic usefulness. Abdominal masses may be identified by displacement of adjacent loops of bowel gas, giving some idea of their location and size. The presence or absence of calcification will be confirmed. *Calcification* of various

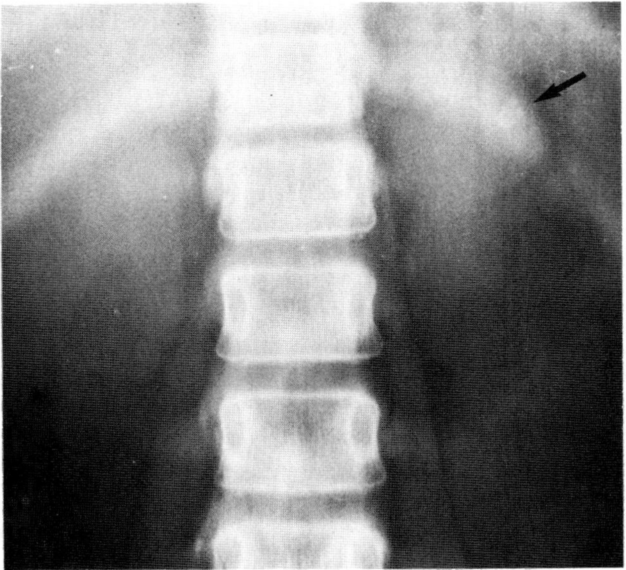

Fig. 37.32 Plain film tomogram showing calcification in the left suprarenal neuroblastoma (arrow).

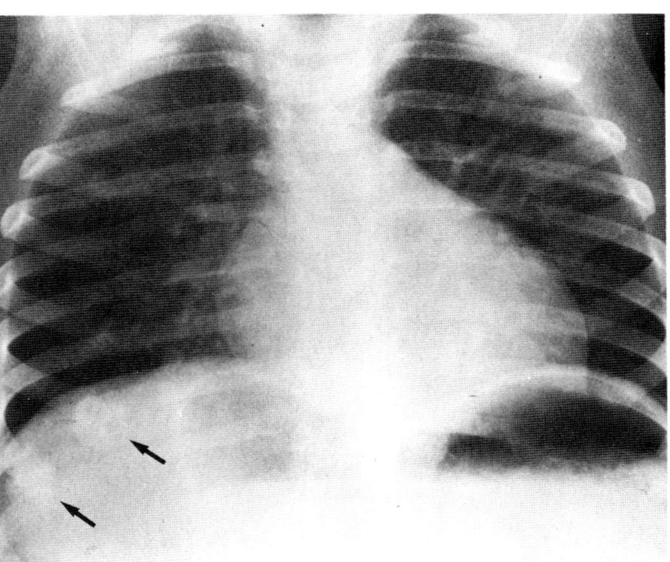

Fig. 37.33 Chest X-ray demonstrating calcification beneath the right hemidiaphragm in a hepatoblastoma.

appearances may be seen in neuroblastomas, teratomas, nephroblastomas and less commonly hepatoblastomas. (Figs 37.32, 37.33). Associated abnormalities in the skeletal system, such as metastases and hemihypertrophy, may be apparent.

Plain radiographs of the chest are also required to demonstrate pulmonary metastases — these are frequently present in cases of nephroblastoma and hepatoblastoma.

Intravenous urography

Until the recent advent of ultrasound scanning and computerized tomography, the intravenous urogram was a routine and important investigation in the diagnostic work-up of an abdominal mass. The majority of these masses are retroperitoneal and often renal in origin. Intravenous urography provides information about renal function, renal position, kidney outline and calyceal abnormalities. A mass may be identified as *extrarenal* when there is displacement of the whole kidney or as *renal* if displacement of the calyces and distortion of the renal outline are seen. Obstructed conditions with *hydronephrosis* secondary to pelviureteric junction obstruction, or posterior urethral valves, and congenital abnormalities such as duplications of the renal tract will be demonstrated (Fig. 37.34). *Non-function* of a kidney may be seen in cases of obstruction, dysplastic multicystic kidney and complete replacement of a kidney by tumour. Tomograms and delayed films may be required.

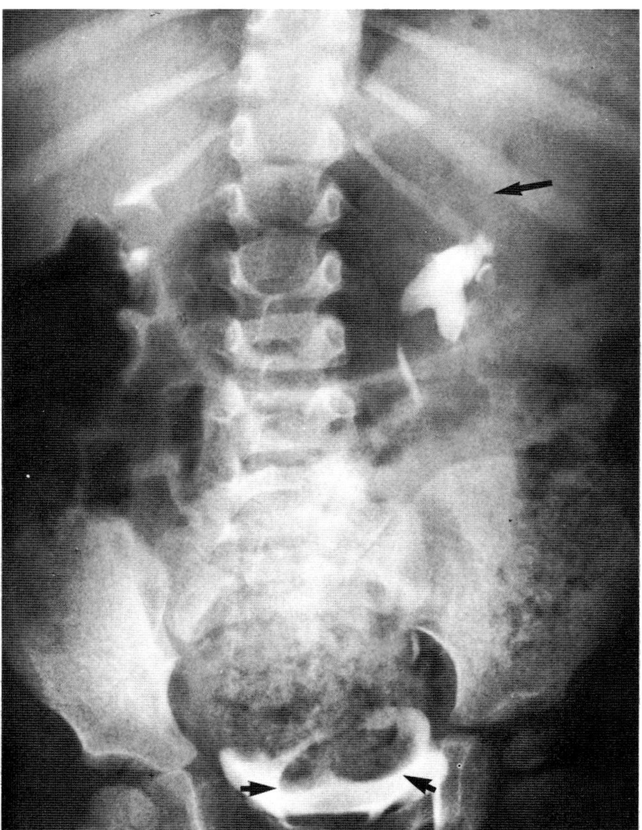

Fig. 37.34 Intravenous urogram of a duplex left kidney with a non-opacified hydronephrotic upper moiety (arrow) and a ureterocele within the bladder (arrows).

Simultaneous inferior vena cavography by injection of contrast medium into a vein in the foot has been used in the investigation of an abdominal mass, as a method of detecting tumour thrombus in the inferior vena cava. However, false positives are not uncommon with non-opacification of the inferior vena cava if the child is crying during the procedure, or if the inferior vena cava is grossly compressed and displaced by a large mass.

In the neonatal age group there are disadvantages in the use of intravenous urography and alternative methods of investigation are preferred. Neonates have immature and relatively poor renal function and are unable to concentrate contrast media, thus resulting in poor quality images. If the neonate is unwell and dehydrated the examination can be hazardous with a significant morbidity.

Ultrasound scanning

The development of this technique and the advent of real-time ultrasonography has resulted in important changes in the investigation of abdominal masses in children. The technique is non-invasive and most children can be examined without sedation. The lack of exposure to radiation is important in children and examinations can be repeated at frequent intervals if required. Scanning can be performed in any plane thus facilitating three-dimensional conceptualization. With real-time scanners major blood vessels are easily identified and their relationship to the mass demonstrated. Unlike CT, the image produced by ultrasound is improved by the lack of abdominal fat.

An ultrasound scan is recommended as the first examination in a child or neonate with an abdominal mass. This will yield much information, and in some cases may be the only imaging technique required to make the diagnosis and assist further management. The localization of the mass and the organ of origin will be demonstrated. The internal structure of the mass, whether cystic or solid, often an indicator of its benign or malignant nature, is easily seen. Non-functioning kidneys, which are not visualized on the intravenous urogram, may be examined, and those which are obstructed and hydronephrotic may be identified and distinguished from other pathologies, such as nephroblastomas and multicystic kidneys. Involvement of other organs can also be assessed, e.g. liver metastases.

Computerized tomography

Although computerized tomography is an excellent method for imaging abdominal masses and can be superior to ultrasound scanning, it has several disadvantages in children. Not only does it require the use of X-rays, but in most children below 5 years of age sedation or a general anaesthetic may be necessary. The lack of abdominal fat may result in images which are difficult to interpret. However, it is very useful in cases where detailed and precise demonstration of anatomy is required. For example, a CT scan is recommended in the investigation of liver masses to assess their lobar involvement. Para-aortic lymphadenopathy in lymphoma and associated with other tumours is more consistently and reliably shown on CT. The size and extent of masses in the pelvis such as rhabdomyosarcoma will be more clearly defined on CT. In cases of nephroblastoma, CT may be the most sensitive method for examining the opposite kidney for bilateral tumour involvement or nephroblastomatosis. Involvement of major blood vessels can be shown with dynamic CT scanning and intravenous contrast.

Angiography

Angiography has been largely replaced by ultrasound and CT scanning in the investigation and diagnosis of an abdominal mass. In particular instances an angiogram is however still indicated. The preoperative assessment of liver tumours should include an angiogram in order to demonstrate the vascular supply of the liver (Fig. 37.35). In certain complicated cases of nephroblastoma, if conservative surgery, such as a partial nephrectomy, is indicated, an angiogram is again necessary to demonstrate the anatomy of the renal arteries.

Angiography is also important when interventional techniques such as embolization of tumours are contemplated. This practice is, however, rare in paediatrics.

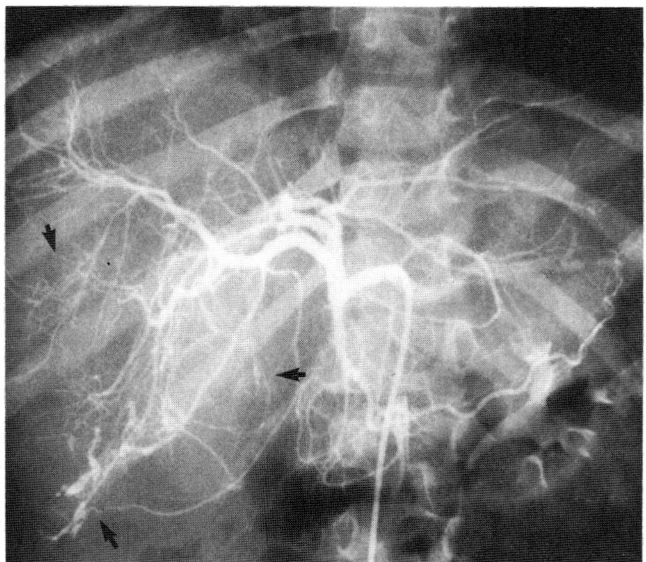

Fig. 37.35 Coeliac axis arteriogram demonstrating the anatomy of the vascular supply to the liver and an abnormal circulation to a hepatoblastoma in the right lobe (arrows).

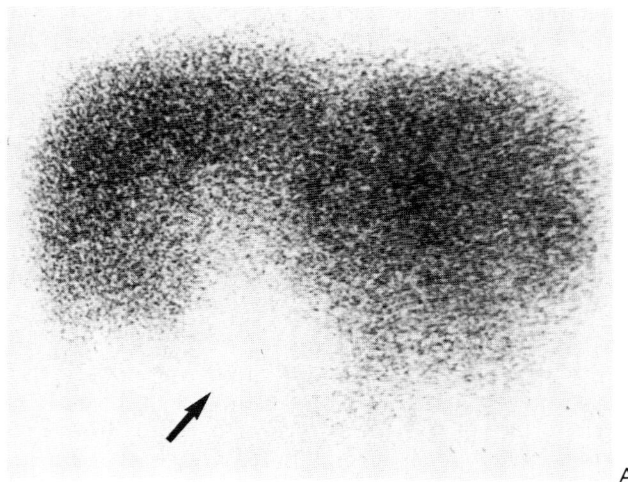

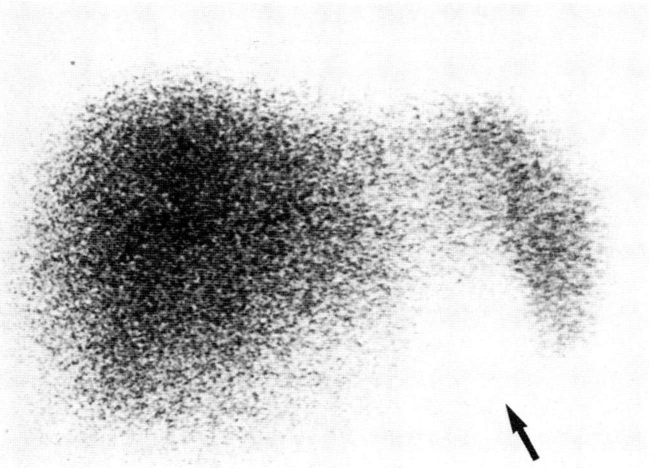

Fig. 37.36 Isotope scan of the liver with a unifocal defect in the right lobe due to a hepatoblastoma. **A.** RAO projection. **B.** LPO projection.

Nuclear medicine

Radioisotope studies have a limited role in the evaluation of abdominal masses. In the investigation of hepatobiliary masses a scan with radiolabelled colloid will demonstrate whether a mass is intrahepatic or extrahepatic. If intrahepatic, it will be shown to be unifocal or multifocal (Fig. 37.36). *Dynamic imaging* will give information on the vascularity of a liver mass and is diagnostic in cases of haemangioendothelioma. Liver scanning is also used to demonstrate secondary deposits in the liver. The use of a $^{99}Tc^{m}$-labelled imino-diacetic acid derivative ($^{99}Tc^{m}$-HIDA) will demonstrate a *choledochal cyst*.

Renal scanning with labelled diethylene-triamine-penta-acetate ($^{99}Tc^{m}$-DTPA) is useful for studying renal function in cases of hydronephrosis, and sometimes in distinguishing between a hydronephrotic kidney due to pelviureteric junction obstruction, and a congenital multicystic kidney.

Abdominal masses in childhood can be divided into predominantly three groups and will be described under these headings:

1. Retroperitoneal
   a. renal
   b. non-renal
2. Hepatobiliary
3. Gastrointestinal.

RETROPERITONEAL MASSES

RENAL

The majority of abdominal masses in childhood are retroperitoneal and renal in origin. Renal masses, which may present as an abdominal mass, include the following:

1. Hydronephrotic kidney
2. Multicystic dysplastic kidneys
3. Polycystic kidneys
4. Nephroblastoma (Wilm's tumour)
5. Mesoblastic nephroma
6. Renal vein thrombosis
7. Miscellaneous renal.

1. Hydronephrotic kidneys

This is the most common abdominal mass in the neonate. Underlying causes of the hydronephrosis will include pelviureteric junction obstruction, posterior urethral valves, duplex kidney with an ectopic ureterocele, prune belly syndrome and ureteral and ureterovesical junction obstruction. Visualization and diagnosis of the hydronephrotic kidney is usually straightforward with ultrasound. The appearances are those of an enlarged kidney, with separation of the central echogenic complex, and one large or several interconnecting echolucent, cystic structures within the kidney (Fig. 37.37). In cases of posterior urethral valves, bilateral hydronephrotic kidneys with dilated ureters and a thickened bladder wall are seen (Fig. 37.38). Scanning through the perineum will demonstrate a dilated posterior urethra (Fig. 37.39). A micturating cystourethrogram is then required to demonstrate the urethral obstruction and presence of vesicoureteric reflux.

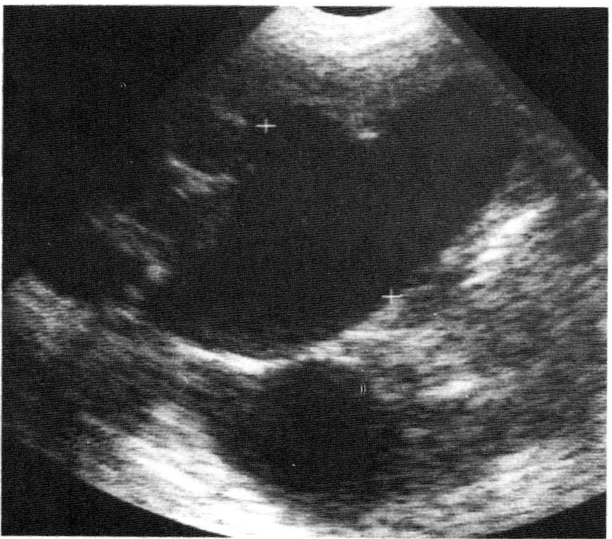

Fig. 37.37 Longitudinal ultrasound scan of a hydronephrotic kidney. (The dilated pelvis is between the markers.)

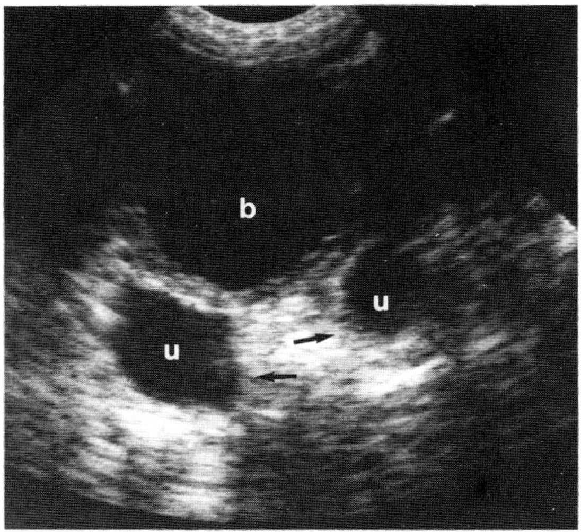

Fig. 37.38 Transverse ultrasound scan of the pelvis showing the bladder (b) with a thickened wall and two dilated ureters (u) posteriorly (arrows).

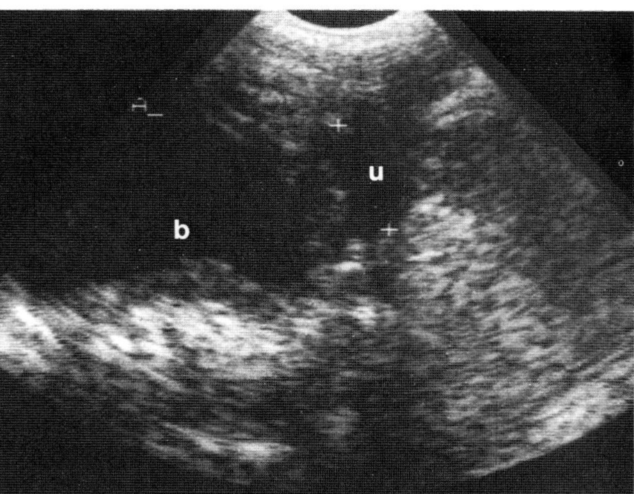

Fig. 37.39 Longitudinal ultrasound scan of the bladder (b) and dilated posterior urethra (u — between markers).

If there is a hydronephrosis of the upper moiety of a duplex kidney with an ectopic ureterocele, both ultrasound and intravenous urography will demonstrate the hydronephrosis, dilated ureter and cystic ureterocele within the bladder.

In cases of pelviureteric junction obstruction, a hydronephrotic kidney without a dilated ureter is seen. This diagnosis may be confirmed with repeat ultrasound scans following a waterload. A DTPA isotope scan with intravenous diuretic is useful for confirmation of the diagnosis, assessment of function and follow-up.

Ultrasound scanning should be able to elucidate most cases of hydronephrosis. If intravenous urography is required delayed films to demonstrate the level of obstruction may be necessary.

2. Multicystic dysplastic kidney

This congenital abnormality is usually discovered in the early neonatal period. The abnormal kidney has an atretic pelvis and is made up of grape-like, smooth-walled, non-intercommunicating cysts of various sizes. Ultrasound scanning will demonstrate the enlarged kidney with multiple echolucent cysts separated by septa (Fig. 37.40). The diagnosis is usually straightforward, although in some cases with few cysts, it may be difficult to distinguish a multicystic kidney from a hydronephrotic kidney with a pelviureteric junction obstruction. Intravenous urography will usually reveal a non-functioning, non-opacified kidney, although there may be 'puddling' of contrast within cysts on delayed films, at 24 hours and 48 hours, depending on the amount of functioning renal tissue present.

3. Nephroblastoma (Wilm's tumour)

This malignant neoplasm of the kidney is one of the more common primary abdominal tumours in childhood. It is associated with various congenital abnormalities including aniridia, horseshoe kidney and Beckwith's syndrome (macroglossia, omphalocele and neonatal hypoglycaemia). It is bilateral in approximately 5% of cases and 65% of these bilateral tumours are apparent at the time of initial diagnosis.

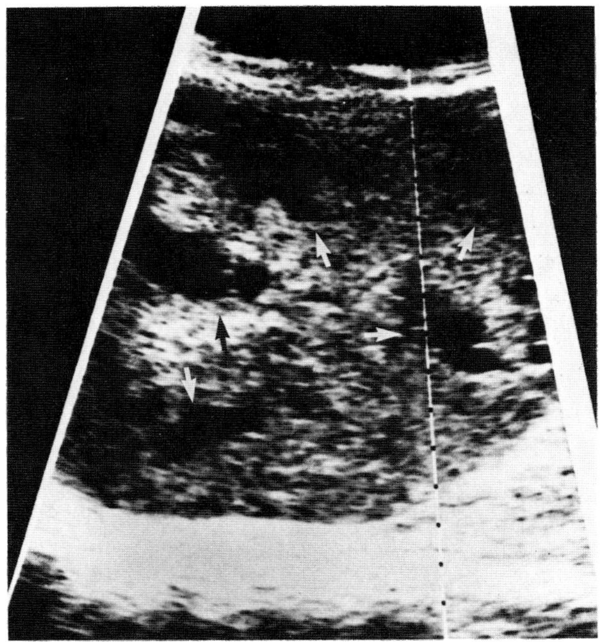

Fig. 37.41 Ultrasound scan of part of a large nephroblastoma with characteristic echolucent lakes (arrows).

The tumour, particularly if involving the right kidney, may extend directly into the renal vein and inferior vena cava. Haematogenous metastases to the lungs are common. A solid, well-circumscribed renal mass is seen on ultrasound scanning. The kidney may be completely replaced by tumour and a normal kidney will not be identified. The echopattern is often non-homogeneous with characteristic echolucent lakes (Fig. 37.41). Calcification is unusual. Ultrasound scanning will also identify tumour thrombus within the inferior vena cava; this will be seen as echogenic, intraluminal material with anterior bowing of the

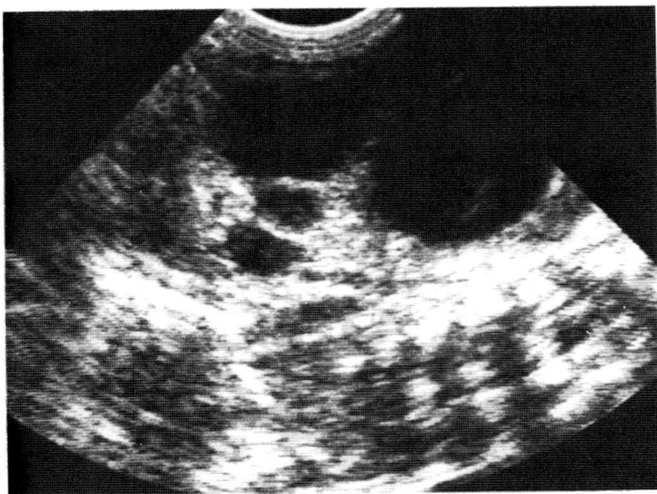

Fig. 37.40 Longitudinal ultrasound scan of a multicystic dysplastic kidney with discrete cysts of varying size.

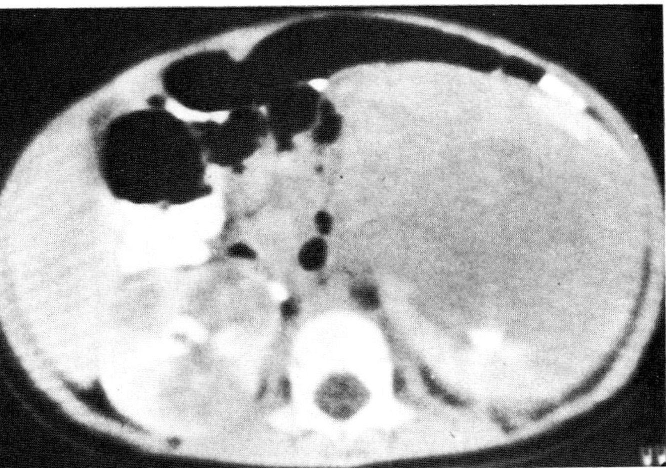

Fig. 37.42 CT scan of the abdomen showing a large nephroblastoma of the left kidney and several small nephroblastomas in the right kidney, showing as low density areas.

inferior vena cava around the thrombus. An intravenous urogram will demonstrate an intrarenal mass with displacement and distortion of the renal outline and pelvicalyceal system. In 10% of cases there is non-function of the involved kidney. CT scanning is useful and will demonstrate a mass of attenuation less than normal renal parenchyma. Extension into adjacent tissues and involvement of para-aortic lymph nodes may be more clearly seen on CT than ultrasound. Bilateral lesions, depending on their size, will be seen with ultrasound scanning, intravenous urography and CT and regular follow-up of the unaffected kidney is required (Fig. 37.42). In conditions with an increased incidence of nephroblastoma, such as Beckwith's syndrome, regular screening of the kidneys with ultrasound scans has been suggested.

4. Mesoblastic nephroma

This benign renal tumour usually presents as an asymptomatic mass in the first weeks of life. The appearances on ultrasound scans are those of a non-homogeneous, echogenic, solid renal mass. On intravenous urography the appearances are identical to those of a nephroblastoma (Fig. 37.43). Diagnosis is made following surgical removal.

5. Renal vein thrombosis

This condition, which can occur in sick and dehydrated neonates, may present as an abdominal mass with haematuria. The ultrasound appearances are characteristic, and show an enlarged kidney with a patchy, bright echogenic pattern (Fig. 37.44). An intravenous urogram is unnecessary, but will show faint or absent opacification of the kidney.

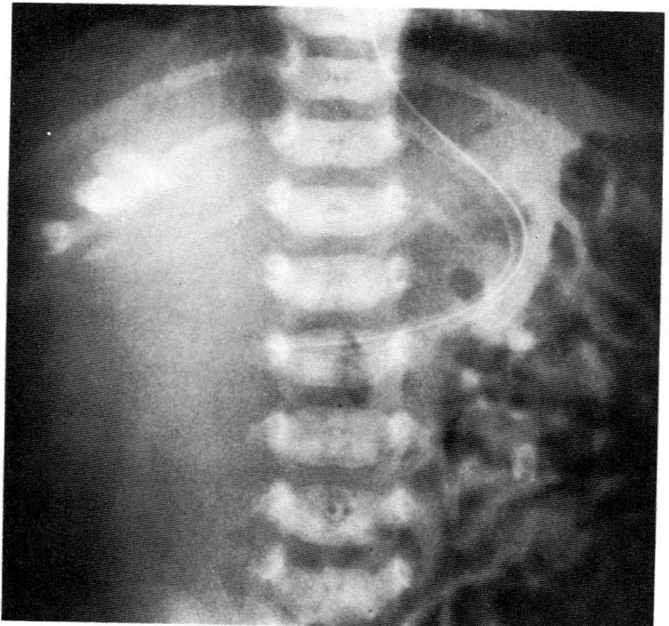

Fig. 37.43 Intravenous urogram of a mesoblastic nephroma of the right kidney, showing R. renal mass with distorted calyces.

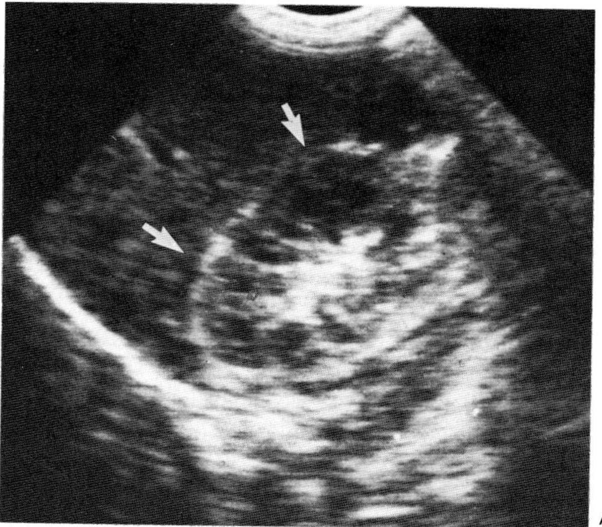

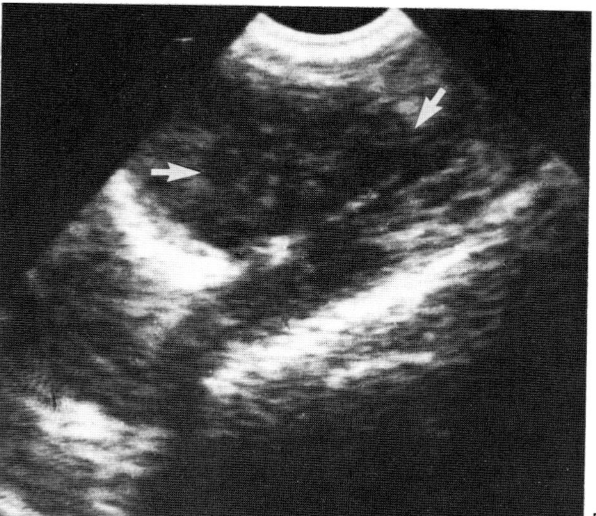

Fig. 37.44 Longitudinal renal ultrasound scans. **A.** A right kidney with renal vein thrombosis. **B.** The normal neonatal left kidney.

6. Polycystic kidneys

Infantile polycystic kidneys may present as bilateral abdominal masses in the neonatal period. This inherited condition can be associated with cysts in the spleen and pancreas and hepatic fibrosis. Bilateral renal enlargement with a diffuse increase in echogenicity throughout the kidneys is seen on ultrasound. If hepatic fibrosis is present, increased echogenicity may be seen in the liver. Bilateral renal enlargement, with poor opacification of the kidneys, is seen on intravenous urography. Characteristically delayed films demonstrate linear streaking of contrast radiating from the renal cortex towards the centre of the kidney (see also Ch. 40).

Rarely, adult polycystic disease of the kidney may present in the neonate as a unilateral or bilateral abdominal mass. The appearances on ultrasound may resemble those

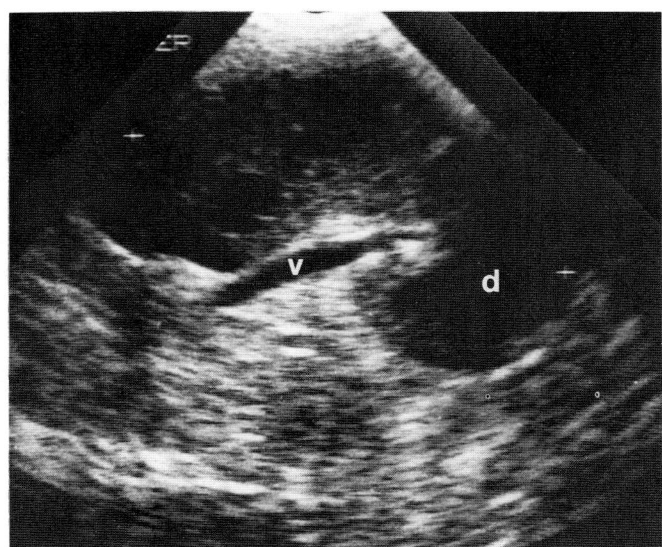

Fig. 37.45 Longitudinal ultrasound scan of the left kidney (between markers) with an echolucent lymphomatous deposit (d) in the lower pole. Renal vein (v) shown at hilum.

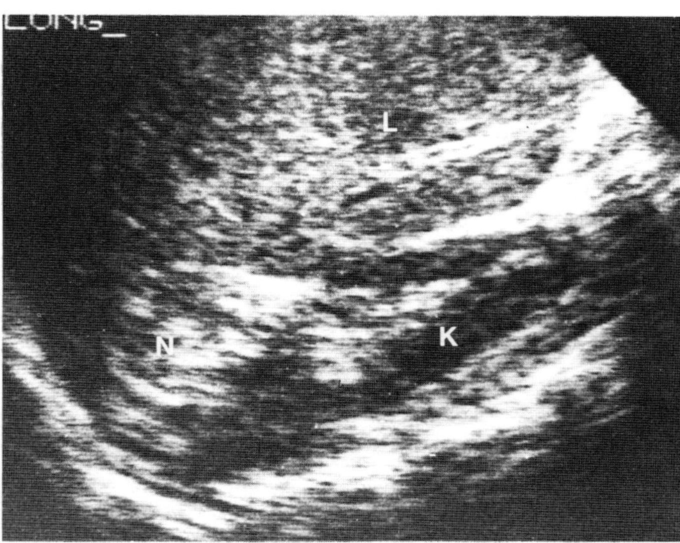

Fig. 37.46 Longitudinal ultrasound scan of liver (L) and right kidney (K) with right suprarenal neuroblastoma (N).

of infantile polycystic kidneys, although sometimes the cysts are large enough to be visualized as discrete echolucent cysts.

7. Miscellaneous renal masses

Infection with renal *abscess* formation may present as a renal mass. An enlarged kidney with an irregular, intrarenal echolucent mass is seen on ultrasound. Intravenous urography will show an intrarenal mass with pelvicalyceal displacement.

Lymphomatous infiltration of the kidneys may be unilateral or bilateral. On ultrasound, the appearances are similar to those of an abscess with an intrarenal, echolucent mass (Fig. 37.45).

NON-RENAL

Neuroblastoma

This is the second most common abdominal malignancy in childhood and is seen most frequently during the first 4 years of life. It may arise in the adrenal medulla or anywhere along the sympathetic chain. Two-thirds occur in the abdomen and 65% of these are suprarenal, with 4% in the pelvis. Tumoral *calcification* which is usually irregular, finely stippled and punctate is seen on plain abdominal films in approximately 60% of cases. If the mass is suprarenal, displacement of the ipsilateral kidney inferiorly and often laterally is seen on the intravenous urogram. Pelvic masses may cause an impression on the bladder and ureteric obstruction. Ultrasound scanning will demonstrate a solid, suprarenal mass with a variable non-homogeneous echopattern. There is usually increased echogenicity with areas of calcification producing intense echoes and acoustic shadowing (Fig. 37.46). The site and extent of the tumour can be seen. Characteristically neuroblastoma will encase and surround the great vessels, resulting in elevation and displacement of the aorta and inferior vena cava (Fig. 37.47). The liver can also be examined for metastases. In cases where the tumour is small, or on the left side, and particularly if surgery is planned, ultrasound may not be sufficient to demonstrate the true

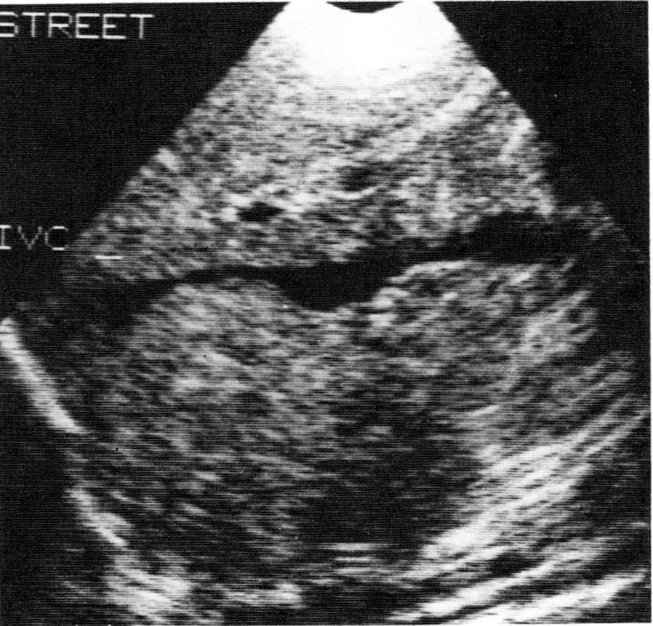

Fig. 37.47 Longitudinal ultrasound scan showing the IVC elevated and indented posteriorly by large solid mass of neuroblastoma.

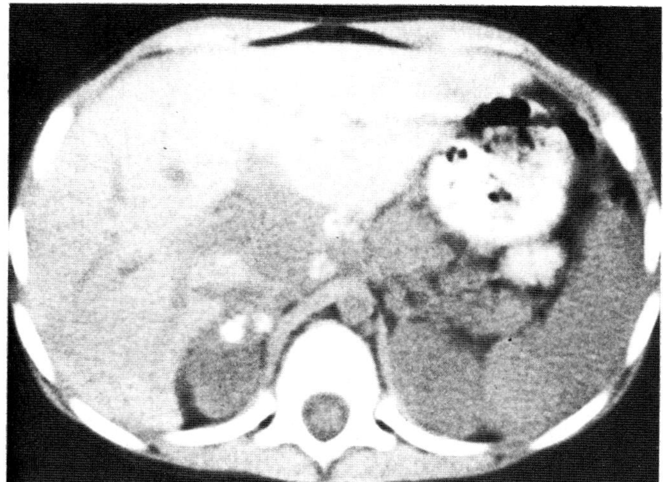

Fig. 37.48 CT scan showing ill-defined mass of neuroblastoma with calcification extending medially and anteriorly from the right suprarenal gland to the porta hepatis.

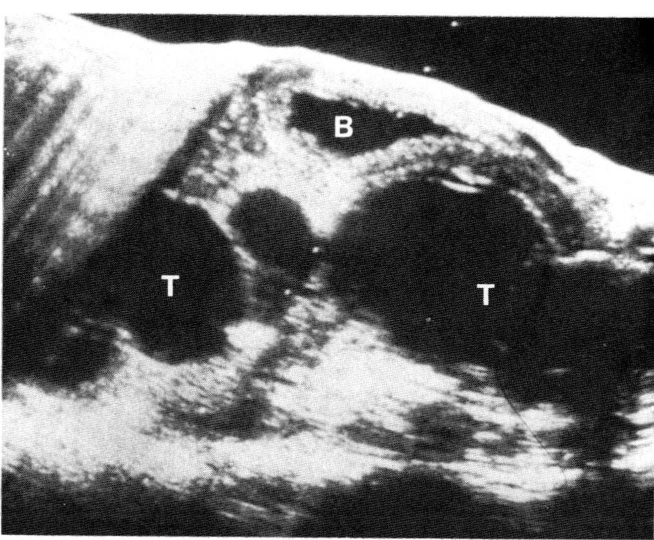

Fig. 37.49 Longitudinal ultrasound scan of a multicystic sacrococcygeal teratoma (T) with displacement of the bladder (B) anteriorly.

extent of the tumour and a CT scan is useful. A lesion of variable density containing calcification is seen (Fig. 37.48). If intravenous contrast is used, displacement and attachment to major vessels is shown.

Adrenal haemorrhage

This condition may present in the neonate following birth trauma and neonatal asphyxia. Ultrasound is very useful in making the diagnosis and in its differentiation from other adrenal masses, such as neuroblastoma. The ipsilateral kidney is displaced inferiorly by a suprarenal mass which will vary in echogenicity depending on the age of the haematoma. Early scans will show a highly echogenic mass and as liquefaction of the haematoma occurs it will become smaller, more echolucent and cystic. Eventually calcification may occur and will be seen on ultrasound and plain films.

Teratomas

These are uncommon abdominal masses in the paediatric age group. In the neonate they may occur in the presacral region and present as a sacrococcygeal mass. Most are benign and readily removed although some have significant extension into surrounding tissues. A soft-tissue mass containing calcification and sometimes recognizable structures, such as teeth, are seen on plain films of the pelvis. Teratomas may also occur in the ovaries and can present as a large abdominal mass. On ultrasound a mass containing a mixture of cystic, echolucent and echogenic elements is seen. Displacement of the bladder and rectum will be demonstrated (Fig. 37.49). Further investigations such as barium studies, intravenous urography, CT scanning and myelography may be necessary to fully define these lesions.

HEPATOBILIARY MASSES

Hepatobiliary masses account for approximately 6% of all abdominal masses in childhood and are the third most common solid abdominal neoplasms after nephroblastomas and neuroblastomas. Most of the masses are hepatic and approximately one-third of these are benign and the remaining two-thirds malignant.

Malignant hepatic tumours are either *hepatoblastomas* or *hepatocellular carcinomas*. Hepatomegaly and calcification can be seen on plain films. Ultrasound will demonstrate a poorly defined intrahepatic mass with an irregular echogenic pattern and calcification. However, the precise anatomic location and lobar extent of the tumour is not

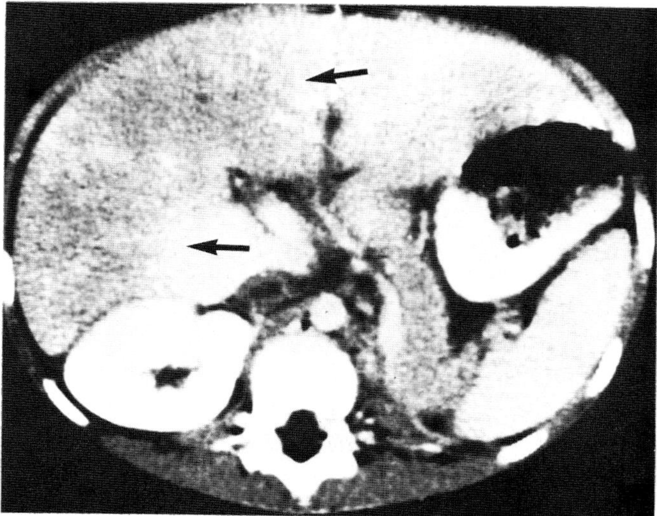

Fig. 37.50 CT scan showing a low attenuation, poorly defined hepatoblastoma in the right lobe of the liver (arrows).

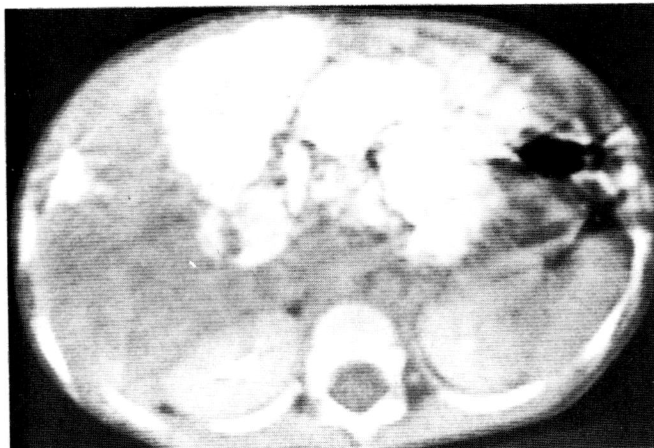

Fig. 37.51 CT scan showing dense calcification in the liver due to a hepatoblastoma.

accurately demonstrated on ultrasound. CT scanning, which will show a low attenuation intrahepatic mass, sometimes with calcification, is required to localize the tumour precisely (Figs 37.50, 37.51). Angiography is necessary if surgery is indicated.

Benign hepatic masses are more common in the neonate and are often vascular in origin. Intrahepatic *haemangiomas* and *haemangioendotheliomas* may be associated with cutaneous haemangiomas. They may cause symptoms with high output congestive cardiac failure, thrombocytopenia and acute intra-abdominal haemorrhage due to rupture. Multiple echolucent tubular structures secondary to

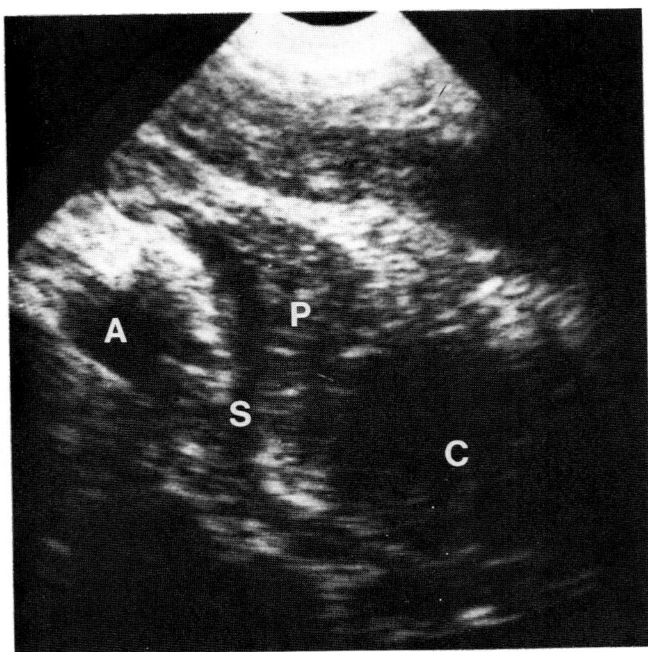

Fig. 37.52 Transverse ultrasound scan of pancreas (P) and splenic vein (S) with a large pseudocyst (C) in the tail of pancreas. A = aorta.

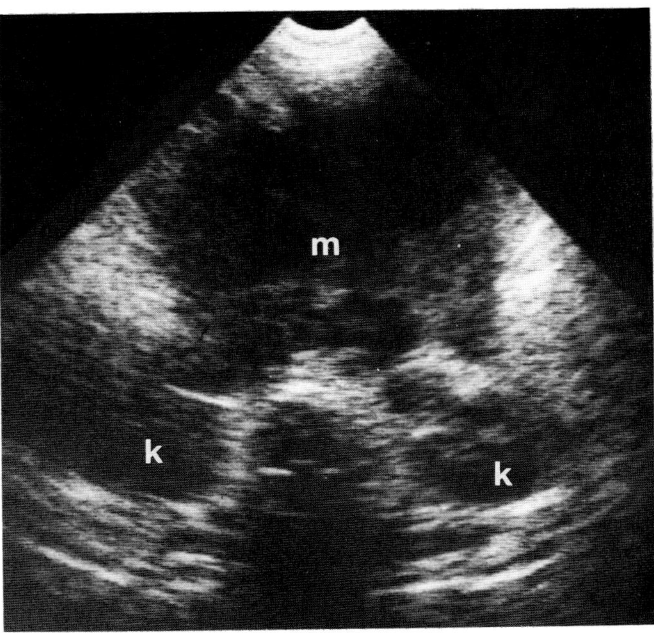

Fig. 37.53 Transverse ultrasound scan of the upper abdomen showing a large echolucent mass of lymphomatous tissue (m) in front of the spine and kidneys (k).

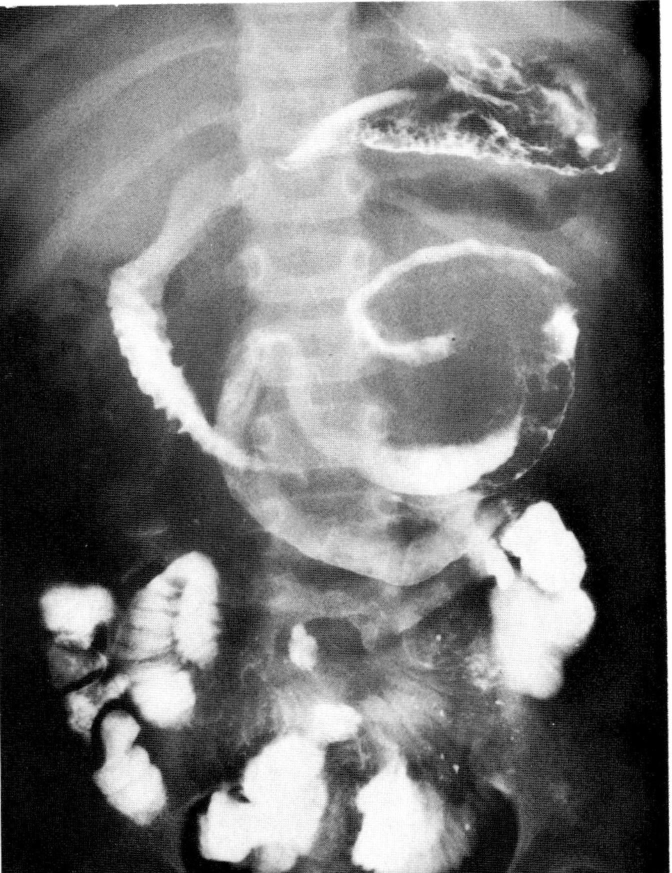

Fig. 37.54 Barium follow-through film of lymphomatous infiltration of small bowel and mesentery.

enlarged vascular channels are seen on ultrasound. Dynamic and static radionuclide scanning is diagnostic of these large vascular haemangiomata. Angiography is required if vascular ligation or transcatheter embolization is planned.

Choledochal cysts may present in the neonate as an upper abdominal mass. A cystic mass in the course of the biliary tree, sometimes with dilatation of the bile ducts will be seen with ultrasound. The diagnostic investigation is a $^{99}Tc^{m}$-HIDA isotope scan. The isotope is excreted by the liver and then accumulates within the choledochal cyst.

Hepatic adenomas are rare tumours in children, but may be seen in cases of glycogen storage disease.

GASTROINTESTINAL MASSES

Duplication cysts

If the plain abdominal radiograph of a neonate with a mass reveals an abnormal gastrointestinal gas pattern with obstruction, the mass is likely to arise from the gastrointestinal tract, and may be a duplication cyst. These are commonly associated with the ileum, but may occur in the stomach, proximal small bowel and rarely, colon. A barium study will demonstrate displacement of normal gut around the mass, and an ultrasound scan will show it to be cystic and echolucent.

Pancreatic masses

Pancreatic tumours are rare in children (see above). However, following trauma a *pancreatic pseudocyst* may arise. This should be diagnosed on ultrasound by its location and cystic, echolucent appearance (Fig. 37.52). It should be differentiated from a duplication cyst associated with the stomach. Barium studies and CT scans will also demonstrate the lesion.

Lymphoma

This may present as a retroperitoneal or mesenteric mass. Characteristically, lymphomatous masses present as well-defined, lobular echolucent masses on ultrasound. They may occur in many sites including the para-aortic region, mesenteries, kidneys, spleen and pelvis (Fig. 37.53). Gastrointestinal involvement is more clearly demonstrated with barium studies (Fig. 37.54). CT scanning is important in demonstrating para-aortic lymph node masses.

REFERENCES AND SUGGESTIONS FOR FURTHER READING

The GI tract

Caffey, J. (1978) *Pediatric X-ray Diagnosis*, 7th ed. Chicago, London: Year Book Medical Publishers Inc.

Gyll, C. (1984) Horizontal versus vertical, or Lying down is better. *British Journal of Radiology* 57, 191–193.

Ratcliffe, J. F. (1984) The use of Ioxaglate in the paediatric gastro-intestinal tract: a report of 25 cases. *Clinical Radiology*, **34**, 579–583.

Singleton, G. B., Wagner, M. L. & Dutton, R. V. (1977) *Radiology of the Alimentary Tract in Infants and Children*, 2nd edn. Philadelphia, London — Toronto; W. B. Saunders Company.

Speidel, B. (1978) Adverse effects of routine procedures in preterm infants. *Lancet*, **i**, 664–685.

Steiner, G. H. (1983) *Essential Paediatric Radiology*. Oxford, London: Blackwell Scientific Publications.

Swischuk, L. E. (1980) *Radiology of the Newborn and Young Infant*, 2nd edn. Baltimore, London: Williams and Wilkins.

Abdominal masses

Caffey, J. (1978) *Paediatric X-ray Diagnosis*, 7th edn. London: Lloyd-Luke.

Cohen, M. D., Siddiqui, A., Weetman, R. et al. (1982) A rational approach to the radiologic evaluation of children with Wilm's tumour. *Cancer*, **50**, 887–892.

Cremin, B. J., Mervis, B. (1983) Paediatric abdominal computed tomography: the technique and use in neuroblastomas and pelvic masses. *British Journal of Radiology*, **56**, 291–298.

Griscom, N. T. (1965) The roentgenology of neonatal abdominal masses. *American Journal of Roentgenology*, **93**, 447–463.

Kirks, D. R., Merten, D., Grossman, H. et al. (1981) Diagnostic imaging of paediatric abdominal masses: An overview. *Radiologic Clinics of North America*, **19**, 527–545.

Lamont, A. C., Stavinsky, R., Cremin, B. J. (1984) Ultrasonic diagnosis of duplication cysts in children. *British Journal of Radiology*, **57**, 463–467.

Lebowitz, R. L., Griscom, N. T. (1977) Neonatal hydronephrosis, 146 cases. *Radiologic Clinics of North America*, **15**, 46–49.

Moore, A. V., Kirks, D. R., Mills, S. R., et al. (1982) Paediatric abdominal angiography: panacea or passé? *American Journal of Roentgenology*, **138**, 433–443.

Parker, B. R., Castellino, R. A. (1977) *Paediatric Oncologic Radiology*, 1st edn. St. Louis: C. V. Mosby.

Pussell, S. J., Cosgrove, D. O. (1981) Ultrasound features of tumour thrombus in the IVC in retropertioneal tumours. *British Journal of Radiology*, **54**, 866–869.

Rosenberg, E. R., Trough, W. S., Kirks, D. R. et al. (1980) Ultrasonic diagnosis of renal vein thrombosis in neonates. *American Journal of Roentgenology*, **134**, 35–38.

Siegel, M. J., Glasier, C. M., Sagel, S. S. (1981) CT of pelvic disorders in children. *American Journal of Roentgenology*, **137**, 1139–1143.

Siegel, M. J., McAlister, W. H., Shackelford, G. D. (1978) Radiographic findings in ovarian teratomas in children. *American Journal of Roentgenology*, **131**, 613–616.

Smith, W. L., Franker, E. A., Mitros, F. A. (1983) Liver tumours in children. *Seminars in Roentgenology*, **18**, 136–148.

INDEX

INDEX